Gordon and Nivatvongs' Principles and Practice of Surgery for the Colon, Rectum, and Anus

Fourth Edition

David E. Beck, MD, FACS, FASCRS
Professor and Chairman Emeritus
Department of Colon and Rectal Surgery
Ochsner Clinic Foundation
The University of Queensland School of Medicine–Ochsner Clinical School
New Orleans, Louisiana

Steven D. Wexner, MD, PhD(Hon), FACS, FASCRS, FRCS, FRCS(Ed), FRCSI(Hon)
Director, Digestive Disease Center
Chair, Department of Colorectal Surgery
Cleveland Clinic Florida
Affiliate Professor, Florida Atlantic University College of Medicine
Clinical Professor, Florida International University College of Medicine
Professor of Surgery, Ohio State University Wexner College of Medicine
Affiliate Professor, Department of Surgery, Division of General Surgery
University of South Florida Morsani College of Medicine
Weston, Florida

Janice F. Rafferty, MD, FACS, FASCRS
Professor of Surgery
Chief, Section of Colon and Rectal Surgery
University of Cincinnati Department of Surgery
Cincinnati, Ohio

748 illustrations

Thieme
New York • Stuttgart • Delhi • Rio de Janeiro

Executive Editor: William Lamsback
Managing Editor: J. Owen Zurhellen IV
Editorial Assistant: Holly Bullis
Director, Editorial Services: Mary Jo Casey
Production Editor: Naamah Schwartz
International Production Director: Andreas Schabert
Editorial Director: Sue Hodgson
International Marketing Director: Fiona Henderson
International Sales Director: Louisa Turrell
Director of Institutional Sales: Adam Bernacki
Senior Vice President and Chief Operating Officer: Sarah Vanderbilt
President: Brian D. Scanlan

Library of Congress Cataloging-in-Publication Data

Names: Beck, David E., author, editor. | Wexner, Steven D., editor. |
    Rafferty, Janice F., editor. | Preceded by (work): Gordon, Philip H.
    Principles and practice of surgery for the colon, rectum, and anus.
Title: Gordon and Nivatvongs' principles and practice of surgery for
    the colon, rectum, and anus / David E. Beck, Steven D. Wexner,
    Janice F. Rafferty, [editors].
Other titles: Principles and practice of surgery for the colon,
    rectum, and anus
Description: Fourth edition. | New York : Thieme, [2019] | Preceded
    by Principles and practice of surgery for the colon, rectum, and
    anus / Philip H. Gordon, Santhat Nivatvongs ; illustrators, Scott
    Thorn Barrows ... [et. al.] 3rd. ed. c2007. | Includes bibliographical
    references and index.
Identifiers: LCCN 2018051035 | ISBN 9781626234291 (hardback)
Subjects: | MESH: Colonic Diseases–surgery | Rectal Diseases–surgery |
    Anus Diseases–surgery | Colorectal Neoplasms–surgery
Classification: LCC RD544 | NLM WI 520 | DDC 617.5/547–dc23 LC
record available at https://lccn.loc.gov/2018051035

© 2019 Thieme Medical Publishers, Inc.

Thieme Publishers New York
333 Seventh Avenue, New York, NY 10001 USA
+1 800 782 3488, customerservice@thieme.com

Thieme Publishers Stuttgart
Rüdigerstrasse 14, 70469 Stuttgart, Germany
+49 [0]711 8931 421, customerservice@thieme.de

Thieme Publishers Delhi
A-12, Second Floor, Sector-2, Noida-201301
Uttar Pradesh, India
+91 120 45 566 00, customerservice@thieme.in

Thieme Publishers Rio de Janeiro, Thieme Publicações Ltda.
Edifício Rodolpho de Paoli, 25º andar
Av. Nilo Peçanha, 50 – Sala 2508,
Rio de Janeiro 20020-906 Brasil
+55 21 3172-2297 / +55 21 3172-1896
www.thiemerevinter.com.br

Cover design: Thieme Publishing Group
Typesetting by DiTech Process Solutions

Printed in   The United States of America by
King Printing Company, Inc.   5 4 3 2 1

ISBN 978-1-62623-429-1

Also available as an e-book:
eISBN 978-1-62623-430-7

Important note: Medicine is an ever-changing science undergoing continual development. Research and clinical experience are continually expanding our knowledge, in particular our knowledge of proper treatment and drug therapy. Insofar as this book mentions any dosage or application, readers may rest assured that the authors, editors, and publishers have made every effort to ensure that such references are in accordance with **the state of knowledge at the time of production of the book**.

Nevertheless, this does not involve, imply, or express any guarantee or responsibility on the part of the publishers in respect to any dosage instructions and forms of applications stated in the book. **Every user is requested to examine carefully** the manufacturers' leaflets accompanying each drug and to check, if necessary in consultation with a physician or specialist, whether the dosage schedules mentioned therein or the contraindications stated by the manufacturers differ from the statements made in the present book. Such examination is particularly important with drugs that are either rarely used or have been newly released on the market. Every dosage schedule or every form of application used is entirely at the user's own risk and responsibility. The authors and publishers request every user to report to the publishers any discrepancies or inaccuracies noticed. If errors in this work are found after publication, errata will be posted at www.thieme.com on the product description page.

Some of the product names, patents, and registered designs referred to in this book are in fact registered trademarks or proprietary names even though specific reference to this fact is not always made in the text. Therefore, the appearance of a name without designation as proprietary is not to be construed as a representation by the publisher that it is in the public domain.

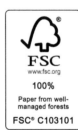

FSC
www.fsc.org
100%
Paper from well-managed forests
FSC® C103101

This fourth edition is dedicated to Philip H. Gordon (13 September 1942 - 11 April 2018) and Santhat Nivatvongs with our utmost respect and affection, and with appreciation for their unmatched contributions to this specialty and their influence on our respective careers.

– DEB, SDW, JFR

Contents

Video Contents

Foreword

The specialty of Colon and Rectal Surgery has a long and distinguished history: we trace our roots to practitioners of proctology and the very beginnings of surgery. Education and teaching has always been a central component of our specialty and textbooks have been central to this activity. Most early textbooks were single authored and described the particular practice of the author. As experience grew and science was brought into Medicine, subsequent textbooks provided evidence and some traditional procedures were abandoned. Unfortunately, most of these texts disappeared with the retirement or death of the author. More recently, multi-authored texts have become the norm. These provide a wider perspective, but often lack unified style or themes. *Principles and Practice of Surgery for the Colon, Rectum, and Anus* was first published in 1992 with the goal to be a comprehensive textbook that would encompass the gamut of colon and anorectal surgery. Authored in the most part by two surgeons, the text emphasized fundamentals of disease, with explanations of etiologies and pathogenesis to guide the reader on why, when and how to institute therapy. The text was a natural extension of their previous text *Essentials of Anorectal Surgery* and was well received by the surgical community; so much so that additional editions were published in 1999 and 2007.

We are pleased that David E. Beck, Steven D. Wexner, and Janice F. Rafferty agreed to continue this legacy and have composed this fully revised fourth edition now entitled *Gordon and Nivatvongs' Principles and Practice of Surgery for the Colon, Rectum, and Anus*. They have produced a new textbook that for the most part retained the organization and style of previous editions. Material that remained current was maintained, but as significant advances have occurred in the last ten years, significant current evidence based material has been added. As this is a textbook written for the busy practicing surgeon, this fourth edition has been streamlined and (with great but careful effort) reduced in bulk.

We hope and expect that our past and future readers (practicing surgeons or those in training) will find this fourth edition as valuable as the previous ones, and we are most grateful that the new authors/editors have continued our commitment to the specialty of Colon and Rectal Surgery.

Philip H. Gordon, MD, FRCS, FACS, FASCRS, FCSCRS(Hon), FRSM(Hon), FACPGBI
Professor of Surgery and Oncology
Director of Colon and Rectal Surgery
McGill University, Jewish General Hospital
Montreal, Québec, Canada

Santhat Nivatvongs, MD, FACS, FASCRS(Hon), FRACS(Hon), FRCST(Thailand)
Emeritus Professor
Department of Surgery
Mayo Clinic College of Medicine and Science
Rochester, Minnesota

Preface

For fifteen years (1992–2007), Dr. Gordon and Dr. Nivatvongs authored the first three editions of *Principles and Practice of Surgery for the Colon, Rectum, and Anus*. They succeeded in producing a comprehensive book that encompassed the gamut of colon and anorectal diseases. The small number of authors and contributors resulted in a uniformity of style rarely seen in the more common multi-authored textbooks. The authors of this fourth edition were honored to be asked by the previous authors to take up the task of producing a new edition.

We are committed to maintaining a small number of authors and specialty contributors and have retained the organization of chapters into 4 main sections. To reflect the significant advances that have occurred in this specialty in the 11 years since the third edition was published, each chapter was reviewed, revised, or rewritten. Some chapters were combined and new ones added, and the text has been condensed by 25% to become easier to handle.

Highlights in this book include an update on the current modalities for anorectal physiology and advances in diagnostic studies such as MRI, CT angiography, and enterography. Perioperative management has seen major changes with adoption of enhanced recovery pathways. The continued migration of outpatient management of anorectal surgery has been highlighted in a new chapter. The limitations of stapled hemorrhoidopexy, and newer options for hemorrhoid treatment, are described. Newer procedures such as ligation of intersphincteric fistula tract (LIFT) have been added to the fistula chapter. The management of sexually transmitted diseases and drug therapies for HIV have been updated. The experience in managing fecal incontinence has been updated, now including the artificial sphincter, hyperbaric oxygen, radiofrequency tissue remodeling, and sacral neuromodulation.

The chapter on the etiology and management of perianal neoplasia and anal carcinoma has been extensively revised reflecting new information, highlighting our current understanding of the role of anal intraepithelial neoplasia (AIN). These additions include new methods of diagnosis and management of high grade AIN of the perianal skin. In the chapter on benign neoplasia, the interest in and better understanding of "serrated" adenoma has been added.

Information on uncommon benign polyps has been expanded and the management of malignant polyps of the low rectum has been updated.

New data regarding the incidence, prevalence, and trends in colorectal carcinoma are presented as well as an update on the genetics of colorectal carcinoma with emphasis on heredity non-polyposis colorectal cancer (HNPCC). Indications for and interpretation of genetic testing and the invaluable role of genetic counseling are highlighted. The significant advances in adjuvant therapy have been documented along with updates on the management of recurrent and metastatic colorectal carcinoma. Operative techniques for sphincter sparing operations (pouch, coloplasty, coloanal anastomosis) and expanded transanal procedures are presented. Screening, surveillance, and follow-up for large bowel carcinoma continue to evolve rapidly with better understanding. A new chapter on large bowel obstruction has been added. The expanded role of medical management in inflammatory bowel has been highlighted along with increased experience with surgical management of Crohn's disease and ulcerative colitis.

The changing paradigm regarding the indications for elective operation in diverticular disease has been revisited along with the most recent data on results of the treatment of diverticulitis. Laparoscopy has evolved to be a standard approach for many procedures, and is discussed from a disease perspective rather than singled out for a separate chapter.

We hope we have summarized the enormous amount of published colorectal literature and shared our personal experience and preferences with our readers. We strived for a book that strikes a balance of being authoritative and detailed while minimizing irrelevant material and minutia. We hope our efforts provide the practicing surgeon and surgeon in training the appropriate information to provide a rational and up-to-date course of action to the benefit of their patients.

David E. Beck, MD, FACS, FASCRS
Steven D. Wexner, MD, PhD(Hon), FACS, FASCRS,
FRCS, FRCS(Ed), FRCSI(Hon)
Janice F. Rafferty, MD, FACS, FASCRS

Acknowledgments

I am highly appreciative of Phil Gordon's and Sandy Nivatvongs' confidence in selecting my coauthors and me for this fourth edition, and allowing us this unique opportunity to update their highly regarded textbook. Throughout my career, Phil has served as a role model and mentor; it has been an honor to carry on one of his singular accomplishments. I thank our specialty contributors for taking time from work and family to produce superb chapters, and I thank my colleagues Steve Wexner and Janice Rafferty for their efforts in authoring and editing this extensive project. Steve and I are lifelong friends and colleagues; our relationship strengthened by the stresses and challenges of projects like this. Janice has added a new perspective and rose to the challenge of such a major project. I thank Elektra McDermott, who did her usual outstanding job as a developmental editor. I remain indebted to my partners, colleagues, and trainees who continue to support and stimulate my clinical and academic efforts. Finally, I reaffirm my love and appreciation for my wife, Sharon, for her support and encouragement for all the nights and weekends spent in my office working on this project.

– DEB

First and foremost, I thank my late dear mentor Phil Gordon for his phenomenal leadership in our field, his important mentorship in my career, and his cherished friendship in my life. I am indebted to him for entrusting me, David, and Jan with the legacy of his decades-long labor of love. I offer the same appreciation to Santhat Nivatvongs for his wisdom and guidance for many decades, and for his trust with this incredible project. I also give my appreciation to Elektra McDermott for her superlative editorial skills without which this text would not have come to timely fruition. In addition, I thank Dave and Jan for their efforts, expertise, time, talent, and friendship; it has been a pleasure working with them on this project. I am appreciative to our chapter contributors for their time and expertise. Lastly, for their wisdom, love, and support I am eternally grateful to the most important people in my life who patiently waited for me each day that I was engaged in academic endeavors: Trevor, Wesley, Mariana, and my parents. Their love, understanding, encouragement, and patience has given me the energy and ability needed during the conception and completion of many scientific endeavors including this formidable textbook.

– SDW

As a trainee and young colorectal surgeon, the textbook by Dr. Gordon and Dr. Nivatvongs was my favorite reference. My later meeting with these scions of our specialty was a highlight of my career. I am immensely honored by the opportunity to participate in this fourth edition of their classic textbook, and appreciate the confidence that Drs. Beck and Wexner have expressed. Their guidance and friendship has been invaluable; I can only aspire to influence the world of surgery as they have done. I have my husband to thank as well, for the patience and space he provides for me to be everything except a traditional spouse.

– JFR

Contributors

David E. Beck, MD, FACS, FASCRS
Professor and Chairman Emeritus
Department of Colon and Rectal Surgery
Ochsner Clinic Foundation
The University of Queensland School of Medicine–Ochsner
    Clinical School
New Orleans, Louisiana

Joshua I.S. Bleier, MD, FACS, FASCRS
Associate Professor
Department of Surgery
Hospital of the University of Pennsylvania/Pennsylvania
    Hospital
Philadelphia, Pennsylvania

**Philip H. Gordon, MD, FRCS, FACS, FASCRS, FCSCRS (Hon),
    FRSM (Hon), FACPGBI**
Director of Colon and Rectal Surgery
Professor of Surgery and Oncology
McGill University, Jewish General Hospital
Montreal, Québec, Canada

Quinton Hatch, MD
Department of Surgery
Madigan Army Medical Center
Tacoma, Washington

David G. Jayne, MD, BSc, MB, BCh, FRCS
Professor of Surgery
Department of Academic Surgery
St. James University Hospital
Leeds, West Yorkshire, England
United Kingdom

Sean J. Langenfeld, MD, FACS, FASCRS
Assistant Professor
Department of Surgery
University of Nebraska Medical Center
Omaha, Nebraska

Lawrence Lee, MD, PhD, FRCSC
Assistant Professor
Department of Surgery
McGill University Health Center
Montreal, Québec, Canada

David J. Maron, MD, MBA, FACS, FASCRS
Director, Colorectal Surgery Residency Program
Vice Chair, Department of Colorectal Surgery
Cleveland Clinic Florida
Weston, Florida

Emily F. Midura, MD
Department of Surgery
University of Cincinnati Medical Center
Cincinnati, Ohio

**John R.T. Monson, MD, MB, BCh, BAO, FRCS[Ire, Eng, Ed
    (Hon), Glas(Hon)], FASCRS, FACS**
Executive Director, Colorectal Surgery
Florida Hospital System
Professor of Surgery
Director of Digestive Health Institute
Florida Hospital
Center for Colon and Rectal Surgery
Orlando, Florida

**Santhat Nivatvongs, MD, FACS, FASCRS(Hon), FRACS(Hon),
    FRCST(Thailand)**
Emeritus Professor
Department of Surgery
Mayo Clinic College of Medicine and Science
Rochester, Minnesota

Rajeev Peravali, BMedSc, MBChB, MCh, FRCS(Ed)
Department of Colorectal Surgery
Sandwell and West Birmingham NHS Trust
Lyndon, England
United Kingdom

Janice F. Rafferty, MD, FACS, FASCRS
Professor of Surgery
Chief, Section of Colon and Rectal Surgery
University of Cincinnati Department of Surgery
Cincinnati, Ohio

W. Ruud Schouten, MD, PhD
Erasmus Medical Center
Department of Surgery
Rotterdam, Netherlands

**Sharmini Su Sivarajah, MBCB, MRCS(Edin), MD(Gla), FRCS
    (Edin)**
Associate Consultant
Department of General Surgery
Sengkang Health
Singapore

Scott R. Steele, MD, FACS, FASCRS
Chairman
Department of Colon and Rectal Surgery
Cleveland Clinic
Cleveland, Ohio

Earl V. Thompson IV, MD
Assistant Professor of Surgery
Department of Colon and Rectal Surgery
University of Cincinnati Medical Center/UC Health
Cincinnati, Ohio

Steven D. Wexner, MD, PhD(Hon), FACS, FASCRS, FRCS, FRCS(Ed), FRCSI(Hon)
Director, Digestive Disease Center
Chair, Department of Colorectal Surgery
Cleveland Clinic Florida

Affiliate Professor, Florida Atlantic University College of Medicine
Clinical Professor, Florida International University College of Medicine
Professor of Surgery, Ohio State University Wexner College of Medicine
Affiliate Professor, Department of Surgery, Division of General Surgery, University of South Florida Morsani College of Medicine
Weston, Florida

Part I

Essential Considerations

1 Surgical Anatomy of the Colon, Rectum, and Anus

Santhat Nivatvongs, Philip H. Gordon, and David E. Beck

Abstract

This chapter will review the surgical anatomy of the colon and rectum, including general configuration, course relations, peritoneal coverings, and ileocecal valve in the colon, and peritoneal relations, fascial attachments, fascia propria, Waldeyer's fascia, Denonvilliers' fascia, lateral ligaments of the rectum, histology, muscles of the anorectal region, anorectal spaces, arterial supply, venous drainage, lymphatic drainage, and innervation.

Keywords: surgical anatomy, colon, rectum, histology, muscles, anorectal region, anorectal spaces, arterial supply, venous drainage, lymphatic drainage, innervation

1.1 Introduction

Although often thought of as a single organ, the colon is embryologically divisible into two parts. The transverse and right colon are derived from the midgut and are supplied by the superior mesenteric artery, while the distal half of the colon is derived from the hindgut and receives blood from the inferior mesenteric artery.

The large bowel begins in the right lower quadrant of the abdomen as a blind pouch known as the cecum. The ileum empties into the medial and posterior aspect of the intestine, a point known as the ileocecal junction. The colon proceeds upward and in its course is designated according to location as: ascending (right) colon, hepatic flexure, transverse colon, splenic flexure, descending (left) colon, sigmoid colon, rectum, and anal canal. The colon is approximately 150 cm long, and its diameter gradually diminishes from the cecum to the rectosigmoid junction, where it widens as the rectal ampulla, only to narrow again as the anal canal.

1.2 Colon

1.2.1 General Configuration

The colon differs from the small bowel in that it is characterized by a saccular or haustral appearance, it contains three taenia bands, and it has appendices epiploicae, a series of fatty appendages located adjacent to the tenae on surface of the colon. The taeniae are thickened bands of longitudinal muscle running along the colon from the base of the appendix. They merge in the distal sigmoid colon, where the longitudinal fibers continue through the entire length of the rectum. A study by Fraser et al[1] demonstrated that the longitudinal muscle forms a complete coat around the colon but is much thicker at the taeniae. The three taenia bands are named according to their relation to the transverse colon: taenia mesocolica, which is attached to the mesocolon or mesentery; taenia omentalis, which is attached to the greater omentum; and taenia libera, which has no attachment. These bands are about one-sixth shorter than the intestine and are believed to be responsible for the sacculations.[2] The transition from the sigmoid colon to the rectum is a gradual one. It is characterized by the taeniae coli spreading out from three distinct bands to a uniformly distributed layer of longitudinal smooth muscle that is thicker on the front and back than on each side, the loss of appendices epiploicae, and change in diameter.

1.2.2 Course and Alterations

The general topography of the colon varies from person to person, and such differences should be taken into account while reading the following discussion (▶ Fig. 1.1).

The vermiform appendix projects from the lowermost part of the cecum. From the ileocecal junction, the colon ascends on the right in front of the quadratus lumborum and transversus abdominis muscles to a level overlying the lower pole of the right kidney, a distance of about 20 cm. It is invested by peritoneum on its anterior, lateral, and medial surfaces. Superior to the colon is the undersurface of the right lobe of the liver, lateral to the gallbladder, and here the colon angulates acutely medially, downward, and forward, forming the hepatic flexure. Occasionally, there is a filmy web of adhesions extending from the right abdominal wall to the anterior taenia of the ascending colon, and this has been referred to as Jackson's membrane.

The transverse colon is the longest (40–50 cm) segment of colon, extending from the hepatic to the splenic flexure. It is

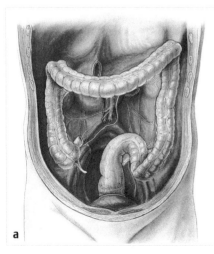
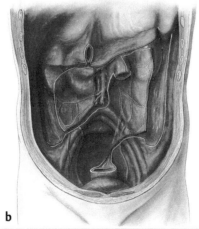

Fig. 1.1 General topography of the large bowel. **(a)** Colon. **(b)** Peritoneum and adjacent structures.

usually mobile and may descend to the level of the iliac crests or even dip into the pelvis. The transverse colon is enveloped between layers of the transverse mesocolon, the root of which overlies the right kidney, the second portion of the duodenum, the pancreas, and the left kidney. It contains the middle colic artery, branches of the right and left colic arteries, and accompanying veins, lymphatic structures, and autonomic nerve plexuses. This posterior relationship is of paramount importance because these structures are subject to injury during a right hemicolectomy if proper care is not exercised. In the left upper quadrant of the abdomen, the colon is attached to the undersurface of the diaphragm at the level of the 10th and 11th ribs by the phrenocolic ligament. The distal transverse colon lies in front of the proximal descending colon. The stomach is immediately above and the spleen is to the left. The greater omentum descends from the greater curvature of the stomach in front of the transverse colon and ascends to the upper surface of the transverse colon. The splenic flexure describes an acute angle, is high in the left upper quadrant, and therefore is less accessible to operative approach. It lies anterior to the midportion of the left kidney.

The descending colon passes along the posterior abdominal wall over the lateral border of the left kidney, turns somewhat medially, and descends in the groove between the psoas and the quadratus lumborum muscles to its junction with the sigmoid at the level of the pelvic brim and the transversus abdominis muscle.[3,4] Its length averages 30 cm. The anterior, medial, and lateral portions of its circumference are covered by peritoneum. The distal portion of the descending colon is usually attached by adhesions to the posterior abdominal wall, and these adhesions require division during mobilization of this portion of the colon.

The sigmoid colon extends from the pelvic brim to the sacral promontory, where it continues as the rectum. Its length varies dramatically from 15 to 50 cm, and it may follow an extremely tortuous and variable course. It often loops to the left but may follow a straight oblique course, loop to the right, or ascend high into the abdomen. It has a generous mesentery and is extremely mobile. The serosal surface has numerous appendices epiploicae. The base of the mesocolon extends from the iliac fossa, along the pelvic brim, and across the sacroiliac joint to the second or third sacral segment; in so doing, it forms an inverted V. Contained within the mesosigmoid are the sigmoidal and superior rectal arteries and accompanying veins, lymphatics, and autonomic nerve plexuses. At the base of the mesosigmoid is a recess, the intersigmoid fossa, which serves as a valuable guide to the left ureter, lying just deep to it. The upper limb runs medially and upward, crossing the left ureter and iliac vessels; this is an extremely important relationship during resection of this part of the colon. The lower limb extends in front of the sacrum and also may be alongside loops of small bowel, the urinary bladder, and the uterus and its adnexa.

1.2.3 Peritoneal Coverings

The antimesenteric border of the distal ileum may be attached to the parietal peritoneum by a membrane (Lane's membrane).[5] The cecum usually is entirely enveloped by peritoneum. The ascending colon is attached to the posterior body wall and is devoid of peritoneum in its posterior surface; thus, it does not have a mesentery. The transverse colon is invested with peritoneum. Its posterosuperior surface, along the taenia band, is attached by the transverse mesocolon to the lower border of the pancreas. The posterior and inferior layers of the greater omentum are fused on the anterosuperior aspect of the transverse colon. To mobilize the greater omentum or to enter the lesser sac, the fusion of the omentum to the transverse colon must be dissected. Because the omental bursa becomes obliterated caudal to the transverse colon and toward the right side, the dissection should be started on the left side of the transverse colon. Topor et al[6] studied 45 cadavers to elucidate surgical aspects of omental mobilization, lengthening, and transposition into the pelvic cavity. They identified that the most important anatomic variables for omental transposition were three variants of arterial blood supply: (1) in 56% of patients, there is one right, one (or two) middle, and one left omental artery; (2) in 26% of patients, the middle omental artery is absent; and (3) in the remaining 18% of patients, the gastroepiploic artery is continued as a left omental artery but with various smaller connections to the right or middle omental artery. The first stage of omental lengthening is detachment of the omentum from the transverse colon mesentery. The second stage is the actual lengthening of the omentum. The third stage is placement of the omental flap into the pelvis. The left colonic flexure is attached to the diaphragm by the phrenocolic ligament, which also forms a shelf for supporting the spleen. The descending colon is devoid of peritoneum posteriorly, where it is in contact with the posterior abdominal wall and thus has no mesentery.

The sigmoid colon begins at about the level of the pelvic brim and is completely covered with peritoneum. The posterior surface is attached by a fan-shaped mesentery. The lateral surface of the sigmoid mesentery is fused to the parietal peritoneum of the lateral abdominal wall and is generally known as the "white line of Toldt." Mobilization of the sigmoid colon requires cutting or incising the lateral peritoneal reflection. The sigmoid colon varies greatly in length and configuration.

1.2.4 Ileocecal Valve

The superior and inferior ileocecal ligaments are fibrous tissue that helps maintain the angulation between the ileum and the cecum. Kumar and Phillips[7] found these structures to be important in the maintenance of competence against reflux at the ileocecal junction. In an autopsy evaluation, the ascending colon was filled with saline solution by retrograde flow, and in 12 of 14 cases the ileocecal junctions were competent to pressures up to 80 mm Hg. Removal of mucosa at the ileocecal junction or a strip of circular muscle did not impair competence to pressures above 40 mm Hg, but division of the superior and inferior ileocecal ligaments rendered the junction incompetent. Operative reconstruction of the ileocecal angle restored competence. It therefore appears that the angulation between the ileum and the cecum determines continence.

1.3 Rectum

Although anatomists traditionally assign the origin of the rectum to the level of the third sacral vertebra, surgeons generally consider the rectum to begin at the level of the sacral promontory. It descends along the curvature of the sacrum and coccyx and ends by passing through the levator ani muscles, at which level it abruptly turns downward and backward to become the anal canal. The rectum differs from the colon in that the outer layer is entirely longitudinal muscle, characterized by the merging of the three taenia bands. It measures 12 to 15 cm in length and lacks a mesentery, sacculations, and appendices epiploicae. These definitions may evolve as magnetic resonance imaging (MRI) is increasingly utilized to define rectal anatomy.

The rectum describes three lateral curves: the upper and lower curves are convex to the right, and the middle is convex to the left. On their inner aspect, these infoldings into the lumen are known as the valves of Houston.[8,9] About 46% of normal persons have three valves, 33% have two valves, 10% have four valves, 2% have none, and the rest have from five to seven valves.[9] The clinical significance of the valves of Houston is that they must be negotiated during successful proctosigmoidoscopic examination and, more importantly, that they are an excellent location for a rectal biopsy, because the inward protrusion makes an easy target. They do not contain all the layers of the bowel wall, and therefore biopsy in this location carries a minimal risk of perforation. The middle fold is the internal landmark corresponding to the anterior peritoneal reflection. Consequently, extra caution must be exercised in removing polyps above this level. Because of its curves, the rectum can gain 5 cm in length when it is straightened (as in performing a low anterior resection); hence, a lesion that initially appears at 7 cm from the anal verge is often found 12 cm from that site after complete mobilization.

In its course, the rectum is related posteriorly to the sacrum, coccyx, levator ani muscles, coccygeal muscles, median sacral vessels, and roots of the sacral nerve plexus. Anteriorly in the male, the extraperitoneal rectum is related to the prostate, seminal vesicles, vasa deferentia, ureters, and urinary bladder; the intraperitoneal rectum may come in contact with loops of the small bowel and sigmoid colon. In the female, the extraperitoneal rectum lies behind the posterior vaginal wall; the intraperitoneal rectum may be related to the upper part of the vagina, uterus, fallopian tubes, ovaries, small bowel, and sigmoid colon. Laterally above the peritoneal reflection, there may be loops of small bowel, adnexa, and sigmoid colon. Below the reflection, the rectum is separated from the sidewall of the pelvis by the ureter and iliac vessels.

1.3.1 Peritoneal Relations

For descriptive purposes, the rectum is divided into upper, middle, and lower thirds. The upper third is covered by peritoneum anteriorly and laterally, the middle third is covered only anteriorly, and the lower third is devoid of peritoneum. The peritoneal reflection shows considerable variation between individuals and between men and women. In men, it is usually 7 to 9 cm from the anal verge, while in women it is 5 to 7.5 cm above the anal verge. The middle valve of Houston roughly corresponds to the anterior peritoneal reflection. The posterior peritoneal reflection is usually 12 to 15 cm from the anal verge (▶ Fig. 1.2).

The location of the peritoneal reflection has not been extensively studied in living patients. Najarian et al[10] investigated the location of the peritoneal reflection in 50 patients undergoing laparotomy. The distance from the anal verge to the peritoneal reflection was measured in each patient via simultaneous intraoperative proctoscopy and intra-abdominal visualization of the peritoneal reflection. The mean lengths of the peritoneal reflection were 9 cm anteriorly, 12.2 cm laterally,

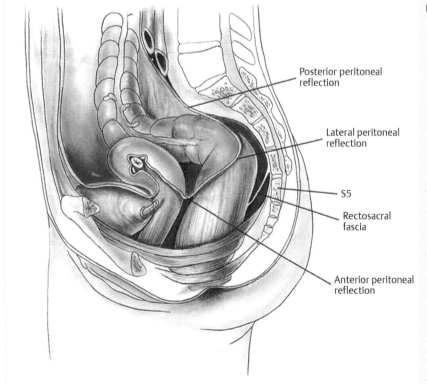

Fig. 1.2 Peritoneal relations of the rectum.

Posterior peritoneal reflection

Lateral peritoneal reflection

S5

Rectosacral fascia

Anterior peritoneal reflection

and 14.8 cm posteriorly for females, and 9.7 cm anteriorly, 12.8 cm laterally, and 15.5 cm posteriorly for males. The lengths of the anterior, lateral, and posterior peritoneal measurements were statistically different from one another, regardless of gender. These authors' data indicated that the peritoneal reflection is located higher on the rectum than reported in autopsy studies, and that there is no difference between males and females. Knowledge of the location and position of a rectal carcinoma in relationship to the peritoneal reflection will help the surgeon optimize the use of peranal techniques of resection.

1.3.2 Fascial Attachments

The posterior part of the rectum, the distal lateral two-thirds, and the anterior one-third are devoid of peritoneum, but they are covered with a thin layer of pelvic fascia, called fascia propria or the investing fascia. At the level of the rectal hiatus, the levator ani is covered by an expansion of the pelvic fascia, which on reaching the rectal wall divides into an ascending

component, which fuses with the fascia propria of the rectum, and a descending component, which interposes itself between the muscular coats forming the conjoint longitudinal coat.[11] These fibroelastic fibers run downward to reach the dermis of the perianal skin and split the subcutaneous striated sphincter into 8 to 12 discrete muscle bundles.

The sacrum and coccyx are covered with a strong fascia that is part of the parietal pelvic fascia. Known as Waldeyer's fascia, this presacral fascia covers the median sacral vessels. The rectosacral fascia is the Waldeyer's fascia from the periosteum of the fourth sacral segment to the posterior wall of the rectum.[12,13] It is found in 97% of cadaver dissections.[13] Waldeyer's fascia contains branches of sacral splanchnic nerves that arise directly from the sacral sympathetic ganglion and may contain branches of the lateral and median sacral vessels. This fascia should be sharply divided with scissors or electrocautery for full mobilization of the rectum (▶ Fig. 1.3). The posterior space below the rectosacral fascia is the supralevator or retrorectal space (▶ Fig. 1.4).

Anteriorly, the extraperitoneal portion of the rectum is covered with a visceral pelvic fascia, the fascia propria, or investing

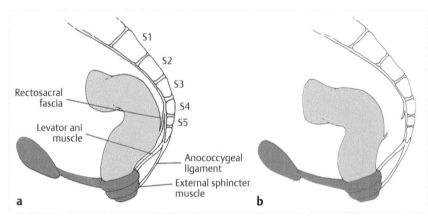

Fig. 1.3 (a) Rectosacral fascia. **(b)** Sharp division of the rectosacral fascia for full mobilization of the rectum.

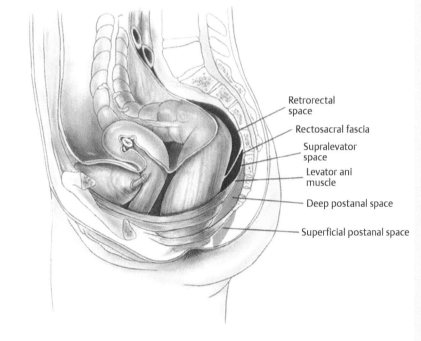

Fig. 1.4 Perianal and perirectal spaces (lateral view).

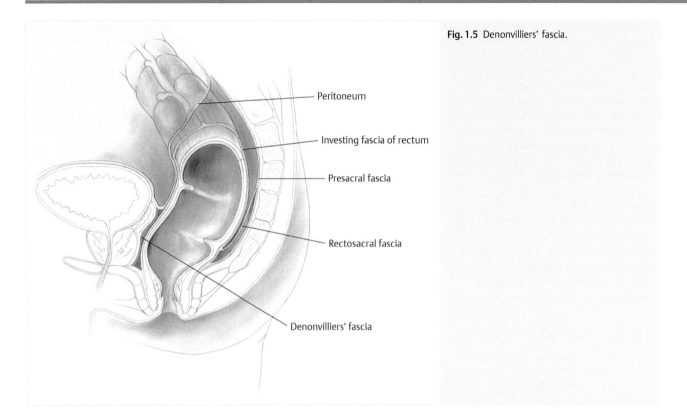

Fig. 1.5 Denonvilliers' fascia.

Peritoneum

Investing fascia of rectum

Presacral fascia

Rectosacral fascia

Denonvilliers' fascia

fascia. Anterior to the fascia propria is a filmy delicate layer of connective tissue known as Denonvilliers' fascia.[14] It separates the rectum from the seminal vesicles and the prostate or vagina (▶ Fig. 1.5). Denonvilliers' fascia has no macroscopically discernible layers. Histologically, it is composed of dense collagen, smooth muscle fibers, and coarse elastic fibers.[15,16] Its attachments have been surrounded by confusion and debates. Some authors believe it is adherent to the rectum,[16,17,18,19] while others note that it is applied to the seminal vesicles and the prostate.[15,20,21,22]

Lindsey et al[23] designed a study to evaluate the anatomic relation of Denonvilliers' fascia: whether it is attached on the anterior fascia propria of the rectum, or on the seminal vesicles and prostate. They prospectively collected 30 specimens from males undergoing total mesorectal excision for mid and low rectal carcinoma, with a deep dissection of the anterior extraperitoneal rectum to the pelvic floor. The anterior aspects of the extraperitoneal rectal sections were examined microscopically for the presence or absence of Denonvilliers' fascia. In patients in whom the carcinoma was anterior, 55% of the specimens had Denonvillier's fascia present. Conversely, when the anterior rectum was not involved with carcinoma 90% of the specimens contained no Denonvilliers' fascia. The authors concluded that "when rectal dissection is conducted on fascia propria in the anatomic plane, Denonvilliers' fascia remains on the posterior aspect of the prostate and seminal vesicles. Denonvilliers' fascia lies anterior to the anatomic fascia propria plane of anterior rectal dissection in total mesorectal excision (TME) and is more closely applied to the prostate than the rectum." This study has put the debates to rest; Denonvilliers' fascia is more closely applied to the seminal vesicles and the prostate than the rectum.

1.3.3 Lateral Ligament

The distal rectum, which is extraperitoneal, is attached to the pelvic sidewall on each side by the pelvic plexus, connective tissues, and middle rectal artery (if present).[24] Histologically, it consists of nerve structures, fatty tissue, and small blood vessels.[25] Recently, the anatomical term *lateral ligament* has been a subject of debate. In dissection of 27 fresh cadavers and 5 embalmed pelves, Nano et al[26] found that lateral ligaments were extension of the mesorectum to the lateral endopelvic fascia. From their experience with anatomic dissection applied to surgery, several conclusions were drawn: lateral ligaments are extensions of the mesorectum and must be cut at their attachment at the endopelvic fascia for TME to take place.

Lateral ligaments contain fatty tissue in communication with mesorectal fat and possibly some vessels and nerve filaments that are of little importance. Insertion of lateral ligaments at the endopelvic fascia is placed under the urogenital bundle. The middle rectal artery courses anteriorly and inferiorly with respect to the lateral ligament. Lateral ligaments can be cut at their insertion on the endopelvic fascia without injuring the urogenital nervous bundle, which, however, should be kept in view during this procedure, because it crosses the middle rectal artery and fans out behind the seminal vesicles. The lateral aspect of the rectum receives the lateral pedicle, which consists of the nervi recti and the middle rectal artery.

A study by Rutegård et al[25] on 10 patients who underwent total mesorectal excision for rectal carcinoma revealed that "the often thin structures, usually referred to as the lateral ligaments, seem to arise from the pelvic plexuses and bridge over into the mesorectum … they can be identified in almost every patient." The authors contend that the lateral ligaments are real anatomical findings. This finding was supported by Sato and Sato[13] in the dissection of 45 cadavers.

Conversely, Jones et al[24] meticulously dissected 28 cadaveric pelves; they found insubstantial thin strands of connective tissues traversing the space between the mesorectum and the pelvic sidewall. These strands of connective tissues were no different from those one would expect to find in any areolar plane. They were often absent altogether. The pelvic plexuses were distinct from the middle rectal artery (if present) and had no association with the connective tissues. Jones et al[24] believed that the lateral ligament was nothing more than a surgical artifact that results from injudicious dissection.

When the rectum is pulled medially, the complex of middle rectal artery and vein, the splanchnic nerves, and their accompanying connective tissues form a bandlike structure extending from the lateral pelvic wall to the rectum.[27] This structure was most likely mistaken as the "lateral ligament" in the past. Whatever one would call the lateral attachment of the low rectum, the tissues need to be divided in full mobilization of the rectum.

1.3.4 Mesorectum

The posterior rectum is devoid of peritoneum and has no mesorectum. The term mesorectum is a misnomer and does not appear in the *Nomina Anatomica*, although it is listed in the *Nomina Embryologica*.[28] The word mesorectum was possibly first used by Maunsell in 1892 and later popularized by Heald of the United Kingdom.[28] In answering the critique of using this word, Heald answered, "... it was a surgical word used by the foremost of my surgical teachers when I was a young registrar. Mr. Rex Lawrice of Guy's Hospital used to describe the process of dividing the mesorectum as was well described in Rob and Smith's textbook of surgery at that time ... no other word seems readily available to describe it."[29]

Total mesorectal excision implies the complete excision of all fat enclosed within the fascia propria, which Heald calls the "mesorectum." This dissection is performed in a circumferential manner down to the levator muscles.[28] Bisset et al[30] preferred the term "extrafascial excision of the rectum." The term mesorectum has now been used worldwide and appears well entrenched.

Canessa et al[31] studied the lymph nodes in 20 cadavers using conventional manual dissection. The starting point was at the bifurcation of the superior rectal artery and ending at the anorectal ring. They found an average of 8.4 lymph nodes per rectum; 71% of the lymph nodes were above the peritoneal reflection and 29% were below it. Dissection of seven fresh cadavers on the mesorectum by Topor et al[32] yielded 174 lymph nodes; over 80% of the lymph nodes were smaller than 3 mm. Fifty-six percent of the nodes were located in the posterior mesentery, and most were located in the upper two-thirds of posterior rectal mesentery. The translational importance of this information is attested to by the need to perform a complete or near complete as compared to incomplete total mesorectal excision (TME) when performing a curative protectomy for rectal cancer.

1.4 Histology

Knowledge of the microscopic anatomy of the large intestine is of paramount importance in understanding the various disease processes. This is especially true in the case of neoplasia, where the depth of penetration will dictate the treatment recommendation.

The innermost layer is the mucosa, which is composed of three divisions. The first is a layer of columnar epithelial cells with a series of crevices or crypts characterized by straight tubules that lie parallel and close to one another and do not branch (glands of Lieberkühn). The surface epithelium around the openings of the crypts consists of simple columnar cells with occasional goblet cells. The tubules are lined predominantly by goblet cells, except at the base of the crypts where undifferentiated cells as well as enterochromaffin and amine precursor uptake and decarboxylation (APUD) cells are found. The epithelial layer is separated from the underlying connective tissue by an extracellular membrane composed of glycopolysaccharides and seen as the lamina densa of the basement membrane when viewed by electron microscopy.[33] Abnormalities classified as defects, multilayering, or other structural abnormalities have been reported in many types of neoplasms, including those of the colon and rectum. These abnormalities are more common in malignant than in benign neoplasms. The second division of the mucosa is the lamina propria, composed of a stroma of connective tissue containing capillaries, inflammatory cells, and lymphoid follicles that are more prominent in young persons. The third division is the muscularis mucosa, a fine sheet of smooth muscle fibers that serves as a critical demarcation in the diagnosis of invasive carcinoma and includes a network of lymphatics.[34]

Beneath the muscularis mucosa is the submucosa, a layer of connective tissue and collagen that contains vessels, lymphatics, and Meissner's plexus. It is the strongest layer of the bowel. The next layer is the circular muscle, which is a continuous sheath around the bowel, including both the colon and the rectum. On the external surface of the circular muscle are clusters of ganglion cells and their ramifications; these make up the myenteric plexus of Auerbach. Unmyelinated postganglionic fibers penetrate the muscle to communicate with the submucosal plexus. The outer or longitudinal muscle fibers of the colon are characteristically collected into three bundles, called the taeniae coli; however, in the rectum these fibers are spread out and form a continuous layer. The muscularis propria is pierced at regular intervals by the main arterial blood supply and venous drainage of the mucosa.

The outermost layer, which is absent in the lower portions of the rectum, is the serosa or visceral peritoneum. This layer contains blood vessels and lymphatics.

1.5 Anal Canal

The anal canal is the terminal portion of the intestinal tract. It begins at the anorectal junction (the point passing through the levator ani muscles), is about 4 cm long, and terminates at the anal verge.[35,36] This definition differs from that of the anatomist, who designates the anal canal as the part of the intestinal tract that extends from the dentate line to the anal verge.

The anal canal is surrounded by strong muscles, and because of tonic contraction of these muscles, it is completely collapsed and represents an anteroposterior slit. The musculature of the anorectal region may be regarded as two tubes, one surrounding the other (▶ Fig. 1.6).[37] The inner tube, being visceral, is smooth muscle and is innervated by the autonomic nervous system, while the outer funnel-shaped tube is skeletal muscle and has somatic innervation. This short segment of the intestinal tract is of

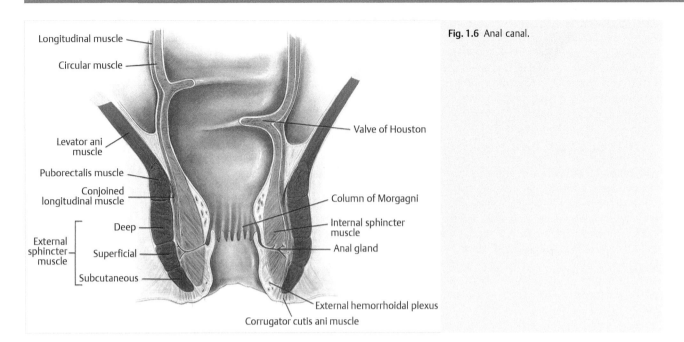

Fig. 1.6 Anal canal.

Labels (clockwise/around figure): Longitudinal muscle; Circular muscle; Levator ani muscle; Puborectalis muscle; Conjoined longitudinal muscle; External sphincter muscle — Deep, Superficial, Subcutaneous; Corrugator cutis ani muscle; External hemorrhoidal plexus; Anal gland; Internal sphincter muscle; Column of Morgagni; Valve of Houston

paramount importance because it is essential to the mechanism of fecal continence and also because it is prone to many diseases.

The anatomy of the anal canal and perianal structures has been imaged using endoluminal magnetic resonance imaging.[38] Investigators found that the lateral canal was significantly longer than its anterior and posterior part. The anterior external anal sphincter was shorter in women than in men and occupied, respectively, 30 and 38% of the anal canal length. The median length and thickness of the female anterior external anal sphincter were 11 and 13 mm, respectively. These small dimensions explain why a relatively small obstetrical tear may have a devastating effect on fecal continence and why it may be difficult to identify the muscle while performing a sphincter repair after an obstetrical injury. The caudal ends of the external anal sphincter formed a double layer. The perineal body was thicker in women than in men and easier to define. The superficial transverse muscles had a lateral and caudal extension to the ischiopubic bones. The bulbospongiosus was thicker in men than in women. The ischiocavernosus and anococcygeal body had the same dimensions in both sexes.

Posteriorly, the anal canal is related to its surrounding muscle and the coccyx. Laterally is the ischioanal fossa with its inferior rectal vessels and nerves. Anteriorly in the male is the urethra, a very important relationship to know during abdominoperineal resection of the rectum. Anteriorly in the female are the perineal body and the lowest part of the posterior vaginal wall.

1.5.1 Lining of Canal

The lining of the anal canal consists of epithelium of different types at different levels (▸ Fig. 1.7). At approximately the midpoint of the anal canal, there is an undulating demarcation referred to as the dentate line. This line is approximately 2 cm from the anal verge. Because the rectum narrows into the anal canal, the tissue above the dentate line takes on a pleated appearance. These longitudinal folds, of which there are 6 to 14, are known as the columns of Morgagni. There is a small pocket or crypt at the lower end of and between adjacent columns of the folds. These crypts are of surgical significance because foreign material may

become lodged in them, obstructing the ducts of the anal glands and possibly resulting in sepsis.

The mucosa of the upper anal canal is lined by columnar epithelium. Below the dentate line, the anal canal is lined with a squamous epithelium. The change, however, is not abrupt. For a distance of 6 to 12 mm above the dentate line, there is a gradual transition where columnar, transitional, or squamous epithelium may be found. This area, referred to as the anal transitional or cloacogenic zone, has extremely variable histology.

A color change in the epithelium is also noted. The rectal mucosa is pink, whereas the area just above the dentate line is deep purple or plum color due to the underlying internal hemorrhoidal plexus. Subepithelial tissue is loosely attached to and radially distensible from the internal hemorrhoidal plexus. Subepithelial tissue at the anal margin, which contains the external hemorrhoidal plexus, forms a lining that adheres firmly to the underlying tissue. At the level of the dentate line, the lining is anchored by what Parks[39] called the mucosal suspensory ligament. The perianal space is limited above by this ligament and below by the attachment of the longitudinal muscle to the skin of the anal verge. The area below the dentate line is not true skin because it is devoid of accessory skin structures (e.g., hair, sebaceous glands, and sweat glands). This pale, delicate, smooth, thin, and shiny stretched tissue is referred to as anoderm and runs for approximately 1.5 cm below the dentate line. At the anal verge, the lining becomes thicker and pigmented and acquires hair follicles, glands, and other histologic features of normal skin.[2] In this circumanal area, there is also a well-marked ring of apocrine glands, which may be the source of the clinical condition called hidradenitis suppurativa. Proximal to the dentate line, the epithelium is supplied by the autonomic nervous system, while distally the lining is richly innervated by the somatic nervous system.[40]

1.5.2 Anal Transitional Zone

The anal transitional zone (ATZ) is interposed between uninterrupted colorectal-type mucosa (columnar) above and uninterrupted

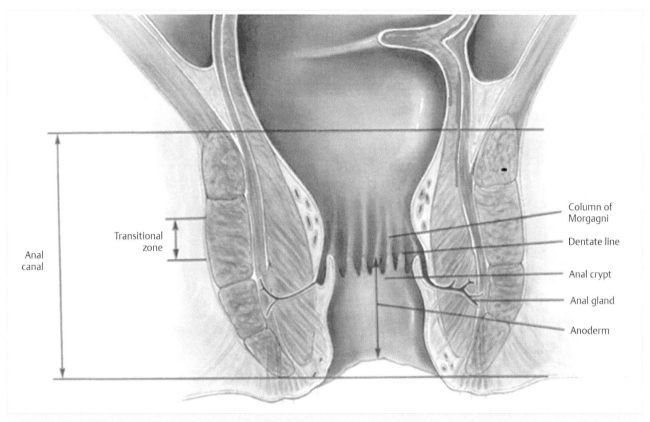

Fig. 1.7 Lining of the anal canal.

Column of Morgagni

Dentate line

Anal crypt

Anal gland

Anoderm

Transitional zone

Anal canal

squamous epithelium (anoderm) below, irrespective of the type of epithelium present in the zone itself.[41] The ATZ usually commences just above the dentate line. Using computer maps of histology, Thompson-Fawcett et al[42] found that the dentate line was situated at a median of 1.05 cm above the lower border of the internal sphincter. This is much smaller than that reported in the study by Fenger,[41] which portrayed the ATZ extending 0.9 cm above the dentate line. Fenger used the traditional alcian blue stain. This results in overestimation of the length of the ATZ because the pale blue staining is due to staining of superficial nuclei of both squamous anoderm and transitional epithelium rather than staining of mucin-producing cells in the transitional epithelium.[42] The ATZ is much smaller than commonly thought.

The histology of the ATZ is extremely variable. Most of the zone is covered by ATZ epithelium, which appears to be composed of four to nine cell layers—the basal cells, columnar, cuboidal, unkeratinized squamous epithelium, and anal glands. The ATZ epithelium contains a mixture of sulfomucin and sialomucin. The mucin pattern in the columnar variant of the ATZ epithelium and in the anal canal is of the same type and differs from that of colorectal-type epithelium. The findings of a similar mucin pattern in mucoepidermoid carcinoma and in some cases of carcinoma arising in anal fistulas as well as in carcinoma suspected of arising in anal glands might indicate a common origin of the neoplasm in the ATZ epithelium.

Histochemical study shows that endocrine cells have been demonstrated in 87% of specimens. Their function is unknown. Melanin is found in the basal layer of the ATZ epithelium in 14%

of specimens. Melanin cannot be demonstrated in the anal gland but is a constant finding in the squamous epithelium below the dentate line, increasing in amount as the perianal skin is approached. The melanin-containing cells in the ATZ seem a reasonable point of origin for melanoma, as do the findings of junctional activity and atypical melanocyte hyperplasia in the ATZ.

The ATZ epithelium has a dominating diploid population, although there was a small hyperdiploid peak representing nuclei with a scattered volume considerably higher than that of the main diploid population. This was present regardless of the histologic variant (columnar or cuboid) of the ATZ epithelium. Tetraploid or octoploid populations are not found.[41]

1.5.3 Anal Glands

The average number of glands in a normal anal canal is six (range, 3–10).[43] Each gland is lined by stratified columnar epithelium with mucus-secreting or goblet cells interspersed within the glandular epithelial lining and has a direct opening into an anal crypt at the dentate line. Occasionally, two glands open into the same crypt, while half the crypts have no communication with the glands. These glands were first described by Chiari in 1878.[44] The importance of their role in the pathogenesis of fistulous abscess was presented by Parks in 1961.[37]

Seow-Choen and Ho[43] found that 80% of the anal glands are submucosal in extent, 8% extend to the internal sphincter, 8% to the conjoined longitudinal muscle, 2% to intersphincteric space, and 1% penetrate the external sphincter. The anal glands are fairly evenly distributed around the anal canal, although the greatest number is found at the anterior quadrant. Mild-to-moderate lymphocytic infiltration is noted around the anal glands and ducts; this is sometimes referred to as "anal tonsil."

In an autopsy study of 62 specimens, Klosterhalfen et al[45] found that nearly 90% of specimens contained anal sinuses. In fetuses and children, more than half of the anal sinuses were accompanied by anal intramuscular glands penetrating the internal anal sphincter, while in adult specimens anal intramuscular glands were rare.

1.6 Muscles of the Anorectal Region and Internal Sphincter Muscle

The downward continuation of the circular, smooth muscle of the rectum becomes thickened and rounded at its lower end and is called the internal sphincter. Its lowest portion is just above the lowest part of the external sphincter and is 1 to 1.5 cm below the dentate line (▶ Fig. 1.6).

1.6.1 Conjoined Longitudinal Muscle

At the level of the anorectal ring, the longitudinal muscle coat of the rectum is joined by fibers of the levator ani and puborectalis muscles. Another contributing source is the pelvic fascia.[11] The conjoined longitudinal muscle so formed descends between the internal and external anal sphincters (▶ Fig. 1.6).[46] Many of these fibers traverse the lower portion of the external sphincter to gain insertion in the perianal skin and are referred to as the corrugator cutis ani.[47] Fine and Lawes[48] described a longitudinal layer of muscle lying on the inner aspect of the internal sphincter and named it the muscularis submucosae ani. These fibers may arise from the conjoined longitudinal muscle. Some fibers that traverse the internal sphincter muscle and become inserted just below the anal valves have been referred to as the mucosal suspensory ligament.[37] Some fibers may traverse the external sphincter to form a transverse septum of the ischioanal fossa (▶ Fig. 1.6). In a review of the anatomy and function of the anal longitudinal muscle, Lunnis and Phillips[49] speculated that this muscle plays a role as a skeleton supporting and binding the internal and external sphincter complex together, as an aid during defecation by everting the anus, as a support to the hemorrhoidal cushions, and as a determining factor in the ramification of sepsis.

1.6.2 External Sphincter Muscle

This elliptical cylinder of skeletal muscle that surrounds the anal canal was originally described as consisting of three distinct divisions: the subcutaneous, superficial, and deep portions.[36] This account was shown to be invalid by Goligher,[50] who demonstrated that a sheet of muscle runs continuously upward with the puborectalis and levator ani muscles. The lowest portion of the external sphincter occupies a position below and slightly lateral to the internal sphincter. A palpable groove at this level has been referred to as the intersphincteric groove. The lowest part (subcutaneous fibers) is traversed by the conjoined longitudinal muscle, with

some fibers gaining attachment to the skin. The next portion (superficial) is attached to the coccyx by a posterior extension of muscle fibers that combine with connective tissue, forming the anococcygeal ligament. Above this level, the deep portion of the external sphincter is devoid of posterior attachment and proximally becomes continuous with the puborectalis muscle. Anteriorly, the high fibers of the external sphincter are inserted into the perineal body, where some merge and are continuous with the transverse perineal muscles. The female sphincter has a variable natural defect occurring along its anterior length.[51,52,53,54,55,56] This makes interpretation of the isolated endoanal ultrasound difficult and explains overreporting of obstetric sphincter defects. The external sphincter is supplied by the inferior rectal nerve and a perineal branch of the fourth sacral nerve. From their embryonic study, Levi et al[52] demonstrated that the external sphincter is subdivided into two parts, one superficial and one deep without any connection with the puborectalis.

Shafik[46] has suggested that the anal sphincter mechanism consists of three **U**-shaped loops and that each loop is a separate sphincter and complements the others to help maintain continence (▶ Fig. 1.8). This concept has not been generally accepted. In fact, more recently, Ayoub[56] found that the external sphincter is one muscle mass, not divided into layers or laminae, and that all fibers of the external sphincter muscles retain their skeletal attachment by the anococcygeal ligament to the coccyx. Clinical experience supports Ayoub's concept; we have not been able to identify Shafik's three-part scheme.[46] Indeed, during postanal repairs for anal incontinence, the external sphincter, puborectalis, and levator ani muscles present as one continuous funnel-shaped sheet of skeletal muscle. The currently accepted perception of the arrangement of the external sphincter is that it is one continuous circumferential mass, a

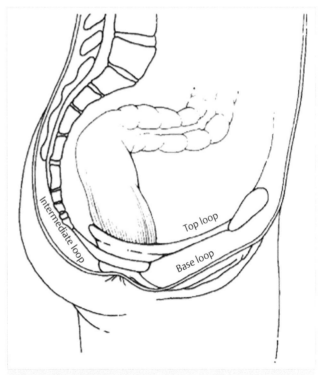

Fig. 1.8 Shafik loops.[46]

concept in accordance with a study in which anal endosonography was used.[53]

1.6.3 Perineal Body

The perineal body is the anatomic location in the central portion of the perineum where the external sphincter, bulbocavernosus, and superficial and deep transverse perineal muscles meet (▶ Fig. 1.9). This tends to be a tendinous intersection and is believed to give support to the perineum and to separate the anus from the vagina. In patients who have sustained a sphincter injury, an effort should be made to rebuild the perineal body as well as to reconstruct the sphincter.

1.6.4 Pelvic Floor Muscles

The levator ani muscle is a broad, thin muscle that forms the greater part of the floor of the pelvic cavity and is innervated by the fourth sacral nerve (▶ Fig. 1.10). This muscle traditionally has been considered to consist of three muscles: the iliococcygeus, the pubococcygeus, and the puborectalis.[3] Oh and Kark[54] and Shafik[55] suggested that it consists only of the iliococcygeus and pubococcygeus muscles and that the puborectalis is part of the deep portion of the external sphincter muscle, since the two are fused and have the same nerve supply, the pudendal nerve.[56] However, the electrophysiologic study by Percy et al[57] concluded that in 19 of 20 patients, stimulation of sacral nerves above the pelvic floor resulted in electromyographic activity in the ipsilateral puborectalis but not in the external sphincter. Results of postmortem innervation studies have favored a perineal nerve supply to the puborectalis, but the weight of evidence in favor of a pudendal nerve supply has been challenged by in vivo studies. Levi et al[52] believe that the puborectalis muscle must be considered part of the levator ani because it is never connected with the external sphincter in different steps of embryonic development.

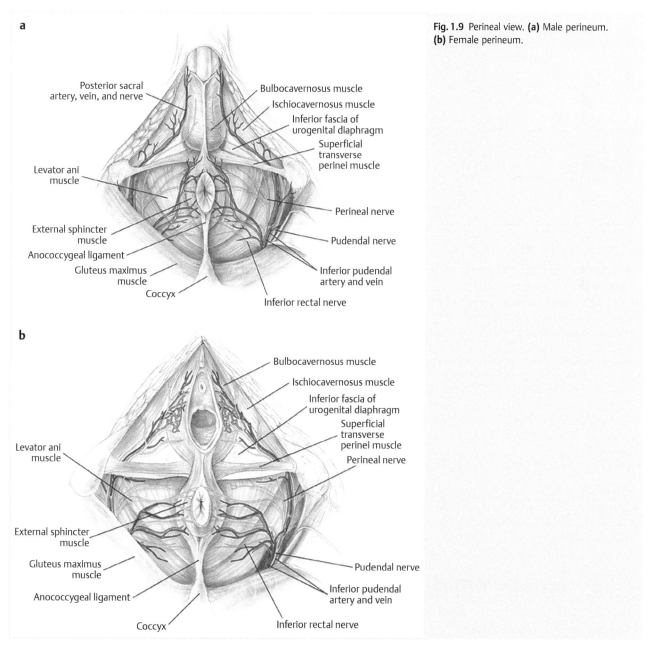

Fig. 1.9 Perineal view. **(a)** Male perineum. **(b)** Female perineum.

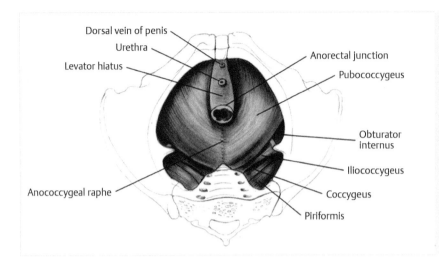

Fig. 1.10 Levator muscles.[46]

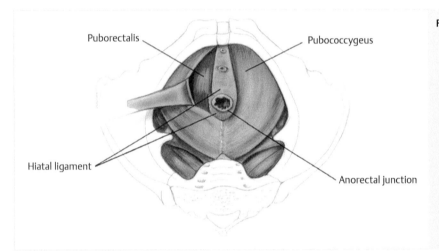

Fig. 1.11 Hiatal ligament.[46]

In a neuroanatomy study, Matzel et al[58] dissected cadavers and traced the sacral nerves from their entrance into the pelvis through the sacral foramina throughout their branching to their final destinations and found that the neural supply of the levator ani was distinct from that of the external anal sphincter. The levator is supplied by branches from the sacral nerves proximal to the sacral plexus and running on the inner surface; the external anal sphincter is supplied by nerve fibers traveling with the pudendal nerve on the levator's undersurface. To document the functional relevance of these anatomic findings, stimulation of the pudendal and sacral nerves was performed. The former increased anal pressure, whereas stimulation of S3 increased anal pressure only slightly but caused an impressive decrease of the rectoanal angle. When S3 was stimulated after bilateral pudendal block, anal pressure did not change, but the decrease in rectoanal angulation persisted. The authors concluded from their anatomic dissection and neurophysiologic study that two different peripheral nerve supplies are responsible for anal continence, that one muscle complex is innervated mainly by the third sacral nerve and another by the pudendal nerve. Further investigation will be required to clarify this point.

Puborectalis Muscle

The puborectalis muscle arises from the back of the symphysis pubis and the superior fascia of the urogenital diaphragm, runs backward alongside the anorectal junction, and joins its fellow muscle of the other side immediately behind the rectum, where they form a **U**-shaped loop that slings the rectum to the pubes (▶ Fig. 1.11).

Iliococcygeus Muscle

The iliococcygeus muscle arises from the ischial spine and posterior part of the obturator fascia, passes downward, backward, and medially, and becomes inserted on the last two segments of the sacrum, the coccyx, and the anococcygeal raphe. There are no connections to the anal canal.[11]

Pubococcygeus Muscle

The pubococcygeus muscle arises from the anterior half of the obturator fascia and the back of the pubis. Its fibers are directed backward, downward, and medially, where they decussate with fibers of the opposite side.[11,56] This line of decussation is called the anococcygeal raphe (▶ Fig. 1.10). Some fibers, which lie more posteriorly, are attached directly to the tip of the coccyx and the last segment of the sacrum. This muscle also sends fibers to share the formation of the conjoined longitudinal muscle (▶ Fig. 1.6). The muscle fibers of the pubococcygeus, while proceeding backward, downward, and medially, form an elliptical space, called the "levator hiatus" (▶ Fig. 1.10), through which pass the lower part of the rectum and either the prostatic urethra and dorsal vein of the penis in men or the vagina and urethra in women. The intrahiatal viscera are bound together by part of the pelvic fascia, which is more condensed at the level of the anorectal junction and has been called the "hiatal ligament" (▶ Fig. 1.11).[56] This ligament is believed to keep the movement of the intrahiatal structures in harmony with the levator ani muscle. The crisscross arrangement of the anococcygeal raphe prevents the constrictor effect on the intrahiatal structures during levator ani contraction and causes a dilator effect.[56] The puborectalis and the levator ani muscles have a reciprocal action. As one contracts, the other relaxes. During defecation, there is puborectalis relaxation accompanied by levator ani contraction, which widens the hiatus and elevates the lower rectum and anal canal. When a person is in an upright position, the levator ani muscle supports the viscera.

1.6.5 Anorectal Ring

"Anorectal ring" is a term coined by Milligan and Morgan[36] to denote the functionally important ring of muscle that surrounds the junction of the rectum and the anal canal. It is composed of the upper borders of the internal sphincter and the puborectalis muscle. It is of paramount importance during the treatment of abscesses and fistulas because division of this ring will inevitably result in anal incontinence.

1.7 Anorectal Spaces

Certain potential spaces in and about the anorectal region are of surgical significance and will be briefly described (▶ Fig. 1.4, ▶ Fig. 1.12, ▶ Fig. 1.13).

1.7.1 Perianal Space

The perianal space is in the immediate area of the anal verge surrounding the anal canal. Laterally, it becomes continuous with the subcutaneous fat of the buttocks or may be confined by the conjoined longitudinal muscle. Medially, it extends into the lower part of the anal canal as far as the dentate line. It is continuous with the intersphincteric space. The perianal space contains the lowest part of the external sphincter, the external

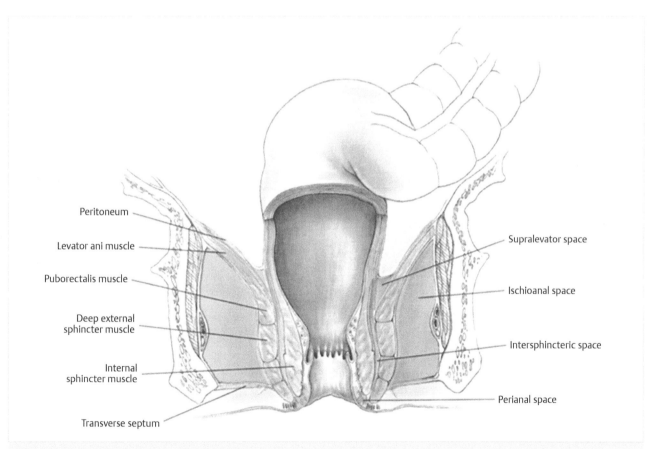

Peritoneum

Levator ani muscle

Puborectalis muscle

Deep external sphincter muscle

Internal sphincter muscle

Transverse septum

Supralevator space

Ischioanal space

Intersphincteric space

Perianal space

Fig. 1.12 Perianal and perirectal spaces (frontal view).

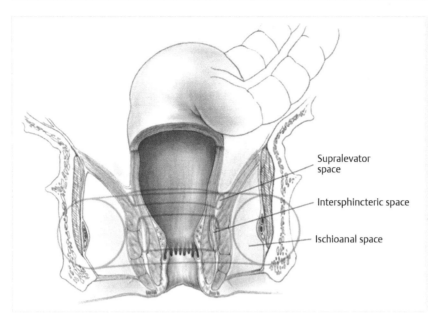

Fig. 1.13 Horseshoe-shaped connections of the anorectal spaces.

Supralevator space

Intersphincteric space

Ischioanal space

hemorrhoidal plexus, branches of the inferior rectal vessels, and lymphatics. The radiating elastic septa divide the space into a compact honeycomb arrangement, which accounts for the severe pain produced by a collection of pus or blood.

1.7.2 Ischioanal Space

The ischioanal fossa is a pyramid-shaped space. The apex is formed at the origin of the levator ani from the obturator fascia, and the inferior boundary is the skin on the perineum. The anterior boundary is formed by the superficial and deep transverse perineal muscles and the posterior boundary of the perineal membrane. The posterior boundary is the gluteal skin. The medial wall is composed of the levator ani and the external sphincter muscles. The lateral wall is nearly vertical and is formed by the obturator internus muscle and the ischium and by the obturator fascia. The base or inferior boundary is the transverse septum, which divides this space from the perianal space.[59] In the obturator fascia, on the lateral wall, is the Alcock canal, which contains the internal pudendal vessels and the pudendal nerve. When the ischioanal and perianal spaces are regarded as a single tissue space, it is called the ischioanal fossa.[60] The contents of the ischioanal fossa consist of a pad of fat, the inferior rectal nerve coursing from the back of the ischioanal fossa forward and medially to the external sphincter, the inferior rectal vessels, portions of the scrotal nerves and vessels in men and the labial nerves and vessels in women, the transverse perineal vessels, and the perineal branch of the fourth sacral nerve running to the external sphincter from the posterior angle of the fossa.[61] Anteriorly, the ischioanal space has an important extension forward, above the urogenital diaphragm, which may become filled with pus in cases of ischioanal abscesses.

1.7.3 Intersphincteric Space

The intersphincteric space lies between the internal and external sphincter muscles, is continuous below with the perianal space, and extends above into the wall of the rectum.

1.7.4 Supralevator Space

Situated on each side of the rectum is the supralevator space, bounded superiorly by the peritoneum, laterally by the pelvic wall, medially by the rectum, and inferiorly by the levator ani muscle. Sepsis in this area may occur because of upward extension of anoglandular origin or from a pelvic origin.

1.7.5 Submucous Space

Between the internal sphincter and the mucosa lies the submucous space. It extends distally to the dentate line and proximally becomes continuous with the submucosa of the rectum. It contains the internal hemorrhoidal plexus. Although abscesses in this space have been described, they are probably of little clinical significance and have been mistaken for what, in fact, were intersphincteric abscesses.

1.7.6 Superficial Postanal Space

The superficial postanal space connects the perianal spaces with each other posteriorly below the anococcygeal ligament.

1.7.7 Deep Postanal Space

The right and left ischioanal spaces are continuous posteriorly above the anococcygeal ligament but below the levator ani muscle these spaces communicate through the deep postanal space (▶ Fig. 1.4), also known as the retrosphincteric space of Courtney.[62] This postanal space is the usual pathway by which purulent infection spreads from one ischioanal space to the other, which results in the so-called horseshoe abscess (▶ Fig. 1.13).

1.7.8 Retrorectal Space

The retrorectal space lies between the upper two-thirds of the rectum and sacrum above the rectosacral fascia. It is limited anteriorly by the fascia propria covering the rectum, posteriorly by the presacral fascia, and laterally by the lateral ligaments (stalks) of the rectum. Superiorly, it communicates with the retroperitoneal space, and inferiorly it is limited by the rectosacral fascia, which passes forward from the S4 vertebra to the rectum, 3 to 5 cm proximal to the anorectal junction.

Below the rectosacral fascia is the supralevator space, a horseshoe-shaped potential space, limited anteriorly by the fascia propria of the rectum and below by the levator ani muscle (▶ Fig. 1.4). The retrorectal space contains loose connective tissue. The presacral fascia protects the presacral vessels that lie deep to it. The presacral veins are part of the extensive vertebral plexus and are responsible for the major bleeding problems encountered in this area during operation. In addition to the usual tissues from which neoplasms can arise, this is an area of embryologic fusion and remodeling; thus, it is the site for persistence of embryologic remnants from which neoplasms also can arise. The perianal, ischioanal, and supralevator spaces on each side connect posteriorly with their counterparts on the opposite side, forming a horseshoe-shaped communication (▶ Fig. 1.13).

1.8 Arterial Supply

Because the arterial supply of the large bowel is variable, the following descriptions are presented with the full recognition that they represent only the most frequently encountered patterns. However, they do serve as a basis on which a host of variations will be observed. In general, the right colon is served by branches of the superior mesenteric artery, while the left colon is served by the inferior mesenteric artery.

1.8.1 Ileocolic Artery

The ileocolic artery is the last branch of the superior mesenteric artery, arising from its right side and running diagonally around the mesentery to the ileocecal junction. It is always present and as a rule has two chief branches. The ascending branch anastomoses with the descending branch of the right colic artery, and the descending branch anastomoses with the ileal artery. Others include anterior and posterior cecal branches and an appendicular branch (▶ Fig. 1.14a).

1.8.2 Right Colic Artery

The origin of the right colic artery varies greatly from person to person. This artery may arise from the superior mesenteric artery, the middle colic artery, or the ileocolic artery (▶ Fig. 1.14a). In the series of Steward and Rankin,[63] the right colic artery was absent in 18% of cases, whereas in the series of Michels et al[64] it was absent in only 2% of cases. In a detailed dissection of 56 human cadavers, García-Ruiz et al[65] found an ileocolic artery in all cases, a middle colic in 55 of 56 cases, and a right colic artery in only 6 (10.7%) cadavers. Conventionally, the right colic artery is described as dividing into a descending branch that anastomoses with colic branches of the ileocolic artery and an ascending branch that anastomoses with the right branch of the middle colic artery.

1.8.3 Middle Colic Artery

The middle colic artery normally arises from the superior mesenteric artery either behind the pancreas or at its lower border

(▶ Fig. 1.14a). It frequently shares a common stem with the right colic artery. The artery curves toward the hepatic flexure, and, at a variable distance from the colonic wall, it divides into a right branch that anastomoses with the ascending branch of the right colic artery and a left branch that anastomoses with the ascending branch of the left colic artery. Although Griffiths[66] found the middle colic artery to be absent in 22% using arteriography and dissection, other investigators using cadaver dissection found it to be present in 96 to 98%.[63,67,68]

1.8.4 Inferior Mesenteric Artery

The inferior mesenteric artery arises from the abdominal aorta approximately 3 to 4 cm above the aortic bifurcation, about 10 cm above the sacral promontory, or 3 to 4 cm below the third part of the duodenum.[66] The first branch is the left colic artery, arising 2.5 to 3 cm from its origin (▶ Fig. 1.14a). It bifurcates, and its ascending branch courses directly toward the splenic flexure and anastomoses with the left branch of the middle colic artery. The descending branch anastomoses with sigmoid vessels. According to Griffiths,[66] the sigmoid arteries exhibit two principal modes of origin. In 36% of cases, they arise from the inferior mesenteric artery, and in 30% of cases the first sigmoid artery arises from the left colic artery. The second and third branches of the sigmoid arteries usually come directly from the inferior mesenteric artery. The number of sigmoidal branches may vary up to six.

1.8.5 Superior Rectal Artery

The inferior mesenteric artery proceeds downward, crossing the left common iliac artery and vein to the base of the sigmoid mesocolon to become the superior rectal artery. The superior rectal artery starts at the last branch of the sigmoid artery. It lies posterior to the right of the sigmoid colon, coming in close contact with the posterior aspect of the bowel at the rectosigmoid junction. It forms a rectosigmoid branch, an upper rectal branch, and then divides into left and right terminal branches. The terminal branches extend downward and forward around the lower two-thirds of the rectum to the level of the levator ani muscle. Tortuous small branches ascend subperitoneally to the anterior aspect of the upper third of the rectum and anastomose with the upper rectal branch (▶ Fig. 1.14b).[67]

The rectosigmoid branch arises at the rectosigmoid junction and divides directly into two diverging branches. One ascends to the sigmoid colon and anastomoses with branches of the last sigmoid artery, and the other descends to the rectum and anastomoses with the upper rectal branch. The upper rectal branch arises from the superior rectal artery before its bifurcation. It makes an extramural anastomosis with the lower branch of the rectosigmoid artery and the terminal branch of the superior rectal artery (▶ Fig. 1.14b).[67]

1.8.6 Middle Rectal Arteries

Most middle rectal arteries arise from the internal pudendal arteries (67%). The rest come from inferior gluteal arteries (17%) and internal iliac arteries (17%).[13] A middle rectal artery of appreciable diameter (1–2 mm) is observed on both sides in only 4.8%, on the right side in 4.8%, and on the left side in 2.4%

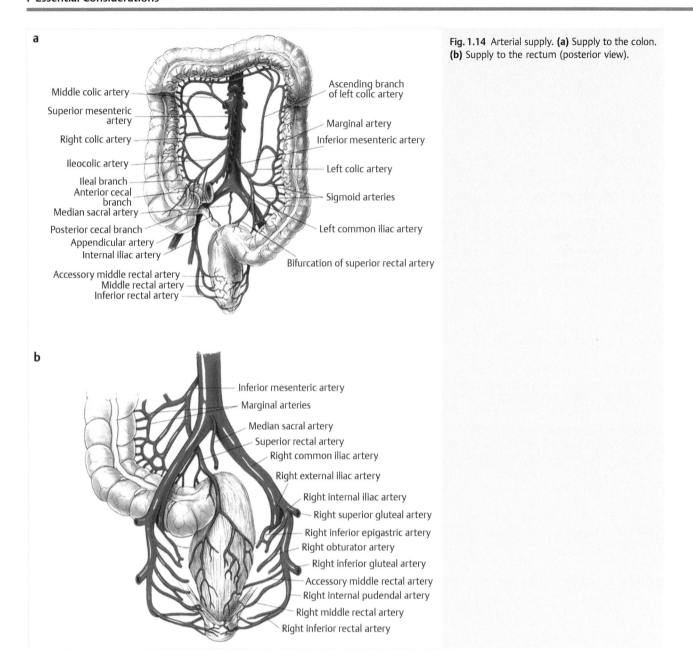

a

Middle colic artery

Superior mesenteric artery

Right colic artery

Ileocolic artery

Ileal branch
Anterior cecal branch
Median sacral artery

Posterior cecal branch
Appendicular artery
Internal iliac artery

Accessory middle rectal artery
Middle rectal artery
Inferior rectal artery

Ascending branch of left colic artery

Marginal artery
Inferior mesenteric artery

Left colic artery

Sigmoid arteries

Left common iliac artery

Bifurcation of superior rectal artery

b

Inferior mesenteric artery

Marginal arteries

Median sacral artery
Superior rectal artery
Right common iliac artery

Right external iliac artery

Right internal iliac artery
Right superior gluteal artery

Right inferior epigastric artery
Right obturator artery
Right inferior gluteal artery

Accessory middle rectal artery
Right internal pudendal artery
Right middle rectal artery
Right inferior rectal artery

Fig. 1.14 Arterial supply. **(a)** Supply to the colon. **(b)** Supply to the rectum (posterior view).

in the cadaver dissection by Ayoub.[68] Sato and Sato[13] find middle rectal arteries in 22% of the specimens. Their terminal branches pierce the wall of the rectum at variable points but usually in the lower third of the rectum. The presence of the middle rectal artery can be anticipated if the diameter of the terminal branches of the superior rectal artery is smaller than usual. Conversely, when the middle rectal arteries are absent, the superior rectal artery has larger size than usual.[68]

There is considerable controversy in the literature regarding the presence and origin of this vessel. Other series found the middle rectal artery to be present in 47 to 100% of cases.[27,69,70] Sato and Sato[13] believe that discrepancies, for the most part, result from incomplete dissection. The origin and course of several arteries, those from inferior vesical arteries, arteries to the ductus deferens, and uterine or vaginal arteries,[13] are almost indistinguishable from the middle rectal arteries, which enter the rectum via the lateral stalks. In the presence of occlusive vascular disease,

Fisher and Fry[71] believe that collateral circulation develops between superior and middle rectal arteries.

1.8.7 Inferior Rectal Arteries

The inferior rectal arteries, which are branches of the inferior iliac arteries, arise from the pudendal artery (in Alcock's canal). They traverse the ischioanal fossa and supply the anal canal and the external sphincter muscles. There is no extramural anastomosis between the inferior rectal arteries and other rectal arteries. However, arteriography demonstrates an abundance of anastomoses among the inferior and superior rectal arteries at deeper planes in the walls of the anal canal and rectum.[68]

The superior rectal artery is the chief blood supply of the rectum. The middle rectal arteries are inconsistent and cannot be relied on after ligation of the superior rectal artery. Although there is no extramural anastomosis among the superior rectal artery, middle rectal arteries, and inferior rectal arteries on cadaver dissection, arteriography shows abundant intramural anastomosis among them, particularly in the lower rectum.[66,67] When a low anterior resection for carcinoma of the rectum is performed in which the superior rectal artery and the middle rectal arteries are ligated, the rectal stump relies on the blood supply from the inferior rectal arteries. It may be safer to perform the anastomosis lower rather than higher, provided there is no tension.

1.8.8 Median Sacral Artery

The median sacral artery arises from the back of the aorta at 1.5 cm above its bifurcation and descends over the last two lumbar vertebrae, the sacrum and the coccyx, and behind the left common iliac vein (▶ Fig. 1.14a). Twigs of arteries form the median sacral artery. The terminal part of the anterior division of the internal iliac artery, the internal pudendal artery, arteries of the levator ani, and the inferior vesical artery in males and the vaginal artery in females are frequently found. These twigs are distributed mainly to pararectal tissues and sparsely to the wall of the rectum. No obvious anastomosis exists between these twigs and other rectal arteries. They are the major source of oozing during mobilization of the rectum.[68] The surgical significance of the median sacral artery is that during rectal excision it is exposed on the front of the sacrum, and when the coccyx is disarticulated, this vessel may demonstrate troublesome bleeding. The presence of this artery is inconsistent (often it is absent), and it probably is insignificant in providing the blood supply to the lower rectum.

1.8.9 Collateral Circulation

The marginal artery, generally known as the marginal artery of Drummond, is a series of arcades of arteries along the mesenteric border of the entire colon. It is the branch that connects the superior and the inferior mesenteric arteries. The arcades begin with the ascending colic branch of the ileocolic artery and continue distally to the sigmoid arteries (▶ Fig. 1.14a). The arcades are constant and rarely incomplete. Ligation of the inferior mesenteric artery in performing a rectosigmoidectomy can keep the left colon viable via the marginal artery.

Slack[72] attributed our current understanding of the distribution of vessels around the colon to the classic paper by Drummond in 1916. That description remains generally accepted today. By using injection studies, Slack determined the exact relationship of the blood vessels supplying the colon to the muscle layers and the position of diverticula. His findings supported those of Drummond. As soon as the vasa recta arise from the marginal artery, they divide into anterior and posterior branches, except in the sigmoid colon, where they may form secondary arcades (▶ Fig. 1.15).[73] They initially run subserosally in the wall, and just prior to the taeniae they penetrate the circular muscle and continue in the submucosa toward the antimesenteric border.[3] The vasa brevia are smaller arteries arising from the vasa recta, and some originate from the marginal artery.[74] They supply the mesocolic two-thirds of the circumference. However, a truly critical point exists at the splenic flexure, where the marginal artery is often small. As noted in 11% of the subjects in a series studied by Sierociński,[74] an area from 1.2 to 2.8 cm in the splenic flexure is devoid of vasa recta. This "weak point" is prone to a compromised blood supply. In the absence of the left colic artery, the marginal artery in this region is larger than usual.[50]

The "arc of Riolan" is found in about 7% of individuals. It is a short loop connecting the left branch of the middle colic artery and the trunk of the inferior mesenteric artery (▶ Fig. 1.16). The term frequently has been misquoted for the marginal anastomosis at the left colic flexure. The arc of Riolan also has been referred to as the "meandering mesenteric artery." It courses in the left colon mesentery roughly parallel to the mesenteric border of the colon. Its size enlarges when a significant arterial occlusion is present. If the arc of Riolan is present in patients undergoing operations to correct aneurysms, consideration

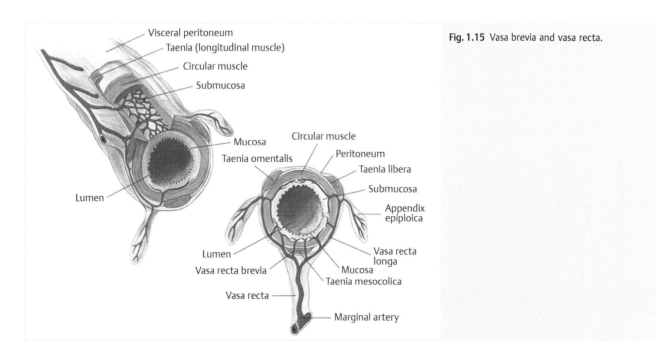

Fig. 1.15 Vasa brevia and vasa recta.

should be given to reimplantation of the inferior mesenteric artery. If the superior mesenteric artery is stenotic, the celiac and inferior mesenteric arteries provide the main collateral flow necessary for viability of the small intestine and the right colon (▶ Fig. 1.17a).[71] If the inferior mesenteric artery is stenotic, the superior mesenteric artery provides the main collateral flow necessary for the viability of the left colon and the rectum (▶ Fig. 1.17b).[71]

The inferior mesenteric artery also can function as an important collateral vessel to the lower extremities.[71] In instances of distal aortic occlusion, the trunk of the inferior mesenteric artery, the internal iliac artery, and the external iliac artery frequently remain patent. In this circumstance, blood flowing antegrade through the meandering mesenteric artery flows into the superior rectal artery, which then forms a collateral network with the middle rectal artery, an anterior division branch of the internal iliac artery. Blood can flow from the middle rectal artery into the internal iliac artery and from there into the

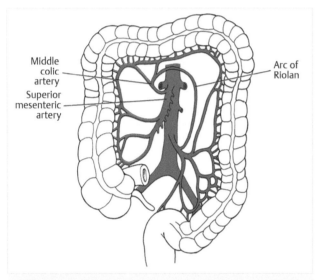

Fig. 1.16 Arc of Riolan.

external iliac artery. Obviously, incorrect ligation of the inferior mesenteric artery or ligation of the meandering mesenteric artery not only would threaten the viability of the rectum but also may cause acute ischemia of the lower extremity (▶ Fig. 1.17c).

The significance of the meandering mesenteric artery is that, during operation on the aorta, if flow is from the superior mesenteric artery to the inferior mesenteric artery, the inferior mesenteric artery may be ligated at its origin; however, if flow direction is the reverse, the inferior mesenteric artery must be reimplanted to avoid necrosis of the left colon (▶ Fig. 1.17a and b). For operations planned on the left colon, major mesenteric resection must be avoided because, by necessity, the meandering mesenteric artery will be divided. If flow is from the superior mesenteric artery to the inferior mesenteric artery,[75] necrosis of the sigmoid or rectum or even vascular insufficiency of the lower limb may occur. If flow is from the inferior mesenteric artery to the superior mesenteric artery, necrosis of the proximal colon and small bowel may occur.

In 1907, Sudeck[76] described an area in the rectosigmoid colon where the marginal artery between the lowest sigmoid and the superior rectal arteries is absent. Under these circumstances, ligation of the last sigmoid artery was believed to account for the occasional necrosis of part of the sigmoid and rectum during a rectal resection through a perineal or presacral approach. Most recent experiences with transabdominal rectosigmoid resection and dye injection studies have shown that the anastomosis between the superior artery and the last sigmoid artery is always adequate.[66,77] Thus, Sudeck's critical point does not have the surgical importance that was previously emphasized. With the use of an aortogram, Lindstrom[78] found that there is an important anastomosis between the superior and middle rectal vessels that potentially can prevent gangrene of pelvic organs when the distal aorta is occluded.

1.9 Venous Drainage

The veins of the intestine follow their corresponding arteries and bear the same terminology.

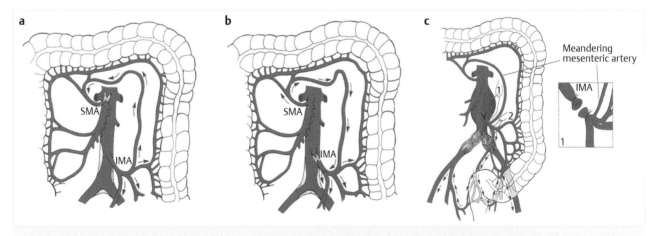

Fig. 1.17 Pathologic anatomy and occlusion of the superior mesenteric artery (SMA) and the inferior mesenteric artery (IMA). **(a)** Occlusion of SMA. **(b)** Occlusion of IMA. **(c)** Location for ligating IMA: (1) correct location of ligation (see inset); (2) incorrect location of ligation.

1.9.1 Superior Mesenteric Vein

The veins from the right colon and transverse colon drain into the superior mesenteric vein. The superior mesenteric vein lies slightly to the right and in front of the superior mesenteric artery. It courses behind the head and neck of the pancreas, where it joins the splenic vein to form the portal vein (▶ Fig. 1.18).

In the cadaver dissection, Yamaguchi et al[79] found highly variable venous anatomy of the right colon: all ileocolic veins drained into the superior mesenteric vein. The right colic vein, if present, joined the superior mesenteric vein in 56% and gastrocolic trunk in 44%. The middle colic vein, which was the most variable, and the right colic vein occasionally formed a common trunk with the right gastroepiploic vein and/or the pancreaticoduodenal vein. This common trunk was defined as the gastrocolic trunk. The middle colic vein drained into the superior mesenteric vein in 85% and the rest drained into the gastrocolic trunk.

1.9.2 Inferior Mesenteric Vein

The inferior mesenteric vein is a continuation of the superior rectal vein. It receives blood from the left colon, the rectum, and the upper part of the anal canal. All the tributaries of the inferior mesenteric vein closely follow the corresponding arteries but are slightly to the left of them. At the level of the left colic artery, the inferior mesenteric vein follows a course of its own and ascends in the extraperitoneal plane over the psoas muscle to the left of the ligament of Treitz. It continues behind the body of the pancreas to enter the splenic vein (▶ Fig. 1.18).

In the conduct of an extended low anterior resection of the rectum or a coloanal anastomosis, division of the inferior mesenteric vein just inferior to the duodenum prior to its union with the splenic vein may be necessary to ensure adequate mobilization of the colon to permit a tension-free anastomosis. Access to

the vessel is facilitated by incising the peritoneum at and just to the left of the ligament of Treitz.

Blood return from the rectum and anal canal is via two systems: portal and systemic. The superior rectal vein drains the rectum and upper part of the anal canal, where the internal hemorrhoidal plexus is situated, into the portal system via the inferior mesenteric vein. The middle rectal veins drain the lower part of the rectum and the upper part of the anal canal into the systemic circulation via the internal iliac veins. The inferior rectal veins drain the lower part of the anal canal, where the external hemorrhoidal plexus is located, via the internal pudendal veins, which empty into the internal iliac veins and hence into the systemic circulation (▶ Fig. 1.18). Controversy exists regarding the presence or absence of anastomoses formed by these three venous systems. Current thinking supports the concepts of free communication among the main veins draining the anal canal and that of no association between the occurrence of hemorrhoids and portal hypertension.[80]

1.10 Lymphatic Drainage

Lymphatic drainage of the large intestine starts with a network of lymphatic vessels and lymph follicles in the lower part of the lamina propria, along the muscularis mucosa, but becomes more abundant in the submucosa and muscle wall.[34] These vessels are connected with and drain into the extramural lymphatics. Although some lymphatic channels exist in the lamina propria above the muscularis mucosa, carcinomas that are confined to the lamina propria have not been known to metastasize.[34,81,82] On this basis, the term "invasive carcinoma" is used only when the malignant cells have invaded through the muscularis mucosae.[34] Knowledge of the lymphatic drainage is essential in planning operative treatment for malignancies of the large intestine.

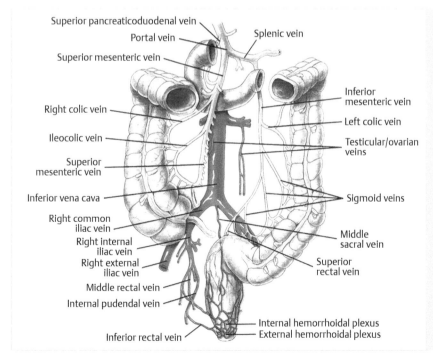

Fig. 1.18 Venous drainage of the colon and rectum. (Dark blue represents systemic venous drainage. Light blue shows portal venous drainage.)

Superior pancreaticoduodenal vein
Portal vein
Splenic vein
Superior mesenteric vein
Inferior mesenteric vein
Right colic vein
Left colic vein
Ileocolic vein
Testicular/ovarian veins
Superior mesenteric vein
Inferior vena cava
Sigmoid veins
Right common iliac vein
Right internal iliac vein
Middle sacral vein
Right external iliac vein
Superior rectal vein
Middle rectal vein
Internal pudendal vein
Internal hemorrhoidal plexus
External hemorrhoidal plexus
Inferior rectal vein

1.10.1 Colon

The extramural lymphatic vessels and lymph nodes follow the regional arteries. Retrograde flow is retarded by numerous semilunar valves. Jamieson and Dobson[83] conveniently classified colonic lymph nodes into four groups: epicolic, paracolic, intermediate, and main (principal) glands (▶ Fig. 1.19).

Epicolic Glands

The epicolic glands lie on the bowel wall under the peritoneum and in the appendices epiploicae. In the rectum, they are situated on the areolar tissue adjacent to the outer longitudinal muscular coat and are known as the "nodules of Gerota." The

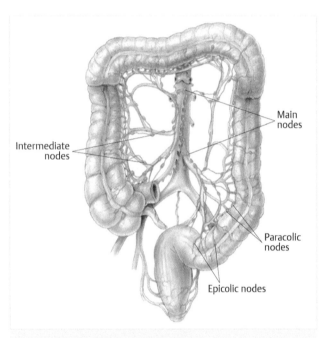

Fig. 1.19 Lymphatic drainage of the colon.

epicolic glands are very numerous in young subjects, but decrease in number in older patients. Although found on any part of the large intestine, they are especially numerous in the sigmoid colon.

Paracolic Glands

The paracolic glands lie along the inner margin of the bowel from the ileocolic angle to the rectum, mainly between the intestine and the arterial arcades along the marginal artery and on the arcades. The paracolic glands are believed to be the most important colonic lymph glands and to have the most numerous filters.

Intermediate Glands

The intermediate glands lie around the main colic arteries before their point of division.

Main Glands

The main (principal) glands lie along the origins of the superior and inferior mesenteric vessels and their middle and left colic branches. The main glands receive the efferents of the intermediate glands, from efferents of the paracolic glands, and frequently from vessels directly from the bowel.

1.10.2 Rectum and Anal Canal

Lymph from the upper and middle parts of the rectum ascends along the superior rectal artery and subsequently drains to the inferior mesenteric lymph nodes. The lower part of the rectum drains cephalad via the superior rectal lymphatics to the inferior mesenteric nodes and laterally via the middle rectal lymphatics to the internal iliac nodes (▶ Fig. 1.20).

Studies of the lymphatic drainage of the anorectum in women have shown that when dye is injected 5 cm above the anal verge, spread of the dye occurs to the posterior vaginal wall,

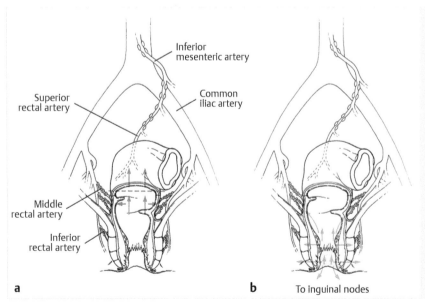

Fig. 1.20 Lymphatic drainage of the rectum **(a)** and anal canal **(b)**.

uterus, cervix, broad ligament, fallopian tubes, ovaries, and cul-de-sac. When the dye is injected at 10 cm above the anal verge, spread occurs only to the broad ligament and cul-de-sac, whereas injection at the 15 cm level shows no spread to the genital organs.[84] It generally has been known that retrograde lymphatic spread in carcinoma of the rectum and anal canal occurs only after there has been extensive involvement of the perirectal structures, serosal surfaces, veins, perineural lymphatics, and proximal lymphatic channels.[85]

The most modern study of lymphatic drainage of the rectum and anal canal has used lymphoscintigraphy. Following injection of a radiocolloid (rhenium sulfide labeled with technetium-99m), lymphatic drainage was detected by means of a computerized gamma camera. The lymphatic drainage of both the intraperitoneal and extraperitoneal rectum occurs along the superior rectal and inferior mesenteric vessels to the lumboaortic nodes. There is no communication between these vessels and the vessels along the internal iliac nodes.[86]

Canessa et al[87] performed a systematic examination of the number and distribution of lateral pelvic lymph nodes using 16 cadaveric dissections.[19] Dissection fields were divided according to the three surgical groups of pelvic wall lymph nodes: presacral, obturator, and hypogastric. A total of 458 lymph nodes were found, with a mean of 28.6 nodes per pelvis (range, 16–46). Lymph node size ranged from 2 to 13 mm. The highest number of lymph nodes was found in the obturator fossa group (mean, 7; range, 2–18). Hypogastric lymph nodes were found lying predominantly above the inferior hypogastric nerve plexus but reaching the deep pelvic veins. Complete excision of hypogastric lymph nodes demands a deep pelvic dissection of neurovascular structures.

Lymphatics from the anal canal above the dentate line drain cephalad via the superior rectal lymphatics to the inferior mesenteric nodes and laterally along both the middle rectal vessels and the inferior rectal vessels through the ischioanal fossa to the internal iliac nodes. Lymph from the anal canal below the dentate line usually drains to the inguinal nodes. It also can drain to the superior rectal lymph nodes or along the inferior rectal lymphatics through the ischioanal fossa if obstruction occurs in the primary drainage (▶ Fig. 1.20).

1.11 Innervation

The large intestine is innervated by the sympathetic and parasympathetic systems, the distribution of which follows the course of the arteries. The peristalsis of the colon and rectum is inhibited by sympathetic nerves and is stimulated by parasympathetic nerves. A third division of the autonomic nervous system is the enteric nervous system, which is described in Chapter 2.

1.11.1 Colon

Sympathetic Innervation

The sympathetic fibers are derived from the lower thoracic and upper lumber segments of the spinal cord. They reach the sympathetic chain via corresponding white rami. The thoracic fibers proceed to the celiac plexus by way of the lesser splanchnic nerves. From here, they proceed to the superior mesenteric plexus. Nerve fibers from the superior mesenteric ganglia supply

the right colon including the appendix. The lumbar sympathetic nerves leave the sympathetic chain via the lumbar splanchnic nerves and join the mesenteric nerves. The fibers to the descending colon, the sigmoid colon, and the upper rectum originate in the inferior mesenteric plexus. A lumbar or sacral sympathectomy is often followed by increased tone and contraction of the colon.

Parasympathetic Innervation

Parasympathetic innervation of the colon derives from two levels of the central nervous system: vagus nerve and sacral outflow.[5] The vagus nerves descend to the preaortic plexus and then are distributed along the colic branches of the superior mesenteric artery that supply the cecum, the ascending colon, and most of the transverse colon.[88] These nerves are secretomotor to the glands, motor to the muscular coat of the gut, but inhibitory to the ileocolic sphincter.[88] Administration of parasympathomimetic drugs such as Prostigmin (Valeant Pharmaceuticals North America, Aliso Viejo, CA) usually causes vigorous intestinal contraction and diarrhea. Fibers of the sacral outflow emerge in the anterior roots of the corresponding sacral nerves, as the nervi erigentes, which in turn join the hypogastric plexuses. The uppermost fibers of the sacral outflow are believed to extend as high as the splenic flexure. The preganglionic parasympathetic fibers entering the colon form synapses in ganglia clustered in the myenteric plexus of Auerbach and Meissner's plexus. There are numerous intricate connections between postganglionic fibers of adjacent myenteric and submucosal ganglia. Postganglionic parasympathetic fibers are cholinergic (▶ Fig. 1.21 and ▶ Fig. 1.22).

1.11.2 Rectum

Sympathetic Innervation

The sympathetic fibers to the rectum are derived from the first three lumbar segments of the spinal cord, which pass through

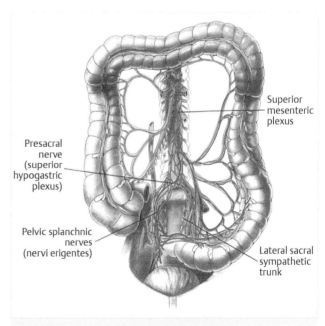

Fig. 1.21 Nerve supply to the rectum (frontal view).

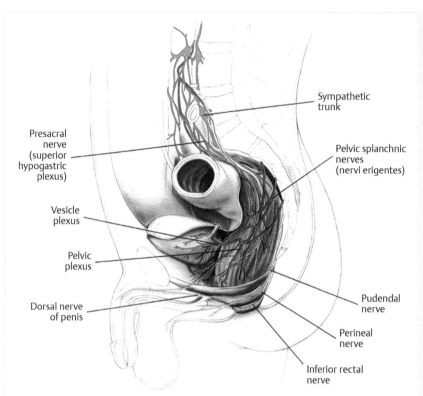

Fig. 1.22 Nerve supply to the rectum (lateral view).

Labels on figure:
- Sympathetic trunk
- Presacral nerve (superior hypogastric plexus)
- Pelvic splanchnic nerves (nervi erigentes)
- Vesicle plexus
- Pelvic plexus
- Dorsal nerve of penis
- Pudendal nerve
- Perineal nerve
- Inferior rectal nerve

the ganglionated sympathetic chains and leave as a lumbar sympathetic nerve that joins the preaortic plexus. From there, a prolongation extends along the inferior mesenteric artery as the mesenteric plexus and reaches the upper part of the rectum. The presacral nerve or superior hypogastric plexus arises from the aortic plexus and the two lateral lumbar splanchnic nerves (▶ Fig. 1.21 and ▶ Fig. 1.22). The plexus thus formed divides into two hypogastric nerves. The hypogastric nerves are identified at the sacral promontory, approximately 1 cm lateral to the midline and 2 cm medial to each ureter on cadaver dissection.[27] The hypogastric nerve on each side continues caudally and laterally following the course of the ureter and the internal iliac artery along the pelvic wall. It joins the branches of the sacral parasympathetic nerves, or nervi erigentes, to form the pelvic plexus.

During mobilization of the rectum after the peritoneum on each side of the rectum is incised, the hypogastric nerves along with the ureters should be brushed off laterally to avoid injury. The key zones of sympathetic nerve damage are during ligation of the inferior mesenteric artery and high in the pelvis during initial posterior rectal mobilization adjacent to the hypogastric nerves.

Parasympathetic Innervation

The parasympathetic nerve supply is from the nervi erigentes, which originate from the second, third, and fourth sacral nerves on either side of the anterior sacral foramina. The third sacral nerve is the largest of the three and is the major contributor.[27] The fibers pass laterally, forward, and upward to join the sympathetic nerve fibers to form the pelvic plexus on the pelvic side walls (▶ Fig. 1.21 and ▶ Fig. 1.22). From here, the two types of nerve fibers are distributed to the urinary and genital organs

and to the rectum. In women, the sympathetic nerve fibers from the presacral nerve pass toward the uterosacral ligament close to the rectum. In men, the nerve fibers from the presacral nerve pass immediately adjacent to the anterolateral wall of the rectum in the retroperitoneal tissue.[89,90]

The pelvic plexus supplies the prostate, seminal vesicles, corpora cavernosa, terminal parts of vasa deferentia, prostatic and membranous urethra, ejaculatory ducts, and bulbourethral glands.[91]

The pelvic plexus also provides visceral branches that innervate the bladder, ureters, seminal vesicles, prostate, rectum, membranous urethra, and corpora cavernosa. In addition, branches that contain somatic motor axons travel through the pelvic plexus to supply the levator ani, coccygeus, and striated urethral musculature. The pelvic plexus on each side is encased in the midportion of the lateral ligament, which is located just above the levator ani muscle. To avoid nerve injury in full mobilization of the rectum, the lateral ligament should be cut close to the rectal sidewall.[90,92]

The branches of the pelvic plexus along with the blood vessels (neurovascular bundle) that supply the male genital organs are located posterolateral to the seminal vesicles (▶ Fig. 1.23).[93]

The nerves innervating the prostate, the membranous urethra, and the corpora cavernosa travel dorsolaterally in the lateral pelvic fascia between the prostate and rectum. The bulk of the pelvic plexus is located lateral and posterior to the seminal vesicles, which can be used as an intraoperative landmark. Near the apex of the prostate, the nerves course slightly anteriorly to travel on the lateral surface of the membranous urethra. After piercing the urogenital diaphragm, they pass behind the dorsal penile artery and dorsal penile nerve before entering the corpora cavernosa.

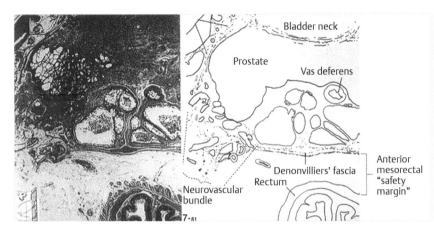

Fig. 1.23 Section shows the avascular areolar space between rectum and seminal vesicles and the location of the neurovascular bundle.[93] (Reproduced with permission from Lepor H, Gregerman M, Crosby R, Mostifi FK, Walsh PC. Precise localization of the autonomic nerves from the pelvic plexus to the corpora cavernosa: A detailed anatomic study of the adult male pelvis. J Urol. 1985;133:207-212.)

Both sympathetic and parasympathetic nervous systems are involved in erection. The nerve impulses from the parasympathetic nerves that lead to erection produce arteriolar vasodilation and increase blood in the cavernous spaces of the penis. Activity of the sympathetic system inhibits vasoconstriction of the penile vessels, thereby adding to vascular engorgement and sustained erection. Moreover, sympathetic activity causes contraction of the ejaculatory ducts, seminal vesicles, and prostate, with subsequent expulsion of semen into the posterior urethra.[94] Depending on which nerves have been damaged, certain deficiencies may occur, including incomplete erection, lack of ejaculation, retrograde ejaculation, or total impotence. Injury to nervi erigentes may occur during division of the lateral ligaments.

Anterior mobilization should start at the avascular plane between the rectum and the seminal vesicles in the midline. The incision is carried laterally to the lateral border of the seminal vesicle. At this point, the incision should curve downward (posteriorly) to avoid injury to the neurovascular bundles. Injury to the neurovascular bundle (▶ Fig. 1.23) probably causes ejaculation problems. Key zones of risk to parasympathetic nerves are during lateral dissection in the pelvis near the pelvic plexus and during the anterolateral dissection deep in the pelvis while mobilizing the rectum from the seminal vesicles and the prostate.

Pudendal Nerve

The pudendal nerve arises from the sacral plexus (S2–S4). It leaves the pelvis through the greater sciatic foramen, crosses the ischial spine, and continues in the pudendal canal (Alcock's canal) toward the ischial tuberosity in the lateral wall of the ischioanal fossa on each side. Three of its important branches are the inferior rectal, perineal, and dorsal nerves of the penis or clitoris (▶ Fig. 1.22). The main pudendal nerve is anatomically protected from injury during mobilization of the rectum. Sensory stimuli from the penis and clitoris are mediated by the branch of the pudendal nerve and are preserved after proctectomy.

1.11.3 Anal Canal

Motor Innervation

The internal anal sphincter is supplied by both sympathetic and parasympathetic nerves that presumably reach the muscle by the same route as that followed to the lower rectum. The parasympathetic nerves are inhibitory to the internal sphincter. The action of

sympathetic nerves to the internal sphincter is conflicting. Shepherd and Wright[95] and Lubowski et al[96] found it to be inhibitory, whereas Carlstedt et al[97] found it to be stimulating.

The external sphincter is supplied by the inferior rectal branch of the internal pudendal nerve and the perineal branch of the fourth sacral nerve. The pudendal nerve passes through the greater sciatic foramen and crosses the sacrospinous ligament accompanied by the internal pudendal artery and vein. The pudendal nerve lies on the lateral wall of the ischioanal fossa, where it gives off the inferior rectal nerve, which crosses the ischioanal fossa with the inferior rectal vessels to reach the external sphincter. Gruber et al[98] studied the topographic relationship of the pudendal nerve to the accompanying pudendal vessels and the ischial spine. In 58 left and 58 right pelves, the course of the pudendal nerve and vessels at the ischial spine were evaluated. Multi-trunked pudendal nerves were found in 40.5% with a left-versus-right ratio of 1:1.5. The diameters of the single-trunked nerves ranged from 1.3 to 6.8 mm. In 75.9%, the pudendal nerve was found medial to the accompanying internal pudendal artery. The distance to the artery ranged from 17.2 mm medial to 8 mm lateral. The distance to the tip of the ischial spine ranged from 13.4 mm medial to 7.4 mm lateral. Knowledge of the close spatial relationship between the pudendal nerve and the internal pudendal artery is important for any infiltration technique and even surgical release. In 31% of cases, an additional direct branch from the fourth sacral nerve innervates the external sphincter. This is important because it helps to explain why a bilateral pudendal block produces complete paralysis of the external sphincter in only about half the subjects, despite loss of sensation in the area innervated by the pudendal nerves.[99] The puborectalis muscle is supplied not by the pudendal nerves, but by a direct branch of the third and fourth sacral nerves, which lie above the pelvic floor.[57] The levator ani muscles are supplied on their pelvic surface by twigs from the fourth sacral nerves, and on their perineal aspect by the inferior rectal or perineal branches of the pudendal nerves.

Sensory Innervation

The sensory nerve supply of the anal canal is the inferior rectal nerve, a branch of the pudendal nerve. The epithelium of the anal canal is profusely innervated with sensory nerve endings, especially in the vicinity of the dentate line. Pain sensation in the anal canal can be felt from the anal verge to 1.5 cm proximal to the dentate line.[40] The anal canal can sense touch, cold, and pressure.

References

[1] Fraser ID, Condon RE, Schulte WJ, DeCosse JJ, Cowles VE. Longitudinal muscle of muscularis externa in human and nonhuman primate colon. Arch Surg. 1981; 116(1):61–63

[2] Morson BC, Dawson IMP. Gastrointestinal Pathology. Oxford: Blackwell Scientific Publications; 1972:603–606

[3] Goligher JC. Surgery of the Anus, Rectum, and Colon. 4th ed. London: Bailliere Tindall; 1980:14–15

[4] Saunders BP, Masaki T, Sawada T, et al. A peroperative comparison of Western and Oriental colonic anatomy and mesenteric attachments. Int J Colorectal Dis. 1995; 10(4):216–221

[5] Haubrich WS. Anatomy of the colon. In: Bockus HL, ed. Gastroenterology. 3rd ed. Philadelphia, PA: WB Saunders; 1976:781–802

[6] Topor B, Acland RD, Kolodko V, Galandiuk S. Omental transposition for low pelvic anastomoses. Am J Surg. 2001; 182(5):460–464

[7] Kumar D, Phillips SF. The contribution of external ligamentous attachments to function of the ileocecal junction. Dis Colon Rectum. 1987; 30(6):410–416

[8] Houston J. Observation on the mucous membrane of the rectum. Dublin Hosp Rep Commun Med Surg. 1830; 5:158–165

[9] Abramson DJ. The valves of Houston in adults. Am J Surg. 1978; 136(3):334–336

[10] Najarian MM, Belzer GE, Cogbill TH, Mathiason MA. Determination of the peritoneal reflection using intraoperative proctoscopy. Dis Colon Rectum. 2004; 47(12):2080–2085

[11] Garavoglia M, Borghi F, Levi AC. Arrangement of the anal striated musculature. Dis Colon Rectum. 1993; 36(1):10–15

[12] Crapp AR, Cuthbertson AM. William Waldeyer and the rectosacral fascia. Surg Gynecol Obstet. 1974; 138(2):252–256

[13] Sato K, Sato T. The vascular and neuronal composition of the lateral ligament of the rectum and the rectosacral fascia. Surg Radiol Anat. 1991; 13(1):17–22

[14] Walsh PC. Anatomic radical retropubic prostatectomy. In: Walsh PC, Gittes RF, Perlmutter AD, Stamey TA, eds. Campbell's Urology. Vol. 3. 5th ed. Philadelphia, PA: WB Saunders; 1986:2754–2755

[15] Lindsey I, Guy RJ, Warren BF, Mortensen NJ. Anatomy of Denonvilliers' fascia and pelvic nerves, impotence, and implications for the colorectal surgeon. Br J Surg. 2000; 87(10):1288–1299

[16] Aigner F, Zbar AP, Ludwikowski B, Kreczy A, Kovacs P, Fritsch H. The rectogenital septum: morphology, function, and clinical relevance. Dis Colon Rectum. 2004; 47(2):131–140

[17] Goligher JC. Surgery of the Anus, Rectum and Colon. 4th ed. London: Baillière-Tindall; 1980:6

[18] Moriya Y, Sugihara K, Akasu T, Fujita S. Nerve-sparing surgery with lateral node dissection for advanced lower rectal cancer. Eur J Cancer. 1995; 31A(7–8):1229–1232

[19] Heald RJ, Moran BJ. Embryology and anatomy of the rectum. Semin Surg Oncol. 1998; 15(2):66–71

[20] Church JM, Raudkivi PJ, Hill GL. The surgical anatomy of the rectum–a review with particular relevance to the hazards of rectal mobilisation. Int J Colorectal Dis. 1987; 2(3):158–166

[21] Nano M, Levi AC, Borghi F, et al. Observations on surgical anatomy for rectal cancer surgery. Hepatogastroenterology. 1998; 45(21):717–726

[22] van Ophoven A, Roth S. The anatomy and embryological origins of the fascia of Denonvilliers: a medico-historical debate. J Urol. 1997; 157(1):3–9

[23] Lindsey I, Warren BF, Mortensen NJ. Denonvilliers' fascia lies anterior to the fascia propria and rectal dissection plane in total mesorectal excision. Dis Colon Rectum. 2005; 48(1):37–42

[24] Jones OM, Smeulders N, Wiseman O, Miller R. Lateral ligaments of the rectum: an anatomical study. Br J Surg. 1999; 86(4):487–489

[25] Rutegård J, Sandzén B, Stenling R, Wiig J, Heald RJ. Lateral rectal ligaments contain important nerves. Br J Surg. 1997; 84(11):1544–1545

[26] Nano M, Dal Corso HM, Lanfranco G, Ferronato M, Hornung JP. Contribution to the surgical anatomy of the ligaments of the rectum. Dis Colon Rectum. 2000; 43(11):1592–1597, discussion 1597–1598

[27] Havenga K, DeRuiter MC, Enker WE, Welvaart K. Anatomical basis of autonomic nerve-preserving total mesorectal excision for rectal cancer. Br J Surg. 1996; 83(3):384–388

[28] Chapuis P, Bokey L, Fahrer M, Sinclair G, Bogduk N. Mobilization of the rectum: anatomic concepts and the bookshelf revisited. Dis Colon Rectum. 2002; 45(1):1–8, discussion 8–9

[29] Morgado PJ. Total mesorectal excision: a misnomer for a sound surgical approach. Dis Colon Rectum. 1998; 41(1):120–121

[30] Bisset IP, Chau KY, Hill GL. Extrafascial excision of the rectum: surgical anatomy of the fascia propria. Dis Colon Rectum. 2000; 43(7):903–910

[31] Canessa CE, Badía F, Fierro S, Fiol V, Háyek G. Anatomic study of the lymph nodes of the mesorectum. Dis Colon Rectum. 2001; 44(9):1333–1336

[32] Topor B, Acland R, Kolodko V, Galandiuk S. Mesorectal lymph nodes: their location and distribution within the mesorectum. Dis Colon Rectum. 2003; 46(6):779–785

[33] Frei JV. Objective measurement of basement membrane abnormalities in human neoplasms of colorectum and of breast. Histopathology. 1978; 2(2):107–115

[34] Fenoglio CM, Kaye GI, Lane N. Distribution of human colonic lymphatics in normal, hyperplastic, and adenomatous tissue. Its relationship to metastasis from small carcinomas in pedunculated adenomas, with two case reports. Gastroenterology. 1973; 64(1):51–66

[35] Nivatvongs S, Stern HS, Fryd DS. The length of the anal canal. Dis Colon Rectum. 1981; 24(8):600–601

[36] Milligan ETC, Morgan CN. Surgical anatomy of the anal canal: with special reference to anorectal fistulae. Lancet. 1934; 2:1150–1156

[37] Parks AG. Pathogenesis and treatment of fistuila-in-ano. BMJ. 1961; 1(5224):463–469

[38] Morren GL, Beets-Tan RGH, van Engelshoven JM. Anatomy of the anal canal and perianal structures as defined by phased-array magnetic resonance imaging. Br J Surg. 2001; 88(11):1506–1512

[39] Parks AG. The surgical treatment of haemorrhoids. Br J Surg. 1956; 43(180):337–351

[40] Duthie HL, Gairns FW. Sensory nerve-endings and sensation in the anal region of man. Br J Surg. 1960; 47:585–595

[41] Fenger C. The anal transitional zone. Acta Pathol Microbiol Immunol Scand Suppl. 1987; 289 Suppl 289:1–42

[42] Thompson-Fawcett MW, Warren BF, Mortensen NJ. A new look at the anal transitional zone with reference to restorative proctocolectomy and the columnar cuff. Br J Surg. 1998; 85(11):1517–1521

[43] Seow-Choen F, Ho JMS. Histoanatomy of anal glands. Dis Colon Rectum. 1994; 37(12):1215–1218

[44] Chiari H. Über die Nalen Divertikel der Rectumschleimhaut und Ihre Beziehung zu den Anal Fisteln. Wien Med Press. 1878; 19:1482

[45] Klosterhalfen B, Offner F, Vogel P, Kirkpatrick CJ. Anatomic nature and surgical significance of anal sinus and anal intramuscular glands. Dis Colon Rectum. 1991; 34(2):156–160

[46] Shafik A. A new concept of the anatomy of the anal sphincter mechanism and the physiology of defecation. The external anal sphincter: a triple-loop system. Invest Urol. 1975; 12(5):412–419

[47] Goligher JC, Leacock AG, Brossy JJ. The surgical anatomy of the anal canal. Br J Surg. 1955; 43(177):51–61

[48] Fine J, Lawes CHW. On the muscle fibres of the anal submucosa with special reference to the pecten band. Br J Surg. 1940; 237:723–727

[49] Lunniss PJ, Phillips RKS. Anatomy and function of the anal longitudinal muscle. Br J Surg. 1992; 79(9):882–884

[50] Goligher JC. The blood-supply to the sigmoid colon and rectum with reference to the technique of rectal resection with restoration of continuity. Br J Surg. 1949; 37(146):157–162

[51] Bollard RC, Gardiner A, Lindow S, Phillips K, Duthie GS. Normal female anal sphincter: difficulties in interpretation explained. Dis Colon Rectum. 2002; 45(2):171–175

[52] Levi AC, Borghi F, Garavoglia M. Development of the anal canal muscles. Dis Colon Rectum. 1991; 34(3):262–266

[53] Nielson MB, Pedersen JF, Hauge C, Rasmussen OO, Christiansen J. Normal endosonographic appearance of the anal sphincter: longitudinal and transverse imaging. Am J Radiol. 1991; 157:1199–1202

[54] Oh C, Kark AE. Anatomy of the external anal sphincter. Br J Surg. 1972; 59(9):717–723

[55] Shafik A. New concept of the anatomy of the anal sphincter mechanism and the physiology of defecation. II. Anatomy of the levator ani muscle with special reference to puborectalis. Invest Urol. 1975; 13(3):175–182

[56] Ayoub SF. Anatomy of the external anal sphincter in man. Acta Anat (Basel). 1979; 105(1):25–36

[57] Percy JP, Neill ME, Swash M, Parks AG. Electrophysiological study of motor nerve supply of pelvic floor. Lancet. 1981; 1(8210):16–17

[58] Matzel KE, Schmidt RA, Tanagho EA. Neuroanatomy of the striated muscular anal continence mechanism. Implications for the use of neurostimulation. Dis Colon Rectum. 1990; 33(8):666–673

[59] Netter F. The Ciba Collection of Medical Illustrations. Digestive System. Part II. Lower Digestive Tract. Vol. 3. New York, NY: Color Press; 1962:32

[60] Lilius HG. Investigation of human fetal anal ducts and intramuscular glands and a clinical study of 150 patients. Acta Chir Scand Suppl. 1968; 383:1–88

[61] Brasch JC, ed. Cunningham's Manual of Practical Anatomy. 12th ed. London: Oxford University Press; 1958:383

[62] Courtney H. The posterior subsphincteric space; its relation to posterior horseshoe fistula. Surg Gynecol Obstet. 1949; 89(2):222–226

[63] Steward JA, Rankin FW. Blood supply of the large intestine. Its surgical considerations. Arch Surg. 1933; 26:843–891

[64] Michels NA, Siddharth P, Kornblith PL, Parks WW. The variant blood supply to the small and large intestines: its importance in regional resections. A new anatomic study based on four hundred dissections, with a complete review of the literature. J Int Coll Surg. 1963; 39:127–170

[65] Garćia-Ruiz A, Milsom JW, Ludwig KA, Marchesa P. Right colonic arterial anatomy. Implications for laparoscopic surgery. Dis Colon Rectum. 1996; 39(8):906–911

[66] Griffiths JD. Surgical anatomy of the blood supply of the distal colon. Ann R Coll Surg Engl. 1956; 19(4):241–256

[67] Sonneland J, Anson BJ, Beaton LE. Surgical anatomy of the arterial supply to the colon from the superior mesenteric artery based upon a study of 600 specimens. Surg Gynecol Obstet. 1958; 106(4):385–398

[68] Ayoub SF. Arterial supply to the human rectum. Acta Anat (Basel). 1978; 100 (3):317–327

[69] Boxall TA, Smart PJG, Griffiths JD. The blood-supply of the distal segment of the rectum in anterior resection. Br J Surg. 1963; 50:399–404

[70] DiDio LJA, Diaz-Franco C, Schemainda R, Bezerra AJC. Morphology of the middle rectal arteries. A study of 30 cadaveric dissections. Surg Radiol Anat. 1986; 8(4):229–236

[71] Fisher DF, Jr, Fry WJ. Collateral mesenteric circulation. Surg Gynecol Obstet. 1987; 164(5):487–492

[72] Slack WW. The anatomy, pathology, and some clinical features of diverticulitis of the colon. Br J Surg. 1962; 50:185–190

[73] Griffiths JD. Extramural and intramural blood-supply of colon. BMJ. 1961; 1 (5222):323–326

[74] Sierociński W. Arteries supplying the left colic flexure in man. Folia Morphol (Warsz). 1975; 34(2):117–124

[75] Moskowitz M, Zimmerman H, Felson B. The meandering mesenteric artery of the colon. Am J Roentgenol Radium Ther Nucl Med. 1964; 92:1088–1099

[76] Sudeck P. Füber die Gefassversorgung des Mastdarmes in Hinsicht auf die Operative Gangran. Munch Med Wochenschr. 1907; 54:1314

[77] Goligher JC. The adequacy of the marginal blood-supply to the left colon after high ligation of the inferior mesenteric artery during excision of the rectum. Br J Surg. 1954; 41(168):351–353

[78] Lindstrom BL. The value of the collateral circulation from the inferior mesenteric artery in obliteration of the lower abdominal aorta. Acta Chir Scand. 1950; 100(4):367–374

[79] Yamaguchi S, Kuroyanagi H, Milsom JW, Sim R, Shimada H. Venous anatomy of the right colon: precise structure of the major veins and gastrocolic trunk in 58 cadavers. Dis Colon Rectum. 2002; 45(10):1337–1340

[80] Bernstein WC. What are hemorrhoids and what is their relationship to the portal venous system? Dis Colon Rectum. 1983; 26(12):829–834

[81] Okike N, Weiland LH, Anderson MJ, Adson MA. Stromal invasion of cancer in pedunculated adenomatous colorectal polyps: significance for surgical management. Arch Surg. 1977; 112(4):527–530

[82] Whitehead R. Rectal polyps and their relationship to cancer. Clin Gastroenterol. 1975; 4(3):545–561

[83] Jamieson JK, Dobson JF. The lymphatics of the colon. Proc R Soc Med. 1909; 2 ((Surg Sect)):149–174

[84] Block IR, Enquist IF. Lymphatic studies pertaining to local spread of carcinoma of the rectum in female. Surg Gynecol Obstet. 1961; 112:41–46

[85] Quer EA, Dahlin DC, Mayo CW. Retrograde intramural spread of carcinoma of the rectum and rectosigmoid; a microscopic study. Surg Gynecol Obstet. 1953; 96(1):24–30

[86] Miscusi G, Masoni L, Dell'Anna A, Montori A. Normal lymphatic drainage of the rectum and the anal canal revealed by lymphoscintigraphy. Coloproctology. 1987; 9:171–174

[87] Canessa CE, Miegge LM, Bado J, Silveri C, Labandera D. Anatomic study of lateral pelvic lymph nodes: implications in the treatment of rectal cancer. Dis Colon Rectum. 2004; 47(3):297–303

[88] Siddharth P, Ravo B. Colorectal neurovasculature and anal sphincter. Surg Clin North Am. 1988; 68(6):1185–1200

[89] Bauer JJ, Gelernt IM, Salky B, Kreel I. Sexual dysfunction following proctocolectomy for benign disease of the colon and rectum. Ann Surg. 1983; 197 (3):363–367

[90] Schlegel PN, Walsh PC. Neuroanatomical approach to radical cystoprostatectomy with preservation of sexual function. J Urol. 1987; 138(6):1402–1406

[91] Weinstein M, Roberts M. Sexual potency following surgery for rectal carcinoma. A followup of 44 patients. Ann Surg. 1977; 185(3):295–300

[92] Pearl RK, Monsen H, Abcarian H. Surgical anatomy of the pelvic autonomic nerves. A practical approach. Am Surg. 1986; 52(5):236–237

[93] Lepor H, Gregerman M, Crosby R, Mostofi FK, Walsh PC. Precise localization of the autonomic nerves from the pelvic plexus to the corpora cavernosa: a detailed anatomical study of the adult male pelvis. J Urol. 1985; 133(2):207–212

[94] Babb RR, Kieraldo JH. Sexual dysfunction after abdominoperineal resection. Am J Dig Dis. 1977; 22(12):1127–1129

[95] Shepherd JJ, Wright PG. The response of the internal anal sphincter in man to stimulation of the presacral nerve. Am J Dig Dis. 1968; 13(5):421–427

[96] Lubowski DZ, Nicholls RJ, Swash M, Jordan MJ. Neural control of internal anal sphincter function. Br J Surg. 1987; 74(8):668–670

[97] Carlstedt A, Nordgren S, Fasth S, Appelgren L, Hultén L. Sympathetic nervous influence on the internal anal sphincter and rectum in man. Int J Colorectal Dis. 1988; 3(2):90–95

[98] Gruber H, Kovacs P, Piegger J, Brenner E. New, simple, ultrasound-guided infiltration of the pudendal nerve: topographic basics. Dis Colon Rectum. 2001; 44(9):1376–1380

[99] Rasmussen OO. Anorectal function. Dis Colon Rectum. 1994; 37(4):386–403

2 Colonic and Anorectal Physiology

W. Ruud Schouten and Philip H. Gordon

Abstract

This chapter will focus on colonic physiology, including function, microflora, and propulsion and storage, and anorectal physiology, including anal continence, investigative techniques, and clinical applications.

Keywords: anorectal physiology, colonic physiology, function, microflora, propulsion, storage, anal continence, investigative techniques, clinical application

2.1 Colonic Physiology

The colon is the final conduit of the digestive tract in which digestive material is stored. Another major function of the large bowel is the absorption of water and salt. The absorption of sodium and chloride is balanced with the secretion of potassium and bicarbonate. This interaction is essential for the maintenance of electrolyte homeostasis. By absorbing most of the water and salt presented to it, the colon responds to body requirements and plays an essential role in protecting the body against dehydration and electrolyte depletion. The absorptive capability enables the colon to reduce the volume of fluid material received from the small bowel and to transform it into a semisolid mass suitable for defecation. The propulsion of feces toward the rectum and the storage of this material between defecations are the result of complex and poorly understood patterns of motility. Other functions of the large bowel include digestion of carbohydrate and protein residues and secretion of mucus.

2.1.1 Functions

Absorption

Physiologic control of intestinal ion transport involves an integrated system of neural, endocrine, and paracrine components.[1] Endogenous mediators, including neurotransmitters and peptides, act on enterocytes through membrane receptors coupled to energy-requiring "pumps" or "channels" through which ions flow passively in response to electrochemical gradients.

In healthy individuals, the colon absorbs water, sodium, and chloride, while secreting potassium and bicarbonate. It receives approximately 1,500 mL of fluid material from the ileum over a 24-hour period. From this input, the large bowel absorbs approximately 1,350 mL of water, 200 mmol of sodium, 150 mmol of chloride, and 60 mmol of bicarbonate.[2] It has been estimated that the colon possesses enough reserve capacity to absorb an additional 3.5 to 4.5 L of ileal effluent, a feature that allows the large bowel to compensate for impaired absorption in the small intestine.[3] Several factors that determine colonic absorption include the volume, composition, and rate of flow of luminal fluid. The success of whole gut irrigation capitalizes on this principle. The absorptive capacity is not homogeneous throughout the large intestine due to significant differences in the colonic segments. It has been shown that more salt and water are absorbed from the right colon than from the distal colon.[3] Thus, a right hemicolectomy is more likely to result in diarrhea than is a left hemicolectomy. Whenever ileocecal flow exceeds the capacity of the colon to absorb fluid and electrolytes, an increase in fecal water excretion (diarrhea) will ensue.

Most electrolytes cannot cross the phospholipid membrane of colonic epithelial cells by simple diffusion. Passing this membrane is only possible using distinct membrane proteins, which act like channels, carriers, and pumps. These proteins are required to facilitate and to speed up the transport across the apical membrane. This transport is passive because it is not energy dependent and because the flow is down the concentration gradient.

Absorption of Salt

The average concentration of sodium in the fluid chyme accepted by the colon from the terminal ileum is 130 to 135 mmol/L and in the stool is approximately 40 mmol/L. When the luminal concentration of sodium is high, more is absorbed; no absorption occurs when the luminal concentration is below 15 to 25 mmol/L.[4] In this way, there is a linear relationship between the luminal concentration of sodium and sodium absorption. The bulk of sodium absorption is electroneutral in exchange for intracellular hydrogen. This electroneutral absorption is facilitated by Na^+/H^+ exchange proteins. To date, three types of Na^+/H^+ exchangers (NHE) have been identified in the colon. NHE3 is the most prominent one. In addition to the electroneutral pathway, the distal colon also exhibits an electrogenic way to enhance the sodium uptake. This electrogenic absorption is facilitated by proteins in the apical membrane, which act like an ion-specific channel, belonging to the family of epithelial Na^+ channels (ENaCs). These ENaC proteins are inhibited by the diuretic amiloride and stimulated by mineralocorticoids. A small proportion of sodium is absorbed with the help of a sodium–glucose linked transporter. This membrane protein acts like a carrier and couples sodium and glucose. The transport of sodium across the apical membrane with the aid of all these distinct proteins is driven by the downhill electrochemical gradient and the negative membrane voltage. The electrochemical gradient is generated by the Na^+, K^+-ATPase at the basolateral membrane, which acts as a pump. This pump is stimulated by mineralocorticoids and has an electrogenic effect, extruding three Na^+ ions in exchange for two K^+ ions, and thereby maintaining relatively low intracellular Na^+ and high intracellular K^+ concentrations compared with concentrations of these electrolytes in the extracellular environment. The Na^+/K^+ pump results in a negative intracellular voltage. Across the colonic mucosa, there is an electrical potential difference of approximately 20 to 60 mV.[2] The basolateral membrane of the mucosal cell is electrically positive, whereas the apical membrane along the luminal border is electrically negative (▸ Fig. 2.1).[5,6] Sodium absorption is also stimulated by short-chain fatty acids (SCFAs) such as acetate, butyrate, and propionate, which are produced by bacterial fermentation.[7,8,9] The absorption of sodium is closely linked to the absorption of chloride. This anion either moves through the paracellular pathway or enters the epithelial cell

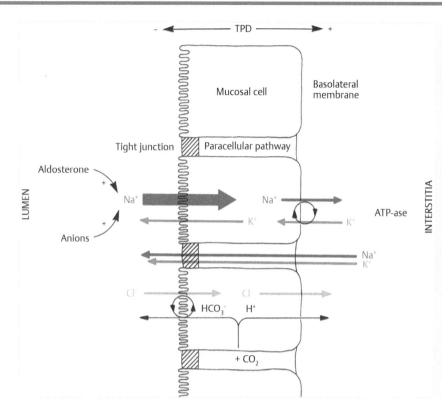

Fig. 2.1 Simplified diagram showing electrolyte transport across colonic epithelium. This diagram does not show the membrane proteins, which are required to facilitate and to speed up this process of electrolyte transport. TPD, transmural potential difference.

through its apical membrane (▶ Fig. 2.1). The transcellular absorption of chloride is electroneutral in exchange for intracellular bicarbonate[10] and is facilitated by Cl^-/HCO_3^- exchange proteins. The absorption of chloride is also driven by a concentration gradient and is increased by a low luminal pH. Chloride concentrations are high in ileal effluent but fall markedly during passage through the large intestine. Although the transport of salt across the colonic mucosal layer is characterized by net absorption, salt can also move backward into the colonic lumen through cellular and paracellular pathways. After basolateral uptake, the cellular pathway ends with apical excretion of chloride through Cl^- channels. The most important one is cystic fibrosis transmembrane conductance regulator. In patients with cystic fibrosis, this apical membrane protein does not function properly, resulting in impaired secretion of both Cl^- and HCO_3^-.[11]

Absorption of Water

Like the small bowel, the colon also absorbs water by simple diffusion. This process does not require membrane proteins and is driven by the osmotic gradient across the colonic mucosa, generated by the absorption of sodium. Water is transported through both paracellular and cellular pathways. Like salt, water also can move backward into the colonic lumen (▶ Fig. 2.1). Water cannot be absorbed if the colonic lumen contains a high concentration of inabsorbable, osmotically active solutes. Any water that remains in the colon will simply be excreted as watery diarrhea. The most common cause of this so-called osmotic diarrhea is lactose intolerance. Lactose must be cleaved into its component monosaccharides by lactase before their absorption. In the absence of lactase, osmotically active lactose cannot be absorbed and remains in the intestinal lumen, thus interfering with water resorption.

Secretion

Bicarbonate

As described earlier, chloride is absorbed in exchange for intracellular bicarbonate. This process is facilitated by Cl^-/HCO_3^- exchange proteins located in the apical membrane. The fact that chloride in the colonic lumen facilitates the secretion of bicarbonate is clinically evident in patients with ureterosigmoidostomy, who may develop hyperchloremia and secrete excessive amounts of bicarbonate.[12] Besides this Cl^--dependent process, there are two other pathways involved in the secretion of bicarbonate. One is through the apical Cl^- channels, mediated by cyclic adenosine monophosphate (cAMP). The other pathway is by exchange with SCFAs. The resulting net secretion of bicarbonate ions into the lumen aids in neutralization of the acids generated by microbial fermentation in the large bowel.[11,13]

Potassium

Potassium may be absorbed or secreted, depending on the luminal concentration. It is absorbed if the concentration exceeds 15 mEq/L, and is secreted if it falls below this value. Since luminal K^+ concentration is usually less than 15 mEq/L, net secretion normally occurs.[5] Potassium moves into the colonic lumen through both cellular and paracellular pathways (▶ Fig. 2.1). In the past, it was thought that this transport was mainly passive, along an electrochemical gradient. At present, it has become clear that colonic epithelial cells also contain membrane proteins, which act as channels to facilitate the uptake and excretion of potassium at their basolateral and apical membrane, respectively.[3,11] Because the distal colon is relatively impermeable to potassium, the luminal concentration may increase by the continued absorption of water. It has been suggested that there may be active secretion of potassium in the human rectum.[8] The presence of potassium in fecal bacteria and colonic mucus, as well as from desquamated cells, also may contribute to the high concentration (50–90 mmol/L) of potassium in human stool.[7,9]

Urea

Urea is another constituent of the fluid secreted into the colonic lumen. Of the urea synthesized by the liver, about 6 to 9 g/day (20%) is metabolized in the digestive tract, mainly in the colon.[2] Because the maximum amount of urea entering the colon from the ileum is about 0.4 g/day,[14] the bulk of urea hydrolyzed in the large bowel by bacterial ureases must be secreted into the lumen. The metabolism of urea in the colon gives rise to 200 to 300 mL of ammonia each day. Since only a small amount of ammonia (1–3 mmol) can be found in the feces, most must be absorbed across the colonic mucosa. Although the production of ammonia in the large bowel can be abolished by neomycin, the absorption of ammonia is not affected by this antibiotic.

Ammonia

Ammonia absorption probably occurs by passive coupled nonionic diffusion in which bicarbonate and ammonium ions form ammonia and carbon dioxide.[2] The nonionized ammonia can freely diffuse across the colonic mucosa. This process is partially influenced by the pH of the luminal contents; as the luminal pH falls, the absorption of ammonia decreases.[2] Although urea is the most important source of ammonia, the ammonia in the colon also may be derived from dietary nitrogen, epithelial cells, and bacterial debris.

Mucus

Mucus is another product secreted into the colonic lumen. Throughout the entire length of the large bowel, the epithelium contains a large number of mucus-secreting cells, and it has been shown that nerve fibers come close to these goblet cells. Stimulation of the pelvic nerves increases mucus secretion from the colonic mucosa, as has been confirmed histologically. There is evidence for such a nerve-mediated secretion of mucus in the large bowel.[15] The colon is able to absorb amino acids and fatty acids, but only by passive mechanisms. Bile acids also can be reabsorbed.

Digestion

A little recognized function of the colon is the role it plays in digestion. Digestion of food begins in the stomach and is almost accomplished when transit to the end of the small intestine is complete. However, a small amount of protein and carbohydrate is not digested during transit through the small bowel. The colon plays a role in salvaging calories from malabsorbed sugars and dietary fiber.[16] In the colon, some of the protein residues are fermented by anaerobic bacteria into products such as indole, skatole (b-methylindole), phenol, cresol, and hydrogen sulfide, which create the characteristic odor of feces. The carbohydrate residues are broken down by anaerobic bacteria into SCFAs such as acetic 60%, propionic 20%, and butyric acid 15%.[17] It has been estimated that 100 mmol of volatile fatty acids are produced for each 20 g of dietary fiber consumed.

Most of these SCFAs, which constitute the major fecal anion in humans,[18] are absorbed in a concentration-dependent way. Their absorption is associated with the appearance of bicarbonate in the lumen, which in turn stimulates the absorption of sodium and water.[1] Other end products of fiber fermentation are hydrogen and methane. About 70% of colonic mucosal energy supply is derived from SCFAs originating in the lumen.[17] The functions of the colonocytes, mainly dependent on the absorption and oxidation of SCFAs, include cellular respiration, cell turnover, absorption, and numerous enzyme activities. Furthermore, SCFAs are used by the colonocytes not only as a source of energy but also as substrates for gluconeogenesis, lipogenesis, protein synthesis, and mucin production.

Propulsion and Storage

The main functions of colonic and anorectal motor activity are to absorb water, to store fecal wastes, and to eliminate them in a socially acceptable manner.[19] The first is achieved by colonic segmentation and motor activity that propels colonic material forward and backward over relatively short distances. The second is facilitated by colonic and rectal compliance and accommodation, whereas the third is regulated by the coordination of anorectal and pelvic floor mechanisms with behavioral and cognitive responses.[19]

Distinct patterns of mechanical activity are required for the normal propulsion and storage of colonic contents. The rate and volume of material moved along a viscus also is related to the pressure differential, the diameter of the tube, and the viscosity of the material. Observation of transit does not necessarily reflect the contractile activity responsible for transit. Although the investigation of colonic motility in vivo has proved to be difficult because of the relative inaccessibility of the colon, new data have been revealed through the use of modern recording techniques. This information provides a better understanding of normal colonic motility in humans.

Assessment and Control of Motility

Radiologic Evaluation

Early efforts to investigate colonic motility involved radiographic studies in which the colon was filled with barium from either above or below. These studies could demonstrate only organized movements of the colon, represented by changes in contour, and were not helpful in the detailed examination of colonic motility. Moreover, the well-known side effects of radiation have limited the possibilities of radiologic observations, even with such sophisticated techniques as time-lapse cinematography.[20]

At the beginning of the 20th century, radiographic studies revealed three types of colonic motility: retrograde movement, segmental nonpropulsive movement, and mass movement. Retrograde movements were identified as contractions originating in the transverse colon and traveling toward the cecum.[21,22] Later, studies with cinematography also demonstrated a retrograde transportation of colonic contents.[23] These retrograde movements are believed to delay the transit in the right colon, resulting in greater exposure of colonic contents to the mucosa to allow sufficient absorption of salt and water.[24]

Segmental nonpropulsive movements are the type more frequently observed during radiologic investigation. These segmental movements are caused by localized, simultaneous contractions of longitudinal and circular muscles, isolating short segments of the colon from one another. Adjacent segments alternately contract, pushing the colonic contents either anterograde or retrograde over a short distance.[20] Although segmental movements occur mainly in the right colon, they also have been observed in the descending colon and the sigmoid colon. Like retrograde movements, segmental contractions also might slow colonic transit.

The third type of colonic motility identified from radiographic observations is mass movement, for the first time described by Hertz.[25] It occurs three or four times a day, primarily in the transverse and descending colon, but it also occurs in the sigmoid colon during defecation. Colonic contents are propelled by mass movement over a long distance at a rate of approximately 0.5–1 cm/s.[26,27] Using a microtransducer placed via a sigmoid colostomy, Garcia et al[28] recorded activity over a 24-hour period. They documented a series of contractions and spiking potentials averaging 5.6 minutes, following which a "big contraction" appeared with mean pressure values of 127 mm Hg and mean electric values of 10.6 mV. The duration of this phenomenon averaged 24.93 seconds and corresponded to an observed intense evacuation via the colostomy. They assumed that this electropressure phenomenon represents the mass movement.

Radiologic assessment can demonstrate only changes in contour. For detailed examination of colonic motility, other techniques must be employed, such as isotope scintigraphy, the measurement of intracolonic pressure, the investigation of colonic and rectal wall contractility with barostat balloons, and the examination of myoelectrical activity of colonic smooth muscle.

Isotope Scintigraphy

Although evacuation proctography and isotope proctography with radiolabeled material inserted into the rectum allow the description of rectal emptying, neither technique provides any information about transport of colonic contents during defecation. Colorectal scintigraphy after oral intake of isotopes is a physiological technique and allows accurate assessment of colorectal transport during defecation. Utilizing this technique, Krogh and co-workers observed an almost complete emptying of the rectosigmoid, the descending colon, and part of the transverse colon after normal defecation.[29]

Measurement of Intracolonic Pressure

Pressure activity of the large bowel has been intensively studied with many different devices, including water- or air-filled balloons, perfused catheters, radiotelemetry capsules, and microtransducers. The measurement of intracolonic pressure presents special problems. First, the colonic contents may interfere with recording by changing the basal physiologic state of the colon or plugging or displacing the recording device. Second, problems of retrograde introduction of recording devices and difficulty in maintaining them at a constant site may be encountered.

Initially, manometric recordings were limited to the rectum and distal sigmoid colon. Most studies were static and manometry was performed with a retrogradely placed assembly in the prepared left hemicolon. To avoid the potential perturbation of motor patterns by colonic cleansing and to permit ambulation, several authors have adopted an antegrade approach via nasocolonic intubation of the unprepared colon. To capture all the relevant activity throughout the entire colon with sufficient spatial resolution, it is necessary to use an assembly with multiple, closely spaced recording sites.[30] Initially, the manometric devices, designed for this purpose, contained a maximum of about 16 recording sites. In order to obtain recordings from the entire length of the colon, the sensors were spaced at intervals of 7 cm or more. Recently, it has been shown that sensor spacing above 2 cm results in misinterpretation of the frequency and polarity of propagating pressure waves.[31] Studies utilizing manometric devices with sensor spacing of 7 cm or more are actually based on low-resolution manometry. This technique has revealed two major pressure wave patterns. The first wave pattern is a very distinctive pattern of high-amplitude propagating sequences (HAPS). Most of these pressure waves with a high amplitude (> 100 mm Hg) arise in the cecum and ascending colon, especially after awaking and after a meal. The other pressure wave pattern, detected by this low-resolution manometry, is difficult to classify and is usually defined as segmental or nonpropagating activity. Recently, Dinning et al introduced high-resolution fiber-optic manometry.[32] The device, utilized in their study, contained 72 sensors spaced at 1-cm intervals. After mechanical bowel preparation, the catheter was introduced with a colonoscope and fastened to the mucosa of the ascending colon with endoclips. An abdominal X-ray was performed to verify the correct placement of the catheter (▶ Fig. 2.2).

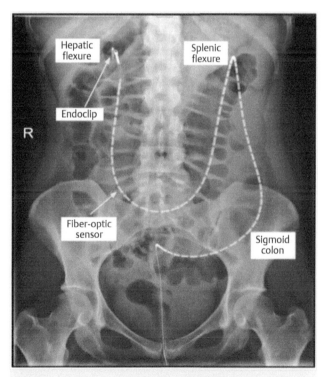

Fig. 2.2 X-ray image of the fiber-optic catheter positioned in the healthy human colon. The tip of the catheter can be seen at the hepatic flexure. The middle of each white segment is the position of each pressure sensor.[32] (With permission © 2004 John Wiley and Sons.)

Manometric recordings were obtained from 10 healthy individuals. The authors were able to identify five distinct motor patterns:

1. High-amplitude propagating sequences. These HAPS occurred in all subjects, started in the proximal colon, and always propagated in an antegrade direction. HAPS represented only 1 to 2% of all detected pressure events. They had a high amplitude (> 116 mm Hg) and their average extent of propagation was 33 ± 12 cm, with a mean velocity of 0.4 ± 0.1 cm per second (▶ Fig. 2.3).

2. Cyclic motor patterns. These patterns are characterized by repetitive propagating pressure events with a cyclic frequency of two to six per minute and an amplitude of 23.1 ± 21.4 mm Hg. These pressure events propagated both antegrade and retrograde with an average extent of < 7 cm. They occurred in all patients and represented almost 70% of all detected activity in the colon. Although observed in all

colonic segments, most cyclic motor patterns were identified in the sigmoid colon (▶ Fig. 2.4).

3. Short single motor patterns. These patterns are characterized by single pressure events, separated by intervals of more than 1 minute, when they occurred repetitively. These pressure events had an amplitude of 58.1 ± 26.7 mm Hg and propagated both antegrade and retrograde with an average extent of < 7 cm. They were observed in all subjects and represented almost a quarter of detected pressure events.

4. Long single motor events. These are also characterized by single pressure events, separated by intervals of more than 1 minute, when they occurred repetitively. In contrast to short single motor events, they propagated only in antegrade direction, over a longer distance and with a greater velocity. These pressure events were detected in 7 of the 10 subjects.

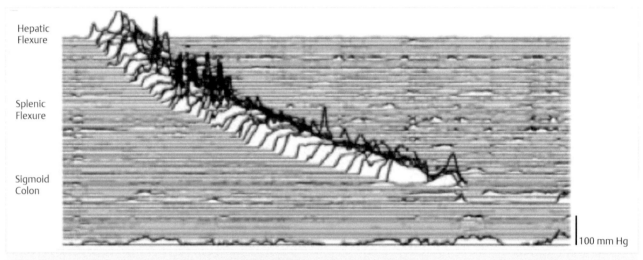

Fig. 2.3 High-amplitude propagating sequence.[32] (With permission © 2004 John Wiley and Sons.)

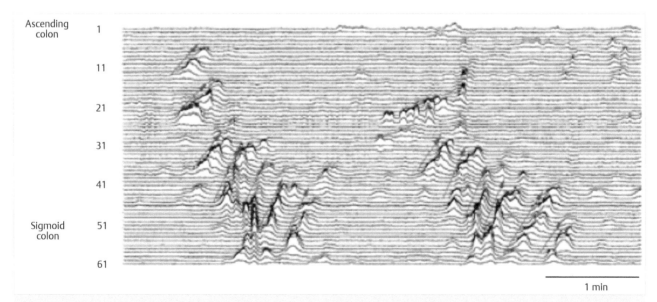

Fig. 2.4 Cyclic retrograde propagating motor pattern.[32] (With permission © 2004 John Wiley and Sons.)

5. Retrograde slowly propagating motor pattern. This pattern was observed in only two patients. This pattern started in the sigmoid colon and propagated backward into the transverse colon.

After a meal, HAPS appeared in 5 of 10 subjects. Apart from these HAPS, the major effect of ingesting a meal was a significant increase in cyclic retrograde motor patterns, especially in the sigmoid colon. According to the authors, the relative scarcity of HAPS (not detected in the fasting state and observed in only five subjects after ingesting a meal) may have been influenced by the study protocol. The recordings started within an hour of catheter placement in a prepared and empty colon and stopped 4 hours later. It has been shown that HAPS are more abundant in an unprepared colon. It seems likely that colonic distension due to large volumes of fecal material triggers the activation of HAPS.

Simultaneous assessment of isotope movement and intracolonic pressure changes has revealed that HAPS represent the manometric equivalent of propulsive mass movements and that fewer than 5% of these pressure events reach the rectum.[33] In contrast to earlier reports, more recent work has revealed that HAPS do not display regional variation in conduction velocity.[30] They can be activated by mechanical colonic distension and by intraluminal chemical stimulation with agents such as glycerol, bisacodyl, oleic acid, chenodeoxycholic acid, and SCFAs. It has been shown that neostigmine, which can be used to relieve distension in acute colonic pseudo-obstruction, also induces HAPS.[34] Colonic distension and chemical stimulation act on underlying enteric circuits. Because HAPS increase upon awakening and appear rapidly after a meal, it seems likely that extrinsic neural input is also important. Crowell et al[35] found that 41% of these pressure waves occur in the hour before defecation. The relationship between high-amplitude pressure waves and defecation has been confirmed by others.[36,37] Bampton et al studied the spatial and temporal organization of pressure patterns throughout the unprepared colon during spontaneous defecation.[38,39] They were able to demonstrate a preexpulsive phase commencing up to 1 hour before stool expulsion. This phase is characterized by a distinctive biphasic spatial and temporal pattern with an early and a late component. The early component is characterized by an array of antegrade propagating sequences. The site of their origin migrates distally with each subsequent sequence. The late component, in the 15 minutes before stool expulsion, is characterized by an array of antegrade propagating sequences. The site of their origin migrates proximally with each subsequent sequence. The amplitude of the pressure waves, occurring in this late phase, increases significantly. Many of them are real high-amplitude pressure waves. They are associated with an increasing sensation of urge to defecate. Some of the last propagating sequences, prior to stool expulsion, commence in the ascending colon (▶ Fig. 2.5). This latter finding illustrates that the entire colon is involved in the process of defecation. Hirabayashi et al investigated colorectal motility in adult mongrel dogs before and during spontaneous defecation with the help of force strain gauge transducers implanted in the proximal, distal, and sigmoid colon, as well as in the rectum and the anal canal. During defecation, giant contractions were detected, running from the distal

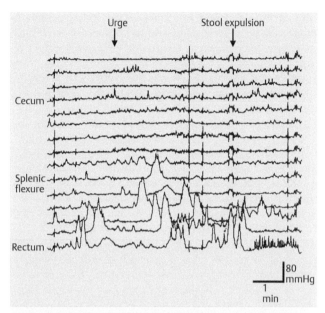

Fig. 2.5 Manometric trace of spontaneous defecation. This trace demonstrates an array of propagating sequences with site of origin becoming more proximal with each subsequent sequence. Note that the propagating pressure waves in the sequences immediately before defecation exhibit a slower velocity and greater amplitude than pressure waves in earlier sequences, and in this example stool expulsion follows immediately after a propagating sequence.[38] (With permission © 2000 Nature Publishing Group.)

colon into the rectum. It seems likely that these giant contractions are the myoelectric equivalent of the high-amplitude pressure waves.[40]

As previously mentioned, the cyclic motor pattern is by far the most common colonic motor pattern. This pattern is characterized by short-extent and low-amplitude contractions with a cyclic frequency of 2 to 6 per minute. In the past, this activity was classified as nonpropagating, based on low-resolution manometry with sensors spaced at intervals of 7 cm or more. However, since the introduction of high-resolution manometry, it has become clear that these cyclic contractions propagate both antegrade and retrograde with an average extent of < 7 cm. Although these contractions occur in all regions of the colon, they are most prevalent in the sigmoid and the rectum. In this region of the colon, these complexes have a predominant retrograde direction. Based on this finding, it has been suggested that they resist anally directed flow and assist in the maintenance of continence and control of defecation.[32] Like HAPS, this type of activity is also suppressed during the night and increases after awakening. Ingesting a meal results in a rapid and large increase in cyclic retrograde propagating contractions, whereas the cyclic antegrade propagating contractions show no change after a meal. Retrograde transport is a major component of normal colonic physiology. It has been postulated that the cyclic retrograde propagating contractions contribute to this retrograde transport, thereby acting as a gatekeeper to keep the rectum empty. It has been suggested that reduction or absence of these contractions may contribute to fecal incontinence. It has been shown that sacral nerve stimulation is associated with an increase in cyclic retrograde patterns. This intriguing finding may explain some of the symptomatic improvement obtained with this type of treatment.[41] The cyclic retrograde motor patterns in the rectum are most likely the same as the rectal motor complexes, as described by Kumar et al.[42] All colonic motor activity is reduced during sleep. Another potent inhibitor of colonic activity is rectal distension. This rectocolonic inhibitory reflex prevents further passage of stool to a loaded rectum and is presumed to be mediated by long colocolonic pathways.[43]

Using low-resolution manometry, some workers were able to demonstrate that constipated subjects display significantly fewer high-amplitude contractions than healthy volunteers.[44,45,46] During the last decade, numerous studies, based on high-resolution manometry, have revealed that slow transit constipation is indeed associated with abnormal colonic motility. It has been convincingly demonstrated that the large bowel of patients with slow transit constipation exhibit little or no HAPS. In these patients, the normal increase of HAPS after a meal is lacking. Almost all patients with slow transit constipation exhibit normal cyclic propagating pressure events in the fasting state. However, the huge increase in the postprandial retrograde propagating cyclic motor pattern, normally seen in healthy subjects, is completely absent in patients with slow transit constipation. Based on this finding, it has been suggested that this phenomenon is due to attenuated neural input to the colon.[47] Similar abnormalities have been observed in children with intractable constipation.[48] Recently, Dinning et al conducted an intriguing study in patients with slow transit constipation before and after subtotal colectomy. Prior to the operation, abnormal colonic motility was recorded in vivo, as described above. Once the colon was removed, ex vivo manometric recordings were obtained with the colonic specimen in an organ bath. Regular propagating motor patterns were recorded at approximately 1 per minute. This activity did not differ from control colon tissue obtained from patients undergoing a low anterior resection. Since the deficits in colonic motility are not apparent ex vivo, the authors suggest that extrinsic parasympathetic input to the colon plays a role in the pathophysiology of slow transit constipation.[49]

Contractile Activity

It has been reported that barostat balloons have the potential to explore variations in the contractile state of the colonic and rectal wall. Barostat balloons are infinitely compliant plastic bags. The barostat assembly moves air in and out to maintain a constant preset pressure in the balloon. Changes in tone are reflected by changes in bag volume. A significant reduction of bag volume has been documented immediately after the ingestion of food, indicating a sustained increase in colonic tone in the postprandial period. During overnight sleep, colonic tone decreases.[50,51] The increase in colonic tone in response to feeding shows remarkable regional differences. Assessing the contractile activity in the transverse and sigmoid colon using a barostat assembly, Ford et al[52] found that the mean increase in colonic tone after the ingestion of food was significantly greater in the transverse than in the sigmoid colon. The contractile responses in the human colon are mediated by a 5HT3 mechanism.[53] It has been reported that hypocapnic hyperventilation produces an increase in colonic tone. This finding suggests that autonomic mechanisms are also involved in the control of the contractile state of the large bowel.[54] Grotz et al[55] reported that changes in

rectal wall contractility in response to feeding, to a cholinergic agonist, and to a smooth muscle relaxant are decreased in constipated patients. Gosselink and Schouten[56] used a barostat assembly to investigate the tonic response of the rectum to a meal in healthy volunteers and in 60 women with obstructed defecation. Total colonic transit time was normal in 30 patients and prolonged in the other 30. Following the meal, all controls showed a significant increase in rectal tone. A similar response was found in the patients with a normal colonic transit time. In the patients with a prolonged colonic transit, the increase in rectal tone was significantly lower. In the past, it has been stated that intracolonic barostat balloons are more sensitive than manometric probes in the detection of nonoccluding contractions. Using a combined barostat–manometry assembly, von der Ohe et al[53] found a significant decrease of bag volume consistent with an increment in colonic tone after the ingestion of a 1,000-kcal meal. This response was not associated with concomitant changes in intracolonic pressure. In addition, they also reported that the barostat balloon measurements indicated 70% more phasic events than the manometric side holes located 2 cm proximal to 7 cm distal to the balloon. However, it should be mentioned that the manometric assembly, used in this and other studies, only provided low-resolution recordings. It seems likely that the modern high-resolution techniques are more suitable for detailed examination of colonic motility.

Myoelectrical Activity

The electrical activity of smooth muscle cells of the colon is characterized by cyclical depolarization and repolarization of their membrane, resulting in slow wave potentials. The frequency of these slow wave potentials varies between 3 and 12 cycles per minute. This basic electrical rhythm is generated by the interstitial cells of Cajal (ICC), in particular the subpopulations of these cells which are located within the myenteric plexus and along the submucosal surface of the circular muscle layer.[57] Experimental studies have revealed that slow waves are absent in animals lacking ICC. Based on these and other studies, it is now abundantly clear that ICC act as pacemakers. Within the ICC, fluctuations in intracellular calcium concentrations appear responsible for the spontaneous changes in membrane polarization. The slow waves generated by ICC conduct passively into neighboring smooth muscle cells. Thereafter, they sweep over many other smooth muscle cells. Slow waves are the manifestation of incomplete depolarization. The baseline membrane potential of smooth muscle cells is usually –70 to –60 millivolts (mV). Under resting conditions, the membrane potential exhibits spontaneous fluctuations, varying between 20 and 30 mV. Complete depolarization (0 mV) cannot be achieved with these small fluctuations. The membrane potential can only come closer to zero mV if the smooth muscle cell is sensitized by excitatory molecules. These substances elevate the baseline membrane potential (bring it closer to zero) and make the cell more excitable. When the membrane potential exceeds the threshold value, Ca^{2+} channels are opened. The inward flow of Ca^{2+} produces a further upward depolarization resulting in action potentials and subsequent contraction of the smooth muscle cell. The frequency of these contractions is equal to or less than the frequency of the slow waves (▶ Fig. 2.6). Because spike potentials cannot occur without slow waves, these spontaneous

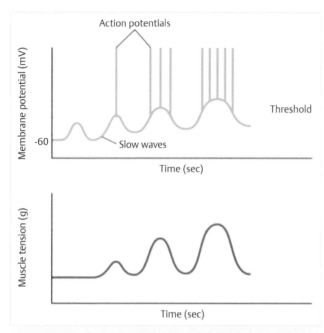

Fig. 2.6 Schematic representation of slow waves (*green*). Spike potentials are superimposed on top of slow waves when they reach a certain threshold. These spike potentials initiate contractions (*blue*).

fluctuations in membrane potential are a prerequisite for contraction of smooth muscle cells. Because these cells are electrically interconnected by gap junctions, the electrical signal responsible for contraction can spread readily from cell to cell. The smooth muscle cells of the colon are arranged in fibers. These fibers are grouped together in bundles. Because fibers and bundles also make connections with one another by gap junctions, the smooth muscle of the colon functions as a syncytium. Because of this syncytial arrangement, an action potential elicited at any point spreads in all directions. The distance depends on the excitability of the smooth muscle, which is regulated by excitatory and inhibitory substances derived from the enteric nervous system (ENS) and from the endocrine/paracrine system. As mentioned above, excitatory substances, such as acetylcholine, elicit smooth muscle cell contraction by elevating the baseline membrane potential, whereas inhibitory substances, such as norepinephrine, inhibit contraction by lowering the baseline. The complex interaction between smooth muscle cells, ENS, and endocrine/paracrine system is also essential for the synchronization of contractions. This is an important aspect of myoelectrical activity. For example, the circular muscle layer of the colon can only act appropriately when all smooth muscle cells in the corresponding section of the circumference contract simultaneously. Therefore, slow waves pass simultaneously over the entire circumference of the circular muscle layer. If that area has been sensitized by an excitatory regulatory molecule, the entire circumference of circular muscle will contract in synchrony.

Most of our knowledge regarding the electrophysiological characteristics of the colon is based on in vitro studies and on studies conducted in animal models. In vivo studies are difficult to perform. The technique most often described for the in vivo

investigation of large bowel myoelectrical activity uses monopolar or bipolar electrodes mounted on intraluminal tubes. After introduction of the tube into the colon, the electrodes are clipped to the mucosa or attached to the mucosal surface by suction. Alternatively, the electrodes can be implanted under the serosal coat. Some researchers have used silver/silver chloride electrodes placed on the skin of the abdominal wall and overlying the large bowel. With this technique, only the frequency and regularity of the colonic slow waves can be determined.[58]

The in vivo investigation of large bowel myoelectrical activity poses many problems. First, it is very difficult with intraluminal recording techniques to obtain a continuous and stable contact between electrode and mucosal surface and to eliminate the effects of colonic contents and/or transit. Second, none of the recording devices is capable of measuring all the activity actually generated. Serosal electrodes record a greater number of spike potentials and a higher proportion of the longitudinal muscle activity than do mucosal electrodes.[59] Third, it is not possible to differentiate between the myoelectrical activity generated by the two muscle layers. Finally, the reliability of the recording techniques and the comparability of methods have yet to be evaluated. Differences in recording techniques undoubtedly account for the conflicting results reported in the literature. Although in vivo studies are inappropriate to unravel all details of colonic myoelectrical activity in humans, they are not futile. Using in vivo techniques, for example, it has been shown that slow waves could be recorded in a continuous manner.[60] Furthermore, two types of slow wave activity have been described: slow waves with a low frequency of 3 to 4 cpm and slow waves with a higher frequency of 6 to 12 cpm, the latter being more common.[58,61,62] In recent years, in vitro studies have revealed that slow waves with a higher frequency are generated by ICC located within the myenteric plexus, whereas slow waves with a lower frequency arise in ICC along the submucosal surface of the circular muscle layer.[57,63] Using in vivo studies, spike potentials can be recorded as short spike bursts (SSBs), lasting only a few seconds, and as long spike bursts (LSBs), which last approximately 30 seconds.[64] SSBs are related to low-frequency slow waves[59] and are associated with low-amplitude contractions.[64] LSBs are related to high-frequency slow waves, which appear in bursts and are likely to represent the electrical control activity of the longitudinal muscle and also periodically the circular muscle.[57,58,59,60,61,62,63,64,65,66] The LSBs are associated with high-amplitude contractions.[64]

It has been postulated that abnormal slow wave activity, as well as changing ratios of SSBs to LSBs, might reflect colonic dysfunction. Myoelectrical investigation of rectosigmoid activity in cases of irritable bowel syndrome has revealed an increased incidence of low-frequency slow waves.[66,67] Furthermore, increased SSBs were found in patients with predominantly constipation-type bowel activity, whereas in patients with predominantly diarrhea-type activity, a considerable decrease in SSB frequency, and LSB frequency to a lesser extent, could be demonstrated.[64] An increased incidence of SSBs also was found in patients with slow-transit constipation, whereas a short colonic transit time (as in patients with diarrhea) seems to be correlated with a preponderance of LSBs (▶ Fig. 2.7).[68,69]

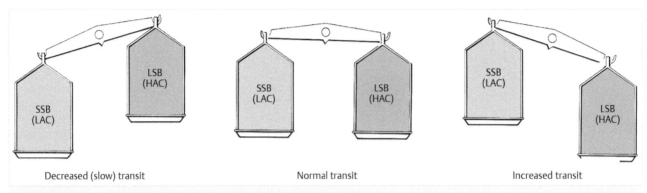

Fig. 2.7 Balance between short and long spike bursts in normal and abnormal colonic transit. HAC, high-amplitude contraction; LAC, low-amplitude contraction; LSB, long spike burst; SSB, short spike burst.

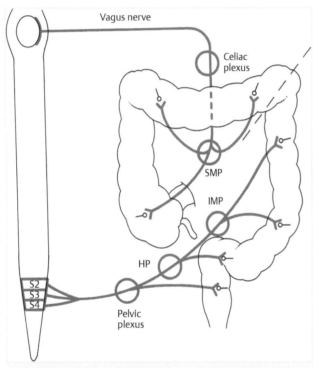

Fig. 2.8 Parasympathetic pathways. HP, hypogastric plexus; IMP, inferior mesenteric plexus; SMP, superior mesenteric plexus.

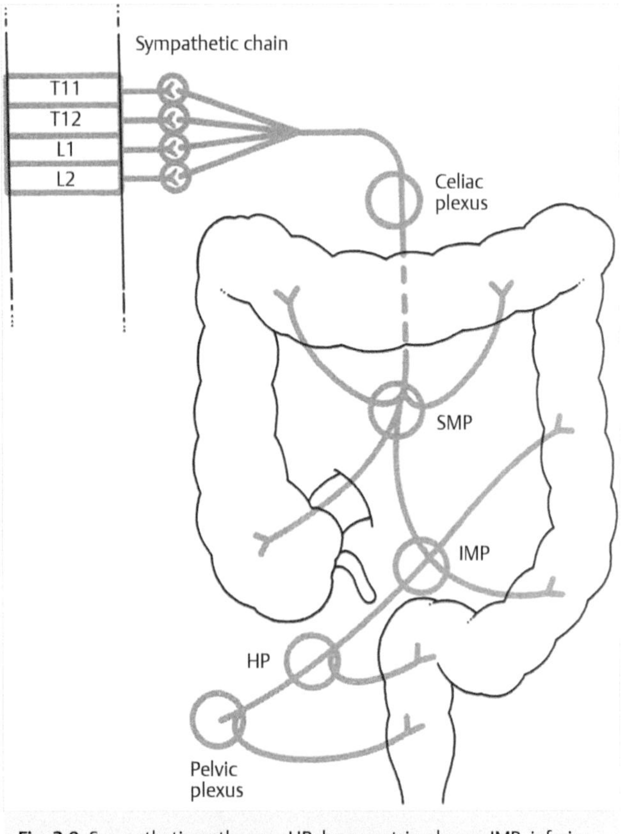

Fig. 2.9 Sympathetic pathways. HP, hypogastric plexus; IMP, inferior mesenteric plexus; SMP, superior mesenteric plexus.

Neurogenic Control of Motility

Colonic motility is controlled by extrinsic and intrinsic neuronal systems. Considering the influence of these systems, it must be remembered that they are acting on a background of fluctuating intrinsic changes in smooth muscle cell membrane excitability.[70] The extrinsic system consists of preganglionic parasympathetic neurons and postganglionic sympathetic neurons. The intrinsic (or enteric) nervous system may be defined as that system of neurons in which the cell body is within the wall of the colon. The extrinsic innervation of the colon is described in Chapter 1. The pathways are summarized in ▶ Fig. 2.8 and ▶ Fig. 2.9.

The ENS plays a major role in the regulation of secretion, motility, immune function, and inflammation in the small and large bowels.[71] The intrinsic nervous system of the colon consists of a number of interconnected plexuses. Within these networks, small groups of nerve cell bodies or enteric ganglia can be seen.

The 80 to 100 million enteric neurons can be classified into functionally distinct subpopulations, including intrinsic primary afferent neurons (IPANs), interneurons, motor neurons, secretomotor and vasomotor neurons. The enteric nerve cells are organized in two main plexuses, the myenteric plexus of Auerbach and the submucosal plexus of Meissner. Within the myenteric plexus, there is an abundant network of separate cells, first described by Cajal. These cells, now commonly referred to as ICC, are neither neurons nor Schwann cells.[72] In the colon, the ICC are also situated within the circular and longitudinal smooth muscle layers and along the submucosal surface of the circular muscle layer. These cells are connected not only with each other, but also with neurons and smooth muscle cells. The main function of ICC is the generation of the autorhythmicity of the circular muscle. They also serve as conductors of excitable events and may be mediators of enteric neurotransmission.[71] Recently, another class of interstitial cells has been described. These fibroblastlike cells have a similar distribution to the ICC and exhibit platelet-derived growth factor receptor α (PDGFRα). These cells are now referred to as PDGFRα + cells. There is growing evidence that these cells play an important role as mediators of purinergic neurotransmission.[57] The interstitial cells (Cajal and PDGFRα) are both interconnected and electrically coupled to neighboring smooth muscle cells through low-resistance gap junctions. They also make synapselike contacts with enteric nerves. The smooth muscle cells, the ICC, and the PDGFRα+ cells form an integrated system, referred to as the SIP syncytium (▶ Fig. 2.10).

Studies with the aid of zinc-iodide osmium-impregnated colon have revealed that the structural organization of the ENS is far more complex than previously thought.[73] In the mucosal plexus, fine nerve fibers were evident in the connective tissue of the lamina propria among the tubular glands, close to the glandular epithelium and encircling their fundus like a nest to form the interglandular, periglandular, and subglandular networks, respectively. No ganglia were found in the mucosal plexus. The muscularis mucosae plexus appeared as a fine felt made up of a nonganglionated nervous network in which nerve bundles ran mostly parallel to the long axes of the smooth muscle cells. Ganglia of the submucosal plexus appeared arranged along three different planes. The innermost network was composed of small-sized, regularly arranged ganglia in a single row immediately below the muscularis mucosae. Nerve strands from these ganglia ran toward the mucosal plexus and the middle part of the submucosa. A second series of ganglia was deeply located, often at the same level as the large blood vessels, and a third was closely opposed to the circular muscle layer. Nerve strands connected all these ganglia to each other. The intramuscular nerve fiber bundles run parallel to the long axes of the smooth muscle cells and form the nonganglionated circular and longitudinal muscular plexuses, respectively. Large-caliber nerve fibers pass through the serosa and penetrate

the longitudinal muscle layer. The subserosal plexus at all colonic levels except the sigmoid has no ganglia, and all nerve fibers are amyelinated.

The ENS functions semi-autonomously. It receives preganglionic fibers from the parasympathetic system and postganglionic fibers from the sympathetic system. The parasympathetic and sympathetic fibers that synapse on neurons within the ENS appear to play a modulatory role, as indicated by the observation that deprivation of input from both autonomic nerve systems does not abolish colonic activity. The ENS also receives sensory input from the luminal side of the colonic wall. Three groups of neurons can be distinguished in the ENS: (1) sensory neurons, (2) interneurons, and (3) motor neurons. The sensory neurons are divided into two groups: IPANs with their cell bodies within the colonic wall and extrinsic primary afferent neurons (EPANs) with their cell bodies outside the colonic wall. The sensory neurons function as a surveillance network. The IPANs transmit sensory information directly to the motor neurons in the same plane or indirectly through an ascending or descending chain of interneurons.[74] The sensory neurons play an important role in local reflex pathways, monitoring the chemical nature of the colonic contents as well as the tension in the wall of the large bowel. For example, localized radial distention of the colon evokes an ascending excitatory reflex (i.e., contraction of the circular muscle on the proximal side) and a descending inhibitory reflex (i.e., relaxation of the circular muscle on the distal side) (▶ Fig. 2.11).[70] These reflexes also can be elicited by mechanical and chemical irritation of the mucosa. Some of the sensory neurons for these reflexes have their endings in the mucosa (▶ Fig. 2.12). The interneurons form a relay system, linking information between enteric neurons.[70] They project more than 10 mm in oral, aboral, and circumferential directions. Interneurons are interconnected with each other and are arranged in chains, enabling the transmission of signals over longer distances. Descending interneurons are more numerous than ascending interneurons. Interneurons synapse on motor neurons. The ascending interneurons are mainly cholinergic, whereas the descending interneurons release a wide variety of neurotransmitters.[75] The most important enteric neurons are the motor neurons, of which different groups can be distinguished: excitatory motor, inhibitory motor, secretomotor, and vasomotor.[70] The motor neurons, innervating the longitudinal and circular muscles and the muscularis mucosae, are either excitatory or inhibitory. By releasing neurotransmitters that provoke

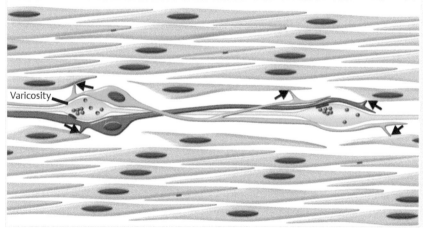

Varicosity

Fig. 2.10 Diagrammatic representation of interstitial cells of Cajal (*red*) and PDGFRα + cells (*green*) between smooth muscle cells. The interstitial cells form gap junctions with the smooth muscle cells (*arrows*) and have synapselike connections with enteric nerves (*light blue*) at their varicosities (*dark line*). These varicosities are filled with vesicles, containing neurotransmitters. These components together constitute the SIP syncytium.[57] (With permission © 2014 The Korean Society of Neurogastroenterology and Motility.)

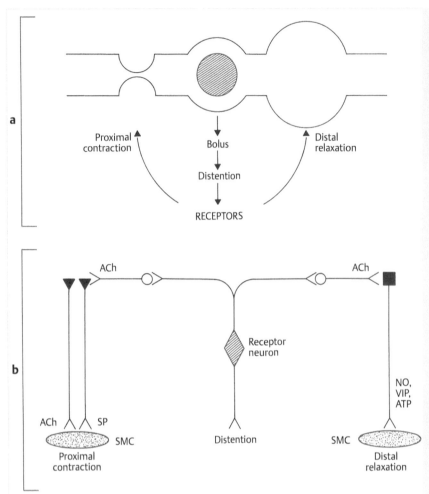

Fig. 2.11 Peristaltic reflex arc. **(a)** Proximal contraction is mediated by acetylcholine and substance P. **(b)** Descending inhibitory phase (distal relaxation) is mediated by nitric oxide, vasoactive intestinal peptide, and adenosine triphosphate. ACh, acetylcholine; ATP, adenosine triphosphate; NO, nitric oxide; SMC, smooth muscle cell; SP, substance P; VIP, vasoactive intestinal polypeptide.

muscle contraction or relaxation, they play an important role in controlling colonic motility (▸ Fig. 2.11). The main neurotransmitters of the excitatory motor neurons are acetylcholine and substance P, of which acetylcholine is the most important one. The receptors for acetylcholine on colonic smooth muscle cells are of the muscarinic subtype. They are blocked by muscarinic antagonists such as atropine and scopolamine, but not by nicotinic antagonists.[70] The receptors for acetylcholine also have been found on the membrane of myenteric ganglion cells. Therefore, acetylcholine might have a direct as well as an indirect effect on colonic motility. Inhibitory motor neurons of the ENS are nonadrenergic and noncholinergic (NANC). The cell bodies of these inhibitory neurons are located in the myenteric plexus (▸ Fig. 2.12). They predominantly supply the circular muscle and to a lesser extent the longitudinal muscle. The neurotransmitters of the inhibitory NANC neurons are nitric oxide (NO), vasoactive intestinal polypeptide (VIP), adenosine triphosphate, and possibly pituitary adenylate cyclase–activating polypeptide, gamma aminobutyric acid (GABA), neuropeptide Y, and carbon monoxide.[76] In the past, NANC neurons have been called purinergic, based on the signaling by adenosine triphosphate and peptidergic, based on the signaling by vasoactive intestinal peptide.[70,77] The inhibitory motor neurons are involved in the mediation of the descending inhibitory phase of the peristaltic reflex (▸ Fig. 2.11 and

▸ Fig. 2.12).[70] The secretomotor and vasomotor neurons, which have their cell bodies in the submucosal plexus, control epithelial transport (mainly secretion) and local blood flow, respectively. These neurons are driven by the IPANs. Chemical and mechanical stimuli result in a release of local mediators, such as 5-hydroxytryptamine (serotonin). These mediators activate the IPANs, which, in turn, stimulate the secretomotor and vasomotor neurons by releasing acetylcholine and vasoactive intestinal peptide.[78] The secretomotor neurons are either cholinergic or noncholinergic. The cholinergic neurons release acetylcholine as transmitter, whereas the noncholinergic neurons utilize nitric oxide and vasoactive intestinal peptide for their signal transmission (▸ Fig. 2.12). It has been reported that the number of colonic neurons declines with age, with the exception of the NANC neurons.[79,80] This finding might be an explanation for the higher incidence of constipation among older people.

2.2 Hormonal Control of Motility

Colonic function is affected by an extensive endocrine system. Approximately 15 different gastrointestinal hormones have been identified.[81] These gut hormones are synthesized in endocrine and paracrine cells. Many of these substances also are found in enteric neurons; therefore, they are potential neurotransmitters.

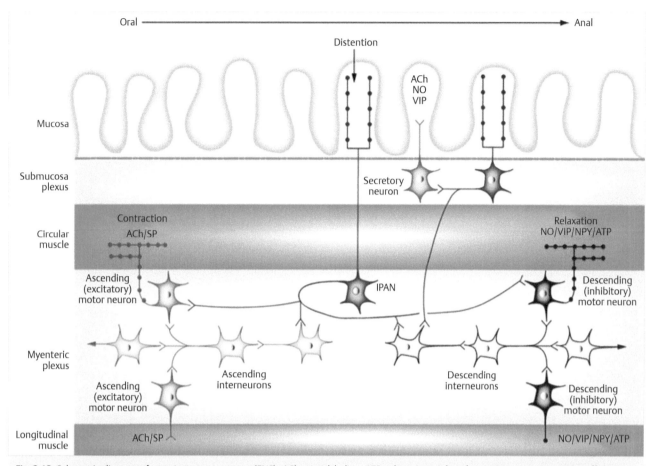

Fig. 2.12 Schematic diagram of enteric nervous system (ENS). ACh, acetylcholine; ATP, adenosine triphosphate; IPAN, intrinsic primary afferent neuron; NO, nitric oxide; NPY, neuropeptide Y; SP, substance P; VIP, vasoactive intestinal peptide.[80] (With permission © Wolters Kluwer Inc.)

The pharmacokinetics, catabolism, and release of these hormones are very complex, and their exact role in the regulation of large bowel motor activity is undetermined. The role of only a few hormones, such as gastrin and cholecystokinin, is known. These hormones are synthesized and released in the upper part of the gastrointestinal tract. Because they can reach the colon through the bloodstream, they might be able to control colonic motility.

Investigators have shown that spike potential activity of the colon does increase following the administration of gastrin and pentagastrin.[61,82] However, the gastrocolic reflex (i.e., increased colonic motility during and after a meal) is unlikely to be due to gastrin, because this reflex is still present in patients with total gastrectomy and because plasma levels of gastrin peak much later than the postprandial increase in colonic motility.[83] More likely, cholecystokinin is the mediator of this postprandial colonic activity. Cholecystokinin is a well-known colonic stimulant, increasing colonic spike activity at physiologic concentrations and in a dose-dependent manner.[84]

Other upper gastrointestinal hormones such as glucagon and somatostatin have inhibitory effects.[82] It has been reported that secretin also inhibits colonic motility,[85] but this effect could not be demonstrated by others.[61] Therefore, it is not clear whether secretin has an inhibitory effect or no effect at all on colonic motility. Present knowledge indicates that these hormones play their major role in the control of secretion and absorption.

2.2.1 Pharmacologic Influence

In a study of the effects of morphine and the opiate antagonist naloxone on human colonic transit, Kaufman et al[86] found that morphine significantly delayed transit in the cecum and ascending colon and decreased the number of bowel movements per 48 hours. Naloxone accelerated transit in the transverse colon and rectosigmoid colon but had no effect on the number of bowel movements per 48 hours. These results suggest that narcotic analgesics may cause constipation in part by slowing colonic transit in the proximal colon and by inhibiting defecation. Acceleration of transit by naloxone suggests that endogenous opiate peptides may play an inhibitory role in the regulation of human colonic transit. Of immediate practical significance is the fact that it thus may be inadvisable to prescribe morphine as a postoperative analgesic following colonic operations.

2.3 Microflora

2.3.1 Common Microflora

The bacterial population of the gastrointestinal tract is a complex collection of aerobic and anaerobic microorganisms. Distal to the ileocecal valve, the bacterial concentrations increase sharply, rising to 10^{11} to 10^{12} colony-forming units (cfu) per milliliter. Nearly one-third of the fecal dry weight consists of

Table 2.1 Colonic flora

Organism	Concentration (cfu/mL)
Aerobic or facultative organisms	
Streptococci	10^7–10^{12}
Microorganisms	10^4–10^{10}
Enterobacteria	10^5–10^{10}
Staphylococci	10^4–10^7
Lactobacilli	10^6–10^{10}
Fungi	10^2–10^6
Anaerobic bacteria	
Bacteroides spp.	10^{10}–10^{12}
Bifidobacterium spp.	10^8–10^{10}
Streptococci[a]	10^8–10^{11}
Clostridium spp.	10^6–10^{11}
Eubacterium spp.	10^9–10^{12}

[a]Includes Peptostreptococcus and Peptococcus.[89]

Table 2.2 Microbial flora found in conventional ileostomies and ileal reservoirs in normal individuals[90]

	Organisms	Aerobes	Anaerobes
Upper small intestine	0–105	0–105	Few
Lower small intestine	104–109	104–109	104–109
Conventional ileostomy			
Upper small intestine	0–105	0–105	Few
Lower small intestine	107–109	104–1,010	104–1,011
Continent ileostomy			
Upper small intestine	0–105	0–105	Few
Lower small intestine	107–109	103–1,010	106–1,010
Ileal ileoanal reservoir			
Upper small intestine	103–105	103–105	102–104
Lower small intestine	106–1,011	106–1,011	107–1,011

viable bacteria, with as many as 10^{11} to 10^{12} microorganisms present per gram of feces.[87,88] Stephen and Cummings[88] reported that bacteria comprise 55% of the total fecal solids. Anaerobic bacteria outnumber aerobes by a factor of 10^2 to 10^4. Typically, *Bacteroides* species are present in numbers of 10^{10} to 10^{12}/g of feces, and *Escherichia coli* are present in numbers of 10^8 to 10^{10}/g of feces. The predominant isolates are listed in ▶ Table 2.1.[89] Dunn[90] has summarized the microbial flora that are found in conventional ileostomies and ileal reservoirs (▶ Table 2.2).[90]

It is self-evident that the nature of colonic bacteria is of paramount importance to the surgeon. Knowledge of the type of resident bacteria serves as a useful guide to the rational selection of appropriate antibiotic therapy, both in the prophylactic and therapeutic settings.

2.3.2 Microflora Activity

Guarner and Malagelada conducted an extensive review of gut flora in health and disease in which they summarize the major functions of the gut microflora, including metabolic activities that result in salvage of energy and absorbable nutrients, important trophic effects on intestinal epithelia and on immune structure and function, and protection of the colonized host against invasion by alien microbes.[91] Much of the following information has been derived from their comprehensive review. Gut microflora might also be an essential factor in certain pathologic disorders including multisystem organ failure, colon carcinoma, and inflammatory bowel diseases. Several hundred grams of bacteria living within the colonic lumen affect host homeostasis. Some of these bacteria are potential pathogens and can be a source of infection and sepsis when the integrity of the bowel barrier is physically or functionally breached. Bacteria are also useful in promotion of human health. The constant interaction between the host and its microbial guests

can infer important health benefits to the human host. Probiotics and prebiotics are known to have a role in the prevention or treatment of some diseases.

2.3.3 Metabolic Functions

A major metabolic function of the colonic microflora is the fermentation of nondigestible dietary residue, which is a major source of energy in the colon. Nondigestible carbohydrates include large polysaccharides (resistant starches, cellulose, hemicellulose, pectins, and gums), some oligosaccharides that escape digestion, and unabsorbed sugars and alcohols. The metabolic end point is generation of SCFAs. Anaerobic metabolism of peptides and proteins (putrefaction) by the microflora also produces SCFAs but, at the same time, it generates a series of potentially toxic substances including ammonia, amines, phenols, thiols, and indoles. Available proteins include elastin and collagen from dietary sources, pancreatic enzymes, sloughed epithelial cells, and lysed bacteria. Substrate availability in the human adult colon is about 20 to 60 g carbohydrates and 5 to 10 g protein per day.

Colonic microorganisms also play a part in vitamin synthesis and in absorption of calcium, magnesium, and iron. Absorption of ions in the cecum is improved by carbohydrate fermentation and production of SCFAs, especially acetate, propionate, and butyrate. All of these fatty acids have important functions in host physiology. Butyrate is almost completely consumed by the colonic epithelium, and it is a major source of energy for colonocytes. Acetate and propionate are found in portal blood and are eventually metabolized by the liver (propionate) or peripheral tissues, particularly muscle (acetate). Acetate and propionate might also have a role as modulators of glucose metabolism: absorption of these SCFAs would result in lower glycemic responses to oral glucose or standard meal—a response consistent with an ameliorated sensitivity to insulin. Foods with a high proportion of nondigestible carbohydrates have a low glycemic index. Vitamin K is produced by intestinal microorganisms.[89]

The enterohepatic circulation of many compounds depends on flora that produce bacterial enzymes, such as B-glucuronidase and sulfatase. Some of the endogenous and exogenous substances that undergo an enterohepatic circulation include bilirubin, bile acids, estrogens, cholesterol, digoxin, rifampin, morphine, colchicine, and diethylstilbestrol.[92] The main role of anaerobes appears to be the provision of catabolic enzymes for organic compounds that cannot be digested by enzymes of eukaryotic origin. They are needed for the catabolism of cholesterol, bile acids, and steroid hormones; they hydrolyze a number of flavonoid glycosides to anticarcinogens; and they detoxify certain carcinogens.[93]

2.3.4 Trophic Functions

All three SCFAs stimulate epithelial cell proliferation and differentiation in the large and small intestine in vivo in rats. A role for SCFAs in prevention of some human pathological states such as chronic ulcerative colitis and colonic carcinogenesis has been long suspected, although conclusive evidence is still lacking.[91] SCFAs butyrate, propionate, and acetate produced during fiber fermentation promote colonic differentiation and can reverse or suppress neoplastic progression. Basson et al[94] sought to identify candidate genes responsible for SCFA activity on colonocytes and to compare the relative activities of independent SCFAs. A total of 30,000 individual genetic sequences were analyzed for differential expression among the three SCFAs. More than 1,000 gene fragments were identified as being substantially modulated in expression by butyrate. Butyrate tended to have the most pronounced effects and acetate the least.

2.3.5 Host Immunity Functions

The intestinal mucosa is the main interface between the immune system and the external environment.[91] Gut-associated lymphoid tissues contain the largest pool of immunocompetent cells in the human body. The dialogue between host and bacteria at the mucosal interface seems to play a part in development of a competent immune system. The immune response to microbes relies on innate and adaptive components, such as immunoglobulin secretion. Most bacteria in human feces are coated with specific IgA units. Innate responses are mediated not only by white blood cells such as neutrophils and macrophages that can phagocytose and kill pathogens, but also by intestinal epithelial cells, which coordinate host responses by synthesizing a wide range of inflammatory mediators and transmitting signals to underlying cells in the mucosa. The innate immune system has to discriminate between potential pathogens from commensal bacteria, with the use of a restricted number of preformed receptors. The system allows immediate recognition of bacteria to rapidly respond to an eventual challenge.

2.3.6 Protective Functions

Anaerobes are usually seen as destructive creatures without any redeeming virtues. Resident bacteria are a crucial line of resistance to colonization by exogenous microbes and, therefore, are highly relevant in prevention of invasion of tissues by pathogens.[91] Colonization resistance also applies to opportunistic bacteria that are present in the gut but have restrictive growth. Use of antibiotics can disrupt the ecological balance and allow overgrowth of species with potential pathogenicity such as toxigenic *Clostridium difficile*, associated with pseudomembranous colitis.

Benefits we derive from anaerobes include their probable function in restraining growth of *C. difficile* in human carriers.[93]

2.3.7 Bacterial Translocation

The passage of viable bacteria from the gastrointestinal tract through the epithelial mucosa is called bacterial translocation. Translocation of endotoxins from viable or dead bacteria in very small amounts probably constitutes a physiologically important boost to the reticuloendothelial system, especially to the Kupffer cells in the liver. However, dysfunction of the gut mucosal barrier can result in the translocation of many viable microorganisms, usually belonging to gram-negative aerobic genera (*Escherichia*, *Proteus*, *Klebsiella*). After crossing the epithelial barrier, bacteria can travel via the lymph to extraintestinal sites, such as the mesenteric lymph nodes, liver, and spleen. Subsequently, enteric bacteria can disseminate throughout the body producing sepsis, shock, multisystem organ failure, or death of the host.[91]

The three primary mechanisms in promotion of bacterial translocation in animals are overgrowth of bacteria in the small intestine, increased permeability of the intestinal mucosal barrier, and deficiencies in host immune defenses. Bacterial translocation can occur in human beings during various disease processes. Indigenous gastrointestinal bacteria have been cultured directly from the mesenteric lymph nodes of patients undergoing laparotomy. Data suggest that the baseline rate of positive mesenteric lymph node culture could approach 5% in otherwise healthy people. However, in disorders such as multisystem organ failure, acute severe pancreatitis, advanced liver cirrhosis, intestinal obstruction, and inflammatory bowel diseases, rates of positive culture are much higher (16–50%).[91]

2.3.8 Colon Carcinogenesis

Intestinal bacteria could play a part in the initiation of colon carcinoma through production of carcinogens, cocarcinogens, or procarcinogens. In healthy people, diets rich in fat and meat but poor in vegetables increase the fecal excretion of N-nitroso compounds, a group of genotoxic substances that are known initiators and promoters of colon carcinoma. Such diets also increase the genotoxic potential of human fecal water. Another group of carcinogens of dietary origin are the heterocyclic aromatic amines that are formed in meat when it is cooked. Some intestinal microorganisms strongly increase damage to DNA in colon cells induced by heterocyclic amines, whereas other intestinal bacteria can uptake and detoxify such compounds.[91] Bacteria of the *Bacteroides* and *Clostridium* genera increase the incidence and growth rate of colonic neoplasms induced in animals, whereas other genera such as lactobacillus and bifidobacteria prevent carcinogenesis. Although the evidence is not conclusive, colonic flora seem to be an environmental factor that modulates risk of colonic carcinoma in human beings.[91]

2.3.9 Role in Inflammatory Bowel Diseases

Resident bacterial flora have been suggested to be an essential factor in driving the inflammatory process in human inflammatory bowel diseases. In patients with Crohn's disease, intestinal

T lymphocytes are hyperactive against bacterial antigens.[91] Patients with Crohn's disease or ulcerative colitis have increased intestinal mucosal secretion of IgG-type antibodies against a broad spectrum of commensal bacteria. Patients with inflammatory bowel diseases have higher amounts of bacteria attached to their epithelial surfaces than do healthy people. Unrestrained activation of the intestinal immune system by elements of the flora could be a key event in the pathophysiology of inflammatory bowel disease. Some patients with Crohn's disease (17–25%) have mutations in the *NOD2/CARD15* gene, which regulates host responses to bacteria.[94,95]

In inflammatory bowel diseases in human beings, direct interaction of commensal microflora with the intestinal mucosa stimulates inflammatory activity in the gut lesions. Fecal stream diversion has been shown to prevent recurrence of Crohn's disease, whereas infusion of intestinal contents to the excluded ileal segments reactivated mucosal lesions.[96] In ulcerative colitis, short-term treatment with an enteric-coated preparation of broad-spectrum antibiotics rapidly reduced mucosal release of cytokines and eicosanoids and was more effective in reduction of inflammatory activity than were intravenous steroids.[97] However, antibiotics have limited effectiveness in clinical management of inflammatory bowel disease, since induction of antibiotic-resistant strains substantially impairs sustained effects.

2.3.10 Probiotics and Prebiotics

Bacteria can be used to improve human health. A bacterium that provides specific health benefits when consumed as a food component or supplement would be called a probiotic. Oral probiotics are living microorganisms that upon ingestion in specific numbers exert health benefits beyond those of inherent basic nutrition.[91] According to this definition, probiotics do not necessarily colonize the human intestine. Prebiotics are nondigestible food ingredients that beneficially affect the host by selectively stimulating growth, or activity, or both, of one or a restricted number of bacteria in the colon. For example, coadministration of probiotics to patients on antibiotics significantly reduced antibiotic-associated diarrhea[98,99] and can be used to prevent such antibiotic-associated diarrhea.[100] Examples of such bacteria include various strains of lactobacillus GG, *Bifidobacterium bifidum*, and *Streptococcus thermophilus*.

Probiotics and prebiotics have been shown to prevent colon carcinoma in several animals, but their role in reduction of risk of colon carcinoma in human beings is not established.[101] However, probiotics have been shown to reduce the fecal activity of enzymes known to produce genotoxic compounds that act as initiators of carcinoma in human beings.[91]

2.4 Intestinal Gas

Intestinal gas may be endogenous or exogenous. Five gases—nitrogen, oxygen, carbon dioxide, hydrogen, and methane—make up 99% of all the gas in the gut. Only nitrogen and oxygen are found in the atmosphere and therefore can be swallowed. Hydrogen, methane, and carbon dioxide are produced by bacterial fermentation of carbohydrates and proteins in the colon. Approximately one-third of the human population produces

methane. Small amounts of hydrogen sulfide are also produced. Levitt,[102] in his extensive studies of this subject, found that patients who complain of excessive flatus almost invariably have high concentrations of hydrogen and carbon dioxide. Hydrogen is cleared by the lungs. Since carbon dioxide is a result of fermentation, therapy consists of diet manipulation with a decrease in the amount of carbohydrate, especially lactose, wheat, and potatoes.

The most dramatic and important point for the surgeon regarding intestinal gas is the fact that explosions may occur during electrocautery in the colon. Because both hydrogen and methane are explosive, intestinal gases should be aspirated before electrocautery is used.

2.5 Anorectal Physiology

During the last decades, detailed investigations have given us a better understanding of anorectal physiology. The methods that are used for the systematic and fundamental study of anorectal physiology include anorectal manometry, defecography, continence tests, electromyography of the anal sphincters and the pelvic floor, and nerve stimulation tests. Moreover, combining proctography with simultaneous pressure recordings and electromyographic measurements permits these investigations to present a more dynamic and physiologic account of the state of the anorectal region. Modern imaging techniques furnish a clearer picture of the mechanisms of anal continence and defecation and demonstrate pathophysiologic abnormalities in patients with disorders of continence and defecation.

2.5.1 Anal Continence

It is difficult to give a clear definition of anal continence. Complete control or complete lack of control is easy to define; however, while varying degrees of lack of control of flatus and fecal soiling may seem like major disabilities to some patients, other less fastidious individuals may be unconcerned by them. Maintaining anal continence is a complex matter because it is controlled by local reflex mechanisms as well as by conscious will. Normal continence depends on a highly integrated series of complicated events. Stool volume and consistency are important because patients who have weakened mechanisms may be continent for a firm stool but incontinent for liquid feces. Also significant is the rate of delivery of feces into the rectum, which emphasizes the reservoir function of the rectum. Other important factors include the sphincteric component, sensory receptors, mechanical factors, and the corpus cavernosum of the anus (see Box 2.1).

2.5.2 Mechanisms of Continence

Stool Volume and Consistency

Stool weight and volume vary from individual to individual, from one time to another in a given individual, and from one geographic region to another. The frequency of passing stool may play some role in continence in that colonic transit time is rapid when the large bowel content is liquid because the left colon does not store fluid well. Stool consistency probably is the most important physical characteristic influencing anal continence.[103] The ability to maintain normal control may depend on whether the rectal contents are solid, liquid, or gas.

Mechanisms of anal continence

- Stool volume and consistency
- Reservoir function
- Sphincteric factors
  - Internal sphincter
  - External sphincter
- Sensory components
  - Rectal sensory perception
  - Anal sensory perception
  - Neuropathways
  - Reflexes
- Mechanical factors
  - Angulation between rectum and anal canal
  - Flutter valve
  - Flap valve
- Corpus cavernosum of anus

Some patients may be continent for solid stool but not for liquid or gas, or continent for stool but not for gas. This fact is important in the management of patients with anal incontinence because the maneuver of changing stool consistency from liquid into solid may be enough to allow the patient to recapture fecal control ("Mechanisms of anal continence" Box).

Reservoir Function of Rectum

The distal part of the large intestine has a reservoir function that is important in the maintenance of anal continence and depends on several factors. First, the lateral angulations of the sigmoid colon and the valves of Houston provide a mechanical barrier and retard progression of stool.[104] The weight of the stool tends to accentuate these angles and enhances their barrier effect (▶ Fig. 2.13).[105]

It has been suggested that a pressure barrier exists at the junction of the rectum and sigmoid colon (a concept referred to as O'Beirne's sphincter); however, evidence for such a pressure barrier is lacking. It also has been proposed that differences in motor activity and myoelectrical activity between the rectum and the sigmoid colon provide a barrier that resists caudad progression of stool.[58] Motor activity is more frequent and contractile waves are of higher amplitude in the rectum than in the sigmoid colon. This mechanism may account for the cephalad movement of retention enemas or suppositories.[105] A more recent study, however, has disputed the pathophysiologic significance of this phenomenon.[59]

The rectum responds to filling by relaxation of its smooth muscle layer to accommodate fecal load. This adaptive compliance of the rectum, along with rectal capacity and distensibility, also is an important factor for effective reservoir function. Differences in pressure patterns between the distal and proximal levels of the anal canal result in the development of a force vector in the direction of the rectum. This continuous differential activity may be important in controlling the retention of small amounts of liquid matter and flatus in the rectum. Furthermore, the angulation between the rectum and anal canal, which is due to the continuous tonic activity of the puborectalis muscle, as well as the high-pressure zone in the anal canal contributes to the reservoir function of the rectum.

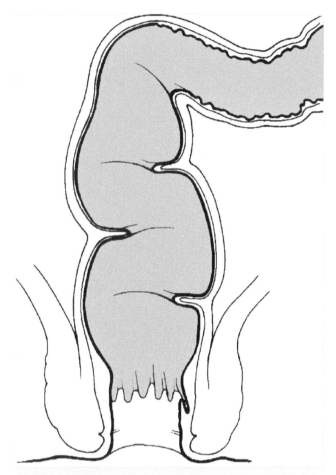

Fig. 2.13 Mechanical reservoir function.

Sphincteric Factors

Activity of the anal sphincters is generally believed to be the most important factor in maintaining anal continence. Within the anal canal, the sphincters are responsible for the high-pressure zone. The maximum anal resting pressure varies between 40 and 80 mm Hg[106] and appears to provide a barrier against intrarectal pressure. The high-pressure zone, as demonstrated by pull-through recordings, has an average length of 3.5 cm[107,108,109] and results mainly from the continuous tonic activity of both sphincters. Variation in sphincter length at rest has been 3.5, 3.0, and 2.8 cm, and with squeeze 4.2, 3.7, and 3.8 cm for males, parous, and nulliparous females, respectively.[110]

Internal Sphincter

The major contribution to the high-pressure zone comes from the internal anal sphincter, estimated to account for 52 to 85% of the pressure recorded (▶ Table 2.3).[110,111,112,113,114] In a detailed study of factors that contribute to anal basal pressure, Lestar et al[114] concluded that when a 0.3-cm-diameter probe was used, 30% of the maximum anal basal pressure is made up by striated sphincter tonic activity, 45% by nerve-induced internal sphincter activity, 10% by purely myogenic internal sphincter activity, and 15% by the expansion of the hemorrhoidal plexus. The overlapping of the sphincters has generated controversy regarding the relative importance of the internal and external sphincters in maintaining

Table 2.3 Contribution of internal anal sphincter (IAS) to high-pressure zone

Author(s)	Recording device	% of IAS
Duthie and Watts (1965)[102,111]	Balloon catheter	60
	Perfused catheter	68
Frenckner and Euler (1975)[103,112]	Balloon catheter	85
Schweiger (1982)[104,113]	Balloon catheter	74
Lestar et al (1989)[105,114]	Balloon catheter	55
Cali et al (1992)[101,110]	Perfused catheter	
	• Males	52
	• Females, parous	59
	• Females, nulliparous	65

anal continence. However, when the external sphincter is paralyzed, the pressure is not significantly changed, so that the resting pressure would seem to be due largely to the internal sphincter.[111] Normally, the internal sphincter is in a continual state of tonic contraction, only relaxing in response to rectal distention. The basal tone of the internal sphincter is controlled by both intrinsic and extrinsic neuronal systems and probably is also myogenic in origin. Frenckner and Ihre[115] believed that internal sphincter tone was controlled only by sympathetic (i.e., hypogastric) pathways, but Meunier and Mollard[116] have shown that the sacral parasympathetic pathways also are involved and clinical evidence supports their findings.[117]

External Sphincter

Continuous tonic activity at rest and even during sleep has been recorded in the pelvic floor muscles and in the external sphincter.[118] The external sphincter is unique in this regard because other striated muscles are electrically silent at rest. Although activity is always present in the external sphincter, its basal tone shows considerable variations, determined by postural changes. For example, external sphincter activity will increase when an individual is in an upright position. The activity also is augmented by perianal stimulation (anal reflex) and by increases in intra-abdominal pressure, such as coughing, sneezing, and the Valsalva maneuver. Rectal distention with initial small volumes also will result in increased activity. The permanent activity of the external sphincter is modulated by the second sacral spinal segment.[119] In patients with tabes dorsalis, the external sphincter shows no activity at all because this spinal reflex pathway is disturbed as a result of degeneration of the posterior root. The same phenomenon has been demonstrated in patients with cauda equina lesions. Although the external sphincter will be completely paralyzed following transection of the spinal cord, the tonic activity of the sphincter will return after a period of spinal shock in cases where transection has occurred above the second sacral spinal segment. The external sphincter is unique in that it does not degenerate even when separated from its nerve supply. Although activity always is present in the external sphincter and the pelvic floor muscles, these muscles can be contracted voluntarily for only 40- to 60-second periods; then both electrical activity and pressure within the anal canal return to basal levels (▶ Fig. 2.13).[120]

In contrast to other skeletal muscles, the fiber distribution in the external sphincter is the result of a developmental process.[121] The predominance of type II (twitching) fibers explains the state of reflex continence of the young infant. With increasing maturation of tonic type I fibers, an additional voluntary component to continence is made possible with the help of the supporting pelvic musculature. This maturation is determined by the increasing strain on the pelvic floor as the child learns to sit and walk. With increasing age, the number of type II fibers again increases, so that at the age of approximately 75 the reflex component of continence again becomes important.

Rectal Sensory Perception

The conscious sensation of urgency is mediated by extrinsic afferent neurons. These neurons are activated by mechanoreceptors. Although it has been suggested that these receptors are located in the pelvic floor,[122] there is growing evidence that the rectal wall itself contains many mechanoreceptors. According to Rühl et al, the sacral dorsal roots contain afferents from low-threshold mechanoreceptors located in the rectal wall. These afferents monitor the filling state and contraction level of the rectum.[123] These receptors are very rare or absent more proximally in the colon.[124] They do not act simply as tension and stretch receptors. They also detect mechanical deformation, such as flattening of myenteric ganglia. Furthermore, they are able to encode the contractile activity of smooth muscle cells. Activation of the rectal mechanoreceptors induces extrinsic and intrinsic reflexes that play a key role in defecation. Some authors distinguish the superficial mucosal mechanoreceptors from the deeper muscular and serosal receptors. It has been suggested that the superficial mechanoreceptors are connected with sacral afferents, which can be stimulated by slow-ramp rectal distensions, and that the deeper mechanoreceptors are connected with splanchnic afferents, which can be stimulated by rapid phasic distensions.[125] Several lines of evidence support this hypothesis. Topical application of lidocaine decreases the sensation elicited by slow-ramp distension, but has no effect on the sensation elicited by rapid phasic distension. In patients with irritable bowel syndrome, abnormal sensory responses have been demonstrated during rapid phasic distension but not during slow-ramp distension. Patients with a complete lesion of the lower spinal cord do not perceive slow-ramp distensions, although they still perceive phasic stimuli.[126] Several workers have tried to modulate rectal sensory perception. The 5-HT1 receptor agonist sumatriptan causes a relaxation of the descending colon, thereby allowing higher volumes to be accommodated before thresholds for perception and discomfort are reached. In contrast to this effect, on the descending colon, sumatriptan has no influence on distension evoked rectal perception. This finding may reflect a difference in 5-HT1 receptor location between descending colon and rectum.[127] The 5-HT4 receptor agonist serotonin seems to be a better candidate for the modulation of rectal sensitivity.[128] It has been shown that neurotensin also has an effect on perception by intensifying rectal sensation.[129] Chenodeoxycholic acid in physiological concentrations reduces sensory thresholds to rectal distension. It is not clear whether this effect is due to chemoreceptor activation or to chemical-induced alterations in tone or compliance.[130] Recently, it has been shown that the cortical representation of rectal distension differs between males and females. Kern et al[131] studied 13 male and 15 female volunteers with functional magnetic resonance imaging during barostat-controlled rectal distension. The volume of cortical activity during rectal distension was significantly higher in women. They also observed that intensity and volume of cortical activity were directly related to the strength of the stimulus and that rectal distension below perception level still results in cortical activity. Most frequently, rectal sensory perception is assessed by distension of an intrarectal balloon, either with air or with water. During this procedure, the subject is asked to indicate the onset of awareness of distension, the first urge to defecate, and finally the maximum tolerable volume, which is characterized by an irresistible and painful urgency. It has been reported that the volumes registered for each sensation do not differ between men and women, irrespective of their age.[132] Sloots et al[133] investigated rectal sensory perception by pressure-controlled distension with a barostat assembly. Although males had larger volumes at the same pressures than females, the sensory perception was found to be equal. It should be taken into account that the intensity of perceived sensation depends on the distension rate. The distension stimulus is poorly defined with an air-filled or water-filled latex balloon because with increasing distension, varying degrees of balloon elongation occur, depending on the compliance of the rectal wall. For the assessment of rectal sensory perception, the use of an electromechanical barostat assembly is more accurate. It enables the measurement of rectal compliance by recording the change in rectal volume per unit change in pressure. It is also important to perform the isobaric distensions in random order and to use a visual analogue scale in order to record the intensity of the perceived sensation in a more objective manner. Reduced rectal sensory perception, diagnosed on the basis of elevated sensory threshold volumes, is not necessarily the result of impaired afferent nerve function alone. In the case of increased rectal compliance, greater distension volumes are required to elicit rectal sensations. Rectal hyposensitivity (RH) in patients with normal rectal compliance reflects impairment of afferent nerve function, whereas this finding in patients with an increased compliance might be due to other factors such as abnormal rectal wall properties.[134] Reduced rectal sensitivity has been demonstrated in patients with slow transit constipation.[135] Rectal afferent fibers travel with the parasympathetic nerves to the dorsal roots of S2, S3, and S4. The parasympathetic pelvic nerves might be injured during pelvic surgery such as rectopexy, when afferent fibers in the lateral ligaments may be divided, and hysterectomy, when division of the uterine-supporting ligaments may result in nerve injury.[136] Gosselink et al assessed rectal compliance and rectal sensory perception in female patients with obstructed defecation, utilizing a barostat assembly. Most of their patients had a normal colonic transit time. About half of their patients reported onset of symptoms following pelvic surgery, such as hysterectomy and rectopexy. Rectal compliance was found to be normal, whereas rectal sensory perception was blunted or absent in the majority of their patients. Both findings indicate that impairment of afferent nerve function contributes to obstructed defecation.[137,138]

Anal Sensory Perception

A more precise perception of the nature of the rectal content is achieved by sensory receptors within the anal canal. Careful histologic studies have demonstrated an abundance of free and organized nerve endings in the epithelium of the anal canal.[139] Several types of sensory receptors have been identified: nerve endings that denote pain (free intraepithelial), touch (Meissner's corpuscles), cold (bulbs of Krause), pressure or tension (Pacini corpuscles and Golgi-Mazzoni corpuscles), and friction (genital corpuscles).[139] These nerve endings are located primarily in the distal half of the anal canal but may extend for 5 to 15 mm above the dentate line (▶ Fig. 2.14). Pain can be felt as far as 1 to 1.5 cm above the anal valves; this corresponds with clinical experience, such as the application of rubber band ligation of hemorrhoids. The rectum is insensitive to stimuli other than stretch.

Whether or not this sensory zone is important for anal continence remains controversial. In a study in which a saline continence test was used, no effect could be demonstrated when the anal canal was anesthetized with lidocaine, leading the authors to conclude that anal canal sensation does not play a crucial role in continence.[140] However, in a more recent study in which a technique to assess anorectal temperature sensation was used, it has been shown that very small changes in temperature can be detected in the anal canal. The lower and middle parts of the canal were found to be much more sensitive to temperature changes than was the upper part.[141] This finding supports the concept of the sampling response and reinforces the role of this sensory zone of the anal canal in maintaining continence.

Neuropathways

The internal anal sphincter has a dual extrinsic innervation containing both sympathetic and parasympathetic nerves. In nonsphincteric areas, the sympathetic nerves are inhibitory and the parasympathetic nerves are excitatory to the gastrointestinal smooth muscle cells. The opposite occurs with the internal anal sphincter.

The sympathetic pathway to the internal anal sphincter emerges from the 12th thoracic lumbar segment and from the first two lumbar spinal segments. The preganglionic sympathetic neurons are cholinergic and form synapses on the cell bodies of postganglionic neurons in prevertebral ganglia, which are located in the sympathetic trunk. The noradrenergic axons of these postganglionic sympathetic neurons run through the sacral splanchnic nerves to the inferior hypogastric plexus and continue through the inferior rectal plexus. The sympathetic nerves have a direct effect on the internal sphincter muscle cells, which possess α- and β-adrenoreceptors (▶ Fig. 2.15). Stimulation of the α-adrenoreceptors results in contraction, whereas stimulation of the β-adrenoreceptors is followed by relaxation.[142] Since there is a dominant population of excitatory α-adrenoreceptors on the smooth muscle fibers of the internal anal sphincter, the overall effect of the sympathetic nervous system on the internal anal sphincter is excitatory. The internal sphincter also is supplied by preganglionic parasympathetic fibers that emerge from the second, third, and fourth sacral spinal segments. These fibers run via the pelvic splanchnic nerves to the inferior hypogastric plexus and continuing downward to the inferior rectal plexus. The cholinergic axons of these preganglionic parasympathetic neurons form synapses on the cell bodies of postganglionic parasympathetic neurons located

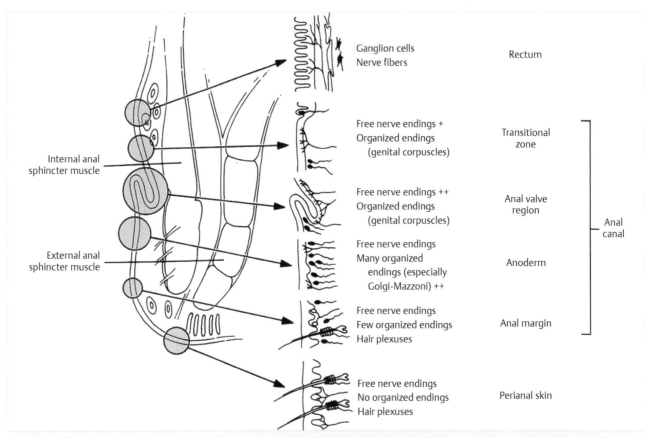

Fig. 2.14 Sensory nerve endings in the anal canal.[139] (With permission from John Wiley and Sons © 1960 British Journal of Surgery Society Ltd.)

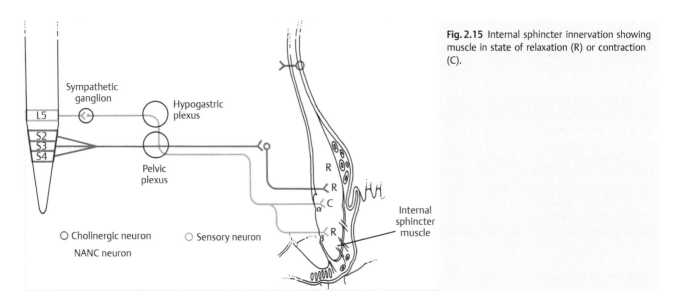

Fig. 2.15 Internal sphincter innervation showing muscle in state of relaxation (R) or contraction (C).

within the anorectal wall, proximal to the aganglionic sphincteric area. The axons of these neurons run downward to reach the internal sphincter (▶ Fig. 2.15). The postganglionic parasympathetic fibers are also cholinergic and produce the neurotransmitter acetylcholine. This neurotransmitter binds with muscarinic receptors on the smooth muscle cells of the internal anal sphincter, resulting in their relaxation.[143] The contractile state of the internal anal sphincter is modified not only by the extrinsic sympathetic and parasympathetic nerve supply, but also by intrinsic nerves belonging to the ENS. As described earlier, the nerves of this ENS are nonadrenergic and noncholinergic. These NANC nerves release several inhibitory neurotransmitters such as nitric oxide (NO), vasoactive intestinal peptide (VIP), and carbon monoxide (CO). Nitric oxide appears to be the main neurotransmitter mediating relaxation of the internal anal sphincter. There is a close interaction between the NANC neurotransmitters. For example, VIP acts directly on the smooth muscle cells but also has a role in regulating the production and release of NO. There also seems to be an interaction between the extrinsic and the intrinsic nerve supply of the internal anal sphincter. It has been shown that muscarinic receptors are also present on the terminals of NO releasing nerves. Stimulation of these receptors by acetylcholine results in activation of nitric oxide synthase (NOS) with subsequent release of NO.[144] The basal tone in the internal anal sphincter is mainly due to intrinsic myogenic properties and extrinsic innervation. Relaxation of the internal anal sphincter in response to rectal distension is mediated by intrinsic NANC nerves. This reflex is independent of the extrinsic nerve supply. NO is by far the most important neurotransmitter involved in this reflex. Factors that affect the tone of the internal anal sphincter are summarized in ▶ Table 2.4. Contraction of smooth muscle cells is dependent on the intracellular concentration of calcium. Stimulation of α-adrenoreceptors on the smooth muscle cell membrane is followed by intracellular mobilization of calcium and an increased influx of calcium through calcium channels, finally resulting in contraction. Blocking of these channels by antagonists such as diltiazem results in relaxation. Stimulation of β-adrenoreceptors causes an increase in cAMP, which results in a return of calcium to the sarcoplasmic reticulum, thereby lowering the intracellular concentration of calcium. Calcium can also be pumped out of the cell. This process is facilitated by cyclic GMP. The production of cyclic GMP is stimulated by NO.

The classic anal reflex is elicited by pricking the perianal skin; the response is contraction of the external sphincter as evidenced by skin dimpling. The reflex has its afferent and efferent pathway in the pudendal nerve and uses sacral segments S1–S4. The reflex responses of both sphincters are essential for the maintenance of anal continence. Rectal distension results in transient relaxation of the internal sphincter and simultaneous contraction of the external sphincter (▶ Fig. 2.16).

The reflex response of the external sphincter represented by a transient increase in activity can be initiated by a number of stimuli, such as postural changes, perianal scratch, and increased intra-abdominal pressure. The reflex response of the internal sphincter, which consists of transient relaxation, can be stimulated by rectal distension or the Valsalva maneuver. Although this reflex occurs almost immediately after material enters the rectum, peristalsis is not involved because the

sphincter relaxes at the moment of rectal distention before the peristaltic wave of contraction reaches the sphincter.[145] The transient relaxation of the internal sphincter allows the rectal contents to come into contact with the sensory epithelium of the anal canal to assess whether the contents are solid, liquid, or gas. During this sampling response, continence will be maintained by synchronous contraction of the external sphincter, which allows time for impulses to reach conscious awareness; thus, having determined the nature of the material, the individual can decide what to do about it and then take appropriate action. Voluntary contraction of the external sphincter can extend the period of continence and allow time for compliance mechanisms within the rectum to provide for adjustment to increased intrarectal volumes. As the rectum accommodates to its new volume, stretch receptors are no longer activated, and afferent stimuli and the sensation of urgency disappear. Further rectal distention leads to inhibition of the external sphincter. Recognizing the nature of the rectal contents is not only a conscious process but also a subconscious one, since flatus can be passed safely during sleep. Conscious sampling is done by slightly increasing intra-abdominal pressure and maintaining, by voluntary control, an increase in the activity of the external anal sphincter. In this way, solids can be retained, while gas can be passed, thereby relieving the intrarectal pressure.

The inhibition induced by rectal distention was thought to be under parasympathetic control via the sacral nerves. However, evidence now suggests that the reflex is predominantly an intramural one,[114] although subject to some sacral control. It is not necessarily abolished by spinal anesthesia, and it disappears in experimental animals after the rectal application of cocaine and after transection of the lower rectum.[115] Internal sphincter relaxation is modulated by the spinal cord, since no reflex is

Table 2.4 Factors that affect the tone of the internal anal sphincter

Factor	Effect
α-Adrenoceptor agonists (phenylephrine, noradrenaline)	Contraction
β-Adrenoceptor agonists	Relaxation
Muscarinic receptor agonists (carbachol)	Relaxation
Nicotinic receptor agonists (nicotine)	Relaxation
Nitric oxide (or an NO donor)	Relaxation
Vasoactive intestinal polypeptide	Relaxation
Carbon monoxide	Relaxation
Purinergic receptor agonists (adenosine triphosphate)	Relaxation

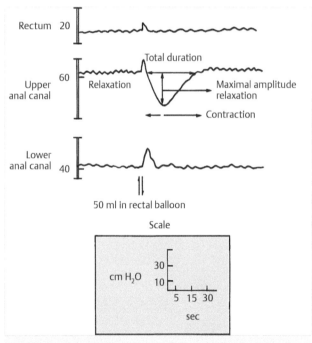

Fig. 2.16 Anorectal reflex.

found in spinal shock and there is no relationship between the degree of distention and the amplitude of relaxation in patients with meningocele.[116] The internal sphincter reflex is a neurogenic response, initiated by sensory neurons located in the rectal wall. The cell bodies of these inhibitory neurons are located in the myenteric plexus, and their axons run downward to the aganglionic part of the internal sphincter where they supply the smooth muscle cells (▶ Fig. 2.15). These inhibitory nerves are non-cholinergic and nonadrenergic. Nitric oxide has been identified as the chemical messenger of the intrinsic, nonadrenergic, and non-cholinergic pathway mediating relaxation of the internal anal sphincter.[146,147,148,149] It has been shown that the axons of nitric oxide–producing nerve cell bodies, located in the distal part of the rectum, descend into the anal canal where they ramify into and throughout the internal anal sphincter.[150] Without these inhibitory neurons, the reflex response of the internal sphincter on rectal distention is impossible, as shown in patients with congenital and acquired aganglionosis. In patients with an anastomosis between the site of distention and the sphincters, the internal sphincter reflex also is abolished. In one study, the internal sphincter reflex could be demonstrated despite such an anastomosis, probably because of regeneration of descending axons of the inhibitory neurons across the anastomosis. It is likely that external sphincter reflexes are initiated by receptors in the levator muscles rather than in the gut. For good functional results, the anatomic relationships must not be distorted by pelvic sepsis.

Ferrara et al[151] studied the relationship between anal canal tone and rectal motor activity. They noted that rectal motor complexes were invariably accompanied by a rise in mean anal canal pressure and contractile activity such that pressure in the anal canal was always greater than pressure in the rectum. Anal canal relaxation never occurred during a rectal motor complex.

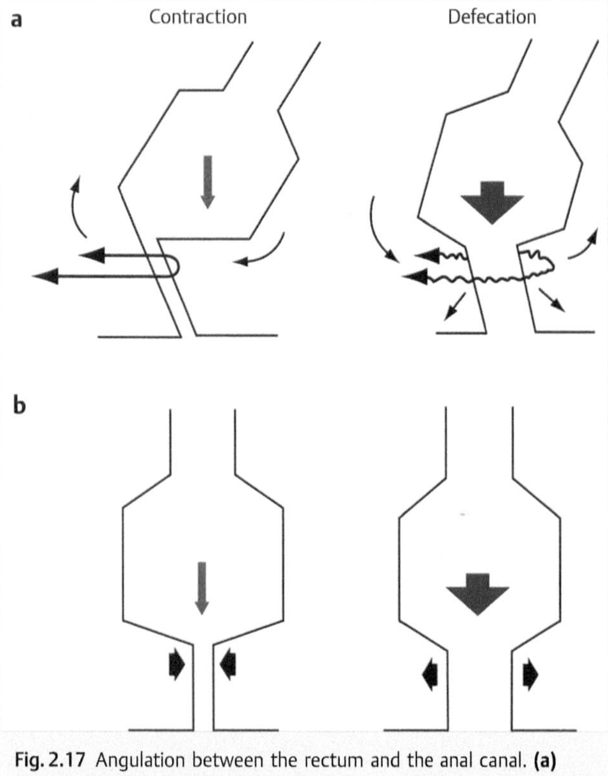

The onset of rectal contractions was accompanied by increased resting pressure and contractile activity of the anal canal. They concluded that this temporal relationship represents an important mechanism preserving fecal continence.

Mechanical Factors

Angulation between Rectum and Anal Canal

Without doubt, the most important component for the conservation of gross fecal continence is the angulation of the anorectal system, which is due to the continuous tonic activity of the puborectalis muscle.

As measured by defecography, the angle between the axis of the anal canal and the rectum in the resting state is about 90 degrees. Radiographic studies have elucidated changes in this angle during defecation (▶ Fig. 2.17).

Flutter Valve

It has been suggested that additional protection of continence might be afforded by intra-abdominal pressure being transmitted laterally to the side of the anal canal just at the level of the anorectal junction. The anal canal is an anteroposterior slitlike aperture, and any increased intra-abdominal pressure tends to compress it in a fashion similar to a flutter valve. This flutter valve mechanism is controversial because the highest pressure is found in the middle part of the anal canal rather than in the upper part, and therefore intra-abdominal forces would need to act at an infralevator level (▶ Fig. 2.18).[152]

Flap Valve Theory

According to the flap valve theory advanced by Parks et al,[153] any increase in intra-abdominal pressure (weight lifting, straining, laughing, coughing) tends to accentuate the anorectal angle and force the anterior rectal wall to lie firmly over the upper end of the anal canal, which produces an occlusion or a flap

Fig. 2.17 Angulation between the rectum and the anal canal. **(a)** Lateral view. **(b)** Anteroposterior view.

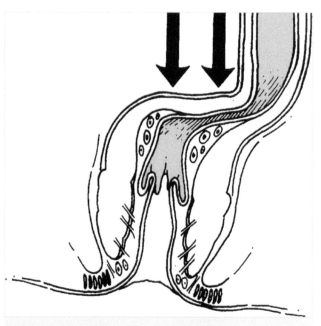

Fig. 2.18 Flutter valve mechanism.

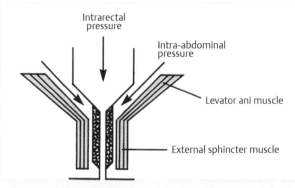

Fig. 2.19 Flap valve mechanism.

valve effect. For defecation to occur, the flap valve must be broken. This breakage takes place by lengthening the puborectalis, lowering the pelvic floor, and obliterating the angle (▶ Fig. 2.19).

The importance of the flap valve mechanism has been questioned. It was pointed out that a valve operates only if it separates compartments of different pressures. Thus, if a flap valve is responsible for preservation of anal continence during increases in intra-abdominal pressure, the anal pressure should be lower than intra-abdominal pressure. A study that measured anal and rectal pressures during serial increases in intra-abdominal pressure found that anal pressure always remained higher than intrarectal pressure, and this pressure gradient was the reverse of what would be found if a flap valve maintained continence. Based on this finding, it was concluded that anal continence is maintained by reflex contraction of the external sphincter rather than by a flap valve mechanism.[154] In another study, anal and rectal pressures were measured simultaneously with external sphincter and puborectalis electromyography and synchronously superimposed on an image intensifier displaying the rectum outlined by barium. The anterior rectal wall always was clearly separated from the upper part of the anal canal despite maximal effort to raise intra-abdominal pressure.[155] The results of this dynamic study also called into question the flap valve theory because during Valsalva maneuvers (while the rectum was filled with liquid contrast material) continence was maintained by sphincteric activity with no evidence of a valve. The authors of this study commented that normal defecation would require the anterior rectal wall to be lifted away from the upper part of the anal canal. Therefore, they consider a valvular occlusion to be more likely to lead to obstructed defecation.[155] Nevertheless, clinical experience with the postanal repair suggests that this mechanism indeed may play some role in continence. However, the modest success this surgical procedure enjoys may be the result of elevated intra-anal pressures.

Corpus Cavernosum of Anus

Stelzner[156] postulated that the vascular architecture in the submucosal and subcutaneous tissues of the anal canal really represents what he called a corpus cavernosum of the rectum. These cushions consist of discrete masses of blood vessels, smooth muscle fibers, and elastic and connective tissue. They have a remarkably constant configuration and are located in the left lateral, right anterolateral, and right posterolateral segments of the anal canal. These vascular cushions have the physiologic ability to expand and contract and to take up "slack," and hence they contribute to the finest degree of anal continence. This theory might be supported by the fact that certain patients who have undergone a formal hemorrhoidectomy have minor alterations in continence, a situation that may be the result of excision of this corpus cavernosum.

Defecation

Usual Sequence of Events

The stimulus for initiating defecation is distention of the rectum. This in turn may be related to a critical threshold of sigmoid and possibly descending colon distention. As long as fecal matter is retained in the descending and sigmoid colon, the rectum remains empty and the individual feels no urge to defecate. This reservoir type of continence does not depend on sphincter function. Distention of the left colon initiates peristaltic waves, which propel the fecal mass downward into the rectum.

Normally, this process occurs once or several times a day. The timing of the act is a balance between environmental factors, since the urge may be suppressed by a complex cortical inhibition of the basic reflexes of the anorectum. Many people establish a pattern whereby the urge is felt either on arising in the morning, in the evening, or after ingestion of food or drink. This balance can be altered by travel, by admission to a hospital, or by changes in diet.

Rectal distention induces relaxation of the internal sphincter, which in turn triggers contraction of the external sphincter. Thus, sphincter continence is induced. If the individual decides to accede to the urge, a squatting position is assumed. This causes the angulation between the rectum and the anal canal to straighten. A Valsalva maneuver is the second semivoluntary stage. This overcomes the resistance to the external sphincter by voluntarily increasing the intrathoracic and intra-abdominal pressure. The pelvic floor descends, and the resulting pressure on the fecal mass in the rectum increases intrarectal pressure. Inhibition of the external sphincter permits passage of the fecal bolus. Once evacuation has been completed, the pelvic floor and the anal canal muscles regain their resting activity, and the anal canal is closed.

Responses to Entry of Material into the Rectum

Duthie[157] conducted extensive studies on the dynamics of the rectum and anus and concluded that most dynamic changes in the anorectum are in response to two stresses: (1) the change in intra-abdominal pressure, and (2) entry of material from the colon into the rectum. There is considerable variation in the rate and timing of the entry of feces and flatus into the rectum in different individuals. Colonic transit is accelerated by engaging in physical activity and by eating meals. Local reflexes may be inhibited by cortical inhibition, which is a feature of social training. Afferent nerve impulses, which signal the entry of material into the rectum, proceed at a subconscious level, with the accommodation and sampling responses taking place reflexly. In support of this contention, clinical findings show that patients admitted for routine clinical examination of the rectum often have, unknown to them, a considerable amount of feces in the rectum.

Accommodation Response

The accommodation response is said to consist of receptive relaxation of the rectal ampulla to accommodate the fecal mass. Studies with a rectal balloon show that after inflation of the balloon to approximately 10 mL, the external anal sphincter shows a transient increase in electromyographic activity, while in the internal sphincter a similar short-lived reduction in its pressure activity can be measured within the lumen. With persistent inflation of the balloon, an increase in pressure within the rectal ampulla is maintained for 1 to 2 minutes and then it decreases to preinflation level. This is the accommodation response. With increasing volume, there is a gradual stepwise increase in rectal pressure, and depending on the age of the patient, an urge to defecate is experienced. This urge abates in a few seconds as the rectum accommodates to the stimulus. When volume increases rapidly over a short period, the accommodation response fails, leading to urgent emptying of the rectum (▸ Fig. 2.20).

The afferent nerve endings for the accommodation reflex are in the rectal ampulla and in the levator ani muscle. The nerve center for the spinal part of the reflex is in the lumbosacral cord with higher center control to permit suppression of the urge to defecate.

Sampling Response

The sampling response consists of transient relaxation of the upper part of the internal sphincter, which permits rectal contents to come into contact with the somatic sensory epithelium of the anal canal for assessment of the nature of the contents. Conscious sampling is done by slightly increasing abdominal tension and maintaining, by voluntary control, an increase in the activity of the external sphincter. Thus, solids can be retained, while gas can be passed, thereby relieving the intrarectal pressure. If fluid is present in the rectum, contact with the sensory area in the anal canal excites conscious activity of the external sphincter to maintain control until the rectal accommodation response occurs, and so continence is maintained.

Commencement of Defecation

The method of beginning the act of defecation varies from person to person. If one is exerting anal control during an urge, merely relinquishing this voluntary control will allow the reflex to proceed. However, if the urge abates, voluntary straining with increased intra-abdominal pressure is necessary before defecation can begin. Once begun, the act will follow either of two patterns: (1) expulsion of the rectal contents, accompanied by mass peristalsis of the distal colon, which clears the bowel in one continuous movement, or (2) passage of the stool piecemeal with several bouts of straining. The pattern followed is largely determined by the habit of the individual and the consistency of the feces. Using scintigraphic assessment, after oral intake of isotopes, Lubowski et al[158] demonstrated that normal defecation is not a process of rectal emptying alone but also includes colonic emptying. This process of colorectal emptying has been quantified by Krogh and coworkers. During normal defecation, colorectal emptying varied between 60% emptying of the rectosigmoid to complete emptying of the rectosigmoid, descending colon, and transverse colon, and 19% emptying of the ascending colon. They observed large inter- and intraindividual variations. They also detected retrograde movements, mainly from transverse and descending colon, during normal defecation. It is not known whether these retrograde movements are caused by contractile activity of the colonic wall or by Valsalva maneuvers supporting the defecation.[29] Kamm et al reported that defecation, evoked by bisacodyl, is preceded by propagating pressure waves arising in the cecum.[159] These pressure waves also occur in dogs prior to defecation evoked by guanethidine, neostigmine, glucose, and castor oil.[160] Bampton et al performed prolonged multipoint recordings of colonic pressure after nasocolonic intubation of the unprepared colon. They were able to demonstrate a preexpulsive phase commencing up to 1 hour before stool expulsion. This phase is characterized by a distinctive biphasic spatial and temporal pattern with an early and a late component. The early component is characterized by an array of antegrade propagating sequences. The site of their origin migrates distally with each subsequent sequence.

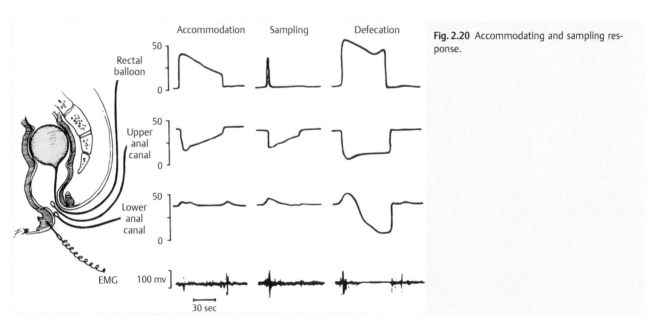

Fig. 2.20 Accommodating and sampling response.

The late component, in the 15 minutes before stool expulsion, is characterized by an array of antegrade propagating sequences. The site of their origin migrates proximally with each subsequent sequence. The amplitude of the pressure waves, occurring in this late phase, increases significantly. Many of them are real high-amplitude pressure waves. They are associated with an increasing sensation of urge to defecate. Some of the last propagating sequences, prior to stool expulsion, commence in the ascending colon. This latter finding illustrates that the entire colon is involved in the process of defecation.[30] Hagger et al also detected clusters of high-amplitude propagated contractions prior to defecation.[161] These contractions were associated with a sensation of an urge to defecate. Similar giant contractions, migrating distally into the rectum, have been observed in mongrel dogs prior to spontaneous defecation.[40] These giant contractions could be evoked by electrical stimulation of the sacral nerves. All these findings indicate that high-amplitude propagating contractions are necessary for an effective expulsion of stool. Recently, it has been shown that patients with obstructed defecation lack the normal predefecatory augmentation in frequency and amplitude of these propagating pressure waves.[45] When fecal material enters the rectum due to HAPS, the rectal wall deforms by circumferential strain and shearing forces. This deformation activates mechanoreceptors, which results in a sense of rectal fullness and ultimately in an urge to defecate. All these events are involuntary. The urge to defecate can only be suppressed by voluntary contraction of the external anal sphincter. By doing so, the call to stool fades away, because intrarectal pressure gradually decreases by accommodation of the rectal wall. After admitting the urge to defecate, expulsion of fecal material is facilitated by an increase in intrarectal pressure and a reduction of anal pressure. Ultimately, intrarectal pressure exceeds anal pressure, resulting in a propulsive force. MacDonald et al conducted a study in 10 healthy female volunteers. During attempted evacuation of an inflated balloon, intrarectal pressure increased to the same extent as intravesical pressure. According to these authors, the true intrarectal pressure (intrarectal minus intravesical) did not rise. Based on this finding, the authors concluded that the rise in intrarectal pressure during attempted evacuation was the result of straining alone.[162] It is doubtful whether this conclusion is justified. Attempted evacuation of an inflated balloon is not the same as defecation at home. A normal bowel movement is always preceded by HAPS. It seems unlikely that these high-amplitude contractions underlie balloon expulsion on command. Furthermore, it should be noted that laboratory conditions are rather embarrassing and may induce inappropriate contractions of the pelvic floor due to the patient's fear of incontinence. At present, it is generally assumed that both rectal contractions and additional straining underlie the increase in intrarectal pressure. However, it is unknown which of these two factors is the most important one. It has been suggested that the relative contribution of each depends on volume and consistency of the stool.[163] Since quite a few people can expel their rectal contents without straining, it seems logical to assume that rectal contractions are the driving force behind the evacuation of fecal material. It is not quite clear whether these rectal contractions are the final part of

HAPS or the manifestation of a local reflex initiated by activation of mechanoreceptors in the rectal wall. Furthermore, it is unknown whether additional straining itself can provoke rectal contractions. Utilizing a specially designed barostat–manometric assembly, Andrews and coworkers demonstrated that rectal ramp distention at 100 mL/min is associated with a marked rectal contractile response.[164] This finding suggests that rectal contractions are the outcome of a local reflex, triggered by rectal distension. Although rectal contractions are referred to in many textbooks, the evidence for their existence is scarce. Unlike detrusor contractions during micturition, rectal contractions are difficult to detect during normal defecation. In an experimental dog model, Tabe and coworkers were able to demonstrate the presence of propulsive rectal contractions during spontaneous defecation. These rectal contractions had a relatively low amplitude and were always preceded by HAPS.[165] Utilizing a specially designed video manometry technique, Ito et al were able to detect rectal contractions during defecation in 15 healthy volunteers.[166] Based on these findings, it seems likely that evacuation of rectal contents is driven by rectal contractions, whether or not supported by additional straining. The weaker these contractions, the more additional straining required. Normal defecation depends not only on appropriate rectal function, but also on the cooperation between colon and rectum, as illustrated by the role of HAPS in the expulsion of stool. Complex reflex pathways are also involved, such as the gastrorectal reflex. It has been shown that rectal tone increases after a meal.[50,57,167] This gastrorectal reflex probably contributes to postprandial defecation. It has been postulated that the increase in rectal tone, as a result of this reflex, results in a greater incremental pressure from the fecal mass on the rectal wall, providing a heightened sensation. This assumption is supported by the observation that distension volumes needed to elicit an urge to defecate are significantly reduced after a meal.[168] This suggests that the increased tension in the rectal wall following a meal results in a change in the set point at which the mechanoreceptors are stimulated. Many women with obstructed defecation apply digital pressure upon their perineum in order to facilitate defecation. Recently, it has been shown that this maneuver results in an increase in rectal tone.[169] This observation has been confirmed by others.[170] All these findings and data illustrate that the act of defecation is far more complex than previously thought.

Urgent Defecation

If large volumes of fecal material are introduced rapidly into the rectum, the accommodation response may be overcome and cortical inhibition may be unavailing. In this situation, the urgency can be controlled for only 40 to 60 seconds by the voluntary external sphincter complex. This may be enough time to allow for some accommodation; if not, leakage will temporarily relieve the situation.

Pathologic Conditions

During the period of "spinal shock," which supervenes for some weeks immediately after transection of the spinal cord above the origin of the fifth lumbar segment, the rectum and sphincters are completely paralyzed and the patient is incontinent. Frenckner[171] revealed that in these patients there is a cessation of all electrical activity from the striated muscles in response to rectal distention and also a less-pronounced inflation reflex. Thereafter, the tonus of the sphincter returns, and defecation occurs reflexly from the lumbosacral center through pelvic and pudendal nerves.

Because voluntary contraction of the external sphincter is no longer possible and because distention of the rectum is no longer perceived, the patient has no control over the act of defecation. This poses a difficult problem in paraplegic patients, in whom defecation generally must be managed by the regular use of enemas and digital evacuation of the rectum. In some of these patients, the defecation mechanism can be triggered by stimulating the somatic innervation, such as by stroking the thigh or the perianal region.

When the cord lesion involves the cauda equina with destruction of the sacral innervation, the reflexes are abolished, and defecation then becomes automatic (i.e., dependent entirely on intrinsic neural mechanisms). In these circumstances, the rectum still responds, although with little force to distention, and the reciprocal relaxation of the already patulous sphincters enables feces to be extruded.

Internal sphincter relaxation can persist with spinal cord transection and occurs if the presacral sympathetic nerves are stimulated. Possibly, this mechanism is some form of local muscular reflex.[157]

The accumulation of a large fecal mass in a greatly dilated rectum (as occurs especially in the elderly) suggests the abnormal condition known as rectal dyschezia, which results from a loss of tonicity of the rectal musculature. It may be due to a long-standing habit of ignoring or suppressing the urge to defecate or to degeneration of the neural pathways concerned with defecation reflexes. When further complicated by weakness of the abdominal muscles, defecation becomes a chronic problem. In these cases, evacuation may be obtained only by a mechanical washing out of the mass with enemas or by the administration of cathartics that keep the stools semiliquid.

Painful lesions of the anal canal, such as ulcers, fissures, and thrombosed hemorrhoids, impede defecation by exciting a spasm of the sphincters and by causing voluntary suppression to avoid the resulting pain.

A constant urge to defecate in the absence of appreciable content in the rectum may be caused by external compression of the rectum, by intrinsic neoplasms, and particularly by inflammation of the rectal mucosa. This mucosa is normally insensitive to cutting or burning; however, when inflamed it becomes highly sensitive to all stimuli, including those acting on the receptors mediating the stretch reflex.

2.5.3 Investigative Techniques

Techniques have been developed to physiologically assess disorders of function of the anal sphincters, rectum, and pelvic floor. These techniques are used to establish a diagnosis, provide an objective assessment of the function, or identify the anatomic site of a lesion. Sophisticated tests are designed to complement but not to substitute for good clinical examination and sound surgical judgment. Well-established laboratories from around the world have made significant contributions in this area.[103,105,157,172] A leader in the field was the late Sir Alan Parks, in whose name a physiology unit was established at St. Mark's Hospital, London.

Manometry

Anorectal manometry is a means of quantifying the function of the internal and external sphincters. A more dynamic and physiologic investigation can be achieved by combining proctography with simultaneous pressure recordings and electromyographic measurements.

There is no standardized method of performing anorectal manometry. Of the many methods available for measuring anorectal pressure, each has its own particular advantages and disadvantages; hence, none has emerged as a gold standard. Until recently, techniques available to perform anorectal manometry have included closed balloon systems and perfused fluid-filled open-tipped catheters. Air-filled balloon systems have a poor frequency response due to the compressibility of air, but one report has suggested that air-filled microballoon manometry gives results similar to those of a water-filled microballoon system.[173] Nevertheless, it is more advisable to use a noncompressible medium such as water. However, even water-filled balloon catheters have disadvantages. The relatively large balloons, varying in diameter from 3 to 15 mm, disturb the resting state of the sphincters to some extent; it is a well-known fact that anal pressure rises with an increase in the diameter of the recording device. Another disadvantage of balloon catheters is that reliability depends on the balloon's elasticity; each balloon catheter shows a considerable baseline drift due to a gradual change in its compliance.[174]

Perfused open-tipped catheters are smaller than balloon catheters and therefore cause less disturbance of the sphincter muscles. Nevertheless, perfused manometry has been criticized on practical and theoretical grounds because it also has disadvantages. The pressure recorded with a perfused system depends on the compliance of the catheter system and the perfusion rate, as well as on the site and location of the opening.[175] In the case of a side opening, the recorded pressure depends on the distance between the opening and the distal end of the tube. Continuous perfusion of water results in leakage from the anal canal with stimulation of the perianal skin, sometimes causing reflex activity of the sphincters. Because the lumen of the anal canal is flattened from side to side rather than circular in cross section, open-tipped tubes are less suitable.[176]

Microtransducers are used to overcome the measurement problems and errors associated with perfused open-tipped catheters and closed balloon systems. These recording devices, which consist of a miniature pressure sensor located at the tip of the catheter, offer many advantages in anorectal manometry (▶ Fig. 2.21). The direct connection to a chart recorder obviates the need for fluid-filled tubes, thereby eliminating all the associated artifacts. The small diameter of the catheter minimizes stimulation of the sphincters because it does not distend the anal canal. Most microtransducers have good thermal stability, and therefore the rise in temperature between calibration and actual measurement does not affect the recording. There is no problem of perianal skin irritation caused by continuous perfusion and leakage from the anal canal. Furthermore, recordings are not influenced by hydrostatic factors, compliance, or perfusion rate. The high-frequency response of the transducer registers sudden pressure changes. However, the microtransducer-tipped catheters are much more expensive than conventional recording devices.

For the assessment of an anal pressure profile, the recording probe must be withdrawn from the rectum, either stepwise or continuously at a constant rate. Although the step-by-step pull-through technique provides reliable measurements of resting anal canal pressure, the continuous pull-through technique allows a more appropriate assessment of the anal pressure profile and functional sphincter length.[109] With the latter technique, the length of the high-pressure zone varies between 2.5 and 5 cm and is shorter in women than in men.[108,109,177,178] Most of the difference in functional sphincter length between men and women is attributed to a shorter length of the anterior axis of the anal canal in women.[109]

The highest pressure of a pull-through profile is defined as the maximal resting anal pressure (MRAP) (▶ Fig. 2.22). Normal values of the MRAP are poorly defined because (1) a variety of techniques have been used, (2) "normal" values have been reported only for small control populations, and (3) there is a large range of MRAP in the normal population. McHugh and Diamant[179] have suggested that normal values for MRAP, as determined in 157 healthy subjects, can be constructed only for each sex on a decade basis. Their study revealed that the process of aging in both men and women is associated with a marked decrease in MRAP and that this age-related reduction is more significant in women than in men.[178,179]

In another study, no change in MRAP could be noted in subjects until the eighth and ninth decade, at which time a sudden decrease occurred.[180] However, because a closed balloon system was used, it may have detected only the more marked decrease in MRAP seen in the very aged population. It has been suggested that the age-related reduction in MRAP that occurs in women might be attributed to previous childbearing.[181] However, such a relationship has not been demonstrated by other researchers.[179] Jameson et al[178] conducted a study to determine the effects of age, sex, and parity on anorectal function. They found that parity leads only to lower squeeze pressure and does not result in a decrease in anal canal resting pressure.

In yet another study in women, maximum resting anal pressure and maximum squeeze pressure declined with age more rapidly after menopause.[182] Closing pressure (i.e., the difference between maximum resting anal pressure and rectal pressure), an important determinant of anal continence, was more markedly reduced with age than was maximum resting anal pressure. Parity and anal pressures were unrelated. Women are more frequently affected by anal incontinence than are men. The more rapid decline of anal pressure after menopause might imply that anal sphincter tissue is a target for estrogen.

Pregnancy itself does not have a significant effect on anal sphincter morphology or function. Sultan et al[183] conducted manometric and anal endosonographic studies on patients during pregnancy and 6 weeks after cesarean section and found no differences in pressures or muscle thickness, indicating that any change in sphincter function is caused by mechanical trauma rather than by hormonal factors.

Resting pressure in the anal canal exhibits regular fluctuations that vary from day to night by the presence or absence of fecal material in the rectum and by posture.[184] Most of these fluctuations present as slow waves with a frequency between

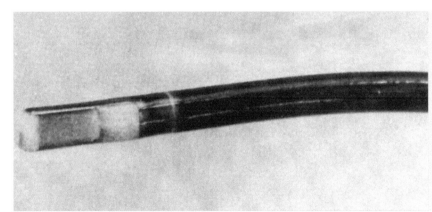

Fig. 2.21 Microtransducer catheter. Note the miniature silicone strain gauge located at the tip.

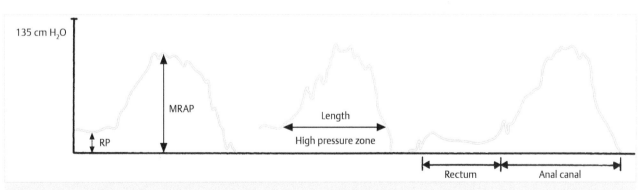

Fig. 2.22 Anal pressure profile recorded by the pull-through technique, repeated three times to obtain mean values. Rectal pressure (RP) and maximal resting anal pressure (MRAP) are indicated.

10 and 20/min and an amplitude varying between 5 and 25 cm H_2O (▸ Fig. 2.23a). Although these slow waves can be found in all normal subjects, they are not present continuously. Less frequently observed are the ultraslow waves, with an amplitude varying between 30 and 100 cm H_2O and a frequency of < 3/min (▸ Fig. 2.23b). These ultraslow waves seem to be associated with high resting anal pressures.[184] Slow and ultraslow waves represent regular fluctuations in internal sphincter activity, as demonstrated by electrical recordings from the internal sphincter.[185]

Based on the results of a manometric study with a rigid recording device and a step-by-step pull-through technique, it has been concluded that intra-anal pressure exhibits longitudinal and radial variations.[181] In the proximal part of the anal canal, the pressure recorded in the dorsal segment is higher than the pressure in the anterior segment. This finding has been ascribed to the activity of the puborectalis muscle. In the middle anal canal, the pressure is equally distributed in all segments, whereas in the lower anal canal the pressure is highest anteriorly.[181] However, a more recent study has not been able to demonstrate this radial asymmetry.[109] In contrast, significant differences in radial symmetry were found between the two sexes. In women, the pressure in the anterior segment of the anal canal was higher distally, while in men the pressure in the anterior and lateral segments was higher proximally.[109]

With the aid of a microcomputer and an eight-channel multilumen probe, Coller[177] determined the pressures at each point along the length of the anal canal. The typical resting pressure profile during continuous pullout describes the length and distribution of pressure along the longitudinal axis of the sphincter. The normal MRAP will range from 65 to 85 mm Hg above the rectal intraluminal pressure and is located 1 to 1.5 cm from the distal end of the sphincter. The range of normal sphincter length is 2.5 to 5 cm. With the same equipment, Coller calculated the radial cross-sectional pressure in five segments of the sphincter and found a gradient of pressure that changes from the posterior to lateral to anterior as one proceeds from the proximal end to the distal end. Williamson et al[186] reported a comparison of simultaneous longitudinal and radial recordings of anal canal pressures. The catheter they used had the capability of making simultaneous linear longitudinal pressure measurements. An asymmetry of basal, squeeze, and relaxation pressures was found. The highest basal pressures were in the middle of the anal canal, regardless of quadrant orientation. With the radial perfusion catheter, the squeeze pressure profile was consistent with a double-loop external sphincter mechanism. With the linear perfusion catheter, the internal sphincter relaxation pressures showed a greater negative deflection at the proximal portions of the sphincter, which was not achieved at points distally in the same quadrant. This implies that during reflex, relaxation pressure is maintained in the distal anal canal; hence, patients remain continent during sensory sampling of rectal contents.

Voluntary contraction of the external sphincter gives an increase in anal pressure that is superimposed on the basal tone. This increase in pressure is maximal in the distal part of the anal canal where the bulk of the external sphincter is situated. To determine the functional activity of the different parts of the external sphincter, the recording device has to be withdrawn stepwise. After each step, the patient is asked to squeeze at full strength. In this way, it is possible to measure the maximal squeeze anal pressure (MSAP) at every level of the anal canal (▸ Fig. 2.24). It has been shown that MSAP is

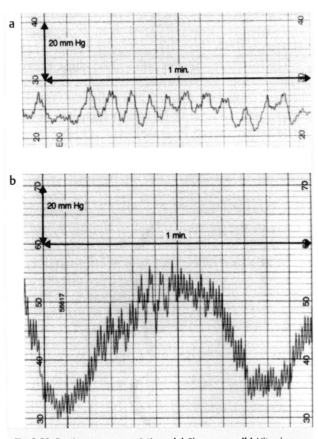

Fig. 2.23 Resting pressure variations. **(a)** Slow waves. **(b)** Ultraslow waves.

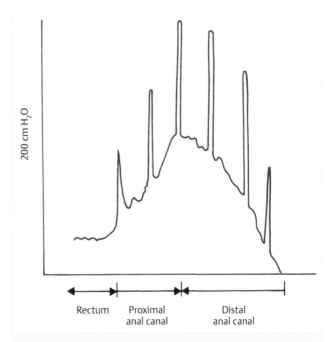

Fig. 2.24 Maximal squeeze anal pressure: maximal voluntary contraction of the external sphincter muscle indicated by increase in pressure superimposed on the anal resting pressure.

higher in male than in female subjects, and is reduced as subjects get older.[179,180,187] This age-related reduction of MSAP is most noticeable in women.[178,179]

The internal sphincter reflex in response to rectal distention can be elicited by inflation of a rectal balloon. Transient inflation of a balloon with relatively small volumes of air results in an initial rise in pressure, caused by a transient contraction of the external sphincter. Almost immediately after this initial increase in pressure, a transient reduction in anal canal pressure can be observed as a result of relaxation of the internal sphincter (▶ Fig. 2.25). It has been reported that the transient inflation of a rectal balloon with 30 mL of air results in a pressure reduction of approximately 50% for a mean duration of 19 seconds.[188] However, as the balloon is inflated with larger volumes, the amplitude as well as the duration of the relaxation reflex increases. Not only does the relaxation of the internal sphincter result in a pressure reduction, but it also abolishes the pressure fluctuations (slow and ultraslow waves) within the anal canal. The effect of body position on anal canal pressures was studied by Johnson et al,[189] who used a probe in which were embedded four transducers oriented radially, 90 degrees apart. They concluded that: (1) transducer manometry recorded similar resting pressures but higher squeeze pressures as compared with perfused manometry; (2) transducer manometry recorded the same radial variation in anal canal resting and squeeze pressures as that recorded by the perfused manometer; and (3) standing and sitting caused a fourfold rise in intrarectal pressure, which was associated with a concomitant rise in resting anal canal pressure.

In an effort to correctly interpret manometric results, Cali et al[110] noted that manometric values for normal patients cover a wide range but categorize definable distinctions among subgroups of patients. They found mean maximal squeeze pressures (MSPs) and length of the anal sphincter at rest and with squeezing are significantly greater in men than women. Parous females have a significant decrease in mean maximal resting pressures compared with nulliparous females. They found no difference in resting pressures of males and nulliparous females. These authors concluded that patients must be compared with their normal subgroups to correctly identify manometric abnormalities. Felt-Bersma et al[106] also tried to determine normal values in anal manometry. They found that

maximal basal pressure (MBP) was not significantly different in men and women (68 vs. 63 mm Hg) but that MSP was significantly different (183 vs. 102 mm Hg). Both MBP and MSP decreased significantly with age. Sphincter length was longer in men than women (4.1 vs. 3.5 cm). In recent years, high-resolution manometry has been introduced. Initially, this technique was used for the examination of esophageal physiology. Sometime later it was also applied in anorectal testing. For high-resolution anorectal manometry (HRAM), a solid-state assembly is required with multiple circumferential-oriented pressure sensors. Each sensor consists of multiple radially dispersed sensing elements. Usually, the probe used in this assembly has a central lumen for inflation of a balloon at the tip (▶ Fig. 2.26). More recently, a three-dimensional (3D) HRAM technique has been developed. This technique enables 3D mapping of anorectal pressure in rest as well as during squeezing and straining.[190] The pressure morphology at rest and the changes during squeezing and straining are shown in ▶ Fig. 2.27. Proponents of this innovative technique underline several advantages of HRAM.[191] The multiple, closely spaced circumferential sensors, each with radially dispersed sensing elements, provide an enhanced spatiotemporal resolution. Unlike conventional techniques, HRAM does not require withdrawal of the recording

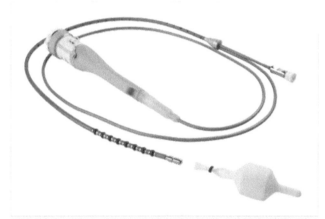

Fig. 2.26 Example of HRAM probe with eight circumferential pressure sensors.

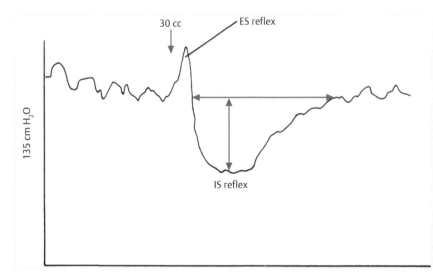

Fig. 2.25 ES reflex in response to rectal distension with 30 mL of air followed by IS reflex. ES, external sphincter; IS, internal sphincter.

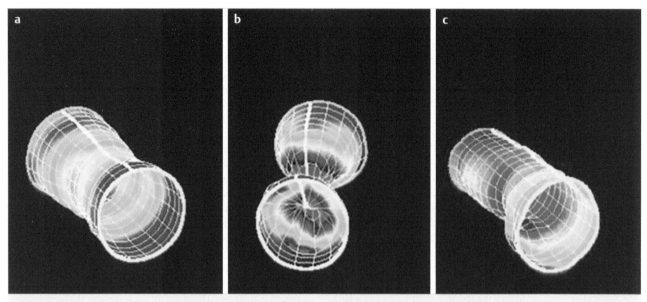

Fig. 2.27 (a) 3D mapping of anorectal pressure during squeezing. The yellow high-pressure ring has turned to a red higher-pressure ring ("sandy clock" shape). **(b)** 3D mapping of anorectal pressure during straining. **(c)** The pressure cylinder has turned to a typical "trumpet" shape, which is due to the increase of intrarectal pressure and the reduction of anal pressure.

device. This stationary examination seems to be more comfortable for the patient. The interpretation of events is not difficult due to the color topographic display. According to the proponents, HRAM can delineate the function and anatomy of the anorectum in greater detail than conventional manometry. It has also been argued that high-resolution manometry can be used for the evaluation of sphincter defects. However, the agreement between HRAM and endoanal ultrasound is rather poor.[192] It is questionable whether the advantages of this new and innovative technique outweigh the costs, fragility, and relatively short lifespan of the recording devices, which are needed. In addition, the clinical relevance of this HRAM has yet to be determined. Although it has been reported that HRAM can be used for the assessment of obstructed defecation, it is questionable whether this technique has added value compared to conventional defecography or MR-defecography.[193]

Defecography, Balloon Proctography, and Dynamic MRI

In the 1960s, cineradiography was developed for the dynamic investigation of the defecation mechanism. Some of the techniques used in that period were complex and time-consuming and required sophisticated radiologic equipment. Now, however, simplified techniques such as defecography and balloon proctography are available.

Defecography can be performed with different contrast media. A liquid barium suspension might be adequate and convenient for demonstrating specific abnormalities, such as rectal prolapse. A semisolid medium is required for detailed investigation of the physiologic aspects of normal continence and defecation. A contrast medium with a semisolid consistency can be prepared by heating potato starch or rolled oats with barium sulfate and water. After this mixture is introduced into the rectum, the subject is seated on a radiolucent commode to void

the contrast medium.[194] It has been argued, however, that such a semisolid mixture does not simulate the inspissated feces frequently seen in patients with obstructed defecation, so it is questioned whether the use of a semisolid paste is relevant for the defecographic investigation of patients with evacuation difficulties.[195]

Defecography can be used to measure the anorectal angle. This angle depends on the tone of the puborectalis muscle and is normally 92 ± 1.5^S at rest and 137 ± 1.5 during straining.[196] Another application of defecography is determination of the position of the pelvic floor by calculating the distance between the anorectal junction and the pubococcygeal line. In this way, perineal descent at rest and during straining can be measured. The pubococcygeal line is drawn from the tip of the coccyx to the posteroinferior margin of the pubic ramus; normally, the pelvic floor lies at a plane approximately 1 cm below that of the pubococcygeal line. Other determinations that can be made include the distance between the anorectal junction and the lower end of the coccyx, the presence of a rectocele, and the ability of the patient to expel rectal contents.

Balloon proctography has been developed to afford a more simplified procedure and make it more acceptable for the patient.[197] It provides a visual assessment of the pelvic floor both in the resting state and during defecation. The examination is conducted by inserting into the rectum a special shaped balloon filled with a barium suspension. With the patient seated on a commode, lateral radiographs are taken and the rectum and anal canal can be outlined at rest and during straining. Evacuation of the balloon rather than feces is more esthetically acceptable for both patient and staff. The examination is well tolerated, is quick and clean, and involves a relatively low dose of radiation. Agachan et al[198] assessed the incidence and clinical significance of defecographic findings in patients with possible evacuation disorders. Of 744 patients, 60% were diagnosed who complained of constipation, 16.5% of fecal incontinence, 5.6% of rectal prolapse, 11% of rectal pain, and 6.9% of a combination of more than one of these diagnoses. Although 12.5% of these evaluations were considered normal, 8% revealed rectal prolapse, 25.7% rectocele, 11% sigmoidocele, 12.6% intussusception, and 30% a combination of these findings. Patients with paradoxical puborectalis contraction had an extremely high frequency of constipation compared with other symptoms. The authors caution against treating patients strictly on the basis of radiographic findings.

A further refinement in the assessment of rectal evacuation was described by Lestar and colleagues.[199] In what they termed "defecometry," they reported the ability to quantify the maximum rectal pressure increase during straining, the duration of effective evacuation, and the work performed to evacuate a simulated stool. Simultaneous anal pressure records (permitted by the incorporation of a catheter into the balloon device) demonstrate the nature of the sphincter activity during simulated defecation. They believe that defecometry permits more adequate identification and characterization of the outlet-obstruction type of constipated patient than does the single-balloon expulsion test.

The largest series from a single institution was reported by Mellgren et al.[200] They analyzed the results of 2,816 patients who underwent defecography for defecation disorders. Their findings included: normal, 23%; rectal intussusception, 31%; rectal prolapse, 13%; rectocele, 27%; and enterocele, 19%. A combination of one or more of these diagnoses was present in 21% of patients studied.

For the evaluation of disorders such as anterior rectal wall prolapse, incomplete or complete rectal prolapse, rectocele, and solitary rectal ulcer syndrome, defecography seems to be more sensitive than balloon proctography. With regard to rectoceles, defecographic criteria are used to select which patients should undergo surgical repair. These criteria are rectocele size and retention of barium within the rectocele at the end of attempted evacuation. Although many surgeons use these proctographic selection criteria, it has been shown that they fail to predict who will and who will not benefit from rectocele repair.[201]

A scintigraphic method using a balloon filled with technetium-99 m (^{99m}Tc)-labeled suspension has been developed. With this method, the anorectal angle can be measured accurately with minimal radiation exposure.[202] To reduce radiation exposure, Hutchinson et al[203] believe this to be the investigation of choice for objective and dynamic assessment of anorectal function.

In summary, defecography is a useful imaging modality for detecting anorectal functional and anatomic abnormalities as possible causes of defecation disturbances and for anatomically guided anorectal surgery.[204] The main contribution of defecography is its specific ability to reveal rectal intussusception and enterocele as well as sigmoidocele. Other diagnoses that can be made by defecography include nonrelaxing puborectalis syndrome, perineal descent, and rectocele.[205]

With the advent of open-configuration magnetic resonance (MR) imaging systems, MR defecography with the patient in the sitting position has become possible. This nonradioactive imaging technique is a promising modality to investigate structural and functional disturbances in patients with defecatory problems.[206] MR defecography permits analysis of the anorectal angle, the opening of the anal canal, the function of the puborectalis muscle, and the descent of the pelvic floor during defecation.[207] Good demonstration of the rectal wall permits visualization of intussusceptions and rectoceles. Excellent demonstration of the perirectal soft tissues allows assessment of spastic pelvic floor syndrome and descending perineum syndrome and visualization of enteroceles. MR defecography with an open-configuration magnet allows accurate assessment of anorectal morphology and function in relation to surrounding structures without exposing the patient to harmful ionizing radiation.

The wide range of morphologic variations among healthy individuals and a large interobserver variation in measurements prevent defecography from being an ideal examination of anorectal defecation disturbance. Nevertheless, some patients with clinically occult disorders of anorectal function can be diagnosed with dynamic defecography.[208]

Another imaging technique is dynamic transperineal ultrasound. Recent studies suggest that this ultrasound modality is an attractive alternative for defecography with opacification of the small bowel, bladder, and vagina.[209,210,211] Beer-Gabel et al compared dynamic transperineal ultrasound with defecography in 33 women with obstructed defecation. In all these patients, the small bowel was opacified following ingestion of Gastrografin. They found good agreement for the assessment of rectocele, intussusception, and rectal prolapse. There was also agreement with regard to the measurement of the anorectal angle at rest, the position of the anorectal junction at rest, and the movement of this junction during straining.[212]

Simultaneous Dynamic Proctography and Peritoneography

It is believed that simultaneous dynamic proctography and peritoneography identifies both rectal and pelvic floor pathologic conditions and provides a qualitative assessment of severity, allowing for better treatment planning in selected patients with obstructed defecation, pelvic fullness and/or prolapse, and/or chronic intermittent pelvic floor pain.[213] As described by Sentovich et al,[213] the method consists of injection of 50 mL of nonionic contrast (Renografin-60, Squibb Diagnostics, Princeton, NJ) intraperitoneally along the lateral border of the rectus muscle using fluoroscopy. Patients are asked to perform Valsalva maneuver, and anteroposterior and lateral pelvic radiographs are obtained. Patients are immediately given 100 to 120 mL of barium and instant mashed potato mixture as an enema and 20 to 25 mL of liquid barium intravaginally. On a radiolucent commode, lateral radiographs are taken with the patient at rest and during maximal anal squeeze. Patients are asked to evacuate the rectal contrast material, which is observed on videotape using fluoroscopy. A final static radiograph is obtained while the patient strains to evacuate any residual rectal contrast. The initial static radiographs are taken when patients have been given only peritoneal contrast to evaluate for pelvic floor hernias. Radiographs taken on the commode at rest, squeeze, and strain are used to determine the anorectal angle and perineal descent. The evacuation videotape is used to identify rectoceles, enteroceles, and rectal prolapse. An enterocele is present if peritoneal contrast separates the rectum from the vagina, either at rest or during strain.

Sentovich et al[213] identified clinically suspected and nonsuspected enterocele in 10 of the 13 patients studied. An enterocele or other pelvic floor hernia was ruled out by the technique in three of the women studied. Findings affected operative treatment planning in 85% of patients studied. Women with rectoceles and suspected enteroceles confirmed by dynamic proctography with peritoneography underwent abdominal rectopexy and colopexy rather than per anal repair of their rectocele. In one woman, dynamic proctography with peritoneography ruled out a clinically suspected enterocele, and subsequently she underwent a successful perineal repair of her rectal prolapse. Operation was avoided in women in whom dynamic proctography and peritoneography identified no enterocele or pelvic floor hernia or only a small, non-obstructing enterocele. Complications occurred in two patients (15%)—a vasovagal reaction and postprocedure abdominal pain.

To identify enterocele, some authors have recommended giving patients oral barium 1 to 3 hours before defecography so that small bowel herniating into an enterocele sac can be easily identified.[214] Other authors have given substantial amounts of barium paste intrarectally so that sigmoidoceles can be identified.[215] Although both these techniques have been found to be useful, neither directly visualizes the enterocele sacs that may, in fact, be filled with omentum rather than with small bowel or sigmoid colon. In addition, neither technique adequately visualizes potential pelvic floor hernias such as obturator, sciatic, or perineal hernias.

Peritoneography outlines both enterocele and pelvic floor hernia sacs and thus more completely and efficiently evaluates pelvic floor anatomy.[213] Other investigators have also found this technique useful.[216] A variation of the theme was reported by Altringer et al,[217] who used complete visceral opacification of the small bowel and bladder and vaginal and rectal contrast to improve diagnostic accuracy beyond that provided by physical examination alone. These authors believe that fluoroscopic assessment of the female pelvis is frequently needed to evaluate chronic pain, urinary tract symptoms, vaginal eversions, rectal prolapse, and obstructed defecation. Therefore, contrast defecography changed the diagnosis in 75% of the 46 patients studied.

Balloon Expulsion Test

Rectal balloon expulsion may be used as an alternative to defecography, as the inability to expel an intrarectal balloon can point to impaired rectal evacuation. This simple method has been adopted by many units as a test for anismus.[218] It is questionable, however, whether the inability to expel a balloon represents paradoxical contraction of the puborectalis muscle during attempted evacuation. Dahl et al[219] reported that 13 of 14 patients with electromyographic evidence of anismus were able to pass an inflated balloon. They concluded that the balloon expulsion test is not a useful marker of inappropriate contraction of the pelvic floor.

In contrast with this finding, Minguez and coworkers reported that 87% of their patients with manometric and defecographic signs of anismus were not able to expel a balloon. Only 12 of 102 patients (11%), admitted with functional constipation without signs of anismus, showed the same inability to expel an intrarectal balloon. According to these authors, the specificity and negative predictive value of the balloon-expulsion test for excluding anismus were 89 and 97%, respectively.[220]

It has been argued that the failure to expel an inflated balloon might be due to structural abnormalities of the rectum. This seems unlikely, since it has been shown that the ability to pass a balloon is not impaired, neither by the presence and size of a rectocele nor by the presence of a rectal intussusception.[195] It might be possible that the inability to expel a balloon represents insufficient colonic and rectal contractility or the failure to adequately increase intrarectal pressure by inappropriate contraction of the diaphragm and abdominal muscles.

Saline Continence Test

The saline continence test provides a more dynamic assessment of the fecal continence mechanism.[221] The ability of an individual to retain 1,500 mL of saline solution infused into the rectum at a rapid rate (60 mL/min) can provide insights into the strength of the sphincteric barrier against the physical stress of fluid in the rectum. Simultaneous measurements of anorectal pressure and electrical activity of the external sphincter have revealed that rectal infusion of saline induces a regular series of events: rectal contractions, relaxations of the internal sphincter, and contractions of the external sphincter.

The initial phasic contraction of the external sphincter in response to rectal infusion occurs both before the deepest relaxation of the internal sphincter and also before rectal peak pressure, which in normal subjects is lower than anal pressure. Based on these findings, it has been concluded that this brief phasic contraction of the external sphincter contributes little to continence during saline infusion. However, the initial response of the external sphincter is followed by an increased activity that remains continuously above basal values as long as the rectum remains distended. It has been suggested that this compensatory activity of the external sphincter is the major contribution to continence during rectal infusion of saline.

In continent patients, two distinct patterns of anorectal activity have been demonstrated using the saline continence test. In some patients, rectal infusion results in normal rectal contractions and internal sphincter relaxations but little or no compensatory activity of the external sphincter. Although this defective response of the external sphincter may be the result of neuropathic weakness, it also may be caused by diminished anorectal sensation.[222] In contrast, other patients with fecal incontinence present a sustained reduction of resting anal pressure soon after saline infusion is begun, whereas the external sphincter of these patients shows irregular contractions, as demonstrated in integrated electromyography.[222] These findings suggest that there is a functional weakness of the internal sphincter in this subgroup of patients.

Colonic Transit Studies

Although constipation is not directly related to anorectal function in all cases, colonic transit studies are helpful in understanding the constipated patient. Details are described in Chapter 33.

Anorectal Electrosensitivity

In recent years, there has been a growing interest in the physiologic significance of anorectal sensation. Roe et al[223] have described a method for the quantitative assessment of anorectal sensation that involves placing a bipolar ring electrode into the rectum or the anal canal and incrementally increasing the current until a threshold of sensation is reported by the patient. They found no significant differences in electrosensitivity thresholds between the two sexes and no relationship between age and anorectal sensory function.[223] In contrast, Jameson et al[178] demonstrated that midanal and rectal electrosensitivity decline with increasing age and that midanal sensitivity is affected by parity. A similar finding has been reported by Broens and Penninckx.[224]

Chan et al[225] found that strong correlation between heat thresholds and balloon distention to maximum tolerable volumes and defecatory desire suggests a common sensory afferent pathway excitation. Heat stimulation is a simple technique that has a high degree of repeatability and may be an objective assessment of polymodal nociceptor function in the rectum. As mentioned before, normal perception of rectal fullness is an essential component of the defecation reflex. Rectal hypersensitivity has been studied extensively, especially in the context of irritable bowel syndrome. In recent years, RH also has gained more interest. Although RH can be defined as diminished sensation to all kind of stimuli, it is generally defined as blunted sensation to mechanical balloon distension. Blunted rectal sensation is a frequent finding in patients with hindgut dysfunction[226] and is probably due to disruption or dysfunction of rectal sensory afferent nerves with or without altered rectal wall properties. Damage to the afferent sensory nerves during pelvic surgery has been classified as one of the underlying causes. Age-related damage to the mechanoreceptors of the rectal wall may also contribute to blunted sensation. According to others, psychosocial factors, such as depression, give rise to RH, probably by aberrant brain processing of sensation.[227] Analyzing rectal evoked potentials and their latencies, Burgell et al[228] observed prolonged peak latencies in patients with constipation associated with RH. This finding provides strong evidence for a primary defect in sensory neuronal function. Recently, it has been reported that RH is linked with obstructed defecation but not with slow transit constipation.[229] Data are emerging that elevated sensory threshold volumes may reflect altered rectal wall properties. Therefore, some authors have proposed to make a distinction between primary and secondary RH. Primary RH is due to impairment of afferent nerve function, whereas secondary RH is linked to altered rectal biomechanical properties. Gladman et al[230] stratified patients with constipation and RH into subgroups on the basis of a systematic evaluation of rectal compliance, rectal diameter, and afferent nerve sensitivity to electrical stimulation. In 33% of the patients, primary RH was found, whereas in all other patients rectal sensitivity was impaired due to altered rectal wall properties, such as increased compliance. It has been reported that compliance is only increased in constipated patients with concomitant impairment of rectal sensation, whereas constipated subjects with normal rectal sensation have normal compliance.[231] Although impaired rectal sensation and increased compliance are closely linked, their relationship is not absolute. At present it is not known whether increased compliance is a precursor of impaired sensation or vice versa. The optimum treatment of patients with RH is currently unclear. Although it

has been reported that biofeedback, intrarectal electrostimulation, and sacral neuromodulation can relieve the symptoms of obstructed defecation, it is unknown whether this beneficial effect is due to normalization of rectal sensitivity.

Rectal Compliance

Rectal compliance reflects the distensibility of the rectal wall (i.e., the volumetric response of the rectum to stretch when subjected to an increase of intraluminal pressure). It has been shown that an ultrathin and infinitely compliant polyethylene bag is the most suitable device with which to measure rectal compliance.[232] The balloon should be tied at both ends to prevent longitudinal extension during distention. After introduction into the rectum, the balloon is continuously inflated to selected pressure plateaus. The volume changes at the various levels of distending pressures are recorded. Next, a volume–pressure curve is plotted. The slope of this curve (dV/dP) represents compliance. There is growing evidence that the elastance and the compliance of the rectum are closely interwoven with rectal sensation.

Measurements of rectal volumes in response to cumulative pressure steps with an electromechanical barostat system have revealed a characteristic triphasic compliance curve.[137] During the first phase, the increase of pressure only gives rise to a small increase of volume, probably reflecting an initial resistance of the rectal wall. The second phase of the compliance curve is characterized by a larger increase of volume, presumably reflecting an adaptive relaxation of the rectal wall. The last phase of the curve is more flattened and probably represents increasing resistance of the rectal wall against further distension (▶ Fig. 2.28). Control subjects experience an initial perception of distension during the first phase of the compliance curve. An urge to defecate is experienced during the second phase. It has been reported that among patients with obstructed defecation the call to stool is encountered much later, at the end of the third phase of the compliance curve.[137] This finding does suggest that rectal sensory perception is interwoven with rectal compliance.

There are some conflicting data regarding rectal compliance in patients with obstructed defecation. Varma observed an increased compliance in women with obstructed defecation after hysterectomy,[234] whereas Rasmussen et al noted a decreased compliance.[235] In another study, conducted by Gosselink et al, no difference was found between controls and patients with obstructed defecation regarding their rectal compliance.[137] Gladman et al[134] reported that, in constipated patients with normal rectal sensitivity, compliance was similar to that in healthy controls. According to these authors, rectal compliance was only increased in constipated patients with RH. The discrepancy among these and other studies is assumed to be the result of variations in recording techniques and differences in defining compliance. This controversy and the reported inter- and intraindividual variations in pressure–volume profiles in normal subjects[236] indicate that compliance measurements should be interpreted with caution. Alstrup et al[233,237] reported an endosonographic method that they believe provides a more precise and reproducible estimation of rectal compliance.

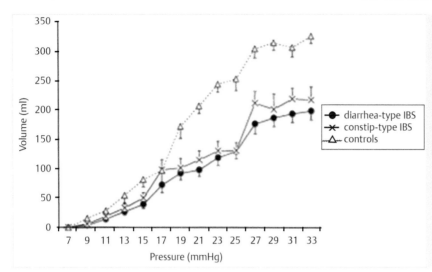

Fig. 2.28 Pressure–volume curve during intermittent isobaric distension (7–33 mm Hg) of the rectum in control subjects (Δ) and in patients with irritable bowel syndrome (•: diarrhea type, x: constipation type). Both in controls and in the IBS patients, the compliance curve exhibits a triphasic pattern. According to Steens et al, rectal compliance, as calculated over the steep part (second phase of the curve), is significantly lower in IBS patients compared with control subjects.[233] (With permission © 2002 John Wiley and Sons.)

Electromyography

Electromyography (EMG) records action potential derived from motor units within contracting muscle. The external sphincter and probably the puborectalis are unique skeletal muscles because they show continuous tonic contractions at rest, with activity present even during sleep. Sphincter activity ceases during defecation.

Conventional Concentric EMG

Various electrophysiologic techniques are available for the investigation of myoelectrical activity generated by the external sphincter and the puborectalis muscle. Some investigators have used silver/silver chloride electrodes applied to the perianal skin. Although these surface electrodes are well tolerated by patients and cause only slight disturbance of the sphincter muscles, they have the disadvantage of recording potentials summated from multiple motor units. Because bipolar concentric needle electrodes have the advantage of recording potentials summated from only a limited number of muscle fibers (±30), they are the type most often used.

Bowel preparation is not necessary before the examination. With the patient lying in the left lateral position, the needle electrode is inserted directly into the external sphincter or the puborectalis muscle without a local anesthetic. The needle is inserted posterior to the anal verge at an angle of 45 degrees. The position of the tip of the needle electrode in the puborectalis can be controlled with a finger hooked into the rectum. Normally, with the muscles at rest, a basal low-frequency activity will be recorded that consists of low-amplitude potentials varying between 2 and 50 mV.[238] This phenomenon usually is not displayed by skeletal muscle, which is characteristically silent at rest. During coughing, a burst of electrical activity, which is the consequence of increased frequency of motor unit firing and recruitment of new motor units, is recorded (▶ Fig. 2.29). Normally, the electrical activity is inhibited during straining. In patients with obstructed defecation, the opposite can be observed (▶ Fig. 2.29). However, one must bear in mind that this paradoxical activity is detected under laboratory conditions after painful insertion of a needle electrode. It is therefore questionable whether this phenomenon is the ultimate evidence for abnormal contraction of the pelvic floor and the external anal sphincter during defecation in the home environment. Contraction of the external sphincter and puborectalis, reflexly induced by balloon distention, saline infusion of the rectum, or perianal pinprick, also can be recorded electromyographically.

Single-Fiber EMG

Single-fiber EMG is an even more sophisticated technique for identifying the muscle action potential from a single muscle fiber. The technique provides a means of assessing innervation and reinnervation of the muscle under investigation.[238] The assessment can be made quantitatively using the fiber density, which represents the mean of a number of muscle fibers supplied by one motor unit within the uptake area of the electrode averaged from 20 different electrode positions.[238] Normal fiber density is 1.51 ± 0.16. A raised fiber density can be used as an index of collateral sprouting and reinnervation of denervated muscle fibers. A raised fiber density has been demonstrated in the majority of patients with primary "idiopathic" anal incontinence and in patients with incontinence secondary to neurologic disorders.[238,239]

In the past, the most useful clinical application of EMG was anal mapping for incontinent patients. Now other techniques such as endoanal sonography and endoanal MRI seem to be more accurate in the detection of sphincter defects. Furthermore, the latter techniques obviate the need for the painful insertion of a needle at several locations around the anal canal.

However, Jost et al[240] reported on the use of surface versus needle electrodes in the determination of motor conduction time to the external anal sphincter. Mean latency in the group with surface electrodes was 19.4 ms, and in the group with needle electrodes, it was 23.4 ms. The authors believe that the surface electrodes are preferable.

Nerve Stimulation Techniques

Even more sophisticated techniques have been described to develop a better understanding of perineal functional abnormalities that may be of neurogenic origin. The techniques of nerve stimulation provide objective assessment of neuromuscular

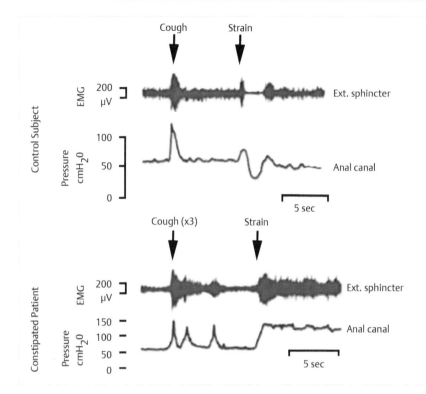

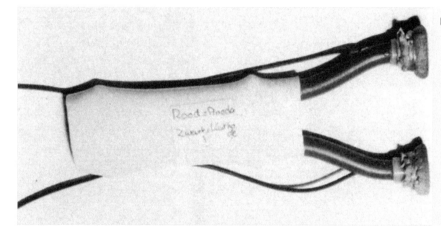

Fig. 2.29 EMG of the external anal sphincter and anal pressure tracings in a healthy control subject and a patient with obstructed defecation. In both the control subject and the constipated patient, a cough produces a rise in anal pressure. When the normal subject strains (upper tracing), EMG activity of the external anal sphincter is inhibited and anal pressure falls. In the patient with obstructed defecation, EMG activity of the external anal sphincter is not inhibited on straining and anal pressure increases (lower tracing). This paradoxical contraction has been termed anismus, dyssynergia, and spastic pelvic floor syndrome.

Fig. 2.30 Spinal cord stimulator.

function as well as more precise identification of the anatomic site of the nerve or muscle lesion. Also, both the distal and proximal motor innervation of the perianal striated sphincter muscle can be evaluated.

Spinal Nerve Latency

The central component of the motor innervation of the pelvic floor can be studied by transcutaneous spinal stimulation. With the patient in the left lateral position, a stimulus electrode is placed vertically across the lumbar spine (▶ Fig. 2.30). This special device stimulates the spinal cord, usually at the level of L1 and L4. The induced response of the puborectalis or external sphincter can be detected either by a surface anal plug electrode located at the top of a finger glove or by an intramuscular needle electrode.[238] The normal values of motor latency following transcutaneous spinal cord stimulation are shown in ▶ Table 2.5.[223]

Table 2.5 Normal values of motor latency after spinal cord and pudendal nerve stimulation[223]

Stimulation	Contraction response	Latency (ms)
L1 nerve	Puborectalis	4.8 ± 0.4
	External sphincter	5.5 ± 0.4
L4 nerve	Puborectalis	3.7 ± 0.5
	External sphincter	4.4 ± 0.4
Pudendal nerve	External sphincter	1.9 ± 0.2

The difference in the latencies from L1 and L4 has been called the spinal latency ratio. This ratio is increased in patients with anal incontinence caused by a proximal lesion in the innervation.[241] Such a proximal lesion may be the result of damage to the motor nerve roots of S3 and S4 from disk disease. Stenosis of the spinal canal from osteoarthritis also may disturb proximal motor conduction. Innervation of the puborectalis probably is not derived from the pudendal nerves but rather from direct branches of the motor roots of S3 and S4.[242] Therefore, latency measurements of this muscle can be performed only by spinal cord stimulation.

External sphincter motor latencies can be recorded after both spinal cord stimulation and pudendal nerve stimulation.

Pudendal and perineal nerve stimulation techniques are used to assess the distal motor innervation of the pelvic floor musculature (i.e., the external anal sphincter and periurethral striated sphincter muscles). The terminal motor latency of the pudendal nerve can be determined by a transrectal stimulation technique, utilizing a specially designed and disposable device. This device is secured to the glove of the investigator and consists of one stimulating electrode located at the tip and two recording electrodes incorporated into its base (▶ Fig. 2.31). With the patient in the left lateral position, the index finger is introduced into the rectum, and the tip of the finger is brought into contact with the ischial spine on each side. After a square wave stimulus is delivered, a tracing is examined for evidence of contraction in the external sphincter as detected by the recording electrodes, thereby indicating accurate localization of the pudendal nerve. A supramaximal stimulus is delivered, and the latency between stimulus and external sphincter contraction is measured (▶ Fig. 2.32). The terminal motor latency of a normal pudendal nerve is of the order of 1.9 ± 0.2 ms (▶ Table 2.5).[223] It

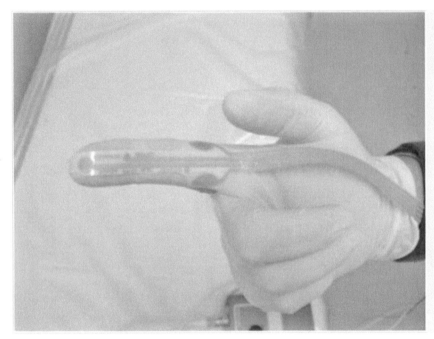

Fig. 2.31 This device is secured to the glove of the investigator and consists of one stimulating electrode located at the tip and two recording electrodes incorporated into its base.

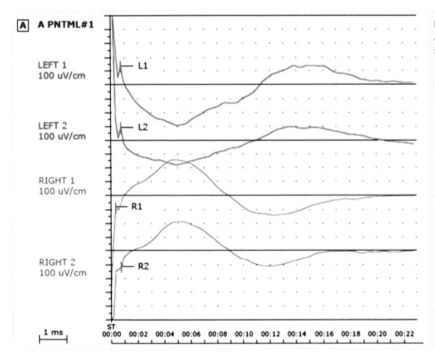

Fig. 2.32 A supramaximal stimulus is delivered, and the latency between stimulus and external sphincter contraction is measured.

is increased in patients with pelvic floor disorders, such as anal incontinence with or without rectal prolapse, solitary rectal ulcer syndrome, and traumatic division of the external sphincter. The same phenomenon has been found in patients with intractable constipation. However, this increase in pudendal nerve latency is most impressive in patients with fecal incontinence.[238] This technique also can detect occult pudendal nerve damage, which usually is symptomless.

Perineal Nerve Terminal Motor Latency

A similar technique can be used to determine the distal motor latency in the perineal branch of the pudendal nerve by measuring the latency from pudendal nerve stimulation to the periurethral striated muscles. The response to the periurethral sphincter muscle is recorded by intraurethral electrodes mounted on a bladder catheter. Nerve stimulation techniques have been used in studies of patients with pelvic floor disorders, especially anal incontinence. They have proved useful in determining the site of conduction delay and in investigating the differential innervation of the puborectalis and the external sphincter.

Ultrasonography

Ultrasonography combined with manometry is another method of assessing anorectal angles and puborectalis function.[243] The technique involves ultrasonographic measurement of the anorectal angles at rest and with maximal voluntary contraction of the puborectalis, using a water-filled Lahr balloon in the rectum as contrast, and a vaginal ultrasound probe on the posterior wall of the vagina. The angles are measured with the patient in the 45-degree supine position on a gynecologic examination table. Significantly different results have been noted in incontinent patients and in control subjects. Advantages of this technique are that it avoids radiation exposure and allows for a longer viewing time. It is less expensive compared with radiographic proctography, and the data are complementary.

Anal endosonography can reveal sphincter defects after anorectal surgery. Felt-Bersma et al[244] studied 50 patients after hemorrhoidectomy ($n = 24$), fistulectomy ($n = 18$), and internal sphincterotomy ($n = 8$). In 23 patients (46%), a defect of the anal sphincter was found (13 patients had an internal sphincter defect, 1 had an external sphincter defect, and 9 had a combined sphincter defect). In 70%, the sphincter defect did not produce symptoms. This has clinical implications in the evaluation of patients with fecal incontinence.

2.5.4 Clinical Application

Physiologic studies of the anorectal region play an increasingly important role in the diagnosis and management of a number of anorectal disorders. Schuster[105] pointed out that rectosphincteric studies can be used (1) to investigate physiology and pathophysiology, (2) as a sensitive tool to detect functional abnormalities that represent early signs of disease, (3) for the differential diagnosis of clinical disorders, (4) to assess immediate response to some clinical modality, (5) to evaluate long-term progress, and (6) as an integral part of treatment itself (as in operant conditioning). On the other hand, it has been argued that anorectal physiology measurements fail to meet the criteria of a useful clinical test because (1) they are not widely available to clinicians, (2) it is not

possible to establish a reproducible normal range, (3) abnormal measurements do not always correlate with disease entities or explain symptoms, (4) the results are often unhelpful in diagnosis and management, and (5) clinical outcome after intervention does not correlate with alteration in the measurements obtained.[245] Furthermore, treatment of a disorder may be empiric or rational. Rational treatment relies on the understanding of basic physiology and pathophysiology. With this in mind, specific applications and potential clinical implications are outlined. Details of abnormalities of specific disorders in which physiologic information may assist in management are described in their respective chapters. Wexner and Jorge[246] assessed the value of physiological tests in 308 patients with functional disorders of defecation. Definitive diagnoses were made after history and physical examination alone in 8% with constipation, 11% with incontinence, and 23% with intractable rectal pain. The figures after physiologic tests were 75, 66, and 42%, respectively. Treatable conditions were diagnosed by physiologic testing in 67% of patients with constipation and in 55% of patients with incontinence.

2.5.5 Anal Incontinence

This socially crippling disorder has been studied via a number of investigative techniques including manometry, electromyography, and nerve stimulation techniques to better define the exact cause of incontinence. For example, anal manometry may distinguish which of the two sphincters is principally responsible for the incontinence. This is important because if symptoms are due to internal sphincter dysfunction alone, a sphincter repair may not benefit the patient.

The clinical value of manometry in patients with fecal incontinence has been questioned. For example, one study found that 43% of incontinent subjects had "normal" values for both MRAP and MSAP. In contrast, a low MSAP was demonstrated in 9% of normal continent individuals.[179] Based on these results, the authors concluded that anal incontinence cannot be assessed by anorectal manometry alone.

Penninckx et al[247] described the balloon-retaining test, which consists of progressive filling of a compliant intrarectal balloon in a patient in the sitting position. The pressure inside the balloon is monitored, and the patient is asked to retain the balloon as long as possible and to report first, constant, and maximal tolerable sensation levels. The balloon is used to simulate semisolid and solid stool. The authors believe this test to be a more realistic approach to the evaluation of fecal continence than the rectal saline infusion test and anal manometry. The test evaluates the rectal reservoir function, sensation, and sphincter competence simultaneously and also permits objective evaluation of the effect of different treatments in incontinent patients.

In a sophisticated computer model, Perry et al[248] developed a manometric technique of anal pressure vectography for the detection of anal sphincter injuries. Abnormal symmetry indices exposed even occult anal sphincter injuries. Perry et al believe that the vector symmetry index may be useful in determining which incontinent patients should have sphincter repair.

Endoanal sonography facilitates the detection of occult sphincter defects. Since the introduction of this investigative technique, opinions about the pathogenesis, investigation, and management of fecal incontinence have changed dramatically.

It is well known that 0.5 to 2% of women delivering vaginally will sustain a third-degree tear. Primary repair of such injury is often inadequate. Sultan et al[249] reported that half the women with a repaired third-degree tear have symptoms of fecal incontinence or urgency and that sphincter defects can be identified with endoanal sonography in 85% of these women. Sonographic investigations have also revealed that one of three primiparas who deliver vaginally develop a permanent defect involving one or both sphincters[250] and that 90% of incontinent women, in whom the only apparent factor is obstetric damage, have a structural abnormality of one or both sphincters.[251] It is now agreed that childbirth is the most common cause of fecal incontinence in healthy adult women. In many patients, biofeedback therapy has been effective in correcting or at least improving anal incontinence.

Constipation

The use of intestinal transit studies and anal manometry has allowed a better definition of the extent of dysfunction of patients having severe chronic constipation, megarectum, megacolon, or Hirschsprung's disease. Biofeedback has been used in the treatment of some patients with constipation.

Rectal Procidentia

A number of manometric and electromyographic abnormalities have been described, but there has not been uniform agreement about their value. Contradictory reports have been discussed by Hiltunen et al.[252]

Rectocele

Cinefluoroscopic studies in women with a rectocele demonstrate a blind pouch that fills up like a hernial sac during efforts at defecation.

Solitary Ulcer Syndrome

Electromyographic abnormalities, characterized by overactivity in the puborectalis and no reflex relaxation during straining, have been demonstrated.

Descending Perineum Syndrome

Several manometric abnormalities have been described. On radiographic examination, the perineal floor can be seen to descend and the anorectal angle is more obtuse. Caution should be exercised in interpreting the results. Skomorowska et al[253] have noted that patients with normal position of the pelvic floor during rest may exhibit considerable descent during straining, whereas those patients who have abnormal position of the perineum during rest may show normal descent during straining. This observation may indicate that the first sign of abnormal function is an increased descent during straining and that only later will it be followed by descent during rest.

Fissure-in-Ano

High anal pressure that is due to increased activity of the internal anal sphincter is found in almost all patients with a chronic anal fissure. Ambulatory anorectal manometry has revealed that the internal anal sphincter hypertonia in fissure patients is sustained during daytime and disappears during sleep.[254] Ultraslow wave pressure fluctuations are another manifestation of increased myogenic activity of the internal anal sphincter. These ultraslow waves disappear when high anal pressure is reduced either by manual dilatation[255] or by lateral internal sphincterotomy.[184] There is mounting evidence that increased internal sphincter tone reduces microvascular perfusion at the fissure site and that reduction of anal pressure improves anodermal blood flow at the posterior midline and eventually results in fissure healing.[256] These findings provide evidence for the ischemic nature of anal fissure.

Hemorrhoids

Electrophysiologic and manometric investigations in patients with internal hemorrhoids have suggested that the pathogenesis of this condition may be due to a dysrhythmia within the internal sphincter.[257]

Anorectal Malformations

Electromyographic techniques have been used preoperatively to determine the location of the external sphincter in infants with imperforate anus and thus can assist in appropriate placement of the rectum if a pull-through operative procedure is planned. Spina bifida and cauda equina lesions may be accompanied by malfunction of visceral and striated muscle.

Aging

Balloon studies have shown a progressive decrease in rectal sensitivity to distention in the aging population.

Coloanal Anastomosis

Sphincter-saving operations with very low anastomoses have been associated with varying degrees of alteration in continence. This has been attributed to a number of factors including decreased bowel distensibility, varying degrees of ischemia, and decreased anal pressures. The fact that incontinence is temporary in some patients has been attributed to the initial loss of the rectoanal inhibitory reflex that reappears later, possibly associated with improved neorectal compliance with time.

Fistula-in-Ano

Anal manometry has been used in studies of patients undergoing operations for fistula-in-ano repair. A significantly lower pressure was measured in patients in whom the external sphincter had been divided when compared with those in whom the muscle had been preserved.

Disturbance of continence was related to abnormally low resting pressures.[258,259]

Trauma

In the planning of a sphincter repair, electromyographic studies and sonographic investigations can be used to determine whether there is adequate muscle mass to accomplish a satisfactory repair.

Pelvic Pouches

Preoperative study of the sphincter mechanism might help determine whether a patient will be continent after a pouch–anal anastomosis. Pouch volumes have been studied and correlated with stool leakage.[260] Defecography (evacuation pouchography) has been used to study postoperative function.[261] Poorer results were caused by rapid pouch filling and impaired pouch evacuation, which led to increased stool frequency.[262] Poor continence after ileoanal anastomosis correlates with an abnormal EMG of the external sphincter.[263] From their studies of patients undergoing ileoanal procedures, Beart et al[264] believe that in the presence of normal sphincter function, which they found to be preserved with this operation, continence is not dependent on the presence of normal mucosa or the anal inhibitory reflex but correlates with reservoir capacity, compliance, and the frequency and strength of intrinsic bowel contractions.

Inflammatory Bowel Diseases

Patients with inflammatory bowel diseases, especially those in the active phase, have a decreased distensibility of the rectum, which could be the result of either decreased muscle compliance or increased sensitivity. Knowledge of this decreased rectal capacity may be of practical value in predicting which patients with Crohn's disease would benefit from an ileorectal anastomosis.[103]

Ischemic Fecal Incontinence

Devroede et al[103] described the disorder of fecal incontinence due to ischemia. They used a combination of patient history, anal manometry, arteriography, barium enema, and biopsy to define this entity.

Spinal Cord Lesions

Bowel dysfunction is common in patients with spinal cord lesions. Tjandra et al[265] studied 12 patients with significant spinal cord lesions who had mixed symptoms of constipation, fecal impaction, and fecal incontinence. None of the patients had a sphincter defect as evaluated by endoanal ultrasonography. Eight of them had traumatic spinal cord injuries, while other lesions included spina bifida, syringomyelia, arachnoid cyst, and spinal cord ischemia after abdominal aortic aneurysm repair. In patients with spinal cord lesions, the mean resting anal canal pressure and maximum squeeze anal canal pressure were 46 and 76 mm Hg, respectively, compared with 62 and 138 mm Hg, respectively, in healthy controls. Eleven patients had prolonged pudendal nerve terminal motor latency (nine bilateral and two unilateral), whereas rectoanal inhibitory reflex was abolished in all nine patients tested.

Miscellaneous

Rare conditions such as scleroderma, dermatomyositis, and myotonic dystrophy also may be studied.

References

[1] Gaginella TS. Absorption and secretion in the colon. Curr Opin Gastroenterol. 1995; 11:2–8
[2] Duthie HL, Wormsley KG. Absorption from the human colon. In: Shields R, ed. Scientific Basis of Gastroenterology. Edinburgh: Churchill Livingstone; 1979
[3] Pemberton JH, Phillips SF. Colonic absorption. Perspect Colon Rectal Surg. 1988; 1(1):89–103
[4] Devroede GJ, Phillips SF. Conservation of sodium, chloride, and water by the human colon. Gastroenterology. 1969; 56(1):101–109
[5] Cummings JH. Colonic absorption: the importance of short chain fatty acids in man. In: Polak JM, Bloom SR, Wright NA, Butler AG, eds. Basic Science in Gastroenterology. Physiology of the Gut. Ware, Herts: Glaxo Group Research Limited, Royal Postgraduate Medical School; 1984
[6] Venkatasubramanian J, Rao MC, Sellin JH. Intestinal electrolyte absorption and secretion. In: Feldman M, Friedman LS, Brandt LJ, eds. Sleisenger and Fordtran's Gastrointestinal and Liver Disease: Pathophysiology/Diagnosis/Management. 9th ed. Philadelphia, PA: Elsevier; 2005:1675–1693
[7] Giller J, Phillips SF. Electrolyte absorption and secretion in the human colon. Am J Dig Dis. 1972; 17(11):1003–1011
[8] Agarwal R, Afzalpurkar R, Fordtran JS. Pathophysiology of potassium absorption and secretion by the human intestine. Gastroenterology. 1994; 107(2):548–571
[9] Binder HJ, Sandle GI. Electrolyte absorption and secretion in the mammalian colon. In: Johnson LR, ed. Physiology of the Gastrointestinal Tract. 2nd ed. New York, NY: Raven Press; 1987:1389–1418
[10] Powell DW. Transport in the large intestine. In: Giebisch G, Tosteson DC, Ussing HH, eds. Membrane Transport in Biology. New York, NY: Springer-Verlag; 1978:781–809
[11] Geibel JP. Secretion and absorption by colonic crypts. Annu Rev Physiol. 2005; 67:471–490
[12] McConnell JB, Murison J, Stewart WK. The role of the colon in the pathogenesis of hyperchloraemic acidosis in ureterosigmoid anastomosis. Clin Sci (Lond). 1979; 57(4):305–312
[13] Binder HJ, Rajendran V, Sadasivan V, Geibel JP. Bicarbonate secretion: a neglected aspect of colonic ion transport. J Clin Gastroenterol. 2005; 39(4) Suppl 2:S53–S58
[14] Gibson JA, Sladen GE, Dawson AM. Proceedings: Studies in the role of the colon in urea metabolism. Gut. 1973; 14(10):816
[15] Phillips TE, Phillips TH, Neutra MR. Regulation of intestinal goblet cell secretion. IV. Electrical field stimulation in vitro. Am J Physiol. 1984; 247(6, Pt 1):G682–G687
[16] Bond JH, Currier BE, Buchwald H, Levitt MD. Colonic conservation of malabsorbed carbohydrate. Gastroenterology. 1980; 78(3):444–447
[17] Latella G, Caprilli R. Metabolism of large bowel mucosa in health and disease. Int J Colorectal Dis. 1991; 6(2):127–132
[18] Kerlin P, Phillips SF. Absorption of fluids and electrolytes from the colon: with reference to inflammatory bowel disease. In: Allan RN, Keighley MRB, Alexander-Williams J, Hawkins C, eds. Inflammatory Bowel Diseases. Edinburgh: Churchill Livingstone; 1983
[19] Wald A. Colonic and anorectal motility testing in clinical practice. Am J Gastroenterol. 1994; 89(12):2109–2115
[20] Ritchie JA. Movement of segmental constrictions in the human colon. Gut. 1971; 12(5):350–355
[21] Cannon WB. The movements of the intestine studied by means of roentgen rays. Am J Physiol. 1902; 6(5):251–277
[22] Elliott TR. Antiperistalsis and other muscular activities of the colon. J Physiol. 1904; 31(3–4):272–304
[23] Ritchie JA, Truelove SC, Ardran GM, Tuckey MS. Propulsion and retropulsion of normal colonic content. Am J Dig Dis. 1971; 16(8):697–703
[24] Cohen S, Snape WJ. Movement of the small and large intestine. In: Fordtran J, Sleisinger M, eds. Gastrointestinal Disease. 3rd ed. New York, NY: McGraw-Hill; 1983:859–873
[25] Hertz AF. Lectures on the passage of food through the human alimentary canal: delivered at Guy's Hospital for London University Advanced Students during October, 1907. Br Med J. 1908; 1(2456):191–196
[26] Ritchie J. Mass peristalsis in the human colon after contact with oxyphenisatin. Gut. 1972; 13(3):211–219
[27] Torsoli A, Ramorino ML, Ammaturo MV, Capurso L, Paoluzi P, Anzini F. Mass movements and intracolonic pressures. Am J Dig Dis. 1971; 16(8):693–696
[28] Garcia D, Hita G, Mompean B, et al. Colonic motility: electric and manometric description of mass movement. Dis Colon Rectum. 1991; 34(7):577–584
[29] Krogh K, Olsen N, Christensen P, Madsen JL, Laurberg S. Colorectal transport in normal defaecation. Colorectal Dis. 2003; 5(2):185–192
[30] Bampton PA, Dinning PG, Kennedy ML, Lubowski DZ, Cook IJ. Prolonged multi-point recording of colonic manometry in the unprepared human

colon: providing insight into potentially relevant pressure wave parameters. Am J Gastroenterol. 2001; 96(6):1838–1848

[31] Dinning PG, Wiklendt L, Gibbins I, et al. Low-resolution colonic manometry leads to a gross misinterpretation of the frequency and polarity of propagating sequences: Initial results from fiber-optic high-resolution manometry studies. Neurogastroenterol Motil. 2013; 25(10):e640–e649

[32] Dinning PG, Wiklendt L, Maslen L, et al. Quantification of in vivo colonic motor patterns in healthy humans before and after a meal revealed by high-resolution fiber-optic manometry. Neurogastroenterol Motil. 2014; 26 (10):1443–1457

[33] Cook IJ, Furukawa Y, Panagopoulos V, Collins PJ, Dent J. Relationships between spatial patterns of colonic pressure and individual movements of content. Am J Physiol Gastrointest Liver Physiol. 2000; 278(2):G329–G341

[34] Law NM, Bharucha AE, Undale AS, Zinsmeister AR. Cholinergic stimulation enhances colonic motor activity, transit, and sensation in humans. Am J Physiol Gastrointest Liver Physiol. 2001; 281(5):G1228–G1237

[35] Crowell MD, Bassotti G, Cheskin LJ, Schuster MM, Whitehead WE. Method for prolonged ambulatory monitoring of high-amplitude propagated contractions from colon. Am J Physiol. 1991; 261(2, Pt 1):G263–G268

[36] Soffer EE, Scalabrini P, Wingate DL. Prolonged ambulant monitoring of human colonic motility. Am J Physiol. 1989; 257(4, Pt 1):G601–G606

[37] Herbst F, Kamm MA, Morris GP, Britton K, Woloszko J, Nicholls RJ. Gastrointestinal transit and prolonged ambulatory colonic motility in health and faecal incontinence. Gut. 1997; 41(3):381–389

[38] Bampton PA, Dinning PG, Kennedy ML, Lubowski DZ, deCarle D, Cook IJ. Spatial and temporal organization of pressure patterns throughout the unprepared colon during spontaneous defecation. Am J Gastroenterol. 2000; 95 (4):1027–1035

[39] Bampton PA, Dinning PG, Kennedy ML, Lubowski DZ, deCarle D, Cook IJ. Spatial and temporal organization of pressure patterns throughout the unprepared colon during spontaneous defecation. Am J Gastroenterol. 2000; 95(4):1027–1035

[40] Hirabayashi T, Matsufuji H, Yokoyama J, et al. Colorectal motility induction by sacral nerve electrostimulation in a canine model: implications for colonic pacing. Dis Colon Rectum. 2003; 46(6):809–817

[41] Patton V, Wiklendt L, Arkwright JW, Lubowski DZ, Dinning PG. The effect of sacral nerve stimulation on distal colonic motility in patients with faecal incontinence. Br J Surg. 2013; 100(7):959–968

[42] Kumar D, Williams NS, Waldron D, Wingate DL. Prolonged manometric recording of anorectal motor activity in ambulant human subjects: evidence of periodic activity. Gut. 1989; 30(7):1007–1011

[43] Bampton PA, Dinning PG, Kennedy ML, Lubowski DZ, Cook IJ. The proximal colonic motor response to rectal mechanical and chemical stimulation. Am J Physiol Gastrointest Liver Physiol. 2002; 282(3):G443–G449

[44] Bassotti G, Gaburri M, Imbimbo BP, et al. Colonic mass movements in idiopathic chronic constipation. Gut. 1988; 29(9):1173–1179

[45] Dinning PG, Bampton PA, Andre J, et al. Abnormal predefecatory colonic motor patterns define constipation in obstructed defecation. Gastroenterology. 2004; 127(1):49–56

[46] Hervé S, Savoye G, Behbahani A, Leroi AM, Denis P, Ducrotté P. Results of 24-h manometric recording of colonic motor activity with endoluminal instillation of bisacodyl in patients with severe chronic slow transit constipation. Neurogastroenterol Motil. 2004; 16(4):397–402

[47] Dinning PG, Wiklendt L, Maslen L, et al. Colonic motor abnormalities in slow transit constipation defined by high resolution, fibre-optic manometry. Neurogastroenterol Motil. 2015; 27(3):379–388

[48] Wessel S, Koppen IJ, Wiklendt L, Costa M, Benninga MA, Dinning PG. Characterizing colonic motility in children with chronic intractable constipation: a look beyond high-amplitude propagating sequences. Neurogastroenterol Motil. 2016; 28(5):743–757

[49] Dinning PG, Sia TC, Kumar R, et al. High-resolution colonic motility recordings in vivo compared with ex vivo recordings after colectomy, in patients with slow transit constipation. Neurogastroenterol Motil. 2016; 28(12):1824–1835

[50] Bell AM, Pemberton JH, Hanson RB, Zinsmeister AR. Variations in muscle tone of the human rectum: recordings with an electromechanical barostat. Am J Physiol. 1991; 260(1, Pt 1):G17–G25

[51] Steadman CJ, Phillips SF, Camilleri M, Haddad AC, Hanson RB. Variation of muscle tone in the human colon. Gastroenterology. 1991; 101(2):373–381

[52] Ford MJ, Camilleri M, Wiste JA, Hanson RB. Differences in colonic tone and phasic response to a meal in the transverse and sigmoid human colon. Gut. 1995; 37(2):264–269

[53] von der Ohe MR, Hanson RB, Camilleri M. Serotonergic mediation of postprandial colonic tonic and phasic responses in humans. Gut. 1994; 35 (4):536–541

[54] Ford MJ, Camilleri MJ, Hanson RB, Wiste JA, Joyner MJ. Hyperventilation, central autonomic control, and colonic tone in humans. Gut. 1995; 37 (4):499–504

[55] Grotz RL, Pemberton JH, Levin KE, Bell AM, Hanson RB. Rectal wall contractility in healthy subjects and in patients with chronic severe constipation. Ann Surg. 1993; 218(6):761–768

[56] Gosselink MJ, Schouten WR. The gastrorectal reflex in women with obstructed defecation. Int J Colorectal Dis. 2001; 16(2):112–118

[57] Blair PJ, Rhee PL, Sanders KM, Ward SM. The significance of interstitial cells in neurogastroenterology. J Neurogastroenterol Motil. 2014; 20(3):294–317

[58] Taylor I, Duthie HL, Smallwood R, Linkens D. Large bowel myoelectrical activity in man. Gut. 1975; 16(10):808–814

[59] Huizinga JD, Daniel EE. Control of human colonic motor function. Dig Dis Sci. 1986; 31(8):865–877

[60] Sarna S, Latimer P, Campbell D, Waterfall WE. Electrical and contractile activities of the human rectosigmoid. Gut. 1982; 23(8):698–705

[61] Snape WJ, Jr, Carlson GM, Cohen S. Human colonic myoelectric activity in response to prostigmin and the gastrointestinal hormones. Am J Dig Dis. 1977; 22(10):881–887

[62] Frieri G, Parisi F, Corazziari E, Caprilli R. Colonic electromyography in chronic constipation. Gastroenterology. 1983; 84(4):737–740

[63] Snape WJ, Jr, Matarazzo SA, Cohen S. Abnormal gastrocolonic response in patients with ulcerative colitis. Gut. 1980; 21(5):392–396

[64] Bueno L, Fioramonti J, Ruckebusch Y, Frexinos J, Coulom P. Evaluation of colonic myoelectrical activity in health and functional disorders. Gut. 1980; 21 (6):480–485

[65] Waterfall WE, Shannon S. Human colonic electrical activity: transverse and human colons [abstr]. Clin Invest Med. 1985; 8:A104

[66] Snape WJ, Jr, Carlson GM, Cohen S. Colonic myoelectric activity in the irritable bowel syndrome. Gastroenterology. 1976; 70(3):326–330

[67] Taylor I, Darby C, Hammond P. Comparison of rectosigmoid myoelectrical activity in the irritable colon syndrome during relapses and remissions. Gut. 1978; 19(10):923–929

[68] Bueno L, Fioramonti J, Frexinos J, Ruckebusch Y. Colonic myoelectrical activity in diarrhea and constipation. Hepatogastroenterology. 1980; 27(5):381–389

[69] Schang JC, Devroede G, Duguay C, Hémond M, Hébert M. Constipation par inertie colique et obstruction distale: étude électromyographique. Gastroenterol Clin Biol. 1985; 9(6–7):480–485

[70] Furness JB, Costa M. The Enteric Nervous System. Edinburgh: Churchill Livingstone; 1987

[71] Mulvihill SJ, Debas HT. Neuroendocrine regulation of intestinal function. Perspect Colon Rectal Surg. 1992; 5:221–234

[72] Sanders KM. A case for interstitial cells of Cajal as pacemakers and mediators of neurotransmission in the gastrointestinal tract. Gastroenterology. 1996; 111(2):492–515

[73] Ibba-Manneschi L, Martini M, Zecchi-Orlandini S, Faussone-Pellegrini MS. Structural organization of enteric nervous system in human colon. Histol Histopathol. 1995; 10(1):17–25

[74] Sarna SK. Colonic Motility: From Bench Side to Bedside. Colloquium Series on Integrated Systems Physiology: From Molecule to Function. New York, NY: Morgan & Claypool Life Sciences; 2010

[75] Hansen MB. The enteric nervous system I: organisation and classification. Pharmacol Toxicol. 2003; 92(3):105–113

[76] Hansen MB. The enteric nervous system III: a target for pharmacological treatment. Pharmacol Toxicol. 2003; 93(1):1–13

[77] Burnstock G. Neural nomenclature. Nature. 1971; 229(5282):282–283

[78] Hansen MB. The enteric nervous system II: gastrointestinal functions. Pharmacol Toxicol. 2003; 92(6):249–257

[79] Bernard CE, Gibbons SJ, Gomez-Pinilla PJ, et al. Effect of age on the enteric nervous system of the human colon. Neurogastroenterol Motil. 2009; 21(7):746–e46

[80] Benarroch EE. Enteric nervous system: functional organization and neurologic implications. Neurology. 2007; 69(20):1953–1957

[81] Bloom SR, Polak JM. Gut Hormones. Edinburgh: Churchill Livingstone; 1981

[82] Taylor I, Duthie HL, Smallwood R, Brown BH, Linkens D. The effect of stimulation on the myoelectrical activity of the rectosigmoid in man. Gut. 1974; 15(8):599–607

[83] Dockray GJ, Taylor IL. Heptadecapeptide gastrin: measurement in blood by specific radioimmunoassay. Gastroenterology. 1976; 71(6):971–977

[84] Weber J, Ducrotte P. Colonic motility in health and disease. Dig Dis. 1987; 5 (1):1–12

[85] Dinoso VP, Jr, Meshkinpour H, Lorber SH, Gutierrez JG, Chey WY. Motor responses of the sigmoid colon and rectum to exogenous cholecystokinin and secretin. Gastroenterology. 1973; 65(3):438–444

[86] Kaufman PN, Krevsky B, Malmud LS, et al. Role of opiate receptors in the regulation of colonic transit. Gastroenterology. 1988; 94(6):1351–1356

[87] Moore WEC, Moore LVH, Cato EP. You and your flora. US Fed Culture Collect Newslett. 1988; 18:7–22

[88] Stephen AM, Cummings JH. The microbial contribution to human faecal mass. J Med Microbiol. 1980; 13(1):45–56

[89] Simon GL, Gorbach SL. Intestinal flora and gastrointestinal function. In: Johnson LR, ed. Physiology of the Gastrointestinal Tract. 2nd ed. New York, NY: Raven Press; 1987:1729–1747

[90] Dunn DL. Autochthonous microflora of the gastrointestinal tract. Perspect Colon Rectal Surg. 1989; 2(2):105–119

[91] Guarner F, Malagelada JR. Gut flora in health and disease. Lancet. 2003; 361 (9356):512–519

[92] Plaa GL. The enterohepatic circulation. In: Gillette JR, ed. Handbook of Experimental Pharmacology. Vol. 28. New York, NY: Springer-Verlag; 1975:130–149

[93] Bokkenheuser V. The friendly anaerobes. Clin Infect Dis. 1993; 16 Suppl 4: S427–S434

[94] Basson MD, Liu YW, Hanly AM, Emenaker NJ, Shenoy SG, Gould Rothberg BE. Identification and comparative analysis of human colonocyte short-chain fatty acid response genes. J Gastrointest Surg. 2000; 4(5):501–512

[95] Hampe J, Cuthbert A, Croucher PJ, et al. Association between insertion mutation in NOD2 gene and Crohn's disease in German and British populations. Lancet. 2001; 357(9272):1925–1928

[96] D'Haens GR, Geboes K, Peeters M, Baert F, Penninckx F, Rutgeerts P. Early lesions of recurrent Crohn's disease caused by infusion of intestinal contents in excluded ileum. Gastroenterology. 1998; 114(2):262–267

[97] Casellas F, Borruel N, Papo M, et al. Antiinflammatory effects of enterically coated amoxicillin-clavulanic acid in active ulcerative colitis. Inflamm Bowel Dis. 1998; 4(1):1–5

[98] McFarland LV, Surawicz CM, Greenberg RN, et al. Prevention of beta-lactam-associated diarrhea by Saccharomyces boulardii compared with placebo. Am J Gastroenterol. 1995; 90(3):439–448

[99] Armuzzi A, Cremonini F, Bartolozzi F, et al. The effect of oral administration of Lactobacillus GG on antibiotic-associated gastrointestinal side-effects during Helicobacter pylori eradication therapy. Aliment Pharmacol Ther. 2001; 15(2):163–169

[100] D'Souza AL, Rajkumar C, Cooke J, Bulpitt CJ. Probiotics in prevention of antibiotic associated diarrhoea: meta-analysis. BMJ. 2002; 324 (7350):1361–1366

[101] Burns AJ, Rowland IR. Anti-carcinogenicity of probiotics and prebiotics. Curr Issues Intest Microbiol. 2000; 1(1):13–24

[102] Levitt MD. Intestinal gas production–recent advances in flatology. N Engl J Med. 1980; 302(26):1474–1475

[103] Devroede G, Arhan P, Schang JC. Orderly and disorderly fecal continence. In: Kodner I, Fry RD, Roc JP, eds. Colon, Rectal and Anal Surgery. St. Louis, MO: CV Mosby; 1985:40–62

[104] Schuster MM, Mendeloff AJ. Characteristics of rectosigmoid motor function; their relationship to continence, defecation and disease. In: Glass CBJ, ed. Progress in Gastroenterology. Vol. 2. New York, NY: Grune & Stratton; 1970

[105] Schuster MM. The riddle of the sphincters. Gastroenterology. 1975; 69 (1):249–262

[106] Felt-Bersma RJF, Gort G, Meuwissen SGM. Normal values in anal manometry and rectal sensation: a problem of range. Hepatogastroenterology. 1991; 38 (5):444–449

[107] Varma JS, Smith AN. Anorectal profilometry with the microtransducer. Br J Surg. 1984; 71(11):867–869

[108] Nivatvongs S, Stern HS, Fryd DS. The length of the anal canal. Dis Colon Rectum. 1981; 24(8):600–601

[109] McHugh SM, Diamant NE. Anal canal pressure profile: a reappraisal as determined by rapid pullthrough technique. Gut. 1987; 28(10):1234–1241

[110] Cali RL, Blatchford GJ, Perry RE, Pitsch RM, Thorson AG, Christensen MA. Normal variation in anorectal manometry. Dis Colon Rectum. 1992; 35 (12):1161–1164

[111] Duthie HL, Watts JM. Contribution of the external anal sphincter to the pressure zone in the anal canal. Gut. 1965; 6:64–68

[112] Frenckner B, Euler CV. Influence of pudendal block on the function of the anal sphincters. Gut. 1975; 16(6):482–489

[113] Schweiger M. Funktionelle Analsphinkteruntersuchungen. Berlin: Springer-Verlag; 1982

[114] Lestar B, Penninckx F, Kerremans R. The composition of anal basal pressure. An in vivo and in vitro study in man. Int J Colorectal Dis. 1989; 4 (2):118–122

[115] Frenckner B, Ihre T. Influence of autonomic nerves on the internal and sphincter in man. Gut. 1976; 17(4):306–312

[116] Meunier P, Mollard P. Control of the internal anal sphincter (manometric study with human subjects). Pflugers Arch. 1977; 370(3):233–239

[117] Gunterberg B, Kewenter J, Petersén I, Stener B. Anorectal function after major resections of the sacrum with bilateral or unilateral sacrifice of sacral nerves. Br J Surg. 1976; 63(7):546–554

[118] Kumar D, Waldron D, Williams NS, Browning C, Hutton MR, Wingate DL. Prolonged anorectal manometry and external anal sphincter electromyography in ambulant human subjects. Dig Dis Sci. 1990; 35(5):641–648

[119] Varma KK, Stephens D. Neuromuscular reflexes of rectal continence. Aust N Z J Surg. 1972; 41(3):263–272

[120] Parks AG, Porter NH, Melzak J. Experimental study of the reflex mechanism controlling the muscle of the pelvic floor. Dis Colon Rectum. 1962; 5:407–414

[121] Lierse W, Holschneider AM, Steinfeld J. The relative proportions of type I and type II muscle fibers in the external sphincter ani muscle at different ages and stages of development–observations on the development of continence. Eur J Pediatr Surg. 1993; 3(1):28–32

[122] Stephens FD, Smith ED. Anorectal Malformations in Children. Chicago, IL: Year Book Medical Publishers; 1971:28

[123] Rühl A, Thewissen M, Ross HG, Cleveland S, Frieling T, Enck P. Discharge patterns of intramural mechanoreceptive afferents during selective distension of the cat's rectum. Neurogastroenterol Motil. 1998; 10(3):219–225

[124] Lynn PA, Olsson C, Zagorodnyuk V, Costa M, Brookes SJ. Rectal intraganglionic laminar endings are transduction sites of extrinsic mechanoreceptors in the guinea pig rectum. Gastroenterology. 2003; 125(3):786–794

[125] Sun WM, Read NW, Prior A, Daly JA, Cheah SK, Grundy D. Sensory and motor responses to rectal distention vary according to rate and pattern of balloon inflation. Gastroenterology. 1990; 99(4):1008–1015

[126] Sabate JM, Coffin B, Jian R, Le Bars D, Bouhassira D. Rectal sensitivity assessed by a reflexologic technique: further evidence for two types of mechanoreceptors. Am J Physiol Gastrointest Liver Physiol. 2000; 279(4): G692–G699

[127] Coulie B, Tack J, Demedts I, Vos R, Janssens J. Influence of sumatriptan on rectal tone and on the perception of rectal distension in man. Neurogastroenterol Motil. 1998; 10:66

[128] Schikowski A, Thewissen M, Mathis C, Ross HG, Enck P. Serotonin type-4 receptors modulate the sensitivity of intramural mechanoreceptive afferents of the cat rectum. Neurogastroenterol Motil. 2002; 14(3):221–227

[129] van der Veek PPJ, Schots EDCM, Masclee AAM. Effect of neurotensin on colorectal motor and sensory function in humans. Dis Colon Rectum. 2004; 47 (2):210–218

[130] Bampton PA, Dinning PG, Kennedy ML, Lubowski DZ, Cook IJ. The proximal colonic motor response to rectal mechanical and chemical stimulation. Am J Physiol Gastrointest Liver Physiol. 2002; 282(3):G443–G449

[131] Kern MK, Jaradeh S, Arndorfer RC, Jesmanowicz A, Hyde J, Shaker R. Gender differences in cortical representation of rectal distension in healthy humans. Am J Physiol Gastrointest Liver Physiol. 2001; 281(6):G1512–G1523

[132] Sørensen M, Rasmussen OO, Tetzschner T, Christiansen J. Physiological variation in rectal compliance. Br J Surg. 1992; 79(10):1106–1108

[133] Sloots CEJ, Felt-Bersma RJF, Cuesta MA, Meuwissen SGM. Rectal visceral sensitivity in healthy volunteers: influences of gender, age and methods. Neurogastroenterol Motil. 2000; 12(4):361–368

[134] Gladman MA, Dvorkin LS, Lunniss PJ, Williams NS, Scott SM. Rectal hyposensitivity: a disorder of the rectal wall or the afferent pathway? An assessment using the barostat. Am J Gastroenterol. 2005; 100(1):106–114

[135] De Medici A, Badiali D, Corazziari E, Bausano G, Anzini F. Rectal sensitivity in chronic constipation. Dig Dis Sci. 1989; 34(5):747–753

[136] Gladman MA, Scott SM, Williams NS, Lunniss PJ. Clinical and physiological findings, and possible aetiological factors of rectal hyposensitivity. Br J Surg. 2003; 90(7):860–866

[137] Gosselink MJ, Hop WCJ, Schouten WR. Rectal compliance in females with obstructed defecation. Dis Colon Rectum. 2001; 44(7):971–977

[138] Gosselink MJ, Schouten WR. Rectal sensory perception in females with obstructed defecation. Dis Colon Rectum. 2001; 44(9):1337–1344

[139] Duthie HL, Gairns FW. Sensory nerve-endings and sensation in the anal region of man. Br J Surg. 1960; 47:585–595

[140] Read MG, Read NW. Role of anorectal sensation in preserving continence. Gut. 1982; 23(4):345–347

[141] Miller R, Bartolo DCC, Cervero F, Mortensen NJ. Anorectal temperature sensation: a comparison of normal and incontinent patients. Br J Surg. 1987; 74 (6):511–515

[142] Mills K, Chess-Williams R. Pharmacology of the internal anal sphincter and its relevance to faecal incontinence. Auton Autacoid Pharmacol. 2009; 29 (3):85–95

[143] Lubowski DZ, Nicholls RJ, Swash M, Jordan MJ. Neural control of internal anal sphincter function. Br J Surg. 1987; 74(8):668–670

[144] Cook TA, Brading AF, Mortensen NJ. The pharmacology of the internal anal sphincter and new treatments of ano-rectal disorders. Aliment Pharmacol Ther. 2001; 15(7):887–898

[145] Burleigh DE, D'Mello A. Physiology and pharmacology of the internal anal sphincter. In: Henry MM, Swash M, eds. Coloproctology and the Pelvic Floor. London: Butterworths; 1985

[146] Tøttrup A, Glavind EB, Svane D. Involvement of the L-arginine-nitric oxide pathway in internal anal sphincter relaxation. Gastroenterology. 1992; 102 (2):409–415

[147] Chakder S, Rattan S. Release of nitric oxide by activation of nonadrenergic noncholinergic neurons of internal anal sphincter. Am J Physiol. 1993; 264 (1, Pt 1):G7–G12

[148] Rattan S, Chakder S. Role of nitric oxide as a mediator of internal anal sphincter relaxation. Am J Physiol. 1992; 262(1, Pt 1):G107–G112

[149] O'Kelly T, Brading A, Mortensen N. Nerve mediated relaxation of the human internal anal sphincter: the role of nitric oxide. Gut. 1993; 34(5):689–693

[150] O'Kelly TJ, Davies JR, Brading AF, Mortensen NJ. Distribution of nitric oxide synthase containing neurons in the rectal myenteric plexus and anal canal. Morphologic evidence that nitric oxide mediates the rectoanal inhibitory reflex. Dis Colon Rectum. 1994; 37(4):350–357

[151] Ferrara A, Pemberton JH, Levin KE, Hanson RB. Relationship between anal canal tone and rectal motor activity. Dis Colon Rectum. 1993; 36(4):337–342

[152] Duthie HL. Progress report. Anal continence. Gut. 1971; 12(10):844–852

[153] Parks AG, Porter NH, Hardcastle J. The syndrome of the descending perineum. Proc R Soc Med. 1966; 59(6):477–482

[154] Bannister JJ, Gibbons C, Read NW. Preservation of faecal continence during rises in intra-abdominal pressure: is there a role for the flap valve? Gut. 1987; 28(10):1242–1245

[155] Bartolo DCC, Roe AM, Locke-Edmunds JC, Virjee J, Mortensen NJ. Flap-valve theory of anorectal continence. Br J Surg. 1986; 73(12):1012–1014

[156] Stelzner F. The morphological principles of anorectal continence. In: Rickham PP, Hecker WCh, Prévot J, eds. Anorectal Malformations and Associated Diseases. Progress in Pediatric Surgery Series. Vol. 9. Munich: Urban und Schwarzenberg; 1976:1–6

[157] Duthie HL. Dynamics of the rectum and anus. Clin Gastroenterol. 1975; 4 (3):467–477

[158] Lubowski DZ, Meagher AP, Smart RC, Butler SP. Scintigraphic assessment of colonic function during defaecation. Int J Colorectal Dis. 1995; 10(2):91–93

[159] Kamm MA, van der Sijp JR, Lennard-Jones JE. Colorectal and anal motility during defaecation. Lancet. 1992; 339(8796):820

[160] Karaus M, Sarna SK. Giant migrating contractions during defecation in the dog colon. Gastroenterology. 1987; 92(4):925–933

[161] Hagger R, Kumar D, Benson M, Grundy A. Periodic colonic motor activity identified by 24-h pancolonic ambulatory manometry in humans. Neurogastroenterol Motil. 2002; 14(3):271–278

[162] MacDonald A, Paterson PJ, Baxter JN, Finlay IG. Relationship between intra-abdominal and intrarectal pressure in the proctometrogram. Br J Surg. 1993; 80(8):1070–1071

[163] Palit S, Lunniss PJ, Scott SM. The physiology of human defecation. Dig Dis Sci. 2012; 57(6):1445–1464

[164] Andrews C, Bharucha AE, Seide B, Zinsmeister AR. Rectal sensorimotor dysfunction in women with fecal incontinence. Am J Physiol Gastrointest Liver Physiol. 2007; 292(1):G282–G289

[165] Tabe Y, Mochiki E, Yanai M, et al. Characterization of special propulsive contractions during rectal evacuation in a canine model of intestinal extrinsic denervation and rectal transection. Int J Colorectal Dis. 2010; 25(1):53–61

[166] Ito T, Sakakibara R, Uchiyama T, Zhi L, Yamamoto T, Hattori T. Videomanometry of the pelvic organs: a comparison of the normal lower urinary and gastrointestinal tracts. Int J Urol. 2006; 13(1):29–35

[167] Leroi AM, Saiter C, Roussignol C, Weber J, Denis P. Increased tone of the rectal wall in response to feeding persists in patients with cauda equina syndrome. Neurogastroenterol Motil. 1999; 11(3):243–245

[168] Musial F, Crowell MD, Kalveram KT, Enck P. Nutrient ingestion increases rectal sensitivity in humans. Physiol Behav. 1994; 55(5):953–956

[169] Gosselink MJ, Schouten WR. The perineo-rectal reflex: The perineorectal reflex in health and obstructed defecation. Dis Colon Rectum. 2002; 45 (3):370–376

[170] Shafik A, Ahmed I, El-Sibai O. Effect of perineal compression on the rectal tone: a study of the mechanism of action. Dis Colon Rectum. 2003; 46 (10):1366–1370

[171] Frenckner B. Function of the anal sphincters in spinal man. Gut. 1975; 16 (8):638–644

[172] Henry MM, Snooks SJ, Barnes PRH, Swash M. Investigation of disorders of the anorectum and colon. Ann R Coll Surg Engl. 1985; 67(6):355–360

[173] Miller R, Bartolo DCC, James D, Mortensen NJ. Air-filled microballoon manometry for use in anorectal physiology. Br J Surg. 1989; 76(1):72–75

[174] Jonas U, Klotter HJ. Study of threee urethral pressure recording devices: theoretical considerations. Urol Res. 1978; 6(3):119–125

[175] Hancock BD. Measurement of anal pressure and motility. Gut. 1976; 17 (8):645–651

[176] Schouten WR, van Vroonhoven TJ. A simple method of anorectal manometry. Dis Colon Rectum. 1983; 26(11):721–724

[177] Coller JA. Clinical application of anorectal manometry. Gastroenterol Clin North Am. 1987; 16(1):17–33

[178] Jameson JS, Chia YW, Kamm MA, Speakman CT, Chye YH, Henry MM. Effect of age, sex and parity on anorectal function. Br J Surg. 1994; 81 (11):1689–1692

[179] McHugh SM, Diamant NE. Effect of age, gender, and parity on anal canal pressures. Contribution of impaired anal sphincter function to fecal incontinence. Dig Dis Sci. 1987; 32(7):726–736

[180] Matheson DM, Keighley MRB. Manometric evaluation of rectal prolapse and faecal incontinence. Gut. 1981; 22(2):126–129

[181] Taylor BM, Beart RW, Jr, Phillips SF. Longitudinal and radial variations of pressure in the human anal sphincter. Gastroenterology. 1984; 86 (4):693–697

[182] Haadem K, Dahlström JA, Ling L. Anal sphincter competence in healthy women: clinical implications of age and other factors. Obstet Gynecol. 1991; 78(5, Pt 1):823–827

[183] Sultan AH, Kamm MA, Hudson CN, Bartram CI. Effect of pregnancy on anal sphincter morphology and function. Int J Colorectal Dis. 1993; 8(4):206–209

[184] Schouten WR, Blankensteijn JD. Ultra slow wave pressure variations in the anal canal before and after lateral internal sphincterotomy. Int J Colorectal Dis. 1992; 7(3):115–118

[185] Bouvier M, Gonella J. Nervous control of the internal anal sphincter of the cat. J Physiol. 1981; 310:457–469

[186] Williamson JL, Nelson RL, Orsay C, Pearl RK, Abcarian H. A comparison of simultaneous longitudinal and radial recordings of anal canal pressures. Dis Colon Rectum. 1990; 33(3):201–206

[187] Read NW, Harford WV, Schmulen AC, Read MG, Santa Ana C, Fordtran JS. A clinical study of patients with fecal incontinence and diarrhea. Gastroenterology. 1979; 76(4):747–756

[188] Schouten WR, van Vroonhoven TJ. Lateral internal sphincterotomy in the treatment of hemorrhoids. A clinical and manometric study. Dis Colon Rectum. 1986; 29(12):869–872

[189] Johnson GP, Pemberton JH, Ness J, Samson M, Zinsmeister AR. Transducer manometry and the effect of body position on anal canal pressures. Dis Colon Rectum. 1990; 33(6):469–475

[190] Li Y, Yang X, Xu C, Zhang Y, Zhang X. Normal values and pressure morphology for three-dimensional high-resolution anorectal manometry of asymptomatic adults: a study in 110 subjects. Int J Colorectal Dis. 2013; 28 (8):1161–1168

[191] Lee YY, Erdogan A, Rao SSC. High resolution and high definition anorectal manometry and pressure topography: diagnostic advance or a new kid on the block? Curr Gastroenterol Rep. 2013; 15(12):360–368

[192] Vitton V, Ben Hadj Amor W, Baumstarck K, Behr M, Bouvier M, Grimaud JC. Comparison of three-dimensional high-resolution manometry and endoanal ultrasound in the diagnosis of anal sphincter defects. Colorectal Dis. 2013; 15(10):e607–e611

[193] Heinrich H, Sauter M, Fox M, et al. Assessment of obstructive defecation by high-resolution anorectal manometry compared with magnetic resonance defecography. Clin Gastroenterol Hepatol. 2015; 13(7):1310–1317.e1

[194] Womack NR, Williams NS, Holmfield JHM, Morrison JFB, Simpkins KC. New method for the dynamic assessment of anorectal function in constipation. Br J Surg. 1985; 72(12):994–998

[195] Halligan S, Thomas J, Bartram C. Intrarectal pressures and balloon expulsion related to evacuation proctography. Gut. 1995; 37(1):100–104

[196] Mahieu P, Pringot J, Bodart P. Defecography: I. Description of a new procedure and results in normal patients. Gastrointest Radiol. 1984; 9 (3):247–251

[197] Preston DM, Lennard-Jones JE, Thomas BM. The balloon proctogram. Br J Surg. 1984; 71(1):29–32

[198] Agachan F, Pfeifer J, Wexner SD. Defecography and proctography. Results of 744 patients. Dis Colon Rectum. 1996; 39(8):899–905

[199] Lestár B, Penninckx FM, Kerremans RP. Defecometry. A new method for determining the parameters of rectal evacuation. Dis Colon Rectum. 1989; 32(3):197–201

[200] Mellgren A, Bremmer S, Johansson C, et al. Defecography. Results of investigations in 2,816 patients. Dis Colon Rectum. 1994; 37(11):1133–1141

[201] Stojkovic SG, Balfour L, Burke D, Finan PJ, Sagar PM. Does the need to self-digitate or the presence of a large or nonemptying rectocoele on proctography influence the outcome of transanal rectocoele repair? Colorectal Dis. 2003; 5(2):169–172

[202] Barkel DC, Pemberton JH, Pezim ME, Phillips SF, Kelly KA, Brown ML. Scintigraphic assessment of the anorectal angle in health and after ileal pouch-anal anastomosis. Ann Surg. 1988; 208(1):42–49

[203] Hutchinson R, Mostafa AB, Grant EA, et al. Scintigraphic defecography: quantitative and dynamic assessment of anorectal function. Dis Colon Rectum. 1993; 36(12):1132–1138

[204] Yang XM, Partanen K, Farin P, Soimakallio S. Defecography. Acta Radiol. 1995; 36(5):460–468

[205] Jorge JM, Habr-Gama A, Wexner SD. Clinical applications and techniques of cinedefecography. Am J Surg. 2001; 182(1):93–101

[206] Fletcher JG, Busse RF, Riederer SJ, et al. Magnetic resonance imaging of anatomic and dynamic defects of the pelvic floor in defecatory disorders. Am J Gastroenterol. 2003; 98(2):399–411

[207] Roos JE, Weishaupt D, Wildermuth S, Willmann JK, Marincek B, Hilfiker PR. Experience of 4 years with open MR defecography: pictorial review of anorectal anatomy and disease. Radiographics. 2002; 22(4):817–832

[208] Karasick S, Karasick D, Karasick SR. Functional disorders of the anus and rectum: findings on defecography. AJR Am J Roentgenol. 1993; 160(4):777–782

[209] Rubens DJ, Strang JG, Bogineni-Misra S, Wexler IE. Transperineal sonography of the rectum: anatomy and pathology revealed by sonography compared with CT and MR imaging. AJR Am J Roentgenol. 1998; 170(3):637–642

[210] Kleinübing H, Jr, Jannini JF, Malafaia O, Brenner S, Pinho TM. Transperineal ultrasonography: new method to image the anorectal region. Dis Colon Rectum. 2000; 43(11):1572–1574

[211] Piloni V. Dynamic imaging of pelvic floor with transperineal sonography. Tech Coloproctol. 2001; 5(2):103–105

[212] Beer-Gabel M, Teshler M, Schechtman E, Zbar AP. Dynamic transperineal ultrasound vs. defecography in patients with evacuatory difficulty: a pilot study. Int J Colorectal Dis. 2004; 19(1):60–67

[213] Sentovich SM, Rivela LJ, Thorson AG, Christensen MA, Blatchford GJ. Simultaneous dynamic proctography and peritoneography for pelvic floor disorders. Dis Colon Rectum. 1995; 38(9):912–915

[214] Ekberg O, Nylander G, Fork FT. Defecography. Radiology. 1985; 155(1):45–48

[215] Jorge JM, Yang YK, Wexner SD. Incidence and clinical significance of sigmoidoceles as determined by a new classification system. Dis Colon Rectum. 1994; 37(11):1112–1117

[216] Bremmer S, Ahlbäck SO, Udén R, Mellgren A. Simultaneous defecography and peritoneography in defecation disorders. Dis Colon Rectum. 1995; 38(9):969–973

[217] Altringer WE, Saclarides TJ, Dominguez JM, Brubaker LT, Smith CS. Four-contrast defecography: pelvic "floor-oscopy". Dis Colon Rectum. 1995; 38(7):695–699

[218] Beck DE. Simplified balloon expulsion test. Dis Colon Rectum. 1992; 35(6):597–598

[219] Dahl J, Lindquist BL, Tysk C, Leissner P, Philipson L, Järnerot G. Behavioral medicine treatment in chronic constipation with paradoxical anal sphincter contraction. Dis Colon Rectum. 1991; 34(9):769–776

[220] Minguez M, Herreros B, Sanchiz V, et al. Predictive value of the balloon expulsion test for excluding the diagnosis of pelvic floor dyssynergia in constipation. Gastroenterology. 2004; 126(1):57–62

[221] Bartolo DCC, Read MG, Read NW. The saline continence test. Dynamic studies in faecal incontinence, haemorrhoids and the descending perineum syndrome. Acta Gastroenterol Belg. 1985; 48(1):39–50

[222] Read NW, Haynes WG, Bartolo DC, et al. Use of anorectal manometry during rectal infusion of saline to investigate sphincter function in incontinent patients. Gastroenterology. 1983; 85(1):105–113

[223] Roe AM, Bartolo DCC, Mortensen NJ. New method for assessment of anal sensation in various anorectal disorders. Br J Surg. 1986; 73(4):310–312

[224] Broens PMA, Penninckx FM. Relation between anal electrosensitivity and rectal filling sensation and the influence of age. Dis Colon Rectum. 2005; 48(1):127–133

[225] Chan CL, Scott SM, Birch MJ, Knowles CH, Williams NS, Lunniss PJ. Rectal heat thresholds: a novel test of the sensory afferent pathway. Dis Colon Rectum. 2003; 46(5):590–595

[226] Gladman MA, Scott SM, Chan CL, Williams NS, Lunniss PJ. Rectal hyposensitivity: prevalence and clinical impact in patients with intractable constipation and fecal incontinence. Dis Colon Rectum. 2003; 46(2):238–246

[227] Lee TH, Lee JS. Psychosocial factors and rectal hyposensitivity. J Neurogastroenterol Motil. 2013; 19(3):418

[228] Burgell RE, Lelic D, Carrington EV, et al. Assessment of rectal afferent neuronal function and brain activity in patients with constipation and rectal hyposensitivity. Neurogastroenterol Motil. 2013; 25(3):260–267, e167–e168

[229] Yu T, Qian D, Zheng Y, Jiang Y, Wu P, Lin L. Rectal hyposensitivity is associated with a defecatory disorder but not delayed colon transit time in a functional constipation population. Medicine (Baltimore). 2016; 95(19):e3667

[230] Gladman MA, Aziz Q, Scott SM, Williams NS, Lunniss PJ. Rectal hyposensitivity: pathophysiological mechanisms. Neurogastroenterol Motil. 2009; 21(5):508–516, e4–e5

[231] Scott SM, van den Berg MM, Benninga MA. Rectal sensorimotor dysfunction in constipation. Best Pract Res Clin Gastroenterol. 2011; 25(1):103–118

[232] Toma TP, Zighelboim J, Phillips SF, Talley NJ. Methods for studying intestinal sensitivity and compliance: in vitro studies of balloons and a barostat. Neurogastroenterol Motil. 1996; 8(1):19–28

[233] Steens J, Van Der Schaar PJ, Penning C, Brussee J, Masclee AAM. Compliance, tone and sensitivity of the rectum in different subtypes of irritable bowel syndrome. Neurogastroenterol Motil. 2002; 14(3):241–247

[234] Varma JS. Autonomic influences on colorectal motility and pelvic surgery. World J Surg. 1992; 16(5):811–819

[235] Rasmussen OO, Sørensen M, Tetzschner T, Christiansen J. Dynamic anal manometry in the assessment of patients with obstructed defecation. Dis Colon Rectum. 1993; 36(10):901–907

[236] Kendall GP, Thompson DG, Day SJ, Lennard-Jones JE. Inter- and intraindividual variation in pressure-volume relations of the rectum in normal subjects and patients with the irritable bowel syndrome. Gut. 1990; 31(9):1062–1068

[237] Alstrup NI, Skjoldbye B, Rasmussen OØ, Christensen NEH, Christiansen J. Rectal compliance determined by rectal endosonography. A new application of endosonography. Dis Colon Rectum. 1995; 38(1):32–36

[238] Snooks SJ, Swash M. Electromyography and nerve latency studies. In: Gooszen HG, ten Cate Hoedemaker HO, Weterman IT, Keighley MRB, eds. Disordered Defecation. Dordrecht, the Netherlands: Nyhoff; 1987

[239] Preston DM, Lennard-Jones JE. Anismus in chronic constipation. Dig Dis Sci. 1985; 30(5):413–418

[240] Jost WH, Ecker KW, Schimrigk K. Surface versus needle electrodes in determination of motor conduction time to the external anal sphincter. Int J Colorectal Dis. 1994; 9(4):197–199

[241] Swash M, Snooks SJ. Slowed motor conduction in lumbosacral nerve roots in cauda equina lesions: a new diagnostic technique. J Neurol Neurosurg Psychiatry. 1986; 49(7):808–816

[242] Percy JP, Neill ME, Swash M, Parks AG. Electrophysiological study of motor nerve supply of pelvic floor. Lancet. 1981; 1(8210):16–17

[243] Pittman JS, Benson JT, Sumners JE. Physiologic evaluation of the anorectum. A new ultrasound technique. Dis Colon Rectum. 1990; 33(6):476–478

[244] Felt-Bersma RJF, van Baren R, Koorevaar M, Strijers RL, Cuesta MA. Unsuspected sphincter defects shown by anal endosonography after anorectal surgery. A prospective study. Dis Colon Rectum. 1995; 38(3):249–253

[245] Carty NJ, Moran B, Johnson CD. Anorectal physiology measurements are of no value in clinical practice. True or false? Ann R Coll Surg Engl. 1994; 76(4):276–280

[246] Wexner SD, Jorge JMN. Colorectal physiological tests: use or abuse of technology? Eur J Surg. 1994; 160(3):167–174

[247] Penninckx FM, Lestár B, Kerremans RP. A new balloon-retaining test for evaluation of anorectal function in incontinent patients. Dis Colon Rectum. 1989; 32(3):202–205

[248] Perry RE, Blatchford GJ, Christensen MA, Thorson AG, Attwood SE. Manometric diagnosis of anal sphincter injuries. Am J Surg. 1990; 159(1):112–116, discussion 116–117

[249] Sultan AH, Kamm MA, Hudson CN, Bartram CI. Third degree obstetric anal sphincter tears: risk factors and outcome of primary repair. BMJ. 1994; 308(6933):887–891

[250] Sultan AH, Kamm MA, Hudson CN, Thomas JM, Bartram CI. Anal-sphincter disruption during vaginal delivery. N Engl J Med. 1993; 329 (26):1905–1911

[251] Deen KI, Kumar D, Williams JG, Olliff J, Keighley MRB. The prevalence of anal sphincter defects in faecal incontinence: a prospective endosonic study. Gut. 1993; 34(5):685–688

[252] Hiltunen KM, Matikainen M, Auvinen O, Hietanen P. Clinical and manometric evaluation of anal sphincter function in patients with rectal prolapse. Am J Surg. 1986; 151(4):489–492

[253] Skomorowska E, Hegedüs V, Christiansen J. Evaluation of perineal descent by defaecography. Int J Colorectal Dis. 1988; 3(4):191–194

[254] Farouk R, Duthie GS, MacGregor AB, Bartolo DCC. Sustained internal sphincter hypertonia in patients with chronic anal fissure. Dis Colon Rectum. 1994; 37(5):424–429

[255] Hancock BD. Internal sphincter and the nature of haemorrhoids. Gut. 1977; 18(8):651–655

[256] Schouten WR, Briel JW, Auwerda JJA, De Graaf EJR. Ischaemic nature of anal fissure. Br J Surg. 1996; 83(1):63–65

[257] Duthie HL. Defaecation and the anal sphincters. Clin Gastroenterol. 1982; 11 (3):621–631

[258] Belliveau P, Thomson JP, Parks AG. Fistula-in-ano. A manometric study. Dis Colon Rectum. 1983; 26(3):152–154

[259] Sainio P, Husa A. A prospective manometric study of the effect of anal fistula surgery on anorectal function. Acta Chir Scand. 1985; 151(3):279–288

[260] Heppell J, Kelly KA, Phillips SF, Beart RW, Jr, Telander RL, Perrault J. Physiologic aspects of continence after colectomy, mucosal proctectomy, and endorectal ileo-anal anastomosis. Ann Surg. 1982; 195(4):435–443

[261] Lindquist K, Liljeqvist L, Sellberg B. The topography of ileoanal reservoirs in relation to evacuation patterns and clinical functions. Acta Chir Scand. 1984; 150(7):573–579

[262] Stryker SJ, Kelly KA, Phillips SF, Dozois RR, Beart RW, Jr. Anal and neorectal function after ileal pouch-anal anastomosis. Ann Surg. 1986; 203(1):55–61

[263] Stryker SJ, Daube JR, Kelly KA, et al. Anal sphincter electromyography after colectomy, mucosal rectectomy, and ileoanal anastomosis. Arch Surg. 1985; 120(6):713–716

[264] Beart RW, Jr, Dozois RR, Wolff BG, Pemberton JH. Mechanisms of rectal continence. Lessons from the ileoanal procedure. Am J Surg. 1985; 149(1):31–34

[265] Tjandra JJ, Ooi BS, Han WR. Anorectal physiologic testing for bowel dysfunction in patients with spinal cord lesions. Dis Colon Rectum. 2000; 43 (7):927–931

3 Diagnosis of Colorectal and Anal Disorders

David E. Beck

Abstract

This chapter will discuss important elements in the diagnosis of colorectal and anal disorders, including patient and family history, symptoms, physical and radiological examination, and examination of stool.

Keywords: diagnosis, colorectal disorders, anal disorders, family history, physical examination, radiological examination, stool examination, occult blood testing

3.1 Patient History

History is important in the diagnosis of colorectal and anal disorders. These conditions produce a myriad of signs and symptoms, and appropriate questions will pinpoint the diagnosis or narrow the differential.

3.1.1 Symptoms

Bleeding Per Anus

The occurrence and clinical significance of overt blood loss per rectum varies according to the clinical situation. Using a Medline literature search, the incidence of rectal bleeding in the general population was estimated to be approximately 20 per 100 people per year; in general practice patients, it was approximately 6 per 1,000, and in referral medical specialists, it was about 0.07 per 1,000 per year.[1] The predictive value of anorectal blood loss for colorectal malignancy was estimated to be less than 1 in 1,000 in the general population, approximately 0.2 per 1,000 in general practice, and as many as 360 per 1,000 in referral patients.

The character of the bleeding often suggests the diagnosis. Blood that drips into the toilet bowl and is bright red, free, and separate from the stool is frequently associated with bleeding internal hemorrhoids. Blood that is on the toilet tissue tends to be associated with anal fissures or an abrasion of the anal canal. Melena can be caused by any pathologic process in the right colon or higher up in the gastrointestinal (GI) tract. The association of blood and mucus usually indicates a low-lying carcinoma or, more frequently, an inflammatory condition, such as ulcerative colitis or Crohn's disease. If blood clots are being passed, the source is usually of colonic origin.

Pain

The lower anal canal obtains its innervation from the somatic nervous system and any pain-producing lesion in the anal canal is likely to be described as sharp, burning, or stinging. Sharp anorectal pain that occurs during and following a bowel movement is usually associated with an anal fissure or an abrasion in the anal canal. Tenesmus, a symptom complex of straining and the urge to defecate, is frequently associated with inflammatory or neoplastic conditions of the anorectum. The pain associated with a perianal abscess usually is described as constant and throbbing in nature. Pain that increases in intensity when the patient coughs or sneezes is often associated with an intersphincteric abscess.

Anorectal pain may be referred to the sacral region but is usually related to bowel movements. Pain associated with levator ani muscle spasm or proctalgia fugax (rectal muscle spasm) will vary from a pressure feeling to a stabbing pelvic pain that is of short duration and is not related to activity or bowel movements. Rectal pain may also be referred from aneurysmal dilatations in the pelvic vascular tree or from retrorectal tumors and usually presents as a feeling of fullness. Coccygeal pain usually results from trauma to the ligaments or periosteum of the coccyx or an inflamed presacral cyst.

Abdominal pain tends to be nonspecific. Pain from the cecum usually is located in the right lower quadrant, while pain from the sigmoid colon is located in the left lower quadrant. Pain experienced in the lower rectum may be referred pain from the sigmoid colon, whereas pain originating in the rectum itself usually is experienced in the perineum and rarely in the hypogastrium. Obstruction of the left colon may manifest as pain in the right lower quadrant because of the distention of the cecum. The character and duration of pain and its relation to meals should be determined.

Abdominal pain that originates from the colon may be crampy in nature when related to an intramural lesion or to excessive colonic contraction or distention, or it may be associated with peritoneal irritation when related to any inflammation in the colon. When the mesentery of the colon is stretched, pain will be experienced, and this can be duplicated in the process of performing a proctosigmoidoscopic or colonoscopic examination. Peritoneal pain may be secondary to colonic disease when there are adhesions between the colon and the parietes. Sites of referred pain to the body surface are determined by the same principles as referred pain elsewhere; pain from the colon is referred to just above the symphysis pubis, and rectal pain can go directly to the sacral area.

Abdominal pain may be a manifestation of anorectal disease when the supralevator space is involved. Because this space has peritoneum as its "roof," a suppurative process may result in signs of peritoneal irritation.

Change in Bowel Habits

Normal bowel movement frequency varies from three per day to three per week.[2,3] To a patient, constipation may mean a variety of conditions, such as stools that are infrequent, hard, small, or difficult to pass. To determine the necessity for further investigation, it is important to know the duration of the constipation, whether the onset is recent, or if the condition is a chronic one. Constipation can also result from a pelvic floor disorder.

Diarrhea is a symptom of many GI diseases. The duration, amount, character, and frequency of the diarrhea should be determined. Clear watery diarrhea may be from a large secretory rectal villous adenoma. A bloody mucous diarrhea may indicate inflammatory bowel disease. Operative procedures such as vagotomy, cholecystectomy, or gastric or small bowel resection may alter GI motility, absorption, and secretion, and consequently will alter bowel habits. Patients who have had a jejunoileal bypass for morbid obesity are subject to many anorectal problems associated with diarrhea.

Discharge

Mucus is secreted by the goblet cells of the colonic and rectal mucosa and may be seen in the stool under many different circumstances. It may be the result of normal production of mucus,[1] the early sign of a villous adenoma of the rectum,[2] the indication of an early colitic condition,[3] or caused by chemical irritants.[4] The packaged buffered phosphate enemas (e.g., Phospho-Soda) can elicit a tremendous response from the bowel and extra mucus may be seen on endoscopic examination of the bowel after administration of such an enema. Mucus associated with bleeding may be a sign of a neoplasm or an inflammatory process.

Mucus should normally not leak through the anus unless the patient is incontinent. Soiling of underwear may be a sign of rectal mucosal prolapse, ectropion from a previous hemorrhoidectomy, or overproduction of mucus, such as occurs with a villous adenoma.

Purulent discharge is indicative of an infectious process. A history of purulent discharge and pain is characteristic for an anorectal abscess, whereas a painless purulent discharge more likely is due to a fistula-in-ano. Passing pus per rectum may indicate a gonococcal proctitis or a spontaneously drained intersphincteric abscess.

Fecal soiling of underwear is usually asymptomatic. However, it may be a consequence of early postoperative anorectal procedures, such as hemorrhoidectomy, internal sphincterotomy, and fistulotomy. Fecal soiling is relatively common in the elderly. Fecal soiling must not be mistaken as fecal incontinence.

Perianal Swelling

One must always determine whether or not a perianal swelling is painful and whether it has discharged blood or pus. The swelling also might be intermittent as would be expected with a prolapsing hypertrophied anal papilla. If the swelling is associated with fever and chills, an anorectal abscess should be suspected. The common swelling at the anal verge usually is a thrombosed external hemorrhoid, which develops rather quickly and, if ulcerated, is associated with pain and occasional bleeding.

Pruritus

Pruritus ani (intense itching) is a common symptom associated with anorectal pathology. Most often, it occurs in patients who have loose stools and are unable to properly cleanse the anal area. Pruritus also may be associated with the healing phase of an anal condition. Severe pruritus ani is usually associated with a mucoid discharge, which may be blood tinged from the open ulceration of the perianal skin. The patient always should be questioned regarding the use of antibiotics, because these drugs may be the cause of the pruritus ani. In rare cases, pruritus ani in adults may be caused by *Enterobius vermicularis* (pinworms). Most of these adults have a history of contact with infected children.

Prolapse

In questioning the patient who presents with a protrusion from the anal aperture, it should be determined whether the prolapse occurs only at the time of defecation or whether it occurs independently. Independent prolapsing is more suggestive of a hypertrophied anal papilla or a complete rectal procidentia. Does the prolapse reduce itself spontaneously, or must it be replaced manually? This may suggest the magnitude of the problem. Frequently, the patient can give an idea of the relative size of the prolapsing mass; this information often helps in making the diagnosis. The most common prolapsing condition is rectal mucosal prolapse associated with prolapsing hemorrhoids. This must be differentiated from true procidentia of the rectum. Large hypertrophied anal papillae also are known to prolapse from the anal canal. Polyps in the rectum can prolapse; however, this usually is seen in a child with juvenile polyposis or in an elderly patient with a massive villous adenoma.

Incontinence

When a patient presents with a history of incontinence following a previous anorectal surgical procedure, the details of that procedure must be elicited to evaluate the complaints completely. In a parous woman, a good obstetric history should be obtained regarding the nature of an episiotomy and any complications associated with it, as well as the nature and type of delivery. In bedridden elderly patients, fecal impaction may be the cause of overflow incontinence.

Loss of Weight

It is important to note the amount of weight loss occurring over a given time period. Rapid loss of weight without obvious reasons (such as dieting) may indicate GI disease or malignancy.

Flatulence

All patients pass gas through the rectum, so it must be determined whether there is actually an excessive passage of flatus or merely an unusual sense of awareness of the normal passage. Gas in the GI tract is either "swallowed" or the result of bacterial action on luminal contents. Most patients with increased flatulence are found to have a dietary indiscretion in the form of excessive intake of gas-producing substances, rather than a specific malady of the GI tract. Patients are not aware that fermentation is taking place all the time in the bowel. A simple test is to have the patient intake only a clear liquid diet for 24 hours and observe the amounts of flatus following this therapeutic test. Frequently, the patient will learn that very little gas is formed when there is not an excessive amount of food in the GI tract. Another simple test is to ask the patient if flatus was experienced on the day of a barium enema study. Often, the patient will indicate that there was freedom from flatus for the first time when the GI tract was cleaned out for the X-ray study.

Studies by Levitt[4] have shown that hydrogen and methane are produced solely by bacteria and are not a product of human cellular metabolism. Levitt also has shown that hydrogen production is negligible in the fasting state; it appears that colonic bacteria are dependent on ingested fermentable substrates (carbohydrates) for hydrogen production. Certain vegetables, particularly legumes, contain a high concentration of indigestible oligosaccharides, which are nonabsorbable even by normal subjects, and these oligosaccharides account for the notorious gaseous properties of legumes. Carbon dioxide can be produced by bacterial fermentation or by the reaction of bicarbonate and acid. Digestion of an average meal could theoretically produce several hundred milliequivalents of acid, thus yielding 4,000 mL of carbon dioxide. Although excessive gas is assumed to be a common cause of "functional abdominal complaints," there are little hard data to support this assumption. Passing gas through the vagina or through the urethra usually is indicative of a fistula to the GI tract. Occasionally, gas-forming organisms in the bladder may give rise to pneumaturia without a fistula, but this is rare except in the diabetic patient. Instrumentation of the bladder by a Foley or cystoscopy may explain transient air. A complete GI evaluation is mandatory if a history of pneumaturia or flatus per vagina is obtained.

Anorexia

Anorexia is a lack or loss of appetite for food. Frequently, this appetite change is psychogenic in origin, as with depression, worry, and boredom, or it may be caused by drugs such as digitalis preparations, sulfasalazine, and antihypertensive agents. Anorexia is a common symptom for patients with an acute viral hepatitis and/or carcinoma. Numerous signals have been implicated in the short-term control of appetite. These include changes in blood glucose, free fatty acid, and amino acid concentrations; altered neuronal activity resulting from distention of the GI tract; or alterations in the concentrations of various hormones such as insulin, glucagon, bombesin, and cholecystokinin.[5] Other clinical factors that may contribute to the development of anorexia and reduced food intake in patients with carcinoma include intestinal obstruction, radiation therapy, chemotherapy-induced nausea and vomiting, altered taste sensitivity, and oral ulceration.

3.1.2 Associated Illnesses

Inflammatory bowel disease is well known for its associated anorectal problems. A history of this condition should be pursued in any patient with an anorectal complaint. Diabetes mellitus occasionally is associated with nocturnal diarrhea. The patient with peptic ulcer disease may be taking antacids, which alter the consistency of stool (harder or looser).

3.1.3 Medications

To evaluate symptoms completely, one must ascertain the medications (both prescribed and over-the-counter) that a patient is ingesting. A detailed laxative history is mandatory for any patient with a bowel complaint. A complete history of drug allergies should also be obtained.

3.1.4 Family History

A patient's bowel habits will often be very similar to those of their parents. Frequently, a familial history of hemorrhoids is seen in patients who are suffering from a rectal mucosal prolapse. A pertinent family history of carcinoma should be sought.

In a case–control study in which data from a Utah population database were used, patients with first-degree relatives with colon carcinoma had an increased risk of developing colon carcinoma[6]; in men, the odds ratio (OR) was 2.51, and in women the OR was 2.90. A second- or third-degree relative with colon carcinoma increased the risk from 25 to 52%. Risk associated with family history was greater in those patients diagnosed before age 50 than in those diagnosed at age 50 or older. Women were at an increased risk of colon carcinoma if they had a first-degree relative with breast (OR = 1.59), uterine (OR = 1.50), ovarian (OR = 1.63), or prostate (OR = 1.49) carcinoma. Men were at increased risk of colon carcinoma if they had a first-degree relative with breast (OR = 1.30), uterine (OR = 1.96), or ovarian (OR = 1.59) carcinoma.

A study from Melbourne, Australia, by St John et al[7] also found that first-degree relatives of patients with colorectal carcinoma had an increased risk for colorectal carcinoma. This risk was greater if the diagnosis was made at an early age and was greater when other first-degree relatives were affected. From the National Polyp Study Work Group[8] in the United States, the relative risk of colorectal carcinoma for siblings of patients in whom adenomas were diagnosed before 60 years of age was 2.59, as compared with the risk for siblings of patients who were 60 years or older at the time of diagnosis. The risk increased with decreasing age at the time of the diagnosis of adenoma (p for trend, < 0.001). The relative risk for the siblings of patients who had a parent with colorectal carcinoma, as compared with those who had no parent with carcinoma, was 3.25. Thus, siblings and parents of patients with colorectal adenomatous polyps are at increased risk for colorectal carcinoma, particularly when the adenoma is diagnosed before the age of 60 or, in the case of siblings, when a parent has had colorectal carcinoma.[8] These data support the recommendations that individuals who have an increased risk of colon and rectal carcinoma should have regular screening.

3.1.5 Bleeding Tendency

If a surgical procedure is necessary, a history of a bleeding tendency should be ruled out. A simple question may reveal a diagnosis of hemophilia. The patient should also be asked if he or she is taking medications that cause bleeding, such as aspirin, warfarin (Coumadin), and nonsteroidal anti-inflammatory drugs.

3.1.6 Exposure

In taking a history, one also must be cognizant of the fact that the patient may have returned recently from a tropical country with exposure to certain parasitic diseases or from areas such as West Africa where infectious diseases such as Ebola are a consideration.

A history of sexual exposure is important, especially if the patient has had anal intercourse. This may lead to the diagnosis of venereal diseases, human immunodeficiency virus (HIV), and/or acquired immunodeficiency syndrome (AIDS).

3.2 Physical Examination

The precise organization of the consulting room, examining room, and endoscopy suite will vary from one institution to another. Some office examining rooms are designed primarily for diagnostic evaluation, while others are equipped for the performance of minor operative procedures. Nevertheless, the appropriate stage must be set to accomplish the required objective of a complete colorectal examination.

3.2.1 Room

The room should be equipped with essential items for the examination: a suction system, a good portable or head light, a toilet, and a washing sink. It is important that instruments be within easy reach of the surgeon, but they should be kept covered and out of view of the patient, who may find them to be a source of unnecessary anxiety.

3.2.2 Equipment

Ideally, a proctoscopic table should be used. The table can be either put in the jackknife position or laid flat, with the height of

the table adjusted as desired. If this is not available, any table (at least 3 feet high) or a litter or stretcher can be used.

A good light is important for an efficient anorectal examination. Several types of lamps are commercially available for this purpose. A headlamp is convenient and saves space; a tall lamp on a stand with wheels also is excellent. Lighted instruments are another option.

A Vernon-David anoscope is an ideal size for anorectal examination (▶ Fig. 3.1). It is not quite as large as a standard anoscope, which stretches the anal canal and hence results in an underestimation of hemorrhoid size. A medium-size Hinkel-James anoscope is an excellent instrument for rubber band ligation of hemorrhoids, but it is less useful for examining the anal canal (▶ Fig. 3.2).[9]

Proctosigmoidoscope

Three sizes of proctosigmoidoscopes are available (▶ Fig. 3.3). A19-mm 25-cm scope is the standard size and should be used

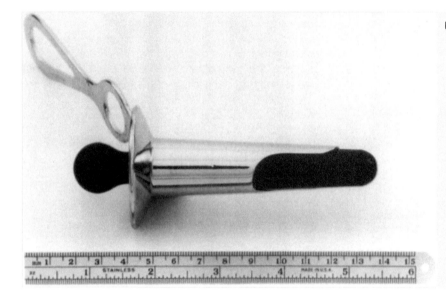

Fig. 3.1 Vernon-David anoscope.

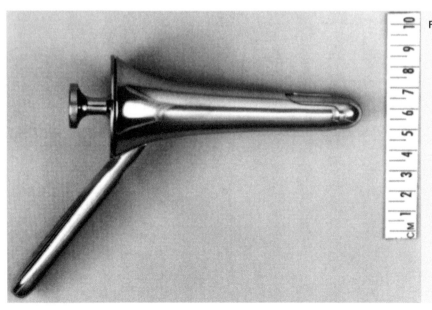

Fig. 3.2 Hinkel-James anoscope.

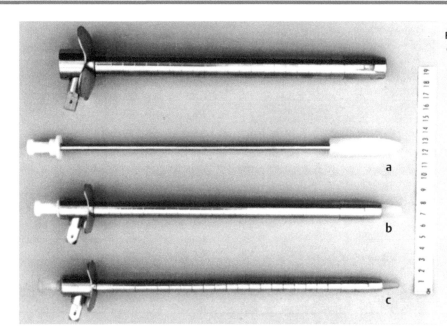

Fig. 3.3 Proctosigmoidoscopes. (a) 19 mm × 25 cm. (b) 15 mm × 25 cm. (c) 11 mm × 25 cm.

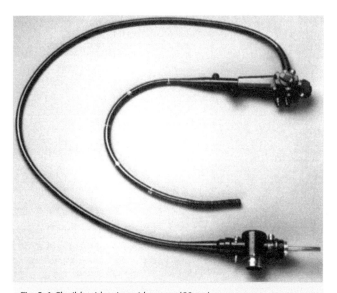

Fig. 3.4 Flexible videosigmoidoscope (60 cm).

for polypectomy or electrocoagulation. A 15-mm 25-cm scope is an ideal size for general examination. It is much better tolerated by the patient, causing less spasm of the rectum and thus minimal air insufflation, yet enables as adequate an examination as the standard-size scope. An 11-mm 25-cm scope should be available for examining the patient who has an anorectal stricture, such as in Crohn's disease. More recently, a disposable standard-size proctosigmoidoscope has become popular for routine examination.

Flexible Sigmoidoscope

The standard flexible fiberoptic sigmoidoscope (FFS) is 60 cm long (▶ Fig. 3.4). It has all the features of a colonoscope. Because of the shorter length of the flexible sigmoidoscope, its cost, maintenance, and durability are considerably better than those of the colonoscope.

Colonoscope

Colonoscopy was introduced to clinical practice in 1970 and has become an established component of colon and rectal surgery. Indications, equipment, and the procedure are discussed in Chapter 4.

Ancillary Equipment

A ball-tip electrode with an insulated shaft works well for coagulating a small rectal or sigmoid polyp (▶ Fig. 3.5a). A suction–coagulation electrode is ideal for coagulating a bleeding area, such as after biopsy of rectal mucosa or a lesion (▶ Fig. 3.5b). It is more versatile because the oozing of blood can be sucked dry during the coagulation, and the gas and smoke that are produced can be readily eliminated. A piece of wire or a needle always should be available to push the plug of tissue or blood out of the insulated shaft.

There are two types of electrocautery snare wires available commercially (▶ Fig. 3.6). A rigid-wire snare, known as the Frankfeldt snare, has been in use for a long time and is good for snaring small- or medium-size polyps. A soft-wire snare has a larger loop and is easier to use, especially for larger polyps or for piecemeal snaring; however, the problem with this type of wire is that it is too soft and bends easily. Several snare wires should be available as spare parts.[10]

There are basically two types of biopsy forceps for use with the proctosigmoidoscope—the cup-shaped forceps and the Turrell biopsy forceps. Both types are excellent for biopsy of lesions or rectal mucosa. The size of the specimen obtained is between 5 and 8 mm. Because of the relatively large size, electrocoagulation usually is required to stop the bleeding. Alligator-type forceps for retrieval of polyps or foreign bodies should be available (▶ Fig. 3.7).

Because anorectal probes for fistula-in-ano or sinus tracts cause considerable pain, they should only be used in the operating room when the patient is under anesthesia. The grooved Lockhart-Mummery fistula probes are suitable for diagnosis and fistula surgery (▶ Fig. 3.8).

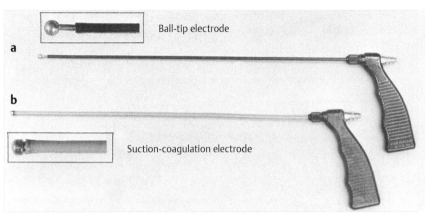

Ball-tip electrode

Suction-coagulation electrode

Fig. 3.5 Electrocoagulation electrodes. **(a)** Ball-tip electrode. **(b)** Suction-coagulation electrode.

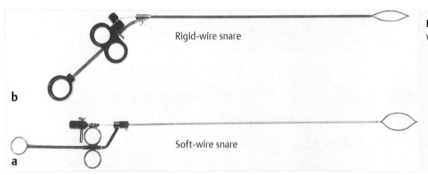

Rigid-wire snare

Soft-wire snare

Fig. 3.6 (a,b) Snaring devices for polypectomy via proctosigmoidoscope.

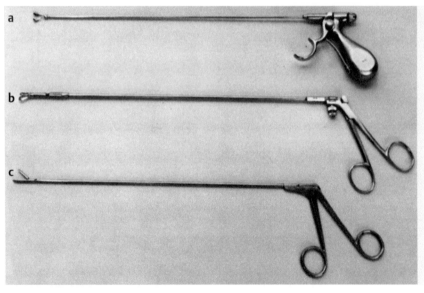

Fig. 3.7 Biopsy instruments. **(a)** Cup-shaped biopsy forceps. **(b)** Turrell biopsy forceps. **(c)** Alligator-type forceps.

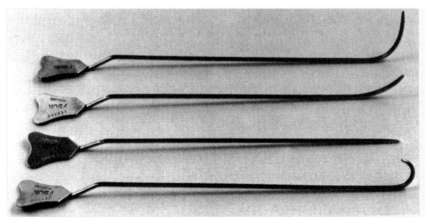

Fig. 3.8 Lockhart-Mummery fistula probes.

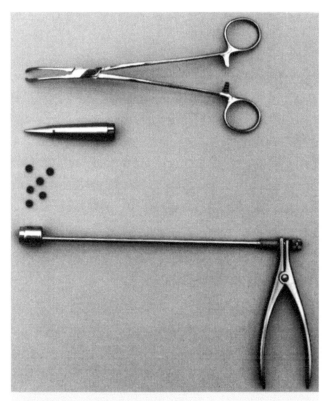

Fig. 3.9 Rubber band ligation equipment.

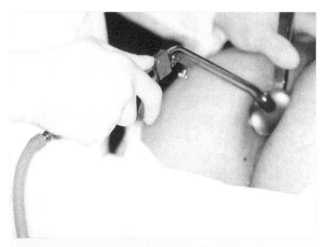

Fig. 3.10 A suction hemorrhoid ligator.

Rubber Band Ligation Equipment

Rubber band ligation equipment, including ligator, O ring, and forceps, should be available for immediate use (▶ Fig. 3.9). Several forceps have been advocated for this technique; however, an Allis forceps may suffice. A suction hemorrhoid ligator is also available. It has the advantage that one can apply the ligation without needing an assistant (▶ Fig. 3.10). Another advantage is that only the redundant mucosa is sucked into the cup for ligation.

Sclerosing Equipment

Sclerosing procedures require a syringe loaded with a solution of either 5% phenol and vegetable oil or 5% quinine and urea hydrochloride. However, sclerosing of hemorrhoids has been replaced largely by rubber band ligation.

Miscellaneous Items

Along with the necessary equipment already described, there are accessories essential for the examination. A good suction system (either water or motor suction) is indispensable. A long metal or plastic suction rod must be available. Lubricant jelly is required in every case. A 2% lidocaine (Xylocaine) jelly also should be available, especially for patients with anal fissures or abrasions. Rubber or plastic gloves are essential. (Some people are allergic to rubber gloves.) A 1.5- to 2-inch 27-gauge needle, a 3-mL syringe, and a local anesthetic should be available. Scalpels, scissors, needle holders, tissue forceps, and suture materials also should be on hand. An irrigating syringe or bottle for irrigating via the proctosigmoidoscope also

is needed. A pulsating water injection device (i.e., Waterpik[1]) can be easily adapted for irrigating via the colonoscope or flexible sigmoidoscope and should be available. An area with proper antiseptic solution must be arranged for cleaning the instruments after they are used. Disposable buffered phosphate enemas should be available for use when the rectum is loaded with stool. Ideally, a toilet should be in or near the examining room. Soft paper tissues are needed to wipe the lubricant jelly from the anal area after the examination. Basic resuscitation equipment should be available, especially when minor surgical procedures are being performed.

3.2.3 General Examination

Abdomen

Inspection of the abdomen may reveal asymmetry suggestive of a neoplastic mass or enlargement of the internal organs. Distended abdominal veins suggest portal hypertension or obstruction of the inferior vena cava. Pulsation from an abdominal aortic aneurysm may be seen in very thin patients. Palpation should be aimed at detecting any tenderness, peritoneal irritation, or abdominal mass. The scar from a previous large bowel resection should be examined for healing, sinus or fistula, and metastatic mass.

Perineum

The most common site of recurrence of rectal carcinoma is the pelvis and perineum. Follow-up examination should encompass the perineal wound to determine if it has healed completely or has any evidence of sinus, mass, or tenderness.

Groin

Anorectal carcinoma that has invaded into or below the dentate line may metastasize to the inguinal lymph nodes. Therefore, the presence or absence of enlarged inguinal nodes should be recorded. Enlargement of these nodes before or after excision of an anorectal lesion requires further management or a change in management approach.

3.2.4 Anorectal Examination

Positioning

Although the inverted prone jackknife position on a proctoscopic table is most popular and is extensively used in the United States (▶ Fig. 3.11a), the left lateral (Sim's) position with the buttocks projecting slightly beyond the edge of the examining table is as good for examination and is much more acceptable to the patient (▶ Fig. 3.11b). The prone jackknife position should not be used in conditions such as acute glaucoma, retinal detachment, severe cardiac arrhythmia, severe debilitation, late pregnancy, and recent abdominal surgery.

Inspection

Inspection of the anal area always should precede any other examination, and for this, good lighting is essential. The shape of the buttocks should be noted, because this information can be useful in determining the position in which to place the patient for the operation and the type of anesthetic to use.[11] The cheeks of the buttocks are gently spread to gain exposure. Skin tags, excoriation, and change in color or thickness of the anal verge and perianal skin can be detected quickly. A scarred, patulous, or irregularly shaped anus may give clues to the cause of anal incontinence. Particularly in multiparous women, the anal verge may be pushed down too far during straining—a feature of the perineal descent syndrome.[12] Prolapse of the rectum (procidentia) is best demonstrated by asking the patient to strain while in a lateral position or sitting on the toilet. When the anal verge is pricked with a needle, the external sphincter visibly contracts because of anal reflex. It is useful for testing the sensibility of the anal canal, which may be absent in areas of a previous scar or defect, or in patients with an underlying neuropathy.

Digital Examination

To begin the digital examination, the index finger should be well lubricated with a lubricant jelly, and the finger pressed on the anal aperture to "warn" the patient. Then, the finger should be gradually inserted and swept all around the anal canal to detect any mass or induration. In men, the prostate should be felt. In women the posterior vaginal wall should be pushed anteriorly to detect any evidence of a rectocele. Anal tone, whether tight or loose, can be easily estimated. A stricture or narrowing

from scarring or a defect in the internal or external sphincters from a previous operation can be felt. A fibrous cord or induration in the anal area and anal canal may indicate a fistulous track. The external sphincter, puborectalis, and levator ani muscles can also be appreciated by digital examination. When the puborectalis is pulled in the posterior quadrant, the anus will gape but will close immediately when the traction is released.[13,14] Persistence of the gaping indicates an abnormal reflex pathway in the thoracolumbar region, commonly seen in paraplegic patients. The finger should press gently on these muscles for signs of tenderness. When a person with good sphincter function is asked to contract the muscles, the examiner not only feels the squeeze of the muscle on the examining finger but also feels the finger pulled forward by the puborectalis muscle.

Anoscopy

Anoscopy, as the name implies, is the examination of the anal canal. The anoderm, dentate line, internal and external hemorrhoids, and lower part of the rectal mucosa can be seen through the anoscope. Anoscopy should not begin until a digital examination has been completed. For most cases, an enema is not required. Insertion of the anoscope always should be done with the obturator in place. The obturator is removed during examination and reinserted to rotate the instrument to another area. If an inverted jackknife position is used, the examination table should not be tipped down more than 10 to 15 degrees. If a left lateral position is used, an assistant needs to pull up the right cheek of the buttocks for exposure. During examination, the patient is asked to strain, with the anoscope sliding out to detect any prolapse of the rectal mucosa and the anal cushion. Excoriation, metaplastic changes, and friable mucosa indicate a prolapsed hemorrhoid.

Proctosigmoidoscopy

Although a standard proctosigmoidoscope is 25 cm in length, the average distance that the scope can be passed is 20 cm. In men, the scope can be passed to 21 to 25 cm half of the time, and in women it can be passed that distance one-third of the time.[15] Proctosigmoidoscopy is suitable only to examine the rectum and, in some persons, the distal sigmoid colon. The pain experienced from proctosigmoidoscopy is from stretching the mesentery of the rectosigmoid colon when the scope is pushed against the rectal wall and from the air insufflation. When

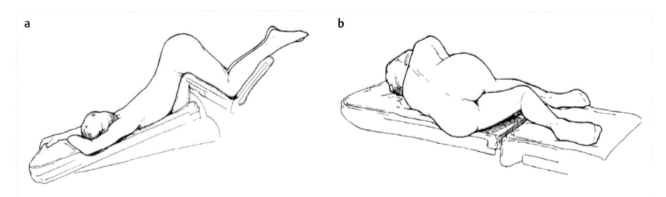

Fig. 3.11 (a) Prone jackknife position. (b) Left lateral position (note that the buttocks project slightly beyond the edge of the examining table).

properly performed, proctosigmoidoscopy should produce no pain at all or only mild discomfort. Most patients are fearful of the examination because of past bad experience with the procedure or from what they have heard. A few words of reassurance will be helpful. Since many patients feel undignified in the "bottom-up" positioning, a left lateral position can be used instead to alleviate this feeling.

Technique: With the obturator in place and held steady with the right thumb, the proctoscope is gently inserted into the anal canal, aiming toward the umbilicus for a distance of about 4 to 5 cm. Then the scope is angled toward the sacrum and advanced another 4 to 5 cm into the rectum. The obturator is removed, and the bowel lumen is negotiated under direct vision. Air insufflation is limited to the amount necessary to open the lumen. When an angle is encountered, the scope is withdrawn 3 to 4 cm and then readvanced. This may be repeated several times to straighten the angulation. If further advancement is unsuccessful, the procedure is terminated at this point. Careful examination is done as the instrument is withdrawn. It usually is necessary to insufflate a small amount of air for good visualization of the lumen. The instrument should be rotated on withdrawal to ensure examination of the entire circumference. The mucosal folds (valves of Houston) can be flattened with the tip of the scope to see the area behind them.

The length of insertion should be measured from the anal verge without stretching the bowel wall. Some physicians measure it in relation to the dentate line. This is more cumbersome because one also needs to measure the distance to the dentate line and subtract from it the distance to the anal verge. The appearance of the mucosa and depth of insertion should be accurately described. If a lesion is seen, the size, appearance, location, and level must be recorded. If a biopsy is performed, the location, level, number of biopsies, and whether electrocoagulation is necessary should be noted.

Ideally, a phosphate enema should be given within 2 hours of the examination. If the patient has had a bowel movement that morning, an enema usually is unnecessary. Mucus and watery stool can be easily aspirated. Even if there is some formed stool, the scope can be slipped between the fecal mass and the colonic wall. However, a large amount of solid or soft stool can impede further passage of the scope; in this situation, a phosphate enema should be given in the examining room, or the patient should return at some later date with better preparation.

Flexible Sigmoidoscopy

A flexible sigmoidoscope is no longer fiberoptic but contains a video chip at the tip of scope. This video chip transmits the image through the processing unit of the monitor. The entire sigmoid colon can be reached by the flexible sigmoidoscope in 45 to 85% of cases, and in a few, the splenic flexure also can be visualized.[16,17] The discrepancies in success depend on patient selection and the experience of the endoscopist. For selective screening examination, flexible sigmoidoscopy has a three to six times greater yield than does proctosigmoidoscopy in detecting colonic and rectal abnormalities, especially neoplasms.[18,19] Because of this higher yield, proponents of flexible sigmoidoscopy have discarded proctosigmoidoscopy.[20] With the advance in technology of colonoscopy and because large bowel carcinomas have shifted proximally during the last few

decades, the role of proctosigmoidoscopy is now limited to examination of the rectum and is no longer adequate for the screening of large bowel neoplasms.

The role of flexible sigmoidoscopy is difficult to define. Although this type of sigmoidoscopy detects more lesions than proctosigmoidoscopy, flexible sigmoidoscopy cannot be considered adequate when a complete colonic examination is indicated. However, it plays a superior role to proctosigmoidoscopy in case finding. Because barium enema studies miss some lesions in the rectosigmoid and sigmoid colon, a successful flexible sigmoidoscopy that is followed by an air-contrast barium enema gives a more accurate examination than an air-contrast study alone or an air-contrast barium enema combined with rigid proctosigmoidoscopy.[21] Although the flexible sigmoidoscope is easier to handle and learn to use than the fiberoptic colonoscope, proper training is nevertheless necessary. The basic principles of technique, the limitations, and the risk of complications must be fully understood.

Technique: Because flexible sigmoidoscopy is designed for examination of the left colon, a formal bowel preparation with laxatives is unnecessary. Normally, one or two phosphate enemas before the examination are adequate.

The examination is best performed with the patient in a left lateral position, although a prone position is sometimes preferred by some examiners. Sedation is unnecessary. The anal canal is lubricated by digital examination. A well-lubricated flexible sigmoidoscope then is inserted. Advancement of the scope is performed under direct vision. Pushing the scope through a bend in the bowel is a poor technique. Instead, the scope should be withdrawn to straighten the bowel. The key to success is short withdrawal and advancement of the scope or a to-and-fro movement, together with rotating the instrument clockwise and/or counterclockwise as needed. Use of air insufflation should be kept to a minimum. The procedure should be completed within 5 to 10 minutes. If a lesion is detected and proved by biopsy to be a neoplasm, a complete colonic investigation may be indicated ideally by total colonoscopy at some later date. A polyp up to 8 mm in size can be sampled with coagulation (hot) biopsy forceps or biopsy and electrocoagulation. A larger polyp should be reserved for colonoscopy and polypectomy. To prevent possible gas explosion due to hydrogen or methane gas in the lumen, air should be exchanged in the colon and rectum with repeated insufflation and suction.

3.3 Radiologic Examination

3.3.1 Plain Films of Abdomen

Radiographic examination of the abdomen is indicated whenever there is clinical evidence of an acute intra-abdominal condition. Although plain X-ray films of the abdomen are generally nonspecific, they often give clues to the underlying problems and lead to further, more specific investigations. Because the intra-abdominal organs change with position, interpretation of the findings must correlate with the position used. The standard techniques are the supine and upright radiographs of the abdomen, with a lateral decubitus included as indicated. Plain abdominal films give useful information regarding the gas pattern in the intestinal tract; masses and fluid also may be appreciated.

Normally, there is a variable amount of gas in the large bowel and only a minimal amount in the small bowel. Interpretation of the plain abdominal film is made by the evidence of an abnormal pattern or amount of gas, as in mechanical bowel obstruction or ileus. Displacement of gas is a sign for a mass effect. The presence of gas in organs in which it does not belong indicates a fistula with the bowel, such as air in the biliary tree in a choledochoduodenal fistula or air in an abscess cavity produced by bacteria. Free air in the abdominal cavity is best seen when the patient is upright. Frequently, upright chest radiography provides a better picture. Chew et al[22] found that patients with severe ulcerative colitis have a poor response to medical treatment if three or more loops of small bowel distended with gas are noted on plain abdominal films.

Intraperitoneal fluid usually collects in the pelvis, which is the most dependent area. With negative pressure from the diaphragm, fluid may ascend along the paracolic gutters to the subphrenic areas.[23] An early roentgenographic sign of peritoneal effusion is fluid density. A large amount of fluid may displace the right and left colon medially or separate loops of small bowel. Extraperitoneal fluid in perirenal and pararenal spaces also can be detected in the same manner.

Organ enlargement (particularly the kidneys, spleen, and liver) can be detected easily by a plain abdominal radiograph. Mass densities in cysts or solid tumors can be outlined or detected by displacement of gas-containing structures such as the stomach, small bowel, and large bowel. Plain abdominal radiographs may reveal calcification in various stones, appendicolith, and calcified atheromatous plaques in abdominal aneurysms.

3.3.2 Computed Tomography

Computed tomography (CT) is a technique that uses a computer to construct an image from radiographic attenuation data. These data are then converted into either a numeric printout or a cross-sectional image of the anatomic part studied. Depending on the attenuation or absorption values, the image produced varies in density (▶ Fig. 3.12). More than 2,000 density differences can be appreciated by CT, rather than the four (air,

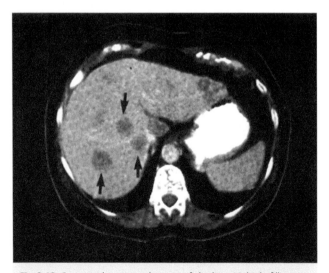

Fig. 3.12 Computed tomography scan of the liver. Multiple filling defects from metastases are shown (*arrows*).

bone, fat, and soft tissue) seen by conventional radiography. This accounts for the exquisite density discrimination of CT, which is fundamental to its ability to detect small lesions. The CT scan uses X-rays but the radiation exposure to the patient is small; it is equivalent to 1 minute of fluoroscopy or one-third to one-fifth the radiation exposure of standard radiographic studies, such as barium enema or excretory urography.[24] Barium contrast will cause artifacts and distort the image. Large numbers of metal clips in the abdominal cavity cause severe streaking and often lead to a nondiagnostic study. Abdominal fat, because of its low computed tomographic number, helps to outline organs. It is helpful, especially in thin patients, to use a diluted oral contrast agent such as 2% diatrizoate meglumine (Gastrografin) to provide sufficient enhancement of the density of the luminal contents. This will allow distinction between loops of bowel and solid structures within the abdomen.

The CT scan is commonly used for the diagnosis of diverticulitis, Crohn's disease, and small and large intestinal obstruction.[25] It has also played an important role in the early detection of strangulation in small intestinal obstruction.[26] CT scan is also useful in diagnosing an intra-abdominal abscess and in investigating carcinoma of the colon and anorectum. With CT as a guide, many intra-abdominal abscesses can be drained percutaneously.[27] For large bowel carcinoma, although the diagnosis should be made by barium enema studies or colonoscopy, CT scanning is of great value because it permits direct visualization of the bowel wall, mesentery, and extension of a malignancy into the surrounding organs. In many instances, a CT scan can be used to stage the disease without the need for exploratory celiotomy.[28]

The most frequent CT finding in primary colonic carcinoma is focal thickening of the colonic wall. Retroperitoneal adenopathy, liver metastasis, and direct invasion of pelvic muscles, prostate, uterus, bladder, ureter, and spine may be seen. The accuracy of CT scan for staging of colorectal carcinoma is between 77 and 100%. The high accuracy rates result from the more advanced cases of the series.[29] The newer technique of CT arterial portography has a positive predictive value of 96% for liver metastases.[30] CT offers comparable potential in detecting recurrent rectal carcinoma. Ideally, a baseline CT scan should be performed 6 to 9 weeks after surgery, and then every 6 to 12 months for 2 to 3 years as indicated. A metastatic lesion to the liver can be detected by CT scan because the lesion has a lower attenuation value than normal hepatic parenchyma. However, in most cases the CT scan is incapable of suggesting a histologic diagnosis. For instance, a primary hepatoma cannot be distinguished from a solitary metastasis.[31] Metastatic lesions are less well circumscribed and less uniform in density than cysts. The prospective study by Smith et al[32] showed that there is no statistical difference in either the sensitivity or overall accuracy among any of the imaging modalities for detecting metastatic lesions in the liver. Liver scintiscan is the most sensitive test (79%), ultrasonography has the greatest specificity (94%), and CT is the most accurate overall (84%). It is interesting to note that the majority of lesions 2 cm in diameter or smaller are missed by all three modalities, while virtually all lesions 4 cm or larger are detected. In spite of technologic advances in CT scanning, no imaging test available today allows accurate resolution of metastatic lesions that are smaller than 2 cm in diameter.

Computed Tomography Angiography

Computed tomography angiography (CTA) uses a multidetector row CT with thin collimation, with intravenous contrast, multiple image postprocedure processing techniques to produce high-quality imaging. Factors influencing the ability to visualize active bleeding at CT are multiple and include the nature of the bleeding lesion (bleeding rate, intermittence), patient factors (hemodynamic status, body mass index), the CT technique (rate of injection, concentration of iodine in contrast material, number of phases, type of scanner, postprocessing), and the experience of the radiologist.[33] The addition of imaging phases to the CTA study may provide more information but also increases the total radiation dose. Findings of recent studies suggest that the highest sensitivity for detecting intestinal bleeding is achieved by means of a dual-phase protocol (arterial and portal venous phases).[34] The two-phase protocol improves depiction of extravasated contrast medium during the arterial phase alone and also provides information about the cause of the bleeding.[35] The preliminary unenhanced scan minimizes misinterpretations of hyperattenuating material that can mimic contrast medium extravasation and can be a cause of false-positive results, such as retained contrast material in diverticula, medications, wall suture material, hemostatic clips, or calcifications.[36]

The inclusion of CTA in the diagnostic algorithm of acute lower intestinal bleeding helps identify patients with active bleeding and accurately determine the site of the bleeding. This information is helpful for directing therapy and, when necessary, for selecting the most appropriate hemostatic intervention: endoscopic, angiographic, or surgical. Precise anatomic localization of the bleeding point allows a targeted endovascular embolization, with a reduction in the number of angiographic series and a resulting savings in time, radiation dose, and the load of contrast material administered.[37] Since even massive GI tract hemorrhage can be intermittent, the finding of active bleeding or a potential hemorrhagic lesion serves to direct the interventional radiologist to the area of concern and increases the success rate of endovascular therapeutic techniques.[38,39] Conversely, a completely negative CT angiogram decreases the likelihood of subsequent angiographic identification of bleeding and might warrant a more conservative treatment and an initial "wait-and-see" strategy, with the possibility of repeating the CT angiogram in cases of re-bleeding.[40]

The identification and anatomic localization of the lesion that is potentially responsible for the hemorrhage and its characterization as vascular, inflammatory, diverticular, or neoplastic (even in a patient who is not actively bleeding) are important for planning the definitive treatment.[41] The accuracy in detecting the bleeding lesion has ranged from 80 to 85%.[41,42,43]

A meta-analysis confirmed a good correlation between conventional angiography and CTA in the identification of the source of bleeding.[33] In some circumstances, the sensitivity of CTA may even exceed that of conventional angiography.[42] One limitation of CTA is the necessity to use intravenous contrast media, which may damage kidney function, limiting its use in patients with renal insufficiency. The ready availability of CTA and its ability to localize the source of bleeding has encouraged many centers to use CTA as the initial test in significant GI bleeds in patients with normal renal function.[44,45]

3.3.3 Computed Tomography Colonography

Computed tomography colonography (CTC) (virtual colonoscopy) is performed with a helical CT scanner to create high-quality axial and reformatted two-dimensional (2D) (▶ Fig. 3.13a) and three-dimensional (3D) (▶ Fig. 3.13b) simulated images of the colon and rectum. A bowel preparation similar to that for colonoscopy is required. Because the average colon length is 1,400 mm, approximately 560 reformatted images are produced (▶ Fig. 3.13).[46] The technique was first described by Vining in 1994 and successfully applied in clinical trials by Hara et al in 1996.[46,47]

Potential advantages for CTC as a screening study for colorectal carcinoma are the possibility that this study one day may be performed without prior bowel preparation, have greater patient acceptability (not yet proven), and have the potential for screening of important disease outside the colon.[48]

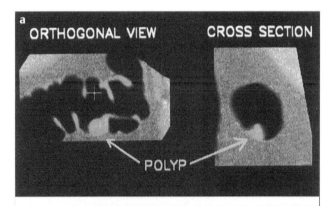

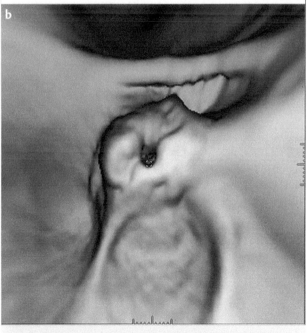

Fig. 3.13 (a) A pedunculated colonic polyp detected by 2-D CT colonography. (Courtesy of C. Daniel Johnson, MD, Mayo Clinic, Rochester, MN.) **(b)** A large, ulcerated carcinoma of the cecum detected by 3D endoluminal CT colonography. (Courtesy of Robert L. MacCarty, MD, Mayo Clinic, Rochester, MN.)

The accuracy of CTC varies widely among reported series depending on how the studies were performed. Pickhardt et al[49] reported a prospective evaluation of CTC as a colorectal carcinoma screening test. The study included 1,233 asymptomatic adults who underwent CTC and same-day colonoscopy. More than 97% of subjects were at average risk for colorectal neoplasia. Radiologists used the 3D endoluminal display for the initial detection of polyps on CTC. They found that the sensitivity of CTC for polyps size of 1 cm, 8 mm, and 6 mm was 93.8, 93.9, and 88.7% compared to 87.5, 91.5, and 92.3%, respectively, for colonoscopy. The authors concluded that CTC with the use of 3D approach is an accurate screening method for the detection of colorectal neoplasia in asymptomatic average risk adults and compares favorably with colonoscopy.

Pineau et al[50] conducted a similar prospective study of 205 patients with average risk of colorectal neoplasia using oral contrast with CTC. They showed the sensitivity of 84.4% and specificity of 83.1% for lesions 6 mm, and 90 and 94.6%, respectively, for lesions 10 mm. Of note was the negative predictive value of 95% for a 6-mm cutoff size and 98.9% for a 10-mm cutoff.

In contrast, Cotton et al found the sensitivity of CTC to be low compared to colonoscopy and the accuracy varied considerably between centers.[51] This was a nonrandomized, noninferiority study by a blinded evaluator of 615 participants aged 50 years or older who were referred for routine clinically indicated colonoscopy in nine major hospital centers. The CTC was performed by using multislice scanners immediately before standard colonoscopy. The results showed that the sensitivity of CTC for detecting lesions size at least 6 mm was 39% (95% confidence interval [CI], 29.6–48.4%), and for lesions at least 10 mm, it was 55% (95% CI, 39.9–70.0%). These results were significantly lower than those for conventional colonoscopy, with sensitivities of 99.0% (95% CI, 97.1–99.9%) and 100%, respectively. Johnson et al prospectively evaluated the performance of CTC in a large asymptomatic population with low disease prevalence.[52] As such, the study population represents a sample of patients likely to undergo CTC screening. In total, 703 asymptomatic persons underwent CTC followed by same-day colonoscopy. Diagnostic review of each study was performed by two of three experienced radiologists in the blind fashion. With colonoscopy serving as gold standard, CTC detected 34, 32, 73, and 63% of the 59 polyps 1 cm for readers 1, 2, 3, and double-reading, respectively; and 35, 29, 57, and 54% of 94 polyps 5 to 9 mm for readers 1, 2, 3, and double-reading, respectively. The results from this low lesion prevalence study (5% of patients had polyps 1 cm) differ from reports of other medical centers including their own previous reports. Technical and perceptual errors accounted for polyps missed by CTC. Causes of error are multifactorial. Technical errors were defined as polyps missed by both observers. This error accounted for 46% of the polyps 5 to 9 mm in diameter and 37% of polyps 1 cm. If a lesion was identified by one observer and missed by another, these were classified as perceptive errors. Perceptive errors accounted for 27% of polyps 5 to 9 mm and 34% of polyps greater than 1 cm. Polyp morphology such as sessile polyps, but not location, influenced detection rates.

Limitation in evaluating the current state of CTC technique includes a wide variation in results of clinical trials. There are as yet insufficient data on the use of CTC in routine clinical practice such as screening colorectal carcinoma.[53]

At present, CTC seems reasonable in the patient with incomplete colonoscopy or who is a poor candidate for colonoscopy, although double-contrast barium enema is also a good choice and costs less. It also makes sense to do CTC (with intravenous contrast) in patients with obstructive colon carcinoma.[54]

3.3.4 Fluoroscopy

Barium Enema

Barium sulfate enema was historically the principal method for detecting large bowel neoplasms. When properly performed, the accuracy is high and the detection of large bowel polyps approaches the rate found at colonoscopy.[55] Most radiologists now agree that the air-contrast barium enema is superior to the single-column enema.[56,57,58] With good bowel preparation and technique, 4- to 5-mm polyps in the large bowel are detectable. Most missed lesions are the result of poor bowel preparation, faulty technique, and inadequate attention to detail rather than invisibility of the lesion. A good-quality air-contrast barium enema also is accurate and useful in diagnosing inflammatory bowel diseases. It is essential that different views and angles at different anatomic areas be taken to produce a complete colonic examination.[59]

Barium enema study generally is safe if there are no contraindications. Cardiac arrhythmia, believed to be caused by stress, occurs in 40% of patients during the procedure,[31] but rarely causes damage. Although the significance of this fact is not known, it suggests that a barium enema should be performed with cautious indications in patients with severe myocardial ischemia. Perforation of the colon and rectum from too much pressure and from the enema tip can be prevented by careful technique. If the patient has had a biopsy specimen taken from a neoplasm, it is not contraindicated to have a barium enema study. However, if a rectal mucosal biopsy is done via a proctosigmoidoscope or a flexible scope, the study should be postponed for at least 1 week.[60] Because the biopsy specimen from colonoscopy or flexible sigmoidoscopy is small and superficial, a barium enema study can be performed safely without delay, provided there is no evidence of inflammatory bowel disease.[61] It should not be performed after a recent snare polypectomy or a hot biopsy. In partial colonic obstruction and acute diverticulitis, the use of a barium sulfate enema is contraindicated; instead, an enema study using water-soluble material should be done. In fulminating colitis and in toxic megacolon, a barium enema study is both unnecessary and unwise.[31] In children, barium enema has been used successfully to reduce an intussusception.

Water-Soluble Contrast

Many acute or subacute conditions, such as sigmoid and cecal volvulus, pseudo-obstruction of the colon, colonic obstruction, and anastomotic leak, require a "rule in" or "rule out" diagnosis, but do not require a detailed evaluation of the colonic mucosa. Because these conditions may necessitate an operation or colonoscopy, it is best that the colon not be full of barium. In such circumstances, a water-soluble contrast medium should be used. These media also have been shown to be safe in evaluating the postoperative anastomotic leak.[62]

The most commonly used water-soluble contrast media are diatrizoate meglumine and diatrizoate sodium (i.e., Gastrografin, Hypaque). These aqueous agents, unlike barium sulfate, are readily absorbed from the peritoneal cavity in the event of perforation and are clear liquids which do not interfere with visualization in colonoscopy or fill the bowel lumen if bowel resection is required.[63] They also help to clean and empty the colon. The potential danger associated with the use of water-soluble contrast media is related to their high osmolarity, which may cause serious dehydration in a dehydrated patient. The aqueous contrast media also have an irritant effect on GI mucosa, which may lead to severe hemorrhage or inflammation.[64,65] Water-soluble contrast media should be used with caution, particularly in cases of partial bowel obstruction, which may lead to a prolonged retention of the medium in the viscus. Water-soluble contrast material has been found to be a helpful diagnostic tool in postoperative small-bowel obstruction; however, it does not help to relieve small bowel obstruction.[66]

The choice between colonoscopy and barium enema has been a subject of debate for years. Prospective studies comparing the two methods for detecting colonic neoplasms have been biased because expertise in radiologic and colonoscopic procedures has not been equal. In the diagnosis of colonic neoplasms, most studies have reported a sensitivity of 76 to 98.5% for barium enema and 86 to 95% for colonoscopy.[67,68,69] Most reports conclude that when properly performed, both barium enema and total colonoscopy are highly sensitive in the detection of colorectal neoplasms.

The advantages of colonoscopy are that when polyps or carcinomas are seen, a biopsy can be done or the neoplasms can be removed; also, stool sometimes can be irrigated or aspirated for an adequate examination. The disadvantages of colonoscopy are its higher cost, its time-consuming nature, its inability to allow passage of the scope all the way to the cecum in all cases, and the risk of complications.

The advantages of barium enema are its lower cost, more rapid performance, and greater suitability for mass screening. The disadvantages are that it is difficult to differentiate between stool and neoplasm, there must be an absolutely clean colon, and it requires proctosigmoidoscopy or flexible sigmoidoscopy for rectum and sigmoid colon examination because these areas are not visualized well on barium enema study.

A prospective study by Rex et al compared examinations of experienced radiologists with those of experienced gastroenterologists.[70] The radiologists were blinded to flexible sigmoidoscopic findings and the colonoscopists were blinded to the barium enema results but not to the flexible sigmoidoscopic findings. The radiologists did not find additional lesions that were not detected during flexible sigmoidoscopy, but 9 of 114 patients (8%) had additional polyps found at colonoscopy that were not detected by flexible sigmoidoscopy and barium enema. All nine carcinomas of the distal colon and rectum were found by both barium enema studies and flexible sigmoidoscopy. With the wide availability of colonoscopy, it has become the first line of diagnostic examination of the colon and rectum. Barium enema is reserved for the situation when a complete colonoscopy could not be accomplished or resources limit the availability of colonoscopy.

Genitourinary Examination

Intravenous Urography

While some series have found significant numbers of urologic abnormalities,[71] others have found a low yield of abnormal findings.[72] However, in selected cases intravenous urogram (IVU) is valuable, and in many cases it is essential. One argument for not doing routine IVU is the small but definite risk of a patient having an anaphylactic reaction to the contrast medium; this can be fatal, particularly in the patient with a history of the reaction.[73]

Use of IVU is highly advisable in cases with a large colonic or rectal mass, such as a carcinoma or a diverticular abscess, where the lesions might become adherent to the ureter, or in cases in which a large lesion is identified in the splenic or hepatic flexure, which may require a concomitant nephrectomy. IVU may show deviations or obstructions of the ureters and may call for the placement of ureteral catheters to promote a safer operation. It also gives useful information on the function of the opposite kidney in the event one ureter is injured. In a large series from the Cleveland Clinic, the incidence of hydroureter and hydronephrosis in patients with Crohn's disease was 5%; IVU is advised in such patients.[74]

Cystography

Urinary symptoms of blood in the urine and of pneumaturia require cystoscopy, followed by a cystogram if indicated. A biopsy should be performed to reveal the nature of the disease and, in particular, to rule out malignancy. The cystogram may reveal the anatomic features of the fistula to the bladder, although, in general, barium enema studies have a higher yield in demonstrating the fistula.

Fistulography

Barium enema studies are highly successful in demonstrating coloenteric fistulas.[75] However, in colocutaneous fistulas, although the underlying pathology usually is revealed by barium enema, the most useful information is obtained from fistulography, provided care is taken to achieve a leakproof seal around the mouth of the fistula and the investigation is carefully planned. For a GI tract fistula, thin barium is superior to water-soluble contrast media. The contrast medium is injected via a soft rubber catheter that can be introduced down the tract or by a bladder catheter in which the balloon can be inflated to occlude the mouth of the orifice. Every orifice that can be found is cannulated, the flow of contrast medium is examined under fluoroscopy, and films are taken in two directions. Fistulography is not worth attempting in patients who have large defects in the abdominal wall and very high outputs; fistulas in such cases usually are better demonstrated by conventional contrast studies.[76]

Simple fistula-in-ano does not require a fistulogram. However, in a highly placed and complicated anorectal fistula, fistulography can reveal the depth and branches of the tracts and is valuable in planning the surgical approach.

3.3.5 Ultrasonography

Ultrasonography is a noninvasive imaging technique that uses high-frequency sound waves. A transducer acts as a receiver to record echoes reflected back from the body. The transducer is applied directly to the skin surface, with mineral oil or a water-soluble gel used as a surface couplant. A striking feature of ultrasonographic imaging is that it distinguishes clearly between solid and fluid-filled structures (▶ Fig. 3.14). The important feature of ultrasonography is its safety; there is no risk of radiation exposure, which makes it ideal for studies in children and pregnant women. Its limitations are the acoustic barriers such as intestinal gas, bone, excessive fat deposits, and barium. Because the sonic probe must be in direct contact with the skin, it is difficult to apply to postoperative patients who have dressings, retention sutures, drains, and open wounds. As with CT and scintigraphy, the accuracy of ultrasonographic detection of liver metastatic carcinoma is high, but it is not better than palpation on celiotomy.[77]

Ultrasonography is an extremely sensitive tool for detecting fluid collections in the abdomen and pelvis; however, its limitations make the findings nonspecific, and its accuracy is inferior to that of the CT scan.[78] At the present time, the limited sensitivity in identifying the large bowel process precludes the use of ultrasonography in screening for abnormalities of the gut. Ultrasonography of the liver is complementary to the CT scan in detecting liver metastasis.

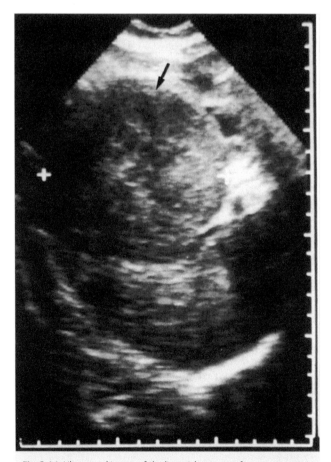

Fig. 3.14 Ultrasound image of the liver. A large mass from metastasis is shown (*arrow*).

Intraoperative sonography has served to detect the liver metastasis that cannot be appreciated by inspection and palpation. The liver is surveyed by placing the ultrasonographic probes directly over the liver. Multiple investigators consider intraoperative sonography to be the modality of choice for hepatic surgery because lesions have been detected that were not identified by preoperative imaging studies or by the surgeon at the time of operation. With the wide use of laparoscopic evaluation and laparoscopic surgery, laparoscopic sonographic probes have been developed and applied in hepatobiliary and GI surgery. It is anticipated that laparoscopic sonography may lead to a less invasive manner of staging colon and rectal carcinoma and to providing pathologic confirmation.[79]

Endorectal Ultrasonography

In 1956, Wild and Reid used an ultrasonographic probe in the rectal lumen to visualize the rectal wall.[80] The equipment at that time was inadequate, and the method was neglected until 1983 when an improved and more powerful transducer became available.[81] Endorectal ultrasonography can identify different layers of the rectum, and it is included in the armamentarium for preoperative staging of rectal carcinoma. Endorectal ultrasonography is more accurate than CT scanning and magnetic resonance imaging (MRI) in preoperative assessment of carcinoma of the rectum.[82] Endorectal ultrasonography, however, cannot evaluate a lesion that causes stenosis or stricture of the rectum. It can determine the depth of malignant infiltration with accuracy of 85 to 95% (▶ Fig. 3.15), and in the detection of lymph node metastasis, with an accuracy of 60 to 85%.[83,84,85]

Currently, endorectal ultrasound is the best tool for preoperative staging of rectal carcinoma. However, endorectal ultrasound identified only one-third of asymptomatic local recurrences that were missed by digital or proctoscopic examination.[86] This is probably due to the interference of postoperative scars or radiation reactions. Poor results are also observed in detection of recurrences after chemoradiation for squamous cell carcinoma of the anal canal.[87] More recently, endorectal ultrasonography has

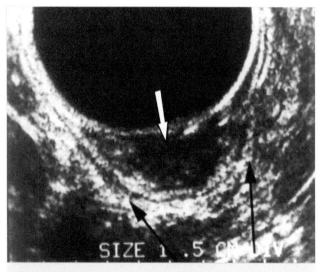

Fig. 3.15 Endorectal ultrasound image showing a lesion limited to the rectal wall (*arrows*). *Note that the muscularis propria is intact.*

been used to identify the anal sphincter defects in cases of anal incontinence and in the evaluation of a fistula-in-ano.[88,89]

3.3.6 Magnetic Resonance Imaging

MRI is a technique for making pictures of internal organs by using the special properties of atoms inside the body and magnetic force. Because no ionizing radiation is used, MRI is potentially safer than studies that use X-rays or injected radionuclides. It is important to note that patients with ferrous metal appliances must be excluded from study.

MRI can detect liver metastases from carcinoma as accurately as contrast-enhanced CT scanning, but it is expensive for routine use. The only advantage of MRI over CT is that it avoids irradiation. The accuracy of MRI for staging of carcinoma of rectum has not reached a clinically useful level.[90] MRI is found to be useful and accurate in demonstrating complicated anal fistulas.[91]

MRI with rectal protocol modification is a reliable staging modality, which is rapidly replacing transrectal ultrasound for staging of rectal cancer.[92] The superior soft-tissue contrast achieved with state-of-the-art rectal protocol MRI allows for measurement of the tumor depth of invasion (T stage), determination of the relationship of the most invasive component of the tumor to the mesorectal fascia, and elucidation of the tumor's relationship to the sphincter complex, peritoneal reflection, and perirectal venous plexus. Furthermore, MRI is able to assess for lymph nodes and tumor deposits in the tissues beyond the mesorectal fascia, including the pelvic sidewall, which, if unaddressed, are a source of residual and/or recurrent disease. MRI is able to identify the location of the tumor with respect to the anterior peritoneal reflection in 75 to 90% of cases.[93] Additional information on this modality is presented in the rectal cancer chapter.

3.3.7 Radionuclide Studies

Radionuclide studies for the detection of GI bleeding were first introduced in 1954, but the early studies did not permit localization of the bleeding source.[94] With improvement in radionuclide imaging techniques, it became possible to detect and localize active GI bleeding.[95,96,97] The technetium-99 m (^{99m}Tc) sulfur colloid scan has since been abandoned and has been replaced by the red blood cell–tagged scan. Bleeding sites in the colon that overlap the liver or spleen may be obscured by the uptake in the reticuloendothelial cells of the organs.

^{99m}Tc-Labeled Red Blood Cells

In this technique, the circulating ^{99m}Tc-labeled red blood cells are extravasated during bleeding (▶ Fig. 3.16). Focal accumulation of the radioactivity is interpreted as the site. The advantage of this technique is that the activity remains in the blood pool for a longer time; therefore, intermittent bleeding in a patient may be detected by performing the imaging over several hours. The disadvantage is that, if imaging is not performed precisely when extravasation occurs, the radioactive agent may move with the bowel peristalsis, which may result in erroneous localization of the bleeding site. For patients who are actively bleeding, ^{99m}Tc sulfur colloid scans, which are now largely abandoned by nuclear radiologists, can identify small amounts of bleeding in a rapid fashion (within 5 minutes). The disadvantage of this imaging technique is that the window of opportunity for diagnosis is short (10–15 minutes) because the agent is rapidly taken up by the liver.

Radionuclide studies are noninvasive procedures. Some authors use them in a secondary role to arteriography, especially in cases of massive lower GI bleeding.[35] Some investigators use them as initial diagnostic procedures for localizing bleeding during conservative therapy of patients with mild or intermittent GI bleeding. When a radionuclide test reveals no bleeding, no further immediate diagnostic studies are required and subsequent elective studies can be scheduled for further management. When, on the other hand, the radionuclide study shows active bleeding, arteriography should be performed immediately to confirm the bleeding site.[48] CTA (discussed previously)

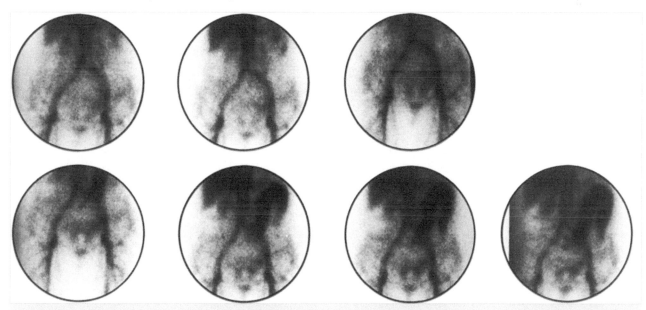

Fig. 3.16 ^{99m}Tc-labeled red blood cell scan shows hyperactivity of the extravasated blood in left transverse colon and descending colon. (Courtesy of Michael McKusick, MD, Rochester, MN.)

has replaced red blood cell scanning in many institutions as it is more readily available and faster, and better localizes to site of bleeding.[35,45]

In addition to CT and MRI, several other procedures are used to detect intra-abdominal diseases. These include liver scintigraphy, ultrasonography, endorectal ultrasonography, positron emission tomography (PET), and radiolabeled antibody imaging.

Liver Scintigraphy

Scintigraphy is widely accepted as a valuable tool for detecting metastatic malignant disease in the liver. The liver scintiscan is obtained after an intravenous injection of ^{99m}Tc sulfur colloid, and the images are collected on nuclear medicine films. Detection of focal masses by this method depends on the lack of uptake of ^{99m}Tc sulfur colloid by the lesions (▶ Fig. 3.17). Most reports demonstrate a sensitivity of 80 to 85%, but a significant false-negative and false-positive rate of 15 to 25% has been observed.[98] Radionuclide scanning is inexpensive and relatively easy to perform, but it is nonspecific. The average size of a metastasis detected by radionuclide scintigraphy is 2 cm or larger. Also, most detectable lesions are peripherally located; a large lesion centrally located may not be detected.[98] A study by Tempero et al suggested that metastatic disease in the liver that causes no biochemical abnormalities may be too subtle or small to create focal changes on the liver scan.[99] For practical purposes, a liver scintiscan should be obtained only when the liver function tests are abnormal.[99] Liver scintiscan is largely replaced by CT.

Positron Emission Tomography

PET is a new method of imaging in which a positron-emitting isotope–labeled compound is used. In PET studies, functional images of colorectal neoplasms are obtained by taking advantage of the increase in anaerobic glycolysis that occurs in malignant cells. Fluorine-18 deoxyglucose (FDG), like glucose, is phosphorylated intracellularly. When injected intravenously, this substance is used by all cells with variable uptake, depending on cellular metabolism. Increased uptake of FDG has been noted in cases of colorectal carcinoma (▶ Fig. 3.18).[79,100] PET is

performed by injecting FDG intravenously. After 1 hour, emission imaging of the abdomen and pelvis is performed. The PET-FDG images are oriented into sagittal, coronal, and transverse views. Qualitative image analysis for the presence of hypermetabolic regions is performed for each of the views.[101] PET scanners are now available in most major metropolitan centers in the United States and PET use is expected to continue to grow despite the expensive equipment.[102] In a pilot study performed by Falk et al, metabolic imaging using PET-FDG appeared to be more sensitive and accurate than CT scanning in the preoperative detection of colorectal carcinoma.[101] PET-FDG can detect both locally recurrent and distant metastatic disease. It may detect additional metastatic disease not seen on CT scan.[103] It is particularly useful for detecting recurrence at the site of resection because CT scans

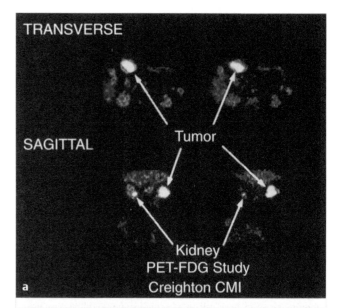
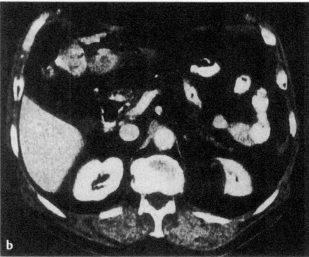

Fig. 3.18 (a) PET transverse and sagittal views detect a lesion in the hepatic flexure of the colon. Normal renal uptake seen. (b) The lesion visualized by PET was not detected on CT scan. CT, computed tomography; PET-FDG, positron emission tomography-fluorine-18 deoxyglucose.[101] (Reproduced with permission from © 1994 Wolters Kluwer.)

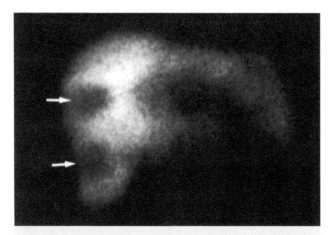

Fig. 3.17 Liver scintiscan showing multiple filling defects from metastasis (arrows).

often show postoperative changes that cannot be differentiated from recurrent carcinoma.[104]

A meta-analysis of 11 published studies showed that PET-FDG had an overall sensitivity for recurrent colorectal carcinoma of 97% and specificity of 76% and that PET-FDG findings led to clinical management changes in 29% of cases.[105] PET-FDG imaging is less sensitive in the assessment of mucinous carcinoma and neuroendocrine neoplasms of the GI tract. This is possibly related to the low metabolic rate of the malignancies. PET is limited by its poor sensitivity for detecting small lesions (<1 cm) and its inability to discriminate between lesions close to one another as well as between malignant necrotic lesions. False-positive lesions may be caused by inflammatory disease, especially granulomatous lesions, which can accumulate significant FDG because of activated macrophage.[105]

One of the important indications for PET-FDG is the rising carcinoembryonic antigen (CEA) and negative CT scans; PET scan detects recurrent disease in 68% of cases.[106] Flanagan et al[107] showed a positive-predictive value for PET of 85% and a negative-predictive value of 100%.

Another usefulness of PET is to follow patients after radiation therapy and after chemotherapy. However, immediately after radiation therapy, FDG uptake may be associated with inflammatory changes and not necessarily residual carcinoma for approximately 6 months.[62]

Radioimmunoscintigraphy

CT scanning and MRI are limited in their ability to detect the location and extent of metastatic disease, particularly extrahepatic metastases. They are unable to detect metastases in lymph nodes of normal size or <2 cm. Furthermore, they cannot distinguish between postoperative changes from scar tissue or postoperative radiation changes from recurrent carcinoma.

Radioimmunoscintigraphy (RIS) uses monoclonal antibody labeled with radionuclides such as [111]indium or [99m]technetium that produces gamma radiation detectable by a gamma camera. The antibody is targeted against antigen sites found on malignant cells, in this instance CEA. Hepatic metastasis may appear as areas of increased isotope activity or photopenic areas. CT is more accurate in the detection of hepatic metastasis.[108]

The major role of RIS is in the detection of metastatic disease. Numerous studies have reported on the usefulness of RIS in identifying pelvic recurrence.[109,110] Both RIS and PEI are useful in detecting occult disease and local recurrence. They offer an important adjuvant to conventional imaging.

3.3.8 Interventional Radiology

Arteriography

Since the introduction of percutaneous catheterization angiography by Seldinger in 1953, tremendous improvements in knowledge, technique, and equipment have been made.[111] Arteriography currently is available in more medical centers for the diagnosis and treatment of GI bleeding.

Bleeding from the colon can be massive and life threatening. At the present time, selective arteriography is the procedure of choice for massive ongoing bleeding. Not only is it highly successful in identifying the exact location of bleeding, but also it can be used to control bleeding with transcatheter emboli to occlude the bleeding vessel or infusion of vasopressin.[112]

Embolization

Refractory hemorrhage may require angiography and transcatheter intervention.[113] Noninvasive imaging such as CTA is useful for characterizing the bleeding source and confirming the presence of active hemorrhage before angiography. If a bleeding source is angiographically identified, superselective catheterization with embolization is typically effective in controlling hemorrhage while minimizing complications. The choice of embolic agent depends on the vascular anatomy, angiographic findings, achievable catheter position, and operator preference. The most common agents are metallic coils, polyvinyl alcohol, gelatin sponge and n-butyl cyanoacrylate. The embolization can be classified as localized (the bleeding point is superselected), proximal (embolization of the parent artery), and segmental (adjacent branch or branches are embolized).[114] With proximal embolization, recanalization of the bleeding point can occur due to distal backflow. With excessive segmental embolization, ischemic complications of the involved bowel can occur.

If embolization is not possible, a vasopressin (Pitressin) drip via a selective arteriographic catheter can control lower GI bleeding.[115] This infusion works by constricting the mesenteric vessels and contraction of the smooth muscle in the bowel wall, thus reducing the blood flow to the site of bleeding and inducing the formation of a stable clot at the bleeding site. Patients should be on continuous cardiac monitoring, since vasopressin can induce coronary vasoconstriction. Infusion is started at 0.1 units/min. Repeat angiography is performed after 20 minutes to ensure that bleeding has stopped and that the vessels are not overconstricted. If bleeding persists, the dose is increased to 0.2 units/min. Infusion is then increased to 0.4 units/min if bleeding persists. Excessive vasoconstriction can lead to bowel infarction. It is known to be effective in patients with microcatheter-inaccessible bleeding or diffuse bleeding (such as hemorrhagic gastritis). However, disadvantages include the rate of rebleeding after discontinuation of the infusion, cardiovascular complications, and the difficulty in maintaining a selective catheter position. In one study, the success rate of 52% for vasopressin was inferior to that of 88% for embolization in major GI bleeding.[116]

Barium enema studies and colonoscopy should not be used in the patient with acute life-threatening bleeding. Barium may obscure the extravasation of contrast medium and must not be used before arteriography. However, once the bleeding has slowed or stopped, the entire large bowel should be examined by colonoscopy. A "blind subtotal colectomy" will not solve the problem if the bleeding site is not in the resected segment.[117] A vigorous attempt should be made to find the precise anatomic site of the bleeding; also, one must not overlook bleeding from the anorectum, which can be verified by proctoscopy or anoscopy.

To be successful in identifying the site of the bleeding, selective arteriography of appropriate vessels is required. Bleeding from the small intestine and the ascending and transverse colon is studied by superior mesenteric arteriography. Bleeding from the descending colon, sigmoid, and rectum is evaluated by inferior mesenteric arteriography. A bleeding aortoenteric fistula is the only type of GI bleeding for which selective arteriography is not appropriate; rather, aortography is needed. Selective arteriography is indicated only if there is continued evidence of bleeding. The rate of bleeding necessary to permit detection by arteriography is at least 0.5 mL/min. Clinically, if a patient requires 500 mL of blood transfusions every 8 hours (1 mL/min) to maintain hemodynamic stability, then selective arteriography is indicated.[115]

Arteriography is an invasive procedure, but the advantages outweigh the risks. In experienced hands and with proper application, arteriography has a small incidence of complications. Fatal complications have been reported in < 0.1% of cases. Major complications such as hematomas, infection, false aneurysms, and arterial thromboses occur in 0.7 to 1.7% of cases and for the most part are localized to the arterial puncture site. Minor complications occur in approximately 5% of cases, and most represent puncture-site hematomas.[115]

Percutaneous Abscess Drainage

Percutaneous abscess drainage (PAD) has virtually eliminated the morbidity and mortality associated with surgical exploration. CT is the most appropriate modality in image-guided PAD.[118] PAD of an intra-abdominal abscess is effective with a single treatment in 70% of patients and this increases to 82% if a second drainage is performed.[119] The overall findings from a large series of 2,311 PADs report a success rate of 80 to 85%.[120] Complication rates of PAD are between none and 10%. Vascular laceration may occur and, if the vessel is small, the bleeding will usually stop spontaneously.[121] PAD may be complicated by bowel perforation from the needle or catheter traversing the bowel. If the patient develops signs of peritonitis after catheter penetration of bowel, then surgical intervention may be required.

Image-Guided Percutaneous Biopsy

The majority of image-guided biopsies can be performed on an outpatient basis. All interventional procedures can result in bleeding, but this complication can be reduced by correction of any coagulopathy before the procedure.[122] Ultrasonography offers the advantages of real-time needle visualization, low cost, portability, and no ionizing radiation. Ultrasonography guidance can be problematic in obese patients because the echogenic needle can be hard to visualize in echogenic fat. Lesions located deep to bone or bowel cannot be biopsied with ultrasound owing to lack of visualization of the lesion. CT can be used to guide biopsy needles to virtually any area of the body. CT provides excellent visualization of lesions and allows accurate identification of organs between the skin and the lesion.[123] Disadvantages of CT include increased cost, ionizing radiation, and longer procedure times. Complications of abdominal, liver, or lung biopsy include bleeding, introducing infection, pneumothorax, and hemoptysis. Postprocedure pneumothorax may occasionally require chest tube placement and observation in the hospital.[124,125]

Radiofrequency Ablation and Chemoembolization of Hepatic Metastasis

Radiofrequency ablations (RFAs) of liver metastasis are performed similarly to image-guided needle biopsy, with the RF probe taking the place of the needle. The RF probe is placed in the hepatic tumor and vibrates at a high frequency, conducting heat into and ablating the tumor.[124] Studies show that the overall 5-year survival rate for colorectal liver metastasis treated by RF ablation is similar to surgical series (25–40%).[126] There are no absolute contraindications, and relative contraindications include low platelets and coagulopathy. RFA of hepatic tumors is associated with very low complication rates, generally below 2%. Complications include pain, pleural effusion, bleeding, and abscess formation.[124]

The treatment of certain tumors (metastatic hepatic lesions) with intravascular delivery of chemotherapeutic agents can be palliative and prolong life, but it is not considered curative.[126] A wide variety of chemotherapeutic regimens are used. These chemotherapeutic medications are usually mixed with an embolic agent that slows flow and allows the drugs to remain in the organ. Metastatic disease to the liver can also be embolized by yttrium-loaded microspheres that emit beta-radiation. Fulminant hepatic failure or liver abscess formation occurs in less than 1% of patients. Gallbladder infarction due to chemoembolization is rare.[126]

3.4 Diagnostic Procedures

3.4.1 Capsule Endoscopy

This is a diagnostic tool to image the entire small bowel. The imaging system consists of a single-use capsule endoscope. Although the capsule measures only 11 × 26 mm, it packs a color camera, light sources, a radio transmitter, and batteries. The patient swallows the capsule, and relies on peristalsis to advance it through the digestive tract. The system allows 5 hours of continuous recording and can be performed on an outpatient basis.[127] In a report by Appleyard et al[128] on four patients with recurrent small bowel bleeding, capsule endoscopy identified angiodysplasias in the stomach and small bowel. All four patients described the capsule as easy to swallow, painless, and preferable to conventional endoscopy.

Selby evaluated 42 patients (24 men, 18 women) who had GI bleeding of obscure origin, and 50 patients (25 men, 25 women) who had anemia alone.[129] Clinical and other data were collected prospectively. Patients had at least upper endoscopy and colonoscopy, which were negative, and were referred for capsule endoscopy. The results showed a definite or probable cause of GI blood loss in 60 of 92 patients (65%). The nature of the abnormality was similar between those who presented with overt bleeding and those with anemia. The majority were angiodysplasia (47 of 60), 45 of which were in the small intestine; the most common site was the jejunum (40 patients). Seven patients had small bowel neoplasms, five presented with anemia alone, and two presented with overt bleeding. Three patients had ulcers in the small intestine (two Crohn's, one anastomotic ulcers). One patient had radiation enteritis with active bleeding.

Two patients had gastric antral vascular ectasia, a finding not identified at prior endoscopies. Given its diagnostic superiority for examination of the small intestine, capsule endoscopy should be used as the next investigation after a nondiagnostic endoscopy and a colonoscopy in patients with GI bleeding of obscure origin. Capsule endoscopy is complementary to other exams such as double-balloon enteroscopy.[130,131]

3.4.2 Double-Balloon Enteroscopy

Double-balloon enteroscopy, also known as push-and-pull enteroscopy, is an endoscopic technique for visualization of the small bowel. The technique involves the use of a balloon at the end of a special enteroscope camera and an overtube, which is also fitted with a balloon.[132] The procedure is usually done under general anesthesia, but may be done with the use of conscious sedation.[133] The enteroscope and overtube are inserted through the mouth and passed in conventional fashion (that is, as with gastroscopy) into the small bowel.[134]

Following this, the endoscope is advanced a small distance in front of the overtube and the balloon at the end is inflated. Using the assistance of friction at the interface of the enteroscope and intestinal wall, the small bowel is accordioned back to the overtube. The overtube balloon is then deployed, and the enteroscope balloon is deflated. The process is then continued until the entire small bowel is visualized.[135] The double-balloon enteroscope can also be passed in retrograde fashion, through the colon and into the ileum to visualize the end of the small bowel.

Double-balloon enteroscopy offers a number of advantages to other small bowel image techniques, including barium imaging, wireless capsule endoscopy, and push enteroscopy: it allows for visualization of the entire small bowel to the terminal ileum, it allows for the application of therapeutics, it allows for the sampling or biopsying of small bowel mucosa, for the resection of polyps of the small bowel, and in the placement of stents or dilatation of strictures of the small bowel, and it allows for access to the papilla in patients with long afferent limbs after Billroth II antrectomy.[136,137]

The key disadvantage of double-balloon enteroscopy is the time required to visualize the small bowel; this can exceed 3 hours, and may require that patients be admitted to hospital for the procedure.[138] There have also been case reports of acute pancreatitis and intestinal necrosis associated with the technique.[139,140]

3.5 Examination of Stool

3.5.1 Guaiac Test

Hemoccult is a commercial guaiac-impregnated filter paper used to detect occult blood in the stool (fecal occult blood test [FOBT]). It has good sensitivity, but poor specificity. The test can be done at home by smearing stool on the paper slides provided. Basically, the test detects peroxidase in the hemoglobin; after application of a reagent, the chemically impregnated filter paper will turn blue. The reason the Hemoccult test is not specific is that many foods also contain peroxidase (raw meat, pheasant, salmon, sardines, turnips, radishes, cherry tomatoes,

and many fruits and vegetables).[141,142] These foods may cause a false-positive result. Vitamin C is known to give a false-negative test, whereas iron and aspirin give false-positive results.[143] During the time of stool collection, these factors must be avoided. A restricted diet is recommended for 2 to 3 days before the test and should be continued during the test. At the present time, Hemoccult II and the more sensitive Hemoccult II Sensa are available. The sensitivity of the Hemoccult test varies from series to series. In the series of Allison et al,[144] the sensitivity of Hemoccult II was 37% compared with a sensitivity of 79% for Hemoccult II Sensa.

3.5.2 Heme-Porphyrin Assays

HemoQuant, which differs from Hemoccult, is a newer test for occult fecal blood. It removes the iron from hemoglobin heme and measures the fluorescence of the derived porphyrin.[145] Although pseudoperoxidase activity does not affect the assay, a strict diet in which nonhuman heme is excluded is essential.[146] The HemoQuant test is quantitative. It measures both degraded and intact hemoglobin, in contrast to a guaiac test. It is more sensitive than the Hemoccult test.[147] HemoQuant has not been widely used for fecal occult blood screening because of its complex processing.

3.5.3 Fecal Immunologic Test

The fecal immunochemical test (FIT), also called an *immunochemical fecal occult blood test* (iFOBT), is an immunologic test based on antihuman hemoglobin. It is specific to human hemoglobin and therefore avoids the problems of dietary interference. The likelihood of false-positive results from upper GI blood loss is also reduced, because the immunoreactive hemoglobin is rapidly degraded before it reaches the large bowel.[146] Only one to two stool samples are required, but as the test requires more lab time, it is more expensive than traditional FOBT. A number of tests are currently available in the United States. Some are quantitative, while others are qualitative.[148] Few have been compared head to head, and reviewing the limited data available, none have been shown to be superior. A systemic review and meta-analysis in 2014 reviewed 19 studies and found a sensitivity of 79%, a specificity of 94%, and an accuracy of 95%.[148] The current available tests include Cologuard (Exact Sciences, Madison, WI), HemeSelect (SmithKline Diagnostics, Inc., San Jose, CA), *OC-Micro/ Sensor* (Eiken Chemical), and *OC-Light* (Polymedco). Several countries in Europe and Asia have adopted widespread colon and rectal surgery (CRS) screening programs using FIT. Patient compliance with FIT appears to be better than FOBT and has a high diagnostic yield.[149,150] However, it lacks a therapeutic option, and in the United States, colonoscopy remains the primary screening modality.

3.5.4 Stool DNA

Fecal (stool) DNA tests have been under development over the past several years.[151] These tests are designed to detect in stool samples any number of DNA markers shown to be associated with colorectal cancer. ColoSure (Laboratory Corporation of America, http://www.labcorp.com) is currently the only commercially or clinically available fecal DNA test marketed for CRC screening in the United States. The at-home test requires that patients collect and mail one whole stool sample. ColoSure is a single-marker test that detects methylation of the vimentin gene. Increased DNA methylation in the promoter region of genes is an epigenetic change that is common in human cancers, including colorectal cancer.[152] Vimentin is a protein characteristically expressed in cells of mesenchymal origin, such as fibroblasts, macrophages, smooth muscle cells, and endothelial cells. Studies have demonstrated that the vimentin gene is not (or rarely) methylated in normal colonic epithelial cells, but is methylated in colorectal cancer and adenomas.[153] Aberrant methylation of vimentin has been detected in 53 to 83% of colorectal cancer tissue, 50 to 84% of adenoma samples, and 0 to 11% of normal colon tissue samples, though one preliminary study detected methylated vimentin in 29% of normal colon tissue.[154] ColoSure requires a prescription for testing. It is currently available from two sources: LabCorp and from DNA Direct's Genomic Medicine Institutes (which only offers referrals to physicians who can prescribe the test).

In order to consider integrating fecal DNA testing into current CRC screening strategies, additional research is needed to establish analytic validity, clinical validity, and clinical utility within the general (average-risk) population. The estimates of DNA marker sensitivity and specificity found from small case–control studies should not be extrapolated to make any estimates of the performance of methylated vimentin or ColoSure in the general population.

In addition, the ongoing development and refinement of stool DNA tests presents some difficulty for the integration of these tests as a CRC screening approach. Currently, only one fecal DNA test is commercially available in the United States, a test that will likely be replaced by a newer version for which FDA approval will be sought.

Other critical matters must also be addressed, including the determination of cost-effectiveness, optimal testing intervals, and strategies for the follow-up evaluation of patients who test positive on a fecal DNA test. The clinical validity of methylated vimentin as a biomarker for CRC screening remains to be determined in a general (average-risk) screening population. Moreover, the willingness of individuals from the general population to adopt fecal DNA test protocols and future screening recommendations is a vital consideration. All of these factors will be crucial in affecting the impact of fecal DNA testing on the overall CRC screening paradigm and on colorectal cancer incidence and mortality.

3.5.5 Diarrheal Stool Examination

Examination of the feces in diarrhea, especially in the acute phase, often gives clues to the underlying disease.

Wet-Mount Examination

Wet-mount examination of diarrheal stool stained with Wright's stain or methylene blue is a rapid and reliable procedure for aiding in the early diagnosis of the cause of diarrhea. A large number of white blood cells suggest inflammation. In acute or traveler's diarrhea, pus in the stool suggests invasion of the large bowel mucosa by bacteria, such as invasive *Escherichia coli*, *Entamoeba histolytica*, *Shigella*, *Salmonella*, *Campylobacter*, gonococci, and other invasive organisms.[155,156,157] Diarrhea caused by noninvasive organisms that produce enterotoxin by viruses and by *Giardia lamblia* is not associated with pus in the stool. Simple Gram staining of direct stool smears frequently can provide an accurate and rapid diagnosis of enteritis caused by *Campylobacter* bacteria. Typically, a vibrio-shaped gram-negative organism is seen.[158] In some health centers, acute diarrhea with wet-mount evidence of fecal leukocytes and darting forms has become pathognomonic of *Campylobacter* enteritis.[157]

Examination of a wet-mount or a stained smear of stool usually is adequate for detecting ova, cysts, or trophozoites of parasites. Because most parasites are passed intermittently with variable numbers into the stool, examining three specimens collected at intervals of 2 to 3 days will improve the yield substantially. Collected intestinal aspirates or soft-to-watery fecal specimens should immediately be placed in a preservative, such as polyvinyl alcohol, to prevent rapid disintegration of fragile protozoan trophozoites and to allow the preparation of permanently stained smears. Protozoan cysts and helminthic ova in formed stool will survive for 1 to 2 days at room temperature and indefinitely if placed in 5% formaldehyde.

The presence of *Candida* organisms in feces of persons with no underlying disease invariably has been considered nonpathogenic. However, *Candida* proliferation in the GI tract may be responsible for diarrhea. The common presentation is multiple loose or watery bowel movements without blood or mucus, but sometimes associated with abdominal cramps, and lasting as long as 3 months. Direct microscopic examination of stool, suspended in saline or iodine solutions, gives precise information. Yeast forms with budding and often mycelial forms are predominant. Once the condition has been diagnosed, antifungal therapy gives a rapid resolution.[159]

Stool Cultures

A stool culture should be obtained in patients with acute and severe diarrhea to determine the common infectious diseases. *Campylobacter* bacteria require a selective isolation medium containing antibiotics, and the plates are grown at 43 °C under carbon dioxide or reduced oxygen condition. *Yersinia* is an important intestinal pathogen that causes a spectrum of severe illness. It requires a special culture condition for its isolation.[160,161] The laboratory must be informed of the suspicion of this organism. Gonococci require Thayer–Martin medium for the culture.

The preferred method of establishing the diagnosis of colitis caused by *Clostridium difficile* is the detection of enzyme immunoarrays for the presence of toxin A and/or B in the stool. The specificity of these tests is very high but false-negative results are not uncommon.[162] Although tissue culture assay is accurate and specific, its use may pose a problem to centers where the testing facilities are not available.

Examination for Steatorrhea

Most patients with clinically relevant malabsorption have steatorrhea. Consequently, documentation of steatorrhea is important and is the cornerstone of diagnostic evaluation.

Steatorrhea is defined as excretion in the stool of > 7% of ingested fat.[163] Steatorrheic stool is bulky and has a grayish cast or silvery sheen. It may have a soft, sticky consistency with a rancid odor; it may be liquid, frothy, and notable for floating oil droplets. However, steatorrheal stool also may be formed and may appear to be normal.[164]

Microscopic examination of the stool for excessive fat has been shown to be a rapid, inexpensive, sensitive, and specific screening test for steatorrhea and pancreatic insufficiency. To detect neutral fat, the stool is stained with Sudan III in 80% alcohol and is examined microscopically. The test is termed positive when 10 or more orange-colored globules that are 10 mm in size are present. To detect split fat, 36% acetic acid is added to the stool along with Sudan III, heated until boiling to melt fatty acid crystals, and then examined under the microscope while still warm. The result is positive if 10 or more orange-colored globules that are 20 mm in size or larger are present.

The only truly reliable means of documenting steatorrhea is with quantitative chemical analysis of fat in a 72-hour stool collection while the patient is ingesting a high-fat diet (at least 100 g/day). On such a diet, normal subjects excrete < 7 g of fat/day (coefficient of absorption of > 93%). Unfortunately, the quantitative fecal fat determination is cumbersome to perform and difficult to obtain in most hospitals. Furthermore, the documentation of steatorrhea indicates only that the patient has the malabsorption syndrome. It does not indicate pathophysiology or confer a specific diagnosis.[156]

The breath test is a more recent approach to the diagnosis of fat malabsorption. This test is based on the measurement of $^{14}CO_2$ in expired air following the ingestion of various ^{14}C-labeled triglycerides (triolein, tripalmitin, and trioctanoin). Steatorrhea from either pancreatic insufficiency or other causes results in a decreased absorption of triglycerides by the digestive system. This in turn results in a decrease in expired CO_2 derived from metabolism of triglyceride fatty acids.[165]

References

[1] Fijten GH, Blijham GH, Knottnerus JA. Occurrence and clinical significance of overt blood loss per rectum in the general population and in medical practice. Br J Gen Pract. 1994; 44(384):320–325

[2] Martelli H, Devroede G, Arhan P, Duguay C. Mechanisms of idiopathic constipation: outlet obstruction. Gastroenterology. 1978; 75(4):623–631

[3] Bartolo DCC. Pelvic floor disorders: incontinence, constipation, and obstructed defecation. Perspect Colon Rectal Surg. 1988; 1(1):1–24

[4] Levitt MD. Intestinal gas production–recent advances in flatology. N Engl J Med. 1980; 302(26):1474–1475

[5] Fearon KCH, Carter DC. Cancer cachexia. Ann Surg. 1988; 208(1):1–5

[6] Slattery ML, Kerber RA. Family history of cancer and colon cancer risk: the Utah Population Database. J Natl Cancer Inst. 1994; 86(21):1618–1626

[7] St John DJB, McDermott FT, Hopper JL, Debney EA, Johnson WRB, Hughes ESR. Cancer risk in relatives of patients with common colorectal cancer. Ann Intern Med. 1993; 118(10):785–790

[8] Winawer SJ, Zauber AG, Gerdes H, et al. National Polyp Study Workgroup. Risk of colorectal cancer in the families of patients with adenomatous polyps. N Engl J Med. 1996; 334(2):82–87

[9] Nivatvongs S, Goldberg SM. An improved technique of rubber band ligation of hemorrhoids. Am J Surg. 1982; 144(3):378–380

[10] Waye JD. Techniques of polypectomy: hot biopsy forceps and snare polypectomy. Am J Gastroenterol. 1987; 82(7):615–618

[11] Nivatvongs S, Fang DT, Kennedy HL. The shape of the buttocks. A useful guide for selection of anesthesia and patient position in anorectal surgery. Dis Colon Rectum. 1983; 26(2):85–86

[12] Oettle GJ, Roe AM, Bartolo DCC, Mortensen NJ. What is the best way of measuring perineal descent? A comparison of radiographic and clinical methods. Br J Surg. 1985; 72(12):999–1001

[13] Porter NH. A physiological study of the pelvic floor in rectal prolapse. Ann R Coll Surg Engl. 1962; 31:379–404

[14] Sullivan ES, Corman ML, Devroede G, Rudd WW, Schuster MM. Symposium: anal incontinence. Dis Colon Rectum. 1982; 25(2):90–107

[15] Nivatvongs S, Fryd DS. How far does the proctosigmoidoscope reach? A prospective study of 1000 patients. N Engl J Med. 1980; 303(7):380–382

[16] Lehman GA, Buchner DM, Lappas JC. Anatomical extent of fiberoptic sigmoidoscopy. Gastroenterology. 1983; 84(4):803–808

[17] Ott DJ, Wu WC, Gelfand DW. Extent of colonic visualization with the fiberoptic sigmoidoscope. J Clin Gastroenterol. 1982; 4(4):337–341

[18] Marks G, Boggs HW, Castro AF, Gathright JB, Ray JE, Salvati E. Sigmoidoscopic examinations with rigid and flexible fiberoptic sigmoidoscopes in the surgeon's office: a comparative prospective study of effectiveness in 1,012 cases. Dis Colon Rectum. 1979; 22(3):162–168

[19] Winnan G, Berci G, Panish J, Talbot TM, Overholt BF, McCallum RW. Superiority of the flexible to the rigid sigmoidoscope in routine proctosigmoidoscopy. N Engl J Med. 1980; 302(18):1011–1012

[20] Traul DG, Davis CB, Pollock JC, Scudamore HH. Flexible fiberoptic sigmoidoscopy–the Monroe Clinic experience. A prospective study of 5000 examinations. Dis Colon Rectum. 1983; 26(3):161–166

[21] Farrands PA, Vellacott KD, Amar SS, Balfour TW, Hardcastle JD. Flexible fiberoptic sigmoidoscopy and double-contrast barium-enema examination in the identification of adenomas and carcinoma of the colon. Dis Colon Rectum. 1983; 26(11):725–727

[22] Chew CN, Nolan DJ, Jewell DP. Small bowel gas in severe ulcerative colitis. Gut. 1991; 32(12):1535–1537

[23] Hau T, Ahrenholz DH, Simmons RL. Secondary bacterial peritonitis: the biologic basis of treatment. Curr Probl Surg. 1979; 16(10):1–65

[24] Isikoff MB, Guter M. Dagnostic imaging of the upper part of the abdomen. Surg Gynecol Obstet. 1979; 149(2):161–167

[25] Taourel P, Pradel J, Fabre J-M, Cover S, Senéterre E, Bruel J-M. Role of CT in the acute nontraumatic abdomen. Semin Ultrasound CT MR. 1995; 16(2):151–164

[26] Ha HK. CT in the early detection of strangulation in intestinal obstruction. Semin Ultrasound CT MR. 1995; 16(2):141–150

[27] Bernini A, Spencer MP, Wong WD, Rothenberger DA, Madoff RD. Computed tomography-guided percutaneous abscess drainage in intestinal disease: factors associated with outcome. Dis Colon Rectum. 1997; 40(9):1009–1013

[28] Gore RM, Moss AA, Margulis AR. The assessment of abdominal and pelvic neoplasia: the impact of CT. Curr Probl Surg. 1982; 19(9):493–552

[29] Thoeni RF, Rogalla P. CT for the evaluation of carcinomas in the colon and rectum. Semin Ultrasound CT MR. 1995; 16(2):112–126

[30] Beasley HS. MR and CT imaging of intraabdominal spread of colorectal cancer. Semin Colon Rectal Surg. 2002; 13:105–118

[31] Amberg JR. Complications of colon radiography. Gastrointest Endosc. 1980; 26(2) Suppl:15S–17S

[32] Smith TJ, Kemeny MM, Sugarbaker PH, et al. A prospective study of hepatic imaging in the detection of metastatic disease. Ann Surg. 1982; 195(4):486–491

[33] Wu LM, Xu JR, Yin Y, Qu XH. Usefulness of CT angiography in diagnosing acute gastrointestinal bleeding: a meta-analysis. World J Gastroenterol. 2010; 16(31):3957–3963

[34] Dobritz M, Engels HP, Schneider A, et al. Evaluation of dual-phase multi-detector-row CT for detection of intestinal bleeding using an experimental bowel model. Eur Radiol. 2009; 19(4):875–881

[35] Martí M, Artigas JM, Garzón G, Álvarez-Sala R, Soto JA. Acute lower intestinal bleeding: feasibility and diagnostic performance of CT angiography. Radiology. 2012; 262(1):109–116

[36] Jaeckle T, Stuber G, Hoffmann MH, Jeltsch M, Schmitz BL, Aschoff AJ. Detection and localization of acute upper and lower gastrointestinal (GI) bleeding with arterial phase multi-detector row helical CT. Eur Radiol. 2008; 18(7):1406–1413

[37] Anthony S, Milburn S, Uberoi R. Multi-detector CT: review of its use in acute GI haemorrhage. Clin Radiol. 2007; 62(10):938–949

[38] Yoon W, Jeong YY, Shin SS, et al. Acute massive gastrointestinal bleeding: detection and localization with arterial phase multi-detector row helical CT. Radiology. 2006; 239(1):160–167

[39] Kennedy DW, Laing CJ, Tseng LH, Rosenblum DI, Tamarkin SW. Detection of active gastrointestinal hemorrhage with CT angiography: a 4(1/2)-year retrospective review. J Vasc Interv Radiol. 2010; 21(6):848–855

[40] Jaeckle T, Stuber G, Hoffmann MH, Freund W, Schmitz BL, Aschoff AJ. Acute gastrointestinal bleeding: value of MDCT. Abdom Imaging. 2008; 33 (3):285–293

[41] Horton KM, Jeffrey RB, Jr, Federle MP, Fishman EK. Acute gastrointestinal bleeding: the potential role of 64 MDCT and 3D imaging in the diagnosis. Emerg Radiol. 2009; 16(5):349–356

[42] Scheffel H, Pfammatter T, Wildi S, Bauerfeind P, Marincek B, Alkadhi H. Acute gastrointestinal bleeding: detection of source and etiology with multi-detector-row CT. Eur Radiol. 2007; 17(6):1555–1565

[43] Ernst O, Bulois P, Saint-Drenant S, Leroy C, Paris JC, Sergent G. Helical CT in acute lower gastrointestinal bleeding. Eur Radiol. 2003; 13(1):114–117

[44] Zink SI, Ohki SK, Stein B, et al. Noninvasive evaluation of active lower gastrointestinal bleeding: comparison between contrast-enhanced MDCT and 99mTc-labeled RBC scintigraphy. AJR Am J Roentgenol. 2008; 191 (4):1107–1114

[45] Jacovides CL, Nadolski G, Allen SR, et al. Arteriography for lower gastrointestinal hemorrhage: role of preceding abdominal computed tomographic angiogram in diagnosis and localization. JAMA Surg. 2015; 150(7):650–656

[46] Hara AK, Johnson CD, Reed JE, et al. Detection of colorectal polyps by computed tomographic colography: feasibility of a novel technique. Gastroenterology. 1996; 110(1):284–290

[47] Vining DJ. Virtual colonoscopy. Gastrointest Endosc Clin N Am. 1997; 7 (2):285–291

[48] Rex DK. Barium studies/virtual colonoscopy: the gastroenterologist's perspective. Gastrointest Endosc. 2002; 55(7) Suppl:S33–S36, discussion S36

[49] Pickhardt PJ, Choi JR, Hwang I, et al. Computed tomographic virtual colonoscopy to screen for colorectal neoplasia in asymptomatic adults. N Engl J Med. 2003; 349(23):2191–2200

[50] Pineau BC, Paskett ED, Chen GJ, et al. Virtual colonoscopy using oral contrast compared with colonoscopy for the detection of patients with colorectal polyps. Gastroenterology. 2003; 125(2):304–310

[51] Cotton PB, Durkalski VL, Pineau BC, et al. Computed tomographic colonography (virtual colonoscopy): a multicenter comparison with standard colonoscopy for detection of colorectal neoplasia. JAMA. 2004; 291(14):1713–1719

[52] Johnson CD, Harmsen WS, Wilson LA, et al. Prospective blinded evaluation of computed tomographic colonography for screen detection of colorectal polyps. Gastroenterology. 2003; 125(2):311–319

[53] van Dam J, Cotton P, Johnson CD, et al. American Gastroenterological Association. AGA future trends report: CT colonography. Gastroenterology. 2004; 127(3):970–984

[54] Rex DK. Is virtual colonoscopy ready for widespread application? Gastroenterology. 2003; 125(2):608–610

[55] Warden MJ, Petrelli NJ, Herrera L, Mittelman A. Endoscopy versus double-contrast barium enema in the evaluation of patients with symptoms suggestive of colorectal carcinoma. Am J Surg. 1988; 155(2):224–226

[56] Kelvin FM. Radiologic approach to the detection of colorectal neoplasia. Radiol Clin North Am. 1982; 20(4):743–759

[57] de Roos A, Hermans J, Shaw PC, Kroon H. Colon polyps and carcinomas: prospective comparison of the single- and double-contrast examination in the same patients. Radiology. 1985; 154(1):11–13

[58] Young J. The double contrast barium enema: why bother? South Med J. 1982; 75(1):46–55

[59] Miller RE. Detection of colon carcinoma and the barium enema. JAMA. 1974; 230(8):1195–1198

[60] Merrill CR, Steiner GM. Barium enema after biopsy: current practice and opinion. Clin Radiol. 1986; 37(1):89–92

[61] Maglinte DD, Strong RC, Strate RW, et al. Barium enema after colorectal biopsies: experimental data. AJR Am J Roentgenol. 1982; 139(4):693–697

[62] Shorthouse AJ, Bartram CI, Eyers AA, Thomson JP. The water soluble contrast enema after rectal anastomosis. Br J Surg. 1982; 69(12):714–717

[63] Ott DJ, Gelfand DW. Gastrointestinal contrast agents. Indications, uses, and risks. JAMA. 1983; 249(17):2380–2384

[64] Gallitano AL, Kondi ES, Phillips E, Ferris E. Near-fatal hemorrhage following gastrografin studies. Radiology. 1976; 118(1):35–36

[65] Lutzger LG, Factor SM. Effects of some water-soluble contrast media on the colonic mucosa. Radiology. 1976; 118(3):545–548

[66] Feigin E, Seror D, Szold A, et al. Water-soluble contrast material has no therapeutic effect on postoperative small-bowel obstruction: results of a prospective, randomized clinical trial. Am J Surg. 1996; 171(2):227–229

[67] Bolin S, Franzén L, Nilsson E, Sjödahl R. Carcinoma of the colon and rectum. Tumors missed by radiologic examination in 61 patients. Cancer. 1988; 61 (10):1999–2008

[68] Reiertsen O, Bakka A, Trønnes S, Gauperaa T. Routine double contrast barium enema and fiberoptic colonoscopy in the diagnosis of colorectal carcinoma. Acta Chir Scand. 1988; 154(1):53–55

[69] Irvine EJ, O'Connor J, Frost RA, et al. Prospective comparison of double contrast barium enema plus flexible sigmoidoscopy v colonoscopy in rectal bleeding: barium enema v colonoscopy in rectal bleeding. Gut. 1988; 29 (9):1188–1193

[70] Rex DK, Mark D, Clarke B, Lappas JC, Lehman GA. Flexible sigmoidoscopy plus air-contrast barium enema versus colonoscopy for evaluation of symptomatic patients without evidence of bleeding. Gastrointest Endosc. 1995; 42(2):132–138

[71] Peel AL, Benyon L, Grace RH. The value of routine preoperative urological assessment in patients undergoing elective surgery for diverticular disease or carcinoma of the large bowel. Br J Surg. 1980; 67(1):42–45

[72] Phillips R, Hittinger R, Saunders V, Blesovsky L, Stewart-Brown S, Fielding P. Preoperative urography in large bowel cancer: a useless investigation? Br J Surg. 1983; 70(7):425–427

[73] Madowitz JS, Schweiger MJ. Severe anaphylactoid reaction to radiographic contrast media. Recurrences despites premedication with diphenhydramine and prednisone. JAMA. 1979; 241(26):2813–2815

[74] Siminovitch JM, Fazio VW. Ureteral obstruction secondary to Crohn's disease: a need for ureterolysis? Am J Surg. 1980; 139(1):95–98

[75] Abcarian H, Udezue N. Coloenteric fistulas. Dis Colon Rectum. 1978; 21 (4):281–286

[76] Alexander-Williams J, Irving M. Intestinal Fistulas. Bristol: John Wright & Sons; 1982:60–61

[77] Grace RH, Hale M, Mackie G, Marks CG, Bloomberg TJ, Walker WJ. Role of ultrasound in the diagnosis of liver metastases before surgery for large bowel cancer. Br J Surg. 1987; 74(6):480–481

[78] Mueller PR, Simeone JF. Intraabdominal abscesses. Diagnosis by sonography and computed tomography. Radiol Clin North Am. 1983; 21(3):425–443

[79] Tempero M, Brand R, Holdeman K, Matamoros A. New imaging techniques in colorectal cancer. Semin Oncol. 1995; 22(5):448–471

[80] Wild JJ, Reid JM. Diagnostic use of ultrasound. Br J Phys Med. 1956; 19 (11):248–257, passim

[81] Hildebrandt U, Feifel G, Schwarz HP, Scherr O. Endorectal ultrasound: instrumentation and clinical aspects. Int J Colorectal Dis. 1986; 1(4):203–207

[82] Thaler W, Watzka S, Martin F, et al. Preoperative staging of rectal cancer by endoluminal ultrasound vs. magnetic resonance imaging. Preliminary results of a prospective, comparative study. Dis Colon Rectum. 1994; 37 (12):1189–1193

[83] Wong WD, Orrom WJ, Jensen LL. Preoperative staging of rectal cancer with endorectal ultrasonography. Perspect Colon Rectal Surg. 1990; 3:315–334

[84] Harewood GC, Wiersema MJ, Nelson H, et al. A prospective, blinded assessment of the impact of preoperative staging on the management of rectal cancer. Gastroenterology. 2002; 123(1):24–32

[85] Yoshida M, Tsukamoto Y, Niwa Y, et al. Endoscopic assessment of invasion of colorectal tumors with a new high-frequency ultrasound probe. Gastrointest Endosc. 1995; 41(6):587–592

[86] de Anda EH, Lee SH, Finne CO, Rothenberger DA, Madoff RD, Garcia-Aguilar J. Endorectal ultrasound in the follow-up of rectal cancer patients treated by local excision or radical surgery. Dis Colon Rectum. 2004; 47(6):818–824

[87] Lund JA, Sundstrom SH, Haaverstad R, Wibe A, Svinsaas M, Myrvold HE. Endoanal ultrasound is of little value in follow-up of anal carcinomas. Dis Colon Rectum. 2004; 47(6):839–842

[88] Gold DM, Halligan S, Kmiot WA, Bartram CI. Intraobserver and interobserver agreement in anal endosonography. Br J Surg. 1999; 86(3):371–375

[89] Cheong DMO, Nogueras JJ, Wexner SD, Jagelman DG. Anal endosonography for recurrent anal fistulas: image enhancement with hydrogen peroxide. Dis Colon Rectum. 1993; 36(12):1158–1160

[90] Hadfield MB, Nicholson AA, MacDonald AW, et al. Preoperative staging of rectal carcinoma by magnetic resonance imaging with a pelvic phased-array coil. Br J Surg. 1997; 84(4):529–531

[91] Lunniss PJ, Barker PG, Sultan AH, et al. Magnetic resonance imaging of fistula-in-ano. Dis Colon Rectum. 1994; 37(7):708–718

[92] dePrisco G. MRI local staging and restaging in rectal cancer. Clin Colon Rectal Surg. 2015; 28(3):194–200

[93] Gollub MJ, Maas M, Weiser M, et al. Recognition of the anterior peritoneal reflection at rectal MRI. AJR Am J Roentgenol. 2013; 200(1):97–101

[94] Owen CA, Jr, Cooper M, Grindlay JH, Bollman JL. Quantitative measurement of bleeding from alimentary tract by use of radiochromium-labeled erythrocytes. Surg Forum. 1955; 5:663–667

[95] Alavi A. Detection of gastrointestinal bleeding with 99mTc-sulfur colloid. Semin Nucl Med. 1982; 12(2):126–138

[96] Markisz JA, Front D, Royal HD, Sacks B, Parker JA, Kolodny GM. An evaluation of 99mTc-labeled red blood cell scintigraphy for the detection and localization of gastrointestinal bleeding sites. Gastroenterology. 1982; 83 (2):394–398

[97] Winzelberg GG, McKusick KA, Froelich JW, Callahan RJ, Strauss HW. Detection of gastrointestinal bleeding with 99mTc-labeled red blood cells. Semin Nucl Med. 1982; 12(2):139–146

[98] Bernardino ME, Thomas JL, Barnes PA, Lewis E. Diagnostic approaches to liver and spleen metastases. Radiol Clin North Am. 1982; 20(3):469–485

[99] Tempero MA, Petersen RJ, Zetterman RK, Lemon HM, Gurney J. Detection of metastatic liver disease. Use of liver scans and biochemical liver tests. JAMA. 1982; 248(11):1329–1332

[100] Kim EE, Tilbury RS, Haynie TR, Podoloff DA, Lamki LM, Dodd GD. Positron emission tomography in clinical oncology. Cancer Bull. 1988; 40:158–164

[101] Falk PM, Gupta NC, Thorson AG, et al. Positron emission tomography for preoperative staging of colorectal carcinoma. Dis Colon Rectum. 1994; 37 (2):153–156

[102] Arulampalam THA, Costa DC, Loizidou M, Visvikis D, Ell PJ, Taylor I. Positron emission tomography and colorectal cancer. Review. Br J Surg. 2001; 88 (2):176–189

[103] Strasberg SM, Dehdashti F, Siegel BA, Drebin JA, Linehan D. Survival of patients evaluated by FDG-PET before hepatic resection for metastatic colorectal carcinoma: a prospective database study. Ann Surg. 2001; 233 (3):293–299

[104] Pham KH, Ramaswamy MR, Hawkins RA. Advances in positron emission tomography imaging for the GI tract. Gastrointest Endosc. 2002; 55(7) Suppl: S53–S63

[105] Huebner RH, Park KC, Shepherd JE, et al. A meta-analysis of the literature for whole-body FDG PET detection of recurrent colorectal cancer. J Nucl Med. 2000; 41(7):1177–1189

[106] Valk PE, Abella-Columna E, Haseman MK, et al. Whole-body PET imaging with [18F]fluorodeoxyglucose in management of recurrent colorectal cancer. Arch Surg. 1999; 134(5):503–511, discussion 511–513

[107] Flanagan FL, Dehdashti F, Ogunbiyi OA, Kodner IJ, Siegel BA. Utility of FDG-PET for investigating unexplained plasma CEA elevation in patients with colorectal cancer. Ann Surg. 1998; 227(3):319–323

[108] Saunders TH, Mendes Ribeiro HK, Gleeson FV. New techniques for imaging colorectal cancer: the use of MRI, PET and radioimmunoscintigraphy for primary staging and follow-up. Br Med Bull. 2002; 64:81–99

[109] Lunniss PJ, Skinner S, Britton KE, Granowska M, Morris G, Northover JMA. Effect of radioimmunoscintigraphy on the management of recurrent colorectal cancer. Br J Surg. 1999; 86(2):244–249

[110] Corman ML, Galandiuk S, Block GE, et al. Immunoscintigraphy with 111 In-satumomab pendetide in patients with colorectal adenocarcinoma: performance and impact on clinical management. Dis Colon Rectum. 1994; 37 (2):129–137

[111] Seldinger SI. Catheter replacement of the needle in percutaneous arteriography; a new technique. Acta Radiol. 1953; 39(5):368–376

[112] Athanasoulis CA. Angiography in the management of patients with gastrointestinal bleeding. In: Maclean LD, ed. Advances in Surgery. Chicago, IL: Year Book Medical Publishers; 1983:1–20

[113] Zurkiya O, Walker TG. Angiographic evaluation and management of nonvariceal gastrointestinal hemorrhage. AJR Am J Roentgenol. 2015; 205(4):753–763

[114] Shin JH. Recent update of embolization of upper gastrointestinal tract bleeding. Korean J Radiol. 2012; 13 Suppl 1:S31–S39

[115] Kadir S, Ernst CB. Current concepts in angiographic management of gastrointestinal bleeding. Curr Probl Surg. 1983; 20(5):281–343

[116] Gomes AS, Lois JF, McCoy RD. Angiographic treatment of gastrointestinal hemorrhage: comparison of vasopressin infusion and embolization. AJR Am J Roentgenol. 1986; 146(5):1031–1037

[117] Gianfrancisco JA, Abcarian H. Pitfalls in the treatment of massive lower gastrointestinal bleeding with "blind" subtotal colectomy. Dis Colon Rectum. 1982; 25(5):441–445

[118] Lambiase RE. Percutaneous abscess and fluid drainage: a critical review. Cardiovasc Intervent Radiol. 1991; 14(3):143–157

[119] Cinat ME, Wilson SE, Din AM. Determinants for successful percutaneous image-guided drainage of intra-abdominal abscess. Arch Surg. 2002; 137 (7):845–849

[120] Catalano OA, Hahn PF, Hooper DC, Mueller PR. Efficacy of percutaneous abscess drainage in patients with vancomycin-resistant enterococci. AJR Am J Roentgenol. 2000; 175(2):533–536

[121] Boland GW, Lee MJ, Dawson SI, et al. Percutaneous abscess drainage complications. Semin Intervent Radiol. 1994; 11:267–275

[122] Bernardino ME. Percutaneous biopsy. AJR Am J Roentgenol. 1984; 142 (1):41–45

[123] Charboneau JW, Reading CC, Welch TJ. CT and sonographically guided needle biopsy: current techniques and new innovations. AJR Am J Roentgenol. 1990; 154(1):1–10

[124] McGhana JP, Dodd GD, III. Radiofrequency ablation of the liver: current status. AJR Am J Roentgenol. 2001; 176(1):3–16

[125] Wood BJ, Ramkaransingh JR, Fojo T, Walther MM, Libutti SK. Percutaneous tumor ablation with radiofrequency. Cancer. 2002; 94(2):443–451

[126] Sullivan KL. Hepatic artery chemoembolization. Semin Oncol. 2002; 29 (2):145–151

[127] Weinstein LS, Timmcke AE. Future technology: colography and the wireless capsule. Clin Colon Rectal Surg. 2001; 14:393–399

[128] Appleyard M, Glukhovsky A, Swain P. Wireless-capsule diagnostic endoscopy for recurrent small-bowel bleeding. N Engl J Med. 2001; 344(3):232–233

[129] Selby W. Can clinical features predict the likelihood of finding abnormalities when using capsule endoscopy in patients with GI bleeding of obscure origin? Gastrointest Endosc. 2004; 59(7):782–787

[130] Lewis BS. The history of enteroscopy. Gastrointest Endosc Clin N Am. 1999; 9(1):1–11

[131] Adler DG, Knipschield M, Gostout C. A prospective comparison of capsule endoscopy and push enteroscopy in patients with GI bleeding of obscure origin. Gastrointest Endosc. 2004; 59(4):492–498

[132] Yamamoto H, Sekine Y, Sato Y, et al. Total enteroscopy with a nonsurgical steerable double-balloon method. Gastrointest Endosc. 2001; 53 (2):216–220

[133] Yamamoto H, Sugano K. A new method of enteroscopy–the double-balloon method. Can J Gastroenterol. 2003; 17(4):273–274

[134] May A, Nachbar L, Wardak A, Yamamoto H, Ell C. Double-balloon enteroscopy: preliminary experience in patients with obscure gastrointestinal bleeding or chronic abdominal pain. Endoscopy. 2003; 35(12):985–991

[135] Yamamoto H, Yano T, Kita H, Sunada K, Ido K, Sugano K. New system of double-balloon enteroscopy for diagnosis and treatment of small intestinal disorders. Gastroenterology. 2003; 125(5):1556; author reply 1556–1557

[136] Nishimura M, Yamamoto H, Kita H, et al. Gastrointestinal stromal tumor in the jejunum: diagnosis and control of bleeding with electrocoagulation by using double-balloon enteroscopy. J Gastroenterol. 2004; 39(10):1001–1004

[137] Ohmiya N, Taguchi A, Shirai K, et al. Endoscopic resection of Peutz-Jeghers polyps throughout the small intestine at double-balloon enteroscopy without laparotomy. Gastrointest Endosc. 2005; 61(1):140–147

[138] Lo SK, Mehdizadeh S. Therapeutic uses of double-balloon enteroscopy. Gastrointest Endosc Clin N Am. 2006; 16(2):363–376

[139] Honda K, Mizutani T, Nakamura K, et al. Acute pancreatitis associated with peroral double-balloon enteroscopy: a case report. World J Gastroenterol. 2006; 12(11):1802–1804

[140] Yen HH, Chen YY, Su WW, Soon MS, Lin YM. Intestinal necrosis as a complication of epinephrine injection therapy during double-balloon enteroscopy. Endoscopy. 2006; 38(5):542

[141] Bassett ML, Goulston KJ. False positive and negative hemoccult reactions on a normal diet and effect of diet restriction. Aust N Z J Med. 1980; 10(1):1–4

[142] Caligiore P, Macrae FA, St John DJB, Rayner LJ, Legge JW. Peroxidase levels in food: relevance to colorectal cancer screening. Am J Clin Nutr. 1982; 35 (6):1487–1489

[143] Lifton LJ, Kreiser J. False-positive stool occult blood tests caused by iron preparations. A controlled study and review of literature. Gastroenterology. 1982; 83(4):860–863

[144] Allison JE, Tekawa IS, Ransom LJ, Adrain AL. A comparison of fecal occult-blood tests for colorectal-cancer screening. N Engl J Med. 1996; 334(3):155–159

[145] Ahlquist DA, Wieand HS, Moertel CG, et al. Accuracy of fecal occult blood screening for colorectal neoplasia. A prospective study using Hemoccult and HemoQuant tests. JAMA. 1993; 269(10):1262–1267

[146] Bennett DH, Hardcastle JD. Early diagnosis and screening. In: Williams NS, ed. Colorectal Cancer. New York, NY: Churchill Livingstone; 1996:21–37

[147] Ahlquist DA, McGill DB, Fleming JL, et al. Patterns of occult bleeding in asymptomatic colorectal cancer. Cancer. 1989; 63(9):1826–1830

[148] Tinmouth J, Lansdorp-Vogelaar I, Allison JE. Faecal immunochemical tests versus guaiac faecal occult blood tests: what clinicians and colorectal cancer screening programme organisers need to know. Gut. 2015; 64 (8):1327–1337

[149] Lee JK, Liles EG, Bent S, Levin TR, Corley DA. Accuracy of fecal immunochemical tests for colorectal cancer: systematic review and meta-analysis. Ann Intern Med. 2014; 160(3):171

[150] Hol L, van Leerdam ME, van Ballegooijen M, et al. Screening for colorectal cancer: randomised trial comparing guaiac-based and immunochemical faecal occult blood testing and flexible sigmoidoscopy. Gut. 2010; 59(1):62–68

[151] Ned RM, Melillo S, Marrone M. Fecal DNA testing for colorectal cancer screening: the ColoSure™ test. PLoS Curr. 2011; 3:RRN1220

[152] Grady WM, Carethers JM. Genomic and epigenetic instability in colorectal cancer pathogenesis. Gastroenterology. 2008; 135(4):1079–1099

[153] Zou H, Harrington JJ, Shire AM, et al. Highly methylated genes in colorectal neoplasia: implications for screening. Cancer Epidemiol Biomarkers Prev. 2007; 16(12):2686–2696

[154] Shirahata A, Sakata M, Sakuraba K, et al. Vimentin methylation as a marker for advanced colorectal carcinoma. Anticancer Res. 2009; 29(1):279–281

[155] Gertler S, Pressman J, Cartwright C, Dharmsathaphorn K. Management of acute diarrhea. J Clin Gastroenterol. 1983; 5(6):523–534

[156] Harris JC, Dupont HL, Hornick RB. Fecal leukocytes in diarrheal illness. Ann Intern Med. 1972; 76(5):697–703

[157] Murray BJ. Campylobacter enteritis. [letter]. Ann Intern Med. 1983; 98 (6):1029–1030

[158] Sazie ES, Titus AE. Rapid diagnosis of campylobacter enteritis. Ann Intern Med. 1982; 96(1):62–63

[159] Kane JG, Chretien JH, Garagusi VF. Diarrhoea caused by Candida. Lancet. 1976; 1(7955):335–336

[160] Kohl S. Yersinia enterocolitica: a significant 'new' pathogen. Hosp Pract. 1978; 13(12):81–85

[161] Saebø A. The Yersinia enterocolitica infection in acute abdominal surgery. A clinical study with a 5-year follow-up period. Ann Surg. 1983; 198 (6):760–765

[162] Fekety R. Pseudomembranous colitis. In: Goldman L, Bennett JC, eds. Cecil Textbook of Medicine. 21st ed. Philadelphia, PA: Saunders JB; 2000:1670–1673

[163] Wilson FA, Dietschy JM. Differential diagnostic approach to clinical problems of malabsorption. Gastroenterology. 1971; 61(6):911–931

[164] Drummey GD, Benson JA, Jr, Jones CM. Microscopical examination of the stool for steatorrhea. N Engl J Med. 1961; 264:85–87

[165] Heisig DG, Threatte GA, Henry JB. Laboratory diagnosis of gastrointestinal and pancreator disorders. In: Henry JB, ed. Clinical Diagnosis and Management by Laboratory Methods. 12th ed. Philadelphia, PA: W.B. Saunders; 2001:462–476

4 Colonoscopy

David E. Beck

Abstract

Colonoscopy was introduced for clinical use in 1970 and was initially used as a diagnostic aid to barium enema studies. Increasing experience and technologic advancements have resulted in colonoscopy becoming a major component of colorectal surgery and the ultimate procedure for the detection of colonic diseases. This chapter reviews various factors related to colonoscopy including indications and contraindications, bowel preparation, sedation and antibiotics, technique, and complications.

Keywords: colonoscopy, indications, contraindications, bowel preparation, sedation, antibiotics, technique, complications

4.1 General Principles

Colonoscopy was introduced for clinical use in 1970 and was initially used as a diagnostic aid to barium enema studies. Lesions or mucosal abnormalities could be visualized and confirmed by biopsy, but early endoscopists reached the cecum in only 30 to 50% of procedures. The first colonoscopic polypectomy was performed by Hiromi Shinya of New York in 1969.[1] Increasing experience and technologic advancements have resulted in colonoscopy becoming a major component of colorectal surgery and the ultimate procedure for the detection of colonic diseases. Current colonoscopies (▶ Fig. 4.1) use high-definition video to produce quality images.

Performed properly, the procedure is well tolerated, the complication rate is low, and the cecum is reached in > 95% of procedures.[2,3,4,5] The colorectal mucosa or lesions can be biopsied and almost all pedunculated polyps can be removed and most large sessile polyps can be removed piecemeal, in more than one session, or with advanced techniques (e.g., endoscopic submucosal dissection).[6,7]

Several studies evaluating large numbers of colonoscopies found that approximately 25% of procedures are easy, 50% are more challenging, and 25% are difficult or impossible.[8,9] The most common cause of difficulty in colonoscopy is recurrent looping or bowing in a long or mobile colon. The colonic length is greater in women (median, 155 cm) compared to men (median, 145 cm) ($p < 0.005$), with most of the difference being in the transverse colon.[9] Many patients also have mobile portions of their colon.[10]

To become a competent colonoscopist, extensive training and hands-on experience in colonoscopy is essential. Although numbers have limitations (performing hundreds of procedures with poor technique does not make one competent), the "learning curve" for colonoscopy is approximately 150 to 200 procedures.[11,12]

4.2 Indications

Colonoscopy is indicated for the diagnosis of colorectal diseases, treatment of colorectal polyps, surveillance of chronic ulcerative colitis and Crohn's colitis, preoperative and postoperative examination in patients with carcinoma of the large bowel, and screening for average and high-risk patients for colorectal carcinoma.[13] Colonoscopy is also an option to decompress acute pseudo-obstruction of the colon if medical management with neostigmine fails or is contraindicated.[14,15,16,17,18]

4.3 Contraindications

There are few contraindications to colonoscopy. A patient with poor bowel preparation should be rescheduled and recleansed. The procedure should not be pursued if there is a fixed angle that cannot be straightened. Patients with acute inflammatory bowel disease or acute diverticulitis may benefit from a distal

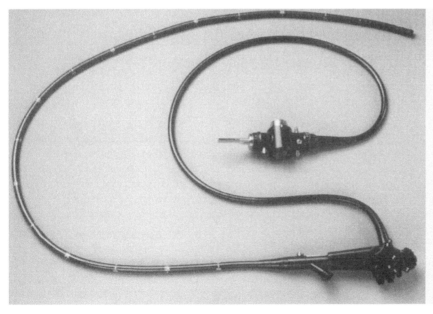

Fig. 4.1 Videocolonoscope (160 cm).

diagnostic exam, but proximal scope passage must be individualized. Colonoscopy is avoided in patients with small bowel obstruction and anal diseases that cause stricture or severe pain. However, patients with large bowel obstruction may benefit from a diagnostic exam or endoscopic placement of a colonic stent.[19,20] Finally, patients who are too weak or unstable to undergo bowel preparation, or those who have experienced a recent myocardial infarction, are poor candidates for colonoscopy. The most common excuses for not doing colonoscopy are the cost of the procedure and the unavailability of experienced colonoscopists.

4.4 Bowel Preparation

Safe and accurate colonoscopy requires a clean colon. Colon cleansing preparations initially were modifications of barium enema preparations, but have evolved extensively over the years. A variety of methods are currently available. Numerous comparison studies have been performed with mixed results. The patient completing the preparation as directed may be more important than the method chosen. All preparations use some form of dietary limitation and can be divided into isosmotic, hyperosmotic, and stimulant preparations.[21]

4.4.1 Isosmotic Preparations

Isosmotic preparations that contain polyethylene glycol (PEG) are osmotically balanced, high-volume, nonabsorbable, and nonfermentable electrolyte solutions (▶ Table 4.1). These solutions became available in the 1980s and cleanse the bowel with minimal water and electrolyte shifts and provide evacuation, primarily by the mechanical effect of large-volume lavage.[22,23] With sodium sulfate preparations, sodium absorption in the small intestine is largely reduced because of the absence of chloride, the accompanying anion necessary for active absorption against electrochemical gradient.[24] The conventional total adult dose is 4 L given orally as 240 mL every 10 minutes until rectal effluent is clear, or it is administered by a nasogastric tube at a rate of 20 to 30 mL/min. Alternatively, split dosing has also been advocated, with a portion taken the evening before and the residual taken the morning of the procedure.[25,26] Low-volume PEG preparations are used in combination with stimulant laxatives or ascorbic acid. For one of these regimens, 10 mg of bisacodyl tablets is followed after the first bowel movement by 240 mL of preparation every 10 minutes until effluent is clear or until a total of 2 L is ingested. In another regimen, the ascorbic acid is included in the 2-L PEG solution, which is also dosed at 240 mL every 10 minutes.[27,28] For this latter regimen, it is recommended that the patient ingest at least an additional 1 L of fluid, which makes the total volume of ingestion 3 L. Another formulation of PEG-3350 (MiraLAX, Schering Plough Healthcare Products, Summit, NJ), which does not contain electrolytes, has been approved and marketed as an agent to treat constipation (▶ Table 4.1). This formulation has been used for colonic cleansing.[29] However, these PEG agents without electrolytes are not approved for bowel preparation, and the volume required and safety for use as a bowel preparation have not been adequately defined.

4.4.2 Hyperosmotic Preparations

Hyperosmotic preparations draw water into the bowel lumen, which stimulates peristalsis and evacuation. These are smaller-volume preparations but, because of their hyperosmotic nature, can cause fluid shifts, accompanied by transient electrolyte alterations.

A low-volume stimulant and osmotic laxative combination of sodium picosulfate, magnesium citrate, and anhydrous citric acid (PM/C) (Prepopik, Ferring Pharmaceuticals, Parsippany, NJ) is administered as a total of 10 oz. of preparation solution and 64 oz. of clear liquids in two divided doses. PM/C doses may be administered the day before colonoscopy (separated by 6 hours) or in a split dose fashion.[30]

Sodium phosphate preparations were developed in an effort to increase patient compliance by offering a lower volume, more palatable option for bowel cleansing. Oral sodium phosphate was available as a solution (Phosphosoda and Fleet Phos-phosoda EZ Prep, Fleet Pharmaceuticals, Lynchburg, VA) and in tablet form (Visicol, InKine Pharmaceutical Co., Inc., Blue Bell, PA; Osmoprep, Salix Pharmaceuticals). Phosphate preparations have been demonstrated to be equally effective to oral gut lavage solutions with regard to cleansing and were superior in patient tolerance.[31,32]

Sodium phosphate preparations are hyperosmotic and work by drawing fluid into the bowel lumen, potentially causing fluid and electrolyte disturbances. In healthy subjects, administration of sodium phosphate has demonstrated hyperphosphatemia, hypocalcemia, increased parathyroid hormone, and increased urinary cyclic adenosine monophosphate (cAMP). These findings raise concern about phosphate preparation use in patients with cardiac, renal, and hepatic disease.[33] The development of acute phosphate nephropathy following phosphate preparation has also been recognized.[34] Accumulating evidence prompted the Food and Drug Administration (FDA) to issue a cautionary note on prescribing phosphate products, including a boxed warning, and restricted the use of over-the-counter phosphates for cleansing preparations. Oral sodium phosphate solution has been withdrawn from the market. A tablet formulation remains available and should be taken in divided doses (OsmoPrep, Salix Pharmaceuticals) with adequate hydration. Sodium phosphate seemed to be an attractive alternative to gut lavage for colon cleansing. However, because of fluid, metabolic, and electrolyte disturbances, it should not be used in pediatric or elderly patients, patients with suspected intestinal obstruction or other intestinal structural abnormalities, gut dysmotility, active colitis, renal insufficiency, liver insufficiency, or heart failure, and those at risk of complications due to electrolyte abnormalities or fluid shifts.[35,36] It has been suggested that adequate hydration could minimize the risk of acute phosphate nephropathy. Pelham et al, however, have shown that hyperphosphatemia can occur in healthy young men when given as much as 4.4 L of hydration, even with no signs of dehydration.[36]

Sodium sulfate (SUPREP, Braintree Laboratories, Braintree, MA) is taken as two doses diluted in water.[37] Multiple comparative studies have demonstrated that this preparation produces equivalent cleansing with minimal patient discomfort. A variation of oral sulfate followed by sulfate-free electrolyte lavage solution (SuClear, Braintree Laboratories, Inc, Braintree, MA) has recently been FDA approved.[30]

Table 4.1 Bowel preparations for colonoscopy

Type	Brand name	Total volume	Flavor(s)	Usual dosing	Comments	Cost
Polyethylene glycol (PEG) solutions	PEG-3350 (generic of CoLyte)	4 L	Regular	8 oz every 10 min until rectal output is clear or 4 L are consumed; or split dose by taking 2–3 L the night before and 1–2 L the morning of procedure	More effective than diet with cathartics, high-volume gut lavage, or mannitol; safer than osmotic laxatives/sodium phosphate for patients with electrolyte or fluid imbalances (e.g., renal/liver insufficiency, congestive heart failure); MoviPrep contains ascorbic acid (avoid in patients with G6PD deficiency); no solid foods at least 2 h before administration	$16.41
	CoLyte	1 gal	Regular, pineapple			$13.89
		4 L	Regular, cherry, citrus-berry, lemon-lime, orange			$25.63
	GoLYTELY	4 L	Regular, pineapple			$18.46 (regular); $29.56 (pineapple)
	MoviPrep	2 L plus 1 L clear liquid	Lemon	8 oz every 15 min until 1 L is consumed, then drink 16 oz of clear liquid, repeat process 90 min later; or repeat dose in the morning of procedure, then drink 16 oz of clear liquids		$48.75
	NuLytely	4 L	Cherry, lemon-lime, orange	8 oz every 10 min until rectal output is clear or 4 L are consumed; or split dose by taking 2–3 L the night before and 1–2 L the morning of procedure	Comparable to PEG in safety, effectiveness, and tolerance; do not contain sodium sulfate (improved taste and smell); no solid foods at least 2 h before administration	$25.65
	TriLyte (generic of NuLytely)	4 L	Cherry, citrus berry, lemon-lime, orange, pineapple			$25.63
	HalfLytely Bowel Prep Kit	2 L plus 2 bisacodyl 5 mg tabs	Cherry, lemon-lime, orange	2 tablets at noon, wait for bowel movement or 6 h, then 8 oz every 10 min until 2 L are consumed	Consume only clear liquids on the day of administration	$48.75
	MiraLAX	2 L plus 4 bisacodyl 5 mg tabs	Regular	4 tablets at noon, wait for bowel movement or 6 h, then 8 oz every 10 min until 2 L are consumed	Does not contain electrolytes; consume only clear liquids on the day of administration; mix entire bottle (238 or 255 g) with 64 oz of Gatorade or Crystal Light (if diabetic) and shake well	$21.73 (255 g); $43.45 (527 g)
	GlycoLax (generic of MiraLax)	2 L plus 4 bisacodyl 5 mg tabs	Regular			$22.78 (14 × 17 g); $19.54 (255 g); $39.06 (527 g)
Sodium phosphate (NaP) agents*	OsmoPrep Visicol	32–40 tabs plus 64–80 oz clear liquid	n/a	20 tablets the night before and 12–20 tablets 3–5 h before procedure; taken as 4 tabs every 15 min with 8 oz of clear liquid	Same contraindications as aqueous NaP; improved taste and palatability of tablet NaP compared with aqueous NaP resulted in improved overall patient tolerance; OsmoPrep is gluten-free	$1.73/tab $3.04/tab
	GlycoLax (generic of MiraLax)	2 L plus 4 bisacodyl 5 mg tabs	Regular			$22.78 (14 × 17 g); $19.54 (255 g); $39.06 (527 g)
Sodium phosphate (NaP) agents*	OsmoPrep Visicol	32–40 tabs plus 64–80 oz clear liquid	n/a	20 tablets the night before and 12–20 tablets 3–5 h before procedure; taken as 4 tabs every 15 min with 8 oz of clear liquid	Same contraindications as aqueous NaP; improved taste and palatability of tablet NaP compared with aqueous NaP resulted in improved overall patient tolerance; OsmoPrep is gluten-free	$1.73/tab $3.04/tab

Table 4.1 continued

Type	Brand name	Total volume	Flavor(s)	Usual dosing	Comments	Cost
Sodium picosulfate, magnesium oxide citric acid	**Prepopik**	2 150 ml doses each followed by 1200 cc clear liquids	Orange Cranberry	Dose 1: 1 st packet in 5 oz of water followed by 40 oz glasses of water Dose 2: 2nd packet in 5 oz of water followed by 24 oz of water	Small volume and good taste. Additional hydration is important	$162
Sodium sulfate, potassium sulfate Magnesium sulfate	**Suprep**	1 liter		Dose 1: Suprep packet with 19 oz water followed by 326 oz of water Dose 2: Suprep packet with 19 oz water followed by 326 oz of water		$27.24
Sodium sulfate, magnesium sulfate with PEG and electrolytes	**Suclear**	240 ml		Dose 1: 6 oz prep with 10 oz water followed by 32 oz water Dose 2: 6 oz prep with 10 oz water followed by 32 oz water		$128

Abbreviations: G6PD, glucose-6-phosphate dehydrogenase.

Note: Split-dose regimens are recommended for patients scheduled for colonoscopy after 10:30am. In most cases, final dose should be taken at least 1 hour before the procedure.

Drug related considerations:
- NaP agents are contraindicated in patients on angiotensin-converting enzyme inhibitors (ACEIs) and angiotension receptor blockers (ARBs), and should be used with caution in patients on diuretics or nonsteroidal anti-inflammatory drugs (NSAIDs). Maintaining adequate hydration is important during the preparation and patients should be advised to drink clear liquids up until 2 hours prior to the procedure.
- Cilostazol, clopidogrel, ticlopidine, and warfarin should be stopped 1 week prior to the procedure to decrease bleeding risk from polypectomy. Bridging with unfractionated heparin or a low-molecular weight heparin may be required if clinically indicated.
- Aspirin should *not* be stopped prior to a colonoscopy if the patient is at risk of an acute myocardial infarction.

* NaP agents have a black-box warning for acute phosphate nephropathy when used for bowel cleansing. This form of acute and potentially permanent renal injury may occur even in patients without identifiable risk factors. Avoid use of NaP agents in patients at increased risk of developing acute phosphate nephropathy (e.g., age ≥ 55 years, hypovolemic, history of renal dysfunction, or concomitant use of ACEIs, ARBs, or NSAIDs).

Sources: (1) American Society of Colon and Rectal Surgeons (ASCRS); American Society for Gastrointestinal Endoscopy (ASGE); Society of American Gastrointestinal and Endoscopic Surgeons (SAGES), Wexner SD, Beck DE, Baron TH, Fanelli RD, Hyman N, Shen B, Wasco KE. A consensus document on bowel preparation before colonoscopy: prepared by a Task Force from the American Society of Colon and Rectal Surgeons (ASCRS), the American Society for Gastrointestinal Endoscopy (ASGE), and the Society of American Gastrointestinal and Endoscopic Surgeons (SAGES). Surg Endosc. 2006 Jul;20(7):1161
(2) A-Rahim YI, Falchuk M. Bowel preparation for colonoscopy. In: UpToDate, Rose, BD (ed). UpToDate, Waltham, MA; 2008
(3) Facts & Comparisons
(4) MicroMedex
(5) Amerisource Price Lookup
(6) Red Book, May 2008, Update 4
(7) Prescription Drug Plan Formularies

4.4.3 Stimulant Preparations

Senna, an anthracene derivative, is processed by colonic bacteria, and its active ingredients, anthraquinones and their glucosides, stimulate colonic peristalsis. A bowel response can be expected approximately 6 hours after the dose ingestion. It has been used as the primary cleansing agent, with a liquid diet, particularly in children.[38]

4.4.4 Adjunctive Agents

Bisacodyl is a diphenylmethane derivative that is poorly absorbed in the small intestine and that is hydrolyzed by endogenous esterases.[39] Its active metabolites stimulate colonic motility, with an onset of action between 6 and 10 hours. There are reports of ischemic colitis related to the use of bisacodyl.[40]

Metoclopramide is a dopamine receptor antagonist that sensitizes tissue to acetylcholine, which results in improved gastric contraction and small bowel peristalsis. It has a half-life of 5 to 6 hours. Various dietary regimens, hydration electrolyte solutions, enemas, and antigas agents are also used as adjuncts for colonoscopy preparation.

It is important that physicians be aware of the comorbid conditions that put patients at risk for complications. Physicians should make the decision about which patients should not undergo a bowel preparation as none of the currently available cleansing agents are without risk.

4.5 Sedation

Colonoscopy can be performed without medications in selected patients, but this technique requires a skillful and gentle colonoscopist who uses good techniques.[13,41] Most colonoscopists, however, prefer to give preprocedural medications. Ideal drugs for endoscopic sedation have a rapid onset and short duration of action, maintain hemodynamic stability, and do not cause major side effects. Commonly used agents include opiates, such as meperidine or fentanyl, benzodiazepines, such as midazolam or diazepam, or a hypnotic, such as propofol (▶ Table 4.2). The choice of agents is often a matter of personal or institutional preference. Combinations of a benzodiazepine and an opiate can be administered by the endoscopist or specially trained nurses. The administration of propofol is governed by state law and facility/hospital rules.

Benzodiazepines induce central nervous system (CNS) depression resulting in anxiolysis, sedation, muscle relaxation, and anterograde amnesia.[42] The principal class side effect is respiratory depression. This effect is intensified when coadministered with opiates, and dose reduction of the benzodiazepine, opiate, or both is often required.[43] Midazolam and diazepam are the most commonly used benzodiazepines. In a nationwide survey, midazolam was preferred over diazepam for endoscopic sedation.[44] Both drugs demonstrate similar efficacy with regard to sedation.[45] Midazolam, however, is associated with greater potency, better amnesic effects, reduced respiratory depression, less injection discomfort, and superior patient satisfaction when compared with diazepam.[46,47,48]

Midazolam has a rapid onset (1–2 minutes), short duration of action (15–60 minutes), and favorable amnesic properties.[49] The initial dose is 1 mg, followed by repeat doses (if needed) of 1 mg in 2-minute intervals until the desired effect is achieved.[50] When given in combination with an opiate or other sedatives, the dose of midazolam should be reduced by 30%.[51] Because it is lipophilic, midazolam can be sequestered in adipose tissue resulting in a prolonged sedative effect.[49] Patients who are obese or elderly or those with impaired hepatic or renal function are at increased risk for delayed drug clearance. In this population, utilization of lower doses and longer intervals of administration should be considered.[49] By comparison, diazepam has less amnesic capabilities, a slower onset of action (2–3 minutes), and prolonged duration of effect (360 minutes).[49] The dose for colonoscopy is 2.5 to 5 mg initially. Additional doses of 2.5 mg every 3 to 5 minutes can be given as needed.

The benzodiazepine receptor antagonist flumazenil should be immediately available for administration in all endoscopy suites. The primary effect of flumazenil is reversal of benzodiazepine-induced sedation and psychomotor impairment. It has minimal effect on reversal of respiratory depression.[51] For this reason, opioid reversing agents (i.e., naloxone) are given prior to flumazenil in situations of benzodiazepine/opioid-induced respiratory depression. The typical flumazenil dose is a 0.2 mg intravenous (IV) bolus and can be repeated three times.[50]

Similar to benzodiazepines, opioids are efficacious for induction of moderate sedation.[52] However, unlike benzodiazepines they provide analgesia as well. This favorable characteristic enhances the overall sedative effect when opioids are adjunctively used with benzodiazepines. Fentanyl and meperidine are two short-acting opioids used for sedation during colonoscopy. Many endoscopists prefer fentanyl due to its pharmacologic profile and reduced incidence of nausea as compared with meperidine.[52] Additionally, fentanyl was associated with a shorter procedure time in a recent study comparing meperidine and fentanyl use during upper endoscopy and colonoscopy.[53]

Fentanyl is a lipid-soluble, synthetic opioid narcotic with a rapid onset (1–2 minutes) and short duration of action (30–70 minutes).[43] For endoscopic procedures, an initial bolus of 50 μg is given. Subsequent doses of 25 μg in 2- to 5-minute intervals can be administered if necessary. Meperidine has a longer onset (3–6 minutes) and duration of effect (3–5 hours) as compared with fentanyl.[43,50] The starting dose of meperidine is usually 25 to 50 mg, followed by 25 mg every 2 to 5 minutes if required.

Table 4.2 Sedation and analgesia medications

Drug	Dosing		Onset	Duration	Comments
	Pediatric	Adult			
Midazolam (Versed)	Initial: 0.05–0.1 mg/kg Titrate: 0.025 mg/kg every 5 min	Initial: 0.5–2.5 mg/kg slowly over 2 min Titrate: 0.5 mg/kg	1–5 min	1–2.5 h	Major side effect is respiratory depression
Diazepam (Valium)	0.1–0.3 mg/kg	Initial: 2.5–10 mg slowly Titrate: 2–5 mg every 5–10 min Max: 20 mg/kg	30 s to 5 min	2–6 h	Painful on injection
Meperidine hydrochloride (Demerol)	Initial: 1–1.5 mg/kg Titrate: 1 mg/kg increments	Initial: 10 mg Titrate: 10 mg increments	1–5 min	1–3 h	
Fentanyl (Sublimaze)	Not recommended	Initial: 0.005–2 μg/kg slowly Titrate: 1 μg/kg every 30 min Max: 4 μg/kg	30–60 s	30–60 min	
Propofol		Initial: 20–60 mg Titrate: 10–30 mg every 30–60 s	30–45 s	4–8 min	Deep sedation possible

Opioids cause synergistic CNS and respiratory depression when used in patients taking other centrally acting medications such as antihistamines, benzodiazepines, narcotics, monoamine oxidase inhibitors, and phenothiazines.[54] All opioids reduce seizure thresholds, and narcotic dose reduction or avoidance should be considered in patients with epilepsy. Chest wall rigidity due to increased skeletal muscle tonicity has been reported with high doses of fentanyl.[54] This may result in difficulty with assisted ventilation. Meperidine is metabolized in the liver to normeperidine, an active metabolite with a half-life of 15 to 20 hours.[43] Patients with renal and hepatic insufficiency are at risk for normeperidine accumulation, which can cause tremors, myoclonus, and seizures.[50] Naloxone does not reverse normeperidine-induced seizures.[55] Unlike meperidine, fentanyl does not cause accumulation of active metabolites.[56]

Naloxone is an opioid receptor antagonist used for reversal of narcotic-induced CNS effects including respiratory depression, sedation, and analgesia. The typical dose is 0.4 mg every 2 to 4 minutes until adequate clinical response has occurred. The duration of effect of naloxone is shorter than that of fentanyl and meperidine, so all patients receiving rescue doses should be closely monitored for relapse of sedation. In such circumstances, repeat administration of naloxone may be required.

Propofol is an ultra-short-acting hypnotic used for induction and maintenance of anesthesia, conscious sedation in minor procedures, and sedation in intensive care unit patients.[43] At doses used during colonoscopy, it provides sedation and mild amnesia but has no analgesic properties.[57] It is usually administered in combination with a short-acting benzodiazepine or opioid to enhance each individual drug's desired effect, a method referred to as "balanced propofol sedation" or "multidrug propofol."[58] Given the lack of analgesic effects, when used alone during endoscopy higher propofol doses may be required to maintain patient comfort. This may result in more profound levels of sedation (i.e., deep sedation) than originally targeted for colonoscopy. Indeed, several studies have demonstrated that utilization of balanced propofol for achieving moderate sedation is associated with fewer instances of deep sedation than when opioids and benzodiazepines are used alone.[58,59]

Propofol is usually given as an initial 20 to 60 mg bolus, followed by repeat doses of 10 to 30 mg in 30- to 60-second intervals as needed.[50] As with benzodiazepines and opioids, use of propofol with other sedatives results in synergistic respiratory depression, and dose reduction of all medications used may be required.[60] It has a rapid onset of action (30–45 seconds) and short duration of effect (4–8 minutes). The primary side effects of propofol are respiratory depression and hemodynamic disturbance, including hypotension, decreased cardiac output, and systemic vascular resistance.[43] Unlike benzodiazepines and opioids, there is no medication available to reverse the effects of propofol.[59] Instances of propofol oversedation are treated supportively with IV fluids and vasopressors as needed for hypotension and maintenance of ventilation until drug effect wears off. Injection site pain during bolus infusion is reported in approximately 30% of patients and can be minimized by using a large vein and avoiding veins in the dorsum of the hand.[52,61] Propofol is formulated in a soybean, egg phosphatide, and glycerol emulsion and is contraindicated in patients who are allergic to soy, egg, or sulfite.[56] Propofol, however, is not contraindicated in patients with sulfonamide allergy.[61]

Propofol is the most frequently used IV anesthetic today.[62] It was originally described in 1977 and subsequently approved for "induction and maintenance of general anesthesia" by the FDA. For this reason, administration of propofol has traditionally been limited to anesthesiologists. However, its utilization and experience by nonanesthesiologists has expanded over the years and now includes a variety of outpatient procedures. A recent survey of gastroenterologists in the United States found that propofol is used in up to 25% of endoscopies; however, 68% of physicians indicated they were reluctant to give propofol due to perceived increased risk of complications.[43]

There is a well-established and growing body of literature to support the safety and efficacy of propofol administration by the endoscopist (termed gastroenterologist-directed propofol) or nurse administration of propofol under the direction of the endoscopist for sedation during colonoscopy.[62,63,64,65,66] Greater than 220,000 cases of gastroenterologist-directed propofol have been reported, with only one reported instance of intubation and no instances of death.[62] A recent meta-analysis comparing the effectiveness of propofol to other sedation regimens for colonoscopy found that propofol sedation was associated with faster recovery and discharge times, and increased patient satisfaction without increased side effects.[67] Given the amount of supporting data, the American College of Gastroenterology (ACG), the American Gastroenterological Association (AGA), and the American Society for Gastrointestinal Endoscopy (ASGE) jointly conclude that "Compared to standard doses of benzodiazepines and narcotics, propofol may provide faster onset and deeper sedation" and that "with adequate training physician-supervised nurse administration of propofol can be done safely and effectively."[68]

4.6 Patient Monitoring

Conscious sedation is commonly used in endoscopic procedures, and it is associated with a small but definitive risk. To minimize this risk, patient monitoring is performed in a variety of ways. Some of these modalities are established; others are evolving and more data are needed prior to their incorporation in everyday endoscopy practice.[69] The term monitoring includes the use of both visual and physiologic measurement of these parameters. Standard monitoring includes measurement of blood pressure, pulse rate, and oxygen saturation, and electrocardiogram (ECG) monitoring. This is usually accomplished by the use of a pulse oximeter, a portable ECG monitor, and automatic sphygmomanometers.

4.6.1 Electrocardiogram

Continuous ECG monitoring is recommended per American Society of Anesthesiologists (ASA) guidelines for patients with a significant history of cardiovascular disease and arrhythmias.[70] Other groups benefiting from this are patients with pulmonary disorders, the elderly, and when prolonged procedures are anticipated. The use of continuous ECG monitoring in low-risk patients is not required.

4.6.2 Oxygen Saturation

Arterial hemoglobin oxygen saturation can be monitored in a noninvasive manner with pulse oximetry. Measurement of oxygen saturation is relatively insensitive to early desaturation and, as such, it is recommended that monitoring of ventilatory function should also include close patient observation. Baseline oxygen saturation of < 95%, a procedure of long duration, difficulty with esophageal intubation, comorbid illnesses, and emergency indication for endoscopic procedure are risk factors for hypoxemia. Both the ASA and ASGE recommend that pulse oximetry be used during all endoscopic procedures.[52,71]

4.6.3 Hemodynamics

Monitoring heart rate and blood pressure is important to assess the circulatory status and properly monitor the effect of sedation. Tachycardia and hypertension may indicate that the patient is sedated inadequately, whereas bradycardia and hypotension may be an indication of oversedation. After baseline measurement of blood pressure and pulse rate, it should be monitored at every 3- to 5-minute interval. Automated noninvasive blood pressure devices are now widely used for this purpose. A recent study advocated using continuous blood pressure monitoring as conventional intermittent blood pressure monitoring of patients receiving sedating agents failed to detect fast changes in blood pressure. The new technique, continuous noninvasive arterial pressure, improved the detection of rapid blood pressure changes, and may contribute to better patient safety for those undergoing interventional procedures.[71]

4.6.4 Capnography

Capnography is a noninvasive technique used to quantitate carbon dioxide in expired gases, providing a measure of ventilatory function. It can detect hypoventilation before pulse oximetry can detect oxygen desaturation.[72] Data also suggest that capnography is more sensitive in detecting alveolar hypoventilation than is visual observation.[73,74]

The principal risk factor for adverse respiratory events during sedation is hypoxia from depressed respiratory activity. Thus, it has been suggested that integrating this modality into patient monitoring protocols may improve patient safety.[74] Currently, there are insufficient data in support of its use during routine sedation for colonoscopy.[52,73] The ASA concludes that carbon dioxide monitoring "should be considered for all patients whose ventilation cannot be observed directly during moderate sedation."[52]

4.7 Antibiotic Prophylaxis

Antibiotic prophylaxis is indicated to reduce the possibility of a significant infectious complication. The value of antibiotic prophylaxis for gastrointestinal (GI) procedures has been debated for many years. Previously, antibiotic prophylaxis was recommended for many GI endoscopic procedures in patients with high-risk cardiac conditions to protect against infective endocarditis and in orthopaedic and vascular patients with implants.[75,76] However, practices have substantially changed, in part due to the low incidence of infective endocarditis following GI procedures and the lack of controlled data supporting the benefit of antibiotic prophylaxis. Furthermore, the indiscriminate use of antibiotics can be associated with the development of resistant organisms, *Clostridium difficile* colitis, unnecessary expense, and drug toxicity.

Updated guidelines for antibiotic prophylaxis were published in 2007 and 2008 by the American Heart Association (AHA) and the ASGE, respectively.[77,78] The recommendations in these guidelines are largely consistent with one another, but substantially different from prior guidelines. Essentially, prophylactic antibiotics are not indicated for almost all colonoscopic procedures.

4.8 Colonoscopic Technique

4.8.1 Insertion and Withdrawal

With the patient in the left lateral position, insertion of the colonoscope is preceded by digital examination of the anal canal. This is important to exclude the presence of neoplasms or structures that might be missed as the scope slides through the anus. The distal 10 to 15 cm tip of the scope is lubricated and inserted. Thereafter, a lubricant jelly should be used liberally. Throughout the entire procedure, the scope should be passed under direct vision. The procedure should be performed in a stepwise manner: advance the scope, straighten the scope, exert abdominal compression, change the patient's position. Not all patients require abdominal compression or a change in position. The ultimate goal of the colonoscopist is to pass the colonoscope to the cecum with minimal looping or bowing. Properly performed, a question mark configuration is achieved (▸ Fig. 4.2). In this situation, the scope can be advanced, withdrawn, torqued left, right, and turned all around on command. The pain caused by colonoscopy is from stretching of the colonic mesentery and/or an excessive amount of air insufflation. Pushing the scope forward may stretch the mesentery, whereas pulling it back may release it. Spasm of the colon often is due to stretching of the mesentery rather than irritability of the colon. This pain will be alleviated if the scope is pulled back to release the stretching.

Air insufflation should be used only to open the collapsed bowel. Not only is a distended bowel painful, but also it makes the angles more acute, and thins out the bowel wall, making it more susceptible to transmural burn when electrocautery is used. Aspiration of air to slightly collapse the colonic lumen, while still providing adequate exposure for snaring, will eliminate this problem.

Passing the tip of the scope into the sigmoid colon by slightly withdrawing the scope and then gradually torquing or rotating it clockwise not only will straighten the sigmoid colon but also will press it against the lateral or posterior abdominal wall. The scope can then be advanced without a looping or bowing formation; the sigmoid-descending angle is best passed by a to-and-fro motion, frequently requiring clockwise torquing of the scope (▸ Fig. 4.3). A "slide by" technique is occasionally necessary. Turning the patient to a supine position after the scope has passed the sigmoid or transverse colon frequently makes passing the scope easier. Sometimes turning the patient on their right side is helpful to advance the scope. If an alpha-loop is formed in the sigmoid colon, it must be reduced before the scope can be advanced beyond the splenic flexure; this is accomplished by withdrawing and gradually rotating the scope clockwise (an alpha-maneuver) (▶ Fig. 4.4).[79] An alpha-loop formation is suspected if advancing the scope causes more pain than it should, or when there is a paradoxical motion at the tip

of the scope (i.e., the tip of the scope advances when it is withdrawn and recedes when it is pushed up). Feeling the scope on the anterior abdominal wall indicates that a looping or bowing of the sigmoid colon is being formed.

The same basic principles are applied to passing the scope into the transverse colon and the right colon. Abdominal compression and changes in patient's positioning are helpful. Pressure is most commonly used when the colonoscope tip is at the splenic flexure followed by when the tip is at the hepatic flexure. Abdominal compression helps splint the colonoscope to prevent a looping or bowing formation. In the right colon, suction of the distended colon often produces an accordion-like bowel, which allows the scope to advance into the cecum. Variable stiffness colonoscopes have not been shown to make a substantial difference in cecal intubation rates or speed of intubation for routine colonoscopy.[80]

4.8.2 Polypectomy

Colonoscopic polypectomy has risks, and good technique is essential. When visualizing the gross appearance of the lesion through the scope, the colonoscopist must decide whether to perform a biopsy, electrocoagulate, excise, or leave the lesion alone. In performing a polypectomy, the snare wire should not be placed around a polyp until the colonoscopist is in complete control of the colonoscope. A looping or a bowing of the scope can be corrected by pulling down the scope and turning it clockwise. Once the scope has been straightened, a 1:1 ratio of movement can be recognized. With the scope under full control, it can be turned to the left and right, advanced, or withdrawn as required. The polyp is best snared at the 5 to 7 o'clock position. The channel for the snare coming out at the tip of the colonoscope is at the 5 o'clock position. It is safer and easier to snare the polyp in the lower half of the bowel lumen. With complete control of the scope, the polyp in the upper half of the bowel lumen can be rotated to the lower half without much difficulty.

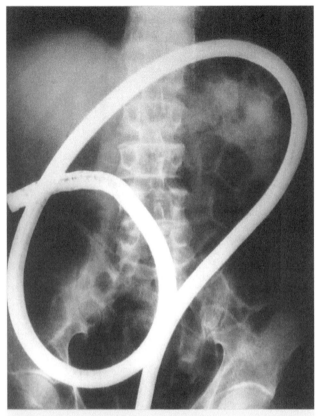

Fig. 4.2 Question mark configuration of a properly performed colonoscopy with tip of colonoscope intubated into the terminal ileum.

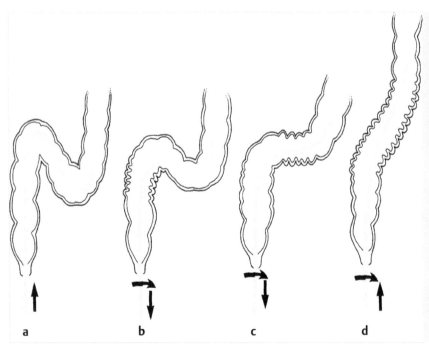

Fig. 4.3 Angulations of the sigmoid colon. (a) Advancement of the colonoscope causing **N**-shaped configuration with sharp angles between rectum and sigmoid and sigmoid and descending colon. (b) Withdrawal of the scope and clockwise rotation to widen the angles. (c) Further withdrawal and clockwise rotation to straighten the sigmoid colon. (d) While clockwise rotation is maintained, the scope can be advanced through the straightened sigmoid colon.

a   b   c   d

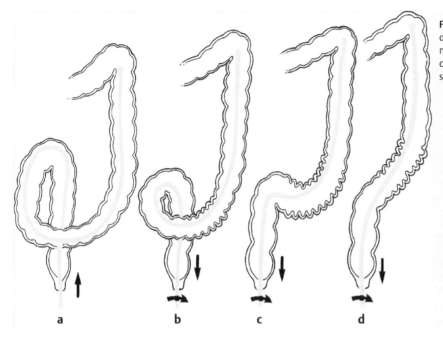

Fig. 4.4 α-Loop of the sigmoid colon. **(a)** An α-loop formation of sigmoid colon during colonoscopy. **(b–d)** Withdrawal of the scope with clockwise rotation will eliminate the α-loop and straighten the sigmoid colon.

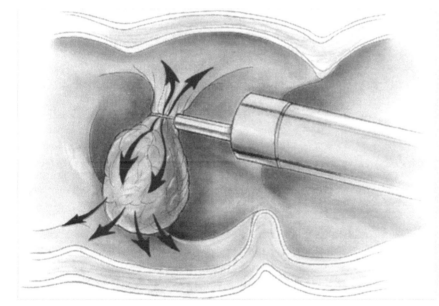

Fig. 4.5 Transmission of heat through polyp to opposite bowel wall.

Different cautery units have different intensities, and the amount of electrocauterization should vary according to the size of the tissue to be snared. A pure coagulation current should usually be used. The larger the tissue to be cut, the higher the intensity. In patients with a juvenile polyp, the heat should be turned down to approximately half. The stalk in a juvenile polyp has no muscularis mucosa, and very little coagulation current is needed to cut through it. On the other hand, entrapment of the snare wire into the substance of the polyp can occur when the current density is set too low, causing charring of the tissue. A lipoma contains 90% water and requires a tremendous amount of heat to transect it. Polypectomy for a large sessile lipoma should be avoided. Sessile polyps with induration, ulceration, or firmness are signs of invasive carcinoma. Once the snare wire is closed

around a carcinoma, it may not be possible to cut through it or disengage the wire. Therefore, avoid trying to remove an obvious carcinoma. These lesions are better biopsied.

In the case of a large polyp, the tip of the polyp frequently touches the opposite bowel wall, and heat from the snare at the base of the polyp can be transmitted to this opposite wall (▶ Fig. 4.5). When such heat transmission occurs, the burn is rarely severe. Jiggling the polyp head to and fro during snaring will prevent this type of damage by moving a small point of contact to various areas on the wall. An alternative method is to allow the entire head of the polyp to touch the bowel wall, thus distributing the heat to a larger area. Sessile polyps with a base larger than 2 cm should be removed piecemeal in 1- to 1.5-cm increments each, occasionally in more than one session.

Pedunculated Polyps

Almost all pedunculated polyps of any size can be safely snared in one piece because the stalk rarely is larger than 1.5 cm. Usually, the snare wire can be manipulated to loop around the polyp, even when it is larger than the size of the wire loop itself. The basic principles of snaring a pedunculated polyp are first to place the snare wire around the head of the polyp and then to manipulate the scope and/or wire toward the stalk. Once the wire is in the desired position just below the head of the polyp, the snare or the scope is advanced so that the base of the wire loop or the plastic sheath is in contact with the stalk. At this point, the snare wire is closed snugly, and the electric current is activated (▶ Fig. 4.6). The level of coagulating current should be set according to the size of the tissue being cut. A large tissue requires a higher setting. For large polyps, it may be wise to cinch the snare around the stalk snugly and wait for a couple of minutes to give the feeding vessels in the stalk a chance to thrombose prior to transection. With optimum setting on the electrocautery machine, the snare wire should cut through the polyp within 4 to 5 seconds. If this is not accomplished, the following should be rechecked: possible malfunction of the machine, too low heat, or too much tissue incorporated in the snare wire. Pure coagulation current is preferred.

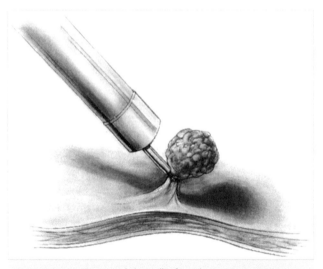

Fig. 4.6 Snare wire around the stalk of a polyp.

Sessile Polyp

Sessile polyps smaller than 2 cm usually can be snared in one piece. The technique is the same as for a pedunculated polyp, except that the wire is placed flush on the mucosa. When the snare wire is closed, the mucosa and the submucosa are squeezed into the snare wire. Before electrocautery is applied, the polyp should be lifted slightly from the bowel wall to minimize the chance of burning into the colonic wall (▶ Fig. 4.7). A larger polyp should be snared piecemeal in 1- to 1.5-cm pieces (▶ Fig. 4.8). It is important that an effort be made to retrieve each piece of the transected polyp for histopathologic examination, because any of these pieces may harbor a focal area of an invasive carcinoma. Depending on the size and difficulty in snaring, some large polyps should be snared in more than one session. Some authors recommend injection of saline with or without epinephrine into the submucosa beneath the polyp.[80] The "saline cushion" elevates the polyp from the muscularis propria and renders it safer and more successfully snared. This technique is recommended for large sessile polyps.[81,82] Hydroxypropyl methylcellulose or artificial tear (Gonak, Akorn, Inc., Buffalo Grove, IL) is excellent for submucosal injection.[83] The bottle of 15 mL should be diluted with 60-mL normal saline solution. Very large polyps (especially those in the right colon) should be reserved for colonic resection.

4.8.3 Advanced Polyp Techniques

Advanced techniques for polypectomy include endoscopic mucosal resection (EMR) and endoscopic submucosal resection (ESD). EMR, first developed in Japan, is an endoscopic technique designed for the removal of sessile or flat neoplasms confined to the superficial layers (mucosa and submucosa) of the GI tract. For many years, conventional EMR and surgery have been the only available therapy for large colorectal tumors. EMR is typically used for removal of lesions smaller than 2 cm or piecemeal removal of larger lesions.[84] EMR removes polyps using snares and saline lifting techniques described previously. For large lesions, incomplete resection is common, which can lead to local recurrence. ESD is a newer method, which has been developed for en bloc removal of large (usually larger than 2 cm), flat GI tract lesions. ESD uses a cautery knife and injection to remove polyps in one piece. Compared with EMR, ESD results in higher en bloc resection rate and lower local recurrence

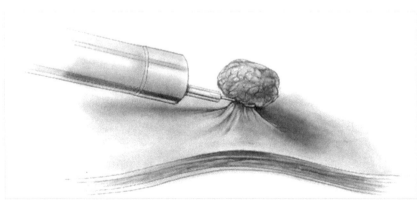

Fig. 4.7 Snare wire at the base of a sessile polyp. Note tenting of the mucosa.

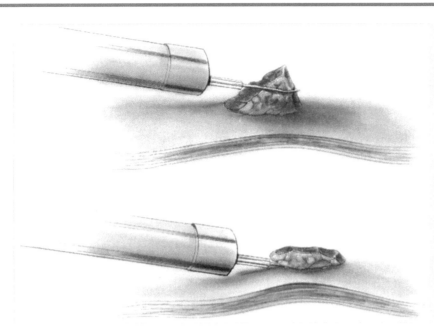

Fig. 4.8 Piecemeal snaring of a large sessile polyp.

rate for the treatment of colorectal tumors. However, ESD is more time-consuming, has a higher rate of procedure-related complications, and is more costly.[85]

Diminutive Polyp

Diminutive polyps are defined as polyps that are smaller than 5 mm in diameter. Contrary to past beliefs that most small polyps of the large bowel were of the hyperplastic type and were confined primarily to the rectum, in the era of colonoscopy, diminutive polyps have been found throughout the entire large bowel, and the incidence of neoplastic types is over 50%. In themselves, diminutive polyps have no clinical significance, and most of them probably grow very slowly.[86,87,88,89] However, it is impossible to predict which ones will grow to sizes that are of clinical significance. A diminutive neoplastic polyp seen in the colon or rectum may be a clue that additional polyps are in the more proximal colon. This calls for a complete colonic examination.

The importance of destroying diminutive polyps of the large bowel is arguable. There are many advantages in removing these small polyps. The histologic type is known from the biopsy, appropriate endoscopic surveillance can be planned, and the follow-up with a barium enema study every 1 or 2 years can be eliminated. Small polyps are treated by a cold or "hot biopsy" forceps.[90] If preferred, the polyp can be excised with a snare wire.[91] For practical purposes, many diminutive polyps can be electrocoagulated without biopsy.[92]

4.9 Intraoperative Colonoscopy

Colonoscopy has become a standard procedure for diagnosing colonic diseases and for removing colonic polyps. In skilled hands, total colonoscopy can be achieved more than 90% of the time. However, certain conditions make total colonoscopy impossible, including severe sigmoid diverticular disease, acute and fixed colonic angles from adhesions, an unusually tortuous colon, pelvic inflammation, and irradiation. The only way for

colonoscopy to be successful in these situations is by performing an intraoperative colonoscopy (i.e., passing the scope through the rectum with the abdomen open). The number of cases in which it has been used is small. The reasons are obvious—the procedure is at best a nuisance, a colonoscopy setup is required in the operating room, the procedure requires two teams of surgeons or a surgeon and an endoscopist, it consumes additional operative time, and there may be considerable colonic distention from air insufflation.

Intraoperative colonoscopy may have a definite place in a small number of cases. One example is to locate the site of the lesion when it cannot be identified by palpation. When properly performed, it is safe.[93,94,95] However, it must be performed with care and by personnel familiar with the technique. Cohen and Forde reported two cases of splenic capsular tear.[96] Other potential dangers are serosal tears of the colon or even perforation.

4.9.1 Polypectomy

Intraoperative colonoscopic polypectomy is indicated if the polyp cannot be reached by conventional colonoscopy. Laparoscopic, hand assisted, or open techniques can be used to manipulate or mobilize sections of the colon to allow a colonoscope to reach the area of the polyp. Once reached, the techniques of polypectomy are the same as those of the conventional method. Another indication for intraoperative colonoscopy is to locate the site from which a malignant polyp was previously removed and for which colonic resection is required. This can be achieved only if the scar from the polypectomy is not completely healed, which usually occurs within 2 week of a polypectomy. An additional option for challenging polyps has been described as laparoscopic-assisted colonoscopy.[97,98] In this technique, the procedure is performed in the operating room. One team places a laparoscopic camera into the abdomen with CO_2 insufflation to observe the segment of colon containing the polyp. The second team inserts a colonoscope into the anus and advances it to the site of the polyp. If necessary, the colon can be mobilized or manipulated. The polypectomy is performed while being observed with the laparoscopic camera. If there is dimpling or perforation during the polypectomy, the colonic wall can be oversewn or repaired with laparoscopic instruments (sutures or staples). Dribbling water over the polypectomy site can also be used to exclude any leakage. This technique has also been used as part of the "learning curve" for ESD.

4.9.2 Bleeding

Chronic blood loss from the GI tract can be very difficult to detect by colonoscopy, barium enema, upper intestinal and small bowel barium studies, and arteriography. Intraoperative enteroscopy in conjunction with intraoperative colonoscopy can help identify the bleeding source.[93] The techniques consist of passing the colonoscope orally and advancing it all the way to the ileocecal junction. An alternative method is to pass a sterile colonoscope via an upper jejunal enterotomy. The mucosa of the entire small bowel is examined. At the same time, the serosa is examined via the transillumination for vascular abnormalities. The final step is to pass the colonoscope through the anal canal and advance it to the cecum. The entire large bowel is examined in the same manner.

Acute or massive colonic bleeding may be another indication for intraoperative colonoscopy, when all other methods, including preoperative colonoscopy, have failed to localize the source of the bleeding. Intraoperative colonoscopy has the advantages of both intraluminal and extraluminal examination.[99] Intraoperative colonic lavage via a catheter inserted into the appendiceal base or a cecostomy has been shown to improve the quality of the examination.[100,101]

4.9.3 Carcinoma

Patients with carcinoma of the large bowel require a complete colonic investigation to detect a synchronous carcinoma or adenoma.[102] Ideally, the examination should be completed before the operation. However, if an examination is not performed, one can proceed with the operation and perform an intraoperative colonoscopy either before the abdomen is opened or after the anastomosis is performed. Intraoperative colonoscopy also is indicated in cases in which the lesion shown on barium enema cannot be palpated at exploration. For patients with obstructive carcinoma in whom preoperative colonoscopy could not be performed, intraoperative colonoscopy immediately following colonic resection may be an option.[93] This indication is limited because colonoscopy may damage the freshly constructed anastomosis.

4.10 Complications

The reported complication rates from colonoscopy are low. The risk of perforation ranges from 0.06 to 0.8% in diagnostic colonoscopy and from 0.7 to 3% in therapeutic colonoscopy.[1,2,103,104] The importance of these rates is magnified by the large number of patients undergoing the procedure. These figures may not represent the true incidence of complications because most reports come from individuals or institutions with extensive experience. Bleeding is the most common serious complication, followed in frequency by transmural burn and perforation.[103,105,106,107,108]

Other complications are snare entrapment, ensnarement of the bowel wall, and incarceration of the scope in a hernia. Early recognition of manifestations and understanding of proper treatment are crucial.

4.10.1 Bleeding

Colonoscopic-related bleeding may be immediate or delayed. Immediate bleeding from removal of a sessile polyp can be controlled with injection of diluted epinephrine solution at the site of the bleeding, fulguration, or the use of hemoclips.[109] Bleeding from a pedunculated polyp is more common with a thick stalk. It is important when doing a polypectomy to leave enough stalk so that if bleeding occurs, the remnant of the stalk can be clipped or resnared and coagulated or strangulated with the snare wire. Holding the snare occluded for 15 to 20 minutes without electrocoagulation will allow a thrombosis to form (▶ Fig. 4.9).[1] Delayed bleeding can occur from a few hours to several days after the procedure. It is thought to occur with premature separation of the coagulation eschar.

Management of delayed postpolypectomy bleeding starts with an assessment of the magnitude of the bleed, fluid resuscitation, and confirming whether the bleeding is ongoing. History of anticoagulant medication use and review of the colonoscopy report are important. Minimal and moderate bleeding is more common and usually stops with bowel rest and support but may require repeat endoscopy to control the bleeding site. For massive bleeding, supportive care should first include acute resuscitation, localization with proctoscopy, and computed tomography angiography (CTA). Proctoscopy confirms that the bleeding is proximal to the anus and distal rectum. CTA is readily available in most hospitals and can quickly confirm ongoing bleeding and suggest localization. A positive CTA is followed by selective arteriography and selective embolization (▶ Fig. 4.10). If anatomy prevents embolization, a vasopressin drip may be considered (▶ Fig. 4.11). The amount of blood in the colonic lumen with massive bleeding usually limits visualization and makes endoscopic control extremely difficult or impossible. On the rare occasions when angiographic control fails, an exploratory celiotomy may be necessary.

4.10.2 Perforation

Transmural burn or microperforation occurs when excessive heat burns through the bowel wall or when the snare wire is too close to the bowel wall. The classic symptoms are fever, localized abdominal pain and peritoneal signs, and leukocytosis. A CT scan will demonstrate colonic wall inflammation or pericolonic inflammation. Patients are managed similarly to diverticulitis with admission, bowel rest, and IV fluids and antibiotics. Close observation and serial exams are necessary as transmural burns may progress to an intra-abdominal abscess, which can be managed with a CT-guided percutaneous drainage.

Perforations associated with diagnostic procedures are usually large and result from forceful passage of the colonoscope through a loop, bowing of the sigmoid colon, narrowing from diverticular disease, or adhesions from previous pelvic operation. The spectrum of perforations ranges from "silent" pneumoperitoneum to serosal tear, extraperitoneal perforation, and

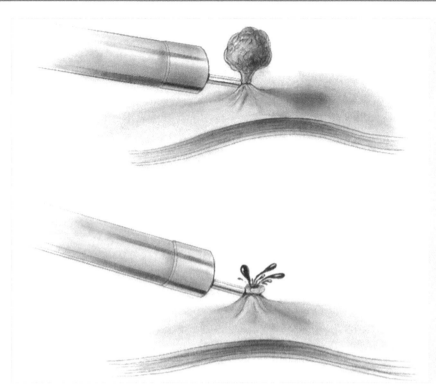

Fig. 4.9 Bleeding stump of a polyp is strangulated by the snare.

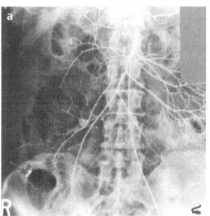
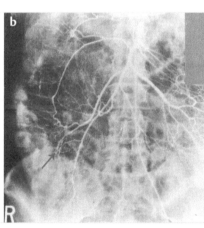

Fig. 4.10 Bleeding in the cecum after colonoscopic polypectomy. **(a)** Superior mesenteric arteriography showing bleeding (*arrow*). **(b)** Bleeding stopped after introduction of Gelfoam emboli (*arrow*).[103] (With permission © 1986 Wolters Kluwer.)

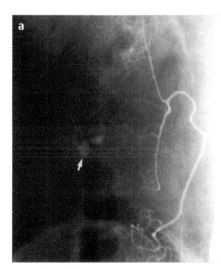
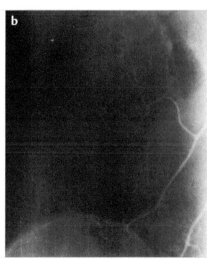

Fig. 4.11 Bleeding in the ascending colon after colonoscopic polypectomy. **(a)** Superior mesenteric arteriography showing bleeding (*arrow*). **(b)** Bleeding stopped after vasopressin drip.[103] (With permission © 1986 Wolters Kluwer.)

intraperitoneal perforation. Retroperitoneal perforations are usually difficult to assess clinically and may not be detected until the appearance of subcutaneous emphysema. The air may track along the retroperitoneal planes, up to the flank, mediastinum, neck, and around the eyes or down to the scrotum. The most frequent site of perforation is in the intraperitoneal sigmoid colon. Although the incidental finding of "silent" pneumoperitoneum can be observed, operation is indicated in most perforations that occur during diagnostic colonoscopy because those perforations are generally large. If the operation for colonoscopic perforation is performed early, a primary repair can be performed. If generalized peritonitis has already occurred, resection without anastomosis is the safest procedure.

Unlike the usually large perforation caused by injury from the colonoscope, perforation from polypectomy may vary from "silent" asymptomatic air under the diaphragm (▶ Fig. 4.12) to a large perforation that causes generalized peritonitis. Management may vary from observation to immediate exploratory celiotomy.

No treatment is needed to correct asymptomatic air under the diaphragm, but the patient must be observed to detect any development of peritonitis.[110] If there is a large symptomatic perforation associated with signs and symptoms of peritonitis, an immediate exploratory celiotomy is required. Perforation in colonoscopic polypectomy is caused by snaring too large a piece, applying too much heat, or snaring tissue that is too deep or too close to the bowel wall.

4.10.3 Snare Entrapment

If the snare wire gets caught in the substance of a polyp, it may be impossible to cut through the polyp or disengage the wire. This problem is caused by too much tissue in the snare, too low a heat setting (causing "charring" of the tissue), or misjudgment in snaring a frank carcinoma. For a benign lesion, the entrapped wire should be tightened and left in place while the colonoscope is removed from the patient. With the strangulation of the wire, the polyp should fall off in a few days. If the entrapment occurs in a frank carcinoma, a colonic resection is done.[103] If care is not taken during polypectomy, the adjacent bowel wall inadvertently may be incorporated into the wire loop, causing perforation to occur (▶ Fig. 4.13). Being aware of this possibility may prevent the complication. Difficulty in transecting the polyp, as evidenced by unusually high current requirements, may indicate that too much tissue is within the wire loop.

4.10.4 Miscellaneous Complications

Hernial incarceration of the colonoscope is an unusual complication. Incarceration can be avoided by considering the presence of a large sliding inguinal or ventral hernia as a relative contraindication to colonoscopy. The risk of incarceration can be minimized by reducing the hernia before the procedure and by maintaining reduction while the colonoscope is advanced. If inadvertent incarceration occurs, simple traction on the colonoscope is avoided and a "pulley" technique, in which the colonoscope is extricated one limb at a time, should be applied (▶ Fig. 4.14).[111]

Splenic injury from colonoscopy is uncommon, most likely occurring from pulling down the colonoscope from the transverse colon with the tip of the scope in a locked position. Abdominal pain is the most common symptom, usually within 24 hours. CT scan of abdomen is helpful to confirm the diagnosis.[112] The complication rate in diagnostic colonoscopy can be kept to a minimum by use of proper technique, knowledge of when to stop the procedure, and appreciation of the causes and mechanisms.

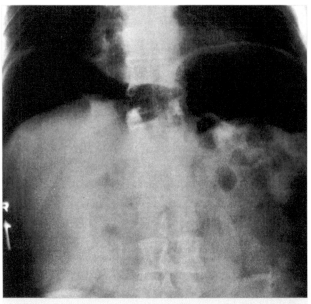

Fig. 4.12 Asymptomatic free air under diaphragm after colonoscopic polypectomy. (Reproduced with permission from Pineau et al.[106])

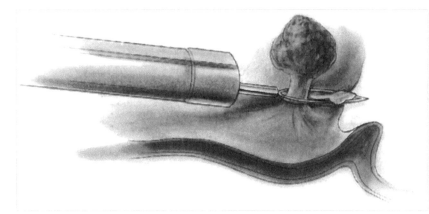

Fig. 4.13 Inadvertent ensnarement of adjacent bowel wall.

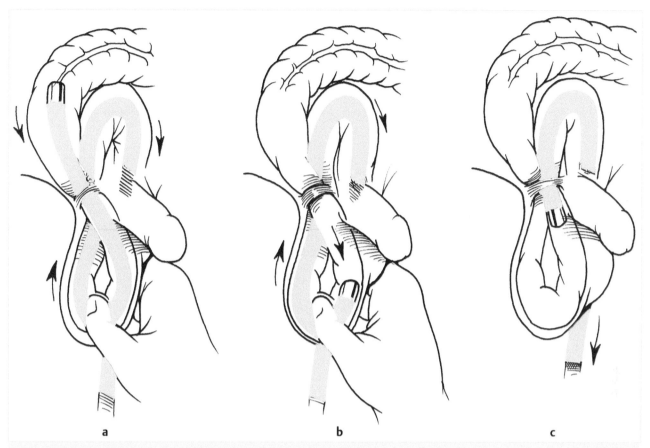

Fig. 4.14 "Pulley" technique of removal. **(a)** Scope held along inner edge of loop. **(b,c)** Instrument exits one limb at a time; thumb and finger are used as the "pulley."

Two explosive gases in the colon are hydrogen and methane, both of which are formed by colonic bacteria. To produce hydrogen, colonic bacteria require a constant supply of exogenous substrate, primarily unabsorbed carbohydrate.[113] Hence, a good bowel cleansing followed by an overnight fast markedly reduces hydrogen production. In contrast, methane is produced from an exogenous carbon source; thus, its production has no clear-cut relation to diet.[114] However, the vigorous bowel cleansing required for colonoscopy reduces by 10-fold the amount of hydrogen and methane liberated in the colon.[115] The risk of bowel gas explosion can be reduced further by exchanging gas and air in the bowel lumen by air insufflation and alternated with several aspirations before the snaring is performed. It is not necessary to use carbon dioxide to prevent gas explosion in the well-prepared colon unless it is done to decrease abdominal distention.[116] The tragic case report of a bowel gas explosion was attributed to preparation of the bowel with mannitol, a potent substrate in which bacteria produce hydrogen.[117] Mannitol preparation should not be used in patients who require snaring or electrocoagulation of a large bowel polyp.

References

[1] Shinya H. Colonoscopy: Diagnosis and Treatment of Colonic Diseases. New York, NY: Igaku-Shoin; 1982

[2] Jentschura D, Raute M, Winter J, Henkel T, Kraus M, Manegold BC. Complications in endoscopy of the lower gastrointestinal tract. Therapy and prognosis. Surg Endosc. 1994; 8(6):672–676

[3] Nivatvongs S. Colonic perforations during colonoscopy. Perspect Colon Rectal Surg. 1988; 1(2):107–112

[4] Nivatvongs S. How to teach colonoscopy. Clin Colon Rectal Surg. 2001; 14:387–392

[5] Waye JD, Bashkoff E. Total colonoscopy: is it always possible? Gastrointest Endosc. 1991; 37(2):152–154

[6] Nivatvongs S, Snover DC, Fang DT. Piecemeal snare excision of large sessile colon and rectal polyps: is it adequate? Gastrointest Endosc. 1984; 30(1):18–20

[7] Shinya H, Wolff WI. Morphology, anatomic distribution and cancer potential of colonic polyps. Ann Surg. 1979; 190(6):679–683

[8] Hull T, Church JM. Colonoscopy-how difficult, how painful? Surg Endosc. 1994; 8(7):784–787

[9] Saunders BP, Fukumoto M, Halligan S, et al. Why is colonoscopy more difficult in women? Gastrointest Endosc. 1996; 43(2, Pt 1):124–126

[10] Saunders BP, Phillips RK, Williams CB. Intraoperative measurement of colonic anatomy and attachments with relevance to colonoscopy. Br J Surg. 1995; 82(11):1491–1493

[11] Ward ST, Mohammed MA, Walt R, Valori R, Ismail T, Dunckley P. An analysis of the learning curve to achieve competency at colonoscopy using the JETS database. Gut. 2014; 63(11):1746–1754

[12] Sedlack RE. Training to competency in colonoscopy: assessing and defining competency standards. Gastrointest Endosc. 2011; 74(2):355–366.e1-2

[13] Nivatvongs S. Diagnosis. In: Gordon PH, Nivatvongs S, eds. Principles and Practice of Surgery for the Colon, Rectum, and Anus. 3rd ed. New York, NY: Informa; 2007:65–98

[14] Nivatvongs S, Vermeulen FD, Fang DT. Colonoscopic decompression of acute pseudo-obstruction of the colon. Ann Surg. 1982; 196(5):598–600

[15] Dorudi S, Berry AR, Kettlewell MGW. Acute colonic pseudo-obstruction. Br J Surg. 1992; 79(2):99–103

[16] Jetmore AB, Timmcke AE, Gathright JB, Jr, Hicks TC, Ray JE, Baker JW. Ogilvie's syndrome: colonoscopic decompression and analysis of predisposing factors. Dis Colon Rectum. 1992; 35(12):1135–1142

[17] Sgambati SA, Armstrong DN, Ballantyne GH. Management of acute colonic pseudo-obstruction. (Ogilvie's syndrome). Perspect Colon Rectal Surg. 1994; 7:77–96

[18] Ponec RJ, Saunders MD, Kimmey MB. Neostigmine for the treatment of acute colonic pseudo-obstruction. N Engl J Med. 1999; 341(3):137–141

[19] Beck DE. Endoscopic colonic stents and dilatation. Clin Colon Rectal Surg. 2010; 23(1):37–41

[20] Sagar J. Colorectal stents for the management of malignant colonic obstructions. Cochrane Database Syst Rev. 2011(11):CD007378

[21] Mamula P, Adler DG, Conway JD, et al. ASGE Technology Committee. Colonoscopy preparation. Gastrointest Endosc. 2009; 69(7):1201–1209

[22] Ernstoff JJ, Howard DA, Marshall JB, Jumshyd A, McCullough AJ. A randomized blinded clinical trial of a rapid colonic lavage solution (Golytely) compared with standard preparation for colonoscopy and barium enema. Gastroenterology. 1983; 84(6):1512–1516

[23] Shawki S, Wexner SD. Oral colorectal cleansing preparations in adults. Drugs. 2008; 68(4):417–437

[24] Wexner SD, Beck DE, Baron TH, et al. A consensus document on bowel preparation before colonoscopy: prepared by a task force from the American Society of Colon and Rectal Surgeons (ASCRS), the American Society of Gastrointestinal Endoscopy (ASGE), and the Society of American Gastrointestinal and Endoscopic Surgeons (SAGES). Surg Endosc. 2006; 20:147–160

[25] Rösch T, Classen M. Fractional cleansing of the large bowel with "Golytely" for colonoscopic preparation: a controlled trial. Endoscopy. 1987; 19 (5):198–200

[26] Aoun E, Abdul-Baki H, Azar C, et al. A randomized single-blind trial of split-dose PEG-electrolyte solution without dietary restriction compared with whole dose PEG-electrolyte solution with dietary restriction for colonoscopy preparation. Gastrointest Endosc. 2005; 62(2):213–218

[27] Ell C, Fischbach W, Bronisch HJ, et al. Randomized trial of low-volume PEG solution versus standard PEG + electrolytes for bowel cleansing before colonoscopy. Am J Gastroenterol. 2008; 103(4):883–893

[28] Bitoun A, Ponchon T, Barthet M, Coffin B, Dugué C, Halphen M, Norcol Group. Results of a prospective randomised multicentre controlled trial comparing a new 2-L ascorbic acid plus polyethylene glycol and electrolyte solution vs. sodium phosphate solution in patients undergoing elective colonoscopy. Aliment Pharmacol Ther. 2006; 24(11–12):1631–1642

[29] Pashankar DS, Uc A, Bishop WP. Polyethylene glycol 3350 without electrolytes: a new safe, effective, and palatable bowel preparation for colonoscopy in children. J Pediatr. 2004; 144(3):358–362

[30] Landreneau SW, Di Palma JA. Colon cleansing for colonoscopy 2013: current status. Curr Gastroenterol Rep. 2013; 15(8):341–347

[31] Belsey J, Epstein O, Heresbach D. Systematic review: oral bowel preparation for colonoscopy. Aliment Pharmacol Ther. 2007; 25(4):373–384

[32] Johanson JF, Popp JW, Jr, Cohen LB, et al. A randomized, multicenter study comparing the safety and efficacy of sodium phosphate tablets with 2 L polyethylene glycol solution plus bisacodyl tablets for colon cleansing. Am J Gastroenterol. 2007; 102(10):2238–2246

[33] DiPalma JA, Buckley SE, Warner BA, Culpepper RM. Biochemical effects of oral sodium phosphate. Dig Dis Sci. 1996; 41(4):749–753

[34] Markowitz GS, Stokes MB, Radhakrishnan J, D'Agati VD. Acute phosphate nephropathy following oral sodium phosphate bowel purgative: an underrecognized cause of chronic renal failure. J Am Soc Nephrol. 2005; 16 (11):3389–3396

[35] Wexner SD, Beck DE, Baron TH, et al. American Society of Colon and Rectal Surgeons, American Society for Gastrointestinal Endoscopy, Society of American Gastrointestinal and Endoscopic Surgeons. A consensus document on bowel preparation before colonoscopy: prepared by a task force from the American Society of Colon and Rectal Surgeons (ASCRS), the American Society for Gastrointestinal Endoscopy (ASGE), and the Society of American Gastrointestinal and Endoscopic Surgeons (SAGES). Gastrointest Endosc. 2006; 63(7):894–909

[36] Pelham R, Dobre A, van Diest K, Cleveland MVB. Oral sodium phosphate bowel preparations: how much hydration is enough? Gastrointest Endosc. 2007; 65(5):AB314

[37] Patel V, Nicar M, Emmett M, et al. Intestinal and renal effects of low-volume phosphate and sulfate cathartic solutions designed for cleansing the colon: pathophysiological studies in five normal subjects. Am J Gastroenterol. 2009; 104(4):953–965

[38] Trautwein AL, Vinitski LA, Peck SN. Bowel preparation before colonoscopy in the pediatric patient: a randomized study. Gastroenterol Nurs. 1996; 19 (4):137–139

[39] Manabe N, Cremonini F, Camilleri M, Sandborn WJ, Burton DD. Effects of bisacodyl on ascending colon emptying and overall colonic transit in healthy volunteers. Aliment Pharmacol Ther. 2009; 30(9):930–936

[40] Baudet JS, Castro V, Redondo I. Recurrent ischemic colitis induced by colonoscopy bowel lavage. Am J Gastroenterol. 2010; 105(3):700–701

[41] Rex DK, Imperiale TF, Portish V. Patients willing to try colonoscopy without sedation: associated clinical factors and results of a randomized controlled trial. Gastrointest Endosc. 1999; 49(5):554–559

[42] Reves JG, Fragen RJ, Vinik HR, Greenblatt DJ. Midazolam: pharmacology and uses. Anesthesiology. 1985; 62(3):310–324

[43] Horn E, Nesbit SA. Pharmacology and pharmacokinetics of sedatives and analgesics. Gastrointest Endosc Clin N Am. 2004; 14(2):247–268

[44] Cohen LB, Wecsler JS, Gaetano JN, et al. Endoscopic sedation in the United States: results from a nationwide survey. Am J Gastroenterol. 2006; 101 (5):967–974

[45] Zakko SF, Seifert HA, Gross JB. A comparison of midazolam and diazepam for conscious sedation during colonoscopy in a prospective double-blind study. Gastrointest Endosc. 1999; 49(6):684–689

[46] Cole SG, Brozinsky S, Isenberg JI. Midazolam, a new more potent benzodiazepine, compared with diazepam: a randomized, double-blind study of preendoscopic sedatives. Gastrointest Endosc. 1983; 29(3):219–222

[47] Lee MG, Hanna W, Harding H. Sedation for upper gastrointestinal endoscopy: a comparative study of midazolam and diazepam. Gastrointest Endosc. 1989; 35(2):82–84

[48] McQuaid KR, Laine L. A systematic review and meta-analysis of randomized, controlled trials of moderate sedation for routine endoscopic procedures. Gastrointest Endosc. 2008; 67(6):910–923

[49] Bahn EL, Holt KR. Procedural sedation and analgesia: a review and new concepts. Emerg Med Clin North Am. 2005; 23(2):503–517

[50] Waring JP, Baron TH, Hirota WK, et al. American Society for Gastrointestinal Endoscopy, Standards of Practice Committee. Guidelines for conscious sedation and monitoring during gastrointestinal endoscopy. Gastrointest Endosc. 2003; 58(3):317–322

[51] Mora CT, Torjman M, White PF. Sedative and ventilatory effects of midazolam infusion: effect of flumazenil reversal. Can J Anaesth. 1995; 42(8):677–684

[52] Lichtenstein DR, Jagannath S, Baron TH, et al. Standards of Practice Committee of the American Society for Gastrointestinal Endoscopy. Sedation and anesthesia in GI endoscopy. Gastrointest Endosc. 2008; 68(5):815–826

[53] Robertson DJ, Jacobs DP, Mackenzie TA, Oringer JA, Rothstein RI. Clinical trial: a randomized, study comparing meperidine (pethidine) and fentanyl in adult gastrointestinal endoscopy. Aliment Pharmacol Ther. 2009; 29(8):817–823

[54] Scholz J, Steinfath M, Schulz M. Clinical pharmacokinetics of alfentanil, fentanyl and sufentanil. An update. Clin Pharmacokinet. 1996; 31(4):275–292

[55] Umans JG, Inturrisi CE. Antinociceptive activity and toxicity of meperidine and normeperidine in mice. J Pharmacol Exp Ther. 1982; 223(1):203–206

[56] Bodenham A, Shelly MP, Park GR. The altered pharmacokinetics and pharmacodynamics of drugs commonly used in critically ill patients. Clin Pharmacokinet. 1988; 14(6):347–373

[57] Graber RG. Propofol in the endoscopy suite: an anesthesiologist's perspective. Gastrointest Endosc. 1999; 49(6):803–806

[58] Cohen LB, Hightower CD, Wood DA, Miller KM, Aisenberg J. Moderate level sedation during endoscopy: a prospective study using low-dose propofol, meperidine/fentanyl, and midazolam. Gastrointest Endosc. 2004; 59 (7):795–803

[59] Sipe BW, Scheidler M, Baluyut A, Wright B. A prospective safety study of a low-dose propofol sedation protocol for colonoscopy. Clin Gastroenterol Hepatol. 2007; 5(5):563–566

[60] Bryson HM, Fulton BR, Faulds D. Propofol. An update of its use in anaesthesia and conscious sedation. Drugs. 1995; 50(3):513–559

[61] Byrne MF, Baillie J. Nurse-assisted propofol sedation: the jury is in! Gastroenterology. 2005; 129(5):1781–1782

[62] Clarke AC, Chiragakis L, Hillman LC, Kaye GL. Sedation for endoscopy: the safe use of propofol by general practitioner sedationists. Med J Aust. 2002; 176(4):158–161

[63] Rex DK, Deenadayalu V, Eid E. Gastroenterologist-directed propofol: an update. Gastrointest Endosc Clin N Am. 2008; 18(4):717–725, ix

[64] Rex DK, Heuss LT, Walker JA, Qi R. Trained registered nurses/endoscopy teams can administer propofol safely for endoscopy. Gastroenterology. 2005; 129(5):1384–1391

[65] Heuss LT, Schnieper P, Drewe J, Pflimlin E, Beglinger C. Safety of propofol for conscious sedation during endoscopic procedures in high-risk patients-a prospective, controlled study. Am J Gastroenterol. 2003; 98(8):1751–1757

[66] Dikman AE, Sanyal S, Aisenberg J, et al. Gastroenterologist-directed, balanced propofol sedation for EGD and colonoscopy: an analysis of safety in 15,286 patients. Gastrointest Endosc. 2008; 67:AB84

[67] Singh H, Poluha W, Cheung M, Choptain N, Baron KI, Taback SP. Propofol for sedation during colonoscopy. Cochrane Database Syst Rev. 2008(4): CD006268

[68] Joint Statement of a Working Group from the American College of Gastroenterology (ACG), the American Gastroenterological Association (AGA), and the American Society for Gastrointestinal Endoscopy (ASGE). Recommendations on the administration of sedation for the performance of endoscopic procedures. Available at: http://www.gastro.org/wmspage.cfm?parm1_371. Accessed October 14, 2009

[69] Wiggins TF, Khan AS, Winstead NS. Sedation, analgesia, and monitoring. Clin Colon Rectal Surg. 2010; 23(1):14–20

[70] Gross JB, Bailey PL, Connis RT, et al. American Society of Anesthesiologists Task Force on Sedation and Analgesia by Non-Anesthesiologists. Practice guidelines for sedation and analgesia by non-anesthesiologists. Anesthesiology. 2002; 96(4):1004–1017

[71] Siebig S, Rockmann F, Sabel K, et al. Continuous non-invasive arterial pressure technique improves patient monitoring during interventional endoscopy. Int J Med Sci. 2009; 6(1):37–42

[72] Poirier MP, Gonzalez Del-Rey JA, McAneney CM, DiGiulio GA. Utility of monitoring capnography, pulse oximetry, and vital signs in the detection of airway mishaps: a hyperoxemic animal model. Am J Emerg Med. 1998; 16 (4):350–352

[73] Vargo JJ, Zuccaro G, Jr, Dumot JA, Conwell DL, Morrow JB, Shay SS. Automated graphic assessment of respiratory activity is superior to pulse oximetry and visual assessment for the detection of early respiratory depression during therapeutic upper endoscopy. Gastrointest Endosc. 2002; 55(7):826–831

[74] Lightdale JR, Goldmann DA, Feldman HA, Newburg AR, DiNardo JA, Fox VL. Microstream capnography improves patient monitoring during moderate sedation: a randomized, controlled trial. Pediatrics. 2006; 117(6): e1170–e1178

[75] Hirota WK, Petersen K, Baron TH, et al. Standards of Practice Committee of the American Society for Gastrointestinal Endoscopy. Guidelines for antibiotic prophylaxis for GI endoscopy. Gastrointest Endosc. 2003; 58 (4):475–482

[76] Oliver G, Lowry A, Vernava A, et al. The American Society of Colon and Rectal Surgeons. Practice parameters for antibiotic prophylaxis–supporting documentation. The Standards Task Force. Dis Colon Rectum. 2000; 43(9):1194–1200

[77] Wilson W, Taubert KA, Gewitz M, et al. American Heart Association Rheumatic Fever, Endocarditis, and Kawasaki Disease Committee, American Heart Association Council on Cardiovascular Disease in the Young, American Heart Association Council on Clinical Cardiology, American Heart Association Council on Cardiovascular Surgery and Anesthesia, Quality of Care and Outcomes Research Interdisciplinary Working Group. Prevention of infective endocarditis: guidelines from the American Heart Association: a guideline from the American Heart Association Rheumatic Fever, Endocarditis, and Kawasaki Disease Committee, Council on Cardiovascular Disease in the Young, and the Council on Clinical Cardiology, Council on Cardiovascular Surgery and Anesthesia, and the Quality of Care and Outcomes Research Interdisciplinary Working Group. Circulation. 2007; 116(15):1736–1754

[78] Banerjee S, Shen B, Baron TH, et al. ASGE STANDARDS OF PRACTICE COMMITTEE. Antibiotic prophylaxis for GI endoscopy. Gastrointest Endosc. 2008; 67(6):791–798

[79] Sakai Y. The technic of colonofiberscopy. Dis Colon Rectum. 1972; 15 (6):403–412

[80] Shumaker DA, Zaman A, Katon RM. A randomized controlled trial in a training institution comparing a pediatric variable stiffness colonoscope, a pedia-

[81] Karita M, Tada M, Okita K, Kodama T. Endoscopic therapy for early colon cancer: the strip biopsy resection technique. Gastrointest Endosc. 1991; 37 (2):128–132

[82] Waye JD. Saline injection colonoscopic polypectomy. Am J Gastroenterol. 1994; 89(3):305–306

[83] Kanamori T, Itoh M, Yokoyama Y, Tsuchida K. Injection-incision–assisted snare resection of large sessile colorectal polyps. Gastrointest Endosc. 1996; 43(3):189–195

[84] Kantsevoy SV, Adler DG, Conway JD, et al. ASGE TECHNOLOGY COMMITTEE. Endoscopic mucosal resection and endoscopic submucosal dissection. Gastrointest Endosc. 2008; 68(1):11–18

[85] Wang J, Zhang X-H, Ge J, Yang CM, Liu JY, Zhao SL. Endoscopic submucosal dissection vs endoscopic mucosal resection for colorectal tumors: a meta-analysis. World J Gastroenterol. 2014; 20(25):8282–8287

[86] Feitoza AB, Gostout CJ, Burgart LJ, Burkert A, Herman LJ, Rajan E. Hydroxypropyl methylcellulose: a better submucosal fluid cushion for endoscopic mucosal resection. Gastrointest Endosc. 2003; 57(1):41–47

[87] Ryan ME, Norfleet RG, Kirchner JP, et al. The significance of diminutive colonic polyps found at flexible sigmoidoscopy. Gastrointest Endosc. 1989; 35 (2):85–89

[88] Tedesco FJ, Hendrix JC, Pickens CA, Brady PG, Mills LR. Diminutive polyps: histopathology, spatial distribution, and clinical significance. Gastrointest Endosc. 1982; 28(1):1–5

[89] Feczko PJ, Bernstein MA, Halpert RD, Ackerman LV. Small colonic polyps: a reappraisal of their significance. Radiology. 1984; 152(2):301–303

[90] Waye JD. Techniques of polypectomy: hot biopsy forceps and snare polypectomy. Am J Gastroenterol. 1987; 82(7):615–618

[91] Tappero G, Gaia E, De Giuli P, Martini S, Gubetta L, Emanuelli G. Cold snare excision of small colorectal polyps. Gastrointest Endosc. 1992; 38 (3):310–313

[92] Spencer RJ, Melton LJ, III, Ready RL, Ilstrup DM. Treatment of small colorectal polyps: a population-based study of the risk of subsequent carcinoma. Mayo Clin Proc. 1984; 59(5):305–310

[93] Bowden TA, Jr. Intraoperative endoscopy of the gastrointestinal tract: clinical necessity or lack of preoperative preparation? World J Surg. 1989; 13 (2):186–189

[94] Saclarides TJ, Wolff BG, Pemberton JH, Devine RM, Nivatvongs S, Dozois RR. Clean sweep of the colon. The use of intraoperative colonoscopy. Dis Colon Rectum. 1989; 32(10):864–866

[95] Whelan RL, Buls JG, Goldberg SM, Rothenberger DA. Intra-operative endoscopy. University of Minnesota experience. Am Surg. 1989; 55(5):281–286

[96] Cohen JL, Forde KA. Intraoperative colonoscopy. Ann Surg. 1988; 207 (3):231–233

[97] Beck DE, Karulf RE. Laparoscopic-assisted full-thickness endoscopic polypectomy. Dis Colon Rectum. 1993; 36(7):693–695

[98] Prohm P, Weber J, Bönner C. Laparoscopic-assisted coloscopic polypectomy. Dis Colon Rectum. 2001; 44(5):746–748

[99] Rossini FP, Ferrari A, Spandre M, et al. Emergency colonoscopy. World J Surg. 1989; 13(2):190–192

[100] Campbell WB, Rhodes M, Kettlewell MG. Colonoscopy following intraoperative lavage in the management of severe colonic bleeding. Ann R Coll Surg Engl. 1985; 67(5):290–292

[101] Scott HJ, Lane IF, Glynn MJ, et al. Colonic haemorrhage: a technique for rapid intra-operative bowel preparation and colonoscopy. Br J Surg. 1986; 73 (5):390–391

[102] Langevin JM, Nivatvongs S. The true incidence of synchronous cancer of the large bowel. A prospective study. Am J Surg. 1984; 147(3):330–333

[103] Nivatvongs S. Complications in colonoscopic polypectomy. An experience with 1,555 polypectomies. Dis Colon Rectum. 1986; 29(12):825–830

[104] Walsh RM, Ackroyd FW, Shellito PC. Endoscopic resection of large sessile colorectal polyps. Gastrointest Endosc. 1992; 38(3):303–309

[105] Waye JD, Lewis BS, Yessayan S. Colonoscopy: a prospective report of complications. J Clin Gastroenterol. 1992; 15(4):347–351

[106] Pineau BC, Paskett ED, Chen GJ, et al. Virtual colonoscopy using oral contrast compared with colonoscopy for the detection of patients with colorectal polyps. Gastroenterology. 2003; 125(2):304–310

[107] Cotton PB, Durkalski VL, Pineau BC, et al. Computed tomographic colonography (virtual colonoscopy): a multicenter comparison with standard colonoscopy for detection of colorectal neoplasia. JAMA. 2004; 291(14):1713–1719

[108] Garbay JR, Suc B, Rotman N, Fourtanier G, Escat J. Multicentre study of surgical complications of colonoscopy. Br J Surg. 1996; 83(1):42–44

[109] Binmoeller KF, Bohnacker S, Seifert H, Thonke F, Valdeyar H, Soehendra N. Endoscopic snare excision of "giant" colorectal polyps. Gastrointest Endosc. 1996; 43(3):183–188

[110] Lo AY, Beaton HL. Selective management of colonoscopic perforations. J Am Coll Surg. 1994; 179(3):333–337

[111] Koltun WA, Coller JA. Incarceration of colonoscope in an inguinal hernia. "Pulley" technique of removal. Dis Colon Rectum. 1991; 34(2):191–193

[112] Ahmed A, Eller PM, Schiffman FJ. Splenic rupture: an unusual complication of colonoscopy. Am J Gastroenterol. 1997; 92(7):1201–1204

[113] Levitt MD. Production and excretion of hydrogen gas in man. N Engl J Med. 1969; 281(3):122–127

[114] Bond JH, Jr, Engel RR, Levitt MD. Factors influencing pulmonary methane excretion in man. An indirect method of studying the in situ metabolism of the methane-producing colonic bacteria. J Exp Med. 1971; 133(3):572–588

[115] Bond JH, Jr, Levitt MD. Factors affecting the concentration of combustible gases in the colon during colonoscopy. Gastroenterology. 1975; 68(6):1445–1448

[116] Phaosawasdi K, Cooley W, Wheeler J, Rice P. Carbon dioxide-insufflated colonoscopy: an ignored superior technique. Gastrointest Endosc. 1986; 32 (5):330–333

[117] Bigard MA, Gaucher P, Lassalle C. Fatal colonic explosion during colonoscopic polypectomy. Gastroenterology. 1979; 77(6):1307–1310

5 Preoperative and Postoperative Management of Colorectal Surgery Patients

David E. Beck

Abstract

The perioperative management of colorectal surgery patients has changed dramatically in recent years. Efforts toward cost reduction, reducing or eliminating hospital stays, and the increasing use of evidence-based practices have all had an influence. The experience gained from minimally invasive procedures has been transitioned to other patients. Many of these practices have been grouped into Enhanced Recovery After Surgery (ERAS) protocols or care paths. As these practices can be applied in almost all patients, Care Paths seems a better term. Initially, a host of activities were grouped and used with good overall results. Specific components of these protocols are only now being subjected to prospective evaluation. Until such evidence is available, it is difficult to know the true value of each component. Perioperative management is arbitrarily divided into three phases: preoperative, intraoperative, and postoperative.

Keywords: preoperative management, postoperative management, patient education, operative risk, mechanical bowel cleansing, antibiotic bowel preparation, analgesia, early ambulation, deep venous thrombosis prevention, resumption of diet, postoperative pain

5.1 General Consideration

The perioperative management of colorectal surgery patients has changed dramatically in recent years. Efforts toward cost reduction, reducing or eliminating hospital stays, and the increasing use of evidence-based practices have all had an influence. In addition, the experience gained from minimally invasive procedures has been transitioned to other patients. Many of these practices have been grouped into Enhanced Recovery After Surgery (ERAS) protocols or care paths. As these practices can be applied in almost all patients, Care Paths seems a better term. Initially, a host of activities were grouped and used with good overall results. Specific components of these protocols have only recently been subject to prospective evaluation. Until such evidence is available, it is difficult to know the true value of each component. Perioperative management is arbitrarily divided into three phases: preoperative, intraoperative, and postoperative. However, some components such as pain management occur in several phases. Important components of each phase are listed in ▶ Table 5.1. An additional discussion of ambulatory anorectal procedures is presented in Chapter 6.

5.2 Preoperative

5.2.1 Patient Education

The patient undergoing an elective colorectal procedure should be given general information regarding their care path, which includes preoperative preparation, in-hospital stay,

postoperative period at home, and overall recovery time. This quantity of information may challenge patients' memories. Best practice is to provide the patient with a handout that summarizes this information.

At the outset, the surgeon should discuss the goals of the proposed intervention. The type of incision, the extent of the wounds to be created, and the anatomy involved should be outlined in addition to various aspects of normal wound healing. Where appropriate, the possibility of a minimally invasive laparoscopic approach and the possibility of intraoperative decision making should be mentioned. The surgeon should also be willing to discuss potential complications. The patient should be afforded the opportunity to ask questions regarding potential risks of the operation, the expected outcome, and any alternative therapy. A discussion of postoperative pain will reassure the patient that the presence of some pain is by itself not an indication that something has gone wrong. At the same time, the patient should be reassured that every effort will be made to minimize their pain with appropriate use of analgesics and that considerate and empathetic nursing care will be offered. Realistic expectations should be given regarding the functional results after "reconstructive" colorectal operations, such as ileoanal procedures, coloanal anastomoses, and anal sphincter repair. If there is a possibility of an ostomy, involvement of a wound and ostomy care nurse is extremely helpful (see Chapter 30).

The patient should be reassured that all measures will be taken to bring about an uneventful postoperative course. At the same time, the patient's need to cooperate with postoperative care, especially with regard to pulmonary care and ambulation, must be stressed. Finally, all aspects of daily activities pertinent to recovery should be discussed.

5.2.2 Assessment and Optimization of Operative Risk

Recommendations for elective colorectal surgery are based on an appropriate clinical history, physical examination, and

Table 5.1 Components of a colorectal surgery care path

Preoperative	Intraoperative	Postoperative
Patient education	Fluid management	Ambulation
Optimizing overall health	Minimally invasive	Oral intake/nutrition
Nutritional assessment	Temperature control	Fluid management
Labs/X-rays/tests	Drain usage	Pain management
Bowel preparation	Pain management	Discharge criteria
Reduction of fasting state and/or nutritional supplementation		
Pain management		

diagnostic evaluation. Before any elective colorectal operation, the patient should be assessed and prepared carefully. Special attention should be given to previous exposure to anesthetic agents and medication and to allergies, personal habits (alcohol and drug abuse), and concurrent systemic illness. Since abnormalities in systemic functions may affect the uptake and action as well as the distribution and elimination of anesthetic drugs, the patient should be in the best possible state of fitness consistent with his systemic disease. Operative risk is assessed in the following areas: cardiovascular status, pulmonary function, renal status, hepatic function, hematologic status, nutritional status, obesity, age, and psychological status.

Cardiovascular Status

Patients with a history of myocardial infarction are prone to experience another infarction during or following subsequent operations. The incidence of perioperative myocardial infarction was reviewed by Roizen and Fleisher,[1] who reported the overall reinfarction rate ranged from 1.9 to 15.9%, mostly in the 7 to 9% range, with mortality ranging from 1.1 to 5.4%, mostly in the 3 to 4% range. In the first 3 months following a myocardial infarction, the numbers are much higher with reported reinfarction rates ranging from 0 to 86%, mostly in the 20 to 40% range, with mortality ranging from 0 to 86%, mostly in the 23 to 38% range. With time, the numbers improve so that at 4 to 6 months following myocardial infarction, reinfarction rates range from 0 to 26%, mostly in the 6 to 16% range, and the corresponding mortality rates range from 0 to 5.9%. After 6 months, reinfarction and mortality rates continue to decrease. Since postoperative myocardial infarction is associated with a high mortality rate, it is best to schedule an elective operation 6 months or longer after a previous infarction.

Several drugs used in the treatment of cardiovascular disorders may interfere with anesthesia. For example, diuretics used in the treatment of hypertension can cause hypokalemia. As a result, the action of nondepolarizing muscle relaxants is prolonged and the heart is more irritable. Therefore, when possible, serum potassium concentrations below 3 mEq/L should be corrected before operation. Interaction between β-adrenergic antagonists and anesthetic drugs can result in bradycardia, hypotension, and congestive heart failure.[2] In preparing patients with hypertension, associated organic dysfunctions such as nephropathy and heart failure should be brought under control. If blood pressure is optimal, patient medication can be continued until the time of the operation because circulatory complications due to interaction between antihypertensive drugs and anesthetic agents are now rare.

Review of the patient's cardiovascular status is especially important when a laparoscopic colorectal procedure is considered, since the maintenance of increased intra-abdominal pressure during prolonged periods of time is not without adverse hemodynamic effects. The extent of the cardiovascular changes depends on several factors such as the level of the insufflation pressure and the volume of carbon dioxide absorbed. Usually, cardiac index and central venous blood pressure remain relatively unchanged.[3] The increased intra-abdominal pressure, however, leads to splanchnic vasoconstriction and a considerable reduction in inferior vena cava, renal, and portal vein blood

flow. Because of these changes, the venous return to the heart decreases, which finally results in reduction in stroke volume.[4] The heart rate will rise to compensate for this reduction in stroke volume. At higher-than-normal insufflation pressures, the cardiac output will decline because of failure of this compensation mechanism. The rise in abdominal venous pressure results in a significant increase in systemic vascular resistance and mean arterial blood pressure.[5]

Pulmonary Function

The pulmonary function of patients with chronic obstructive lung disease may deteriorate further as a result of ventilatory depression and ventilation–perfusion disturbances occurring during anesthesia. Moreover, postoperative hypoventilation due to residual anesthetic effects and the recumbency and diminished breathing resulting from a painful operative wound may result in pulmonary complications such as retention of secretions, atelectasis, and pulmonary infection. Patients with significant chronic obstructive lung disease might benefit from admission for pulmonary preparation in advance of the operation. Preoperative examination of these patients might include obtaining chest radiographs, arterial blood gas measurements, and pulmonary function tests. Breathing exercises, postural drainage, inhalation therapy with a mucolytic agent or bronchodilator, and administration of corticosteroids may be helpful in improving respiratory function.

Patients with chronic respiratory disease are also at risk during laparoscopic colorectal surgery. The pneumoperitoneum pushes the diaphragm upward and leads to a reduction in pulmonary function. This situation is aggravated when the Trendelenburg position is used. The physiologic dead space will increase and a ventilation–perfusion mismatch will occur.[6] During insufflation with carbon dioxide, the arterial partial pressure of carbon dioxide ($PaCO_2$) rises with a resultant respiratory acidosis. The decrease in pH can be compensated by increasing the ventilation rate. A rise in $PaCO_2$, however, may occur in patients with chronic respiratory disease despite an increase in ventilation, causing a reduction in stroke volume and cardiac arrhythmia.[7] Finally, the patient's smoking status and history should be documented, and smokers are advised to quit and offered cessation material and programs.

Renal Status

Patients with renal insufficiency are prone to sustain intraoperative and postoperative complications, especially if the renal disorder is associated with hypertension, severe anemia, and electrolyte disturbances. Fortunately, many affected patients tolerate chronic anemia of renal origin relatively well. The introduction and clinical use of erythropoietin has facilitated a more effective treatment of this type of anemia. Therefore, in this group of patients, anemia is not a contraindication to anesthesia and operation. In patients with hyperkalemia, the administration of succinylcholine may result in a further increase in serum potassium concentration. Anesthetic drugs, which are entirely dependent on the kidney for elimination, and nephrotoxic agents are contraindicated in patients with chronic renal insufficiency. Dialysis patients may need to be scheduled the day after their outpatient dialysis, with subsequent treatments performed while an inpatient. Obviously, nephrotoxic drugs (e.g., antibiotics) should be used with increased caution in these patients.

Hepatic Function

Although intravenous (IV) anesthetics and narcotic analgesics are largely eliminated by the liver, the detoxification and excretion of these agents is still adequate in most patients with liver disease, unless liver damage is severe. Special attention should be given to biochemical abnormalities such as hyperbilirubinemia, hypoalbuminemia, and elevated levels of liver enzymes and ammonia. The hypoalbuminemia and the reversed albumin/globulin ratio in liver disease are associated with altered sensitivity to drugs bound to albumin and to globulin. Attention should be directed to the correction of electrolyte disturbances such as dilutional hyponatremia in patients with ascites and hypokalemia due to excessive urinary loss resulting from secondary aldosteronism. In many patients, chronic liver disease is associated with anemia that is due to hemolysis or blood loss from esophageal varices. Thrombocytopenia caused by hypersplenism secondary to portal hypertension may occur in addition to decreased levels of clotting factors II, V, VII, IX, and X. Both abnormalities result in a coagulopathy, which should be corrected by platelet transfusion and administration of fresh frozen plasma. Finally, it should be noted that potentially hepatotoxic agents such as halothane are best avoided.

Hematologic Status

Patients with a low hemoglobin concentration have a decreased oxygen transport capacity. To maintain adequate oxygen delivery, cardiac output is increased in patients with anemia. However, many anemic patients tolerate an operation quite well, unless they present with a concurrent systemic disorder. Furthermore, in many patients admitted for a colorectal operation, a low hemoglobin concentration may be the manifestation of the underlying disease itself, and the proposed intervention may be curative. Although it has been advocated to correct anemia before operation in patients with a hemoglobin concentration below 10 g, many patients with lower values will tolerate operation. Although arbitrary, surgically acceptable ranges for hematocrit are 29 to 57% for men and 27 to 54% for women, and for white blood counts 2,400 to 16,000/mm³ for both men and women.[8]

Obesity

Obesity may be associated with endocrine abnormalities, hypertension, heart failure, a smaller-than-normal functional residual capacity, and other complications. Therefore, for markedly obese patients, arterial blood gas and pulmonary function studies and examination for endocrine dysfunction should be part of the preoperative evaluation. Because the obese patient is at increased risk for postoperative complications such as deep vein thrombosis (DVT), pulmonary embolism, and respiratory failure, adequate preoperative and postoperative measures are necessary to minimize these complications. Such measures are effective only in patients who are willing to cooperate, and therefore the potential complications and the necessity to cooperate should be explained to patients prior to operation.

Age

In assessing operative risk, age is another aspect that needs to be taken into account since an increasing number of older patients are requiring major operations. On admission, older patients frequently present with concurrent systemic disorders and inadequate nutrition. As already mentioned, both factors have a negative impact on intraoperative and postoperative morbidity and mortality. Age alone, however, is not a contraindication to operation. Nevertheless, in an older patient with less than optimal fitness, the surgeon may, for example, modify a recommendation for an abdominoperineal resection and opt for a local procedure. With greater age, for example, "reconstructive" procedures such as ileoanal and coloanal anastomoses are relatively contraindicated because both procedures are associated with a functional outcome that is not as good in older patients compared to younger ones.

Physiologic Status

Most patients who have had an operation recommended to them will become anxious. Sometimes, the degree of anxiety will be out of all proportion to the magnitude of the proposed operation. For example, a patient may be offered an anal operation when he or she expects a simple pill or cream to solve the problem. Alternatively, the patient may be seeking help for hemorrhoids and, after examination, learn that the problem is a carcinoma of the rectum for which a proctectomy is being recommended. Clearly, a patient in the latter situation requires considerable reassurance about the change in lifestyle that a stoma may create, along with potential complications such as impotence. Explanation of reasonable expectations from the operation, such as duration of hospitalization and estimated time off from work, as well as reassurance that the patient can return to his former type of work, may do much to calm the patient confronted with this totally unexpected diagnosis.

Nutritional Assessment and Optimization

A patient's nutritional status has significant influence on postoperative morbidity.[9] In addition, malnutrition is common, with reported rates up to 50% in certain populations of hospitalized patients.[10] Nutritional assessment identifies patients at risk and starts with a history of nutritional intake and weight status. Moderate or severe malnutrition is associated with body weight loss > 10% within 6 months of presentation and a body mass index (BMI) under 18.5 to 22 kg/m². Physical examination in patients with fat or muscle wasting identifies a low triceps skinfold thickness and a decreased midarm muscle circumference. Other criteria include biochemical parameters such as anemia, low serum albumin level (< 35 g/L), low prealbumin, low serum transferrin level, and deficiencies of vitamins, minerals, and trace elements.

Nutritional support may be indicated for malnourished patients requiring surgical intervention, or for healthy patients undergoing major surgery with an anticipated lengthy recovery time to return of normal gastrointestinal function; however, it is unclear when it is appropriate to intervene. Several studies have demonstrated that 7 to 10 days of preoperative parenteral nutrition improves postoperative outcome in patients with severe undernutrition who cannot be adequately orally or enterally fed. Conversely, its use in well-nourished or mildly undernourished patients is associated either with no benefit or with increased morbidity.[10,11] Postoperative parenteral nutrition is recommended in patients who cannot meet their caloric requirements within 7 to 10 days orally or enterally. In patients who require postoperative artificial nutrition, enteral feeding or a combination of enteral and supplementary parenteral feeding is the first choice.

A major consideration when administering fat and carbohydrates in parenteral nutrition is not to overfeed the patient. The commonly used formula of 25 kcal/kg ideal body weight furnishes an approximate estimate of daily energy expenditure and requirements. Under conditions of severe stress, requirements may approach 30 kcal/kg ideal body weights. In those patients who are unable to be fed via the enteral route after surgery, and in whom total or near-total parenteral nutrition is required, a full range of vitamins and trace elements should be supplemented on a daily basis.

A newer aspect of enteral nutrition is immunonutrition (IN) supplements, which may reduce postoperative complications. Braga et al reported that preoperative oral arginine and *n*-fatty acids improve the immunometabolic response and decrease the infection rate from 32 to 12%.[12] Postoperative supplementation has not shown additional benefits. Many studies included pre- and postoperative regimens and have utilized inconsistent controls. A recent review and meta-analysis reviewed 561 patients in eight randomized controlled trials (RCT) of preoperative IN versus standard oral nutritional supplements (ONS) and 895 patients in nine RCT of IN vs no supplements.[13] There was no difference between IN and ONS, but IN was associated with decreased infectious complications when compared to no supplements.

Several preoperative aspects have been combined into the Strong for Surgery program.[14] This program, initiated in Washington state, brings a presurgery checklist to doctor's offices to help with education, communication, and standardization of best practices. The program currently focuses on four areas: nutrition, glycemic control, smoking cessation, and medications.

For nutritional screening, four questions are asked: Is the patient's BMI less than 19? Has the patient had intentional weight loss of over 8 pounds in the last 3 months? Has the patient had a poor appetite—eating less than half or fewer than two meals per day? Is the patient unable to take food orally? If any of these questions are yes, the patient may be referred for evaluation by a dietician or considered for nutritional therapy. A serum albumin is obtained for risk stratification and patients having complex surgery are considered for evidence-based immune modulating supplements.

For blood sugar control, patients with diabetes, age > 45, or BMI > 30 have a fasting blood sugar drawn the morning of surgery. If the glucose level is > 200, then an insulin drip is suggested during the case. Diabetic patients also have a hemoglobin A 1C drawn. If that level is greater than 7% or any finger stick was > 200 in the last 2 weeks, the patients are referred for better diabetic management.

Medications

Medications such as warfarin, clopidogrel, and acetylsalicylic acid are documented with special attention to patients with bleeding risks, beta blockers, and problematic herbal medications, including *Echinacea*, garlic, ginkgo, ginseng, kava, saw palmetto, St. John's wort, and valerian.

Laboratory Tests

Screening laboratory studies should be considered before a major surgical procedure. In the past, multiple studies were routinely ordered. Recent critical evaluation of this policy has resulted in significantly fewer studies being performed. Unneeded tests result in unnecessary cost and morbidity. Many of these result from the workup suggested by an abnormal value obtained on "screening tests." Currently, in the absence of symptoms or disease processes that require evaluation, the studies listed in ▶ Table 5.2 are recommended.

Chest X-Rays

Routine chest radiography obtained on admission to hospital or in the preoperative setting was a common practice. However, significant evidence and national guidelines argue against such a policy.[15] In 2005, a meta-analysis of manuscripts published between 1966 and 2004 addressed the value of screening preoperative chest radiographs.[16] In this analysis, the diagnostic yield of the preoperative chest radiograph was found to increase with age. However, most of the abnormalities consisted of chronic disorders such as cardiomegaly and chronic obstructive pulmonary disease, which were already identified clinically. The proportion of patients who had a change in management was low (10% of investigated patients). Postoperative pulmonary complications were similar between patients who had preoperative chest radiographs (12.8%) and those who did not (16%). The authors concluded that preoperative screening chest radiographs did not decrease morbidity and mortality. Preoperative chest radiographs should not be performed on patients younger than 70 years and without risk factors. For patients older than 70 years, there is insufficient evidence against performance of routine chest radiographs. Routine preoperative and admission chest radiographs are not recommended except when acute cardiopulmonary disease is suspected on the basis of history and physical examination or there is a history of stable chronic cardiopulmonary disease in an elderly patient (older than 70 years) without a recent chest radiograph within the past 6 months.

5.3 Colorectal Operations

5.3.1 Preoperative Preparation

Mechanical Bowel Cleansing

Colorectal operations are associated with a high potential for septic complications that most commonly manifest as surgical site infections (SSIs), wound infections, or as intra-abdominal sepsis. Endogenous bacterial contamination is the most important

Table 5.2 Preoperative laboratory evaluations

Age (y)	Men	Women
< 40	No laboratory tests required	Hemoglobin and hematocrit
> 40	ECG	ECG

Abbreviation: ECG, electrocardiogram.

factor in the development of postoperative wound infection after elective colorectal procedures. However, exogenous contamination and patient-related factors such as age, nutritional status, and other disorders also can contribute to the development of wound infection.

Intra-abdominal sepsis after a colorectal operation is most commonly due to anastomotic dehiscence. Uneventful anastomotic healing depends on many variables, such as the skill of the surgeon and the use of excellent operative techniques. The method by which the anastomosis is made (staples, suture with one vs. two layers), the use or nonuse of drains, the construction of a defunctioning stoma, and the use of peritoneal lavage are other factors that may influence the outcome.

It is generally agreed that antimicrobial preparation is required in order to reduce the incidence of septic complications after elective colorectal surgery. Since many surgeons believed that fecal loading interfered with healing of colonic anastomoses, mechanical bowel preparation (MBP) was a traditional ritual. Proponents of mechanical cleansing justify their practice by referring to a paper published by Irvin and Goligher in 1973.[17] Based on their retrospective study, these authors concluded that poor MBP is associated with a significantly higher incidence of anastomotic dehiscence. They assumed that mechanical cleansing minimizes the risk of fecal impaction at the anastomotic site, thereby reducing undue

tension and local ischemia at the suture line. An early randomized clinical trial questioned this view and concluded that vigorous MBP was not necessary.[18] In 1987, Irving and Scrimgeour also questioned the efficacy of mechanical bowel cleansing.[19,20] They argued that preoperative bowel cleansing is time-consuming, expensive, unpleasant for the patient, and even dangerous on occasion. More recent concerns involve the fact that an empty colon is easier to manipulate during laparoscopic surgery and a clean colon is helpful if a surgeon needs to palpate a small lesion or use intraoperative colonoscopy.

While many surgeons continue to routinely use MBP for patients undergoing elective colorectal surgeries, some reports suggest that this practice may be abandoned for many procedures and patients. Both clinical trials and retrospective reviews have found a trend toward increased infectious complications in patients who underwent MBP when compared to those who did not.[21,22] There have also been reports of earlier return of bowel function and shorter hospital stays among patients who did not have MBP prior to surgery.[21,23,24,25] The most recent large, multicenter trial, however, found that there was no difference between MBP and no-MBP groups in rate of anastomotic leak or severity of infectious complications.[26] ▶ Table 5.3 summarizes the randomized clinical trials on the MBP versus no-MBP issue.[26,27,28,29,30,31,32,33,34,35,36,37,38,39] A 2011 Cochrane

Table 5.3 Comparison of randomized clinical trials of mechanical bowel prep versus nonmechanical bowel prep on anastomotic leaks and wound infections (2000–2011)

Study	No. of patients	MBP agent	Anastomotic leaks with MBP (%)	Anastomotic leaks without MBP (%)	p-Value	Wound infections with MBP (%)	Wound infections without MBP (%)	p-Value
Miettinen et al 2000[28]	267	PEG	3.8	2.5	0.72	3.6	2.3	0.72
Young Tabusso et al 2002[29]	47	Mannitol or PEG	20.8	0	0.004	8.3	0	0.49
Bucher et al 2005[43]	153	PEG	6.4	1.3	0.21	12.8	4	0.07
Ram et al 2005[30]	329	NaP	0.6	1.3	1	9.8	6.1	0.22
Fa-Si-Oen et al 2005[31]	250	PEG	5.6	4.8	0.78	7.2	5.6	0.79
Zmora et al 2003[20]	249	PEG	4.2	2.3	0.48	6.7	10.1	0.36
Pena-Soria et al 2007[33]	97	PEG	8.3	4.1	0.005	12.5	12.2	1
Jung et al 2007[25]	1,343	PEG, NaP, enema	1.9	2.6	0.46	7.9	6.4	0.34
Contant et al 2007[34]	1,354	PEG + bisacodyl or NaP	4.8	5.4	0.69	13.4	14	0.75
Leiro et al (Argentina) 2008[35]	129	PEG or NaP	5.7	15.2	0.183	21.9	21.5	1
Alcantara Moral et al 2009 (Spain)[36]	139	PEG or NaP or aqueous NaP	7.2	5.7	0.75	11.6	5.7	0.24
van't Sant et al 2011[26]	449	PEG + bisacodyl or NaP	7.6	6.6	0.8	9	7	0.43
Scabini et al 2010[38]	244	PEG	5.8	4	0.52	9.2	4.8	0.18
Bretagnol et al 2010[39]	178	Oral senna solution and povidone-iodine enema	11	19	0.09	1	3	NS

Abbreviations: MPB, mechanical bowel prep; NaP, sodium phosphate; NS, nonsignificant; PEG, polyethylene glycol.

review on MBP in elective colorectal procedures (18 randomized trials with 5,805 patients) did not detect any differences in rates of anastomotic leak or wound infections following colorectal procedures.[40] Based on these conclusions, some experts and national groups had called for the omission of MBP prior to elective colorectal procedures.[41,42]

There may be exceptions to this recommendation. In cases where a colonoscopy will be performed immediately before the resection, a bowel preparation may still be warranted. This is particularly true in patients with small (< 2 cm) and nonpalpable tumors that may need to be located intraoperatively with a scope. These patients were frequently excluded from trials and therefore conclusions cannot be drawn on the safety of abandoning MBP in these circumstances.[20,43]

Despite the numerous reports supporting the safety of colorectal procedures without MBP, physicians around the world have been slow to abandon the practice. In a 2002 survey of surgeons in the United States, 99% reported routinely prescribing an MBP prior to colorectal surgery, with 47% using oral sodium phosphate and 32% oral polyethylene glycol solution.[20] A study of almost 300 hospitals in Europe and the United States also found that 96% of patients admitted for a colorectal procedure underwent preoperative MBP.[44] Recent reports from Switzerland and New Zealand are more in line with the recommendations to abandon MBP, with less than half of physicians reporting MBP use in colon procedures. However, even in these countries, MBP use is common during anorectal procedures (60–80%).[42,45] Of note, more recent survey studies have found that younger physicians, board-certified colorectal surgeons, and high volume of colorectal surgeons are more likely to have abandoned the practice of MBP prior to elective colorectal procedures.[45,46] However, this trend toward abandoning mechanical preparation has been reconsidered in light of several large database studies that have looked at mechanical preparation used with oral antibiotic preparations. This experience is discussed in greater detail in the antibiotic preparation section. In addition, few of the studies looking at MBP for surgery have focused on rectal surgery (e.g., low anterior resections), and most did not evaluate the role of oral antibiotics.[47] Although no significant effect was found, it has been suggested that MBP could be used selectively in rectal surgery below the peritoneal verge in which bowel continuity is restored.

If a mechanical prep is used, it may be a variation of those discussed in Chapter 4. None of the current commercially available colon cleansing preparations has received Federal Drug Administration approval as a preoperative preparation. The author currently uses a limited, low-volume mechanical preparation in most patients: clear liquids the day prior to surgery and two doses (17 g) of polyethylene glycol 3350 (MiraLax) the afternoon prior to surgery. Patients undergoing distal left colon or rectal procedures or those who may need intraoperative colonoscopy receive a polyethylene glycol 3350 preparation (see Box 5.1).

Bowel cleansing preparation

On the day before the procedure, the patient is instructed as follows:
1. Clear liquids
2. 0900: take 10–20 mg bisacodyl (Dulcolax)
3. 1300: take 1 g of neomycin and 250 mg of metronidazole
4. 1400: take 1 g of neomycin and 250 mg of metronidazole
5. 1600: 240 mL (8 oz) clear liquids
6. 2200: take 1 g of neomycin and 250 mg of metronidazole
7. Drink plenty of additional clear liquids all day
8. Nothing by mouth at least 4 h prior to the procedure

Antibiotic Bowel Preparation

The aim of antibiotic prophylaxis is to facilitate the function of the host immune defense system by decreasing or suppressing bacterial growth at the surgical site.[47] The surgical opening of the large bowel causes contamination of the surgical field by endogenous bacteria, so patients undergoing elective colon and rectal surgery are at a high risk of postoperative wound infection. Without antibiotic prophylaxis, SSI after colon and rectal surgery can be as high as 40%.[48] This percentage decreases to approximately 11% with the use of prophylactic antibiotics.[49]

In response to the health and financial issues associated with SSIs, the Centers for Disease Control and Prevention (CDC), the Centers for Medicare and Medicaid Services (CMS), and representatives from other established health care organizations are working together on the Surgical Care Improvement Project (SCIP) to reduce surgical morbidity and mortality by targeting several components of surgical care including antibiotic prophylaxis.[50,51] SCIP has an infection prevention component for elective surgical procedures, which covers the administration of antibiotics within 1 hour before the surgical incision, appropriate antibiotic selection, and the discontinuation of antibiotics within 24 hours following the surgery end time. Based on these principles, hospitals and physicians are monitoring and implementing adherence with these recommendations. Unfortunately, adoption of these processes has not uniformly resulted in reduced infections.[52]

An ideal antibiotic regimen used for prophylaxis during elective colon and rectal surgery should provide broad suppression of fecal flora with activity against aerobic and anaerobic microorganisms. It should be cost effective, provide minimal toxicity, and avoid the emergence of resistant organisms. Furthermore, the choice of antibiotics to be used for prophylaxis should take into account both the microorganisms usually found in the surgical suite and hospital-specific microbiologic epidemiology. Currently, the recommended antibiotic regimen for elective colon and rectal surgery includes an oral or parenteral antimicrobial, or a combination of both. The regimen should include coverage against enteric gram-negative bacilli, anaerobes, and enterococci. The SCIP issued guidelines for the use of prophylactic antibiotics in colorectal surgery.[53,54] Cefoxitin (a second-generation cephalosporin) is recommended as the parenteral prophylactic antibiotic of choice; however, the combination of cefazolin and metronidazole can be used as a cost-effective alternative. In cases where gram-negative bacilli have become resistant to cefoxitin, reasonable alternatives include cefazolin plus metronidazole or monotherapy with ampicillin-sulbactam. In patients with confirmed allergies or adverse reactions to beta-lactams, use of clindamycin with gentamicin, aztreonam, or ciprofloxacin, or metronidazole with gentamicin or ciprofloxacin is recommended. A single dose of ertapenem is acceptable for colon and rectal surgery. However, its use has been discouraged, since its widespread use may result in increased rates of resistance.[53]

A systematic review of RCTs to evaluate the efficacy of antimicrobial prophylaxis and different regimens in colon and rectal surgery was conducted in 1998.[49] It concluded that the use of prophylactic antibiotics is efficacious in the prevention of SSIs in colon and rectal surgery. With the exception of a few inadequate regimens, there is no significant difference in the rate of SSIs between the regimens studied. Moreover, the use of a multiple-dose regimen may be unnecessary for the prevention of SSIs since single-dose regimens have been demonstrated to be as efficacious as multiple dosing, and may be associated with less toxicity, fewer adverse effects, less risk of developing bacterial resistance, and lower costs. Similarly, no convincing evidence supported the idea that the new-generation cephalosporins were more efficacious than first-generation cephalosporins in preventing SSIs in colon and rectal surgery. In 2009, the same group published a systematic Cochrane review that included 182 trials (30,880 participants).[54] The results were similar to the 1998 study in regard to the fact that no statistically significant differences were shown when comparing short- and long-term duration of prophylaxis or single dose versus multiple dose antibiotics. Statistically significant improvements in the rate of SSIs were noted with the use of combined oral and IV antibiotic prophylaxis when compared to IV alone or oral alone. It concluded that antibiotics covering aerobic and anaerobic bacteria should be delivered orally and intravenously prior to colon and rectal surgery with the resultant risk reduction of SSIs by at least 75%.

The most recent questionnaire regarding the use of prophylactic antibiotics before colon and rectal surgery showed that the use of oral antibiotic prophylaxis was still practiced by 75% of surgeons. IV antibiotic prophylaxis was almost invariably used (98% of the respondents).[20]

Prophylactic antibiotics should be administered within 60 minutes of incision to ensure adequate drug tissue levels at the time of the initial incision. If vancomycin or a fluoroquinolone is used, they should be administered within 120 minutes before incision. This timing of administration also reduces the likelihood of antibiotic-associated reactions during induction of anesthesia.[51,54,55,56]

A 2007 survey regarding the use of prophylactic antibiotics showed that 75% of colorectal surgeons used oral antibiotics and 98% used IV antibiotics.[55] In regard to redosing of prophylactic antibiotics during surgery, for procedures lasting less than 4 hours, a single dose of IV antibiotics is appropriate.[53] For procedures lasting more than 4 hours or in the setting of major blood loss, repeating dosing is indicated every one to two half-lives of the drug in patients with normal renal function. This recommendation is supported by a retrospective study in 1,548 patients who underwent cardiac surgery lasting more than 240 minutes after preoperative administration of cefazolin. Intraoperative redosing of cefazolin was associated with a 16% reduction in the overall risk for SSI after cardiac surgery, including procedures lasting less than 240 minutes.[57] There has been no evidence that a continuous administration of antibiotics for more than 24 hours after elective colon and rectal surgery decreases the risk of wound infection and that extended dosing may increase the risk of resistant organisms and development of *Clostridium difficile* colitis.[53,54,58]

Three recent studies have provided insight into the role of MBPs combined with preoperative oral antibiotics. A review of 499 patients from the 2012 Colectomy-Targeted American College of Surgeons National Surgical Quality Improvement Program (ACS NSQIP) who underwent elective colorectal resections found that patients who received preparation with mechanical cleansing and oral antibiotics had a significantly lower incidence of incisional SSIs, anastomotic leakage, and hospital readmission than patients who received no preparation.[59] A second analysis of 5,021 colon cancer patients from the NSQIP database who underwent scheduled colon resections during 2012–2013 found that solitary MBP and solitary oral bowel preparation had no significant effects on major postoperative complications. However, a combination of mechanical and oral antibiotic preparations showed significant decrease in postoperative morbidity.[60] Finally, a meta-analysis reviewed seven RCTs consisting of 1,769 patients undergoing elective colorectal surgery.[61] Patients who received oral systemic antibiotics and MBP had significantly reduced incisional SSIs compared to patients receiving systemic antibiotics and mechanical preparation (4.6 vs. 12.1%, $p < 0.00001$). Organ/space SSIs were not significantly different (4.0 vs. 4.8%, $p = 0/56$).[62,63,64]

These studies along with the Veterans Affairs Surgical Quality Improvement Program (VASQIP) and Michigan Surgical Quality Collaborative (MSQC) provide clear support for combined administration of mechanical cleansing with oral antibiotic preparation before elective colorectal resections.[64,65] In the absence of a randomized trial of oral antibiotics alone compared to oral antibiotics and MBP, the combined regimen should be recommended.

A 2016 email survey of American Society of Colon and Rectal Surgeons found that an MBP was used routinely by 59% and selectively by 36%.[65] Oral antibiotics were used routinely by 48% and selectively by 18%. IV antibiotics were always used by 94% and the remaining 6% used them selectively. Thus, the majority of surgeons responding to this survey continue to use a mechanical preparation along with oral and IV antibiotics. The editors routinely employ both mechanical cathartic and oral antibiotic bowel preparation for elective colorectal operations.

Reduction of Fasting State and Carbohydrate Supplementation

Traditionally, patients fasted from midnight on the night before elective surgery. With the adoption of enhanced recovery programs, patients have been allowed to continue solids up to 6 hours prior to surgery and clear liquids up to 2 hours prior to surgery. Additional experience suggested that nutritional supplements in the immediate preoperative period would enhance postoperative recovery. A literature review of 11 English language articles in 2011 found that the use of carbohydrate drinks preoperatively was safe and effective.[66] There was no increased risk of aspiration, and it resulted in a shorter hospital stay, quicker return of bowel function, and less loss of muscle mass. The authors felt that preoperative carbohydrate drinks should be standard in elective colorectal surgery. A meta-analysis of 21 randomized studies of 1,685 patients also found that preoperative carbohydrate treatment was associated with a reduced length of stay in patients undergoing major abdominal surgery.[67] Most studies have used a 50-g carbohydrate drink such as 240 mL of Gatorade. Other studies have used a carbohydrate and protein solution. ▸ Table 5.4 lists common preoperative beverage options.

Table 5.4 Preoperative beverages for enhanced recovery programs

	Manufacturer	Total carb (g)	Simple sugars	Protein (g)	% carb	Calories	Volume (mL)	Osmolality
Clearfast	BevMD	50	6	0	14.0	200	355	270
Gatorade 01	PepsiCo	25	23.8	0	27.1	100	118	650
Gatorade 02	PepsiCo	14	14	0	5.8	50	240	360
Gatorade 03	PepsiCo	14	14	16	2.8	230	500	360
Boost	Nestle	41	41	10	17.3	240	237	610
Breeze	Nestle	54	34	9	22.8	250	237	750
Impact AR	Nestle	45	45	18	18.9	3340	237	930
Ensure Clear	Abbott	43	43	7	21.5	200	200	700
Pedialyte	Abbott	6	6	0	2.5	25	237	270

5.3.2 Intraoperative

Normothermia

SSI rates in patients undergoing surgery are significantly decreased when operative normothermia is maintained to a temperature less than 36.0 °C. In a study that included 200 patients undergoing colon and rectal surgery, SSIs were found in 19% of patients assigned to hypothermia, but in only 6% of patients assigned to normothermia intraoperatively ($p = 0.009$).[68] Another study involving 421 patients evaluated whether warming patients before short duration clean surgery would reduce the rate of SSIs. They identified 19 wound infections in 139 nonwarmed patients (14%), but only 13 in 277 patients who received warming (5%; $p = 0.001$).[69]

Increased Oxygen Delivery

Several studies have addressed the potential favorable impact in the prevention of wound infection by increasing oxygen delivery.[70] In a prospective randomized trial that assigned 500 patients undergoing colorectal surgery to receive 30 or 80% inspired oxygen during the operation and for 2 hours afterward along with prophylactic antibiotics, rates of SSIs were compared between groups. Among the patients who received 80% oxygen, 13 (5.2%, 95% confidence interval [CI]) had surgical-wound infections, compared with 28 patients given 30% oxygen (11.2%; 95% CI; $p = 0.01$).[71] However, the optimal inspired oxygen concentration still needs to be evaluated.[72]

Intraoperative Goal-Directed Fluid Therapy

In support of enhanced surgical recovery programs, there has been renewed interest in optimizing surgical fluid regimens. The historical debate between liberal versus restrictive fluid regimens has been re-evaluated and the idea of individualized goal-directed therapy has been introduced and subjected to a number of RCTs. While untreated hypovolemia can be detrimental to patients, fluid overload can be just as (if not more) hazardous. By tailoring fluid administration to an individual patient's needs using a treatment algorithm based on closely monitored flow variables, postoperative recovery can be improved with reduced morbidity, less gastrointestinal dysfunction, and reduced hospital stay.[73]

Wound Protectors and Closing Trays

Wound protectors are devices that are used during laparotomy to protect the abdominal wound edges from contamination. The evidence for the efficacy in reducing SSI rates has been discrepant.[74] In a recent meta-analysis of RCTs evaluating the use of wound protectors in gastrointestinal and biliary surgical procedures and the impact on SSIs, the researchers found that the use of a wound protector was associated with nearly a 50% decrease in SSIs (relative risk, 0.55; 95% CI, 0.31–0.98; $p = 0.04$).[75]

Another surgical technique to reduce superficial SSIs is changing gloves, gowns, and instruments just prior to incisional closure.[76]

Drains

The routine placement of drains in the abdominal cavity and postoperative nasogastric suction (as discussed later) has largely been abandoned by colorectal surgeons.[77] The selective use of closed suction drains in the areas such as the pelvis is discussed along with each specific surgical technique (e.g., low anterior resection).

5.3.3 Postoperative Care

Analgesia

Adequate pain relief is an important aspect of postoperative care and leads to shortened hospital stays, reduced hospital costs, and increased patient satisfaction.[78] Postoperative pain management is an increasingly monitored quality measure. The Hospital Consumer Assessment of Health Providers and Systems (HCAHPS) scores measure patient satisfaction with in-hospital pain management and may have implications in regard to reimbursements.

Opioid Analgesia

Opioids have been the mainstay of postoperative pain control. Morphine and hydromorphone (Dilaudid) can be given via oral, transdermal, parenteral, neuraxial, and rectal routes. All opioids have side effects that limit their use. The most important side effect is respiratory depression that could result in hypoxia and respiratory arrest. Hence, regular monitoring of respiration and oxygen saturation is essential in patients on opioids postoperatively. In addition, nausea, vomiting, pruritus, and reduction in bowel motility leading to ileus and constipation are also common side effects of these medications.[79,80] Longer-term use of opioids can lead to dependence and addiction. Once the patient is able to tolerate oral intake, oral opioids can be initiated and continued after discharge from the hospital. With the development of enhanced recovery protocols, particularly in colorectal surgery, primarily opioid-based regimens are being challenged by other agents and approaches to postoperative pain management.[81,82]

Intravenous Patient-Controlled Analgesia

The concept of continuous intravenous (IV) analgesia and subsequently of patient-controlled analgesia (PCA) came into practice in the 1970s.[83,84] Morphine, hydromorphone, and fentanyl can be administered through the PCA pump. This method of analgesia requires special equipment and gives the patient better autonomy and control over the amount of medication used. However, both patients and staff setting up the equipment require training for proper use. A meta-analysis of 15 RCTs comparing IV PCA and intramuscular-administered opioids showed that patients preferred IV PCA and obtained better pain control with no increase in side effects.[85] A subsequent Cochrane review comparing IV opioid PCA with conventional IV "as needed" opioid administration reported that IV PCA had more analgesic effect and was preferred by patients based on satisfaction scores. However, the amount of opioid used, pain scores, length of hospital stay, and incidence of opioid-related side effects were similar between the groups, concluding that PCA is an efficacious alternative to conventional systemic analgesia when managing postoperative pain.[86]

Patient-Controlled Transdermal Delivery System

A new device delivery system (fentanyl hydrochloride patient-controlled transdermal delivery system [PCTS]) is a needle-free, credit-card-sized device that delivers analgesics by iontophoresis.[87] When the system is activated by the patient pressing a recessed button twice in 3 seconds, an imperceptible, low-intensity electric current generated by a battery housed within the system transfers fentanyl from a hydrogel reservoir across the skin and into the systemic circulation. The unit has an adhesive backing and is placed either on the upper outer arm or on the chest. The system is self-contained; therefore, in contrast to IV PCA, additional materials, such as tubing, pumps, and power cables, are not necessary for operation. When the button is pressed on the self-contained PCTS device, an audible beep and a red light from a light-emitting diode (LED) indicate that delivery of a dose has been initiated. The system is preprogrammed to deliver a 40-µg fentanyl hydrochloride dose over a 10-minute period. Patients can initiate up to six doses per hour for up to 24 hours from the time the first dose was initiated or a maximum of 80 doses, whichever occurs first. At that point, the unit will no longer generate the electric current necessary for drug delivery and becomes unresponsive to additional requests for medication. It should be removed and replaced with a new system if continued PCA is indicated. A system-initiated lockout prevents the patient from activating the system for additional drug during the 10-minute delivery period. This delivery period is preprogrammed by the manufacturer; administration cannot be accelerated or extended beyond the 10-minute interval. After each dose is delivered, the LED flashes to indicate the cumulative number of doses the patient has received, with each flash signifying delivery of a range of five doses (one flash = 1–5 doses delivered, two flashes = 6–10 doses, etc.).

In an RCT, PCTS was equianalgesic to IV PCA (morphine) in 636 patients who had undergone major surgery, including abdominal, orthopaedic, and thoracic procedures.[88] This and other trials demonstrate the comparable efficacy and safety of PCTS to PCA with morphine.

Epidural and Spinal Analgesia

Epidural and spinal analgesia act as neuraxial regional blocks and are used extensively in thoracic, abdominal, and pelvic surgery. In epidural analgesia, a catheter is inserted into the epidural space in the thoracic or lumbar spine, and continuous infusion of local anesthetic agent along with opioids results in postoperative analgesia. A Cochrane database review of nine RCTs comparing IV PCA and continuous epidural analgesia (CEA) showed the latter to achieve better pain control in the first 72 hours after abdominal surgery.[89] There was no difference in length of hospital stay and adverse events between the two routes. Patients with CEA had a higher incidence of pruritus related to opioids. Subsequent meta-analysis of RCTs comparing the two modes of opioid delivery in colorectal surgery showed that CEA significantly reduced post-op pain and ileus but was associated with pruritus, hypotension, and urinary retention.[90] A combination of local anesthetic and opioid can be administered via a patient-controlled epidural pump, which lowers the dose requirements for each individual drug as well as the frequency of side effects.[91]

Insertion of epidural catheters is technically challenging and failure of adequate analgesia is seen in 27% of patients after lumbar and 32% after thoracic epidural, despite adequate catheter placement.[92] In patients with successful analgesia from CEA, hypotension can be a problem requiring administration of additional IV fluids.[90] In addition, most patients with epidurals need to retain their urinary drainage catheters to prevent urinary retention, and administration of prophylactic anticoagulants may need to be scheduled or held to accommodate epidural catheter removal.

Intrathecal administration of opioid and local anesthetic (0.5% bupivacaine) at induction of anesthesia results in good postoperative analgesia for up to 24 hours. Administration of intrathecal analgesia takes the same time as epidural analgesia during anesthetic process before surgery but does not need the skilled postoperative care required for epidural analgesia.

A recent observational study showed that single-dose intrathecal opioid followed by IV PCA resulted in better pain control than CEA in patients undergoing colorectal surgery.[93] In addition, time to mobility and consequently hospital stay was shorter in the intrathecal analgesia group. A subsequent RCT comparing CEA, intrathecal analgesia, and IV PCA in laparoscopic colorectal surgery showed that duration of nausea, return of bowel function, and total hospital stay were higher in the CEA group than the other two groups. The pain scores were significantly higher in the IV PCA group than the other two groups.[84] This positive effect of intrathecal analgesia in laparoscopic colorectal surgery was further confirmed in a subsequent randomized study.[94,95]

Nonopioid Analgesia

Opioid-sparing techniques using different analgesic mechanisms of action are recognized as an important component of strategy for postoperative pain management. Nonsteroidal anti-inflammatory drugs (NSAIDs) are useful in reducing the amount of opiates requested and administered to the patient, thus reducing opioid side effects.[96] They are useful in mild-moderate levels of pain. NSAIDs act by inhibiting the enzyme cyclooxygenase (COX), thereby blocking the production of prostaglandins, resulting in an anti-inflammatory response. NSAIDs are classified by their selectivity of the COX isoenzymes. There is a risk of bleeding with these agents, so use of NSAIDs is dependent on the individual patient's risk factors. Nonselective agents such as ibuprofen do have an increased side effect profile (bleeding, antiplatelet effect); however, general consensus in the literature is that COX-1 inhibitors are preferred over selective COX-2 inhibitors such as celecoxib, given the recent evidence of cardiovascular risks associated with COX-2 agents.[96,97]

Ketorolac is an injectable NSAID with analgesic properties. It predominantly affects COX-1 and can be used as preemptive analgesia and as an adjunct to other agents.[97] Ketorolac reduces narcotic consumption by 25 to 45%, and is a common adjunct in colorectal surgery postoperative protocols.[97,98,99,100] The usual dose is 30 mg given intravenously. In a prospective randomized clinical trial in postoperative colorectal surgery patients, the addition of ketorolac to morphine PCA had an opioid-sparing effect with a resultant decrease in postoperative ileus.[101]

IV ibuprofen is an NSAID that acts by inhibiting the enzymes Cox 1 and 2, thereby blocking the production of prostaglandins resulting in an anti-inflammatory response. IV ibuprofen (Caldolor, Cumberland Pharmaceuticals, Nashville, TN) is administered as 800 mg every 6 hours.[102] In a prospective randomized study, Cataldo et al compared the effect of intramuscular ketorolac in combination with PCA (morphine) to that of PCA alone. Narcotic requirements were decreased by 45%.[103] They suggested that this combination may be particularly beneficial in patients especially prone to narcotic-related complications.

Acetaminophen is a centrally acting analgesic but lacks peripheral anti-inflammatory effects. Oral acetaminophen is widely used for acute pain relief. Acetaminophen is a common ingredient in many combination oral pain medications, so it is vital to counsel the patient not to exceed the 4,000 mg daily maximum dose due to the risk of hepatotoxicity. Systematic reviews of RCTs confirm the efficacy of oral acetaminophen for acute pain.[104] However, acetaminophen has a slow onset of analgesia and until recently the nonavailability of the oral route immediately after surgery limited its value in treating immediate postoperative pain. An IV form of acetaminophen is now commercially available (Ofirmen, Mallinkrodt Pharmaceuticals, St. Louis, MO). Major advantages of acetaminophen over NSAIDs are its lack of interference with platelet function and safe administration in patients with a history of peptic ulcers or asthma. Opioid-sparing effects have been associated with acetaminophen administered intravenously.[105] A mixed trial comparison found a decrease in 24-hour morphine consumption when acetaminophen, NSAIDs, or COX-2 inhibitors are given in addition to PCA morphine after surgery with a reduction in morphine-related adverse effects. However, the study did not find any clear differences between the three nonopioid agents.[106] A systematic review identified 21 studies comparing acetaminophen alone or in combination with other NSAIDs and reported increased efficacy with the combination of two agents than with either alone.[106] Current dosing is 1,000 g IV.

Peripheral Nerve Blocks

The transversus abdominis plane (TAP) block is a peripheral nerve block, which results in anesthesia of the abdominal wall.[107] The technique was first described in 2001 as a refined abdominal field block with a single shot into the plane between the internal oblique and transabdominal muscles.[82] This plane represents an anatomical potential space with nerves leaving the plane to innervate the abdominal muscles and skin. Local anesthetic is injected into this plane either uni- or bilaterally. The site of injection can be modified according to the anticipated site of incision. The technique can be blind or laparoscopic- or ultrasound-guided. Furthermore, the TAP block is thought by its proponents to have a lower risk of complications and greater acceptability to patients than epidural analgesia. There are a number of heterogeneous studies looking at the effect of TAP rectus sheath blocks on pain relief after abdominal surgery, with insufficient data on method of localization, timing, doses, and volumes of local anesthetics. TAP blocks are clearly subject to operator variability and skill.

A Cochrane review that included eight studies with 358 participants with moderate risk of bias showed that TAP block patients had significantly less postoperative requirement for morphine at 24 and 48 hours compared with no TAP or saline placebo.[107] There was no significant impact on nausea, vomiting, or sedation scores. Recent studies have looked at the use of TAP in colorectal surgery. In an enhanced recovery protocol, TAP plus IV acetaminophen in laparoscopic colorectal surgery resulted in earlier resumption of diet and discharge from hospital compared with morphine PCA.[82] One study from 2012 compared TAP plus PCA versus subcutaneous local infiltration plus PCA in open right hemicolectomies.[108] This study showed reduced PCA morphine use at 24 hours and decreased sedation in the TAP arm. Similarly, Conaghan et al reported decreased IV opioid use in laparoscopic colorectal resections with TAP + PCA versus PCA alone.[109] While there is limited evidence to suggest improvement in pain scores and opioid consumption after abdominal surgery, further studies are needed to evaluate the role of TAP blocks compared with other modalities of pain management such as epidural anesthesia.

Local Infiltration

Colon and rectal surgeons have used infiltration of local anesthetics throughout the history of the specialty. Many cases such as anorectal procedures can be accomplished with local anesthetics and IV sedation.[110] A limitation of the anesthetics previously available (Xylocaine and bupivacaine) was their short duration (minutes to a few hours). Recently, a new formulation of liposomal bupivacaine (Exparel, Pacira

Pharmaceuticals, Parsippany, NJ) has received approval from the U.S. Food and Drug Administration and can provide analgesia for up to 72 hours. It was approved for injection into the surgical site to produce postsurgical analgesia. The two pivotal studies leading to approval were in hemorrhoidectomy and bunionectomy patients.[111,112] The drug is provided in a 20-mL vial that contains 266 mg of liposomal bupivacaine. It can be diluted up to 14 times if desired. Since its release, this drug has seen increasing adoption, but the reported experience has been limited to date.[113] A series of four consecutive patients undergoing loop ileostomy closure were successfully managed with multimodality postoperative pain management (including liposomal bupivacaine, IV paracetamol, and ibuprofen) as 23-hour procedures. Utilization of local infiltration as part of a multimodality approach appears to have great potential.

Many of the pain management options described previously have been grouped into multimodality pain management programs. In patients undergoing major colorectal operations, Beck and colleagues compared 66 patients who received multimodality pain management to 167 patients managed with opioid PCA and found that the multimodality patients had lower pain scores, used less opioids, had less opioid-related adverse events, and decreased lengths of postoperative hospital stay (average 1.8 days).[114] A sample multimodality pain management regimen is presented in ▶ Table 5.5.

Early Ambulation and Deep Venous Thrombosis Prevention

Colorectal surgery is associated with a significant incidence of thromboembolic complications. Immobilization is considered an important causative factor in the pathogenesis of postoperative DVT. The incidence of pulmonary emboli in patients with DVT varies from 10 to 30%, depending on the location and morphology of the thrombus. One of 10 patients with pulmonary embolism dies within the first hour.[115] Therefore, ambulation is mandatory as early as possible. Postoperative ambulation can be efficacious only when pain relief is adequate and physiotherapy is added.

Table 5.5 Sample multimodality pain management

Preoperative

- Acetaminophen (paracetamol) 1,000 mg IV

- Ibuprofen 800 mg IV

Intraoperative

- Liposomal bupivacaine 266 mg wound infiltration

Postoperative

- Acetaminophen (paracetamol) 1,000 mg IV every 6 h until patient taking oral meds

- Ibuprofen 800 mg IV every 8 h until patient taking oral meds

- PCA (morphine or Dilaudid) for severe pain (scale 6–10) until patient taking oral meds

- Oxycodone 10 mg orally every 4 h for moderate pain when taking oral medication

Abbreviations: IV, intravenously; PCA, patient-controlled anesthesia.

Administration of low-dose heparin is another measure found to be effective in preventing thromboembolic complications.[116] Using iodine-125-labeled fibrinogen, Törngren and Rieger could detect DVT in 17% of the patients receiving low-dose heparin, whereas the DVT rate was 42% among untreated patients.[117] Although it has been assumed that rectal dissection is associated with an increased risk of DVT, these authors could not demonstrate a significant difference in the frequency of DVT between patients who underwent resections of the colon and those who underwent rectal resections. The incidence of DVT was significantly higher in patients with postoperative infection than among uninfected patients (37 vs. 12%). Based on these findings, Törngren and Rieger concluded that measures aimed at reducing postoperative infection combined with low-dose heparin and adequate ambulation will reduce the incidence of postoperative DVT.[117]

Heparin administration may be associated with an increased incidence of postoperative bleeding. Nevertheless, in high-risk patients, such as those with a previous history of DVT and/or pulmonary embolus, consideration should be given to the subcutaneous administration of low-dose heparin (5,000 U every 12 hours). Intermittent pneumatic compression also has been found to be effective in diminishing the incidence of DVT.[117]

Resumption of Diet

Like most abdominal procedures, colorectal operations are associated with some paralytic ileus in the early postoperative period. Intestinal motor dysfunction is a physiologic response to operative trauma.

There is growing evidence that postoperative ileus is related to the degree of surgical manipulation and the magnitude of the inflammatory response within the muscle layers of the bowel wall. It has been shown that the activation of macrophages within the muscularis during abdominal surgery initiates an inflammatory cascade of events, finally resulting in extravasation of leukocytes into the circular muscle layer. Various potent leukocytic products, such as nitric oxide, prostaglandins, and oxygen radicals, contribute to the inhibition of muscularis function.[118] For many years, Taché and coworkers have focused their attention on another mechanism.[119] They have found that surgical stress and manipulation of the large bowel initiate the central release of corticotropin-releasing factor (CRF) in the paraventricular nucleus of the hypothalamus. The subsequent stimulation of efferent inhibitory sympathetic pathways, mediated by the CRF release, seems to be a major contributing factor to the motor alterations induced by abdominal surgery. According to others, plasma changes in motilin and substance P are related to depressed gastrointestinal motility after the operation.[120]

Somatovisceral and viscerovisceral reflexes also contribute to postoperative ileus. Afferent, inhibitory sympathetic reflexes, involving the spinal cord, are of major importance, and these reflexes can be modified by epidural blockade. It has also been suggested that postoperative ileus is related to complications such as anastomotic dehiscence. Based on these data, it is obvious that the pathogenesis of postoperative ileus is multifactorial. Traditionally, the mean duration of the paralytic state was felt to vary between 0 and 24 hours in the small bowel, 24 and

48 hours in the stomach, and 48 and 72 hours in the colon. Therefore, the effective duration of postoperative ileus is mainly dependent on the return of colonic motility.[121,122,123]

Postoperative ileus is associated with significant discomfort. Furthermore, it delays the resumption of a regular diet as well as the mobilization of the patient, thereby resulting in a prolonged hospital stay. The morbidity associated with postoperative ileus is widely acknowledged and its economic burden has been estimated at $1 billion per year in the United States.[124]

Most surgeons have their own idea of when to feed patients after a laparotomy for colorectal disease. Some favor resumption of oral intake at the first sign of a bowel sound. Others would like to witness the return of organized peristalsis, which is recognized by the passage of flatus or a bowel movement. In the absence of enhanced recovery interventions, this usually has occurred by the fifth postoperative day. The rationale of such a period of starvation is to prevent nausea and vomiting and to protect the anastomosis, allowing it time to heal. This policy is not really evidence based.

Contrary to the previous widespread opinion, there is growing evidence suggesting that early feeding is advantageous. The advent of laparoscopic colorectal surgery has prompted a shift toward early feeding. Several RCTs comparing laparoscopic and open colonic resections have revealed that minimally invasive surgery is associated with a faster resolution of postoperative ileus, an earlier tolerance of diet, and a faster discharge from the hospital.[125] This beneficial effect is probably due to reduction in surgical trauma, resulting in reduced activation of inhibitory reflexes and local inflammation. It has been questioned, however, whether this advantageous effect is a result of the laparoscopic procedure alone or merely reflects a change in postoperative care principles with allowance of earlier transition to a regular diet. Milsom et al conducted a randomized trial comparing the ileus patterns after laparoscopic and open colorectal surgery and found a significantly shorter time to first flatus for patients who underwent laparoscopic surgery, but no significant difference in time to first bowel movement.[126] The length of hospital stay was similar in both groups. Bufo et al reported on a prospective study of 38 patients undergoing elective open colorectal operations.[127] They found early feeding (ad lib) was tolerated in 86% of patients. They noted that longer operative time and increased blood loss intraoperatively may indicate a more difficult procedure and identify those patients who will not tolerate early feeding. Early feeding also led to shortened length of hospital stay.

Binderow and coworkers randomized 64 patients undergoing open colorectal surgery to either receive a regular diet on the first postoperative day or have their diet held until resumption of bowel movements.[128] There were no differences in the incidence of nasogastric tube reinsertion, vomiting, and the duration of the postoperative ileus. In a subsequent group of an additional 161 consecutive patients, similar results were demonstrated.[129] However, the patients in the early feeding group tolerated a regular diet significantly earlier than the patients in the regular feeding group (2.6 vs. 5 days). It might be noted that the early feeding did not result in any significant shortening of the hospital stay.

Ortiz et al also conducted a prospective randomized trial and found that 80% of patients tolerated early feeding but 21.5% developed vomiting and required reinsertion of a nasogastric tube.[130] The time until the first bowel movement was similar. Based on these data, it has been suggested that an early oral feeding regimen consisting of clear liquids on the first postoperative day, followed by a regular diet as tolerated within the next 24 to 48 hours, is safe. Additional studies also demonstrated that early oral feeding is indeed permissible after elective open colorectal surgery. Early oral feeding is tolerated by 70 to 80% of the patients.[131,132] Lewis et al performed a systematic review and conducted a meta-analysis of RCTs comparing any type of enteral feeding started within 24 hours after the operation with nil by mouth management in elective gastrointestinal surgery.[133] Eleven studies, including 837 patients, met their inclusion criteria. Early feeding reduced the risk of any type of infection and the mean hospital stay. Risk reductions were also seen for anastomotic dehiscence, pneumonia, wound infection, intra-abdominal abscess, and mortality. However, these risk reductions failed to reach significance. The risk of vomiting was increased among patients fed early. Even in elderly patients, aged 70 years and older, early postoperative feeding is feasible and beneficial, as shown by DiFronzo et al.[134] Reviewing the literature, it is apparent that 10 to 20% of the patients do not tolerate early feeding.

Kehlet, from Copenhagen, Denmark, pioneered a more fundamental and multimodal approach to enhance the overall recovery rate after open abdominal surgery.[135] His regimen includes a plan for discharge from the hospital at 48 hours after the operation, optimal pain relief with thoracic epidural anesthesia, limited surgical incision, early postoperative oral intake, and early postoperative mobilization. Bradshaw and coworkers, from the United States, utilized a comparable perioperative regimen, resulting in a faster return of bowel function and a shorter length of hospital stay.[136] With the multimodal approach developed by Kehlet, Basse et al were able to discharge 32 of 60 patients at 48 hours after open colorectal surgery.[137] In a subsequent report, Basse et al evaluated the postoperative outcome after colonic resection of 130 consecutive patients receiving conventional care compared with 130 consecutive patients receiving multimodal fast-track rehabilitation.[138] American Society of Anesthesiologist score was significantly higher in the fast-track group. Defecation occurred on day 4.5 in the conventional group and day 2 in the fast-track group. Median hospital stay was 8 days in the conventional group and 2 days in the fast-track group. The use of nasogastric tube was longer in the conventional group. The overall complication rate (26.9%) was lower in the fast-track group, especially cardiopulmonary complications (3.8%). Readmission was necessary in 12% of cases for the conventional group and 20% in the fast-track group. Although other workers were not able to achieve such a short hospital stay, some of them have demonstrated that this approach results in a faster readiness for discharge. In an RCT, Delaney et al demonstrated that patients assigned to a pathway of controlled rehabilitation with early ambulation and early feeding spent less time in the hospital than patients who were assigned to traditional postoperative care (5 vs. 7 days).[139] Fearon and Luff reported that, in their unit, hospital stay has been reduced from approximately 10 days with traditional care to 7 days with an enhanced recovery program.[140] Smedh et al were able to discharge their patients after a median postoperative hospital stay of 3.5 days, by using a similar program.[141] Henriksen et al reported a longer ambulation time and better muscle function after the operation by using this program.[142] The benefits of the multimodal rehabilitation approach cannot be achieved with a unimodal intervention based on early postoperative feeding alone.[143,144]

The custom of starting patients on clear fluids and progressing to full fluids and then a "soft" diet seems unnecessary. Once it is deemed permissible to allow oral intake, full fluids may be started and followed shortly thereafter by regular food and a bulk-forming agent such as one of the psyllium seed preparations. This regimen should ensure the passage of a soft stool without straining.

Pulmonary Function

Abdominal surgical procedures are associated with a high risk of postoperative pulmonary complication. The development of fever in the first 24 to 48 hours after operation often points to atelectasis as the source, and vigorous chest physiotherapy should be instituted. Prevention or lessening the severity of pulmonary complications is possible with treatments designed to encourage inspiration and lung volume. Incentive spirometers are mechanical devices developed to help people take long, deep, and slow breaths to increase lung inflation. Deep breathing is helpful in maintaining postoperative pulmonary function. A Cochrane systematic review of 12 studies with a total of 1,834 patients found that there was low-quality evidence to support the use of incentive inspirometers.[145] However, as the cost of the device is relatively low, it may remain in clinical use until large RCTs are performed.

Postoperative Laboratory Tests

In the early postoperative period, fluid and electrolyte balance must be monitored. The preoperative fasting and the operative procedure itself may be associated with a significant loss of fluid and electrolyte, which need to be restored. Special attention should be given to hemodynamic parameters such as pulse rate, blood pressure, hemoglobin concentration, and urine output to detect early signs of intra-abdominal hemorrhage or sepsis. The frequency of the laboratory work will depend on the complexity of the operation performed and any preexisting associated medical conditions.

Perioperative Fluid Management

Perioperative fluid management of the colorectal surgical patient has evolved significantly over the last five decades.[146] Older notions espousing aggressive hydration have been shown to be associated with increased complications. Newer data regarding fluid restriction have shown an association with improved outcomes. Management of perioperative fluid administration can be considered in three primary phases: preoperative, intraoperative, and postoperative.

In the preoperative phase, as described previously, data suggest that limiting or avoiding preoperative bowel preparation and avoidance of preoperative dehydration can improve outcomes. Intraoperative fluid is administered to ensure adequate circulating volume for tissue perfusion and oxygenation.

Although the type of intraoperative fluid given does not have a significant effect on outcome, data do suggest that a restrictive fluid regimen results in improved outcomes. Patient-specific or goal-directed therapy has also improved outcomes; however, it has not been compared to fluid restriction.[147]

Finally, in the postoperative phase of fluid management, a fluid-restrictive regimen, coupled with early enteral feeding, also seems to result in improved outcomes. Brandstrup et al investigated the effect of a restricted IV fluid regimen on complications after colorectal resection.[148] In a randomized observer-blinded multicenter trial, 172 patients were allocated to either restricted or a standard intraoperative and postoperative IV fluid regimen. The restricted regimen aimed at maintaining preoperative body weight; the standard regimen resembled everyday practice. The restricted IV fluid regimen significantly reduced postoperative complications by both intention-to-treat (33 vs. 51%) and per-protocol (30 vs. 56%) analyses. The numbers of both cardiopulmonary (7 vs. 24%) and tissue healing complications (16 vs. 31%) were significantly reduced. No patients died in the restricted group compared with four deaths in the standard group (0 vs. 4.7%). No harmful adverse effects were observed.

Nasogastric Intubation

Nasogastric or orogastric tubes are used intraoperatively to decompress the stomach. Since its introduction by Levin, the use of a nasogastric tube became a routine aspect of postoperative care for most surgeons.[149] It was thought to relieve postoperative discomfort and to shorten the duration of ileus, thereby decreasing the length of hospital stay. It was also thought to decrease the incidence of complications. However, nasogastric tubes, which are unpleasant at best and usually distressing to the patient, may cause tube-related complications such as vomiting, nasopharyngeal soreness, coughing, wheezing, and sinusitis.[150]

In the 1980s, surgeons started to question the efficacy of the use of nasogastric tubes. From a prospective study comparing the postoperative course in patients with and without a nasogastric tube, Bauer et al concluded that routine use of a nasogastric tube was not needed.[151] In their study, most patients with a nasogastric tube suffered discomfort, and the incidence of postoperative complications was not increased in the patients without a nasogastric tube. Furthermore, only 6% of the patients in whom nasogastric tubes were not routinely used required nasogastric intubation during the postoperative period.

Clevers and Smout evaluated the restoration of gastrointestinal motility following abdominal operations in 50 patients.[152] Bowel sounds were heard at auscultation on postoperative day 1 or 2. The passage of flatus was first noted in almost all patients on postoperative day 2, and the first defecation occurred on postoperative day 4 or 5. These physical signs, occurring at relatively predictable times, were not influenced by the type of operation, nor were they predicative of postoperative nausea and vomiting. Because the period of intestinal decompression and the volume of gastric aspirate in patients with postoperative nausea did not differ from those of the patients without nausea, the authors concluded that prolonged gastric decompression is not necessary.

In a prospective randomized trial, Colvin et al compared use of a long intestinal tube (Cantor) placed preoperatively, a nasogastric tube placed intraoperatively, and no tube at all.[153] With respect to the length of hospital stay, duration of postoperative ileus, adequacy of intraoperative intestinal decompression, gastric dilatation, and operative complications, there was no significant difference between the patients with tubes and those without tubes. The authors concluded that the routine practice of employing nasointestinal tubes should be abandoned in elective colonic operations. Others have come to the same conclusion.[154,155]

In 1995, Cheatham et al performed a meta-analysis of the results obtained from 26 trials including almost 4,000 patients.[156] These trials compared selective versus routine nasogastric decompression. Although patients managed without a nasogastric tube more frequently encountered abdominal distension, nausea, and vomiting, this was not associated with an increased number of complications or a prolonged hospital stay. They also showed that for every patient who needed postoperative gastric decompression, 20 patients did not. Based on these data, the authors concluded that routine use of a nasogastric tube was not supported by their meta-analysis. In an RCT comparing early versus regular feeding, Reissman et al also demonstrated that after elective colorectal surgery patients can be safely managed without nasogastric tubes.[157] In the early feeding group and in the regular feeding group, the tube reinsertion rate was almost equal (11 vs. 10%). In a similar study, Feo et al observed that tube reinsertion was necessary in 20% of their patients because of vomiting.[158] Based on all these data, it is apparent that routine use of a nasogastric tube is not needed following elective colorectal surgery.

Bladder Catheter

Most patients undergoing abdominal colorectal operations and especially laparoscopic operations require a urethral catheter for intraoperative decompression and for postoperative monitoring. Following hemicolectomy and segmental colectomies, the bladder catheter was usually left in place for 1 to 2 days and for 2 to 3 after proctectomy. Recent experience with accelerated care paths, multimodality pain management, and the interest in preventing urinary tract infections has challenged these traditional teachings. The urinary catheter is currently removed within 1 or 2 days in almost all patients.

It is well established that the risk of catheter-associated urinary tract infection (CAUTI) increases with increasing duration of indwelling urinary catheterization. A pooled analysis of 10 prospective trials dating from 1983 to 1995 published in 2000 estimated that bacteriuria will develop in 26% of patients after 2 to 10 days of catheterization.[159] Additional analyses demonstrated that 24% of those patients will develop symptomatic UTI and bacteremia will develop in 3.6%. Postoperative patients discharged to subacute care with urinary catheters were more likely to be readmitted to the hospitals with a UTI compared with those who had catheters removed prior to hospital discharge.[160,161] Among selected major surgical patients in the Surgical Infection Project (SIP) cohort, Wald et al demonstrated that 85% had perioperative indwelling catheters placed and half of those patients had catheters for greater than 2 days postoperatively. These patients were twice as likely to develop UTIs prior to hospital discharge. On multivariate analysis, those who had indwelling bladder catheters for more than 2 days postoperatively were 21% more likely to develop UTI, significantly less likely to be discharged to home, and had a significant increase in mortality at 30 days. Additional analyses suggest there is sizeable variation in the duration of postoperative catheterization among hospitals and that hospital factors may account for this variation. A multifaceted intervention study in 2006 of orthopaedic surgery patients in which protocols limited the use and duration of postoperative catheterization reported a resultant 60% reduction in UTI incidence-density.[162] These data were used to support the SCIP criteria calls for urinary catheters to be removed on postoperative day 1 or 2.

Retention or incontinence after catheter removal may require continuous bladder drainage for another 3- to 5-day period until the patient is fully mobile. Opiates may cause urinary retention by inhibition of detrusor contraction and impaired bladder sensation, resulting in an increased maximum bladder capacity and overdistention.[163] The changes are rapidly reversed by therapeutic doses of IV naloxone. When retention persists, urologic examination, including cystoscopy and urodynamic investigation, is indicated. Micturition difficulties after colorectal operations most frequently occur in elderly men because of obstruction by prostatic hypertrophy. Bladder dysfunction as a result of pelvic nerve injury during rectal excision is another potential causative factor. The reported incidence of urinary dysfunction following conventional procedures for rectal carcinoma varies between 30 and 70%.[164] In many patients with postoperative urinary dysfunction, sexual function is also affected. In male patients, impotence and/or disturbed ejaculation occur in about 30 to 40%.[165] In female patients, sexual function may be affected, resulting in dyspareunia, loss of lubrication of the vagina, and the inability to achieve orgasm.[166] In contrast to voiding disturbances, sexual difficulties rarely disappear. To reduce the incidence of these disabling complications, nerve-sparing operation techniques have been developed that do not compromise adequate clearance of the malignancy.[167]

Repeated removal and reinsertion of a transurethral catheter is unpleasant and may be associated with increased risk of urethral trauma and urinary tract infection. Nevertheless, some urologists currently prefer repeated straight catheterization rather than prolonged bladder catheterization. Patients can be taught to catheterize themselves. To overcome these problems, in special circumstances, consideration can be given to the use of a catheter inserted into the bladder through the lower abdominal wall. A percutaneous catheter facilitates bladder training since it simply can be clamped when left in situ but this option is rarely adopted today.

Pharmacologic Treatment of Postoperative Ileus

Postoperative ileus is a significant side effect of abdominal surgery. Without specific prevention or treatment, major abdominal surgery causes a predictable gastrointestinal dysfunction, which endures for 4 to 5 days and results in an average hospital stay of 7 to 8 days. Ileus occurs because of initially absent and subsequently abnormal motor function of the stomach, small bowel, and colon. This disruption results in delayed transit of gastrointestinal content, intolerance of food, and gas retention.

The etiology of ileus is multifactorial, and includes autonomic neural dysfunction, inflammatory mediators, narcotics, gastrointestinal hormone disruptions, and anesthetics.[168] In the past, treatment has consisted of nasogastric suction, IV fluids, correction of electrolyte abnormalities, and observation. Currently, the most effective treatment is a multimodal approach. Median stays of 2 to 3 days after removal of all or part of the colon have now been reported.

Opioid Receptor Antagonists

Taguchi at al studied the effects of an investigational μ-opioid antagonist with limited oral absorption and limited ability to cross the blood–brain barrier, on postoperative gastrointestinal function and length of hospital stay. In a randomized, placebo-controlled study, they were able to demonstrate that selective inhibition of gastrointestinal opioid receptors by this antagonist speeds recovery of bowel function and shortens the duration of hospitalization.[169]

Cisapride

Cisapride acts as a serotonin receptor agonist. There is growing evidence that IV administration of cisapride reduces the duration of postoperative ileus. However, the reported adverse cardiac effects will probably limit the widespread use of this agent.[170]

Ceruletide

This peptide acts as a cholecystokinin antagonist and may stimulate gastrointestinal activity. In two placebo-controlled studies, only a slight effect on postoperative ileus was observed. This finding and the reported side effects such as nausea and vomiting have limited the use of this agent.[171,172]

Erythromycin

This antibiotic acts as a motilin receptor agonist and might be a candidate for the reduction of postoperative ileus. However, such an advantageous effect could not be demonstrated in an RCT.[173]

Metoclopramide

Metoclopramide acts as a dopamine antagonist and a cholinergic stimulant. Holte and Kehlet have reviewed six controlled trials assessing the effect of metoclopramide. None of these studies has demonstrated a significant effect of this agent on the resolution of postoperative ileus.[174]

References

[1] Roizen MF, Fleisher LA. Anesthetic implication of concurred diseases. In: Miller RD, ed. Miller's Anesthesia. 6th ed. Philadelphia. PA: Elsevier; 2005:1062–1063

[2] Chang DC, Lam AM, Mezan BJ, eds. Essentials of Anesthesiology. Philadelphia, PA: WB Saunders; 1983

[3] Liu SY, Leighton T, Davis I, Klein S, Lippmann M, Bongard F. Prospective analysis of cardiopulmonary responses to laparoscopic cholecystectomy. J Laparoendosc Surg. 1991; 1(5):241–246

[4] Ho HS, Gunther RA, Wolfe BM. Intraperitoneal carbon dioxide insufflation and cardiopulmonary functions. Laparoscopic cholecystectomy in pigs. Arch Surg. 1992; 127(8):928–932, discussion 932–933

[5] Rasmussen IB, Berggren U, Arvidsson D, Ljungdahl M, Haglund U. Effects of pneumoperitoneum on splanchnic hemodynamics: an experimental study in pigs. Eur J Surg. 1995; 161(11):819–826

[6] McMahon AJ, Baxter JN, Kenny G, O'Dwyer PJ. Ventilatory and blood gas changes during laparoscopic and open cholecystectomy. Br J Surg. 1993; 80 (10):1252–1254

[7] Baxter JN, O'Dwyer PJ. Pathophysiology of laparoscopy. Br J Surg. 1995; 82 (1):1–2

[8] Roizen MF. Preoperative evaluation. In: Miller RD, ed. Miller's Anesthesia. 6th ed. Philadelphia, PA: Elsevier; 2005:954

[9] Braga M, Ljungqvist O, Soeters P, Fearon K, Weimann A, Bozzetti F, ESPEN. ESPEN Guidelines on parenteral nutrition: surgery. Clin Nutr. 2009; 28 (4):378–386

[10] Bruun LI, Bosaeus I, Bergstad I, Nygaard K. Prevalence of malnutrition in surgical patients: evaluation of nutritional support and documentation. Clin Nutr. 1999; 18(3):141–147

[11] Reilly JJ, Jr, Gerhardt AL. Modern surgical nutrition. Curr Probl Surg. 1985; 22(10):1–81

[12] Braga M, Gianotti L, Vignali A, Carlo VD. Preoperative oral arginine and n-3 fatty acid supplementation improves the immunometabolic host response and outcome after colorectal resection for cancer. Surgery. 2002; 132 (5):805–814

[13] Hegazi RA, Hustead DS, Evans DC. Preoperative standard oral nutrition supplements vs immunonutrition: results of a systematic review and meta-analysis. J Am Coll Surg. 2014; 219(5):1078–1087

[14] Strong for Surgery. Available at: https://www.facs.org/quality-programs/strong-for-surgery. Accessed June 16, 2018

[15] Mohammed TL, Kirsch J, Amorosa JK, et al, Expert Panel on Thoracic Imaging. ACR Appropriateness Criteria® Routine Admission and Preoperative Chest Radiography. [Online publication]. Reston, VA: American College of Radiology (ACR); 2011:6

[16] Joo HS, Wong J, Naik VN, Savoldelli GL. The value of screening preoperative chest x-rays: a systematic review. Can J Anaesth. 2005; 52(6):568–574

[17] Irvin TT, Goligher JC. Aetiology of disruption of intestinal anastomoses. Br J Surg. 1973; 60(6):461–464

[18] Hughes ESR. Asepsis in large-bowel surgery. Ann R Coll Surg Engl. 1972; 51 (6):347–356

[19] Irving AD, Scrimgeour D. Mechanical bowel preparation for colonic resection and anastomosis. Br J Surg. 1987; 74(7):580–581

[20] Zmora O, Wexner SD, Hajjar L, et al. Trends in preparation for colorectal surgery: survey of the members of the American Society of Colon and Rectal Surgeons. Am Surg. 2003; 69(2):150–154

[21] Howard DD, White CQ, Harden TR, Ellis CN. Incidence of surgical site infections postcolorectal resections without preoperative mechanical or antibiotic bowel preparation. Am Surg. 2009; 75(8):659–663, discussion 663–664

[22] Bretagnol F, Alves A, Ricci A, Valleur P, Panis Y. Rectal cancer surgery without mechanical bowel preparation. Br J Surg. 2007; 94(10):1266–1271

[23] McKenna T, Macgill A, Porat G, Friedenberg FK. Colonoscopy preparation: polyethylene glycol with Gatorade is as safe and efficacious as four liters of polyethylene glycol with balanced electrolytes. Dig Dis Sci. 2012; 57 (12):3098–3105

[24] Leys CM, Austin MT, Pietsch JB, Lovvorn HN, III, Pietsch JB. Elective intestinal operations in infants and children without mechanical bowel preparation: a pilot study. J Pediatr Surg. 2005; 40(6):978–981, discussion 982

[25] Jung B, Påhlman L, Nyström PO, Nilsson E, Mechanical Bowel Preparation Study Group. Multicentre randomized clinical trial of mechanical bowel preparation in elective colonic resection. Br J Surg. 2007; 94 (6):689–695

[26] van't Sant HP, Weidema WF, Hop WC, Lange JF, Contant CM. Evaluation of morbidity and mortality after anastomotic leakage following elective colorectal surgery in patients treated with or without mechanical bowel preparation. Am J Surg. 2011; 202(3):321–324

[27] Duncan JE, Quietmeyer CM. Bowel preparation: current status. Clin Colon Rectal Surg. 2009; 22(1):14–20

[28] Miettinen RPJ, Laitinen ST, Mäkelä JT, Pääkkönen ME. Bowel preparation with oral polyethylene glycol electrolyte solution vs. no preparation in elective open colorectal surgery: prospective, randomized study. Dis Colon Rectum. 2000; 43(5):669–675, discussion 675–677

[29] Young Tabusso F, Celis Zapata J, Berrospi Espinoza F, Payet Meza E, Ruiz Figueroa E. Mechanical preparation in elective colorectal surgery, a useful practice or a necessity? [in Spanish]. Rev Gastroenterol Peru. 2002; 22 (2):152–158

[30] Ram E, Sherman Y, Weil R, Vishne T, Kravarusic D, Dreznik Z. Is mechanical bowel preparation mandatory for elective colon surgery? A prospective randomized study. Arch Surg. 2005; 140(3):285–288

[31] Fa-Si-Oen P, Roumen R, Buitenweg J, et al. Mechanical bowel preparation or not? Outcome of a multicenter, randomized trial in elective open colon surgery. Dis Colon Rectum. 2005; 48(8):1509–1516

[32] Zmora O, Mahajna A, Bar-Zakai B, et al. Is mechanical bowel preparation mandatory for left-sided colonic anastomosis? Results of a prospective randomized trial. Tech Coloproctol. 2006; 10(2):131–135

[33] Pena-Soria MJ, Mayol JM, Anula-Fernandez R, Arbeo-Escolar A, Fernandez-Represa JA. Mechanical bowel preparation for elective colorectal surgery with primary intraperitoneal anastomosis by a single surgeon: interim analysis of a prospective single-blinded randomized trial. J Gastrointest Surg. 2007; 11(5):562–567

[34] Contant CM, Hop WC, van't Sant HP, et al. Mechanical bowel preparation for elective colorectal surgery: a multicentre randomised trial. Lancet. 2007; 370(9605):2112–2117

[35] Leiro F., Barredo C., Latif J., et al. Preparación mecánica en cirugía electiva del colon y recto. Rev Argent Cirug. 2008; 95(3–4):154–167

[36] Alcantara Moral M, Serra Aracil X, Bombardó Juncá J, et al. A prospective, randomised, controlled study on the need to mechanically prepare the colon in scheduled colorectal surgery [in Spanish]. Cir Esp. 2009; 85(1):20–25

[37] Van't Sant HP, Weidema WF, Hop WCJ, Oostvogel HJM, Contant CM. The influence of mechanical bowel preparation in elective lower colorectal surgery. Ann Surg. 2010; 251(1):59–63

[38] Scabini S, Rimini E, Romairone E, et al. Colon and rectal surgery for cancer without mechanical bowel preparation: one-center randomized prospective trial [retracted in:World J Surg Oncol 2012;10:196]. World J Surg Oncol. 2010; 8:35

[39] Bretagnol F, Panis Y, Rullier E, et al. French Research Group of Rectal Cancer Surgery (GRECCAR). Rectal cancer surgery with or without bowel preparation: The French GRECCAR III multicenter single-blinded randomized trial. Ann Surg. 2010; 252(5):863–868

[40] Güenaga KF, Matos D, Wille-Jørgensen P. Mechanical bowel preparation for elective colorectal surgery. Cochrane Database Syst Rev. 2011(9):CD001544

[41] Harris LJ, Moudgill N, Hager E, Abdollahi H, Goldstein S. Incidence of anastomotic leak in patients undergoing elective colon resection without mechanical bowel preparation: our updated experience and two-year review. Am Surg. 2009; 75(9):828–833

[42] Businger A, Grunder G, Guenin MO, Ackermann C, Peterli R, von Flüe M. Mechanical bowel preparation and antimicrobial prophylaxis in elective colorectal surgery in Switzerland–a survey. Langenbecks Arch Surg. 2011; 396(1):107–113

[43] Bucher P, Gervaz P, Soravia C, Mermillod B, Erne M, Morel P. Randomized clinical trial of mechanical bowel preparation versus no preparation before elective left-sided colorectal surgery. Br J Surg. 2005; 92(4):409–414

[44] Kehlet H, Büchler MW, Beart RW, Jr, Billingham RP, Williamson R. Care after colonic operation–is it evidence-based? Results from a multinational survey in Europe and the United States. J Am Coll Surg. 2006; 202(1):45–54

[45] Peppas G, Alexiou VG, Falagas ME. Bowel cleansing before bowel surgery: major discordance between evidence and practice. J Gastrointest Surg. 2008; 12(5):919–920

[46] Kahokehr A, Robertson P, Sammour T, Soop M, Hill AG. Perioperative care: a survey of New Zealand and Australian colorectal surgeons. Colorectal Dis. 2011; 13(11):1308–1313

[47] Poggio JL. Perioperative strategies to prevent surgical-site infection. Clin Colon Rectal Surg. 2013; 26(3):168–173

[48] Ludwig KA, Carlson MA, Condon RE. Prophylactic antibiotics in surgery. Annu Rev Med. 1993; 44:385–393

[49] Song F, Glenny AM. Antimicrobial prophylaxis in colorectal surgery: a systematic review of randomized controlled trials. Br J Surg. 1998; 85(9):1232–1241

[50] Bratzler DW, Hunt DR. The surgical infection prevention and surgical care improvement projects: national initiatives to improve outcomes for patients having surgery. Clin Infect Dis. 2006; 43(3):322–330

[51] Edmiston CE, Spencer M, Lewis BD, et al. Reducing the risk of surgical site infections: did we really think SCIP was going to lead us to the promised land? Surg Infect (Larchmt). 2011; 12(3):169–177

[52] Bratzler DW, Houck PM, Surgical Infection Prevention Guidelines Writers Workgroup, American Academy of Orthopaedic Surgeons, American Association of Critical Care Nurses, American Association of Nurse Anesthetists, American College of Surgeons, American College of Osteopathic Surgeons, American Geriatrics Society, American Society of Anesthesiologists, American Society of Colon and Rectal Surgeons, American Society of Health-System Pharmacists, American Society of PeriAnesthesia Nurses, Ascension Health, Association of periOperative Registered Nurses, Association for Professionals in Infection Control and Epidemiology, Infectious Diseases Society of America, Medical Letter, Premier, Society for Healthcare Epidemiology of America, Society of Thoracic Surgeons, Surgical Infection Society. Antimicrobial prophylaxis for surgery: an advisory statement from the National Surgical Infection Prevention Project. Clin Infect Dis. 2004; 38(12):1706–1715

[53] Antimicrobial prophylaxis for surgery. Treat Guidel Med Lett. 2009; 7(82):47–52

[54] Nelson RL, Glenny AM, Song F. Antimicrobial prophylaxis for colorectal surgery. Cochrane Database Syst Rev. 2009(1):CD001181

[55] Dellinger EP. Prophylactic antibiotics: administration and timing before operation are more important than administration after operation. Clin Infect Dis. 2007; 44(7):928–930

[56] Weber WP, Marti WR, Zwahlen M, et al. The timing of surgical antimicrobial prophylaxis. Ann Surg. 2008; 247(6):918–926

[57] Zanetti G, Giardina R, Platt R. Intraoperative redosing of cefazolin and risk for surgical site infection in cardiac surgery. Emerg Infect Dis. 2001; 7(5):828–831

[58] McDonald M, Grabsch E, Marshall C, Forbes A. Single- versus multiple-dose antimicrobial prophylaxis for major surgery: a systematic review. Aust N Z J Surg. 1998; 68(6):388–396

[59] Scarborough JE, Mantyh CR, Sun Z, Migaly J. Combined mechanical and oral antibiotic bowel preparation reduces incisional surgical site infection and anastomotic leak rates after elective colorectal resection: an analysis of colectomy-targeted ACS NSQIP. Ann Surg. 2015; 262(2):331–337

[60] Moghadamyeghaneh Z, Hanna MH, Carmichael JC, Mills SD, Pigazzi A, Nguyen NT, Stamos MJ. Nationwide analysis of outcomes of bowel preparation in colon surgery. J Am Coll Surg. 2015; 220:912–920

[61] Chen M, Song X, Chen LZ, Lin ZD, Zhang XL. Comparing mechanical bowel preparation with both oral and systemic antibiotics versus mechanical bowel preparation and systemic antibiotics alone for the prevention of surgical site infection after elective colorectal surgery: a meta-analysis of randomized controlled clinical trials. Dis Colon Rectum. 2016; 59(1):70–78

[62] Cannon JA, Altom LK, Deierhoi RJ, et al. Preoperative oral antibiotics reduce surgical site infection following elective colorectal resections. Dis Colon Rectum. 2012; 55(11):1160–1166

[63] Toneva GD, Deierhoi RJ, Morris M, et al. Oral antibiotic bowel preparation reduces length of stay and readmissions after colorectal surgery. J Am Coll Surg. 2013; 216(4):756–762, discussion 762–763

[64] Kim EK, Sheetz KH, Bonn J, et al. A statewide colectomy experience: the role of full bowel preparation in preventing surgical site infection. Ann Surg. 2014; 259(2):310–314

[65] Beck DE, McCoy AB. Perioperative management of the colorectal surgery patient. An ASCRS Survey. Dis Colon Rectum. In press

[66] Jones C, Badger SA, Hannon R. The role of carbohydrate drinks in pre-operative nutrition for elective colorectal surgery. Ann R Coll Surg Engl. 2011; 93(7):504–507

[67] Awad S, Varadhan KK, Ljungqvist O, Lobo DN. A meta-analysis of randomised controlled trials on preoperative oral carbohydrate treatment in elective surgery. Clin Nutr. 2013; 32(1):34–44

[68] Kurz A, Sessler DI, Lenhardt R, Study of Wound Infection and Temperature Group. Perioperative normothermia to reduce the incidence of surgical-wound infection and shorten hospitalization. N Engl J Med. 1996; 334(19):1209–1215

[69] Melling AC, Ali B, Scott EM, Leaper DJ. Effects of preoperative warming on the incidence of wound infection after clean surgery: a randomised controlled trial. Lancet. 2001; 358(9285):876–880

[70] Knighton DR, Halliday B, Hunt TK. Oxygen as an antibiotic. A comparison of the effects of inspired oxygen concentration and antibiotic administration on in vivo bacterial clearance. Arch Surg. 1986; 121(2):191–195

[71] Greif R, Akça O, Horn EP, Kurz A, Sessler DI, Outcomes Research Group. Supplemental perioperative oxygen to reduce the incidence of surgical-wound infection. N Engl J Med. 2000; 342(3):161–167

[72] Kabon B, Kurz A. Optimal perioperative oxygen administration. Curr Opin Anaesthesiol. 2006; 19(1):11–18

[73] Noblett SE, Horgan AF. Perioperative fluid management. Semin Colon Rectal Surg. 2010; 21:160–164

[74] Gheorghe A, Calvert M, Pinkney TD, et al. West Midlands Research Collaborative, ROSSINI Trial Management Group. Systematic review of the clinical effectiveness of wound-edge protection devices in reducing surgical site infection in patients undergoing open abdominal surgery. Ann Surg. 2012; 255(6):1017–1029

[75] Edwards JP, Ho AL, Tee MC, Dixon E, Ball CG. Wound protectors reduce surgical site infection: a meta-analysis of randomized controlled trials. Ann Surg. 2012; 256(1):53–59

[76] Cima R, Dankbar E, Lovely J, et al. Colorectal Surgical Site Infection Reduction Team. Colorectal surgery surgical site infection reduction program: a national surgical quality improvement program–driven multidisciplinary single-institution experience. J Am Coll Surg. 2013; 216(1):23–33

[77] Samaiya A. To drain or not to drain after colorectal cancer surgery. Indian J Surg. 2015; 77 Suppl 3:1363–1368

[78] Garimella V, Cellini C. Postoperative pain control. Clin Colon Rectal Surg. 2013; 26(3):191–196

[79] Barletta JF, Asgeirsson T, Senagore AJ. Influence of intravenous opioid dose on postoperative ileus. Ann Pharmacother. 2011; 45(7–8):916–923

[80] Goettsch WG, Sukel MP, van der Peet DL, van Riemsdijk MM, Herings RM. In-hospital use of opioids increases rate of coded postoperative paralytic ileus. Pharmacoepidemiol Drug Saf. 2007; 16(6):668–674

[81] Levy BF, Tilney HS, Dowson HM, Rockall TA. A systematic review of postoperative analgesia following laparoscopic colorectal surgery. Colorectal Dis. 2010; 12(1):5–15

[82] Zafar N, Davies R, Greenslade GL, Dixon AR. The evolution of analgesia in an 'accelerated' recovery programme for resectional laparoscopic colorectal surgery with anastomosis. Colorectal Dis. 2010; 12(2):119–124

[83] Keeri-Szanto M, Remington B. Drug levels on continuous intravenous infusion. Lancet. 1971; 2(7724):601

[84] Evans JM, Rosen M, MacCarthy J, Hogg MI. Apparatus for patient-controlled administration of intravenous narcotics during labour. Lancet. 1976; 1 (7949):17–18

[85] Ballantyne JC, Carr DB, Chalmers TC, Dear KB, Angelillo IF, Mosteller F. Postoperative patient-controlled analgesia: meta-analyses of initial randomized control trials. J Clin Anesth. 1993; 5(3):182–193

[86] Hudcova J, McNicol E, Quah C, Lau J, Carr DB. Patient controlled opioid analgesia versus conventional opioid analgesia for postoperative pain. Cochrane Database Syst Rev. 2006(4):CD003348

[87] Koo PJS. Postoperative pain management with a patient-controlled transdermal delivery system for fentanyl. Am J Health Syst Pharm. 2005; 62 (11):1171–1176

[88] Viscusi ER, Reynolds L, Chung F, Atkinson LE, Khanna S. Patient-controlled transdermal fentanyl hydrochloride vs intravenous morphine pump for postoperative pain: a randomized controlled trial. JAMA. 2004; 291 (11):1333–1341

[89] Werawatganon T, Charuluxanun S. Patient controlled intravenous opioid analgesia versus continuous epidural analgesia for pain after intra-abdominal surgery. Cochrane Database Syst Rev. 2005(1):CD004088

[90] Marret E, Remy C, Bonnet F, Postoperative Pain Forum Group. Meta-analysis of epidural analgesia versus parenteral opioid analgesia after colorectal surgery. Br J Surg. 2007; 94(6):665–673

[91] Mann C, Pouzeratte Y, Boccara G, et al. Comparison of intravenous or epidural patient-controlled analgesia in the elderly after major abdominal surgery. Anesthesiology. 2000; 92(2):433–441

[92] Hermanides J, Hollmann MW, Stevens MF, Lirk P. Failed epidural: causes and management. Br J Anaesth. 2012; 109(2):144–154

[93] Virlos I, Clements D, Beynon J, Ratnalikar V, Khot U. Short-term outcomes with intrathecal versus epidural analgesia in laparoscopic colorectal surgery. Br J Surg. 2010; 97(9):1401–1406

[94] Levy BF, Scott MJ, Fawcett W, Fry C, Rockall TA. Randomized clinical trial of epidural, spinal or patient-controlled analgesia for patients undergoing laparoscopic colorectal surgery. Br J Surg. 2011; 98(8):1068–1078

[95] Wongyingsinn M, Baldini G, Stein B, Charlebois P, Liberman S, Carli F. Spinal analgesia for laparoscopic colonic resection using an enhanced recovery after surgery programme: better analgesia, but no benefits on postoperative recovery: a randomized controlled trial. Br J Anaesth. 2012; 108(5):850–856

[96] Lowder JL, Shackelford DP, Holbert D, Beste TM. A randomized, controlled trial to compare ketorolac tromethamine versus placebo after cesarean section to reduce pain and narcotic usage. Am J Obstet Gynecol. 2003; 189 (6):1559–1562, discussion 1562

[97] Dajani EZ, Islam K. Cardiovascular and gastrointestinal toxicity of selective cyclo-oxygenase-2 inhibitors in man. J Physiol Pharmacol. 2008; 59 Suppl 2:117–133

[98] De Oliveira GS, Jr, Agarwal D, Benzon HT. Perioperative single dose ketorolac to prevent postoperative pain: a meta-analysis of randomized trials. Anesth Analg. 2012; 114(2):424–433

[99] Pavy TJ, Paech MJ, Evans SF. The effect of intravenous ketorolac on opioid requirement and pain after cesarean delivery. Anesth Analg. 2001; 92 (4):1010–1014

[100] Chen JY, Wu GJ, Mok MS, et al. Effect of adding ketorolac to intravenous morphine patient-controlled analgesia on bowel function in colorectal surgery patients–a prospective, randomized, double-blind study. Acta Anaesthesiol Scand. 2005; 49(4):546–551

[101] Chen JY, Ko TL, Wen YR, et al. Opioid-sparing effects of ketorolac and its correlation with the recovery of postoperative bowel function in colorectal surgery patients: a prospective randomized double-blinded study. Clin J Pain. 2009; 25(6):485–489

[102] Southworth S, Peters J, Rock A, Pavliv L. A multicenter, randomized, double-blind, placebo-controlled trial of intravenous ibuprofen 400 and 800 mg every 6 hours in the management of postoperative pain. Clin Ther. 2009; 31 (9):1922–1935

[103] Cataldo PA, Senagore AJ, Kilbride MJ. Ketorolac and patient controlled analgesia in the treatment of postoperative pain. Surg Gynecol Obstet. 1993; 176 (5):435–438

[104] Toms L, McQuay HJ, Derry S, Moore RA. Single dose oral paracetamol (acetaminophen) for postoperative pain in adults. Cochrane Database Syst Rev. 2008(4):CD004602

[105] Maund E, McDaid C, Rice S, Wright K, Jenkins B, Woolacott N. Paracetamol and selective and non-selective non-steroidal anti-inflammatory drugs for the reduction in morphine-related side-effects after major surgery: a systematic review. Br J Anaesth. 2011; 106(3):292–297

[106] Ong CK, Seymour RA, Lirk P, Merry AF. Combining paracetamol (acetaminophen) with nonsteroidal antiinflammatory drugs: a qualitative systematic review of analgesic efficacy for acute postoperative pain. Anesth Analg. 2010; 110(4):1170–1179

[107] Charlton S, Cyna AM, Middleton P, Griffiths JD. Perioperative transversus abdominis plane (TAP) blocks for analgesia after abdominal surgery. Cochrane Database Syst Rev. 2010(12):CD007705

[108] Brady RR, Ventham NT, Roberts DM, Graham C, Daniel T. Open transversus abdominis plane block and analgesic requirements in patients following right hemicolectomy. Ann R Coll Surg Engl. 2012; 94(5):327–330

[109] Conaghan P, Maxwell-Armstrong C, Bedforth N, et al. Efficacy of transversus abdominis plane blocks in laparoscopic colorectal resections. Surg Endosc. 2010; 24(10):2480–2484

[110] Scott NB. Wound infiltration for surgery. Anaesthesia. 2010; 65 Suppl 1:67–75

[111] Haas E, Onel E, Miller H, Ragupathi M, White PF. A double-blind, randomized, active-controlled study for post-hemorrhoidectomy pain management with liposome bupivacaine, a novel local analgesic formulation. Am Surg. 2012; 78(5):574–581

[112] Golf M, Daniels SE, Onel E. A phase 3, randomized, placebo-controlled trial of DepoFoam® bupivacaine (extended-release bupivacaine local analgesic) in bunionectomy. Adv Ther. 2011; 28(9):776–788

[113] Cohen SM. Extended pain relief trial utilizing infiltration of Exparel(®), a long-acting multivesicular liposome formulation of bupivacaine: a Phase IV health economic trial in adult patients undergoing open colectomy. J Pain Res. 2012; 5:567–572

[114] Beck DE, Margolin DA, Babin SF, Russo CT. Benefits of a multimodal regimen for postsurgical pain management in colorectal surgery. Ochsner J. 2015; 15 (4):408–412

[115] Benotti JR, Dalen JE. The natural history of pulmonary embolism. Clin Chest Med. 1984; 5(3):403–410

[116] Nicolaides AN, Miles C, Hoare M, Jury P, Helmis E, Venniker R. Intermittent sequential pneumatic compression of the legs and thromboembolism-deterrent stockings in the prevention of postoperative deep venous thrombosis. Surgery. 1983; 94(1):21–25

[117] Törngren S, Rieger A. Prophylaxis of deep venous thrombosis in colorectal surgery. Dis Colon Rectum. 1982; 25(6):563–566

[118] Kalff JC, Türler A, Schwarz NT, et al. Intra-abdominal activation of a local inflammatory response within the human muscularis externa during laparotomy. Ann Surg. 2003; 237(3):301–315

[119] Taché Y, Martinez V, Million M, Wang L. Stress and the gastrointestinal tract III. Stress-related alterations of gut motor function: role of brain corticotropin-releasing factor receptors. Am J Physiol Gastrointest Liver Physiol. 2001; 280(2):G173–G177

[120] Cullen JJ, Eagon JC, Kelly KA. Gastrointestinal peptide hormones during postoperative ileus. Effect of octreotide. Dig Dis Sci. 1994; 39(6):1179–1184

[121] Waldhausen JH, Shaffrey ME, Skenderis BS, II, Jones RS, Schirmer BD. Gastrointestinal myoelectric and clinical patterns of recovery after laparotomy. Ann Surg. 1990; 211(6):777–784, discussion 785

[122] Condon RE, Cowles VE, Ferraz AA, et al. Human colonic smooth muscle electrical activity during and after recovery from postoperative ileus. Am J Physiol. 1995; 269(3, Pt 1):G408–G417

[123] Shibata Y, Toyoda S, Nimura Y, Miyati M. Patterns of intestinal motility recovery during the early stage following abdominal surgery: clinical and manometric study. World J Surg. 1997; 21(8):806–809, discussion 809–810

[124] Prasad M, Matthews JB. Deflating postoperative ileus. Gastroenterology. 1999; 117(2):489–492

[125] Sands DR, Wexner SD. Nasogastric tubes and dietary advancement after laparoscopic and open colorectal surgery. Nutrition. 1999; 15(5):347–350

[126] Milsom JW, Böhm B, Hammerhofer KA, Fazio V, Steiger E, Elson P. A prospective, randomized trial comparing laparoscopic versus conventional techniques in colorectal cancer surgery: a preliminary report. J Am Coll Surg. 1998; 187(1):46–54, discussion 54–55

[127] Bufo AJ, Feldman S, Daniels GA, Lieberman RC. Early postoperative feeding. Dis Colon Rectum. 1994; 37(12):1260–1265

[128] Binderow SR, Cohen SM, Wexner SD, Nogueras JJ. Must early postoperative oral intake be limited to laparoscopy? Dis Colon Rectum. 1994; 37 (6):584–589

[129] Reissman P, Teoh TA, Cohen SM, et al. Is early oral feeding safe after elective colorectal surgery? A prospective randomized trial. Ann Surg. 1995; 222 (1):73–77

[130] Ortiz H, Armendariz P, Yarnoz C. Is early postoperative feeding feasible in elective colon and rectal surgery? Int J Colorectal Dis. 1996; 11(3):119–121

[131] Di Fronzo LA, Cymerman J, O'Connell TX. Factors affecting early postoperative feeding following elective open colon resection. Arch Surg. 1999; 134 (9):941–945, discussion 945–946

[132] Petrelli NJ, Cheng C, Driscoll D, Rodriguez-Bigas MA. Early postoperative oral feeding after colectomy: an analysis of factors that may predict failure. Ann Surg Oncol. 2001; 8(10):796–800

[133] Lewis SJ, Egger M, Sylvester PA, Thomas S. Early enteral feeding versus "nil by mouth" after gastrointestinal surgery: systematic review and meta-analysis of controlled trials. BMJ. 2001; 323(7316):773–776

[134] DiFronzo LA, Yamin N, Patel K, O'Connell TX. Benefits of early feeding and early hospital discharge in elderly patients undergoing open colon resection. J Am Coll Surg. 2003; 197(5):747–752

[135] Kehlet H. Multimodal approach to control postoperative pathophysiology and rehabilitation. Br J Anaesth. 1997; 78(5):606–617

[136] Bradshaw BGG, Liu SS, Thirlby RC. Standardized perioperative care protocols and reduced length of stay after colon surgery. J Am Coll Surg. 1998; 186 (5):501–506

[137] Basse L, Hjort Jakobsen D, Billesbølle P, Werner M, Kehlet H. A clinical pathway to accelerate recovery after colonic resection. Ann Surg. 2000; 232 (1):51–57

[138] Basse L, Thorbøl JE, Løssl K, Kehlet H. Colonic surgery with accelerated rehabilitation or conventional care. Dis Colon Rectum. 2004; 47(3):271–277, discussion 277–278

[139] Delaney CP, Zutshi M, Senagore AJ, Remzi FH, Hammel J, Fazio VW. Prospective, randomized, controlled trial between a pathway of controlled rehabilitation with early ambulation and diet and traditional postoperative care after laparotomy and intestinal resection. Dis Colon Rectum. 2003; 46 (7):851–859

[140] Fearon KCH, Luff R. The nutritional management of surgical patients: enhanced recovery after surgery. Proc Nutr Soc. 2003; 62(4):807–811

[141] Smedh K, Strand E, Jansson P, et al. Rapid recovery after colonic resection. Multimodal rehabilitation by means of Kehlet's method practiced in Vasteras [in Swedish]. Lakartidningen. 2001; 98(21):2568–2574

[142] Henriksen MG, Jensen MB, Hansen HV, Jespersen TW, Hessov I. Enforced mobilization, early oral feeding, and balanced analgesia improve convalescence after colorectal surgery. Nutrition. 2002; 18(2):147–152

[143] Bisgaard T, Kehlet H. Early oral feeding after elective abdominal surgery—what are the issues? Nutrition. 2002; 18(11–12):944–948

[144] Mythen MG. Postoperative gastrointestinal tract dysfunction. Anesth Analg. 2005; 100(1):196–204

[145] do Nascimento Junior P, Módolo NS, Andrade S, Guimarães MM, Braz LG, El Dib R. Incentive spirometry for prevention of postoperative pulmonary complications in upper abdominal surgery. Cochrane Database Syst Rev. 2014 (2):CD006058

[146] Bleier JIA, Aarons CB. Perioperative fluid restriction. Clin Colon Rectal Surg. 2013; 26(3):197–202

[147] Doherty M, Buggy DJ. Intraoperative fluids: how much is too much? Br J Anaesth. 2012; 109(1):69–79

[148] Brandstrup B, Tønnesen H, Beier-Holgersen R, et al. Danish Study Group on Perioperative Fluid Therapy. Effects of intravenous fluid restriction on postoperative complications: comparison of two perioperative fluid regimens: a randomized assessor-blinded multicenter trial. Ann Surg. 2003; 238 (5):641–648

[149] Levin AL. A new gastroduodenal catheter. JAMA. 1921; 76:1007

[150] Burg R, Geigle CF, Faso JM, Theuerkauf FJ, Jr. Omission of routine gastric decompression. Dis Colon Rectum. 1978; 21(2):98–100

[151] Bauer JJ, Gelernt IM, Salky BA, Kreel I. Is routine postoperative nasogastric decompression really necessary? Ann Surg. 1985; 201(2):233–236

[152] Clevers GJ, Smout AJ. The natural course of postoperative ileus following abdominal surgery. Neth J Surg. 1989; 41(5):97–99

[153] Colvin DB, Lee W, Eisenstat TE, Rubin RJ, Salvati EP. The role of nasointestinal intubation in elective colonic surgery. Dis Colon Rectum. 1986; 29 (5):295–299

[154] Wolff BG, Pemberton JH, van Heerden JA, et al. Elective colon and rectal surgery without nasogastric decompression. A prospective, randomized trial. Ann Surg. 1989; 209(6):670–673, discussion 673–675

[155] Petrelli NJ, Stulc JP, Rodriguez-Bigas M, Blumenson L. Nasogastric decompression following elective colorectal surgery: a prospective randomized study. Am Surg. 1993; 59(10):632–635

[156] Cheatham ML, Chapman WC, Key SP, Sawyers JL. A meta-analysis of selective versus routine nasogastric decompression after elective laparotomy. Ann Surg. 1995; 221(5):469–476, discussion 476–478

[157] Reissman P, Teoh TA, Cohen SM, Weiss EG, Nogueras JJ, Wexner SD. Is early oral feeding safe after elective colorectal surgery? A prospective randomized trial. Ann Surg. 1995; 222(1):73–77

[158] Feo CV, Romanini B, Sortini D, et al. Early oral feeding after colorectal resection: a randomized controlled study. ANZ J Surg. 2004; 74(5):298–301

[159] Saint S. Clinical and economic consequences of nosocomial catheter-related bacteriuria. Am J Infect Control. 2000; 28(1):68–75

[160] Stéphan F, Sax H, Wachsmuth M, Hoffmeyer P, Clergue F, Pittet D. Reduction of urinary tract infection and antibiotic use after surgery: a controlled, prospective, before-after intervention study. Clin Infect Dis. 2006; 42(11):1544–1551

[161] Wald H, Epstein A, Kramer A. Extended use of indwelling urinary catheters in postoperative hip fracture patients. Med Care. 2005; 43(10):1009–1017

[162] Wald HL, Ma A, Bratzler DW, Kramer AM. Indwelling urinary catheter use in the postoperative period: analysis of the national surgical infection prevention project data. Arch Surg. 2008; 143(6):551–557

[163] Wight R, Kennedy H, Abdelal A, Fulton JD. Postoperative urinary retention. BMJ. 1991; 302(6785):1151

[164] Petrelli NJ, Nagel S, Rodriguez-Bigas M, Piedmonte M, Herrera L. Morbidity and mortality following abdominoperineal resection for rectal adenocarcinoma. Am Surg. 1993; 59(7):400–404

[165] Havenga K, Welvaart K. Sexual dysfunction in male patients after surgical treatment of rectosigmoid cancer [in Dutch]. Neth J Med. 1991; 135:710–713

[166] van Driel MF, Weymar Schultz WC, van de Wiel HBM, Hahn DE, Mensink HJ. Female sexual functioning after radical surgical treatment of rectal and bladder cancer. Eur J Surg Oncol. 1993; 19(2):183–187

[167] Scholefield JH, Northover JMA. Surgical management of rectal cancer. Br J Surg. 1995; 82(6):745–748

[168] Miedema BW, Johnson JO. Methods for decreasing postoperative gut dysmotility. Lancet Oncol. 2003; 4(6):365–372

[169] Taguchi A, Sharma N, Saleem RM, et al. Selective postoperative inhibition of gastrointestinal opioid receptors. N Engl J Med. 2001; 345(13):935–940

[170] Holte K, Kehlet H. Postoperative ileus: a preventable event. Br J Surg. 2000; 87(11):1480–1493

[171] Sadek SA, Cranford C, Eriksen C, et al. Pharmacological manipulation of adynamic ileus: controlled randomized double-blind study of ceruletide on intestinal motor activity after elective abdominal surgery. Aliment Pharmacol Ther. 1988; 2(1):47–54

[172] Madsen PV, Lykkegaard-Nielsen M, Nielsen OV. Ceruletide reduces postoperative intestinal paralysis. A double-blind placebo-controlled trial. Dis Colon Rectum. 1983; 26(3):159–160

[173] Bonacini M, Quiason S, Reynolds M, Gaddis M, Pemberton B, Smith O. Effect of intravenous erythromycin on postoperative ileus. Am J Gastroenterol. 1993; 88(2):208–211

[174] Holte K, Kehlet H. Fluid therapy and surgical outcomes in elective surgery: a need for reassessment in fast-track surgery. J Am Coll Surg. 2006; 202 (6):971–989

Part II

Anorectal Disease

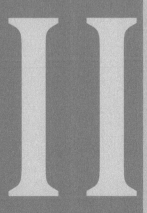

6 Ambulatory and Anorectal Procedures

David E. Beck

Abstract

Ambulatory procedures are those in which the patient returns home on the day of the operation, regardless of the type of anesthesia or location. An increasing number of colorectal procedures are being performed on an outpatient basis, especially those involving the anus and rectum. Factors contributing to this increase include the development of improved local and general anesthetics, the public's increased interest in and knowledge of medical matters, the willingness of ambulatory patients and their families to participate in nursing, spiraling health care costs, and the desire of insurance carriers to minimize surgery-related expenses. To accommodate these changes better, outpatient postoperative care systems were developed. Not suited for the outpatient environment are those patients who may have postoperative pain unrelieved by oral analgesics, those whose operations are likely to be followed by postoperative bleeding, patients who have severe emotional objections to the idea, those who live alone, patients with significant medical comorbidities requiring postoperative observation, individuals unable to tolerate oral intake, and patients at significant risk for complications requiring immediate care (such as hemorrhage).

Keywords: ambulatory procedures, outpatient procedures, operative management, local anesthesia, patient preparation, postoperative care, pain control, anorectal preparations

6.1 Introduction

By definition, ambulatory procedures are those in which the patient returns home on the day of the operation, regardless of the type of anesthesia or location (physician's office, emergency department, hospital operating room, or a freestanding, independent ambulatory surgery unit). Other terms that have been used to apply to this situation include one-day surgery, same-day surgery, office-based surgery, and outpatient surgery.

An increasing number of colorectal procedures are being performed on an outpatient basis, especially those involving the anus and rectum. Factors contributing to this increase include the development of improved local and general anesthetics, the public's increased interest in and knowledge of medical matters, ambulatory patients' willingness to participate in nursing themselves, as well as the willingness of their families, spiraling health care costs, and the desire of insurance carriers to minimize surgery-related expenses. The changes have been achieved through technological advances, sustained by patient and provider preference, and driven largely by payment system changes.[1] In the United States, it has been estimated that over 90% of anorectal cases can be performed on an outpatient basis.[2]

To accommodate these changes better, outpatient postoperative care systems were developed. This begins with patient and family education. Discharge personnel inform family members what to expect with regard to diet, pain, bowel function, medications, activity, and wound care. Home health and visiting nurses are available to provide expert care in the patient's homes, and to act as liaisons to the physician should any questions or problems arise.

Not suited for the outpatient environment are those patients who may have postoperative pain unrelieved by oral analgesics, those whose operations are likely to be followed by postoperative bleeding, patients who have severe emotional objections to the idea, those who live alone, patients with significant medical comorbidities requiring postoperative observation, individuals unable to tolerate oral intake, and patients at significant risk for complications requiring immediate care (such as hemorrhage).[3]

6.2 Preoperative Assessment and Patient Evaluation

For patients having procedures under local anesthesia, a simple history about bleeding diatheses and allergies to local anesthesia or medications such as anticoagulants should be obtained. Particular attention should be focused on comorbid medical conditions and medications (such as cardiac medications and anticoagulants), which may need to be manipulated to maximize patient safety. In addition, disabilities limiting an individual's ability to care for him- or herself (such as blindness, stroke, or dementia) should be evaluated. Patients receiving a general procedure should be evaluated as described in Chapter 5. A preoperative discussion with the patient should describe the procedure and include any of the patient's concerns, such as pain control, complications, and recommended activity at home. Bowel preparation will vary from nothing for an anal fissure, to an enema for hemorrhoids to a full mechanical preparation for a transanal minimally invasive surgical procedure.

6.3 Patient Preparation

In addition to being diagnosed and evaluated for operation, individuals should be prepared for postoperative discharge at their preoperative visit. Patients and families should be informed as to the nature of the operation including alternative approaches, benefits, and potential complications. The postoperative home course should be detailed, including normal pain, wound, and drainage expectations. Alterations in bowel habits (particularly medication-induced constipation) should be predicted and remedies provided. In addition, individuals and families should be educated regarding events which should prompt calls to their physician, such as high fever, excessive vomiting, inability to void, intractable pain, and significant bleeding. Ideally, all of this information should be available in a preprinted postoperative instruction sheet or booklet, and should include a number to call 24 hours a day in case of emergency.

In addition to patient education, office and perioperative medical personnel should be educated regarding their roles in outpatient surgical procedures. Office assistants and nurses will be the first points of contact when patients develop problems or have questions following operation. Therefore, they too should be informed of the normal postoperative course and worrisome complaints that might indicate a significant postoperative complication. Perioperative nursing specialists may also provide follow-up phone calls the evening of the operation. The patient is also instructed about preoperative dietary limitations, as described in Chapter 5.

6.4 Operative Management

Procedures are often performed in the prone jackknife or left lateral (Sims') position. Anesthesia should be effective and should allow rapid recovery with minimal side effects. Anesthetic techniques should have little impact on the ability to discharge patients following anorectal operations, with the exception of issues described in the following.

Regional anesthesia presents a special set of considerations.[4] Spinal, epidural, and caudal anesthesia have the following problems in common: time consumed during the block, potential technical difficulties with the block, variability in degree of block produced, and problems during the recovery period. Any degree of motor paralysis significantly prolongs time in the recovery room. Although it is possible to send a patient from the recovery room to the surgical ward with a small amount of residual block, the ambulatory patient must be able to walk to his or her car. The problem of post–lumbar puncture headache is always a consideration and can significantly complicate the ambulatory surgical patient's course of recovery and early return to work.

Long-acting spinal anesthetics, particularly combined with large, intraoperative fluid administration, will increase urinary retention rates and delay discharge.[5] Alpha-adrenergic blockers have been administered prophylactically in this setting to decrease the spasm of the autonomically innervated internal sphincter at the bladder neck in attempts to decrease urinary retention, but have not met with success.[6] Limiting postoperative fluids in combination with short-acting spinal anesthetic has, however, decreased urinary retention rates.[7] General anesthesia with heavy emphasis on narcotics may cause postoperative nausea and vomiting, leading to prolonged recovery room stay or even overnight hospitalization.

Perianal shaving is not necessary except for patients with pilonidal disease.

6.5 Procedures

The majority of anorectal cases can be performed on an outpatient basis. Procedures related to specific disease processes are discussed in the respective chapter, while other outpatient procedures are discussed in the following sections.

6.5.1 Examination under Anesthesia

An examination under anesthesia is valuable in a number of conditions. These include patients whose anus is too painful to adequately examine, patients with complex fistulas, and patients with a nonhealing perineal wound.

6.5.2 Rectal Biopsy

A biopsy is essential for the diagnosis of neoplasms, particularly malignant ones, and in the diagnosis of inflammatory conditions, including specific infections such as amebic dysentery. Serial biopsies can be valuable in the diagnosis of ulcerative colitis and Crohn's disease and can be useful in judging the response to treatment. Biopsy may detect changes not apparent to the endoscopist. The correlation between proctosigmoidoscopic observations and the histology of biopsies of the rectal mucosa is not always accurate. For this reason, biopsy can, in certain circumstances, add refinement to the clinical opinion. It also confirms the presence of normal rectal mucosa.

Unusual local conditions that can be identified by rectal biopsy include pneumatosis cystoides intestinalis, mucoviscidosis, melanosis coli, oleogranuloma, and parasitic infections such as schistosomiasis.[8] Rectal biopsy may be useful in detecting certain systemic conditions such as neurolipidoses, metachromatic leukodystrophy, Hurler's syndrome, amyloidosis, the arteritis of rheumatoid arthritis, periarteritis nodosa, malignant hypertension, cystinosis, and Whipple's disease.[8]

Various forceps and suction biopsy apparatus are available for obtaining specimens from the rectum for histologic evaluation. For the pathologist to provide maximal information to the clinician, a correct anatomic orientation is necessary. The specimen is submitted with the submucosal surface downward against a flat, ground-glass slide or on paper to which it adheres by its own stickiness or sutured in place.

6.5.3 Foreign Body Removal

A host of foreign bodies may be found in the rectum. They often can be removed with the aid of local anesthesia. Occasionally, a general or regional anesthetic is necessary. Patients are usually discharged after a short period of observation. Selected patients may require observation for 24 hours to ensure that no bowel perforation has occurred (see Chapter 34).

6.6 Local Anesthesia

Local anesthetic agents produce a loss of sensation and muscle paralysis in a circumscribed area of the body by a localized effect on peripheral nerve endings or fibers.[9] The anal canal and the perianal skin can be anesthetized with minimal pain or discomfort, and become fully relaxed.

6.6.1 Selection of Patients

A highly nervous and apprehensive patient or one with a very painful anal canal is not a good candidate for local anesthesia. Success requires a cooperative patient, who should be given a thorough explanation of the procedure and be told what to expect and be apprised of the advantages and disadvantages of local anesthesia.

Almost all kinds of simple anorectal conditions are suitable for local anesthesia. These conditions include hemorrhoids (even thrombosed, strangulated, or gangrenous), anal fissure, simple intersphincteric anal fistula, small perianal abscess, pilonidal abscess and sinus, low rectal adenoma, and perianal and anal condyloma acuminatum, as well as in carefully selected cases of sphincter repair and many other anorectal conditions.[10]

Most perianal abscesses can be drained with the patient under local anesthesia, especially with catheter drainage.

However, patients with very large abscesses require an excessive amount of the anesthetic agent because the tissue is acidotic, which causes slower diffusion of the anesthetic solution through the nerve sheath. Patients with significant scar tissue such as that found in cases of a complicated anal fistula also do not respond well to a local anesthetic. Anorectal procedure expected to exceed 2 hours may not be suitable for a local anesthetic because of positional discomfort.

6.6.2 Actions of Local Agents

Local anesthetic agents inhibit the excitatory process in nerve endings or fibers. Their location of action is in the nerve membrane, which has a lipid and protein structure. The anesthetic potency of different agents is a function of their lipid solubility, while protein binding is the primary determinant of anesthetic duration.[9]

Local anesthetics exist in both a charged and an uncharged (free base) form, with the equilibrium determined by the pH of the surrounding medium. As the pH of the solution decreases (hydrogen ion concentration increases), the equilibrium shifts toward the charged cation form. Conversely, as the pH increases, the equilibrium shifts toward the free-base form. The uncharged (free) base form diffuses more readily through the nerve sheath and is reflected clinically in the onset of anesthesia.[9] This explains why local anesthesia is less effective for large abscesses, because the tissue is acidotic.

The susceptibility of nerve fibers to local anesthetics is related to the size of the fiber and its myelin coating. Smaller nerves are blocked first, and lightly myelinated nerves are more susceptible than more heavily coated nerves. In general, the first nerves blocked are the last ones to recover. Sensory nerves are blocked before motor nerves. The usual order of sensory loss is pain, temperature, touch, and deep pressure.

6.6.3 Disposition of Agent

Knowing the vascular absorption, tissue distribution, metabolism, and excretion of local anesthetic agents is important in understanding their potential toxicity. Absorption varies according to site of injection, dosage, addition of a vasoconstrictor agent, and specific agent used.[9]

After their absorption from the injection site, local anesthetic agents distribute themselves throughout total body water. An initial rapid disappearance from blood (alpha phase) occurs because of uptake by tissues with a high vascular perfusion. A secondary slower disappearance rate (beta phase) reflects distribution to slowly perfused tissues and metabolism and excretion of the compound. Although all tissues will take up local anesthetics, the highest concentrations are found in the more highly perfused organs such as the lungs and kidneys. The greater percentage of an injected dose of a local anesthetic agent is distributed to skeletal muscle because of the large mass of tissue in the body.[9]

The metabolism of local anesthetic agents varies according to their chemical classification. The ester- or procainelike agents undergo hydrolysis in plasma by the enzyme pseudocholinesterase. The amide- or lidocainelike agents undergo enzymatic degradation primarily in the liver. Lidocaine (Xylocaine), mepivacaine (Carbocaine), and etidocaine (Duranest) are intermediate in terms of rate of degradation, whereas bupivacaine (Marcaine) is metabolized most slowly.[9]

6.6.4 Choice of Agent

Although several local anesthetic agents are available for clinical use in anorectal surgery, lidocaine and bupivacaine are most suitable and most widely used.[11] Both lidocaine and bupivacaine are amide compounds that undergo enzymatic degradation in the liver. On the other hand, ester compounds such as procaine are metabolized to para-aminobenzoic acid. Unlike the ester compounds, the amide groups rarely produce an allergic phenomenon. Lidocaine and bupivacaine are available in various concentrations. The lowest effective concentration should be selected; thus, 0.5% lidocaine and 0.25% bupivacaine are the concentrations of choice.

6.6.5 Epinephrine

All local anesthetic agents except cocaine cause peripheral vasodilatation by producing a direct relaxant effect on the musculature of the blood vessels. The degree of vasodilator activity appears related to intrinsic anesthetic potency. The more potent and longer-acting local anesthetic agents produce a greater degree and longer duration of vasodilatation. Epinephrine incorporated into local anesthetic solutions constricts blood vessels, thereby slowing absorption and minimizing any toxic reaction. Epinephrine accomplishes three purposes: (1) it reduces capillary bleeding; (2) it prevents rapid absorption of the local anesthetic agent, thus avoiding a high blood level of the anesthetic agent while minimizing any toxic reaction; and (3) it prolongs analgesia during surgery. Systemic toxic reactions may occur when the epinephrine in the blood reaches a high level. The common signs and symptoms of these reactions are pallor, tachycardia, perspiration, palpitation, apprehension, dyspnea, rapid respiration, and hypertension.[12] The side effects are rare when the dilution of 1:200,000 is used.

There are several useful methods of administration that minimize the pain. The needle should be small and the injecting pressure should be low. For practical purposes and availability, a 1.5-inch (3.5 cm) 27- to 30-gauge needle with 3-mL disposable syringe works well. The lower the concentration of the anesthetic solution, the less painful it is. Superficial wheal-producing dermal injection is uniformly much more painful than that into the deep dermal-subcutaneous tissue. Rapid injection almost always hurts more than slow infiltration.[13,14]

Most local anesthetic solutions are quite acidic, with a pH ranging from 5.0 to 7.0. Lidocaine has a pH of 6.8 and bupivacaine is 5.5. Local anesthetic is more soluble and has a shelf life of 3 to 4 years. Raising the pH to 7.2 to 7.4 would substantially reduce effective storage shelf life and solubility. Raising the pH above 7.4 increases the risk of precipitation of local anesthetic out of solution. A study by Christoph et al showed that infiltration of 1% lidocaine is 5 times more painful than buffered 1% lidocaine, 1% lidocaine with epinephrine is 2.8 times more painful than buffered 1% lidocaine without epinephrine, and 1% mepivacaine (an intermediate action local anesthetic) is 5.7 times more painful than buffered mepivacaine.[15] These results are statistically highly significant. Buffering can be easily and safely accomplished by the addition of sodium bicarbonate solution so that the resultant ratio of local anesthetic to sodium bicarbonate equals 10:1. In doing so, the efficacy of the local anesthetic is not compromised. Local anesthetic buffering should be performed immediately before its use to eliminate concerns regarding shortened shelf life of the anesthetic caused by the alkalinization.[15]

6.6.6 Adverse Reactions

Toxicity of different anesthetic agents varies, usually in parallel with potency. To some extent, the rate of biotransformation will affect toxicity. The rate of absorption also will influence toxicity, and this may be determined by the route of administration. ▶ Table 6.1 lists the signs and symptoms of local anesthetic toxicity. There are two types of adverse reaction to local anesthetic agents: allergic reaction and toxic reaction.

Allergic reaction, a rare occurrence, may be systemic or local. More than 80% of reactions are cell mediated, resulting in contact dermatitis. The remaining reactions are caused by circulating antibodies that give rise to systemic anaphylaxis. Acute anaphylactic reactions are rare, but they are invariably fatal unless promptly treated. Localized systemic anaphylactic reactions manifested by urticaria, laryngeal edema, and extrinsic asthma are less serious and are amenable to treatment. There is no foolproof test for screening susceptible persons. The intradermal test is of no value in determining possible systemic sensitivity. The patch test is useful in the detection of contact allergy.[16]

Toxic reactions to local anesthetic agents are far more common than allergic sequelae. The majority of adverse reactions to local anesthetics are due to high plasma levels resulting from the administration of excessive quantities of the drug. The major manifestations of local anesthetic toxicity occur in the central nervous system (CNS) and the cardiovascular system.

All local anesthetics have the capacity to stimulate the CNS at low toxic doses and suppress the CNS at high toxic doses. Initial signs and symptoms of a high toxic dose are CNS excitation, resulting from the suppression of inhibitory cortical neurons, which permits unopposed functioning of facilitatory pathways.

Table 6.1 Signs and symptoms of local anesthetic toxicity

Central nervous system effects	Cardiovascular effects
Mild	
Lightheadedness	↑ PR interval
Dizziness	↑ QRS duration
Tinnitus	↓ Cardiac output
Drowsiness	↓ Blood pressure
Disorientation	
Severe	
Muscle twitching	↑↑ PR interval
Tremors of face and extremities	↓↓ QRS duration
	• Sinus bradycardia
Unconsciousness	• Atrioventricular block
Generalized convulsions	↓↓ Cardiac output
Respiratory arrest	↓↓ Hypotension
	• Asystole

Subsequent signs and symptoms of a high toxic dose include lightheadedness, dizziness, nystagmus, sensory disturbances (e.g., visual difficulties, tinnitus, perioral tingling, metallic taste), restlessness, and disorientation or psychosis. Slurred speech and muscle twitching or tremors may immediately precede seizures. If serum levels of the drug continue to increase, generalized depression of the entire CNS occurs, with resultant drowsiness, coma, and respiratory arrest.[9,17]

The cardiovascular system is relatively resistant to local anesthetic toxicity in comparison with the CNS and does not exhibit toxic reactions until blood levels are much higher. Cardiovascular complications result from negative inotropism, peripheral vasodilatation, and slowing of the myocardial conductive system. The end results of local anesthetic toxicity are hypotension, bradycardia, prolonged electrocardiographic intervals, and cardiac arrest.[9,17]

Anaphylactic shock is the least common yet most serious of the allergic reactions. It is characterized by a sudden circulatory and respiratory collapse, loss of consciousness, laryngeal edema, and urticaria. Anaphylaxis must be dealt with promptly. The immediate treatment consists of the subcutaneous injection of 0.5 mL of 1:1,000 epinephrine. To increase the rate of absorption, the injection site should be vigorously massaged. Meanwhile, ventilation should be maintained with oxygen under pressure. If the patient does not show rapid improvement, the administration of epinephrine can be repeated in 5 to 15 minutes. If severe bronchospasm persists, 250 to 500 mg of aminophylline should be administered intravenously. Once an improvement has been noted, corticosteroids and an antihistamine can be administered intramuscularly to prevent recurrence of symptoms and avoid the use of additional epinephrine.[16,18]

Toxic reactions must be recognized and treated as follows without delay:

1. Clear airway (if patient is unconscious).
2. Prevent aspiration.
3. Administer oxygen.
4. Induce intravenous fluid (for administration of intravenous medication).
5. Stop convulsion.
   a) Administration of oxygen alone may stop convulsion.
   b) If oxygen does not stop convulsion, intravenous medications such as thiopental (50–100 mg), midazolam (2–5 mg), and propofol (1 mg/kg) can terminate seizures.[19] If seizures fail to respond to such treatment, short-acting neuromuscular blocking agents such as succinylcholine (Anectine) or vecuronium (Norcuron) should be administered until serum levels of local anesthetic agents fall.[20]
6. Raise blood pressure by giving a vasopressive drug.
7. Perform cardiac massage if patient's heart has arrested.

6.6.7 Prevention of Adverse Reactions

Preventing or minimizing the risk of complications is the most important aspect in giving local anesthetic agents. The lowest effective concentration should be used. In anorectal surgery, 0.5% lidocaine and 0.25% bupivacaine are ideal. Unless contraindicated, an addition of 1:200,000 epinephrine should be used to prolong the action and minimize the absorption. The amount injected should not exceed the maximum dose—500 mg lidocaine with 1:200,000 epinephrine (100 mL) and 225 mg bupivacaine with 1:200,000 epinephrine (90 mL). Dosage should be reduced for elderly patients and debilitated patients with cardiac or liver disease. Rapid injection with a large volume of the anesthetic should be avoided; fractional doses should be used when feasible.

Having the patient breathe oxygen during the procedure and avoiding heavy preoperative sedation are helpful. Hypercarbia and acidosis decrease the threshold of local anesthetic agents for convulsive activity. Similarly, hypercarbia, acidosis, and hypoxia tend to increase the cardiodepressant effect of local anesthetic agents.[9]

6.6.8 Hyaluronidase

Hyaluronic acid found in interstitial spaces normally prevents the diffusion of invasive substances. Hyaluronidase (Wydase), a mucolytic enzyme, allows anesthetic solutions to spread in the tissues by inactivating the hyaluronic acid.[21] It also tends to reduce swelling and increase the absorption of blood in the subcutaneous tissues. Hyaluronidase is not toxic to tissues and will not cause them to slough. Allergic reactions to hyaluronidase may occur but are insignificant.

Hyaluronidase, 150 IU, can be added to 20 mL of anesthetic solution. Clark and Mellette[22] found that the addition of hyaluronidase reduces tissue edema, enlarges the area of anesthesia, and augments the onset of anesthesia. In a randomized controlled study on the use of peribulbar block during intraocular surgery, the addition of hyaluronidase produced no advantages.[23] The disadvantage of using hyaluronidase is that it shortens the duration of analgesia because it enhances absorption, thus defeating the purpose of adding epinephrine to prolong the anesthetic action and to slow down clearance. Therefore, there is no reason to add hyaluronidase to the anesthetic solution.

6.6.9 Induction of Anesthesia

Rules that must be observed in inducing local anesthesia.
1. Do not exceed the recommended maximum dosage of the local anesthetic drugs.
2. Do not rely on premedication to prevent systemic toxic reactions.
3. Carefully observe the patient after completion of the injection.
4. Objectively evaluate any type of reaction, no matter how mild. Do not treat a reaction without making a definite diagnosis; give only the necessary indicated therapy.
5. Be prepared to treat any type of reaction, for example, convulsion, respiratory collapse, or cardiovascular collapse.
6. Do not overtreat or undertreat the reaction. Some reactions require no treatment; on the other hand, intensive treatment and even closed cardiac massage may be necessary to save the patient's life.

Modified from Petros and Bradley.[5]

6.6.10 Techniques of Local Anesthesia: General Considerations

For good-risk patients, preoperative medication should be given. Both diazepam (Valium) and midazolam (Versed) are excellent agents for blunting consciousness during the procedure. In addition, fentanyl (Sublimaze), a potent but short-acting narcotic drug, may be used as a supplement. For ambulatory short-duration procedures, preoperative sedation is usually not necessary.

A 27-gauge needle with a 3-mL disposable syringe is used for the injection. For most patients, the anesthetic solution causes considerable burning pain during the injection. The key is to slowly infiltrate the subdermal plane. Buffering the anesthetic solution with sodium bicarbonate, as described earlier, helps.

6.6.11 Conventional Technique

The anesthetic solution is infiltrated around the perianal skin and the anal verge (▸ Fig. 6.1 and ▸ Fig. 6.2). Next, the anal canal is injected subdermally and submucosally in a circumferential manner (▸ Fig. 6.3). Complete sphincteric relaxation is achieved without having to inject the anesthetic solution

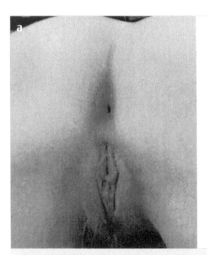
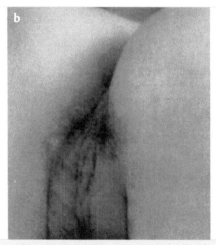
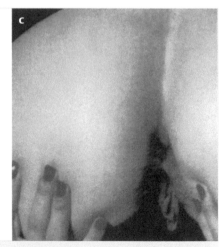

Fig. 6.1 Shape of the buttock. **(a)** Flat cheeks, ideal for anesthesia. **(b)** Deep, prominent cheeks, the anal canal is deep, less suitable for local anesthesia. **(c)** Flat cheeks but the anus is more anterior than normal, still suitable for local anesthesia.

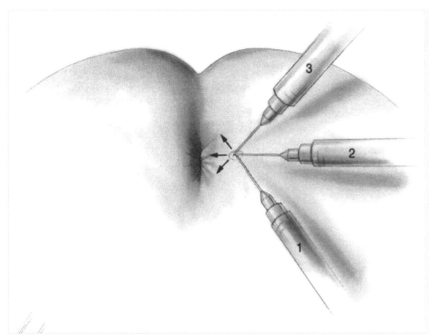

Fig. 6.2 Infiltration of the perianal skin and anal verge in a subcutaneous plane.

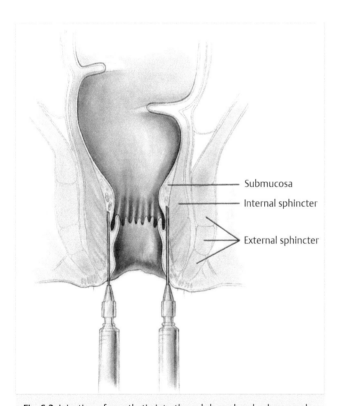

— Submucosa
— Internal sphincter
— External sphincter

Fig. 6.3 Injection of anesthetic into the subdermal and submucosal tissue.

6.6.12 Alternative Techniques

Intra-anal Injection

Because the mucosa of the anal canal above the dentate line is less sensitive to pain, injection of anesthetic solution into this area is almost painless. An improved technique has been developed based on this fact.[25]

Mild sedation may be used but is not necessary in some patients. Following digital examination of the anal canal with 2% lidocaine jelly, a small anoscope (ideally a Vernon-David anoscope) is inserted into the anal canal. Injection of 2 to 3 mL of the anesthetic solution makes a submucosal wheal 2 mm above the dentate line (▸ Fig. 6.4a). If injection at this level still causes pain, the injection site is moved 2 mm higher. The injection is made in four quadrants. The index finger is then inserted into the anal canal, and each wheal of the anesthetic solution is milked into the subdermal plane below the dentate line. This is best accomplished by bending the finger like a hockey stick over the anesthetic wheal and withdrawing it distally (▸ Fig. 6.4b). The anal canal at this point will be well relaxed to accommodate a large Hill-Ferguson or other suitable anal speculum with ease and without discomfort. Next, with the Hill-Ferguson anal speculum in place for exposure, at 2 mm below the dentate line the anoderm is infiltrated (in the subcutaneous plane) with 2 mL of the anesthetic solution in four quadrants (▸ Fig. 6.4c). The anal verge and perianal skin are next injected circumferentially.

The same technique can be applied for a patient with a painful anal fissure, but the injection should start in the quadrant that has the fissure. Such a patient may require heavier sedation.

Posterior Perineal Block

This technique involves infiltration of the anesthetic solution to the inferior rectal nerves, the perineal nerves, and the anococcygeal nerves.[26]

directly into the sphincter muscles.[24] Some surgeons prefer to inject the muscle and/or the ischioanal fossa directly, but this is not necessary. In most cases, 20 to 25 mL of the anesthetic solution is used.

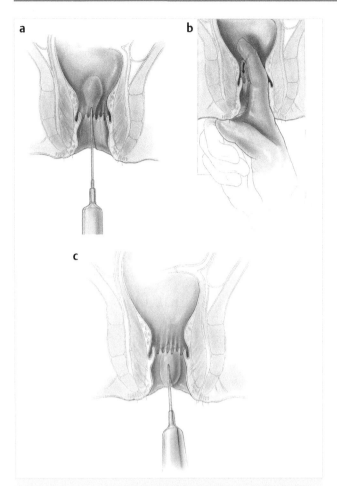

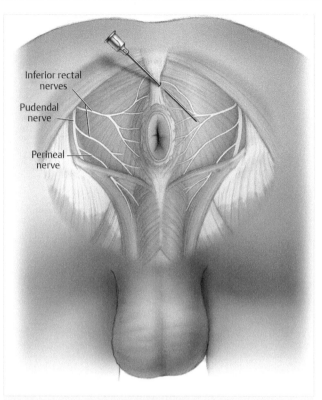

Fig. 6.5 Infiltration of the nerves in ischioanal fossa.

Fig. 6.4 Intra-anal injection. (a) Injection 5 mm above the dentate line in the submucosal plane. (b) Milking the anesthetic wheal to below the dentate line. (c) Injection 2 mm below the dentate line in the subcutaneous plane.

First, the surgeon injects 2 mL of the anesthetic solution in the posterior midline of the perianal skin. The needle is then angled 45 degrees, 8 to 10 cm into each ischioanal fossa to block the inferior rectal and the perineal nerves (▶ Fig. 6.5). Next, the needle is aimed at the presacral fascia, injecting 5 mL of the anesthetic solution into the presacral space to block the anococcygeal nerves. Finally, about 15 mL of the anesthetic solution are injected into the perianal skin circumferentially to anesthetize the sensitive branches of the superficial perineal nerves. Gabrielli et al[26] used this technique in 400 hemorrhoidectomies with excellent results.

6.7 Postoperative Care

Patients undergoing procedures under local anesthesia usually can be discharged immediately. Patients having a general anesthetic are monitored in a recovery room, and when vital signs are stable and the level of consciousness returns to normal, they may be discharged. In either case, they should be given simple instructions about diet, activity, wound care, and medication. In general, there are no dietary restrictions. Patients are advised to take nonconstipating analgesics and bulk stool softeners. Sitz baths are advised for local comfort. Patients are instructed about how to obtain help if any questions or problems arise.

6.7.1 Pain Control

Adequate pain control is essential to discharge a patient.

6.7.2 Discharge Criteria

In order to ensure a safe and comfortable transition from the postanesthesia care unit to home, certain criteria must be met. Many units use an Aldrete score or modified Aldrete score to evaluate a patient's readiness for discharge (▶ Table 6.1).[27,28] This score is comprised of vital signs, level of consciousness, and activity level, with each category being scored from 0 to 2. When a patient's total score is greater than 11 (with no 0 scores in any category), the patient meets the criteria for discharge to an inpatient unit. A second set of "outpatient discharge criteria" must be met prior to discharge home (▶ Table 6.2). These are comprised of vital signs, level of consciousness, activity level, and logistic arrangements to ensure that the family (and/or professional support services) will be ready to care for postoperative needs once the patient is home. These criteria act as guidelines and are helpful in minimizing unexpected readmissions or repeat outpatient evaluations.

Table 6.2 Discharge criteria

Inpatient discharge criteria	Outpatient discharge criteria
1. Respiratory/airway	**1. Vital signs**
0: Apnea/dyspnea or limited	• Within 20% of pre-op status
2: Deep breath/cough/NL respiratory rate	**2. Activity and mental status**
2. Circulation	• Oriented ×3 and a steady gaze
0: BP ± 50% pre-op	• Consistent with developmental age/or pre-op status
1: BP ± 20–50%	**3. Nausea and/or vomiting**
2: BP ± 20% pre-op	• Minimal
3. Level of consciousness	**4. Surgical bleeding**
0: Nonresponsive	• Minimal—no evidence of progression
1: Sleepy but arousable	**5. Tolerating PO fluids**
2: Awake/alert, responds appropriately	**6. Void if spinal anes, or as per surgeon's order (N/A if GU appliance)**
4. Spinal/activity level	**7. Responsible adult for transport and to accompany home.** *Exception*: Local anesthesia/no sedation
0: Unable to lift extremities or head on command/T9 or above	**8. Verbal/written Instructions**
2: Move four extremities/or T10 spinal level or below	• Given/reviewed with patient and family/significant other
5. O₂ saturation level	**9. Arrangements made for post-op prescriptions**
0: < 93%	**10. Arrangements made for follow-up appointment**
2: > 93% with O₂	**11. Adequate neurovascular status of operative extremity**
6. Temperature	**12. Pain assessment > 4/10 comment**
0: < 36 °C (86.8–97 °F)	
1: 36–36.5 °C (96.8–97 °F)	
2: < 36.5 °C (97.7 °F)	
7. Pain assessment > 4/10 comment	
Total score = 12	

6.7.3 Complications

Ambulatory procedure can be performed safely with high quality. Several authors have reported on the safety of ambulatory surgery.[19,20,29,30,31,32,33] In the Surgicenter in Tucson Medical Center, more than 47,000 patients have been treated safely without a single death.[2] In fact, the types of surgical problems treated have become progressively complex. In another report by Ford,[32] in more than 40,000 cases, no deaths or serious medical emergencies have occurred. Mezei and Chung[29] determined the overall and complication-related readmission rates within 30 days after ambulatory surgery at a major ambulatory surgical center. Preoperative, intraoperative, and postoperative data were collected on 17,638 consecutive patients undergoing ambulatory surgery at a major ambulatory surgical center in Toronto, Ontario. With the use of the database of the Ontario Ministry of Health, the authors identified all return hospital visits and hospital readmissions occurring in Ontario within 30 days after ambulatory surgery. There were 193 readmissions within 30 days after ambulatory surgery (readmission rate, 1.1%). Six patients returned to the emergency room, 178 patients were readmitted to the ambulatory surgical unit, and 9 patients were readmitted as inpatients. Twenty-five readmissions were the result of surgical complications, and one resulted from a medical complication (pulmonary embolism). The complication-related readmission rate was 0.15%. Their results support the view that ambulatory surgery is a safe practice.

Encouraging reports about the performance of anorectal surgery on an ambulatory basis have been made.[20] Friend and Medwell,[20] who championed the drive toward ambulatory anorectal surgery, reviewed over 6,000 outpatient anorectal operations performed since 1975. They noted that approximately 1 patient in every 200 is admitted to the hospital from the day-surgery recovery room because of cardiac arrhythmias, anesthetic complications or drug reactions, or postoperative pain or bleeding. Of the first 1,433 consecutive patients, only 14 (1%) required catheterization within 24 hours of operation. They found no correlation between catheterization and volume of intravenous fluids, type of anesthesia, age, sex, pathologic condition, or operation. There is no clear explanation for this low rate of urinary retention. In their series of 6,000 patients, they never had to extract a fecal impaction. Smith[34] reported that less than 1% of the ambulatory population required admission to the hospital after anorectal surgery. The usual reason for admissions is either pain control or urinary retention. Other possible reasons are hemorrhage and infection. In Europe, where ambulatory surgery has not yet been well accepted, Marti and Laverriere[33] reported on 1,947 procedures carried out between 1978 and 1990 without any mortality. Complications were observed in 5 of 966 cases—bleeding. No postoperative infection or urinary retention requiring catheterization was seen, and only one case required hospital admission.

Conaghan et al[19] randomized 100 patients with minor and intermediate surgical emergency conditions to receive standard inpatient care or day surgery. There was a reduction in the number of nights spent in hospital in the day case group (median, 0 vs. 2 nights). The median time from diagnosis to treatment was 1 day in both groups. There was no significant difference in postoperative outcome or patient and general practitioner satisfaction. The day-case option had no increased impact on primary care services but was associated with a significant saving of about US$200 per patient.

6.8 Benefits

6.8.1 Patient

For the patient, the advantages of ambulatory operations are numerous. There is no need for a formal hospital admission with its attendant psychologic trauma. Patients may not be as frightened or anxious about an operation if they know they will be home the same day and will not have to spend the night in the hospital. The daily routines and schedules of both patients and their families are less disrupted. Patients have greater accessibility and scheduling convenience, the waiting time for operation is markedly decreased, and there is a considerable cost saving. Patients are not likely to be "bumped" from the operating schedule for "more important" or emergency procedures such as may occur with cases scheduled in the main operating theater.

In general, patients probably convalesce better and are more comfortable in the familiar surroundings of their own homes. In the home environment, patients become mobile, enter the daily routine more rapidly, and return to work sooner. Furthermore, they circumvent exposure to the potential iatrogenic hazards of hospitalization.[1]

6.8.2 Surgeon

Ambulatory surgery allows surgeons to use their time better. Fewer hospital visits are required, and less time is needed to complete chart work. In addition, accessibility and scheduling convenience are greater. The turnover time between cases in an outpatient setting is dramatically less than in a hospital setting.[32] This factor alone would allow a surgeon to accomplish more in the same time.

6.8.3 Hospital

With ambulatory procedures, hospitals can make better use of their facilities. Because the demand for hospital beds is lessened, use of expensive health care facilities can be handled more efficiently. Pressure on overloaded operating rooms is relieved, thereby freeing more time and space to devote to more complicated procedures. In addition, the need for postoperative nursing care is decreased.

6.8.4 Insurer

Although the list of benefits for third-party carriers is short, the cost for insurance companies has definitely decreased. The daily charge represents the largest single expense saved by same-day operations. This cost saving has led private and public payers to cover ambulatory surgery. In the 1970s, only 35% of payers covered such surgery, but by the 1980s fully 96% of payers provided coverage.[1] Moreover, third-party payers began to create financial incentives to encourage ambulatory surgery.[1] These include reduced reimbursement if the procedure is performed on an inpatient basis and compilation of lists of procedures that will be reimbursed only if they are provided on an ambulatory basis.

6.8.5 Cost

Financial incentives have spurred the growth of same-day surgery. At a time when costs for medical care are increasing steadily, great savings can be afforded to the patient, third-party carriers, and institutions by performing many anorectal procedures in the office or at least on an ambulatory basis.

Although the adoption of ambulatory surgery will decrease the costs per case, it will also lead to greater throughput of patients and thus to added total costs.[19] This so-called efficiency trap is one greater reason hospital administrators in European countries have been reluctant to adopt ambulatory surgery. This also puts a strain on institutions located in a health care system such as that of Canada, where global budgets are the order of the day. A hospital does not reap any financial reward for improving efficiency. Moving cases to the ambulatory setting and replacing inpatient beds with new and potentially more expensive admissions may provide care for more patients but inevitably creates a budget deficit.[35] In certain localities where hospital bed shortages occur, waiting periods are eliminated or reduced by outpatient operations.

Cost analysis is always a difficult subject to evaluate because costs vary considerably from region to region. However, if patients are recovering at home, the cost of hospitalization and ambulatory services is eliminated, and tremendous savings are accrued by both patient and third-party carriers. The exact saving, of course, is difficult to determine. Using the number of inpatient procedures in 1982, obtained from the National Hospital Discharge Survey of the National Center for Health Care Statistics in Hyattsville, Maryland, along with the average cost per day for a hospital bed obtained from the American Hospital Association, Smith[34] estimated that for the procedures hemorrhoidectomy, fistula repair, and fissure operations, a savings of approximately $200 million would have been obtained. A reduction in hospital charges of 25 to 50% has been noted.[36]

In a cost analysis, Rhodes[37] calculated that there was a 67% reduction in the cost of a hemorrhoidectomy performed on an ambulatory basis compared with an inpatient procedure. It is, however, clearly stated that a cost comparison between ambulatory surgery and inpatient surgery is confounded by numerous factors that make comparisons difficult to assess.

In a commentary on insights on outpatient surgery, Cannon[38] noted that the dramatic increase in the use of outpatient surgical facilities has been good for society in general and the patient in particular. Outpatient surgery has been the most dramatic cost-saving change the medical profession has initiated, and Cannon believes that all areas should be encouraged to introduce this concept to their community. As evidence grows to support the fact that an ever-widening scope of anorectal procedures can be performed safely on an ambulatory basis, this method of management will and in many cases already has become the norm for many patients with anorectal disorders requiring operative intervention. Davis[39] cited four forces that drive this expansion: (1) improved and better operated facilities, (2) new surgical techniques, (3) improved anesthetic agents and practices, and (4) regulations influencing ambulatory surgery. All these forces are strong and appear to be gaining momentum. He believes growth of ambulatory surgery will increase phenomenally in the years ahead.

6.9 Anorectal Preparations

Self-treatment occurs more frequently in the anorectal region than any other part of the human body. This is explained by the ready availability of over-the-counter preparations along with the fear and embarrassment associated with this part of the anatomy. In addition, the troubled individual is often influenced by the unsupported advertising claims that some manufacturers make for the efficacy of their medications. Undue reliance on these preparations, combined with the universal belief that almost all symptoms originate from hemorrhoidal disease, leads to failure or delay in seeking medical advice with potential serious consequences.

Indications for the use of anorectal preparations include the relief of pain and discomfort after anorectal surgery, hemorrhoids (whether or not complicated by thromboses and prolapse), pruritus ani, proctitis, fissures, fistulas, and other congestive, allergic, or inflammatory conditions. Anorectal preparations are also useful in rectal examination to anesthetize an area that is too tender or spasmatic to admit the examining finger. Pharmaceutical preparations are available in several forms: creams, ointments, and suppository. The number of each type exceeds 100 products. It is estimated several hundred million dollars are spent each year on these products.

Available preparations contain combinations of traditional ingredients, including topical anesthetics and analgesics, antiseptics, mild astringents, anti-inflammatory agents, emollients, and vasoconstrictors in a host of bases and preservatives. Unfortunately, little evidence is available about the efficacy of these drugs alone or in combination in relieving the symptoms of anorectal disease.

6.9.1 Topical Anesthetics and Analgesics

Topical analgesics are included in many ointments and suppositories. Pramoxine hydrochloride provides surface analgesia within 2 to 3 minutes, lasts up to 4 hours, and is less toxic and less sensitizing than other agents. Provided they are active on broken skin and mucous membranes and are present in sufficient concentrations, topical anesthetics can be useful in relieving anal pain and pruritus. Surface or topical anesthetics block the sensory nerve endings in the skin, but to reach these structures the drug must have good powers of penetration. Local anesthetics found in commercial preparations include benzocaine (5–20%), tetracaine, pramoxine, diperodon, dibucaine, and lidocaine.[40] These agents should not be administered intrarectally because mucosal absorption may be quite rapid and can precipitate toxic systemic effects. The risk of contact sensitization and hypersensitivity common to nearly all the drugs must be considered. Of the topical anesthetics used, tetracaine, dibucaine, and benzocaine have caused sensitization most often.[40]

The main systemic toxic effect of topical agents is excitation of the CNS, manifested by yawning, restlessness, excitement, nausea, and vomiting, and may be followed by depression, muscular twitching, convulsions, respiratory failure, and coma.[41] There is simultaneous depression of the cardiovascular system, with pallor, sweating, and hypotension. Arrhythmias may occur. Repeated application to the skin is more likely than systemic administration to give rise to allergic reactions.

6.9.2 Antiseptics

Many preparations include antiseptics such as phenol, menthol, boric acid, oxyquinoline, or benzethonium chloride. Antiseptics are used to destroy or inhibit the growth of pathogenic microorganisms. The inclusion of these agents in low concentrations has only a marginal effect on the constantly renewed bacterial

population of the anus and rectum. These agents are probably harmless, but the risk of contact sensitization must be taken into consideration.

6.9.3 Astringents

Astringents include substances such as bismuth subgallate, hamamelis water (witch hazel), tannic acid, zinc oxide, calamine, or balsam of Peru. When applied to mucous membranes or to damaged skin, these agents precipitate proteins and form a protective layer, which is not absorbed.[41] They are designed to contract tissue, harden the skin, and check exudative secretions and minor hemorrhage.

6.9.4 Protectants

Protectants act to prevent irritation of the anorectal area and water loss from the skin by forming a physical barrier.[42] Protection of the perianal area from irritants such as fecal matter may lead to a reduction in irritation and itching. Absorbents, adsorbents, demulcents, and emollients are included in the protectant classification. Recommended protectants include aluminum hydroxide gel, calamine, cocoa butter, cod liver oil, glycerin, kaolin, lanolin, mineral oil, petrolatum, shark liver oil, starch, wood alcohols, and zinc oxide. Petrolatum is probably the most effective protectant.[42]

Emollients are fats or oils used for their local action on the skin and occasionally on the mucous membranes.[43] They are used for protection and as agents for softening the skin and rendering it more pliable, but chiefly they act as vehicles for more active drugs. Cocoa butter is a solid that melts at body temperature and hence is widely used as a suppository and an ointment base. Liquid paraffin and other oils also have been included in many products. Because these substances may lubricate the anal canal during defecation, especially in the presence of painful conditions of the anus, they may have some value as soothing agents.

6.9.5 Vasoconstrictors

Agents such as ephedrine and phenylephrine are intended to reduce bleeding from hemorrhoids, but clinical evidence to support this claim is lacking. These vasoconstrictors produce capillary and arterial constrictions, but conclusive evidence that they reduce swollen hemorrhoids is lacking.[42] In large doses, ephedrine can cause side effects such as giddiness, headache, nausea, vomiting, sweating, thirst, tachycardia, hypertension, arrhythmia, precordial pain, palpitations, difficulty in micturition, muscular weakness and tremors, anxiety, restlessness, and insomnia. Some patients exhibit these symptoms with the usual therapeutic dose.[41] Manufacturers caution against the use of vasoconstrictors in patients who are sensitive to one of the ingredients and in patients with severe cardiac disease, diabetes mellitus, glaucoma, hypertension, or hyperthyroidism. Vasoconstrictors should not be given to patients being treated with a monoamine oxidase inhibitor.

6.9.6 Wound-Healing Agents

Several ingredients in nonprescription hemorrhoidal products claim to be effective in promoting wound healing or tissue repair in anorectal disease.[42,44] In particular, considerable controversy surrounds the substance skin respiratory factor (SRF), a water-soluble extract of brewer's yeast also referred to as live yeast cell derivative. Although some tests have supported the manufacturers' claims, there is no conclusive evidence that products containing SRF promote the healing of diseased anorectal tissue. The Food and Drug Administration advisory review panel on nonprescription hemorrhoidal drug products studied data on live yeast cell derivative as well as cod liver oil, balsam of Peru, shark liver oil, vitamin A, and vitamin D and found them lacking in demonstrated effectiveness as wound healers. One study suggested that SRF could be shown to increase the rate of wound healing in artificially created ulcers in humans, but that study did not address the clinical situation in which the agent is used.[37]

6.9.7 Corticosteroids

Numerous steroid preparations are currently available and are often used in combination with some of the ingredients already mentioned. There is no clinical evidence that corticosteroids relieve hemorrhoids, anal fissures, or posthemorrhoidectomy pain. These agents are available in the following forms for anorectal disease: ointments and creams, suppositories, and enemas and foams.

6.9.8 Steroid Ointments and Creams

Steroid ointments and creams frequently are prescribed topically to provide symptomatic relief in the treatment of pruritus ani. However, the side effects of these agents must be recognized.[45]

The long-term use of potent topical corticosteroids in the perianal region may produce an itchy dermatosis. Stopping the medication may produce a temporary increase in the rash and itching, encouraging reinstitution of the medication. Atrophy and telangiectasia may take months or years to develop, and their extent and degree vary. In general, the long-term use of fluorinated steroid preparations should be avoided to prevent this complication.

The anti-inflammatory action of steroids removes or decreases the erythema and other findings in conditions such as scabies and taenia corporis. This effect can make identification of such conditions difficult unless a high index of suspicion is maintained.

After lengthy use of steroids over large areas of the body, systemic absorption may occur, but application of the steroids to the perianal region probably is of limited significance. Since the safety of using topical corticosteroids during pregnancy has not been confirmed, these should not be used in large amounts or for prolonged periods of time by pregnant women.

Jackson[45] classified topical steroids into three groups: weak, medium, and strong. Jackson believes that almost all side effects can be avoided completely by restricting the use of potent topical corticosteroids to small areas for short periods. In many conditions, maintenance therapy with 0.5% hydrocortisone or another weak steroid preparation is adequate. Triamcinolone is more effective than hydrocortisone.[41] Jackson points out that potent steroids should not be used to treat undiagnosed conditions.

Corticosteroid suppositories may prove of value in treating patients who suffer from distal proctitis. This nonspecific inflammatory condition of the rectum, which involves the distal 8 to 10 cm of bowel, frequently responds to the administration of hydrocortisone suppositories. Factitial (postirradiation) proctitis may be another indication for the use of such suppositories, although no controlled studies have been done.[46]

Patients who suffer from distal proctitis and do not respond to hydrocortisone suppositories may be helped by steroid enemas. These proprietary enemas are aqueous suspensions of either hydrocortisone or prednisolone. They are administered as retention enemas or foams once or twice daily. They may be effective in treating both distal proctitis and left-sided nonspecific ulcerative colitis. Some systemic absorption occurs with these agents.[47] Only a small part of a rectal dose of hydrocortisone acetate foam is absorbed (the mean bioavailability is 2%).[48]

General precautions usually mentioned in the pharmaceutical compendia for the use of these agent mixtures include avoidance by patients with a sensitivity to any of the components. Hydrocortisone preparations must not be used in the presence of existing tuberculosis or fungal or viral lesions of the skin.

6.9.9 5-Aminosalicylic Acid Products

5-Aminosalicylic acid has been used topically in enema or suppository form for some years for the treatment of distal proctitis or proctosigmoiditis.[49] It produces good clinical response; the medication is well tolerated and safe, and few or no side effects are reported. In suppository form, spread is limited to the rectum, but in enema form, when administered as recommended clinically, it routinely flows retrograde as far as the splenic flexure.[49,50]

6.9.10 Nitroglycerin

Nitric oxide has emerged as one of the most important neurotransmitters mediating internal anal sphincter relaxation. The effect of glyceryl trinitrate, a nitric oxide donor, on anal tone was examined by Loder et al.[51] They found a 27% decrease in sphincter pressure 20 minutes after application of a 0.2% glyceryl trinitrate ointment. Gorfine[52] found that following the topical application of 0.5% nitroglycerin ointment, patients with thrombosed external hemorrhoids and anal fissures reported dramatic relief of anal pain. Side effects were limited to transient headache in 7 of 20 patients. Nitroglycerin has also been found to significantly reduce upper anal sphincter pressure in patients with terminal constipation.[53]

6.9.11 Miscellaneous

A host of bases and preservatives generally are included in anorectal preparations, and little is known about their effects. Adeps solidus (a mixtures of monoglycerides, diglycerides, and triglycerides of saturated fatty acid), theobroma oil, beeswax, and cetyl alcohol are often used.

6.9.12 Dosage Forms

Although from a pharmaceutical point of view there are considerable differences among ointments, creams, pastes, and gels, the therapeutic differences are not significant. These preparations serve as vehicles for drug use and possess inherent protectant and emollient properties.

Suppositories may ease straining at stool by providing a lubricating effect. Because they must melt to release the active ingredient, they are relatively slow acting. Occasionally, insertion of suppositories has produced local trauma.

A hydrocortisone acetate foam enema is effective in the treatment of distal ulcerative colitis and proctitis. Some patients prefer a foam enema to a liquid enema because it causes less interference with social, sexual, and occupational activities. There is systemic absorption when the hydrocortisone foam is administered intrarectally and the potential for adrenal suppression exists, especially if the foam is used as a long-term treatment.[54]

Steroid enemas have become an established form of therapy for patients with distal ulcerative colitis and distal proctitis. Different steroid preparations have been advocated, but all result in systemic absorption to some degree. An enema preparation that contains a poorly absorbed steroid is preferred to avoid the possibility of systemic steroid effects in patients requiring long-term steroid treatment.[55] 5-Aminosalicylic acid is also available in enema form and has been used in the treatment of distal proctosigmoiditis.

6.9.13 Product Considerations

The patient's general condition and associated diseases should enter the decision-making process. For example, caution should be exercised in prescribing products with vasoconstrictors to patients suffering from cardiovascular disease, diabetes mellitus, hypertension, and hyperthyroidism or patients experiencing difficulty in urination or taking monoamine oxidase inhibitors.[5] Patients taking phenothiazines should avoid taking products containing ephedrine. The presence of specific allergies should be determined. The literature has a paucity of definitive information about the efficacy of any proprietary medications.

The continued use of the numerous available agents and the credit given to them for their effectiveness are almost certainly functions of the self-limiting nature of the diseases they are treating. The natural history of a thrombosed hemorrhoid is one of resolution, with decreasing pain after 2 or 3 days. Patients frequently relate that the suppository or ointment did not work for the first 2 or 3 days. By the same token, patients may use a given preparation for 2 or 3 days and then switch to a second preparation, which they then praise; again, this healing is almost certainly a function of the natural history of the disease. Had they used the preparations in reverse order, the praise and disdain for the two preparations almost certainly would have been reversed.

References

[1] Detmer DE, Gelijns AC. Ambulatory surgery. A more cost-effective treatment strategy? Arch Surg. 1994; 129(2):123–127

[2] Detmer DE. Sounding board. Ambulatory surgery. N Engl J Med. 1981; 305 (23):1406–1409

[3] Reed WA. The concept of the surgicenter. In: Brown BR Jr, ed. Outpatient Anesthesia. Philadelphia, PA: FA Davis; 1978:15–19

[4] Putnam LP, Landeen FH. Outpatient anesthesia at the ambulatory surgery center, Tucson Medical Center. In: Brown BR Jr, ed. Outpatient Anesthesia. Philadelphia, PA: FA Davis; 1978:1–5

[5] Petros JG, Bradley TM. Factors influencing postoperative urinary retention in patients undergoing surgery for benign anorectal disease. Am J Surg. 1990; 159(4):374–376

[6] Cataldo PA, Senagore AJ. Does alpha sympathetic blockade prevent urinary retention following anorectal surgery? Dis Colon Rectum. 1991; 34 (12):1113–1116

[7] Bailey HR, Ferguson JA. Prevention of urinary retention by fluid restriction following anorectal operations. Dis Colon Rectum. 1976; 19(3):250–252

[8] Day DW, Jass JR, Price AB, et al., eds. Morson and Dawson's Gastrointestinal Pathology. 4th ed. Malden, MA: Blackwell Science; 2008

[9] Philip BK, Covino BG. Local and regional anesthesia. In: Wetchler BV, ed. Anesthesia for Ambulatory Surgery. Philadelphia, PA: JB Lippincott; 1991:309–365

[10] Read TE, Henry SE, Hovis RM, et al. Prospective evaluation of anesthetic technique for anorectal surgery. Dis Colon Rectum. 2002; 45(11):1553–1558, discussion 1558–1560

[11] Moore DC, Bridenbaugh LD, Thompson GE, Balfour RI, Horton WG. Bupivacaine: a review of 11,080 cases. Anesth Analg. 1978; 57(1):42–53

[12] Moore DC. Regional Block. 4th ed. Springfield, IL.: Charles C Thomas; 1978:19–43

[13] Arndt KA, Burton C, Noe JM. Minimizing the pain of local anesthesia. Plast Reconstr Surg. 1983; 72(5):676–679

[14] Kaplan PA, Lieberman RP, Vonk BM. Does heating lidocaine decrease the pain of injection? AJR Am J Roentgenol. 1987; 149(6):1291

[15] Christoph RA, Buchanan L, Begalla K, Schwartz S. Pain reduction in local anesthetic administration through pH buffering. Ann Emerg Med. 1988; 17 (2):117–120

[16] Adriani J, Zepernick R. Allergic reactions to local anesthetics. South Med J. 1981; 74(6):694–699, 703

[17] Norris RL, Jr. Local anesthetics. Emerg Med Clin North Am. 1992; 10 (4):707–718

[18] Laskin DM. Diagnosis and treatment of complications associated with local anaesthesia. Int Dent J. 1984; 34(4):232–237

[19] Conaghan PJ, Figueira E, Griffin MA, Ingham Clark CL. Randomized clinical trial of the effectiveness of emergency day surgery against standard inpatient treatment. Br J Surg. 2002; 89(4):423–427

[20] Friend WG, Medwell SJ. Outpatient anorectal surgery. Perspect Colon Rectal Surg. 1989; 2:167–173

[21] Clery AP. Local anaesthesia containing hyaluronidase and adrenaline for anorectal surgery: experiences with 576 operations. Proc R Soc Med. 1973; 66 (7):680–681

[22] Clark LE, Mellette JR, Jr. The use of hyaluronidase as an adjunct to surgical procedures. J Dermatol Surg Oncol. 1994; 20(12):842–844

[23] Crawford M, Kerr WJ. The effect of hyaluronidase on peribulbar block. Anaesthesia. 1994; 49(10):907–908

[24] Ramalho LD, Salvati EP, Rubin RJ. Bupivacaine, a long-acting local anesthetic, in anorectal surgery. Dis Colon Rectum. 1976; 19(2):144–147

[25] Nivatvongs S. An improved technique of local anesthesia for anorectal surgery. Dis Colon Rectum. 1982; 25(3):259–260

[26] Gabrielli F, Cioffi U, Chiarelli M, Guttadauro A, De Simone M. Hemorrhoidectomy with posterior perineal block: experience with 400 cases. Dis Colon Rectum. 2000; 43(6):809–812

[27] Aldrete JA, Kroulik D. A postanesthetic recovery score. Anesth Analg. 1970; 49(6):924–934

[28] Aldrete JA. The post-anesthesia recovery score revisited. J Clin Anesth. 1995; 7(1):89–91

[29] Mezei G, Chung F. Return hospital visits and hospital readmissions after ambulatory surgery. Ann Surg. 1999; 230(5):721–727

[30] Bruns K, Freestanding Ambulatory Surgical Association. FASA statistics reveal top 10 procedures. Same Day Surg. 1981; 5(4):47–49

[31] Natof HE. Complications associated with ambulatory surgery. JAMA. 1980; 244(10):1116–1118

[32] Ford JL. Outpatient surgery: present status and future projections. South Med J. 1978; 71(3):311–315

[33] Marti MC, Laverriere C. Proctological outpatient surgery. Int J Colorectal Dis. 1992; 7(4):223–226

[34] Smith LE. Ambulatory surgery for anorectal diseases: an update. South Med J. 1986; 79(2):163–166

[35] Maloney S, Helyar C. Measuring opportunities to expand ambulatory surgery in Canada. J Ambul Care Manage. 1993; 16(3):1–7

[36] Place R, Hyman N, Simmang C, et al. Standards Task Force, American Society of Colon and Rectal Surgeons. Practice parameters for ambulatory anorectal surgery. Dis Colon Rectum. 2003; 46(5):573–576

[37] Rhodes RS. Ambulatory surgery and the societal cost of surgery. Surgery. 1994; 116:938–940

[38] Cannon WB. Insights on outpatient surgery. Bull Am Coll Surg. 1986; 71(7):9–12

[39] Davis JE. Ambulatory surgery ... how far can we go? Med Clin North Am. 1993; 77(2):365–375

[40] Andrusiak OI. Hemorrhoids. In: Clarke C, ed. Self medication. A Reference for Health Professionals. Ottawa: Canadian Pharmaceutical Association; 1988:347–354

[41] Reynolds JEF, ed. Martindale: The Extra Pharmacopoeia. 30th ed. London: Pharmaceutical Press; 1993

[42] Hodes B. Hemorrhoidal products. In: American Pharmacy Association, ed. Handbook of Nonprescription Drugs. 8th ed. Washington, DC: American Pharmaceutical Association; 1986:689–702

[43] Gilman AG, Goodman LS, Rail TW, Murad F, eds. Goodman and Gilman's the Pharmacological Basis of Therapeutics. 7th ed. New York, NY: MacMillan Publishing; 1985

[44] Goodson W, Hohn D, Hunt TK, Leung DYK. Augmentation of some aspects of wound healing by a "skin respiratory factor". J Surg Res. 1976; 21(2):125–129

[45] Jackson R. Side effects of potent topical corticosteroids. Can Med Assoc J. 1978; 118(2):173–174

[46] Sherman LF, Prem KA, Mensheha NM. Factitial proctitis: a restudy at the University of Minnesota. Dis Colon Rectum. 1971; 14(4):281–285

[47] Rodrigues C, Lennard-Jones JE, English J, Parsons DG. Systemic absorption from prednisolone rectal foam in ulcerative colitis. Lancet. 1987; 1(8548):1497

[48] Möllmann H, Barth J, Möllmann C, Tunn S, Krieg M, Derendorf H. Pharmacokinetics and rectal bioavailability of hydrocortisone acetate. J Pharm Sci. 1991; 80(9):835–836

[49] Williams CN, Haber G, Aquino JA. Double-blind, placebo-controlled evaluation of 5-ASA suppositories in active distal proctitis and measurement of extent of spread using 99mTc-labeled 5-ASA suppositories. Dig Dis Sci. 1987; 32(12) Suppl:71S–75S

[50] Chapman NJ, Brown ML, Phillips SF, et al. Distribution of mesalamine enemas in patients with active distal ulcerative colitis. Mayo Clin Proc. 1992; 67 (3):245–248

[51] Loder PB, Kamm MA, Nicholls RJ, Phillips RKS. 'Reversible chemical sphincterotomy' by local application of glyceryl trinitrate. Br J Surg. 1994; 81(9):1386–1389

[52] Gorfine SR. Treatment of benign anal disease with topical nitroglycerin. Dis Colon Rectum. 1995; 38(5):453–456, discussion 456–457

[53] Guillemot F, Leroi H, Lone YC, Rousseau CG, Lamblin MD, Cortot A. Action of in situ nitroglycerin on upper anal canal pressure of patients with terminal constipation. A pilot study. Dis Colon Rectum. 1993; 36 (4):372–376

[54] Cann PA, Holdsworth CD. Systemic absorption from hydrocortisone foam enema in ulcerative colitis. Lancet. 1987; 1(8538):922–923

[55] McIntyre PB, Macrae FA, Berghouse L, English J, Lennard-Jones JE. Therapeutic benefits from a poorly absorbed prednisolone enema in distal colitis. Gut. 1985; 26(8):822–824

7 Hemorrhoids

David E. Beck

Abstract

The term hemorrhoid has, from the patient's perspective, always signified a variety of anal complaints varying from minor itching to acute disabling pain. As the presence of some hemorrhoidal tissue is normal, hemorrhoidal disease should be thought of as hemorrhoidal tissue that causes significant symptomatology. Large sums of money are spent on products to control these symptoms, and the amount of work lost because of hemorrhoids is economically important. Our understanding of etiology and symptoms helps us to make recommendations for therapy. This chapter discusses the anatomy, pathophysiology, and methods of treatment of symptomatic hemorrhoids.

Keywords: hemorrhoids, anatomy, pathophysiology, treatment, symptomatic hemorrhoids

7.1 Introduction

Hemorrhoids and the symptoms they produce have plagued mankind throughout recorded history.[1] In the Bible, the Old Testament passage of I Samuel, Chapters 5 and 6 describes the Philistines after taking the ark of the covenant from the Israelites as being smitten by God with *aphelim* or *techorim*. Both words are believed by scholars to relate to hemorrhoids.[2,3] Many centuries ago, Maimonides described a variety of soothing medications, ointments, and even suppositories for the treatment of hemorrhoids and argued against surgery as a treatment for the condition.[4]

The term hemorrhoid has, from the patient's perspective, always signified a variety of anal complaints varying from minor itching to acute disabling pain. As the presence of some hemorrhoidal tissue is normal, hemorrhoidal disease should be thought of as hemorrhoidal tissue that causes significant symptomatology. Large sums of money are spent on products to control these symptoms, and the amount of work lost because of hemorrhoids is economically important.[5] Our understanding of etiology and symptoms helps us to make recommendations for therapy. This chapter discusses the anatomy, pathophysiology, and methods of treatment of symptomatic hemorrhoids.

7.2 Anatomy

Hemorrhoids are cushions of vascular tissue found in the anal canal.[2] Hemorrhoidal tissue is present at birth and in nonpathologic conditions. Microscopically, this tissue contains vascular structures whose walls do not contain muscle. Thus, hemorrhoids are not veins (which have muscular walls) but are sinusoids (▶ Fig. 7.1).[6] In addition to the vascular structures, the anal cushions are composed of smooth muscle (Treitz's muscle) and elastic connective tissue in the submucosa. Studies have also demonstrated that hemorrhoidal bleeding is arterial and not venous. When these sinusoids are injured (disrupted), hemorrhage occurs from presinusoidal arterioles. The arterial nature of the bleeding explains why hemorrhoidal hemorrhage is bright red and has an arterial pH.[7]

Cutaneous sensation in the perianal area is mediated through the pudendal nerve and the sacral plexus, both arising from sacral nerve roots 2 through 4, as described in Chapter 1. Some of the pressure sensation in this area may also be mediated by sacral nerve endings (S2–S4) located in the lower rectum and pelvic floor.[5]

In humans, hemorrhoidal tissue is thought to contribute to anal continence by forming a spongy bolster, which cushions the anal canal and prevents damage to the sphincter mechanism during defecation.[2] In addition, this tissue acts as a compressible lining, which allows the anus to close completely. The three main cushions (or bundles) lie at the left lateral, right anterolateral, and right posterolateral portion of the anal canal.

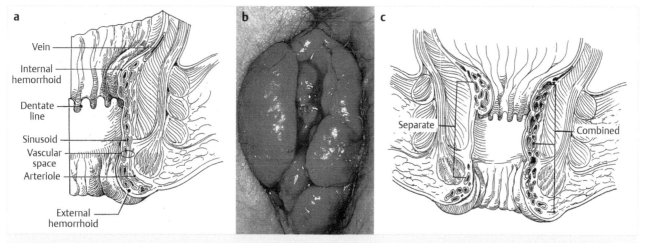

Fig. 7.1 Hemorrhoidal anatomy. **(a)** Arteriovenous anastomosis (AV shunts) forming hemorrhoidal plexus. **(b)** Fourth-degree hemorrhoids. **(c)** Usual position of the hemorrhoids. Separate external and internal hemorrhoids are seen on the left and a combined internal-external hemorrhoidal complex is seen on the right.

Smaller secondary cushions may occasionally lie between these main cushions. Each bundle starts superiorly (cranially) in the anal canal and extends inferiorly (caudally) to the anal margin. The superior portion of the hemorrhoidal tissue (above the dentate line) is covered by anal mucosa and the inferior portion (below the dentate line) is covered by anoderm or skin. The configuration of the anal cushions bears no relationship to the terminal branching of the superior rectal artery.

Return of blood from the anal canal is via two systems: the portal and the systemic. A connection between the two occurs in the region of the dentate line. The submucosal vessels situated above the dentate line constitute the internal hemorrhoidal plexus from which blood is drained through the superior rectal veins into the inferior mesenteric vein and subsequently into the portal system. Elevations in portal venous pressure may manifest as engorgement and gross dilatation of this internal hemorrhoidal plexus. Vessels situated below the dentate line constitute the external hemorrhoidal plexus from which blood is drained, in part through the middle rectal veins terminating in the internal iliac veins, but mainly through the inferior rectal veins into the pudendal veins, which are tributaries of the internal iliac veins. The veins constituting this external hemorrhoidal plexus are normally small; however, in situations of straining, because communication exists between internal and external hemorrhoidal plexuses, these veins become engorged with blood. If allowed to persist, this condition can lead to the development of combined internal and external hemorrhoids.

New concepts of the pathophysiology of hemorrhoids have been defined during the past 30 years, yet medical education at the undergraduate and graduate levels has not kept pace with the newer concepts. The traditional concepts of varicose veins are perpetuated in all medical dictionaries and in most textbooks of surgery, medicine, anatomy, and pathology.

7.3 Pathophysiology

7.3.1 Prevalence

Assessing the true prevalence of hemorrhoids is virtually impossible, with reported prevalence rates varying from 1 to 86%, depending on the method of ascertainment and the definition of "hemorrhoids."[8] Using the data from the National Center for Health Statistics, Johanson and Sonnenberg found that 10 million people in the United States complained of hemorrhoids, a prevalence rate of 4.4%.[9] Of them, approximately one-third went to a physician for evaluation, and an average 1.5 million prescriptions were written annually for hemorrhoidal preparations. The rate of hospitalization for patients with hemorrhoids was 12.9 per million people. The age distribution of hemorrhoids demonstrated a hyperbolic pattern, with a peak between age 45 and 65 years and a subsequent decline after age 65 years. The presence of hemorrhoids in patients younger than 20 years old was unusual.[9] All these figures could have been easily exaggerated, since they are based on complaint. Obviously, not all the complaints are true hemorrhoids.

National Hospital Discharge Survey data indicate that, on average, 49 hemorrhoidectomies per 100,000 people in the United States were performed annually from 1983 to 1987. Hemorrhoidectomies are performed 1.3 times more commonly in males than in females. Most hemorrhoidectomies are performed in patients 45 to 64 years old. According to National Hospital Discharge Survey data, a threefold decrease in the number of hemorrhoidectomies is observed, from a peak of 117 per 100,000 in the United States in 1974 to a low of 37 per 100,000 in 1987.[10] This decline may not reflect a decrease in the occurrence of hemorrhoidal disease, but may be a response to the increase in nonoperative and outpatient procedures.

7.3.2 Etiology

Enlargement or pathologic changes in hemorrhoidal tissue result in symptoms of the "hemorrhoidal syndrome." Proposed etiologic factors for these changes include constipation, prolonged straining, pregnancy, and derangement of the internal sphincter.[2] Constipation and the associated straining with defecation, as suggested by Burkitt and Graham-Stewart,[11] are related to eating habits, specifically to a low-residue diet. The typical American low-fiber diet may explain the high prevalence of constipation, straining, and hemorrhoidal symptoms in America.[12] With time (aging), the anatomic structures supporting the muscularis submucosae weaken, which leads to slippage or prolapsing of the hemorrhoidal tissue. Haas et al confirmed microscopically that anal supporting tissues deteriorate by the third decade of life.[13] Finally, many studies have consistently shown higher anal resting pressures in patients with hemorrhoids.[14,15,16] An increase in resting pressure is reduced to normal after hemorrhoidectomy. Internal sphincter, external sphincter, and pressure within the anal cushions can all account for the increased resting tone. However, it is not possible to distinguish their contributions.[17,18] Patients with enlarged hemorrhoids have been found on electromyography to have increased activity.[18] Another abnormality found in many of these patients is an ultraslow pressure wave caused by the contraction of the internal sphincter as a whole, but its significance is not known.[18] Anal electrosensitivity and temperature sensation are reduced in patients with hemorrhoids. The greatest change is noted in the proximal anal and midanal canals, perhaps because of prolapse of the less-sensitive rectal mucosa. This may also contribute to decreased continence. Rectal sensation to balloon distention is no different from that observed in control subjects.[19]

Although chronic constipation has been considered the cause of hemorrhoids, Gibbons et al cast doubt on this hypothesis.[20] Their studies show that patients with hemorrhoids are not necessarily constipated but tend to have abnormal anal pressure profiles and anal compliance. It is well known, however, that constipation aggravates symptoms of hemorrhoids. A case–control study on the risk factors for hemorrhoids by Johanson and Sonnenberg questions the influence of chronic constipation but supports diarrhea as a potential risk factor.[20] The tenesmus from diarrhea does cause straining.

Many other factors have been implicated in the causation of hemorrhoidal disease, notably heredity, erect posture, absence of valves in the hemorrhoidal plexuses and draining veins, and obstruction of venous return from raised intra-abdominal pressure. All these factors may contribute to causing the disease, but these anatomic factors do not account for the differences found in epidemiologic studies. Pregnancy undoubtedly aggravates preexisting disease and, by mechanisms not well understood, predisposes to the development of disease in patients who were previously asymptomatic. Furthermore, such patients usually become asymptomatic after delivery, which suggests that hormonal changes, in addition to direct pressure effects, may be involved.

In addition to the hemorrhoidal plexuses lying superficial to the sphincter mechanism, it has been theorized that a dysfunctional sphincter could lead to venous outflow obstruction and congestion, followed by engorgement of the hemorrhoids and subsequent symptoms.[13] All of these conditions contribute toward stretching and slippage of the hemorrhoidal tissue. The overlying skin or mucosa is stretched and additional fibrous and sinusoidal tissue develops. The extra tissue tends to move caudally toward the anal verge, making it susceptible to injury and causing symptoms to develop. A survey into the prevalence of benign anorectal disease demonstrated that 9% of adults had previous treatment of hemorrhoidal disease and 8% had hemorrhoidal symptoms.[14]

Hemorrhoids are not related to portal hypertension.[7] With increased portal venous pressure, the body develops portosystemic communications in several locations. In the pelvis, communications enlarge between the superior and middle hemorrhoidal veins, which results in development of rectal varices. These varices are located in the lower rectum, not the anus. Because of the rectum's large capacity, they rarely bleed. Older literature suggested a relationship between portal hypertension and hemorrhoids partly due to the fact that hemorrhoids are common and therefore many portal hypertensive patients will have hemorrhoids. If portal hypertension was an etiologic factor, hemorrhoidal bleeding would be venous blood rather than arterial bleeding, as described earlier. Hemorrhoidal symptoms may be difficult to manage in patients with portal hypertension as their liver disease frequently is associated with coagulation and platelet problems.

7.3.3 Classification

For anatomic and clinical reasons, hemorrhoidal tissue has been divided into two types: external and internal. External hemorrhoids are located in the distal one-third of the anal canal (distal to the dentate line) and are covered by anoderm (modified squamous epithelium that bears no skin appendages) or skin (▶ Fig. 7.1). As this overlying tissue is innervated by somatic nerves, it is sensitive to touch, temperature, stretch, and pain. Symptoms from external hemorrhoids usually result from thrombosis of the hemorrhoidal plexus. The rapid tissue expansion produced by the clots and edema causes pain. Physical effort is felt to be an etiologic factor in thrombosis of external hemorrhoids. Physical examination reveals one or more tender blue colored masses at the anus; additional symptoms are discussed below.

Internal hemorrhoids are located proximal (cranial) to the dentate line and covered by columnar mucosa or transitional epithelium. Based on size and clinical symptoms, internal hemorrhoids can be further subdivided by grades.[2,21,22,23] **Grade 1** hemorrhoids protrude into, but do not prolapse out of, the anal canal. **Grade 2** hemorrhoids prolapse out of the anal canal with bowel movements or straining, but spontaneously reduce. **Grade 3** hemorrhoids prolapse during the maneuvers described above and must be manually reduced by the patient. **Grade 4** hemorrhoids are prolapsed out of the

anus and cannot be reduced (▶ Fig. 7.1b). Hemorrhoids that remain prolapsed may develop ischemia, thrombosis, or gangrene. Patients may have both internal and external hemorrhoids (mixed or combined; ▶ Fig. 7.1c).

7.4 Evaluation

7.4.1 Symptoms

Patients with any anal complaints commonly present to physicians complaining of "hemorrhoids." Careful exploration of their symptoms will often lead to the correct diagnosis.

Symptoms associated with hemorrhoidal disease include: mucosal protrusion, pain, bleeding, a sensation of incomplete evacuation, mucous discharge, difficulties with perianal hygiene, and cosmetic deformity. General disorders of bowel function such as diarrhea and constipation, and associated disorders such as bleeding problems should be considered. A dietary and medication history should always be taken.

Except when thrombosis or edema occurs, hemorrhoids are painless. Painless bleeding occurs from internal hemorrhoids, is usually bright red, and is associated with bowel movements. The blood will occasionally drip into the commode and stain the toilet water bright red. After trauma by firm stools or forceful bowel movements, bleeding may continue to occur with bowel movements for several days. The bleeding will often then resolve for a variable period of time. It is unusual for hemorrhoidal bleeding to be severe enough to cause anemia but this has been reported to occur in 0.5 patients per 100,000 population.[24]

Prolapse may be appreciated by the patient as an anal mass, a feeling of incomplete evacuation, or a mucous discharge. The patient's requirement to manually reduce prolapsed hemorrhoids should be ascertained. If thrombosis or gangrene occurs, it will be apparent on physical examination and may be associated with systemic symptoms.

7.4.2 Examination

Examination of the anal area is usually undertaken with the patient in a prone position on a special proctologic table. If the patient is elderly or uncomfortable in this position, however, the modified left lateral decubitus (Sims') position is an acceptable alternative. Inspection of the anus should be done slowly, with calm reassurance by the examiner. The skin about the perineum, genitalia, and sacrococcygeal areas should be scrutinized. Gentle, steady spreading of the buttocks will allow for close inspection of the majority of the squamous portion of the anal canal.

Straining while sitting on the toilet is the useful examination in patients with grades 2, 3, and 4 hemorrhoids. The severity of the prolapse can be easily seen and the degree of descending perineum can be evaluated. It can also differentiate hemorrhoid from rectal prolapse particularly when the true rectal prolapse comes to but not through the anus. By asking the patient to strain while the examiner's index finger is in the anorectum, an enterocele can be detected.

Digital examination gives the examiner an appreciation for the amount and location of any pain in the anal canal. It enables assessment of the sphincter tone and helps exclude other diseases such as palpable tumors or abscesses in the lower rectum and anal canal. Hemorrhoids are not generally palpable unless quite large or thrombosed.

Anoscopy, usually done with a side-viewing instrument, permits visualization of the condition of the anoderm and internal hemorrhoidal complexes. As the patient strains, the hemorrhoids bulge into the lumen of the anoscope. The degree of prolapse may be assessed by gently withdrawing the anoscope as the patient strains.

Rigid proctosigmoidoscopy and flexible sigmoidoscopy form an important part of the initial examination and are performed to exclude more proximal disease. If the patient is younger than 40 years and hemorrhoidal disease compatible with symptoms is seen on physical examination, most authors feel that no additional workup is required. If the patient is older than 40 years, hemorrhoidal disease is not observed, or additional symptoms are present, a barium enema or colonoscopy is obtained to identify other etiologies for bleeding not observed by the proctoscopy.

7.4.3 Differential Diagnosis

It is extremely important that other causes of bleeding, itching, or discharge be considered, as listed in ▶ Table 7.1. Although patients invariably attribute anal pain to hemorrhoids, acute anal pain is almost always caused by either anal fissure or anorectal abscess. Pain from hemorrhoids occurs only in association with thrombosis or prolapse.

7.5 Treatment

7.5.1 General Principles

Treatments are many and varied, with some treatments, as described earlier, dating back to biblical times.[17] Modern therapy includes identification and correction of gastrointestinal tract dysfunction, minimization of symptoms, and, in some patients, correction of anal abnormalities, excision of excess hemorrhoidal tissue, and prevention of slippage or prolapse. Treatment can be nonoperative or operative. Nonoperative techniques include dietary modifications, topical medications, and measures (such as sitz baths) to reduce symptoms. Operative techniques, many of which can be performed in an office setting, include tissue fixation, major tissue excision, or physiologic alterations of the anal canal (Lord's dilation or lateral internal sphincterotomy). The method chosen is usually related to the type of hemorrhoidal tissue causing symptoms, and the experience and judgment of the treating physician.[2]

7.5.2 Internal Hemorrhoids

Diet and Stool Bulking Agents

Dietary modification is a mainstay for any therapy for hemorrhoidal disease.[25] If the patient is constipated or straining, a diet high in fiber (usually at least 20–30 g/day) with adequate oral fluid intake is recommended, striving for a soft-formed compressible stool that is easy to pass.

This type of stool reduces the requirement to strain with bowel movements and lessens the chance of hemorrhoidal injury. Moesgaard and colleagues[26] conducted a prospective

Table 7.1 Differential diagnosis in hemorrhoidal disease

Symptoms	Other diseases	Hemorrhoidal problems
Acute pain	Fissure Abscess/fistula	Thrombosed Prolapsed thrombosed
Chronic pain	Fissure Abscess/fistula Perianal Crohn's disease	
Bleeding	Fissure Colorectal polyp Colorectal cancer	Internal hemorrhoid Thrombosed external hemorrhoid
Itching/ discharge	Hypertrophic anal papilla Fistula Condylomata (anal warts) Rectal prolapse Anal incontinence	Prolapse
Lump or mass	Hypertrophic anal papilla Abscess Anal tag Crohn's disease	Thrombosed Prolapsed
Unusual	Anal or rectal tumor (benign or malignant) Ulcerative colitis	

double-blind trial, which demonstrated that psyllium fiber, when added to the diet of patients with anal bleeding and pain with defecation, improved their symptoms over a 6-week period. Patients with diarrhea and hemorrhoidal disease, after an evaluation of the underlying cause of their loose stools, should also receive dietary manipulation with fiber and antidiarrheals as indicated.

Dietary fiber is more appropriately referred to as a stool normalizer rather than a stool softener. It is uncommon for dietary fiber to cause complications, and allergic reactions to the active or inactive ingredients are exceptionally rare. The most common clinical difficulty is noncompliance due to problems with taste or symptoms of bloating and crampy abdominal pain. Fiber products currently available are listed in ▶ Table 7.2. Manufacturers have attempted to improve the palatability of these products in several ways. Adding flavoring and sweeteners has improved taste but usually at a higher cost and less fiber per unit volume. The different fiber sources may produce variable effects in different patients. It is advisable, therefore, to try alternate products if the first selection does not produce the desired results. To minimize symptoms, many providers find it helpful to start patients at a lower dose of the fiber supplement and to slowly increase the amount of fiber ingested until the desired stool consistency is achieved. It is also important to counsel patients to ingest an appropriate amount of water with their fiber, generally 80 to 120 oz (240–360 mL) per day. Fiber consumption of greater than 35 g/day with inadequate water intake can predispose to bezoar formation. Polyethylene glycol supplementation (e.g., Miralax, Bayer Health Care, Whippany, NJ) aids in the retention of water in the stool. It can be helpful in patients who are less compliant with fiber, especially females. If dietary manipulations fail to relieve symptoms, additional therapy is indicated (▶ Table 7.3).

Table 7.2 Fiber products

Type of fiber	Amount of fiber	Trade name	Manufacturer
Bran			
Psyllium	3.5 g	Metamucil	Procter & Gamble Cincinnati, OH
	6.0 g	Konsyl	Konsyl Pharmaceuticals Fort Worth, TX
Methylcellulose		Citrucel	Merrell Dow Pharmaceuticals Cincinnati, OH
Calcium polycarbophil		Fibercon	Lederle Laboratories American Cyanamid Company Pearl River, NY
		Konsyl Fiber Tablets	Konsyl Pharmaceuticals Fort Worth, TX
Inulin		Gummy Fiber	
		Benefiber	

Flavonoids

Flavonoids are plant products that have been prescribed to reduce hemorrhoidal bleeding. A meta-analysis of 14 randomized trials (1,514 patients) found limitations in methodological quality, heterogeneity, and potential publication bias.[27] The authors had questions on the beneficial effects in the treatment of hemorrhoids. These products have not been used widely in North America.

Topical Medications and Measures

Sitz baths, a bidet, or soaks in a warm tub are used to soothe the acutely painful anal area. Dodi and associates[28] demonstrated a significant reduction in anal pressure after patients with anorectal disorders soaked in warm (40°C) water. Soaking time should be limited as prolonged exposure to water can lead to edema of the perineal skin and subsequent pruritus. Some patients prefer to apply ice packs to the anal area. Again, as long as contact is not prolonged, this option is acceptable if it reduces symptoms.

The pharmaceutical industry has actively promoted multiple products such as creams, foams, and suppositories. One percent hydrocortisone may temporarily reduce the symptoms caused by pruritus associated with hemorrhoidal disease. However, prolonged use of topical steroids may attenuate the skin, predisposing it to further injury. Suppositories, after insertion, end up in the lower rectum rather than in the anal canal where hemorrhoids are located. Outside of providing a little lubrication of the stool, they have little to no pharmacologic rationale in the management of hemorrhoidal disease.[29] Ointments can cause or exacerbate pruritus ani, and again, except for those that contain a topical anesthetic (e.g., 1% pramoxine hydrochloride), offer little benefit except for thrombosed external hemorrhoids. Success in reducing symptoms associated with thrombosed external hemorrhoids has also been reported with

Table 7.3 Treatment of internal hemorrhoids by degree of prolapse

Severity	Treatment
First degree (no prolapse)	Dietary Infrared coagulation, *or* banding or sclerotherapy
Second degree (spontaneously reducible)	Dietary plus banding, *or* infrared coagulation, or sclerotherapy
Third degree (manual reduction necessary)	Dietary plus banding, *or* infrared coagulation, or sclerotherapy, *or* excisional hemorrhoidectomy[a]
Fourth degree (irreducible)	Excisional hemorrhoidectomy; rarely, multiple rubber band ligations
Acutely prolapsed and thrombosed	Emergency hemorrhoidectomy

[a]Excisional hemorrhoidectomy is recommended if external tags are also present.

topical nitroglycerin.[28] Effective marketing of over-the-counter medications, the placebo effect of any medication placed on the bothersome area, and the intermittent nature of hemorrhoidal symptoms explain the large volumes of these products purchased in the United States.

Rubber Band Ligation

Rubber band ligation was originally described by Blaisdell in 1958[30] and refined and popularized by Barron in 1963.[31] Placement of a tight rubber band around excess hemorrhoidal tissue constricts the blood supply to the contained tissue, which sloughs over 5 to 7 days. This leaves a small ulcer which heals fixing the tissue to the underlying muscle. Because of its simplicity, safety, and effectiveness, rubber band ligation is currently the most widely used technique in the United States for treating first-, second-, and some third-degree internal hemorrhoids.[5]

To accomplish this procedure, informed consent is obtained and an anoscope is inserted into the anus (the author prefers a slotted lighted scope; ▶ Fig. 7.2). A hemorrhoid bundle is identified, and through the anoscope, a band is placed using one of two types of ligators (▶ Fig. 7.3). A suction ligator (McGown, Pembroke Pines, FL) draws the hemorrhoid bundle into the ligator barrel and, closing the handle, places the band around the hemorrhoidal tissue. With a Barron or McGivney ligator (Electro-Surgical Instrument Co, Rochester, NY), an atraumatic clamp (▶ Fig. 7.4) is used to retract mucosa and redundant hemorrhoidal tissue at the apex of the bundle into the applicator and a small rubber band is placed. This tight band causes ischemia of the enclosed tissue. After it necroses, the tissue sloughs, forming a small ulcer. Excess tissue is eliminated, and as healing occurs, the remaining lining becomes fixed in the anal canal. Rubber band ligation works best for grade 2 to 3 internal hemorrhoids.

Several points require additional elaboration. First, it is crucial that the bands be placed on tissue entirely covered by anal mucosa. If bands are placed too distal and include any somatically enervated skin, the patient will develop excruciating pain. The pain is usually so severe that the patient will

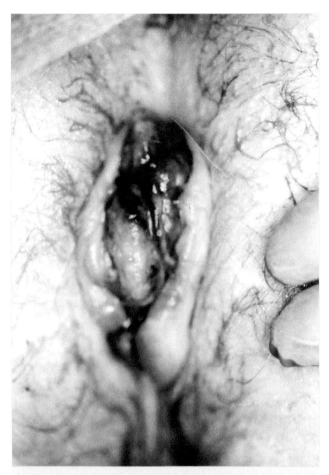

Fig. 7.2 Prolapsed thrombosed internal hemorrhoids that have caused swelling of the external hemorrhoids as well.

demand removal of the band. To prevent this from occurring, it is recommended that bands be placed at the apex of the hemorrhoid bundle or just cranial to it. As an additional check, the proposed site of banding is tested by placing a clamp on the mucosa. If the patient feels the pain, the procedure should be abandoned. It is important that the clamp not be pulled after being applied. As the anal and rectal mucosa is sensitive to stretch, traction on the mucosa will produce inappropriate pain.

A second consideration, when using a Barron-type ligator, is to resist too forceful retraction of the hemorrhoidal tissue. If pulled too hard, the hemorrhoidal tissue may be torn, resulting in hemorrhage that is sometimes difficult to control. This type of bander also requires two hands and an assistant to stabilize the anoscope during the procedure. The McGown ligator can be used with one hand, but it is more difficult to control the amount of tissue drawn into the bander. Finally, some providers preload two bands on the applicator to ensure tissue constriction and guard against slippage and breakage.[5] Other providers have advocated injecting the pedicle of tissue contained within the band with saline or xylocaine. This injection causes the pedicle to swell, which reduces the chance of the bands slipping off prematurely.

Controversy exists about the appropriate number of hemorrhoidal bundles that can be banded at one session.[32] The author prefers to treat one or two bundles at a time. Banding this number eliminates symptoms in most patients, does not produce too large an amount of banded tissue in the anal canal or cause excessive discomfort, and probably leads to efficient care.[33,34]

Before leaving the office, patients are instructed both verbally and in writing that after banding they may experience a feeling of incomplete evacuation. The sensation of fullness is from the bunched tissue in the anal canal. If the urge to defecate or urinate is noted, patients are instructed to sit and try to pass the

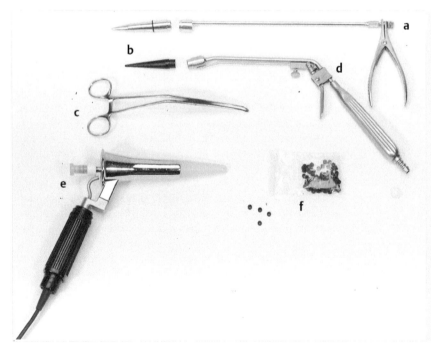

Fig. 7.3 Hemorrhoidal banders. **(a)** Band ligator (McGivney type). **(b)** Band loaders. **(c)** Avascular clamp. **(d)** Suction ligator (McGown). **(e)** Fiberoptic anoscope. **(f)** Rubber bands. (Reproduced with permission from Beck DE. Hemorrhoids. In Beck DE, ed. Handbook of Colorectal Surgery. 3rd ed. London: J.P. Medical; 2013.)

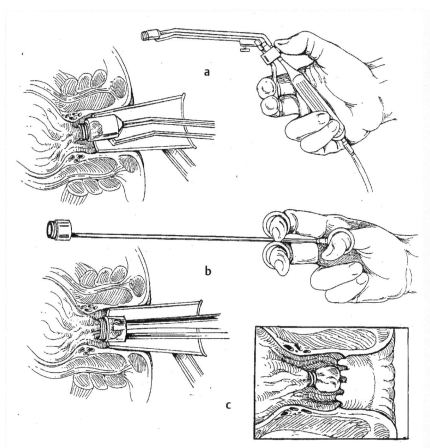

Fig. 7.4 Banding an internal hemorrhoid. The internal hemorrhoid is teased into the barrel of the ligating gun with **(a)** a suction (McGown) ligator or **(b)** a McGivney ligator. **(c)** The apex of the banded hemorrhoid is well above the dentate line in order to minimize pain.

stool. If no stool is produced, they should refrain from prolonged straining. At 5 to 7 days after treatment, the bands and necrotic tissue will slough, which may be associated with a small amount of bleeding. If the symptoms have not resolved at reexamination 2 to 6 weeks later, additional bands are placed. Normal activities can otherwise be resumed immediately after banding.

Complications are infrequent with rubber band ligation (< 2%).[25] They vary from transient problems such as a vasovagal response on placement of the bands, to anal pain, or rarely pelvic sepsis. The vasovagal response to banding includes diaphoresis, bradycardia, nausea, and mild hypotension. Reassuring the patient, elevating their feet, and applying a cold compress to the patient's forehead are frequently all that is necessary. Symptoms should resolve in 10 to 15 minutes. Despite the rarity of pelvic sepsis, its devastating sequela makes it worthwhile to explain the heralding symptoms as part of the office discharge instructions. Accordingly, patients must know that if the pain increases instead of decreasing or urinary retention or fever develops, they should immediately contact their physician.

Pain occurs due to incorporation of somatically enervated tissue into the band. This occurs when the band is placed too close to the dentate line or the internal sphincter muscle is included into the band (i.e., too much tissue included within the band). In this case, the pain is acute in onset at the time of banding. Mild pain can be managed with analgesics such as propoxyphene napsylate and acetaminophen or injection of a local anesthetic (e.g., 0.5% xylocaine hydrochloride or 0.25% bupivacaine hydrochloride). More intense pain is best managed by removal of the band by hooked scissors or a hooked cutting probe (▶ Fig. 7.5). Most

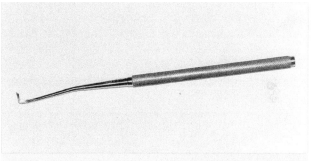

Fig. 7.5 Hooked probe for use in cutting misplaced rubber bands.

patients will require injection of local anesthetic in order to remove the band. Pain and swelling that develop several hours after banding may be due to edema and thrombosis distal to the banded area, which can usually be managed by conservative measures. Increasing rather than decreasing pain may require emergency evaluation by the surgeon.

Not infrequently, younger patients with high anal tone may experience mild to severe anismus. Also, fear of pain may cause patients to delay defecation as long as possible, leading to harder stools that are more difficult to pass. For these reasons, patients should be carefully counseled as to what to expect after banding. Fecal impaction is best avoided by limiting narcotic use, adding stool softeners, and maintaining adequate hydration.

Secondary thrombosis of external hemorrhoids may occur in 2 to 11% of patients.[35] As with spontaneous thrombosis, mild symptoms can be treated with topical preparations and sitz baths. More severe complaints may require excision. Urinary retention is not common with rubber band ligation. When it does occur, onset is shortly after banding and will often resolve spontaneously, or may require one time catheterization. The development of difficult urination or urinary retention days after the procedure may herald pelvic sepsis, as described below.

Delayed hemorrhage may also occur, usually 7 to 10 days postprocedure as the banded tissue sloughs. Patients should be cautioned that they may notice a small amount of bleeding, which usually requires no treatment. Major bleeding is fortunately very rare, 0.5% out of 600 patients reviewed by Rothberg et al and others.[35,36] Significant bleeding demands immediate attention and may require suture ligation in the operating room. To minimize the risk of hemorrhage after banding, some providers ask their patients to refrain from any aspirin products before and after banding. However, little prospective data are available on the risks associated with aspirin use and postbanding hemorrhage. The experience with other anticoagulants such as warfarin is even less. With the increasing use of and need for anticoagulants, individual decisions must be made on the risks of stopping the anticoagulant and potential thrombosis compared to the risk of bleeding while remaining on the medication. The author currently bands patients on anticoagulation and has not seen significant postbanding bleeding.

The most serious complication is postbanding sepsis, believed to be related to necrosis from the banded tissue allowing adjacent soft tissue to become infected.[2] First reported in 1980, it is associated with fever, perineal or pelvic pain, or both, and difficulty urinating.[37,38] Development of these symptoms after banding mandates urgent evaluation. A pelvic computed tomography (CT) scan will often demonstrate changes compatible with pelvic sepsis. Some patients may require an anesthetic to adequately evaluate the perineum. Large doses of broad-spectrum antibiotics to include clostridial coverage are indicated for empirical treatment to reduce the risk of potentially fatal sepsis.

Operative debridement (drainage of any abscess and excision of necrotic tissue) and removal of the bands is reasonable, and in cases of overwhelming infections, a diverting colostomy may also be required.[25]

Success rates of rubber band ligation vary depending on the grade of hemorrhoids treated, length of follow-up, and the criteria for success. The results with rubber band ligation have been excellent with patient satisfaction of 80 to 91% in large series, but probably only 60 to 70% of patients have been completely cured of symptoms by one treatment session.[39,40,41] Recurrence at 4 to 5 years of follow-up is as high as 68% but symptoms usually respond to repeat ligations; only 10% of such patients require excisional hemorrhoidectomy.[42] If two or three banding sessions do not ameliorate the symptoms, an alternative form of therapy (e.g., hemorrhoidectomy) should be contemplated.

Infrared Photocoagulation

A newer technique, first described by Neiger,[43] is photocoagulation. Infrared radiation, generated by a tungsten-halogen lamp, is focused onto the hemorrhoidal tissue from a gold-plated reflector housing through a solid quartz glass light guide (Redfield Corporation, Montvale, NJ) using technology similar to laser devices.[2] The infrared coagulator (IRC; ▶ Fig. 7.6) light penetrates tissue to the submucosal level and is converted to heat, leading to inflammation, destruction, and eventual scarring of the treated area.[44] The tip of the instrument is applied to the base of the hemorrhoid and a 1.5- to 1.8-second pulse of energy is delivered. This produces an immediate area of coagulation of 3 to 4 mm² in diameter. This area ulcerates and eventually scars over the subsequent 2 weeks. Three or four applications are applied to the base of each treated hemorrhoid (▶ Fig. 7.7). One to three bundles may be treated per visit. Additional treatment, if necessary, can be performed every 3 to 4 weeks. However, clinicians need to be aware that Medicare has placed a 90-day global on reimbursement for IRC.

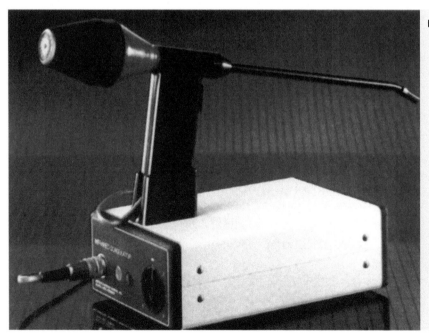

Fig. 7.6 Infrared photocoagulator.

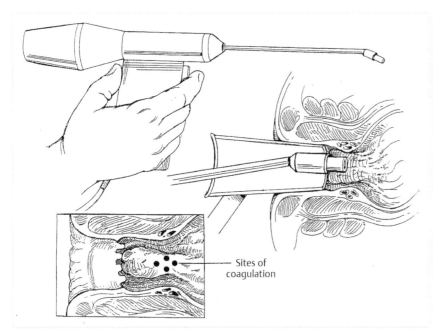

Sites of
coagulation

Fig. 7.7 The infrared photocoagulator creates a small thermal injury. Thus, several applications are required for each hemorrhoidal column. (Reproduced with permission from Beck DE. Hemorrhoids. In Beck DE, ed. Handbook of Colorectal Surgery. 3rd ed. London: J.P. Medical; 2013.)

Complications with this technique have been infrequent. Pain can occur if the energy is inappropriately delivered to the anoderm rather than the base of the hemorrhoid. Excessive application can also lead to bleeding. Most authors report the incidence of bleeding is considerably less with photocoagulation compared with banding.[5] In one study of 51 patients, 3 developed anal fissures after treatment, and no other complications were noted after a median follow-up of 8 months.[45] As mentioned, ulcer formation is an expected result of both rubber band ligation and IRC. The resultant scarring creates fixation. However, large ulcers may rarely be associated with fissure formation and persistent complaints.

The IRC works best on patients with small bleeding hemorrhoids (first or second degree). An advantage of this technique is that the maximum discomfort occurs at the time of IRC treatment and not at a later time, as seen with incorrectly placed bands. Disadvantages of this technique are that the cost of the instrument is significantly higher than a bander and this method is less effective in eliminating bulky hemorrhoids.[25]

Sclerotherapy

Sclerotherapy, one of the oldest forms of therapy, aims to cause scarring, thereby fixation and eventual shrinking of hemorrhoidal tissue. Sclerotherapy works by obliterating the vascularity of the hemorrhoids, fixing them to the adjacent anorectal muscularis propria and preventing prolapse. In 1869, John Morgan described injection of iron persulfate into external hemorrhoids.[46] Since then, various substances have been used.[47] Quinine and urea (5% solution), phenol (5% in almond oil), and sodium tetradecyl sulfate (1–3% solution) are the agents currently in use. Most practitioners inject 3 to 5 mL of the sclerosing solution into the submucosa of each hemorrhoidal bundle, 1 cm or more above the dentate line using a 25-gauge spinal needle or a specialized hemorrhoid (Gabriel) needle. The proper site of injection is just proximal to the hemorrhoidal plexus and the injection should be sufficiently deep to not blanch the mucosa, but not too deep so

as to injure the underlying muscle. Pain occurs if the needle is too deep causing spasm of the sphincter muscle or too distal in the anal canal with sclerosant irritating the sensitive somatic nerves distal to the dentate line.[2] Contraindications to sclerotherapy include inflammatory bowel disease, portal hypertension, immunocompromised states, anorectal infection, and prolapsed thrombosed hemorrhoids.[2]

Complications of sclerotherapy are related to incorrect placement or excess injection of sclerosing agent.[17] The most frequent problem is superficial sloughing of the hemorrhoidal mucosa, which generally heals without treatment. Excessive sloughing may lead to scarring and stricture. Sclerotherapy may also precipitate thrombosis of an adjacent hemorrhoidal complex. If the thrombosis is severe, it may require excision. Most patients, however, can be managed with sitz baths, a high-fiber diet, and local measures. Because of the potential for scarring and stricture, repetitive use of sclerotherapy is not recommended. More unusual complications of sclerotherapy are abscess or oleoma, a granulomatous reaction to an oil-based sclerosant.[38] A case of necrotizing fasciitis after injection sclerotherapy for hemorrhoids requiring debridement and defunctioning colostomy has been reported.[48]

Results of sclerotherapy have been sparsely reported and difficult to compare to other forms of treatment.[2] Alexander-Williams and Crapp[49] compared injection to freezing and rubber band ligation and found it "satisfactory" over short-term follow-up in grade 1 (first degree) hemorrhoids. Dencker and associates[50] compared sclerotherapy to a variety of other treatments and found it to be satisfactory in only 21% of patients. Although the results produced by this method are similar to IRC, sclerotherapy is being used with less frequency. Similar to IRC, sclerotherapy works best for grade 1 or 2 hemorrhoids.[6]

Cryotherapy

Cryotherapy is discussed for completeness, but it is infrequently used. Through a cryoprobe inserted into the anus, cold nitrous oxide (–60 °C to –80 °C) or liquid nitrogen (–196°C) is delivered to freeze a hemorrhoidal bundle. One disadvantage is the inability to control the amount of destruction that occurs. A prolonged, necrotic tissue slough results, causing increased pain and an unpleasant anal discharge.[36]

Cryotherapy is based on rapid freezing and thawing of tissue, which theoretically causes analgesia and tissue destruction. The "ice ball" that forms around the cryoprobe approximates the extent of tissue destruction. Although initial reports were optimistic,[51,52] subsequent experience demonstrated significant problems.[2,25] After therapy, patients experienced significant pain and a profuse foul discharge from the treatment sites. Healing frequently took 6 weeks or more.[53] Smith and colleagues[54] randomly treated 26 hemorrhoid patients with cryotherapy on one side of the anus and a closed hemorrhoidectomy on the other side. Pain was more prolonged and a foul-smelling discharge persisted on the cryotherapy side, and six of the seven patients who required additional treatment needed it at the cryosurgical site.[54] If cryotherapy is not performed properly, destruction of the anal sphincter muscle can cause anal stenosis and incontinence. The expensive cumbersome equipment and significant side effects have led to almost total abandonment of this technique.

Electrocoagulation

Bipolar and direct current devices are currently available for electrocautery. Bipolar diathermy uses a bipolar radio frequency electric current to generate a coagulum of tissue at the end of a cautery-tipped applicator (Circon ACMI, Stamford, CT). Patient grounding is not necessary and a 2-second pulse is applied to the base of each hemorrhoid. Yang and colleagues treated 25 patients with bipolar electrocautery in a prospective controlled trial.[55] Ulcerations developed in six patients (24%) and caused minor rectal pain and self-limited fever. One patient experienced prolonged pain lasting greater than 1 day after therapy and two patients (8%) developed uncontrolled bleeding. In another study of 51 patients, fissures were seen in 2 patients (4%).[45] This technique has not been widely accepted because of the expense of the equipment and lack of results superior to results with other methods.

Direct current therapy uses a special probe (Ultroid, Microvasive, Watertown, MA) to deliver an electrical current (of up to 16 mA) to the internal hemorrhoid. The technique entails delivering the current for up to 10 minutes to each hemorrhoid. In the randomized study of 25 patients by Yang et al, 5 patients (20%) had to have the procedure terminated due to pain, 4 patients (16%) had prolonged pain after the procedure, and 1 patient (4%) had uncontrolled bleeding.[55] The equipment for both methods is expensive, and neither method offers any advantage over the methods previously described.[25]

A variation is the use of a ball-tip or spatula-tip monopolar electrocoagulation to treat second- and early third-degree hemorrhoids. The equipment is readily available in any colon and rectal clinic. The key to success is to coagulate the tops of the internal hemorrhoids until they are charred. The mucosa will be ulcerated as in rubber band ligation and fixed onto the anorectal ring. Because of extensive vascularity, the degree of electrocoagulation must be rather extensive to produce the desired destruction of the submucosa.

Anal Stretch Dilatation

In 1968, Lord described his technique of anal dilatation for the treatment of symptomatic hemorrhoids.[56,57] The treatment is based on the premise that increased anal pressure or a narrowing of the lower canal contributes to hemorrhoid symptoms.[23] The narrowing is caused by a fibrosis deposit that Lord called the "pectin band." The procedure entails careful but firm dilatation of the anal canal. Two lubricated fingers of the surgeon's hand are inserted into the anorectum and the anus is pulled laterally; then, two fingers of the other hand are inserted and countertraction is applied. With increasing dilatation and traction, additional fingers are inserted until the lower rectum can accommodate up to eight of the operator's fingers. The amount of dilation varies: the purpose is to dilate and "iron out" the anorectum until no "constrictors" remain. Lord cautions that it is safer to do too little than too much. Patients were also instructed to use a dilating cone after the procedure. The necessity of this postoperative dilation has been questioned.[21] Although used extensively in Europe with excellent results, some patients complain of incontinence after the procedure. An unacceptably high rate of incontinence occurred in 40% of patients during the first month after dilatation in one study.[58] Fortunately, most episodes were minor and resolved with additional follow-up. This treatment option has not gained wide acceptance in North America.[21] A new variation on dilatation uses a hydrostatic balloon dilator, which allows the operator to control the pressure and volume in a more graduated and reproducible fashion.

Internal Anal Sphincterotomy

This treatment has been recommended for hemorrhoids for precisely the same theories to which Lord subscribed. A sphincterotomy seems an inherently more controlled technique to lower anal pressure.[59] The technique may be done under local anesthesia, but in 25% of cases, some degree of minor transient incontinence may occur.[60] However, sphincterotomy does not address associated tags or external hemorrhoids.

A controlled study by Arabi and colleagues showed no improvement in results when an internal anal sphincterotomy was compared to rubber band ligation in early hemorrhoids,[60] and Schouten and van Vroonhoven[61] demonstrated only a 75% success rate with sphincterotomy alone. Leong and colleagues found no improvement when internal sphincterotomy was combined with other procedures such as hemorrhoidectomy.[62] Although sphincterotomy may be reasonable in the surgical treatment of hemorrhoids with concomitant anal fissure, neither the author nor editors recommend its use as the sole treatment for isolated hemorrhoidal disease.[2] In addition, most surgeons would be very hesitant to perform a sphincterotomy in patients with lax sphincters or in elderly patients for hemorrhoidal symptoms.

Stapled Rectopexy or Procedure for Prolapsing Hemorrhoids

Stapled rectopexy, also referred to as procedure for prolapse and hemorrhoids (PPH), involves transanal, circular stapling of redundant anorectal mucosa with a modified circular stapling instrument (Proximate PPH 03, Ethicon Endosurgery, Cincinnati, OH; or HEM 3348, Covidien, Minneapolis, MN). There is continued debate about the mechanisms by which this procedure relieves symptoms. As hemorrhoids are thought to be redundant fibrovascular cushions, most treatments reduce blood flow and remove redundant tissue. Stapled rectopexy is thought to work by similar mechanisms. Redundant mucosa is drawn into the instrument and excised within the "stapled doughnut." Additionally, mucosal and submucosal blood flow is interrupted by the circular staple line. No incisions are made in the somatically innervated, highly sensitive anoderm which significantly reduces postoperative pain. The procedure involves techniques that are different from more common surgical procedures. Proper technique with meticulous attention to detail is required to get a successful result and avoid the serious complications that have been reported.

Patients are prepared as for a standard hemorrhoidectomy with partial or complete mechanical bowel preparation. General, spinal, and local anesthesia have all been described. Patients may be positioned in prone, lithotomy, or Sims position depending on the surgeon's preference.

After thorough examination of the anal canal and perianal tissues, a specially designed anoscope in inserted and a purse-string suture is placed. The purse-string should be 4 to 5 cm proximal to the dentate line and include only mucosa and submucosa. Suture "bites" should be close together as large gaps will allow redundant mucosa to evade the stapler resulting in persistent hemorrhoids. Most surgeons place eight bites of the purse-string suture. The circular stapling instrument is then introduced (usually at 33 mm), fully opened into the anal canal, and the suture tightened between the anvil and shaft of the instrument. Ends of the suture are drawn through slots of the stapler drawing distal redundant mucosa proximally into the jaws of the stapler. After tightening the stapler, a finger is placed transvaginally in females to assure that the anovaginal septum has not been included within the stapler. The stapler is then fired and removed (▶ Fig. 7.8). Following this, the staple line is inspected for gaps and particularly for bleeding points, which can then be cauterized or oversewn. Some authors routinely place three figure-of-eight sutures at the location of the primary hemorrhoidal bundles to minimize the chances of postoperative bleeding.[63,64]

A meta-analysis of all randomized controlled trials assessing two or more treatment modalities for symptomatic hemorrhoids, from 1966 to January 2001, was conducted by Macrae et al.[65] The main outcome measures were response to therapy, need for further therapy, complications, and pain. Twenty-three trials were available for analysis. With short-term follow-up, stapled hemorrhoidopexy was found to be associated with significantly less pain than conventional hemorrhoidectomy, with no significant difference in complication rate or response to treatment. A multicenter prospective controlled trial with long-term follow-up compared stapled rectopexy to a modified Ferguson technique.[66] The authors demonstrated that stapled rectopexy offered less postoperative pain, less requirement for analgesics, and less pain at first bowel movement, while providing similar control of symptoms and need for additional hemorrhoid treatment at 1-year follow-up from surgery.

Peng et al conducted a randomized controlled trial comparing rubber band ligation to stapled hemorrhoidopexy for symptomatic grade 3 or small grade 4 hemorrhoids.[67] For the rubber band ligation group, three piles were banded, all in one session. There were 25 patients in the rubber band ligation group and 30 patients in the hemorrhoidopexy group. All rubber bands

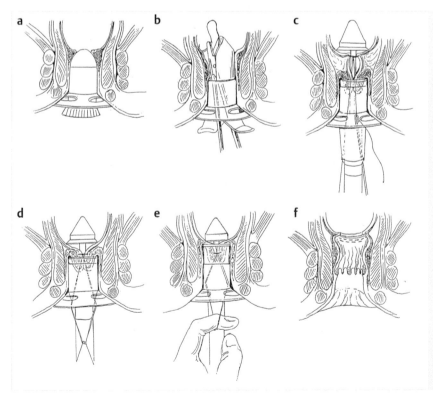

Fig. 7.8 Stapled rectopexy (procedure for prolapse and hemorrhoids [PPH]). (a) Retracting anoscope and dilator inserted. (b) Monofilament purse-string suture (eight bites) placed using operating anoscope approximately 3–4 cm above anal verge. (c) Stapler inserted through purse-string. Purse-string suture tied and ends of suture manipulated through stapler. (d) Retracting on suture pulls anorectal mucosa into stapler. (e) Stapler closed and fired. (f) Completed procedure.

were performed as an outpatient, whereas 29 of 30 stapled hemorrhoidopexies stayed in the hospital for 24 hours and 1 patient stayed longer because of urinary retention. The study demonstrated that both rubber band ligation and stapled hemorrhoidopexy were suitable techniques for the treatment of grade 3 and early grade 4 hemorrhoids. There was no difference between the two groups in terms of patient satisfaction or quality of life for the 6-month follow-up.

A second meta-analysis of randomized trials between 2000 and 2013, comparing Milligan-Morgan to PPH, identified 1,343 patients.[66] The PPH had shorter operative time, duration of hospitalization, and return to normal activity. PPH had better patient satisfaction, but higher rate of prolapse and need for subsequent surgery. Lehur et al[68] evaluated the cost effectiveness of Doppler-guided hemorrhoidal artery ligation with hemorrhoidopexy (DGHAL) compared to stapled hemorrhoidopexy (SH) in a multicentre randomized controlled trial. 393 patients with grades II or III hemorrhoids were randomized between 2010 and 2013 to either undergo SH (n = 196) or DGHAL (n = 197). The DGHAL procedures required a mean of 44 minutes as compared to a mean of 30 minutes in the SH group (p < 0.001). Although the DGHAL group resulted in less postoperative pain at the 2-week point and a shorter sick leave (12.3 vs. 14.8 days, respectively [p = 0.045]), it led to more residual grade III hemorrhoidal disease than did SH (15% vs. 5%, respectively) and a higher reoperation rate of 8% vs. 4%, respectively. Despite these differences, patient satisfaction was in excess of 90% for each group. Cost comparison of the two approaches demonstrated that the DGHAL was more costly compared to SH at 90-day and 1-year follow-up, while at the same time being less effective at the 1-year mark.

Another Austrian randomized controlled trial of 40 patients compared DGHAL to suture hemorrhoidopexy alone.[69] Although the patients in the DGHAL with mucopexy group reported less pain during the first two weeks than did the mucopexy alone group at the 12-month follow-up, there was no difference in recurrent grade III hemorrhoids. Moreover, the authors also conducted transperineal contrast enhanced ultrasound. Using this tool they were unable to identify any significant morphological differences between the preoperative and 6 months postoperative assessment in either group. The authors concluded that the mucopexy rather than the DG-HAL was the reason for successful outcome.

In summary, stapled rectopexy is a technique available to patients otherwise requiring surgical hemorrhoidectomy. Stapled rectopexy is associated with significantly less pain and similar complication rates when compared to conventional treatment. Considering the technique, however, the potential for disastrous complications may be higher (rectovaginal or rectourethral fistula due to including too much tissue within the purse-string). Bleeding also remains a problem, and cases of perforation and leaks have been reported. Finally, a small number of patients have developed significant chronic anorectal pain following the procedure. The etiology of the pain is not well understood and it has been challenging to manage.[70,71]

Transanal Hemorrhoidal Dearterialization

A newer addition to surgical armamentarium is **Doppler-guided arterial ligation with hemorrhoidopexy** (▶ Fig. 7.9).[72] The technique has evolved and currently uses a Doppler-guided ligation of hemorrhoidal arterial inflow with a suture rectopexy. There are currently two commercial products available in the United States[73]: transanal hemorrhoidal dearterialization (THD America, Ankeny, IA) and hemorrhoidal artery ligation and rectoanal repair (HAL/RAR, A.M.I, Inc., Natick, MA). These nonexcisional techniques rely on detection and ligation of the branches of the superior hemorrhoidal artery in the mucosa that lacks sensation well above the dentate line. The associated suture rectopexy reduces the redundant prolapsing mucosa and internal hemorrhoids.

The procedure is performed in the operating room and requires anesthesia similar to a traditional hemorrhoidectomy. A specially designed anoscope with a removable Doppler ultrasound probe and a slot for suture placement is used. After insertion, the anoscope is rotated until one of the arterial branches is located. Through the anoscope slot, the vessel is suture ligated (2–3 cm above the dentate line). Loss of the Doppler signal confirms accurate placement of the ligating suture. After ligating the vessel, the suture is used to oversew the internal

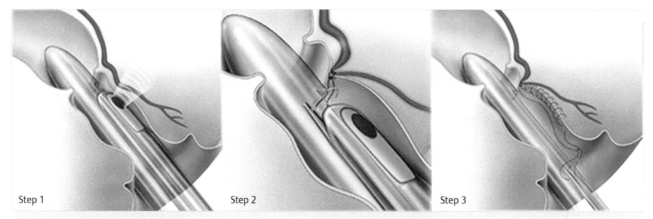

Fig. 7.9 Transanal hemorrhoidal dearterialization (THD). Step 1: THD uses a Doppler ultrasound, placed into the rectum, to locate the specific arteries which cause bleeding. Step 2: once the arteries have been located, the surgeon sutures the problematic artery(s) closed, resulting in an immediate reduction in swelling and bleeding. This is completed without cutting or removal of any tissue. Step 3: last, the surgeon will reposition any prolapsed or hanging tissue outside the anus to its natural anatomical position inside the anal canal with self-absorbing sutures.

hemorrhoid with a running technique from proximal to distal direction. The suture is completed proximal to the dentate line to minimize pain. Usually, four to six arteries are ligated and depending on the patient's anatomy and two to four hemorrhoids are fixated.

The operation has a short operating time and purports to accomplish the same goals as a stapled hemorrhoidopexy.[72] It is an operative procedure which includes anesthesia risks, operating room expense, and surgical risks of bleeding, infection, urinary retention, hematoma, and postoperative pain. The specialized anoscope and Doppler probe are disposable and add to the cost of the procedure, which is somewhat less than a stapled hemorrhoidopexy. A variety of publications have documented safety, reduced pain, and short recovery with the technique.[74] It appears effective for grades 2 and 3 hemorrhoids, but long-term results and cost–benefit analysis need additional study.

7.5.3 External Hemorrhoids

Acute Thrombosis

The management of thrombosed external hemorrhoids depends on when in the course of the disease the patient presents.[5] The natural course of this condition starts with thrombosis of an external hemorrhoid. This event is sometimes associated with effort or straining (moving or lifting furniture, heavy exercise, etc.). The tissue around these clots swells, causing moderate to severe pain. The pain is usually described as burning rather than throbbing, and the degree usually, but not always, depends on the size of the thrombus. Histopathologic studies reveal an intravascular thrombus of the capillaries that can be stretched to 1 cm in diameter or larger. The thrombus is confined to the anoderm and does not cross proximally beyond the dentate line.

The natural history of thrombosed external hemorrhoids is an abrupt onset of an anal mass and pain that usually peaks within 48 to 72 hours. The pain then reduces and the thrombus will shrink and dissolve in 2 to 4 weeks. Occasionally, the skin overlying the thrombus becomes thinned and residual clot is extruded with associated bleeding. A large thrombus can result

in a skin tag. Since thrombosed external hemorrhoids are self-limited, the treatment should be aimed at relief of severe pain, prevention of recurrent thromboses, and residual skin tags. If not treated, in 2 to 4 weeks, the clot in the thrombosed vessels will either spontaneously drain through the thinned overlying skin or be gradually resorbed and the discomfort will gradually diminish. After resolution, redundant anal skin will remain, which is usually asymptomatic and requires no treatment. If a tag causes irritation or difficulty in cleansing the anal area, a conservative excision under local anesthesia can be performed in the office.

If the patient presents early, the procedure of choice is excision (▶ Fig. 7.10). The remaining wound may be left open or closed. The goal with excision is to remove the clots and leave a cosmetically pleasing wound. The procedure can be performed in the office with local anesthesia. Incision and drainage has no role as it removes only a portion of the clot, may not adequately relieve symptoms, and leaves excess skin when healing occurs. The relief of pain usually is immediate provided the wound is closed without tension. Postoperative care is aimed at keeping the wound clean. Warm sitz baths of 10 to 15 minutes three to four times daily are used only for throbbing pain. An analgesic drug may be required during the first 24 hours.

Greenspon et al retrospectively studied 231 patients with thrombosed external hemorrhoids.[75] Fifty-one percent were managed conservatively. This study showed that most patients treated conservatively had resolution of their symptoms. Excision of thrombosed external hemorrhoids resulted in more rapid symptom resolution, lower incidence of recurrence, and longer remission intervals.

A conservative treatment of thrombosed external hemorrhoids has been successful using nifedipine gel. Perrotti et al conducted a prospective, randomized trial in which 46 patients received topical 0.3% nifedipine and 1.5% lidocaine gel every 12 hours for 2 weeks.[76] The control group, consisting of 44 patients, received 1.5% lidocaine and 1% hydrocortisone acetate gel. Relief of pain occurred in 85% in nifedipine group as opposed to 50% of controls after 7 days of therapy ($p < 0.01$); oral analgesics were used by 9% of patients in nifedipine group as opposed to 55% of the control group ($p < 0.01$); resolution of thrombosed external hemorrhoids occurred after 14 days of

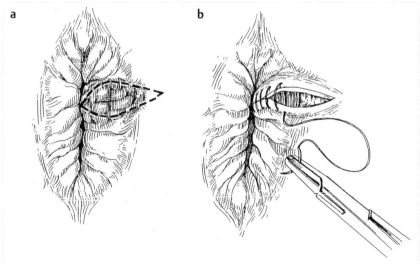

a   **b**

Fig. 7.10 Thrombosed external hemorrhoid. **(a)** Site of incision. **(b)** Running stitch for wound closure. (Reproduced with permission from Beck DE. Hemorrhoids. In Beck DE, ed. Handbook of Colorectal Surgery. 3rd ed. London: J.P. Medical; 2013.)

therapy in 91% of nifedipine-treated patients, as opposed to 45% of the controls ($p < 0.01$). No systemic side effects or significant anorectal bleeding was observed in patients treated with nifedipine.

Operative Hemorrhoidectomy

For symptomatic combined external and internal hemorrhoids, a hemorrhoidectomy is indicated.[77,78] Hemorrhoidectomy should be considered when (1) hemorrhoids are severely prolapsed and require manual replacement, (2) patients fail to improve after multiple applications of nonoperative treatments, or (3) hemorrhoids are complicated by associated pathology, such as ulceration, fissure, fistula, large hypertrophied anal papilla, or extensive skin tags. Several different **operative techniques** have been described.[21] Each of these procedures can be performed with general, spinal, or local anesthesia. The choice must be individualized for each patient, but the national trend is toward local anesthesia. With a general anesthetic, the author prefers the Sims' (left lateral decubitus) position, although the editors prefer the prone jackknife position. With all other anesthetics, the prone jackknife position is used. A bowel preparation is not used and the anus is prepared with a povidone-iodine solution. If a local anesthetic (1% xylocaine with 1:100,000 epinephrine) is not being used, the anal submucosa is infiltrated with plain 1:100,000 epinephrine solution. The perineum is re-prepped and draped. An examination confirms the preoperative findings and determines the number of hemorrhoidal bundles to be excised.

The author's preferred procedure is a modified closed Ferguson technique.[21,79] A medium or large Hill-Ferguson or Fansler retractor placed in the anus exposes a hemorrhoidal bundle. A double elliptical incision is made in the mucosa (▶ Fig. 7.11). For a pleasing cosmetic result, the incision should be at least three times as long as it is wide, but the width should almost never be wider that 1.5 cm. The distal edge is grasped with a fine-toothed pickup and the dissection is performed with scissors. Dissection in the proper plane results in elevation of all the varicosities with the specimen, while the sphincter muscles remain in their normal anatomic position. With the previously scored mucosa as a guide, the dissection is continued into the anal canal.

At the superior edge of the hemorrhoidal bundle, the remaining vascular pedicle is clamped and the hemorrhoid is detached. The hemorrhoid specimen should be sent for pathologic evaluation. In the absence of suspicion or some abnormality, it may be unnecessary to separately label each bundle (i.e., left lateral, right posterior, etc.).[21,80] Any bleeding vessels are cauterized with the electrocautery. An absorbable suture (e.g., 4–0 Vicryl or 3–0

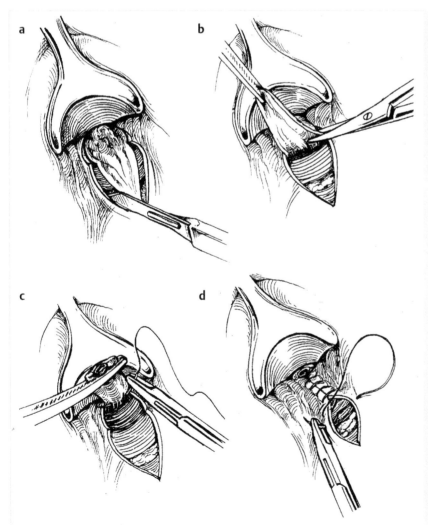

Fig. 7.11 Excisional hemorrhoidectomy. **(a)** Double elliptical incision made in mucosa and anoderm around hemorrhoid bundle with a scalpel. **(b)** The hemorrhoid dissection is carefully continued cephalad by dissecting the sphincter away from the hemorrhoid. **(c)** After dissection of the hemorrhoid to its pedicle, it is either clamped, or secured, or excised. The pedicle is suture ligated. **(d)** The wound is closed with a running stitch. Excessive traction on the suture is avoided to prevent forming dog ears or displacing the anoderm caudally.

chromic) is utilized to suture ligate the pedicle beneath the clamp. The pedicle should not be advanced toward the anus as it may lead to an ectropia. This suture is then used to reapproximate the mucosal edges. It is important to take small bites at the edge of the mucosa and a small bite of the sphincter with every other bite. The sutures should be placed about 2 mm apart. Too large an advancement will contribute toward bleeding from the mucosal edge. This running suture is continued to close the wound and eliminate dead space. As sutures are placed, the mucosa is advanced in a cranial direction to reestablish the normal anal anatomy and result in a "plastic" closure. At the outer edge, the suture is loosely tied to itself to provide an escape for any hematoma developing after surgery. The other hemorrhoidal bundles are handled in a similar manner. The number of bundles that are excised will depend on the amount of excess tissue but usually should not involve more than three columns. To minimize the chance of postoperative anal stenosis, the residual mucosal edges should be able to be approximated over a medium Hill-Ferguson retractor with minimal tension. The procedure preserves bridges of anoderm between the major bundles and maintains the dentate line in its anatomic position. Technique variations include the use of electrocautery instead of scissor excision and elimination of the pedicle stitch.

At St. Marks Hospital, Milligan et al[81] popularized an **open technique** of hemorrhoidectomy, which was widely adopted. The procedure starts with gentle anal canal dilatation to two or three fingers. The hemorrhoidal complex is then everted by traction on a forceps placed just beyond the mucocutaneous junction. Additional forceps can then be placed toward the level of the anorectal ring, producing the "triangle of exposure." The hemorrhoid is excised from the subjacent sphincter and the proximal pedicle is ligated with strong suture material (3–0 chromic catgut). The rest of the wound is left open. Three quadrants are usually removed. Hemostasis is accomplished and an anal dressing is applied. Care must be taken to ensure that adequate islands of anoderm are retained to prevent anal stenosis with healing of the open hemorrhoid wounds.[21]

Another operative technique described by Whitehead,[82] used a circumferential incision made at the level of the dentate line. Submucosal and subdermal hemorrhoidal tissue was dissected out and excised. After redundant rectal mucosa was removed, the proximal rectal mucosa was sutured circumferentially to the anoderm. While Whitehead described good results with his procedure, many surgeons who attempted the procedure encountered problems. When performed improperly, the procedure was associated with high rates of stricture, loss of normal sensation, and the development of ectropion commonly referred to as the "Whitehead deformity" (▶ Fig. 7.12). These postoperative complications are often challenging to correct. Common mistakes in performing the Whitehead procedure include excising excess anoderm and failing to recreate the dentate line in the correct location. Despite its poor reputation, some surgeons have obtained good results after modifying and simplifying the procedure.[83,84]

The type of hemorrhoidectomy a surgeon performs is based primarily on that surgeon's experience and training; few comparative trials are available. Seow-Choen and Low compared a modified Whitehead hemorrhoidectomy to a modified Ferguson technique (four bundles excised with retention of anodermal bridges) in 28 patients.[85] The four-bundle technique was found to be easier and required less operative time to perform. At 6 months, there was no difference in patient perception of success. Recent experience has been directed toward performing hemorrhoidal surgery as outpatient surgery. With the proper support systems, patient preparation, and appropriate technique, hemorrhoidectomy can safely be performed as an outpatient procedure.[86]

Acute, incapacitating hemorrhoids consisting of prolapse, thrombosis, and strangulation of hemorrhoidal tissue can involve one or all three primary complexes.[21] Although conservative therapy with bed rest, ice packs, and analgesics has been used with success, an emergency (acute) hemorrhoidectomy is preferred by most experienced surgeons. This provides rapid resolution of symptoms and prevents recurrence of hemorrhoidal symptoms. A closed hemorrhoidectomy, as described previously, is performed. Injection of an epinephrine solution (1:100,000) with 150 units of hyaluronidase (Wydase, Wyeth-Ayerst Laboratories, Philadelphia, PA) into the hemorrhoidal

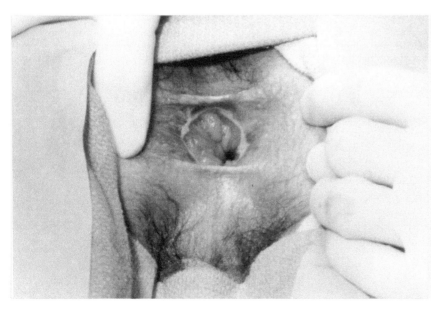

Fig. 7.12 Completely circumferential anal ectropion (classic "Whitehead" deformity).

complex produces considerable shrinkage of the tissue and reduction of the edema. This simplifies the operation. Care must again be taken to preserve adequate anoderm. Recovery for these patients is similar to those with less acute disease.

Alternate Energy Sources

Laser hemorrhoidectomy (using a laser rather than a scalpel or scissors to remove the hemorrhoidal tissue) has received a lot of attention. Proponents have claimed that this technique involves less pain and has a better cosmetic result. Both the carbon dioxide (CO2) and the neodymium:yttrium-aluminum-garnet (Nd:YAG) have been used to surgically manage hemorrhoids.[21] Unfortunately, there are very few articles available in the English literature describing excisional hemorrhoidectomy with the laser, and the relatively small number of well-controlled prospective studies have demonstrated no advantage of a laser over traditional techniques.[11,30] Senagore et al[87] reported a prospective, randomized study comparing the Nd:YAG to a cold scalpel in 86 patients. Each method resulted in similar degrees of postoperative discomfort, requirements for postoperative analgesia, and time away from work.

Wang et al[88] reported a randomized trial comparing Nd:YAG laser hemorrhoidectomy to a closed technique in 88 patients. Overall complications were similar, but prolonged wound healing was noted in the laser-treated group. Based on the available evidence, the Standards of Practice Task Force of the American Society of Colon and Rectal Surgeons produced the following statement.[89]

"No controlled trials have yet been completed to demonstrate superiority or even equivalence of the laser to more traditional treatment methods. Isolated reports suggest that the laser can be used with success, but there is as yet no reason to believe that results will be superior to current techniques. The additional cost and safety requirements of the laser equipment along with the lack of significantly better results argue against its routine use."

Other energy devices (e.g., Ligasure, Covidien, Minneapolis, MN; and harmonic scalpel, Ethicon, Cincinnati, OH) have been evaluated to reduce blood loss and pain in hemorrhoidectomy. A Cochrane Systematic Review in 2009 evaluated 12 studies with 1,142 patients who were randomized to either a hemorrhoidectomy with conventional diathermy or a Ligasure technique.[90] The authors concluded that the Ligasure technique resulted in less postoperative pain without adverse effect on postoperative complications. A randomized study of 151 patients randomized to harmonic scalpel and Ferguson's with electrocautery found that the harmonic scalpel was safe and effective and resulted in less blood loss and postoperative pain than the Ferguson's with electrocautery.[91] However, none of these studies addressed the cost of the alternate energy devices (several hundred dollars) or their utilization with modern multimodality pain management (described below). In the author's experience, the cost of these devices far outweighs any potential advantages.

Postoperative care after hemorrhoidectomy focuses on two areas: prevention of potential complications and relief of pain. Preparing the patients mentally as well as physically aids in both areas. Truthful descriptions of the postoperative recovery allow the patient to develop a sense of relief as well as confidence. Patients are told that pain will occur, but depending on the type of anesthesia, it will not occur for several hours after the procedure and medication will be given to minimize their discomfort.

Several actions have been shown to reduce the incidence of postoperative urinary retention, which has varied from 0.5 to 17%.[92] Intravenous fluids are kept to a minimum during the intraoperative and postoperative period (< 250 mL). The patient is asked to attempt to void soon after surgery. An adequate dose of the parasympathomimetic drug bethanechol (10 mg subcutaneously) has been shown to increase the likelihood of spontaneous voiding.[93] Patients who live close to the medical facility and are reliable may be discharged after surgery. They are instructed to return if bleeding or urinary retention occurs. An adequate amount of a strong, preferably nonconstipating, oral narcotic is given for outpatient pain control. An alternative is patient controlled anesthesia using a subcutaneous morphine pump.[94] Bulking agents and thrice-daily sitz baths are also prescribed. If constipation occurs, the patient may be administered a 500-mL warm tap water enema or gentle laxative. Most patients are seen 5 to 10 days after discharge.

Postoperative complications after hemorrhoid surgery are unusual (▶ Table 7.4).[2,95,96] Hemorrhage, usually at one of the pedicles, represents the most acute problem and occurred in 4% of 500 patients in a study by Buls and Goldberg,[97] with a 1% incidence of bleeding severe enough to warrant a return trip to the operating room for suture ligation of a vessel. This agrees with a study from the Ferguson Clinic in which over 2,000 hemorrhoidectomies were reviewed.[98] Major hemorrhage usually requires an adequate examination and suture ligation of the bleeding vessel. A 1- to 2-mL submucosal injection of 1/10,000 adrenaline at the bleeding point has also been successful.[99]

Table 7.4 Posthemorrhoidectomy complications

	Incidence, %[2]
Acute (first 48 h)	
• Bleeding	2–4
• Bleeding requiring reoperation	0.8–1.3
• Urinary retention	10–32
Early (first week)	
• Fecal impaction	< 1
• Wound infection	< 1
• Thrombosed hemorrhoids	< 1
Late	
• Skin tags	6.00
• Anal stenosis	1.00
• Anal fissure	1–2.6
• Incontinence	< 0.4
• Anal fistula	< 0.5
• "Recurrent" hemorrhoids	< 1

Note: Over 2,500 patients.

Sepsis related to the wound itself is extremely rare. It is not unusual, however, to see erythema and drainage from the wound edges. If there is suspicion of infection (fever, increased pain, difficulty voiding) and no obvious other source, the patient should be empirically started on antibiotics and watched carefully. Metronidazole, 500 mg orally three times a day for 5 days, has been shown to combat inflammation or infection and minimize pain.[92] This should be prescribed to patients in cases where the closed wound breaks down causing swelling and pain.

Outpatient observation is acceptable if the patient manifests no signs of toxicity, but severe pain or worsening symptoms should prompt consideration for in-hospital management and careful examination, under anesthesia if necessary.

Postoperative pain is generally moderate in the first 24 to 48 hours, and traditionally controllable by oral or parenteral narcotics. Patients were encouraged to take oral medications such as oxycodone or propoxyphene as soon as possible and informed that while bowel movements will be uncomfortable, they will not be as painful as they have heard from other patients. The use of multimodality pain management has significantly reduced the pain associated with hemorrhoidectomy. A multicenter randomized, double blind placebo-controlled trial of 186 patients undergoing hemorrhoidectomy found that patients receiving an extended-release bupivacaine (Exparel, Pacira, Parsippany, NJ) had significantly less pain through 72 hours, decreased opioid requirements, and improved patient satisfaction.[100] The addition of intravenous acetaminophen and ibuprofen further reduces the need for narcotics and improves the patient experience.[101] The use of warm soaks and stool normalizers (fiber bulking agents), as described in previous sections, is also helpful.

Fecal impaction may occur in the first 7 to 10 days after hemorrhoidectomy and should be suspected if the patient reports watery feculent discharge, rectal pressure, and constipation during the early postoperative period. This problem is best avoided by giving the patient a high-fiber diet with added psyllium or another bulking agent two or three times per day for the first several weeks after surgery.[102] An added mild laxative such as mineral oil or milk of magnesia can be offered to help stimulate the first evacuation. Treatment of an impaction should consist of two or three gentle, warm, 500-mL tap water enemas given through a soft latex catheter until the impaction is cleared. Anal pain or inability to clear the impaction by these methods may require manual disimpaction under anesthesia.

If external thrombosis or swelling of the external hemorrhoids occurs subsequent to hemorrhoidectomy, the usual cause is a subcutaneous bleeding vessel. Gentle compression should be applied to the wound for 10 minutes if it appears to be enlarging. Comfort measures such as sitz baths, analgesics, and local application of a topical soothing cream may then be used. The thrombotic area will generally resolve spontaneously, and only rarely require any additional therapy. Tense edema and swelling may require excision of the external hemorrhoid as described earlier, again erring on the side of very conservative removal of the anoderm.

Edematous skin tags, often of concern to patients, should be left alone for 3 to 4 months since they usually shrink significantly over that time and usually require no treatment beyond reassurance. If tags remain after that time that are bothersome to the patient, they can usually be excised in the office using local anesthesia.

Anal stenosis, although rare, may be the most troublesome long-term complication and should nearly always be preventable by conservative removal of anoderm at hemorrhoidectomy. Retention of adequate anoderm to prevent stenosis is confirmed by the ability to close all of the hemorrhoidectomy incisions without tension while a medium Hill-Ferguson retractor remains in the anal canal. Anal stenosis may be treated by simple anal sphincterotomy,[103] leaving the longitudinally oriented wound open if scarring is so severe that a closed-type procedure is not possible. When stenosis is severe (will not allow insertion of a lubricated index finger or small Hill-Ferguson retractor at surgery), a plastic surgical correction of the stenosis may be required. Several of these techniques are described in detail in Chapter 8. The author's preference is one or two "House" advancement flaps along with a partial sphincterotomy as needed.

Ectropion may occur by inadvertent removal of anoderm and subsequent caudal displacement of rectal mucosa into the anal canal (▶ Fig. 7.10). This can be avoided by remembering the rule that anoderm may always be safely advanced above the dentate line, but rectal mucosa should rarely be advanced below it. If ectropion does occur postoperatively, the patient may report wetness, itching, and irritation.[104] Most patients, unless entirely asymptomatic, require surgical correction. Treatment, if confined to only one half or less of the anal circumference, may be performed by merely excising the ectopic rectal mucosa, but the author nearly always prefers to perform an anoplasty. One or more "House" advancement flaps, as described in Chapter 8, work well to close the defect created after the ectopic rectal mucosa is excised.

In cases of circumferential mucosa ectropion, the classic "Whitehead deformity," or in cases where more than 50% of the circumference is involved, the S-anoplasty remains the procedure of choice.[105] As described in Chapter 8, it may be performed on one or both sides of the anus.

Anal fissure may develop in the postoperative period, heralded by pain or burning bowel movements. Often, a degree of stenosis is an associated finding. If fissures occur in the first 3 to 4 weeks after surgery and are of mild to moderate severity, conservative measures such as sitz baths, dietary fiber, and topical creams should be adopted. The patient is reassured and advised that soft, bulky stools are necessary to dilate the anal passage naturally and that watery, loose stools can contribute to narrowing of the area. If symptoms are severe, or if conservative measures are not helpful, a careful examination under anesthesia with a planned sphincterotomy, possibly with an advancement flap anoplasty, may be needed.

Fecal incontinence is an unusual but potentially disastrous complication after hemorrhoidectomy and may occur more frequently than reported in the literature (< 1%). Patients at higher risk include the elderly, especially women, and patients who have had prior anal surgery.[2] These patients required a detailed and carefully documented inquiry regarding anal continence. Digital rectal examination at rest and during maximum voluntary squeeze to ascertain sphincter tone, and anal manometry should be used to quantify anal pressures. Patients should be counseled about goals of the surgery, and nonoperative measures reconsidered if bowel control is impaired. At surgery, it is acceptable to perform a one- or two-quadrant hemorrhoidectomy, conserving anoderm, and to rubber-band ligate the other quadrants or leave them alone. The underlying sphincter should be carefully protected. While this conservative approach may lead to a slightly greater chance for recurrence, patients will understand the concern to protect continence.

Minor incontinence is rare unless an open sphincterotomy is performed concomitantly with hemorrhoidectomy as a "pain-relieving" measure. A sphincterotomy should be avoided unless some degree of stenosis is present or when a concomitant fissure is present.

Recurrence of significant hemorrhoidal disease following a closed hemorrhoidectomy is unusual—only 1% in the 2,038 patients surveyed by Ganchrow and colleagues.[98] Most symptoms that patients equate with recurrence are either skin tags or small external hemorrhoids, or are related to bleeding of small superficial veins near the hemorrhoidectomy wounds. Tags can be excised in the office under local anesthesia. Bleeding from the internal hemorrhoids is nearly always treatable with rubber band ligation, infrared coagulation, or sclerotherapy.

7.6 Special Considerations

Hemorrhoidal disease in human immunodeficiency virus (HIV) patients deserves additional comment. As discussed in Chapter 13, HIV infection can manifest initially with minimal alterations in health and physiology to complete immunologic failure. The major fear in these patients has been failure to heal and infection. Experience has demonstrated that early stage patients can be treated and expected to respond similarly to uninfected patients. Late-stage patients even with newer medical treatment for their HIV remain at significant risk of problems and should be managed as conservatively as possible.[106,107] Most symptoms can be minimized with dietary manipulations or topical medications. If this fails, infrared coagulation has been used in selected patients with reasonable results.

There is no contraindication to hemorrhoid treatment during any stage of pregnancy.[21] However, an operative hemorrhoidectomy is usually avoided during pregnancy unless the patient is suffering from acute disease. With acute disease, treatment as described elsewhere is accomplished along with special attention afforded to the fetus. Saleeby et al[108] reported on 12 of 12,455 pregnant women (0.2%) who had surgical hemorrhoidectomy. Most were in their third trimester of pregnancy and all did well.

Inflammatory bowel disease patients also develop hemorrhoidal disease. Symptoms of the two conditions must be differentiated. In known inflammatory bowel disease patients, hemorrhoidal symptoms are usually related to their abnormal bowel movements. The presence of anorectal diseases increases concern about Crohn's disease. Crohn's disease patients should not have hemorrhoidectomies unless absolutely necessary, but in selected patients good results can be obtained.[109] In ulcerative colitis patients, a safe hemorrhoidectomy can be performed if the colitis is under control.[21]

Hemorrhoidal symptoms commonly occur and intensify during **pregnancy** and delivery. In most instances, however, hemorrhoids that intensify during delivery resolve. Hemorrhoidectomy is indicated during pregnancy only if acute prolapse and thrombosis occur. It should be performed with the patient under local anesthesia. In the second and third trimester, a left anterolateral position can be used.[110]

Prolapse and thrombosis of hemorrhoids occurring during delivery is an indication for operation in the immediate postpartum period. Similarly, operation is indicated for patients in whom hemorrhoidal disease has been symptomatic before pregnancy, is aggravated during pregnancy, and persists after delivery. In such patients, hemorrhoidectomy is performed best in the immediate postpartum period. Most patients have relief of symptoms the day after the operation.[108]

Abramowitz et al[111] prospectively studied 165 pregnant women during the last 3 months of pregnancy and after delivery (within 2 months). Patients underwent perineal and proctoscopic examinations. The results showed that 13 patients (8%) developed external hemorrhoids before delivery. The problems were more frequently observed in females with constipation ($p = 0.023$) than those without constipation.

Thirty-three patients developed thrombosed external hemorrhoids after delivery; 91% of the external hemorrhoids were observed during the first day after delivery. Constipation and late deliveries were independent risk factors. The most important risk factor was constipation, with an odds ratio of 5.7 (95% confidence interval [CI], 2.7–12). Mild laxatives such as milk of magnesia should be given during the last 3 months of pregnancy and postpartum period for patients with constipation problems. Late delivery had an odds ratio of 1.4 (95% CI, 1.05–1.9). Patients who delivered after 39.7 weeks of pregnancy were more likely to have thrombosed external hemorrhoids than those who delivered before that time. Traumatic deliveries, such as perineal tear and heavy babies, were associated with thrombosed external hemorrhoids. Cesarean section appears to protect against this problem.

Patients with leukemia or lymphoma or other conditions involving immunosuppression may present with hemorrhoidal disease. In these circumstances, treatment is difficult because the risks from operative intervention are great and poor wound healing and abscesses are common.

Although anorectal problems in patients with leukemia are not uncommon, hemorrhoidal problems are rare. In a series reported from Memorial Sloan-Kettering Cancer Center of 2,618 patients hospitalized with leukemia, 151 (6%) had anorectal diseases.[112] Of the 54 patients with leukemia and severe neutropenia, 9 patients had hemorrhoidal disease. Two had surgery with a 50% mortality, and the remaining seven resolved with nonoperative management. In these very high-risk patients, surgery should be performed as a last resort to relieve pain and sepsis. *Escherichia coli* and *Pseudomonas aeruginosa* are the most common bacteria isolated from both blood and anorectal cultures.[112] Correction of any coexisting coagulation disorder and administration of appropriate antibiotics are important parts of the management of hemorrhoidal disease in that patient population.

Anal infections in these patients lack classical signs of abscess formation. Fever and local pain along with local tenderness are the most common findings.[112] The infected area usually has no pus but rather a cavity of necrotic tissue.

7.7 Summary

Understanding of the pathophysiology of hemorrhoidal disease guides treatment selection. The author's preferred treatment plan is summarized in ▶ Table 7.5. A meta-analysis of hemorrhoidal treatment modalities supports this approach.[113] Appropriate treatments provide symptom resolution in a safe and cost-effective manner.

Table 7.5 Author's treatment plan

Symptomatic internal hemorrhoids (bleeding)

1. Trial of supplemental fiber (e.g., Konsyl, Citrucel, Fibercon)

2. If symptoms not resolved, then perform rubber band ligation

3. Repeat ligation in 1 to 6 months if symptoms improving and minimal discomfort with previous banding

4. If discomfort with banding, consider infrared photocoagulation

5. If symptoms persist, consider operative hemorrhoidectomy

Symptomatic external or combined hemorrhoids

1. Operative hemorrhoidectomy (modified Ferguson technique) with local or regional anesthesia

References

[1] Beck DE. Hemorrhoids. In: Beck DE, Welling DR, eds. Patient Care in Colorectal Surgery. Boston, MA: Little, Brown and Company, Inc.; 1991:213–224

[2] Milsom JW. Hemorrhoidal disease. In: Beck DE, Wexner SD, eds. Fundamentals of Anorectal Surgery. New York, NY: McGraw-Hill; 1992:192–214

[3] Dirckx JH. The biblical plague of "hemorrhoids". An outbreak of bilharziasis. Am J Dermatopathol. 1985; 7(4):341–346

[4] Maimonides M, Rosner F, Munter S, trans. Treatise on Hemorrhoids. Philadelphia, PA: JB Lippincott; 1969

[5] Beck DE. Hemorrhoids. In: Beck DE, ed. Handbook of Colorectal Surgery. St Louis, MO: Quality Medical Publishing; 1997:299–311

[6] Thomson WH. The nature of haemorrhoids. Br J Surg. 1975; 62(7):542–552

[7] Thulesius O, Gjöres JE. Arterio-venous anastomoses in the anal region with reference to the pathogenesis and treatment of haemorrhoids. Acta Chir Scand. 1973; 139(5):476–478

[8] Nelson RL. Editorial comment on time trends of hemorrhoids. Dis Colon Rectum. 1991; 34:591–593

[9] Johanson JF, Sonnenberg A. The prevalence of hemorrhoids and chronic constipation. An epidemiologic study. Gastroenterology. 1990; 98(2):380–386

[10] Johanson JF, Sonnenberg A. Temporal changes in the occurrence of hemorrhoids in the United States and England. Dis Colon Rectum. 1991; 34 (7):585–591, discussion 591–593

[11] Burkitt DP, Graham-Stewart CW. Haemorrhoids–postulated pathogenesis and proposed prevention. Postgrad Med J. 1975; 51(599):631–636

[12] Sonnenberg A, Koch TR. Epidemiology of constipation in the United States. Dis Colon Rectum. 1989; 32(1):1–8

[13] Haas PA, Fox TA, Jr, Haas GP. The pathogenesis of hemorrhoids. Dis Colon Rectum. 1984; 27(7):442–450

[14] Hiltunen KM, Matikainen M. Anal manometric findings in symptomatic hemorrhoids. Dis Colon Rectum. 1985; 28(11):807–809

[15] Sun WM, Peck RJ, Shorthouse AJ, Read NW. Haemorrhoids are associated not with hypertrophy of the internal anal sphincter, but with hypertension of the anal cushions. Br J Surg. 1992; 79(6):592–594

[16] Hancock BD. Internal sphincter and the nature of haemorrhoids. Gut. 1977; 18(8):651–655

[17] Sun WM, Read NW, Shorthouse AJ. Hypertensive anal cushions as a cause of the high anal canal pressures in patients with haemorrhoids. Br J Surg. 1990; 77(4):458–462

[18] Waldron DJ, Kumar D, Hallan RI, Williams NS. Prolonged ambulant assessment of anorectal function in patients with prolapsing hemorrhoids. Dis Colon Rectum. 1989; 32(11):968–974

[19] Loder PB, Kamm MA, Nicholls RJ, Phillips RKS. Haemorrhoids: pathology, pathophysiology and aetiology. Br J Surg. 1994; 81(7):946–954

[20] Gibbons CP, Bannister JJ, Read NW. Role of constipation and anal hypertonia in the pathogenesis of haemorrhoids. Br J Surg. 1988; 75(7):656–660

[21] Mazier WP. Hemorrhoids. In: Maxier WP, Levin DH, Luchtefeld MA, Senagore AJ, eds. Surgery of the Colon, Rectum and Anus. Philadelphia, PA: W.B. Saunders Co; 1995:229–254

[22] Nelson RL, Abcarian H, Davis FG, Persky V. Prevalence of benign anorectal disease in a randomly selected population. Dis Colon Rectum. 1995; 38(4):341–344

[23] Corman ML. Colon and Rectal Surgery. 2nd ed. Philadelphia, PA: J.B. Lippincott; 1989:49–105

[24] Kluiber RM, Wolff BG. Evaluation of anemia caused by hemorrhoidal bleeding. Dis Colon Rectum. 1994; 37(10):1006–1007

[25] Larach S, Cataldo TE, Beck DE. Nonoperative treatment of hemorrhoidal disease. In: Hicks TC, Beck DE, Opelka FG, Timmcke AE, eds. Complications of Colon and Rectal Surgery. Baltimore, MD: Williams & Wilkins; 1997:173–180

[26] Moesgaard F, Nielsen ML, Hansen JB, Knudsen JT. High-fiber diet reduces bleeding and pain in patients with hemorrhoids: a double-blind trial of Vi-Siblin. Dis Colon Rectum. 1982; 25(5):454–456

[27] Alonso-Coello P, Zhou Q, Martinez-Zapata MJ, et al. Meta-analysis of flavonoids for the treatment of haemorrhoids. Br J Surg. 2006; 93(8):909–920

[28] Dodi G, Bogoni F, Infantino A, Pianon P, Mortellaro LM, Lise M. Hot or cold in anal pain? A study of the changes in internal anal sphincter pressure profiles. Dis Colon Rectum. 1986; 29(4):248–251

[29] Gorfine SR. Treatment of benign anal disease with topical nitroglycerin. Dis Colon Rectum. 1995; 38(5):453–456, discussion 456–457

[30] Blaisdell PC. Prevention of massive hemorrhage secondary to hemorrhoidectomy. Surg Gynecol Obstet. 1958; 106(4):485–488

[31] Barron J. Office ligation treatment of hemorrhoids. Dis Colon Rectum. 1963; 6:109–113

[32] Lee HH, Spencer RJ, Beart RW, Jr. Multiple hemorrhoidal bandings in a single session. Dis Colon Rectum. 1994; 37(1):37–41

[33] Lau WY, Chow HP, Poon GP, Wong SH. Rubber band ligation of three primary hemorrhoids in a single session. A safe and effective procedure. Dis Colon Rectum. 1982; 25(4):336–339

[34] Khubchandani IT. A randomized comparison of single and multiple rubber band ligations. Dis Colon Rectum. 1983; 26(11):705–708

[35] Rothberg R, Rubin RJ, Eisenstat T, Salvati EP. Rubber band ligation hemorrhoidectomy. Long-term results. Am Surg. 1983; 49(3):167

[36] Corman ML, Veidenheimer MC. The new hemorrhoidectomy. Surg Clin North Am. 1973; 53(2):417–422

[37] O'Hara VS. Fatal clostridial infection following hemorrhoidal banding. Dis Colon Rectum. 1980; 23(8):570–571

[38] Russell TR, Donohue JH. Hemorrhoidal banding. A warning. Dis Colon Rectum. 1985; 28(5):291–293

[39] Bartizal J, Slosberg PA. An alternative to hemorrhoidectomy. Arch Surg. 1977; 112(4):534–536

[40] Steinberg DM, Liegois H, Alexander-Williams J. Long term review of the results of rubber band ligation of haemorrhoids. Br J Surg. 1975; 62(2):144–146

[41] Wrobleski DE, Corman ML, Veidenheimer MC, Coller JA. Long-term evaluation of rubber ring ligation in hemorrhoidal disease. Dis Colon Rectum. 1980; 23(7):478–482

[42] Madoff RD, Fleshman JW, Clinical Practice Committee, American Gastroenterological Association. American Gastroenterological Association technical review on the diagnosis and treatment of hemorrhoids. Gastroenterology. 2004; 126(5):1463–1473

[43] Neiger A. Hemorrhoids in everyday practice. Proctology. 1979; 2:22–28

[44] O'Connor JJ. Infrared coagulation of hemorrhoids. Pract Gastroenterol. 1979; 10:8–14

[45] Dennison A, Whiston RJ, Rooney S, Chadderton RD, Wherry DC, Morris DL. A randomized comparison of infrared photocoagulation with bipolar diathermy for the outpatient treatment of hemorrhoids. Dis Colon Rectum. 1990; 33(1):32–34

[46] Gabriel WB. The Principles and Practice of Rectal Surgery. London: Lewis; 1963:131

[47] Andrews E. The treatment of hemorrhoids by injection. Med Rec. 1879; 15:451

[48] Kaman L, Aggarwal S, Kumar R, Behera A, Katariya RN. Necrotizing fasciitis after injection sclerotherapy for hemorrhoids: report of a case. Dis Colon Rectum. 1999; 42(3):419–420

[49] Alexander-Williams J, Crapp AR. Conservative management of haemorrhoids. Part I: injection, freezing and ligation. Clin Gastroenterol. 1975; 4 (3):595–618

[50] Dencker H, Hjorth N, Norryd C, Tranberg KG. Comparison of results obtained with different methods of treatment of internal haemorrhoids. Acta Chir Scand. 1973; 139(8):742–745

[51] Wilson MC, Schofield P. Cryosurgical haemorrhoidectomy. Br J Surg. 1976; 63(6):497–498

[52] Savin S. Hemorrhoidectomy-how I do it: results of 444 cryorectal surgical operations. Dis Colon Rectum. 1977; 20(3):189–196

[53] Goligher JC. Cryosurgery for hemorrhoids. Dis Colon Rectum. 1976; 19 (3):213–218

[54] Smith LE, Goodreau JJ, Fouty WJ. Operative hemorrhoidectomy versus cryo-destruction. Dis Colon Rectum. 1979; 22(1):10–16

[55] Yang R, Migikovsky B, Peicher J, Laine L. Randomized, prospective trial of direct current versus bipolar electrocoagulation for bleeding internal hemorrhoids. Gastrointest Endosc. 1993; 39(6):766–769

[56] Lord PH. A new regime for the treatment of haemorrhoids. Proc R Soc Med. 1968; 61(9):935–936

[57] Lord PH. Diverse methods of managing hemorrhoids: dilatation. Dis Colon Rectum. 1973; 16(3):180–183

[58] McCaffrey J. Lord treatment of haemorrhoids. Four-year follow-up of fifty patients. Lancet. 1975; 1(7899):133–134

[59] Allgower M. Conservative management of haemorrhoids, III: partial internal sphincterotomy. Clin Gastroenterol. 1975; 4:608–618

[60] Arabi Y, Gatehouse D, Alexander-Williams J, Keighley MR. Rubber band ligation or lateral subcutaneous sphincterotomy for treatment of haemorrhoids. Br J Surg. 1977; 64(10):737–740

[61] Schouten WR, van Vroonhoven TJ. Lateral internal sphincterotomy in the treatment of hemorrhoids. A clinical and manometric study. Dis Colon Rectum. 1986; 29(12):869–872

[62] Leong AFP, Husain MJ, Seow-Choen F, Goh HS. Performing internal sphincterotomy with other anorectal procedures. Dis Colon Rectum. 1994; 37(11):1130–1132

[63] Longo A. Treatment of hemorrhoidal disease by reduction of mucosa and hemorrhoidal prolapse with a circular suturing device: a new procedure. In: Proceedings of the 6th World Congress of Endoscopic Surgery; 1998; Rome. 777–784

[64] Esser S, Khubchandani I, Rakhmanine M. Stapled hemorrhoidectomy with local anesthesia can be performed safely and cost-efficiently. Dis Colon Rectum. 2004; 47(7):1164–1169

[65] Macrae HM, Teruple LKF, McLeod RS. A meta-analysis of hemorrhoidal treatments. Semin Colon Rectal Surg. 2002; 13:77–83

[66] Senagore AJ, Singer M, Abcarian H, et al. Procedure for Prolapse and Hemorrhoids (PPH) Multicenter Study Group. A prospective, randomized, controlled multicenter trial comparing stapled hemorrhoidopexy and Ferguson hemorrhoidectomy: perioperative and one-year results. Dis Colon Rectum. 2004; 47(11):1824–1836

[67] Peng BC, Jayne DG, Ho YH. Randomized trial of rubber band ligation vs. stapled hemorrhoidectomy for prolapsed piles. Dis Colon Rectum. 2003; 46(3):291–297, discussion 296–297

[68] Lehur PA, Didnée AS, Faucheron JL, et al. LigaLongo Study Group. Cost-effectiveness of New Surgical Treatments for Hemorrhoidal Disease: A Multicentre Randomized Controlled Trial Comparing Transanal Doppler-guided Hemorrhoidal Artery Ligation With Mucopexy and Circular Stapled Hemorrhoidopexy. Ann Surg. 2016; 264(5):710–716

[69] Aigner F, Kronberger I, Oberwalder M, et al. Doppler-guided haemorrhoidal artery ligation with suture mucopexy compared with suture mucopexy alone for the treatment of Grade III haemorrhoids: a prospective randomized controlled trial. Colorectal Dis. 2016; 18(7):710–716

[70] Wang GQ, Liu Y, Liu Q, et al. A meta-analysis on short and long term efficacy and safety of procedure for prolapse and hemorrhoids [in Chinese]. Zhonghua Wai Ke Za Zhi. 2013; 51(11):1034–1038

[71] Thaha MA, Irvine LA, Steele RJC, Campbell KL. Postdefaecation pain syndrome after circular stapled anopexy is abolished by oral nifedipine. Br J Surg. 2005; 92(2):208–210

[72] Morinaga K, Hasuda K, Ikeda T. A novel therapy for internal hemorrhoids: ligation of the hemorrhoidal artery with a newly devised instrument (Moricorn) in conjunction with a Doppler flowmeter. Am J Gastroenterol. 1995; 90(4):610–613

[73] Singer M. Hemorrhoids. In: Beck DE, Wexner SD, Roberts PL, Sacclarides TJ, Senagore A, Stamos M, eds. ASCRS Textbook of Colorectal Surgery. 2nd ed. New York, NY: Springer; 2011:175–202

[74] Giordano P, Overton J, Madeddu F, Zaman S, Gravante G. Transanal hemorrhoidal dearterialization: a systematic review. Dis Colon Rectum. 2009; 52(9):1665–1671

[75] Greenspon J, Williams SB, Young HA, Orkin BA. Thrombosed external hemorrhoids: outcome after conservative or surgical management. Dis Colon Rectum. 2004; 47(9):1493–1498

[76] Perrotti P, Antropoli C, Noschese G, et al. Topical Nifedipine(®) for conservative treatment of acute haemorrhoidal thrombosis. Colorectal Dis. 2000; 2(1):18–21

[77] Ferguson JA, Mazier WP, Ganchrow MI, Friend WG. The closed technique of hemorrhoidectomy. Surgery. 1971; 70(3):480–484

[78] Mazier WP, Halleran DR. Excisional hemorrhoidectomy. In: Kodner IJ, Fry RD, Roe JP, eds. Colon, Rectal, and Anal Surgery. St. Louis, MO: C.V. Mosby, Co.; 1985:3–14

[79] Ferguson JA, Heaton JR. Closed hemorrhoidectomy. Dis Colon Rectum. 1959; 2(2):176–179

[80] Cataldo PA, MacKeigan JM. The necessity of routine pathologic evaluation of hemorrhoidectomy specimens. Surg Gynecol Obstet. 1992; 174(4):302–304

[81] Milligan ETC, Morgan CN, Jones LE, Officer R. Surgical anatomy of the anal canal and the operative treatment of hemorrhoids. Lancet. 1937; 2:1119–1124

[82] Whitehead W. The surgical treatment of haemorrhoids. Br Med J. 1882; 1(1101):148–150

[83] Bonello JC. Who's afraid of the dentate line? The Whitehead hemorrhoidectomy. Am J Surg. 1988; 156(3, Pt 1):182–186

[84] Wolff BG, Culp CE. The Whitehead hemorrhoidectomy. An unjustly maligned procedure. Dis Colon Rectum. 1988; 31(8):587–590

[85] Seow-Choen F, Low HC. Prospective randomized study of radical versus four piles haemorrhoidectomy for symptomatic large circumferential prolapsed piles. Br J Surg. 1995; 82(2):188–189

[86] Patel N, O'Connor T. Suture haemorrhoidectomy: a day-only alternative. Aust N Z J Surg. 1996; 66(12):830–831

[87] Senagore A, Mazier WP, Luchtefeld MA, MacKeigan JM, Wengert T. Treatment of advanced hemorrhoidal disease: a prospective, randomized comparison of cold scalpel vs. contact Nd:YAG laser. Dis Colon Rectum. 1993; 36(11):1042–1049

[88] Wang JY, Chang-Chien CR, Chen JS, Lai CR, Tang RP. The role of lasers in hemorrhoidectomy. Dis Colon Rectum. 1991; 34(1):78–82

[89] Standards Task Force, American Society of Colon and Rectal Surgeons. Practice parameters for the treatment of hemorrhoids. Dis Colon Rectum. 1990; 33:7A–8A

[90] Nienhuijs S, de Hingh I. Conventional versus LigaSure hemorrhoidectomy for patients with symptomatic hemorrhoids. Cochrane Database Syst Rev. 2009; 21(1):CD006761

[91] Bulus H, Tas A, Coskun A, Kucukazman M. Evaluation of two hemorrhoidectomy techniques: harmonic scalpel and Ferguson's with electrocautery. Asian J Surg. 2014; 37(1):20–23

[92] Carapeti EA, Kamm MA, McDonald PJ, Phillips RK. Double-blind randomised controlled trial of effect of metronidazole on pain after day-case haemorrhoidectomy. Lancet. 1998; 351(9097):169–172

[93] Gottesman L, Milsom JW, Mazier WP. The use of anxiolytic and parasympathomimetic agents in the treatment of postoperative urinary retention following anorectal surgery. A prospective, randomized, double-blind study. Dis Colon Rectum. 1989; 32(10):867–880

[94] Goldstein ET, Williamson PR, Larach SW. Subcutaneous morphine pump for postoperative hemorrhoidectomy pain management. Dis Colon Rectum. 1993; 36(5):439–446

[95] Smith LE. Current therapy on colon and rectal surgery. In: Fazio VW, ed. Current Therapy in Colon and Rectal Surgery. Philadelphia, PA: B.C. Decker, Inc.; 1990:9–14

[96] Dean KI, Wong WD. Hemorrhoidal surgery. In: Hicks TC, Beck DE, Opelka FG, Timmcke AE, eds. Complications of Colon and Rectal Surgery. Baltimore, MD: Williams & Wilkins; 1997:163–172

[97] Buls JG, Goldberg SM. Modern management of hemorrhoids. Surg Clin North Am. 1978; 58(3):469–478

[98] Ganchrow MI, Mazier WP, Friend WG, Ferguson JA. Hemorrhoidectomy revisited–a computer analysis of 2,038 cases. Dis Colon Rectum. 1971; 14(2):128–133

[99] Nyam DCNK, Seow-Choen F, Ho YH. Submucosal adrenaline injection for posthemorrhoidectomy hemorrhage. Dis Colon Rectum. 1995; 38(7):776–777

[100] Gorfine SR, Onel E, Patou G, Krivokapic ZV. Bupivacaine extended-release liposome injection for prolonged postsurgical analgesia in patients undergoing hemorrhoidectomy: a multicenter, randomized, double-blind, placebo-controlled trial. Dis Colon Rectum. 2011; 54(12):1552–1559

[101] Beck DE, Margolin DA, Babin SF, Russo CT. Benefits of a multimodal regimen for postsurgical pain management in colorectal surgery. Ochsner J. 2015; 15(4):408–412

[102] Corman ML. Management of postoperative constipation in anorectal surgery. Dis Colon Rectum. 1979; 22(3):149–151

[103] Milsom JW, Mazier WP. Classification and management of postsurgical anal stenosis. Surg Gynecol Obstet. 1986; 163(1):60–64

[104] Granet E. Hemorrhoidectomy failures: causes, prevention and management. Dis Colon Rectum. 1968; 11(1):45–48

[105] Ferguson JA. Repair of Whitehead deformity of the anus. Surg Gynecol Obstet. 1959; 108(1):115–116

[106] Wexner SD. AIDS: What the colorectal surgeon needs to know. Perspect Colon Rectal Surg. 1989; 2:19–54

[107] Morandi E, Merlini D, Salvaggio A, Foschi D, Trabucchi E. Prospective study of healing time after hemorrhoidectomy: influence of HIV infection, acquired immunodeficiency syndrome, and anal wound infection. Dis Colon Rectum. 1999; 42(9):1140–1144

[108] Saleeby RG, Jr, Rosen L, Stasik JJ, Riether RD, Sheets J, Khubchandani IT. Hemorrhoidectomy during pregnancy: risk or relief? Dis Colon Rectum. 1991; 34(3):260–261

[109] Wolkomir AF, Luchtefeld MA. Surgery for symptomatic hemorrhoids and anal fissures in Crohn's disease. Dis Colon Rectum. 1993; 36(6):545–547

[110] Nivatvongs S. Alternative positioning of patients for hemorrhoidectomy. Dis Colon Rectum. 1980; 23(5):308–309

[111] Abramowitz L, Sobhani I, Benifla JL, et al. Anal fissure and thrombosed external hemorrhoids before and after delivery. Dis Colon Rectum. 2002; 45(5):650–655

[112] Grewal H, Guillem JG, Quan SHQ, Enker WE, Cohen AM. Anorectal disease in neutropenic leukemic patients. Operative vs. nonoperative management. Dis Colon Rectum. 1994; 37(11):1095–1099

[113] MacRae HM, McLeod RS. Comparison of hemorrhoidal treatment modalities. A meta-analysis. Dis Colon Rectum. 1995; 38(7):687–694

8 Fissure-In-Ano and Anal Stenosis

David J. Maron and Steven D. Wexner

Abstract

Fissure-in-ano, or anal fissure, is a linear ulcer in the anal canal extending from below the dentate line to the level of the anal verge. They can be acute or chronic, and often cause symptoms and suffering out of proportion to the size and extent of the lesion. Fissures are a common reason that patients visit a colorectal surgeon, and recurrence rates are high following spontaneous healing. Anal stenosis occurs due to a loss of the physiologic capacity of the anal canal. Stenosis develops when the normally pliable tissues of the anus are replaced with scarred, fibrotic tissue. Although anal stenosis may occur in some congenital syndromes, the overwhelming majority of cases are secondary in nature, most of which are due to surgical trauma.

Keywords: anal stenosis, anal fissure, fissure-in-ano, anal canal, scarring, surgical trauma

8.1 Fissure-In-Ano

Fissure-in-ano, or anal fissure, is a linear ulcer in the anal canal extending from below the dentate line to the level of the anal verge. They can be acute or chronic, and often cause symptoms and suffering out of proportion to the size and extent of the lesion. Fissures are a common reason that patients visit a colorectal surgeon, and recurrence rates are high following spontaneous healing.

8.1.1 Clinical Features

Fissures are more commonly encountered in younger and middle-aged adults, but may also occur in children and the elderly.[1] Both sexes are affected equally. Because many patients with acute fissures do not seek medical advice and improve without intervention, the exact incidence of fissures is not known. It has been suggested, however, that the lifetime incidence is 11%.[2]

The vast majority of fissures occur as a single tear in the midline. Most (75–90%) occur in the posterior midline. In a review of 876 patients with fissure-in-ano, Hananel and Gordon[3] found the equal sex distribution (women, 51.1%; men, 49.9%) with a mean age of 39.9 years. The fissure was located in the posterior midline in 73.5%, the anterior midline in 16.4%, and in both in 2.6%. The fissure was located in the anterior midline in 12.6% of women and 7.7% of men. Other authors have also found that anterior fissures occur more commonly in female patients.[4] Up to 10% of acute anal fissures occur in the postpartum period, and many of these are located in the anterior midline.[5] In patients presenting with fissure that occurs off the midline, other underlying conditions must be considered (▶ Fig. 8.1).

8.1.2 Pathology

Acute anal fissures appear as a longitudinal or elliptical tear in the mucosal lining of the anal canal. While many fissures will heal spontaneously or with conservative treatment, some show considerable reluctance to heal. When symptoms are present for more than 8 to 12 weeks, the fissure often develops chronic features. This may include edema of the distal end of the fissure, which results in a tag or "sentinel pile." The tag often has an inflamed, tense, and edematous appearance. Later, it may undergo fibrosis and persist as a permanent fibrous skin tag, even if the fissure heals. At the proximal end of the fissure at the level of the dentate line, swelling caused by edema and fibrosis may result in a hypertrophied anal papilla.

In longstanding cases, fibrous induration frequently develops in the lateral edges of the fissure. After several months without healing, the base of the ulcer, which is the internal sphincter, may become fibrosed, resulting in a spastic, fibrotic, tightly contracted internal sphincter. Infrequently, frank suppuration may occur and extend into the surrounding tissues, forming an intersphincteric or perianal abscess that may discharge through the anal canal or burst spontaneously externally and produce a low intersphincteric fistula. Usually, the external opening of this fistula is close to the midline and a short distance from the anus.

8.1.3 Etiology

The exact etiology of anal fissures is not completely understood; however, it is generally agreed that the initiating factor is trauma to the anal canal. This is often due to passage of a large or hard stool that tears the anal mucosa. In a case–control

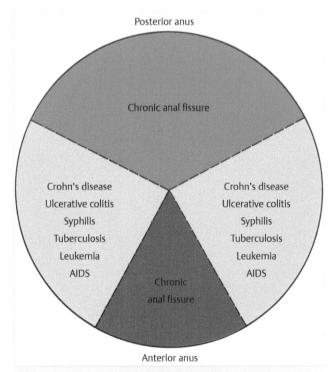

Fig. 8.1 Common locations of chronic anal fissure and other anal conditions.

study, Jensen[6] found evidence to indicate that anal fissure is likely to result at least partly from an inappropriate diet and that dietary manipulation might reduce the incidence. A significantly decreased risk was associated with frequent consumption of raw fruits, vegetables, and whole-grain bread, and a significantly increased risk was related to frequent consumption of white bread, sauces thickened with roux, and bacon or sausages. Risk ratios for consumption of coffee, tea, and alcohol were not significantly different.

While most patients with anal fissure report constipation and hard stool, fissures may also develop following a bout of diarrhea or frequent defecation. Individuals with a longstanding condition of loose stools, usually resulting from chronic laxative abuse, may develop an anal stenosis with scarring, again predisposing to fissure formation. Fissures may also occur in the postpartum period and are thought to be secondary to shearing forces from the fetus on the anal canal. Perineal trauma leads to scarring and abnormal tethering of the anal submucosa, thus rendering it more susceptible to trauma because of its loss of laxity and mobility.

Secondary fissures may occur as a result of either an anatomic anal abnormality or inflammatory bowel disease, particularly Crohn's disease.[7] When a fissure is encountered in a lateral location, the clinician should consider underlying inflammatory bowel disease or other inflammatory conditions such as tuberculosis, syphilis, and HIV infection. Previous anal surgery, especially hemorrhoidectomy, may result in anal scarring, skin loss, and stenosis. Fistula surgery may result in distortion of the anal canal with scarring and fixation of the anal skin. This decreased elasticity of the anal canal may then predispose to fissure formation. The presence of hemorrhoids is not likely a predisposing factor; it is more likely that an abnormality of the internal sphincter predisposes the patient to the formation of both hemorrhoids and fissures.

8.1.4 Pathogenesis

Many patients who suffer from an acute anal fissure will heal without any or with minimal intervention. If the concept that trauma to the anal canal is the initiating factor in the establishment of a fissure-in-ano is accepted, then why certain fissures proceed to and persist in a chronic state must be asked. Perpetuating factors might include infection, for example, but it is unlikely since sepsis is no more common in chronic fissures than in acute fissures. Persistently hard or large bowel movements, in addition to initiating the process, may continuously aggravate the anal canal and result in perpetuation of the fissure. This factor must be taken into account when planning treatment.

Studies have demonstrated that after the initiation of a tear in the anal canal, chronicity is perpetuated by an abnormality in the internal anal sphincter. Most investigators have found that resting pressures within the internal anal sphincter are higher in patients with fissures than in normal controls.[8,9,10,11,12,13,14,15,16] Nothmann and Schuster[13] demonstrated that after rectal distention there is a normal reflex relaxation of the internal sphincter. In patients with anal fissures, this relaxation is followed by an abnormal "overshoot" contraction. This may explain the pain that results from rectal stimulation during defecation and account for the sphincter spasm found in most patients with anal fissure. Furthermore, the authors demonstrated that after successful treatment of the fissure, the abnormal reflex contraction of the internal sphincter vanishes, a finding confirmed by others.[17]

Keck et al[11] were not able to identify an overshoot contraction but did demonstrate hypertonic contraction of the internal sphincter. Several authors[9,15,17] have reported a significant reduction in mean resting pressure within the internal sphincter following lateral sphincterotomy and that the results persist for up to 1 year. Adequate internal sphincterotomy appears to permanently reduce anal canal pressure, which suggests that abnormal activity in the sphincter contributes to the development and persistence of a fissure. Farouk et al[10] found that following lateral internal sphincterotomy the number of internal sphincter relaxations increased, lending further evidence to the hypothesis that internal sphincter hypertonia may be relevant to the pathogenesis of this disorder. Abcarian et al[8] have suggested that the beneficial effect of internal sphincterotomy might be due to the anatomic widening of the anal canal, a concept supported by Olsen et al,[18] who failed to find a reduction in resting pressures after lateral sphincterotomy. Xynos et al[16] also found that following internal sphincterotomy, preoperative elevated resting pressures returned to normal. Patients with unhealed fissures showed the same pathologic manometric features as those before operation.

It has also been hypothesized that an inverse relationship exists between anal canal pressure and perfusion of the anoderm. This was first suggested by Gibbons and Read,[19] who documented increased resting pressures within the anal canal, whereas maximal pressures recorded during a voluntary contraction of the sphincter were no higher than in control subjects. They noted that it was unlikely that high resting pressures recorded in patients with chronic anal fissures were caused by spasm but probably represented a true increase in basal sphincter tone. They further proposed that elevated sphincter pressures may cause ischemia of the anal lining, resulting in the pain of anal fissures and failure to heal.

In an effort to define perfusion of the anal canal, Klosterhalfen et al[20] performed angiography of the inferior rectal artery in a cadaver model. The authors demonstrated that in 85% of specimens, the posterior commissure is less perfused than the remainder of the anal canal, and postulated that this finding may play a role in the pathogenesis of fissure-in-ano. They also suggested that vessels passing through the sphincter muscle are subject to compression during periods of increased sphincter tone and that the resulting decrease in blood supply might lead to ischemia at the posterior commissure. In a landmark study, Schouten et al[21] used laser Doppler flowmetry to study perfusion of the anoderm in healthy subjects and demonstrated that perfusion of the posterior anal canal was lower than the rest of the anus. In addition, patients with fissure were evaluated and were found to have elevated mean maximum anal resting pressure and significantly lower anodermal blood flow at the fissure site when compared with flow at the posterior commissure of the healthy subjects. Both measurements were repeated 6 weeks after lateral internal sphincterotomy and compared with the measurements of the controls. In the patients with fissures, a significant decrease in resting pressure was noted (35%) that was accompanied by a consistent rise in blood flow (65%) at the previous fissure site. It is therefore believed that reduction of anal pressure by sphincterotomy improves anodermal blood flow at the posterior midline, resulting in fissure healing.

A primary internal anal sphincter disturbance may also be an etiologic factor. Internal anal smooth muscle relaxation occurs with stimulation of the β-adrenoreceptor, which induces the return of cytosolic calcium to the sarcoplasmic reticulum via cyclic adenosine monophosphate. Internal anal sphincter supersensitivity to β2 (beta-2) agonists has been observed in patients with chronic anal fissure.[22] Relaxation is also induced by nonadrenergic noncholinergic nitric oxide (NO), which is mediated via cyclic guanosine monophosphate (cGMP).[22,23] Sphincter contraction depends on an increase in cytoplasmic calcium and is enhanced by sympathetic adrenergic stimulation. Blocking direct influx of extracellular calcium through the membranes of the calcium channels may help inhibit contraction.

8.1.5 Symptoms

The most common symptom of a fissure is anal pain during and after defecation. Patients will often describe the pain as a sharp, cutting, "knifelike," or tearing sensation during the passage of stool. Following defecation, the pain may be less severe and may be described as a burning or gnawing discomfort that may persist from a few minutes to several hours. Because of the anticipated pain, many patients may not defecate when the natural urge occurs. Such procrastination leads to harder stools, causing subsequent bowel movements to be more painful. A relentless cycle may ensue with the individual living from one bowel movement to the next.

Bleeding is very common with fissure but is not invariably present. The blood is typically bright red and is usually seen after wiping or may coat the outside of the stool. Some patients have a large sentinel pile and present complaining of a painful external hemorrhoid. Perianal itch is also very common in patients with fissure. Constipation is often an accompanying symptom as well as an initiating symptom of anal fissure. Infrequently, patients with an acutely painful fissure can develop urinary symptoms including dysuria, retention, or frequency.

8.1.6 Diagnosis

Examination

The diagnosis of a fissure is usually straightforward and is often made from the patient's history alone. Physical examination confirms the suspicion of fissure and rules out other associated disease. The association between fissures and inflammatory bowel disease should always be remembered, and a careful history should be taken and followed, if indicated, by appropriate radiologic, hematologic, and biochemical investigations.

Inspection is the most important step in the examination for anal fissure (▶ Fig. 8.2). Because anal fissures are such extremely painful lesions, special care must be taken to make the examination as gentle as possible. Careful separation of the buttocks usually reveals the fissure; however, patient apprehension and involuntary spasm of the sphincter may keep the anal orifice closed. The coexistence of large hemorrhoids or skin folds may also hide the ulcer, and when the lesion cannot be visualized, the diagnosis may be made more by history and palpation than by visual appearance.

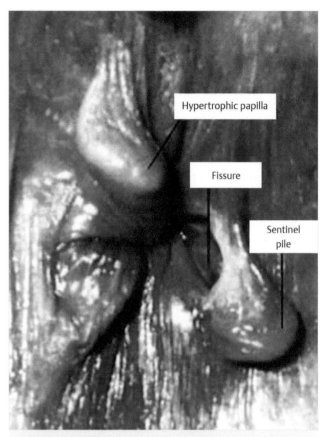

Fig. 8.2 A chronic posterior anal fissure with skin tag and hypertrophied anal papilla.

In patients with acute anal fissure, palpation often confirms the presence of sphincter spasm. The digital examination is uncomfortable, with maximal tenderness usually elicited in the posterior midline. If the diagnosis of fissure is made by inspection, digital examination may be omitted as the pain may be so intense. However, it is essential that the examination be performed at a later date to exclude other lesions of the lower rectum such as carcinoma or a polyp. With an acute fissure, anoscopic examination is usually impossible because of the severe pain.

The triad of a chronic fissure includes a sentinel pile, an anal ulcer, and a hypertrophied anal papilla. The sentinel pile is visible externally, and can sometimes be very large. The ulcer is often deep, with fibers of the internal anal sphincter visible at the base and induration of the base and the lateral edges. Just proximal to the ulcer, the hypertrophied anal papilla may be identified. A chronic fissure may be associated with anal stenosis of varying severity, especially if the patient has had a previous anal surgery such as a hemorrhoidectomy. Although there is no specific duration that defines a fissure as chronic, evaluation of the chronicity of the process is important. Once the entire internal sphincter is bared with scarring and fibrosis, and the history of problems is longstanding, the fissure is unlikely to heal without surgical intervention. Patients with chronic anal fissure tend to have less pain, which may permit anoscopy to rule out other conditions such as internal hemorrhoids or proctitis.

Sigmoidoscopy likewise may be impossible to perform during the initial examination, but it must be performed at a subsequent visit (or colonoscopy) to rule out an associated carcinoma or inflammatory bowel disease.

A biopsy should be performed on any fissure that fails to heal after treatment. Such biopsy may reveal unsuspected Crohn's disease or an implanted adenocarcinoma. Squamous carcinoma of the anal canal may also be confused with fissure-in-ano.

Differential Diagnosis

Anal pain, swelling, and bleeding are common complaints that prompt evaluation by a colorectal surgeon. Many conditions may result in symptoms similar to those of a fissure. Thrombosed hemorrhoids or perianal abscesses are readily seen; however, certain other conditions may require more careful discrimination.

Anorectal Suppuration

Symptoms of an intersphincteric abscess may closely mimic those of a fissure. An intersphincteric fistulous abscess without an external opening is usually situated posteriorly in the mid-anal canal between the internal and external sphincter. It causes great pain that may last for many hours after defecation. A diagnostic clue that may help to identify an intersphincteric abscess is that unlike with a fissure, the pain associated with an abscess often does not completely go away. Little, if anything, is seen externally, but during the examination exquisite tenderness will be elicited over the abscess, which itself may not be palpable.

Pruritus Ani

Discerning pruritus ani with superficial cracks in the anal skin from anal fissure may sometimes prove difficult as many patients with anal fissure develop pruritus as a result of the discharge irritating the perianal skin. The skin in pruritus ani, however, shows only superficial cracks extending radially from the anus, and these cracks never extend up to the dentate line. Therefore, digital examination of the rectum does not elicit pain, and there is no true anal spasm or tenderness as seen in patients with fissure.

Fissures in Patients with Inflammatory Bowel Disease

Anal fissures may develop in patients with ulcerative colitis. These fissures are often situated off the midline and may be multiple. As well as being broad, the fissures are surrounded by inflamed skin. This inflammation should alert the surgeon to an associated proctocolitis, which can be diagnosed by sigmoidoscopy or colonoscopy.

Anal and perianal ulceration frequently occurs in patients with Crohn's disease. The ulcer seen in Crohn's is often much more extensive than an idiopathic fissure, and again may occur off the midline. Despite the opinion of some authors, Crohn's fissures are not always painless. If a lesion is suspect, biopsy frequently reveals the histologic features of Crohn's disease. Evaluation of the entire gastrointestinal tract is necessary, as sigmoidoscopy alone may, in fact, be normal because the involved intestine may be more proximal.

Anal Carcinoma

Squamous cell carcinoma of the anus or adenocarcinoma of the rectum may involve the anal skin, and patients may present with anal pain and bleeding. Palpation, however, may detect a greater degree of induration, and a biopsy of any suspect lesion along with endoscopic evaluation of the colon should be performed.

Specific Infectious Perianal Conditions

Syphilitic fissures may be caused by either primary chancres or condylomata lata. In its initial stage, a chancre may closely resemble an ordinary fissure but subsequently develops significant induration at its margin, and inguinal lymph nodes become enlarged. History of anoreceptive intercourse, location of the fissure off the midline, and a more external location away from the anal verge or internally above the dentate line help distinguish these lesions from idiopathic anal fissures. In addition, patients with syphilitic fissures may have multiple lesions that have irregular borders and appear opposite one another in a mirror image ("kissing"). Suspect lesions can be diagnosed by a dark-field examination. Anal condylomata lata may occur at the anal orifice, as well as in the perianal region, and may cause multiple anal fissures.

A tuberculous ulcer in the anal region is rare. When it occurs, it tends to enlarge and develop undermined edges. Differentiating this lesion from Crohn's disease may be very difficult; however, the tuberculous ulcer is often associated with pulmonary tuberculosis. Performing a biopsy may be necessary. If the fissure remains after antituberculous chemotherapy has been administered, treatment is the same as with an idiopathic fissure.

8.1.7 Treatment

Acute Fissure

Avoidance of constipation is probably the single most important nonoperative treatment. The aim of treatment of an acute fissure-in-ano is to break the cycle of a hard stool, pain, and reflex spasm. This result often can be accomplished with simple measures such as addition of bulk-forming agents, increase in water intake, and warm baths to help relieve the sphincter spasm. Ingestion of bulk-forming foods (e.g., adequate amounts of unprocessed bran) or stool softeners such as psyllium seed preparations can be used to create a soft stool that hopefully will not further tear the anal canal. In addition, a large bulky stool may result in physiologic dilatation of the anal sphincter. Warm sitz baths several times a day as well as following bowel movements may help with symptomatic relief and may result in relaxation of the sphincter muscles.[24]

Shub et al[25] followed 393 patients with fissure-in-ano for 5 years and found that 44% healed within 4 to 8 weeks with nonoperative treatment consisting of an emollient suppository, a psyllium seed preparation, and sitz baths. The recurrence rate was 27%, and one-third of those lesions healed after further nonoperative treatment. Hananel and Gordon[3] reviewed 876 patients who presented with fissure-in-ano with a mean follow-up of 26 months (range, 0.5–215 months). Forty-four percent of patients responded to nonoperative therapy (consisting of bulk-forming agents and sitz baths), 62.4% of them in the first 2 months. Recurrent symptoms developed in 18.6% of patients whose fissures healed; 60% responded to further medical therapy. Of the patients who initially did not respond to medical treatment, lateral internal sphincterotomy was recommended. The authors found that of those patients that responded to nonoperative treatment, there was an increase in healing rates from 62.4% at 2 months to 86.2% at 6 months. Therefore, depending upon the severity of the patient's symptoms, it may be worthwhile to continue medical treatment for up to 6 months if the patient demonstrates steady improvement.

In a double-blind, placebo-controlled trial, Jensen[26] found that the use of unprocessed bran in doses of 5 g three times per day resulted in a decreased recurrence rate. Patients were randomized to receive three daily doses of a placebo or unprocessed bran at 2.5- or 5-g doses. After a 1-year follow-up, the recurrence rate in patients receiving 5 g of bran was 16%, 60% in patients receiving 2.5 g, and 68% in the placebo group ($p < 0.01$). Patients in this study were also followed for 6 months after therapy was stopped. Recurrent fissures developed in 25% of patients, suggesting that maintenance therapy of fiber should be continued for life.

Topical anesthetic agents and hydrocortisone have also been used in the treatment of acute anal fissures. In a prospective trial, patients with acute fissure were randomized into one of three treatment categories: lidocaine ointment, hydrocortisone ointment, or warm sitz baths combined with an intake of unprocessed bran.[27] After 1 and 2 weeks of treatment, symptomatic relief was significantly better among patients treated with sitz baths and bran than among patients in the other treatment arms. After 3 weeks, there was no significant difference in symptomatic relief among the three groups, but patients treated with lidocaine had significantly fewer healed fissures (60%) than did patients treated with hydrocortisone (82.4%) or warm sitz baths and bran (87%).

Chronic Anal Fissure

A fissure that persists for at least 6 to 8 weeks is typically considered a chronic fissure. Unlike acute fissures, the majority of chronic fissures will not heal spontaneously or with conservative treatment.[1] In fact, a recent Cochrane review of 70 randomized trials of nonoperative treatment for chronic anal fissure demonstrated a combined healing rate in the placebo group of only 35%.[28] Anatomic features of chronicity include exposure of the internal sphincter at the base of the fissure, induration of the fissure edges, development of a large sentinel pile, and hypertrophied anal papilla. Lock and Thomson[2] reported that once these features were present, it was unlikely that spontaneous healing will occur and early recognition of these associated problems was very important for the institution of the correct treatment.

Sphincter Relaxants

Because of the relationship between hypertonicity of the anal sphincter and anal fissure, pharmacologic therapies have been used to create a reversible reduction in sphincter pressure until the fissure has healed. Topical agents include nitroglycerin and calcium channel blockers (diltiazem or nifedipine) that aim to cause relaxation of the muscle, and injectable botulinum toxin

that results in chemical denervation of the muscle. A wide variation of results have been reported with the use of these agents, in part due to the fact that some studies have included acute fissures, some chronic fissures, and often both. The dosage of medication, the frequency of administration of the medication, and the length of follow-up also account for the wide variation of results.

Nitroglycerin

Nitric oxide is the principal nonadrenergic, noncholinergic neurotransmitter mediating neurogenic relaxation of the internal sphincter. Glyceryl trinitrate (GTN) acts as a nitric oxide donor that promotes healing of anal fissure by two mechanisms. Nitric oxide stimulates guanylate cyclase, leading to formation of cGMP, which in turn activates protein kinases that then dephosphorylate myosin light chains, resulting in muscle fiber relaxation.[23] When applied as a topical ointment, it diffuses across the skin barrier and causes a reduction in internal sphincter pressure as well as improving anodermal blood flow through its vasodilatory effect on the anal vessels.

Studies have shown that GTN effectively reduces mean resting anal pressure.[29,30,31] In a controlled trial, Loder et al[30] demonstrated a significant reduction in anal sphincter pressure from the topical application of 0.2% GTN, a finding confirmed by others.[32] Lund and Scholefield[31] conducted a prospective randomized double-blind, placebo-controlled study to determine the efficacy of topical GTN 0.2% applied twice a day. After 8 weeks, healing was observed in 68% of patients compared to 8% of controls, and maximum anal resting pressures fell significantly from 115.9 to 75.9 cm H_2O in the treatment group. Schouten et al[33] evaluated the influence of the topical application of isosorbide dinitrate on anal anodermal blood flow and fissure healing. Before treatment and at 3 and 6 weeks, 22 patients underwent conventional anal manometry and laser Doppler flowmetry of the anoderm. Maximum resting anal pressures were significantly reduced, there was a significant increase in anodermal blood flow, and fissure healing occurred in 88% of patients at 12 weeks.

McLeod and Evans[34] reviewed the literature with respect to the use of nitroglycerin in the management of patients with anal fissure. A total of nine randomized controlled trials have studied the efficacy of GTN in chronic anal fissure. In four out of five trials, GTN was significantly more effective than placebo in healing fissures.[29,31,32,35,36] The healing rates in the GTN group varied from 46 to 70% and healing in the placebo group ranged from 8 to 51%. Two trials have reported results of long-term follow-up with symptomatic recurrence rates ranging from 27 to 62%.[29,37] Three trials compared 0.2 to 0.5% GTN to lateral sphincterotomy.[38,39,40] Sphincterotomy was superior in two of these trials.

Conflicting results with the use of GTN have been reported in the literature with respect to healing rate, recurrence rate, and side effects (▶ Table 8.1). Differences in reported healing rates may relate to the difficulty in administering a standardized dose to all patients. Most published studies of topical GTN have used 0.2 to 0.3% preparations. Dosing frequencies varied from two to three times a day and durations varied from 4 to 8 weeks. Healing rates may well be affected by alteration of any of these dosing variables.

Table 8.1 Use of glyceryl trinitrate in treatment of anal fissure

Author	Year	n	Dose	Frequency	Follow-up (in months)	Healing rate	Recurrence rate	Side effects
Bacher et al[36]	1997	20	0.20%	Thrice daily	1	80%	–	20%
Lund and Scholefield[31]	1997	38	0.20%	Twice daily	2	68%	–	58%
Oettlé[39]	1997	12	–	–	22	83%	0%	–
Lysy et al[41]	1998	41	1.25–2.5 mg	Thrice daily	11	83%	15%	–
Brisinda et al[42]	1999	50	0.20%	Twice daily	15	60%	–	10%
Carapeti et al[32]	1999	70	0.1–0.6%	Thrice daily	–	67%	33%	72%
Dorfman et al[43]	1999	31	0.20%	Twice daily	6	56%	27%	78%
Hyman and Cataldo[44]	1999	33	0.30%	Thrice daily	–	48%	–	75%
Jonas et al[45]	1999	49	0.20%	Twice daily	1.5	43%	2%	4%
Kennedy et al[29]	1999	43	0.20%	–	29	46–59%	63%	29%
Altomare et al[35]	2000	59	0.20%	Twice daily	12	49%	19%	34%
Richard et al[40]	2000	44	0.25%	Thrice daily	6	27%	38%	84%
Evans et al[38]	2001	33	0.20%	Thrice daily	–	61%	45%	–
Gecim[46]	2001	30	0.30%	Thrice daily	18	80%	25%	7%
Graziano et al[47]	2001	22	0.25%	Twice daily	0.5–12	77%	53%	–
Pitt et al[48]	2001	64	0.20%	–	16	41%	46%	–
Bailey et al[49]	2002	304	0.1–0.4%	Twice daily to thrice daily	2	50%	–	3%
Kocher et al[50]	2002	29	0.20%	Twice daily	2	86%	7%	72%
Parellada[51]	2004	27	0.20%	Thrice daily	24	89%	11%	30%
Gagliardi et al[52]	2010	153	0.40%	Twice daily	–	58%	–	23%
Pérez-Legaz et al[53]	2012	52	0.40%	Twice daily	6	77%	–	15%

The major drawback of treatment with GTN is that a significant proportion of patients experience adverse effects. The high incidence of side effects interferes with quality of life and may result in poor patient compliance. Headaches are the primary adverse event and have been reported in 29 to 72% of patients.[29,32] Most were transient (lasting roughly 15 minutes) and dose related, and only 3 to 20% of patients discontinued treatment because of headaches.[29,31,39] Educating patients prior to initiation of treatment, beginning with a lower dose and escalating over several days, using a glove during application to avoid absorption through the skin of the finger, and remaining in a recumbent position for 15 minutes after application may help to reduce symptoms.[54,55]

Pitt et al[48] conducted a study to identify factors associated with treatment failure of GTN. The authors cited risk factors of constipation, recent childbirth, colonoscopy, and anal receptive intercourse. Fissures in patients who had an associated sentinel pile were significantly less likely to heal initially, more likely to recur, and more likely to remain unhealed in the long term. Fissures with a history of more than 6 months were also less likely to heal initially.

Although GTN is effective in healing one-half to two-thirds of patients with chronic anal fissure, long-term follow-up symptoms may recur in 15 to 63% (▶ Table 8.1). The risk of long-term recurrence, in addition to poor patient compliance, has diminished the role of nitrates in the treatment of anal fissure. In addition, randomized trials have demonstrated that GTN is inferior to both botulinum toxin[42] and lateral internal sphincterotomy in providing symptomatic relief and fissure healing.[38,40]

Calcium Channel Blockers

Calcium channel blockers inhibit voltage-dependent calcium channels within the plasma membrane of electrically excitable muscle cells. This results in a decrease in the calcium ion concentration within the sarcoplasmic reticulum, which interferes with calcium-mediated signal transduction and phosphorylation. This disruption decreases contraction of the muscle cells and results in relaxation of the muscle fibers.[23] Both diltiazem and nifedepine have been used in the treatment of chronic anal fissures.

Nifedipine, a dihydropyridine, is a calcium antagonist that causes smooth muscle relaxation and vasodilatation. Chrysos et al[56] demonstrated that anal resting pressure was reduced by 30% following a sublingual dose of 20 mg. Other studies have also demonstrated a reduction in mean resting pressures between 21 and 36% in healthy volunteers[57,58,59] and 11 to 36% in patients with fissures.[57,59,60] Topical application has also been shown to lower resting pressure, relieve pain, and heal acute fissures.[57] Perrotti et al[60] performed a prospective randomized double-blind study in 110 patients to test the efficacy of local application of nifedipine and lidocaine ointment in healing chronic anal fissure. Patients treated with nifedipine used topical 0.3% nifedipine and 1.5% lidocaine ointment every 12 hours for 6 weeks. The control group received topical 1.5% lidocaine and 1% hydrocortisone acetate ointment during therapy. After a median follow-up of 18 months, healing of chronic anal fissure was achieved after 6 weeks of therapy in 94.5% of the nifedipine-treated patients in comparison to 16.4% of the controls. Mean anal resting pressure decreased by 11%. Recurrence of the fissure was observed in 3 of 52 patients in the nifedipine group within 1 year of treatment, and 2 of these patients healed with an additional course of topical nifedipine ointment. Antropoli et al[57] showed very similar results.

Ezri and Susmallian compared the use of 0.2% topical nifedipine to 0.2% topical GTN.[61] Healing of fissures was higher in the nifedipine group (89 vs. 58%) and side effects of headache and flushing were lower (5 vs 40%). Recurrence rates were similar between the two groups. Results with the use of nifedipine in the treatment of fissure-in-ano both in the cream form and in the oral form are noted in ▶ Table 8.2.

Diltiazem is another calcium channel blocker that reduces resting anal sphincter pressures. This agent was introduced because of the previously noted side effects of the topical GTN. Jonas et al[66] evaluated the efficacy of diltiazem for fissures that failed to heal with GTN. Diltiazem 2% was applied twice daily for 8 weeks or until the fissure healed. Fissures healed in 49% of patients within 8 weeks. Side effects occurred in 10% of patients and included perianal itching, but they continued with treatment as they were generally well tolerated. Knight et al[67] treated 71 patients with 2% diltiazem gel and reported healing in 75% of these patients. Carapeti et al[58] compared the use of diltiazem 2% with 0.1% bethanechol thrice daily. Fissures healed in 67% of patients with diltiazem and 60% of those treated with 0.1% bethanechol gel. Both diltiazem and bethanechol substantially reduced anal sphincter pressure and achieved fissure healing in a similar degree reported with topical nitrates but without side effects. Results with the use of diltiazem are listed in ▶ Table 8.3.

Jonas et al[74] further assessed the effectiveness of oral versus topical diltiazem in the healing of chronic fissures. Healing was noted to be complete in 38% of patients who received 60 mg of oral diltiazem compared to 65% of those receiving 2% topical gel. Oral diltiazem caused side effects of headaches, nausea, vomiting, and reduced smell and taste, whereas no side effects were seen in those receiving topical therapy. The authors concluded that topical diltiazem is more effective, achieving healing rates comparable to those reported with topical nitrates with significantly fewer side effects. Kocher et al[50] conducted a prospective double-blind randomized trial to compare the incidence of side effects with 0.2% GTN ointment and 2% DTZ cream in the treatment of chronic anal fissure. Treatments were applied perianally, twice daily for 6 to 8 weeks. There were more side effects with GTN (72%) than with DTZ (42%). In particular, more headaches occurred with GTN (59%).

Botulinum Toxin

Botulinum toxin, a product of clostridium botulinum, is an endopeptidase that blocks acetylcholine release at the neuromuscular junction, producing a potent neuromuscular blockade.[75] It does not block storage or synthesis of acetylcholine, but interferes with its delivery by blocking vesicle transport.[23] Once injected into the neuromuscular junction, paralysis occurs within hours, and its effect persists for 3 to 4 months until axonal regeneration occurs with formation of new nerve terminals.[1] While the effect of botulinum toxin on skeletal muscle fibers is well documented, the exact mechanism of the toxin on smooth muscle is unclear, as these fibers lack neuromuscular synapses. Despite this, injection of botulinum toxin into the internal sphincter (smooth muscle) is associated with sphincter relaxation and improvement in blood flow.[76,77]

Table 8.2 Use of nifedipine in treatment of anal fissure

Author	Year	n	Dose	Frequency	Follow-up (in months)	Healing rate	Recurrence rate	Side effects
Antropoli et al[57]	1999	141	0.2% cream	Twice daily	1	95%	–	–
Cook et al[59]	1999	15	25 mg orally	Twice daily	2	60%	–	–
Perrotti et al[60]	2002	55	0.3% + 1.5% lidocaine	Twice daily	18	95%	6%	–
Ansaloni et al[62]	2002	21	6 mg orally	Daily	2	90%	–	33%
Ezri and Susmallian[61]	2003	26	0.5%	Twice daily	6	89%	42%	5%
Ağaoğlu et al[63]	2003	10	20 mg orally	Twice daily	–	50%	–	10%
Ho and Ho[64]	2005	41	20 mg orally	Twice daily	4	17%	10%	–
Golfam et al[65]	2010	60	0.5%	Twice daily	12	70%	26%	–

Table 8.3 Use of diltiazem in treatment of anal fissure

Author	Year	n	Dose	Frequency	Follow-Up (in months)	Healing rate	Recurrence rate	Side effects
Carapeti et al[58]	2000	15	2%	Thrice daily	–	67%	–	–
Knight et al[67]	2001	71	2%	Twice daily	8	88%	34%	3%
Jonas et al[66]	2001	39	2%	Twice daily	–	49%	–	10%
Kocher et al[50]	2002	31	2%	Twice daily	3	77%	0%	42%
DasGupta et al[68]	2002	23	2%	Thrice daily	3	48%	0%	0%
Bielecki and Kolodziejczak[69]	2003	22	2%	Twice daily	2	86%	–	0%
Shrivastava et al[70]	2007	31	2%	Twice daily	–	80%	12%	0%
Sanei et al[71]	2009	51	2%	Twice daily	–	66%	–	–
Jawaid et al[72]	2009	40	2%	Twice daily	–	77%	–	32%
Ala et al[73]	2012	36	2%	Twice daily	–	91%	–	0%

Table 8.4 Use of botulinum toxin in treatment of anal fissure

Author	Year	n	Dose	Follow-up (in months)	Healing rate	Recurrence rate	Temporary incontinence
Jost[78]	1997	100	2.5–5.0 units	6	79%	8%	7%
Fernández López et al[79]	1999	76	80 units	–	67%	–	3%
González Carro et al[80]	1999	40	15 units	6	50%	–	–
Maria et al[81]	2000	50	40 units	–	60%	–	0%
Gecim[46]	2001	27	5 units	18	86%	25%	–
Brisinda et al[82]	2002	75	30 units	2	96%	4%	3%
Menteş et al[75]	2003	61	30 units	12	75%	11%	–
Arroyo et al[83]	2005	40	25 units	36	45%	–	0%
Massoud et al[84]	2005	25	25 units	6	60%	20%	–
Iswariah et al[85]	2005	17	20 units	26	41%	53%	0%
De Nardi et al[86]	2006	15	20 units	6	57%	33%	0%
Brisinda et al[87]	2007	50	30 units	20	92%	20%	6%
Festen et al[88]	2009	37	20 units	6	38%	13%	5%
Nasr et al[89]	2010	40	20 units	6	62%	40%	0%
Samim et al[90]	2012	60	20 units	39	43%	39%	5%
Berkel et al[91]	2014	27	60 units	2	66%	28%	–

Many authors have reported on the use of botulinum toxin in the treatment of fissure-in-ano and their results are summarized in ▶ Table 8.4. Temporary incontinence has been reported between 0 and 12%, with complications ranging 0 to 11% and recurrence rates 0 to 52%.[42] Varied dose regimens, different injection sites, and follow-up protocols make the data difficult to interpret.

In a comparison study of injection of botulinum toxin and topical GTN ointment for the treatment of chronic anal fissure, Brisinda et al[42] found botulinum toxin more effective (96% vs. 60% healing rate). In a follow-up study,[87] the authors randomized 100 patients to receive either 30 U of botulinum toxin or 0.2% GTN three times daily for 8 weeks. The healing rate in the GTN group in this study was 70%, compared with a healing rate of 90% in the botulinum toxin group. Sixteen nonhealing fissures in both groups (4 botulinum toxin and 16 GTN) underwent cross-over therapy, and all healed. Seven fissures relapsed in the GTN group, whereas all healed in the botulinum toxin group.

Minguez et al[92] analyzed the long-term outcome of patients in whom an anal fissure had healed after botulinum toxin injection and the factors contributing to recurrence. After 42 months of follow-up, recurrence developed in 42% of the 57 patients in whom the fissures had initially healed. Statistical differences between the permanently healed and the relapsed group were detected when analyzing the anterior location of the fissure (6 vs. 45%), a longer duration of disease (38 vs. 68%), the need for reinjection (26 vs. 59%), a higher total dose injected to achieve definitive healing (13 vs. 45%), and the percentage decrease of maximum squeeze pressure after injection (–28 vs. –13%).

Patients who fail to heal their anal fissure with a single modality may benefit from combination therapy. Lysy et al[93] evaluated 30 patients who had previously failed to heal with isosorbide dinitrate (ISDN). Patients were randomized to receive either ISDN (2.5 mg three times daily for 3 months) plus injection of 20 U of botulinum toxin or botulinum toxin injection alone. The authors found that ISDN application induced a greater reduction in the resting pressure of the anal sphincter following botulinum toxin injection than when the toxin was used alone. Healing rates at 12 weeks were similar between the groups at 60 and 66%. In a randomized controlled trial, Jones et al[94] compared the use of botulinum toxin alone or in combination therapy with GTN. There was a nonsignificant trend to better outcomes in the combination group compared with botulinum toxin alone in terms of fissure healing (47 vs. 27%), symptomatic improvement (87 vs. 67%), and the need for surgery (27 vs. 47%).

Combining botulinum toxin with surgery has also been reported. Lindsey et al[95] treated 30 patients who failed single therapy (19 GTN and 11 botulinum toxin) with botulinum toxin injection combined with fissurectomy. At a median follow-up of 16 weeks, 93% of patients healed their fissure and the remaining 7% reported an improvement in their symptoms. For patients who have failed to heal following lateral internal sphincterotomy, use of botulinum toxin may also be of use. Brisinda et al[96] treated 80 patients with persistent fissure following sphincterotomy with injection of 30 U of botulinum toxin and found that 74% of these patients healed at 2 months. Those patients who failed were treated with 50 U and all healed. Ten percent of patients treated in this study reported incontinence to flatus; however, symptoms were transient and resolved spontaneously.

Many trials have compared injection of botulinum toxin with lateral internal sphincterotomy in patients with fissure that have failed to heal with medical therapy. In a randomized controlled study of 80 patients, Arroyo et al[83] evaluated treatment outcomes and manometric investigations in patients undergoing botulinum toxin or sphincterotomy. Healing rates were significantly higher in the surgery group (92 vs. 45%); however, the authors commented that treatment with botulinum toxin remained their preference due to the increased risk of incontinence following surgery, particularly in patients over the age of 50. Chen et al[97] conducted a meta-analysis of 489 patients in seven randomized controlled trials comparing botulinum toxin to internal sphincterotomy. Patients undergoing lateral internal sphincterotomy had a higher healing rate, but the rates of incontinence were also higher. Patients treated with lateral internal sphincterotomy also had a significantly lower recurrence rate than the patients treated with botulinum toxin injection.

8.1.8 Surgical Treatment

Operative repair of a fissure-in-ano is indicated when the fissure does not respond to medical management and the patient has persistent pain and bleeding after 6 to 8 weeks of treatment. The surgical approach relies on similar principles used in medical management: reversing hypertonia of the sphincter and improving perfusion of the anal mucosa. Surgical options include anal dilation and sphincterotomy for fissures without a significant papilla, and fissurectomy or V–Y anoplasty for fissures with a significant external component or other associated anal conditions.

Anal Dilation

Recamier[98] is credited with first describing anal dilation, and the procedure was championed by Lord[99] for various forms of anorectal disease. This technique involves the forceful stretching of the anal sphincter with as many as six or eight fingers. The effect on the internal and external sphincters is to produce a temporary paralysis, usually lasting several days or a week, and there may be some incontinence during this time. Because of the nature of the procedure, sphincter fibers are torn, resulting in extravasation of blood and leading to perianal bruising and discoloration, which may be quite extensive. Advantages of this technique are that there is no anal wound and that the patients often have a quick return to normal function. Disadvantages include the incidence of recurrent fissures (10–56%) and the potential risk of permanent sphincter damage leading to incontinence. Anal dilatation may also be complicated by bleeding, perianal bruising, strangulation of prolapsed hemorrhoids, perianal infection, Fournier's gangrene, bacteremia, and rectal procidentia.

Isbister and Prasad[100] reported on a 15-year experience with a four-finger anal dilatation in 104 patients. There were five failures but no complaints of incontinence. Sohn et al[101] recommended a more precise dilatation performed with a Parks retractor opened to 4.8 cm or with a 40 mm rectosigmoid balloon. In 105 patients, the authors found a success rate of 93% with no reports of incontinence. Nielsen et al[102] performed anal ultrasound to assess the risk of sphincter damage and anal incontinence after anal dilatation for fissure-in-ano. Anal ultrasound demonstrated sphincter defects in 65% of patients studied; however, only minor anal incontinence was reported by 12% of patients.

Renzi et al[103] evaluated the clinical, anatomic, and functional pattern in a group of 33 patients with anal fissure treated by pneumatic balloon dilatation. Dilation was accomplished by means of an endoanal 40-mm balloon inflated with a pressure of 1.4 atm that was left in place for 6 minutes under local anesthesia. Fissures healed between the third and fifth weeks in 94% of patients who became asymptomatic 2.5 days after treatment, and the first postdilatation defecation was painless in 82% of cases. Six percent of the patients complained of minor transient anal incontinence. Manometry demonstrated that the preoperative anal resting pressure decreased from 91 to 70.5 and to 78 mm Hg, 6 and 12 months after pneumatic balloon dilatation, respectively.

In a review by Lund and Scholefield[104] of 16 trials examining the use of anal dilatation, reported recurrence rates ranged from 2 to 56% and tended to be higher with longer follow-up. Disturbance of continence ranged from 0 to 39% for incontinence of flatus or fecal soiling, and fecal incontinence was reported in up to 16%. Although reasonable success and complication rates have been reported by some authors, very few centers continue to employ this technique.

Lateral Internal Sphincterotomy

Sphincterotomy was originally described by Brodie[105] in 1835. The method originally favored was division of the lower half of the internal sphincter in the posterior midline through the fissure itself. This procedure resulted in satisfactory results but had two significant disadvantages: the opened wound in the anal canal took a long time to heal (up to 6–7 weeks) and there was a disturbingly high incidence of incontinence and fecal soiling. Some of the fecal soiling and minor imperfections in continence were due to the "keyhole" deformity created by a posterior sphincterotomy, which allows fecal-stained mucus and possibly stool to escape. Melange et al[106] studied 76 patients who underwent fissurectomy with posterior midline sphincterotomy for anal fissure. The fissure healed in all cases, but sporadic loss of continence for flatus or liquid stool occurred in 21 patients (27.6%), and soiling was present in seven other patients (9.2%).

The possibility that a lateral sphincterotomy might cause a less prominent groove than a posterior one and be followed by less disturbance of function was suggested by Eisenhammer in 1959.[107] Parks[108] also strongly recommended a lateral approach to a sphincterotomy. There are variations in the exact details of current forms of performing lateral sphincterotomy.

The procedure may be done with the patient under local, regional, or general anesthesia, through a radial or circumferential incision, or using a subcutaneous technique. The muscle may be divided medially to laterally or vice versa.

Open Technique (▶ Fig. 8.3)

The great advantage of the open technique for internal sphincterotomy is that it avoids an intra-anal wound. The internal sphincter is divided under direct visual control because the thickness and length of the internal sphincter vary from patient to patient. Bleeding sites can also be seen and directly controlled.

After the anesthetic is administered, the patient is placed in either the lithotomy or prone jack-knife position. A fine needle is used to infiltrate the area of the fissure with an anesthetic solution of 0.5% xylocaine in 1:200,000 epinephrine. The anesthetic solution is next infiltrated into the lateral aspect near the anal verge, which ensures that the solution is directed to the level of the dentate line. The entire perianal region may be anesthetized. A Pratt bivalve or Hill Ferguson speculum is inserted and the anal pathology is evaluated. A short incision is made overlying the intersphincteric groove, which can usually be palpated easily. The anoderm is lifted from the underlying internal sphincter to the level of the dentate line, and the intersphincteric plane is developed. The full thickness of the internal sphincter is divided from its lower edge to the level of the dentate line or to the depth of the anal fissure with either a pair of Metzenbaum scissors or a scalpel. A definite "give" will be noted, and this should correct any element of anal stenosis and cure the fissure. Any adjacent hemorrhoidal tissue can be excised as indicated. Since prolapsing hemorrhoids are a recognized complication after lateral internal sphincterotomy, judicious use of concomitant hemorrhoidectomy should be made in patients with large hemorrhoids to avoid this complication. Hemostasis is obtained with cautery, and the wound can be closed with two or three interrupted sutures of 3–0 absorbable suture.

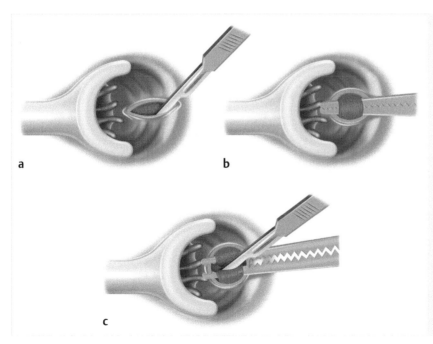

Fig. 8.3 (a–c) The technique of open sphincterotomy.

Postoperatively, patients are discharged home and are advised to eat a regular diet and to take sitz baths and a psyllium seed preparation as a bulk-forming agent. A narcotic oral analgesic also is prescribed; however, many patients describe less pain immediately after the procedure than just prior to it. Patients are typically seen one month after the procedure.

Closed Technique (▶ Fig. 8.4)

The closed technique modification is the method of lateral subcutaneous internal sphincterotomy described by Notaras.[109] This procedure leaves virtually no wound. The operation can be performed in the lithotomy, left lateral, or semi-prone position. An anal speculum such as the Pratt bivalve or Hill Ferguson is inserted; when the blades are opened, the anus is placed in a slight stretch. The intersphincteric groove and lower edge of the internal sphincter are then palpable. A narrow-bladed scalpel, flat side adjacent to muscle, is introduced through the skin in either lateral position and the tip is advanced submucosally to the dentate line. The sharp edge of the blade is then turned toward the internal sphincter, and the sphincterotomy is performed. Alternatively, the scalpel blade can be advanced in the intersphincteric plane and turned toward the lumen, thus accomplishing the sphincterotomy. When this step is accomplished, a "give" will result in release of the tension of the blades of the anal speculum. Pressure will arrest any bleeding, and the wound is left open to allow any drainage to escape. Again, a large sentinel pile and hypertrophied anal papillae can be dealt with appropriately.

8.1.9 Results

Healing rates and postoperative complications following lateral internal sphincterotomy are summarized in ▶ Table 8.5. Although complications after internal sphincterotomy are known to occur, their numbers are few and include ecchymosis and hemorrhage, perianal abscess, fistula-in-ano, prolapsed hemorrhoids, and, very rarely, minor alterations in continence. Clinical experience has shown that operative division of the internal sphincter may result in defects of fine anal continence. Careful technique will reduce these complications to a minimum.

Few studies have been conducted comparing the different options, especially comparing lateral internal sphincterotomy with fissurectomy. One study compared the results of lateral internal sphincterotomy to those of fissurectomy and posterior midline sphincterotomy.[110] Each group contained 150 patients. The lateral internal sphincterotomy group fared better with regard to faster pain relief (1–2 weeks vs. 2–3 weeks) and quicker wound healing (2–3 weeks vs. 6–7 weeks). Although early and temporary loss of continence occurred in 30% of patients with lateral internal sphincterotomy and 40% of patients with fissurectomy and posterior midline sphincterotomy, normal function returned in the lateral sphincterotomy group. Five percent of patients in the fissurectomy and posterior midline sphincterotomy group reported persistent loss of control of flatus, and another 5% experienced fecal soiling. The recurrence rate was the same in both groups (1.3%).

Saad and Omer[129] conducted a prospective randomized study in which anal dilatation, posterior internal sphincterotomy, and lateral internal sphincterotomy were compared. Lateral internal sphincterotomy fared the best with immediate relief of pain, the lowest incidence of complications, and the earliest return to work. Anal dilatation fared the poorest with the main disadvantage being the high rate of postoperative anal incontinence (24.3%).

Garcia-Aguilar et al[120] compared the healing rate and long-term effects on continence of open and closed lateral internal sphincterotomy in 549 patients with chronic fissure-in-ano. Differences in persistence of symptoms, recurrence of the fissure, and need for reoperation were statistically not significant. However, statistically significant differences were seen in the percentage of patients with permanent postoperative difficulty controlling gas (30.3 vs. 23.6%; $p < 0.062$), soiling underclothing (26.7 vs. 16.1%; $p < 0.001$), and accidental bowel movements (11.8 vs. 3.1%; $p < 0.001$) between those who underwent open internal sphincterotomy and those who had closed internal sphincterotomy. The authors concluded that lateral internal sphincterotomy is highly effective in the treatment of chronic anal fissure but is associated with significant permanent alterations in continence and that the closed technique is preferable to open technique because it effects a similar rate of cure with less impairment of control.

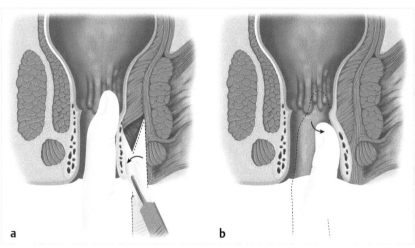

Fig. 8.4 (a,b) The technique of closed sphincterotomy.

Table 8.5 Lateral internal sphincterotomy

| Author | Year | n | Healing | Incontinence | | |
				Flatus	Stool	Soiling
Abcarian[110]	1980	150	98%	30%	0%	0%
Lewis et al[111]	1988	350	94%	16%	0%	–
Hiltunen and Matikainen[112]	1991	65	87%	0%	0%	0%
Frezza et al[113]	1992	134	99%	0%	0%	0%
Xynos et al[16]	1993	42	95%	–	–	–
Leong et al[114]	1994	97	97%	8%	0%	0%
Pernikoff et al[115]	1994	500	97%	3%	1%	4%
Romano et al[116]	1994	44	100%	5%	5%	5%
Neufeld et al[117]	1995	112	97%	13%	1%	9%
Oh et al[118]	1995	1313	98%	2%	0%	0%
Usatoff and Polglase[119]	1995	98	97%	7%	1%	11%
Garcia-Aguilar et al[120]	1996	324	86%	30%	12%	27%
Hananel and Gordon[121]	1997	265	98%	1%	1%	1%
Jonas et al[45]	1999	26	100%	0%	0%	0%
Nyam and Pemberton[122]	1999	487	92%	31%	23%	39%
Argov and Levandovsky[123]	2000	2108	99%	2%	0%	0%
Richard et al[40]	2000	38	92%	0%	0%	0%
Evans et al[38]	2001	27	97%	7%	0%	0%
Menteş et al[75]	2003	50	94%	16%	0%	–
Arroyo et al[124]	2004	80	91%	0%	4%	–
Parellada[51]	2004	27	100%	15%	0%	0%
Casillas et al[125]	2005	298	90%	30%	0%	8%
Algaithy[126]	2008	50	100%	0%	2%	0%
Hancke et al[127]	2010	21	100%	24%	21%	43%
Sileri et al[128]	2010	72	98%	0%	0%	0%

Khubchandani and Reed[130] also reported on the sequelae of internal sphincterotomy for chronic fissure-in-ano. Their series of 1,102 patients from whom surgical data were obtained also noted a complication rate not in keeping with most reports. Alteration in control of flatus occurred in 35.1%, soiling of underclothing in 22%, and accidental bowel movements in 5.3%. Their series contained patients who underwent lateral, posterior, or bilateral sphincterotomy, but the authors state that there were no significant differences between the different groups.

In a prospective study of the extent of internal sphincterotomy, Sultan et al[131] performed anal ultrasonography before and two months after operation. In 9 of the 10 female patients, the defect involved the full length of the internal sphincter; however, this was not true in males. It may be that the high incidence of alterations in continence reported by some of the authors may be related to a more extensive division of the muscle than intended. It is therefore important to tailor the amount of muscle divided to each individual patient. Furthermore, combining the sphincterotomy with other anorectal procedures may explain the increased complication rate.

Factors that may contribute to the wide variation of results include the retrospective analysis used in some studies, the unspecified duration of follow-up, and the lack of a precise definition of incontinence (i.e., for solid stool, liquid stool, or flatus, and whether the problem was temporary or permanent). Some series include patients who have undergone additional anorectal procedures. Thus, the summaries of reports in ▶ Table 8.2 and ▶ Table 8.3 are not strictly comparable but present a general overview and acknowledgment of the efficacy of lateral internal sphincterotomy.

Caution should be exercised before performing internal sphincterotomy in patients with diarrhea, irritable bowel syndrome, diabetes, and in the elderly.[132] Before operation is contemplated, consideration should be given to obtaining resting anal pressures and visualizing the anal sphincter by intra-anal ultrasonography in women who have previously undergone an episiotomy or suffered a third-degree tear during labor. Cassilas et al[125] assessed the long-term outcomes and quality of life of patients who had undergone sphincterotomy for chronic anal fissure using the Fecal Incontinence Quality of Life and Fecal Incontinence Severity Index in 298 patients. Recurrence of the fissure occurred in 5.6% of patients of whom 52% were female. Significant factors that resulted in recurrence were initial sphincterotomy performed in the office and the use of local anesthesia only. Twenty-nine percent of females who had a vaginal delivery recorded problems with incontinence to flatus. Temporary incontinence was reported in 31% of patients and persistent incontinence to gas occurred in 30%. Stool incontinence was not a significant finding. The overall quality of life scores were in the normal range, whereas the median Fecal Incontinence Severity Index score was 12. The authors recommended that females who have two or more previous vaginal deliveries should be warned about possible incontinence.

The incidence of recurrence may be related to the amount of internal sphincter divided. With this in mind, Littlejohn and Newstead[133] proposed the tailored lateral sphincterotomy, by which they meant that the amount of sphincter division is tailored exactly to the height of the fissure with some recognition of the degree of anal tone, if excessive. In most cases, the vertical height of the sphincter division is between 5 and 10 mm. In a review of 287 patients treated, recorded complications included imperfect control of flatus, 1.4%; minor staining, 0.35%; and urgency, 0.7%. No patients experienced incontinence of feces or leakage of stool. Five patients underwent repeat sphincterotomy, four for recurrence, and one for persistent fissure.

In a small percentage of patients in whom the fissure fails to heal or recurrence develops, a number of options are available to the surgeon. In some patients, a recurrent fissure will heal with nonoperative treatment such as stool softeners and sitz baths, or treatment with injection of botulinum toxin. Since a persistence or recurrence of the fissure is generally attributed to an inadequate sphincterotomy, the surgeon should investigate to ensure that a complete internal sphincterotomy was accomplished.

Farouk et al[10] used endoanal ultrasonography and anal manometry to assess 13 patients with persistent anal fissure after sphincterotomy. Endoluminal ultrasonography revealed partial division of the internal sphincter in two patients. The remaining 11 patients had an intact internal anal sphincter but had ultrasonographic evidence of division of the external sphincter at the site of the previous operation. All 13 patients subsequently underwent a second lateral internal sphincterotomy, with resolution of their symptoms. Median preoperative resting pressures of 115 cm H_2O fell to 89 cm H_2O postoperatively. The authors concluded that failure of the original sphincterotomy appears to be related to an inadequate internal sphincterotomy or to inadvertent division of the external anal sphincter. Xynos et al[16] also reported that fissures that fail to heal after lateral internal sphincterotomy can be successfully treated by performing an additional internal sphincterotomy on the opposite side.

Advancement Flaps

Advancement flaps may be an alternative option in patients who have failed lateral internal sphincterotomy, patients who may be at high risk for postoperative incontinence, or patients with anal fissure without evidence of hypertonia. A method using excision of the fissure combined with an advancement flap of anoderm has been referred to as V–Y anoplasty. A triangular skin flap based outside the anal canal is elevated in continuity with the excised fissure. A broad base with adequate blood supply to the flap must be ensured. The flap is adequately mobilized to avoid tension on the suture line. Meticulous attention is paid to hemostasis to prevent hematoma formation, which increases tension and the chance of infection. The flap is then advanced, and the defect of the skin and anal canal is closed.

Extensive experience with this technique has been reported by Samson and Stewart.[134] According to these authors, excision of a chronic fissure-in-ano and coverage of the defect with a sliding, broad-based skin graft offer several advantages over the classic excision, including less postoperative pain, decreased need for postoperative wound care, and lower rate of postoperative complications. Of 2,072 patients treated with a V–Y advancement flap, recurrent fissures occurred in 10, and there were only seven cases of mild anal stenosis. Postoperative bleeding occurred in two cases, and the slough rate of the flap was 2.4%. The major disadvantages to this method are that it involves considerable dissection and requires increased operative time.

Leong and Seow-Choen[135] conducted a randomized, prospective study to compare the use of a rhomboid anal advancement flap and a lateral internal anal sphincterotomy for the treatment of chronic fissure-in-ano. Twenty patients were assigned to each group. The authors found that healing occurred in all patients in the group who underwent sphincterotomy, while there were three failures in the group treated with an advancement flap. Nevertheless, the authors concluded that the flap is an alternative to the sphincterotomy.

Nyam et al[136] recommended the use of island advancement flaps in the management of anal fissures in patients with weak sphincters, including those with a failed lateral sphincterotomy, previous obstetric trauma, previous perianal surgery, and other low-pressure fissures-in-ano. The authors found significantly lower resting pressures in 21 such patients, of which 15 had sphincter defects on endoanal ultrasound. All of these patients underwent flap repair, and healing occurred primarily with preservation of sensation, maintenance of continence, and no serious complications. Hanke et al[127] used a rectangular dermal advancement flap and compared the results to patients who underwent a lateral internal sphincterotomy. The authors found that the chronic fissure wounds healed in both groups regardless of surgical technique; however, the incidence of anal incontinence was significantly higher in patients who underwent lateral internal sphincterotomy (47.5 vs 5.8%, $p < 0.05$).

8.2 Anal Stenosis

Anal stenosis occurs due to a loss of the physiologic capacity of the anal canal. Stenosis develops when the normally pliable tissues of the anus are replaced with scarred, fibrotic tissue. Although anal stenosis may occur in some congenital syndromes, the overwhelming majority of cases are secondary in nature, most of which are due to surgical trauma. In fact, 90% of cases of anal stenosis occur following surgery for hemorrhoids.[137,138] The incidence of posthemorrhoidectomy stenosis ranges from 1.5 to 4%,[139] and occurs when adequate skin bridges are not preserved. Stenosis may also occur following excision of perianal lesions, fistulectomy, fulguration of condyloma, low rectal anastomoses (ileal pouch, coloanal), radiation therapy, trauma, anorectal inflammatory bowel disease, chronic laxative use, sexually transmitted diseases, and chronic diarrhea.[140]

8.2.1 Symptoms

The most common complaint of patients with anal stenosis is difficulty with evacuation and narrow caliber of stools. Patients may complain of constipation, anal pain with bowel movements, rectal bleeding, and abdominal cramping. Occasionally, patients may present with incontinence secondary to overflow constipation. If ectropion is present, patients may also complain of anal seepage. Many patients with stenosis will rely on daily laxatives or enemas to prevent constipation.

8.2.2 Diagnosis

Physical examination is often all that is needed to diagnose anal stenosis. In many patients, it may not be possible to perform digital examination or anoscopy. This may necessitate an examination under anesthesia, particularly in patients with severe or painful strictures.[137] If the etiology of the stenosis is unknown, it is important to evaluate the remainder of the colon with colonoscopy or barium enema.

Frequently, the onset of symptoms can be associated with a prior hemorrhoidectomy or other anorectal procedure. In patients with no surgical history, the cause of the stenosis must be sought as the treatment may be different. While anoplasty

may be indicated in patients with postsurgical stenosis, patients with stenosis secondary to anal Crohn's disease or radiation may require proctectomy or fecal diversion.

8.2.3 Treatment

Nonoperative Management

Conservative therapy may be sufficient in patients with mild anal stenosis or stenosis that only involves the distal anal canal. Treatment includes stool softeners, enemas, and suppositories. Patients with persistent symptoms despite the addition of stool softeners may benefit from anal dilation. Initial dilation is typically performed under sedation, followed by daily self-digital or mechanical dilation at home.[141] This treatment is preferred in patients with anal stenosis where surgical intervention may be associated with potential healing complications (stenosis due to Crohn's disease or radiation).[142]

Operative Management

Surgical treatment is recommended for the treatment of patients with moderate to severe anal stenosis, or in those patients in which medical management fails to significantly improve symptoms. The aim of any intervention is to increase the diameter and pliability of the anal canal either by simply incising the scar, or by excising the fibrotic area and replacing it with a flap of healthy tissue. The choice of procedure is based on the degree of the stenosis and the experience of the surgeon.

Stricturotomy/Stricturoplasty

For patients with mild to moderate short anal stenosis, division of the stricture and excision of the eschar (with or without concomitant sphincterotomy) may be useful. Simply dividing the stricture alone may temporarily relieve symptoms; however, the scar will typically reform. The stricture is incised longitudinally for approximately 3 to 4 cm, leaving the underlying sphincter muscle intact. A Hill-Ferguson retractor can then typically be inserted. The distal cut edge of the rectal mucosa can then be sutured to the underlying sphincter at the level of the dentate line in a transverse fashion, thereby widening the anal canal. This can be done in multiple quadrants if a single stricturotomy does not relieve the stenosis. Several authors have reported favorable outcomes following this procedure[143,144]; however, most surgeons prefer the use of flaps to repair anal stenosis.

Advancement Flaps

For patients with stenosis of the upper or midanal canal, mucosal advancement flaps may be an option. The goal is to bring healthy rectal mucosa down to the area of the stenosis, and it may be combined with sphincterotomy after the stenotic area has been excised. A flap of anal and rectal mucosa and submucosa is developed in similar fashion to flaps for anal fistulas. The flap maintains its blood supply through

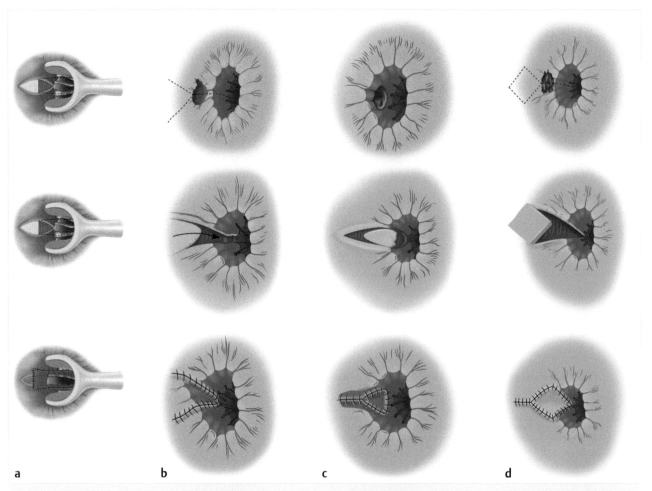

Fig. 8.5 Operative procedures for anal stenosis. **(a)** Mucosal advancement flap. **(b)** Y-V advancement flap. **(c)** House advancement flap. **(d)** Diamond advancement flap.

submucosal plexuses and is advanced into the anal canal where it is sutured to the distal edge of the anal sphincter. This is done as close to the dentate line as possible with the goal of advancing the flap beyond the strictured area. If the flap is advanced to the level of the anal verge, patients may develop an ectropion and develop leakage or incontinence. Several authors have reported success of greater than 90% in patients with stenosis treated with mucosal advancement flaps.[145,146]

Anoplasty with perianal skin flap advancement can be used to correct stenosis in patients with distal stenoses and loss of anal canal tissue. With the patient placed in the prone jack-knife position, the stricture is incised, and a sphincterotomy may also be performed. A flap of anal skin in the posterior midline is mobilized in a full-thickness fashion, ensuring that the underlying blood supply is left intact. The flap is then advanced into the anal canal at the site of the stricturotomy to create a new anal lining. Various options for advancement flaps have been described, including V–Y flaps, diamond or

house flaps, rotational flaps (▶ Fig. 8.5), and endorectal advancement flaps (▶ Fig. 8.6).

The choice of which flap to employ is based on the anatomic findings and the experience of the surgeon. V–Y flaps may be best suited for shorter stenosis, whereas house or diamond flaps are often used for longer stenosis and rotational flaps are reserved for large or complex defects. Numerous case series demonstrate significant improvement in symptoms regardless of the type of flap used.[141,142,145,146,147,148,149,150]

Farid et al conducted a prospective randomized study comparing the use of house flap, rhomboid flap, or Y–V anoplasty in 60 patients with anal stenosis at a single institution.[151] Clinical improvement (no straining, no sense of anorectal obstruction) was significantly better in patients who underwent a house flap (95%) versus those who underwent a rhomboid flap (80%) or Y–V anoplasty (65%). These results persisted at 1 year and were also reflected in improved GI Quality of Life scores in the house flap group.

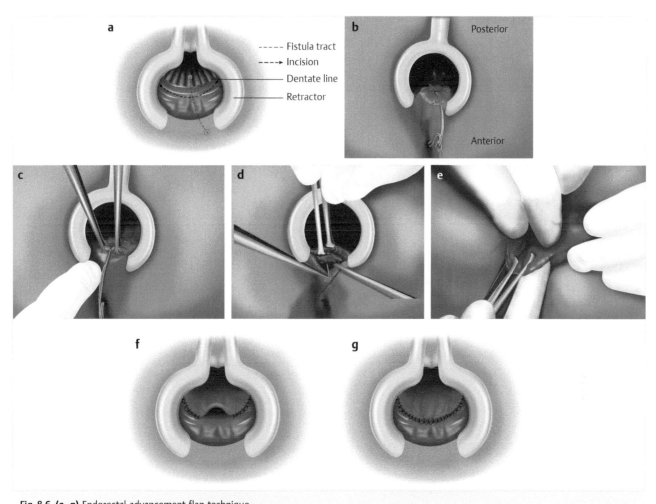

Fistula tract
Incision
Dentate line
Retractor

Posterior

Anterior

Fig. 8.6 (a–g) Endorectal advancement flap technique.

References

[1] Jonas M, Scholefield JH. Anal fissure. Gastroenterol Clin North Am. 2001; 30 (1):167–181

[2] Lock MR, Thomson JP. Fissure-in-ano: the initial management and prognosis. Br J Surg. 1977; 64(5):355–358

[3] Hananel N, Gordon PH. Re-examination of clinical manifestations and response to therapy of fissure-in-ano. Dis Colon Rectum. 1997; 40(2):229–233

[4] Costedio M, Cataldo PA. Anal fissures. In: Cameron JL, ed. Current Surgical Therapy. 9th ed. Philadelphia, PA: Elsevier; 2008:268–271

[5] Martin JD. Postpartum anal fissure. Lancet. 1953; 1(6754):271–273

[6] Jensen SL. Diet and other risk factors for fissure-in-ano. Prospective case control study. Dis Colon Rectum. 1988; 31(10):770–773

[7] Crapp AR, Alexander-Williams J. Fissure-in-ano and anal stenosis. Part I: conservative management. Clin Gastroenterol. 1975; 4(3):619–628

[8] Abcarian H, Lakshmanan S, Read DR, Roccaforte P. The role of internal sphincter in chronic anal fissures. Dis Colon Rectum. 1982; 25(6):525–528

[9] Chowcat NL, Araujo JG, Boulos PB. Internal sphincterotomy for chronic anal fissure: long term effects on anal pressure. Br J Surg. 1986; 73(11):915–916

[10] Farouk R, Duthie GS, MacGregor AB, Bartolo DC. Sustained internal sphincter hypertonia in patients with chronic anal fissure. Dis Colon Rectum. 1994; 37 (5):424–429

[11] Keck JO, Staniunas RJ, Coller JA, Barrett RC, Oster ME. Computer-generated profiles of the anal canal in patients with anal fissure. Dis Colon Rectum. 1995; 38(1):72–79

[12] McNamara MJ, Percy JP, Fielding IR. A manometric study of anal fissure treated by subcutaneous lateral internal sphincterotomy. Ann Surg. 1990; 211(2):235–238

[13] Nothmann BJ, Schuster MM. Internal anal sphincter derangement with anal fissures. Gastroenterology. 1974; 67(2):216–220

[14] Prohm P, Bönner C. Is manometry essential for surgery of chronic fissure-in-ano? Dis Colon Rectum. 1995; 38(7):735–738

[15] Williams N, Scott NA, Irving MH. Effect of lateral sphincterotomy on internal anal sphincter function. A computerized vector manometry study. Dis Colon Rectum. 1995; 38(7):700–704

[16] Xynos E, Tzortzinis A, Chrysos E, Tzovaras G, Vassilakis JS. Anal manometry in patients with fissure-in-ano before and after internal sphincterotomy. Int J Colorectal Dis. 1993; 8(3):125–128

[17] Cerdán FJ, Ruiz de León A, Azpiroz F, Martín J, Balibrea JL. Anal sphincteric pressure in fissure-in-ano before and after lateral internal sphincterotomy. Dis Colon Rectum. 1982; 25(3):198–201

[18] Olsen J, Mortensen PE, Krogh Petersen I, Christiansen J. Anal sphincter function after treatment of fissure-in-ano by lateral subcutaneous sphincterotomy versus anal dilatation. A randomized study. Int J Colorectal Dis. 1987; 2(3):155–157

[19] Gibbons CP, Read NW. Anal hypertonia in fissures: cause or effect? Br J Surg. 1986; 73(6):443–445

[20] Klosterhalfen B, Vogel P, Rixen H, Mittermayer C. Topography of the inferior rectal artery: a possible cause of chronic, primary anal fissure. Dis Colon Rectum. 1989; 32(1):43–52

[21] Schouten WR, Briel JW, Auwerda JJ, De Graaf EJ. Ischaemic nature of anal fissure. Br J Surg. 1996; 83(1):63–65

[22] Bhardwaj R, Vaizey CJ, Boulos PB, Hoyle CH. Neuromyogenic properties of the internal anal sphincter: therapeutic rationale for anal fissures. Gut. 2000; 46(6):861–868

[23] Madalinski M, Kalinowski L. Novel options for the pharmacological treatment of chronic anal fissure–role of botulin toxin. Curr Clin Pharmacol. 2009; 4(1):47–52

[24] Dodi G, Bogoni F, Infantino A, Pianon P, Mortellaro LM, Lise M. Hot or cold in anal pain? A study of the changes in internal anal sphincter pressure profiles. Dis Colon Rectum. 1986; 29(4):248–251

[25] Shub HA, Salvati EP, Rubin RJ. Conservative treatment of anal fissure: an un-selected, retrospective and continuous study. Dis Colon Rectum. 1978; 21 (8):582–583

[26] Jensen SL. Maintenance therapy with unprocessed bran in the prevention of acute anal fissure recurrence. J R Soc Med. 1987; 80(5):296–298

[27] Jensen SL. Treatment of first episodes of acute anal fissure: prospective rando-mised study of lignocaine ointment versus hydrocortisone ointment or warm sitz baths plus bran. Br Med J (Clin Res Ed). 1986; 292(6529):1167–1169

[28] Nelson RL, Thomas K, Morgan J, Jones A. Non surgical therapy for anal fis-sure. Cochrane Database Syst Rev. 2012; 2(2):CD003431

[29] Kennedy ML, Sowter S, Nguyen H, Lubowski DZ. Glyceryl trinitrate ointment for the treatment of chronic anal fissure: results of a placebo-controlled trial and long-term follow-up. Dis Colon Rectum. 1999; 42(8):1000–1006

[30] Loder PB, Kamm MA, Nicholls RJ, Phillips RK. 'Reversible chemical sphincter-otomy' by local application of glyceryl trinitrate. Br J Surg. 1994; 81 (9):1386–1389

[31] Lund JN, Scholefield JH. A randomised, prospective, double-blind, placebo-controlled trial of glyceryl trinitrate ointment in treatment of anal fissure. Lancet. 1997; 349(9044):11–14

[32] Carapeti EA, Kamm MA, McDonald PJ, Chadwick SJ, Melville D, Phillips RK. Randomised controlled trial shows that glyceryl trinitrate heals anal fis-sures, higher doses are not more effective, and there is a high recurrence rate. Gut. 1999; 44(5):727–730

[33] Schouten WR, Briel JW, Auwerda JJ, Boerma MO, Graatsma BH, Wilms EB. In-tra-anal application of isosorbide dinitrate in chronic anal fissure. Ned Tijdschr Geneeskd. 1995; 139(28):1447–1449

[34] McLeod RS, Evans J. Symptomatic care and nitroglycerin in the management of anal fissure. J Gastrointest Surg. 2002; 6(3):278–280

[35] Altomare DF, Rinaldi M, Milito G, et al. Glyceryl trinitrate for chronic anal fis-sure–healing or headache? Results of a multicenter, randomized, placebo-controled, double-blind trial. Dis Colon Rectum. 2000; 43(2):174–179, dis-cussion 179–181

[36] Bacher H, Mischinger HJ, Werkgartner G, et al. Local nitroglycerin for treat-ment of anal fissures: an alternative to lateral sphincterotomy? Dis Colon Rectum. 1997; 40(7):840–845

[37] Lund JN, Scholefield JH. Follow-up of patients with chronic anal fissure treated with topical glyceryl trinitrate. Lancet. 1998; 352(9141):1681

[38] Evans J, Luck A, Hewett P. Glyceryl trinitrate vs. lateral sphincterotomy for chronic anal fissure: prospective, randomized trial. Dis Colon Rectum. 2001; 44(1):93–97

[39] Oettlé GJ. Glyceryl trinitrate vs. sphincterotomy for treatment of chronic fis-sure-in-ano: a randomized, controlled trial. Dis Colon Rectum. 1997; 40 (11):1318–1320

[40] Richard CS, Gregoire R, Plewes EA, et al. Internal sphincterotomy is superior to topical nitroglycerin in the treatment of chronic anal fissure: results of a randomized, controlled trial by the Canadian Colorectal Surgical Trials Group. Dis Colon Rectum. 2000; 43(8):1048–1057, discussion 1057–1058

[41] Lysy J, Israelit-Yatzkan Y, Sestiere-Ittah M, Keret D, Goldin E. Treatment of chronic anal fissure with isosorbide dinitrate: long-term results and dose determination. Dis Colon Rectum. 1998; 41(11):1406–1410

[42] Brisinda G, Maria G, Bentivoglio AR, Cassetta E, Gui D, Albanese A. A compar-ison of injections of botulinum toxin and topical nitroglycerin ointment for the treatment of chronic anal fissure. N Engl J Med. 1999; 341(2):65–69

[43] Dorfman G, Levitt M, Platell C. Treatment of chronic anal fissure with topical glyceryl trinitrate. Dis Colon Rectum. 1999; 42(8):1007–1010

[44] Hyman NH, Cataldo PA. Nitroglycerin ointment for anal fissures: effective treatment or just a headache? Dis Colon Rectum. 1999; 42(3):383–385

[45] Jonas M, Lobo DN, Gudgeon AM. Lateral internal sphincterotomy is not re-dundant in the era of glyceryl trinitrate therapy for chronic anal fissure. J R Soc Med. 1999; 92(4):186–188

[46] Gecim I. Comparison of glyceryl trinitrate and botulinum toxin a in treat-ment of chronic anal fissure: a prospective, randomized study. Dis Colon Rectum. 2001; 44:A5–A26

[47] Graziano A, Svidler López L, Lencinas S, Masciangioli G, Gualdrini U, Bisisio O. Long-term results of topical nitroglycerin in the treatment of chronic anal fissures are disappointing. Tech Coloproctol. 2001; 5(3):143–147

[48] Pitt J, Williams S, Dawson PM. Reasons for failure of glyceryl trinitrate treat-ment of chronic fissure-in-ano: a multivariate analysis. Dis Colon Rectum. 2001; 44(6):864–867

[49] Bailey HR, Beck DE, Billingham RP, et al. Fissure Study Group. A study to de-termine the nitroglycerin ointment dose and dosing interval that best pro-mote the healing of chronic anal fissures. Dis Colon Rectum. 2002; 45 (9):1192–1199

[50] Kocher HM, Steward M, Leather AJ, Cullen PT. Randomized clinical trial as-sessing the side-effects of glyceryl trinitrate and diltiazem hydrochloride in the treatment of chronic anal fissure. Br J Surg. 2002; 89(4):413–417

[51] Parellada C. Randomized, prospective trial comparing 0.2 percent isosorbide dinitrate ointment with sphincterotomy in treatment of chronic anal fissure: a two-year follow-up. Dis Colon Rectum. 2004; 47(4):437–443

[52] Gagliardi G, Pascariello A, Altomare DF, et al. Optimal treatment duration of glyceryl trinitrate for chronic anal fissure: results of a prospective random-ized multicenter trial. Tech Coloproctol. 2010; 14(3):241–248

[53] Pérez-Legaz J, Arroyo A, Moya P, et al. Perianal versus endoanal application of glyceryl trinitrate 0.4% ointment in the treatment of chronic anal fissure: results of a randomized controlled trial. Is this the solution to the head-aches? Dis Colon Rectum. 2012; 55(8):893–899

[54] Altomare DF, Binda GA, Canuti S, Landolfi V, Trompetto M, Villani RD. The management of patients with primary chronic anal fissure: a position paper. Tech Coloproctol. 2011; 15(2):135–141

[55] Perez-Legaz J, Arroyo A, Ruiz-Tovar J, et al. Treatment of chronic anal fissure with topical nitroglycerin ointment 0.4%: a prospective clinical study. Tech Coloproctol. 2011; 15(4):475–476

[56] Chrysos E, Xynos E, Tzovaras G, Zoras OJ, Tsiaoussis J, Vassilakis SJ. Effect of nifedipine on rectoanal motility. Dis Colon Rectum. 1996; 39(2):212–216

[57] Antropoli C, Perrotti P, Rubino M, et al. Nifedipine for local use in conserva-tive treatment of anal fissures: preliminary results of a multicenter study. Dis Colon Rectum. 1999; 42(8):1011–1015

[58] Carapeti EA, Kamm MA, Phillips RK. Topical diltiazem and bethanechol de-crease anal sphincter pressure and heal anal fissures without side effects. Dis Colon Rectum. 2000; 43(10):1359–1362

[59] Cook TA, Humphreys MM, McC Mortensen NJ. Oral nifedipine reduces rest-ing anal pressure and heals chronic anal fissure. Br J Surg. 1999; 86 (10):1269–1273

[60] Perrotti P, Bove A, Antropoli C, et al. Topical nifedipine with lidocaine oint-ment vs. active control for treatment of chronic anal fissure: results of a pro-spective, randomized, double-blind study. Dis Colon Rectum. 2002; 45 (11):1468–1475

[61] Ezri T, Susmallian S. Topical nifedipine vs. topical glyceryl trinitrate for treat-ment of chronic anal fissure. Dis Colon Rectum. 2003; 46(6):805–808

[62] Ansaloni L, Bernabè A, Ghetti R, Riccardi R, Tranchino RM, Gardini G. Oral lacidipine in the treatment of anal fissure. Tech Coloproctol. 2002; 6 (2):79–82

[63] Ağaoğlu N, Cengiz S, Arslan MK, Türkyilmaz S. Oral nifedipine in the treat-ment of chronic anal fissure. Dig Surg. 2003; 20(5):452–456

[64] Ho KS, Ho YH. Randomized clinical trial comparing oral nifedipine with lat-eral anal sphincterotomy and tailored sphincterotomy in the treatment of chronic anal fissure. Br J Surg. 2005; 92(4):403–408

[65] Golfam F, Golfam P, Khalaj A, Sayed Mortaz SS. The effect of topical nife-dipine in treatment of chronic anal fissure. Acta Med Iran. 2010; 48 (5):295–299

[66] Jonas M, Speake W, Simpson J, Varghese T, Scholefield JH. Diltiazem heals glyceryl nitrate (GTN)-resistant chronic anal fissures. Dis Colon Rectum. 2001; 44:A5–A26

[67] Knight JS, Birks M, Farouk R. Topical diltiazem ointment in the treatment of chronic anal fissure. Br J Surg. 2001; 88(4):553–556

[68] DasGupta R, Franklin I, Pitt J, Dawson PM. Successful treatment of chronic anal fissure with diltiazem gel. Colorectal Dis. 2002; 4(1):20–22

[69] Bielecki K, Kolodziejczak M. A prospective randomized trial of diltiazem and glyceryltrinitrate ointment in the treatment of chronic anal fissure. Colorec-tal Dis. 2003; 5(3):256–257

[70] Shrivastava UK, Jain BK, Kumar P, Saifee Y. A comparison of the effects of dil-tiazem and glyceryl trinitrate ointment in the treatment of chronic anal fis-sure: a randomized clinical trial. Surg Today. 2007; 37(6):482–485

[71] Sanei B, Mahmoodieh M, Masoudpour H. Comparison of topical glyceryl tri-nitrate with diltiazem ointment for treatment of chronic anal fissure. A randomized clinical trial. Ann Ital Chir. 2009; 80(5):379–383

[72] Jawaid M, Masood Z, Salim M. Topical diltiazem hydrochloride and glyceryl trinitrate in the treatment of chronic anal fissure. J Coll Physicians Surg Pak. 2009; 19(10):614–617

[73] Ala S, Saeedi M, Hadianamrei R, Ghorbanian A. Topical diltiazem vs. top-ical glyceril trinitrate in the treatment of chronic anal fissure: a prospec-tive, randomized, double-blind trial. Acta Gastroenterol Belg. 2012; 75 (4):438–442

[74] Jonas M, Neal KR, Abercrombie JF, Scholefield JH. A randomized trial of oral vs. topical diltiazem for chronic anal fissures. Dis Colon Rectum. 2001; 44 (8):1074–1078

[75] Menteş BB, Irkörücü O, Akin M, Leventoğlu S, Tatlicioğlu E. Comparison of botulinum toxin injection and lateral internal sphincterotomy for the treatment of chronic anal fissure. Dis Colon Rectum. 2003; 46(2):232–237

[76] Brisinda G, Cadeddu F, Brandara F, Brisinda D, Maria G. Treating chronic anal fissure with botulinum neurotoxin. Nat Clin Pract Gastroenterol Hepatol. 2004; 1(2):82–89

[77] Jost WH, Schimrigk K. Therapy of anal fissure using botulin toxin. Dis Colon Rectum. 1994; 37(12):1321–1324

[78] Jost WH. One hundred cases of anal fissure treated with botulin toxin: early and long-term results. Dis Colon Rectum. 1997; 40(9):1029–1032

[79] Fernández López F, Conde Freire R, Rios Rios A, García Iglesias J, Caínzos Fernández M, Potel Lesquereux J. Botulinum toxin for the treatment of anal fissure. Dig Surg. 1999; 16(6):515–518

[80] González Carro P, Pérez Roldán F, Legaz Huidobro ML, Ruiz Carrillo F, Pedraza Martín C, Sáez Bravo JM. The treatment of anal fissure with botulinum toxin. Gastroenterol Hepatol. 1999; 22(4):163–166

[81] Maria G, Brisinda G, Bentivoglio AR, Cassetta E, Gui D, Albanese A. Influence of botulinum toxin site of injections on healing rate in patients with chronic anal fissure. Am J Surg. 2000; 179(1):46–50

[82] Brisinda G, Maria G, Sganga G, Bentivoglio AR, Albanese A, Castagneto M. Effectiveness of higher doses of botulinum toxin to induce healing in patients with chronic anal fissures. Surgery. 2002; 131(2):179–184

[83] Arroyo A, Pérez F, Serrano P, Candela F, Lacueva J, Calpena R. Surgical versus chemical (botulinum toxin) sphincterotomy for chronic anal fissure: long-term results of a prospective randomized clinical and manometric study. Am J Surg. 2005; 189(4):429–434

[84] Massoud BW, Mehrdad V, Baharak T, Alireza Z. Botulinum toxin injection versus internal anal sphincterotomy for the treatment of chronic anal fissure. Ann Saudi Med. 2005; 25(2):140–142

[85] Iswariah H, Stephens J, Rieger N, Rodda D, Hewett P. Randomized prospective controlled trial of lateral internal sphincterotomy versus injection of botulinum toxin for the treatment of idiopathic fissure in ano. ANZ J Surg. 2005; 75(7):553–555

[86] De Nardi P, Ortolano E, Radaelli G, Staudacher C. Comparison of glycerine trinitrate and botulinum toxin-a for the treatment of chronic anal fissure: long-term results. Dis Colon Rectum. 2006; 49(4):427–432

[87] Brisinda G, Cadeddu F, Brandara F, Marniga G, Maria G. Randomized clinical trial comparing botulinum toxin injections with 0.2 per cent nitroglycerin ointment for chronic anal fissure. Br J Surg. 2007; 94(2):162–167

[88] Festen S, Gisbertz SS, van Schaagen F, Gerhards MF. Blinded randomized clinical trial of botulinum toxin versus isosorbide dinitrate ointment for treatment of anal fissure. Br J Surg. 2009; 96(12):1393–1399

[89] Nasr M, Ezzat H, Elsebae M. Botulinum toxin injection versus lateral internal sphincterotomy in the treatment of chronic anal fissure: a randomized controlled trial. World J Surg. 2010; 34(11):2730–2734

[90] Samim M, Twigt B, Stoker L, Pronk A. Topical diltiazem cream versus botulinum toxin a for the treatment of chronic anal fissure: a double-blind randomized clinical trial. Ann Surg. 2012; 255(1):18–22

[91] Berkel AE, Rosman C, Koop R, van Duijvendijk P, van der Palen J, Klaase JM. Isosorbide dinitrate ointment vs botulinum toxin A (Dysport) as the primary treatment for chronic anal fissure: a randomized multicentre study. Colorectal Dis. 2014; 16(10):O360–O366

[92] Minguez M, Herreros B, Espi A, et al. Long-term follow-up (42 months) of chronic anal fissure after healing with botulinum toxin. Gastroenterology. 2002; 123(1):112–117

[93] Lysy J, Israelit-Yatzkan Y, Sestiery-Ittah M, Weksler-Zangen S, Keret D, Goldin E. Topical nitrates potentiate the effect of botulinum toxin in the treatment of patients with refractory anal fissure. Gut. 2001; 48(2):221–224

[94] Jones OM, Ramalingam T, Merrie A, et al. Randomized clinical trial of botulinum toxin plus glyceryl trinitrate vs. botulinum toxin alone for medically resistant chronic anal fissure: overall poor healing rates. Dis Colon Rectum. 2006; 49(10):1574–1580

[95] Lindsey I, Cunningham C, Jones OM, Francis C, Mortensen NJ. Fissurectomy-botulinum toxin: a novel sphincter-sparing procedure for medically resistant chronic anal fissure. Dis Colon Rectum. 2004; 47(11):1947–1952

[96] Brisinda G, Cadeddu F, Brandara F, et al. Botulinum toxin for recurrent anal fissure following lateral internal sphincterotomy. Br J Surg. 2008; 95(6):774–778

[97] Chen HL, Woo XB, Wang HS, et al. Botulinum toxin injection versus lateral internal sphincterotomy for chronic anal fissure: a meta-analysis of randomized control trials. Tech Coloproctol. 2014; 18(8):693–698

[98] Recemier JCA. Extension, massage et percussion cadence dansle traitement des contractures musculaires. Revue Medicale. 1838; 1:74–89

[99] Lord PH. Diverse methods of managing hemorrhoids: dilatation. Dis Colon Rectum. 1973; 16(3):180–183

[100] Isbister WH, Prasad J. Fissure in ano. Aust N Z J Surg. 1995; 65(2):107–108

[101] Sohn N, Eisenberg MM, Weinstein MA, Lugo RN, Ader J. Precise anorectal sphincter dilatation-its role in the therapy of anal fissures. Dis Colon Rectum. 1992; 35(4):322–327

[102] Nielsen MB, Rasmussen OO, Pedersen JF, Christiansen J. Risk of sphincter damage and anal incontinence after anal dilatation for fissure-in-ano. An endosonographic study. Dis Colon Rectum. 1993; 36(7):677–680

[103] Renzi A, Brusciano L, Pescatori M, et al. Pneumatic balloon dilatation for chronic anal fissure: a prospective, clinical, endosonographic, and manometric study. Dis Colon Rectum. 2005; 48(1):121–126

[104] Lund JN, Scholefield JH. Aetiology and treatment of anal fissure. Br J Surg. 1996; 83(10):1335–1344

[105] Brodie JC. Preternatural contraction of the sphincter ani. London Med Gaz. 1835; 16:26–31

[106] Melange M, Colin JF, Van Wymersch T, Vanheuverzwyn R. Anal fissure: correlation between symptoms and manometry before and after surgery. Int J Colorectal Dis. 1992; 7(2):108–111

[107] Eisenhammer S. The evaluation of the internal anal sphincterotomy operation with special reference to anal fissure. Surg Gynecol Obstet. 1959; 109:583–590

[108] Parks AG. The management of fissure-in-ano. Br J Hosp Med. 1967; 1:737–738

[109] Notaras MJ. The treatment of anal fissure by lateral subcutaneous internal sphincterotomy-a technique and results. Br J Surg. 1971; 58(2):96–100

[110] Abcarian H. Surgical correction of chronic anal fissure: results of lateral internal sphincterotomy vs. fissurectomy–midline sphincterotomy. Dis Colon Rectum. 1980; 23(1):31–36

[111] Lewis TH, Corman ML, Prager ED, Robertson WG. Long-term results of open and closed sphincterotomy for anal fissure. Dis Colon Rectum. 1988; 31(5):368–371

[112] Hiltunen KM, Matikainen M. Closed lateral subcutaneous sphincterotomy under local anaesthesia in the treatment of chronic anal fissure. Ann Chir Gynaecol. 1991; 80(4):353–356

[113] Frezza EE, Sandei F, Leoni G, Biral M. Conservative and surgical treatment in acute and chronic anal fissure. A study on 308 patients. Int J Colorectal Dis. 1992; 7(4):188–191

[114] Leong AF, Husain MJ, Seow-Choen F, Goh HS. Performing internal sphincterotomy with other anorectal procedures. Dis Colon Rectum. 1994; 37(11):1130–1132

[115] Pernikoff BJ, Eisenstat TE, Rubin RJ, Oliver GC, Salvati EP. Reappraisal of partial lateral internal sphincterotomy. Dis Colon Rectum. 1994; 37(12):1291–1295

[116] Romano G, Rotondano G, Santangelo M, Esercizio L. A critical appraisal of pathogenesis and morbidity of surgical treatment of chronic anal fissure. J Am Coll Surg. 1994; 178(6):600–604

[117] Neufeld DM, Paran H, Bendahan J, Freund U. Outpatient surgical treatment of anal fissure. Eur J Surg. 1995; 161(6):435–438

[118] Oh C, Divino CM, Steinhagen RM. Anal fissure. 20-year experience. Dis Colon Rectum. 1995; 38(4):378–382

[119] Usatoff V, Polglase AL. The longer term results of internal anal sphincterotomy for anal fissure. Aust N Z J Surg. 1995; 65(8):576–578

[120] Garcia-Aguilar J, Belmonte C, Wong WD, Lowry AC, Madoff RD. Open vs. closed sphincterotomy for chronic anal fissure: long-term results. Dis Colon Rectum. 1996; 39(4):440–443

[121] Hananel N, Gordon PH. Lateral internal sphincterotomy for fissure-in-ano-revisited. Dis Colon Rectum. 1997; 40(5):597–602

[122] Nyam DC, Pemberton JH. Long-term results of lateral internal sphincterotomy for chronic anal fissure with particular reference to incidence of fecal incontinence. Dis Colon Rectum. 1999; 42(10):1306–1310

[123] Argov S, Levandovsky O. Open lateral sphincterotomy is still the best treatment for chronic anal fissure. Am J Surg. 2000; 179(3):201–202

[124] Arroyo A, Pérez F, Serrano P, Candela F, Calpena R. Open versus closed lateral sphincterotomy performed as an outpatient procedure under local anesthesia for chronic anal fissure: prospective randomized study of clinical and manometric longterm results. J Am Coll Surg. 2004; 199(3):361–367

[125] Casillas S, Hull TL, Zutshi M, Trzcinski R, Bast JF, Xu M. Incontinence after a lateral internal sphincterotomy: are we underestimating it? Dis Colon Rectum. 2005; 48(6):1193–1199

[126] Algaithy ZK. Botulinum toxin versus surgical sphincterotomy in females with chronic anal fissure. Saudi Med J. 2008; 29(9):1260–1263

[127] Hancke E, Rikas E, Suchan K, Völke K. Dermal flap coverage for chronic anal fissure: lower incidence of anal incontinence compared to lateral internal sphincterotomy after long-term follow-up. Dis Colon Rectum. 2010; 53(11):1563–1568

[128] Sileri P, Stolfi VM, Franceschilli L, et al. Conservative and surgical treatment of chronic anal fissure: prospective longer term results. J Gastrointest Surg. 2010; 14(5):773–780

[129] Saad AM, Omer A. Surgical treatment of chronic fissure-in-ano: a prospective randomised study. East Afr Med J. 1992; 69(11):613–615

[130] Khubchandani IT, Reed JF. Sequelae of internal sphincterotomy for chronic fissure in ano. Br J Surg. 1989; 76(5):431–434

[131] Sultan AH, Kamm MA, Nicholls RJ, Bartram CI. Prospective study of the extent of internal anal sphincter division during lateral sphincterotomy. Dis Colon Rectum. 1994; 37(10):1031–1033

[132] Perry WB, Dykes SL, Buie WD, Rafferty JF, Standards Practice Task Force of the American Society of Colon and Rectal Surgeons. Practice parameters for the management of anal fissures (3rd revision). Dis Colon Rectum. 2010; 53 (8):1110–1115

[133] Littlejohn DR, Newstead GL. Tailored lateral sphincterotomy for anal fissure. Dis Colon Rectum. 1997; 40(12):1439–1442

[134] Samson RB, Stewart WR. Sliding skin grafts in the treatment of anal fissures. Dis Colon Rectum. 1970; 13(5):372–375

[135] Leong AF, Seow-Choen F. Lateral sphincterotomy compared with anal advancement flap for chronic anal fissure. Dis Colon Rectum. 1995; 38(1):69–71

[136] Nyam DC, Wilson RG, Stewart KJ, Farouk R, Bartolo DC. Island advancement flaps in the management of anal fissures. Br J Surg. 1995; 82(3):326–328

[137] Brisinda G, Vanella S, Cadeddu F, et al. Surgical treatment of anal stenosis. World J Gastroenterol. 2009; 15(16):1921–1928

[138] Milsom JW, Mazier WP. Classification and management of postsurgical anal stenosis. Surg Gynecol Obstet. 1986; 163(1):60–64

[139] Bonello JC. Who's afraid of the dentate line? The Whitehead hemorrhoidectomy. Am J Surg. 1988; 156(3, Pt 1):182–186

[140] Shawki S, Costedio M. Anal fissure and stenosis. Gastroenterol Clin North Am. 2013; 42(4):729–758

[141] Khubchandani IT. Anal stenosis. Surg Clin North Am. 1994; 74 (6):1353–1360

[142] Liberman H, Thorson AG. How I do it. Anal stenosis. Am J Surg. 2000; 179 (4):325–329

[143] Malgieri JA. Anoplasty to correct anal stricture. Dis Colon Rectum. 1961; 4:289–291

[144] Shropshear G. Posterior and anterior aal prototomy: a simplified technic for postoperative aal stensis. Dis Colon Rectum. 1971; 14(1):62–66

[145] Carditello A, Milone A, Stilo F, Mollo F, Basile M. Surgical treatment of anal stenosis following hemorrhoid surgery. Results of 150 combined mucosal advancement and internal sphincterotomy. Chir Ital. 2002; 54(6):841–844

[146] Ramajunan PS. Y-V anoplasty for severe anal stenosis. Contemp Surg. 1988; 33:62–68

[147] Habr-Gama A, Sobrado CW, de Araújo SE, et al. Surgical treatment of anal stenosis: assessment of 77 anoplasties. Clinics (Sao Paulo). 2005; 60 (1):17–20

[148] Maria G, Brisinda G, Civello IM. Anoplasty for the treatment of anal stenosis. Am J Surg. 1998; 175(2):158–160

[149] Rosen L. Anoplasty. Surg Clin North Am. 1988; 68(6):1441–1446

[150] Sentovich SM, Falk PM, Christensen MA, Thorson AG, Blatchford GJ, Pitsch RM. Operative results of House advancement anoplasty. Br J Surg. 1996; 83 (9):1242–1244

[151] Farid M, Youssef M, El Nakeeb A, Fikry A, El Awady S, Morshed M. Comparative study of the house advancement flap, rhomboid flap, and y-v anoplasty in treatment of anal stenosis: a prospective randomized study. Dis Colon Rectum. 2010; 53(5):790–797

9 Anorectal Abscess and Fistula-In-Ano

Janice F. Rafferty and Earl V. Thompson IV

Abstract

A majority of abscesses are of nonspecific cryptoglandular origin but may also be due to a variety of processes, which are primarily inflammatory or traumatic. A fistula typically begins in the middle of the anal canal at the level of the crypts and extends downward to the anal verge. Penetration through the external sphincter will lead to an abscess into the ischioanal fossa, while upward extension by way of the intersphincteric plane will course along the rectal wall or penetrate beyond the rectum. High upward extension can enter the true pelvis. The most common presenting symptoms for anorectal abscess are pain and swelling. Presentation of fistula-in-ano may be subtle, but most patients will give a history of prior abscess or anorectal procedures. This chapter focuses on etiology and pathology, avenues of extension, diagnosis, investigations, treatment, and complications related to anorectal abscess and fistula-in-ano.

Keywords: anorectal abscess, fistula-in-ano, anal fistula, etiology, pathogenesis, diagnosis, anoscopy, proctoscopy, treatment, fistulotomy

9.1 Anatomy

A thorough understanding of pelvic floor anatomy is a critical prerequisite in the evaluation and management of anorectal abscess and fistula. A comprehensive discussion of the relevant anatomy is provided elsewhere in this text (Chapter 1). For our purposes, the anal sphincter complex and its immediate environment can be thought of as two funnels of muscle surrounding the distal rectum and anal lumen. The internal anal sphincter is the thickened and rounded distal extent of the inner circular smooth muscle layer of the rectum. It terminates just distal to the dentate line and remains in a constant tonic contraction, contributing to continence. The internal sphincter

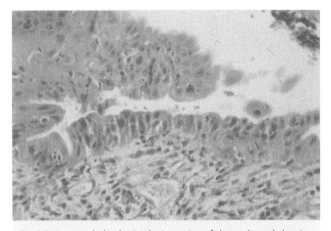

Fig. 9.1 Anorectal gland. Histologic section of the anal canal showing the duct of an anal gland entering at the level of the dentate line. Transition from squamous epithelium to transitional epithelium to columnar epithelium can be noted.

is nested within a broad funnel of striated muscle consisting of the external anal sphincter, levator ani, and puborectalis. The external anal sphincter extends slightly more caudad than the internal sphincter, and the intersphincteric groove between them can be visualized and palpated. At the level of the dentate line, a variable number of anal glands empty into crypts (▶ Fig. 9.1).

9.2 Etiology and Pathogenesis

A majority of abscesses are of nonspecific cryptoglandular origin. The remainder are due to a variety of processes, which are primarily inflammatory or traumatic. The specific processes that can lead to anorectal abscesses are as follows:

- Infectious/inflammatory
  - Cryptoglandular abscess
  - Inflammatory bowel disease
  - Diverticulitis
  - Pelvic abscess
  - Tuberculosis
  - Actinomycosis
  - Lymphogranuloma venereum
- Malignancy
  - Carcinoma
  - Lymphoma
  - Leukemia
- Trauma
  - Impalement
  - Penetrating trauma
  - Episiotomy
  - Hemorrhoidectomy
  - Prostatectomy
  - Enemas
- Radiation

The cryptoglandular origin theory was first described by Eisenhammer in 1958 and further supported by Parks' anatomic studies in 1961.[1,2] These anatomic studies demonstrated that anal glands provide a passage from crypts in the lumen of the bowel, through the internal sphincter, and into the intersphincteric space. Parks wrote that bacterial infection becomes established in glands that are either cystic or whose lumen is obstructed. While some glands may become obstructed due to stool, foreign bodies, trauma, or inflammation, there is no clear source of obstruction for most patients. Once infection is established, the epithelialized gland remains patent to the bowel lumen, while pus drains to the skin via any path of least resistance, thereby forming a fistula.

9.3 Avenues of Extension

A fistula typically begins in the middle of the anal canal at the level of the crypts and then most often extends downward in the intersphincteric plane to the anal verge. Penetration through the external sphincter will lead an abscess into the ischioanal fossa, while upward extension by way of the intersphincteric plane will course along the rectal wall or penetrate beyond the rectum. High upward extension can enter the true pelvis (▶ Fig. 9.2).

Pus may also track circumferentially around the anus in one of three tissue planes. The most common of these is known as a posterior horseshoe and begins with an abscess in the posterior midline that penetrates the sphincter complex into the deep postanal space and tracks into the bilateral ischioanal fossae. Circumferential spread may also occur in the intersphincteric plane or the pararectal tissue above the levator muscles.

9.4 Diagnosis

9.4.1 History

The most common presenting symptoms for anorectal abscess are pain and swelling.[3] While the patient will most often complain of perianal pain, the clinician should also be wary of supralevator abscess in the patient who complains of generalized pelvic or gluteal pain. Other symptoms of abscess include swelling, purulent drainage, odor, difficulty urinating, bleeding, and fevers. Patients who are immunocompromised by disease or medication may have subtle presentations with fevers and malaise without pain or swelling. Patients who give a history of prior anorectal abscess, inflammatory bowel disease, or anal trauma often have more complex abscess, and early consideration should be given to adjunct means of evaluation including examination under anesthesia and imaging.

Presentation of fistula-in-ano may be subtle, but most patients will give a history of prior abscess or anorectal procedures. Symptoms of fistula include drainage, bleeding, pain, and swelling. The fistula tract may intermittently occlude, leading to recurrent abscess formation.

9.4.2 Physical Examination

Findings on physical examination of the patient with acute abscess will vary depending on the location of the abscess. A superficial perianal or ischioanal abscess may be characterized by erythema, induration, fluctuance, tenderness, and occasionally purulent drainage. Evaluation of an intersphincteric abscess deserves special mention as the patient may present without erythema, induration, or swelling of the perineum. The patient will complain of severe perianal pain and tenderness with attempted rectal examination but no external signs of inflammation. Supralevator abscesses may also present with pain and tenderness without physical examination findings. Whereas patients with an intersphincteric abscess may not tolerate digital rectal examination due to discomfort, patients with a supralevator abscess, beyond the sphincter complex, may allow passage of an examining finger to elicit tenderness more cephalad in the pelvis.

The most common physical examination finding of a fistula-in-ano without acute suppuration is the external opening. This is characterized as a small elevated sinus with granulation tissue. With compression, this may express serous or purulent fluid. Palpation may reveal the firm cord of the fistula tract within the perianal tissue. Anoscopy on the awake patient rarely reveals the internal fistula opening.

Goodsall's rule is an often-cited method for identifying a fistula's internal opening based on the location of its external opening (▶ Fig. 9.3). According to the first published account of Goodsall's observation in 1887, "For fistulae having their external orifices situate behind a plane passing transversely through the center of the anus usually have their internal aperture in the middle line dorsally, while those with their external orifice in front of this plane generally terminate in an internal opening immediately opposite, thus forming a simple, straight, complete fistula."[4] Several studies have cast doubt on the utility of Goodsall's rule. In one, Goodsall's rule accurately predicted the site of the internal opening in approximately 59% of fistula tracts. It was most accurate at identifying anterior openings (72%) compared to posterior openings (41%).[5] Interestingly, an earlier but larger study of 216 patients suggested that Goodsall's rule was 90% accurate for identifying posterior fistulas that track to the midline but only 49% accurate for identifying the internal opening of an anterior fistula.[6]

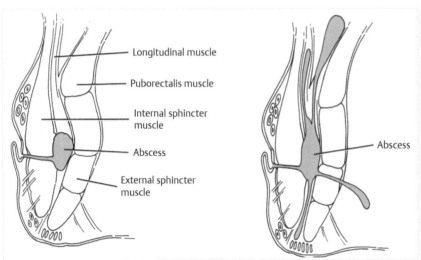

Fig. 9.2 Avenues of extension for an anal abscess or fistula.

Longitudinal muscle

Puborectalis muscle

Internal sphincter muscle

Abscess

External sphincter muscle

Abscess

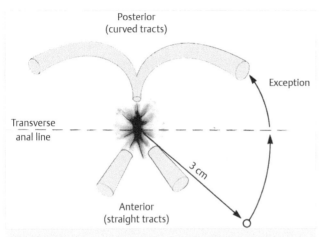

Fig. 9.3 Goodsall's rule. Anterior fistula runs straight to the nearest crypt while a posterior fistula will curve to a crypt at the posterior midline. An exception is that anterior fistulas more than 3 cm from the anus may track to the posterior midline.

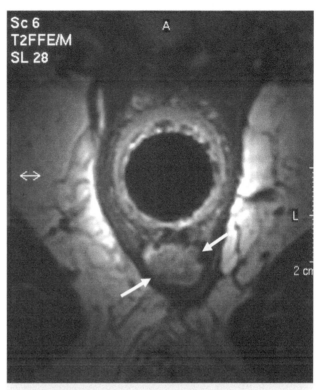

Fig. 9.4 MR image of an intersphincteric fistula with supralevator extension. Arrows point to an intersphincteric abscess. (Courtesy of Ruud Schouten, MD.)

9.4.3 Anoscopy and Proctoscopy

Examination under anesthesia with a patient comfortable and optimally positioned, and with ideal lighting and necessary equipment, provides an opportunity for the most complete evaluation of anorectal abscess and fistula. These procedures are easily performed in the prone position, although occasionally examination in the lithotomy or lateral decubitus position is necessary. General or local anesthesia sufficient to allow an unhurried examination should be administered. Anoscopy may allow identification of a crypt associated with an internal opening draining pus. Intersphincteric abscesses may be identified by palpation or passage of an 18-gauge finder needle.

Evaluation of fistula-in-ano requires identification of the internal opening whenever possible. Inserting a fistula probe into a chronic, mature fistula tract is an acceptable method for delineating the path of the fistula but must be done with caution to avoid formation of false channels. With an examining finger in the anus, the probe is gently advanced as long as resistance is not met. If the probe does not pass easily, dilute methylene blue or hydrogen peroxide can be instilled in the external opening to highlight an internal opening. Another method is to enlarge the external opening and dissect following the granulation tissue of the fistula tract, again taking care not to create false passages.

Anoscopy and proctoscopy or flexible sigmoidoscopy are also important if the abscess or fistula could be attributed to an underlying disease such as inflammatory bowel disease, malignancy, ischemia, or foreign body. Every patient undergoing treatment for fistula-in-ano should, at a minimum, be evaluated for proctitis.

9.4.4 Investigation

Magnetic Resonance Imaging

The ability of MRI to noninvasively evaluate distorted anatomy in patients with complex fistulas or prior perineal surgery makes it a useful tool in the management of selected patients with anorectal abscess or fistula (▶ Fig. 9.4, ▶ Fig. 9.5, ▶ Fig. 9.6). Initial interest in endoanal MRI coil has been tempered by its lack of availability and patient discomfort. The majority of studies therefore rely on body coil imaging. Pelvic MRI is described as the gold standard imaging technique for perianal fistulas associated with the complex anatomic disruption often found with Crohn's disease.[7]

An early study of MRI for fistula-in-ano using surgical findings as the gold standard in 35 patients demonstrated concordance of 86% for the presence and course of the primary tract, 93% for the presence and site of secondary extensions, and 80% for the position of the internal opening. This included two patients in whom an initial examination under anesthesia was unable to locate fistula tracts previously identified by blinded MRI but then required repeat surgical drainage after developing perianal sepsis at the site indicated by MRI.[8] Recent studies using more powerful MRI magnets have supported these findings and have particularly confirmed the ability of MRI to reliably identify secondary tracts. Sensitivity for extension or secondary tracts was 80 to 94%, and specificity was 94 to 100%.[9,10] Meta-analysis of four studies reported combined sensitivity and specificity of MRI for overall fistula detection of 87 and 69%. This was compared to sensitivity and specificity of 87 and 43% for endoanal ultrasound.[11]

One study by Buchanan et al compared clinical examination, endoanal ultrasonography, and MRI to an outcome-derived reference standard in 104 patients. In this study, clinical examination, ultrasonography, and MRI were able to correctly classify

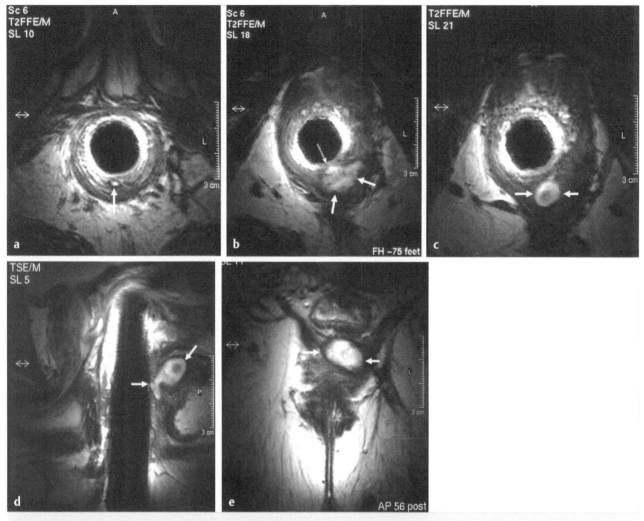

Fig. 9.5 MR image of an intersphincteric fistula with a high blind tract ending at the level of the puborectalis muscle. **(a)** Low level—arrow points to intersphincteric tract in posterior midline. **(b)** Higher level—thin arrow points to internal opening, thick arrows point to intersphincteric abscess. **(c)** Higher level—upward extension of the fistulous tract. **(d)** Sagittal plane—arrows point to fistulous tract ending in an abscess cavity in the posterior midline at the level of the puborectalis muscle. **(e)** Coronal plane—upper end of abscess cavity with excellent demonstration of the pelvic floor. (Courtesy of Ruud Schouten, MD.)

61, 81, and 91% of possible fistula tracts and 36, 70, and 88% of abscesses, respectively.[12]

Fistulography

Fistulography involves cannulation of the external fistula opening and injection of water-soluble contrast material while multiple fluoroscopic images are obtained. Its utility is limited as there is poor visualization of soft-tissue anatomy including the absence of landmarks to localize internal openings.

Recent global consensus guidelines for fistula management in Crohn's disease state that fistulography and CT are outdated modalities as they provide poor anatomic relationship between the fistula and the pelvic floor muscles.[7] There may be a role for fistulography in certain exceptionally complex fistulas as it may change operative strategy in some.[13] A more recent study utilizing radiopaque markers to delineate anatomy for fistulography found this modality to be 74% accurate in identifying the presence or absence of an internal opening.[14] Other authors have shown that the rate of fully correlating fistulography with operative findings is only 16%.[15]

Ultrasonography

Endoanal ultrasound is a useful alternative to MRI for evaluation of fistulas as it may be more readily available and has similar accuracy. Its usefulness is limited by smaller field of view and by its inability to adequately visualize abscesses in the supralevator or ischioanal spaces. Hydrogen peroxide and saline fistulography are useful adjuncts to improve visualization.[7] Using definitive surgical findings as the reference standard, Toyonaga et al found endoanal ultrasound to be 88% accurate at detecting a primary fistula tract, 85.7% accurate at describing horseshoe extension, and 85.5% accurate

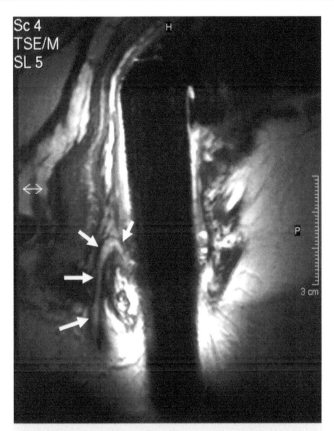

Fig. 9.6 MR image in the sagittal plane of an anteriorly located transsphincteric fistula in a female patient. Arrows point to the tract in the rectovaginal septum. (Courtesy of Ruud Schouten, MD.)

for localizing the primary fistula opening in 401 patients.[16] This study selectively used hydrogen peroxide injected into the fistula opening to enhance visualization (4.9%). Other studies have shown similar results using peroxide-enhanced ultrasound.[17] Directly comparing peroxide-enhanced ultrasound and MRI has demonstrated close correlation between the findings of these two modalities. In one study, the agreement between ultrasound and MRI was 90% for classification of the primary tract, 71% for secondary tracts, and 90% for location of internal openings.[18]

Computed Tomography

The utilization of CT imaging for evaluation of anorectal fistula has been limited due to the inability to provide sufficient soft-tissue resolution around the anal sphincter. The entry of multi-planar CT imaging systems with improved resolution has re-kindled interest in CT fistulography as a less expensive and more readily available alternative to MRI. One recent study compared CT fistulography and MRI to operative findings in 41 patients. CT was able to correctly predict fistula classification in 73% of patients, number of secondary extensions in 85% of patients, and quadrant of the internal opening in 68.2% of patients compared to 92.7, 87.8, and 85.3%, respectively, for MRI. These authors concluded that MRI is superior to CT fistulography in most cases, but CT fistulography could be considered the first choice in uncomplicated cases.[19] As uncomplicated fistulas rarely require radiologic evaluation, this study provides little

support for invasive imaging involving ionizing radiation for simple fistulas.

Endoanal ultrasonography and pelvic MRI may add useful information in the evaluation of anorectal abscess and fistula in selected, complex patients. Fistulography is not widely practiced and few published studies support its use. The widespread availability of CT scan and the speed with which it can be obtained may make it useful in the evaluation of an acute anorectal abscess. However, MRI and ultrasonography are the preferred modality for evaluation of complex fistulas or small abscess due to superior resolution of sphincter complex anatomy without exposure to radiation.

9.5 Anorectal Abscess

9.5.1 Microbiology

Bacterial isolates from anorectal abscesses typically represent a mix of aerobic and anaerobic normal bowel flora and are rarely resistant to common antibiotics. Organisms typically isolated include *Escherichia coli, Bacteroides fragilis, Klebsiella pneumoniae,* coagulase-negative *Staphylococci,* and *Enterococcus* species.[20,21,22] There may be an association between bowel-related organisms cultured from acute abscess and fistula formation. One study reported that 54% of patients whose anorectal abscess cultures grew bowel-derived organisms developed fistulas, compared to 0% of 34 patients whose cultures grew skin-derived organisms, and therefore the authors advocate for a second surgical evaluation to search for fistula in those patients whose anal abscess grows bowel-derived organisms.[23] Most conclude that aggressive pursuit of a fistula based on microbiologic data is unnecessary, as the majority of patients with bowel-derived organisms will not develop a fistula.[24] They suggest that a delayed fistula procedure be performed later if necessary. Microbiologic evaluation of anorectal abscess has been largely absent from recent studies as it is felt to be a somewhat sensitive but not specific means of evaluating for fistulas and inferior to careful anatomic evaluation.[25] One study from 2014 found that 98% of bacteria isolated from anorectal abscesses were sensitive to common oral antibiotics, while 2/172 cultures grew methicillin-resistant *Staphylococcus aureus.*[26] Our practice is to limit the collection of anorectal abscess cultures to those patients who may harbor multidrug-resistant bacteria due to extensive prior antibiotic exposure.

9.5.2 Incidence and Classification

The exact incidence of anorectal abscess is unknown as no national registries exist for outpatient or in-office procedures. Nelson performed a fascinating extrapolation of abscess incidence based on historical data on fistula incidence and an assumption that a defined percentage of abscesses will result in fistulas. His analysis suggests that in the United States the incidence of anorectal abscess is 68,000 to 96,000 cases per year.[27] Several large series have shown a higher incidence in males than females, with ratios ranging from 2:1 to 5:1.[3,28,29,30]

Anorectal abscesses are classified based on anatomic location within potential spaces: perianal, ischioanal, intersphincteric, and supralevator (▶ Fig. 9.7). Posterior abscesses that enter the deep postanal space by penetrating the posterior

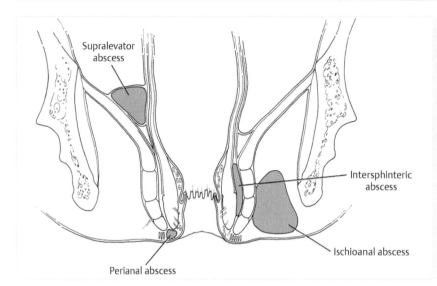

Fig. 9.7 Classification of anorectal abscess.

midline conjoint longitudinal muscle and extend to one or both ischioanal spaces are described as a horseshoe abscess. These are often discussed as a separate classification of abscess as their management can be complex. In a review of 1,023 patients with anorectal abscess at Cook County Hospital, Ramanujam et al found the following frequency of anatomic distribution: perianal, 42.7%; ischioanal, 22.8%; intersphincteric, 21.4%; supralevator, 7.3%; submucous (high intermuscular), 5.8%.[3]

9.5.3 Treatment

Role of Antibiotics

The use of antibiotics in anorectal abscess should be limited to a few specific clinical scenarios as there is no evidence that their use improves healing time or decreases complications. Seow-En and Ngu retrospectively reviewed 172 patients who underwent drainage of anorectal abscess; 63% were prescribed postoperative antibiotics. Despite the fact that the mean abscess size was significantly larger in the group that received antibiotics, there was no difference in abscess recurrence.[26] A randomized, double-blinded, placebo-controlled, multicenter trial of antibiotics after anorectal abscess drainage failed to reveal an improvement in rate of fistula formation in patients randomized to postoperative antibiotics. Rate of fistula formation was lower in patients randomized to placebo, when compared to those given antibiotics (22.4 vs. 37.3%).[31]

The Clinical Practice Guidelines from the American Society of Colon and Rectal Surgeons state: "… the addition of antibiotics to routine incision and drainage of uncomplicated anorectal abscess does not improve healing time or reduce recurrences, and it is therefore not indicated." However, there are specific circumstances for which antibiotics might complement incision and drainage: cellulitis, immunosuppression, concomitant systemic illness, prosthetic heart valves, prior bacterial endocarditis, congenital heart disease, or heart transplant with valvular disease.[32]

Perianal Abscess

The majority of simple perianal abscesses can be drained under local anesthesia in the office or when seen in the emergency department. Generous injection of local anesthetic with epinephrine at and around the point of maximum fluctuance allows complete drainage and can improve hemostasis. A cruciate incision may be created and the skin edges excised (▶ Fig. 9.8) or an ellipse of skin may be excised. Some overlying skin must be removed, as simple stab incision may allow pus to reaccumulate as the skin edges heal closed. We typically place packing if hemostasis is needed, or place a small bulb-tipped catheter if the cavity is large.

In general, there is no need for prolonged packing or repeated dressing changes of the abscess cavity as this is uncomfortable for the patient and provides no long-term benefits. Two small randomized studies have compared packing versus not packing these wounds. In each study, after incision and drainage of perianal abscess, a hemostatic packing was placed. Patients were then randomized to daily nursing packing changes or no packing. One study evaluated 43 patients and found no difference in time to healing, recurrent abscess formation, rate of fistula formation, pain scores, or length of stay.[33] A more recent study evaluated 14 patients and found faster mean time to healing in the nonpacking group (19.5 vs. 26.8 days, $p = 0.047$) along with lower pain scores at 2 weeks in the nonpacking group. There was no difference in recurrence rates, and a single fistula was reported in the packing group.[34]

Ischioanal Abscess

Ischioanal abscesses can typically be managed using the same general principles as perianal abscesses. A smaller abscess in a compliant patient can often be incised and drained under local anesthesia. A larger abscess may require drainage under anesthesia to allow complete evaluation for loculations and counterincisions as needed to completely drain the cavity. Again, excision of a sufficient amount of skin to allow complete drainage is advised and packing is unnecessary.

We will often supplement incision and drainage of a large ischioanal abscess with drainage catheter insertion into the abscess cavity. In the initial description of this technique by Isbister, 91 patients were managed with simple Pezzer catheter insertion. The procedure was generally well tolerated and 22/91 (24.2%) patients developed fistulas.[29] In a large anorectal abscess, it has

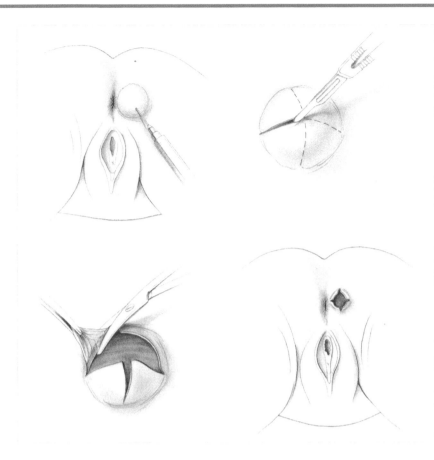

Fig. 9.8 Incision and drainage of a simple perianal or ischioanal abscess. A cruciate incision is created and skin edges are trimmed to prevent early skin healing.

been our practice to secure a Pezzer catheter in the abscess cavity for several weeks as the cavity collapses. The catheter is then removed in the office and ongoing drainage or recurrent suppuration is evaluated for fistula.

Intersphincteric Abscess

As previously discussed, the diagnosis of an intersphincteric abscess often requires a high degree of clinical suspicion as patients may present with pain but no external signs of inflammation. Focal tenderness and fluctuance on digital rectal examination can direct the health care provider to the abscess. Incision and drainage of an intersphincteric abscess will often require general or regional anesthesia for patient comfort and to allow adequate exposure. Treatment consists of drainage of the abscess internally, including division of internal anal sphincter fibers overlying the abscess cavity.

Supralevator Abscess

Like intersphincteric abscess, supralevator abscess can often be difficult to diagnose as findings on physical examination can be few and subtle. The patient may complain of severe perianal pain with no external evidence of inflammation. The source of a supralevator abscess determines its proper management and should therefore be determined whenever possible before treatment begins. The three possible origins of a supralevator abscess are: cephalad extension of an intersphincteric abscess, cephalad extension of an ischioanal abscess, or caudad extension of a pelvic abscess caused by diverticulitis, appendicitis, Crohn's disease, or other source. A combination of evaluation

under anesthesia and radiographic examination may be necessary to determine the abscess origin. Both CT and MRI have proven valuable in the evaluation of supralevator abscess.[35,36]

If the supralevator abscess is a result of intersphincteric or ischioanal abscess, then it should be drained as would be appropriate for its progenitor abscess. That is, a supralevator abscess of intersphincteric origin should be drained internally by dividing internal sphincter overlying the abscess cavity. Drainage of an intersphincteric-derived supralevator abscess via the ischioanal fossa may produce a suprasphincteric fistula. A supralevator abscess of ischioanal origin should be drained through the ischioanal fossa and not via internal drainage with division of internal sphincter fibers. Internal drainage of an ischioanal-derived supralevator abscess may produce an extrasphincteric fistula (▶ Fig. 9.9). Management of the third type of supralevator abscess, one created from downward extension of a pelvic process, is determined by the original disease process. Typically, image-guided catheter drainage of the pelvic abscess provides the least morbid means of treatment. However, surgical drainage through the rectal lumen, through the ischioanal fossa, or through the abdominal wall may be necessary.

Horseshoe Abscess

Lateral extension of an anorectal abscess is commonly described as a horseshoe abscess. This description may be applied to an intersphincteric abscess that has simply extended from the anterior or posterior midline to involve the lateral potential intersphincteric space. This is managed like other intersphincteric abscesses by dividing internal sphincter and allowing internal drainage. The more complex horseshoe abscess is one that has penetrated the conjoint longitudinal muscle at the posterior midline, involved the deep postanal space, and may have spread to one or both ischioanal fossae. The location of the deep postanal space, deep to the external sphincter but superficial to the levator muscles, is important to appreciate as it is relevant to both the formation of these abscesses and their management.

Management of the deep postanal space horseshoe abscess must focus on adequate drainage of this space and was famously described by Hanley. Hanley's original technique includes performing a fistulotomy by inserting a fistula probe in the posterior midline primary fistula opening and dividing the overlying superficial external sphincter in the posterior midline between the primary fistula opening and the coccyx. This allows access to the deep postanal space. Counterincisions may

then be created in the ischioanal fossa on either side to allow complete drainage of the lateral extensions of the horseshoe abscess (▶ Fig. 9.10).[37] Instead of completely laying open the posterior midline external sphincter, Hamilton described a series of 65 patients in whom the deep postanal space was accessed by making a skin incision in the posterior midline and spreading the sphincter fibers. To avoid incontinence, some patients with deep or complex abscesses underwent staged procedures with seton placement. Follow-up data were available for 57 of these patients and 4 recurrences were reported.[38] In later years, Hanley described this modification of his lay-open procedure by placing a cutting seton in the primary fistula tract instead of performing an immediate fistulotomy (▶ Fig. 9.11).[39] As cutting setons have largely fallen from favor, our practice has been to place a loose seton and defer management of the fistula to one of the myriad of less destructive options that have proliferated in recent years.

Recurrent Abscess

Diagnostic evaluation and management of a recurrent abscess can be challenging. Patients may have undergone multiple drainage procedures before referral to a specialist and the resultant anatomic disruptions can complicate evaluation. Early recurrence should raise concern for inadequate drainage. In a study of 500 patients who underwent incision and drainage of anorectal abscess, Onaca et al reported 48 early reoperations within 10 days of the index procedure. As several patients required more than one reoperation, the overall reoperation rate per procedure was 7.6%. Early reoperation was due to inadequate drainage in 23/48 (48%) or missed loculations in 15/48 (32%). Reoperation rate was highest for supralevator abscesses (33%) and low for perianal, ischiorectal, and intersphincteric abscesses (6.9, 7.8, and 7.3%, respectively). Only age older than 21 was a significant risk factor for reoperation, while diabetes, steroids, time from symptom onset to surgery, primary or recurrent abscess, associated fistula, and Crohn's disease were not significant risk factors. Interestingly, there was no difference in the reoperation rate for procedures by junior residents compared to those performed by senior residents or attending surgeons.[40]

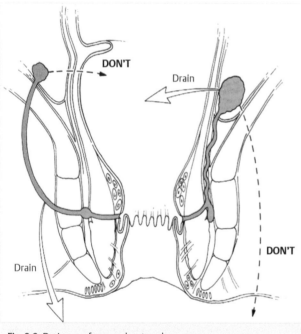

Fig. 9.9 Drainage of a supralevator abscess.

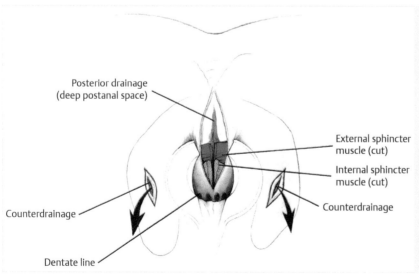

Fig. 9.10 Hanley's original technique for incision and drainage of a horseshoe abscess. Note division of both internal and external sphincter muscle.

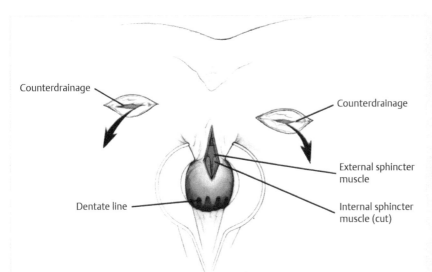

Fig. 9.11 Modification of Hanley's technique for incision and drainage of horseshoe abscess. Note division of internal sphincter muscle with preservation of external sphincter.

A more recent study of recurrent abscesses reported the need for early reoperation in 2.4% and a 36.1% long-term recurrence at a mean of 20 months' follow-up. Fistula was diagnosed in 20% of patients with recurrence. Shorter time from onset of symptoms to drainage was the only factor associated with recurrence with a hazard ratio of 0.4 (95% confidence interval [CI] = 0.23–0.68, p = 0.001). Gender, age, BMI (body mass index), method of anesthesia, abscess location, anatomic classification, drain use, and diabetes were not significant.[41] Ramanujam et al reported 25 recurrences out of 663 patients who underwent incision and drainage of anorectal abscess, and the majority (22/25) were found to have a fistula.[3]

Primary Fistulotomy

Fistulotomy when draining the index abscess is controversial. Proponents of the search for and destruction of a fistula tract at the time of abscess drainage cite a decrease in the rate of recurrence and the need for future surgery. Opponents argue that the majority of anorectal abscesses treated with incision and drainage will not recur or form a fistula, and the search for a fistula converts a simple drainage procedure to an unnecessarily complex procedure. In addition, the presence of acute inflammation may increase incidence of false passages in the search for a fistula, or increased risk of incontinence upon division of excessive sphincter muscle.

Large retrospective series have shown that fistula develops in approximately one-third of patients who undergo incision and drainage of anorectal abscess and another 10% suffer from recurrent abscess.[24,28] Results of these selected series are shown in ▶ Table 9.1. These authors have concluded that primary fistulotomy at the time of abscess drainage is unnecessary as less than 50% of patients who undergo incision and drainage go on to require further procedures. The remainder, in whom incision and drainage is sufficient treatment, derive no benefit from primary fistulotomy and risk complications.

However, a recent meta-analysis evaluated 479 patients from six studies randomized to drainage or drainage with primary fistulotomy. The majority of these trials excluded patients with prior fistula surgery, Crohn's disease, suprasphincteric fistulas,

Table 9.1 Recurrence or persistence of abscess after drainage: selected studies

Study	Number of patients	Abscess recurrence	Fistula formation	Overall recurrence or persistence
Hämäläinen and Sainio[24]	146	10%	37%	47%
Vasilevsky and Gordon[28]	83	11%	37%	48%

or extrasphincteric fistulas. Meta-analysis showed a significant reduction in recurrence after primary fistulotomy (risk ratio [RR] = 0.13, 95% CI = 0.07–0.24) and a trend toward increased incontinence at 1 year (RR = 3.06, 95% CI = 0.7–13.45). Because of significant heterogeneity in the incontinence data, these authors conclude that patients overall benefit from decreased recurrence and the risk of harm is minimal when low fistulas are treated with primary fistulotomy.[42] With these results in mind, we suggest that there is a role for primary fistulotomy in properly selected patients, such as those who have a clearly identifiable internal opening of a low intersphincteric or transsphincteric fistula without significant comorbid conditions or prior anorectal surgery.

9.5.4 Postoperative Care

After abscess drainage, the patient can typically be discharged home directly from the office, emergency room, or postoperative recovery room. The patient should be counseled on the risk of abscess recurrence or fistula formation and given a reasonable timeline for wound healing. The risk of recurrence after drainage of an abscess is summarized in ▶ Table 9.1.

Nonhealing wounds or persistent drainage should prompt evaluation for a fistula. Sitz baths, stool softeners, fiber preparations, and narcotic or nonnarcotic analgesia should be recommended as appropriate. As previously discussed, prolonged wound packing and antibiotics are rarely indicated.

9.6 Fistula-In-Ano

9.6.1 Incidence

As with anorectal abscess, fistula-in-ano is a condition more commonly identified in the male population. Male-to-female ratios are generally reported around 2:1.[43,44,45] Overall incidence has been estimated to range from 1.04 to 2.32 cases per 10,000 population/year based on large, anonymous European databases.[46]

9.6.2 Indications for Operation

In general, the presence of a symptomatic fistula-in-ano is in itself sufficient indication for surgical repair as spontaneous healing is uncommon. Symptoms typically include persistent drainage, recurrent abscesses, or discomfort. Although the majority of fistulas are associated with prior cryptoglandular abscess, the surgeon should also be wary of rare causes of fistulas including Crohn's disease, hidradenitis suppurativa, tuberculosis, or malignancy. Patients presenting with a draining anorectal sinus tract without a prior history of abscess should be carefully evaluated for these conditions before planning repair.

Relative contraindications to fistula repair include medical risk factors for general or regional anesthesia, fecal incontinence, and unmanaged inflammatory bowel disease. In each of these cases, the surgeon must weigh the risks of the procedure against the patient's symptoms. Often, recurrent abscess due to persistent fistula can be managed with long-term seton placement until underlying disease can be controlled.

9.6.3 Principles of Treatment

The principles of fistula surgery are individually simple but can present a complex challenge when considered as a whole. The goal is to heal the fistula in a reasonable amount of time, with the lowest possible recurrence rate, without disrupting continence. To accomplish these goals, several principles should be adhered to as described in ► Table 9.2.

9.6.4 Classification and Treatment

Multiple classification systems have been proposed to describe the anatomic relationships of fistulas-in-ano. The most beneficial system is one that allows communication between surgeons and helps inform treatment of the fistula. Therefore, precise description of the primary tract along with the fistula's relationship to the muscular anatomy of the pelvic floor is necessary. The description by Parks et al is complex but provides this level of detail.[47] Four main classifications are determined

Table 9.2 Principles of fistula surgery

1. Evaluation for underlying disease that may impede wound healing

2. Identification of the primary (internal) opening

3. Delineation of the relationship between the fistula tract and the anatomy of the patient's pelvic floor muscles and sphincter complex

4. Evaluation for blind or side tracts

5. Division of as little sphincter muscle as possible

by relationship between the sphincter muscle and the primary tract of the fistula: intersphincteric, transsphincteric, suprasphincteric, and extrasphincteric. Each of these can be modified based on secondary ramifications and extensions:

- Intersphincteric fistulas
  - Simple low tract
  - High blind tract
  - High tract with rectal opening
  - Rectal opening without a perineal opening
  - Extrarectal extension
  - Secondary to pelvic disease
- Transsphincteric fistulas
  - Uncomplicated
  - High blind tract
- Suprasphincteric fistulas
  - Uncomplicated
  - High blind tract
- Extrasphincteric fistulas
  - Secondary to anal fistula
  - Secondary to trauma
  - Secondary to anorectal disease
  - Caused by pelvic inflammation

What follows is a brief description of each type of fistula along with an illustration of the fistula. Each illustration contains the disease process on the left and the excisional treatment option on the right. These illustrations should be considered a general guide to management and the reader is reminded to refer to the following sections of this chapter for other management options that involve division of less sphincter muscle and may provide equal fistula healing rates. Surgical treatment of fistulas requiring resection of large amounts of sphincter muscle may result in permanent incontinence.

Intersphincteric Fistula

The intersphincteric fistula is the most common type of fistula and involves only the intersphincteric plane. It is often the precursor to other types of fistulas and has multiple possible extensions or secondary ramifications. A simple low tract intersphincteric fistula penetrates the internal sphincter and then passes to the anoderm. It can be treated with division of the distal internal sphincter muscle with little risk to continence (► Fig. 9.12). An intersphincteric fistula with a high blind tract adds an additional upward extension between the internal sphincter and the longitudinal muscle of the rectal wall. Identification and management of the high blind tract by division of more proximal sphincter muscle will decrease the chances of recurrence without adding significantly to the risk of incontinence (► Fig. 9.13). If this high blind tract penetrates back into the lower rectum, a second rectal opening may be produced. As with a high blind tract, this second opening must be identified and treated with division of further internal sphincter to prevent recurrence (► Fig. 9.14). If an intersphincteric abscess forms without draining to the perineum, it is considered an intersphincteric fistula without a perineal opening. These must also be treated with division of the lower portion of the internal sphincter to eliminate the causative crypt (► Fig. 9.15). Finally, an intersphincteric cryptoglandular abscess can extend into the pelvic cavity or a pelvic abscess caused by a primary intestinal

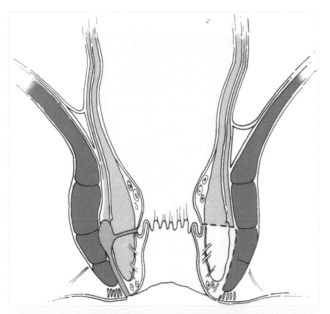

Fig. 9.12 Intersphincteric fistula with low simple tract treated with division of the lower internal sphincter.

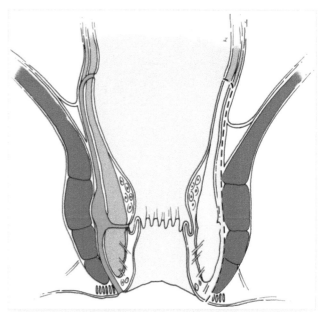

Fig. 9.14 Intersphincteric fistula with high tract and rectal opening treated with division of internal sphincter to the level of the proximal rectal opening.

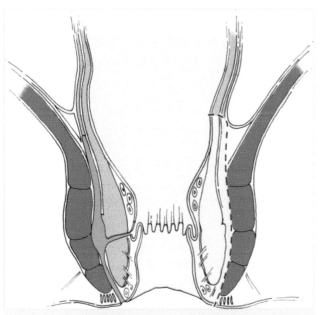

Fig. 9.13 Intersphincteric fistula with high blind tract treated with division of the lower internal sphincter to the proximal extent of the high blind tract.

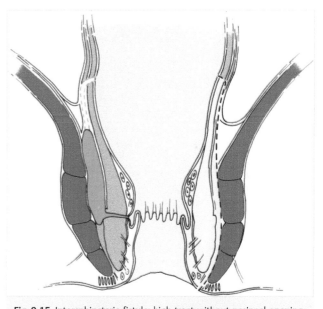

Fig. 9.15 Intersphincteric fistula: high tract without perineal opening.

process can spontaneously drain through the intersphincteric plane. Management is different in each of these cases as division of sphincter muscle plays no role in management of intersphincteric fistula caused by bowel perforation but is important in an intersphincteric fistula that extends proximally from a cryptoglandular abscess (▶ Fig. 9.16, ▶ Fig. 9.17).

Transsphincteric Fistula

An uncomplicated transsphincteric fistula penetrates both the internal and external sphincter and drains through the ischioanal fossa. The level at which the fistula tract crosses the sphincter complex determines options for management. A low transsphincteric fistula can often be treated simply by division

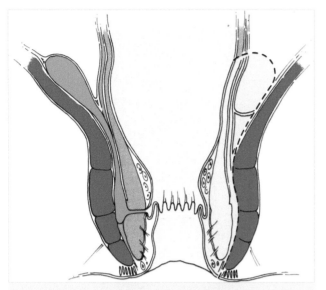

Fig. 9.16 Intersphincteric fistula with extrarectal extension treated with division of internal sphincter to the proximal extent of the fistula.

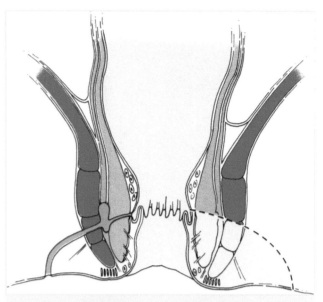

Fig. 9.18 Uncomplicated transsphincteric fistula can be treated with division of a small amount of distal internal and external sphincter or less destructive measures.

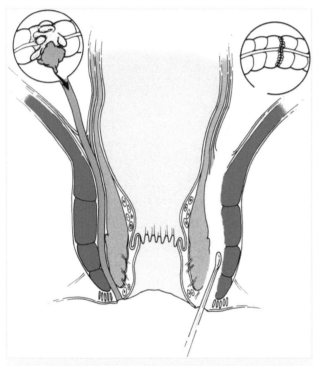

Fig. 9.17 Intersphincteric fistula secondary to pelvic abscess. Management of the bowel injury is necessary but sphincter muscle need not be divided.

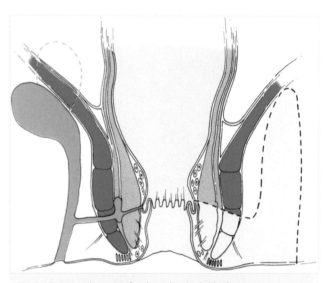

Fig. 9.19 Transsphincteric fistula with a high blind tract.

of the lowest portion of the external sphincter without risk of incontinence (▶ Fig. 9.18). Higher transsphincteric fistulas may be best addressed by some of the less destructive techniques described in the following sections. A high blind tract of a transsphincteric fistula is important to recognize as its improper management can cause complications. Injudicious probing of the high blind tract may create a second opening into the rectum,

thus forming an iatrogenic extrasphincteric fistula. As long as this complication is not encountered, management of the primary transsphincteric fistula will adequately drain the high blind tract (▶ Fig. 9.19). As with an uncomplicated transsphincteric fistula, division of distal internal and external sphincter may not cause significant incontinence but treatment options that do not destroy large amounts of tissue can also be considered.

Suprasphincteric Fistula

An uncomplicated suprasphincteric fistula extends upward from the intersphincteric space to cross above the puborectalis muscle and then tracks downward outside of the sphincter into

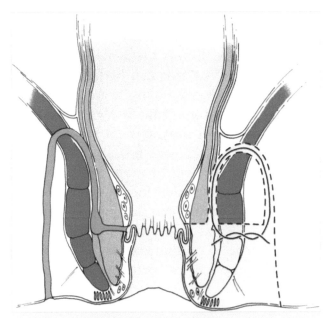

Fig. 9.20 Uncomplicated suprasphincteric fistula.

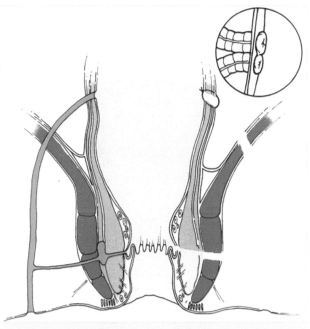

Fig. 9.22 Extrasphincteric fistula secondary to extension of anal fistula of cryptoglandular origin. Treatment includes division of distal internal sphincter, closure of the rectal wall defect, and may require fecal diversion.

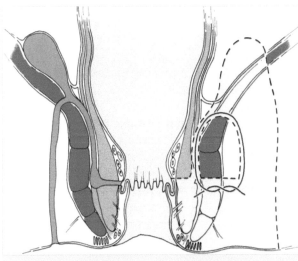

Fig. 9.21 Suprasphincteric fistula with a high blind tract.

the ischioanal fossa. Laying open the entire fistula tract would divide excessive sphincter muscle and likely lead to incontinence. Therefore, excisional management of this fistula should be performed in stages and setons used liberally (▶ Fig. 9.20). Alternative methods such as fistula plug or fibrin glue should also be considered. A high blind tract of a suprasphincteric fistula is very uncommon but may extend into the supralevator space (▶ Fig. 9.21). Treatment is similar to that of an uncomplicated suprasphincteric fistula but the superior extension must be adequately drained and none of the less destructive methods such as plug or fistula glue should be attempted in the face of ongoing infection.

Extrasphincteric Fistula

An extrasphincteric fistula passes from the skin, through the ischioanal fossa, through the levator muscle, and into the

bowel wall within the pelvis. These are challenging to manage as their course is outside the sphincter complex and lay-open technique will lead to incontinence. Also, the high pressure of the rectum forces mucus and debris into the proximal opening and holds the fistula open. Etiology of an extrasphincteric fistula can be spontaneous upward extension of a transsphincteric fistula, iatrogenic perforation of the rectum during probing of a transsphincteric fistula, or secondary to trauma to the perineum that penetrates the rectum. An extrasphincteric fistula may also form by downward extension of an abdominal process such as diverticulitis, Crohn's disease, or perforated malignancy.

Treatment of an extrasphincteric fistula depends on both eliminating the source of contamination and decreasing the high-pressure flow of debris from the rectum. If the source is a transsphincteric fistula, the lower half of the internal sphincter is divided to eliminate the primary tract and the opening in the rectal wall is sutured closed. Temporary fecal diversion must be considered in this case. Treatment of extrasphincteric fistulas caused by downward extension of a pelvic process begins with controlling the underlying disease. This may also require fecal diversion but division of sphincter muscle is unnecessary (▶ Fig. 9.22, ▶ Fig. 9.23, ▶ Fig. 9.24).

9.6.5 Technique (Operative Options)

Simple Low Fistula

When possible, this procedure is performed with the patient under deep monitored sedation in the prone jackknife position. Comorbid conditions such as obesity, sleep apnea, or

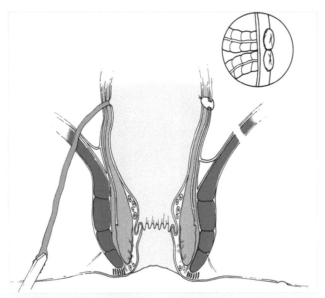

Fig. 9.23 Extrasphincteric fistula secondary to trauma. Treatment consists of eliminating the foreign body and fecal diversion. Division of sphincter muscle is not necessary.

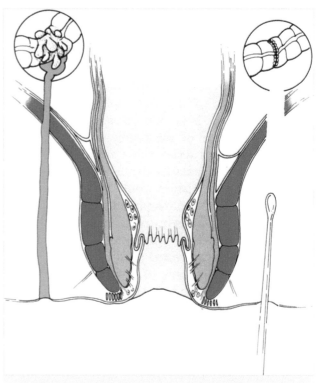

Fig. 9.24 Extrasphincteric fistula secondary to pelvic disease. Treatment of the inciting colon or rectal process will eliminate the fistula. Division of sphincter muscle is unnecessary and ill-advised.

pulmonary disease may preclude this approach and mandate general anesthesia in the lateral decubitus, prone, or lithotomy position. The perianal region is infiltrated with local anesthetic containing epinephrine. Digital examination and anal speculum are used to evaluate the fistula anatomy and identify internal openings or inflammation. A probe is inserted through the external opening and gently passed through the tract to an internal opening. Attempts should be made to identify any secondary openings or side branches and the fistula anatomy should be determined. If a simple intersphincteric or low transsphincteric fistula is present, the tissue overlying the fistula probe can be divided. Bleeding is controlled by electrocautery (▶ Fig. 9.25).

Marsupialization of the fistula tract is often performed by running an absorbable suture to approximate the skin edges to the tract. Two randomized trials have supported marsupialization over completing the procedure with an entirely open wound. Ho et al randomized 103 patients who underwent fistulotomy for intersphincteric or low transsphincteric fistula to marsupialization or open wounds. Marsupialized wounds healed in a mean of 6 weeks compared to 10 weeks for wounds left open ($p < 0.001$). Also, maximum anal squeeze pressure measured by manometry was lower at 3 months in the wounds left open compared to those marsupialized. There was a 2% incidence of incontinence in the marsupialization group compared to 12% in the group left open, but this was not statistically significant.[49] In a more recent trial, Pescatori et al randomized 46 patients to marsupialization or open wounds after fistulotomy or fistulectomy. This trial included patients with high, recurrent, and horseshoe fistula. Measured wound size was smaller in the marsupialization group both intraoperatively (1,749 vs. 819 mm^2) and at a 4-week follow-up (543 vs. 217 mm^2) and bleeding risk was lower in the marsupialization group (36 vs. 46%, $p < 0.05$). No difference was found in postoperative pain.[48]

If the primary opening cannot be identified or the probe cannot be easily passed, we inject hydrogen peroxide into the external opening. This may be expressed as bubbles from the internal opening. Other dyes such as dilute methylene blue or betadine may be used as well. If the internal opening is still not evident, laying open the tract from the external opening to the extent that it can be identified by a fistula probe may alter the exposure of the tract such that its course becomes evident.

Horseshoe Fistula

As previously described, circumferential spread of a posterior abscess in the deep postanal space can result in a horseshoe fistula, which may have multiple lateral secondary openings. Preoperative evaluation of the suspected horseshoe fistula with MRI or ultrasound may allow identification of the multiple complex tracts and increase the probability of a successful repair. Surgeon and patient should be aware that the management of horseshoe abscess and fistula often requires multiple procedures and is particularly challenging in the patient with Crohn's disease. Rosen et al reported 143 operations on 31 patients (mean, 2.5) referred to their facility for management of horseshoe abscess and fistula. Only 47% of patients with Crohn's disease were healed or asymptomatic at follow-up compared to 75% of patients without Crohn's disease.[50]

Surgical management of the horseshoe fistula is conceptually similar to that of the acute abscess and must involve adequate drainage of any lateral secondary tracts along with management of the primary posterior midline fistula tract. An

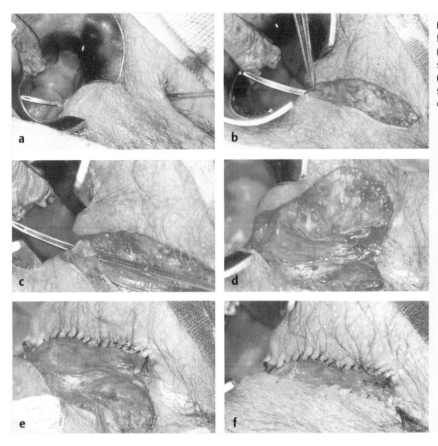

Fig. 9.25 Technique for laying open a low simple fistula. **(a)** Lockhart–Mummery probe in fistula. **(b)** Skin and anoderm incised. **(c)** External sphincter incised and internal sphincter exposed. **(d)** Entire tract unroofed and curetted. **(e)** One side of tract marsupialized. **(f)** Marsupialization completed.

aggressive management strategy begins with laying open the lateral limbs of the horseshoe tract. The primary fistula opening at the crypt in the posterior midline is identified and a probe is passed through it. Identification of the primary fistula opening at the dentate line is important to prevent recurrence. Once the primary opening has been identified, the overlying posterior sphincter muscle can be divided and the exposed fistula tracts curetted of debris. Marsupialization of the wound edges can facilitate healing of the resulting large tissue defect (▶ Fig. 9.26). While this technique is successful at eradicating the fistula, it also produces a large wound and carries a risk of incontinence.

A less locally destructive approach to horseshoe fistula management is similar to the modified procedure Hanley described for treatment of the acute abscess. This technique involves isolating the midline fistula by incising the space between the superficial external sphincter and the coccyx and thereby entering the deep postanal space. Once the fistula tract is identified, Hanley's initial description involved excising a "T" portion of the fistula tract within the deep postanal space and carrying the fistulotomy through the posterior sphincter complex to the primary opening (▶ Fig. 9.27).[37] In the later modification, placement of a cutting seton was preferred to fistulotomy of the primary tract. The seton allowed preservation of the external and distal internal sphincter muscles overlying the primary fistula tract.[39] In either case, the lateral secondary openings are enlarged to allow curettage and adequate drainage. Performing an internal sphincterotomy over the primary fistula tract while leaving the external

sphincter complex intact may provide adequate eradication of the fistula while preserving continence. For high fistula tracts, one should also consider less destructive techniques such as fibrin glue, fistula plugs, or the ligation of intersphincteric fistula tract (LIFT) procedure, described in the following pages.

Division of the sphincter muscles in management of anterior horseshoe fistulas carries a high risk of incontinence as there is no puborectalis muscle. Therefore, seton drain placement is preferred over primary fistulotomy for the anterior abscess. Definitive fistula management may include division of the internal sphincter muscle with adequate drainage of the external openings. Again, less destructive alternatives such as fibrin glue, fistula plugs, or LIFT should be considered when appropriate for a high anterior fistula.

Use of Seton

A seton is any foreign material inserted into a fistula tract to encircle the sphincter muscle. Materials used historically have included vessel loops, silk suture, penrose drains, and wire. In cases of high transsphincteric or suprasphincteric fistulas, enough sphincter muscle may be involved that simple division can lead to unacceptably high risk to continence and therefore seton placement may be required. The technique for inserting the seton is relatively straightforward once the fistula tract has been clearly identified. The material selected is secured to the probe, which is then passed through the fistula tract and the seton is then pulled through the fistula. The seton is then secured to itself (▶ Fig. 9.28).

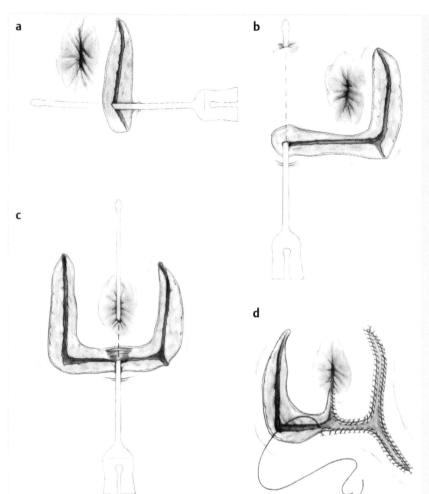

Fig. 9.26 Technique for laying open a horseshoe fistula. **(a)** Probe is inserted in lateral extension and used to identify the fistula crossing midline. **(b)** Contralateral tracts are identified and divided as needed. **(c)** The posterior midline primary fistula is identified and overlying sphincter muscle is divided. **(d)** Wound edges are marsupialized.

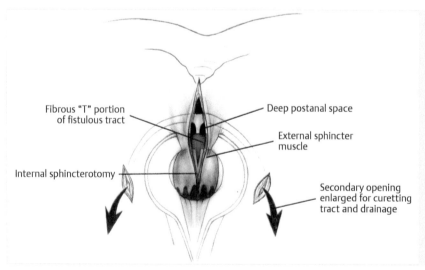

Fibrous "T" portion of fistulous tract

Deep postanal space

External sphincter muscle

Internal sphincterotomy

Secondary opening enlarged for curetting tract and drainage

Fig. 9.27 Modification of Hanley's treatment of a horseshoe fistula.

There are several benefits of seton placement and specific clinical situations in which it is particularly useful. First, even loose setons placed for drainage alone stimulate fibrosis and scar formation in the underlying sphincter muscle. This may allow later division of overlying sphincter without a large gap in the muscle. It may be left in place in an inflamed abscess cavity to allow resolution of the suppuration and future fistula management. This approach is also beneficial in patients with poor wound healing or Crohn's disease as it prevents premature skin healing before resolution of the abscess cavity. Also, prolonged seton placement and formation of fibrosis may allow more clear delineation of the fistula tract and the amount of overlying

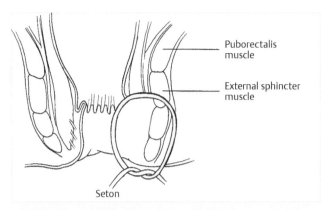

Fig. 9.28 Placement of seton.

sphincter muscle on follow-up evaluation. Finally, we perform LIFT after a seton has been in place for a sufficient amount of time to allow the epithelialized tract to be more easily identified and manipulated.

In the interest of preserving sphincter muscle and thereby continence, a seton can be used as the sole means of management of a high transsphincteric fistula without dividing further muscle. A seton is initially placed in a high transsphincteric fistula, the underlying subcutaneous tissue and internal sphincter are divided, and the external sphincter is preserved. If the wounds heal well, the seton is simply removed. Parks and Stitz reported alteration in continence in 17% of patients who had a seton removed without division of external sphincter compared to 39% of patients whose sphincter was divided.[51] Kennedy and Zegarra reported results in 32 patients managed similarly. Primary healing after seton removal occurred in 78% of patients with 33% complaining of some form of incontinence.[52] Eitan et al reported long-term results in 41 patients (87.8% male) managed with only seton placement without sphincter division over 5 years. Rate of fistula persistence was 19.5% and alteration in continence was 14.6%. Of note, all patients whose fistula did not initially heal had complete, durable healing after a second attempt with the same technique.[53]

The use of cutting setons has been largely abandoned in recent years due to concerns about incontinence and quality of life. A cutting seton is any seton which is initially placed loosely but then serially tightened to advance it through the sphincter muscle by pressure necrosis. This has been thought to result in less incontinence than primary fistulotomy as the divided muscle is able to form scar instead of gaping widely apart. One large review of published studies reported an overall incontinence rate of 12% in 1,490 patients. In studies that reported type of incontinence, 46% reported incontinence to flatus, 1% to mucus, 69% to liquid stool, and 18% to solid stool. Many patients had incontinence to multiple types of stool, hence a total greater than 100%. These authors suggest that this rate of incontinence should stimulate interest in other, sphincter-sparing procedures.[54]

Others have suggested that the rate of incontinence after cutting seton use is acceptably low. For example, Patton et al reported 93% primary healing and 98% secondary healing in 59 patients who were treated with cutting seton. At a mean of 9.4 years of follow-up, 32% reported perfect continence, 46% reported mild incontinence, 13.5% reported moderate incontinence, and 8.5% reported severe incontinence based on the St.

Marks scale. The patient perception of bowel control after cutting seton compared to before showed that 63% perceived no change or improved control, while 37% experienced worsened continence. These authors conclude that, while further study is required, cutting seton may be superior to advancement flap or LIFT.[55] The use of a cutting seton is likely best suited to the male patient with a low transsphincteric fistula although it is unclear that this method is superior to any other described and tightening of the seton is often poorly tolerated.

Fibrin Glue

The use of fibrin glue for fistula management has been appealing as the technique is simple and does not require division of sphincter muscle. In the operating room, the primary and secondary fistula openings are identified. The patient is evaluated for ongoing suppuration; the procedure is abandoned if purulence is discovered as perianal sepsis can develop if fibrin glue is applied in the setting of ongoing infection. The fistula tract is cleaned of granulation tissue using a curette or fistula brush and the glue is instilled through the external opening until it is seen extruding through the internal opening. A semi-occlusive dressing of petroleum gauze is applied and the patient can be discharged from the recovery room.[56] The addition of a rectal advancement flap over the internal opening has been advocated as an adjunct to fibrin glue placement.[57,58] Other surgeons prefer to close the internal opening with suture before instilling glue.[59]

Tyler et al reported results for 89 patients treated with fibrin glue in the largest retrospective, nonrandomized study encountered in a literature search. Fifty-five of 89 (65%) patients experienced primary healing after 6 to 12 weeks of follow-up. Of those who failed initial treatment but had repeat instillation of fibrin glue, 57% healed. The remaining patients who failed treatment with fibrin glue were successfully treated with rectal advancement flap.[59] The largest prospective, nonrandomized study to date of fibrin glue for anal fistula reported results of 79 patients. Success was defined as no drainage from the previously existing fistula. Overall success rate was 61% with a mean of 12-month follow-up (range, 6–18 months). Success in patients with Crohn's, HIV, or rectovaginal fistula was achieved in only 36%. Average time to recurrence was 3.3 months, with one recurrence as late as 11 months.[56]

There have been few randomized trials using fibrin glue for anal fistulas. A small randomized trial compared fibrin glue to conventional therapy with fistulotomy or seton placement in 13 simple and 29 complex fistulas. At 12-week follow-up, fibrin glue healed 3 of 6 simple fistulas and 9 of 13 complex fistulas. This compared to conventional therapy healing 7 of 7 simple and 2 of 16 complex fistulas. The difference in healing complex fistulas was statistically significant.[60] Ellis and Clark reported 58 patients randomized to rectal advancement flap alone or rectal advancement flap with fibrin glue obliteration of the fistula tract. At a mean of 22-month follow-up, patients treated with flap and glue had a higher fistula recurrence rate than those treated with flap alone (46.4 vs. 20%, $p < 0.05$).[61] These authors elected not to debride the fistula tract, which may explain the lack of improvement with fibrin glue.

Length of fistula tract may be an important predictor of success when fibrin glue is used. In one trial, fistulas less than 3.5 cm recurred in 54% of patients treated with fibrin glue compared to 11% recurrence in patients with fistulas longer than 3.5 cm.[62] Although not always successful, the use of fibrin glue is associated with minimal complications and is generally well tolerated by patients. It also does not preclude future fistula management by other means.

Anal Fistula Plug

The moderate success of fibrin glue generated interest in other less invasive management techniques for fistula-in-ano with low risk of incontinence that could more reliably accomplish fistula healing. Anal fistula plugs are believed to occlude the fistulous tract by providing a scaffold for native tissue regeneration. Commercially available brands include: Surgisis (Cook Surgical, Inc., Bloomington, IN) and GORE BIO-A (W.L. Gore & Associates, Inc., Flagstaff, AZ). The Surgisis plug is a porcine intestinal submucosa xenograft formed into a conical shape, while the Gore Bio-A plug is composed of absorbable synthetic materials: polyglycolic acid:trimethylene carbonate. The initial description of this technique by Johnson et al reported 87% fistula closure at 13-week follow-up.[63] Enthusiasm for this technique has been somewhat tempered as larger, more recent studies have shown success rates of 24 to 52%, but the ability to treat a high fistula with minimal risk of injury to sphincter muscle continues to be appealing.[64,65,66,67,68]

Insertion of the fistula plug is best accomplished with the patient in prone jackknife position after the administration of an enema and preoperative antibiotics. Internal and external fistula openings must be clearly identified and a probe is passed through the tract. The plug is pulled from the internal opening through the tract toward the external opening. When the plug is seated tightly within the internal opening, the plug is secured to the internal opening and any excess material is trimmed. This allows occlusion of the internal opening while allowing drainage from the external opening.

In a recent review of 84 patients from 12 studies evaluating the use of anal fistula plug for treatment of fistula associated with Crohn's disease, Nasseri et al reported an overall fistula healing rate of 58.3% with a median follow-up time of 9 months. This study did not report complication rates. These authors note that evaluation of the fistula plug in Crohn's disease is limited by a lack of standardized studies, small patient numbers in published studies, short and variable follow-up time, and lack of reporting of confounding variables or reason for plug failures. However, this review does describe use of anal fistula plug in Crohn's disease as safe with little morbidity and reasonable success.[69] A different trial randomized patients with fistulizing perianal Crohn's disease to fistula plug or simple seton removal. Fistula closure after 12 weeks of follow-up was reported in 31.5% of 54 patients randomized to fistula plug and 23.1% of 52 patients randomized to seton removal. This difference was not significant and these authors describe fistula plug as an ineffective means to manage anal fistula in Crohn's disease.[70]

9.6.6 Ligation of Intersphincteric Fistula Tract

The LIFT procedure was conceived as an option to minimize risk of incontinence while successfully resolving transsphincteric fistulas. First described by Rojanasakul, LIFT is performed by creating an incision over the intersphincteric groove and circumferentially dissecting around the fibrous fistula tract as it traverses the intersphincteric plane. Once the tract is isolated, it is divided and the two cut ends within the intersphincteric plane are securely ligated using absorbable suture. Complete obliteration of the tract is confirmed using saline or hydrogen peroxide injected into the internal and external fistula openings and reinforcing the suture ligation at any leak. Granulation tissue is curetted from the fistula tract. In this initial technical description, patients were maintained on oral antibiotics for 2 weeks postoperatively.[71] Of the first 18 patients treated by this group, 17 had fistula healing with no reported complications.[72] The initial reports of larger series of patients treated by LIFT revealed somewhat lower success rates (57–82%) but confirmed the low rate of postoperative complications.[73,74,75]

The largest meta-analysis of LIFT outcomes performed to date accumulated 1,025 patients from 15 published articles and 9 nonpublished abstracts presented at national meetings. After a weighted mean follow-up duration of 10.3 months, overall success rate of fistula healing was 76.4%. The overall postoperative complication rate was 5.5%. There was relatively large heterogeneity of outcomes in the included studies and these authors therefore advocate for further studies to elucidate factors contributing to failure of LIFT to resolve a fistula.[76]

Comparison of LIFT to mucosal advancement flap for transsphincteric fistula was performed in a randomized controlled trial involving 70 patients. There were more postoperative complications in the mucosal advancement flap (two urinary retention and two flap suture disruption) compared to the LIFT group (one perianal hematoma), and higher visual analog scale pain scores in the mucosal advancement flap group at 1 week (4.8 vs. 3.1, $p = 0.002$). However, pain scores were equal at 4 weeks and overall quality of life scores were equivalent between groups. The authors do report a trend toward worsening of baseline incontinence in the mucosal advancement flap group, but this did not reach statistical significance. This study was unable to detect a significant difference between mucosal advancement flap and LIFT for the primary outcome of fistula healing at 1 year (74.3% in LIFT, 65.7% for mucosal advancement flap, $p = 0.58$). These authors suggest that the technical simplicity of LIFT compared to mucosal advancement flap would make it the procedure of choice if outcomes are similar.[77]

Several modifications of LIFT have been described in recent years. Ellis described reinforcing the closure of the external sphincter defect in the intersphincteric groove with a bioprosthetic graft. There were two treatment failures out of 31 patients after a minimum 12-month follow-up with this technique.[78]

A combination procedure utilizing both the LIFT technique and a fistula plug has been described. These authors perform the LIFT procedure as previously described and then obliterate the isolated section of fistula tract coursing through the external sphincter by securing a fistula plug in it. Early results of this technique were promising, with a 95% fistula closure rate at a median of 14-month follow-up.[79] A randomized, controlled trial included 239 patients with transsphincteric fistulas equally randomized to LIFT, or LIFT plus plug. For the primary outcome of fistula healing after 6 months, LIFT-plug was significantly superior to LIFT alone (94 vs. 83.9%, $p < 0.001$). Secondary outcomes such as postoperative pain and fecal incontinence were equivalent between groups and essentially negligible. There were two wound infections reported in the LIFT-plug group with no complications reported in the LIFT group.[80] As with any first report of a new technique, these impressive results await confirmation in further studies.

Rectal Advancement Flap

Rectal advancement flap is another option for treatment of a high transsphincteric or suprasphincteric fistula. This technique allows the fistula to be addressed without the disturbances in continence that can be associated with division of significant sphincter muscle. The steps of the procedure differ somewhat from surgeon to surgeon but meticulous attention to detail is advocated to improve rates of success. The fistula tract is identified and the external opening enlarged to allow drainage and then debrided using a curette. A full-thickness flap of rectal wall is raised proximal to the internal opening. We recommend a broad-based flap, historically twice as wide as the length of the flap, to allow sufficient flap perfusion. The length of the flap should allow some overlap with the mucosa distal to the internal opening. Absorbable suture is used to close the fistula defect in the underlying muscle. The tip of the flap containing the mucosal defect is amputated, and the flap is sutured into place (▶ Fig. 9.29).

Several large series have demonstrated excellent success with minimal complications in patients treated using advancement flap. Aguilar et al reported a series of 189 patients who underwent mucosal advancement flap. Follow-up information was available for 80% and ranged from 8 months to 7 years. Minor fecal soiling, incontinence to flatus, or incontinence to loose stools was reported in 10%, while only 1.5%

had a recurrent fistula.[81] Mizrahi et al reported success in 59.6% of patients at a mean follow-up of 40.3 months. This study population contained 29.8% fistulas caused by Crohn's disease with a 57.1% recurrence rate, compared to 33.3% recurrence in non-Crohn's fistulas. Overall median time to recurrence was 8 months.[82]

A review of 1,654 patients from 35 studies published between 1978 and 2008 evaluated rates of success and incontinence. At an average follow-up of 28.9 months, success rates varied from 36.6 to 98.5% with an average of 76.2%. Incontinence rates varied from 0 to 35% with a weighted average rate of incontinence of 13.3% in fistulas of cryptoglandular origin and 9.4% in fistulas of Crohn's origin.[83]

Dermal Island Flap Anoplasty

Similar in concept to rectal advancement flap is dermal island flap anoplasty. A variety of specific techniques have been described for this procedure, but the common steps are excision of the involved internal opening and surrounding anoderm, eradication of the fistula tract, advancement of a wide-based anal skin flap to cover the defect, and opening the external opening to allow drainage (▶ Fig. 9.30). The most common scenario for choosing dermal island flap anoplasty over endorectal advancement flap is those patients in whom a relatively low internal opening may require advancement of the mucosal advancement flap low in the anal canal, resulting in mucosal ectropion. Other authors referenced below have cited the technical challenge and bleeding risk of mucosal advancement flap as reasons for preferring dermal island flap anoplasty.

Nelson et al described their technique and results in 65 patients. After excision of the originating crypt, a teardrop-shaped

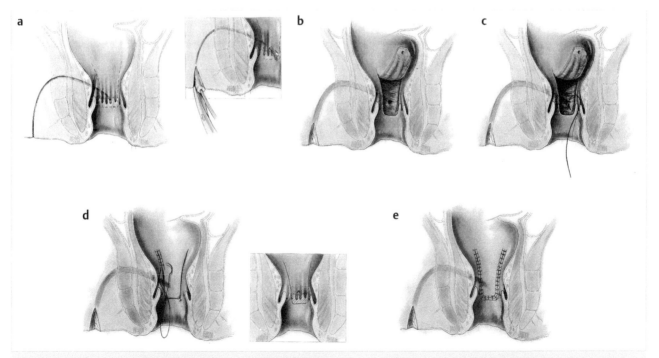

Fig. 9.29 Advancement rectal flap. **(a)** Dotted line outlines flap to be raised in repair of high transsphincteric fistula-in-ano. Inset indicates beginning of coring-out procedure. **(b)** Fistula is cored out and flap of mucosa, submucosa, and internal sphincter is elevated. **(c)** Opening in anal canal is sutured. **(d)** Flap is drawn down and distal end is excised (inset). **(e)** Flap is sutured in place.

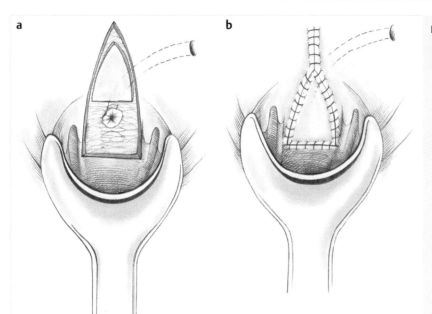

Fig. 9.30 (a,b) V–Y dermal island flap anoplasty.

flap centered on the fistula tract and ending beyond the external fistula opening is designed. The defect in the internal sphincter is closed and the flap is sutured to the rectal mucosa. The external opening is left in place and not debrided. Using this technique, a success rate of 80% at a mean of 28.4 months of follow-up was seen. The majority of recurrences occurred in less than 1 year with the latest recurrence recorded at 20 months. Of note, fibrin glue was used to obliterate the fistula tract in some patients, but this technique was abandoned when it was found to significantly increase the risk of recurrence.[84]

The technique described by Amin et al includes a V–Y advancement flap. The initial "V" incision is designed so that the external opening is included in one lateral side and the internal opening is included in the base. The internal and external openings are excised, the tract is debrided, and the defect in the internal sphincter is closed. The flap is then sutured to the rectum and the skin is closed, leaving open most of the side formerly containing the external opening. Overall, 15 of 18 patients were reported to have healed using this technique with no deterioration of continence.[85] Using a similar technique, Sungurtekin et al reported successful outcome in 59 of 65 patients with no deterioration in continence at a mean follow-up of 32 months.[86]

A randomized trial of advancement flap versus conventional management of transsphincteric fistulas by Ho and Ho evaluated 20 consecutive patients. These authors found no difference in pain, bleeding, incontinence, or quality of life at 16 weeks and no recurrences in either group at a mean of 63.3-week follow-up.[87]

Fistoloscopy

Evaluation and management of fistula-in-ano has been described utilizing a technique called video-assisted anal fistula treatment (VAAFT). The fistuloscope is an 18 cm long by 3.3 to 4.7 mm wide rigid, tapered endoscope, which contains optical, working, and irrigation channels. Constant irrigation is used to distend the fistula tract as the fistuloscope is advanced and the

fistula's course, secondary ramifications, and abscess cavities are evaluated. Cautery can then be used to directly eradicate the fistula tract from the inside.

Large series evaluating this technique have shown some success in fistula management. In the first report, Meinero and Mori described 98 patients who were followed for a minimum of 6 months after VAAFT. Operative time improved from 2 hours to 30 minutes as the learning curve was overcome and failure to resolve the fistula was reported in 26.5%.[88] Kochhar et al reported a later series of 82 patients who underwent fistuloscopy. Mean operative time was 45 minutes (range, 30–90 minutes) and recurrence rate was 15.85%.[89] In a study of 203 patients, many of whom were included in Meinero and Mori's initial report, no postoperative reduction in continence was reported using continence questionnaires. The 6-month cumulative probability of freedom from fistula estimated according to a Kaplan–Meier analysis was 70% in this larger series.[90] These reports suggest that VAAFT has an acceptable success rate compared to other sphincter-sparing fistula management techniques but initial equipment cost and lack of widespread experience with the technique are likely barriers to adoption.

9.6.7 Causes of Recurrence

Although some fistulas will recur in spite of the most meticulous surgical technique and attention to detail, there are some common pitfalls to avoid. The most common reason for anal fistula recurrence is failure to identify and obliterate the internal opening. If the causative infected gland is left untreated, recurrence can be expected. In addition, failure to detect and treat lateral or upward extension may also lead to recurrence. Premature skin healing over fistulotomy wounds can result in recurrence. Formation of new fistulas in a patient previously treated is not unexpected in patients with Crohn's disease.

In a review of 375 patients who had undergone fistula surgery and responded to a mailed questionnaire, Garcia-Aguilar et al reported the following as statistically significant risk factors for recurrence: complex fistula, failure to identify internal opening, internal opening on a lateral side compared to anterior or posterior midline, and fistulas with horseshoe extension. Type of treatment, prior fistula surgery, and less surgeon experience all showed a trend toward worse outcome but were not statistically significant.[91]

9.6.8 Causes of Anal Incontinence after Operation for Anal Fistula

Multiple patient factors have been implicated in postoperative incontinence after anal fistula surgery. In the same review of 375 patients who underwent fistula surgery, Garcia-Aguilar et al also reported risk factors for disturbances in continence. Overall, they reported that 45% of patients complained of some degree of incontinence. Thirty-two percent of this study population self-reported staining of undergarments, 31% incontinence to gas, and 13% accidental bowel movements. The rate of incontinence was related to type of fistula with 37% of patients with an intersphincteric fistula reporting incontinence compared to 83% with a history of extrasphincteric fistula. There was a statistically significant increase in risk for female patients compared to male patients (64 vs. 39%, $p < 0.01$). Other significant factors were amount of external sphincter muscle divided and prior fistula surgery. There was also increased risk with two-stage or cutting seton compared to primary fistulotomy but the authors attribute this to more complex fistulas treated by the former modality.[91]

Operative technique can impact incontinence. In addition to the amount of external sphincter muscle divided, the surgeon must be aware of the inferior rectal nerves providing motor innervation of the rectum. Damage to one nerve may be tolerated but division of bilateral nerves leads to incontinence. As previously mentioned, prolonged packing does not improve wound healing and may increase risk of incontinence.

9.6.9 Postoperative Care

Time to complete healing may be prolonged, and both patient and surgeon must be reassured that complex fistulas can take several months to resolve. Careful postoperative care may improve wound healing and decrease the chance of recurrence. Good care of the postoperative fistula must begin with good surgery. Early recurrence is often attributed to premature closure of the skin edges over a fistula site and fistulotomy must therefore be sufficiently aggressive to prevent this complication. Patients may be advised to take warm baths for comfort and perineal toilet. Stool softeners and bulking agents are advisable to improve hygiene and decrease discomfort with bowel movements.

Time to complete healing depends on the type of fistula and the complexity of the procedure. In addition, patients with underlying conditions such as Crohn's disease or immunosuppression can expect prolonged wound healing. A simple fistulotomy can be expected to heal in several weeks, whereas a more complex procedure may require several months to complete healing.

9.7 Special Considerations

9.7.1 Fistulotomy versus Fistulectomy

Debate continues over the appropriate use of fistulectomy in the management of anal fistula-in-ano. In comparison to fistulotomy, which includes only excision of tissue overlying the fistula tract, fistulectomy requires excision of all inflamed tissue surrounding the tract (▶ Fig. 9.31). Fistulectomy has generally been discouraged as it leads to larger wounds, larger sphincter defects, and presumably prolonged wound healing with higher risk of incontinence.

In a trial of 47 patients randomized to fistulectomy or fistulotomy, Kronborg found that healing time after fistulectomy was prolonged (41 vs. 34 days, $p < 0.02$) with similar recurrence rates at 1 year.[92] In a recent meta-analysis comparing fistulectomy and fistulotomy, Xu et al evaluated 6 randomized controlled trials containing 565 patients. These studies only included patients with low fistulas. There was no significant difference between the two techniques for any variables analyzed. No significant difference was reported in operative time or healing time, but each was reported in only three of six studies. Complications including pain, infection, and bleeding were also not different. Finally, rates of fecal incontinence and recurrence were not significantly different between the two methods.[93]

While these results do not demonstrate significant harm from fistulectomy for low fistula, they also do not demonstrate any benefit. It is therefore difficult to advocate for fistulectomy as it will produce a larger wound without improving outcome.

9.7.2 Necrotizing Perineal Infection

Necrotizing soft-tissue infections of the perineum carry a high risk of mortality and a certain significant morbidity. As this is a relatively rare condition, lack of experience and delay in diagnosis contribute to poor outcomes, and overall morbidity is

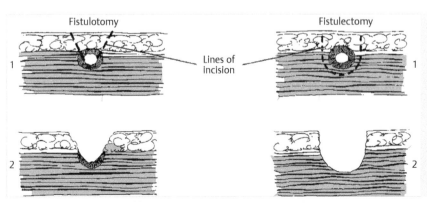

Fig. 9.31 Fistulotomy versus fistulectomy.

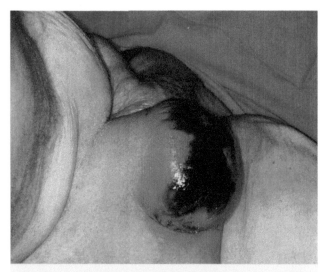

Fig. 9.32 Typical Fournier's gangrene with blackened, necrotic scrotal skin.

86%—with nosocomial infections, ventilator-dependent respiratory failure, and acute renal failure occurring in over 25% of patients.[94] Overall annual incidence of necrotizing soft-tissue infection in the United States is estimated to be 0.04 cases per 1,000 person-years resulting in 500 to 1,500 cases/year.[95] Infection of the perineum comprises a subset of this population and includes Fournier's gangrene with the classically described blackened necrosis of the scrotal skin (▶ Fig. 9.32).

Risk factors for necrotizing soft-tissue infection include any condition that alters normal immune function or tissue perfusion. Diabetes, peripheral vascular disease, obesity, chronic renal failure, HIV, alcohol abuse, IV drug use, surgical incisions, and trauma have all been implicated. Up to 50% of patients, however, will have no specific inciting event.[94]

Evaluation and management of necrotizing soft-tissue infection are dependent on a high degree of clinical suspicion and rapid initiation of multimodal treatment. Clinical practice guidelines drive home the point that any rapidly progressive soft-tissue infection should be presumed to be a necrotizing soft-tissue infection and treated accordingly. Appropriate treatment includes source control, broad-spectrum antibiotics, and supportive care most often requiring admission to a critical care setting.[96]

Source control by aggressive surgical debridement is the cornerstone of management. Multiple studies have shown dramatic increases in mortality if debridement is inadequate or delayed. For example, Mok et al reported that risk of death was 7.5 times higher when initial debridement was inadequate, and Wong et al found that mortality increased nine times if surgical management was delayed more than 24 hours from hospital admission.[97,98] Resection includes all nonviable tissue and should extend to normal, healthy tissue. Consideration should be given to saving life over functional or cosmetic outcome. Early return to the operating room for repeat evaluation and debridement is to be thought of as the standard of care and should only be omitted in patients who show clear clinical evidence of improvement. Management of the resulting large wounds can be complex and is especially difficult with perineal infections. Negative pressure wound therapy devices have been shown to improve tissue granulation, hospital length of stay, and patient's pain compared to wet-to-dry dressings.[99,100] Patients with extensive perineal wounds may require fecal and urinary diversion to facilitate wound hygiene and dressing changes but this is an individualized decision based on patient needs.

Antimicrobial therapy is complex and may best be managed with the assistance of a specialist. Early empiric therapy with activity against gram-positive, gram-negative, and anaerobic organisms should be initiated as soon as the diagnosis of necrotizing soft-tissue infection is suspected. This includes appropriate coverage against methicillin-resistant *Staphylococcus aureus* and often includes antiribosomal agents such as clindamycin, linezolid, or tetracyclines as rapidly progressive infection can be potentiated by exotoxins.[96]

9.7.3 Carcinoma Associated with Chronic Fistula-in-Ano

Anal carcinoma associated with chronic fistula-in-ano is uncommon and often misdiagnosed. The etiology of these malignancies also remains a subject of debate and it is likely that there is no one source for these cancers. Malignancy may begin within the anal crypts and fistulize toward the skin, be spread from other GI malignancies and become implanted in a chronic benign fistula, or may begin in a longstanding fistula tract. On the question of whether the chronic inflammation of the fistula led to the carcinoma or the carcinoma led to the fistula, Skir offered the suggestion that to implicate the fistula as the source of the malignancy, it must have preceded the malignancy by a sufficient amount of time to rule out even the most slowly growing malignancy. Ten years is offered as an arbitrary amount of time.[101] One case series described 11 patients who developed anal adenocarcinoma after 10 to 26 years of anal fistulas. The majority of these patients had Crohn's disease and had undergone prior anorectal surgery and the authors suggest that the chronic, deep fistula tracts associated with Crohn's disease are particularly high risk for malignant degeneration.[102]

A penetrating malignancy of the anal glands has also been theorized as one source of a malignant fistula. This is also an uncommon malignancy and is primarily described in case reports, but a large series of 34 patients treated at University of Texas, MD Anderson Cancer Center, described evaluation and management of anal adenocarcinoma over 21 years. The most common presenting symptoms were bleeding (53%) followed by mass or "hemorrhoids" (32%). These authors make no mention of patients presenting with fistula, underscoring the infrequency of this process. Stage at presentation was T1 in 8.8%, T2 in 53%, T3 in 26%, and T4 in 12%. Outcomes were generally poor with median disease-free survival of 22 months and actuarial 5-year survival of 31%.[103]

There have been multiple case reports of synchronous proximal colorectal cancer in a patient with adenocarcinoma in an existing fistula.[104,105,106,107] It has been theorized that shed tumor cells implant in the chronic granulation tissue of the fistula tract. These reports underscore the importance of evaluating the entire gastrointestinal tract for malignancy if carcinoma is discovered associated with fistula. Management of anal adenocarcinoma is similar to that of low rectal cancer. Locally advanced disease may be treated with neoadjuvant chemotherapy and radiation followed by resection, while local resection alone may be appropriate for earlier stage tumors.[103]

9.7.4 Septic Complications in Immunocompromised Patients

In the patient with hematologic malignancies or other source of severe immunocompromise, management of anorectal abscess or fistula can be particularly challenging. The incidence of perianal sepsis in patients with hematologic malignancies has been estimated to be 8 to 9%. Presenting symptoms can range from the typical pain, swelling, and induration in more immunocompetent hosts to subtle presentations of fevers or discomfort without clear findings on examination.[108,109] Mortality rates have historically been high in this patient population with earlier series reporting mortality of 45 to 80%, although this is all-cause mortality and anorectal suppuration is likely a marker for overall poor prognosis in these severely ill patients rather than a proximate cause of their death.[110,111,112,113,114] Larger, more recent series have reported mortality rates of 0 to 25%.[115,116,117]

The infection is typically polymicrobial with *Escherichia coli* the most commonly recovered organism, followed by *Pseudomonas aeruginosa* and other enteric organisms. Barnes et al reported an average of 2.1 different organisms recovered per patient.[109]

Controversy exists on the best way to manage this complication as both surgical and nonsurgical intervention have shown success. In a retrospective review of 81 patients with symptomatic anorectal disease and leukemia, Grewal et al reported equivalent outcomes between patients treated with nonoperative or operative management. A total of 52 (64%) patients underwent operative management, while the remaining patients were treated without surgery. These authors further analyzed 54 patients from this population who were severely neutropenic (absolute neutrophil count [ANC] < 500/mm^3). In 20 patients who underwent operative therapy, there were 4 deaths (20%) compared to 6 deaths in the 34 patients managed nonoperatively (18%). Because there was no increase in mortality, they concluded that anorectal sepsis in the severely neutropenic patient can be safely drained.[116]

In a more recent series, Lehrnbecher et al evaluated 64 patients who presented with 82 episodes of anorectal sepsis and a variety of malignancies. ANC was less than 500 during 43 (52%) of these encounters, and 22 of 64 (34%) patients had leukemia or lymphoma. The majority of these episodes (63%) were treated with antibiotics alone and surgery was reserved for those patients with extending cellulitis, increasing pain or fluctuance, formation of a clinically apparent abscess, or necrosis. These authors report no complications directly attributed to the surgical procedure. While there were two deaths in the study population, there were no deaths that could be attributed to the anorectal infection. These authors attribute the low mortality to judicious use of broad-spectrum antibiotics (third-generation cephalosporins and carbapenems) and suggest that surgery should be reserved for those patients with the findings described above.[117]

9.7.5 Anoperineal Tuberculosis

Anoperineal tuberculosis is an uncommon finding in the developed world and can be easily misdiagnosed as an abscess or fistula of cryptoglandular origin. Incidence is reported to be less than 1% of anorectal fistulas but may be much higher in the developing world. Most information is gathered from case reports and small series. Sultan et al described seven patients accumulated over 17 years in Paris. All were male with a median age of 55 years, all had pulmonary tuberculosis, and five of seven were not of French origin. All were managed with antituberculosis drugs in addition to surgery and all healed without recurrence.[118] Tai et al reported on 17 patients recruited from a single hospital in Taiwan over 15 years. Fourteen of 17 were male, mean age was 44.8 years, and 13 of 17 had coexisting pulmonary disease. Fifteen of 17 received a full course of antituberculosis drugs and all healed without recurrence.[119] In both studies, tuberculosis was diagnosed based on histologic findings of giant cell granulomas, caseous necrosis, or acid-fast bacilli.

Clinical manifestations of anoperineal tuberculosis can vary widely but the most common presentation is a nonhealing anal fistula. Other examination findings can include ulceration, recurrent perianal growths, fissures, or strictures. Fistulas can be complex and may have multiple secondary tracts at presentation but there is no clinical sign that can easily differentiate between tuberculous and cryptoglandular fistulas.[120]

9.7.6 Rectourethral Fistulas

Rectourethral fistula is an increasingly common complication of treatment for prostate cancer. Radical prostatectomy, external beam radiation therapy, and brachytherapy are all treatment modalities used in prostate cancer and all carry a risk of fistula. Keller et al recently published an excellent review of the management of rectourethral fistula and much of the information here is gathered from their work.[121]

Incidences of rectourethral fistula are reported to be less than 2% from radical retropubic prostatectomy, 0.2% from brachytherapy, 2.9% from combined brachytherapy and external beam therapy, and 0.4 to 1.2% from cryotherapy or high-frequency ultrasound. Symptoms typically consist of fecaluria, pneumaturia, recurrent urinary tract infections, and urine leaking from the rectum during urination. Evaluation of symptoms concerning for rectourethral fistula includes anoscopy and flexible sigmoidoscopy to assess the rectum along with cystoscopy and cystourethrogram to evaluate the morphology of the fistula, urethral strictures, and bladder capacity. Patients with symptoms or signs of ongoing infection should be evaluated with CT scan to evaluate for abscess.

The treatment algorithm described by Keller et al is based on symptoms and the nature of the fistula. All patients underwent drainage of any underlying abscess along with maintenance of an indwelling urinary catheter. Diverting stoma was performed in patients with severe symptoms, fistula > 1 cm in size, significant tissue scarring, severe urethral stricture, or pelvic sepsis. Patients whose fistulas healed within 3 months after these interventions were offered stoma closure. Definitive surgery was offered to those patients whose fistulas did not heal. Patients with nonfunctional bladder or positive oncologic margins were offered pelvic exenteration or cystectomy with ileal conduit. All others were offered transperineal gracilis interposition flap or local flap repair.

Of 30 patients treated using this algorithm, 20 required fecal diversion. Fourteen patients healed with or without fecal diversion but no other surgical intervention. Thirteen of the remaining 16 patients consented to definitive repair with transperineal or transabdominal surgical approach and all healed. After a mean follow-up of 72 months, there was no recurrence of healed fistulas. There was urinary incontinence in 11 of 30 patients (37%).[121] Another large series of gracilis flap interposition repair of rectourethral fistula reported similar results. At a mean follow-up of 28 months, 25 of 25 patients experienced successful fistula closure with no recurrence. Urinary incontinence was reported in 48% of patients including four who required permanent urinary diversion and three who were lost to follow-up.[122] Success rates in excess of 70% have been reported.[123],[124]

Harris et al reported the largest study to date of patients who were treated for rectourethral fistula after prostate cancer treatment. A retrospective cohort of 210 patients was accumulated from four centers in the United States. Repair was performed through a transperineal approach in 79% of patients and a combined transperineal and transabdominal approach in the remainder. Fecal diversion was performed in 83.6% of patients and muscle interposition flaps were used in 91.9% of procedures. Overall final success rate was 92.9% for all patients. When analyzed by initial treatment modality for prostate cancer, final fistula repair rate was higher in patients who underwent radical prostatectomy than in those who underwent energy ablation therapy (99 vs. 86.5%, $p < 0.001$). These authors advocate for placement of a muscle interposition flap such as the gracilis flap and emphasize that none of the patients in this cohort underwent transsphincteric (York-Mason) approach.[125]

With the evolving application of natural orifice and minimally invasive surgery, repair of rectourethral fistulas can possibly be approached using transanal minimally invasive surgery (TAMIS) or transanal endoscopic microsurgery (TEMS).[126],[127],[128] Nicita et al retrospectively evaluated 12 patients with rectourethral fistula after prostatectomy who underwent transanal repair using laparoscopic instruments introduced through a Parks' anal retractor. They were able to identify and suture the urothelial wall via the fistula tract and then suture the rectal wall closed. No recurrence was identified at a median of 21-month follow-up.[129] Kanehira et al described a similar approach using TEMS equipment to suture repair both the urothelial wall and the rectal wall in 10 patients who had undergone prostatectomy. Seven of 10 patients healed and one of the recurrent fistulas was in a patient who had undergone radiation therapy and two prior failed repairs.[130]

References

[1] Eisenhammer S. A new approach to the anorectal fistulous abscess based on the high intermuscular lesion. Surg Gynecol Obstet. 1958; 106(5):595–599
[2] Parks AG. Pathogenesis and treatment of fistuila-in-ano. BMJ. 1961; 1 (5224):463–469
[3] Ramanujam PS, Prasad ML, Abcarian H, Tan AB. Perianal abscesses and fistulas. A study of 1023 patients. Dis Colon Rectum. 1984; 27(9):593–597
[4] Edwards FS. On some of the rarer forms of rectal fistulae. BMJ. 1887; 2 (1383):13–15
[5] Gunawardhana PA, Deen KI. Comparison of hydrogen peroxide instillation with Goodsall's rule for fistula-in-ano. ANZ J Surg. 2001; 71(8):472–474
[6] Cirocco WC, Reilly JC. Challenging the predictive accuracy of Goodsall's rule for anal fistulas. Dis Colon Rectum. 1992; 35(6):537–542
[7] Gecse KB, Bemelman W, Kamm MA, et al. World Gastroenterology Organization, International Organisation for Inflammatory Bowel Diseases IOIBD, European Society of Coloproctology and Robarts Clinical Trials, World Gastroenterology Organization International Organisation for Inflammatory Bowel Diseases IOIBD European Society of Coloproctology and Robarts Clinical Trials. A global consensus on the classification, diagnosis and multidisciplinary treatment of perianal fistulising Crohn's disease. Gut. 2014; 63 (9):1381–1392
[8] Barker PG, Lunniss PJ, Armstrong P, Reznek RH, Cottam K, Phillips RK. Magnetic resonance imaging of fistula-in-ano: technique, interpretation and accuracy. Clin Radiol. 1994; 49(1):7–13
[9] Mahjoubi B, Haizadch Kharazi H, Mirzaei R, Moghimi A, Changizi A. Diagnostic accuracy of body coil MRI in describing the characteristics of perianal fistulas. Colorectal Dis. 2006; 8(3):202–207
[10] Singh K, Singh N, Thukral C, Singh KP, Bhalla V. Magnetic resonance imaging (MRI) evaluation of perianal fistulae with surgical correlation. J Clin Diagn Res. 2014; 8(6):RC01–RC04
[11] Siddiqui MR, Ashrafian H, Tozer P, et al. A diagnostic accuracy meta-analysis of endoanal ultrasound and MRI for perianal fistula assessment. Dis Colon Rectum. 2012; 55(5):576–585
[12] Buchanan GN, Halligan S, Bartram CI, Williams AB, Tarroni D, Cohen CR. Clinical examination, endosonography, and MR imaging in preoperative assessment of fistula in ano: comparison with outcome-based reference standard. Radiology. 2004; 233(3):674–681
[13] Weisman RI, Orsay CP, Pearl RK, Abcarian H. The role of fistulography in fistula-in-ano. Report of five cases. Dis Colon Rectum. 1991; 34(2):181–184
[14] Pomerri F, Dodi G, Pintacuda G, Amadio L, Muzzio PC. Anal endosonography and fistulography for fistula-in-ano. Radiol Med (Torino). 2010; 115 (5):771–783
[15] Kuijpers HC, Schulpen T. Fistulography for fistula-in-ano. Is it useful? Dis Colon Rectum. 1985; 28(2):103–104
[16] Toyonaga T, Tanaka Y, Song JF, et al. Comparison of accuracy of physical examination and endoanal ultrasonography for preoperative assessment in patients with acute and chronic anal fistula. Tech Coloproctol. 2008; 12 (3):217–223
[17] Nagendranath C, Saravanan MN, Sridhar C, Varughese M. Peroxide-enhanced endoanal ultrasound in preoperative assessment of complex fistula-in-ano. Tech Coloproctol. 2014; 18(5):433–438
[18] West RL, Zimmerman DD, Dwarkasing S, et al. Prospective comparison of hydrogen peroxide-enhanced three-dimensional endoanal ultrasonography and endoanal magnetic resonance imaging of perianal fistulas. Dis Colon Rectum. 2003; 46(10):1407–1415
[19] Soker G, Gulek B, Yilmaz C, et al. The comparison of CT fistulography and MR imaging of perianal fistulae with surgical findings: a case-control study. Abdom Radiol (NY). 2016; 41(8):1474–1483
[20] Liu CK, Liu CP, Leung CH, Sun FJ. Clinical and microbiological analysis of adult perianal abscess. J Microbiol Immunol Infect. 2011; 44(3):204–208
[21] Ulug M, Gedik E, Girgin S, Celen MK, Ayaz C. The evaluation of bacteriology in perianal abscesses of 81 adult patients. Braz J Infect Dis. 2010; 14(3):225–229
[22] Leung E, McArdle K, Yazbek-Hanna M. Pus swabs in incision and drainage of perianal abscesses: what is the point? World J Surg. 2009; 33 (11):2448–2451
[23] Grace RH, Harper IA, Thompson RG. Anorectal sepsis: microbiology in relation to fistula-in-ano. Br J Surg. 1982; 69(7):401–403
[24] Hämäläinen KP, Sainio AP. Incidence of fistulas after drainage of acute anorectal abscesses. Dis Colon Rectum. 1998; 41(11):1357–1361, discussion 1361–1362
[25] Lunniss PJ, Phillips RK. Surgical assessment of acute anorectal sepsis is a better predictor of fistula than microbiological analysis. Br J Surg. 1994; 81 (3):368–369
[26] Seow-En I, Ngu J. Routine operative swab cultures and post-operative antibiotic use for uncomplicated perianal abscesses are unnecessary. ANZ J Surg. 2017; 87(5):356–359
[27] Nelson R. Anorectal abscess fistula: what do we know? Surg Clin North Am. 2002; 82(6):1139–1151, v–vi
[28] Vasilevsky CA, Gordon PH. The incidence of recurrent abscesses or fistula-in-ano following anorectal suppuration. Dis Colon Rectum. 1984; 27 (2):126–130
[29] Isbister WH. A simple method for the management of anorectal abscess. Aust N Z J Surg. 1987; 57(10):771–774
[30] Oliver I, Lacueva FJ, Pérez Vicente F, et al. Randomized clinical trial comparing simple drainage of anorectal abscess with and without fistula track treatment. Int J Colorectal Dis. 2003; 18(2):107–110
[31] Sözener U, Gedik E, Kessaf Aslar A, et al. Does adjuvant antibiotic treatment after drainage of anorectal abscess prevent development of anal fistulas? A randomized, placebo-controlled, double-blind, multicenter study. Dis Colon Rectum. 2011; 54(8):923–929
[32] Steele SR, Kumar R, Feingold DL, Rafferty JL, Buie WD, Standards Practice Task Force of the American Society of Colon and Rectal Surgeons. Practice parameters for the management of perianal abscess and fistula-in-ano. Dis Colon Rectum. 2011; 54(12):1465–1474

[33] Tonkin DM, Murphy E, Brooke-Smith M, et al. Perianal abscess: a pilot study comparing packing with nonpacking of the abscess cavity. Dis Colon Rectum. 2004; 47(9):1510–1514

[34] Perera AP, Howell AM, Sodergren MH, et al. A pilot randomised controlled trial evaluating postoperative packing of the perianal abscess. Langenbecks Arch Surg. 2015; 400(2):267–271

[35] Garcia-Granero A, Granero-Castro P, Frasson M, et al. Management of cryptoglandular supralevator abscesses in the magnetic resonance imaging era: a case series. Int J Colorectal Dis. 2014; 29(12):1557–1564

[36] Ortega AE, Bubbers E, Liu W, Cologne KG, Ault GT. A novel classification, evaluation, and treatment strategy for supralevator abscesses. Dis Colon Rectum. 2015; 58(11):1109–1110

[37] Hanley PH, Ray JE, Pennington EE, Grablowsky OM. Fistula-in-ano: a ten-year follow-up study of horseshoe-abscess fistula-in-ano. Dis Colon Rectum. 1976; 19(6):507–515

[38] Hamilton CH. Anorectal problems: the deep postanal space–surgical significance in horseshoe fistula and abscess. Dis Colon Rectum. 1975; 18(8):642–645

[39] Hanley PH. Reflections on anorectal abscess fistula: 1984. Dis Colon Rectum. 1985; 28(7):528–533

[40] Onaca N, Hirshberg A, Adar R. Early reoperation for perirectal abscess: a preventable complication. Dis Colon Rectum. 2001; 44(10):1469–1473

[41] Yano T, Asano M, Matsuda Y, Kawakami K, Nakai K, Nonaka M. Prognostic factors for recurrence following the initial drainage of an anorectal abscess. Int J Colorectal Dis. 2010; 25(12):1495–1498

[42] Malik AI, Nelson RL, Tou S. Incision and drainage of perianal abscess with or without treatment of anal fistula. Cochrane Database Syst Rev. 2010(7): CD006827

[43] Isbister WH. Fistula in ano: a surgical audit. Int J Colorectal Dis. 1995; 10(2):94–96

[44] Malouf AJ, Buchanan GN, Carapeti EA, et al. A prospective audit of fistula-in-ano at St. Mark's hospital. Colorectal Dis. 2002; 4(1):13–19

[45] Nwaejike N, Gilliland R. Surgery for fistula-in-ano: an audit of practise of colorectal and general surgeons. Colorectal Dis. 2007; 9(8):749–753

[46] Zanotti C, Martinez-Puente C, Pascual I, Pascual M, Herreros D, García-Olmo D. An assessment of the incidence of fistula-in-ano in four countries of the European Union. Int J Colorectal Dis. 2007; 22(12):1459–1462

[47] Parks AG, Gordon PH, Hardcastle JD. A classification of fistula-in-ano. Br J Surg. 1976; 63(1):1–12

[48] Pescatori M, Ayabaca SM, Cafaro D, Iannello A, Magrini S. Marsupialization of fistulotomy and fistulectomy wounds improves healing and decreases bleeding: a randomized controlled trial. Colorectal Dis. 2006; 8(1):11–14

[49] Ho YH, Tan M, Leong AF, Seow-Choen F. Marsupialization of fistulotomy wounds improves healing: a randomized controlled trial. Br J Surg. 1998; 85(1):105–107

[50] Rosen SA, Colquhoun P, Efron J, et al. Horseshoe abscesses and fistulas: how are we doing? Surg Innov. 2006; 13(1):17–21

[51] Parks AG, Stitz RW. The treatment of high fistula-in-ano. Dis Colon Rectum. 1976; 19(6):487–499

[52] Kennedy HL, Zegarra JP. Fistulotomy without external sphincter division for high anal fistulae. Br J Surg. 1990; 77(8):898–901

[53] Eitan A, Koliada M, Bickel A. The use of the loose seton technique as a definitive treatment for recurrent and persistent high trans-sphincteric anal fistulas: a long-term outcome. J Gastrointest Surg. 2009; 13(6):1116–1119

[54] Ritchie RD, Sackier JM, Hodde JP. Incontinence rates after cutting seton treatment for anal fistula. Colorectal Dis. 2009; 11(6):564–571

[55] Patton V, Chen CM, Lubowski D. Long-term results of the cutting seton for high anal fistula. ANZ J Surg. 2015; 85(10):720–727

[56] Cintron JR, Park JJ, Orsay CP, et al. Repair of fistulas-in-ano using fibrin adhesive: long-term follow-up. Dis Colon Rectum. 2000; 43(7):944–949, discussion 949–950

[57] van Koperen PJ, Wind J, Bemelman WA, Slors JF. Fibrin glue and transanal rectal advancement flap for high transsphincteric perianal fistulas; is there any advantage? Int J Colorectal Dis. 2008; 23(7):697–701

[58] Zmora O, Mizrahi N, Rotholtz N, et al. Fibrin glue sealing in the treatment of perineal fistulas. Dis Colon Rectum. 2003; 46(5):584–589

[59] Tyler KM, Aarons CB, Sentovich SM. Successful sphincter-sparing surgery for all anal fistulas. Dis Colon Rectum. 2007; 50(10):1535–1539

[60] Lindsey I, Smilgin-Humphreys MM, Cunningham C, Mortensen NJ, George BD. A randomized, controlled trial of fibrin glue vs. conventional treatment for anal fistula. Dis Colon Rectum. 2002; 45(12):1608–1615

[61] Ellis CN, Clark S. Fibrin glue as an adjunct to flap repair of anal fistulas: a randomized, controlled study. Dis Colon Rectum. 2006; 49(11):1736–1740

[62] Patrlj L, Kocman B, Martinac M, et al. Fibrin glue-antibiotic mixture in the treatment of anal fistulae: experience with 69 cases. Dig Surg. 2000; 17(1):77–80

[63] Johnson EK, Gaw JU, Armstrong DN. Efficacy of anal fistula plug vs. fibrin glue in closure of anorectal fistulas. Dis Colon Rectum. 2006; 49(3):371–376

[64] Adamina M, Ross T, Guenin MO, et al. Anal fistula plug: a prospective evaluation of success, continence and quality of life in the treatment of complex fistulae. Colorectal Dis. 2014; 16(7):547–554

[65] Blom J, Husberg-Sellberg B, Lindelius A, et al. Results of collagen plug occlusion of anal fistula: a multicentre study of 126 patients. Colorectal Dis. 2014; 16(8):626–630

[66] Cintron JR, Abcarian H, Chaudhry V, et al. Treatment of fistula-in-ano using a porcine small intestinal submucosa anal fistula plug. Tech Coloproctol. 2013; 17(2):187–191

[67] Herold A, Ommer A, Fürst A, et al. Results of the Gore Bio-A fistula plug implantation in the treatment of anal fistula: a multicentre study. Tech Coloproctol. 2016; 20(8):585–590

[68] Stamos MJ, Snyder M, Robb BW, et al. Prospective multicenter study of a synthetic bioabsorbable anal fistula plug to treat cryptoglandular transsphincteric anal fistulas. Dis Colon Rectum. 2015; 58(3):344–351

[69] Nasseri Y, Cassella L, Berns M, Zaghiyan K, Cohen J. The anal fistula plug in Crohn's disease patients with fistula-in-ano: a systematic review. Colorectal Dis. 2016; 18(4):351–356

[70] Senéjoux A, Siproudhis L, Abramowitz L, et al. Groupe d'Etude Thérapeutique des Affections Inflammatoires du tube Digestif [GETAID]. Fistula Plug in Fistulising Ano-Perineal Crohn's Disease: a Randomised Controlled Trial. J Crohn's Colitis. 2016; 10(2):141–148

[71] Rojanasakul A. LIFT procedure: a simplified technique for fistula-in-ano. Tech Coloproctol. 2009; 13(3):237–240

[72] Rojanasakul A, Pattanaarun J, Sahakitrungruang C, Tantiphlachiva K. Total anal sphincter saving technique for fistula-in-ano; the ligation of intersphincteric fistula tract. J Med Assoc Thai. 2007; 90(3):581–586

[73] Aboulian A, Kaji AH, Kumar RR. Early result of ligation of the intersphincteric fistula tract for fistula-in-ano. Dis Colon Rectum. 2011; 54(3):289–292

[74] Bleier JI, Moloo H, Goldberg SM. Ligation of the intersphincteric fistula tract: an effective new technique for complex fistulas. Dis Colon Rectum. 2010; 53(1):43–46

[75] Shanwani A, Nor AM, Amri N. Ligation of the intersphincteric fistula tract (LIFT): a sphincter-saving technique for fistula-in-ano. Dis Colon Rectum. 2010; 53(1):39–42

[76] Hong KD, Kang S, Kalaskar S, Wexner SD. Ligation of intersphincteric fistula tract (LIFT) to treat anal fistula: systematic review and meta-analysis. Tech Coloproctol. 2014; 18(8):685–691

[77] Madbouly KM, El Shazly W, Abbas KS, Hussein AM. Ligation of intersphincteric fistula tract versus mucosal advancement flap in patients with high transsphincteric fistula-in-ano: a prospective randomized trial. Dis Colon Rectum. 2014; 57(10):1202–1208

[78] Ellis CN. Outcomes with the use of bioprosthetic grafts to reinforce the ligation of the intersphincteric fistula tract (BioLIFT procedure) for the management of complex anal fistulas. Dis Colon Rectum. 2010; 53(10):1361–1364

[79] Han JG, Yi BQ, Wang ZJ, et al. Ligation of the intersphincteric fistula tract plus a bioprosthetic anal fistula plug (LIFT-Plug): a new technique for fistula-in-ano. Colorectal Dis. 2013; 15(5):582–586

[80] Han JG, Wang ZJ, Zheng Y, et al. Ligation of intersphincteric fistula tract vs ligation of the intersphincteric fistula tract plus a bioprosthetic anal fistula plug procedure in patients with transsphincteric anal fistula: early results of a multicenter prospective randomized trial. Ann Surg. 2016; 264(6):917–922

[81] Aguilar PS, Plasencia G, Hardy TG, Jr, Hartmann RF, Stewart WR. Mucosal advancement in the treatment of anal fistula. Dis Colon Rectum. 1985; 28(7):496–498

[82] Mizrahi N, Wexner SD, Zmora O, et al. Endorectal advancement flap: are there predictors of failure? Dis Colon Rectum. 2002; 45(12):1616–1621

[83] Soltani A, Kaiser AM. Endorectal advancement flap for cryptoglandular or Crohn's fistula-in-ano. Dis Colon Rectum. 2010; 53(4):486–495

[84] Nelson RL, Cintron J, Abcarian H. Dermal island-flap anoplasty for transsphincteric fistula-in-ano: assessment of treatment failures. Dis Colon Rectum. 2000; 43(5):681–684

[85] Amin SN, Tierney GM, Lund JN, Armitage NC. V-Y advancement flap for treatment of fistula-in-ano. Dis Colon Rectum. 2003; 46(4):540–543

[86] Sungurtekin U, Sungurtekin H, Kabay B, et al. Anocutaneous V-Y advancement flap for the treatment of complex perianal fistula. Dis Colon Rectum. 2004; 47(12):2178–2183

[87] Ho KS, Ho YH. Controlled, randomized trial of island flap anoplasty for treatment of trans-sphincteric fistula-in-ano: early results. Tech Coloproctol. 2005; 9(2):166–168

[88] Meinero P, Mori L. Video-assisted anal fistula treatment (VAAFT): a novel sphincter-saving procedure for treating complex anal fistulas. Tech Coloproctol. 2011; 15(4):417–422

[89] Kochhar G, Saha S, Andley M, et al. Video-assisted anal fistula treatment. JSLS. 2014; 18(3):e2014.00127

[90] Meinero P, Mori L, Gasloli G. Video-assisted anal fistula treatment: a new concept of treating anal fistulas. Dis Colon Rectum. 2014; 57(3):354–359

[91] Garcia-Aguilar J, Belmonte C, Wong WD, Goldberg SM, Madoff RD. Anal fistula surgery. Factors associated with recurrence and incontinence. Dis Colon Rectum. 1996; 39(7):723–729

[92] Kronborg O. To lay open or excise a fistula-in-ano: a randomized trial. Br J Surg. 1985; 72(12):970

[93] Xu Y, Liang S, Tang W. Meta-analysis of randomized clinical trials comparing fistulectomy versus fistulotomy for low anal fistula. Springerplus. 2016; 5(1):1722

[94] Sarani B, Strong M, Pascual J, Schwab CW. Necrotizing fasciitis: current concepts and review of the literature. J Am Coll Surg. 2009; 208(2):279–288

[95] Anaya DA, Dellinger EP. Necrotizing soft-tissue infection: diagnosis and management. Clin Infect Dis. 2007; 44(5):705–710

[96] Sartelli M, Malangoni MA, May AK, et al. World Society of Emergency Surgery (WSES) guidelines for management of skin and soft tissue infections. World J Emerg Surg. 2014; 9(1):57

[97] Mok MY, Wong SY, Chan TM, Tang WM, Wong WS, Lau CS. Necrotizing fasciitis in rheumatic diseases. Lupus. 2006; 15(6):380–383

[98] Wong CH, Chang HC, Pasupathy S, Khin LW, Tan JL, Low CO. Necrotizing fasciitis: clinical presentation, microbiology, and determinants of mortality. J Bone Joint Surg Am. 2003; 85-A(8):1454–1460

[99] Assenza M, Cozza V, Sacco E, et al. VAC (Vacuum Assisted Closure) treatment in Fournier's gangrene: personal experience and literature review. Clin Ter. 2011; 162(1):e1–e5

[100] Huang WS, Hsieh SC, Hsieh CS, Schoung JY, Huang T. Use of vacuum-assisted wound closure to manage limb wounds in patients suffering from acute necrotizing fasciitis. Asian J Surg. 2006; 29(3):135–139

[101] Skir I. Mucinous carcinoma associated with fistulas of long-standing. Am J Surg. 1948; 75(2):285–289

[102] Gaertner WB, Hagerman GF, Finne CO, et al. Fistula-associated anal adenocarcinoma: good results with aggressive therapy. Dis Colon Rectum. 2008; 51(7):1061–1067

[103] Chang GJ, Gonzalez RJ, Skibber JM, Eng C, Das P, Rodriguez-Bigas MA. A twenty-year experience with adenocarcinoma of the anal canal. Dis Colon Rectum. 2009; 52(8):1375–1380

[104] Gravante G, Delogu D, Venditti D. Colosigmoid adenocarcinoma anastomotic recurrence seeding into a transsphincteric fistula-in-ano: a clinical report and literature review. Surg Laparosc Endosc Percutan Tech. 2008; 18(4):407–408

[105] Hyman N, Kida M. Adenocarcinoma of the sigmoid colon seeding a chronic anal fistula: report of a case. Dis Colon Rectum. 2003; 46(6):835–836

[106] Ishiyama S, Inoue S, Kobayashi K, et al. Implantation of rectal cancer in an anal fistula: report of a case. Surg Today. 2006; 36(8):747–749

[107] Wakatsuki K, Oeda Y, Isono T, et al. Adenocarcinoma of the rectosigmoid colon seeding into pre-existing anal fistula. Hepatogastroenterology. 2008; 55(84):952–955

[108] Baker B, Al-Salman M, Daoud F. Management of acute perianal sepsis in neutropenic patients with hematological malignancy. Tech Coloproctol. 2014; 18(4):327–333

[109] Barnes SG, Sattler FR, Ballard JO. Perirectal infections in acute leukemia. Improved survival after incision and debridement. Ann Intern Med. 1984; 100(4):515–518

[110] Birnbaum W, Ahlquist R. Rectal infections and ulcerations associated with blood dyscrasias. Am J Surg. 1955; 90(2):367–372

[111] Blank WA. Anorectal complications in leukemia. Am J Surg. 1955; 90(5):738–741

[112] Schimpff SC, Wiernik PH, Block JB. Rectal abscesses in cancer patients. Lancet. 1972; 2(7782):844–847

[113] Sehdev MK, Dowling MD, Jr, Seal SH, Stearns MW, Jr. Perianal and anorectal complications in leukemia. Cancer. 1973; 31(1):149–152

[114] Vanhueverzwyn R, Delannoy A, Michaux JL, Dive C. Anal lesions in hematologic diseases. Dis Colon Rectum. 1980; 23(5):310–312

[115] Badgwell BD, Chang GJ, Rodriguez-Bigas MA, et al. Management and outcomes of anorectal infection in the cancer patient. Ann Surg Oncol. 2009; 16(10):2752–2758

[116] Grewal H, Guillem JG, Quan SH, Enker WE, Cohen AM. Anorectal disease in neutropenic leukemic patients. Operative vs. nonoperative management. Dis Colon Rectum. 1994; 37(11):1095–1099

[117] Lehrnbecher T, Marshall D, Gao C, Chanock SJ. A second look at anorectal infections in cancer patients in a large cancer institute: the success of early intervention with antibiotics and surgery. Infection. 2002; 30(5):272–276

[118] Sultan S, Azria F, Bauer P, Abdelnour M, Atienza P. Anoperineal tuberculosis: diagnostic and management considerations in seven cases. Dis Colon Rectum. 2002; 45(3):407–410

[119] Tai WC, Hu TH, Lee CH, Chen HH, Huang CC, Chuah SK. Ano-perianal tuberculosis: 15 years of clinical experiences in Southern Taiwan. Colorectal Dis. 2010; 12(7 Online):e114–e120

[120] Gupta PJ. Ano-perianal tuberculosis–solving a clinical dilemma. Afr Health Sci. 2005; 5(4):345–347

[121] Keller DS, Aboseif SR, Lesser T, Abbass MA, Tsay AT, Abbas MA. Algorithm-based multidisciplinary treatment approach for rectourethral fistula. Int J Colorectal Dis. 2015; 30(5):631–638

[122] Ghoniem G, Elmissiry M, Weiss E, Langford C, Abdelwahab H, Wexner S. Transperineal repair of complex rectourethral fistula using gracilis muscle flap interposition–can urinary and bowel functions be preserved? J Urol. 2008; 179(5):1882–1886

[123] Wexner SD, Ruiz DE, Genua J, Nogueras JJ, Weiss EG, Zmora O. Gracilis muscle interposition for the treatment of rectourethral, rectovaginal, and pouch-vaginal fistulas: results in 53 patients. Ann Surg. 2008; 248(1):39–43

[124] Takano S, Boutros M, Wexner SD. Gracilis muscle transposition for complex perineal fistulas and sinuses: a systematic literature review of surgical outcomes. J Am Coll Surg. 2014; 219(2):313–323

[125] Harris CR, McAninch JW, Mundy AR, et al. Rectourethral fistulas secondary to prostate cancer treatment: management and outcomes from a multi-institutional combined experience. J Urol. 2017; 197(1):191–194

[126] Atallah SB, deBeche-Adams TC, Larach S. Transanal minimally invasive surgery for repair of rectourethral fistula. Dis Colon Rectum. 2014; 57(7):899

[127] Bochove-Overgaauw DM, Beerlage HP, Bosscha K, Gelderman WA. Transanal endoscopic microsurgery for correction of rectourethral fistulae. J Endourol. 2006; 20(12):1087–1090

[128] Quinlan M, Cahill R, Keane F, Grainger R, Butler M. Transanal endoscopic microsurgical repair of iatrogenic recto-urethral fistula. Surgeon. 2005; 3(6):416–417

[129] Nicita G, Villari D, Caroassai Grisanti S, Marzocco M, Li Marzi V, Martini A. Minimally invasive transanal repair of rectourethral fistulas. Eur Urol. 2017; 71(1):133–138

[130] Kanehira E, Tanida T, Kamei A, Nakagi M, Iwasaki M, Shimizu H. Transanal endoscopic microsurgery for surgical repair of rectovesical fistula following radical prostatectomy. Surg Endosc. 2015; 29(4):851–855

10 Pilonidal Disease

David E. Beck

Abstract

The proximity of pilonidal disease to the anus has prompted the referral of many patients with this problem to colon and rectal surgeons. Pilonidal sinus is a chronic subcutaneous abscess in the natal cleft, which spontaneously drains through the openings. It is not a "cyst," as frequently referred to. This chapter discusses the pathophysiology, clinical presentation, diagnosis, and treatment of pilonidal disease.

Keywords: pilonidal disease, sinus, complex disease, recurrent disease, clinical presentation, diagnosis, treatment

10.1 Introduction

Although not technically a gastrointestinal tract problem, the proximity of pilonidal disease to the anus has prompted the referral of many patients with this problem to colon and rectal surgeons. The first report of pilonidal disease is attributed to Anderson in 1847[1] and the first series of patients to Warren.[2] In 1880, Hodges[3] coined the term "pilonidal sinus" from the Latin pilus, meaning hair, and nidus, meaning nest, to describe the chronic sinus containing hair and found between the buttocks. The intent of this term was to note the association of trapped hair in this unusual form of natal cleft skin infection. Pilonidal

sinus is a chronic subcutaneous abscess in the natal cleft, which spontaneously drains through the openings. It is not a "cyst," as frequently referred to in many textbooks and articles.[4]

10.2 Pathophysiology

The origin of the pilonidal sinus is controversial with two main theories. The congenital theory was initially popular and suggested that a remnant of the medullary canal with infolding of the surface epithelium or a faulty coalescence of the cutaneous covering in early embryonic life led to pilonidal sinus development.[5,6] The acquired theory is now widely accepted, but its mechanisms are speculative and varied. Bascom[7] believes the affected hair follicles become distended with keratin and subsequently infected, leading to folliculitis and the formation of an abscess that extends down into the subcutaneous fat (▶ Fig. 10.1). Examination of a section of a pit reveals a distended hair follicle with inflammation (▶ Fig. 10.2). Once the abscess cavity is formed, hairs can enter through the tiny pit

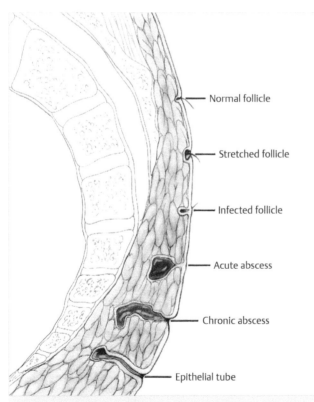

Fig. 10.1 Pathogenesis of pilonidal abscess and sinus.[7] (With permission © 1980 Elsevier.)

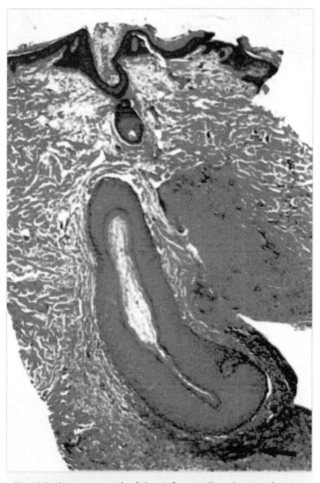

Fig. 10.2 Photomicrograph of the pit from midline showing chronic inflammation from infected hair follicle. (Courtesy of Andrew R. McLeish, MD.)

and lodge in the abscess cavity from the suction created by movement of the gluteal area (▶ Fig. 10.3). Karydakis,[8] on the other hand, believes the shaft of loose hair, because of its scales with chisel-like root ends, inserts into the depth of the natal cleft in the midline of sacrococcygeal area (▶ Fig. 10.4). Once one hair inserts successfully, other hairs can insert more easily. Foreign body tissue reaction and infection follow, and the primary sinus of pilonidal disease forms. Secondary openings often occur because of the self-propelling ability of hair to burrow through the skin or spontaneous rupture of the abscess. The author leans toward Karydakis's explanation.

Isolated reports of pilonidal sinus occurring in unusual locations, such as the umbilicus, a healed amputation stump, and interdigital clefts, and the recurrence of the disease in an adequately excised area support the acquired theory of this disease and Karydakis's concept of hair insertion.

Pilonidal disease and its treatment were significant issues during World War II.[9] Seventy-nine thousand U.S. servicemen were hospitalized, each for an average of 55 days. The frequent reactivation of the quiescent sacrococcygeal sinuses among military personnel who entered training for combat duty, with rugged lifestyle and stresses of driving trucks, tanks, and jeeps, led Buie[10] to call it "jeep disease."

The main feature of a pilonidal sinus is the subcutaneous fibrous tract that may be lined with squamous epithelium. This subcutaneous tract extends for a variable distance, usually 2 to 5 cm. A small abscess cavity and branching tracts may come off the primary tract (▶ Fig. 10.5). Often, hairs that are usually disconnected from the surrounding skin are seen entering the midline pit (▶ Fig. 10.6). As a rule, hair follicles are not identified. The secondary openings have a different appearance from the primary midline ones in that they are marked by elevations of granulation tissue and discharge of seropurulent material. Hairs, if seen, sticking out of the secondary opening are in the abscess cavity that the body tries to spit out (▶ Fig. 10.6). Most sinus tracts (93%) run cephalad; the rest (7%) run caudad and may be confused with a fistula-in-ano or with hidradenitis suppurativa.[11]

Pilonidal sinus is a chronic disease with a natural regression.[12] The disease usually manifests in puberty and seldom occurs after the third or fourth decade of life. However, pilonidal sinus may occur at any age.[8,13,14]

10.2.1 Predisposing Factors

Tiny skin dimples in the sacrococcygeal area are common in the normal population (9%), but most never become a problem.[15] Because of the common problems of infected pilonidal sinuses among Army and Navy officers, it was speculated that trauma to the sacrococcygeal area was the primary predisposing factor. However, the acquired theory of folliculitis[7] and the spontaneous insertion of hair in the natal cleft[8] refute this theory as the primary cause.

Akinci et al[16] examined 1,000 Turkish soldiers including information on their characters and habits. Eighty-eight (8.8%) of the soldiers had pilonidal sinuses; 48 were symptomatic and 40 were asymptomatic. The factors associated with the presence of a pilonidal sinus were: obesity (weight over 90 kg) ($p < 0.0001$); being the driver of a vehicle ($p < 0.0001$); incidence of folliculitis or furuncle at another site on the body ($p < 0.0001$); and family history of pilonidal sinus ($p < 0.0001$). The history of pilonidal sinus in the family does not mean a congenital tendency but rather indicates the similar body habitat and hair characteristics.

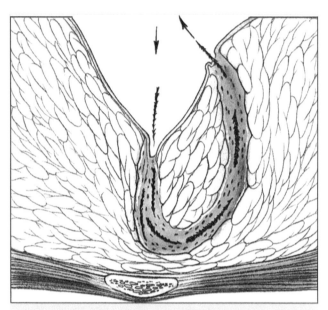

Fig. 10.4 Pathogenesis. Insertion of a shaft of loose hair.

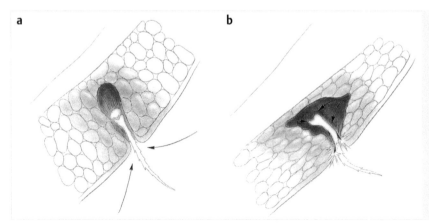

Fig. 10.3 Ingestion of hair by a chronic pilonidal abscess cavity. Scales of hair direct the inward movement of hair. Motion causes movement in the cavity. (a) Standing, (b) sitting.[7] (With permission © 1980 Elsevier.)

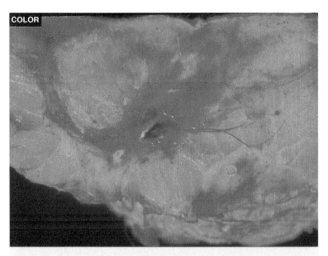

Fig. 10.5 Section of an en bloc specimen shows hairs in a chronic abscess cavity and a sinus tract leading to a secondary opening. (Courtesy of Clyde Culp, MD.)

10.3 Clinical Presentations and Diagnosis

The average patients with pilonidal disease are hirsute and moderately obese in their second decade.[17] While hirsute people or people with dark hairs may have an increased tendency to develop pilonidal disease, the disease is also seen in people without these features.[18] People of both sexes and any age can be affected. Pilonidal disease initially may be seen as an acute abscess in the sacrococcygeal area. It frequently ruptures spontaneously, leaving unhealed sinuses with chronic drainage. Once the sinus develops, pain is usually minimal. About 71 to 85% of patients with pilonidal infection are men.[5,14]

The diagnosis is usually suggested by the patient's history with three common presentations. Nearly all patients have an episode of acute abscess formation, characterized as a painful and indurated swelling or cellulitis in the gluteal cleft. When this abscess resolves, either spontaneously or with medical assistance, many patients develop a pilonidal sinus. This chronic state is confirmed by the sinus opening or dermal pit in the intergluteal fold approximately 5 cm above the anus (▶ Fig. 10.7). Although many sinus tracts resolve, some patients go on to have chronic or recurrent disease after treatment. Treatment methods vary for each stage in pilonidal disease, and will be discussed in detail.

The differential diagnoses include any furuncle in the skin, an anal fistula, specific granulomas (e.g., syphilitic or tuberculous), and osteomyelitis with multiple draining sinuses in the skin. Actinomycosis in the sacral region has been described as virtually indistinguishable from pilonidal disease.

10.4 Treatment

10.4.1 Pilonidal Abscess

Although the infected epithelial sinus is in the midline, the abscess is usually lateral on either side and cephalad. As a midline

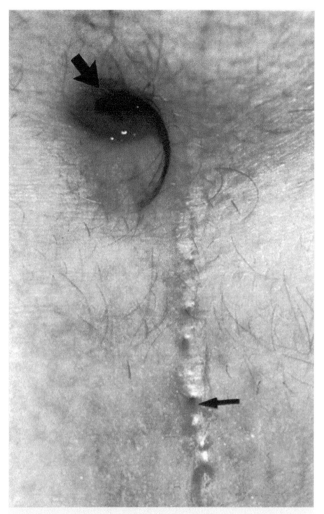

Fig. 10.6 Numerous noninflamed midline pits, the primary source of the disease (small arrow). Hairs extrude from the secondary sinus (large arrow).

wound in the intergluteal cleft heals poorly and slowly, every attempt is made to keep the wound small and off the midline. Drainage of a pilonidal abscess can almost always be performed under local anesthesia in the clinic or emergency room. A longitudinal incision is made lateral to the midline in the coccygeal area (▶ Fig. 10.8). The incision is deepened into the subcutaneous tissue, entering the abscess cavity. Hair, if present in the abscess cavity, must be removed. All the infected granulation tissues and necrotic debris are thoroughly curetted. The skin edges are trimmed to make the abscess cavity an open wound. The wound is lightly packed with fine mesh gauge. Antibiotics are unnecessary. The patient is instructed to irrigate the wound with diluted hydrogen peroxide (dilution 1:4) twice a day for a few days, if possible. This will effectively remove the residual debris. At the very least, the wound should be washed with soap and water in the shower twice a day. The most important aspect is to prevent hairs from getting into the wound and to remove them from the wound. The hairs around the wound should be shaved or plucked for at least a couple of months. A Cytette brush (Birchwood Laboratories, Inc., Eden Prairie, MN), which is commonly used for obtaining Papanicolaou (Pap) smears, is an excellent tool for swabbing the hairs and debris from the wound (▶ Fig. 10.9). During office visits, excess granulation tissue is removed. With diligent wound care, complete healing is common.

10.4.2 Pilonidal Sinus

Treatment of pilonidal sinus can be done in one of several ways: nonoperative treatment, incision and curettage, lateral incision (▶ Fig. 10.10) and excision of midline pits, wide local excision with or without primary closure, excision and Z-plasty, or advancing flap operations (Karydakis procedure).

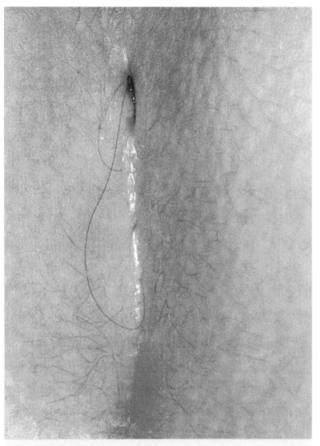

Fig. 10.7 A midline pit. Note hairs entering the pit.

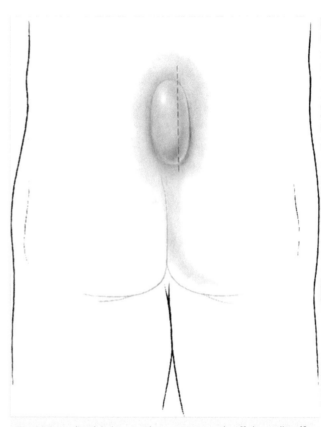

Fig. 10.8 A pilonidal abscess. The incision is made off the midline.[18]

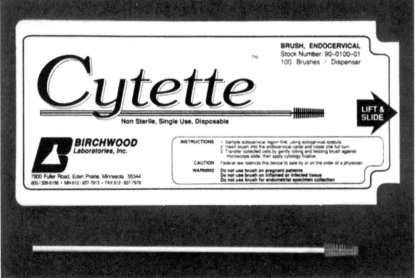

Fig. 10.9 Cytette brush, an excellent tool to clean the wound.

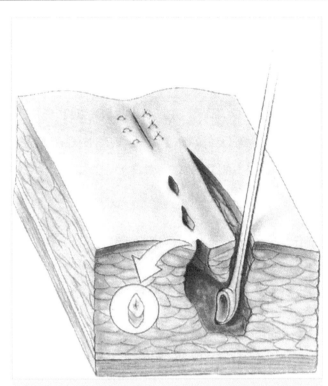

Fig. 10.10 Lateral incision to the sinus tract. Granulated tissues are scraped with a curette.[7] (With permission © 1980 Elsevier.)

Nonoperative Treatment

Klass[15] believed that the immediate cause of the infection in a pilonidal sinus is a collection of loose hairs and fecal residue in the internatal cleft and that, when an abscess has developed, incision and drainage are all that is required. He thus treated his patients with strict hygiene by washing with soap and water in the perineal and sacrococcygeal area (▶ Fig. 10.11). An abscess is drained, the sinus is kept open, and the area is cleaned. In a series of 15 patients with chronic discharge from the sinuses, 11 were cured, with follow-up of 3 years or longer. In another group of 12 patients who required incision and drainage of the abscess, 10 patients healed, and 2 patients required a second incision and drainage. The follow-up was at least 3 years.

The most important conservative treatment comes from Tripler Army Medical Center, Hawaii. Armstrong and Barcia[19] treated pilonidal disease mainly by shaving all hairs within the natal cleft, 5 cm from the anus to the presacrum. Visible hairs within the sinus are removed, but no attempt is made to probe for hairs within the sinus. If there is an abscess, a lateral incision for drainage is made. This conservative method was applied to 101 consecutive patients during a 1-year period. The wounds healed in all patients. Unfortunately, the length of follow-up and the recurrence rate were not stated in the study.

Injecting phenol into the sinus tract has been advocated by some authors. Schneider et al[20] studied 45 patients with pilonidal sinuses treated with 1 to 2 mL of 80% phenol injected into the sinus. The injection was performed under local anesthesia. Only 60% of the patients completely healed, and it took 6 weeks on average. Besides, 11% develop abscess requiring excision and

drainage, and other patients frequently develop local inflammation caused by the phenol. This method of treatment should not be used.

Conversely, Dogru et al[21] used crystallized phenol with success. First, they cleaned out and removed hairs from the abscess cavity and sinus tracts. The surrounding skin was protected before applying the crystals into the wound. The crystallized phenol turned into liquid form quickly at body temperature and filled the sinus. It was left in situ for 2 minutes and then expressed out. The procedure may be repeated thereafter as indicated. Of 41 patients so treated, 2 patients had recurrences at 5 and 8 months. The median follow-up was 24 months. The mean recovery time was 43 days. This noninvasive technique may sound good but crystallized phenol is not readily available in most hospitals.

Incision and Curettage

Laying open (unroofing, not excision) and curettage is a minimally invasive procedure to treat pilonidal disease. A meta-analysis in 2015 of 13 studies and 1,445 patients demonstrated that laying open (unroofing) and curettage had high success rates (4.47% recurrence), 1.44% rate of complications, a healing time of 21 to 72 days, and return to work of 8.4 days.[22]

A variation of this was advocated by Buie[10] and later by Culp.[25] The technique consists of opening the sinus tract in the midline. The debris and granulation tissues are scraped with a curette. The fibrous tissue in the tract is saved and is sutured to the edges of the wound. This technique not only minimizes the size and depth of the wound but also prevents the wound from premature closure. In addition, it is easy to pack and clean the wound (▶ Fig. 10.12). In doing so, the size of the wound is reduced 50 to 60%.[23] The average healing time is 4 to 6 weeks, with prolonged healing (12–20 weeks) in 2 to 4% and recurrence in 8%.[8,24] Although this technique is simple, it is still more extensive than the lateral incision and lay open of the sinus tracts.

Lateral Incision and Lay Open of Midline Sinus Tracts

Lord and Bascom advocate excision of the midline pits or sinuses and thorough cleansing of hair and debris from the sinus tract.[6,7] Bascom[7] emphasizes avoiding midline wounds by using a longitudinal incision off the midline to enter the sinus tract (▶ Fig. 10.10). In a follow-up of 149 patients, with a mean follow-up of 3.5 years (longest, 9 years), the cure rate was 84%.[25] Senapati et al[24] reported a success rate of 90%, with a mean follow-up of 12 months (range, 1–60) in 218 patients.

Advantages of this technique are minimal surgery and small wounds. It can be done on an outpatient basis. Excisions of the midline pits are frequently slow to heal. A better way is to lay open the midline pits toward the lateral incision. This is an important technique to minimize recurrence.

Proper care of the open wound is essential for healing.[26] The patient should be examined 1 week after surgery. Hypertrophic granulation signifies improper packing and requires cauterization with silver nitrate sticks. The gauze packing should not be tight but the mesh gauze should touch on the entire subcutaneous wound.

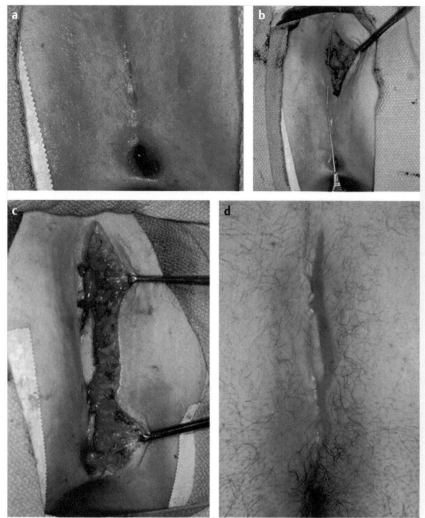

Fig. 10.11 (a) Several openings in midline sacrococcygeal area. (b) An incision is made about 1 cm lateral to the midline, and then dissected to connect with the chronic abscess cavity. A lacrimal probe is used to identify the sinus tracts from the midline pits. (c) Note the shaggy edges of the wound resulting from laying open of the sinus tracts. (d) Complete wound healing at 3 weeks.

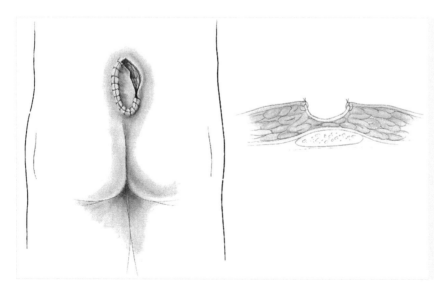

Fig. 10.12 Marsupialization. Fibrotic wall at the base of the wound is sutured to the edges of the skin all around with continuous absorbable suture. (Reproduced with permission from Garg et al.[22])

Wide Local Excision with or without Primary Closure

An en bloc excision is made around the midline pilonidal, deep down to the sacrococcygeal fascia. The wound is packed with moist saline gauze. In a series of 50 patients, al-Hassan et al[27] found that the mean time of healing was 13 weeks (range, 4–78 weeks) and that the recurrence rate was 12% with a mean follow-up of 25 months.

Søndenaa et al[28] performed a radical excision in 153 patients who had chronic pilonidal sinus. Seventy-eight of those patients received a single dose of 2 g cefoxitin intravenously, and 75 patients received no antibiotic. There was no difference in the rate of wound healing between the two groups. The wounds healed within 1 month in 69% of patients who received cefoxitin and in 64% of patients who received no antibiotic. The complication rates were 44 and 43%, respectively. Other studies have seen similar problems.[29,30] Despite this radical operation, some authors find it to be satisfactory and advocate its use.[31,32,33] In a randomized trial with a 3-year follow-up, Kronborg et al[34] found that excision with primary closure of the wound resulted in a shorter healing time than excision with an open wound, and that the recurrence rate varied from 0 to 38%.[35] A randomized trial by Testini et al[36] also showed a quicker wound healing and a quicker return to normal activity in the primary closure group versus an open technique. A meta-analysis in 2010 of 26 studies and 2,530 patients compared healing by primary versus secondary intention.[37] No clear benefit was shown for open healing over surgical closure, but a clear benefit was shown in favor of off-midline rather than midline closure.

Excision and Z-Plasty

Excision of pilonidal sinuses with primary closure of the wound is simple but has a high recurrence rate. The use of primary closure, however, is appealing because successful wound healing can be accomplished within 7 to 10 days. To avoid recurrence or breakdown of the midline wound, the anatomy of the natal crease must be altered. Z-plasty can be done to achieve this goal. Excision of pilonidal sinuses with primary Z-plasty fills out and flattens the natal crease, directs the hair points away from the midline, largely prevents maceration, reduces suction effects in the soft tissues of the buttocks, and minimizes friction between their adjacent surfaces. The excision is carried down to the subcutaneous tissue. The limbs of the Z are cut to form a 30-degree angle with the long axis of the wound. Subcutaneous skin flaps are raised, and the flaps are transposed and sutured (▶ Fig. 10.13). A closed suction drain is placed under the full-thickness flaps. Z-plasty thus avoids the midline wound, which is the main cause of slow healing and recurrences. In a series of 110 patients treated with Z-plasty by Toubanakis,[38] there were no recurrences. Mansoory and Dickson[39] reported similar good results. The main disadvantage of this procedure is that it is a rather extensive one for a noncomplicated pilonidal sinus and is not suitable for performance on an outpatient basis. Besides, part of the wound is still in the midline.

Flap Operations

Karydakis Procedure

Karydakis[8] believes that pilonidal sinuses occur because of the entry of hair into the midline of the intergluteal fold. The hairs are then forced by friction into the depth of the fold. He designed an operative technique to avoid these problems. A "semilateral" excision is made over the sinuses all the way down to the presacral fascia (▶ Fig. 10.14). Mobilization is carried to the opposite side so that the entire flap can be advanced toward the other side on closure. A closed suction drain is placed. This technique avoids the midline wound. In a series of 7,471 patients who received the advancing flap procedure, the complication rate was 8.5%, mainly infection and fluid collection. The mean hospital stay was 3 days, with many patients requiring 1-day hospitalization or the procedure performed on an outpatient basis. The recurrence rate was 1%, with follow-up ranging from 2 to 20 years. In each recurrence, reinsertion of

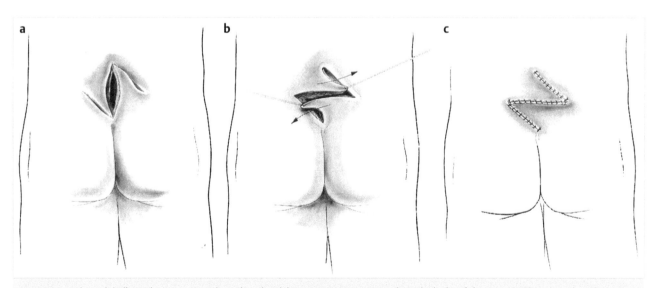

Fig. 10.13 Z-plasty. **(a)** Elliptical excision is made to the pilonidal sinuses. Incisions are made at the limbs of the Z at a 30-degree angle with the long axis of the wound. **(b)** Subcutaneous skin flaps are raised and transposed. **(c)** Skin is closed.

hairs was observed. The Karydakis flap procedure has proved to be effective, but it is a moderately extensive procedure.[8,40,41]

Rhomboid Excision with Transposition of Flap

This technique was first reported in French by Dufourmentel et al[42] in 1966 for a sacrococcygeal cyst. Subsequently, in 1984, Azab et al[43] accurately described its construction and used it for the treatment of pilonidal sinuses. A rhomboid is outlined to encompass the pilonidal sinuses in the midline (▶ Fig. 10.15a). The lines ab = bc = cd = ad. The line de is drawn to bisect the angle made by bd and cd. The lines de and ef are the same length as ad. The d-e-f angle is the same as the b-a-d angle.

The rhomboid excision is made down to the sacral periosteum in the midline and to the gluteal fascia laterally. The d-e-f flap is made deep to the gluteal fascia to release any tension. The flap is then transposed to cover the rhomboid wound (▶ Fig. 10.15b). A suction drain is placed under the flap and the wound is closed with sutures (▶ Fig. 10.15c).

Using rhomboid excision and flap in 67 patients with pilonidal sinuses, Milito et al[44] reported no recurrence after a mean follow-up of 74 months (range, 8–137 months); primary healing was obtained in all patients except two who developed a seroma and one who had a partial dehiscence of the wound due to a hematoma, which necessitated a drainage. The average hospital stay was 5 days (range, 1–16 days).

Daphan et al[45] reported a recurrence of 5% in 147 patients, after a mean follow-up of 13 months (range, 1–40 months); 2% of the patients developed a postoperative seroma and 4% had a wound separation. Urhan et al[46] and Arumugam et al[47] reported recurrences of 5 and 7% after a mean follow-up of 36 and 24 months, respectively. Topgül et al[48] reported 200 cases, including 13 cases for recurrences, using this technique. Minimal flap necrosis occurred in 3%, seroma in 2%, wound infection in 1.5%, and recurrence in 0.5%; the mean follow-up was 5 years. Rhomboid excision with transposition of flap is appealing because it is easy to perform and the results are as good as any other more complicated flaps.

Petersen et al[49] performed a Medline search in February 2001 for a survey of results of different surgical approaches with primary closure techniques. The search identified 74 publications including 1,090 patients for primary closure in midline and 35 publications with 2,034 patients evaluated; the results of asymmetric or oblique technique (e.g., Karydakis's, Bascom's) were described in 6,812 patients of 16 publications, whereas for the rhomboid technique 739 patients in 16 articles were found. For V-Y plasty, 73 patients and 4 publications, and finally for the Z-flap technique, 432 patients in 11 articles were included.

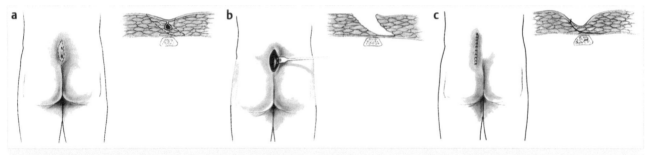

Fig. 10.14 Karydakis sliding flap. (a) Elliptical excision is made around the pilonidal sinuses deep to the presacral fascia and off the midline to one side. (b) Wound on one side is undermined, creating a full-thickness flap. (c) Flap is slid and closed to the edges of the wound on the opposite side. Closed wound is off the midline.

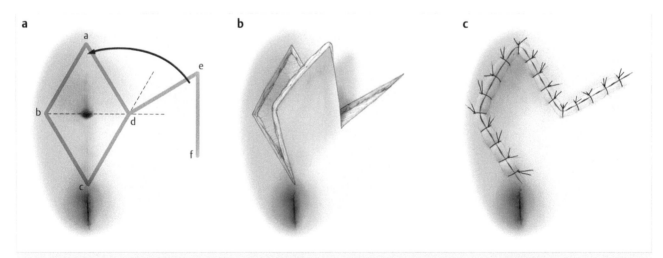

Fig. 10.15 (a) Outline of rhomboid excision: ab = bc = cd = da; de bisects the angle made by bd and cd. de = ef = ad. (b) The flap is made deep into gluteal fascia. The flap is rotated and transposed to cover the rhomboid wound. (c) At completion.[40] (With permission © 1996 John Wiley and Sons.)

The results showed that overall wound infection occurred in up to 38.5%. The highest pooled infection rate of 12.4% (95% confidence interval [CI], 11.1–13.8) was observed in the midline closure group, and the lowest in the V-Y group. The wound failure appeared in up to 52.4% of all procedures. The lowest pooled failure rates of 3.5% (95% CI, 2.6–4.7) and 3.4% (95% CI, 2.3–4.9) were observed in asymmetric oblique technique group and the rhomboid group, respectively. Recurrence was observed in up to 26.8%, with highest in the midline closure group and lowest in asymmetric oblique group and rhomboid group. An additional pooled analysis of six randomized controlled studies with 641 patients in 2012 supported a rhomboid excision and Limberg flap repair over primary midline suture techniques.[50]

10.4.3 Complex or Recurrent Disease

The length of time needed for the pilonidal wound to heal depends on the type of operation and the extent of the disease. The recurrence rate varies widely from series to series (0–37%).[8,14,30] Recurrence is caused by reinsertion of the loose hairs into the natal cleft. The mechanism is the same as for primary pilonidal disease, and the treatment is also the same.

Not uncommonly, the wound does not heal after operation for a pilonidal sinus. Most often, the base of the wound is filled with gelatinous granulation tissue, which is usually the result of improper postoperative wound care. Hairs may grow into the edges of the wound, preventing complete healing. Some wounds are kept clean and yet do not heal. Almost all unhealed wounds are in the midline natal cleft area. The lateral incision technique usually avoids this problem.

Curettage, Re-excision, and Saucerization

The hairs around the unhealed wound must be shaved and plucked, after which a complete curettage of the granulation tissue is done. If the shape of the wound appears to fold together causing "pocketing," it should be refashioned and saucerization performed to avoid accumulation of discharge. If the wound is infected with anaerobic bacteria, administering an antibiotic can improve healing. Using a water-pulsating device (e.g., WaterPik[1]) offers a simple method for irrigation of the wound.[51]

Reverse Bandaging

Some pilonidal wounds heal well initially but fail to form epithelium. The problem is mainly mechanical when the patients involved are obese and have a narrow intergluteal cleft. The motion of the buttocks traumatizes the wound constantly. Rosenberg[52] has used reverse bandaging with success. A wide piece of adhesive tape is placed on each side of the wound, stretching it outward. The tapes are tied in front of the abdomen (▶ Fig. 10.16). The net effect is to flatten the wound and remove most of the angle of the intergluteal cleft.

Gluteus Maximus Myocutaneous Flap

If the wound is extensive and conservative management fails, the wound should be excised. In this situation, use of a gluteus maximus myocutaneous flap offers a secure repair. However, the procedure is rather extensive for a simple disease.

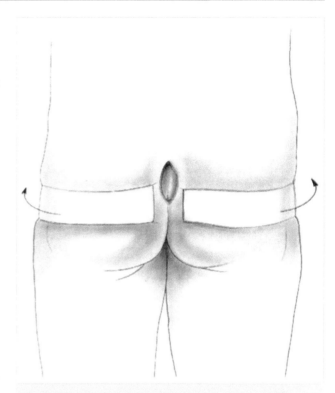

Fig. 10.16 Patient's buttocks are strapped with tape in a reverse direction, spreading the wound open.

Under general anesthesia, the patient is placed in the prone position. The unhealed wound, along with a scar and the granulation tissue, is excised to reach normal surrounding fat and presacral fascia. A rotational buttock flap is raised, incorporating skin and the underlying superior portion of the gluteus maximus muscle (▶ Fig. 10.16). After the skin and subcutaneous tissue of the buttock have been traversed, the upper portion of the gluteus maximus is transected to the level of the gluteus medius and piriformis muscles, with care taken to protect the sciatic nerve. The myocutaneous flap is then rotated into place, a closed suction drain is inserted, and the wound is closed in layers.[53] The patient is not allowed to lie on the flap for 1 week. This technique is seldom necessary since I prefer a simpler Bascom's flap as described below. Z-plasty, V-Y sliding flaps, and rhomboid excision with transposition of flap can also be applied.[38,48,54]

Bascom's Flap (Cleft Closure)

This unique method for treating the unhealed wound was devised by Bascom.[55] The basic concept is to excise the unhealed skin and the underlying subcutaneous tissue. The natal cleft is eliminated by replacing the defect at the depth of the cleft with a skin flap over the wound. This operation is easier than it appears and is less extensive than the gluteus maximus myocutaneous and other types of flaps. The subcutaneous fat is not mobilized. The flap is a full-thickness skin flap. It is the operation of choice for extensive recurrent pilonidal disease or an unhealed midline wound.

The procedure is performed with the patient under general or spinal anesthesia. A broad-spectrum antibiotic is administered

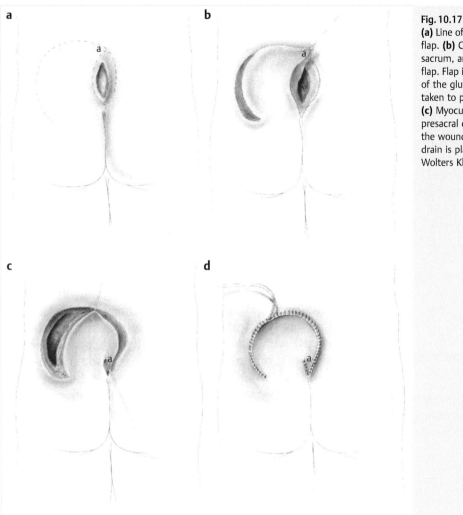

Fig. 10.17 Gluteus maximus myocutaneous flap. **(a)** Line of incision for the gluteus myocutaneous flap. **(b)** Chronic wound is excised down to the sacrum, and the flap is created; a is apex of the flap. Flap is raised, incorporating superior portion of the gluteus maximus muscle, with great care taken to protect the gluteal vessels and nerve. **(c)** Myocutaneous flap is rotated to cover the presacral defect; a is rotated to inferior part of the wound. **(d)** Wound is closed, and a suction drain is placed.[49] (With permission © 2002 Wolters Kluwer.)

when the patient is called to the operating room and continued until the drain is removed 4 to 5 days later. The patient is placed in the prone jackknife position.

With the patient's buttocks pressed together, the lines of contact of the cheeks of the buttocks are marked with a felt-tipped pen (▶ Fig. 10.17a). The cheeks of the buttocks are then taped apart, and the skin is prepared and draped (▶ Fig. 10.17b). The skin in this region is infiltrated with 0.25% bupivacaine (Marcaine) containing 1:200,000 epinephrine to decrease bleeding. A triangle-shaped section of skin overlying the unhealed wound is excised, extending above and lateral to the apex of the cleft. The lower end of the incision is curved medially toward the anus to avoid a "dog-ear" upon closure (▶ Fig. 10.17c). The granulation tissue and hairs are removed. No fat or muscle is mobilized.

After the skin flap (dissected only into the dermis) is raised out to the previously marked line on the left side, the tapes are released. The skin flap is positioned to overlap the edges of the wound on the right side. The excess skin is excised. A closed suction drain is placed in the subcutaneous tissue. The subcutaneous tissue is closed with 3–0 chromic catgut, and the skin is closed with subcuticular 3–0 synthetic monofilament absorbable suture (▶ Fig. 10.18d, e). The suture line can be reinforced with a running suture, or Steri-Strips can be applied. The key to this operation is to create the skin flap so that the suture line is off the midline, as seen in ▶ Fig. 10.18e.

It should be noted that Bascom described this technique to treat unhealed wound or recurrent pilonidal sinuses, although it is possible to use it for a complex primary disease. Unlike all other flaps, which are myocutaneous or subcutaneous, Bascom's flap is a full-thickness skin flap. It may look complex, but actually if one follows Bascom's description and drawings, it is quite simple technically.

10.4.4 Pilonidal Sinus and Carcinoma

Carcinoma arising in a chronic pilonidal sinus is rare. In a review of the world literature from 1900 to 1994, only 44 patients were described (▶ Table 10.1).[56] Thirty-nine cases are squamous cell carcinomas, three are basal cell carcinomas, one is an adenocarcinoma (sweat gland type), and one is an unspecified carcinoma. The cause of pilonidal carcinoma appears to be the same as that by which other chronic inflamed wounds such as scars, skin ulcers, and fistulas undergo malignant degeneration. The average duration of pilonidal disease in the patients is 23 years. Pilonidal carcinoma has a distinctive appearance, and the diagnosis can usually be made on inspection of the patient. A central ulceration is often present,

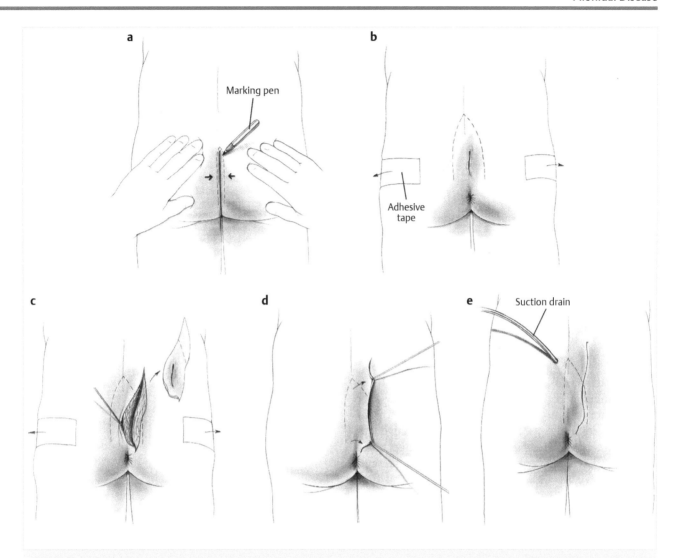

Fig. 10.18 **(a)** Natural lines of contact of cheeks of buttock are marked. **(b)** Cheeks of buttock are taped apart. **(c)** Unhealed wound is excised in a triangular shape. **(d)** After skin flap is raised out to marked line, tapes are released. Skin flap is positioned to overlap edges of wound on opposite side. Excess skin is excised. Closed suction drain is placed in subcutaneous tissue, which is approximated with 3–0 chromic catgut. **(e)** Skin is closed with subcuticular 3–0 synthetic monofilament absorbable suture.[50] (With permission © 2011 The Authors. Colorectal Disease © 2011 The Association of Coloproctology of Great Britain and Ireland.)

Table 10.1 World literature on pilonidal carcinoma (*n* = 44)

Male:female ratio	35:9	Mean follow-up	29 mo
Age at presentation	50 y	Recurrence	34%
Mean duration of symptoms	23 y	Time to recurrence	16 mo
Inguinal adenopathy treatment	5 (11%)	Total deceased	12 (27%)
Excision	35	Total deceased with disease	8 (18%)
Chemotherapy only	1		
Radiation only	0		
No treatment	2		
Excision and radiation	4		
Excision and chemotherapy	1		
Excision, chemotherapy, and radiation	1		

with a friable, indurated, erythematous, and fungating margin. Biopsy confirms the diagnosis. It is usually a well-differentiated squamous cell carcinoma, frequently with focal areas of keratinization and rare mitosis. The carcinoma grows locally before metastasizing to inguinal nodes. Preoperative evaluation of patients with pilonidal carcinoma should include examination of the inguinal areas, perineum, and anorectum. Treatment involves wide local excision to include the presacral fascia. For an extensive wound, a V-Y myocutaneous flap can be performed.[57]

According to the review of the literature, the recurrence rate is 34%, and death from the disease occurs in 18% of patients on follow-up of 29 months.[56]

10.5 Summary

Many operations for pilonidal disease end up worse than the disease itself. The treatment of pilonidal disease should be simple and most, if not all, can be performed on an outpatient basis. A simple incision and drainage off the midline of the abscess, with complete removal of hairs and debris, and shaving hairs around the wound are all that is necessary for an acute pilonidal abscess. The central pit should be searched for and, if identified, should be laid open to the lateral incision. Perineal hair removal helps prevent subsequent problems. For a chronic pilonidal sinus, the method of choice is a lateral incision into the chronic abscess cavity, with removal of all hairs and granulation tissues. It is to be done along with laying open of the midline pits with their tracts to the lateral wound. If a flap is necessary, the rhomboid excision with transposition of subcutaneous skin flap is the simplest technique to do.

A meta-analysis of 25 randomized controlled trials and 2,949 patients in 2014 recommended unroofing or en bloc resection with off midline primary closure.[58]

The surgeon must make it clear to the patients and their families that they are responsible for the second half of the treatment. The open wounds must be irrigated or cleaned in the shower with soap and water. Hairs and debris in the wound must be removed. The wound should be lightly packed to prevent premature closure. The skin around the wound should be shaved, the hairs plucked, or a depilatory cream used every 10 to 21 days. The surgeon should check the wound every 1 to 2 weeks and cauterize the hypertrophic granulation tissues until proper wound care has been achieved.

References

[1] Anderson AW. Hair extracted from an ulcer. Boston Med Surg J. 1847; 36:74
[2] Warren JM. Abscess containing hair on the nates. Am J Med Sci. 1854; 28:112
[3] Hodges RM. Pilonidal sinus. Boston Med Surg J. 1880; 103:485–486
[4] Nivatvong S. Pilonidal disease. In: Gordon PH, Nivatvongs S, eds. Principles and Practice of Surgery for the Colon, Rectum, and Anus. 3rd ed. New York, NY: Informa; 2007:235–246
[5] Kooistra HP. Pilonidal sinuses, review of the literature and report of three hundred fifty cases. Am J Surg. 1942; 55:3–17
[6] Lord PH. Anorectal problems: etiology of pilonidal sinus. Dis Colon Rectum. 1975; 18(8):661–664
[7] Bascom J. Pilonidal disease: origin from follicles of hairs and results of follicle removal as treatment. Surgery. 1980; 87(5):567–572
[8] Karydakis GE. Easy and successful treatment of pilonidal sinus after explanation of its causative process. Aust N Z J Surg. 1992; 62(5):385–389
[9] Abramson DJ. Outpatient management of pilonidal sinuses: excision and semiprimary closure technic. Mil Med. 1978; 143(11):753–757
[10] Buie LA. Jeep disease. South Med J. 1944; 37:103–109
[11] Notaras MJ. A review of three popular methods of treatment of postanal (pilonidal) sinus disease. Br J Surg. 1970; 57(12):886–890
[12] Clothier PR, Haywood IR. The natural history of the post anal (pilonidal) sinus. Ann R Coll Surg Engl. 1984; 66(3):201–203
[13] Sagi A, Rosenberg L, Greiff M, Mahler D. Squamous-cell carcinoma arising in a pilonidal sinus: a case report and review of the literature. J Dermatol Surg Oncol. 1984; 10(3):210–212
[14] Solla JA, Rothenberger DA. Chronic pilonidal disease. An assessment of 150 cases. Dis Colon Rectum. 1990; 33(9):758–761
[15] Klass AA. The so-called pilo-nidal sinus. Can Med Assoc J. 1956; 75(9):737–742
[16] Akinci OF, Bozer M, Uzunköy A, Düzgün SA, Coşkun A. Incidence and aetiological factors in pilonidal sinus among Turkish soldiers. Eur J Surg. 1999; 165 (4):339–342
[17] Søndenaa K, Andersen E, Nesvik I, Søreide JA. Patient characteristics and symptoms in chronic pilonidal sinus disease. Int J Colorectal Dis. 1995; 10 (1):39–42
[18] Nivatvongs S, Becker ER. The colon, rectum, and anus. In: James EC, Corry KJ, Perry JF Jr., eds. Basic Surgical Practice. Philadelphia, PA: Hanley & Belfus; 1987:339
[19] Armstrong JH, Barcia PJ. Pilonidal sinus disease. The conservative approach. Arch Surg. 1994; 129(9):914–917, discussion 917–919
[20] Schneider IHF, Thaler K, Köckerling F. Treatment of pilonidal sinuses by phenol injections. Int J Colorectal Dis. 1994; 9(4):200–202
[21] Dogru O, Camci C, Aygen E, Girgin M, Topuz O. Pilonidal sinus treated with crystallized phenol: an eight-year experience. Dis Colon Rectum. 2004; 47 (11):1934–1938
[22] Garg P, Menon GR, Gupta V. Laying open (deroofing) and curettage of sinus as treatment of pilonidal disease: a systematic review and meta-analysis. ANZ J Surg. 2016; 86(1–2):27–33
[23] Bascom J. Pilonidal disease: long-term results of follicle removal. Dis Colon Rectum. 1983; 26(12):800–807
[24] Senapati A, Cripps NPJ, Thompson MR. Bascom's operation in the day-surgical management of symptomatic pilonidal sinus. Br J Surg. 2000; 87(8):1067–1070
[25] Culp CE. Pilonidal disease and its treatment. Surg Clin North Am. 1967; 47:1007–1014
[26] Bissett IP, Isbister WH. The management of patients with pilonidal disease–a comparative study. Aust N Z J Surg. 1987; 57(12):939–942
[27] al-Hassan HKL, Francis IM, Neglén P. Primary closure or secondary granulation after excision of pilonidal sinus? Acta Chir Scand. 1990; 156 (10):695–699
[28] Søndenaa K, Nesvik I, Gullaksen FP, et al. The role of cefoxitin prophylaxis in chronic pilonidal sinus treated with excision and primary suture. J Am Coll Surg. 1995; 180(2):157–160
[29] Isbister WH, Prasad J. Pilonidal disease. Aust N Z J Surg. 1995; 65(8):561–563
[30] Allen-Mersh TG. Pilonidal sinus: finding the right track for treatment. Br J Surg. 1990; 77(2):123–132
[31] Spivak H, Brooks VL, Nussbaum M, Friedman I. Treatment of chronic pilonidal disease. Dis Colon Rectum. 1996; 39(10):1136–1139
[32] Füzün M, Bakir H, Soylu M, Tansuğ T, Kaymak E, Harmancioğlu O. Which technique for treatment of pilonidal sinus–open or closed? Dis Colon Rectum. 1994; 37(11):1148–1150
[33] Dalenbäck J, Magnusson O, Wedel N, Rimbäck G. Prospective follow-up after ambulatory plain midline excision of pilonidal sinus and primary suture under local anaesthesia–efficient, sufficient, and persistent. Colorectal Dis. 2004; 6(6):488–493
[34] Kronborg O, Christensen K, Zimmermann-Nielsen C. Chronic pilonidal disease: a randomized trial with a complete 3-year follow-up. Br J Surg. 1985; 72(4):303–304
[35] Duchateau J, De Mol J, Bostoen H, Allegaert W. Pilonidal sinus. Excision–marsupialization–phenolization? Acta Chir Belg. 1985; 85(5):325–328
[36] Testini M, Piccinni G, Miniello S, et al. Treatment of chronic pilonidal sinus with local anaesthesia: a randomized trial of closed compared with open technique. Colorectal Dis. 2001; 3(6):427–430
[37] Al-Khamis A, McCallum I, King PM, Bruce J. Healing by primary versus secondary intention after surgical treatment for pilonidal sinus. Cochrane Database Syst Rev. 2010; 20(1):CD006213
[38] Toubanakis G. Treatment of pilonidal sinus disease with the Z-plasty procedure (modified). Am Surg. 1986; 52(11):611–612
[39] Mansoory A, Dickson D. Z-plasty for treatment of disease of the pilonidal sinus. Surg Gynecol Obstet. 1982; 155(3):409–411
[40] Kitchen PRB. Pilonidal sinus: experience with the Karydakis flap. Br J Surg. 1996; 83(10):1452–1455
[41] Akinci OF, Coskun A, Uzunköy A. Simple and effective surgical treatment of pilonidal sinus: asymmetric excision and primary closure using suction drain and subcuticular skin closure. Dis Colon Rectum. 2000; 43(5):701–706, discussion 706–707 (commentary by Bascom J in 706–707)
[42] Dufourmentel C, Mouly R, Baruch J, Banzet P. Sacrococcygeal cysts and fistulas. Pathogenic and therapeutic discussion [in French]. Ann Chir Plast. 1966; 11(3):181–186
[43] Azab AS, Kamal MS, Saad RA, Abou al Atta KA, Ali NA. Radical cure of pilonidal sinus by a transposition rhomboid flap. Br J Surg. 1984; 71(2):154–155
[44] Milito G, Cortese F, Casciani CU. Rhomboid flap procedure for pilonidal sinus: results from 67 cases. Int J Colorectal Dis. 1998; 13(3):113–115

[45] Daphan C, Tekelioglu MH, Sayilgan C. Limberg flap repair for pilonidal sinus disease. Dis Colon Rectum. 2004; 47(2):233–237

[46] Urhan MK, Kücükel F, Topgul K, Ozer I, Sari S. Rhomboid excision and Limberg flap for managing pilonidal sinus: results of 102 cases. Dis Colon Rectum. 2002; 45(5):656–659

[47] Arumugam PJ, Chandrasekaran TV, Morgan AR, Beynon J, Carr ND. The rhomboid flap for pilonidal disease. Colorectal Dis. 2003; 5(3):218–221

[48] Topgül K, Ozdemir E, Kiliç K, Gökbayir H, Ferahköşe Z. Long-term results of limberg flap procedure for treatment of pilonidal sinus: a report of 200 cases. Dis Colon Rectum. 2003; 46(11):1545–1548

[49] Petersen S, Koch R, Stelzner S, Wendlandt TP, Ludwig K. Primary closure techniques in chronic pilonidal sinus: a survey of the results of different surgical approaches. Dis Colon Rectum. 2002; 45(11):1458–1467

[50] Horwood J, Hanratty D, Chandran P, Billings P. Primary closure or rhomboid excision and Limberg flap for the management of primary sacrococcygeal pilonidal disease? A meta-analysis of randomized controlled trials. Colorectal Dis. 2012; 14(2):143–151

[51] Hoexter B. Use of Water Pik lavage in pilonidal wound care. Dis Colon Rectum. 1976; 19(5):470–471

[52] Rosenberg I. The dilemma of pilonidal disease: reverse bandaging for cure of the reluctant pilonidal wound. Dis Colon Rectum. 1977; 20 (4):290–291

[53] Perez-Gurri JA, Temple WJ, Ketcham AS. Gluteus maximus myocutaneous flap for the treatment of recalcitrant pilonidal disease. Dis Colon Rectum. 1984; 27(4):262–264

[54] Schoeller T, Wechselberger G, Otto A, Papp C. Definite surgical treatment of complicated recurrent pilonidal disease with a modified fasciocutaneous V-Y advancement flap. Surgery. 1997; 121(3):258–263

[55] Bascom JU. Repeat pilonidal operations. Am J Surg. 1987; 154(1):118–122

[56] Davis KA, Mock CN, Versaci A, Lentrichia P. Malignant degeneration of pilonidal cysts. Am Surg. 1994; 60(3):200–204

[57] Pekmezci S, Hiz M, Saribeyoglu K, et al. Malignant degeneration: an unusual complication of pilonidal sinus disease. Eur J Surg. 2001; 167 (6):475–477

[58] Enriquez-Navascues JM, Emparanza JI, Alkorta M, Placer C. Meta-analysis of randomized controlled trials comparing different techniques with primary closure for chronic pilonidal sinus. Tech Coloproctol. 2014; 18 (10):863–872

11 Perianal Dermatologic Disease

David E. Beck

Abstract

Patients' perianal dermatologic conditions are initially seen with a variety of symptoms and macroscopic appearances. Perianal skin conditions may be classified as pruritic and nonpruritic. When no underlying cause for pruritus can be identified, the condition is termed "idiopathic pruritus ani," the most common type. The dermatologist and the surgeon frequently work in concert. This chapter reviews the dermatologic conditions with emphasis on diagnosis and treatment from the surgeon's perspective.

Keywords: pruritus ani, hygiene, nonpruritic lesions, hidradenitis suppurativa, neoplastic lesions, inflammatory bowel disease, treatment, etiology, skin disease, systemic disease

11.1 Introduction

Patients with primary perianal dermatologic conditions and secondary perianal involvement in systemic diseases are initially seen with a variety of symptoms and macroscopic appearances. Even though patients may have painful, friable, indurated, ulcerated, or raised skin lesions, their most frequent symptom is pruritus.[1] For practical purposes, the perianal skin conditions may be classified as pruritic and nonpruritic. When no underlying cause for pruritus can be identified, the condition is termed "idiopathic pruritus ani," the most common type. Consequently, it serves as the basis for much of this discussion. In treating this group of conditions, the dermatologist and the surgeon frequently work in concert. The dermatologist, because of his or her visual training, is equipped to diagnose, scrape, culture, and prepare microscopic preparations and perform a biopsy in the office, and the surgeon is able to examine and culture and to perform a biopsy on anorectal pathology through anoscopes and proctoscopes. This chapter reviews the dermatologic conditions with emphasis on diagnosis and treatment from the surgeon's perspective.

11.2 Pruritic Conditions

11.2.1 Idiopathic Pruritus Ani

Pruritus ani is an unpleasant cutaneous sensation characterized by varying degrees of itching. Men are affected more often than women in a ratio of 4:1.[1] Idiopathic forms of pruritus ani occur in approximately 50 to 90% of the cases.[2,3] The remaining cases of pruritus are symptomatic presentations of either localized or systemic diseases (e.g., hemorrhoids, diabetes), which are considered later in this chapter.

History

Symptoms, which usually start insidiously, are characterized by the occasional awareness of an uncomfortable perianal sensation. The anal skin is richly endowed with sensory nerves, but the perceptions of individual patients vary. Some patients feel an itch, whereas others sense burning. Often, the patient is more aware of the problem at night or in hot, humid weather, although this is not always the case. The itching also may be exaggerated by friction from clothing, wool, and perspiration; on the other hand, applying cool compresses counters irritation, and heat avoidance, mental distraction, and lubrication of the skin surface ease the itching. With time, the condition may progress to an unrelenting, intolerably tormenting, burning soreness compounded by the insurmountable urge to scratch, claw, and otherwise irritate the area in a futile effort to obtain relief. The severely afflicted patient is eventually exhausted, and a few have been driven to suicide as a means of obtaining relief.

The patient has usually resorted to self-treatment with over-the-counter medications. The patient often overtreats; so a first step for the physician is to stop the acute, contact dermatitis. Poor anal hygiene is often a contributing factor; therefore, questions about the patient's cleansing habits may be important. Specific dietary ingredients and neurogenic, psychogenic, and idiosyncratic reactions with pruritus should be suspected whenever another factor is not readily identified (see specific causes below).[1,4,5,6] Since the diagnosis is made by exclusion, inquiries about diabetes, psoriasis, family history of atopic eczema, use of local topical medications, seborrhea on other sites on the body, children with similar itching reminiscent of pinworms, antibiotic use, vaginal discharge or infection, acholic stools, dark urine, or anal intercourse may establish the factor or factors responsible for the symptom.

Stress and anxiety may exaggerate pruritus ani. Often, personal factors in life are omitted by the patient. When taking a history, the physician may have to encourage the patient to "open up" and to express or consider factors that may be contributing to the discomfort. Common complaints revolve around family, work, and finances.[7] Laurent et al used the Mini-Mult personality test for psychological assessment of patients with idiopathic pruritus ani versus normal controls. They found that the mean hypomania and depression scales were greater and smaller, respectively, in the idiopathic pruritus group. However, the conclusion was that psychological factors are only predisposing factors.[8]

Physical Findings

In the early stages of the condition, examination may reveal only minimal erythema and excoriations. As the symptoms progress, the perianal skin becomes thin, friable, tender, blistered, ulcerated, and "weeping" (▶ Fig. 11.1). In the later stages, the skin is raw, red, lichenified, and oozing or pale (▶ Fig. 11.2), with exaggeration of the radiating folds of anal skin. Often, a secondary bacterial or fungal infection is present. A clinical classification from Washington Hospital Center, Washington, DC, is based on the appearance of the skin. Stage 0 skin appears normal. Stage 1 skin is red and inflamed. Stage 2 has white lichenified skin. Stage 3 has lichenified skin as well as coarse ridges of skin and often ulcerations secondary to scratching.

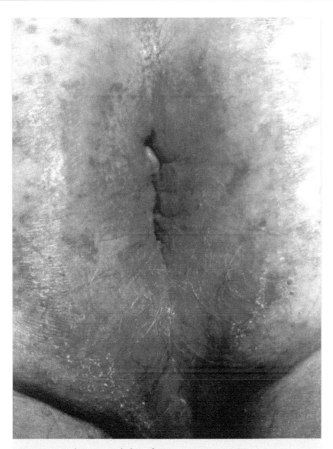

Fig. 11.1 Red excoriated skin of stage 1 pruritus ani.

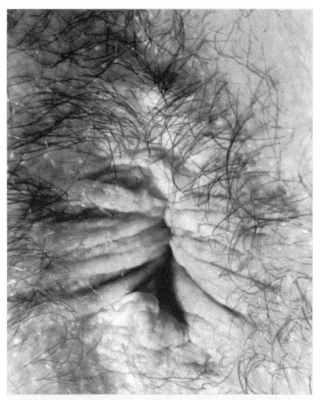

Fig. 11.2 Lichenified skin of stage 3 pruritus ani.

Careful local anorectal examination may distinguish an inciting factor, but a detailed skin examination of the entire body may provide the diagnosis. Adjunctive laboratory and radiologic testing (e.g., determining blood glucose and electrolyte levels or performing a barium enema) may be required to diagnose a primary cause. If a treatment program is begun before the factors that may result in pruritus have been ruled out, a primary cause may be overlooked. Rather than decreasing the misery of the patient, this approach may cause the condition to become worse.

Physiologic Testing

Physiologic studies of patients with pruritus ani have been performed to determine whether disordered function is a causative factor. Manometry, compliance, sensation to rectal balloon, and perineal descent have been measured and were found to be the same as those of controls.[9] The exception was a significantly greater fall in anal pressure with rectal balloon distention.[2,9] Farouk et al[10] used computerized ambulatory electromyography and manometry to demonstrate that patients with pruritus ani have an abnormal transient internal sphincter relaxation, one that is greater and prolonged. Thus, occult fecal leakage with subsequent perianal itching results. Others have shown a decreased resting anal pressure by manometric comparison before and after coffee consumption.[4] Thus, coffee may contribute to a leak.

Saline infusion tests showed early leakage (after 600 mL) as compared to control subjects (after 1,300 mL).[9] There is an inverse relationship between the severity of symptoms and the volume of first leakage. Again, leaking and soiling seem to be major factors.

Histopathology

In acute pruritus, epithelial intercellular edema and vesiculation are present. In chronic cases, hyperkeratosis and acanthosis are noted. Atrophy of the outer layers of the epidermis, sebaceous glands, and hair follicles may occur, but in part this may be due to use of potent steroids. Finally, ulceration may supervene.

Treatment

Therapy for idiopathic pruritus ani is nonspecific and often involves changes over the course of time. The treatment is directed at regaining a clean, dry, and intact perianal skin. The following discussion outlines a broad approach to this symptom complex, including reassurance, education, local treatment, and follow-up.

Reassurance

Since, by definition, idiopathic pruritus ani has no identifiable primary cause, treatment is mainly symptomatic and directed toward decreasing moisture in the perianal area. Reassurance to the patient that there is no underlying pathology, particularly carcinoma, is often as effective in producing a "cure" as any of the physical or medicinal modalities used. Often, these patients have a long, protracted course of treatment, and a sympathetic, reassuring approach is necessary to achieve ultimate success.

Education and Local Treatment

Providing patient education is very important. Patients are instructed to cleanse several times daily, especially after bowel movements. Although cleanliness is stressed, the use of medicated soaps in the perianal region is discouraged. In the acute, excoriated, weeping, crusting stage, warm wet packs may aid in debridement. The patient can dry himself or herself gently with either a soft towel or, preferably, a hair dryer. A combination of Kerodex 71 and 2.5% hydrocortisone ointment is used as a barrier on the perianal skin and to reduce inflammation. Fluorinated steroid topical preparations should not be used over long periods of time because skin atrophy will ensue and perhaps incite a more unpleasant skin condition. Anesthetic preparations such as Xylocaine ointment may mask the disease or contribute to an allergic dermatitis; thus, the use of soothing topical medications is preferred. As the condition improves, or is in milder forms, creams and lotions are replaced with cornstarch powder or talc. A small wisp of absorbent cotton or absorbent paper tissue may be tucked into the anal cleft to help keep the area dry.

Coffee (including decaffeinated blends), tea, colas, chocolate, beer, citrus fruits, alcohol, dairy products, and tomatoes may contribute to idiopathic pruritus.[6] Serial elimination of each item for 2 weeks may help identify the offending substance. If the pruritus disappears, deleted foods are returned to the diet one at a time. If the pruritus recurs, the offending ingredient is withdrawn. Daniel et al[11] found that there is a direct correlation between the severity of perianal irritation and the amount of coffee consumed daily. If the patient has "after leak, " characterized by stinging, burning, or a perianal "crawling" sensation superimposed on the itch after a bowel movement, the patient is instructed to irrigate the rectal ampulla with a small tap-water enema. Following this procedure, the patient needs to cleanse the area with a wet tissue while straining down and opening the anal canal. This process is continued until there is no brown stain left on the tissue. A mucosal prolapse, a rectocele, or a hidden rectal prolapse might be suspected and observed during the physical examination.

Other nonspecific therapy includes shaving hirsute patients. However, as the hair grows back, the short stubble can be a source of irritation and increase the urge to scratch, defeating the original gains. Extreme cases may require sedation and/or antihistamines such as diphenhydramine hydrochloride (Benadryl), 25 mg, four to six times per day. Estrogens may be useful in postmenopausal women. Wearing loose-fitting clothes and undergarments made of cotton may be helpful. Softened fabrics have been shown to reduce frictional effect on skin, especially irritated skin.[12] Underwear made of synthetic fibers does not absorb perspiration. If a secondary bacterial or fungal infection is present, topical antibiotics or fungicides may be instituted based on the results from cultures and sensitivity testing. If medical therapy is failing, a biopsy to identify Bowen's disease or Paget's disease is in order.

In the past, various methods such as tattooing with mercury sulfide, sclerotherapy, radiation therapy, and surgical procedures have been used. These methods are generally condemned because permanent cure is seldom reported. However, Eusebio et al[13] treated 23 patients over a 9.5-year period with one intracutaneous injection treatment of the anodermal and perianal skin using intravenous sedation, local anesthesia, and up to 30 mL of 0.5% methylene blue. Of the 23 patients, 10 had complete long-term relief, 4 had complete relief but were lost to follow-up after 12 weeks, and 4 had relief for 12 weeks but experienced varying degrees of recurrence. The use of methylene blue was verified by Farouk and Lee[14] in six patients.

Follow-Up

Initially, patients with severe disease may need to be seen as frequently as twice per week. Providing reassurance and visible concern is often the most important part of therapy at this time. As symptoms improve, the time between visits can be gradually lengthened until the patient is seen once every 3 to 4 weeks. It is important not to discontinue seeing a patient using a steroid cream because chronic use can lead to the development of atrophic skin, superinfection, and a secondary pruritus or burning sensation.

Often, the symptoms wax and wane, and a cure is based more on a flexible therapy plan coupled with positive psychologic reinforcement than on the actual agent or agents used. Constant reiteration of the desired goals and the methods used to achieve them may be necessary. Finally, the physician should be willing to reassess the patient whenever there is any suggestion that a more specific entity may be responsible for the pruritus.

11.2.2 Primary Etiologies

Poor Hygiene

Poor hygiene is often associated with the diseases discussed in this section. Frequently, this is the only factor identified with cases labeled as "idiopathic." The anatomy of a patient (e.g., a deep intergluteal cleft) may render the perianal region inaccessible to proper cleansing. In other cases, the patient is not fastidious in cleansing, and retained mucus, perspiration, and feces initiate the local irritation process.[4] Some disabled patients, such as those with arthritis, strokes, or multiple sclerosis, are physically incapable of performing adequate perianal hygiene. Likewise, the elderly who have even mild incontinence may not cleanse well, such that irritation and pruritus will ensue.[15]

Anorectal Lesions

Any lesion in the gastrointestinal tract that can cause excessive moisture in the perianal region may result in pruritus. Hemorrhoids, anal fissures and fistulas, hypertrophied papillae, prolapse, and neoplasms are some of the more frequent anorectal offenders. Rubber band ligation often controls pruritus associated with hemorrhoids.[16] Treatment should be directed toward the specific pathology.

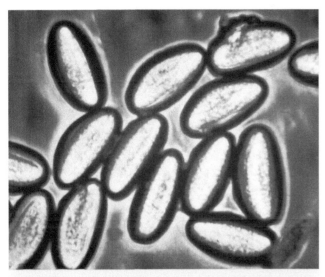

Fig. 11.3 Eggs of *Enterobius vermicularis* on clear adhesive tape.

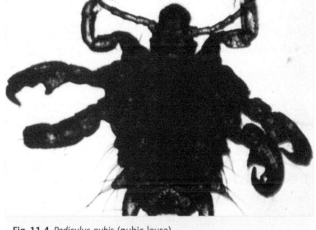

Fig. 11.4 *Pediculus pubis* (pubic louse).

Infections

Infections can be caused by parasites, viruses, bacteria, fungi, or yeasts. These pathologies are considered in the following discussion.

Parasites

A common cause of perianal itching in children is infestation with *Enterobius vermicularis*, or pinworms. The child can be the source of infestation in the family. The worms emerge from the anal canal at night and early morning; consequently, pruritus is worst at those times. Scratching tends to scatter the eggs in the bed and wherever the patient disrobes. The diagnosis is made by microscopically identifying the *E. vermicularis* eggs or adult worms (▶ Fig. 11.3). The specimen is collected by applying clear, adhesive cellulose tape across the anus when symptoms are worst. The tape is then attached to a microscopic slide for examination. The use of lactophenol cotton blue stain enhances the detection of the colorless eggs.[17]

If *E. vermicularis* is found, treatment consists of piperazine citrate (Antepar) in doses varied according to the patient's age and weight or, preferably, mebendazole (Vermox), 100 mg for all ages, in a single dose.[18] Unfortunately, all family members must be treated because of the frequent cross-spread of eggs to family members. The eggs are everywhere in the household; therefore, after treatment, cleaning all floors, furniture, linens, and beds to eradicate the eggs is important to avoid reinfestation.

Pediculus pubis, a louse, is a parasite visible to the naked eye; under magnification, it resembles a crab (▶ Fig. 11.4). The nits of eggs embedded on the pubic hair can readily be observed. Treatment consists of malathion 0.5% lotion applied to the pubic and perianal hair and then rinsed off after at least 2 hours. An alternative is permethrin cream 1% applied and washed off after 10 minutes, carbaryl 1% applied and washed out 12 hours later, and phenothrin 0.2% applied and washed out 2 hours later.[19] A second application can be made a week later.[20] All sexual partners must be treated. Clothing and bedding can be sterilized by washing in very hot water.

Scabies is estimated to infect over 300,000,000 people worldwide.[21] It is a parasitic infestation characterized by itching on the arms, legs, and scrotum before the development of pruritus ani (▶ Fig. 11.5).[17] As the itch mite, *Sarcoptes scabiei*, burrows, it creates dark punctate lesions, which are readily identified on the trunk and particularly between the fingers and ventral surface of the wrists. The diagnosis depends on demonstration of the parasite in a potassium hydroxide preparation (▶ Fig. 11.6). Treatment includes topical application of 5% permethrin or 1% lindane (applied as creams or lotions from the neck down, and then washed off in 8–12 hours).[20,22] Oral ivermectin (150–200 mg/kg of body weight) given as an initial dose and again in 2 weeks cures 95%. Good hygiene and cleansing of all clothing and bedding by washing in hot water is necessary to avoid reinfestation. Some itching may persist for weeks, due to dead scabies parts, but mild topical steroids and systemic antihistamines control the itching.[23] In children, the head also must be treated. Care must be taken to avoid open wounds because absorption may cause convulsions.

Viruses

The most common viral infection in the perianal region is condyloma acuminatum, which is discussed in Chapter 12.

Perianal presentation of herpes simplex virus (HSV-2) is rare compared to its frequent presentation as genital infection (herpes genitalis) and even less frequently when compared to herpes simplex virus (HSV-1), which presents as the familiar "cold sore" and "fever blister." The mode of infection is usually sexual, but the virus may be spread by direct contact from parent to infant or from the mouth and through the gastrointestinal tract to the perianal site. Unfortunately, HSV-1, the nasolabial cold sore type, is becoming a progressively larger proportion of the perineal herpes infections.[24]

The incubation time is usually 2 to 7 days, but it may last up to 3 weeks, with prodromal symptoms consisting of minimal burning, irritation, or paresthesias. The infection is characterized by severe pain and pruritus, with a serous or purulent discharge. Tenesmus and secondary spasm are common. The pain may radiate to the groin, thighs, and buttocks.

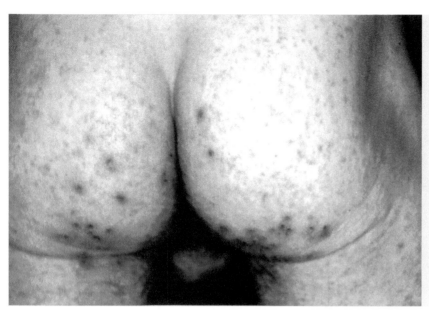

Fig. 11.5 Lesions of scabies. (The image is provided courtesy of Milton Orkin, MD, Minneapolis, MN.)

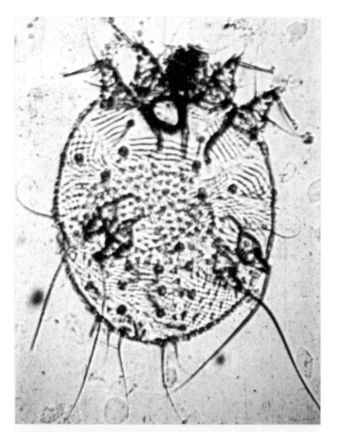

Fig. 11.6 *Sarcoptes scabiei* (scabies parasite). (The image is provided courtesy of Milton Orkin, MD, Minneapolis, MN.)

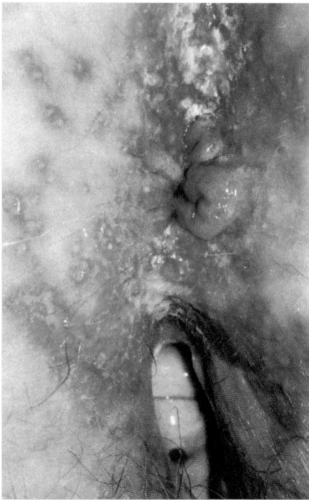

Fig. 11.7 Herpes genitalis. Acute vesicles.

The initial lesion is a small vesicle with a surrounding erythematous areola (▶ Fig. 11.7). Within 24 to 48 hours, the surface ruptures, and an ulcer results (▶ Fig. 11.8). In the immunosuppressed patient, ulcers may become confluent, appearing as ulcerating cellulitis. The lesions are distributed equally between the perianal skin and the anal canal. If the patient has never had a herpes infection, systemic symptoms (e.g., fever, chills, malaise) are common. Healing leaves scalloped scars. A recurrence may involve only some scattered vesicles.

The diagnosis usually is made by history and physical examination alone. Adjunctive methods include cytology, immunofluorescence, viral culture, and the Tzanck test. Currently, there are commercial companies vying for a faster, more accurate test, using the new glycoprotein G-based, type-specific HSV serologies.[25] If a vesicle or the margin of an ulcer is scraped, the scrapings may be smeared on a slide, heat fixed, stained with methylene blue, and rinsed. Multinucleated giant cells may be seen with this viral disease. Other viral diseases such as herpes zoster or chickenpox also have giant cells.

The disease is usually self-limiting in 1 to 3 weeks if there is no secondary bacterial infection. Symptomatic treatment (see discussion of idiopathic pruritus ani) is the basis for relief. Acyclovir may be used to abort the first attack. The usual dose is 400 mg five times per day for 10 days.[26] New antiviral agents, famciclovir 250 mg three times per day for 5 to 10 days and valacyclovir 1 g two times per day for 10 days, offer more convenient treatment schedules.[26] Recurrence is the rule, and acyclovir, valacyclovir, and famciclovir reduce the duration of viral shedding and time to lesion healing.[19] If recurrences are frequent, prescribing these drugs may be tried as prophylaxis.

The prophylactic regimen is acyclovir 400 mg two times per day, valacyclovir 500 mg orally daily, or famciclovir 250 mg orally two times per day for 6 months. The immunosuppressed patient must be hospitalized for intravenous acyclovir treatment.[27] Steroids are never used because they may potentiate the infection. Other specific treatment such as immunization with vaccines has been shown to be largely ineffective in the treatment of genital herpes.[28]

Lumbosacral dermatomes are involved in 11% of patients infected by herpes zoster.[29] The causative virus is *Herpesvirus varicellae*, which has a variable incubation period. The first manifestations are fever, pain, and malaise. After 3 to 4 days, the characteristic closely grouped red papules appear along dermatomes, and they become vesicular and pustular quickly. Lymphadenopathy is common.

Sacral herpes zoster may result in urinary retention and sensory loss in both the bladder and rectum.[29] These results can be seen even with unilateral skin involvement, which is somewhat perplexing since hemisection of the cord does not result in detectable sphincter dysfunction.

Treatment is mainly symptomatic. Oral acyclovir and steroids may give early relief and minimize neurologic sequelae.[29] Complete spontaneous recovery over 3 to 4 weeks is the usual course. Postherpetic neuralgia is the most common adverse sequela.

Bacteria

Erythrasma caused by *Corynebacterium minutissimum* may affect the perianal, perineal, and axillary regions but is most common in the toe webs. The characteristic pruritic perianal lesion is a large round patch, initially pink and irregular, but subsequently turning brown and scaly (▶ Fig. 11.9). The diagnosis is made by examining the lesions under ultraviolet light and observing the characteristic coral-red to salmon-pink fluorescence secondary to porphyrin production by the bacteria (▶ Fig. 11.10). Occasionally, the visible lesion is nonfluorescent; however, the diagnosis can be made by biopsy of the lesion.[30] Treatment consists of 250 mg of erythromycin by mouth, four times per day for a 10- to 14-day period, or chloramphenicol ointment.[30]

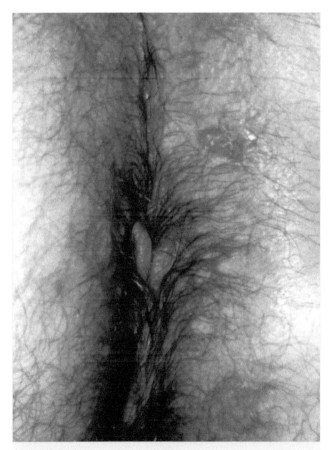

Fig. 11.8 Herpes genitalis. Open ulcers.

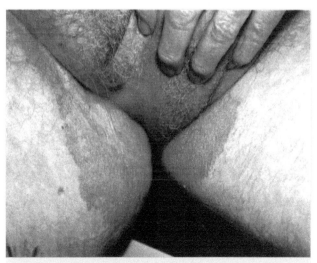

Fig. 11.9 Lesions of erythrasma (*Corynebacterium minutissimum*).

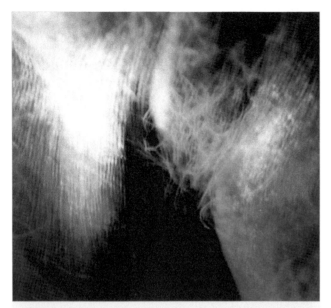

Fig. 11.10 Pink fluorescence of erythrasma when viewed under the ultraviolet lamp.

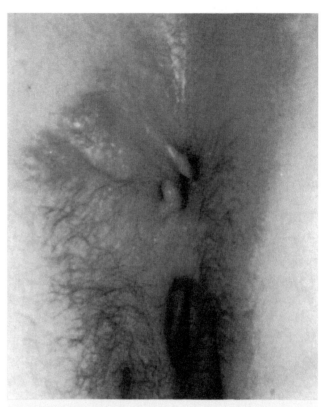

Fig. 11.11 Primary chancre of syphilis on white skin. (The image is provided courtesy of Maria Turner, MD.)

Patients with syphilis may have pruritus caused by irritation secondary to exudates from the primary chancre or the secondary condyloma latum (▶ Fig. 11.11). Pruritus is uncommon in the tertiary stage, when there usually is no gross lesion. This disease is more fully discussed in Chapter 14.

Though rare, perianal tuberculosis may be seen initially either as an ulcer with a sharp irregular outline and a grayish granular base or as a purulent ulcerated verrucous lesion. It also may be seen as an extensive perianal inflammation with areas of healing and breakdown, subcutaneous nodules, sinuses, and deformity. Pain is minimal, but local soreness and pruritus are common. Generally, the colon is also involved, and the diagnosis is made by having an antecedent history of tuberculosis or a positive chest radiograph or by identifying acid-fast organisms in scrapings from the lesions. With modern-day treatments, these lesions are relatively rare, but when present they can be readily conquered. The reader is referred to a standard textbook of medicine for details of antituberculosis drug management.

Streptococcus may cause a perianal dermatitis in both children and adults. That dermatitis is a well-defined erythema of the perianal skin that does not respond to the usual topical treatments for anal complaints. Culture of the perianal dermatitis might verify this diagnosis. In therapy-resistant anal redness, streptococcus dermatitis should be considered.[31,32] In children, cure is usually obtained by oral penicillin or erythromycin for 10 to 14 days.[33] Adults are more difficult to cure, but there has been success with erythromycin, clindamycin, or a dicloxacillin.[34]

Fungi and Yeast

Candida albicans, a saprophytic yeast, is normally present in the gut. This yeast can become pathogenic with a change in the patient's resistance or in the normal skin, such as with uncontrolled diabetes mellitus, prolonged antibiotic treatment, or prolonged use of steroids. The infected skin appears moist, red, and macerated (▶ Fig. 11.12). Pustules form and become confluent, bright red, and scaly, with poorly defined margins and satellite lesions. Under microscopic scrutiny, mycelian forms and spores can be identified from scrapings of the lesion. The microscopic slide is prepared by placing 20% potassium hydroxide on the scrapings and gently warming them; then the slide is examined with 10 and 40 times magnification. Organisms may be grown on Sabouraud's culture medium.

Treatment consists of applying nystatin (Mycostatin) powder or ointment or imidazole compound several times daily, along with controlling or eliminating the precipitating cause (e.g., control of diabetes, withdrawal of antibiotics and/or steroids). For resistant cases, fluconazole (Diflucan) 150 mg orally may be tried, and it may be repeated.

Epidermophyton floccosum, *Trichophyton mentagrophytes*, and *Trichophyton rubrum* are fungal infections that are usually seen unilaterally with a scaly, well-defined, circinate margin (▶ Fig. 11.13). The presence of dermatophytes is always associated with prutitus.[35] The dermatophytes begin as a red bump that spreads centrifugally, eventually to give a ring-within-a-ring, or "ringworm," appearance. Often, a similar lesion is seen between the toes. Diagnosis is confirmed by culturing scrapings on Sabouraud's medium or by examining them as a potassium hydroxide preparation under the microscope. On low power, strands of fungus may be seen (▶ Fig. 11.14). Treatment is achieved with various fungicidal preparations such as tolnaftate (Tinactin) or topical imidazole if the lesion is superficial. Deep invasion of the follicles may warrant oral therapy with griseofulvin ultrafine, 250 mg twice a day for 3 to 4 weeks; a complete response sometimes requires 6 to 8 weeks of treatment. This drug should be taken with

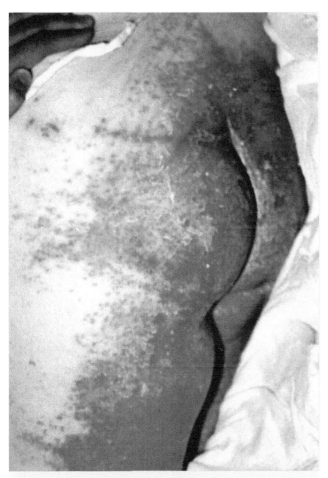

Fig. 11.12 Moist, red, macerated lesions of *Candida albicans*. (The image is provided courtesy of Maria Turner, MD.)

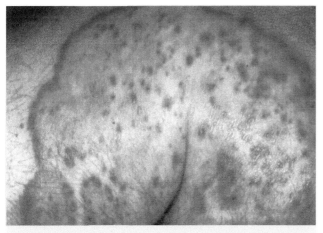

Fig. 11.13 Tinea circinata (ringworm). (The image is provided courtesy of Maria Turner, MD.)

food to minimize gastrointestinal distress and nausea. Ketoconazole (Nizoral) is effective, but occasional deaths resulting from hepatic toxicity have occurred after 5 months. Any interdigital lesions must also be eradicated to achieve a cure. Terbinafine used orally has been shown to be safe and efficacious.[36]

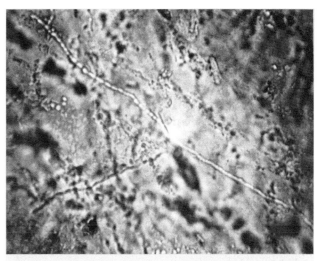

Fig. 11.14 Hyphae of a fungus seen in potassium hydroxide preparation. (The image is provided courtesy of Mervyn Elgart, MD.)

Skin Diseases

Skin lesions may be localized to the perianal region or may be systemic. The patient's entire body must be examined for evidence of further lesions whenever a dermatologic condition is being investigated.

Seborrhea

Seborrhea, or dandruff, may be found on the perineum. The red color is not bright, but fissuring may be seen. Pruritus is the chief complaint. Other parts of the body, such as the scalp, chest, ears, suprapubic area, and beard, should be inspected (▸ Fig. 11.15). Studies of the etiology of seborrheic dermatitis (SD) concentrate on the role of *Pityrosporum ovale* and sebaceous lipids.

Patients with SD have lower levels of free fatty acids and higher triglycerides in their skin as compared to patients without SD.[37] The treatment is 2% sulfur with hydrocortisone lotion or miconazole lotion, or 2% ketoconazole shampoo.[38] Terbinafine solution or 250 mg tablets have been efficacious.[39,40] If the patient is immunocompromised, ketoconazole may be used. The response to treatment is usually good.

Contact Dermatitis

The anogenital region is subject to many products that may cause a contact dermatitis, such as douches, dusting powders, contraceptives, colored toilet paper, poison ivy, and strong topical medications. The history should include questions about over-the-counter medications and home remedies. The highly irritating, eczematous, ill-defined lesions of contact dermatitis may result from prolonged exposure to topical medications such as lanolin, neomycin, and parabens. Parabens is a preservative that is used in topical preparations; unfortunately, it evokes an allergic reaction in some patients. Topical anesthetics of the "-caine" family may be especially irritating (▸ Fig. 11.16).[41] Both amide (e.g., lidocaine) and ester (e.g., procaine) topical anesthetics may cause a reaction. A patch test or perhaps intradermal injection tests will show an allergy to lidocaine and a cross-reaction to bupivacaine.[42] Quinolones in the anesthetic ointment may result in contact

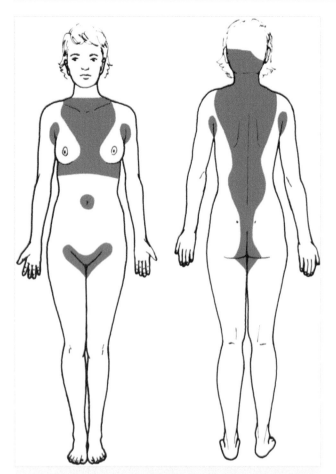

Fig. 11.15 Body pattern of seborrhea.

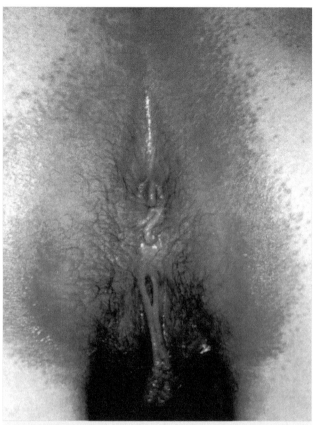

Fig. 11.16 Contact dermatitis caused by use of lidocaine.

dermatitis. Often, the hand with which the patient applies the offending agent is similarly affected. The skin appears intensely erythematous with vesicles and is fragile and macerated.

A common over-the-counter hemorrhoidal preparation that has little efficacy for hemorrhoids causes dermatitis (▶ Fig. 11.17). Common spices used in cooking may result in anal irritation and inflammation.

Toilet paper can cause an allergy. Euxyl K 400 is a preservative system for cosmetics and toiletries that contains methyldibromo glutaronitrile. This ingredient is a newly recognized allergen contained in moistened toilet paper. Thus, anal dermatitis might be tested for with a patch test of 0.3 to 0.5% methyldibromo glutaronitrile in petrolatum.

Cashew nuts, a favorite snack, and oil used to make other foods, unfortunately, belong to the poison oak and poison ivy family. Sensitive people may develop eruptions on the hands, lips, and perianal area when exposed to the cardol oil.[43]

The overuse of topical steroids is a problem that results in "steroid skin" (▶ Fig. 11.18).[44] The perianal skin develops marked striae. Overgrowth with *Candida* organisms is common but can be prevented by limiting the duration of use of and the strength of the steroid ointment. Prolonged use of the fluorinated steroid preparations results in atrophy of the perianal skin, which leads to worse symptoms than those few for which the preparation was initially prescribed.[44] Nystatin (Mycolog), a commonly prescribed medication, formerly contained ethylenediamine as a

preservative, which frequently caused an allergic reaction. Up to 25% of people exposed to neomycin, which is a constituent of Neosporin, may have an allergic reaction. Poison ivy, sumac, or oak may be the source of acute anogenital eruption if the person has knelt or squatted in the outdoors with an exposed perineum. The vesicles may be debrided.

A patient with severe contact dermatitis may require bed rest for a few days. The skin should be open to air; underwear is not to be worn. A solution of one-fourth cup of vinegar in a gallon of tepid water as a sitz bath or applied with a cloth for 1 hour three times per day will dry, cool, and cleanse the skin. A hair dryer on a cool setting is a good dryer. Applying 1% hydrocortisone or 0.05% flurandrenolide (Cordran) lotion is helpful. Ointments are occlusive and should be avoided. For severe contact dermatitis, oral corticosteroids may be employed. A high dose is rapidly tapered, using 50, 40, 30, 20, and 10 mg for 2 days each. Antihistamines, such as 4-mg chlorpheniramine maleate tablets three times a day, initially aid in reduction of the inflammation. If the patient follows these instructions, the skin should revert to normal in 2 weeks.

Unfortunately, topical corticosteroids used specifically on anal skin have been shown to be an increasingly recognized cause of contact dermatitis and should be suspected when recalcitrant dermatitis is encountered after application of steroids.[45]

Psoriasis

This affliction has no known cause, but genetics may play a role, since 30% of patients have a family history of psoriasis. The lesion

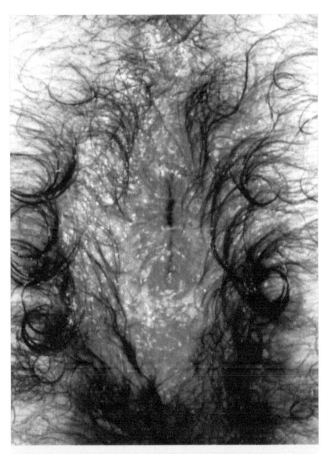

Fig. 11.17 Contact dermatitis caused by use of a common over-the-counter hemorrhoidal ointment preparation.

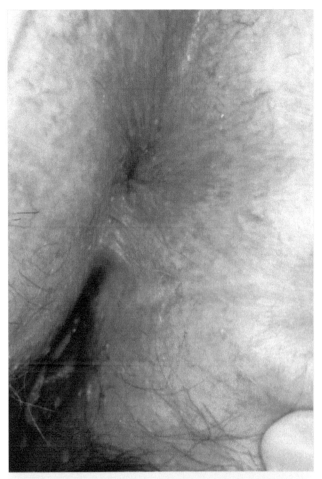

Fig. 11.18 Contact dermatitis caused by long-term use of topical steroids.

is usually a full, red, sharply demarcated, often macerated, scaling plaque. The scales are thick and white and bleeding results if they are removed. Sometimes fissuring is found. The skin may be thickened, and pruritus is common. Because of the moisture in the intergluteal region, the characteristic psoriatic plaque may not be present. Instead, a paler, more poorly defined, nonscaling lesion may result (▶ Fig. 11.19). A search for diagnostic lesions on other parts of the body should be conducted (▶ Fig. 11.20). The scalp, penis, elbows, knees, and knuckles should be inspected. The nails may be onycholytic and hyperkeratotic, and pitting and an "oil drop" appearance may be present.

Psoriasis is not curable, but it can be controlled. Applying 1% hydrocortisone and 2% precipitated sulfur lotion in the intergluteal area may be effective. Creams and ointments often cause maceration where the skin is opposed by the gluteal muscles. Anthralin 0.1% salve applied locally twice a day to a site is effective. The lesions also may respond to fluocinolone acetonide 0.025% cream, flurandrenolide, or fluocinolone cream in a coal tar base.[46]

Lichen Simplex Chronicus (Neurodermatitis)

Recalcitrant pruritus is a hallmark of lichen simplex, a localized variant of atopic dermatitis. Lichenification is a thickening of all layers of the epidermis. Initially, the skin appears red and edematous. In the later stages after cycles of itching and scratching, often at night, the skin lesion evolves into a well-demarcated, erythematous, scaly thickening. The diagnosis is confirmed by performing a biopsy. There is no specific treatment other than the symptomatic methods. Antihistamines reduce itching, and topical steroids reduce inflammation. Unlike atopic dermatitis, there are no familial links.

Atopy

Atopy is an individual's genetic predisposition to develop allergic diseases in response to environmental allergens. Atopic individuals and relatives may have manifestations such as asthma, hay fever, or eczema. Scaling of the face, neck, dorsum of the hands, popliteal fossae, and antecubital fossae may harbor similar eruptions. Soap should be avoided because it is an irritant. Aid is obtained from 5% coal tar solution and 1% hydrocortisone applied topically. Since itching and scratching are worse at night, 50 mg of hydroxyzine should be tried for 2 weeks; then a bland ointment such as A and D ointment or an ointment mixture of cod liver oil, 40% zinc oxide, and talc in a petrolatum-lanolin base (e.g., Desitin ®, Johnson & Johnson) might be used as a barrier. If there is a relapse, the therapy should be reinstituted.

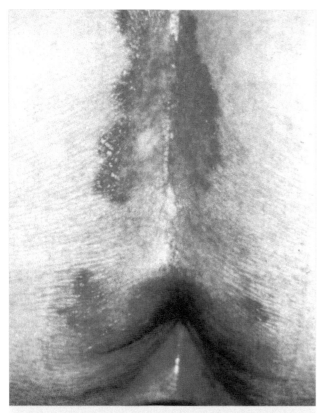

Fig. 11.19 Psoriasis. Note intergluteal fold extension.

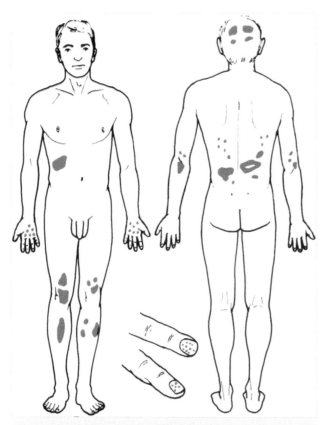

Fig. 11.20 Pattern of lesions in psoriasis.

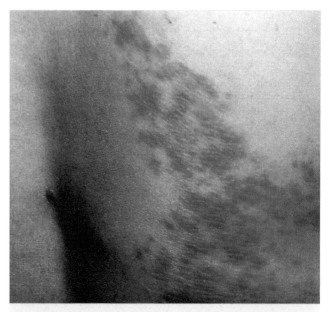

Fig. 11.21 Lichen planus on white skin. (The image is provided courtesy of Maria Turner, MD.)

Lichen Planus

This condition has a peak incidence between 30 and 60 years of age. It may have an association with hepatitis; thus, there may be an immunologic basis. This dermatologic condition begins on the genitals and perianal region and subsequently spreads to distant regions in later stages.[47] The lesions are shiny, flat-topped papules with a darker pigmentation than are usually seen in the more distant lesions (▶ Fig. 11.21, ▶ Fig. 11.22). The mouth is checked for white patches, and plaques often are found on the volar aspects of the wrists and forearms. An application of mineral oil to the plaques may demonstrate the intersecting, small gray lines called "Wickham's striae."

The etiology of the lines is not known. Treatment is with bland, wet dressings, sitz baths, and a low-concentration steroid cream. For heavy patches, triamcinolone acetonide (Kenalog), 10 mg/mL mixed one to one with 1% lidocaine hydrochloride (Xylocaine), may be injected into the lesions. Occasionally, very severe eruptions require the use of short courses of systemic corticosteroids. Starting doses of prednisone are 40 to 60 mg/day.[48]

Lichen Sclerosus et Atrophicus

This disease predominates in women over men in a ratio of 5:1.[49] Its etiology is unknown; however, a preceding history of vaginitis is often present. Ivory-colored, atrophic papules may break down, exposing a red, edematous, raw surface that causes intense pruritus and soreness.[49]

As the edema subsides, it is replaced by sclerosis and chronic inflammation (▶ Fig. 11.23, ▶ Fig. 11.24). Sclerosis around the anus may narrow the stool diameter. The clitoris and labia minora may be absorbed and flattened in the process. White patches in the figure-eight form may be seen over the vulva and anus. The diagnosis is confirmed by performing a skin biopsy. The condition is chronic with exacerbations and remissions, and there is no known effective cure. Potent steroid-containing creams used in short courses

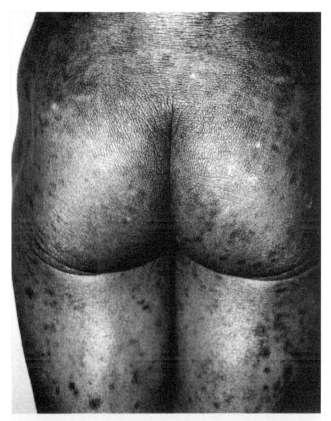

Fig. 11.22 Lichen planus on black skin. (The image is provided courtesy of Maria Turner, MD.)

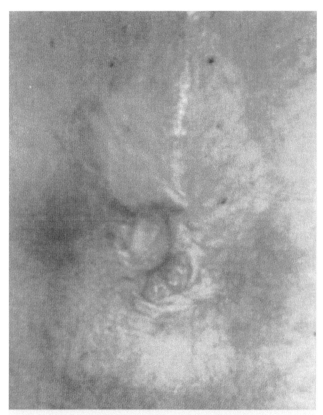

Fig. 11.24 Narrowed area of perianal involvement in lichen sclerosus et atrophicus. (The image is provided courtesy of Maria Turner, MD.)

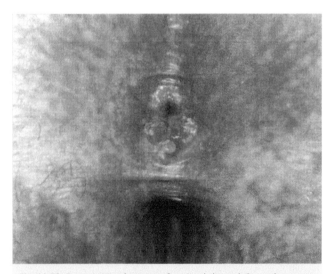

Fig. 11.23 Extensive involvement of perianal skin in lichen sclerosus et atrophicus. (The image is provided courtesy of Maria Turner, MD.)

along with the usual symptomatic treatments may aid in relieving the pruritus.[50] Unfortunately, long-term use of steroids may further thin the skin. Using 2% testosterone cream topically for 6 weeks allows relief of itching. However, the side effects may be hoarseness, hair growth, acne, and increased libido.

Pemphigus Vegetans

Pemphigus vulgaris is a systemic and usually fatal disease without therapy. It may begin in intertriginous areas as pemphigus vegetans. This variant of pemphigus may be seen initially as either early bullae, later giving way to hypertrophic granulations studded with pustules and blisters, or early pustules, later developing into warty vegetations. The former presentation, which is always accompanied by oral lesions, is known as the Hallopeau type. Both types are treated with oral steroids, with the dosage titrated to the response of the disease and the patient's tolerance.

Familial Benign Chronic Pemphigus

This is a hereditary dyskeratotic process. The condition is initially seen as erosions and blisters in intertriginous areas and sometimes as perianal irritation. A biopsy showing a pemphigus split in the epidermis and dyskeratotic cells is diagnostic. Local or systemic antibiotics are helpful. Diaminodiphenylsulfone (Dapsone) is frequently effective.

Diarrheal States

Multiple loose stools can produce pruritus by causing a localized skin irritation secondary to the chemistry of the liquid stool itself. Also, trauma from frequent and vigorous cleansing further results in production of excoriating, weeping, itching lesions.

Dietary Factors

Ingredients such as cola, coffee (decaffeinated and caffeinated), chocolate, tomatoes, beer, and tea have been implicated as inciting factors of pruritus.[6] Certainly, individual allergies to certain foods can result in itching in various portions of the anatomy.[6] Occasionally, it is merely the volume of the ingredient ingested that produces loose watery stools and mucous discharge rather than any inherent characteristic of the individual ingredient. This is seen more with liquids than with solids. In a manometric study done by Smith et al,[4] coffee was shown to decrease anal pressure, which might result in soiling.

Gynecologic Conditions

Any inflammatory or ulcerative lesion of the vulva (e.g., Bartholin's adenitis, lymphogranuloma venereum, granuloma inguinale, syphilis, lichen sclerosus et atrophicus, or carcinoma) can lead to pruritus. Kraurosis vulvae, a condition in which there is loss of the vulvar fat, is often characterized by itching.[50] Irritation secondary to an increased vaginal discharge may lead to pruritus and mandate a workup to identify the underlying cause (e.g., infection, foreign body such as an intrauterine device, or neoplasm).

Antibiotics

The use of antibiotics may lead to pruritus either because of an allergic reaction or by altering the indigenous flora of the bowel or vagina, resulting in an overgrowth of otherwise harmless bacteria or fungi and leading to diarrhea, increased vaginal discharge, or a perianal superinfection, usually candidiasis. Tetracycline is a notable offender.[51]

Systemic Diseases

Occasionally, pruritus will be the presenting symptom of an otherwise distant or systemic disease. Severe jaundice from any cause is notoriously associated with itching.[47] Diabetes, by virtue of its association with candidiasis, frequently has pruritus as its presenting symptom.

Miscellaneous Causes

Any factor that results in irritation to the perianal skin can lead to pruritus. These factors may be quite apparent, such as irradiation, or more nebulous, such as neurogenic, psychogenic, or idiosyncratic reactions.[50]

11.3 Nonpruritic Lesions

Although pruritus ani is the most common presenting symptom of perianal dermatologic conditions, many lesions do not initially present with pruritus, or the pruritus is of minor importance. Some of these diseases are discussed in the following sections.

11.3.1 Infections

Hidradenitis Suppurativa

An infection of the apocrine glands, hidradenitis suppurativa is fully described in Chapter 35.

Leprosy

Leprosy is endemic in the southern United States and tropical areas the world over. In patients with good resistance to

Mycobacterium leprae, infection may be confined to local cooler regions of the body. Leprous lesions appear as macules or plaques with healed central areas surrounded by erythematous or copper-colored extensions.[51] The lesions usually appear on the face, exterior surfaces of the limbs, the buttocks, and the back and are often preceded by anesthesia secondary to early nerve damage. Recently, molecular mechanisms that are responsible for neuropathy have been discovered. Identification of the endoneural laminin-2 isoform and its receptor alpha-dystroglycan as neural targets of *M. leprae* has opened up scientific inquiry into the pathogenesis of neurological damage.[52]

If the individual has poor resistance, the skin lesions can occur anywhere (including the perineum) and appear as small, circular, erythematous or copper-colored, smooth, shiny macules. Nerves are damaged late; consequently, anesthesia follows the development of the skin lesions.[51]

The diagnosis is confirmed by skin biopsy. Biologic false-positive tests for syphilis are common. Treatment is with 4–4' diaminodiphenyl sulfone (Dapsone), clofazimine (Lamprene), or rifampin (Rifamate).[53] The genome sequence of *M. leprae* is now understood, which will enable better use of current chemotherapy and lead to new drug targets.[53] The reader is referred to textbooks on tropical medicine for further details.

Amebiasis

Amebiasis is caused by the protozoan *Entamoeba histolytica*. Perianal manifestations consist of painful serpiginous ulcers with red, dirty, foul-smelling bases covered by a white pseudomembrane.[54] Wet mounting is the simplest and easiest technique to examine the feces for parasites. Lactophenol cotton blue added to the mounting medium stains the trophozoites, cysts, and ova.[55] A difficult differential diagnosis is herpes simplex in acquired immunodeficiency syndrome. Therapy is instituted with metronidazole, 750 mg orally three times daily for 10 days. This should be followed by iodoquinol, 650 mg three times daily for 20 days, or paromomycin, 25 mg/kg/day in three doses for 7 days, to ensure intestinal cure.[18] See Chapter 14 for further details.

Actinomycosis

This rare lesion, actinomycosis, is caused by *Actinomyces israelii*, an anaerobic, non–acid-fast organism. A brawny infiltration of the skin accompanied by proctitis, abscesses, and fistulas is seen. A high degree of suspicion is necessary to recognize an atypical fistula as having an actinomycotic etiology.[56,57] The diagnosis is confirmed by identifying characteristic "sulfur" bodies with club-shaped rays in the discharges from the sinus. Treatment consists of penicillin and local symptomatic measures.

Lymphogranuloma Venereum

Lymphogranuloma venereum is caused by a sexually transmitted virus. In the advanced stage of the disease, the perianal region is deformed with widespread scarring and vegetating lesions. Periproctitis often results in a stricture 5 to 10 cm from the anal margin, around which fistulas develop (see Chapter 13).

11.3.2 Neoplastic Lesions

A variety of neoplastic lesions are found in the perianal region. The reader is referred to Chapter 17 for a discussion of specific therapies.

Acanthosis Nigricans

Acanthosis nigricans sometimes may be associated with an underlying bowel carcinoma, obesity, and/or hyperinsulinemia, severe atopic dermatitis, and Down's syndrome.[58,59,60] It appears as a velvety black, acantholytic papillomatous lesion and is found in the axillary region, neck, knuckles, tongue, and perianal region (▶ Fig. 11.25). It may be benign or malignant. The malignant variety is usually sudden-onset and is rapidly progressive, but is clinically indistinguishable from the benign form. There is a report of the successful use of a combination of 12% ammonium lactate cream and 0.05% tretinoin cream to treat acanthosis nigricans associated with obesity.[61] A complete gastrointestinal workup is warranted to rule out any underlying neoplasm.

High-Grade Squamous Intraepithelial Neoplasia (Bowen's Disease)

High-grade squamous intraepithelial neoplasia (Bowen's disease) is an intraepidermal carcinoma that appears as a yellowish scale that is easily detached, leaving a reddened granular surface.[62] However, there are also reports of hyperpigmented velvety surfaces and well-defined hyperpigmented verrucous patches (▶ Fig. 11.11, ▶ Fig. 11.26) (see Chapter 17).[44]

Squamous Cell Carcinoma

Squamous cell carcinoma can be misdiagnosed as condyloma acuminatum. It is a warty nodular plaque that may or may not be ulcerated. Maceration and secondary infection are common, often disguising the true nature of the disease. The diagnosis is confirmed by performing a biopsy (see Chapter 17).

Melanoma

Melanoma rarely may occur in the perianal region, the anus, or the rectum. The classic malignant melanoma is a black or purple nodule, but it may be flat or pedunculated. Colors vary from pink to red, tan, brown, or black or, more difficult, it may have no color, i.e., amelanotic. Beware of changes in shape, size, color, erythema, induration, friability, or ulceration. The prognosis, with wide local excision or abdominoperineal resection, is dismal.[63,64,65] More complete discussion of melanoma is found in Chapter 18.

Perianal Paget's Disease

This extramammary presentation of Paget's disease is rare. Helwig and Graham[66] reported an 86% association of perianal Paget's disease with subadjacent or bowel carcinomas.[67,68] The disease tends to occur later in life, frequently in the seventh decade. The lesion is seen as a progressive, erythematous, eczematoid plaque (▶ Fig. 11.27). Because of the frequent association of the disease with underlying neoplasms, the prognosis is not good. However, if after wide excision no adjacent or bowel malignancy is found, the prognosis is good, but local recurrence is common.[69] Because wide local excision leaves wide defects, special surgical techniques such as V-Y flaps and staged excisions with split-thickness grafts are being used.[70,71] Close follow-up should continue forever because recurrences have occurred up to 8 years after treatment.[68]

11.3.3 Inflammatory Bowel Disease

Anal lesions are present in approximately 25% of patients with Crohn's ileitis and in 75% of patients with Crohn's colitis; they may precede the intestinal manifestation by several years.

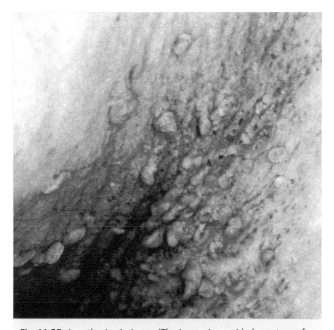

Fig. 11.25 Acanthosis nigricans. (The image is provided courtesy of Maria Turner, MD.)

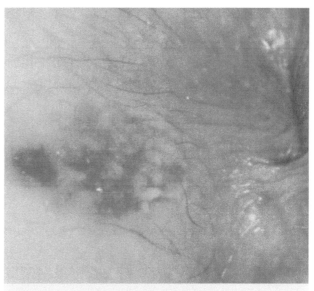

Fig. 11.26 High-grade squamous intraepithelial neoplasia (Bowen's disease).

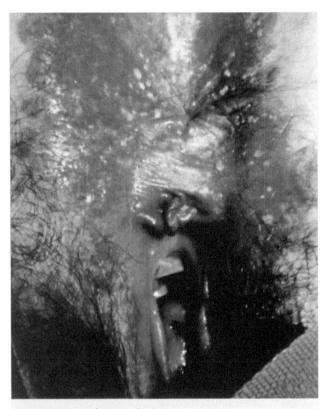

Fig. 11.27 Perianal Paget's disease.

Dusky perianal sinuses with undermining ulcers or edema, indolent single or multiple fissures, and fistulas may be some of the early signs. Diagnosis can be made by biopsy, but performing extensive surgical procedures in the presence of active disease is strongly condemned because the healing is notoriously poor (see Chapter 24 on Crohn's disease and Chapter 9 on fistulas for details).

References

[1] Wexner SD, Dailey TH. Pruritus ani: diagnosis and management. Curr Concepts Skin Disord. 1986; 7:5–9

[2] Eyers AA, Thomson JPS. Pruritus ani: is anal sphincter dysfunction important in aetiology? BMJ. 1979; 2(6204):1549–1551

[3] Goldman L, Kitzmiller KW. Perianal atrophoderma from topical corticosteroids. Arch Dermatol. 1973; 107(4):611–612

[4] Smith LE, Henrichs D, McCullah RD. Prospective studies on the etiology and treatment of pruritus ani. Dis Colon Rectum. 1982; 25(4):358–363

[5] Alexander-Williams J. Causes and management of anal irritation. Br Med J (Clin Res Ed). 1983; 287(6404):1528

[6] Friend WG. The cause and treatment of idiopathic pruritus ani. Dis Colon Rectum. 1977; 20(1):40–42

[7] Mazier WP. Hemorrhoids, fissures, and pruritus ani. Surg Clin North Am. 1994; 74(6):1277–1292

[8] Laurent A, Boucharlat J, Bosson JL, Derry A, Imbert R. Psychological assessment of patients with idiopathic pruritus ani. Psychother Psychosom. 1997; 66(3):163–166

[9] Allan A, Ambrose NS, Silverman S, Keighley MRB. Physiological study of pruritus ani. Br J Surg. 1987; 74(7):576–579

[10] Farouk R, Duthie GS, Pryde A, Bartolo DCC. Abnormal transient internal sphincter relaxation in idiopathic pruritus ani: physiological evidence from ambulatory monitoring. Br J Surg. 1994; 81(4):603–606

[11] Daniel GL, Longo WE, Vernava AM, III. Pruritus ani. Causes and concerns. Dis Colon Rectum. 1994; 37(7):670–674

[12] Piérard GE, Arrese JE, Rodríguez C, Daskaleros PA. Effects of softened and unsoftened fabrics on sensitive skin. Contact Dermat. 1994; 30(5):286–291

[13] Eusebio EB, Graham J, Mody N. Treatment of intractable pruritus ani. Dis Colon Rectum. 1990; 33(9):770–772

[14] Farouk R, Lee PW. Intradermal methylene blue injection for the treatment of intractable idiopathic pruritus ani. Br J Surg. 1997; 84(5):670

[15] Gupta A. Pruritus in the elderly. Practitioner. 1999; 243(1596):203–207

[16] Murie JA, Sim AJ, Mackenzie I. The importance of pain, pruritus and soiling as symptoms of haemorrhoids and their response to haemorrhoidectomy or rubber band ligation. Br J Surg. 1981; 68(4):247–249

[17] Parija SC, Sheeladevi C, Shivaprakash MR, Biswal N. Evaluation of lactophenol cotton blue stain for detection of eggs of Enterobius vermicularis in perianal surface samples. Trop Doct. 2001; 31(4):214–215

[18] Speck WT. Enterobiasis. In: Behrman RE, Vaughan VC, eds. Textbook of Pediatrics. 13th ed. Philadelphia, PA: WB Saunders; 1987

[19] Clinical Effectiveness Group (Association of Genitourinary Medicine and the Medical Society for the Study of Venereal Diseases). National guideline for the management of Phthirus pubis infestation. Sex Transm Infect. 1999; 75 Suppl 1:S78–S79

[20] Wendel K, Rompalo A. Scabies and pediculosis pubis: an update of treatment regimens and general review. Clin Infect Dis. 2002; 35 Suppl 2:S146–S151

[21] Hogan DJ, Schachner L, Tanglertsampan C. Diagnosis and treatment of childhood scabies and pediculosis. Pediatr Clin North Am. 1991; 38(4):941–957

[22] Chouela E, Abeldaño A, Pellerano G, Hernández MI. Diagnosis and treatment of scabies: a practical guide. Am J Clin Dermatol. 2002; 3(1):9–18

[23] Abramowitz M. Drugs for parasitic infections. Med Lett Drugs Ther. 1993; 35 (911):111–122

[24] Brugha R, Keersmaekers K, Renton A, Meheus A. Genital herpes infection: a review. Int J Epidemiol. 1997; 26(4):698–709

[25] Ashley RL. Sorting out the new HSV type specific antibody tests. Sex Transm Infect. 2001; 77(4):232–237

[26] Stanberry L, Cunningham A, Mertz G, et al. New developments in the epidemiology, natural history and management of genital herpes. Antiviral Res. 1999; 42(1):1–14

[27] Balfour HH, Jr, Bean B, Laskin OL, et al. Acyclovir halts progression of herpes zoster in immunocompromised patients. N Engl J Med. 1983; 308 (24):1448–1453

[28] Stanberry LR. Control of STDs–the role of prophylactic vaccines against herpes simplex virus. Sex Transm Infect. 1998; 74(6):391–394

[29] Krusinski PA. Herpes zoster. In: Demis DJ, ed. Clinical Dermatology. Vol. 3. Philadelphia, PA: JB Lippincott; 1989

[30] Mattox TF, Rutgers J, Yoshimori RN, Bhatia NN. Nonfluorescent erythrasma of the vulva. Obstet Gynecol. 1993; 81(5, Pt 2):862–864

[31] Paradisi M, Cianchini G, Angelo C, Conti G, Puddu P. Perianal streptococcal dermatitis [in Italian]. Minerva Pediatr. 1994; 46(6):303–306

[32] Neri I, Bardazzi F, Marzaduri S, Patrizi A. Perianal streptococcal dermatitis in adults. Br J Dermatol. 1996; 135(5):796–798

[33] Kroal AL. Perianal streptococcal dermatitis. Pediatr Dermatol. 1981; 27:518

[34] Weismann K, Sand Petersen C, Røder B. Pruritus ani caused by beta-haemolytic streptococci. Acta Derm Venereol. 1996; 76(5):415

[35] Dodi G, Pirone E, Bettin A, et al. The mycotic flora in proctological patients with and without pruritus ani. Br J Surg. 1985; 72(12):967–969

[36] Abdel-Rahman SM, Nahata MC. Oral terbinafine: a new antifungal agent. Ann Pharmacother. 1997; 31(4):445–456

[37] Ostlere LS, Taylor CR, Harris DW, Rustin MH, Wright S, Johnson M. Skin surface lipids in HIV-positive patients with and without seborrheic dermatitis. Int J Dermatol. 1996; 35(4):276–279

[38] Piérard-Franchimont C, Piérard GE, Arrese JE, De Doncker P. Effect of ketoconazole 1% and 2% shampoos on severe dandruff and seborrhoeic dermatitis: clinical, squamometric and mycological assessments. Dermatology. 2001; 202(2):171–176

[39] Johnson BA, Nunley JR. Treatment of seborrheic dermatitis. Am Fam Physician. 2000; 61(9):2703–2710, 2713–2714

[40] Scaparro E, Quadri G, Virno G, Orifici C, Milani M. Evaluation of the efficacy and tolerability of oral terbinafine (Daskil) in patients with seborrhoeic dermatitis. A multicentre, randomized, investigator-blinded, placebo-controlled trial. Br J Dermatol. 2001; 144(4):854–857

[41] Fregert S, Tegner E, Thelin I. Contact allergy to lidocaine. Contact Dermat. 1979; 5(3):185–188

[42] Hardwick N, King CM. Contact allergy to lignocaine with cross-reaction to bupivacaine. Contact Dermat. 1994; 30(4):245–246

[43] Rosen T, Fordice DB. Cashew nut dermatitis. South Med J. 1994; 87 (4):543–546

[44] Adams BB, Sheth PB. Perianal ulcerations from topical steroid use. Cutis. 2002; 69(1):67–68

[45] Wilkinson SM. Hypersensitivity to topical corticosteroids. Clin Exp Dermatol. 1994; 19(1):1–11

[46] Medansky RS, Bressinck R, Cole GW, Deeken JH, Ellis CN, Guin JD, Herndon JH, Lasser AE, Leibsohn E, Menter MA, et al. Mometasone furoate ointment and cream 0.1 percent in treatment of psoriasis: comparison with ointment and cream formulations of fluocinolone acetonide 0.025 percent and triamcinolone acetonide 0.1 percent. Cutis. 1988; 42(5):480–485

[47] Kilaimy M. Lichen planus subtropicus. Arch Dermatol. 1976; 112(9):1251–1253

[48] Oliver GF, Winkelmann RK. Treatment of lichen planus. Drugs. 1993; 45 (1):56–65

[49] Rowell NR, Goodfield JMD. The connective tissue diseases. In: Champion RH, Burton JL, Ebling FJG, eds. Textbook of Dermatology. Oxford: Blackwell Scientific; 1992:2269–2275

[50] Jorizzo JL. The itchy patient. A practical approach. Prim Care. 1983; 10(3):339–353

[51] Goligher JC. Pruritus ani. In: Surgery of the Anus, Rectum, and Colon. 4th ed. Springfield, IL.: Charles C Thomas; 1980

[52] Rambukkana A. How does Mycobacterium leprae target the peripheral nervous system? Trends Microbiol. 2000; 8(1):23–28

[53] Grosset JH, Cole ST. Genomics and the chemotherapy of leprosy. Lepr Rev. 2001; 72(4):429–440

[54] Stanley SL, Jr. Amoebiasis. Lancet. 2003; 361(9362):1025–1034

[55] Khubnani H, Sivarajan K, Khubnani AH. Application of lactophenol cotton blue for identification and preservation of intestinal parasites in faecal wet mounts. Indian J Pathol Microbiol. 1998; 41(2):157–162

[56] Alvarado-Cerna R, Bracho-Riquelme R. Perianal actinomycosis–a complication of a fistula-in-ano. Report of a case. Dis Colon Rectum. 1994; 37(4):378–380

[57] Posnik MR, Potesman I, Abrahamson J. Primary perianal actinomycosis. Eur J Surg. 1996; 162(2):153–154

[58] Schwartz RA. Acanthosis nigricans. J Am Acad Dermatol. 1994; 31(1):1–19, quiz 20–22

[59] Stuart CA, Driscoll MS, Lundquist KF, Gilkison CR, Shaheb S, Smith MM. Acanthosis nigricans. J Basic Clin Physiol Pharmacol. 1998; 9(2–4):407–418

[60] Muñoz-Pérez MA, Camacho F. Acanthosis nigricans: a new cutaneous sign in severe atopic dermatitis and Down syndrome. J Eur Acad Dermatol Venereol. 2001; 15(4):325–327

[61] Blobstein SH. Topical therapy with tretinoin and ammonium lactate for acanthosis nigricans associated with obesity. Cutis. 2003; 71(1):33–34

[62] Kossard S, Rosen R. Cutaneous Bowen's disease. An analysis of 1001 cases according to age, sex, and site. J Am Acad Dermatol. 1992; 27(3):406–410

[63] Antoniuk PM, Tjandra JJ, Webb BW, Petras RE, Milsom JW, Fazio VW. Anorectal malignant melanoma has a poor prognosis. Int J Colorectal Dis. 1993; 8 (2):81–86

[64] Cagir B, Whiteford MH, Topham A, Rakinic J, Fry RD. Changing epidemiology of anorectal melanoma. Dis Colon Rectum. 1999; 42(9):1203–1208

[65] Bullard KM, Tuttle TM, Rothenberger DA, et al. Surgical therapy for anorectal melanoma. J Am Coll Surg. 2003; 196(2):206–211

[66] Helwig EB, Graham JH. Anogenital (extramammary) Paget's disease. A clinicopathological study. Cancer. 1963; 16:387–403

[67] Grow JR, Kshirsagar V, Tolentino M, Gramling J, Schutte AG. Extramammary perianal Paget's disease: report of a case. Dis Colon Rectum. 1977; 20 (5):436–442

[68] Jensen SL, Sjølin KE, Shokouh-Amiri MH, Hagen K, Harling H. Paget's disease of the anal margin. Br J Surg. 1988; 75(11):1089–1092

[69] McCarter MD, Quan SHQ, Busam K, Paty PP, Wong D, Guillem JG. Long-term outcome of perianal Paget's disease. Dis Colon Rectum. 2003; 46 (5):612–616

[70] Hassan I, Horgan AF, Nivatvongs S. V-Y island flaps for repair of large perianal defects. Am J Surg. 2001; 181(4):363–365

[71] Lam DT, Batista O, Weiss EG, Nogueras JJ, Wexner SD. Staged excision and split-thickness skin graft for circumferential perianal Paget's disease. Dis Colon Rectum. 2001; 44(6):868–870

12 Condyloma Acuminatum

David E. Beck

Abstract

Condyloma acuminatum is a common sexually transmitted disease managed by colorectal surgeons that results from a human papillomavirus infection. This chapter discusses clinical features, diagnosis, treatment, and follow-up of condyloma acuminatum.

Keywords: condyloma acuminatum, human papillomavirus, sexually transmitted diseases, treatment, diagnosis, pathology, cryotherapy, laser therapy, surgical excision, electrocoagulation

12.1 Introduction

There are many sexually transmitted diseases that colorectal surgeon must manage. Common among these is human papillomavirus (HPV) infection, which results in condyloma acuminatum. Condyloma acuminatum is rarely a serious medical problem, but frequently causes emotional distress to patient and physician because of its marked tendency to recur.

12.2 Clinical Features

The causative agent in condyloma acuminatum is a papillomavirus that is autoinoculable, filterable, and transmissible.[1] Multiple types of HPV have been identified, and at least 40 can cause genital infections.[2,3] Certain types of HPV, HPV-6 and HPV-11, are found in benign genital warts.[4,5,6] Syrjänen et al,[7] using a sophisticated in situ hybridization method, detected HPV agents in 76% of patients with condyloma acuminatum. Furthermore, HPV-16 and HPV-18 behave more aggressively and are more frequently associated with dysplasia and malignant transformation. Handley et al[8] detected HPV deoxyribonucleic acid (DNA) (either 6 or 11, 16 or 18, or 31 or 33 or 35) in 53.3% of anogenital warts. The incubation period for this virus is anywhere from 1 to 6 months but may be longer.[9]

The prevalence of condylomata acuminata in the anorectal and urogenital regions points toward a sexual mode of transmission. However, transmission at birth and by close contact with infected individuals has been described.[10] These warts occur with greatest frequency in male homosexual patients but also may be seen in heterosexual men, women, and even children (▶ Fig. 12.1).[10,11] Swerdlow and Salvati[12] reported that 46% of their male patients with condylomata acuminata were homosexual.

A study by Carr and William[13] in a population of homosexual men in New York City revealed anal warts to be more frequent among men who practiced anal-receptive intercourse. Of the patients studied, 72% had internal warts during the course of their illness. Anal warts were several times more common than penile warts in homosexual men. A possible explanation for this discrepancy may be that the moist, warm, perirectal area is more conducive to the growth of warts than the drier, cool penile epidermis. Anal intercourse may introduce the virus into the anal region, and concurrent local trauma may impair local defenses. In a study of 58 patients with anogenital warts, Handley et al[8] found that 37% of men and 25% of women also had warts in the anal canal.

Condylomata acuminata occur more often in immunosuppressed patients than in nonimmunosuppressed patients. Following renal transplantation, the incidence has been reported to be 2.4 to 4%.[14] In this clinical situation, treatment becomes especially difficult. Breese et al[15] found a strong relationship between the occurrence of anal HPV infections and HIV-associated immunosuppression. Overall, 61% of HIV-positive and 17% of HIV-negative men had anal HPV detected. HPV types 16/18 accounted for more than 50% of infections. Among HIV-positive men, HPV prevalence increased with declining CD4 cell counts: 33% with counts > 750, 56% with counts from 200 to 750, and 86% with counts < 200. HPV infection was also associated with younger age and increasing numbers of lifetime sexual partners for all men.

Condyloma acuminatum continues to be a significant health problem, with 1 million new cases seen yearly.[16] Most sexually active persons will have detectable HPV at least once in their lifetime.[17] Condyloma acuminatum may be the third most common sexually transmitted disease in the United States after gonorrhea and nongonococcal urethritis. It is the most commonly diagnosed sexually transmitted viral disease in the United States.[18] It has been estimated that 1% of sexually active adults in the United States have visible genital warts[19]; however, numerous studies predict an incidence of general HPV infection in women ranging from 15 to 50% as determined by HPV DNA detection.[20,21,22] The highest frequencies of HPV and genital warts have consistently been observed in young adults aged 18 to 28 years old, particularly young females.[19,23,24,25] In the past few decades, the incidence of genital warts appears to have increased, based on studies showing

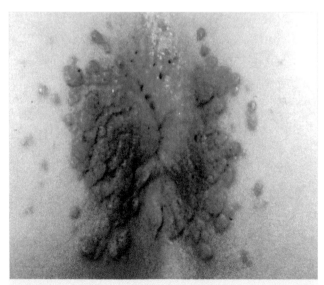

Fig. 12.1 Condylomata acuminata in a child.

an approximately eightfold increase in the incidence of genital warts from the 1950s to the 1970s and a similar fold increase again from the 1970s to the 1990s.[23,26]

12.2.1 Location

Anatomic locations in which condylomata acuminata are found include the perianal region and anal canal, as well as other parts of the perineum, vulva, vagina, and penis. Treatment of perianal condylomata acuminata without treatment of concomitant anal canal condylomata acuminata is doomed to failure. More than three-fourths of the group of patients studied by Schlappner and Shaffer[27] were found to have internal condylomata acuminata. Thus, failure of the examiner to study the anorectum with an anoscope could have resulted in the failure to diagnose intra-anal lesions in 94% of the patients. Carr and William[13] also found a high percentage of internal warts in men with external warts. In a group of immunocompromised patients, de la Fuente et al[28] found that condylomata were limited to the anoderm in 27%, located in the anal canal in 20%, and located in both the anoderm and anal canal in 53%. In men, anal canal condylomata acuminata are frequently associated with penile condylomata; in women, associated condylomata may be found in the vagina, vulva, urethra, and cervix.

12.2.2 Pathology

Condylomata acuminata vary from pinhead-size lesions to projecting cauliflowerlike masses. Their surface is papilliform, and they are pink or white in color (▶ Fig. 12.2a). Individual warts, which may be sessile or pedunculated, have a tendency to grow in radial rows that may become confluent and form almost an entire sheet, around the anal orifice (▶ Fig. 12.2b). They are almost invariably multiple and may be so numerous as to obscure the anal aperture. In addition, these warts frequently extend into the anal canal and even the rectum. Vulvar warts can grow so luxuriantly as to conceal the introitus. Because of the moisture and warmth in the anal region, the warts may become sodden and white. They may produce an irritating discharge with a disagreeable odor. Anal warts are often soft and friable and therefore may bleed.

Microscopically, anal warts show marked acanthosis of the epidermis with hyperplasia of prickle cells, parakeratosis, and an underlying chronic inflammatory cell infiltration. Vacuolation of the cells of the upper prickle layer is present (▶ Fig. 12.3).[29]

12.2.3 Symptoms

Patients with condyloma acuminatum present with relatively minor complaints. Almost all note visible perianal warts. Two-thirds of the patients experience pruritus ani, which may be caused by the irritation of the warts themselves or the patient's inability to cleanse the anal area properly after defecation. Approximately one-half of the patients experience some bleeding with defecation because of the friability of some of these warts. Other patients complain of anal wetness. A majority of patients with condyloma acuminatum experience discomfort or pain. Female patients may present with a vaginal discharge.

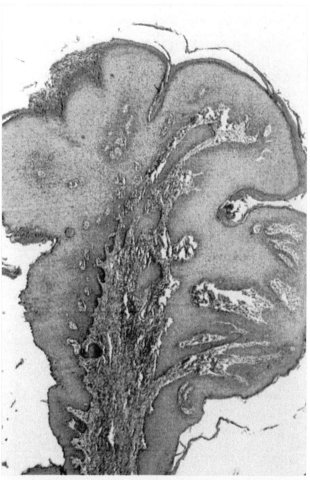

Fig. 12.3 Microscopic features of condylomata acuminata. (The image is provided courtesy of H. Srolovitz, MD.)

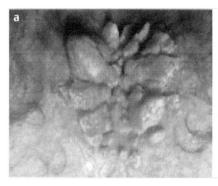
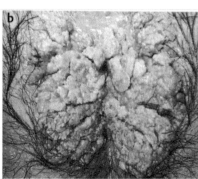

Fig. 12.2 Condylomata acuminata in an adult. **(a)** Scattered condylomata. **(b)** A large crop of condylomata encircling the anus.

12.3 Diagnosis

In most cases, the clinical appearance of the lesions makes the diagnosis obvious. However, prior treatment with podophyllin may alter the gross morphology of the lesions, and this may adversely affect correct diagnosis. The application of 5% acetic acid may reveal subclinical evidence of HPV infection by the demonstration of acetowhite epithelium.[30] It should be stressed that all sexual contacts of the patient should be examined for the presence of warts.

Because of the free association of numerous diseases with the frequent occurrence of condylomata acuminata, other sexually transmitted diseases must be excluded. In addition to the history and physical examination, proctosigmoidoscopy, stool cultures for bacterial pathogens, stool studies for ova and parasites, blood for syphilis serology, and pharyngeal, rectal, and urethral smears for gonococci should be considered. Hillman et al[31] detected HPV DNA in 96.6% of 116 wart specimens and 22.4% of the men had urethral infection with HPV.

Included in the differential diagnosis are condylomata lata, the lesions of secondary syphilis. However, these are usually fewer in number, smoother, flatter, whiter, and usually more moist than those of condylomata acuminata. It must be remembered that the two lesions may occur concomitantly. A definitive diagnosis is made by the dark-field examination, which will demonstrate the spirochetes. Another condition that may require differentiation is the squamous cell carcinoma of the anus, but this is more indurated. A biopsy will establish this diagnosis. A biopsy of condylomata is reasonable, especially in immunosuppressed patients, if the diagnosis is uncertain, the lesions do not respond to standard therapy, or the disease worsens during therapy.

12.4 Treatment

The presence of condyloma acuminatum mandates treatment. The clinical significance of untreated anogenital HPV includes: (1) the transmission of disease to sexual partners, (2) the transmission of viruses to neonates by infected mothers, and (3) the risk of developing invasive squamous cell carcinoma. Many methods of treating condyloma acuminatum have been employed (Box 12.1 and ▸ Table 12.1).[32,33,34,35,36,37,38,39,40,41,42,43,44,45,46] The topical application of caustic agents such as podophyllin or bichloroacetic or trichloroacetic acid has been the therapeutic modality of choice for several decades, but such agents have been used with different degrees of enthusiasm. Various methods of local destruction have included surgical excision, electrodesiccation, cryotherapy, and ultrasonography. The different modes of therapy attempted, in addition to the ones itemized in Box 12.1, have been listed by Billingham and Lewis[36] and include the use of Fowler's solution, autovaccine, vaccinia, bismuth sodium triglycollamate, ammoniated mercury, chloroquine, sulfonamide cream, tetracycline ointment (3%), dinitrochlorobenzene, phenol, colchicine, idoxuridine, dimethyl sulfoxide, and bacille Calmette–Guérin vaccine. Only very rarely will condylomata acuminata regress spontaneously.

Box 12.1 Treatment of condyloma acuminatum

- Caustic agents
- Cryotherapy
  - Podophyllin
- Liquid air
  - Bichloroacetic acid
- Liquid nitrogen
  - Trichloroacetic acid
- Surgical excision
  - Nitric acid
- Antineoplastic preparations
- Imiquimod
- 5-Fluorouracil
- Fulguration
- Laser therapy
- Cidofovir
- Interferon

Table 12.1 Summary of treatment modalities for condylomata acuminata

Treatment	Advantages	Disadvantages	Results
Podophyllin	Ease of application; no anesthesia; inexpensive	Skin burns; cannot use in anal canal; multiple visits necessary; dysplasia with prolonged use; systemic toxicity	Disappointing; recurrence rate high (30–65%)
Bichloroacetic acid	Ease of application; no anesthesia; inexpensive; can be used in anal canal	Skin burn; multiple visits	25% recurrence
Imiquimod 5% cream	Self-administered; fewer office visits	Local skin reaction, mild to moderate; expensive	13% recurrence
Electrocoagulation	Single-session treatment; effective in anal canal	Anesthesia required; postoperative pain; fumes	May require repeated coagulations; 9% failure rate
Cidofovir topical 1%	Can be used with recurrent condylomata	Mild erosive dermatitis	32% cured; 60% partial regression
Cryotherapy	Single-session treatment; can be used in anal canal	Requires expensive equipment; may require anesthesia	24–37% recurrence rate
Surgical excision	Precise removal; tissue for pathologic study	Anesthesia required; postoperative pain	9–42% recurrence
Laser therapy	Effective for extensive warts; can be used during pregnancy	Requires expensive equipment; requires anesthesia	3–14% recurrence
Interferon	Treatment of recurrent disease	Therapy duration: 2–3 mo; systemic side effects; very expensive; discomfort; labor-intensive treatment	36–82% remission

12.4.1 Podophyllin

Podophyllin is a cytotoxic agent applied locally in a vehicle such as liquid paraffin or tincture of benzoin, the latter having the advantage that it adheres better to the warts. Concentrations from 5 to 50% have been used, but a 25% suspension is the one generally employed. The method of application is to paint the warts accurately, avoiding the adjacent skin because podophyllin is intensely irritating. Dusting powder is then applied to the surrounding skin. Patients are instructed to wash the treated area 6 to 8 hours after each application to prevent damage to the surrounding skin. This treatment is repeated at weekly intervals as required. Single applications are rarely effective. In some cases, treatment with podophyllin must be abandoned because of the soreness and irritation of the perianal skin.

Podophyllin has several disadvantages.[47] It is not a pure compound, and therefore batches may vary in potency. It cannot be applied to perianal or anal warts by patients themselves, so repeated visits to the office may be necessary. Local reactions may be severe and penetration into keratinized warts is poor, so only recently acquired lesions may respond to treatment. In a review, Miller[48] summarized the local side effects reported with the use of podophyllin; these included severe necrosis and scarring of the anogenital area, fistula-in-ano, and dermatitis. The application of large amounts of podophyllin may result in severe systemic toxic effects, which include the hematologic, hepatic, renal, gastrointestinal, respiratory, and central nervous systems.[49,50] Karol et al[51] have recommended the avoidance of treatment with podophyllin during pregnancy because of the possible teratogenic effect and even intrauterine death.[49] Finally, prolonged courses of treatment with podophyllin are probably undesirable since it does produce dysplasia. Moreover, treatment with podophyllin may induce temporary cell changes that are difficult to differentiate histologically from carcinoma (▶ Fig. 12.4). The effects of local application of podophyllin on condylomata are typified by the presence of enlarged, swollen cells with pale, basophillic cytoplasm, dispersed chromatin material, and large perinuclear and paranuclear vacuolation. Other changes include eosinophilic cells with pyknotic nuclei and various types of nuclear alterations. These histologic abnormalities are temporary and will reverse completely within a few weeks after discontinuation of the drug.[10]

Podophyllotoxin, one of the active compounds of podophyllin, has been found to be effective in wart clearance in 45 to 53% of cases, but wart recurrence has been observed to be as high as 91%.[52] The agent is relatively safe and can be self-administered, but the availability of other medications has hindered its use.

12.4.2 Bichloroacetic and Trichloroacetic Acid

Swerdlow and Salvati[12] proposed the caustic agent bichloroacetic acid. The technique involves cleansing and drying the perianal region with cotton and witch hazel. The caustic agent is spread on with an applicator, with care taken not to apply the chemical to adjacent skin because a burn will result. If too much acid is applied, it should be wiped off, the area should be washed with water, and sodium bicarbonate should be applied as a local antidote if necessary. The lesions that are cauterized change from pink to a frosty white color. Lesions within the anal canal are treated similarly but dabbed gently with a cotton ball before the walls of the anal canal are allowed to fall back together.

Analgesic agents are prescribed routinely, but they are necessary only when massive involvement is present. Patients are instructed to keep the perianal area clean and dry. The caustic agent is applied at intervals of 7 to 10 days to achieve maximum benefit from the treatment. The patient's sexual partners also should be treated.

Approximately 25% of the patients in Swerdlow and Salvati's[12] report had recurrences. These patients were treated with further short courses of therapy. The number of treatments needed varied according to the size and number of warts. It ranged from 1 to 13 treatments, with most patients receiving 4 or fewer.

Swerdlow and Salvati[12] noted that when patients treated with bichloroacetic acid as an office procedure were compared to patients treated with other modes of therapy, the former were more comfortable, did not develop posttreatment scars

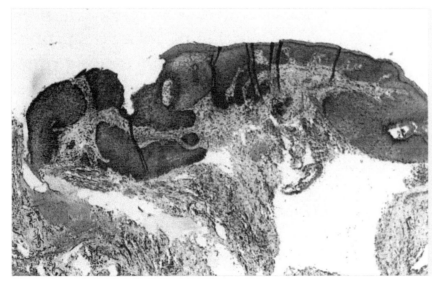

Fig. 12.4 Microscopic features of condylomata acuminata with podophyllin changes. (The image is provided courtesy of H. Srolovitz, MD.)

and strictures, and had prompt resolution of warts without losing time from work. The limited availability of bichloroacetic acid has led to use of trichloroacetic acid, which is less caustic.

12.4.3 Imiquimod

Imiquimod (Aldara; Valeant Pharmaceuticals, Bridgewater, NJ) is an imidazoquinoline, a synthetic compound, which is an immune response stimulator, enhancing both innate and acquired immune pathways (particular T helper cell type 1–mediated immune responses) resulting in antiviral, antineoplastic, and immunoregulatory activities.[53] The mechanism of action of imiquimod involves cytokine induction in the skin, which then triggers the host's immune system to recognize the presence of a viral infection or malignancy, ultimately to eradicate the associated lesion. Imiquimod, a patient-applied topical 5% cream, is clinically efficacious and safe in the management of condylomata acuminata and other warty manifestations of HPV infections. In a randomized, vehicle-controlled, clinical trial conducted in the United States, 50% of patients treated three times per week for up to 16 weeks experienced complete clearance.[54] The clinical outcome of imiquimod therapy in this condition is dependent on gender, with a superior efficacy in females compared to males. This is believed to be attributable to the higher degree of keratinization of the skin on the penis compared to the vulva, the most common locations for genital warts in male and female patients, respectively. In this study, 72% of females treated for up to 16 weeks with imiquimod cleared their warts compared to 33% of males, the majority of whom were circumcised. In a recent phase IIIB, international, open-label trial, Garland et al[55] studied 943 patients from 114 clinic sites in 20 countries with the application of imiquimod 5% cream three times per week for up to 16 weeks. Complete clinical clearance was observed in 47.8% of patients during the initial treatment period, with clearance in an additional 5.5% of patients during the extended treatment period beyond 16 weeks. The overall clearance rate for the combined treatment period was 53.3%. In a treatment failure analysis, the overall clearance rate was 65.5% (females 75.5%, and males 56.9%). Low recurrence rates of 8.8 and 23% were observed at the end of the 3- and 6-month follow-up periods, respectively. The sustained clearance rates (patients who cleared during treatment and remained clear at the end of the follow-up period) after 3 and 6 months were 41.6 and 33.3%, respectively. Local erythema occurred in 67% of patients. The lower degree of keratinization and the semiocclusive effect of the foreskin in uncircumcised males are proposed as possible reasons for the higher clearance rates (62%) observed in a study of uncircumcised males who applied imiquimod three times a week for up to 16 weeks compared to efficacy (33%) in the predominantly circumcised male population in the U.S. trial.[56]

Another study reported a 50% clearance rate (72% females, 33% males).[57] The low recurrence rate of 13% in the 3-month follow-up period after imiquimod treatment is favorable compared to the physician-administered therapies, i.e., cryotherapy, trichloroacetic acid, and podophyllin, and the patient-applied therapy podophyllotoxin.[54,58]

Recently, the FDA has approved a 3.75% cream (Zyclara; Valeant Pharmaceuticals, Bridgewater, NJ) for daily use. Safety and efficacy have not been evaluated in pregnant, breastfeeding, or immunosuppressed patients, or in patients with intravaginal,

cervical, rectal, or intra-anal warts. FDA approval was based on two randomized, double-blinded, placebo-controlled trials involving 601 adult patients with external genital warts treated with vehicle or imiquimod 3.75% cream daily for up to 8 weeks. Sixteen weeks after the start of the study period, treated patients had a clearance rate of 27 to 29%, while patients receiving the vehicle had a clearance rate of 9 to 10%.[59] Treatment-related adverse effects that occurred in > 1% of those treated with imiquimod 3.75% cream included application site pain, pruritus, irritation, erythema, bleeding, and discharge.[60]

12.4.4 Electrocoagulation

Electrocoagulation, which necessitates the use of local anesthesia, is an effective means of destroying the small lesions of condyloma acuminatum. The benefits and complications vary according to the skill of the operator, who must control the depth and width of the wound. The aim is to obtain a white coagulum that generally corresponds to a second-degree burn. Such a wound should heal without any significant scarring. However, a black eschar is likely to represent a third-degree burn, which will probably heal with scarring; if such a burn is created circumferentially, a stricture may result. When working on the vital anoderm, the operator must be alert to the potential problems of stenosis and damage to the underlying sphincter. Special care must be taken not to miss any of the warts lying in the anal canal. Extensive warts, both perianal and intra-anal, might require the use of a general anesthetic agent. Smoke produced by electrocoagulation may contain large viral particles. Therefore, smoke evacuation and special mask filtration for the surgical team has been recommended. Postoperative care follows the conventional lines described in Chapters 5 and 6.

12.4.5 Cidofovir

Coremans et at[61] studied the efficacy of the topical application of the antiviral agent cidofovir at 1%. Twenty patients treated with coagulation were compared with 27 patients treated with cidofovir. Lesions refractory to cidofovir were cleared up with additional coagulations. Cidofovir alone cured the lesions in 32% of patients and induced partial regression in 60%. However, in smokers, complete resolution of the condylomata occurred only in 16.6% compared with 66% of nonsmokers. The number of coagulation sessions was much lower in the cidofovir-treated group (1 vs. 2.9%). The relapse rate was significantly lower in the cidofovir-treated group (3.7 vs. 55%). All recurrences in the electrocoagulation group occurred within 4 months of confirmed lesion clearance. Thirty-three percent of the patients reported only mild pain caused by erosive dermatitis. In contrast, coagulations caused painful ulcerations that necessitated the use of analgesics in all patients treated this way.

12.4.6 Cryotherapy

Another destructive method used for treatment of condyloma acuminatum is cryotherapy. Various techniques have been advocated, including the use of liquid nitrogen, carbon dioxide snow, and liquefied air. Again, the depth and width of the wound must be carefully controlled. The postoperative course is similar to that of electrocoagulation. A reputed advantage is the lack of need for anesthesia, but this has not been the overall experience. O'Connor[62] reported on 936 patients treated and a total of 2,246 cryotherapy sessions. Patients were advised to take sitz baths twice daily. Secondary bacterial infection was not encountered. Recurrences developed in 226 patients, but most patients admitted to re-exposure.

12.4.7 Surgical Excision

When massive involvement is present, surgical excision can be carried out with the use of general or regional anesthesia. A simple enema given the evening before or the morning of treatment is adequate bowel preparation. This method avoids the use of cautery except for controlling bleeding points.

A solution of 1:200,000 adrenaline in saline or 0.25% Marcaine with epinephrine is injected subcutaneously and submucosally. This separates the warts and allows as much healthy skin and mucosa as possible to be preserved when the individual warts are removed with a pair of fine-toothed forceps and fine-pointed scissors. Good judgment is necessary to gauge the amount of anoderm that may be removed and yet protect the underlying sphincter mechanism. Similarly, the warts are removed from the anal mucosa. The resulting small wounds heal rapidly, but the severity of postoperative pain varies, and prolonged convalescence is common. In the majority of patients, it is possible to remove all the warts in one step, but if there are too many warts, removal may be done in two stages at an interval of approximately 1 month.

Thomson and Grace[34] reported the results in 75 patients in whom surgical excision was used. Over 75% of these patients had lesions within the anal canal. In 80%, the warts were removed in one procedure. Postoperative complications occurred in four patients: bleeding (two), hematoma (one), and previously undetected coagulation defect (one). Relatively little discomfort was experienced, but a 42% recurrence rate was noted. In the majority of patients, recurrent wart formation was detected by the end of the second postoperative month. Gollock et al,[33] in a series of 34 patients treated in the same manner, had a primary success rate of 71.4% and a recurrence rate of 9.3%. Handley et al[63] reported a 26.3% recurrence rate in 19 children so treated.

Anal stenosis is a well-known complication that may result from removal of anal and perianal warts. However, if adequate normal skin and mucosa are left between the wounds, stenosis should not occur. A potential advantage of surgical excision over electrocoagulation is that the postoperative wound weeps less, producing a smaller amount of moisture, which is believed to enhance the growth of condylomata.

12.4.8 Laser Therapy

The development of laser technology presents another possible method for decreasing the problem of persistence and recurrence of warts after treatment. Advocates of laser therapy have suggested that there is less postoperative pain and fewer recurrences with this type of therapy. Advantages of laser therapy include the fact that it is rapid and easy to use and that it does not require cleansing of the tip (as does electrical

cautery). Significant disadvantages are the fact that the instrument is very expensive, somewhat cumbersome, and requires special instruction in its use.

Ferenczy[37] reported only a 5% failure rate and a 14% recurrence rate of treating genital condylomata during pregnancy with CO_2 laser. In a review of the literature, Schaeffer[38] reported recurrence rates ranging from 3 to 13% after one to three CO_2 laser treatments of urogenital and anal condylomata acuminata, with follow-up periods ranging from 2 to 12 months. Schaeffer concluded that the CO_2 laser is the treatment of choice for condylomata acuminata that are extensive, recurrent, or present during pregnancy. A cure rate of 80% has been reported with the CO_2 laser, with up to four laser vaporizations required.[64]

In a novel study to evaluate the claims of advocates of laser therapy, Billingham and Lewis[36] undertook to compare laser therapy with conventional electrical cautery. In 38 patients with extensive warts, all warts on the right half of the anus were treated with conventional electrical cautery, while those on the left side of the anus were cauterized with the CO_2 laser; close follow-up was done. When the patients were questioned postoperatively, it was noted that the laser was associated with either more pain or the same amount of pain in comparison with electrical cautery. Recurrences were first seen more often on the laser side. Billingham and Lewis concluded that laser therapy offered no advantage and, indeed, was less effective in control of the condylomata acuminata.

Bergbrant et al[65] studied the contamination of personnel and operating theatres with HPV DNA during treatment sessions with the CO_2 laser or electrocoagulation. HPV DNA was found in 32% of specimens collected from nasolabial folds and 16% of nostril cytobrushes. The authors recommend the use of facemasks and the evacuation of air in the vicinity of the treatment field.

12.4.9 Interferon

It has been suggested that interferon may be used to treat refractory anogenital warts.[39] Schonfeld et al[40] treated 22 patients in a double-blind study of intramuscularly administered natural interferon. Patients with previously untreated condylomata acuminata received 2 million units of interferon beta or placebo for 10 consecutive days. Response to the interferon was measured by decrease in wart size; improvement with complete remission generally was not apparent until 5 to 8 weeks after treatment. Complete remission occurred in 82% of patients who received interferon but in only 18% of the placebo-treated patients, with follow-up done at 10 to 12 months. Gall et al[41] treated refractory condylomata acuminata with intramuscular and intralesional lymphoblastoid interferon. With 5 million units of interferon administered daily for 28 days and then three times a week for 2 weeks, complete responses were obtained in 69% of the patients, partial responses in approximately 25%, and no or minimal response in 6% of patients. Androphy[39] noted that if complete remission is achieved, recurrence rates are very low. The duration of therapy may need to be prolonged to 2 to 3 months. Schonfeld et al[40] reported slow response for complete remission.

Eron et al[42] conducted a randomized, double-blind trial to compare interferon alpha-2b with placebo in the treatment of condylomata acuminata. The placebo or interferon (1 million IU) was injected directly into one to three warts three times weekly for 3 weeks. Side effects of fever, chills, myalgia, headache, fatigue, and leukopenia rarely disrupted daily routines. Of 257 patients evaluated at 13 weeks, the mean of the wart area decreased 40% below initial size, whereas in the placebo group it increased 46%. All treated warts cleared completely in 36% of interferon recipients and in 17% of placebo recipients, while treated warts progressed in 13% of interferon recipients and in 50% of placebo recipients. Despite the low response rate, the authors concluded that interferon was an effective form of therapy.

Friedman-Kien et al[66] reviewed 158 patients who received injections of either interferon alpha or placebo into the base of the wart twice weekly for a maximum of 8 weeks or until all treated warts disappeared. Complete elimination of warts was achieved in 62% of patients treated with interferon alpha compared with 21% of placebo-treated patients. Approximately 25% of patients in each group had relapses. A randomized, double-blind, placebo-controlled, international multicenter trial[67] found no difference in efficacy between interferon alpha-2a and placebo treatment groups.

Fleshner and Freilich[68] conducted a prospective randomized trial with 43 patients comparing surgical excision and fulguration immediately followed by an injection of 500,000 IU (0.1 mL) of interferon alpha-n3 or saline into each quadrant of the anal canal. After a mean follow-up of 3.8 months, 12% of the patients treated with interferon and 39% of the patients treated with saline developed recurrences.

There is growing literature to support the use of interferon in combination with other therapeutic modalities.[18] In the treatment of extensive primary or recalcitrant condyloma acuminatum, interferon combined with locally destructive therapy (laser or electrocautery followed by interferon alpha [1–5 million units injected three times a week for 4–8 weeks]) results in a 50 to 80% response rate. However, the Condylomata International Collaborative Study Group found CO_2 laser ablation combined with systemic recombinant interferon alpha-2a to be ineffective for anogenital condylomata.[69] In a randomized, triple-blind, placebo-controlled trial involving 250 patients, Armstrong et al[70] failed to show any therapeutic advantage of adding interferon alpha-2a to placebo and ablative procedures.

Mayeaux et al[71] compiled information from the literature regarding the efficacy of various forms of therapy. A summary of their findings is presented in ▶ Table 12.2. Each modality of therapy has its advocates, but surprisingly few studies have been conducted comparing different methods of treatment. From the data available in the literature, it is difficult to make firm recommendations as to the optimal form of therapy.

Alam and Stiller[72] conducted a study to determine which treatment modalities for condyloma acuminatum are associated with the lowest direct medical costs in an ambulatory private practice. They constructed a cost-effectiveness model. From a literature review, extraction of commonly accepted guidelines regarding duration and frequency, as well as reports of the efficacy of typical treatment regimens; from Medicare physician fee schedules, costs of physician visits, and physician-administered treatments; and from published data and average wholesale prices of medication was performed. They found that the mean direct medical costs

Table 12.2 Comparison of therapies for condyloma acuminatum[69]

Method	Success rate %	Recurrence rate <6 mo (%)
Cryotherapy	83	28
Podophyllum resin	65	39
Trichloroacetic/ bichloroacetic acid	81	36
CO_2 laser	89	8
Electrocautery	93	24
Excision	93	24
5-Fluorouracil	71	13
Interferon alpha	52	25

per complete clearance were lowest for surgical excision ($285). Other low-cost modalities are loop electrosurgical excision procedure ($316), electrodesiccation ($347), carbon dioxide laser ($416), podofilox ($424), and pulsed-dye laser ($479). Higher cost modalities are cryotherapy ($951), trichloroacetic acid ($986), imiquimod ($1,255), podophyllum resin ($1,632), and interferon alpha-2b ($6,665).

The author uses a number of treatments depending on the extent of the patient's disease. Patients with two to three small warts will have them excised on the office. Four to eight warts are treated with trichloroacetic acid or imiquimod. More extensive warts are managed in the operating room with fulguration or excision. If the condylomata are recurrent, imiquimod is used postoperatively.

12.5 Follow-Up

Because of the frequency of recurrence, follow-up visits at 4- to 6-week intervals for at least 3 months while the patient is free of warts are recommended. Small recurrent warts can be treated easily in the office. Provided that condoms are used prophylactically, sexual activity may be resumed when the patient so desires. Without the use of condoms, sexual intercourse probably may be resumed safely after a 3-month disease-free period has elapsed.

12.5.1 Recurrence

Numerous therapeutic modalities have been used in the treatment of anal condylomata acuminata, with a failure rate ranging from 25 to 70%.[12] This recalcitrance to therapy has been associated with several factors, including repeat infection from sexual contact, localization of virus away from lymphatics, and deep or missed lesions.[73] Recurrence may also be caused by specific biologic factors, such as a long incubation period for HPV and interactions between HPV and tissue-related local immunity. Indeed, numerous reports have shown that HPV destabilizes local immunity by depleting and altering morphologic aspects of Langerhans cells.[74] In HIV-seropositive patients, the infection is further perpetuated by depletion of CD4 cells, CD16 (macrophages/natural killer) cells, and CD1a (Langerhans) cells from the HPV-infected areas, and this local phenomenon correlates well with the systemic immunosuppression characteristic of these patients.[75] These patients also may change sexual partners and acquire new infections. Therefore, their partners also should be treated in order to obtain an effective cure. The potentially long incubation period of condylomata acuminata may cause reinfection of sexual partners or delayed recurrence of a new generation of warts. Patients should be forewarned of the marked tendency of the warts to reappear.

de la Fuente et al[28] investigated risk factors and recurrence rates in immunocompromised patients requiring operation for medically intractable anal condyloma. A retrospective review was performed on 63 consecutive patients who underwent operative intervention for medically intractable anal condyloma. Patient cohorts included immunosuppressed patients (e.g., HIV-seropositive, leukemia, idiopathic lymphopenic syndrome, or transplant patients; $n = 45$) and immunocompetent patients ($n = 18$). Anal condyloma recurred in 66% of the immunosuppressed patients compared with 27% of the immunocompetent group. Recurrence time was shorter in immunosuppressed patients than in immunocompetent patients (6.8 vs. 15 months). In the subpopulation of HIV-seropositive patients, no association was found between recurrence rates and viral loads; however, CD4 counts were significantly lower in those who had recurrence than in those who did not (226 vs. 401 cells/mL).

12.6 Special Circumstances

12.6.1 HIV-Positive Patients

Puy-Montbrun et al[76] analyzed the anorectal lesions found in 148 HIV-positive patients and found anal condylomata to be the most frequent manifestation, affecting 30% of the patients.

Beck et al[77] found that anal condylomata are common (18%) in patients who test positive for HIV, and that these patients can be expected to do well with appropriate treatment. With a follow-up of 4 to 26 months, the recurrence rate for anal condylomata was 26% after local treatment with podophyllin and 4% after fulguration and excision. In patients with symptomatic HIV infection, conservative treatment of condylomata acuminata has been advised because postoperative healing was historically poor.[78] However, with modern highly active antiretroviral therapy (HAART), responding patients have normal healing.

12.6.2 Children

Condylomata acuminata are known to occur in children, perhaps as a consequence of sexual abuse. They have been reported to be associated with the same HPV types found in adults.[79,80] However, Fairley et al[81] conducted a study of prevalence data to support hand–genital transmission of genital warts. They observed a relatively high proportion of genital warts in children that contain HPV types 1 and 4 (15% in children and 2% in adults): If hand–genital transmission does not occur, the observed difference could only be explained by an eightfold greater probability of transmission to children of types 1–4 than of types 6–11, or by an eightfold greater duration of infection with types 1 and 4. Handley et al,[82] in a study of 42 prepubertal children, suggested that the majority of children with anogenital warts do not acquire these sexually and that vertical transmission is an important means by which

young children acquire anogenital warts. Nevertheless, Gutman et al[83] believe that considerable evidence suggests that anogenital HPV disease in children that appears after infancy is usually acquired through abusive sexual contact. Derksen[84] also supports that view. Transmission may also be by fomites. HPV typing may help clarify the mode of transmission.

12.6.3 Verrucous Carcinoma

In 1948, Ackerman[85] published his classic description of a slow-growing, locally aggressive, essentially nonmetastasizing variant of a well-differentiated squamous cell carcinoma and designated it a verrucous carcinoma. Ackerman's original report described the lesion in the oral cavity, but authors subsequently have reported this histologic carcinoma in a wide variety of anatomic locations, including the perianal region and the rectum.[86,87,88]

In 1925, Buschke and Löwenstein[89] described a penile lesion that appeared cytologically benign but behaved in a malignant manner. Because of its histologic similarity to the benign condyloma acuminatum, the lesion was termed a giant condyloma acuminatum or a Buschke–Löwenstein tumor. Although no universal agreement has been reached, there is a growing consensus that this entity probably represents a verrucous carcinoma.[90,91,92,93,94] What many authors in the past have described as condyloma acuminatum with malignant transformation is now believed to be verrucous carcinoma from the onset.

Creasman et al[95] summarized the salient features of 20 cases of giant condyloma acuminatum reported in the literature. They found an average age of 43 years, a male-to-female ratio of 2.3:1.0, a recurrence rate of 65%, an overall mortality rate of 30%, an incidence of malignant transformation of 30%, and a mortality rate of 20% in the malignant group.

In a more recent review of the literature, Trombetta and Place[96] identified 51 reported cases of giant condyloma acuminatum. Giant condyloma acuminatum presents with a 2.7:1 male-to-female ratio. For patients younger than 50 years of age, this ratio was increased to 3.5:1.

The mean age at presentation is 43.9 years, 42.9 in males and 46.6 in females. The most common presenting symptoms are perianal mass (47%), pain (32%), abscess or fistula (32%), and bleeding (18%). Giant condyloma acuminatum has been linked to HPV and has distinct histologic features. Foci of invasive carcinoma are noted in 50% of the reports, "carcinoma in situ" in 8%, and no invasion in 42%.

Macroscopically, the lesion presents as an exophytic, warty, gray-white, soft-to-firm mass varying in size from 1 to 10 cm. The cauliflowerlike mass may arise in the perianal skin, anal canal, or distal rectum and is frequently indistinguishable from benign lesions. The clinical course of this growth is one of relentless progression and expansion of the neoplasm by extensive erosion and pressure necrosis of surrounding tissues with invasion of the ischioanal fossa, perirectal tissues, and even the pelvic cavity. The invasive nature of the lesion may cause multiple sinuses or fistulous tracts that may invade fascia, muscle, or rectum and may cause inflammation, infection, and hemorrhage. Extent of involvement can be precisely determined by CT examination (▶ Fig. 12.5a).[97]

Microscopically, the lesion bears a strong resemblance to condyloma acuminatum. It exhibits marked papillary proliferation of well-differentiated, maturing squamous epithelium that

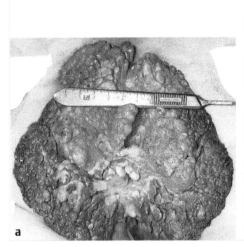
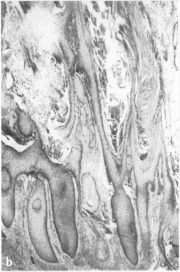

Fig. 12.5 Verrucous carcinoma. **(a)** Macroscopic features of a verrucous carcinoma. (The image is provided courtesy of Charles Orsay, MD.) **(b)** Microscopic features of a verrucous carcinoma demonstrating acanthosis, papillary fronds with rounded bottoms, lack of cytologic atypia, keratin, and lymphoplasma cell infiltrate around bulbous ends of neoplasm. (The image is provided courtesy of H. Srolovitz, MD.)

projects above the skin or mucosal surface and displays extensive surface keratinization. There is extensive acanthosis, parakeratosis, and vacuolation of the superficial layers.[96] Individual cells or groups of cells can have koilocytotic changes as found in condyloma acuminatum. Scattered dyskeratotic and/or slightly atypical squamous cells occur, but a major degree of cytologic atypia or malignancy is not present. There is no evidence of invasion of lymphatics, blood vessels, or other histopathologic criteria of malignancy. The lower borders of proliferating squamous cells are rounded and of the pushing type rather than the kind that infiltrate in narrow cellular cords. Those borders extend below the level of normal adjacent surface epithelium. A heavy inflammatory cellular infiltrate made up of lymphocytes and plasma cells lies close to and often permeates the advancing lesion (▶ Fig. 12.5b).

The extent of operation should be determined for each individual patient. Gingrass et al,[92] who described the lesion as a verrucous carcinoma, recommend wide local excision, with care taken to make certain that the depths of the excision are histologically clear. If the carcinoma involves the anal sphincter, abdominoperineal resection with extended perineal dissection should be performed. Other authors believe that radical surgical excision, which usually means abdominoperineal resection, offers the only hope of eradication of the neoplasm and permanent cure.[91] Creasman et al[95] believe that giant condyloma acuminatum represents an intermediate lesion in a pathologic continuum from condyloma acuminatum to squamous cell carcinoma. They recommend early and radical local excision; in cases of recurrence, invasion, or malignant transformation, they recommend abdominoperineal resection. In the review by Trombetta and Place,[96] treatment varied greatly from simple excision to complex courses of excisions, fecal diversions, radiation therapy, and chemotherapy. Forty-five of 52 cases underwent primary surgical excision of some kind to include simple excision, wide local excision, wide local excision with fecal diversion, and abdominoperineal resection. Of the seven patients who underwent initial nonsurgical management, two underwent primary radiation therapy, three primary topical therapy with podophyllin, one primary chemotherapy, and one primary

interferon therapy. Follow-up period was stated in 41 of 52 cases, and ranged from 3 months to 44 years. Recurrence of giant condyloma acuminatum was documented in 26 of the 52 cases. Five of the seven patients initially treated with nonsurgical therapy had documented recurrence.

The use of multimodality therapy in the treatment of verrucous carcinoma may obviate the need for radical extirpative surgery. Björck et al[98] reported on a case successfully treated with a combination of sphincter-sparing operation, radiotherapy, and adjuvant chemotherapy.

Prasad and Abcarian[9] have termed the clinical situation characterized by ulceration, infiltration, and proliferation into deeper tissues without malignant histologic change as malignant behavior of condylomata. They believed that it was significant that all of their patients with condylomata showing malignant behavior had anal fistulas and that this made the treatment quite difficult. An example of condylomata acuminata growing in a fistulous tract is seen in ▶ Fig. 12.6.

12.6.4 Condyloma Acuminatum and Squamous Cell Carcinoma

The association between anorectal HPV infection and high-grade anal dysplasia and squamous carcinoma has been well established. Carcinoma is common in males with a history of homosexual intercourse, with estimated incidences as high as 37 per 100,000.[99] The relative risk of anal malignancy among homosexuals with genital warts has been estimated to be 12.6.[100] The risk of anal carcinoma in HIV-seropositive patients is 84-fold higher than in the normal population.[101] Prospective cohort studies have shown that among HIV-seropositive patients, the most important risk factors for incidence of anal high-grade squamous intraepithelial lesions are low CD4 cell counts, persistent anal HPV infection, anal infection with multiple HPV types, and higher levels of oncogenic HPV types.[102] Malignant transformation, or at least the association of malignancy, with condylomata acuminata has been reported by several authors.[9,92,93,103,104] Prasad and Abcarian[9] reported that 1.8% of their 330 patients with anal condylomata acuminata demonstrated malignant potential.

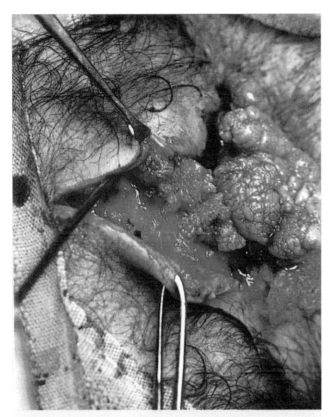

Fig. 12.6 Example of condylomata acuminata growing in a fistulous tract.

Metcalf and Dean[105] investigated the incidence of dysplasia and risk factors for premalignant and malignant changes in patients with anal condyloma acuminatum. Their study population consisted of 59 heterosexuals and 32 homosexuals or bisexuals. Two heterosexuals (3%) had invasive squamous cell carcinoma, and four (6%) had dysplasia. One homosexual or bisexual (3%) had squamous cell carcinoma in situ, and nine (28%) had dysplasia. The authors concluded that homosexual orientation, disease above the dentate line, and HIV seropositivity increase the risk of dysplasia in perianal condyloma.

The incidence of anal intraepithelial neoplasia was studied in a group of 210 homosexual and bisexual men.[106] The overall incidence was 35%. Anal intraepithelial neoplasia was found in 45% of patients with anal warts and only 7% of patients without anal warts. The relative risk of anal warts on anal intraepithelial neoplasia was 4.70. Although the natural history of anal intraepithelial neoplasia remains unknown, parallels with changes seen in the cervix suggest that, if left untreated, a percentage of patients with high-grade dysplasia will ultimately develop invasive carcinoma. The high relative risk of anal intraepithelial neoplasia in patients with condylomata acuminata is in keeping with the epidemiologic evidence linking condylomata and anal carcinoma.[100]

In the most recent report addressing this issue, de la Fuente et al[28] observed no statistical significance in the incidence of dysplasia or carcinoma between immunocompetent and immunosuppressed patients. Dysplasia was revealed in 23% of the former and 19% of the latter; carcinoma in situ in 5.8% of the former and 11.9% of the latter; and invasive carcinoma in 5.8% of the former and 7.1% of the latter.

Several studies have reported the association of HPV infection with anal carcinoma.[107] Beckmann et al[108] found HPV DNA in 35% of squamous neoplasms of the anus. Palmer et al[109] found HPV-16 DNA in 56% and HPV-18 DNA in 5% of 45 anal squamous cell carcinomas. No HPV 6 or 11 DNA was detectable. Nonmalignant anal epithelium and malignant rectal mucosa obtained from patients undergoing hemorrhoidectomy and abdominoperineal excision of the rectum did not contain any detectable HPV DNA. In direct contrast, Kirgan et al[110] found the HPV antigen in 23% of normal colon specimens, 60% of benign neoplasms, and 97% of carcinomas. They believe that HPV also affects the columnar mucosa of the colon, and that an association exists between HPV and colon neoplasia.

In 1986, Longo et al[111] reported the 14th case of squamous cell carcinoma in situ developing in perianal condylomata acuminata. Salient clinical features of the reported cases included an average age of 39 years and the fact that all patients but one were men, 10 of whom were homosexual. Symptom duration ranged from 3 weeks to 5 years, and five patients had AIDS or developed AIDS shortly after onset of symptoms. Local excision was the recommended treatment.

Operation has been the traditional modality of treatment for carcinoma that arises in condylomata acuminata.[9,91,103] Sawyers[112] reported the treatment of four patients with condylomata acuminata who had histologic evidence of squamous cell carcinoma arising in venereal warts. Those patients underwent abdominoperineal resection. Even after aggressive surgical management, local recurrence or distant spread may result in significant morbidity and mortality.

Radiation and chemotherapy also have been used, sometimes in conjunction with operation.[90] Butler et al[113] reported a case of an unresectable squamous cell carcinoma associated with condylomata acuminata rendered operable with chemotherapy (5-fluorouracil and mitomycin C) plus radiation to the primary lesion. An abdominoperineal resection was performed, and it was noted that the surgical specimen contained no residual carcinoma. This is in keeping with similar findings in patients with squamous cell carcinoma of the anal canal that is not associated with condylomata acuminata treated by combination chemoradiotherapy.[114] Therefore, it would appear that combination therapy should be the first line of treatment that is considered for squamous cell carcinoma associated with condyloma acuminatum.

References

[1] Oriel JD. Genital warts. Sex Transm Dis. 1981; 8(4) suppl:326–329

[2] Sykes NL, Jr. Condyloma acuminatum. Int J Dermatol. 1995; 34(5):297–302

[3] Kin C, Welton ML. Sexually transmitted infections. In: Steele SR, Hull TL, Read TE, Saclarides TJ, Senagore AJ, Whitlow CB, eds. The ASCRS Textbook of Colon and Rectal Surgery. 3rd ed. New York, NY: Springer; 2016:325–342

[4] Gissmann L, Schwarz E. Persistence and expression of human papillomavirus DNA in genital cancer. Ciba Found Symp. 1986; 120:190–207

[5] Parker BJ, Cossart YE, Thompson CH, Rose BR, Henderson BR. The clinical management and laboratory assessment of anal warts. Med J Aust. 1987; 147(2):59–63

[6] Labropoulou V, Balamotis A, Tosca A, Rotola A, Mavromara-Nazos P. Typing of human papillomaviruses in condylomata acuminata from Greece. J Med Virol. 1994; 42(3):259–263

[7] Syrjänen SM, von Krogh G, Syrjänen KJ. Detection of human papillomavirus DNA in anogenital condylomata in men using in situ DNA hybridisation applied to paraffin sections. Genitourin Med. 1987; 63(1):32–39

[8] Handley JM, Maw RD, Lawther H, Horner T, Bharucha H, Dinsmore WW. Human papillomavirus DNA detection in primary anogenital warts and

cervical low-grade intraepithelial neoplasias in adults by in situ hybridization. Sex Transm Dis. 1992; 19(4):225–229

[9] Prasad ML, Abcarian H. Malignant potential of perianal condyloma acuminatum. Dis Colon Rectum. 1980; 23(3):191–197

[10] Williams TS, Callen JP, Owen LG. Vulvar disorders in the prepubertal female. Pediatr Ann. 1986; 15(8):588–589, 592–601, 604–605

[11] Baruah MC, Lal S, Selvaraju M, Veliath AJ. Perianal condylomata acuminata in a male child. Br J Vener Dis. 1984; 60(1):60–61

[12] Swerdlow DB, Salvati EP. Condyloma acuminatum. Dis Colon Rectum. 1971; 14(3):226–231

[13] Carr G, William DC. Anal warts in a population of gay men in New York City. Sex Transm Dis. 1977; 4(2):56–57

[14] Landsberg K, Bear RA. Severe condylomata acuminata in a renal transplant recipient. Am J Nephrol. 1986; 6(4):325–326

[15] Breese PL, Judson FN, Penley KA, Douglas JM, Jr. Anal human papillomavirus infection among homosexual and bisexual men: prevalence of type-specific infection and association with human immunodeficiency virus. Sex Transm Dis. 1995; 22(1):7–14

[16] Greene I. Therapy for genital warts. Dermatol Clin. 1992; 10(1):253–267

[17] Hernandez BY, Wilkens LR, Zhu X, et al. Transmission of human papillomavirus in heterosexual couples. Emerg Infect Dis. 2008; 14(6):888–894

[18] Rockley PF, Tyring SK. Interferons alpha, beta and gamma therapy of anogenital human papillomavirus infections. Pharmacol Ther. 1995; 65(2):265–287

[19] Koutsky L. Epidemiology of genital human papillomavirus infection. Am J Med. 1997; 102(5A):3–8

[20] Bauer HM, Hildesheim A, Schiffman MH, et al. Determinants of genital human papillomavirus infection in low-risk women in Portland, Oregon. Sex Transm Dis. 1993; 20(5):274–278

[21] Ho GY, Bierman R, Beardsley L, Chang CJ, Burk RD. Natural history of cervicovaginal papillomavirus infection in young women. N Engl J Med. 1998; 338(7):423–428

[22] Sellors JW, Mahony JB, Kaczorowski J, et al. Survey of HPV in Ontario Women (SHOW) Group. Prevalence and predictors of human papillomavirus infection in women in Ontario, Canada. CMAJ. 2000; 163(5):503–508

[23] Chuang TY, Perry HO, Kurland LT, Ilstrup DM. Condyloma acuminatum in Rochester, Minn, 1950–1978. II. Anaplasias and unfavorable outcomes. Arch Dermatol. 1984; 120(4):476–483

[24] Persson G, Andersson K, Krantz I. Symptomatic genital papillomavirus infection in a community. Incidence and clinical picture. Acta Obstet Gynecol Scand. 1996; 75(3):287–290

[25] Simms I, Fairley CK. Epidemiology of genital warts in England and Wales: 1971 to 1994. Genitourin Med. 1997; 73(5):365–367

[26] Lyttle PH. Surveillance report: disease trends at New Zealand sexually transmitted disease clinics 1977–1993. Genitourin Med. 1994; 70(5):329–335

[27] Schlappner OLA, Shaffer EA. Anorectal condylomata acuminata: a missed part of the condyloma spectrum. Can Med Assoc J. 1978; 118(2):172–173

[28] de la Fuente SG, Ludwig KA, Mantyh CR. Preoperative immune status determines anal condyloma recurrence after surgical excision. Dis Colon Rectum. 2003; 46(3):367–373

[29] Morson BD, Dawson IMP. Gastrointestinal Pathology. Cambridge, MA: Blackwell Scientific Publications; 1972:623

[30] Sand Petersen C, Albrectsen J, Larsen J, et al. Subclinical human papilloma virus infection in condylomata acuminata patients attending a VD clinic. Acta Derm Venereol. 1991; 71(3):252–255

[31] Hillman RJ, Botcherby M, Ryait BK, Hanna N, Taylor-Robinson D. Detection of human papillomavirus DNA in the urogenital tracts of men with anogenital warts. Sex Transm Dis. 1993; 20(1):21–27

[32] Park IU, Introcaso C, Dunne EF. Human papillomavirus and genital warts: a review of the evidence for the 2015 Centers for Disease Control and Prevention sexually transmitted diseases treatment guidelines. Clin Infect Dis. 2015; 61 Suppl 8:S849–S855

[33] Gollock JM, Slatford K, Hunter JM. Scissor excision of anogenital warts. Br J Vener Dis. 1982; 58(6):400–401

[34] Thomson JPS, Grace RH. The treatment of perianal and anal condylomata acuminata: a new operative technique. J R Soc Med. 1978; 71(3):180–185

[35] Figueroa S, Gennaro AR. Intralesional bleomycin injection in treatment of condyloma acuminatum. Dis Colon Rectum. 1980; 23(8):550–551

[36] Billingham RP, Lewis FG. Laser versus electrical cautery in the treatment of condylomata acuminata of the anus. Surg Gynecol Obstet. 1982; 155(6):865–867

[37] Ferenczy A. Treating genital condyloma during pregnancy with the carbon dioxide laser. Am J Obstet Gynecol. 1984; 148(1):9–12

[38] Schaeffer AJ. Use of the CO2 laser in urology. Urol Clin North Am. 1986; 13(3):393–404

[39] Androphy EJ. Papillomaviruses and interferon. Ciba Found Symp. 1986; 120:221–234

[40] Schonfeld A, Nitke S, Schattner A, et al. Intramuscular human interferon-beta injections in treatment of condylomata acuminata. Lancet. 1984; 1(8385):1038–1042

[41] Gall SA, Hughes CE, Whisnant J, Weck P. Therapy of resistant condyloma acuminata with lymphoblastoid interferon. J Cell Biochem Suppl. 1985; 9C:91–92

[42] Eron LJ, Judson F, Tucker S, et al. Interferon therapy for condylomata acuminata. N Engl J Med. 1986; 315(17):1059–1064

[43] Krebs HB. Treatment of genital condylomata with topical 5-fluorouracil. Dermatol Clin. 1991; 9(2):333–341

[44] Handley JM, Maw RD, Horner T, Lawther H, McNeill T, Dinsmore WW. Nonspecific immunity in patients with primary anogenital warts treated with interferon alpha plus cryotherapy or cryotherapy alone. Acta Derm Venereol. 1992; 72(1):39–40

[45] Heaton CL, Lichti HF, Weiner M. The revival of nitric acid for the treatment of anogenital warts. Clin Pharmacol Ther. 1993; 54(1):107–111

[46] Damstra RJ, van Vloten WA. Cryotherapy in the treatment of condylomata acuminata: a controlled study of 64 patients. J Dermatol Surg Oncol. 1991; 17(3):273–276

[47] Oriel D. Letter to the editor. Proc R Soc Med. 1978; 71:234

[48] Miller RA. Podophyllin. Int J Dermatol. 1985; 24(8):491–498

[49] Moher LM, Maurer SA. Podophyllum toxicity: case report and literature review. J Fam Pract. 1979; 9(2):237–240

[50] Montaldi DH, Giambrone JP, Courey NG, Taefi P. Podophyllin poisoning associated with the treatment of condyloma acuminatum: a case report. Am J Obstet Gynecol. 1974; 119(8):1130–1131

[51] Karol MD, Conner CS, Watanabe AS, Murphrey KJ. Podophyllum: suspected teratogenicity from topical application. Clin Toxicol. 1980; 16(3):283–286

[52] Bonnez W, Elswick RK, Jr, Bailey-Farchione A, et al. Efficacy and safety of 0.5% podofilox solution in the treatment and suppression of anogenital warts. Am J Med. 1994; 96(5):420–425

[53] Garland SM. Imiquimod. Curr Opin Infect Dis. 2003; 16(2):85–89

[54] Edwards L, Ferenczy A, Eron L, et al. Self-administered topical 5% imiquimod cream for external anogenital warts. HPV Study Group. Human PapillomaVirus. Arch Dermatol. 1998; 134(1):25–30

[55] Garland SM, Sellors JW, Wikstrom A, et al. Imiquimod Study Group. Imiquimod 5% cream is a safe and effective self-applied treatment for anogenital warts–results of an open-label, multicentre Phase IIIB trial. Int J STD AIDS. 2001; 12(11):722–729

[56] Gollnick H, Barasso R, Jappe U, et al. Safety and efficacy of imiquimod 5% cream in the treatment of penile genital warts in uncircumcised men when applied three times weekly or once per day. Int J STD AIDS. 2001; 12(1):22–28

[57] Beutner KR, Wiley DJ. Recurrent external genital warts: a literature review. Papillomavirus Rep. 1997; 8:69–74

[58] Sauder DN, Skinner RB, Fox TL, Owens ML. Topical imiquimod 5% cream as an effective treatment for external genital and perianal warts in different patient populations. Sex Transm Dis. 2003; 30(2):124–128

[59] Zyclara [package insert]. Scottsdale, AZ: Medicis, The Dermatology Company; 2012

[60] Baker DA, Ferris DG, Martens MG, et al. Imiquimod 3.75% cream applied daily to treat anogenital warts: combined results from women in two randomized, placebo-controlled studies. Infect Dis Obstet Gynecol. 2011; 2011:806105

[61] Coremans G, Margaritis V, Snoeck R, Wyndaele J, De Clercq E, Geboes K. Topical cidofovir (HPMPC) is an effective adjuvant to surgical treatment of anogenital condylomata acuminata. Dis Colon Rectum. 2003; 46(8):1103–1108, discussion 1108–1109

[62] O'Connor JJ. Perianal and anal condylomata acuminata. J Dermatol Surg Oncol. 1979; 5(4):276–277

[63] Handley JM, Maw RD, Horner T, Lawther H, Bingham EA, Dinsmore WW. Scissor excision plus electrocautery of anogenital warts in prepubertal children. Pediatr Dermatol. 1991; 8(3):243–245, 248–249

[64] Sand Petersen C, Menné T. Ano-genital warts in consecutive male heterosexual patients referred to a CO2-laser clinic in Copenhagen. Acta Derm Venereol. 1993; 73(6):465–466

[65] Bergbrant IM, Samuelsson L, Olofsson S, Jonassen F, Ricksten A. Polymerase chain reaction for monitoring human papillomavirus contamination

of medical personnel during treatment of genital warts with CO2 laser and electrocoagulation. Acta Derm Venereol. 1994; 74(5):393–395

[66] Friedman-Kien AE, Eron LJ, Conant M, et al. Natural interferon alfa for treatment of condylomata acuminata. JAMA. 1988; 259(4):533–538

[67] Condylomata International Collaborative Study Group. Recurrent condylomata acuminata treated with recombinant interferon alpha-2a. A multicenter double-blind placebo-controlled clinical trial. Acta Derm Venereol. 1993; 73(3):223–226

[68] Fleshner PR, Freilich MI. Adjuvant interferon for anal condyloma. A prospective, randomized trial. Dis Colon Rectum. 1994; 37(12):1255–1259

[69] The Condylomata International Collaborative Study Group. Randomized placebo-controlled double-blind combined therapy with laser surgery and systemic interferon-alpha 2a in the treatment of anogenital condylomata acuminatum. J Infect Dis. 1993; 167(4):824–829

[70] Armstrong DKB, Maw RD, Dinsmore WW, et al. Combined therapy trial with interferon alpha-2a and ablative therapy in the treatment of anogenital warts. Genitourin Med. 1996; 72(2):103–107

[71] Mayeaux EJ, Jr, Harper MB, Barksdale W, Pope JB. Noncervical human papillomavirus genital infections. Am Fam Physician. 1995; 52(4):1137–1146, 1149–1150

[72] Alam M, Stiller M. Direct medical costs for surgical and medical treatment of condylomata acuminata. Arch Dermatol. 2001; 137(3):337–341

[73] Congilosi SM, Madoff RD. Current therapy for recurrent and extensive anal warts. Dis Colon Rectum. 1995; 38(10):1101–1107

[74] Viac J, Chardonnet Y, Euvrard S, Chignol MC, Thivolet J. Langerhans cells, inflammation markers and human papillomavirus infections in benign and malignant epithelial tumors from transplant recipients. J Dermatol. 1992; 19(2):67–77

[75] Arany I, Tyring SK. Systemic immunosuppression by HIV infection influences HPV transcription and thus local immune responses in condyloma acuminatum. Int J STD AIDS. 1998; 9:268–271

[76] Puy-Montbrun T, Denis J, Ganansia R, Mathoniere F, Lemarchand N, Arnous-Dubois N. Anorectal lesions in human immunodeficiency virus-infected patients. Int J Colorectal Dis. 1992; 7(1):26–30

[77] Beck DE, Jaso RG, Zajac RA. Surgical management of anal condylomata in the HIV-positive patient. Dis Colon Rectum. 1990; 33(3):180–183

[78] Scholefield JH, Northover JMA, Carr ND. Male homosexuality, HIV infection and colorectal surgery. Br J Surg. 1990; 77(5):493–496

[79] Yun K, Joblin L. Presence of human papillomavirus DNA in condylomata acuminata in children and adolescents. Pathology. 1993; 25(1):1–3

[80] Obalek S, Misiewicz J, Jablonska S, Favre M, Orth G. Childhood condyloma acuminatum: association with genital and cutaneous human papillomaviruses. Pediatr Dermatol. 1993; 10(2):101–106

[81] Fairley CK, Gay WJ, Forbes A, Abramson M, Garland SM. Hand–genital transmission of genital warts? An analysis of prevalence data. Epidemiol Infect. 1995; 115:169–176

[82] Handley J, Dinsmore W, Maw R, et al. Anogenital warts in prepubertal children; sexual abuse or not? Int J STD AIDS. 1993; 4(5):271–279

[83] Gutman LT, Herman-Giddens ME, Phelps WC. Transmission of human genital papillomavirus disease: comparison of data from adults and children. Pediatrics. 1993; 91(1):31–38

[84] Derksen DJ. Children with condylomata acuminata. J Fam Pract. 1992; 34(4):419–423

[85] Ackerman LV. Verrucous carcinoma of the oral cavity. Surgery. 1948; 23(4):670–678

[86] Grassegger A, Höpfl R, Hussl H, Wicke K, Fritsch P. Buschke-Loewenstein tumour infiltrating pelvic organs. Br J Dermatol. 1994; 130(2):221–225

[87] Goodman P, Halpert RD. Invasive squamous cell carcinoma of the anus arising in condyloma acuminatum: CT demonstration. Gastrointest Radiol. 1991; 16(3):267–270

[88] Kibrité A, Zeitouni NC, Cloutier R. Aggressive giant condyloma acuminatum associated with oncogenic human papilloma virus: a case report. Can J Surg. 1997; 40(2):143–145

[89] Buschke A, Löwenstein L. Uber Carcinomahnliche Condylomata Acuminata des Penis. Klin Wochenschr. 1925; 4:1726–1728

[90] Headington JT. Verrucous carcinoma. Cutis. 1978; 21(2):207–211

[91] Elliot MS, Werner ID, Immelman EJ, Harrison AC. Giant condyloma (Buschke–Loewenstein tumor) of the anorectum. Dis Colon Rectum. 1979; 22(7):497–500

[92] Gingrass PJ, Bubrick MP, Hitchcock CR, Strom RL. Anorectal verrucose squamous carcinoma: report of two cases. Dis Colon Rectum. 1978; 21(2):120–122

[93] Lee SH, McGregor DH, Kuziez MN. Malignant transformation of perianal condyloma acuminatum: a case report with review of the literature. Dis Colon Rectum. 1981; 24(6):462–467

[94] Prioleau PG, Santa Cruz DJ, Meyer JS, Bauer WC. Verrucous carcinoma: a light and electron microscopic, autoradiographic, and immunofluorescence study. Cancer. 1980; 45(11):2849–2857

[95] Creasman C, Haas PA, Fox TA, Jr, Balazs M. Malignant transformation of anorectal giant condyloma acuminatum (Buschke-Loewenstein tumor). Dis Colon Rectum. 1989; 32(6):481–487

[96] Trombetta LJ, Place RJ. Giant condyloma acuminatum of the anorectum: trends in epidemiology and management: report of a case and review of the literature. Dis Colon Rectum. 2001; 44(12):1878–1886

[97] Balthazar EJ, Streiter M, Megibow AJ. Anorectal giant condyloma acuminatum (Buschke-Loewenstein tumor): CT and radiographic manifestations. Radiology. 1984; 150(3):651–653

[98] Björck M, Athlin L, Lundskog B. Giant condyloma acuminatum (Buschke-Loewenstein tumour) of the anorectum with malignant transformation. Eur J Surg. 1995; 161(9):691–694

[99] Daling JR, Weiss NS, Klopfenstein LL, Cochran LE, Chow WH, Daifuku R. Correlates of homosexual behavior and the incidence of anal cancer. JAMA. 1982; 247(14):1988–1990

[100] Holly EA, Whittemore AS, Aston DA, Ahn DK, Nickoloff BJ, Kristiansen JJ. Anal cancer incidence: genital warts, anal fissure or fistula, hemorrhoids, and smoking. J Natl Cancer Inst. 1989; 81(22):1726–1731

[101] Melbye M, Coté TR, Kessler L, Gail M, Biggar RJ, The AIDS/Cancer Working Group. High incidence of anal cancer among AIDS patients. Lancet. 1994; 343(8898):636–639

[102] Palefsky JM, Holly EA, Ralston ML, Jay N, Berry JM, Darragh TM. High incidence of anal high-grade squamous intra-epithelial lesions among HIV-positive and HIV-negative homosexual and bisexual men. AIDS. 1998; 12(5):495–503

[103] Ejeckam GC, Idikio HA, Nayak V, Gardiner JP. Malignant transformation in an anal condyloma acuminatum. Can J Surg. 1983; 26(2):170–173

[104] Smedley F, Taube M, Ruston M. Malignant change in perianal condylomata acuminata. J R Coll Surg Edinb. 1988; 33(5):282

[105] Metcalf AM, Dean T. Risk of dysplasia in anal condyloma. Surgery. 1995; 118(4):724–726

[106] Carter PS, de Ruiter A, Whatrup C, et al. Human immunodeficiency virus infection and genital warts as risk factors for anal intraepithelial neoplasia in homosexual men. Br J Surg. 1995; 82(4):473–474

[107] Bradshaw BR, Nuovo GJ, DiCostanzo D, Cohen SR. Human papillomavirus type 16 in a homosexual man. Association with perianal carcinoma in situ and condyloma acuminatum. Arch Dermatol. 1992; 128(7):949–952

[108] Beckmann AM, Daling JR, Sherman KJ, et al. Human papillomavirus infection and anal cancer. Int J Cancer. 1989; 43(6):1042–1049

[109] Palmer JG, Scholefield JH, Coates PJ, et al. Anal cancer and human papillomaviruses. Dis Colon Rectum. 1989; 32(12):1016–1022

[110] Kirgan D, Manalo P, Hall M, McGregor B. Association of human papillomavirus and colon neoplasms. Arch Surg. 1990; 125(7):862–865

[111] Longo WE, Ballantyne GH, Gerald WL, Modlin IM. Squamous cell carcinoma in situ in condyloma acuminatum. Dis Colon Rectum. 1986; 29(8):503–506

[112] Sawyers JL. Squamous cell cancer of the perianus and anus. Surg Clin North Am. 1972; 52(4):935–941

[113] Butler TW, Gefter J, Kleto D, Shuck EH, III, Ruffner BW. Squamous-cell carcinoma of the anus in condyloma acuminatum. Successful treatment with preoperative chemotherapy and radiation. Dis Colon Rectum. 1987; 30(4):293–295

[114] Nigro ND. An evaluation of combined therapy for squamous cell cancer of the anal canal. Dis Colon Rectum. 1984; 27(12):763–766

13 Other Sexually Transmitted Illnesses

David E. Beck

Abstract

Sexually transmitted diseases are likely to be encountered by colorectal surgeons who must maintain a high level of suspicion to avoid delays or errors in diagnosis. A frank discussion of sexual history helps direct testing and therapy.

Keywords: sexually transmitted infections, screening, evaluation, genital lesions, perianal lesions, proctitis, enteritis, bacterial infection, viral infection, parasitic infection

13.1 Introduction

"Sexually transmitted diseases" and "sexually transmitted infections" (STIs) are interchangeably used terms, but the latter has been increasingly adopted to emphasize that infections may not cause symptoms or develop into diseases.[1] STIs are likely to be encountered by colorectal surgeons who must maintain a high level of suspicion to avoid delays or errors in diagnosis. A frank discussion of sexual history helps direct testing and therapy.

13.2 Screening Guidelines

Risk factors for STIs are high-risk sexual behavior, concurrent infection with STIs, and human immunodeficiency virus (HIV) seropositivity. Men who have sex with men (MSM), especially those who participate in unprotected anoreceptive intercourse, are at great risk and should undergo regular universal testing. Others at high risk are those in high-risk sexual networks (e.g., swingers and prostitutes). Testing at multiple anatomic sites (anorectal, oropharyngeal, and urogenital) found that over 10% of MSM had chlamydia and 6% had gonorrhea, while 7% of female prostitutes and swingers had chlamydia and 3% had gonorrhea.[2] A universal testing policy would help reduce the prevalence of STIs in these networks.[3]

13.3 Evaluation of Symptomatic Patients

Symptoms of STIs may include painless or painful perianal or genital lesions, rectal, vaginal, or urethral discharge, proctitis, proctocolitis, or enteritis. A summary of suspected etiologies, testing, and empiric therapy by symptom class is provided in ▶ Table 13.1 and ▶ Table 13.2.

13.3.1 Perianal or Genital Lesions

Anal and perianal lesions may be mistaken for other conditions such as fissures, hemorrhoids, fistulas, abscesses, hidradenitis, or pruritus ani, delaying appropriate therapy. Thus, inspection, digital exam, and anoscopy are indicated in any patient who can tolerate it.

In young sexually active patients, herpes and syphilis are the most common lesions followed by chancroid and donovanosis. Patients should undergo serologic testing for syphilis and herpes simplex virus (HSV) culture or polymerase chain reaction (PCR), as well as HIV testing. Empiric treatment of the most likely pathogen should be started. Genital lesions of molluscum contagiosum may cause pruritus.

13.3.2 Proctitis

Proctitis produces anorectal pain, tenesmus, and discharge. Etiologic agents include *Neisseria gonorrhoeae*, *Chlamydia trachomatis*, *Treponema pallidum*, and HSV. Intra-anal swabs should be performed prior to a rectal exam using bacteriostatic lubricant. A proctoscopic exam along with a clear sexual history helps distinguish between inflammatory bowel disease and anorectal cancer.

13.3.3 Proctocolitis

Symptoms include those of proctitis as well as diarrhea and abdominal cramps. Lower endoscopy reveals inflammation of the rectal and distal colonic mucosa. Stool studies reveal fecal leukocytes. Transmission is felt to be oral or oral-anal, and etiologic agents include *Campylobacter*, *Shigella*, *Entamoeba histolytica*, and lymphogranuloma venereum serovars on *C. trachomatis*.

13.3.4 Enteritis

Symptoms include diarrhea and abdominal cramps. Transmission is via oral-anal route and the most common etiology is *Giardia lamblia*.

13.4 Diagnosis and Management

13.4.1 Bacterial

Neisseria Gonorrhoeae

Gonorrhea is the second most commonly reported infectious disease in the United States. In 2014, 350,062 cases of gonorrhea were reported in the United States.[4] The true incidence is likely higher due to underreporting and underdiagnosis, as many patients are asymptomatic.

In males, the urethra is the most common site of infection with dysuria and a creamy yellow urethral discharge. Women experience an erythematous cervix and vaginal discharge and pelvic inflammatory disease. Proctitis is more common in those who engage in anal receptive intercourse.

Diagnosis is best made with a nucleic acid amplification test (NAAT) due to its high sensitivity and specificity.[5] First-catch urine or urethral swabs in men and vaginal or endocervical swabs in women are recommended. Rectal and oropharyngeal specimens can also be tested with NAATs. Identification of gram-positive diplococci in the discharge is highly suggestive.[6,7]

Table 13.1 Sexually transmitted and infectious organisms that cause anorectal pathology

Organism	Symptoms	Anoscopy and proctoscopy	Laboratory test	Treatment
Bacterial				
Gonorrhea (*Neisseria gonorrhea*)	Rectal discharge	Proctitis, mucopurulent discharge	NAAT, Thayer-Martin culture of discharge	Ceftriaxone 250 mg IM for 1 day and azithromycin 1 g orally or doxycycline 100 mg orally twice a day for 7 days
Chlamydia and lymphogranuloma venereum (LGV)	Tenesmus	Friable, often ulcerated rectal mucosa with or without rectal mass	NAAT, serologic antibody titer, biopsy for culture	Azithromycin 1 g orally or doxycycline 100 mg orally twice a day for 7 days
Campylobacter jejuni	Diarrhea, cramps, bloating	Erythema, edema, grayish-white ulcerations of rectal mucosa	Culture stool using selective media	Erythromycin 500 mg orally four times a day for 7 days
Shigella	Abdominal cramps, fever, tenesmus, bloody diarrhea	Erythema, edema, grayish-white ulcerations of rectal mucosa	Stool culture	Ciprofloxacin 500 mg orally twice a day for 7 days
Chancroid (*Haemophilus ducreyi*)	Anal pain	Anorectal abscesses and ulcers	Culture	Azithromycin 1 g orally or ceftriaxone 250 mg IM for 1 day
Donovanosis (*Klebsiella granulomatis*)	Perianal mass	Hard, shiny perianal masses	Biopsy of mass	Trimethoprim-sulfamethoxazole orally twice a day for 7 days and azithromycin 1 g orally for 21 days
Syphilis	Rectal pain	Painful anal ulcer	Dark-field exam of fresh scrapings, serologic tests	Benzathine penicillin 2.4 million units IM
Viral				
Herpes simplex	Anorectal pain, pruritus	Perianal erythema, vesicles, ulcers, diffusely inflamed, friable rectal mucosa	Cytologic exam of scrapings or viral culture of vesicular fluid	Acyclovir 200 mg five times daily for 5 days
Hepatitis	Generalized symptoms		Serologic testing, NAAT	B immune globulin, C antiviral therapy
Human papillomavirus (HPV) (condylomata acuminata)	Pruritus, bleeding, discharge, pain	Perianal warts	Excisional biopsy with viral analysis	Destruction. See Chapter 9
Molluscum contagiosum	Painless dermal lesions	Flattened round umbilicated lesions	Excisional biopsy	Excision, cryotherapy
Human immunodeficiency virus (HIV)	See text	See text	Western blot	AZT, HAART
Cytomegalovirus (CMV)	Rectal bleeding	Multiple small white ulcers	Biopsy, viral culture, antigen assay of ulcers	Intravenous ganciclovir
Isospora	Vomiting, fever, abdominal pain	Normal	Acid-fast stain of stool; endoscopic biopsy	Trimethoprim-sulfamethoxazole (double strength) orally twice a day for 7 days
Parasitic				
Amebiasis (*Entamoeba histolytica*)	Bloody diarrhea	Friable rectal mucosa; shallow ulcers with yellowish exudate and ring of erythema	Fresh stool exam (microscopy)	Metronidazole 750 mg orally three times a day for 10 days, then diiodohydroxyquinoline 650 mg orally three times a day for 20 days
Giardia lamblia	Nausea, bloating, cramps, diarrhea	Normal	Fresh stool exam (microscopy)	Metronidazole 250 mg orally three times a day for 7 days
Lice (*Phthirus pubis*)	Pruritus	Identification of lice	Observations	Permethrin 1% cream

Abbreviations: AZT, azidothymidine; HAART, highly active antiretroviral therapy; IM, intramuscular; NAAT, nucleic acid amplification test.

Culture of the discharge on modified Thayer–Martin medium allows sensitivity testing, which is helpful in treatment failures or persistent NAAT positivity.[8]

Gonococcal proctitis results from anogenital sexual exposure. Presenting symptoms include anal itching and irritation, painful defecation, a sensation of rectal fullness, discharge, and constipation. On anal examination, most patients will have erythema and edema of the crypts from which thick yellow pus may be expressed.[9] Sigmoidoscopy may help to exclude ulcerative colitis and Crohn's colitis. Complications of gonorrhea include Bartholin's gland abscess, epididymitis, pelvic inflammatory disease, pharyngitis, cutaneous abscess, and disseminated infection with chills, fever, joint pain (arthritis), and macular rash. Before the advent of antibiotics, local complications were common and included anal stricture, fistula, fissure, abscess, and rectovaginal fistula.

Treatment for proctitis is ceftriaxone, 250 mg administered intramuscularly once, plus a single dose of oral azithromycin 1 g, or a 7-day course of oral doxycycline, 100 mg twice daily for 7 days.[10] Patients allergic to cephalosporins can be treated with a single oral dose of azithromycin 2 g. Patients who have undergone treatment for gonorrhea should be referred to programs to reduce STI risk and undergo retesting for gonorrhea at 3 months. Sexual partners of infected patients in the preceding 2 months should also undergo treatment.[11] Patients with gonorrhea are at higher risk of HIV and should be tested. N. gonorrhoeae has developed resistance to penicillin, tetracycline, fluoroquinolones, and cephalosporins. Clinicians need to maintain a high suspicion for treatment failure and report those that occur.[12] As drug resistance continues to occur, clinicians who do not treat STIs on a regular basis should review current treatment recommendations when STIs are encountered (▶ Table 13.3 and ▶ Table 13.4).

Chlamydia Trachomatis

Chlamydia infection is the most commonly reported STI in the United States with 1,441,789 U.S. cases in 2014.[13] There are 15 immunotypes of C. trachomatis.[14,15] Trachoma is associated with immunotypes A, B, B-A, and C. Serovars D, E, and F are the most prevalent C. trachomatis strains worldwide.[16] Types D and K are found most often in patients with genital and anal infections. The more serious venereal lymphogranulomatosis can be linked to serotypes L1, L2, and L3. Infection with these serotypes produces a small vesicular lesion followed by enlarged inguinal lymph nodes, which progress to an indurated mass. Chronic infection may lead to lymphedema or rectal structure.

Patients with the more common serotypes of chlamydia are asymptomatic or have minimal symptoms, making screening crucial to disease control. Men with chlamydia experience

Table 13.2 Diagnostic tests for enteric STDs

Pathogen	Test
Spirochete	
Treponema pallidum	Dark-field microscopy, FTA VDRL, serology
Bacteria	
Neisseria gonorrhoeae	Gram's stain, culture
Chlamydia trachomatis	Monoclonal antibody, culture
Shigella spp.	Stool culture
Campylobacter fetus	Stool culture
Salmonella typhimurium	Stool culture, blood culture
Mycobacterium avium	Mucosal biopsy and culture, acid-fast stain of stool
Virus	
Condylomata acuminata	Clinical identification, biopsy
Herpes simplex	Biopsy, culture, monoclonal antibody
Cytomegalovirus	Biopsy, culture
Human immunodeficiency	ELISA, Western blot
Yeast	
Candida	Culture
Cryptosporidiosis	Biopsy: acid-fast stain of stool
Isospora	Biopsy: acid-fast stain of stool
Protozoa	
Entamoeba histolytica	Stool examination
Giardia lamblia	Stool examination

Abbreviations: ELISA, enzyme-linked immunosorbent assay; FTA, fluorescent treponemal antibody; VDRL, venereal disease research laboratory.

Table 13.3 Areas and populations for which fluoroquinolones (FQs) are not recommended for the treatment of gonorrhea

Areas
Asia Pacific Islands (including Hawaii)
India
Israel
Australia
United Kingdom
United States: California, Washington State, Arizona (Maricopa County), Michigan (Ingham, Clinton, Eaton, Jackson, Livingston, and Shiawassee counties)
Areas in Canada experiencing rates of FQ resistance greater than 3–5%: check with local public health officials to learn about FQ resistance in your area
Any area with rates of FQ-resistant N. gonorrhoeae greater than 3–5%
Populations
Men who have sex with men who are epidemiologically linked to the United States[3]
People with sexual contacts from the areas listed above

Note: Hence, a more up-to-date recommendation is treatment with regimens active against the most resistant gonococci. Resistance has been found to penicillin.

Table 13.4 Recommended treatment of urethral, endocervical, rectal, or pharyngeal gonorrhea in patients 9 years of age and older (except pregnant or nursing mothers)

If there is no suspected resistance to FQs and patient has no cephalosporin allergy or history of immediate or anaphylactic reactions to penicillin:

Cefixime 400 mg orally in single dose

Ceftriaxone[a] 125 mg intramuscularly in single dose

Ciprofloxacin 500 mg orally in single dose

Ofloxacin 400 mg orally in single dose

If use of FQs is not recommended:

Cefixime 400 mg orally in single dose

Ceftriaxone[a] 125 mg intramuscularly in single dose

If use of FQs is not recommended and patient has cephalosporin allergy or history of immediate or anaphylactic reactions to penicillin:

Azithromycin[b] 2 g orally in single dose

Spectinomycin[c] 2 g intramuscularly in single dose (available only through Special Access Programme)

If use of FQs is not recommended but all other treatments are not tolerated or available, FQs may be used. Treatment with FQs must be followed by a test of cure and is acceptable only for patients likely to present for follow-up testing:

Ciprofloxacin[d] 500 mg orally in single dose

Ofloxacin[d] 400 mg orally in single dose

Abbreviation: FQs, fluoroquinolones.

[a]The preferred diluent for ceftriaxone is 1% lidocaine without epinephrine (0.9 mL/250 mg, 0.45 mL/125 mg) to reduce discomfort.

[b]A 2-g dose of azithromycin is associated with a significant incidence of gastrointestinal adverse effects. Taking the tablet with food may minimize such adverse effects. Antiemetics may be needed.

[c]If spectinomycin is used, a test of cure is recommended. Spectinomycin should not be used to treat pharyngeal infections.

[d]Ciprofloxacin and ofloxacin are contraindicated in pregnant and nursing women. The safety of FQs in children has not been established. Articular damage has been observed in studies of young animals exposed to FQs, although this has not been shown to date in humans. FQs should not be used in prepubertal children. Clinical judgment should be exercised when considering FQ use in postpubertal adolescents under the age of 18.

urethritis, epididymitis, pharyngitis, or proctitis. In women, chlamydial infections present as cervicitis, urethral syndrome, endometritis, and salpingitis. Long-term complications include infertility, chronic pelvic pain, and ectopic pregnancy. Proctitis produces pain, tenesmus, fever, and an erythematous rectal mucosa, but rarely with ulcerations. Inguinal lymph nodes may be large and matted. On endoscopic examination, the rectal mucosa appears more inflamed and ulcerated with production of purulent and bloody discharge. Biopsy shows crypt abscesses and granulomas.[17] As a result of the granulomas, the diagnosis may be confused with that of Crohn's disease. If the disease is untreated, the severity extends by deeper ulcerations, rectovaginal or rectovesical fistulas, abscesses, and rectal stricture.[18] Surgery may be necessary to correct fistulas and strictures if these problems do not respond to appropriate antibiotic therapy.

The diagnosis is confirmed with NAAT testing. Screening is recommended for sexually active women and men in high-risk groups (e.g., patients in STI clinics, infection with another STI, MSM, and men under 30 in the military or jail).[19]

Suspected or confirmed treatment is with an oral dose of 1 g azithromycin or a 7-day course of doxycycline, 100 mg twice a day.[20] Erythromycin, ofloxacin, and levofloxacin also have been shown to be effective.[21]

Campylobacter

Campylobacter species are recognized as a frequent cause of acute diarrhea. *Campylobacter jejuni* and *Campylobacter coli* cause fever, watery diarrhea, tenesmus, and abdominal pain. *Campylobacter fetus* is more likely to cause intravascular, meningeal, or localized infections such as arthritis, cellulitis, and abscess as well as urinary, placental, and pleural infection. *Campylobacter* infections occur predominantly in men, perhaps related to homosexual activity, but whether the source of infection is by sexual transmission is uncertain.[22] The *Campylobacter* organism is found in cattle, sheep, swine, fowl, and rodents, but it may be cultured from 4.1% of humans with diarrhea.[23] Others sharing the household are exposed and often found to be positive by culture, suggesting a person-to-person transmission. The diagnosis is based on a history of exposure, examination of stool for leukocytes, and stool culture.

Sigmoidoscopy reveals a proctitis. Biopsy shows crypt abscesses and an inflammatory cell infiltration suggestive of ulcerative colitis. With supportive therapy, most cases of diarrhea resolve spontaneously within 1 week. Severe cases may be treated with erythromycin, 500 mg four times a day for 7 days.[24] Other antibiotics that eradicate *Campylobacter* infections include tetracycline, chloramphenicol, clindamycin, and aminoglycosides. For severe systemic infections, 2 to 4 weeks of parenteral antibiotic therapy is warranted.

Shigella

In up to 50% of the homosexual population, shigellosis has been recognized as an STD.[25,26,27] The enteric *Shigella* pathogens may be transferred during anilingus or fellatio. The infective dose of this highly communicable organism is less than 10,[3] and the incubation time is only 1 to 2 days.

Shigella infections are limited to the gastrointestinal tract, where the mucosa is invaded.[28] Crypt abscesses lead to local mucosal necrosis, in turn leading to ulcers (► Fig. 13.1), bleeding, and "pseudomembrane" formation, which may be seen by endoscopy. The clinical picture includes abdominal pain, fever, and watery diarrhea. The diarrhea is likely due to an exotoxin. Straining and tenesmus characterize bowel movements. Culturing with a fresh stool specimen is a key to diagnosis. PCR techniques are being refined and will become tests of choice.[29]

The patient should be rehydrated routinely. Opiates should be avoided, because the diarrhea may be a defense mechanism that may decrease exposure of exotoxin to the bowel mucosa.[27] Antibiotics are suppressive and often fail to eradicate the organisms. Reports of resistance of *Shigella* to antibiotics have come from many countries. The resistance was to ampicillin, trimethoprim/sulfamethoxazole, chloramphenicol, cephalothin, and amoxicillin/clavulanic acid.[30] The current preferred antibiotics are ciprofloxacin, aminoglycosides, and the second- and third-generation cephalosporins. Cultures should be followed until the pathogens are eradicated. A vaccine for *Shigella* is under development.[31]

Haemophilus Ducreyi

Chancroid, caused by *Haemophilus ducreyi*, has declined worldwide, but is a common cause of genital ulcer disease and

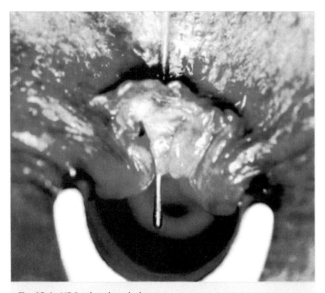

Fig. 13.1 AIDS-related anal ulcers.

is a risk factor for HIV transmission. Ulcers characteristic of chancroid are multiple and painful. They progress through pustular and ulcerative stages on the genitals or the anorectum. The ulcers can be difficult to differentiate from herpes. Painful lymphadenopathy is present in 50% of patients; some of the lymph nodes may become fluctuant with abscesses (bobo formation).[32] Culture of the organism is sometimes possible, but the diagnosis is usually made based on painful genital ulcerations and regional adenopathy in the absence of syphilis and HSV.[33]

The recommended treatment is azithromycin, 1 g orally in a single dose, or ceftriaxone, 250 mg administered intramuscularly as a single dose, ciprofloxacin, 500 mg orally twice daily for three days, or erythromycin base, 500 mg orally three times a day for 7 days.[21,33] If the organism is sensitive, symptoms improve in 3 days and the ulcers resolve markedly in 7 days. Bobo formation may require drainage and usually requires a 2-week course of antibiotic therapy. Follow-up is important and failure to improve necessitates a change in antibiotic. Any sexual partner who had contact with the patient within the 10 days preceding the onset of symptoms should also be treated.

Klebsiella Granulomatis (Donovanosis)

Granuloma inguinale is the chronic granulomatous infection associated with the gram-negative rod *Klebsiella granulomatis* (previously known as *Donovania* or *Calymmatobacterium granulomatis*). Transmission is by sexual contact or fecal contamination. Red, shiny exuberant masses appear on the genitals or around the anorectum that progress to painless ulcers. Because of slow onset, infection time may have occurred months before appearance of the masses. In time, scarring may lead to marked stenosis of the anorectum. Confusion in diagnosis includes secondary syphilis, amebiasis, and carcinoma. Tissue smears or biopsy allows identification of characteristic intracytoplasmic inclusion bodies (Donovan bodies). Treatment is with trimethoprim-sulfamethoxazole (double strength tablet; twice daily), doxycycline (100 mg twice daily), ciprofloxacin (750 mg twice daily), erythromycin base (500 mg twice daily), and azithromycin (1 g per week for 3 weeks or until all ulcers have healed).[21,34]

Syphilis

Syphilis, one of the oldest infectious diseases, remains common with 19,999 cases reported in the United States in 2014.[35] The rate of 6.3/100,000 in 2014 was a 15% increase over 2013. *T. pallidum*, a spirochete, is the causative agent.[36] The infection is transmitted by sexual contact with introduction of the spirochetes through the intact mucous membrane or a break in the skin. The mouth, genitals, and anus are common sites of infections and harbor the primary lesion, the chancre. In 10 to 20% of cases, the primary lesion may be hidden within an orifice. After infection, the chancre appears within 2 to 10 weeks. The chancre may be either painful or painless. In the differential diagnosis, there may be confusion with fissure. However, a lesion situated off the midline, too far out on the anal skin, or too high on the dentate line in addition to irregular configuration is not consistent with the diagnosis of fissure (► Fig. 13.2). Compared with HIV-uninfected patients, HIV-infected patients with primary

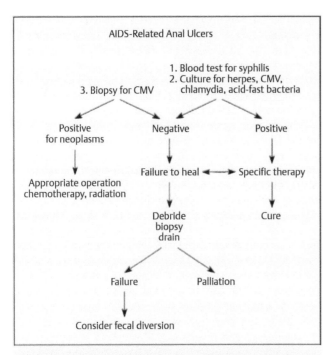

AIDS-Related Anal Ulcers

1. Blood test for syphilis
2. Culture for herpes, CMV, chlamydia, acid-fast bacteria

3. Biopsy for CMV

Positive for neoplasms — Negative — Positive

Appropriate operation chemotherapy, radiation

Failure to heal ◄——► Specific therapy

Debride biopsy drain — Cure

Failure — Palliation

Consider fecal diversion

Fig. 13.2 Anal disease with AIDS. Note condylomata, scars, and ulcerations. (The image is provided courtesy of Bruce Orkin, MD.)

syphilis present more frequently with multiple ulcers.[37] Lymphadenopathy is significantly notable. The primary ulcer proceeds to heal spontaneously. However, in 2 to 10 more weeks, secondary lesions appear as a red maculopapular rash anywhere on the body. Flat, pale lesions, condylomata lata, may be found around the genitals or the anus. Both primary and secondary lesions are infectious. The exudate of lesions in the early stages (i.e., within 1 year) may be tested by dark-field examination. The multiple motile spirochetes can be seen through oil emersion technique.

With antibiotic therapy, the spirochetes disappear from lesions in only a few hours and thus may interfere with early diagnosis. In one-third of patients, the condition will proceed to spontaneous cure, and in another one-third it will remain latent. Unfortunately, the remaining one-third of cases will go on to late or tertiary syphilis. Latent or late syphilis, occurring over 1 year after infection, is detected only by serologic testing because the recognizable primary and secondary lesions are absent. Late disease may lead to cardiovascular, central nervous system, nephritic, and hepatic syphilis. Pregnant women with latent syphilis can pass the disease on to the fetus. Homosexuals develop proctitis and rectal masses, and these lesions are frequently misdiagnosed as lymphomas or neoplasms.[38,39] HIV-infected patients more often present with secondary syphilis and persistent chancres.[40]

Presumptive diagnosis of syphilis is made by two serologic tests. The antibody tests remain positive for life, and titers do not correlate with disease activity. Thus, they are reported as positive or negative. The most often used specific antibody tests are the fluorescent treponemal antibody absorption test (FTA-ABS) and the microhemagglutination assay for antibody to *T. pallidum* (MHATP). These tests become positive earlier than other blood tests; hence, they should be used in cases suspected to be early. Nontreponemal tests most commonly employed for

screening are the Venereal Disease Research Laboratory (VDRL) test and the rapid plasma reagin (RPR). Since both tests vary according to disease activity, titers reflect worsening or response to treatment. Sequential testing to determine disease activity is based on changes of titers of these two tests. Patients who are HIV positive are less likely to experience serologic improvement after recommended therapy than those who are HIV negative.[41] A PCR method has been developed, which is 95.8% sensitive and 95.7% specific.[42]

Treatment is with penicillin G benzathine, 2.4 million units given intramuscularly.[43] The Jarisch–Herxheimer reaction occurs in half of the treated patients as the spirochetes are destroyed. The reaction may begin in 6 hours and be over within 24 hours. The usual manifestations are fever, skin lesions, arthralgia, and adenopathy; these conditions may be treated with analgesics. Patients who are allergic to penicillin may be treated with tetracycline or erythromycin, 500 mg four times a day, or doxycycline, 100 mg twice daily for 2 weeks.

13.4.2 Viral

Herpes

The HSV may include several clinical syndromes. HSV type I causes dermatitis, eczema, keratoconjunctivitis, encephalitis, and labialis. HSV type II causes genital, anal, and neonatal infections. Recently, more HSV-1 infections have been identified on genitals, correlating with more orogenital sex.[44,45] Seroprevalence of 54% for HSV-1 and 15.7% for HSV-2 has been reported.[46] Manifestations at primary infection include fever, malaise, and lymphadenopathy. Primary infections are usually worse than subsequent recurrent infections.

In homosexuals who present with severe proctitis, 6 to 30% will have a positive culture for HSV.[47] In addition, fever is present in 48%, difficulty in urination in 48%, sacral paresthesias in 26%, inguinal adenopathy in 57%, anorectal pain in 100%, tenesmus in 100%, constipation in 78%, and skin ulcerations in 70%.[48] A lumbosacral radiculopathy after the acute infection may leave residual deficits such as impotence, bladder dysfunction, and pain in the buttocks and legs.

Recurrences are far different from the primary infection and appear to be due to reactivation of latent HSV. External inspection and sigmoidoscopic examination of the distal 10 cm reveal vesicles and pustules that break and coalesce to become ulcers. The definitive diagnostic laboratory test is viral isolation and tissue culture. A direct fluorescent monoclonal antibody technique will confirm the diagnosis.[49,50] In one series, serologic testing showed 95% of homosexuals to have been infected with HSV type II.[51]

Acyclovir was the first oral antiherpes agent. It is effective, but it is poorly bioavailable. Oral acyclovir, 200 mg five times a day for 5 days, shortens the duration of virus shedding and thus aids in clearing of the lesions.[52,53] Herpes proctitis, likewise, responds to a larger dose of acyclovir, 400 mg, given orally five times a day. Topical acyclovir may be added, but it is less effective than either oral or intravenous administration. Some herpes viruses have become resistant to acyclovir. Recent reports suggest that foscarnet works as an alternative therapy.[54] Valacyclovir, using 1 g twice a day for 10 days, was developed to overcome the poor bioavailability of acyclovir.[21] Famciclovir is also more bioavailable and may be dosed at 250 mg three times a day for 7 to 10 days.[55]

Frequently, recurrent herpes may be suppressed by long-term treatment with acyclovir, 400 mg twice a day.[56] Recently, famciclovir 250 mg twice daily and valacyclovir 500 mg twice daily have been shown to be effective alternatives.[55] However, untreated herpes proctitis is self-limited, resolving completely in approximately 3 weeks.

Hepatitis

Hepatitis is common and can be transmitted sexually. In 2014, there were 1,239 cases of hepatitis A, 2,953 cases of hepatitis B, and 2,194 cases of hepatitis C reported to the Centers for Disease Control and Prevention (CDC).[57] Hepatitis A virus (HAV) infection produces a self-limited disease that does not result in chronic infection or chronic liver disease (CLD). Acute liver failure from hepatitis A is rare (overall case-fatality rate: 0.5%). Antibody produced in response to HAV infection persists for life and confers protection against reinfection. The presence of immunoglobulin M (IgM) antibody to HAV is diagnostic of acute HAV infection. A positive test for total anti-HAV indicates immunity to HAV infection but does not differentiate current from previous HAV infection. Patients with acute hepatitis A usually require only supportive care, with no restrictions in diet or activity. Vaccination is the most effective means of preventing HAV transmission among persons at risk for infection (e.g., MSM, drug users, and persons with CLD). IG administered intramuscularly can provide postexposure prophylaxis against HAV.

The highest concentrations of hepatitis B virus (HBV) are found in blood, with lower concentrations found in other body fluids including wound exudates, semen, vaginal secretions, and saliva.[58,59] HBV is more infectious and more stable in the environment than other blood-borne pathogens (e.g., hepatitis C virus [HCV] and HIV). HBV infection can be self-limited or chronic. In adults, approximately half of newly acquired HBV infections are symptomatic, and approximately 1% of reported cases result in acute liver failure and death.[60] Risk for chronic infection is inversely related to age at acquisition. HBV is efficiently transmitted by percutaneous or mucous membrane exposure to HBV-infected blood or body fluids that contain HBV. The primary risk factors associated with infection among adolescents and adults are unprotected sex with an infected partner, multiple partners, MSM, history of other STDs, and injection-drug use. In addition, several studies have demonstrated other modes of HBV transmission, including premastication and lapses in health care infection-control procedures, as less common sources of transmission.[61,62,63,64]

Diagnosis of acute or chronic HBV infection requires serologic testing. Because HBsAg is present in both acute and chronic infection, the presence of IgM antibody to hepatitis B core antigen (IgM anti-HBc) is diagnostic of acute or recently acquired HBV infection. Antibody to HBsAg (anti-HBs) is produced after a resolved infection and is the only HBV antibody marker present after vaccination. The presence of HBsAg and total anti-HBc, with a negative test for IgM anti-HBc, indicates chronic HBV infection. The presence of anti-HBc alone might indicate acute, resolved, or chronic infection or a false-positive result.

No specific therapy is available for persons with acute hepatitis B; treatment is supportive. Persons with chronic HBV infection should be referred for evaluation to a provider experienced in the management of chronic HBV infection. Therapeutic agents cleared by FDA for treatment of chronic hepatitis B can achieve sustained suppression of HBV replication and remission of liver disease.[65] Two products have been approved for hepatitis B prevention: hepatitis B immune globulin for postexposure prophylaxis and hepatitis B vaccine.

HCV infection is the most common chronic blood-borne infection in the United States, with an estimated 2.7 million persons living with chronic infection.[66] HCV is not efficiently transmitted through sex, and studies of HCV transmission between heterosexual or homosexual couples have yielded mixed results. Testing for HCV infection should include use of an FDA-cleared test for antibody to HCV (i.e., immunoassay, enzyme immunoassay, or enhanced chemiluminescence immunoassay and, if recommended, a supplemental antibody test) followed by NAAT to detect HCV RNA for those with a positive antibody result.[67] As the management of hepatitis C continues to evolve, providers should consult a specialist or recent guidelines (www.hcvguidelines.org).

Reducing the burden of HCV infection and disease in the United States requires implementation of both primary and secondary prevention activities. Primary prevention reduces or eliminates HCV transmission, whereas secondary prevention activities are aimed at reducing CLD and other chronic diseases in persons with HCV infection by first identifying them and then providing medical management and antiviral therapy.

Human Papillomavirus

Human papillomavirus and anal condylomata are discussed in Chapter 12.

Molluscum Contagiosum

Molluscum contagiosum is a common cutaneous viral infection caused by *Molluscipoxvirus*, a virus of the pox group. It is transmitted by direct body contact. After an incubation period of 3 to 6 weeks, 3 mm, painless, flattened, round, umbilicated lesions develop. Diagnosis can be made by visual inspection but is confirmed by biopsy with viral analysis or PCR.[68] Although the disease is benign and self-limiting, treatment is used to prevent spread and for cosmetic purposes. Options include local destruction with phenol, surgical removal, and cryotherapy. Antiviral and immunomodulatory therapies include topical imiquimod and cidofovir.[69,70]

Human Immunodeficiency Virus (HIV) and Acquired Immunodeficiency Syndrome (AIDS)

HIV is an RNA retrovirus that infects human T-lymphocytes. The virus is spread by contaminated body fluids, and after a variable latent period of up to 2 years, it produces diminished immunologic function.[71] In 2014, an estimated 44,073 people were diagnosed with HIV infection in the United States and more than 1.2 million Americans are living with HIV.[72] Proctologic conditions are common in HIV patients, and in the absence of routine screening, these complaints may be the patient's primary reason for seeking medical help.[73] A systematic approach allows appropriate management of these patients.

The initial evaluation should include a history, physical examination, and review of laboratory studies (HIV status, CD4 count, viral load, etc.). An adequate history is essential to obtain the correct diagnosis for any proctologic complaints. The presenting symptoms should be explored with particular attention given to bowel activity, sexual history, and overall health. A patient's risk for HIV infection or AIDS should be explored with specific questions about sexual preference, intravenous drug usage, and exposure to blood products or to HIV-positive individuals. Alterations in body functions or symptoms may direct the investigations toward specific diseases. HIV-positive patients have been classified by the CDC (▶ Table 13.5).[74] Early-stage patients have minimal alterations in their gross immunologic or healing ability. Patients with later disease stages have significant immunologic dysfunction, resulting in increased morbidity and mortality. Some authors have attempted to use the absolute T helper cell count to predict healing. Others have not found this helpful.[75] This discrepancy may be explained by the use of newer medications used to treat HIV infection, which may improve a patient's ability to heal despite a low T helper cell count.

In HIV-positive patients with gastrointestinal symptoms, it is essential to evaluate the stool for pathogens by cultures and stains.[76,77] In addition, a biopsy should be performed on any abnormal lesion of the perirectal area or rectal mucosa to complete the evaluation. Since the HIV is transmitted sexually, by use of contaminated needles, or by contact with infected body fluids and perhaps tissue, infection control measures are very important. Examiners should observe universal precautions, and any activity with the potential for body fluid contact requires eye and skin protection. Gloves, goggles, mask, and barrier gowns provide the necessary shielding for the examiner. Most patients require only a proctoscopic or anoscopic examination for an adequate evaluation; for convenience, the author uses disposable instruments. Traditional sterilization measures are used should nondisposable instruments be required.

Table 13.5 Centers for Disease Control and Prevention HIV staging

A case definition that incorporates three levels of CD4 counts and three groups of clinical disease states as follows:

CD4 + T Lymphocytes

1. ≥ 500 cells/mL

2. 200–499 cells/mL

3. ≤ 200 cells/mL

Clinical

A: Symptomatic

- Generalized adenopathy

- Acute HIV infection

B: Symptomatic diseases not listed in category C. Examples include but are not limited to:

- Bacillary angiomatosis

- Candidiasis, oropharyngeal (thrush)

Table 13.5 continued

A case definition that incorporates three levels of CD4 counts and three groups of clinical disease states as follows:

- Candidiasis, vulvovaginal; persistent, frequent, or poorly responsive to therapy

- Cervical dysplasia (moderate or severe)/cervical carcinoma in situ

- Constitutional symptoms, such as fever (38.5 °C) or diarrhea lasting greater than 1 month

- Hairy leukoplakia, oral

- Herpes zoster (shingles), involving at least two distinct episodes or more than one dermatome

- Idiopathic thrombocytopenic purpura

- Listeriosis

- Pelvic inflammatory disease, particularly if complicated by tubo-ovarian abscess

- Peripheral neuropathy

C: Clinical conditions of AIDS

- Candidiasis of bronchi, trachea, or lungs

- Candidiasis, esophageal

- Cervical cancer (invasive)

- Coccidioidomycosis, disseminated or extrapulmonary

- Cryptococcosis, extrapulmonary

- Cryptosporidiosis, chronic intestinal for longer than 1 month

- *Cytomegalovirus* disease (other than liver, spleen or lymph nodes)

- Encephalopathy (HIV-related)

- Herpes simplex: chronic ulcer(s) (for more than 1 month); or bronchitis, pneumonitis, or esophagitis

- Histoplasmosis, disseminated or extrapulmonary

- Isosporiasis, chronic intestinal (for more than 1 month)

- Kaposi's sarcoma

- Lymphoma: Burkitt's, immunoblastic, or primary brain

- *Mycobacterium avium* complex

- Mycobacterium, other species, disseminated or extrapulmonary

- *Pneumocystis carinii* pneumonia

- Pneumonia (recurrent)

- Progressive multifocal leukoencephalopathy

- Salmonella septicemia (recurrent)

- Toxoplasmosis of the brain

- Tuberculosis

- Wasting syndrome due to HIV

Source: From http://www.cdc.gov/mmwr/preview/mmwrhtml/00018871.htm and https://www.cdc.gov/mmwr/preview/mmwrhtml/rr5710a1.htm

The diseases identified in HIV-positive patients can be grouped into three categories. The first group includes the common proctologic conditions (e.g., hemorrhoids, fissures, pruritus) routinely discovered in the general population.[78] Second are diseases associated with high-risk groups. Diseases associated with homosexuality in males include candidiasis, cryptosporidiosis, cytomegalic inclusion disease, pneumonia (*Pneumocystis carinii*), herpes simplex, and herpes zoster, whereas intravenous drug use is associated with hepatitis (HBV). The third group are those illnesses associated with HIV infections, such as unusual opportunistic infections, Kaposi's sarcoma (KS), and lymphoma.

The exact incidence of these conditions is not accurately known because of the absence of routine screening and selection biases in the published series. The experience reported by Beck et al[78] in 1990 included 677 HIV-positive patients, most of whom had early-stage disease and were male (95%). Of these patients, 6% had nonsexually related anorectal conditions, whereas more than 60% had at least one other sexually transmitted disease.

Chlamydia and hepatitis were the most common conditions, with serology proving positive in 51 and 31%, respectively, followed by anal condylomata (18%). Combining patients with nonsexually related anorectal diseases and those with anal condylomata, 24% had treatable anorectal conditions. Another report of 1,117 HIV-positive patients treated at the University of Amsterdam[79] found 7.4% had anorectal disease that required a surgical consultation. Many of these 83 patients had more than one problem, including perianal sepsis (55%), condylomata acuminata (34%), anorectal ulcers (33%), hemorrhoids (17%), invasive anorectal carcinoma (17%), and polyps (11%). Finally, in 1998 Barrett et al[80] reported their experience with 260 consecutive HIV-positive patients with perianal disease between 1989 and 1996. The most common disorders were condyloma (42%), fistula (34%), fissure (32%), and abscess (25%). Neoplasms were present in 7% of patients. Sixty-six percent of patients had more than one disorder.

The management of these anorectal conditions in the HIV-positive patient deserves additional comment. Unlike in normal patients, the primary therapeutic goal in HIV-positive patients is to eliminate or reduce symptoms. A secondary goal is resolution of the condition and healing of the wound.

Abscesses with pus usually present with pain and require drainage. Efforts are directed toward keeping the wounds small. Drainage with a latex Pezzer's catheter is very effective.[81] In early-stage patients, symptomatic fistulas are treated in the normal fashion (Chapter 9) and can be expected to heal.[79] Late-stage patients are treated to minimize symptoms. This usually entails establishing adequate drainage. Performing an extensive procedure to resolve the fistula is contraindicated. These fistulas rarely heal and often result in larger nonhealing wounds.

Anal ulcers (▶ Fig. 13.3) can be caused by a number of the infectious agents described in this chapter. The ulcers caused by HIV are deep chronic ulcers with overhanging edges. They are often eccentric or multiple, cavitating, and edematous with a bluish-purple hue. It is important to differentiate these HIV anal ulcers from benign anal fissures and neoplasms. Routine anal fissures are either posterior or anterior, accompanied by skin

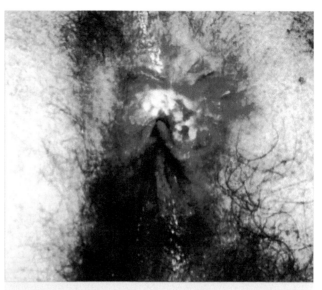

Fig. 13.3 Anal disease in AIDS. Note a deep posterior ulcer, herpes, a skin tag, and a fistula. (The image is provided courtesy of Bruce Orkin, MD.)

tags, and readily visible when the buttocks are retracted. Anal ulcers usually cause pain when there is "pocketing" or inadequate drainage of the associated ulcer cavity. Any HIV-positive patient with anal pain should receive an examination under anesthesia to exclude undrained pus. If a deep cavitating ulcer is identified, it should be unroofed to establish drainage, which usually resolves the pain. Gottesman[82] has also recommended injection of a long-acting steroid into the base of the ulcer to relieve symptoms.

HIV patients are afflicted with a variety of neoplastic disorders related to their immunocompromised state.[82,83] KS, non-Hodgkin's lymphoma, and epidermoid anal carcinoma all present as anal masses or ulcers. An incisional biopsy confirms the diagnosis. Unfortunately, the associated immunodeficiency limits therapeutic options, and the prognosis remains poor.

Management of the HIV patient has changed over the years. Early studies of HIV-infected patients with perianal disease noted poor healing and high morbidity rates. Recent changes in the systemic treatment of HIV infection and newer drug regimens that include combinations of protease inhibitors, nucleoside analogs, and highly active antiretroviral therapy (HAART) have greatly improved the prognosis for HIV-infected patients.[80] Certain measures directed at control of infectious organisms are beneficial.

AIDS-Related Malignancies

KS is caused by infection with human herpesvirus 8 (HHV-8) and was one of the AIDS-defining illnesses in the 1980s. There are four subtypes, one of which is AIDS-related KS. After an initial rapid increase, the proportion of AIDS patients with KS steadily declined from nearly half of those with diagnosed AIDS in 1981 to 15% in 1986 in the United States[84] Patients coinfected with HIV-1 and HHV-8 are at accelerated risk for developing KS.[85,86] The skin is the most frequent site, and the lesions are multicentric. The nodules are usually 0.5 to 2.0 cm in size and vary in color from purple to black. When the gastrointestinal tract is involved, usually there are few symptoms. However, obstructive symptoms and bleeding have been reported. The gastrointestinal lesions are red, raised, sessile nodules. Since the rectum may be involved, sigmoidoscopy and biopsy should be part of the workup.

Once the diagnosis of KS has been made, treatment is based on the subtype and the presence of localized versus systemic disease. Localized cutaneous disease can be treated with cryotherapy, intralesional injections of *vinblastine*, *alitretinoin* gel, radiotherapy, topical immunotherapy (*imiquimod*), or surgical excision. Extensive cutaneous disease and/or internal disease may require intravenous chemotherapy and immunotherapy. Discontinuation or reduction of immunosuppressive therapy is recommended when KS arises in the setting of iatrogenic immunosuppression. However, with AIDS-related KS, HAART has been shown to prevent or induce regression of KS. Some AIDS patients have complete resolution of the lesions and prolonged remission while continuing the therapy. Therefore, HAART should be considered first-line treatment for these patients, though they may require other treatments at the same time.[87,88]

AIDS-Related Infections

AIDS has allowed *Cryptosporidium*, *Isospora belli*, and *Cyclospora* to flourish in the immunocompromised patient and thus become known as a pathogen for man.[89,90,91] Diarrhea is the symptom that may be profound enough to result in fluid and electrolyte imbalance, finally ending in malnutrition and weight loss. The bacterial and parasitic causes of diarrhea must be suspected and ruled out as well. Cramps, weight loss, anorexia, malaise, vomiting, and myalgia are frequent complaints. Cryptosporidia may be found in the stool specimen when an acid-fast staining technique is applied.[92] A new immunofluorescent assay using a monoclonal antibody seems to be more sensitive and specific for detecting the oocytes. A PCR study may be even more sensitive.[93] Unfortunately, there is no specific treatment for cryptosporidiosis. The most common medications used are paromomycin (aminosidine) and azithromycin. On the other hand, isosporiasis responds well to oral trimethoprim-sulfamethoxazole.[94]

Cytomegalovirus (CMV) infects 90% of AIDS patients during their illness.[95] However, this rate may reflect the high incidence of CMV identified in homosexuals, a very high-risk group.[94] The infection may take the form of chorioretinitis, pneumonia, esophagitis, colitis, encephalitis, adrenalitis, or hepatitis.[96] Perianal ulcers may be caused by CMV. CMV colitis is found in up to 10% of AIDS patients.[97] Symptoms of diarrhea, hematochezia, fever, and weight loss are predominant.[98,99] Diffuse submucosal hemorrhage and mucosal ulcerations as dictated by endoscopy typify the proctocolitis. For the differential diagnosis, consideration must be given to *Clostridium difficile*, ulcerative colitis, and granulomatous colitis, especially if the AIDS diagnosis is uncertain. Biopsy shows CMV inclusions and inflammatory reactions. However, in recent years major progress has been made in developing quantitative detection methods, using PCRs.[100,101]

The best drugs for use against CMV are ganciclovir or cidofovir. Although similar in formula to acyclovir, ganciclovir is more effective against CMV. Unfortunately, resistance has developed to ganciclovir and cross resistance to cidofovir. Thus, foscarnet may be used in resistant cases.[102] On the horizon is a vaccine against CMV.[103]

Pathology due to CMV is the most common indication for emergency laparotomy in AIDS patients (▶ Table 13.6). In 1986, Nugent and O'Connell[104] reported on five major abdominal operations in AIDS patients; two of the conditions, a perforation of the colon and a toxic megacolon, were due to CMV. Surgical treatments were colectomy with colostomy and total colectomy. Robinson et al[105] performed seven emergency operations, and the two celiotomies were for CMV. Colectomy with end colostomy was employed in both cases. Deaths occurred at 2 weeks and 5 months in these patients. Eleven AIDS patients underwent 13 emergency celiotomies by Wexner et al[106]; 7 of these procedures were due to CMV. Four of the seven had lower gastrointestinal hemorrhage from proctocolitis, and three had perforations. Surgical procedures included three subtotal colectomies, two segmental resections, and two diverting stomas. The mortality rate was 68% in 6 months. Söderlund et al[107] reported eight patients with advanced HIV disease and severe CMV enterocolitis. These patients had right ileocolectomies; six had complete or partial palliation for a mean of 14 months, one died of hemorrhage from a KS, and one died 3 weeks later from unrelated causes.

Table 13.6 Laparotomy in AIDS patients

Author(s)	No. of patients	Operations for acute conditions	Complications associated with acute operations	Deaths associated with acute operations
Wolkomir et al[108]	20	3	0 (0%)	0 (0%)
Deziel et al[109]	20	10	4 (40%)	2 (20%)
Diettrich et al[110]	58	12	3 (25%)	3 (25%)
Davidson et al[111]	28	28	–	3 (11%)
Whitney et al[112]	57	57	15 (26%)	7 (12%)
Bizer et al[113]	40	15	20 (50%)	15 (38%)
Samantaray and Walker[114]	24	–	12 (50%)	7 (30%)

13.4.3 Parasitic

Entamoeba Histolytica

Reports of amebiasis in homosexual patients are numerous.[115,116] Screening stools of homosexual patients has confirmed the presence of amebic cysts in 20 to 30%, thus identifying another STD.[116] Fecal–oral transmission by anilingus is the likely cause. When cysts are swallowed, the trophozoite emerges in the stomach and divides to produce eight smaller trophozoites. These pass to the cecum, where more are produced. The intestinal mucosa is invaded, resulting in clinical disease in 10% of cases. The amebas penetrate through tiny ulcers in the mucosa and dissect laterally above the muscularis mucosa, creating "collar button" ulcers. Eventually, there may be healing or extension deeper into the wall may occur, sometimes leading to perforation. Chronic infection with a resultant inflammatory mass, the ameboma, may form on the intestinal wall. The rectum and the sigmoid often are involved. Mild disease may present with symptoms of diarrhea, urgency, and cramps. The more serious illness has symptoms of severe abdominal pain and dehydrating diarrhea, which may begin as early as the fourth day after exposure. Microemboli of trophozoites may be carried via the portal vein to the liver, where an abscess may begin.

The diagnosis can be made fastest by examination of a fresh stool sample for trophozoites and cysts. Serologic tests are available, but a highly specific antigen is not always present. The indirect hemagglutination test is employed when stools are not positive and extraintestinal amebiasis is suspected.

Metronidazole, 750 mg three times a day for 10 days, is the drug of choice followed by a course of diloxanide furoate, 500 mg three times a day for 10 days, or iodoquinol, 650 mg three times a day for 20 days. For severe disease, emetine, oxytetracycline, and diloxanide furoate followed by chloroquine may be used if the metronidazole fails or is not tolerated.

Giardia Lamblia

Giardiasis may be contracted by ingesting fecally contaminated food or water. Homosexuals who practice oral–anal contact often are infected.[115] Phillips et al[115] found *G. lamblia* or *E. histolytica* in 21% of homosexuals examined for parasites. Symptoms of malaise, weakness, weight loss, cramps, and flatulence result. The distinctive cysts may be identified in fresh stool samples. The parasites attach to the mucosa of the duodenum and the jejunum. Therefore, sometimes aspiration of the duodenum may be necessary to find the organisms. Metronidazole (250 mg three times a day for 5–7 days) is the best form of treatment[117] but it is not approved by the FDA for use in giardiasis. The approved drug is furazolidone, 100 mg four times a day for 7 to 10 days. ▶ Table 13.1 summarizes the treatments for STDs.

Pubic Lice

Pubic lice (*Phthirus pubis*) are obligate blood-sucking parasites and infestation is diagnosed by observing lice on pubic hair. The lice are transmitted by close contact and the diagnosis should prompt testing for other STIs. Treatment is with permethrin 1% cream or pyrethrins 0.3% piperonyl butoxide 4% cream.

Table 13.7 Diagnosis of AIDS

Cryptosporidiosis

Cytomegalovirus

Isosporiasis

Kaposi's sarcoma

Lymphoma

Lymphoid pneumonia or hyperplasia

Pneumocystis carinii pneumonia

Progressive multifocal leukoencephalopathy

Toxoplasmosis

Candidiasis

Coccidioidomycosis

Cryptococcus

Herpes simplex

Histoplasmosis

Tuberculosis

Other mycobacteriosis

Salmonellosis

HIV encephalopathy

HIV wasting syndrome

Pulmonary tuberculosis

Recurrent pneumonia

Invasive cervical cancer

CD4 T-lymphocyte count < 200

Note: Diagnosis of AIDS is based on HIV infection plus one of the above diseases or conditions.[89]

References

[1] Welton L, Kin C. Sexually transmitted infections. In: Steele SR, Hull TL, Read TE, Saclarides TJ, Senagore AJ, Whitlow CB, eds. The ASCRS Textbook of Colon and Rectal Surgery. 3rd ed. Cham: Springer; 2016:325–342

[2] van Liere GA, Hoebe CJ, Niekamp AM, Koedijk FD, Dukers-Muijrers NH. Standard symptom- and sexual history-based testing misses anorectal Chlamydia trachomatis and neisseria gonorrhoeae infections in swingers and men who have sex with men. Sex Transm Dis. 2013; 40(4):285–289

[3] van Liere GA, Hoebe CJ, Dukers-Muijrers NH. Evaluation of the anatomical site distribution of chlamydia and gonorrhoea in men who have sex with men and in high-risk women by routine testing: cross-sectional study revealing missed opportunities for treatment strategies. Sex Transm Infect. 2014; 90(1):58–60

[4] Centers for Disease Control and Prevention. Gonorrhea. Available at: http://www.cdc.gov/std/stats14/gonorrhea.htm. Accessed September 27, 2016

[5] Zakher B, Cantor AG, Pappas M, Daeges M, Nelson HD. Screening for gonorrhea and Chlamydia: a systematic review for the U.S. Preventive Services Task Force. Ann Intern Med. 2014; 161(12):884–893

[6] Deheragoda P. Diagnosis of rectal gonorrhoea by blind anorectal swabs compared with direct vision swabs taken via a proctoscope. Br J Vener Dis. 1977; 53(5):311–313

[7] William DC, Felman YM, Riccardi NB. The utility of anoscopy in the rapid diagnosis of symptomatic anorectal gonorrhea in men. Sex Transm Dis. 1981; 8(1):16–17

[8] Centers for Disease Control and Prevention. Recommendations for the laboratory-based detection of Chlamydia trachomatis and Neisseria gonorrhoeae–2014. MMWR Recomm Rep. 2014; 63 RR-02:1–19

[9] Schwartz S, Zenilman J, Schnell D, et al. National surveillance of antimicrobial resistance in Neisseria gonorrhoeae. The Gonococcal Isolate Surveillance Project. JAMA. 1990; 264(11):1413–1417

[10] Centers for Disease Control and Prevention (CDC). Update to CDC's Sexually transmitted diseases treatment guidelines, 2010: oral cephalosporins no longer a recommended treatment for gonococcal infections. MMWR Morb Mortal Wkly Rep. 2012; 61(31):590–594

[11] Bolan GA, Sparling PF, Wasserheit JN. The emerging threat of untreatable gonococcal infection. N Engl J Med. 2012; 366(6):485–487

[12] Kovari H, de Melo Oliveira MD, Hauser P, et al. Decreased susceptibility of Neisseria gonorrhoeae isolates from Switzerland to Cefixime and Ceftriaxone: antimicrobial susceptibility data from 1990 and 2000 to 2012. BMC Infect Dis. 2013; 13:603

[13] Centers for Disease Control and Prevention. Chlamydia. Available at: http://www.cdc.gov/std/stats14/chlamydia.htm. Accessed September 28, 2016

[14] Levine JS, Smith PD, Brugge WR. Chronic proctitis in male homosexuals due to lymphogranuloma venereum. Gastroenterology. 1980; 79(3):563–565

[15] Quinn TC, Goodell SE, Mkrtichian E, et al. Chlamydia trachomatis proctitis. N Engl J Med. 1981; 305(4):195–200

[16] Dean D, Millman K. Molecular and mutation trends analyses of omp1 alleles for serovar E of Chlamydia trachomatis. Implications for the immunopathogenesis of disease. J Clin Invest. 1997; 99(3):475–483

[17] Amaral E. Current approach to STD management in women. Int J Gynaecol Obstet. 1998; 63 Suppl 1:S183–S189

[18] McMillan A, Sommerville RG, McKie PM. Chlamydial infection in homosexual men. Frequency of isolation of Chlamydia trachomatis from the urethra, ano-rectum, and pharynx. Br J Vener Dis. 1981; 57(1):47–49

[19] Geisler WM. Diagnosis and management of uncomplicated Chlamydia trachomatis infections in adolescents and adults: summary of evidence reviewed for the 2010 Centers for Disease Control and Prevention Sexually Transmitted Diseases Treatment Guidelines. Clin Infect Dis. 2011; 53 Suppl 3:S92–S98

[20] Stamm WE, Hicks CB, Martin DH, et al. Azithromycin for empirical treatment of the nongonococcal urethritis syndrome in men. A randomized double-blind study. JAMA. 1995; 274(7):545–549

[21] Centers for Disease Control and Prevention. Sexually transmitted diseases treatment guidelines 2002. MMWR Recomm Rep. 2002; 51 RR-6:1–78

[22] Blaser MJ, Wells JG, Feldman RA, Pollard RA, Allen JR. Campylobacter enteritis in the United States. A multicenter study. Ann Intern Med. 1983; 98 (3):360–365

[23] Walker RI, Caldwell MB, Lee EC, Guerry P, Trust TJ, Ruiz-Palacios GM. Pathophysiology of Campylobacter enteritis. Microbiol Rev. 1986; 50(1):81–94

[24] Guerrant RL, Bobak DA. Bacterial and protozoal gastroenteritis. N Engl J Med. 1991; 325(5):327–340

[25] Drusin LM, Genvert G, Topf-Olstein B, Levy-Zombek E. Shigellosis. Another sexually transmitted disease? Br J Vener Dis. 1976; 52(5):348–350

[26] Dritz SK, Back AF. Letter: Shigella enteritis venereally transmitted. N Engl J Med. 1974; 291(22):1194

[27] DuPont HL, Hornick RB. Adverse effect of lomotil therapy in shigellosis. JAMA. 1973; 226(13):1525–1528

[28] Adam T. Exploitation of host factors for efficient infection by Shigella. Int J Med Microbiol. 2001; 291(4):287–298

[29] Houng HS, Sethabutr O, Echeverria P. A simple polymerase chain reaction technique to detect and differentiate Shigella and enteroinvasive Escherichia coli in human feces. Diagn Microbiol Infect Dis. 1997; 28(1):19–25

[30] Jamal WY, Rotimi VO, Chugh TD, Pal T. Prevalence and susceptibility of Shigella species to 11 antibiotics in a Kuwait teaching hospital. J Chemother. 1998; 10(4):285–290

[31] Mani S, Wierzba T, Walker RI. Status of vaccine research and development for Shigella. Vaccine. 2016; 34(26):2887–2894

[32] Catterall RD. Sexually transmitted diseases of the anus and rectum. Clin Gastroenterol. 1975; 4(3):659–669

[33] Workowski KA, Berman S, Centers for Disease Control and Prevention (CDC). Sexually transmitted diseases treatment guidelines, 2010. MMWR Recomm Rep. 2010; 59 RR-12:1–110

[34] Basta-Juzbašić A, Čeović R. Chancroid, lymphogranuloma venereum, granuloma inguinale, genital herpes simplex infection, and molluscum contagiosum. Clin Dermatol. 2014; 32(2):290–298

[35] CDC Fact Sheet. Reported STDs in the United States: 2014 national data for chlamydia, gonorrhea, and syphilis. Available at: http://www.cdc.gov/std/stats14/std-trends-508.pdf. Accessed October 9, 2016

[36] Clyne B, Jerrard DA. Syphilis testing. J Emerg Med. 2000; 18(3):361–367

[37] Rompalo AM, Joesoef MR, O'Donnell JA, et al. Syphilis and HIV Study Group. Clinical manifestations of early syphilis by HIV status and gender: results of the syphilis and HIV study. Sex Transm Dis. 2001; 28 (3):158–165

[38] Faris MR, Perry JJ, Westermeier TG, Redmond J, III. Rectal syphilis mimicking histiocytic lymphoma. Am J Clin Pathol. 1983; 80(5):719–721

[39] Drusin LM, Singer C, Valenti AJ, Armstrong D. Infectious syphilis mimicking neoplastic disease. Arch Intern Med. 1977; 137(2):156–160

[40] Hutchinson CM, Hook EW, III, Shepherd M, Verley J, Rompalo AM. Altered clinical presentation of early syphilis in patients with human immunodeficiency virus infection. Ann Intern Med. 1994; 121(2):94–100

[41] Yinnon AM, Coury-Doniger P, Polito R, Reichman RC. Serologic response to treatment of syphilis in patients with HIV infection. Arch Intern Med. 1996; 156(3):321–325

[42] Liu H, Rodes B, Chen CY, Steiner B. New tests for syphilis: rational design of a PCR method for detection of Treponema pallidum in clinical specimens using unique regions of the DNA polymerase I gene. J Clin Microbiol. 2001; 39 (5):1941–1946

[43] Mattei PL, Beachkofsky TM, Gilson RT, Wisco OJ. Syphilis: a reemerging infection. Am Fam Physician. 2012; 86(5):433–440

[44] Lowhagen GB, Tunback P, Anderson K, Bergstrom T, Johannissou F. First episodes of genital herpes in a Swedish STD population: a study of epidemiology and transmission by the use of herpes simplex virus (HSV) typing and specific serology. Sex Transm Infect. 2000; 76(3):179–182

[45] Schacker T. The role of HSV in the transmission and progression of HIV. Herpes. 2001; 8(2):46–49

[46] Bradley H, Markowitz LE, Gibson T, McQuillan GM. Seroprevalence of herpes simplex virus types 1 and 2–United States, 1999–2010. J Infect Dis. 2014; 209(3):325–333

[47] Peppercorn MA. Enteric infections in homosexual men with and without AIDS. Contemp Gastroenterol. 1989; 2:23–32

[48] Goodell SE, Quinn TC, Mkrtichian E, Schuffler MD, Holmes KK, Corey L. Herpes simplex virus proctitis in homosexual men. Clinical, sigmoidoscopic, and histopathological features. N Engl J Med. 1983; 308 (15):868–871

[49] Samarasinghe PL, Oates JK, MacLennan IPB. Herpetic proctitis and sacral radiomyelopathy–a hazard for homosexual men. BMJ. 1979; 2(6186):365–366

[50] Ashley RL. Sorting out the new HSV type specific antibody tests. Sex Transm Infect. 2001; 77(4):232–237

[51] Nerurkar L, Goedert J, Wallen W, et al. Study of antiviral antibodies in sera of homosexual men. J Fed Proc. 1983; 42:6109

[52] de Ruiter A, Thin RN. Genital herpes. A guide to pharmacological therapy. Drugs. 1994; 47(2):297–304

[53] Rompalo AM, Mertz GJ, Davis LG, et al. Oral acyclovir for treatment of first-episode herpes simplex virus proctitis. JAMA. 1988; 259 (19):2879–2881

[54] Chatis PA, Miller CH, Schrager LE, Crumpacker CS. Successful treatment with foscarnet of an acyclovir-resistant mucocutaneous infection with herpes simplex virus in a patient with acquired immunodeficiency syndrome. N Engl J Med. 1989; 320(5):297–300

[55] Stanberry L, Cunningham A, Mertz G, et al. New developments in the epidemiology, natural history and management of genital herpes. Antiviral Res. 1999; 42(1):1–14

[56] Mertz GJ, Jones CC, Mills J, et al. Long-term acyclovir suppression of frequently recurring genital herpes simplex virus infection. A multicenter double-blind trial. JAMA. 1988; 260(2):201–206

[57] Centers for Disease Control and Prevention. Surveillance for Viral Hepatitis – United States, 2014. Available at: http://www.cdc.gov/hepatitis/statistics/2014surveillance/commentary.htm#summary. Accessed October 11, 2016

[58] Alter HJ, Purcell RH, Gerin JL, et al. Transmission of hepatitis B to chimpanzees by hepatitis B surface antigen-positive saliva and semen. Infect Immun. 1977; 16(3):928–933

[59] Villarejos VM, Visoná KA, Gutiérrez A, Rodríguez A. Role of saliva, urine and feces in the transmission of type B hepatitis. N Engl J Med. 1974; 291 (26):1375–1378

[60] Busch K, Thimme R. Natural history of chronic hepatitis B virus infection. Med Microbiol Immunol (Berl). 2015; 204(1):5–10

[61] Thompson ND, Perz JF, Moorman AC, Holmberg SD. Nonhospital health care-associated hepatitis B and C virus transmission: United States, 1998–2008. Ann Intern Med. 2009; 150(1):33–39

[62] Davis LG, Weber DJ, Lemon SM. Horizontal transmission of hepatitis B virus. Lancet. 1989; 1(8643):889–893

[63] Martinson FE, Weigle KA, Royce RA, Weber DJ, Suchindran CM, Lemon SM. Risk factors for horizontal transmission of hepatitis B virus in a rural district in Ghana. Am J Epidemiol. 1998; 147(5):478–487

[64] CDC. Healthcare-associated hepatitis B and C outbreaks reported to the Centers for Disease Control and Prevention (CDC) in 2008–2013. 2010. Available at: www.cdc.gov/hepatitis/Outbreaks/HealthcareHepOutbreakTable.htm

[65] Lok AS, McMahon BJ. Chronic hepatitis B: update 2009. Hepatology. 2009; 50(3):661–662

[66] Denniston MM, Jiles RB, Drobeniuc J, et al. Chronic hepatitis C virus infection in the United States, National Health and Nutrition Examination Survey 2003 to 2010. Ann Intern Med. 2014; 160(5):293–300

[67] Centers for Disease Control and Prevention (CDC). Testing for HCV infection: an update of guidance for clinicians and laboratorians. MMWR Morb Mortal Wkly Rep. 2013; 62(18):362–365

[68] Hošnjak L, Kocjan BJ, Kušar B, Seme K, Poljak M. Rapid detection and typing of Molluscum contagiosum virus by FRET-based real-time PCR. J Virol Methods. 2013; 187(2):431–434

[69] Simonart T, De Maertelaer V. Curettage treatment for molluscum contagiosum: a follow-up survey study. Br J Dermatol. 2008; 159(5):1144–1147

[70] Liota E, Smith KJ, Buckley R, Menon P, Skelton H. Imiquimod therapy for molluscum contagiosum. J Cutan Med Surg. 2000; 4(2):76–82

[71] Lifson AR, Rutherford GW, Jaffe HW. The natural history of human immunodeficiency virus infection. J Infect Dis. 1988; 158(6):1360–1367

[72] Centers for Disease Control and Prevention. HIV in the United States: at a glance. Available at: http://www.cdc.gov/hiv/statistics/overview/ataglance.html. Accessed October 12, 2016

[73] Gelb A, Miller S. AIDS and gastroenterology. Am J Gastroenterol. 1986; 81 (8):619–622

[74] Schneider E, Whitmore S, Glynn KM, Dominguez K, Mitsch A, McKenna MT, Centers for Disease Control and Prevention (CDC). Revised surveillance case definitions for HIV infection among adults, adolescents, and children aged < 18 months and for HIV infection and AIDS among children aged 18 months to < 13 years — United States, 2008. MMWR Recomm Rep. 2008; 57(RR-10):1–12

[75] Wexner SD, Beck DE. Sexually transmitted and infectious diseases. In: Beck DE, Wexner SD, eds. Fundamentals of Anorectal Surgery. New York, NY: McGraw-Hill; 1992:402–422

[76] Wexner SD, Beck DE. Acquired immunodeficiency syndrome. In: Beck DE, Wexner SD, eds. Fundamentals of Anorectal Surgery. New York, NY: McGraw-Hill; 1992:423–439

[77] Goldberg GS, Orkin BA, Smith LE. Microbiology of human immunodeficiency virus anorectal disease. Dis Colon Rectum. 1994; 37(5):439–443

[78] Beck DE, Jaso RG, Zajac RA. Proctologic management of the HIV-positive patient. South Med J. 1990; 83(8):900–903

[79] Consten ECJ, Slors FJM, Noten HJ, Oosting H, Danner SA, van Lanschot JJ. Anorectal surgery in human immunodeficiency virus-infected patients. Clinical outcome in relation to immune status. Dis Colon Rectum. 1995; 38 (11):1169–1175

[80] Barrett WL, Callahan TD, Orkin BA. Perianal manifestations of human immunodeficiency virus infection: experience with 260 patients. Dis Colon Rectum. 1998; 41(5):606–611, discussion 611–612

[81] Beck DE, Fazio VW, Lavery IC, Jagelman DG, Weakley FL. Catheter drainage of ischiorectal abscesses. South Med J. 1988; 81(4):444–446

[82] Gottesman L. Treatment of anorectal ulcers in the HIV positive patient. Perspect Colon Rect Surg. 1991; 4:19–33

[83] Beck DE, Ramirez RT. Sexually transmitted diseases and the anorectum. In: Phillips RKS, ed. Colorectal Surgery. 2nd ed. London: Harcourt; 2001:365–395

[84] Monfardini S, Tirelii V, Vacchert E. Treatment of acquired immunodeficiency syndrome (AIDS)-related cancer. Cancer Treat Rev. 1994; 20(2):149–172

[85] Jacobson LP, Jenkins FJ, Springer G, et al. Interaction of HIV type 1 and human herpes virus type 8 infections on the incidence of Kaposi's sarcoma. J Infect Dis. 2000; 181:9

[86] Hengge UR, Ruzicka T, Tyring SK, et al. Update on Kaposi's sarcoma and other HHV8 associated diseases. Part 2: pathogenesis, Castleman's disease, and pleural effusion lymphoma. Lancet Infect Dis. 2002; 2(6):344–352

[87] Antman K, Chang Y. Kaposi's sarcoma. N Engl J Med. 2000; 342 (14):1027–1038

[88] Cattelan AM, Calabrò ML, De Rossi A, et al. Long-term clinical outcome of AIDS-related Kaposi's sarcoma during highly active antiretroviral therapy. Int J Oncol. 2005; 27(3):779–785

[89] DeHovitz JA, Pape JW, Boncy M, Johnson WD, Jr. Clinical manifestations and therapy of Isospora belli infection in patients with the acquired immunodeficiency syndrome. N Engl J Med. 1986; 315(2):87–90

[90] Faust EC, Giraldo LE, Caicedo G, Bonfante R. Human isosporosis in the western hemisphere. Am J Trop Med Hyg. 1961; 10:343–349

[91] Sorvillo FJ, Lieb LE, Kerndt PR, Ash LR. Epidemiology of cryptosporidiosis among persons with acquired immunodeficiency syndrome in Los Angeles County. Am J Trop Med Hyg. 1994; 51(3):326–331

[92] Ma P, Soave R. Three-step stool examination for cryptosporidiosis in 10 homosexual men with protracted watery diarrhea. J Infect Dis. 1983; 147 (5):824–828

[93] Zhu G, Marchewka MJ, Ennis JG, Keithly JS. Direct isolation of DNA from patient stools for polymerase chain reaction detection of Cryptosporidium parvum. J Infect Dis. 1998; 177(5):1443–1446

[94] Ma P, Kaufman D, Montana J. Isospora belli diarrheal infection in homosexual men. AIDS Res. 1983–1984; 1(5):327–338

[95] Lange M, Klein EB, Kornfield H, Cooper LZ, Grieco MH. Cytomegalovirus isolation from healthy homosexual men. JAMA. 1984; 252(14):1908–1910

[96] Armstrong D, Gold JWM, Dryjanski J, et al. Treatment of infections in patients with the acquired immunodeficiency syndrome. Ann Intern Med. 1985; 103(5):738–743

[97] Blanshard C, Gazzard BG. Natural history and prognosis of diarrhoea of unknown cause in patients with acquired immunodeficiency syndrome (AIDS). Gut. 1995; 36(2):283–286

[98] DeRodriguez CV, Fuhrer J, Lake-Bakaar G. Cytomegalovirus colitis in patients with acquired immunodeficiency syndrome. J R Soc Med. 1994; 87 (4):203–205

[99] Evans MRW, Booth JC, Wansbrough-Jones MH. Cytomegalovirus viraemia in HIV infection: association with intercurrent infection. J Infect. 1995; 31 (1):21–26

[100] Ehrnst A. The clinical relevance of different laboratory tests in CMV diagnosis. Scand J Infect Dis Suppl. 1996; 100:64–71

[101] Boeckh M, Boivin G. Quantitation of cytomegalovirus: methodologic aspects and clinical applications. Clin Microbiol Rev. 1998; 11(3):533–554

[102] Pérez JL. Resistance to antivirals in human cytomegalovirus: mechanisms and clinical significance. Microbiologia. 1997; 13(3):343–352

[103] Gonczol E, Plotkin S. Development of a cytomegalovirus vaccine: lessons from recent clinical trials. Expert Opin Biol Ther. 2001; 1(3):401–412

[104] Nugent P, O'Connell TX. The surgeon's role in treating acquired immunodeficiency syndrome. Arch Surg. 1986; 121(10):1117–1120

[105] Robinson G, Wilson SE, Williams RA. Surgery in patients with acquired immunodeficiency syndrome. Arch Surg. 1987; 122(2):170–175

[106] Wexner SD, Smithy WB, Trillo C, Hopkins BS, Dailey TH. Emergency colectomy for cytomegalovirus ileocolitis in patients with the acquired immune deficiency syndrome. Dis Colon Rectum. 1988; 31(10):755–761

[107] Söderlund C, Bratt GA, Engström L, et al. Surgical treatment of cytomegalovirus enterocolitis in severe human immunodeficiency virus infection. Report of eight cases. Dis Colon Rectum. 1994; 37(1):63–72

[108] Wolkomir AF, Barone JE, Hardy HW, III, Cottone FJ. Abdominal and anorectal surgery and the acquired immune deficiency syndrome in heterosexual intravenous drug users. Dis Colon Rectum. 1990; 33(4):267–270

[109] Deziel DJ, Hyser MJ, Doolas A, Bines SD, Blaauw BB, Kessler HA. Major abdominal operations in acquired immunodeficiency syndrome. Am Surg. 1990; 56(7):445–450

[110] Diettrich NA, Cacioppo JC, Kaplan G, Cohen SM. A growing spectrum of surgical disease in patients with human immunodeficiency virus/acquired immunodeficiency syndrome. Experience with 120 major cases. Arch Surg. 1991; 126(7):860–865, discussion 865–866

[111] Davidson T, Allen-Mersh TG, Miles AJG, et al. Emergency laparotomy in patients with AIDS. Br J Surg. 1991; 78(8):924–926

[112] Whitney TM, Macho JR, Russell TR, Bossart KJ, Heer FW, Schecter WP. Appendicitis in acquired immunodeficiency syndrome. Am J Surg. 1992; 164 (5):467–470, discussion 470–471

[113] Bizer LS, Pettorino R, Ashikari A. Emergency abdominal operations in the patient with acquired immunodeficiency syndrome. J Am Coll Surg. 1995; 180 (2):205–209

[114] Samantaray DK, Walker ML. Surgery in AIDS patients. Contemp Surg. 1996; 49:207–209

[115] Phillips SC, Mildvan D, William DC, Gelb AM, White MC. Sexual transmission of enteric protozoa and helminths in a venereal-disease-clinic population. N Engl J Med. 1981; 305(11):603–606

[116] Pomerantz MB, Marr JS, Goldman WD. Amebiasis in New York City 1958–1978: identification of the male homosexual high risk population. Bull N Y Acad Med. 1980; 56(2):232–244

[117] Gardner TB, Hill DR. Treatment of giardiasis. Clin Microbiol Rev. 2001; 14 (1):114–128

14 Fecal Incontinence

Joshua I.S. Bleier and Steven D. Wexner

Abstract

Fecal incontinence (FI) is not only prevalent but socially devastating. In any of its manifestations, from mild soilage and inadvertent flatus, to frank stool loss, it can be intolerable. The competent surgeon must therefore be familiar with all treatment options. This chapter focuses on the etiology, diagnosis, management, and outcomes of fecal incontinence.

Keywords: fecal incontinence, soiling, sphincter damage, childbirth, etiology, quality of life, fecal incontinence scales, prior anal operations, sphincter-saving procedures, trauma

14.1 Background

Fecal incontinence (FI) is a socially crippling disorder. Soiling, the escape of flatus, and the inadvertent passage of stool are embarrassing situations few people can tolerate. It therefore behooves surgeons who care for these individuals to be familiar with any treatment options that might be available. Anal continence is dependent on a complex series of learned and reflex responses to colonic and rectal stimuli, and the considerable individual variation in bowel habits makes clear distinction of derangement of continence difficult. Normal continence depends on a number of factors: mental function, stool volume and consistency, colonic transit, rectal distensibility, anal sphincter function, anorectal sensation, and anorectal reflexes.[1] The patient who has lost complete control of solid feces has complete incontinence. The patient who complains of inadvertent soiling or escape of liquid or flatus has partial incontinence. Less fastidious individuals may not complain of partial incontinence; therefore, careful questioning of the patient may be necessary. In an effort to classify the severity of symptoms, Browning and Parks[2] proposed the following criteria: category A, patients continent of solid and liquid stool and flatus (i.e., normal continence); B, patients continent of solid and usually liquid stool but not flatus; C, acceptable continence of solid stool but no control over liquid stool or flatus; and D, continued fecal leakage. Numerous other grading scales exist. All these severity scores are simple to use. However, they mainly reflect sphincter function. The worse the function is, the higher the score. Thus, incontinence to solid stool is always considered worse than incontinence for liquid stool. Unfortunately, this assumption does not necessarily reflect the subjective experience of the patient. Furthermore, the reliability and validity of these grading scales are questionable. Because of these drawbacks and the lack of precision of the grading scales, they are no longer recommended as the sole method of categorizing patients and monitoring outcome of treatment.[3] Some of the deficiencies of grading scales can be addressed by summary scales. These scales produce multilevel summative scores. The values for each type of incontinence are assigned according to the frequency of incontinent episodes, as frequency is one of the factors contributing to the severity of incontinence. Several scales also include items such as cleaning difficulties, the use of pads, and lifestyle alterations. Numerous summary scales have been designed, such as those according to Rockwood, Wexner/Cleveland Clinic Florida Fecal Incontinence Score (CCF-FIS), Pescatori, Vaizey/St. Marks, and many others. Some scales also attempt to assess parameters unrelated to the sphincter, such as urgency and use of antidiarrheal medication. The assignment of values to types and frequencies of incontinence varies between scales. The most frequently cited CCF-FIS is outlined in ▶ Table 14.1.[4] This scale has been globally validated in numerous languages. Moreover, a statistically significant correlation exists between scores > 10 and decreased quality of life (QOL).[5]

In some summary systems, equal values are assigned to the same frequencies of the different types of incontinence, whereas in other scales variable weights are given. However, the lack of patient perspective in this assignment of values compromises the comparability and validity of these summary scales. To address this problem, Rockwood et al developed the Fecal Incontinence Severity Index (FISI). This index assigns values to various frequencies and types of incontinence on the basis of subjective ratings of severity.[6] The matrix includes four types of leakage commonly found in the fecal incontinent population—gas, mucus, and liquid and solid stool—and six frequencies—never, one to three times per month, once per week, twice per week, once per day, and twice per day.

Table 14.1 Cleveland Clinic Florida Fecal Incontinence Continence Score[4]

Type of incontinence	Never	Rarely	Sometimes	Usually	Always
Solid	0	1	2	3	4
Liquid	0	1	2	3	4
Gas	0	1	2	3	4
Wears pad	0	1	2	3	4
Lifestyle alteration	0	1	2	3	4

Note: 0 = perfect; 20 = complete incontinence.

The continence score is determined by adding points from the table, which takes into account the frequency of incontinence and the extent to which it alters the patient's life. Never 0 (never); rarely < 1/mo; sometimes < 1/wk to ≥ 1/mo; usually < 1 day to ≥ 1/wk; always ≥ 1/day

Given the subjective nature of incontinence, the incorporation of patient values into severity measurement has been a major step forward. Although it is important to know the severity of FI, it is also important to measure the impact of incontinence and its treatment on QOL. To assess QOL for patients with FI, generic QOL scales such as the SF-36 and condition-specific scales such as the Fecal Incontinence Quality of Life Scale (FIQLS).[7] The FIQLS, developed by the American Society of Colon and Rectal Surgeons (ASCRS), is an instrument that has been studied well and seems to be very useful.

The FIQLS is composed of a total of 29 items; these items form four scales: lifestyle (10 items), coping/behavior (9 items), depression/self-perception (7 items), and embarrassment (3 items). Detailed questions are listed in ▶ Table 14.2.

Table 14.2 Items in the Fecal Incontinence Quality of Life Scale[7]

Scale 1: Lifestyle

I cannot do many of the things I want to do (agreement, 4 points)

I am afraid to go out (frequency, 4 points)

It is important to plan my schedule (daily activities) around my bowel pattern (frequency, 4 points)

I cut down on how much I eat before I go out (frequency, 4 points)

It is difficult for me to get out and do things like going to a movie or church (frequency, 4 points)

I avoid traveling by plane or train (agreement, 4 points)

I avoid traveling (frequency, 4 points)

I avoid visiting friends (frequency, 4 points)

I avoid going out to eat (agreement, 4 points)

I avoid staying overnight away from home (frequency, 4 points)

Scale 2: Coping behavior

I have sex less often than I would like to (agreement, 4 points)

The possibility of bowel accidents is always on my mind (agreement, 4 points)

I feel I have no control over my bowels (frequency, 4 points)

Whenever I go somewhere new, I specifically locate where the bathrooms are (agreement, 4 points)

I worry about not being able to get to the toilet in time (frequency, 4 points)

I worry about the bowel accidents (agreement, 4 points)

I try to prevent bowel accidents by staying very near a bathroom (agreement, 4 points)

I cannot hold my bowel movement long enough to get to the bathroom (frequency, 4 points)

Whenever I am away from home, I try to stay near a restroom as much as possible (frequency, 4 points)

Scale 3: Depression

In general, would you say your health is ... (excellent–poor, 5 points)

I am afraid to have sex (agreement, 4 points)

I feel different from other people (agreement, 4 points)

I enjoy life less (agreement, 4 points)

I feel like I am not a healthy person (agreement, 4 points)

I feel depressed (agreement, 4 points)

During the past month, have you felt so sad, discouraged, hopeless, or had so many problems that you wondered if anything was worthwhile? (Extremely so–not at all, 6 points)

Scale 4: Embarrassment

I leak stool without even knowing it (frequency, 4 points)

I worry about others smelling stool on me (agreement, 4 points)

I feel ashamed (agreement, 4 points)

Note: Scoring is calculated by addition of each of the individual items.

Each of the four scales of the FIQLS is capable of discriminating between patients with FI and patients with other gastrointestinal problems. The scales in the FIQLS demonstrated significant correlations with the subscales in the SF-36. The psychometric evaluation of the FIQLS showed that this FI-specific QOL measure produces both reliable and valid measurement. However, unfortunately, there was discord between items deemed important by clinicians versus variables felt to be important by patients. Due to this disconnect between clinicians and patients, the well-intended FIQOL is not as widely used as had initially been envisioned. Major incontinence has considerable social consequences and demands an effort at some form of definitive therapy.

The exact incidence of FI is unknown. However, recent reviews estimate that this disorder is much more prevalent than previously believed. Some literature suggests that this may affect up to 18% of the adult population, and is a major factor in nursing home admissions.[8,9] Brown et al, in conjunction with the Nielsen group, queried over 5,800 U.S. women 45 years or older and found a prevalence of nearly 20% when asked about at least one episode of FI within the previous year. A further questionnaire surveyed what specific issues regarding the FI were most prevalent as well as what was most bothersome. Unsurprisingly, 97% of the women surveyed were bothered by the frequency of the leakage, but the most troublesome symptom was not the leakage itself, but rather the associated urgency.[10] Groups of individuals at high risk for incontinence include the elderly, the mentally ill, institutionalized patients, those with neurologic disorders, and parous women. In order to characterize factors associated with the negative impact of accidental bowel leakage (ABL) on QOL, Brown et al conducted an internet survey aimed at identifying the most important factors involved. Issues related to frustration, emotional health, and ability to interact socially showed the greatest negative impact, with over 39% identifying this as "severe."[11] When characterizing factors associated with seeking care in women with ABL, less than 30% of women with ABL sought care, and if they did, the majority spoke to their primary care physicians. Such discussions were more likely to occur if the CCF-FIS was > 10.[12]

In hospitalized geriatric and psychiatric patients, an incidence of 26 and 31%, respectively, has been reported. In 30 residential homes for the elderly, FI occurred at least once weekly in 10.3% of the residents, of whom 94% had evidence of organic brain damage.[13] Thirty-nine percent of Wisconsin nursing home residents have FI,[14] while a 46% incidence was reported from a Canadian long-term hospital.[15] Incontinence of stool is the second most common cause for institutionalizing an elderly person.[16,17]

Macmillan et al[18] conducted a systematic review to investigate FI in the community. A total of 16 studies met the inclusion criteria. These could be grouped into the definitions of incontinence that included or excluded incontinence of flatus. The estimated prevalence of FI (including flatus incontinence) varied from 2 to 24%, and the estimated prevalence of FI (excluding flatus incontinence) varied from 0.4 to 18%. The prevalence estimate of FI from these studies was 11 to 15%.

Most discussions of etiology of FI have been based on the assumption that women, particularly women younger than 65 years of age, are more at risk for FI than men. Obstetric injury to the pudendal nerve or sphincter muscle is described as the primary risk factor, irritable bowel syndrome as second (a disease thought to be more prevalent in women), and other etiologies such as diabetes were listed as a distant third.[14] Yet, each population-based survey of FI prevalence, including that by Nelson et al, has shown a high prevalence in men. Clearly, etiologies other than childbirth must be sought.

In an excellent review of the subject, Sangwan and Coller[16] detail the tremendous socioeconomic and psychological burden of FI on society. Their comprehensive but often not discussed list of concerns includes the annual cost to patient, the prevention and management of skin breakdown, the increased incidence of female genital infection, social alienation, a personal sense of inadequacy with depression, pessimism, and low self-esteem, embarrassment about odor, and fear of coital incontinence with decreased libido and sexual dysfunction. The combination of these factors produces a social impact that is impossible to quantify. In a long-term care hospital, it was estimated that the annual cost of incontinence per patient was $9,771.[15] It was reported that, even in 1996, over $400,000,000 was spent each year for adult diapers.[19] In the United States, in 1994, the economic impact was estimated at $16 to $26 billion annually. More recent calculation placed the annual average total cost for FI at $4,110 per person.[20] Any discussion of the impact of this disabling disorder must address not only the prevalence and impact of the problem, but also the fact that it is disabling and prevalent, as well as that we are probably only seeing the tip of the iceberg; more than two-thirds of patients with FI do not even seek care, in some cases as few as 15%,[12,21,22] and of those that do, more than one-half are speaking only with their primary care physicians—clinicians who may not have a complete understanding of the full capabilities for treatment.[11]

Therapeutic recommendations for incontinence can be made best when the anatomy and physiology of the anorectal region are understood, as detailed in Chapters 1 and 2.

14.2 Etiology

The exact percentage of incontinence attributable to each of the various causes is unknown. In one series, the most common causes of FI were injury sustained to muscles and nerves during operation (48%) and peripheral nerve injuries associated with systemic disease such as diabetes. Spinal cord injuries or defects involving spinal cord injuries accounted for 22% of cases.[23] In most series, obstetric and operative injuries account for most cases of incontinence.[24,25] The variation often depends on the type of referral practice and the special interests of the authors.

14.2.1 Previous Operative Procedures

Previous Anal Operations

Lindsey et al[26] characterized the patterns of anal sphincter injury in 93 patients with FI after manual dilatation, internal sphincterotomy, fistulotomy, and hemorrhoidectomy. The internal sphincter was almost universally injured, in a pattern specific to the underlying procedure. One-third of patients had a related surgical external sphincter injury. Two-thirds of women had an unrelated obstetric external sphincter injury. The distal resting pressure was typically reduced with reversal of the normal resting pressure gradient of the anal canal in 89% of patients. Maximum squeeze pressure was normal in 52%. They concluded incontinences after anal operations are characterized by the virtually universal presence of an internal sphincter injury, which is distal to the high-pressure zone, resulting in reversal of the normal resting pressure gradient in the anal canal.

Internal Sphincterotomy

Lateral internal sphincterotomy is highly effective in the treatment of chronic anal fissure. However, this procedure results in a permanent defect in the internal anal sphincter, which may lead to impairment of fecal continence. The exact incidence of this complication is not known. During the first two decades, after the introduction of lateral internal sphincterotomy, several studies were conducted, aimed at evaluating the sequelae of this procedure. Impaired continence was observed in only a minority of the patients, most of them having temporary incontinence to flatus. In these retrospective studies, the patients were followed by chart review or telephone interview and not by mailed questionnaire. The duration of the follow-up was short and neither grading scales nor QOL scales were used. Some reviews, emphasizing the importance of long-term follow-up, have shown higher incontinence rates. In the series of Khubchandani and Reed, lack of control of flatus was the most common complaint (35%), followed by soiling of underclothing (22%) and accidental bowel movements (5%).[27] A significantly higher proportion of patients who had accidental bowel movements were aged over 40 years. Similar figures have been reported by Garcia-Aguilar et al.[28] A significantly lower incidence of continence disturbances has been reported by others. Pernikoff et al observed an overall incidence of 8%.[29] In their series of 265 patients, Hananel and Gordon encountered impairment of continence in 1.2% of the patients, most of them having only temporary problems.[30] In a prospective study among 35 patients, Hyman assessed continence prior to and 6 weeks after lateral internal sphincterotomy using the FISI.[31] The FIQLS was administered to patients with a FISI score > 0. Three patients had worsening of their FISI score after surgery. Only one of them reported an evident deterioration in FIQLS. Based on these data, the author concluded that lateral internal sphincterotomy is a safe procedure. Anecdotal reports illustrate that incontinence for solid stool, although very rare, can occur after lateral internal sphincterotomy. This complication is often attributed to division of an excessive amount of internal anal sphincter or inadvertent injury to the external anal sphincter. Most recently, Liang and Church reported on a prospective series of 57 patients undergoing lateral internal sphincterotomy for chronic fissure. Only 2 (4%) reported any changes incontinence and overall satisfaction in this cohort was 9.7 ± 0.9 out of 10 ($p < 0.001$).[32]

Coexisting occult defects of the external anal sphincter in multiparous women seem to be another risk factor.[33] When comparing office records and response to a postal survey, Casillas et al found that significantly more patients had incontinence to gas after lateral internal sphincterotomy than that reported in their medical records. This problem was encountered by 29% of the multiparous female patients who underwent this procedure. Incontinence for solid stool was not observed. Among their patients, the overall QOL scores were in the normal range.[34] Sultan et al performed anal endosonography before and 2 months after lateral internal sphincterotomy. They found that this procedure in most females tends to be more extensive than intended in contrast to division of the internal anal sphincter in males. According to the authors, this problem is probably related to the shorter anal canal in females. They also found that lateral internal sphincterotomy may further compromise continence, especially in females with occult sphincter defects.[35]

Fistula Surgery

Fistula surgery is the anorectal procedure most commonly followed by postoperative incontinence. Significant FI may be avoided if the anorectal ring is preserved. However, minor defects in continence may follow if even a small amount of sphincter muscle is severed. This complication can be reduced by avoiding wide separation of the severed ends of the sphincter mechanism. This goal is accomplished either by placing a seton or by "coring out" the fistulous tract, with subsequent sparing of the sphincter mechanism or, in the case of tracts crossing the sphincter mechanism at a high level, by the adoption of the advancement flap technique (see Chapter 10).

Although the transanal advancement flap repair is designed to minimize damage to the anal sphincters, impairment of continence after this procedure has been documented. The reported incidence of this complication varies between 8 and 35%.[36,37,38,39] It has been suggested that anal stretch caused by the use of a Parks retractor is a major contributing factor.[40] It has been demonstrated that the use of a Parks retractor has indeed a deteriorating effect on fecal continence.

Because this side effect is not observed after the use of a Scott retractor, this type of retractor has been advised in fistula repairs.[41] The last decade has seen a significant shift in sphincter-sparing approaches to fistula surgery. The development of these techniques has been driven specifically by the need to develop safer approaches to fistula surgery. The development of the anal fistula plug, a scaffolding of porcine intestinal submucosa, was greeted with high initial enthusiasm, with a near-impeccable safety profile and initial success rates in the mid 80% range.[42] However, more mature data have shown a much lower durable success, with rates as low as 14%.[43] Similarly, the use of fibrin glue to seal fistulas has essentially a zero chance of worsening continence; however, success rates are poor, as low as 14%.[44] In 2007, Rojanasakul et al[45] published their series on the LIFT procedure (ligation of the internal fistula tract), and in 2009, Rojanasakul published a large series[46] with an impressive success rate of over 90% and no reported incidence of incontinence. Seven years and more than 50 publications later, this technique continues to show reliable success, ranging from 60 to 94%, and almost no reported risk of decreased continence.[43,44,45,46,47,48,49]

Hemorrhoidectomy

In modern surgery for hemorrhoids, incontinence is a rare complication. However, if the sphincter mass is inadvertently injured (in a blind-clamping technique in which the internal sphincter is grasped by a clamp), incontinence may result. Minor alterations in continence may be due to the removal of the hemorrhoidal tissue, a tissue that has been described as possibly functioning as a corpus cavernosum of the anus.[50] When incorrectly performed, the Whitehead operation leads to eversion of the rectal mucosa onto the anoderm. This abnormal anatomy results in incontinence through destruction of the normal sensory mechanism and mucosal leak from the exposed mucosal surface onto the perineum. Rarely, a circumferential scar will form after hemorrhoidectomy, which may lead to improper closure of the anal canal, causing some degree of FI.

Manual Dilatation of Anus

Forceful dilatation of the anal canal for the treatment of any anorectal pathology can result in varying degrees of incontinence. The disadvantages and consequences of this form of treatment are discussed fully in Chapter 8.

Sphincter-Saving Procedures

In the usual anterior resection, normal continence for flatus, liquid, or solid feces is generally maintained. However, when a distal anastomosis is performed, impairment of normal continence is not unusual. Incontinence of liquid or flatus often follows, and the patient may be unaware of a sudden bolus of stool. These problems are frequent in the early postoperative period, but they subside within 6 months in the great majority of patients. The lower limit at which an anastomosis can be created without interfering with the mechanism of incontinence is the uppermost level of the anal canal at the top of the anorectal ring, which in most individuals is approximately 4 cm from the anal verge. The circular stapler has made it technically possible to perform extremely low rectal anastomoses. However, if the anorectal ring is disturbed, partial or total incontinence may result. The severity and duration of the dysfunction are not predictable.

Goligher et al[51] reported that of 62 patients who underwent a low anterior resection, all of the 12 patients with the anastomosis less than 7 cm from the anal verge initially had less than perfect continence. With time, however, five developed perfect continence and three nearly perfect continence, but four remained with imperfect continence. Abdominoanal pull-through resection of the rectum, as popularized by Hughes, results in a high incidence of partial incontinence. In a review of his results with this procedure, he found that only 29% of the patients had normal function postoperatively, 23% had severe incontinence, and the remaining 48% had minor incontinence.[52]

Parks and Percy[53] described a coloanal sleeve anastomosis for the treatment of rectal lesions. Of 70 patients who underwent this operation, 1 was incontinent, whereas 30 others experienced increased frequency of stool. Enker et al[54] reported that 64% of patients who could be evaluated in their series of 41 patients who underwent coloanal anastomosis had good or excellent function. Vernava et al[52] reported that 87% of their 16 patients were normally continent. Intersphincteric resection (ISR), designed to push the envelope for sphincter presentation by establishing adequate distal margins with partial sacrifice of the internal sphincter followed by handsewn coloanal anastomosis, exemplifies the adage: "Just because we CAN doesn't mean we always SHOULD." In a prospective comparison of 77 patients who underwent ultralow low anterior resection (LAR) with coloanal anastomoses, Bretagnol et al compared 37 patients with conventional anastomosis to 40 who underwent ISR. They found that compared to the conventional approach, while there was no difference in stool frequency, fragmentation, or urgency, patients with ISR had significantly worse CCF-FIS scores (10.8 vs. 6.9, p <0.001). In addition, QOL was significantly decreased when using FIQL scoring.[55]

After ileorectal and ileoanal anastomosis, varying degrees of incontinence may develop. In the former case, the cause is usually the loss of reservoir function, but the situation may be compounded by a weakened sphincter. In the latter case, intraoperative manipulation by necessity may stretch the sphincter mechanism.

14.2.2 Childbirth

FI has a female-to-male preponderance of 8:1, consistent with childbirth as the principal causative factor. In 1993, Sultan et al published their well-known article entitled "Anal-sphincter disruption during vaginal delivery." In their paper, they described the results of an endosonographic study among 79 primiparous women. Endoanal ultrasound (EAUS) was performed 6 weeks before and 6 months after routine vaginal delivery. After childbirth, sphincter defects were detected in 35% of these females. A similar study was performed in 23 primiparous women who underwent a cesarean section. None of these women had a sphincter defect after delivery.[56] In a study by Eason et al[57] of 949 pregnant women 3 months after delivery, 3.1% reported incontinence of stool and 25.5% had involuntary escape of flatus. Incontinence of stool was more frequent among women who had delivered vaginally and who had third- or fourth-degree perineal tears than among those who had delivered vaginally but had no anal sphincter tears (7.8 vs. 2.9%). Forceps delivery (relative risk, 1.45) and sphincter tears (relative risk, 2.09) were independent risk factors for incontinence of flatus or stool or both. Anal sphincter injury was strongly and independently associated with first vaginal births (relative risk, 39.2), median episiotomy (relative risk, 9.6), forceps delivery (relative risk, 2.3), and vacuum-assisted delivery (relative risk, 7.4), but not with birth weight (relative risk for birth weight 4,000 g or more, 1.4) or length of stage of the second labor (relative risk for second stage 1.5 hours or longer compared with less than 0.5 hours, 1.2).

The reported incidence of occult sphincter defects after normal vaginal delivery varies between 7 and 41% (▶ Table 14.3). Oberwalder et al conducted a meta-analysis in order to determine the incidence of anal sphincter defects after vaginal delivery. Their Medline search yielded five studies with more than 100 women who underwent endoanal ultrasonography after childbirth. All these women were also questioned about symptoms of FI, not including urgency. The incidence of sphincter defects in primiparous women was found to be 27%. In multiparous women, the incidence of new sphincter defects was 8.5%. Overall, 30% of the defects were symptomatic. Only 3% of the women experienced impairment of continence without any sphincter defects. Based on the results of this study, it is clear that sphincter damage during vaginal delivery is quite common in primiparous women. In 70% of these women, the sphincter defects are asymptomatic in the postpartum period.[58] The question is whether women with an occult and asymptomatic sphincter defect are at increased risk for FI with aging. According to Rieger and Wattchow, it seems likely that many women remain asymptomatic, because the number of occult sphincter defects is far greater than the documented prevalence of FI in the community.[59] Oberwalder et al examined elderly females with late-onset incontinence, all of whom had vaginal deliveries. The authors observed sphincter defects in more than 70% of their patients.[60] A similar finding has been reported by others.[21] Despite these findings, it is still not possible to determine the exact risk for asymptomatic women with a sphincter defect to develop FI later in life. More studies, including control groups of equal parity and age, are mandatory. During the last decade, attention has also been focused on the risk factors for obstetric sphincter defects. Donnelly et al conducted a prospective study among primiparous women. After caesarian section, even when performed late in labor, none of the women experienced impairment of continence. Neither induction of labor nor its augmentation with oxytocin influenced the risk of sphincter injury or postpartum impairment of continence. Instrumental delivery was associated with a more than eightfold increased risk of anal sphincter damage and a more than sevenfold increased risk of symptoms when compared with unassisted delivery.[61] The increased risk of sphincter defects after instrumental

Table 14.3 Incidence of occult sphincter defects after normal vaginal delivery in primiparous women

Author(s)	Year	No. of patients	Occult sphincter defects (%)
Sultan et al[56]	1993	79	35
Campbell et al[63]	1996	88	13
Rieger et al[64]	1998	53	41
Zetterström et al[65]	1999	38	20
Varma et al[66]	1999	105	7
Fynes et al[67]	1999	59	34
Faltin et al[68]	2000	150	28
Damon et al[69]	2000	197	34
Abramowitz et al[70]	2000	202	17
Chaliha et al[71]	2001	161	38
Belmonte-Montes et al[72]	2001	98	29
Willis et al[73]	2002	42	19
Nazir et al[74]	2002	86	19
Peschers et al[75]	2003	100	15

vaginal delivery, especially after the use of a forceps, has also been reported by others (▶ Table 14.4). Not all studies confirm the previous observations that anal sphincter injury is common after forceps delivery. de Parades et al observed sphincter defects in only 13% of 93 females after their first forceps delivery. According to the authors, this observation gives support to the conclusion that forceps delivery is still a safe technique.[62] However, recruitment bias might be a possible explanation for their contradictory finding, because 60% of their patients did not return for postpartum assessment. Except for this single study, all other reports provide substantial evidence for the detrimental effect of forceps delivery on anal sphincter integrity.

FI among primiparous women increases over time and is affected by further childbirth.[79] FI at 9 months postpartum is an important predictor of persistent symptoms. In the study by Pollack et al among women with sphincter tears, 44% reported FI at 9 months and 53% at 5 years. Twenty-five percent of women without a sphincter tear reported FI at 9 months, and 32% had symptoms at 5 years. Risk factors for FI at 5 years were age (odds ratio [OR], 1.1), sphincter tear (OR, 2.3), and subsequent childbirth (OR, 2.4). As a predictor of FI at 5 years after the first delivery, FI at both 5 months (OR, 3.8) and 9 months (OR, 4.3) was identified. Among women with symptoms, the majority had infrequent incontinence to flatus, whereas FI was rare.

Besides instrumental delivery, other obstetric events are also associated with an increased risk of anal sphincter injury. Prolongation of the second stage of labor due to epidural analgesia, midline episiotomy, and perineal tears are well known independent risk factors. After primary repair of third- or fourth-degree perineal tears, persistent sphincter defects have been reported in up to 85% of the cases.[80,81] Nine months after primary repair of perineal tears, Pollack et al observed impairment of continence in 44% of the women. Five years later, 53% of the women suffered from continence disturbances.[79] These findings indicate that the damage sustained during third- and fourth-degree tears is much greater than is generally appreciated. Furthermore, it is clear that primary repair does not provide lasting integrity of the anal sphincters. Fernando et al conducted a systemic review and a national practice survey regarding the

Table 14.4 Incidence of sphincter defects after various modes of delivery

Author(s)	Year	Unassisted (%)	Vacuum (%)	Forceps (%)	Cesarean section (%)
Sultan et al[76]	1998	NS	48	81	0
Varma et al[66]	1999	12	NS	83	NS
Abramowitz et al[70]	2000	NS	NS	63	0
Damon et al[69]	2000	29	NS	44	NS
Belmonte-Montes et al[72]	2001	16	50	76	NS
Bollard et al[77]	2003	22	NS	44	0
Peschers et al[75]	2003	10	28	NS	NS
de Parades et al[62]	2004	NS	NS	13	NS
Pinta et al[78]	2004	23	45	NS	0

management of obstetric anal sphincter injury. They identified 11 studies with long-term follow-up (mean duration: 41 months) after primary repair of third-degree tears. In these studies, symptoms of FI were reported by 20 to 59% of the women.[82]

Sze[83,84] found the proportion of women who had severe incontinence was significantly higher among women who had undergone at least two additional deliveries after sustaining a fourth-degree sphincter tear as a nullipara. Sze[83] also found the rate of FI and severe incontinence similar among women who had zero, one, and two or more additional deliveries after sustaining a third-degree perineal laceration and between women who had one sphincter tear and no additional delivery versus those with two tears and more than two subsequent deliveries.

Increasing awareness among women and health professionals about the sequelae of obstetric sphincter injury has given rise to a debate regarding the protective role of cesarean delivery. It has been postulated that elective cesarean section at term before the onset of labor protects the anal sphincters and prevents FI.[85,86] Although cesarean section performed during labor also protects the anal sphincters, it does not prevent FI. This finding indicates neurologic injury to the sphincters during labor. A 2010 Cochrane review of almost 32,000 women, over 6,000 of whom underwent delivery by cesarean section, was performed. This review comprised 21 studies, and in only 1 was there any difference in preservation of anal continence. They concluded that preservation of anal continence should not be used as a criterion for electing cesarean section for delivery.[87]

It is certainly noteworthy that women with transient FI or occult sphincter injury after their first delivery are at higher risk of FI after a second delivery, but from a practical point of view, no change of obstetrical recommendation will be made as women will not be advised to avoid having children based on this information nor would it seem reasonable to recommend a cesarean section on the basis of fear of further alteration in continence. Despite the potential for cumulative sphincter injury or pudendal neuropathy, help is available for those individuals who suffer sphincter damage, and it must be remembered that cesarean section has its own potential immediate complications for mother and baby as well as possible late complications of a laparotomy such as adhesive small-bowel obstruction. Modifying this course of action may be the recognition that injury during the second delivery is primarily neurological with prolonged pudendal nerve terminal motor latency (PNTML). Intra-anal ultrasound has recently been touted as the most accurate method of determining occult injury to the sphincter mechanism, but in the absence of symptoms, a battery of investigative modalities that include intrarectal ultrasound, anorectal manometry, and PNTML would not likely be enthusiastically endorsed by most postpartum women. Nevertheless, understanding the potential for injury is useful knowledge for the clinician.

Previous Hysterectomy

Patients undergoing abdominal hysterectomy may have an increased risk for developing mild-to-moderate postoperative FI; this risk is increased by simultaneous bilateral salpingo-oophorectomy. In a study by Altman et al,[88] an increased risk of FI symptoms could not be identified in patients undergoing vaginal hysterectomy.

14.2.3 Aging

A very common form of FI is that associated with old age and general debilitation. Elderly patients with a longstanding history of straining at defecation may cause a stretch injury to the pudendal nerve as well. This often is described as incontinence of neurogenic origin.

14.2.4 Procidentia

Procidentia, or complete rectal prolapse, may chronically impair the internal and external sphincter mechanism. Procidentia is associated with incontinence in more than 50% of cases,[89] usually attributed in part to nerve injury. Repair of the procidentia results in improvement of the incontinence in approximately 50% of patients. Various treatments have been applied in the past, including waiting and hoping that sphincter tone would return, electrical stimulation of the sphincter mechanisms, and various plicating operations.

None of these methods, including the well-known Parks postanal repair, has met with uniform success. Biofeedback might be worthwhile in the treatment of persistent incontinence after repair of rectal prolapse. If biofeedback fails, sacral neuromodulation (SNM) is an alternative.[90] If incontinence remains a problem, a colostomy is the final option.

14.2.5 Trauma

In the case of impalement injuries, the sphincter mechanism is often disrupted. Depending on the extent of the injury, primary repair may be achieved without performing a protective colostomy. However, if the tissues are badly destroyed and there has been a delay in recognition, performing a protective colostomy with later definitive repair is preferable. Insertion of foreign bodies or alternative sexual practices may result in sphincter injury.

14.2.6 Primary Disease

Diarrheal states from any cause at times may overwhelm the normal continence mechanisms and result in temporary transient episodes of FI. Chronic inflammatory processes of the anorectal region, such as those that occur in patients with ulcerative colitis, amebic colitis, lymphogranuloma venereum, progressive systemic sclerosis, infections, or laxative abuse, can result in local sensory derangement, interference of the sphincter mechanism, and/or mucosal irritability, resulting in a loss of the rectal reservoir function. A patient with carcinoma of the anal canal may also present with incontinence caused by either infiltration into the sphincter mechanism or failure of the anal canal to close adequately.

14.2.7 Radiation

A main component of treatment of cervical and uterine carcinomas is by extracavitary and intracavitary irradiation. Similarly, external beam and brachyradiotherapy are frequently employed for prostate and rectal neoplasms.[91] Varying degrees of destruction of the muscular components of the rectum and anal canal occur, resulting in radiation proctitis. A radiation-induced lumbosacral plexopathy has been reported.[92] Initial conservative management with two or three daily cleansing enemas is generally recommended along with a high-bulk diet. SNM, to be discussed later in this chapter, has shown profound success for incontinence, even in cases of radiation-induced sphincter and nerve damage. If the condition becomes intolerable, colostomy is the last recourse. If severe bleeding remains a problem, therapeutic options include the topical application of short-chain fatty acids or 4% formalin. Laser therapy may also prove helpful. In recalcitrant cases, proctectomy may be necessary.

14.2.8 Neurogenic Causes

In cases of myelomeningocele, both the sensory and motor nerve supplies are disturbed in a variety of ways, leading to incontinence. Any form of trauma, neoplasm, vascular accident, infection, or demyelinating disease to the central nervous system or spinal cord can interfere with normal sensation or motor function, leading to incontinence.

Diabetic patients with autonomic neuropathy may have impaired reflex relaxation of the internal sphincter.[93] Diabetics with FI have a higher threshold of conscious sensation than do continent diabetic patients. Late onset of rectal sensation is one cause of FI in diabetics. Pinna Pintor et al[94] reported that somatic neuropathy plays an important role in FI in diabetic patients, combined with sensation threshold impairment as a feature of autonomic involvement.

14.2.9 Idiopathic Incontinence

Clinically, it is possible to identify those incontinent patients who have a sphincter defect. This can be accomplished by careful physical exam, EAUS, and MRI. Disruption of the external anal sphincter is the most common surgically correctable cause of FI. The prevalence of sphincter defects in patients with FI has been assessed with the use of EAUS. Deen et al examined 42 women and 4 men with FI. They found sphincter defects in 87% of their patients.[95] Karoui et al observed sphincter defects in 65% of 335 incontinent patients.[96] Comparable figures have been reported by others.[97,98] Based on these data, it is obvious that sphincter defects are present in at least two-thirds of incontinent patients. Less than one-third of the patients do not have any evidence of sphincter defects or other anorectal abnormalities. Their incontinence, formerly termed "idiopathic," is thought to be secondary to pudendal neuropathy, characterized by a slowed conduction in the pudendal nerve. It is most likely that this prolonged latency is due to stretching of the nerve during straining. The question is whether such pudendal neuropathy is the principal cause of "idiopathic" FI.

Súilleabháin and coworkers reported a prolonged latency in only 60% of the incontinent patients without sphincter defects. Furthermore, they were not able to demonstrate a correlation between the PNTML and the maximum squeeze pressure in this group of patients. According to these authors, the etiology of "idiopathic" incontinence is more complex than damage to the pudendal nerve alone. This nerve is probably not the only one to sustain trauma during vaginal delivery. Neuropathic changes in the internal anal sphincter and abnormal sensation in the anal canal as well as in the rectum have been observed in patients with "idiopathic" incontinence. These findings indicate

that the neurologic damage associated with vaginal delivery is not limited to the pudendal nerve, but may also involve damage to the autonomic inferior hypogastric nerves.[99,100,101,102]

14.2.10 Congenital Abnormalities

The various operative procedures designed for treating an imperforate anus are based on the type of deformity. The ultimate goal is to establish a perineal opening with adequate sensory and motor control. Rarely are sensory mechanisms preserved; therefore, some defect in continence usually results. Gross incontinence usually can be avoided by careful placement of the colon or rectum through residual sphincter mechanisms such as the puborectalis sling.

14.2.11 Miscellaneous

Overflow secondary to fecal impaction is a frequent cause of incontinence. This problem often is missed because the patient complains of profuse diarrhea. Digital examination usually reveals a rectum full of stool. This problem generally occurs in elderly or debilitated patients, or in young children recovering from surgical procedures (usually anorectal). Thus, physicians must be aware of this potential problem and should routinely institute early preventive measures. In general, hospital patients should be administered a bulk-forming stool softener of a psyllium seed derivative. If impaction occurs, gentle enemas with a combination of tap water, phosphate soda, and hydrogen peroxide may be used. If these measures fail, disimpaction (either with or without administering anesthesia) is the treatment of choice.

In patients with diarrhea, from whatever cause, the normal mechanisms of continence may be overwhelmed, and the patient may experience incontinence.

Soiling rather than complete involuntary loss of rectal contents may occur. For example, large prolapsing third- or fourth-degree hemorrhoids can cause partial incontinence by interfering with the normal closure mechanism of the internal sphincter. This situation can result in the escape of either flatus or liquid feces or in mucosal irritation. After operations for fistula-in-ano or fissures, soiling may occur as well.

A variety of pelvic floor disorders, including descending perineum syndrome, solitary rectal ulcer syndrome, and a nonrelaxing puborectalis muscle, may be associated with varying degrees of incontinence. Psychiatric problems may predispose the patient to the clinical problem of FI.

14.3 Diagnosis and History

As in the investigation of any pathologic condition, obtaining a careful history is necessary. Indeed, treatment recommendations are based on the particular cause of the incontinence together with the assessment of the sphincter status. Particular attention must be paid to the characteristics of the incontinence. Complete incontinence is defined as the uncontrolled passage of solid feces, whereas partial incontinence is defined as the uncontrolled passage of liquid or flatus. True incontinence should be distinguished from perianal leakage, which may be associated with a variety of anorectal disorders. Incontinence also must be distinguished from urgency, in which the patient's diet or individual bowel habits lead to frequent passage of liquid stool accompanied by a great sense of urgency. In such cases, simple dietary change may be all that is necessary. In addition to consistency, knowing the patient's frequency of bowel movements helps determine whether an antidiarrheal agent is required. Urge incontinence has been reported to be a marker of external anal sphincter dysfunction.[103] However, because urge incontinence may be due to any and all proctitides, its attempted quantification in the Vaizey/St. Marks incontinence scores obfuscates the quantification of FI based on sphincter insufficiency. Again, the inclusion of antidiarrheal agent use in the St. Marks/Vaizey score hurts its utility, as diarrhea is not related to sphincter integrity or function. Female patients should be asked about childbirth and type of delivery. It is very important to know whether the delivery was instrumental assisted or not. It is also necessary to obtain a history with regard to episiotomy, perineal tears, and continence in the postpartum period. The patient also should be asked about associated problems or conditions such as urinary incontinence, prolapsing tissue, diabetes mellitus, medications, or radiation treatment. Patients with congenital abnormalities such as Hirschsprung's disease generally present with some form of constipation and megacolon. An accurate history is necessary to distinguish the condition from acquired megacolon in the adolescent and adult age groups. In a patient with acquired megacolon, soiling of the perineum from the overflow incontinence often is secondary to fecal impaction. With Hirschsprung's disease, incontinence of liquid or flatus is rare because of the constantly closed internal sphincter.

Whether the patient has had a previous anorectal operation or low colon anastomosis must be noted, because these procedures can lead to FI. Also, beverages such as coffee or beer can lead to frequent loose bowel movements. Any history of remote or recent trauma to the anorectal area may aid in establishing the cause of incontinence. Associated motor or sensory symptoms may point to a neurologic lesion.[104] A clue to the severity of the problem is to determine the frequency of the incontinence and the necessity to wear a protective pad.

Grading and scoring the severity of the problem is another important aspect of a careful history. It is worthwhile to know the severity of FI as well as the impact of this problem and its treatment on the QOL. Several aspects of grading scales and QOL scales are discussed in more detail elsewhere in this chapter.

14.3.1 Physical Examination

It must be noted whether a patient's incontinence is a manifestation of a generalized disease or neurologic disorder or whether it is a local phenomenon. Undergarments should be inspected for staining by stool, mucus, or pus. In addition, the perineum must be inspected. In female patients with a history of vaginal delivery, it is helpful to measure the length of the perineum between anus and vagina. A decreased length of the perineum is frequently associated with a defect of the external anal sphincter. By simple retraction of the gluteal muscles, the large patulous anus that occurs with rectal procidentia can be recognized easily. Also, any large prolapsing hemorrhoids or evidence of pruritus may point to the fact that local anatomic factors may be responsible for the minor soiling by liquid or flatus. Scars from previous operations or episiotomies may also

be identified. Sensation to pinprick and the anocutaneous reflex should be checked. The anocutaneous reflex can be checked by stroking the perianal skin and observing the sphincter "wink." On straining, perineal descent or mucosal or full-thickness rectal prolapse may become obvious. Examination while the patient squats may be necessary to demonstrate prolapse.

Digital rectal examination reveals the strength (resting tone and augmentation on squeeze) or discontinuity of the sphincter muscle. Palpation points out any "keyhole" deformity of the anal canal, which might lead to soiling that may be misinterpreted as partial incontinence. The assessment of anal tone is, at best, a very indistinct barometer of sphincter function. The ability to assess the strength of voluntary sphincter contraction is subjective. Contraction of the puborectalis at the tip of the finger versus contraction of the external sphincter over the midportion of the finger may be distinguished. The anorectal angle can be assessed. The patient's complaints should provide a more reliable index of incontinence. Anoscopic and proctosigmoidoscopic examinations reveal any inflammatory process or neoplasm contributing to the patient's complaint.

Many tests are available for the assessment of FI. However, need for those tests has recently been controversial. In daily practice, most investigations do not influence the choice of treatment. In many centers, for example, the initial steps in the treatment of FI consist of medical therapy or biofeedback, irrespective of the underlying cause. However, from a surgical point of view, it is helpful to know whether the external anal sphincter is damaged or not. Physical examination is unreliable for the detection of sphincter defects. In the past, needle electromyography (EMG) has been used to identify defects of the external anal sphincter. The potential discomfort and the inability to identify internal anal sphincter defects are drawbacks of this type of investigation. The use of EAUS has largely supplanted this technique.

14.3.2 Special Investigations
Anal Endosonography

As stated earlier, EAUS has supplanted electromyographic mapping as it is easily available and more comfortable for the patient. It has been shown to be superior for the evaluation of sphincter defects with a sensitivity of detecting defects of 100%, compared with 89% for electromyographic mapping, 67% for anorectal manometry, and 56% for physical examination.[105] Based on these and other findings, EAUS is now considered to be the gold standard diagnostic tool for the assessment of FI (▶ Fig. 14.1). However, interpretation of ultrasound images of the external anal sphincter is rather subjective, operator dependent, and confounded by normal anatomical variations. Because the external anal sphincter and the perianal fat are both echogenic, it can be difficult to assess the thickness of the external anal sphincter and to identify atrophy of this muscle. Discrimination of normal variants from sphincter defects is also difficult, especially in the upper part of the anal canal in female patients, due to asymmetry of the external anal sphincter at that level.[106] In 75% of asymptomatic nulliparous women, Bollard et al found a natural gap in the anterior part of the external anal sphincter, just below the level of the puborectalis sling. According to these authors, this gap explains the

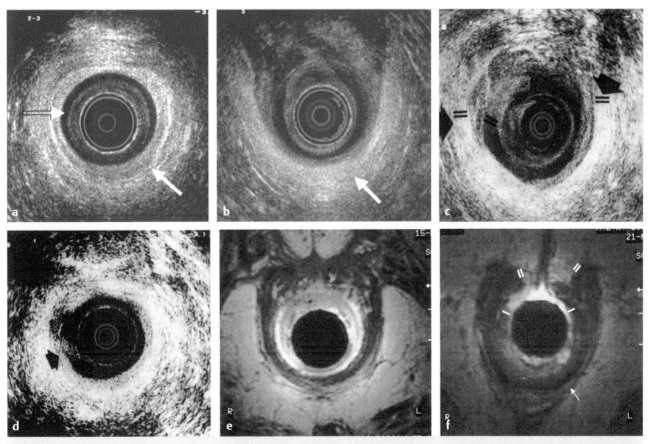

Fig. 14.1 Examples of defects demonstrable by endoanal ultrasonography. **(a)** Endoanal ultrasound of the distal part of the anal canal. Internal anal sphincter (*open arrow*) and external anal sphincter (*closed arrow*). **(b)** Endoanal ultrasound of the proximal part of the anal canal. Puborectalis muscle (*closed arrow*). **(c)** Endoanal ultrasonography in patient with fecal incontinence due to obstetric injury. Internal (*black*) and external (*white*) anal sphincter defect. Margins of each defect are outlined (*slashes and arrows*). **(d)** Endoanal ultrasonography in patient presenting with fecal soiling after lateral internal sphincterotomy. Internal (*black*) anal sphincter defect (*arrow*). **(e)** Endoanal MRI in control subject shows normal internal (*light gray*) and external (*dark gray*) anal sphincter. **(f)** Endoanal MRI in patient with fecal incontinence due to obstetric injury. Internal (*light gray*) anal sphincter defect (*single slashes*) and external (*dark gray*) anal sphincter defect (*double slashes*). Note the rather atrophic external anal sphincter (*arrow*). (The images are provided courtesy of W. Ruud Schouten, MD.)

difficulties in the interpretation of postpartum ultrasounds.[107] Sentovich et al evaluated the accuracy and reliability of EAUS for anterior sphincter defects.[108] In incontinent, parous women, the sphincter defects, detected by ultrasound, were confirmed at operation in 100% of the cases. A similar accuracy has been reported by others.[95] In continent, nulliparous women, the two ultrasonographers identified sphincter defects in 55 and 75%, respectively. This high false-positive rate could be decreased to 40 and 60% by using the video recording of the ultrasounds. The false identification of defects in normal, intact sphincters might be explained by the existence of a natural gap, as described by Bollard et al. It has been suggested that the false-positive rate might be reduced by the measurement of perineal body thickness. Zetterström et al reported that the perineal body thickness was 6 ± 2 mm in patients with an anterior sphincter defect and 1 ± 3 mm in asymptomatic subjects.[109] A similar finding has been reported by others.[110] EAUS is associated with a substantial interobserver variability with regard to the thickness of the sphincters. It has been shown, however, that the interobserver assessment

of sphincter defects is very good.[111] Despite several disadvantages, EAUS is to date the most optimum diagnostic tool for the assessment of FI. During the last decade, the use of three-dimensional (3D) techniques has become more commonplace. Studies have shown that compared to 2D-EAUS, 3D-EAUS (▶ Fig. 14.2, ▶ Fig. 14.3) has an improved concordance with operative anatomic findings.[112] The value and clinical relevance of other tests have been questioned. According to some authors, most of these investigations lack clinical usefulness because they add little additional information to a complete clinical patient assessment. Furthermore, it is thought to be unlikely that these tests result in a significant alteration in a patient's management plan. Frequently, abnormal values do not correlate with the severity of symptoms. Despite these limitations, several tests are still frequently applied. They have been reported to predict the outcome after medical or surgical treatment, thereby permitting the clinician to provide the patient with sound recommendations and allowing the patient to have realistic expectations.[113] In this section, the investigations that are most frequently used are highlighted.

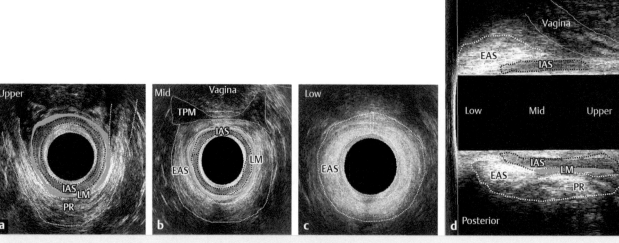

Fig. 14.2 3D ultrasound showing normal ultrasound anatomy (female anal canal). **(a)** Upper, **(b)** mid, **(c)** low anal canal (axial plane). **(d)** Distribution of the sphincter muscles in sagittal plane. EAS, external anal sphincter; IAS, internal anal sphincter; LM, longitudinal muscles; PR, puborectalis muscles; TPM, transverse perineal muscles. (The images are provided courtesy of Sthela Regadas, MD.)

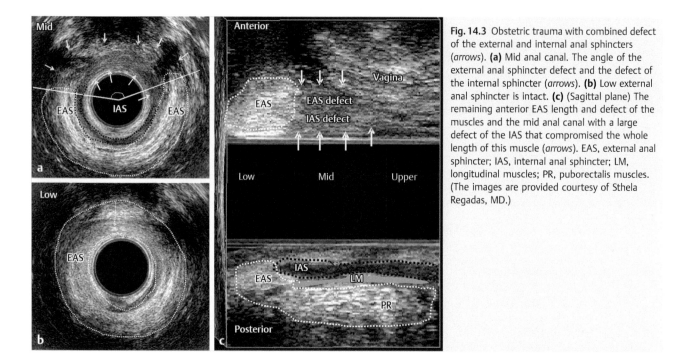

Fig. 14.3 Obstetric trauma with combined defect of the external and internal anal sphincters (*arrows*). **(a)** Mid anal canal. The angle of the external anal sphincter defect and the defect of the internal sphincter (*arrows*). **(b)** Low external anal sphincter is intact. **(c)** (Sagittal plane) The remaining anterior EAS length and defect of the muscles and the mid anal canal with a large defect of the IAS that compromised the whole length of this muscle (*arrows*). EAS, external anal sphincter; IAS, internal anal sphincter; LM, longitudinal muscles; PR, puborectalis muscles. (The images are provided courtesy of Sthela Regadas, MD.)

The "Enema Challenge"

The simplest and most unsophisticated test for incontinence is administration of an enema. The ability to retain a disposable enema is a very useful clinical guide in the assessment of incontinence. If the patient is able to retain a 100-mL water enema, any surgical correction or prolonged treatment plan is likely unnecessary. Reassurance that there is not a more serious problem is all that may be indicated for such a patient.

Anorectal Manometry

Information derived from manometry includes assessment of the resting and squeeze pressures and the anorectal inhibitory reflex. The presence of the reflex eliminates suspicion of Hirschsprung's

disease. Basal pressure is reported to represent mainly the activity of the internal sphincter, and the spontaneous activity of the external sphincter affects maximal basal pressure.[114] Squeeze pressure is reported to be the voluntary function of the external sphincter and the pelvic floor muscles. If both basal and squeeze pressures are low, patients are prone to be totally incontinent. If only the voluntary function is low, the patients are probably partially incontinent.[114] External sphincter function is critical for maintaining continence of solid stool.[115]

Penninckx et al[116] studied the relationship between symptoms and the results of manometric data in incontinent patients. Discriminatory values of greater than 40 mm Hg for maximum basal pressure and greater than 92 mm Hg for squeeze pressure could identify continent patients with 96%

and incontinent patients with 88% accuracy. The uncontrollable evacuation of a balloon, progressively filled with water at 60 mL/min before the maximum tolerable sensation level was reached, was related to the degree of clinical incontinence. Also, the maximum retained volume and the interval between the first sensation volume and the maximum retained volume ("perceived rectal capacity") were related to the clinical symptoms. The balloon-retaining test proved to be superior to the rectal saline infusion test for the determination of the severity of incontinence.

Unfortunately, there is a 10% overlap between the manometric values obtained from incontinent and normal persons.[115] Following childbirth, pudendal nerve damage increases the risk of FI in women with anal sphincter rupture, but manometric findings indicate damage to the sphincter apparatus in both continent and incontinent patients.[117] However, overlap in anorectal physiologic data between continent and incontinent patients is so great as to make accurate prediction of FI impossible. Furthermore, the values do not correlate with the severity of incontinence, nor do they predict postoperative results. No correlation exists between the outcome of the operation and the preoperative anorectal manometric studies.[118] Normal manometric findings do not exclude incontinence entirely.[114]

In recent years, the relationship between anorectal manometry and EAUS has been studied extensively. de Leeuw et al applied both tests in 34 patients at least 10 years after primary repair of a perineal tear and in 12 asymptomatic women with a history of normal, uncomplicated vaginal delivery. Impaired continence was reported by 22 patients (65%). A persistent sphincter defect was found in 86% of these patients. Because maximum anal squeeze pressure and maximum anal resting pressure showed a considerable overlap between the different groups (with and without impaired continence and with and without a sphincter defect), anorectal manometry provided little additional information.[119]

Nazir et al conducted an observational cohort study among 132 patients after primary repair of a third- or fourth-degree perineal tear. The mean time interval between delivery and evaluation was 5 months. All women underwent EAUS and vector volume manometry. They found no difference in manometric values between females without a defect and those with a less extensive defect. Only in women with a large, extensive defect were the manometric values significantly lower. Although they observed a correlation between incontinence scores and manometric variables, there was a large overlap between continent and incontinent females regarding manometric values. No cutoff point could be defined to distinguish continent from incontinent females.[120] Liberman et al designed a study to determine whether anorectal physiology testing alters the management of patients with FI. Manometric findings did not change the pretest management plans. No association was found between manometric results and ultrasound findings. EAUS was the test most likely to change the patient's treatment plan.[113] Voyvodic et al observed a strong correlation between maximum anal squeeze pressure and the presence or absence of an external sphincter defect. The authors classified the defects into partial versus full-length and narrow versus wide-open. This classification appeared to be of little benefit in defining further functional disability because the squeeze pressures

in these subgroups were not significantly different. This might imply that the loss of integrity due to disruption of the external sphincter ring is the most important factor in loss of function rather than the degree of separation of the muscle margins.[121] Bordeianou et al conducted a prospective study aimed at determining the relationship between anal resting pressure and FISI scores in the presence of endosonographic sphincter defects and found that FISI scoring was less sensitive in discriminating between patients with and without sphincter defects; however, the patient had a sphincter defect and a significant decrease in resting pressures.[122]

Defecography

The anorectal angle is postulated to be more obtuse in patients with incontinence[118]; however, voiding defecography or balloon proctography can easily demonstrate this increased angle. This examination will probably add little information regarding the cause of incontinence except perhaps the demonstration of an occult rectal internal procidentia, which may or may not be contributing to the FI.

Pudendal Nerve Terminal Motor Latency

Although the severity of denervation does not appear to influence the severity of incontinence, it seems to affect the outcome of sphincter repair. Assessment of the PNTML provides a useful tool in defining pathology of the pudendal nerves. Prolongation of PNTML is indicative for pudendal neuropathy and is considered to be a hallmark of "idiopathic" incontinence. Roig et al[123] found pudendal neuropathy in 70% of their patients with FI (59% in patients with a sphincter defect and 94% in patients without a sphincter defect). Based on this finding, it seems likely that pudendal neuropathy is an etiologic or associated factor in FI. It is not clear whether a prolonged conduction velocity of the pudendal nerve affects its functional integrity. It has been shown that one out of three patients with bilateral prolonged PNTML has squeeze pressures in the normal range and that almost half of those with a normal PNTML have squeeze pressures below the normal range.[124] Although it has been stated that the information obtained by PNTML testing does not contribute to the management of incontinence in individual patients, it might be of prognostic value when surgical treatment is being considered. Laurberg et al were the first to demonstrate that pudendal neuropathy affects surgical treatment. In their series, the outcome of sphincter repair was successful in 80% of the patients without neuropathy and in only 10% of the patients with neuropathy.[125] This finding has been confirmed by others.[126] Sangwan et al reported that the outcome of sphincter repair was good in patients in whom both pudendal nerves were normal, whereas only one out of six patients with a unilateral pudendal neuropathy had such an outcome. According to these authors, both pudendal nerves must be intact to achieve normal continence after sphincter repair.[127] The relationship between pudendal nerve integrity and successful outcome after surgical repair is not universally accepted. Rasmussen et al, Chen et al, and Young et al were unable to identify any relationship between pudendal neuropathy and a poor outcome after sphincteroplasty.[128,129,130]

Osterberg et al[131] questioned the routine use of PNTML in the assessment of patients with FI. They found pudendal neuropathy and increased fiber density are common in patients with FI. Fiber density but not PNTML was correlated with clinical and manometric variables. The severity of nerve injury correlated with anal motor and sensory function in patients with neurogenic or idiopathic incontinence.

Rectal Compliance

Rasmussen et al[132] studied rectal compliance in 31 patients with FI. The patients experienced a constant defecation urge at a lower rectal volume and also had a lower maximal tolerable volume and a lower rectal compliance than control subjects (median 126 vs. 155 mL, 170 vs. 220 mL, and 9 vs. 15 mm Hg, respectively). There was no difference in the parameters between patients with idiopathic fecal continence and patients with incontinence of traumatic origin, indicating that a poorly compliant rectum in patients with FI may be secondary to FI caused by lack of normal reservoir function. The role of compliance is controversial, because some authors have found a decreased rectal compliance and others have not.[133,134]

Magnetic Resonance Imaging

Regarding the visualization of anal sphincter defects, magnetic resonance imaging (MRI) is comparable to EAUS. However, detailed examination of sphincter morphology is only possible with MRI (▶ Fig. 14.4a,b). Denervation of the external anal sphincter is associated with fiber type changes and atrophy, characterized by muscle fiber loss with subsequent fat and fibrous tissue replacement. In contrast with ultrasound, MRI allows good distinction between muscle fibers, fibrous tissue, and fat. Williams et al performed MRI with an endocoil in women with intact sphincters on EAUS. Continent women with a normal squeeze pressure had a larger external anal sphincter cross-sectional area with a lower fat content than the incontinent women with a low squeeze pressure. Women with a thin internal anal sphincter and/or a poorly defined external anal sphincter on ultrasound were more likely to have atrophy.[135] Briel et al performed EAUS and endoanal MRI in incontinent women with an anterior sphincter defect due to obstetric trauma. Atrophy of the external anal sphincter could only be demonstrated on MRI and was observed in 8 of the 20 patients. The outcome of sphincter repair was significantly better in those without atrophy.[136] During sphincter repair,

performed in another group of patients, the same authors took biopsy specimens from the left and right lateral parts of the external anal sphincter. Endoanal MRI revealed external anal sphincter atrophy in 36% of the patients. This was confirmed by histopathologic examination in all but one. In detection of atrophy, endoanal MRI showed 89% sensitivity, 94% specificity, 89% positive predictive value, and 94% negative predictive value.[137] Based on these and other findings, it is apparent that MRI provides a powerful tool to detect external anal sphincter atrophy, thereby predicting the outcome of sphincter repair.

14.4 Treatment

Specific disorders are treated on their own merits (i.e., whatever is appropriate for inflammatory bowel disease, carcinoma, or rectal procidentia). Regardless of etiology, however, initial conservative management is almost always appropriate. In 2015, the American Society of Colon and Rectal Surgeons published its Clinical Practice Guidelines for the management of FI.[138] In it, the various interventions are evaluated using the GRADE system.[139] We will refer to the associated recommendations for treatment where available. These will be indicated in **bold**.

14.4.1 Nonoperative Options

Medical Treatment

Conservative management is the mainstay of initial treatment. Dietary changes and perineal exercises are often recommended for patients with FI, but generally have proved disappointing in patients with incontinence to solid stool. In those with predominantly loose stool, such management is often efficacious. Rosen et al[140] reviewed the various antidiarrheal agents that might be considered in the management of patients with incontinence associated with frequent loose stools. Substances such as kaolin, activated charcoal, pectin, and bulk-forming agents act on the intestinal contents in an effort to solidify them. Agents such as bismuth salts and astringents such as aluminum hydroxide may produce a barrier between intestinal contents and the intestinal wall. Anticholinergic agents such as atropine act as potent inhibitors of intestinal secretion and gut motility. At therapeutic doses, these drugs may produce disconcerting side effects. The opium derivatives such as tincture of opium, paregoric, and codeine act

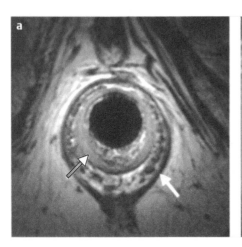
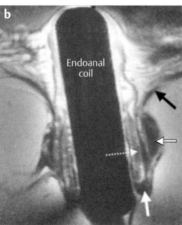

Fig. 14.4 (a) Endoanal magnetic resonance image, transverse image. Internal anal sphincter (*open arrow*) and external anal sphincter (*closed arrow*). (b) Endoanal magnetic resonance image, sagittal image. Levator ani (*black arrow*), puborectalis muscle (*open arrow*), distal border of the external anal sphincter, curving around the distal end of the internal anal sphincter (*closed arrow*), and internal anal sphincter (*dotted arrow*).

directly on the smooth muscle of the intestinal wall, but the risk of addiction makes them less suitable for long-term use. Diphenoxylate hydrochloride (Lomotil) also has been used. One of the most frequently used drugs is loperamide (Imodium), which inhibits intestinal motility by a direct effect on the circular and longitudinal muscles of the intestinal wall. It solidifies the stool and increases rectal compliance, thereby decreasing urgency. It has also been found to increase resting anal pressures[141] and thus improve anal sphincter function and continence after restorative proctocolectomy.[142] For patients with certain neurologic deficiencies, the regular administration of enemas may achieve a certain level of social continence by simply emptying the left colon of stool.

Amitriptyline, a tricyclic antidepressant agent with anticholinergic and serotoninergic properties, has been used empirically in the treatment of idiopathic FI. Santoro et al[143] conducted an open study to test the response of amitriptyline 20 mg daily for 4 weeks by 18 patients with idiopathic FI. Amitriptyline improved incontinence scores (median pretreatment score 16 vs. median posttreatment score 3) and reduced the number of bowel movements per day. Amitriptyline improved symptoms in 89% of patients with FI. The data support that the major change with amitriptyline is a decrease in the amplitude and frequency of rectal motor complexes. The second conclusion is that the drug increases colonic transit time and leads to the formation of a firmer stool that is passed less frequently. These in combination may be the source of the improvement in continence.

Dietary and medical management are recommended as first-line therapy for patients with FI. Grade of recommendation: Strong recommendation based on low- or very low-quality evidence, 1C.[138]

Biofeedback/Pelvic Floor Retraining

Engel et al[144] first described biofeedback training for FI, which is achieved by screening patients for incontinence and selecting well-motivated, alert patients for a three-phase instruction of voluntary control mechanisms.

There are at least three components to biofeedback treatment: exercise of the external sphincter muscle, training in the discrimination of rectal sensations, and training synchrony of the internal and external sphincter responses during rectal distention.[145] Each of these components may be effective for some patients. The method involves placing a balloon in the rectum and connecting pressure transducers to a graph to give the patient a visual feedback corresponding to his or her sphincter responses to command. Initially, large amounts of air are injected into the rectal balloon; gradually, the volume of distention is reduced until the patient can contract the external anal sphincter to small distentions. Subsequently, visual feedback is eliminated, but the patient is assessed by a trained observer to see if she/he can respond to rectal sensations alone.

Training occurs at 4- to 8-week intervals and is supplemented by sphincter exercises to increase muscle strength. The goals of this training are to increase the strength of external sphincter contraction and to teach the patient to detect and respond to small volumes of rectal distention.

One major disadvantage is the time involved. Each session requires at least 1 to 2 hours and involves a significant amount of sophisticated physiologic monitoring apparatus.

Wald[146] reported that diabetic patients exhibit multiple abnormalities of anorectal sensory and motor functions. Pharmacologic treatment and dietary interventions to modulate diarrhea, as well as biofeedback to improve rectal sensory thresholds and striated muscle responsiveness, may prove successful in the reestablishment of bowel control.

Several authors have reviewed the literature in an effort to determine the efficacy of biofeedback treatment in the management of FI. Norton et al conducted a Cochrane review of controlled studies of biofeedback and sphincter exercises for FI. Only five trials met the inclusion criteria of being a randomized or quasi-randomized trial, including a total of 109 participants. The Cochrane review concluded that there is not enough evidence from these trials to judge whether sphincter exercises or biofeedback are effective in reducing FI.[147] Heymen et al searched the Medline database for papers published between 1973 and 1999 including the terms "biofeedback and FI." Thirty-five studies were reviewed. Only six studies used a parallel treatment design and just three of those randomized subjects to treatment groups. A meta-analysis comparing the treatment outcome of studies using coordination training (coordinating pelvic floor muscle contraction with the sensation of rectal filling) to studies using strength training (pelvic floor muscle contraction alone) failed to show any advantage for one treatment strategy over another. The mean success rates were 67 and 70%, respectively. Despite these positive results, the authors state that the conclusions of the reviewed studies are limited by the absence of clearly identified criteria for determining success and by inconsistencies regarding selection criteria, severity of symptoms, duration of treatment, type of biofeedback, and factors predicting outcome.[148] Reviewing the literature, Palsson et al found only a few controlled trials.[149] The largest randomized controlled trial has been conducted by Norton et al. They randomly assigned 171 patients with FI into four treatment arms: (1) standard care; (2) standard care plus instruction in sphincter exercises; (3) same as "2" plus computer-assisted biofeedback involving coordination techniques; (4) same as "3" plus daily use of an EMG home trainer device. Approximately half of the participants in all four groups who completed their treatment protocol showed improvement. This benefit was maintained at 1-year follow-up. These data indicate that improvement can be realized without sphincter exercises and without biofeedback. Patient–therapist interaction and the development of better coping strategies seem to be important factors.[150] Another randomized controlled study, conducted by Solomon et al, revealed that instrument-guided biofeedback offers no advantage over simple pelvic floor retraining with digital guidance alone.[151] The mechanisms by which biofeedback is effective are still not clear. It has been suggested that biofeedback is beneficial by improving the contraction of the external anal sphincter and the pelvic floor muscles due to strength training. Initial attempts to demonstrate objective manometric changes secondary to biofeedback have proved difficult. Fynes et al conducted a randomized controlled trial to compare the effects of biofeedback alone with those of biofeedback combined with electrical stimulation. The manometric parameters did not change after the biofeedback alone, whereas anal resting and squeeze pressures increased after combined biofeedback and electrical stimulation.[67] Beddy et al observed a significant improvement in anal resting pressure, duration of the squeeze, and amplitude of the squeeze after EMG-guided bio-feedback. There was no improvement in the squeeze pressure.[152]

Biofeedback might also work by enhancing the ability to perceive and respond to rectal distensions, known as sensory training. Chiarioni et al reported that sensory retraining is indeed the key to biofeedback treatment of FI. Although they observed an increase of maximum squeeze pressure and squeeze duration after biofeedback, the sphincter strength did not separate responders from nonresponders. However, responders had lower thresholds for first sensation at the end of the treatment.[153] A better coordination between rectal sensory perception and sphincter activity might also contribute to the effectiveness of biofeedback. Critics of this treatment modality argue that the improvement is a result of the supportive interaction between the physiotherapist and the patient, resulting in decreased anxiety and increased confidence. Despite many unanswered questions, it seems obvious that biofeedback is beneficial for more than half of the patients with FI, at least in the short term. Data regarding whether or not the outcome of biofeedback can be predicted are scarce. One study showed that manometric parameters, except for increased cross-sectional asymmetry, do not predict response to biofeedback therapy.[154] Another study revealed that incomplete anal relaxation during straining, especially in patients younger than age 55, adversely affects the outcome of biofeedback.[155] The long-term results after biofeedback are also questionable. Most studies offer a follow-up of less than 2 years. Enck et al posted a questionnaire to patients who were treated by biofeedback 5 to 6 years earlier. The same questionnaire was also sent to patients who had not entered the treatment program. In both groups, 78% of the patients experienced episodes of incontinence. However, the severity of incontinence was significantly less in the treatment group. Five to six years after the treatment, the severity of incontinence was similar to that immediately reported after therapy.[156] In contrast with this finding, two other studies revealed deterioration over time.[157,158] Ryn et al reported an overall success rate of 60% immediately after the treatment. This dropped to 41% after a median follow-up of 44 months.[159] Based on this deterioration over time, it has been suggested that it could be useful to reinitiate biofeedback training. Pager et al were not able to demonstrate this worsening with time. At a median of 42 months after completion of the training program, 75% of their patients still perceived a symptomatic improvement and 83 reported improved QOL. They also observed that patients continued to improve during the years following the training, possibly due to the strong emphasis placed on them to continue the exercises on their own.[160] Biofeedback treatment is multimodal. More studies are needed to establish selection criteria, to compare different biofeedback techniques, and to establish valid end points. Although biofeedback is time consuming and labor intensive, it is noninvasive and utterly safe. Based on the reported outcomes, it can be considered as initial treatment in patients with FI. It has been suggested that biofeedback is also beneficial as an adjuvant therapy following anal sphincter repair. Davis et al evaluated this aspect in a randomized controlled trial. Thirty-eight patients were assigned at random into sphincter repair or sphincter repair plus biofeedback. Shortly after surgery, there was no difference in functional outcome between the two groups. More studies are warranted to elucidate the role of adjuvant biofeedback.[161]

Biofeedback should be considered as an initial treatment for patients with incontinence and some preserved voluntary sphincter contraction. Grade of recommendation: Strong recommendation based on moderate-quality evidence, 1B.[138]

14.4.2 Operative Procedures

All operative techniques involve preparing the patient by evacuation of the large bowel with laxatives and enemas or oral lavage solutions. If an indwelling urethral catheter is placed, it should remain in place until decreased pain permits voluntary voiding. Perioperative broad-spectrum antibiotics are administered. Broadly speaking, we divide operative repairs into one of five categories of classification: (1) repair, (2) replacement, (3) augmentation, (4) stimulation, and (5) diversion.[162]

Repair

Anterior Anal Sphincter Repair

Postobstetric external anal sphincter defects, most frequently located at the anterior anal sphincter, are the principal cause of FI. These anatomic defects can be treated by an anterior anal sphincter repair. Most surgeons use an overlapping technique to repair the divided external anal sphincter; however, a primary or end-to-end repair may be employed early after sphincter injury, as there is no significant scar and muscle tissue is healthy.

The technique of sphincteroplasty, as applied by Fang et al[163] and Parks and McPartlin,[164] provides good-to-excellent results in most patients who have adequate residual muscle mass. Wexner et al added the modification of separate internal and external sphincter repair. The operation is performed with the patient in the prone jackknife position, with the buttocks elevated over a 6-inch roll. Anesthesia may be either regional or general; the entire operative site is infiltrated with local anesthetic and 1:200,000 epinephrine in order to relax the muscles and improve hemostasis (▶ Fig. 14.5a).[165]

The first step is the mobilization of the anoderm from the underlying sphincter mechanism and scar. The incision is curvilinear and parallels the outer edge of the external sphincter. The incision should extend no more than 180 degrees of arc, depending on the amount of scar tissue present as further posterolateral incision risks injury to the pudendal nerves (▶ Fig. 14.5b). Cephalad mobilization should extend approximately to the distal edge of the anorectal ring (▶ Fig. 14.5c) but the cephalad part is dictated by the need to reach the areolar unscarred tissue. The entire sphincter mechanism is then widely dissected from its bed (▶ Fig. 14.5d). Care must be taken to preserve the branches of the pudendal nerves as they enter into the muscle posterolaterally. Wide dissection permits approximation without tension. It is often easiest to begin at the normal muscle and to advance to the scarred area, once a proper plane has been established. In one approach, the entire sphincter mechanism is sectioned transversely through the middle of the scar tissue, with preservation of this area for suture placement (▶ Fig. 14.5e). The puborectalis muscle and internal anal sphincter can be plicated with long-term absorbable sutures. The muscle ends are then overlapped to decrease the anal aperture until it fits snugly over the index finger (▶ Fig. 14.5f).

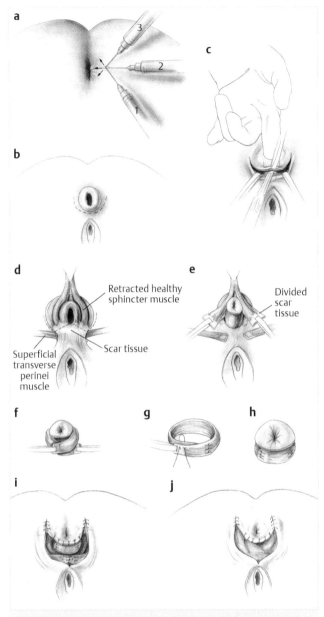

Fig. 14.5 Technique of sphincteroplasty. (a) Infiltration of local anesthesia. (b) Placement of circular incision. (c) Mobilization of anoderm. (d) Dissection of sphincter muscle. (e) Mobilization of severed ends of the sphincter muscle. (f) Muscle ends are overlapped. (g) Mattress sutures are applied. The scar must be left at each end of the muscle to hold the sutures. (h) At completion of suturing, anal canal should admit one finger snugly. (i) Perineal body reconstruction is done anterior to the anal canal, and anoderm is sutured to sphincter muscle. Skin edges are partially closed to decrease the size of wound. (j) Wound is packed open.

Multiple mattress sutures are placed carefully to maintain the desired aperture (▸ Fig. 14.5g). The material used is generally a 2–0 synthetic absorbable suture. The tendency of the sphincter ends to pull apart must be minimal, because separation of the ends is a sign of inadequate mobilization of the muscle from its bed and will predispose to separation at the suture line. When all sutures have been placed, they are pulled tight, and the orifice is checked again to ensure proper placement of the sutures, which

are then tied (▸ Fig. 14.5h). A second approach involves preservation of midline scar, and imbrication of the tissue, and performance of overlapping repair.

If the perineal body is diminutive, attempts should be made to repair it. This is effected by an anterior levatorplasty and internal anal sphincteroplasty. Tissues from each side of the perineum (transverse perinei muscles and/or scar tissue) are approximated in the midline (▸ Fig. 14.5i). This reconstruction lends support to the anovaginal area and effectively separates the anal orifice from the introitus. The anoderm is carefully sutured over the sphincter with interrupted or running absorbable 3–0 chromic catgut or polyglactin sutures. The horseshoe-shaped defect outside the muscle is partially closed, and the remainder is packed open with fine gauze or over a drain (▸ Fig. 14.5j) or a gauze mesh can simply be placed over the wound.

Postoperative management has varied from surgeon to surgeon. The recent trend has been toward early feeding. A randomized controlled trial between bowel confinement and immediate feeding ad lib found no difference in complications when compared to bowel confinement.[166] Although there is concern for the later need for laxatives, we administer opiates to decrease the pain and frequency of bowel movements. Mahony et al[167] conducted a randomized trial designed to compare a laxative regimen with a constipating regimen in early postoperative management after primary obstetric and anal sphincter repair. A total of 105 females were randomized after primary repair of a third-degree tear to receive lactulose (laxative group, 56) or codeine phosphate (constipated group, 49) for 3 days postoperatively. The first postoperative bowel action occurred at a median of 4 days in the constipated group and 2 days in the laxative group. Patients in the constipated group had a significantly more painful first evacuation compared with the laxative group. The mean duration of hospital stay was 3.7 days in the postpartum. The mean duration of hospital stay was 3.7 days in the constipated group and 3.1 days in the laxative group. Continence scores, anal manometry, and EAUS findings were similar in the two groups at 3 months postpartum. Patients in the laxative group had a significantly earlier and less painful bowel motion and earlier postnatal discharge. Sitz baths are given two to three times a day for comfort and to wash away secretions. Some surgeons are concerned about skin maceration and prefer to irrigate the wound with warm saline solution or even diluted hydrogen peroxide (dilute 1:4) to provide both comfort and cleanliness. A pulsatile hand-held shower, bidet, or sitz bath apparatus is a very useful adjunct to maintaining perineal wound cleanliness. Patients are preoperatively counseled that healing will require at least 4 to 6 weeks and that some degree of wound dehiscence is common. With the introduction of food, a psyllium seed preparation is administered twice a day to eliminate any straining at defecation. Performing a covering colostomy is not required. Patients usually leave the hospital in 5 to 6 days. An alternative strategy is to teach patient to irrigate their rectums by sliding a catheter posteriorly along the natal cleft and into the anal canal, away from the surgical site. This may avoid issues of delayed constipation or impaction at home.

Numerous reports have been published on the short-term outcomes of sphincter repair, and overall, initial success is positive, with approximately 60% of patients achieving significant benefit. However, long-term success has not been as durable. In one of the larger studies published, Karoui et al evaluated 86 patients undergoing sphincteroplasty; at 3 months postoperatively, one-third of patients were totally continent, and an additional 33% were incontinent only to gas. However, at 40-month follow-up, less than one-third remained fully continent and over 70% of patients were incontinent to either gas or feces.[168] Malouf et al evaluated 55 consecutive patients undergoing overlapping sphincteroplasty as a result of obstetric injury. At 15 months postoperatively, 42/55 patients were continent to both solid and liquid stool. At 5-year follow-up, no patient was fully continent to both solid and liquid stool, emphasizing the deterioration of continence over time.[169] Similarly, Halverson and Hull reported on a series of 71 consecutive patients undergoing sphincteroplasty who were assessed at a median of 69 months after surgery. Forty-nine (69%) were available for follow-up. Four patients were diverted, and 54% were incontinent to liquid or solid stool. Only six patients (14%) remained fully continent.[170]

Attempts at determining predictive factors for success have looked at age, pudendal nerve injury, and type of repairs. Yet, despite the wealth of literature, clear answers are elusive. The patient's age at the time of sphincter repair has been assessed by several authors. Simmang et al evaluated 14 patients with ages ranging from 55 to 81 years. Almost all of the patients reported improvement in their symptoms and half reported complete continence. In this admittedly small series, advanced age did not seem to predict failure.[171] Rasmussen et al assessed postoperative continence in 24 women under the age of 40 years and in 14 women over 40 years; there was a significant difference in postoperative continence in the older cohort. This was hypothesized to be related to weakening of the pelvic floor.[172] In contrast, Young et al evaluated 57 women undergoing overlapping sphincter repair. They found that 78% of patients younger than 40 years deemed the repair a success compared to 93% of patients in the older group. Formal incontinence scores improved equally in both groups.[129]

Pudendal nerve injury as evidenced by prolonged terminal motor latency has often been cited as one of the causal etiologies in postobstetric injury incontinence. Numerous publications have attempted to assess this, and data are decidedly divided. This is supported by studies of Barisic et al, Londono-Schimmer et al, and Gilliland et al[173,174,175] comparing groups with and without pudendal neuropathy, showing a significant difference in incontinence scoring after sphincteroplasty between the groups; however, this is refuted by multiple contemporaneous studies including those by Bravo Gutierrez et al, Halverson and Hull, Malouf et al, and Karoui et al.[168,169,170,176] Tjandra et al attempted to evaluate whether repair technique, overlapping versus end-to-end repair, was associated with functional outcomes. In this study, 23 patients with anterior defects underwent sphincter repair in this randomized trial; 12 patients were randomized to end-to-end repair and 11 to overlapping repair at a median follow-up of 18 months. CCF-FIS scores were identical in both groups. Resting pressures and maximal squeeze pressures were no different and subjective success scores were no different.[177]

Briel et al conducted a prospective study looking at whether bulk overlapping repair was superior to separate internal and external sphincter repair. In this study, 31 patients underwent separate internal and external sphincter repair and were compared to 24 patients who underwent standard overlapping repair. There is no statistically significant difference in these two groups.[178]

Hasegawa et al[179] conducted a randomized trial to assess whether fecal diversion would improve primary wound healing and functional outcome after sphincter repair. Patients were randomly assigned to a defunctioning stoma ($n = 13$) or no stoma ($n = 14$). They were assessed by the CCF-FIS (0–20). Incontinence score improved significantly in both groups (stoma, 13.5–7.8; no stoma, 14–9.6). No difference was found between the two groups. Maximum resting pressure and maximum squeeze pressure increased significantly only in the no-stoma group. There was no significant difference in the functional outcome or the number of complications of sphincter repair. However, stoma-related complications occurred in 7 of 13 patients having a stoma (parastomal hernia, 2; prolapsed stoma, 1; incisional hernia at the stoma site requiring repair, 5; and wound infection at the closure site, 1). They concluded fecal diversion in sphincter repair is unnecessary, because it gives no benefit in terms of wound healing or functional outcome and it is a source of morbidity.

Lewicky et al[180] evaluated sexual function following anal sphincteroplasty in 32 women with third- and fourth-degree perineal tear secondary to birth trauma who elected to undergo sphincteroplasty for FI. Sexual function is compromised in women with third- and fourth-degree perineal tears. For their patients with this degree of perineal tearing who underwent sphincteroplasty after primary repair, their survey showed consistent improvement in several parameters of sexual function. After sphincteroplasty, physical sensation was higher (much higher in 40%), sexual satisfaction was better (much better in 33.3%), and 28.6% of the patients were much more likely to reach orgasm. Libido was improved in 37.5% of the study population, and 20% reported increased partner satisfaction. Before surgery, 23.5% of patients were physically and 31.2% emotionally unable to participate in sexual activity because of fear of incontinence on intimacy; after surgery, only 6.3% were physically unable and 0% were emotionally unable to engage in sexual activity.

Despite mixed data, sphincteroplasty should remain a viable approach to address continence in damaged sphincters, especially for primary repair after obstetric injury. Reid et al conducted a study of 344 women who underwent primary repair after obstetric injury. In only 18% were there long-term (3-year follow-up) issues with incontinence. Interestingly, of 31 women who had issues at early follow-up (9 weeks), 28 were asymptomatic at 3 years. Predictors of long-term problems were: urgency at 9 weeks (OR, 4.65) and a higher St. Marks score (OR, 1.4).[181]

Glasgow and Lowry performed a systematic review which seems to encapsulate the key findings with regard to long-term outcomes of sphincter repair. They found, in a review of 16 studies, comprising nearly 900 repairs, that in most series, patients remain satisfied over time with surgical outcome. Even in light of more current techniques, the potential of a good sphincter repair should not be overlooked.[182] However, patients should be counseled that even if short-term success is realized, recurrence of symptoms with increasing length of follow-up is expected. Patients may be counseled that sphincter repair is likely the first step in a multiphase therapeutic algorithm. ▶ Table 14.5 was constructed to provide a general idea of what can be expected with an overlapping repair.

Sphincter repair (sphincteroplasty) may be offered to symptomatic patients with a defined defect of the external anal sphincter. Grade of recommendation: Strong recommendation based on moderate-quality evidence, 1B.[138]

Postanal Repair

Prior to the introduction of EAUS, most cases of FI were classified as "idiopathic" or neurogenic. For the treatment of patients presenting with this type of incontinence, Parks devised the postanal repair. He believed that this procedure works by restoring the anorectal angle and increasing the length of the anal canal. Several studies, however, have revealed that a postanal repair does not result in a significant change of the anorectal angle.[196,197,198,199,200] Several studies have revealed an increase in the length of the anal canal after successful postanal repair.[2,196,201] Conflicting data have been reported regarding the impact of postanal repair on anal pressure. Some have found that resting and squeeze anal pressure increase after successful postanal repair.[183,197,198,199,202] According to others, postanal repair does not affect anal pressure.[203,204] Because of the lack of consistent changes in anatomy and physiology, it is unclear why postanal repair is effective in some patients. Clinical improvement might

be the result of lengthening and narrowing of the anal canal. van Tets and Kuijpers even suggested that this procedure might improve continence by a placebo effect and not by enhanced muscle function.[205]

As Parks described the operation, a posterior angular incision is made through the anoderm and proceeds through the intersphincteric plane between the external and internal sphincters. This intersphincteric plane is pursued upward until the puborectalis muscle is reached. The pelvic cavity is entered by dividing the rectosacral fascia, and the perirectal fat is swept off the levator ani muscles. At this point, most of the levator ani muscle can be seen, and sutures can be placed from one side of the pelvis to the other, initially incorporating the ischiococcygeus muscle in the first layer of repair and the pubococcygeus muscle in the second layer. These muscles will not meet; the sutures only form a lattice. A 0 polyglactin (Vicryl) suture is used.

Next, a row of sutures is placed to oppose the two limbs of the puborectalis muscle, further buttressing the anorectal angle. This also makes the pull of the puborectalis muscle more efficient. A suction drain is placed in the presacral space and is brought out through a separate stab wound. Plicating sutures are placed in the external sphincter muscles to narrow their arc of action. By placing a finger in the anal canal, it is possible to determine if the whole area is somewhat stenosed, a state essential for achieving a successful result. The wound is closed

Table 14.5 Results of overlapping sphincteroplasty

Author(s) (year)	No. of patients	Grade of continence (%)[a]		
		1	2	3
Browning and Motson[b] (1984)[183]	83	78	13	9
Fang et al (1984)[163]	76	58	38	4
Hawley[b] (1985)[184]	100	52	30	18
Christiansen and Pedersen (1987)[185]	23	65	30	5
Morgan et al[b] (1987)[186]	45	82	9	9
Ctercteko et al (1988)[24]	44	54	32	14
Abcarian et al[c] (1989)[187]	43	100		
Yoshioka and Keighley (1989)[188]	27	26	48	26
Jacobs et al[c] (1990)[189]	30	83	17	
Fleshman et al (1991)[190]	55	51	44	5
Gibbs and Hooks (1993)[191]	33	30	58	12
Engel et al (1994)[192]	28	57	22	21
Engel et al (1994)[193]	53	79	17	4
Londono-Schimmer et al (1994)[174]	94	50	26	24
Sangalli and Marti (1994)[194]	36	78	19	3
Simmang et al (1994)[171]	14	71	29	–
Oliveira et al[d] (1996)[195]	55	29	47	29

[a]Grades of continence: 1, continent for solid and liquid stool; 2, continent for solid but not always for liquid stool; and 3, little or no continence.
[b]Most patients had a covering colostomy.
[c]Patients had a supplemental anterior puborectalis muscle approximation.
[d]According to study, 55% of patients had previous sphincter repair.

with 3–0 chromic catgut sutures for the subcutaneous tissues, and the skin is approximated with 3–0 subcuticular Vicryl sutures. Systemic antibiotics are administered, one dose preoperatively and two doses postoperatively. Although Parks recommended purging the patient with magnesium sulfate for a 10-day period to ensure liquid stools, we recommend restriction of the patient's intake orally for 5 days, during which time the patient is given loperamide and codeine-containing analgesics to quiet the bowel. When diet is reinstituted, the patient is placed on a psyllium seed preparation twice daily.

Browning and the late Sir Alan Parks were the first to describe the functional outcome after postanal repair. According to these authors, 86% of their patients became continent for solid stool. In the 1980s and early 1990s, the reported success rates varied between 66 and 94%. However, in those days outcome was considered successful not only if patients regained continence for solid and liquid stool, but also if patients experienced improvement despite sporadic episodes of incontinence. Furthermore, most of the studies conducted in that period were retrospective. The definition of incontinence and the method of data collection differed from study to study. In almost all studies, the outcome was assessed without the use of a standardized incontinence scoring system. Furthermore, the duration of follow-up was relatively short or not recorded. During the last decade, several studies have revealed that the long-term results after postanal repair fall short of the short-term results reported in earlier days. This observation is illustrated by the data summarized in ▶ Table 14.6.

These more recent data illustrate that postanal repair is not as good as patients or surgeons would like it to be. The early results are rather disappointing. Moreover, they deteriorate over time. Overall success rates are generally poor, in the range of 35%.[201,208] In general, this technique, though innovative in its time, has been mostly abandoned. However, despite this conventional wisdom, some recent data indicate that in a selected population, there is still some efficacy; Mackey et al reported on 57 patients with a mean follow-up of 9.1 years and found that 79% were still satisfied with the outcome.[209]

Plication of the external anal sphincter (Parks' postanal repair) is not recommended. Grade of recommendation: Strong recommendation based on moderate-quality evidence, 1B.[138]

Replacement

Muscle Transposition

Several advanced techniques have been employed using pedicled muscle flaps to replace a damaged or nonfunctional sphincter. In general, due to technical difficulty and high rates of morbidity, as well as the profound success of newer, less invasive techniques, such modalities are rarely employed, and may only be accessible in select situations and at specialized centers where expertise and experience may maximize results. We detail some of these briefly in the following.

Gracilis Muscle Transposition (Graciloplasty)

This technique was first described more than a century ago by Chetwood and renewed as a technique for use in pediatric FI by Pickrell et al.[210] More recently, it was championed by Wexner et al as a salvage treatment in the setting of catastrophic sphincter damage in otherwise healthy patients. In this technique, patients undergo initial fecal diversion, usually with loop ileostomy. Next, the gracilis muscle is harvested as a proximally pedicled flap. The muscle is tunneled around the sphincter complex and sutured in place (▶ Fig. 14.6). Initially described as a muscle transposition alone, the wrapped graft functions as a biologic cerclage, akin to a Thiersch procedure. In addition, patients learn techniques to voluntarily contract this muscle to augment control.[211] Adductor splinting is employed postoperatively for 3 days. Finally, after complete healing, the ileostomy is closed.

To augment the procedure, electrostimulation was employed in order to convert the more easily fatigued fast-twitch skeletal muscle fibers to slow twitch via neuromodulation, resulting in relatively tonic contraction (▶ Fig. 14.7). Isolated series of dynamic (or stimulated) gracioplasty produced favorable results; however, due to surgical difficulty and high complication rates, it was rarely performed. Wexner et al, reporting on one of the largest series, in a multinational dynamic gracioplasty study group, showed that at 2 years, > 60% of patients had a significant improvement in QOL and incontinence scores.[213] However, unfortunately, long-term success was less favorable: Thornton and others showed a significant decrease in success at 5 years, with only 16% maintaining continence, and overall complication

Table 14.6 Relationship between length of follow-up and outcome after postanal repair

Author(s)	Year	Successful outcome with years of follow-up (%)							
		0.5	1	2	3	3.5	4	6	8
Setti Carraro et al[201]	1994	41						26	
Engel et al[192]	1994					21			
Jameson et al[202]	1994	50		28					
Athanasiadis et al[199]	1995					6			
Briel and Schouten[206]	1995		65		46				
Rieger et al[207]	1997								37
Matsuoka et al[208]	2000				35				

Note: Successful outcome: continent for solid and liquid stool with or without incontinence for gas.

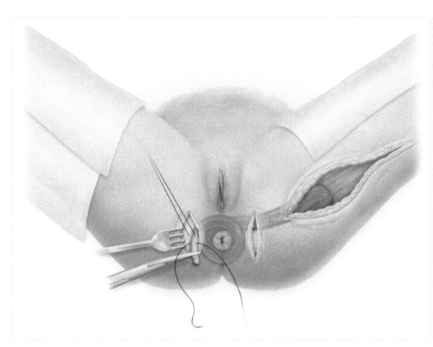

Fig. 14.6 Graciloplasty. The gracilis muscle is harvested as a proximally pedicled flap. The muscle is tunneled around the sphincter complex and sutured in place.[212] (With permission © 2012 Wolters Kluwer.)

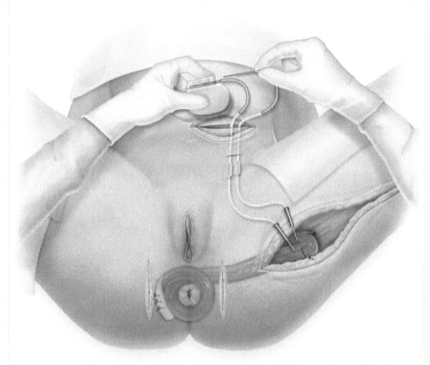

Fig. 14.7 Graciloplasty. Electrostimulation is employed in order to convert the more easily fatigued fast-twitch skeletal muscle fibers to slow twitch via neuromodulation, resulting in relatively tonic contraction.[212] (With permission © 2012 Wolters Kluwer.)

rates reaching 70%. Complications included surgical site infection, stimulator malfunction, and pain.[214]

Geerdes et al[215] reported on the complications and management of patients who underwent dynamic graciloplasty. Dynamic graciloplasty was performed in 67 patients, with a mean follow-up of 2.7 years. Continence was defined as being continent to solid and liquid stool. The technique was successful in 52 patients (78%), whereas failure occurred in 15 patients (22%). Complications resulted from technical difficulties, infection, and problems attributable to an abnormal physiology of the muscle or an anorectal functional imbalance. In total, 53 complications were identified in 36 patients. Most technical problems concerning the transposition and stimulation of the gracilis muscle could be treated. Failures were attributable to a bad contraction of the distal part of the muscle (four) and perforation of the anal canal during stimulation (one). In eight patients, infection of the stimulator and leads required explantation. Three patients did not regain continence after reimplantation. Apart from moderate constipation, physiologic complications were very hard to treat and resulted in failures in five patients because of overflow incontinence, soiling, a nondistending rectum, strong peristalsis, and strong constipation. In two patients, the technique failed despite a well-contracting graciloplasty; no clear reason for the failure was found. The authors concluded that complications associated with the technique of dynamic graciloplasty such as loss of contraction, infection, bad contraction in the distal part of the muscle, and constipation can often be prevented or treated. Difficulties related to an impaired sensation and/or motility, attributable to a congenital cause or degeneration, are impossible to treat. Thus, a good selection of patients is essential to prevent disappointment.[215]

A report from Penninckx, on behalf of the Belgian Section of Colorectal Surgery, indicated that the outcomes were even less favorable. After a median follow-up of 48 months, dynamic graciloplasty had failed in 45% of the patients. The highest rate of failure was observed during the first year after surgery. However, there were also a significant number of subsequent failures.[216]

In fact, both companies who previously manufactured the devices (NICE Technologies, Ft. Lauderdale, FL, and Medtronic Inc., Minneapolis, MN) ceased device distribution in the United States. This stimulator is no longer FDA approved for this indication in the United States. Nonstimulated graciloplasty is still available at limited centers, and is still occasionally the best option in patients after trauma and with FI associated with imperforate anus. This operation is only performed in patients after fecal diversion has been established.

Gluteal Muscle Transposition

Transposition of the gluteus maximus muscle has been used in situations in which a normally functioning sphincter muscle is absent.[217,218,219,220] This operation can be used after accidents in which the perineal tissues are avulsed. An excellent review of the subject was conducted by Fleshner and Roberts, and the following description is drawn from their dissertation.[221]

The gluteus maximus muscle is ideally suited for transposition to the perianal region. It is a well-vascularized muscle supplied by the inferior gluteal artery (▶ Fig. 14.8a). It is innervated by the L5 and S1 nerve roots through the inferior gluteal nerve and thus functions despite denervation of the anal sphincter mechanism, which is supplied by the S2–S4 nerve roots. A potential advantage in using the gluteus maximus muscle rather than the gracilis muscle lies in the fact that it is a large, strong muscle. Its proximity to the anal area eliminates the need for disfiguring thigh incisions. However, because the gluteus maximus muscle is a hip extensor, some theoretical concerns have arisen regarding the impact on hip extension, even though only the inferior portion of the muscle is used.

As with other muscle transposition procedures, transposition of the gluteus maximus muscle is an option of virtually last resort. It is best suited for relatively young, motivated patients with neurogenic FI, multiple failed sphincteroplasties, and severe sphincter defects that preclude primary repair. Needless to say, a functioning gluteus maximus muscle is necessary; this may be ascertained by asking the patient to squeeze the muscle. When the integrity of the muscle is in doubt, particularly in a patient who has had a severe traumatic injury or a necrotizing infection requiring debridement, EMG should be performed. Preoperative anal manometry, although not essential, may precisely measure the improvement in anal pressures.

Technique

After preoperative mechanical and antibiotic bowel preparation, the patient is placed in the prone jackknife position. Bilateral oblique incisions are made lateral to the midline and extending to the ischial tuberosity (▶ Fig. 14.8b). The inferior border of the gluteus maximus muscle is identified and followed to its sacrococcygeal insertion. The inferior (caudal) portion of the muscle is detached from its sacrococcygeal attachment, ensuring that the dense fascia attaching the muscle

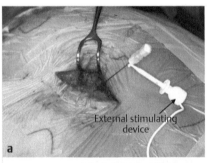
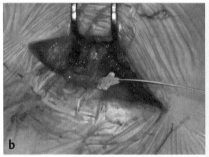
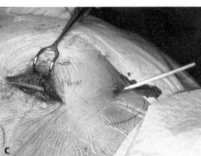
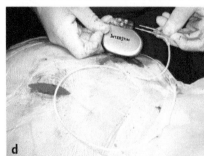

External stimulating device

Fig. 14.8 Gluteoplasty. **(a)** Anatomy of the gluteal region. **(b)** Bilateral incisions are made, and the inferior border of the gluteus muscle is identified. **(c)** Muscle is detached from the sacrococcygeal attachment, with care to preserve the neurovascular supply. The muscle is split into two sections. **(d)** The muscle is tunneled from each side and passed around the anus, overlapped, and sutured.[220] (With permission © 1992 Wolters Kluwer.)

to the sacrum is included. The muscle is mobilized laterally, with care to preserve the inferior gluteal artery and nerve (▶ Fig. 14.8c). A stimulator may be helpful in identifying the nerve.[222] The muscle is divided along the direction of its fibers into two equal segments. A similar procedure is carried out on the opposite side. An important caveat is that no more than 50% of the bulk of this formidable muscle should be mobilized. Any larger amount will not be able to fit in the circular anal tunnel.

Two curvilinear incisions are made several centimeters from the anal verge over the left and right ischioanal space. Subcutaneous tunnels are developed anteriorly and posteriorly around the anus. Space is also developed to tunnel the muscle to the perianal area. The ends of the inferior muscle from the right and left side are passed inferiorly toward the perineum, overlapped, and sutured. Similarly, the ends of the superior muscle are passed posteriorly around the rectum, overlapped, and secured, thus creating a valvelike diaphragm around the anus (▶ Fig. 14.8d). The wounds are closed, and suction drains are left in place.

Postoperative care is routine. Early ambulation is permitted, but sitting is not allowed for several weeks, and the patient should avoid climbing stairs for 2 to 3 weeks.

According to a review of the literature by Fleshner and Roberts, the most common complication after transposition of the gluteus maximus muscle is infection of the wound (24%). Other complications include skin separation and/or necrosis in 8% and fecal impaction in 8%. Their review of the scant literature on the subject revealed complete continence in 60%, partial continence in 36%, and total failure in 4%.[221] Pearl et al[223] reported on seven patients who underwent bilateral gluteus maximus transposition for complete FI. The indications for operation were sphincter destruction secondary to multiple fistulotomies (four), bilateral pudendal nerve damage (two), and high imperforate anus (one). This procedure was performed without the use of a diverting colostomy. The inferior portion of the origin of each gluteus maximus is detached from the sacrum and coccyx, bifurcated, and tunneled subcutaneously to encircle the anus. The ends are then sutured together to form two opposing slings of voluntary muscle. Postoperatively, six patients regained continence to solid stool, two to liquid stool as well, and only one patient in this group was able to control flatus.

Hultman et al reported a retrospective series of 25 patients who underwent unilateral gluteoplasty. At 20 months of follow-up, continence was significantly improved in more than 70% of patients. However, morbidity in this series was significant—in 64% of patients; there were significant complications reported, including donor site infection and perianal sepsis.[224] Devesa et al reported on a series of 20 patients who underwent bilateral gluteoplasty, and while more than 50% showed improved manometric measurements during physiologic testing and with control of solid stool, little to no success was seen in terms of liquid or gas control.[225]

Artificial Sphincter Implantation

The artificial bowel sphincter (ABS), developed by American Medical Systems (Minnetonka, MN), employs an inflatable cuff that is tunneled around the native sphincter complex, and controlled by a fluid-filled pressure-regulated balloon which is implanted anterior to the bladder and controlled manually by an actuator implanted in the scrotum or labia majora, first reported on by Christiansen and Sparsø.[226] Twelve patients with FI due to neurologic disease or failure of previous incontinence surgery underwent implantation of an artificial anal sphincter. The system used was a modification of the AMS 800 artificial urinary sphincter. In two patients, infection necessitated removal of the system, and in four patients, eight revisional procedures had to be performed because of mechanical failure. Only one case of mechanical failure has occurred. Erosion through the anal canal did not occur. Among 10 patients with the system in function for more than 6 months, the result was considered excellent in 5, with only occasional leakage of flatus, good in 3, who occasionally leaked liquid feces and flatus, and acceptable in 2, in whom the cuff obstructed defecation. The authors concluded that implantation of an artificial anal sphincter is a valid alternative to permanent colostomy in patients with FI due to neurologic disorders and in patients in whom other types of incontinence surgery have failed. Since the initial report, more data cast a cautionary tale. Mundy et al published a systematic review in 2004,[227] showing encouraging initial functional success in two-thirds of patients; however, complications were unacceptably high. Infection rates greater than 20% as well as mechanical failures resulted in explantation in more than half of patients. Darnis et al published an even more ominous series showing a greater than 75% complication rate.[228] Wong et al published a more balanced series of 52 patients with a > 5-year follow-up. In this series, there was a revision rate of 50%, but explantation in only 27%, and more than two-thirds of patients had a significant improvement in FI scores and QOL scores in those who still retained their implants at 5 years.[229] In order to better determine predictors of success, Wexner et al followed a cohort of 51 patients over a 9-year period. In this study, there was a 41% rate of infection, most of which were early post-op (18/23). Multivariate analysis showed that prior perianal infection, and time between implant and first bowel movement were predictive of infection.[230] Overall, despite success in a highly select population, the overwhelming technical and infectious complications have resulted in the device being withdrawn by the manufacturer (AMS, see above) from distribution in the United States.

Implantation of an artificial bowel sphincter remains an effective tool for select patients with severe FI. Grade of recommendation: Strong recommendation based on low- or very low-quality evidence, 1C.[138]

Magnetic Anal Sphincter

As the success of neuromodulation is so profound, the group of patients who still fail has become smaller and more difficult to treat. Not surprisingly, new wisdom has looked to the past for inspiration, and so was born the magnetic anal sphincter (MAS). This is a modern update of the cerclage technique popularized by Thiersch. This technique involved the implantation of a string of titanium beads with magnetic cores linked together by wire, named the Fenix device (Torax Medical, St. Paul, MN). As in the Thiersch procedure, this wire is tunneled around the native sphincter complex and sewn in place. At rest, the magnetic cores are drawn together, providing an occlusive force. The technology was first used (and abandoned) for esophageal closure to prevent reflux. Force generated in the rectum during Valsalva is enough to overcome the magnetic forces, and allow passage of stool. Lehur et al first published a feasibility study in 2010, reporting on 14 patients. Complications were reported in 7/14 patients: two devices required explantation secondary to infection, and three were removed for other reasons, one eroded through the anal canal and was extruded. Of those who maintained their implants, five patients at 6-month follow-up had a > 90% reduction in the number of FI episodes, and a significant improvement in CCF-FIS (17.8 to 7.8).[231] Barussaud et al published a prospective study on 23 patients implanted with the MAS with an 18-month follow-up. They reported a significant success: median incontinence scores decreased from 15.2 to 6.9 at 6 months. With follow-up as long as 36 months, reported FI scores remained low, with a CCF-FIS of 5.3. Only two patients required explantation due to infection.[232] This device is currently undergoing a trial in the United States.

Current data are insufficient to support the use of the magnetic sphincter for FI. Grade of recommendation: Weak recommendation based on low- or very low-quality evidence, 2C.[138]

Reversed Pylorus Interposition

A brief mention is deserved of a novel approach for sphincter replacement in patients who have undergone abdominal perineal resection. Reversed pylorus interposition was first described by Chandra et al in 2013.[233] This treatment involves perineal transposition of the antropyloric valve immediately following abdominoperineal resection as an alternative to permanent end colostomy. The technique involves resection of the antropyloric valve with maintenance of a vascular pedicle based on the right gastroepiploic artery and innervation based on the vagus nerve. The graft is sutured proximally to the descending colon conduit, and the distal end is sutured to the anus. In the first publication in humans, Chandra et al reported on a series of eight patients who underwent reversed pylorus interposition. The vagus nerve pedicle was anastomosed to the inferior rectal nerve. Manometric studies postoperatively showed increases in resting and squeeze pressures in all patients, compared to initial postoperative baseline. St. Marks scores ranged between 7 and 12. Interestingly, no major surgical complications were reported.[234] At this time, no other authors have reported on their use of this technique

Augmentation

Injectables

One of the more recent modalities that has been used to treat FI is injectable bulking agents. These synthetic and biological materials are injected into the submucosal or intersphincteric space in order to bulk the area and cause a relative physical obstruction. Numerous materials have been tested in this regard. Examples include autologous fat, collagen, and slowly absorbable bio materials including hydrogel cross-linked with polyacrylamide synthetic calcium hydroxyapatite ceramic microspheres, silicone biospheres (PTQ, Cogentix Medical Incorporated, Minnetonka, MN), carbon-coated beads (Durasphere EXP, Coloplast Corporation, Minneapolis, MN) and non–animal stabilized dextranomer in hyaluronic acid (NASHA Dx – Solesta, Salix Pharmaceuticals, Raleigh, NC).

The majority of published data surrounding the use of NASHA/Dx, under the trade name Solesta, has been regarding studies of this injectable. The seminal study, a randomized double blind trial, compared a treatment arm with a sham saline injection arm. In this study, 52% of patients in the treatment group experienced a 50% or more reduction in the number of incontinent episodes; however, in the sham group 31% also had success.[235] Some significant adverse events were reported including rectal and prostatic abscesses. Maeda et al performed a recent systematic review looking at all trials of injectable bulking agents. Not surprisingly, as the majority of these were industry funded, many were found to be at high risk for bias. Only the Solesta trial showed a statistically significant improvement in continence. One of the trials comparing silicone biospheres (PTQ) to carbon-coated beads (Durasphere) did show some short-term advantages.[236]

Some of the key questions that have yet to be well answered include optimum dose and delivery method. In Maeda et al's review, ultrasound-guided delivery was found to be superior to manually guided injection.

A more recent study of Solesta conducted by La Torre and de la Portilla[237] assessed longer-term results and found some durable efficacy at 24 and 36 months with just over half of patients still maintaining a greater than 50% reduction in fecal incontinent episodes. In order to identify predictors for failure, Hussain et al conducted a systematic review of all injectable materials and found that the only significant predictor for failure was the use of local anesthetic for injection as well as the failure to use laxatives in the postoperative period.[238] This problem may be related to high rates of implant extrusion early after injection.

There are little positive data reflecting any durable success with this modality. Guerra et al followed a cohort of 19 patients with a mean follow-up of 7 years who underwent treatment with Durasphere, PTQ, or Solesta. Patients underwent clinical assessment anal manometry and ultrasound evaluation. In this group, the vast majority of implants were no longer detectable or effective.[239]

In general, it seems that the use of bulking agents has largely been abandoned by colorectal surgeons as an effective modality for the treatment of FI. Theoretically, this therapy may still serve a need in those patients with minor soiling issues or after anorectal surgery that has resulted in anorectal scarring and mild anatomic deformity.

Injection of biocompatible bulking agents into the anal canal may help to decrease episodes of passive FI. Grade of recommendation: Weak recommendation based on moderate-quality evidence, 2B.[138]

Radiofrequency Therapy

Radiofrequency (RF) therapy is a technique that was originally described as the Stretta technique for treating gastroesophageal reflux disease. The adaptation for use in the anal sphincter has been termed the Secca (Mederi Therapeutics, Greenwich, CT) procedure. This technique is based on the use of submucosally applied RF energy to induce tissue remodeling. The Secca procedure can be performed on an ambulatory basis using conscious sedation and local anesthesia. The patient is positioned in the prone jackknife position. The RF instrument comprises an anoscopic barrel with four nickel–titanium curved needle electrodes. Within the tip and at the base of each electrode, thermocouples are present to monitor tissue and mucosal temperature during RF delivery. The instrument is introduced into the anal canal under direct visualization, so that the needle electrodes start to penetrate the tissue 1 cm distal to the dentate line. Additional lesions are created up to 1.5 cm above the dentate line in all four quadrants (▶ Fig. 14.9). Mucosal temperature is cooled by surface irrigation. In this way, thermal lesions are created in the muscle below the mucosa, while preserving the mucosal integrity. In contrast to the belief that RF therapy would cause scarring and tightening of the anal canal, essentially causing mild obstruction akin to cerclage, new or histologic assessment of RF-treated tissue reveals that nonablative RF energy causes morphologic changes in damaged sphincter muscle to become more histologically normal.[240] In an experimental porcine model, RF ablation treatment of the sphincter complex demonstrated an increase in the smooth muscle/connective tissue ratios and increased type 1 collagen (vs. type 3) when compared to controls. The RF treatment group also exhibited greater smooth muscle thickness compared to the control group. Importantly, posttreatment manometry showed significantly higher basal and squeeze pressures, compared to

the control group.[240] Efron published some of the earliest clinical data in a multicenter trial involving 50 patients. In this cohort, mean CCFFI scores improved from a baseline of 14.5 to 11.1 at 6 months. All QOL parameters were also improved and only minor complications were noted.[241] Five-year data were reported by Takahashi-Monroy showing that mean FI scores remained significantly improved from baseline of 14 to 8, with nearly 85% of patients showing a greater than 50% improvement.[242] Ruiz et al reported on more modest results at 2-year follow-up showing mild improvement in incontinence scores from 15.6 to 12.9.[243] Frascio et al conducted a systematic review in 2013 inclusive of 10 studies and 220 patients. They found that in the majority of the studies, RF treatment is an effective treatment of mild-to-moderate FI, and that good patient selection maximizes outcomes, with clinically significant improvement in CCF-FIS and QOL scores.[244] Currently, a few centers are employing this modality.

Application of temperature-controlled radiofrequency energy to the sphincter complex may be used to treat FI. Grade of recommendation: Weak recommendation based on moderate-quality evidence, 2B.[138]

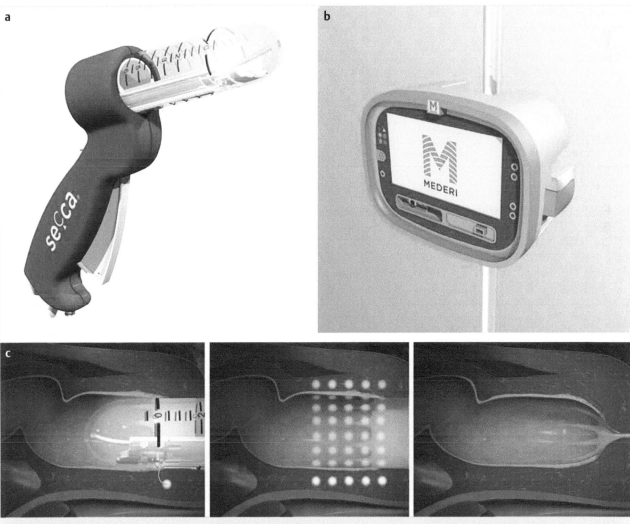

Fig. 14.9 (a) SECCA device. **(b)** Power source. **(c)** Schematic of how SECCA works. (With permissoin © 2015 Informa Healthcare)

Transanal/Transvaginal Plugs and Slings

Another type of diversion procedure entails keeping the stool in the rectum rather than letting it challenge the anal sphincters. A variety of novel transanal and transvaginal plug devices have been employed to fulfill this goal. Lukacz et al reported on a multicenter, prospective, single-arm study of the Renew anal insert device (Renew Medical Inc., Foster City, CA). Seventy-three patients completed the study, and of this cohort, 77% achieved a minimum of a 50% reduction in incontinence frequency. Mean incontinence scores improved by over 32%, and 78% of patients were highly satisfied with the result.[245,246] The Procon-2 device was reported on by Giamundo et al in 2002,[247] and consisted of a catheter with an infrared sensor and an inflatable balloon tip. This device was inserted into the rectum and inflated, obstructing the passage of stool, but allowing the passage of flatus via vent holes. It notified the user when coming in contact with stool, allowing time to go to the bathroom, deflate the catheter, and evacuate. The initial study comprised seven patients, and resulted in a significant reduction in incontinence scores and improvement in QOL scores. Other modalities currently being tested include the TOPAS device (American Medical Systems), which is a polypropylene mesh sling implanted to reinforce the puborectalis angle, as well as the LIBERATE trial (Pelvilon, Inc.), which employs an inflatable vaginal insert used to occlude the anal canal. In addition, the use of an occlusive anal plug has been employed as a minimally invasive option.

Stimulation

Sacral Neuromodulation

Sacral nerve stimulation (SNS) has emerged as the most promising new modality in the treatment of medically refractory FI. The term "new modality" is a misnomer, however, because this technique has been around for almost 20 years. It was originally developed for the treatment of urinary incontinence, but its efficacy for the treatment of FI quickly emerged due to the high incidence of mixed urinary incontinence and FI. Clinically, it seems to be much more efficacious for the treatment of FI compared to its effects on urinary leakage.[244,248] Subsequent to the 2010 American Society of Colon and Rectal Surgeons presentation and subsequent publications,[245,247,249,250] based on multi-institutional trial data, this therapy was approved by the FDA in 2011 for the indication of FI patients who have failed best conservative therapy. The basis of this technique is a quadripolar lead electrode placed transcutaneously and situated adjacent to the S3 nerve root via a transsacral foraminal approach. An initial test phase is incorporated whereby after lead placement, a temporary external pacer is used and efficacy is monitored. The minimum definition of success is based on a 50% reduction in the number of fecal incontinent episodes over the test period. Two separate test phases can be used. An office-based temporary unipolar nontined lead is placed either using anatomic landmarks or with fluoroscopic guidance. As this is a nontined lead, this test phase lasts for a maximum of 3 to 7 days, because of the high likelihood of lead dislodgment. This test is best suited for patients with frequent FI episodes, often one or more per day. An alternative test involves operative placement of the permanent tined quadripolar lead under fluoroscopic guidance into the S3 sacral foramen (▶ Fig. 14.10). This lead will remain in place if the test is positive. With the operatively placed lead, the test lasts for a minimum of 1 week and a maximum of 3 weeks. This test is better suited for patients with less frequent episodes of incontinence, since the test is longer. Patients with one to two fecal incontinent episodes per week can be better assessed for therapeutic success over a longer interval. Stimulation programming is based on best motor responses obtained in the operating room. A successful lead placement causes bellowing of the levators and toe turning of the great toe indicating specific S3 stimulation. In either test, if a greater than 50% improvement in the number of fecal incontinent episodes is achieved, the patient can move on to stimulator implantation. Stimulator is placed in a subcutaneous pocket just inferior to the posterior superior iliac spine. At typical settings, the current stimulator model has a battery life of approximately 5 years.

The seminal prospective trial validating SNS (InterStim Trademark, Medtronic, Minneapolis, MN) was conducted by Tjandra et al and published in 2008. This study compared SNS to best medical therapy. The test population included patients with FI of almost any etiology and included patients with sphincter defects of up to 120 degrees. There were 120 patients in the initial cohort, 60 in the control group and 60 in the SNS group. Remarkably, 90% of patients reported success with initial testing and moved on to implantation. Of this group, almost 50% achieved perfect continence, compared to no improvement in the control group.[248,252] The FDA qualifying trial echoed Tjandra et al's results, with an 87% success rate and an over 40% rate of patients achieving perfect continence. Interim follow-up at 3 years was conducted by Mellgren et al, and found that success was sustained: 83% of patients still reported overall success with a mean decrease in the number of fecal incontinent episodes from a baseline of 9.4 to 1.7.[245,249,253] Forty percent of this cohort still reported perfect continence. Complications in this trial were minimal, the most frequent complication being implant site pain in 25%, with a 10% infection rate noted. Hull et al reported on 5-year follow-up in this cohort in 2013. Impressively, 89% of patients still reported success with therapy and 36% still reported maintenance of perfect continence.[250,254] It should be noted that in this trial, patients with sphincter defects of up to 60 degrees were included, and this had no effect on overall success. Longer-term data for this therapy have been published by numerous groups, primarily from Europe. In the Italian SNS registry, Altomare et al published 5-year follow-up on 52 patients. Mean CCF-FIS decreased from a baseline of 15 to 5. Seventy-four percent of patients had at least a 50% improvement in the number of FI episodes with full continence maintained in 20% of patients.[252,255] Lim et al published 5-year follow-up for the Australian experience in 53 patients.[253,256] Mean CCF-FIS scores improved from a baseline of 11.5 to 8. Michelsen et al published the Danish experience with a 6-year follow-up of 126 patients. At 6 years, mean CCF-FIS score had improved from a baseline of 20 to 7.[254,257] The European SNS outcomes study group reported on 7-year outcomes in a multinational study incorporating 10 European centers and 407 patients with a mean follow-up of 84 months.[255,258] Side-by-side comparisons of multiple incontinence scoring parameters including number of incontinent episodes, CCF-FIS score, and St. Marks score all showed dramatic and significant improvements persisting to 7 years of follow-up. George et al[256,259] published a 10-year follow-up study of 25 patients. Ninety-two percent of patients still had a greater than 50% improvement and full continence was maintained in almost 50%. In an attempt to define predictive variables for success, Brouwer and Duthie evaluated a cohort of patients with 4 years of follow-up looking at variables including sphincter defect, neuropathy, and prior sphincter repair. The therapy was overwhelmingly positive in all groups, irrespective of these variables[257,260] (▶ Table 14.7).

Mechanism of action is incompletely understood in SNM. Normal neural mechanisms of continence rely, at least in part, on inhibition of the defecation reflex in the central pontine center.

Various afferent inputs modulate how the brain perceives when it is time to defecate. Pudendal nerve afferents whose receptors originate in the anal canal and are involved in the sampling reflex help to inhibit colonic activity and activate the internal sphincter. The various ways that these reflexes may be disordered is manifold; however, Gourcerol et al, in a comprehensive systematic review of the literature regarding potential mechanisms of action for SNS, proposed three hypotheses: SNS acts by (1) initiating a somatovisceral reflex, (2) a modulation of the perception of afferent information,

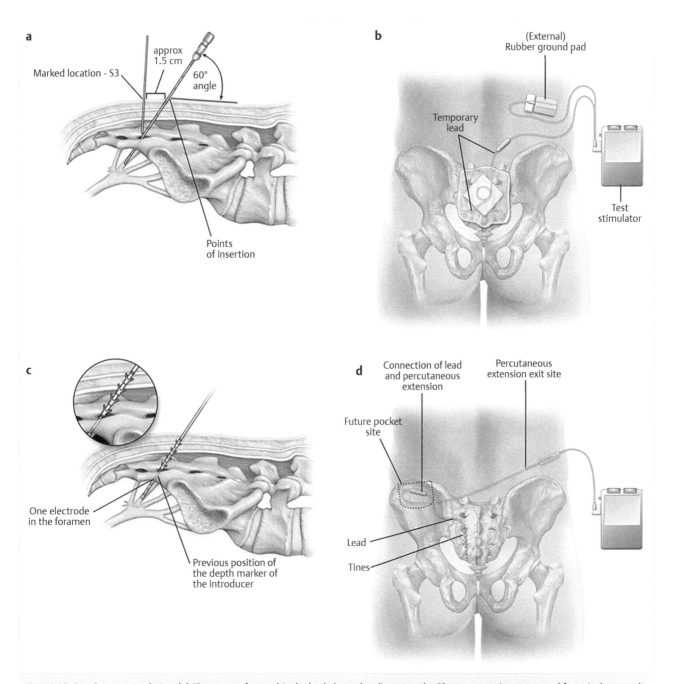

Fig. 14.10 Sacral nerve stimulation. **(a)** Placement of a quadripolar lead electrode adjacent to the S3 nerve root via a transsacral foraminal approach. **(b)** The initial test phase can be performed in the office using a temporary, unipolar, nontined lead, which is placed using either anatomic landmarks or fluoroscopic guidance. **(c)** An alternative test involves operative placement of the permanent quadripolar tined lead under fluoroscopic guidance. **(d)** The patient is then tested with an external battery, programmed to the same settings that the permanent battery would use. (*Continued*)

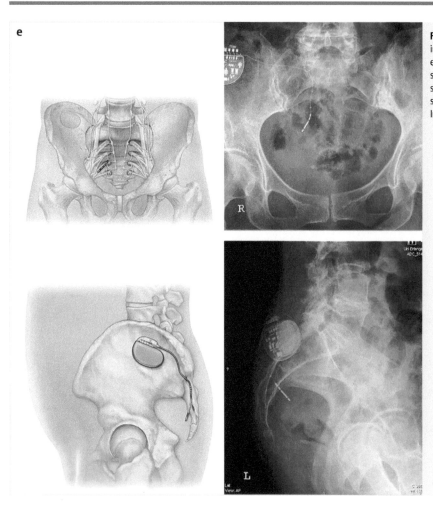

e

Fig. 14.10 (*Continued*) **(e)** If at least a 50% improvement in the number of fecal incontinent episodes is achieved, the test is considered a success, and a permanent device is placed in a subcutaneous pocket just below the posterior superior iliac spine.[251] (With permission © 2015 Informa Healthcare and © 2012 Wolters Kluwer.)

Table 14.7 Results of sacral neuromodulation

Authors	Year	No. of patients	Last follow-up (mo)	% success (based on a minimum decrease of 50% in no. of incontinent episodes)	Perfect continence
Tjandra et al[252]	2008	60	12	90	47.2
Wexner et al[250]	2010	120	12	83	41
Mellgren et al[253]	2011	83	37	86	40
Hull et al[254]	2013	72	60	89	36
Altomare et al[255]	2009	52	60	74	20
Altomare et al[258]	2015	228	84	71	50
George et al[259]	2012	25	114	90	48

and (3) an increase in external anal sphincter activity. The key factor underlying the majority of the mechanism of action seems to depend on the modulation of spinal and/or supraspinal afferent inputs.[258,261]

SNM **may be considered as a first-line surgical option for incontinent patients with and without sphincter defects. Grade of recommendation: Strong recommendation based on moderate-quality evidence, 1B.**[138]

Posterior Tibial Nerve Stimulation (PTNS)

Posterior tibial nerve stimulation (PTNS) was first used for the treatment of urinary incontinence in 1983 by Nakamura et al.[259,262] As with SNS, it was serendipitously found to have efficacy for the use of FI as well. During the application of this treatment, either transcutaneous or percutaneous electrodes are applied over the posterior tibial nerve. Stimulation is

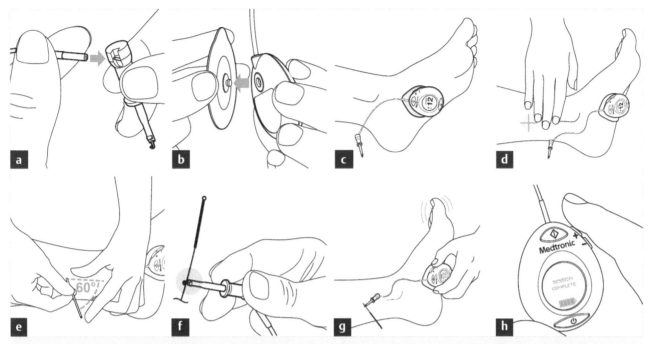

Fig. 14.11 Posterior tibial nerve stimulation (PTNS). **(a)** Use alcohol pad to clean surface of device and cable. Firmly insert device cable to needle holder. **(b)** Snap ground pad to back of NURO device. **(c)** Remove ground pad adhesive and attach to instep of foot. **(d)** Clean skin with alcohol pad. Locate needle insertion site on inner portion of lower leg. **(e)** Insert needle at 60-degree angle. Gently tap needle to pierce skin. Remove guide tube. Advance approximately 2 cm using rotating motion. **(f)** Connect J hook of needle holder to needle. **(g)** Hold power button to turn on device. Press the power button again to get to the Stimulation Level Adjust Mode. Increase stimulation level and observe for patient response. Then reduce setting by one level and press "Start" to begin session. **(h)** Once 30 minutes have elapsed, Therapy Mode will automatically end. Remove needle. Unsnap and remove ground pad. Turn off device. (With permission © Medtronic, Inc.)

typically performed twice daily, for 20-minute sessions over a 3-month period (▸ Fig. 14.11).

An early series employing the percutaneous technique in 2003 was published by Shafik et al. In this study, 32 patients with medically refractory FI were treated with percutaneous stimulation. In over 78% of patients, significant improvement in FI was achieved.[260,263] A more recent systematic review identified nearly 300 patients treated with tibial nerve stimulation. Success, defined as at least a 50% improvement in incontinence scores, was achieved by between 63 and 82% of patients.[261,264] Thin et al also performed a randomized clinical trial comparing tibial nerve stimulation to SNS. Although SNS showed greater success than tibial nerve stimulation, both treatments did show clinical efficacy.[262,265] Knowles et al reported on the largest randomized sham-controlled trial including 227 patients. Compared to 31% in the sham group, 38% of patients in the treatment group achieved a greater than 50% reduction in the number of weekly incontinent episodes. Furthermore, patients with obstructed defecation are more likely to benefit from placebo therapy, whereas patients with obstructed defecation are more likely to benefit from PTNS. This curious finding suggests that if PTNS has any role, it would be in patients who do not report obstructed defecation.[263,266,267,268,]

Transcutaneous stimulation employs a similar therapeutic schedule, but enjoys the advantage of avoidance of skin perforation with electrodes, instead employing inductive electrodes taped to the skin. Leroi et al, using a transcutaneous technique, performed a randomized prospective trial on 144 patients. The treatment group showed improvement in FI scores compared to only 27% of sham, though this did not reach statistical significance.[264,269] These results were echoed in a recent study by Lecompte et al in a series of eight children with various causes of FI including four with congenital anorectal malformations, three with neurogenic causes, and one with Hirschsprung's disease. They found that after 6 months, five patients were totally cured, two significantly improved, and only one had no response. The authors report a plan for a larger, prospective trial.[265,270]

Edenfield et al recently published a systematic review inclusive of 15 studies. The group was comprised of a total of 745 patients, and although the majority of the studies were low quality, both percutaneous and transcutaneous approaches showed significant improvement over controls.[266,271]

PTNS remains an interesting potential option for motivated patients who may be otherwise ineligible for standard SNM, and may be a good option in the pediatric population.

Percutaneous tibial nerve stimulation may be considered because it provides short-term improvement in episodes of FI. Grade of recommendation: Weak recommendation based on low- or very low-quality evidence, 2C.[138]

Diversion/Obstruction

Antegrade Continence Enema (ACE Procedure)

The ACE procedure was first described by Malone in 1990.[269,272] This treatment was developed for patients with disabling colonic motility disorders and difficulty with evacuation of solid stool. In this description, the appendix is reversed and tunneled into the wall of the cecum, creating a one-way valve. The proximal end is brought through the abdominal wall as a small stoma in the right lower quadrant, flush with the skin. In order to eliminate, the appendicostomy is intubated, with tubing in the colon flushed in an antegrade manner with fluid, daily, in order to clear the colon of stool. This has been employed primarily in the pediatric population, afflicted with congenital motility disorders. It is rarely used in adults. Several modifications of this procedure have been described in order to simplify the technical rigors. Some recent adaptations include laparoscopic approaches as well as direct appendicostomy without reversal. Several reports have shown good results.[273,274] Worsøe et al reported long-term results on a series of 80 patients with a mean follow-up of 75 months. In this cohort, there was an overall success rate of 74%, with very positive subjective results.[246,272]

Colostomy

For patients with FI so severe that they are disabled by their problem and unable to control their elimination pattern by conservative means, such as medication, diet, and enemas, and in the failure of any of the above surgical modalities, construction of a colostomy may become necessary. Despite the assumed negative associations with a stoma, the patient's QOL may be significantly enhanced and self-imposed isolation corrected. A colostomy is especially appropriate in patients with profound incontinence related to anorectal disease or tumor, and in whom other surgical approaches are contraindicated, perhaps due to significant comorbidities, or in situations where reconstruction is impossible. Norton et al[273,275] reviewed the formation of a permanent stoma as a last resort when all other interventions for FI have failed. Questionnaires were sent asking about the stoma, previous incontinence, anxiety and depression, and QOL. A total of 69 replies were received. Respondents were 11 males and 58 females with a median age of 64 years and a median of 59 months since the operation. Rating their ability to live with their stoma now on a scale of 0 to 10, the median response was 8. The majority (83%) felt that the stoma restricted their life "a little" or "not at all," a significant improvement from perceived restriction from former incontinence. Satisfaction with the stoma was a median of 9. Eighty-four percent would "probably" or "definitely" choose to have the stoma again. QOL (SF-36) was poor, but neither depression nor anxiety was a prominent feature. They concluded the majority of previously incontinent people were positive about the stoma and the difference it had made to their life. However, a few had not adapted and disliked the stoma intensely.

A novel modification of a colostomy was described by Hughes and Williams.[274,276] A transverse colonic conduit incorporating an intussusception valve and a skin-flapped cutaneous aperture was constructed in nine patients with combined FI and disordered evacuation. Intestinal continuity was restored with a colonic anastomosis. The median follow-up was 4 months (range, 2–15 months), and daily irrigation with a median 1.2 L (range, 0.3–2.0 L) of water resulted in evacuation in less than 1 hour. At 1 month after operation, there was no leakage of solid or liquid feces from the anus between irrigations. The valve was continent to feces and irrigation fluid, and no stoma appliances were required.

Creation of a colostomy is an excellent surgical option for patients who have failed or do not wish to pursue other therapies for FI. Grade of recommendation, 1C.[138]

14.5 Conclusion

The last two decades have seen an unparalleled explosion in the development of options for the treatment of FI. Especially with respect to the success of SNM, there has been a profound paradigm shift in the more conservative, yet profoundly effective, management of all but the most extreme cases of FI. Despite the wide range of surgical options, most patients with FI can be treated very successfully with appropriate conservative management and the use of stool-bulking agents and antidiarrheal medications. For those who failed conservative treatment, there are a wide variety of surgical options. The classical historical gold standard of sphincter repair has been largely supplanted with much more effective techniques, with SNM leading the way. Nevertheless, a thorough and deep understanding of all of the surgical options for management of FI is incumbent on all surgeons who may see these patients.

References

[1] Madoff RD, Williams JG, Caushaj PF. Fecal incontinence. N Engl J Med. 1992; 326(15):1002–1007

[2] Browning GG, Parks AG. Postanal repair for neuropathic faecal incontinence: correlation of clinical result and anal canal pressures. Br J Surg. 1983; 70(2):101–104

[3] Baxter NN, Rothenberger DA, Lowry AC. Measuring fecal incontinence. Dis Colon Rectum. 2003; 46(12):1591–1605

[4] Jorge JM, Wexner SD. Etiology and management of fecal incontinence. Dis Colon Rectum. 1993; 36(1):77–97

[5] Rothbarth J, Bemelman WA, Meijerink WJ, et al. What is the impact of fecal incontinence on quality of life? Dis Colon Rectum. 2001; 44(1):67–71

[6] Rockwood TH, Church JM, Fleshman JW, et al. Patient and surgeon ranking of the severity of symptoms associated with fecal incontinence: the fecal incontinence severity index. Dis Colon Rectum. 1999; 42(12):1525–1532

[7] Rockwood TH. Incontinence severity and QOL scales for fecal incontinence. Gastroenterology. 2004; 126(1) Suppl 1:S106–S113

[8] Luppa M, Luck T, Weyerer S, König HH, Brähler E, Riedel-Heller SG. Prediction of institutionalization in the elderly. A systematic review. Age Ageing. 2010; 39(1):31–38

[9] Bharucha AE, Dunivan G, Goode PS, et al. Epidemiology, pathophysiology, and classification of fecal incontinence: state of the science summary for the National Institute of Diabetes and Digestive and Kidney Diseases (NIDDK) workshop. Am J Gastroenterol. 2015; 110(1):127–136

[10] Brown HW, Wexner SD, Segall MM, Brezoczky KL, Lukacz ES. Accidental bowel leakage in the mature women's health study: prevalence and predictors. Int J Clin Pract. 2012; 66(11):1101–1108

[11] Brown HW, Wexner SD, Segall MM, Brezoczky KL, Lukacz ES. Quality of life impact in women with accidental bowel leakage. Int J Clin Pract. 2012; 66(11):1109–1116

[12] Brown HW, Wexner SD, Lukacz ES. Factors associated with care seeking among women with accidental bowel leakage. Female Pelvic Med Reconstr Surg. 2013; 19(2):66–71

[13] Tobin GW, Brocklehurst JC. Faecal incontinence in residential homes for the elderly: prevalence, aetiology and management. Age Ageing. 1986; 15(1):41–46

[14] Nelson R, Norton N, Cautley E, Furner S. Community-based prevalence of anal incontinence. JAMA. 1995; 274(7):559–561

[15] Borrie MJ, Davidson HA. Incontinence in institutions: costs and contributing factors. CMAJ. 1992; 147(3):322–328

[16] Sangwan YP, Coller JA. Fecal incontinence. Surg Clin North Am. 1994; 74(6):1377–1398

[17] Whitehead WE, Schuster MM. Behavioral approaches to the treatment of gastrointestinal motility disorders. Med Clin North Am. 1981; 65(6):1397–1411

[18] Macmillan AK, Merrie AE, Marshall RJ, Parry BR. The prevalence of fecal incontinence in community-dwelling adults: a systematic review of the literature. Dis Colon Rectum. 2004; 47(8):1341–1349

[19] Johanson JF, Lafferty J. Epidemiology of fecal incontinence: the silent affliction. Am J Gastroenterol. 1996; 91(1):33–36

[20] Xu X, Menees SB, Zochowski MK, Fenner DE. Economic cost of fecal incontinence. Dis Colon Rectum. 2012; 55(5):586–598

[21] Damon H, Henry L, Barth X, Mion F. Fecal incontinence in females with a past history of vaginal delivery: significance of anal sphincter defects detected by ultrasound. Dis Colon Rectum. 2002; 45(11):1445–1450, discussion 1450–1451

[22] Perry S, Shaw C, McGrother C, et al. Leicestershire MRC Incontinence Study Team. Prevalence of faecal incontinence in adults aged 40 years or more living in the community. Gut. 2002; 50(4):480–484

[23] Cerulli MA, Nikoomanesh P, Schuster MM. Progress in biofeedback conditioning for fecal incontinence. Gastroenterology. 1979; 76(4):742–746

[24] Ctercteko GC, Fazio VW, Jagelman DG, Lavery IC, Weakley FL, Melia M. Anal sphincter repair: a report of 60 cases and review of the literature. Aust N Z J Surg. 1988; 58(9):703–710

[25] Keighley MR, Fielding JW. Management of faecal incontinence and results of surgical treatment. Br J Surg. 1983; 70(8):463–468

[26] Lindsey I, Jones OM, Smilgin-Humphreys MM, Cunningham C, Mortensen NJ. Patterns of fecal incontinence after anal surgery. Dis Colon Rectum. 2004; 47(10):1643–1649

[27] Khubchandani IT, Reed JF. Sequelae of internal sphincterotomy for chronic fissure in ano. Br J Surg. 1989; 76(5):431–434

[28] Garcia-Aguilar J, Belmonte C, Wong WD, Lowry AC, Madoff RD. Open vs. closed sphincterotomy for chronic anal fissure: long-term results. Dis Colon Rectum. 1996; 39(4):440–443

[29] Pernikoff BJ, Eisenstat TE, Rubin RJ, Oliver GC, Salvati EP. Reappraisal of partial lateral internal sphincterotomy. Dis Colon Rectum. 1994; 37(12):1291–1295

[30] Hananel N, Gordon PH. Lateral internal sphincterotomy for fissure-in-ano—revisited. Dis Colon Rectum. 1997; 40(5):597–602

[31] Hyman N. Incontinence after lateral internal sphincterotomy: a prospective study and quality of life assessment. Dis Colon Rectum. 2004; 47(1):35–38

[32] Liang J, Church JM. Lateral internal sphincterotomy for surgically recurrent chronic anal fissure. Am J Surg. 2015; 210(4):715–719

[33] Tjandra JJ, Han WR, Ooi BS, Nagesh A, Thorne M. Faecal incontinence after lateral internal sphincterotomy is often associated with coexisting occult sphincter defects: a study using endoanal ultrasonography. ANZ J Surg. 2001; 71(10):598–602

[34] Casillas S, Hull TL, Zutshi M, Trzcinski R, Bast JF, Xu M. Incontinence after a lateral internal sphincterotomy: are we underestimating it? Dis Colon Rectum. 2005; 48(6):1193–1199

[35] Sultan AH, Kamm MA, Nicholls RJ, Bartram CI. Prospective study of the extent of internal anal sphincter division during lateral sphincterotomy. Dis Colon Rectum. 1994; 37(10):1031–1033

[36] Aguilar PS, Plasencia G, Hardy TG, Jr, Hartmann RF, Stewart WR. Mucosal advancement in the treatment of anal fistula. Dis Colon Rectum. 1985; 28(7):496–498

[37] Golub RW, Wise WE, Jr, Kerner BA, Khanduja KS, Aguilar PS. Endorectal mucosal advancement flap: the preferred method for complex cryptoglandular fistula-in-ano. J Gastrointest Surg. 1997; 1(5):487–491

[38] Ortíz H, Marzo J. Endorectal flap advancement repair and fistulectomy for high trans-sphincteric and suprasphincteric fistulas. Br J Surg. 2000; 87(12):1680–1683

[39] Schouten WR, Zimmerman DD, Briel JW. Transanal advancement flap repair of transsphincteric fistulas. Dis Colon Rectum. 1999; 42(11):1419–1422, discussion 1422–1423

[40] van Tets WF, Kuijpers JH, Tran K, Mollen R, van Goor H. Influence of Parks' anal retractor on anal sphincter pressures. Dis Colon Rectum. 1997; 40(9):1042–1045

[41] Zimmerman DD, Gosselink MP, Hop WC, Darby M, Briel JW, Schouten WR. Impact of two different types of anal retractor on fecal continence after fistula repair: a prospective, randomized, clinical trial. Dis Colon Rectum. 2003; 46(12):1674–1679

[42] Champagne BJ, O'Connor LM, Ferguson M, Orangio GR, Schertzer ME, Armstrong DN. Efficacy of anal fistula plug in closure of cryptoglandular fistulas: long-term follow-up. Dis Colon Rectum. 2006; 49(12):1817–1821

[43] Safar B, Jobanputra S, Sands D, Weiss EG, Nogueras JJ, Wexner SD. Anal fistula plug: initial experience and outcomes. Dis Colon Rectum. 2009; 52(2):248–252

[44] Limura E, Giordano P. Modern management of anal fistula. World J Gastroenterol. 2015; 21(1):12–20

[45] Rojanasakul A, Pattanaarun J, Sahakitrungruang C, Tantiphlachiva K. Total anal sphincter saving technique for fistula-in-ano; the ligation of intersphincteric fistula tract. J Med Assoc Thai. 2007; 90(3):581–586

[46] Rojanasakul A. LIFT procedure: a simplified technique for fistula-in-ano. Tech Coloproctol. 2009; 13(3):237–240

[47] Bleier JI, Moloo H, Goldberg SM. Ligation of the intersphincteric fistula tract: an effective new technique for complex fistulas. Dis Colon Rectum. 2010; 53(1):43–46

[48] Bleier JI, Kann BR. Surgical management of fecal incontinence. Gastroenterol Clin North Am. 2013; 42(4):815–836

[49] Kontovounisios C, Tekkis P, Tan E, Rasheed S, Darzi A, Wexner SD. Adoption and success rates of perineal procedures for fistula-in-ano: a systematic review. Colorectal Dis. 2016; 18(5):441–458

[50] Stelzner F. The morphological principles of anorectal continence. Prog Pediatr Surg. 1976; 9:1–6

[51] Goligher JC, Lee PW, Macfie J, Simpkins KC, Lintott DJ. Experience with the Russian model 249 suture gun for anastomosis of the rectum. Surg Gynecol Obstet. 1979; 148(4):516–524

[52] Vernava AM, III, Robbins PL, Brabbee GW. Restorative resection: coloanal anastomosis for benign and malignant disease. Dis Colon Rectum. 1989; 32(8):690–693

[53] Parks AG, Percy JP. Resection and sutured colo-anal anastomosis for rectal carcinoma. Br J Surg. 1982; 69(6):301–304

[54] Enker WE, Stearns MW, Jr, Janov AJ. Peranal coloanal anastomosis following low anterior resection for rectal carcinoma. Dis Colon Rectum. 1985; 28(8):576–581

[55] Bretagnol F, Rullier E, Laurent C, Zerbib F, Gontier R, Saric J. Comparison of functional results and quality of life between intersphincteric resection and conventional coloanal anastomosis for low rectal cancer. Dis Colon Rectum. 2004; 47(6):832–838

[56] Sultan AH, Kamm MA, Hudson CN, Thomas JM, Bartram CI. Anal-sphincter disruption during vaginal delivery. N Engl J Med. 1993; 329(26):1905–1911

[57] Eason E, Labrecque M, Marcoux S, Mondor M. Anal incontinence after childbirth. CMAJ. 2002; 166(3):326–330

[58] Oberwalder M, Connor J, Wexner SD. Meta-analysis to determine the incidence of obstetric anal sphincter damage. Br J Surg. 2003; 90(11):1333–1337

[59] Rieger N, Wattchow D. The effect of vaginal delivery on anal function. Aust N Z J Surg. 1999; 69(3):172–177

[60] Oberwalder M, Dinnewitzer A, Baig MK, et al. The association between late-onset fecal incontinence and obstetric anal sphincter defects. Arch Surg. 2004; 139(4):429–432

[61] Donnelly V, Fynes M, Campbell D, Johnson H, O'Connell PR, O'Herlihy C. Obstetric events leading to anal sphincter damage. Obstet Gynecol. 1998; 92(6):955–961

[62] de Parades V, Etienney I, Thabut D, et al. Anal sphincter injury after forceps delivery: myth or reality? A prospective ultrasound study of 93 females. Dis Colon Rectum. 2004; 47(1):24–34

[63] Campbell DM, Behan M, Donnelly VS, O'Herlihy C, O'Connell PR. Endosonographic assessment of postpartum anal sphincter injury using a 120 degree sector scanner. Clin Radiol. 1996; 51(8):559–561

[64] Rieger N, Schloithe A, Saccone G, Wattchow D. A prospective study of anal sphincter injury due to childbirth. Scand J Gastroenterol. 1998; 33(9):950–955

[65] Zetterström J, Mellgren A, Jensen LL, et al. Effect of delivery on anal sphincter morphology and function. Dis Colon Rectum. 1999; 42(10):1253–1260

[66] Varma A, Gunn J, Gardiner A, Lindow SW, Duthie GS. Obstetric anal sphincter injury: prospective evaluation of incidence. Dis Colon Rectum. 1999; 42(12):1537–1543

[67] Fynes MM, Marshall K, Cassidy M, et al. A prospective, randomized study comparing the effect of augmented biofeedback with sensory biofeedback alone on fecal incontinence after obstetric trauma. Dis Colon Rectum. 1999; 42(6):753–758, discussion 758–761

[68] Faltin DL, Boulvain M, Irion O, Bretones S, Stan C, Weil A. Diagnosis of anal sphincter tears by postpartum endosonography to predict fecal incontinence. Obstet Gynecol. 2000; 95(5):643–647

[69] Damon H, Henry L, Bretones S, Mellier G, Minaire Y, Mion F. Postdelivery anal function in primiparous females: ultrasound and manometric study. Dis Colon Rectum. 2000; 43(4):472–477

[70] Abramowitz L, Sobhani I, Ganansia R, et al. Are sphincter defects the cause of anal incontinence after vaginal delivery? Results of a prospective study. Dis Colon Rectum. 2000; 43(5):590–596, discussion 596–598

[71] Chaliha C, Sultan AH, Bland JM, Monga AK, Stanton SL. Anal function: effect of pregnancy and delivery. Am J Obstet Gynecol. 2001; 185(2):427–432

[72] Belmonte-Montes C, Hagerman G, Vega-Yepez PA, Hernández-de-Anda E, Fonseca-Morales V. Anal sphincter injury after vaginal delivery in primiparous females. Dis Colon Rectum. 2001; 44(9):1244–1248

[73] Willis S, Faridi A, Schelzig S, et al. Childbirth and incontinence: a prospective study on anal sphincter morphology and function before and early after vaginal delivery. Langenbecks Arch Surg. 2002; 387(2):101–107

[74] Nazir M, Carlsen E, Nesheim BI. Do occult anal sphincter injuries, vector volume manometry and delivery variables have any predictive value for bowel symptoms after first time vaginal delivery without third and fourth degree rupture? A prospective study. Acta Obstet Gynecol Scand. 2002; 81(8):720–726

[75] Peschers UM, Sultan AH, Jundt K, Mayer A, Drinovac V, Dimpfl T. Urinary and anal incontinence after vacuum delivery. Eur J Obstet Gynecol Reprod Biol. 2003; 110(1):39–42

[76] Sultan AH, Johanson RB, Carter JE. Occult anal sphincter trauma following randomized forceps and vacuum delivery. Int J Gynaecol Obstet. 1998; 61 (2):113–119

[77] Bollard RC, Gardiner A, Duthie GS, Lindow SW. Anal sphincter injury, fecal and urinary incontinence: a 34-year follow-up after forceps delivery. Dis Colon Rectum. 2003; 46(8):1083–1088

[78] Pinta TM, Kylänpää ML, Teramo KA, Luukkonen PS. Sphincter rupture and anal incontinence after first vaginal delivery. Acta Obstet Gynecol Scand. 2004; 83(10):917–922

[79] Pollack J, Nordenstam J, Brismar S, Lopez A, Altman D, Zetterstrom J. Anal incontinence after vaginal delivery: a five-year prospective cohort study. Obstet Gynecol. 2004; 104(6):1397–1402

[80] Sultan AH, Kamm MA, Hudson CN, Bartram CI. Third degree obstetric anal sphincter tears: risk factors and outcome of primary repair. BMJ. 1994; 308 (6933):887–891

[81] Davis K, Kumar D, Stanton SL, Thakar R, Fynes M, Bland J. Symptoms and anal sphincter morphology following primary repair of third-degree tears. Br J Surg. 2003; 90(12):1573–1579

[82] Fernando RJ, Sultan AH, Radley S, Jones PW, Johanson RB. Management of obstetric anal sphincter injury: a systematic review & national practice survey. BMC Health Serv Res. 2002; 2(1):9

[83] Sze EH. Anal incontinence among women with one versus two complete third-degree perineal lacerations. Int J Gynaecol Obstet. 2005; 90(3):213–217

[84] Sze EH. Prevalence and severity of anal incontinence in women with and without additional vaginal deliveries after a fourth-degree perineal laceration. Dis Colon Rectum. 2005; 48(1):66–69

[85] Faridi A, Willis S, Schelzig P, Siggelkow W, Schumpelick V, Rath W. Anal sphincter injury during vaginal delivery–an argument for cesarean section on request? J Perinat Med. 2002; 30(5):379–387

[86] Fynes M, Donnelly VS, O'Connell PR, O'Herlihy C. Cesarean delivery and anal sphincter injury. Obstet Gynecol. 1998; 92(4, Pt 1):496–500

[87] Nelson RL, Furner SE, Westercamp M, Farquhar C. Cesarean delivery for the prevention of anal incontinence. Cochrane Database Syst Rev. 2010(2): CD006756

[88] Altman D, Zetterström J, López A, Pollack J, Nordenstam J, Mellgren A. Effect of hysterectomy on bowel function. Dis Colon Rectum. 2004; 47(4):502–508, discussion 508–509

[89] Parks AG. Royal Society of Medicine, Section of Proctology; Meeting 27 November 1974. President's Address. Anorectal incontinence. Proc R Soc Med. 1975; 68(11):681–690

[90] Jarrett ME, Matzel KE, Stösser M, Baeten CG, Kamm MA. Sacral nerve stimulation for fecal incontinence following surgery for rectal prolapse repair: a multicenter study. Dis Colon Rectum. 2005; 48(6):1243–1248

[91] Loganathan A, Schloithe AC, Hutton J, et al. Pudendal nerve injury in men with fecal incontinence after radiotherapy for prostate cancer. Acta Oncol. 2015; 54(6):882–888

[92] Iglicki F, Coffin B, Ille O, et al. Fecal incontinence after pelvic radiotherapy: evidences for a lumbosacral plexopathy. Report of a case. Dis Colon Rectum. 1996; 39(4):465–467

[93] Schiller LR, Santa Ana CA, Schmulen AC, Hendler RS, Harford WV, Fordtran JS. Pathogenesis of fecal incontinence in diabetes mellitus: evidence for internal-anal-sphincter dysfunction. N Engl J Med. 1982; 307(27):1666–1671

[94] Pinna Pintor M, Zara GP, Falletto E, et al. Pudendal neuropathy in diabetic patients with faecal incontinence. Int J Colorectal Dis. 1994; 9(2):105–109

[95] Deen KI, Kumar D, Williams JG, Olliff J, Keighley MR. The prevalence of anal sphincter defects in faecal incontinence: a prospective endosonic study. Gut. 1993; 34(5):685–688

[96] Karoui S, Savoye-Collet C, Koning E, Leroi AM, Denis P. Prevalence of anal sphincter defects revealed by sonography in 335 incontinent patients and 115 continent patients. AJR Am J Roentgenol. 1999; 173(2):389–392

[97] Damon H, Henry L, Valette PJ, Mion F. Incidence of sphincter ruptures in anal incontinence: ultrasound study [in French]. Ann Chir. 2000; 125(7):643–647

[98] Nielsen MB, Hauge C, Pedersen JF, Christiansen J. Endosonographic evaluation of patients with anal incontinence: findings and influence on surgical management. AJR Am J Roentgenol. 1993; 160(4):771–775

[99] Rogers J, Henry MM, Misiewicz JJ. Combined sensory and motor deficit in primary neuropathic faecal incontinence. Gut. 1988; 29(1):5–9

[100] Speakman CT, Hoyle CH, Kamm MM, Henry MM, Nicholls RJ, Burnstock G. Abnormalities of innervation of internal anal sphincter in fecal incontinence. Dig Dis Sci. 1993; 38(11):1961–1969

[101] Swash M, Gray A, Lubowski DZ, Nicholls RJ. Ultrastructural changes in internal anal sphincter in neurogenic faecal incontinence. Gut. 1988; 29 (12):1692–1698

[102] Súilleabháin CB, Horgan AF, McEnroe L, et al. The relationship of pudendal nerve terminal motor latency to squeeze pressure in patients with idiopathic fecal incontinence. Dis Colon Rectum. 2001; 44(5):666–671

[103] Gee AS, Durdey P. Urge incontinence of faeces is a marker of severe external anal sphincter dysfunction. Br J Surg. 1995; 82(9):1179–1182

[104] Henry MM. Pathogenesis and management of fecal incontinence in the adult. Gastroenterol Clin North Am. 1987; 16(1):35–45

[105] Sultan AH, Nicholls RJ, Kamm MA, Hudson CN, Beynon J, Bartram CI. Anal endosonography and correlation with in vitro and in vivo anatomy. Br J Surg. 1993; 80(4):508–511

[106] Bharucha AE. Outcome measures for fecal incontinence: anorectal structure and function. Gastroenterology. 2004; 126(1) Suppl 1:S90–S98

[107] Bollard RC, Gardiner A, Lindow S, Phillips K, Duthie GS. Normal female anal sphincter: difficulties in interpretation explained. Dis Colon Rectum. 2002; 45(2):171–175

[108] Sentovich SM, Wong WD, Blatchford GJ. Accuracy and reliability of transanal ultrasound for anterior anal sphincter injury. Dis Colon Rectum. 1998; 41 (8):1000–1004

[109] Zetterström JP, Mellgren A, Madoff RD, Kim DG, Wong WD. Perineal body measurement improves evaluation of anterior sphincter lesions during endoanal ultrasonography. Dis Colon Rectum. 1998; 41(6):705–713

[110] Oberwalder M, Thaler K, Baig MK, et al. Anal ultrasound and endosonographic measurement of perineal body thickness: a new evaluation for fecal incontinence in females. Surg Endosc. 2004; 18(4):650–654

[111] Gold DM, Halligan S, Kmiot WA, Bartram CI. Intraobserver and interobserver agreement in anal endosonography. Br J Surg. 1999; 86(3):371–375

[112] Xue Y, Ding S, Ding Y, Liu F. Comparison of two-dimensional ultrasound and three-dimensional endoanal ultrasound in the diagnosis of perianal fistula [in Chinese]. Zhonghua Wei Chang Wai Ke Za Zhi. 2014; 17(12):1187–1189

[113] Liberman H, Faria J, Ternent CA, Blatchford GJ, Christensen MA, Thorson AG. A prospective evaluation of the value of anorectal physiology in the management of fecal incontinence. Dis Colon Rectum. 2001; 44(11):1567–1574

[114] Hiltunen KM. Anal manometric findings in patients with anal incontinence. Dis Colon Rectum. 1985; 28(12):925–928

[115] Read NW, Bartolo DC, Read MG. Differences in anal function in patients with incontinence to solids and in patients with incontinence to liquids. Br J Surg. 1984; 71(1):39–42

[116] Penninckx F, Lestàr B, Kerremans R. Manometric evaluation of incontinent patients. Acta Gastroenterol Belg. 1995; 58(1):51–59

[117] Tetzschner T, Sørensen M, Rasmussen OO, Lose G, Christiansen J. Pudendal nerve damage increases the risk of fecal incontinence in women with anal sphincter rupture after childbirth. Acta Obstet Gynecol Scand. 1995; 74 (6):434–440

[118] Bartolo DC, Jarratt JA, Read MG, Donnelly TC, Read NW. The role of partial denervation of the puborectalis in idiopathic faecal incontinence. Br J Surg. 1983; 70(11):664–667

[119] de Leeuw JW, Vierhout ME, Struijk PC, Auwerda HJ, Bac DJ, Wallenburg HC. Anal sphincter damage after vaginal delivery: relationship of anal endosonography and manometry to anorectal complaints. Dis Colon Rectum. 2002; 45(8):1004–1010

[120] Nazir M, Carlsen E, Jacobsen AF, Nesheim BI. Is there any correlation between objective anal testing, rupture grade, and bowel symptoms after primary repair of obstetric anal sphincter rupture?: an observational cohort study. Dis Colon Rectum. 2002; 45(10):1325–1331

[121] Voyvodic F, Rieger NA, Skinner S, et al. Endosonographic imaging of anal sphincter injury: does the size of the tear correlate with the degree of dysfunction? Dis Colon Rectum. 2003; 46(6):735–741

[122] Bordeianou L, Lee KY, Rockwood T, et al. Anal resting pressures at manometry correlate with the Fecal Incontinence Severity Index and with presence of sphincter defects on ultrasound. Dis Colon Rectum. 2008; 51(7):1010–1014

[123] Roig JV, Villoslada C, Lledó S, et al. Prevalence of pudendal neuropathy in fecal incontinence. Results of a prospective study. Dis Colon Rectum. 1995; 38 (9):952–958

[124] Kouraklis G, Andromanakos N. Evaluating patients with anorectal incontinence. Surg Today. 2004; 34(4):304–312

[125] Laurberg S, Swash M, Henry MM. Delayed external sphincter repair for obstetric tear. Br J Surg. 1988; 75(8):786–788

[126] Baig MK, Wexner SD. Factors predictive of outcome after surgery for faecal incontinence. Br J Surg. 2000; 87(10):1316–1330

[127] Sangwan YP, Coller JA, Barrett RC, et al. Unilateral pudendal neuropathy. Impact on outcome of anal sphincter repair. Dis Colon Rectum. 1996; 39 (6):686–689

[128] Rasmussen OO, Colstrup H, Lose G, Christiansen J. A technique for the dynamic assessment of anal sphincter function. Int J Colorectal Dis. 1990; 5 (3):135–141

[129] Young CJ, Mathur MN, Eyers AA, Solomon MJ. Successful overlapping anal sphincter repair: relationship to patient age, neuropathy, and colostomy formation. Dis Colon Rectum. 1998; 41(3):344–349

[130] Chen AS, Luchtefeld MA, Senagore AJ, Mackeigan JM, Hoyt C. Pudendal nerve latency. Does it predict outcome of anal sphincter repair? Dis Colon Rectum. 1998; 41(8):1005–1009

[131] Osterberg A, Graf W, Edebol Eeg-Olofsson K, Hynninen P, Påhlman L. Results of neurophysiologic evaluation in fecal incontinence. Dis Colon Rectum. 2000; 43(9):1256–1261

[132] Rasmussen O, Christensen B, Sørensen M, Tetzschner T, Christiansen J. Rectal compliance in the assessment of patients with fecal incontinence. Dis Colon Rectum. 1990; 33(8):650–653

[133] Read NW, Haynes WG, Bartolo DC, et al. Use of anorectal manometry during rectal infusion of saline to investigate sphincter function in incontinent patients. Gastroenterology. 1983; 85(1):105–113

[134] Womack NR, Morrison JF, Williams NS. The role of pelvic floor denervation in the aetiology of idiopathic faecal incontinence. Br J Surg. 1986; 73 (5):404–407

[135] Williams AB, Bartram CI, Modhwadia D, et al. Endocoil magnetic resonance imaging quantification of external anal sphincter atrophy. Br J Surg. 2001; 88(6):853–859

[136] Briel JW, Zimmerman DD, Stoker J, et al. Relationship between sphincter morphology on endoanal MRI and histopathological aspects of the external anal sphincter. Int J Colorectal Dis. 2000; 15(2):87–90

[137] Briel JW, Stoker J, Rociu E, Laméris JS, Hop WC, Schouten WR. External anal sphincter atrophy on endoanal magnetic resonance imaging adversely affects continence after sphincteroplasty. Br J Surg. 1999; 86(10):1322–1327

[138] Paquette IM, Varma MG, Kaiser AM, Steele SR, Rafferty JF. The American Society of Colon and Rectal Surgeons' Clinical Practice Guideline for the Treatment of Fecal Incontinence. Dis Colon Rectum. 2015; 58(7):623–636

[139] Guyatt GH, Cook DJ, Jaeschke R, Pauker SG, Schünemann HJ. Grades of recommendation for antithrombotic agents: American College of Chest Physicians Evidence-Based Clinical Practice Guidelines (8th Edition). Chest. 2008; 133(6) Suppl:123S–131S

[140] Rosen L, Khubchandani IT, Sheets JA, Stasik JJ, Riether RD. Management of anal incontinence. Am Fam Physician. 1986; 33(3):129–137

[141] Bannister JJ, Read NW, Donnelly TC, Sun WM. External and internal anal sphincter responses to rectal distension in normal subjects and in patients with idiopathic faecal incontinence. Br J Surg. 1989; 76(6):617–621

[142] Hallgren T, Fasth S, Delbro DS, Nordgren S, Oresland T, Hultén L. Loperamide improves anal sphincter function and continence after restorative proctocolectomy. Dig Dis Sci. 1994; 39(12):2612–2618

[143] Santoro GA, Eitan BZ, Pryde A, Bartolo DC. Open study of low-dose amitriptyline in the treatment of patients with idiopathic fecal incontinence. Dis Colon Rectum. 2000; 43(12):1676–1681, discussion 1681–1682

[144] Engel BT, Nikoomanesh P, Schuster MM. Operant conditioning of rectosphincteric responses in the treatment of fecal incontinence. N Engl J Med. 1974; 290(12):646–649

[145] Loening-Baucke V. Biofeedback therapy for fecal incontinence. Dig Dis. 1990; 8(2):112–124

[146] Wald A. Incontinence and anorectal dysfunction in patients with diabetes mellitus. Eur J Gastroenterol Hepatol. 1995; 7(8):737–739

[147] Norton C, Hosker G, Brazzelli M. Biofeedback and/or sphincter exercises for the treatment of faecal incontinence in adults. Cochrane Database Syst Rev. 2000(2):CD002111

[148] Heymen S, Jones KR, Ringel Y, Scarlett Y, Whitehead WE. Biofeedback treatment of fecal incontinence: a critical review. Dis Colon Rectum. 2001; 44 (5):728–736

[149] Palsson OS, Heymen S, Whitehead WE. Biofeedback treatment for functional anorectal disorders: a comprehensive efficacy review. Appl Psychophysiol Biofeedback. 2004; 29(3):153–174

[150] Norton C, Chelvanayagam S, Wilson-Barnett J, Redfern S, Kamm MA. Randomized controlled trial of biofeedback for fecal incontinence. Gastroenterology. 2003; 125(5):1320–1329

[151] Solomon MJ, Pager CK, Rex J, Roberts R, Manning J. Randomized, controlled trial of biofeedback with anal manometry, transanal ultrasound, or pelvic floor retraining with digital guidance alone in the treatment of mild to moderate fecal incontinence. Dis Colon Rectum. 2003; 46(6):703–710

[152] Beddy P, Neary P, Eguare EI, et al. Electromyographic biofeedback can improve subjective and objective measures of fecal incontinence in the short term. J Gastrointest Surg. 2004; 8(1):64–72, discussion 71–72

[153] Chiarioni G, Bassotti G, Stanganini S, Vantini I, Whitehead WE. Sensory retraining is key to biofeedback therapy for formed stool fecal incontinence. Am J Gastroenterol. 2002; 97(1):109–117

[154] Sangwan YP, Coller JA, Barrett RC, Roberts PL, Murray JJ, Schoetz DJ, Jr. Can manometric parameters predict response to biofeedback therapy in fecal incontinence? Dis Colon Rectum. 1995; 38(10):1021–1025

[155] Fernández-Fraga X, Azpiroz F, Aparici A, Casaus M, Malagelada JR. Predictors of response to biofeedback treatment in anal incontinence. Dis Colon Rectum. 2003; 46(9):1218–1225

[156] Enck P, Däublin G, Lübke HJ, Strohmeyer G. Long-term efficacy of biofeedback training for fecal incontinence. Dis Colon Rectum. 1994; 37 (10):997–1001

[157] Guillemot F, Bouche B, Gower-Rousseau C, et al. Biofeedback for the treatment of fecal incontinence. Long-term clinical results. Dis Colon Rectum. 1995; 38(4):393–397

[158] Glia A, Gylin M, Akerlund JE, Lindfors U, Lindberg G. Biofeedback training in patients with fecal incontinence. Dis Colon Rectum. 1998; 41(3):359–364

[159] Ryn AK, Morren GL, Hallböök O, Sjödahl R. Long-term results of electromyographic biofeedback training for fecal incontinence. Dis Colon Rectum. 2000; 43(9):1262–1266

[160] Pager CK, Solomon MJ, Rex J, Roberts RA. Long-term outcomes of pelvic floor exercise and biofeedback treatment for patients with fecal incontinence. Dis Colon Rectum. 2002; 45(8):997–1003

[161] Davis KJ, Kumar D, Poloniecki J. Adjuvant biofeedback following anal sphincter repair: a randomized study. Aliment Pharmacol Ther. 2004; 20(5):539–549

[162] Wexner SD. Percutaneous tibial nerve stimulation in faecal incontinence. Lancet. 2015; 386(10004):1605–1606

[163] Fang DT, Nivatvongs S, Vermeulen FD, Herman FN, Goldberg SM, Rothenberger DA. Overlapping sphincteroplasty for acquired anal incontinence. Dis Colon Rectum. 1984; 27(11):720–722

[164] Parks AG, McPartlin JF. Late repair of injuries of the anal sphincter. Proc R Soc Med. 1971; 64(12):1187–1189

[165] Wexner SD, Marchetti F, Jagelman DG. The role of sphincteroplasty for fecal incontinence reevaluated: a prospective physiologic and functional review. Dis Colon Rectum. 1991; 34(1):22–30

[166] Nessim A, Wexner SD, Agachan F, et al. Is bowel confinement necessary after anorectal reconstructive surgery? A prospective, randomized, surgeon-blinded trial. Dis Colon Rectum. 1999; 42(1):16–23

[167] Mahony R, Behan M, O'Herlihy C, O'Connell PR. Randomized, clinical trial of bowel confinement vs. laxative use after primary repair of a third-degree obstetric anal sphincter tear. Dis Colon Rectum. 2004; 47(1):12–17

[168] Karoui S, Leroi AM, Koning E, Menard JF, Michot F, Denis P. Results of sphincteroplasty in 86 patients with anal incontinence. Dis Colon Rectum. 2000; 43(6):813–820

[169] Malouf AJ, Norton CS, Engel AF, Nicholls RJ, Kamm MA. Long-term results of overlapping anterior anal-sphincter repair for obstetric trauma. Lancet. 2000; 355(9200):260–265

[170] Halverson AL, Hull TL. Long-term outcome of overlapping anal sphincter repair. Dis Colon Rectum. 2002; 45(3):345–348

[171] Simmang C, Birnbaum EH, Kodner IJ, Fry RD, Fleshman JW. Anal sphincter reconstruction in the elderly: does advancing age affect outcome? Dis Colon Rectum. 1994; 37(11):1065–1069

[172] Rasmussen OO, Puggaard L, Christiansen J. Anal sphincter repair in patients with obstetric trauma: age affects outcome. Dis Colon Rectum. 1999; 42 (2):193–195

[173] Gilliland R, Altomare DF, Moreira H, Jr, Oliveira L, Gilliland JE, Wexner SD. Pudendal neuropathy is predictive of failure following anterior overlapping sphincteroplasty. Dis Colon Rectum. 1998; 41(12):1516–1522

[174] Londono-Schimmer EE, Garcia-Duperly R, Nicholls RJ, Ritchie JK, Hawley PR, Thomson JP. Overlapping anal sphincter repair for faecal incontinence due to

sphincter trauma: five year follow-up functional results. Int J Colorectal Dis. 1994; 9(2):110–113

[175] Barisic GI, Krivokapic ZV, Markovic VA, Popovic MA. Outcome of overlapping anal sphincter repair after 3 months and after a mean of 80 months. Int J Colorectal Dis. 2006; 21(1):52–56

[176] Bravo Gutierrez A, Madoff RD, Lowry AC, Parker SC, Buie WD, Baxter NN. Long-term results of anterior sphincteroplasty. Dis Colon Rectum. 2004; 47 (5):727–731, discussion 731–732

[177] Tjandra JJ, Han WR, Goh J, Carey M, Dwyer P. Direct repair vs. overlapping sphincter repair: a randomized, controlled trial. Dis Colon Rectum. 2003; 46 (7):937–942, discussion 942–943

[178] Briel JW, de Boer LM, Hop WC, Schouten WR. Clinical outcome of anterior overlapping external anal sphincter repair with internal anal sphincter imbrication. Dis Colon Rectum. 1998; 41(2):209–214

[179] Hasegawa H, Yoshioka K, Keighley MR. Randomized trial of fecal diversion for sphincter repair. Dis Colon Rectum. 2000; 43(7):961–964, discussion 964–965

[180] Lewicky CE, Valentin C, Saclarides TJ. Sexual function following sphincteroplasty for women with third- and fourth-degree perineal tears. Dis Colon Rectum. 2004; 47(10):1650–1654

[181] Reid AJ, Beggs AD, Sultan AH, Roos AM, Thakar R. Outcome of repair of obstetric anal sphincter injuries after three years. Int J Gynaecol Obstet. 2014; 127(1):47–50

[182] Glasgow SC, Lowry AC. Long-term outcomes of anal sphincter repair for fecal incontinence: a systematic review. Dis Colon Rectum. 2012; 55(4):482–490

[183] Browning GG, Motson RW. Anal sphincter injury. Management and results of Parks sphincter repair. Ann Surg. 1984; 199(3):351–357

[184] Hawley PR. Anal sphincter reconstruction. Langenbecks Arch Chir. 1985; 366:269–272

[185] Christiansen J, Pedersen IK. Traumatic anal incontinence. Results of surgical repair. Dis Colon Rectum. 1987; 30(3):189–191

[186] Morgan S, Bernard D, Tasse D. Results of Parks' sphincteroplasty for post traumatic anal incontinence. Can J Surg. 1987; 30:299

[187] Abcarian H, Orsay CP, Pearl RK, Nelson RL, Briley SC. Traumatic cloaca. Dis Colon Rectum. 1989; 32(9):783–787

[188] Yoshioka K, Keighley MR. Sphincter repair for fecal incontinence. Dis Colon Rectum. 1989; 32(1):39–42

[189] Jacobs PP, Scheuer M, Kuijpers JH, Vingerhoets MH. Obstetric fecal incontinence. Role of pelvic floor denervation and results of delayed sphincter repair. Dis Colon Rectum. 1990; 33(6):494–497

[190] Fleshman JW, Peters WR, Shemesh EI, Fry RD, Kodner IJ. Anal sphincter reconstruction: anterior overlapping muscle repair. Dis Colon Rectum. 1991; 34(9):739–743

[191] Gibbs DH, Hooks VH, III. Overlapping sphincteroplasty for acquired anal incontinence. South Med J. 1993; 86(12):1376–1380

[192] Engel AF, van Baal SJ, Brummelkamp WH. Late results of anterior sphincter plication for traumatic faecal incontinence. Eur J Surg. 1994; 160 (11):633–636

[193] Engel AF, Kamm MA, Sultan AH, Bartram CI, Nicholls RJ. Anterior anal sphincter repair in patients with obstetric trauma. Br J Surg. 1994; 81 (8):1231–1234

[194] Sangalli MR, Marti MC. Results of sphincter repair in postobstetric fecal incontinence. J Am Coll Surg. 1994; 179(5):583–586

[195] Oliveira L, Pfeifer J, Wexner SD. Physiological and clinical outcome of anterior sphincteroplasty. Br J Surg. 1996; 83(4):502–505

[196] Womack NR, Morrison JF, Williams NS. Prospective study of the effects of postanal repair in neurogenic faecal incontinence. Br J Surg. 1988; 75(1):48–52

[197] Miller R, Bartolo DC, Locke-Edmunds JC, Mortensen NJ. Prospective study of conservative and operative treatment for faecal incontinence. Br J Surg. 1988; 75(2):101–105

[198] Orrom WJ, Miller R, Cornes H, Duthie G, Mortensen NJ, Bartolo DC. Comparison of anterior sphincteroplasty and postanal repair in the treatment of idiopathic fecal incontinence. Dis Colon Rectum. 1991; 34(4):305–310

[199] Athanasiadis S, Sanchez M, Kuprian A. Long-term follow-up of Parks posterior repair. An electromyographic, manometric and radiologic study of 31 patients [in German]. Langenbecks Arch Chir. 1995; 380(1):22–30

[200] Healy JC, Halligan S, Bartram CI, Kamm MA, Phillips RK, Reznek R. Dynamic magnetic resonance imaging evaluation of the structural and functional results of postanal repair for neuropathic fecal incontinence. Dis Colon Rectum. 2002; 45(12):1629–1634

[201] Setti Carraro P, Kamm MA, Nicholls RJ. Long-term results of postanal repair for neurogenic faecal incontinence. Br J Surg. 1994; 81(1):140–144

[202] Jameson JS, Speakman CT, Darzi A, Chia YW, Henry MM. Audit of postanal repair in the treatment of fecal incontinence. Dis Colon Rectum. 1994; 37 (4):369–372

[203] Keighley MR. Postanal repair. Int J Colorectal Dis. 1987; 2(4):236–239

[204] Laurberg S, Swash M, Henry MM. Effect of postanal repair on progress of neurogenic damage to the pelvic floor. Br J Surg. 1990; 77(5):519–522

[205] van Tets WF, Kuijpers JH. Pelvic floor procedures produce no consistent changes in anatomy or physiology. Dis Colon Rectum. 1998; 41(3):365–369

[206] Briel JW, Schouten WR. Disappointing results of postanal repair in the treatment of fecal incontinence [in Dutch]. Ned Tijdschr Geneeskd. 1995; 139 (1):23–26

[207] Rieger NA, Sarre RG, Saccone GT, Hunter A, Toouli J. Postanal repair for faecal incontinence: long-term follow-up. Aust N Z J Surg. 1997; 67(8):566–570

[208] Matsuoka H, Mavrantonis C, Wexner SD, Oliveira L, Gilliland R, Pikarsky A. Postanal repair for fecal incontinence–is it worthwhile? Dis Colon Rectum. 2000; 43(11):1561–1567

[209] Mackey P, Mackey L, Kennedy ML, et al. Postanal repair–do the long-term results justify the procedure? Colorectal Dis. 2010; 12(4):367–372

[210] Pickrell K, Georgiade N, Maguire C, Crawford H. Correction of rectal incontinence; transplantation of the gracilis muscle to construct a rectal sphincter. Am J Surg. 1955; 90(5):721–726

[211] Wexner SD, Gonzalez-Padron A, Rius J, et al. Stimulated gracilis neosphincter operation. Initial experience, pitfalls, and complications. Dis Colon Rectum. 1996; 39(9):957–964

[212] Matzel KE. Sacral nerve stimulation. In: Wexner SD, Fleshman JD, eds. Master Techniques in Surgery. Colon and Rectal Surgery: Anorectal Operations. Philadelphia, PA: Wolters Kluwer; 2012:135-148

[213] Wexner SD, Baeten C, Bailey R, et al. Long-term efficacy of dynamic graciloplasty for fecal incontinence. Dis Colon Rectum. 2002; 45(6):809–818

[214] Thornton MJ, Kennedy ML, Lubowski DZ, King DW. Long-term follow-up of dynamic graciloplasty for faecal incontinence. Colorectal Dis. 2004; 6 (6):470–476

[215] Geerdes BP, Heineman E, Konsten J, Soeters PB, Baeten CG. Dynamic graciloplasty. Complications and management. Dis Colon Rectum. 1996; 39 (8):912–917

[216] Penninckx F, Belgian Section of Colorectal Surgery. Belgian experience with dynamic graciloplasty for faecal incontinence. Br J Surg. 2004; 91 (7):872–878

[217] Bruining HA, Bos KE, Colthoff EG, Tolhurst DE. Creation of an anal sphincter mechanism by bilateral proximally based gluteal muscle transposition. Plast Reconstr Surg. 1981; 67(1):70–73

[218] Hentz VR. Construction of a rectal sphincter using the origin of the gluteus maximus muscle. Plast Reconstr Surg. 1982; 70(1):82–85

[219] Orgel MG, Kucan JO. A double-split gluteus maximus muscle flap for reconstruction of the rectal sphincter. Plast Reconstr Surg. 1985; 75(1):62–67

[220] Devesa JM, Vicente E, Enríquez JM, et al. Total fecal incontinence–a new method of gluteus maximus transposition: preliminary results and report of previous experience with similar procedures. Dis Colon Rectum. 1992; 35 (4):339–349

[221] Fleshner PR, Roberts PL. Encirclement procedure for fecal incontinence. Perspec Colon Rectal Surg. 1991; 4:280

[222] Chen YL, Zhang XH. Reconstruction of rectal sphincter by transposition of gluteus muscle for fecal incontinence. J Pediatr Surg. 1987; 22(1):62–64

[223] Pearl RK, Prasad ML, Nelson RL, Orsay CP, Abcarian H. Bilateral gluteus maximus transposition for anal incontinence. Dis Colon Rectum. 1991; 34 (6):478–481

[224] Hultman CS, Zenn MR, Agarwal T, Baker CC. Restoration of fecal continence after functional gluteoplasty: long-term results, technical refinements, and donor-site morbidity. Ann Plast Surg. 2006; 56(1):65–70, discussion 70–71

[225] Devesa JM, Madrid JM, Gallego BR, Vicente E, Nuño J, Enríquez JM. Bilateral gluteoplasty for fecal incontinence. Dis Colon Rectum. 1997; 40(8):883–888

[226] Christiansen J, Sparsø B. Treatment of anal incontinence by an implantable prosthetic anal sphincter. Ann Surg. 1992; 215(4):383–386

[227] Mundy L, Merlin TL, Maddern GJ, Hiller JE. Systematic review of safety and effectiveness of an artificial bowel sphincter for faecal incontinence. Br J Surg. 2004; 91(6):665–672

[228] Darnis B, Faucheron JL, Damon H, Barth X. Technical and functional results of the artificial bowel sphincter for treatment of severe fecal incontinence: is there any benefit for the patient? Dis Colon Rectum. 2013; 56(4):505–510

[229] Wong MT, Meurette G, Wyart V, Glemain P, Lehur PA. The artificial bowel sphincter: a single institution experience over a decade. Ann Surg. 2011; 254(6):951–956

[230] Wexner SD, Jin HY, Weiss EG, Nogueras JJ, Li VK. Factors associated with failure of the artificial bowel sphincter: a study of over 50 cases from Cleveland Clinic Florida. Dis Colon Rectum. 2009; 52(9):1550–1557

[231] Lehur PA, McNevin S, Buntzen S, Mellgren AF, Laurberg S, Madoff RD. Magnetic anal sphincter augmentation for the treatment of fecal incontinence: a preliminary report from a feasibility study. Dis Colon Rectum. 2010; 53 (12):1604–1610

[232] Barussaud ML, Mantoo S, Wyart V, Meurette G, Lehur PA. The magnetic anal sphincter in faecal incontinence: is initial success sustained over time? Colorectal Dis. 2013; 15(12):1499–1503

[233] Chandra A, Kumar A, Noushif M, et al. Feasibility of neurovascular antropylorus perineal transposition with pudendal nerve anastomosis following anorectal excision: a cadaveric study for neoanal reconstruction. Ann Coloproctol. 2013; 29(1):7–11

[234] Chandra A, Kumar A, Noushif M, et al. Neurovascular antropylorus perineal transposition using inferior rectal nerve anastomosis for total anorectal reconstruction: preliminary report in humans. Tech Coloproctol. 2014; 18(6):535–542

[235] Graf W, Mellgren A, Matzel KE, Hull T, Johansson C, Bernstein M, NASHA Dx Study Group. Efficacy of dextranomer in stabilised hyaluronic acid for treatment of faecal incontinence: a randomised, sham-controlled trial. Lancet. 2011; 377(9770):997–1003

[236] Maeda Y, Laurberg S, Norton C. Perianal injectable bulking agents as treatment for faecal incontinence in adults. Cochrane Database Syst Rev. 2013; 2 (2):CD007959

[237] La Torre F, de la Portilla F. Long-term efficacy of dextranomer in stabilized hyaluronic acid (NASHA/Dx) for treatment of faecal incontinence. Colorectal Dis. 2013; 15(5):569–574

[238] Hussain ZI, Lim M, Stojkovic SG. Systematic review of perianal implants in the treatment of faecal incontinence. Br J Surg. 2011; 98(11):1526–1536

[239] Guerra F, La Torre M, Giuliani G, et al. Long-term evaluation of bulking agents for the treatment of fecal incontinence: clinical outcomes and ultrasound evidence. Tech Coloproctol. 2015; 19(1):23–27

[240] Herman RM, Berho M, Murawski M, et al. Defining the histopathological changes induced by nonablative radiofrequency treatment of faecal incontinence–a blinded assessment in an animal model. Colorectal Dis. 2015; 17 (5):433–440

[241] Efron JE. The SECCA procedure: a new therapy for treatment of fecal incontinence. Surg Technol Int. 2004; 13:107–110

[242] Takahashi-Monroy T, Morales M, Garcia-Osogobio S, et al. SECCA procedure for the treatment of fecal incontinence: results of five-year follow-up. Dis Colon Rectum. 2008; 51(3):355–359

[243] Ruiz D, Pinto RA, Hull TL, Efron JE, Wexner SD. Does the radiofrequency procedure for fecal incontinence improve quality of life and incontinence at 1-year follow-up? Dis Colon Rectum. 2010; 53(7):1041–1046

[244] Frascio M, Mandolfino F, Imperatore M, et al. The SECCA procedure for faecal incontinence: a review. Colorectal Dis. 2014; 16(3):167–172

[245] Lukacz ES, Segall MM, Wexner SD. Evaluation of an anal insert device for the conservative management of fecal incontinence. Dis Colon Rectum. 2015; 58 (9):892–898

[246] Worsøe J, Christensen P, Krogh K, Buntzen S, Laurberg S. Long-term results of antegrade colonic enema in adult patients: assessment of functional results. Dis Colon Rectum. 2008; 51(10):1523–1528

[247] Giamundo P, Welber A, Weiss EG, Vernava AM, III, Nogueras JJ, Wexner SD. The procon incontinence device: a new nonsurgical approach to preventing episodes of fecal incontinence. Am J Gastroenterol. 2002; 97(9):2328–2332

[248] Chodez M, Trilling B, Thuillier C, Boillot B, Barbois S, Faucheron JL. Results of sacral nerve neuromodulation for double incontinence in adults. Tech Coloproctol. 2014; 18(12):1147–1151

[249] Wexner SD, Coller JA, Devroede G, et al. Sacral nerve stimulation for fecal incontinence: results of a 120-patient prospective multicenter study. Ann Surg. 2010; 251(3):441–449

[250] Wexner SD, Coller JA, Devroede G, et al. Sacral nerve stimulation for fecal incontinence: results of a 120-patient prospective multicenter study. Ann Surg. 2010; 251(3):441–449

[251] Wexner SD, Bleier J. Current surgical strategies to treat fecal incontinence. Expert Rev Gastroenterol Hepatol. 2015; 9(12):1577–1589

[252] Tjandra JJ, Chan MK, Yeh CH, Murray-Green C. Sacral nerve stimulation is more effective than optimal medical therapy for severe fecal incontinence: a randomized, controlled study. Dis Colon Rectum. 2008; 51(5):494–502

[253] Mellgren A, Wexner SD, Coller JA, et al. SNS Study Group. Long-term efficacy and safety of sacral nerve stimulation for fecal incontinence. Dis Colon Rectum. 2011; 54(9):1065–1075

[254] Hull T, Giese C, Wexner SD, et al. SNS Study Group. Long-term durability of sacral nerve stimulation therapy for chronic fecal incontinence. Dis Colon Rectum. 2013; 56(2):234–245

[255] Altomare DF, Ratto C, Ganio E, Lolli P, Masin A, Villani RD. Long-term outcome of sacral nerve stimulation for fecal incontinence. Dis Colon Rectum. 2009; 52(1):11–17

[256] Lim JT, Hastie IA, Hiscock RJ, Shedda SM. Sacral nerve stimulation for fecal incontinence: long-term outcomes. Dis Colon Rectum. 2011; 54 (8):969–974

[257] Michelsen HB, Thompson-Fawcett M, Lundby L, Krogh K, Laurberg S, Buntzen S. Six years of experience with sacral nerve stimulation for fecal incontinence. Dis Colon Rectum. 2010; 53(4):414–421

[258] Altomare DF, Giuratrabocchetta S, Knowles CH, Muñoz Duyos A, Robert-Yap J, Matzel KE, European SNS Outcome Study Group. Long-term outcomes of sacral nerve stimulation for faecal incontinence. Br J Surg. 2015; 102 (4):407–415

[259] George AT, Kalmar K, Panarese A, Dudding TC, Nicholls RJ, Vaizey CJ. Long-term outcomes of sacral nerve stimulation for fecal incontinence. Dis Colon Rectum. 2012; 55(3):302–306

[260] Brouwer R, Duthie G. Sacral nerve neuromodulation is effective treatment for fecal incontinence in the presence of a sphincter defect, pudendal neuropathy, or previous sphincter repair. Dis Colon Rectum. 2010; 53 (3):273–278

[261] Gourcerol G, Vitton V, Leroi AM, Michot F, Abysique A, Bouvier M. How sacral nerve stimulation works in patients with faecal incontinence. Colorectal Dis. 2011; 13(8):e203–e211

[262] Nakamura M, Sakurai T, Tsujimoto Y, Tada Y. Transcutaneous electrical stimulation for the control of frequency and urge incontinence [in Japanese]. Hinyokika Kiyo. 1983; 29(9):1053–1059

[263] Shafik A, Ahmed I, El-Sibai O, Mostafa RM. Percutaneous peripheral neuromodulation in the treatment of fecal incontinence. Eur Surg Res. 2003; 35 (2):103–107

[264] Thomas GP, Dudding TC, Rahbour G, Nicholls RJ, Vaizey CJ. A review of posterior tibial nerve stimulation for faecal incontinence. Colorectal Dis. 2013; 15 (5):519–526

[265] Thin NN, Taylor SJ, Bremner SA, et al. Neuromodulation Trial Study Group. Randomized clinical trial of sacral versus percutaneous tibial nerve stimulation in patients with faecal incontinence. Br J Surg. 2015; 102(4):349–358

[266] Knowles CH, Horrocks EJ, Bremner SA, et al. CONFIDeNT study group. Percutaneous tibial nerve stimulation versus sham electrical stimulation for the treatment of faecal incontinence in adults (CONFIDeNT): a double-blind, multicentre, pragmatic, parallel-group, randomised controlled trial. Lancet. 2015; 386(10004):1640–1648

[267] Wexner SD. Percutaneous tibial nerve stimulation in faecal incontinence. Lancet. 2015; 386(10004):1605–1606

[268] Horrocks EJ, Chadi SA, Stevens NJ, Wexner SD, Knowles CH. Factors Associated With Efficacy of Percutaneous Tibial Nerve Stimulation for Fecal Incontinence, Based on Post-Hoc Analysis of Data From a Randomized Trial. Clin Gastroenterol Hepatol. 2017; 15(12):1915–1921.e2

[269] Leroi AM, Siproudhis L, Etienney I, et al. Transcutaneous electrical tibial nerve stimulation in the treatment of fecal incontinence: a randomized trial (CONSORT 1a). Am J Gastroenterol. 2012; 107(12):1888–1896

[270] Lecompte JF, Hery G, Guys JM, Louis-Borrione C. Evaluation of transcutaneous electrical posterior tibial nerve stimulation for the treatment of fecal and urinary leaks in children: preliminary results. J Pediatr Surg. 2015; 50 (4):630–633

[271] Edenfield AL, Amundsen CL, Wu JM, Levin PJ, Siddiqui NY. Posterior tibial nerve stimulation for the treatment of fecal incontinence: a systematic evidence review. Obstet Gynecol Surv. 2015; 70(5):329–341

[272] Malone PS, Ransley PG, Kiely EM. Preliminary report: the antegrade continence enema. Lancet. 1990; 336(8725):1217–1218

[273] Lawal TA, Rangel SJ, Bischoff A, Peña A, Levitt MA. Laparoscopic-assisted Malone appendicostomy in the management of fecal incontinence in children. J Laparoendosc Adv Surg Tech A. 2011; 21(5):455–459

[274] Ellison JS, Haraway AN, Park JM. The distal left Malone antegrade continence enema–is it better? J Urol. 2013; 190(4) Suppl:1529–1533

[275] Norton C, Burch J, Kamm MA. Patients' views of a colostomy for fecal incontinence. Dis Colon Rectum. 2005; 48(5):1062–1069

[276] Hughes SF, Williams NS. Continent colonic conduit for the treatment of faecal incontinence associated with disordered evacuation. Br J Surg. 1995; 82 (10):1318–1320

15 Rectovaginal and Rectourethral Fistulas

Janice F. Rafferty and Emily F. Midura

Abstract

Rectovaginal fistulas are congenital or acquired epithelial-lined tract between the rectum and vagina. Although an uncommon percentage of anorectal fistulas, they are significant challenges for patients and providers. This chapter looks at the definition and classification, etiology, presentation, evaluation, and management of rectovaginal fistula.

Keywords: rectovaginal fistula, classification, etiology, obstetric injury, neoplasia, clinical presentation, surgical repair, fistulotomy, excision, muscle interposition

15.1 Introduction

A rectovaginal fistula (RVF) is a congenital or acquired epithelial-lined tract between the rectum and vagina. RVFs comprise 5% of all anorectal fistulas and lead to significant morbidity in women. Because of the significant variation in presentation and anatomy, successful treatment can be very complex.

15.1.1 Definition and Classification

RVFs are classified based on location, size, and etiology—a classification system that helps guide both diagnosis and operative intervention. RVF can occur anywhere along distal two-thirds of the anterior rectal wall where it is adjacent to the posterior vaginal wall, and is defined as a communication between the vagina and the rectum above the dentate line; in comparison, an anovaginal fistula is located below the dentate line. The terms "low" RVF and "anovaginal" fistula are sometimes interchangeably used. Most RVFs form between the dentate line and the posterior vaginal fornix.[1] RVFs are further classified as "low" when they are at or slightly above the dentate line, "high" when the vaginal opening is behind or near the cervix, and "middle" if the fistula lies between these two areas (▶ Fig. 15.1). Regarding size, "small" fistulas are typically < 0.5 cm, "medium" are from 0.5 to 2.5 cm, and "large" fistulas are > 2.5 cm in diameter. Other classification schemes have been suggested based on etiology rather than location.[1] The fistula may also be described as "simple" if it is small and direct, or "complex" if it is high, or due to radiation, malignancy, inflammatory bowel disease, or unintended complication of a pelvic anastomosis. The reality is that given the difficulty in curing some of these fistulas, the categorization of some of them as "simple" seems a misnomer.

15.2 Etiology

RVFs can result from congenital malformations or a variety of acquired disorders. Many acquired fistulas arise from obstetric injuries,[2] with neoplasms, radiation injury, inflammatory bowel disease,[3] infections, and trauma contributing as well.

15.2.1 Obstetric Injuries

RVF can acutely develop with a perineal tear or surgical episiotomy, or as a delayed complication of traumatic vaginal delivery. Risk factors for development of obstetric fistulas include episiotomy, third- and fourth-degree lacerations, prolonged labor, and high forceps deliveries.[4] It is estimated that episiotomy and third- and fourth-degree perineal lacerations occur in up to 5% of vaginal births.[5] About 10% of defects repaired in the acute setting fail; two-thirds of those that fail require reoperative intervention.[5] Approximately 0.05 to 0.1% of midline episiotomies lead to RVF, whereas up to 1% of third- and fourth-degree lacerations will be complicated by RVF often due to missed injuries, inadequate repair of an identified injury, or secondary infection of a repaired wound.[5] Prolonged labor results in persistent pressure on the rectovaginal septum resulting in ischemia of the septum, which can fistulize in the postpartum period.[4,6] The development of anal ulcers, anorectal abscesses after delivery, and sphincter injuries during delivery are also possible etiologies. When considering operative repair of RVF resulting from traumatic vaginal delivery, it is important to remember that almost half of obstetric injuries also involve the anal sphincter.[7]

15.2.2 Neoplasm and Pelvic Radiation

Malignant RVF can be the result of a primary, recurrent, or metastatic neoplasm. Common solid neoplasms that cause RVF include colorectal, anal, cervical, uterine, and vaginal cancers. Blood cancers such as leukemia, aplastic anemia, and agranulocytosis can cause RVF but are rare.[8] Gynecologic malignancies treated with pelvic radiation can lead to RVF,[9,10,11]

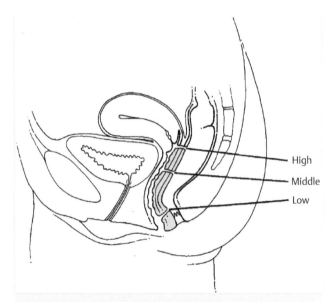

High

Middle

Low

Fig. 15.1 Classification of rectovaginal fistulas by location.

typically presenting 6 months to 2 years after treatment is completed; incidence is related to the dose of radiation delivered,[12] but risk is increased in the setting of hypertension, diabetes mellitus, and previous abdominopelvic surgery.[11] Radiation-induced proctitis can lead to mucosal ulceration with eventual erosion through the full thickness of the rectal and eventually vaginal wall. Patients with radiation proctitis typically describe rectal pressure and a constant urge to defecate; this tends to abate when the fistula forms, at which time complaints transition to feculent drainage from the vagina and persistent vaginitis.

15.2.3 Inflammatory Bowel Disease

The incidence of RVF in inflammatory bowel disease ranges from 6 to 23%.[3,13,14] Crohn's disease, and specifically Crohn's proctitis, is a more common cause when compared to ulcerative colitis, due to transmural inflammation and associated perianal disease.[15] Some success with medical management of RVF has been achieved in Crohn's patients with use of metronidazole,[16] chemotherapeutic agents such as methotrexate[17] and cyclosporine,[18] and more recently with remicade[19] and other anti-TNF agents. The rate of failure to heal the fistula with any medical therapy remains high, and treatment is usually aimed at control of symptoms and stabilization of acute flares to optimize patients for eventual surgical intervention.[20] There are reports of adenocarcinoma developing in the setting of chronic inflammation due to Crohn's disease that may result in fistula formation,[13] as well as adenocarcinoma developing in chronic Crohn's fistulas. Patients with longstanding fistulas-in-ano due to Crohn's disease who do not heal with medical or surgical therapy are at risk for malignant degeneration and should be carefully examined in this setting. Behçet's disease, while rare, can also cause RVF.[21]

15.2.4 Infection

Pelvic infectious processes including diverticulitis, perirectal abscess due to cryptoglandular abscess, venereal disease, abdominal tuberculosis, and pelvic inflammatory disease can lead to RVF. Bartholin's abscesses, as well as infections collecting in the pouch of Douglas, can drain through the rectovaginal septum. Colovaginal fistulas due to diverticulitis, masquerading as high RVFs, occur and are more prevalent in women who have undergone hysterectomy.

15.2.5 Trauma and Miscellaneous Causes

Operative trauma can lead to the inadvertent development of RVF. Both vaginal and rectal operations complicated by infections, wound breakdown, or anastomotic leak can lead to tissue infection, abscess development, ischemia, and fistula development. Low colorectal or coloanal anastomoses, specifically circular stapled anastomoses,[22] the procedure for prolapse and hemorrhoids, and stapled transanal rectal resections,[23] run the risk of including the posterior vaginal wall in the anastomosis if the operating surgeon is not careful. Urogynecologic operations that involve mesh placement adjacent to the rectum and vagina also carry a risk of infection, with subsequent inflammation

and fistula formation. Trauma to the vagina or anus from blunt and penetrating injuries can disrupt healthy tissue resulting in development of a fistula. Fecal impaction resulting in stercoral ulcer and pressure necrosis,[24] prolonged pessary usage,[25] and ergotamine suppositories[26] have also been cited as causes of RVF.

15.3 Clinical Presentation and Evaluation

Symptoms and presentation of RVFs vary based on the etiology. Presentation ranges from chronic vaginitis with foul or feculent smelling discharge to obvious passage of flatus or stool from the vagina. Women may also present with recurrent urinary tract infections, perineal pain, and/or dyspareunia. Patients may complain of passing blood or mucus from the anus, diarrhea, or fecal incontinence from associated sphincter injury.

Physical examination and imaging evaluation should confirm the presence of a fistula. Most low fistulas are palpable on rectovaginal examination, and can be visualized with vaginal speculum evaluation or proctosigmoidoscopy. The darker red, smooth vaginal mucosa often contrasts with the lighter rectal mucosa. Stool may also be found in the vagina on speculum exam. For small fistulas, a probe may be necessary to locate the tract as the openings often appear as a small depression or pit-like defect. Hydrogen peroxide–enhanced exams under anesthesia with or without transanal ultrasound can assist with difficult diagnoses.[27,28] If one is unable to identify a clear fistula tract on exam, water can be instilled into the vagina, the rectum insufflated with a sigmoidoscope or a bulb syringe; the presence of bubbles will confirm the diagnosis. A tampon test may be useful with a difficult diagnosis as well. Specifically, a tampon is inserted into the vagina, and methylene blue instilled in the rectum and held for 15 to 20 minutes. Tampon staining is diagnostic of RVF. On rare occasions, extensive clinical testing will fail to confirm the presence of a fistula, despite highly suspicious signs and symptoms. In this situation, certain imaging studies may be useful, and include hydrogen peroxide–enhanced transanal ultrasound, limited barium enemas, contrast vaginography, CT scans, and MRI. Magnetic resonance imaging has a high sensitivity in the diagnosis of fistulas in the anorectal region,[29] and may be the most practical imaging study to obtain when searching for the origin and characteristics of a fistula. Clinical presentation and physical exam findings often guide the decision for appropriate imaging techniques. If necessary, an examination under anesthesia may be the only method by which the fistula can be identified.

Once the presence of a fistula has been confirmed, it is essential to determine size and location, and evaluate for associated infections, overall tissue health, need for abscess drainage, and sphincter integrity. This goal can often be accomplished by physical exam; however, imaging, as described above and including endoscopy, may be required. While associated sphincter injury can often be suspected based on history, anal manometry and endoanal ultrasound can be useful adjuncts to assess sphincter competence,[7,30] and can influence choice of repair.[31] Evaluation should also exclude the involvement of contiguous organs and assess for the presence of acute infections, inflammatory bowel disease, radiation injury, and neoplasm. For example, the finding of nodular or friable tissue adjacent to a fistula may be suggestive of malignancy; uniform or diffuse tissue friability is more likely consistent with radiation-induced changes or inflammatory bowel disease. Appropriate biopsies and metastatic evaluation should be performed if there is concern for new or recurrent neoplasia, and CT or MR enterography should be considered in patients with a history or suspicion for inflammatory bowel disease.

15.4 Surgical Management

Prior to surgical intervention, underlying pathologies that require medical management should be addressed. Patients with Crohn's or other inflammatory conditions should be medically optimized; patients with a history of pelvic malignancy need a full metastatic assessment. A trial of nonoperative management for obstetric injuries should include sitz baths, perineal wound care, and bowel regimens. While hyperbaric oxygen has been suggested as treatment for infection-related fistulas,[32] the majority of symptomatic fistulas require operative intervention.

15.4.1 Operative Timing

Timing and need for operative repair is guided by both the size and etiology of the RVF. More than half of small fistulas from obstetric trauma will heal spontaneously. Therefore, it is recommended to wait 3 to 6 months after delivery prior to operative repair[33,34] to allow resolution of acute inflammation, which may promote spontaneous healing the majority of the time.[35] However, if a large tear is noted at the time of delivery, repair should be undertaken in the delivery room.[36] If there is an infectious or inflammatory component to an RVF, draining seton placement may be beneficial to help clear the infection and allow contraction and fibrosis of the tract. Seton placement will allow time for medical optimization in patients with inflammatory bowel disease, provide symptomatic relief for poor operative candidates, or provide an interval of time needed for treatment of neoplasia as well.

15.4.2 Operative Approach

Operative repair can be performed through abdominal or local procedures, including perineal, vaginal, rectal, transsphincteric, or transsacral approaches. Regardless of the approach used, adequate mobilization of the vagina and rectum must be ensured to prevent undue tension on the repair and to avoid direct apposition of suture lines to try to limit recurrence. Fecal diversion can also help control symptoms and infection, promote healing, and may even be used for definitive management in poor operative candidates. Sphincter function should also be assessed and taken into consideration when planning a strategy for repair.

15.4.3 Perioperative Management

Smoking and Crohn's disease are the most common risk factors for recurrence of RVF following operative repair, so preoperative smoking cessation and medical control of inflammatory bowel disease are encouraged.[37] Mechanical bowel prep, vaginal cleansing, and perioperative antibiotics are recommended for both local and abdominal procedures. The bladder is decompressed with a catheter, and ureteral stent placement should be considered if difficult pelvic dissection is anticipated. Hospital stays are dependent on the extent of repair, operative blood loss, patient age, and comorbidities. Patients should postoperatively abstain from any vaginal penetration for 6 to 8 weeks.

15.4.4 Management of Recurrence

Approach to repairing recurrent RVF is guided by both the etiology of the fistula and the previous operative technique. Key to success is the introduction of new healthy tissue with adequate blood supply and debridement of all nonviable and infected tissues. Success rates approaching 90% can often be achieved despite the need for multiple repairs.[37]

15.5 Operative Repairs

15.5.1 Simple Fistulotomy

Anovaginal fistulas that do not have extensive involvement of the sphincter mechanism can be managed with laying open of the fistula tract and healing by secondary intention. This approach has been abandoned for higher RVFs as it is likely to impair fecal continence.

15.5.2 Conversion to Complete Perineal Laceration

One local approach for repair of fistulas with extensive anal sphincter defects and fecal incontinence is episioproctotomy with reconstruction of the anorectal-vaginal septum. This procedure should include excision of the fistula tract, division of the adjacent sphincters and perineal body, and then layered closure of all the tissues (▶ Fig. 15.2). This method is similar to the classic technique for closure of fourth-degree perineal lacerations following obstetric trauma, and leads to a high rate of healing of the fistula and improved fecal continence.[38] This procedure is generally performed in lithotomy position, with a full-thickness incision made between the anus and vagina. The rectal mucosa, internal and external sphincters, and the vaginal mucosa are each closed separately. The sphincters may be closed in a single layer if dissection is difficult. Healing of this extensive repair may be promoted by proximal diversion of the fecal stream.

The Musset technique is a two-stage procedure in which a perineoproctotomy is performed followed by a layered closure 8 weeks later. Healing rates of 98 to 100% are reported and 75% of patients maintain sphincter function with this approach.[39,40] Patients who present with a cloacal defect can also be managed with a similar layered repair.[41] Some authors advocate sphincterotomy in the 5 o'clock position opposing the anterior repair if sphincter reconstruction is performed,[42] and others describe X-flap anoplasty to recreate the perineal body.[41]

15.5.3 Fistula Excision with Layered Closure

Excision of the fistula with layered closure can be completed through a vaginal, rectal, perineal, or transsphincteric approach.

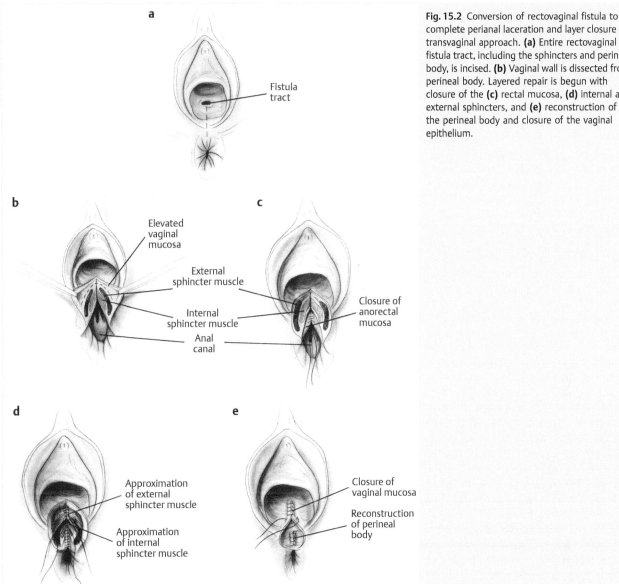

Fig. 15.2 Conversion of rectovaginal fistula to complete perianal laceration and layer closure via transvaginal approach. **(a)** Entire rectovaginal fistula tract, including the sphincters and perineal body, is incised. **(b)** Vaginal wall is dissected from perineal body. Layered repair is begun with closure of the **(c)** rectal mucosa, **(d)** internal and external sphincters, and **(e)** reconstruction of the perineal body and closure of the vaginal epithelium.

Fistulas associated with sphincter defects are often approached through these techniques and muscle flaps utilized if there is significant tissue loss or damage.

In the perineal approach, the patient is in prone jackknife and a 180-degree curvilinear perianal incision just anterior to the anal verge, or Schuchardt incision, is used. The vagina is opened to the level of the lateral fornix and perineal dissection extended to healthy tissue at least 1 to 2 cm above the fistula and associated scar. Once the fistula tract is identified and transected, the levators are plicated, and the vagina, sphincter fibers, and rectal mucosa are closed in layers. Care should be taken to avoid direct apposition of suture lines; the vaginal side may be left open for drainage. The curvilinear incision is then closed in a V–Y flap fashion, reconstructing the breadth of a normal perineal body.[6] A transrectal approach has also been described which avoids the need for a perineal incision[8] but may require advancement of rectal mucosa to cover the defect left by excision of the fistula.

A transsphincteric approach can also be used. While first described to close rectourethral fistulas (RUFs), this technique can be used to fully expose more proximal tracts and reduce the need for transabdominal repairs.[43] The patient is placed in prone jackknife position and the buttocks retracted laterally with adhesive tape. The incision extends from the anal margin to the midsacrum just to the left of midline. The mucocutaneous junction and sphincter muscles are marked with stay sutures. The rectal mucosa is then divided to expose the fistula, the fistula and surrounding scar tissue excised, and the vaginal opening is closed primarily. The incision in the anterior rectal wall is then transversely extended, full-thickness flaps are mobilized, and the rectum is closed using a "vest over pants" technique. The sphincter muscles are then reapproximated and the skin closed.

15.5.4 Muscle Interposition Grafts

Muscle and other interposition grafts are typically reserved for the treatment of recurrent or complex RVF, such as those that develop after coloanal anastomoses or construction of a neorectum. The bulbocavernosus or Martius flap is one of the most commonly utilized tissue interposition techniques used to repair RVF, but only small series are reported in the literature.[44,45,46,47] Healing rates exceed 60% but are lower in patients with Crohn's disease.[44,45] Patients are positioned in lithotomy and a mediolateral perineal incision used. The fistula tract is identified and excised, and the rectal side closed. An incision is then made along the opposing labia majora to allow exposure of the labial fat pad and bulbocavernosus muscle (▶ Fig. 15.3). The mobilized muscle is then tunneled subcutaneously to cover the rectal repair site and the vaginal fistula opening is closed.[48] One can also use the fat pad without muscle with similar success rates to reduce operative morbidity.[46] A diverting ostomy is routinely recommended as an adjunct to allow healing. Modifications using full-thickness flaps from the labia majora[49] and the labia majora and minora[50] have also been used with success rates above 80% for complex fistulas.[47] Complications of this procedure include dyspareunia, numbness, and decreased sensation at the graft site and aesthetic concerns.[51,52]

The gracilis muscle can also be used as a pedicle flap for the closure of large or recurrent RVF. One series of 24 patients, 8 of whom had Crohn's disease, reported an overall healing rate of 79%.[2] Other series have confirmed high rates of healing, but a concurrent high rate of wound infection.[53] The patient is positioned in modified lithotomy or lithotomy and a transverse perineal incision made. The fistula is identified and ligated, the tract excised or curetted, and the vaginal and rectal openings closed. A medial thigh incision over the gracilis muscle is then made and the muscle pedicle harvested. Preservation of the neurovascular bundle during this dissection and subcutaneous tunneling must be ensured. The graft is placed between the vagina and rectum and should be secured 2 cm above the fistula defect. If not secured high above the fistula, the pedicle may retract and the repair may fail. Drains are usually left in place along the graft in the perineum and in the thigh.[53] This technique has been described in multiple

small series with and without fecal diversion and successful closure rates range from 50 to 92%.[53,54,55,56,57] Despite successful closure, a quarter of patients still experience dyspareunia and quality-of-life metrics postprocedure remain low.[53] One of the editors (S. D. W.) prefers to harvest the muscle with the patient in the modified lithotomy position and then perform the perineal dissection and muscle interposition in the prone jackknife position.

15.5.5 Advancement Flaps

Endorectal advancement flap has benefits of minimal tissue mobilization, preservation of the external sphincter, lowered risk of impact upon continence when compared to other techniques, avoidance of perineal wound, and low incidence of flap retraction. This technique was first credited to Noble in 1902 and has been modified over time to optimize repairs for small, low fistulas.[58] It has good success with first-time operations (41–78% healing)[59,60] but a higher rate of failure following previous repairs.[61,62] The patient is given a mechanical bowel prep and intravenous antibiotics and placed in the prone jackknife position; exposure is achieved by taping the buttocks and positioning a Lonestar retractor (Cooper Surgical, Inc., Trumbull, CT). A broad-based flap is outlined, with the fistula located near the distal tip of the flap. Endorectal flaps include mucosa, submucosa, and, in some cases, the circular muscle (▶ Fig. 15.4).[63] The flap should be undermined at least several centimeters cephalad to the fistula, as adequate mobilization to ensure tension-free advancement is key. The base of the flap should be twice the width of the tip near the fistula, to ensure adequate blood supply. The fistula tract is divided during mobilization of the rectal wall, and the tip of the flap including the fistula is excised and sent for pathology. Surrounding sphincter fibers are plicated over the fistula opening, and the circular muscle reapproximated. Finally, the flap is secured around its periphery with absorbable suture to close the defect. The vaginal side can be left open for drainage, or closed with sutures that dissolve within a few days. Inclusion of the internal sphincter as a layer in the flap has been described[63] and is advocated in Crohn's patients having RVF repair with endorectal advancement flap.[64] Concurrent sphincteroplasty should be planned in women with

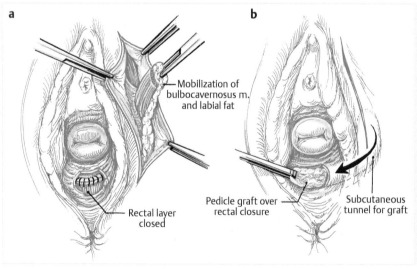

a   b

Fig. 15.3 Martius flap. **(a)** Rectal side of fistula is closed and bulbocavernosus muscle and fat pad are mobilized through a labial incision. **(b)** Fat pad and muscle are interposed between the repair and vaginal mucosa.

Mobilization of bulbocavernosus m. and labial fat

Rectal layer closed

Pedicle graft over rectal closure

Subcutaneous tunnel for graft

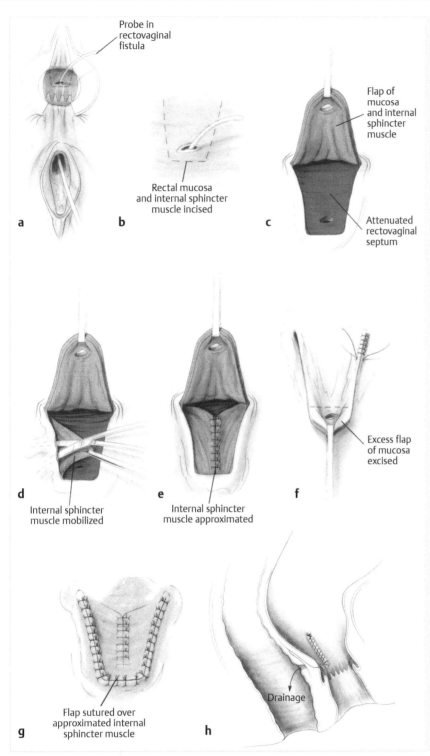

Probe in rectovaginal fistula

a

Rectal mucosa and internal sphincter muscle incised

b

Flap of mucosa and internal sphincter muscle

Attenuated rectovaginal septum

c

Internal sphincter muscle mobilized

d

Internal sphincter muscle approximated

e

Excess flap of mucosa excised

f

Flap sutured over approximated internal sphincter muscle

g

Drainage

h

Fig. 15.4 Endorectal advancement flap. **(a)** Probe is placed in the vaginal fistula opening and the rectal opening identified. **(b)** Rectal flap is outlined around the fistula opening. **(c)** Flap mobilization including the mucosa, submucosa, and circular muscle is completed. **(d)** Internal and external sphincters are both mobilized. **(e)** The internal sphincter is then reapproximated. **(f)** Excess flap including the fistula opening is excised. **(g)** Flap is advanced and sutured in place to cover the rectal wall defect. **(h)** Vagina is left open for drainage.

preexisting fecal incontinence.[65] Complications include tissue ischemia and hematoma formation, both of which can lead to flap failure. One of the editors (S. D. W.) prefers an elliptical slide flap without any incisions extending cephalad toward the rectum.

Transvaginal sliding flap can also be utilized, especially in patients with inflammatory bowel disease or previous rectal reservoir construction that would complicate perineal or transanal approaches. With the patient in lithotomy, the vaginal and rectal sides of the fistula tract are identified. A flap is then created in the posterior vaginal wall using similar principles to those described above with lateral mobilization extending to the ischial tuberosities to ensure a tensionless closure. The levator ani muscles can be approximated in the midline to separate the vaginal and rectal defects, although it should be done with care as dyspareunia may result. The rectal mucosa is then closed. The vaginal fistula site is then excised and the flap anchored to the perineal skin. Closure of the levators as well as consideration of diverting ostomy are believed to improve the success of this approach, especially in patients with Crohn's disease.[66]

Anocutaneous flaps have been described for low rectovaginal and anovaginal fistulas, where mucosal advancement would result in ectropion with wet anus and pruritus ani.[67] With the patient in lithotomy, the fistula tract is completely excised from the vaginal opening to the internal opening in the anal canal; a curette is used to excise any remaining epithelialized tissue in the tract. A wide-based flap is then created from anoderm, the sphincter fibers are reapproximated, and the cutaneous flap anastomosed to the rectal mucosa to close the defect. All patients in one study received diverting ostomy to assist with healing.[68]

15.5.6 Rectal Sleeve Advancement

Rectal sleeve advancement can be considered for fistulas that involve more than one-third of the circumference of the rectum, or those with tissue injury not amenable to primary closure (▸ Fig. 15.5). It involves resection of the rectum proximal to the fistula and mucosectomy of the fistulized segment of rectum, with pull-through of healthy proximal rectum and anastomosis to the dentate line. From the perineal approach, the patient is placed in the prone jackknife position and a curvilinear incision is made extending from the left side of the sacrococcygeal joint to the external anal sphincter, exposing the pelvic floor. The incision exposes the distal rectum and allows proximal circumferential dissection. The distal rectum is transected and a mucosectomy performed from the dentate line to the transection point. The fistula tract is then excised, the rectovaginal septum closed in two layers and the vagina left open for postoperative drainage. The transected rectum is then anastomosed to the dentate line, and the pelvic floor and skin closed.[69]

15.5.7 Transabdominal Repair

High RVFs often require transabdominal repair due to their difficult location. Some surgeons prefer the transabdominal approach in patients with concomitant abdominal pathology such as neoplasms or inflammatory bowel disease regardless of the location. Abdominal approach begins with the patient

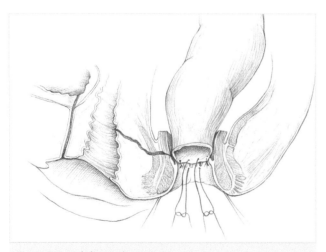

Fig. 15.5 Rectal sleeve advancement.

in lithotomy and an open or minimally invasive approach is performed. The sigmoid colon is mobilized, the presacral space entered, and the peritoneum incised at the inferior portion of the pouch of Douglas. The rectovaginal septum is opened to the pelvic floor, dividing the fistula, and the lateral attachments to the rectum are mobilized. The rectum is transected distally, and the vagina is repaired; the remainder of the procedure is transanally completed as described above (▸ Fig. 15.6).[70] A colonic J-pouch is an option performed to restore intestinal continuity, as is a staged coloanal procedure (Turnbull–Cutait).[71]

Interposition of a tissue flap such as omentum or levators to buttress the repair is also possible from the abdominal approach. Concurrent resection of diseased bowel can be performed. More extensive resections including colectomy and proctectomy with coloanal anastomoses may be indicated in highly selected cases of inflammatory bowel disease. Abdominoperineal resection and pelvic exenteration can be considered in cases of locally advanced neoplasms, usually following neoadjuvant chemoradiation. Fecal diversion alone should be considered for palliation or in poor operative candidates.

15.5.8 Miscellaneous Local Approaches

Local approaches including fibrin glue injections and collagen fistula plugs have prohibitively poor outcomes and are not advocated for repair of RVF,[72,73] although fibrin glue has had some success with longer fistula tracts and has been combined with other local techniques to try and ensure closure and scarring of the tract to prevent recurrence.[74,75,76,77] Similarly, modifications to traditional fistula plugs have been made in an effort to improve success, but results are difficult to reproduce.[78] Bioprosthetic mesh has been used to augment advancement flap or tissue transfer techniques with some improvement in outcomes. Unfortunately, these studies are small and the heterogeneous populations make any definitive conclusions regarding outcomes difficult.[79,80] Minimally invasive approaches have been described, including transanal endoscopic microsurgical repair; however, these reports have been small case series without long-term outcomes.[81]

15.6 Rectourethral Fistula

The etiology of RUFs parallels that of RVFs with urinary and rectal operations, inflammatory bowel disease, pelvic irradiation, trauma, and infectious or inflammatory conditions being the main causes. Rates of fistula formation for patients undergoing treatment for prostate cancer with both surgical resection and radiation treatment are around 3%,[82,83,84,85] and salvage radiation therapy is complicated by fistula formation in almost 10% of patients.[86,87,88] Anorectal procedures after pelvic irradiation have increased risk of RUFs[89] and malignancies related to fistulae are more difficult to treat.[90] Clinical presentation includes pneumaturia, fecaluria, leakage of urine from the rectum, and pain. Diagnosis can be confirmed with rectal exam, urethrocystoscopy, and sigmoidoscopy. Potentially helpful imaging studies include secretory or retrograde urethrography, voiding cystourethrography, CT, or MRI with rectal contrast. Like RVFs, assessment of the size, location, surrounding tissue integrity, anal sphincter function, and underlying etiology impacts decisions

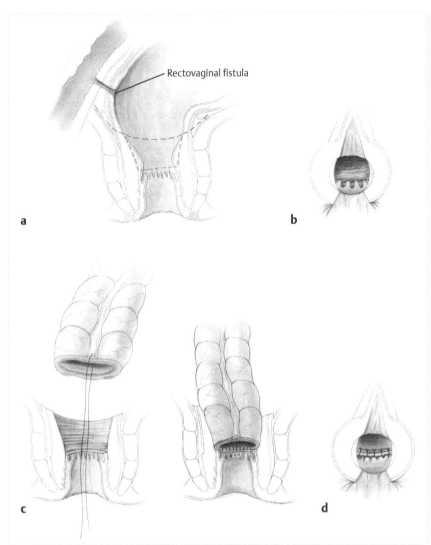

a

b

c

d

Fig. 15.6 Coloanal anastomosis. **(a)** Mobilization of rectum distal to level of the rectovaginal fistula and transection of the rectum distally. **(b)** Removal of mucosa from the anorectal stump. **(c)** Anastomosis between proximal bowel and anal canal at the level of the dentate line. **(d)** Final arrangement of colon within the anal canal.

Rectovaginal fistula

regarding treatment of RUFs. Complicated RUFs include those greater than 2 cm, failure of previous repair, radiation-induced fistulas, and those that lie in an infected operative field.

As with RVFs, there are a variety of operative approaches to repair RUFs. Up to one-quarter of patients suffer recurrence after initial repair, and increasing complexity and failure rates complicate subsequent repairs.[84,91] Fecal and urinary diversion can allow spontaneous closure in some patients[92]; however, most require operative intervention.[91] Similar approaches are used for RUFs as are used for RVF repair and include perineal, transsphincteric, muscle transposition, and rectal advancement flaps. A permanent stoma with or without abdominoperineal resection can also be utilized. All patients should receive perioperative antibiotics and bladder catheter placement. Urinary catheters are usually left in place until healing has been proven. Urinary and fecal diversion can both be utilized, but fecal diversion should be strongly considered in complex closures; loop ileostomy is a common diversion technique. Prior to ostomy closure, voiding cystogram, rectal contrast study, cystoscopy, and examination under anesthesia should be performed to ensure successful fistula closure. If the patient does not have a stoma, an oral mechanical cathartic and antibiotic bowel preparation should be employed.

Perineal approach can be accompanied by use of a dartos muscle flap to buttress the repair.[93,94,95,96] Concerns with this approach are visualization, scarred tissue that is not ideal for closure, and compromise of urinary or fecal continence. The patient is placed in lithotomy position and a curved perineal incision used to expose the anterior perineal space. The rectourethral plane is entered and dissection carried to the peritoneal reflection to expose the entire fistula tract. The tract is excised, the rectal defect is closed primarily, and urethral defects less than 2 cm are also closed primarily. For larger urethral defects, a buccal mucosal graft can be used to prevent stricture. An interposition muscle flap, often the gracilis flap, is used to separate suture lines and protect the repair.[95] A modification of the perineal approach via an anterior transanorectal technique has also been described.[97] The midline perineal incision is extended through all structures superficial to the prostatic capsule including the internal and external anal sphincters. This mobilization improves exposure to fistulas in the prostatic urethra and can result in acceptable continence and erectile preservation.

Another local approach is the posterior midline transanosphincteric approach, or the York-Mason approach, which offers the benefit of dissection through naïve tissue planes.[43]

Successful closure is seen in over 85% of patients. One of the most feared complications is postoperative incontinence.[98,99] With the patient in prone jackknife, an incision is made from the anal margin to the midsacrum just lateral to midline. The layers of the pelvic floor and anal sphincters are opened and the rectal opening identified (▶ Fig. 15.7). The fistula tract is excised (▶ Fig. 15.8), the urethra is closed with absorbable sutures, the rectal flaps are closed in a vest-over-pants technique (▶ Fig. 15.9), and the sphincters and pelvic musculature are reapproximated (▶ Fig. 15.10).

Rectal advancement flaps can be used for repair of RUFs, with success rates as high as 83% and low morbidity rates.[100] Patients are placed in a prone flexed position and rectal retractors used to expose the fistula opening. A full- or partial-thickness rectal flap is first created to include the rectal side of the fistula, and the tract is then opened toward the urethra and excised; then, granulation tissue is excised. The urethral defect is closed with absorbable suture, and the internal and external sphincters reapproximated. The fistula opening is then excised from the tip of the rectal flap, and the flap sutured in place around the periphery with absorbable suture. A tension-free repair is important to success, so wide mobilization of the flap should be performed. Transanal flap repair can be undertaken using transanal endoscopic surgical platforms.[101]

A transabdominal repair can be considered, as it offers the benefit of using omental flaps rather than incurring the morbidity of a muscle flap. This approach is complicated by difficult exposure of the urethral defect in the pelvis, increased operative time due to frequent need for adhesiolysis, and prolonged postoperative recovery.

15.7 Conclusion

Rectovaginal and rectourethral fistulas have a significant negative impact on patients' quality of life. Preoperative planning, including review of the etiology, consideration of the anatomy, and assessment of available healthy tissue for repair, is paramount, but must be combined with meticulous surgical

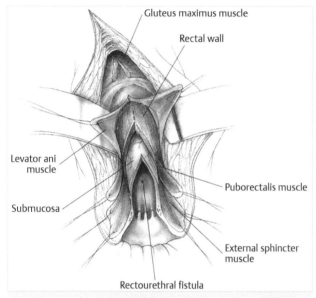

Fig. 15.7 Posterior midline transanosphincteric approach to repair of RVF and RUF. Tissue layers are marked with sutures as they are created.

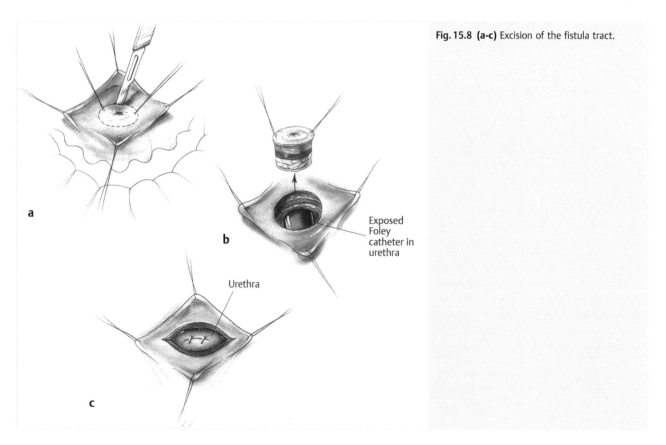

Fig. 15.8 (a-c) Excision of the fistula tract.

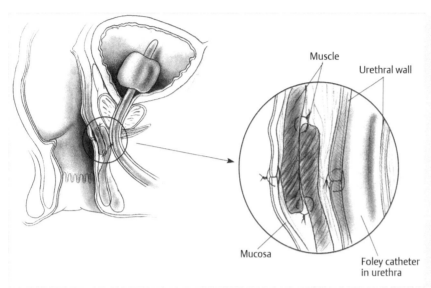

Fig. 15.9 Closure of the urethra over urinary catheter, with approximation of rectal flaps in a vest-over-pants technique.

Muscle

Urethral wall

Mucosa

Foley catheter in urethra

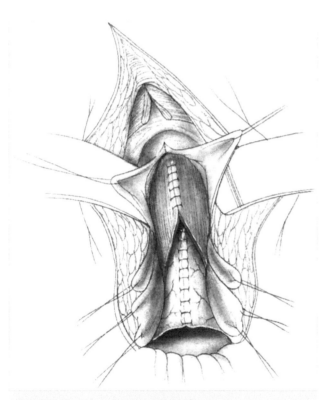

Fig. 15.10 Tissue layers are approximated.

technique to achieve high rates of success. Understanding the options for repair, the outcomes of each, and the benefits of the various surgical approaches allows the surgeon to choose the optimal repair for each patient.

References

[1] Saclarides TJ. Rectovaginal fistula. Surg Clin North Am. 2002; 82 (6):1261–1272

[2] Ommer A, Herold A, Berg E, Fürst A, Schiedeck T, Sailer M. German S3-Guideline: rectovaginal fistula. Ger Med Sci. 2012; 10:Doc15

[3] Radcliffe AG, Ritchie JK, Hawley PR, Lennard-Jones JE, Northover JM. Anovaginal and rectovaginal fistulas in Crohn's disease. Dis Colon Rectum. 1988; 31(2):94–99

[4] Goldaber KG, Wendel PJ, McIntire DD, Wendel GD, Jr. Postpartum perineal morbidity after fourth-degree perineal repair. Am J Obstet Gynecol. 1993; 168(2):489–493

[5] Venkatesh KS, Ramanujam PS, Larson DM, Haywood MA. Anorectal complications of vaginal delivery. Dis Colon Rectum. 1989; 32(12):1039–1041

[6] Lawson J. Rectovaginal fistulae following difficult labour. Proc R Soc Med. 1972; 65(3):283–286

[7] Tsang CB, Madoff RD, Wong WD, et al. Anal sphincter integrity and function influences outcome in rectovaginal fistula repair. Dis Colon Rectum. 1998; 41(9):1141–1146

[8] Hoexter B, Labow SB, Moseson MD. Transanal rectovaginal fistula repair. Dis Colon Rectum. 1985; 28(8):572–575

[9] Kasibhatla M, Clough RW, Montana GS, et al. Predictors of severe gastrointestinal toxicity after external beam radiotherapy and interstitial brachytherapy for advanced or recurrent gynecologic malignancies. Int J Radiat Oncol Biol Phys. 2006; 65(2):398–403

[10] Allen-Mersh TG, Wilson EJ, Hope-Stone HF, Mann CV. The management of late radiation-induced rectal injury after treatment of carcinoma of the uterus. Surg Gynecol Obstet. 1987; 164(6):521–524

[11] Anseline PF, Lavery IC, Fazio VW, Jagelman DG, Weakley FL. Radiation injury of the rectum: evaluation of surgical treatment. Ann Surg. 1981; 194 (6):716–724

[12] Sandeman TF. Radiation injury of the anorectal region. Aust N Z J Surg. 1980; 50(2):169–172

[13] Buchmann P, Allan RN, Thompson H, Alexander-Williams J. Carcinoma in a rectovaginal fistula in a patient with Crohn's disease. Am J Surg. 1980; 140 (3):462–463

[14] Greenstein AJ, Kark AE, Dreiling DA. Crohn's disease of the colon. I. Fistula in Crohn's disease of the colon, classification presenting features and management in 63 patients. Am J Gastroenterol. 1974; 62(5):419–429

[15] Faulconer HT, Muldoon JP. Rectovaginal fistula in patients with colitis: review and report of a case. Dis Colon Rectum. 1975; 18(5):413–415

[16] Bernstein LH, Frank MS, Brandt LJ, Boley SJ. Healing of perineal Crohn's disease with metronidazole. Gastroenterology. 1980; 79(2):357–365

[17] Mahadevan U, Marion JF, Present DH. Fistula response to methotrexate in Crohn's disease: a case series. Aliment Pharmacol Ther. 2003; 18(10):1003–1008

[18] Present DH, Lichtiger S. Efficacy of cyclosporine in treatment of fistula of Crohn's disease. Dig Dis Sci. 1994; 39(2):374–380

[19] Present DH, Rutgeerts P, Targan S, et al. Infliximab for the treatment of fistulas in patients with Crohn's disease. N Engl J Med. 1999; 340(18):1398–1405

[20] Poritz LS, Rowe WA, Koltun WA. Remicade does not abolish the need for surgery in fistulizing Crohn's disease. Dis Colon Rectum. 2002; 45(6):771–775

[21] Teh LS, Green KA, O'Sullivan MM, Morris JS, Williams BD. Behçet's syndrome: severe proctitis with rectovaginal fistula formation. Ann Rheum Dis. 1989; 48(9):779–780

[22] Sugarbaker PH. Rectovaginal fistula following low circular stapled anastomosis in women with rectal cancer. J Surg Oncol. 1996; 61(2):155–158

[23] Pescatori M, Gagliardi G. Postoperative complications after procedure for prolapsed hemorrhoids (PPH) and stapled transanal rectal resection (STARR) procedures. Tech Coloproctol. 2008; 12(1):7–19

[24] Schwartz J, Rabinowitz H, Rozenfeld V, Leibovitz A, Stelian J, Habot B. Rectovaginal fistula associated with fecal impaction. J Am Geriatr Soc. 1992; 40(6):641

[25] Arias BE, Ridgeway B, Barber MD. Complications of neglected vaginal pessaries: case presentation and literature review. Int Urogynecol J Pelvic Floor Dysfunct. 2008; 19(8):1173–1178

[26] Pfeifer J, Reissman P, Wexner SD. Ergotamine-induced complex rectovaginal fistula. Report of a case. Dis Colon Rectum. 1995; 38(11):1224–1226

[27] Maconi G, Parente F, Bianchi Porro G. Hydrogen peroxide enhanced ultrasound- fistulography in the assessment of enterocutaneous fistulas complicating Crohn's disease. Gut. 1999; 45(6):874–878

[28] Poen AC, Felt-Bersma RJ, Eijsbouts QA, Cuesta MA, Meuwissen SG. Hydrogen peroxide-enhanced transanal ultrasound in the assessment of fistula-in-ano. Dis Colon Rectum. 1998; 41(9):1147–1152

[29] Garcia-Granero A, Granero-Castro P, Frasson M, et al. Management of cryptoglandular supralevator abscesses in the magnetic resonance imaging era: a case series. Int J Colorectal Dis. 2014; 29(12):1557–1564

[30] Yee LF, Birnbaum EH, Read TE, Kodner IJ, Fleshman JW. Use of endoanal ultrasound in patients with rectovaginal fistulas. Dis Colon Rectum. 1999; 42(8):1057–1064

[31] El-Gazzaz G, Hull TL, Mignanelli E, Hammel J, Gurland B, Zutshi M. Obstetric and cryptoglandular rectovaginal fistulas: long-term surgical outcome; quality of life; and sexual function. J Gastrointest Surg. 2010; 14(11):1758–1763

[32] Dohgomori H, Arikawa K, Nobori M, Tonari M. Hyperbaric oxygenation for rectovaginal fistula: a report of two cases. J Obstet Gynaecol Res. 1999; 25(5):343–344

[33] Homsi R, Daikoku NH, Littlejohn J, Wheeless CR, Jr. Episiotomy: risks of dehiscence and rectovaginal fistula. Obstet Gynecol Surv. 1994; 49(12):803–808

[34] Fazio VWCJ, Delaney CP. Current Therapy in Colon and Rectal Surgery. 2nd ed. Philadelphia, PA: Elsevier Mosby; 2005

[35] Oakley SH, Brown HW, Yurteri-Kaplan L, et al. Practice patterns regarding management of rectovaginal fistulae: a multicenter review from the Fellows' Pelvic Research Network. Female Pelvic Med Reconstr Surg. 2015; 21(3):123–128

[36] Halverson AL, Hull TL, Fazio VW, Church J, Hammel J, Floruta C. Repair of recurrent rectovaginal fistulas. Surgery. 2001; 130(4):753–757, discussion 757–758

[37] Pinto RA, Peterson TV, Shawki S, Davila GW, Wexner SD. Are there predictors of outcome following rectovaginal fistula repair? Dis Colon Rectum. 2010; 53(9):1240–1247

[38] Hull TL, El-Gazzaz G, Gurland B, Church J, Zutshi M. Surgeons should not hesitate to perform episioproctotomy for rectovaginal fistula secondary to cryptoglandular or obstetrical origin. Dis Colon Rectum. 2011; 54(1):54–59

[39] Mazier WP, Senagore AJ, Schiesel EC. Operative repair of anovaginal and rectovaginal fistulas. Dis Colon Rectum. 1995; 38(1):4–6

[40] Soriano D, Lemoine A, Laplace C, et al. Results of recto-vaginal fistula repair: retrospective analysis of 48 cases. Eur J Obstet Gynecol Reprod Biol. 2001; 96(1):75–79

[41] Kaiser AM. Cloaca-like deformity with faecal incontinence after severe obstetric injury–technique and functional outcome of ano-vaginal and perineal reconstruction with X-flaps and sphincteroplasty. Colorectal Dis. 2008; 10(8):827–832

[42] Tancer ML, Lasser D, Rosenblum N. Rectovaginal fistula or perineal and anal sphincter disruption, or both, after vaginal delivery. Surg Gynecol Obstet. 1990; 171(1):43–46

[43] Mason AY. Transsphincteric approach to rectal lesions. Surg Annu. 1977; 9:171–194

[44] Pitel S, Lefevre JH, Parc Y, Chafai N, Shields C, Tiret E. Martius advancement flap for low rectovaginal fistula: short- and long-term results. Colorectal Dis. 2011; 13(6):e112–e115

[45] Songne K, Scotté M, Lubrano J, et al. Treatment of anovaginal or rectovaginal fistulas with modified Martius graft. Colorectal Dis. 2007; 9(7):653–656

[46] Elkins TE, DeLancey JO, McGuire EJ. The use of modified Martius graft as an adjunctive technique in vesicovaginal and rectovaginal fistula repair. Obstet Gynecol. 1990; 75(4):727–733

[47] Boronow RC. Repair of the radiation-induced vaginal fistula utilizing the Martius technique. World J Surg. 1986; 10(2):237–248

[48] Martius H. Die operative Wiederherstellug der vollkommen fehlenden Harnrohre und des Schliessmuskels derselben. Zentralbl Gynakol. 1928; 52:480

[49] Hoskins WJ, Park RC, Long R, Artman LE, McMahon EB. Repair of urinary tract fistulas with bulbocavernosus myocutaneous flaps. Obstet Gynecol. 1984; 63(4):588–593

[50] Symmonds RE, Hill LM. Loss of the urethra: a report on 50 patients. Am J Obstet Gynecol. 1978; 130(2):130–138

[51] Zimmerman DD, Gosselink MP, Briel JW, Schouten WR. The outcome of transanal advancement flap repair of rectovaginal fistulas is not improved by an additional labial fat flap transposition. Tech Coloproctol. 2002; 6(1):37–42

[52] Petrou SP, Jones J, Parra RO. Martius flap harvest site: patient self-perception. J Urol. 2002; 167(5):2098–2099

[53] Lefèvre JH, Bretagnol F, Maggiori L, Alves A, Ferron M, Panis Y. Operative results and quality of life after gracilis muscle transposition for recurrent rectovaginal fistula. Dis Colon Rectum. 2009; 52(7):1290–1295

[54] Wexner SD, Ruiz DE, Genua J, Nogueras JJ, Weiss EG, Zmora O. Gracilis muscle interposition for the treatment of rectourethral, rectovaginal, and pouch-vaginal fistulas: results in 53 patients. Ann Surg. 2008; 248(1):39–43

[55] Rius J, Nessim A, Nogueras JJ, Wexner SD. Gracilis transposition in complicated perianal fistula and unhealed perineal wounds in Crohn's disease. Eur J Surg. 2000; 166(3):218–222

[56] Zmora O, Tulchinsky H, Gur E, Goldman G, Klausner JM, Rabau M. Gracilis muscle transposition for fistulas between the rectum and urethra or vagina. Dis Colon Rectum. 2006; 49(9):1316–1321

[57] Fürst A, Schmidbauer C, Swol-Ben J, Iesalnieks I, Schwandner O, Agha A. Gracilis transposition for repair of recurrent anovaginal and rectovaginal fistulas in Crohn's disease. Int J Colorectal Dis. 2008; 23(4):349–353

[58] Laird DR. Procedures used in treatment of complicated fistulas. Am J Surg. 1948; 76(6):701–708

[59] Joo JS, Weiss EG, Nogueras JJ, Wexner SD. Endorectal advancement flap in perianal Crohn's disease. Am Surg. 1998; 64(2):147–150

[60] Sonoda T, Hull T, Piedmonte MR, Fazio VW. Outcomes of primary repair of anorectal and rectovaginal fistulas using the endorectal advancement flap. Dis Colon Rectum. 2002; 45(12):1622–1628

[61] MacRae HM, McLeod RS, Cohen Z, Stern H, Reznick R. Treatment of rectovaginal fistulas that has failed previous repair attempts. Dis Colon Rectum. 1995; 38(9):921–925

[62] Lowry AC, Thorson AG, Rothenberger DA, Goldberg SM. Repair of simple rectovaginal fistulas. Influence of previous repairs. Dis Colon Rectum. 1988; 31(9):676–678

[63] Ozuner G, Hull TL, Cartmill J, Fazio VW. Long-term analysis of the use of transanal rectal advancement flaps for complicated anorectal/vaginal fistulas. Dis Colon Rectum. 1996; 39(1):10–14

[64] Marchesa P, Hull TL, Fazio VW. Advancement sleeve flaps for treatment of severe perianal Crohn's disease. Br J Surg. 1998; 85(12):1695–1698

[65] Wise WE, Jr, Aguilar PS, Padmanabhan A, Meesig DM, Arnold MW, Stewart WR. Surgical treatment of low rectovaginal fistulas. Dis Colon Rectum. 1991; 34(3):271–274

[66] Sher ME, Bauer JJ, Gelernt I. Surgical repair of rectovaginal fistulas in patients with Crohn's disease: transvaginal approach. Dis Colon Rectum. 1991; 34(8):641–648

[67] Chew SS, Rieger NA. Transperineal repair of obstetric-related anovaginal fistula. Aust N Z J Obstet Gynaecol. 2004; 44(1):68–71

[68] Hesterberg R, Schmidt WU, Müller F, Röher HD. Treatment of anovaginal fistulas with an anocutaneous flap in patients with Crohn's disease. Int J Colorectal Dis. 1993; 8(1):51–54

[69] Nowacki MP, Szawlowski AW, Borkowski A. Parks' coloanal sleeve anastomosis for treatment of postirradiation rectovaginal fistula. Dis Colon Rectum. 1986; 29(12):817–820

[70] Schouten WR, Oom DM. Rectal sleeve advancement for the treatment of persistent rectovaginal fistulas. Tech Coloproctol. 2009; 13(4):289–294

[71] Remzi FH, El Gazzaz G, Kiran RP, Kirat HT, Fazio VW. Outcomes following Turnbull-Cutait abdominoperineal pull-through compared with coloanal anastomosis. Br J Surg. 2009; 96(4):424–429

[72] Sentovich SM. Fibrin glue for anal fistulas: long-term results. Dis Colon Rectum. 2003; 46(4):498–502

[73] Swinscoe MT, Ventakasubramaniam AK, Jayne DG. Fibrin glue for fistula-in-ano: the evidence reviewed. Tech Coloproctol. 2005; 9(2):89–94

[74] Abel ME, Chiu YS, Russell TR, Volpe PA. Autologous fibrin glue in the treatment of rectovaginal and complex fistulas. Dis Colon Rectum. 1993; 36(5):447–449

[75] Venkatesh KS, Ramanujam P. Fibrin glue application in the treatment of recurrent anorectal fistulas. Dis Colon Rectum. 1999; 42(9):1136–1139

[76] Cintron JR, Park JJ, Orsay CP, Pearl RK, Nelson RL, Abcarian H. Repair of fistulas-in-ano using autologous fibrin tissue adhesive. Dis Colon Rectum. 1999; 42(5):607–613

[77] Mizrahi N, Wexner SD, Zmora O, et al. Endorectal advancement flap: are there predictors of failure? Dis Colon Rectum. 2002; 45(12):1616–1621

[78] Gonsalves S, Sagar P, Lengyel J, Morrison C, Dunham R. Assessment of the efficacy of the rectovaginal button fistula plug for the treatment of ileal pouch-vaginal and rectovaginal fistulas. Dis Colon Rectum. 2009; 52(11):1877–1881

[79] Ellis CN. Outcomes after repair of rectovaginal fistulas using bioprosthetics. Dis Colon Rectum. 2008; 51(7):1084–1088

[80] Schwandner O, Fuerst A, Kunstreich K, Scherer R. Innovative technique for the closure of rectovaginal fistula using Surgisis mesh. Tech Coloproctol. 2009; 13(2):135–140

[81] D'Ambrosio G, Paganini AM, Guerrieri M, et al. Minimally invasive treatment of rectovaginal fistula. Surg Endosc. 2012; 26(2):546–550

[82] Harpster LE, Rommel FM, Sieber PR, et al. The incidence and management of rectal injury associated with radical prostatectomy in a community based urology practice. J Urol. 1995; 154(4):1435–1438

[83] McLaren RH, Barrett DM, Zincke H. Rectal injury occurring at radical retropubic prostatectomy for prostate cancer: etiology and treatment. Urology. 1993; 42(4):401–405

[84] Thomas C, Jones J, Jäger W, Hampel C, Thüroff JW, Gillitzer R. Incidence, clinical symptoms and management of rectourethral fistulas after radical prostatectomy. J Urol. 2010; 183(2):608–612

[85] Chrouser KL, Leibovich BC, Sweat SD, et al. Urinary fistulas following external radiation or permanent brachytherapy for the treatment of prostate cancer. J Urol. 2005; 173(6):1953–1957

[86] Ahmed HU, Ishaq A, Zacharakis E, et al. Rectal fistulae after salvage high-intensity focused ultrasound for recurrent prostate cancer after combined brachytherapy and external beam radiotherapy. BJU Int. 2009; 103(3):321–323

[87] Stone NN, Stock RG. Complications following permanent prostate brachytherapy. Eur Urol. 2002; 41(4):427–433

[88] Theodorescu D, Gillenwater JY, Koutrouvelis PG. Prostatourethral-rectal fistula after prostate brachytherapy. Cancer. 2000; 89(10):2085–2091

[89] Marguet C, Raj GV, Brashears JH, et al. Rectourethral fistula after combination radiotherapy for prostate cancer. Urology. 2007; 69(5):898–901

[90] Muñoz M, Nelson H, Harrington J, Tsiotos G, Devine R, Engen D. Management of acquired rectourinary fistulas: outcome according to cause. Dis Colon Rectum. 1998; 41(10):1230–1238

[91] Hechenbleikner EM, Buckley JC, Wick EC. Acquired rectourethral fistulas in adults: a systematic review of surgical repair techniques and outcomes. Dis Colon Rectum. 2013; 56(3):374–383

[92] Harris CR, McAninch JW, Mundy AR, et al. Rectourethral Fistulas Secondary to Prostate Cancer Treatment: Management and Outcomes from a Multi-Institutional Combined Experience. J Urol. 2017; 197(1):191–194

[93] Muñoz-Duyos A, Navarro-Luna A, Pardo-Aranda F, et al. Gracilis Muscle Interposition for Rectourethral Fistula After Laparoscopic Prostatectomy: A Prospective Evaluation and Long-term Follow-up. Dis Colon Rectum. 2017; 60(4):393–398

[94] Takano S, Boutros M, Wexner SD. Gracilis transposition for complex perineal fistulas: rectovaginal fistula and rectourethral fistula. Dis Colon Rectum. 2014; 57(4):538

[95] Vanni AJ, Buckley JC, Zinman LN. Management of surgical and radiation induced rectourethral fistulas with an interposition muscle flap and selective buccal mucosal onlay graft. J Urol. 2010; 184(6):2400–2404

[96] Ruiz D, Bashankaev B, Speranza J, Wexner SD. Graciloplasty for rectourethral, rectovaginal and rectovesical fistulas: technique overview, pitfalls and complications. Tech Coloproctol. 2008; 12(3):277–281, discussion 281–282

[97] Gecelter L. Transanorectal approach to the posterior urethra and bladder neck. J Urol. 1973; 109(6):1011–1016

[98] Dal Moro F, Mancini M, Pinto F, Zanovello N, Bassi PF, Pagano F. Successful repair of iatrogenic rectourinary fistulas using the posterior sagittal transrectal approach (York-Mason): 15-year experience. World J Surg. 2006; 30 (1):107–113

[99] Renschler TD, Middleton RG. 30 years of experience with York-Mason repair of recto-urinary fistulas. J Urol. 2003; 170(4, Pt 1):1222–1225, discussion 1225

[100] Garofalo TE, Delaney CP, Jones SM, Remzi FH, Fazio VW. Rectal advancement flap repair of rectourethral fistula: a 20-year experience. Dis Colon Rectum. 2003; 46(6):762–769

[101] Pigalarga R, Patel NM, Rezac C. Transanal endoscopic microsurgery-assisted rectal advancement flap is a viable option for iatrogenic rectourethral fistula repair: a case report. Tech Coloproctol. 2011; 15(2):209–211

16 Retrorectal Tumors

Sean J. Langenfeld and Steven D. Wexner

Abstract

This chapter will discuss the most common retrorectal tumors, including their etiology and incidence, but will focus on a practical clinical approach to these tumors based on the best available evidence.

Keywords: retrorectal tumors, anatomy, classification, incidence, pathology, cyst, teratoma, chordoma, meningocele, clinical presentation

16.1 Introduction

The presacral or retrorectal region is an area of embryologic fusion and remodeling, and thus it is a common site for embryologic remnants from which a heterogeneous group of neoplasms can develop. When compared to most other diseases that a colorectal surgeon will encounter, retrorectal tumors are rare and, as a result, poorly studied. Most publications detailing the diagnosis and treatment of these cysts and neoplasms are retrospective and small.

Additionally, there has been very little research in recent years on the subject, with many of the classical teachings stemming from studies that were published over 40 years ago. Within these older studies is a great deal of heterogeneity in available imaging and the extent of preoperative evaluation. The operative approach was also variable, with high rates of margin positivity. This problem likely led to higher rates of recurrence and lower rates of long-term survival.

Since then, there have been significant advances in imaging, record-keeping, and adjuvant therapy, so certain interventions that were previously felt to be contraindicated have re-emerged as viable treatment options. Perhaps the most controversial of these possibilities is the role for preoperative biopsy of solid tumors, which now has a very well-defined role for select tumors. Additionally, there is emerging evidence that observation of benign-appearing lesions may be safe.

This chapter will discuss the most common retrorectal tumors, including their etiology and incidence, but will focus on a practical clinical approach to these tumors based on the best available evidence.

16.2 Anatomy

The retrorectal space lies between the upper two-thirds of the rectum and the sacrum, above the rectosacral fascia. It is anteriorly limited by the fascia propria covering the rectum, posteriorly by the presacral fascia, and laterally by the lateral ligaments (stalks) of the rectum, the ureters, and the iliac vessels. Superiorly, it is bounded by the peritoneal reflection of the rectum and communicates with the retroperitoneal space. Inferiorly, it is limited by the rectosacral (Waldeyer's) fascia, which passes forward from the S4 vertebra to the rectum 3 to 5 cm proximal to the anorectal junction.

Below the rectosacral fascia is the supralevator space, a horseshoe-shaped potential space anteriorly limited by the fascia propria of the rectum and inferiorly by the levator ani muscle (▶ Fig. 16.1). This more inferior area is often included along with the true retrorectal space when describing presacral tumors.

The retroperitoneal space contains loose connective tissue. The presacral fascia protects the presacral vessels that lie deep to it. These vessels are part of the extensive vertebral plexus and are responsible for the major bleeding problems encountered in this area during surgery.

16.3 Classification

Uhlig and Johnson,[1] aided by the composite classification of Freier et al,[2] have proposed the classification outlined in the accompanying ▶ Table 16.1. In general, these tumors are divided into (1) congenital, including developmental cysts, chordomas, and anterior sacral meningoceles, (2) inflammatory, including anal fistulas, (3) neurogenic, (4) osseous, and (5) "miscellaneous" including several sarcomatous lesions and metastatic tumors.

When making clinical decisions, a more practical way to classify these tumors is into the broad categories of solid and cystic. Another practical distinction is between tumors that arise during infancy and early childhood versus those that arise in adulthood, as these tumors often behave quite differently.

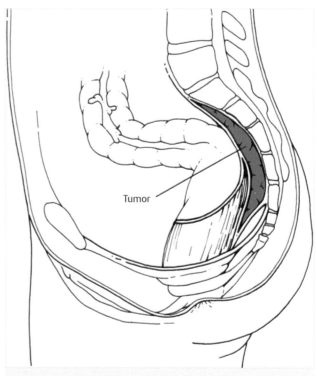

Fig. 16.1 Tumor in the retrorectal space.

Table 16.1 Differential diagnosis of retrorectal tumors and cysts[2]

Congenital

- Developmental cysts (epidermoid, dermoid, and mucus-secreting cysts; teratoma)
- Chordoma
- Teratocarcinoma
- Adrenal rest tumor
- Anterior sacral meningocele
- Duplication of rectum

Inflammatory

- Foreign body granuloma
- Perineal abscess
- Internal fistula
- Retrorectal abscess
- Chronic infectious granuloma

Neurogenic

- Neurofibroma and sarcoma
- Neurilemoma
- Ependymoma
- Ganglioneuroma
- Neurofibrosarcoma

Osseous

- Osteoma
- Osteogenic sarcoma
- Simple bone cyst, sacrum
- Ewing's tumor
- Chondromyxosarcoma
- Aneurysmal bone cyst
- Giant cell tumor

Miscellaneous

- Metastatic carcinoma
- Liposarcoma
- Hemangioendothelial sarcoma
- Lymphangioma
- Extra-abdominal desmoid tumor
- Plasma cell myeloma
- Malignant neoplasm of unknown type
- Lipoma
- Fibroma
- Fibrosarcoma

- Leiomyoma
- Leiomyosarcoma
- Hemangioma
- Pericytoma
- Endothelioma

16.4 Incidence

The true incidence of retrorectal tumors is unknown. It may be underestimated as these tumors likely remain undetected in a large percentage of asymptomatic individuals, and even when discovered, they are often mistaken for other anorectal pathologies such as abscesses and fistulas.

Most case series are quite small, and come from specialty centers that may see a disproportionate number of cases compared to the surrounding population. However, the most quoted incidence is about 1 in 40,000 hospital admissions,[3,4,5] derived from a 1985 case series involving 120 patients treated at the Mayo Clinic.[6]

The relative incidence of this heterogeneous group of tumors is difficult to estimate, as most case series would inherently suffer from sample bias. In general, congenital lesions account for slightly more than half of all presacral tumors, and two-thirds of these lesions are developmental cysts. Neurogenic neoplasms account for 5 to 15% of lesions as well.[3,5] Thankfully, most retrorectal neoplasms are benign, but the most common malignant neoplasms are sacrococcygeal chordomas, followed by sarcomas.[6,7]

16.5 Pathology

An exhaustive review of the pathology of this area is not given in this chapter. Many of the tumors have common symptoms and present in a similar manner; the reader is referred to any standard pathology text. However, the pertinent pathologic features of the most common tumors will be briefly reviewed.

16.5.1 Developmental Cysts

Developmental cysts may arise from any of the germ layers (▶ Table 16.2). All congenital cysts occur with a female predominance,[6] with a female-to-male ratio of incidence of 5:1. The majority of cysts are asymptomatic and, because tension in the cyst is low, their presence may be easily missed on rectal examination. The average age at cyst appearance is in the fourth decade. The duration of symptoms, if they exist, is frequently measured in years. A postanal dimple is associated with some congenital cysts and may be a clue to the diagnosis. While the exact rate of malignancy is not known, up to 12% of cystic lesions can develop into a malignancy.[8,9]

While reported rates of these cysts have been higher in females, they were often asymptomatic, and were found during the reproductive years, when pelvic examinations are most frequent. Thus, the female predominance may be artificial to some extent. This fact also may impact the calculations which will be discussed later that show that men tend to have more malignant lesions.

Table 16.2 Germ layer origin of developmental cysts

	Epidermoid	Dermoid	Enterogenous	Teratomatous
Tissue of origin	Ectoderm	Ectoderm	Endoderm	All three layers
Histologic characteristics	Stratified squamous	Stratified squamous with skin appendages (sweat glands, sebaceous glands, hair follicles)	Columnar or cuboidal lining; may have secretory function	Varying degrees of differentiation between cysts and cell layers of single cyst
General state	Benign	Benign	Benign	Benign or malignant

Epidermoid and Dermoid Cysts

Epidermoid and dermoid cysts result from closure defects of the ectodermal tube with heterotopic inclusions of skin, sometimes with accessory skin appendages. The epidermoid cyst is lined with stratified squamous epithelium with keratohyaline granules and intracellular bridges. In addition to the stratified squamous epithelium seen in epidermoid cysts, dermoid cysts have sweat glands, hair follicles, sebaceous glands, or all three. These appendages characterize dermoid cysts.

Both epidermoid and dermoid cysts tend to be rounded and circumscribed, have a thin connective tissue outer layer, and contain viscid green-yellow material. These cysts can communicate with the skin surface, where they appear as a postanal dimple. The cysts have a 30% rate of infection.[10] In the infected state, they may appear as a retrorectal abscess or perirectal suppuration. When the postanal dimple communicates with an infected cyst, a mistaken diagnosis of anal fistula is commonly made.

Enterogenous Cysts

Enterogenous cysts result from sequestration of the developing hindgut, and may include squamous or transitional epithelium within the lining of an otherwise mucus-secreting cyst. Generally, these are thin-walled cysts lined by columnar epithelium, and they tend to be multilocular, usually with one dominant cyst and a series of minor or "daughter" cysts. In the uninfected state, they are filled with a clear to green mucoid material. Enterogenous cysts also have a tendency to become infected, but they remain asymptomatic in the majority of cases.

Rectal Duplication Cysts

Intestinal duplications are rare developmental anomalies, most commonly occurring in females and associated with other congenital defects, especially genitourinary and vertebral anomalies. The diagnosis depends on the fulfillment of three anatomic criteria, namely the cyst must be attached to the alimentary tract, it must be lined by mucous membrane similar to that part of the alimentary tract, and it must possess a smooth muscle coat.

Patients with rectal duplication cysts may be asymptomatic or may present with a perineal mass, constipation, tenesmus, prolapse, lower back pain, urinary symptoms, or recurrent perianal sepsis or fistula formation. Malignant change in a rectal duplication in an adult has been reported but is rare.[11]

Tailgut Cysts

These cysts, also called cystic hamartomas, occur predominantly in women and cause symptoms of mass effect or pain in half of patients,[12] which is higher than what is seen with other developmental cysts. These cysts are derived from remnants of the embryonic tailgut and differ from teratomas, which always contain elements of three germ cell layers.

Hjermstad and Helwig[12] collected 53 examples of developmental tailgut cysts in the retrorectal space. The lesions were usually circumscribed, unencapsulated, and multicystic, often filled with a colorless to yellow or gray fluid and had no communication with the rectal lumen. Inflammation occurred in 50% of the patients, one of whom had a poorly differentiated adenocarcinoma.

A 2000 literature review identified 10 cases of malignancy including 6 adenocarcinomas and 4 carcinoids, and also added 5 further cases, 1 of which was a neuroendocrine carcinoma.[13] Complete excision of the multilocular and multicystic process is thus warranted to prevent recurrent draining sinuses and eliminate the possibility of malignant change, which is rare.

16.5.2 Teratoma

These are true neoplasms arising from totipotential cells. Classically, they have representative tissue from each germ cell layer, although the degree of differentiation may vary among the elements. Malignancy tends to arise from one of the germ cells; however, in the anaplastic variety, it may be impossible to distinguish the tissue of origin. The more mature the tissue appears, the more benign the neoplasm tends to be, but all neoplasms should be viewed as potentially malignant.

The malignant potential of sacrococcygeal teratomas varies greatly based on patient age at presentation, with these tumors following a more aggressive course in children, and malignancy being much less common beyond the second decade.[3,4] Teratomas tend to be more aggressive when discovered later in childhood. For children, the incidence of malignancy in a 1974 American Academy of Pediatric Surgical Section Survey[14] was only 7% for teratomas present on the first day of life as opposed to 37% for lesions developing at 1 year of age and 50% for those appearing at 2 years of age. Simpson et al[15] reported on 26 sacrococcygeal teratomas in adults. Of these, 21 were benign and 19 occurred in females.

Macroscopic features and the growth pattern of sacrococcygeal teratomas have been described in detail by Pantoja and Rodriguez-Ibanez.[16] The lesions are well encapsulated and may be solid or cystic. They may contain all kinds of tissues, the most prominent ones being respiratory, nervous, and gastrointestinal. Teratomas maintain a strong attachment to the coccyx and sometimes the sacrum, but they rarely adhere to pelvic viscera unless previous inflammation has resulted in secondary adhesions.

16.5.3 Chordoma

Chordoma represents the most common malignant neoplasm in the retrorectal region. It arises from the remnants of the fetal notochord. Although it can occur anywhere from the hypophysis cerebri to the coccyx, the sacrococcygeal area is the site in approximately 50% of cases.[17] These neoplasms may arise in either sex at any age but are more frequent in men (2:1 to 5:1), and the greatest incidence occurs between 40 and 70 years of age.[5,6,18]

Macroscopically, the chordoma is typically a slow-growing, lobulated, well-defined structure composed of soft gelatinous tissue, often with areas of hemorrhage. It invades, distends, and destroys neighboring bone and extends into adjacent regions. Microscopically, the chordoma is said to resemble the various stages of notochordal development. The cells usually are aggregated in irregular groups separated by stromal tissue. Peripheral cells contain mucous droplets in the cytoplasm. As these cells mature, the droplets coalesce, creating single large vacuoles that comprise the physaliphorous cell typical of chordoma. Toward the center of the neoplasms, cords of cells appear to float in mucus, cell boundaries are indistinct, and the appearance is that of a syncytium.

Patients with chordomas experience rectal or perineal pain that is often aggravated by sitting and alleviated by standing or walking. Advanced lesions may be associated with constipation, fecal incontinence, urinary incontinence, or impotence.[19] Physical examination usually reveals a smooth extrarectal mass with intact overlying mucosa.

16.5.4 Anterior Sacral Meningocele

The meningocele is located in the presacral space and contains cerebrospinal fluid. It is more common in women.[20] Patients may experience constipation, urinary difficulties, low back or abdominal pain, headaches, meningitis, or dystocia.[21] Characteristic physical findings include a pelvic mass and almost unmistakable radiologic changes, but diagnoses tend to be delayed for months or years.[22]

The finding of a "scimitar" sacrum, characterized by a rounded, concave border without bone destruction, is pathognomonic (▶ Fig. 16.2). In modern medicine, sacral meningoceles are best characterized by magnetic resonance imaging (MRI). Aspiration should be avoided because of the risk of meningitis. Treatment consists of obliterating the neck of the meningocele. Operative approaches include posterior transsacral by laminectomy, perineal, and anterior transabdominal approaches.[20,23]

16.5.5 Other Entities

Several other retrorectal tumors exist, but an exhaustive list would distract from this chapter's utility. To summarize, several neurogenic neoplasms exist, with the most common being the ependymoma.[5] Primary osseous neoplasms have been well described, but are exceedingly rare and not typically addressed by the colorectal surgeon.

Although connective tissue sarcomas are rare, they represent the second most common malignancy in this area behind chordomas.[7] Another important consideration is retrorectal lesions

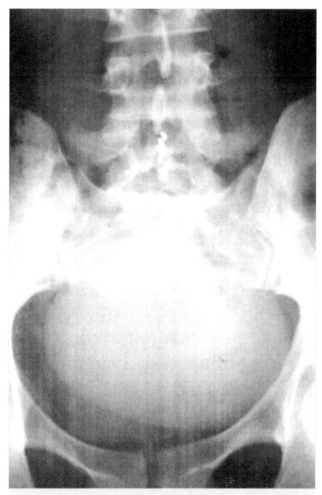

Fig. 16.2 "Scimitar" sign of sacrum. (Courtesy of Charles O. Finne III, MD.)

that are metastatic from another primary site, including lymphoma and adenocarcinoma. For this reason, an appropriate workup to identify other sites of disease is appropriate when clinical suspicion is high.

16.6 Clinical Presentation

16.6.1 Symptoms

The symptoms caused by retrorectal lesions are related to their site, size, and, in the case of retrorectal cysts, the presence or absence of infection. Benign lesions tend to be asymptomatic and may be detected by complete physical examination or, in the case of women, during childbirth. Malignant lesions are more likely to produce symptoms.

Pain

Pain is common in patients with neoplastic lesions and with infected cysts. It is generally poorly localized as low back or perianal pain, rectal ache, or deep rectal pain. If the sacral plexus is involved, patients may experience referred pain in the legs or buttocks. It is unusual for the pain to be accompanied by paralysis in the early stages. Characteristically, the pain experienced with retrorectal neoplasms is frequently postural. The patient associates pain with sitting or standing, and often the onset of pain relates to local trauma such as a fall on the sacrum or coccyx.

Infection

Infection may range from an isolated event with fever, chills, rigors, and pain to recurrent episodes of perianal suppuration, frequently with a history of recurrent surgical attempts at treatment. The latter history in a female should always precipitate a careful search to exclude a retrorectal cyst.

Interference with Pelvic Outlet

Constipation

Large masses may interfere with the passage of stool or give the feeling of unsatisfied defecation. Straining may result in the appearance of hemorrhoids, sometimes with rectal bleeding, but as a rule the tumors do not bleed.

Incontinence

Whether from paradoxical diarrhea secondary to obstruction or to interference with sphincter nerve supply, incontinence is an occasional symptom. In the early stages of tumor growth, gross perianal soiling may be the only manifestation of an early loss of fecal control.

Obstructed Labor

Many solid neoplasms first come to light during pregnancy.[24] Occasionally, a missed retrorectal tumor appears for the first time as a cause of obstructed labor.

Urinary Symptoms

Disturbances in bladder function are not uncommon and may be caused by interference with the pelvic parasympathetic supply, direct pressure on the bladder or urethra, or obstruction of the pelvic ureters.

Central Nervous System Manifestations

Although rare, anterior sacral meningoceles may present as central nervous system problems. In adults, headache and recurrent episodes of meningitis have been reported to result from recurrent infections of a meningocele.[21] The meningomyelocele is a gross disorder of sacral neurogenic and osseous formation, and it occurs with varying degrees of neurogenic disorder in infants.

16.6.2 Previous Surgery

A history of repeated local operations for perianal suppuration is important in the context of retrorectal cysts. In addition, a history of operations for malignant neoplasms of the genitourinary or gastrointestinal tract—in particular, the bladder, prostate, or rectum—is highly significant in terms of recurrence. The retrorectal space is a common site for metastatic spread.

16.6.3 Examination

The potential operability of a tumor and the operative approach required can usually be determined on rectal examination. The examination begins with inspection of the perianal area. A postanal dimple may suggest the presence of a developmental cyst. Soiling and a pouting anus may indicate interference with the nerve supply to the anal sphincters. Laxity of the anal sphincters and saddle anesthesia of the perineum further support involvement of coccygeal nerves.

As the finger passes into the rectum, a solid retrorectal mass should be obvious. In the early Mayo Clinic series, 97% of retrorectal tumors were palpable.[6] High retrorectal tumors may escape detection unless careful assessment of the sacral curve is made, a sudden anterior angulation being the first indication.

Location of the mass should be recorded, as well as whether it is lobulated or solitary, and whether it is possible to define its upper limits. In particular, the mass must be assessed for its relationship to the sacrum and the coccyx. This assessment is important because the location will determine the operative approach (▶ Fig. 16.3).

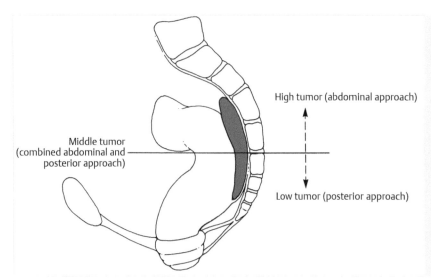

Fig. 16.3 Location of retrorectal tumors and operative approach to their treatment.

High tumor (abdominal approach)

Middle tumor (combined abdominal and posterior approach)

Low tumor (posterior approach)

Cystic neoplasms may be more difficult to detect since, if flaccid, they tend to feel like mucosal folds. However, if the finger is swept across the posterior mucosal surface, fluid within the cyst will be pushed before the finger into the lateral aspect of the cyst, which becomes tense and distended, thus allowing clear delineation. With tense cysts, it is sometimes difficult to distinguish between a supralevator abscess and a deep posterior space infection. Associated features such as a postanal dimple should be sought in these cases. An anterior meningocele can be mistaken for a simple cyst.

In an infant, pressure over the cysts can cause a rise in fontanelle pressure, which can be palpated. Once the fontanelle has closed, Valsalva's maneuver demonstrates spinal canal cyst continuity.

During office examination, anoscopy and proctosigmoidoscopy should also be performed to visualize the surrounding tissue and determine rectal wall involvement. An indentation denoting extrinsic compression may be seen. A note should be made of the state of the overlying rectal mucosa, in particular, the presence of submucosal edema, which may indicate underlying infection. Usually, the mucosa is totally normal.

16.7 Diagnostic Measures

16.7.1 Endoscopy

All patients with retrorectal tumors should undergo endoscopic evaluation of the overlying rectal mucosa. Although most older textbooks recommend flexible sigmoidoscopy,[3,5] colonoscopy is often warranted if the patient has not had recent endoscopic evaluation of the proximal colon, as this will rule out concomitant pathology, which is especially important if the tumor resection will include an abdominal approach.

16.7.2 Imaging

Many different imaging modalities have been employed in the past, some of which have characteristic findings. For instance, bony destruction on a plain X-ray is definitely suggestive of a malignant retrorectal process, and as previously mentioned, the "scimitar sign" is pathognomonic for a meningocele. However, the modern assessment of retrorectal tumors has evolved to the point where plain X-rays, barium enemas, fistulograms, angiograms, and even computed tomography do not provide an adequate amount of tumor detail that will independently affect the treatment plan.

Endorectal Ultrasound (ERUS)

ERUS is a test of choice for many colorectal surgeons due to the high degrees of availability and familiarity, as it is often employed to evaluate fecal incontinence. It is well tolerated, and certainly an appropriate test for initial evaluation if it is freely available within the surgeon's clinic or institution. Its main utility would be to determine if the retrorectal structure is solid or cystic, and if it communicates via fistula with the anal canal. It can also detect invasion of the rectal wall and/or sphincter complex.[4,25]

Magnetic Resonance Imaging (MRI)

In the current era of retrorectal tumor management, pelvic MRI has become the essential component of the evaluation and treatment plan as it is for rectal cancer. MRI provides a detailed image of the anatomic relationship of neoplasms to the muscular and bony structures of the pelvis. It not only determines if the mass is cystic or solid, but also can assess for loculations and mass heterogeneity which may suggest hemorrhage. This modality can determine central nervous system involvement. It has multiplanar capacity and improved soft tissue resolution when compared to CT, which helps to define a plane between the lesion and the presacral fascia.[26] MRI defines sacral invasion and rectal involvement, and can help determine the potential for resectability and/or need for neoadjuvant therapy. MRI has replaced ERUS for the evaluation of both rectal cancer and retrorectal tumors.

16.8 Management

16.8.1 Observation

In general, observation of retrorectal tumors is discouraged. Even benign-appearing cystic lesions have malignant potential, although admittedly most of these smaller tumors will never become a problem for asymptomatic patients. There are certainly some patients in whom the operative morbidity and functional outcomes from resection outweigh the potential benefits. This is especially true in frail, debilitated patients. Alternatively, young healthy patients with a presacral cyst should typically undergo resection as a 10% or more risk of malignant degeneration is substantial.

There has been a single publication detailing nonoperative management of select retrorectal tumors.[27] The authors reported on 69 patients with retrorectal tumors, where 42 were managed nonoperatively with reportedly good outcomes. However, their data included heterogeneous imaging, tissue diagnoses, and follow-up. It appears that they were really reporting on five cystic lesions which were observed with acceptable follow-up and repeat imaging, of which four were stable and one of which regressed. In truth, these lesions are likely observed by many practitioners, but there is no proof as to the advisability of this approach.

16.8.2 Biopsy

Preoperative biopsy of retrorectal tumors has been historically discouraged because of the hypothetical potential to cause tumor seeding along the biopsy tract[3,4,5] and the possibility of triggering infection of cystic lesions. There is concern that biopsy of meningoceles could lead to meningitis. In fact, the previous edition of this textbook stated that "there is no place for preoperative biopsy of a lesion considered to be operable."[3] Additionally, most authors agreed that if a biopsy could not be avoided, a transperineal approach was superior to a transrectal approach, and the biopsy tract should be excised during surgery.

One of the main reasons biopsies have been discouraged, beyond the above-mentioned concerns, is that most experts believed the information obtained from a biopsy would not impact surgical decision making,[3] thus placing the patient at risk for complications without any benefit. However, recent case series have provided justification for biopsies in select patients when it will impact the treatment plan.[28,29,30]

In 2013, Merchea et al from the Mayo Clinic evaluated the value and safety of preoperative biopsy.[30] They reported on 76 biopsies in 73 patients from 1990 to 2010, all of which were obtained via a transperineal or transsacral approach (77% percutaneous vs. 23% open). To address concerns for tumor seeding, the biopsy tract was excised during the surgical procedure.

The authors found biopsy to be well tolerated with only two hematomas and no other major complications. Additionally, they found that biopsy results were more sensitive and specific than noninvasive imaging, and impacted their surgical approach. Specifically, neoadjuvant radiation was employed for nonchordoma malignant lesions, and intraoperative radiation therapy was used for bulky, high-grade, locally advanced lesions.[29] Solid lesions found to be benign on biopsy were treated with nerve-sparing approaches that focused on function preservation rather than wide margins.

Another important case series originated from the Cleveland Clinic, where the authors reported a case series of 87 patients with retrorectal tumors from 1981 to 2011.[28] These authors stressed the importance of individualizing the workup due to the heterogenic nature of these tumors. They performed biopsy of 24 tumors (28%), and reported no recurrence within the biopsy tract with a median follow-up of 37 months, despite only 4/24 undergoing tract excision.

In summary, the risks of biopsy have likely been overstated. Simple cystic lesions do not require biopsy. However, select multiloculated lesions in which malignancy is suspected as well as solid tumors may warrant preoperative biopsy on an individualized basis. When biopsy is employed, it is still recommended that a transperineal approach be utilized, and that the tract be excised at the time of surgery. The tract can often be tattooed at the time of biopsy to aid with later identification.

16.8.3 Neoadjuvant Therapy

As previously stated, there is a well-defined role for preoperative radiation therapy for large solid tumors that are borderline resectable, with the utility being better demonstrated for sarcoma than for chordoma.[29] The role of neoadjuvant chemotherapy remains more poorly defined, but it may be appropriate depending on tumor histology. It may be particularly appropriate for large gastrointestinal stromal tumors and select sarcomas.

16.8.4 Operative Approach

As previously mentioned and outlined in ▶ Fig. 16.3, the extent of disease will determine the best operative approach. For large and locally advanced lesions, a multidisciplinary approach is advisable, including the help of an orthopaedic surgeon or neurosurgeon when appropriate. Complete mechanical and antibiotic bowel preparation is indicated for operations in the retrorectal space because of the significant risk of rectal injury.

Abdominal Approach

Indications for an abdominal approach include the high retrorectal tumors where presacral safe access is unlikely. This approach is also indicated for extraspinal neurogenic neoplasms. The abdomen is entered through a transverse or midline incision. The sigmoid colon is mobilized, and the rectum is placed on stretch so that the pelvis can be examined and the relationship of the tumor to the rectum determined (▶ Fig. 16.4). The presacral sympathetic nerves are identified, and the retrorectal space is entered through a plane anterior to these structures. In this way, the rectum and mesorectum are displaced forward and the tumor defined with a minimum of bleeding. The middle sacral vessels are often significantly enlarged in the case of solid retrorectal tumors, and these should be ligated before mobilization is attempted.[5]

The presacral veins produce the most difficult type of hemorrhage to control because the veins retract when cut and are thus difficult to isolate. Careful dissection with particular attention to hemostasis is essential, and protection of nerve structures should be attempted at all times. By slow and meticulous dissection, the tumor is mobilized; hemoclips are useful in this procedure. The tumor is then removed. This simplified description should in no way play down the difficulties encountered during dissection.

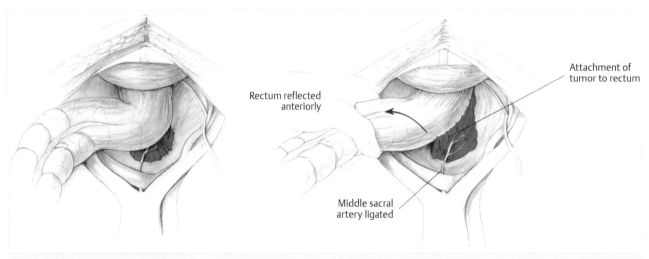

Rectum reflected anteriorly

Attachment of tumor to rectum

Middle sacral artery ligated

Fig. 16.4 Abdominal approach to high retrorectal tumors.

Presacral bleeding is usually best managed with sacral thumb tacks. This procedure can be accomplished provided the tumor is high and the sacrum uninvolved. Malignancies involving the rectal wall require a rectal resection. Depending on the extent of the neoplasm, completion of the operation may require the patient to be repositioned in the prone jackknife position so that the remainder of the excision can be carried out through a posterior approach. If a biopsy has been performed, the excision should include the skin through which the biopsy was performed.

The proximal and lateral extent of the dissection will be determined by the location of the primary lesion. Various bony and nerve structures will be sacrificed, again depending on the location of the lesion. The help of a neurosurgeon or orthopaedic surgeon may prove invaluable in these circumstances.

Posterior Approach

If the examiner's finger can reach the upper extent of the lesion, the posterior approach should prove successful. If even half of the lesion can be palpated, the lesion can usually be posteriorly approached. The patient is placed in the prone jackknife position (▶ Fig. 16.5). Preoperative mechanical cathartic oral and parenteral antibiotic prophylaxis are undertaken. A midline parasacrococcygeal, curvilinear, or horizontal incision is made and deepened to define the sacrum, coccyx, and anococcygeal ligament. The anococcygeal ligament is detached from the coccyx and displaced, revealing the levator ani muscle with the central decussating fibers passing from the rectum to the coccyx. The levator ani muscle is divided, and the supralevator space is entered. The coccyx is disarticulated from the S5 vertebra, allowing entrance into the supralevator space. Varying amounts of levator ani muscle are incised to gain adequate access. The surgeon can double-glove the left hand and insert the index finger in the rectum to push the lesion outward to facilitate excision without injury to the rectal wall.

At this point, a decision about whether the distal one or two sacral segments require excision must be made. The decision depends on the size of the lesion, its relationship to the sacrum, and the exposure required. If removing sacral segments is necessary, the gluteus maximus muscle can be detached from each side, and a portion of the sacroiliac ligaments may be incised. The sacral nerves related to the lowest two sacral vertebrae can be divided without fear of significant neurologic deficit. Neither is sacral instability a problem. Bleeding is frequently a problem until the bone has been completely removed. The jackknife position reduces bleeding to some extent.

In all cases of retrorectal tumors and cysts, it is recommended that the coccyx be sacrificed, not only to achieve better exposure but because the most common factor in recurrence is failure to remove this bone.[1] Other authors support this view.[4,5] All cystic lesions in this area should be assumed to originate in the coccyx; hence, its removal is believed to be mandatory (▶ Fig. 16.5c).

The posterior approach is best suited for the removal of cystic lesions, especially precoccygeal cysts. This approach is ideal for all low tumors and for many midlevel tumors below the sacral promontory. Preoperative examination is obviously important since a mistake in assessing the upward extent of the lesion can be very difficult to correct in the operating room. Maneuverability through this incision is limited. If significant uncontrolled hemorrhage occurs from deep within the wound, pressure packs should be applied. If hemostasis still cannot be achieved, the patient should be repositioned and the abdominal approach used. After removal of the tumor, wound closure is performed in layers around suction catheters. These catheters ensure elimination of the dead space left when the tumor is removed.

Combined Anteroposterior Approach

When large lesions such as chordomas extend above S3, a combined anterior and posterior approach may be employed. The

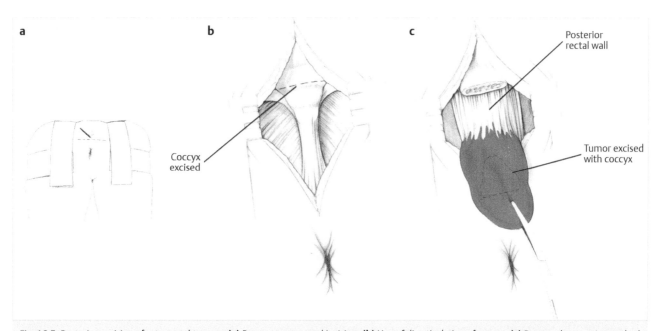

Fig. 16.5 Posterior excision of retrorectal tumors. **(a)** Parasacrococcygeal incision. **(b)** Line of disarticulation of coccyx. **(c)** Removed coccyx is attached to mass.

technique was well described by Dozois.[19] With the patient in the prone jackknife position, an incision is made over the sacrum and coccyx. The anococcygeal ligament is transected and the levator ani muscles retracted laterally. The chordoma is separated from the rectum and the gluteus maximus muscles on both sides, the sacrospinous and sacrotuberous ligaments are detached, and the piriformis muscles are serially divided on each side to expose the sciatic nerve. An osteotomy is performed at the S3 level, and the S3 roots are protected.

The lesion is removed en bloc, and the wound is closed over suction drainage. It is important at the time of sacral excision to recognize dural injury. This may occur in patients with intraspinal extension of the lesion and can lead to a cerebrospinal fluid leak or life-threatening intradural infection. When undertaking sacral resection in the region of S2–S3 or higher, the dural sac should be searched for and closed with an absorbable suture.

For lesions above the S3 level, the presacral space is approached through a laparotomy, and the rectum is mobilized anteriorly. If both S3 roots must be sacrificed, the rectum is transected and an end colostomy is fashioned. Blood loss is reduced by ligation of the middle sacral vessels and the internal iliac vessels on the side of greatest extension of the chordoma. If one S3 root can be preserved, the rectum is left in place. The pelvic floor is reconstructed. The abdomen is closed and the patient repositioned in the prone position. The posterior phase is conducted as previously described.

Postoperative functional outcome and its correlation with nerve root preservation were reported by Baratti et al.[31] No patients with bilateral preservation of S3 experienced urinary or bowel symptoms. The bilateral preservation of S2, although followed in most cases by temporary urinary retention, fecal incontinence, or both, was then characterized by recovery of normal bowel and urinary function in most cases. The preservation of only one S2 root was followed in all cases by urinary and/or bowel symptoms, which were only occasionally recovered. All of the patients in whom only the S1 roots were preserved experienced permanent bowel and urinary dysfunction.

16.9 Outcomes

Outcomes after resection of retrorectal tumors are mostly based on tumor histology and on whether or not an R0 resection was achieved. In general, outcomes after resection of benign solid and cystic lesions are excellent, with rare tumor-specific deaths and recurrence rates of 3 to 15% depending on the series and the quality of resection.[3]

Survival after resection of malignant lesions is more difficult to predict, and there have been discordant reports in the literature. As expected, malignant lesions that are larger and those that are incompletely resected are associated with high rates of local and distant recurrence.[32]

Messick et al reported a local recurrence rate of 11% for benign tumors and 30% for malignant tumors.[28] A 2001 review of the Surveillance, Epidemiology, and End Results (SEER) database looked at chordomas, and found 5- and 10-year overall survival rates of 74 and 32%,[4,33] which is better than previous reports. Dozois et al reported a relatively impressive survival after resection of sacrococcygeal sarcomas,[7] many of whom

required preoperative therapy and multivisceral resections. They achieved an R0 resection in 31/37 patients, with local recurrence rates of 49% at 5 years, but overall 5- and 10-year survival rates of 55 and 47%, respectively.

16.10 Conclusion

Retrorectal tumors are rare and heterogeneous. Diagnosis and treatment require extensive planning and expertise to ensure the best functional and oncologic outcome for the patient. In recent years, pelvic MRI and preoperative biopsy have played larger roles in the treatment plan. Despite their rarity, most colorectal surgeons will encounter these tumors in their practice, and they must possess a strong understanding of the anatomy and the potential for malignancy in order to provide the best possible care for the modern patient.

References

[1] Uhlig BE, Johnson RL. Presacral tumors and cysts in adults. Dis Colon Rectum. 1975; 18(7):581–589

[2] Freier DT, Stanley JC, Thompson NW. Retrorectal tumors in adults. Surg Gynecol Obstet. 1971; 132(4):681–686

[3] Gordon PH. Retrorectal tumors. In: Principles and Practice of Surgery for the Colon, Rectum, and Anus. 3rd ed. New York, NY: Informa; 2007:353–368

[4] Migaly J, Mantyh CR. Presacral tumors. In: The ASCRS Textbook of Colon and Rectal Surgery. 3rd ed. New York, NY: Springer; 2016:373–382

[5] Grundfest-Broniatowski S, Marks K, Fazio VW. Diagnosis and management of sacral and retrorectal tumors. In: Current Therapy in Colon and Rectal Surgery. 2nd ed. Philadelphia, PA: Elsevier; 2005:153–160

[6] Jao SW, Beart RW, Jr, Spencer RJ, Reiman HM, Ilstrup DM. Retrorectal tumors. Mayo Clinic experience, 1960–1979. Dis Colon Rectum. 1985; 28(9):644–652

[7] Dozois EJ, Jacofsky DJ, Billings BJ, et al. Surgical approach and oncologic outcomes following multidisciplinary management of retrorectal sarcomas. Ann Surg Oncol. 2011; 18(4):983–988

[8] Kim JH, Jin SY, Hong SS, Lee TH. A carcinoid tumour arising within a tailgut cyst: a diagnostic challenge. Scott Med J. 2014; 59(1):e14–e17

[9] Toh JW, Morgan M. Management approach and surgical strategies for retrorectal tumours: a systematic review. Colorectal Dis. 2016; 18(4):337–350

[10] Abel ME, Nelson R, Prasad ML, Pearl RK, Orsay CP, Abcarian H. Parasacrococcygeal approach for the resection of retrorectal developmental cysts. Dis Colon Rectum. 1985; 28(11):855–858

[11] Michael D, Cohen CR, Northover JM. Adenocarcinoma within a rectal duplication cyst: case report and literature review. Ann R Coll Surg Engl. 1999; 81(3):205–206

[12] Hjermstad BM, Helwig EB. Tailgut cysts. Report of 53 cases. Am J Clin Pathol. 1988; 89(2):139–147

[13] Prasad AR, Amin MB, Randolph TL, Lee CS, Ma CK. Retrorectal cystic hamartoma: report of 5 cases with malignancy arising in 2. Arch Pathol Lab Med. 2000; 124(5):725–729

[14] Altman RP, Randolph JG, Lilly JR. Sacrococcygeal teratoma: American Academy of Pediatrics Surgical Section Survey-1973. J Pediatr Surg. 1974; 9(3):389–398

[15] Simpson PJ, Wise KB, Merchea A, et al. Surgical outcomes in adults with benign and malignant sacrococcygeal teratoma: a single-institution experience of 26 cases. Dis Colon Rectum. 2014; 57(7):851–857

[16] Pantoja E, Rodriguez-Ibanez I. Sacrococcygeal dermoids and teratomas: historical review. Am J Surg. 1976; 132(3):377–383

[17] Rosai J, ed. Ackerman's Surgical Pathology. Vol. 2. St. Louis, MO: CV Mosby; 1989:1507–1509

[18] Gray SW, Singhabhandhu B, Smith RA, Skandalakis JE. Sacrococcygeal chordoma: Report of a case and review of the literature. Surgery. 1975; 78(5):573–582

[19] Dozois RR. Retrorectal tumors: spectrum of disease, diagnosis, and surgical management. Perspect Colon Rectal Surg. 1990; 3(2):241–255

[20] Kovalcik PJ, Burke JB. Anterior sacral meningocele and the scimitar sign. Report of a case. Dis Colon Rectum. 1988; 31(10):806–807

[21] Oren M, Lorber B, Lee SH, Truex RC, Jr, Gennaro AR. Anterior sacral meningocele: report of five cases and review of the literature. Dis Colon Rectum. 1977; 20(6):492–505

[22] Anderson FM, Burke BL. Anterior sacral meningocele. A presentation of three cases. JAMA. 1977; 237(1):39–42

[23] Simpson BA, Glass RE, Mann CV. Anterior sacral meningocoele: magnetic resonance imaging and surgical management. Br J Surg. 1987; 74(12):1185

[24] Sobrado CW, Mester M, Simonsen OS, Justo CR, deAbreu JN, Habr-Gama A. Retrorectal tumors complicating pregnancy. Report of two cases. Dis Colon Rectum. 1996; 39(10):1176–1179

[25] Böhm B, Milsom JW, Fazio VW, Lavery IC, Church JM, Oakley JR. Our approach to the management of congenital presacral tumors in adults. Int J Colorectal Dis. 1993; 8(3):134–138

[26] Wolpert A, Beer-Gabel M, Lifschitz O, Zbar AP. The management of presacral masses in the adult. Tech Coloproctol. 2002; 6(1):43–49

[27] Hopper L, Eglinton TW, Wakeman C, Dobbs BR, Dixon L, Frizelle FA. Progress in the management of retrorectal tumours. Colorectal Dis. 2016; 18(4):410–417

[28] Messick CA, Hull T, Rosselli G, Kiran RP. Lesions originating within the retrorectal space: a diverse group requiring individualized evaluation and surgery. J Gastrointest Surg. 2013; 17(12):2143–2152

[29] Merchea A, Dozois EJ. Lesions originating within the retrorectal space. J Gastrointest Surg. 2014; 18(12):2232–2233

[30] Merchea A, Larson DW, Hubner M, Wenger DE, Rose PS, Dozois EJ. The value of preoperative biopsy in the management of solid presacral tumors. Dis Colon Rectum. 2013; 56(6):756–760

[31] Baratti D, Gronchi A, Pennacchioli E, et al. Chordoma: natural history and results in 28 patients treated at a single institution. Ann Surg Oncol. 2003; 10 (3):291–296

[32] Buchs NC, Gosselink MP, Scarpa CR, et al. A multicenter experience with perirectal tumors: The risk of local recurrence. Eur J Surg Oncol. 2016; 42 (6):817–822

[33] McMaster ML, Goldstein AM, Bromley CM, Ishibe N, Parry DM. Chordoma: incidence and survival patterns in the United States, 1973–1995. Cancer Causes Control. 2001; 12(1):1–11

17 Perianal and Anal Canal Neoplasms

David E. Beck

Abstract

Perianal and anal canal neoplasms are uncommon and can be divided into malignant and premalignant lesions. A biopsy confirms the diagnosis. Anal margin lesions can often be treated with local excision while anal canal lesions usually require more aggressive treatments.

Keywords: perianal neoplasia, anal margin, anal intraepithelial neoplasia, Bowen's disease, squamous cell carcinoma, Paget's disease, basal cell carcinoma, verrucous carcinoma, anal canal neoplasia, adenocarcinoma

17.1 Introduction

Perianal and anal canal malignancies are uncommon, and the use of terminology and classification in clinical reports has not been uniform. This has limited interpretation of results. Knowledge of anal anatomy is important to manage these patients.

17.2 Anatomy

The anal area, although small, is rather complex with varied histologic features, characteristics, and lymphatic spread. In addition, many reports have used different terminologies to define the location of the malignancy. To overcome this confusion, the World Health Organization (WHO) and the American Joint Committee on Cancer (AJCC) have developed a universally accepted descriptive terminology for the histologic typing of intestinal neoplasms of the anal region.[1,2] According to their terminology, "The **anal canal** is defined as the terminal part of the large intestine, beginning at the upper surface of the anorectal ring and passing … to the anal verge."[1] This is essentially the "surgical anal canal." The anal margin runs from the anal verge to approximately 5 to 6 cm circumanally where skin appendages (such as hairs) can be identified.[1,3,4] This definition is in contrast to many series in the literature that use the dentate line as the dividing line describing the anal canal as the area above the dentate line, and the anal margin as the area below the dentate line.[5,6,7,8,9] Numerous other reports never define the landmarks.

The area above the dentate line up to the anorectal ring (the first 6–10 mm referred to as the transitional zone) has primarily cephalad lymphatic drainage via the superior rectal lymphatics to the inferior mesenteric nodes. It also has lesser drainage laterally along both the middle rectal vessels and inferior rectal vessels through the ischioanal fossa to the internal iliac nodes. Lymphatic drainage from the anal canal below the dentate line drains to the inguinal nodes. However, secondary drainage can follow the inferior rectal lymphatics to the ischioanal nodes and internal iliac nodes, and along the superior rectal nodes (see ▶ Fig. 1.20). Lymphatic drainage of the perianal skin is entirely to the inguinal nodes. The new edition of the WHO classification, which is similar to the AJCC, has started to emerge but probably will take years before it is widely used and becomes standardized. Until then, a meaningful comparison of the anal carcinoma presented in different reports in the literature is difficult. WHO also recommends that the generic term "squamous carcinoma" be used for all subtypes of anal squamous cell.[1]

17.3 Incidence

In 2015, there were an estimated 7,270 new cases of anal carcinomas (anus, anal canal, and anorectum) in the United States (4,630 female, 2,640 male).[10] These lesions accounted for 2.5% of carcinomas of the large bowel.

The anal canal extends from the anorectal ring to the anal verge, and using WHO criteria, 85% of anal carcinomas arise in the anal canal.[11] The mean age of the patient at presentation varies from 58 to 67 years, and the age range is wide: 64 years of age and older, 58%; 45 to 64 years, 37%; and 25 to 44 years, 5%. Anal canal carcinomas show a marked female predominance, with the female-to-male ratio proximately 5:1. However, in areas with a large proportion of male patients at high risk, the female-to-male ratio may approach 1:1. In contrast, perianal carcinomas are more common in men, with a male-to-female ratio of approximately 4:1.[11]

In the United States, the incidence of squamous carcinoma of the anal canal and perianal skin in homosexual men has been estimated to be 11 to 34 times higher than the general male population. Human immunodeficiency virus (HIV)–infected homosexual men appear to be at particular risk. Other factors strongly associated with anal squamous carcinoma include the number of sexual partners, receptive anal intercourse, coexistence of sexually transmitted diseases, history of cervical, vulvar, or vaginal carcinoma, and use of immunosuppression after solid-organ transplantation.[1,12]

17.4 Etiology and Pathogenesis

There is strong evidence that human papilloma virus (HPV) infection causes anal carcinoma in a manner that closely parallels the role of HPV infection in the genesis of cervical carcinoma.[13,14] Evidence supporting this observation includes the fact that many patients have simultaneous anal and genital viral infections and share common demographic characteristics, including an increased number of sexual partners. Furthermore, both anal and cervical carcinomas are associated with the specific "high-risk" HPV genotypes 16 and 18.[15,16,17]

Over 60 different HPV genotypes have been identified, approximately 20 of which are known to infect the anogenital region. HPV types 6 and 11 are generally associated with benign lesions such as warts and a low-grade anal intraepithelial neoplasia (AIN) that rarely progress to carcinoma. In contrast, HPV types 16, 18, 31, 33, 34, and 35 are most commonly associated with high-grade dysplastic AIN, carcinoma in situ, and carcinoma of anus and cervix. HPV-6 and HPV-11 are maintained as extrachromosomal episomes, whereas HPV-16 and HPV-18 are integrated into host DNA, thus explaining the different propensity to initiate the development of carcinoma.[15,18]

The study by Palmer et al,[16] examining patients with invasive squamous cell carcinoma of the anus, demonstrated that the majority of lesions in these patients contained HPV-16 and HPV-18 DNA, which is confined to the nuclei of carcinoma cells and is predominantly integrated into the host cell DNA. Their study showed that none of the 56 control samples examined and none of the 4 nonsquamous cell primary anal malignancies contained any detectable HPV DNA. These observations add considerable weight to the concept of a specific association between HPV-16 and HPV-18 and the development of anal squamous cell carcinoma. The observation that six of seven carcinomas of the upper anal canal contained HPV-16 or HPV-18 DNA, while only 8 of 18 carcinomas of the lower anal canal contained HPV-16 or HPV-18 DNA is of interest because the epithelium of the transitional zone of the anal canal has both embryonic and histologic similarities with the transitional zone of the cervix. This study has also demonstrated a significant relationship between the absence of keratin and the presence of HPV DNA. The authors noted that all six carcinomas containing HPV-16 or HPV-18 arising in the anal canal were nonkeratinizing. In contrast, only one of eight heavily keratinized lesions arising in the anal canal below the dentate line contained HPV-16 or HPV-18 DNA. It is possible that these observations indicate a predilection of HPV-16 and HPV-18 for the environment of the less stable epithelium of the upper anal canal rather than the modified skin of the lower anal canal. None of the cases of anal adenocarcinoma contains HPV-16 or HPV-18 DNA.[17,19]

Immunocompromised patients such as those with renal transplantation, cardiac allograft recipients, and patients with carcinoma after chemotherapy have increased risk of HPV infection and increased progression to anal squamous cell carcinoma.[20,21] They occur at a younger age, are multifocal, persistent, and recurrent, and progress rapidly. Approximately 50% of patients positive for HIV have detectable HPV DNA.[11] Penn[22] noted 65 anogenital (anal canal, perianal skin, or external genitalia) carcinomas in 2,150 renal transplant recipients occurring at an average of 7 years after transplantation. Two-thirds of the patients were women and one-third men. These patients were much younger than those with similar malignancies in the general population, with the average age of 37 years for women and 45 years for men. Generally, the carcinomas are varieties of squamous cell carcinomas. Thirty-two percent of the neoplasms are in situ lesions. Such carcinomas are biologically aggressive despite being histologically low grade. A study by Gervaz et al[23] on molecular biology of squamous cell carcinoma of the anus between HIV-positive and HIV-negative patients revealed that allelic imbalances on chromosomes 17p, 18q, and 5q markedly differ. The data also demonstrated that DCC and p53 mutations were not required for anal squamous cell carcinoma progression in HIV-positive patients. These data suggest that immunosuppression may promote anal squamous cell carcinoma progression through an alternate pathway and that persistence of HPV infection within the anal canal may play a central role in this process.

In a study on anal squamous cell carcinoma, 47% of patients have a positive history for genital warts. In patients without a history of warts, the carcinoma is associated with a history of gonorrhea, herpes simplex type II virus, and *Chlamydia trachomatis*. Smoking is also a substantial risk factor.[24]

Anal intercourse itself does not carry an increased risk of anal squamous carcinomas. Rather, anal sex at young age carries an increased risk. However, most men and women with anal squamous carcinoma do not engage in anal sex. Thus, if HPV is truly a causative agent in anal squamous carcinoma, other modes of transmission to the anal area should be considered.[17] Current evidence suggests that the etiology of anal carcinoma is a multifactorial interaction between environmental factors, HPV infection, immune status, and suppressive genes.[11]

17.5 Staging

The prognosis for survival in anal carcinoma deteriorates as the primary carcinoma enlarges. It worsens when the carcinoma metastasizes to the regional lymph nodes and to extrapelvic sites.[25] Unlike carcinoma of the colon and rectum, the Dukes staging system and its subsequent modifications are irrelevant because part of the lymphatic drainage is in the inguinal region and is outside the extent of the resection. The tumor, node, metastases (TNM) classification system has become the standard. It is important to note that the WHO and AJCC systems determine the T category by the largest diameter of the primary carcinoma measured in centimeters. Additional criteria for the TNM system are summarized in Box 17.1.[1]

The best means of staging anal carcinoma remains a careful examination and, if necessary, under general anesthesia, supplemented by endorectal ultrasonography, computed tomography (CT), or magnetic resonance imaging (MRI) scanning. These procedures enable good biopsies to be taken and an appropriate decision to be made on the best mode of treatment. If the patient receives radiotherapy (RT) or chemoradiotherapy (CHT), further staging may be carried out 8 to 10 weeks after completing treatment to assess the results.[26]

17.6 Perianal Neoplasms (Anal Margin)

17.6.1 Anal Intraepithelial Neoplasia (AIN) of Perianal Skin (Bowen's Disease)

High-grade AIN of perianal skin is synonymous with the old term perianal Bowen's disease because of their indistinguishable histologic and immunohistochemical features.[27] Bowen[28] described an intraepidermal squamous cell carcinoma (carcinoma in situ) in 1912 as a chronic atypical epithelial proliferation.

The term *anal canal intraepithelial neoplasia* was proposed by Fenger and Nielsen in 1986.[29] Fenger, in 1990,[30] used the term *perianal skin intraepithelial neoplasia* in lieu of perianal Bowen's disease. Most authors at the present time regard only high-grade AIN as Bowen's disease, which is mostly caused by HPV-16 and HPV-18, in contrast to low-grade AIN, which is mostly caused by HPV-6 and HPV-11.[27,31,32] Scholefield et al[33] found that high-grade AIN had a relatively low potential for malignant transformation in immunocompetent patients.

The natural history of perianal AIN is unknown.[34] Most data came from the study of HPV infection. Results from cross-sectional analyses before the era of highly active antiretroviral therapy (HAART) show that nearly all HIV-positive men as well as a substantial proportion of HIV-negative homosexual men harbor the infection.[35]

Box 17.1 TNM cancer staging system

Anal canal

Primary carcinoma (T)

Tis	Carcinoma in situ
T0	No evidence of primary carcinoma
T1	Carcinoma 2 cm or less in greatest dimension
T2	Carcinoma more than 2 cm but not more than 5 cm in greatest dimension
T3	Carcinoma more than 5 cm in greatest dimension
T4	Carcinoma of any size invading adjacent organ(s) (e.g., vagina, urethra, bladder); involvement of the sphincter muscle(s) alone is not classified as T4
TX	Primary carcinoma cannot be assessed

Regional lymph node(s) (N)

N0	No regional lymph node metastasis
N1	Metastasis in perirectal lymph node(s)
N2	Metastasis in unilateral internal iliac and/or inguinal lymph node(s)
N3	Metastasis in perirectal and inguinal lymph nodes and/or bilateral internal iliac and/or inguinal lymph nodes
NX	Regional lymph nodes cannot be assessed

Distant metastasis (M)

M0	No distant metastasis
M1	Distant metastasis
MX	Presence of distant metastasis cannot be assessed

Stage grouping

Stage			
Stage 0	Tis	N0	M0
Stage I	T1	N0	M0
Stage II	T2	N0	M0
	T3	N0	M0
Stage IIIA	T1–T3	N1	M0
	T4	N0	M0
Stage IIIB	T4	N1	M0
	Any T	N2	M0
	Any T	N3	M0
Stage IV	Any T	Any N	M1

Histopathologic grade (G)

G1	Well differentiated
G2	Moderately differentiated
G3	Poorly differentiated
G4	Undifferentiated
GX	Grade cannot be assessed

Perianal skin

Primary carcinoma (T)

T0	No evidence of primary carcinoma
Tis	Carcinoma in situ
T1	Carcinoma 2 cm or less in greatest dimension
T2	Carcinoma more than 2 cm but not more than 5 cm in greatest dimension
T3	Carcinoma more than 5 cm in greatest dimension
T4	Carcinoma invades deep extradermal structure (e.g., cartilage, skeletal muscle, or bone)
TX	Primary carcinoma cannot be assessed

Regional lymph node(s) (N)

N0	No lymph node metastasis
N1	Regional lymph node metastasis
NX	Regional lymph nodes cannot be assessed

Distant metastasis (M)

M0	No distant metastasis
M1	Distant metastasis
MX	Presence of distant metastasis cannot be assessed

Stage grouping

Stage			
Stage 0	Tis	N0	M0
Stage I	T1	N0	M0
Stage II	T2	N0	M0
Stage III	T4	N0	M0
	Any T	N1	M0
	Any T	Any N	M1

Histopathologic grade (G)

G1	Well differentiated
G2	Moderately differentiated
G3	Poorly differentiated
G4	Undifferentiated
GX	Grade cannot be assessed

Whether perianal Bowen's disease has higher incidence of malignancy in other organs, particularly internal organs, than the normal population is not clear. Although the studies by Arbesman and Ransohoff[36] and Chute et al[37] found no increased subsequent risk of internal malignancy, these studies were on Bowen's disease of the skin in general and not perianal Bowen's disease. A survey by Marfing et al[38] among members of the American Society of Colon and Rectal Surgery in 1987 yielded 106 cases of perianal Bowen's disease. There were two cases of carcinoma of the colon and one case of carcinoma of the anus. Margenthaler et al[39] reviewed 167 cases (age 34–56 years) of perianal Bowen's disease in the literature; there were 31 (19%) associated carcinomas (not limited to internal organs) diagnosed concomitantly or after treatment for the perianal Bowen's disease, with a follow-up of 1 to 5 years.

Clinical Features

Grossly, high-grade perianal AIN or Bowen's disease appears as discrete, erythematous, occasionally pigmented, noninfiltrating, scaly, or crusted plaques, which sometimes have a moist surface. Foci of ulceration indicate that an invasive carcinoma has developed. Patients may complain of itching, which often is intense, burning, or spotted bleeding, but only a biopsy will confirm the diagnosis. In a series by Marchesa et al,[40] 25.5% of the cases of perianal Bowen's disease were incidental findings, diagnosed after pathologic evaluation of tissue removed from different perianal diseases. The histologic picture is that of in situ squamous cell carcinoma that may have characteristic bowenoid cells, which are multinucleated giant cells with some vacuolization, giving a "halo" effect (▸ Fig. 17.1).

Diagnosis

Perianal high-grade AIN can involve perianal skin, anal verge, anoderm, and vulva. A circumferential involvement of the disease is common.[41] Although the gross lesions can be biopsied, their boundary and extent cannot be ascertained. This problem can be overcome by painting the anal canal and perianal region, and in women, including the vulva, with 3 or 5% acetic acid. The abnormal skin and mucosa will be demarcated by whitening of

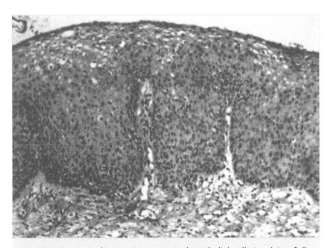

Fig. 17.1 Bowen's disease. Note atypical epithelial cells involving full thickness of the epidermis.

the tissue that should be biopsied. Chang and Welton[27] performed the examination in the operating room under sedation and perianal block. They examined the painted tissue through the operating microscope attached to a real-time video display. Changes in the vascular pattern suggestive of high-grade dysplasia are identified. The same tissue is then painted with Lugol's solution (10% iodine). High-grade AIN does not take up the iodine solution because of the lack of glycogen in the dysplastic cells and they appear yellow or tan, whereas normal tissue or low-grade AIN appears dark brown or black. Lesions suspicious for high-grade AIN are biopsied. As discussed later, this technique is currently referred to as high-resolution anoscopy or HRA.

Treatment

Treatment of Bowen's disease or high-grade AIN has changed dramatically. Although the natural history of high-grade AIN is still not known, recent information has played an important role in the current management. High-grade AIN is preinvasive and requires further management. At the time of surgical treatment, 2 to 28% of patients already have an invasive squamous cell carcinoma.[32,40,41] It is well known that the extent of the disease is usually beyond the gross demarcation of the lesion and can only be detected microscopically. Preoperative mappings were used in the past but were plagued with residual disease.[31,40,41] Currently, the biopsies are performed with the aid of staining the perianal skin, perineum, and anal canal with 3 or 5% acetic acid.[27,42] For low-grade AIN, treatment is not necessary if it is asymptomatic, but the patients should be followed periodically. There are several options on the treatment of high-grade AIN.

Application of Imiquimod

Imiquimod (Aldara, 3 M Pharmaceuticals, St. Paul, MN) is an immune response modifier with potent antiviral and antitumor activity in animal models. It was approved by the FDA in 1997 for topical treatment of external genital and perianal warts in adults.[43] The topical application has also been used for other skin conditions such as basal cell carcinoma, vulva intraepithelial neoplasms, invasive squamous cell carcinoma of skin, herpes simplex virus, and others, with excellent results.[37,38,39] Pehoushek and Smith[44] reported treating an HIV-positive patient with squamous cell carcinoma in situ of perianal skin and the anal canal, with a combination of 5% imiquimod cream three times a week combined with 5% fluorouracil daily with complete remission of the disease, and had no recurrence after a 3-month follow-up. Imiquimod should be used as a preliminary treatment for perianal high-grade AIN.[45,46]

Imiquimod is formulated as 5% cream packaged as one box of 12 single-use sachets, each containing 250 mg of cream to cover an area of 20 cm². A thin layer should be rubbed in until the cream is no longer visible. The application site should not be occluded. The recommended dosage is three times a week on nonconsecutive days (e.g., Monday, Wednesday, and Friday) at night for up to 16 weeks.[43,47]

Most patients tolerate the treatment well. Systemic reactions are rare but may cause fatigue, fever, influenzalike symptoms, headache, diarrhea, nausea, and myalgia. Local reactions are uncommon for applications of three times a week. It may cause itching, burning, and pain at the site of the application.[43] In order to minimize local reactions and yet not compromise the therapeutic effects, Chen and Shumack[48] recommended application of imiquimod three times weekly for 3 weeks, followed by a rest period of 4 weeks, to be repeated as necessary. The rest period allows any local skin reactions to subside.

Local application of imiquimod to a variety of skin diseases is safe and effective but it is new for perianal high-grade AIN. It remains to be seen whether it will become the treatment of choice; the prospect is promising.

Topical 5-Fluorouracil

Topical 5% 5-fluorouracil (5-FU) therapy has been found to be a safe and effective method to treat anal Bowen's disease. Graham et al[49] conducted a prospective study in 11 patients over a 6-year period. For one-half circumferential disease or greater, patients underwent topical 5% 5-FU therapy for 16 weeks. For smaller involvement, wide surgical excision was performed. All patients underwent anal mapping biopsy 1 year after the completion of therapy. Of 11 patients, 8 (5 males) received 16 weeks of topical 5% 5-FU therapy. Three patients (three females) underwent surgical excision for localized disease. All but one patient who was HIV-positive were free of Bowen's disease 1 year after completion of therapy. One patient underwent total excision of a residual microinvasive squamous carcinoma after circumferential Bowen's disease had resolved. One patient received 8 additional weeks of topical 5-FU therapy for incomplete resolution. All patients were followed yearly, with a mean follow-up of 39 months and the range of 12 to 74 months, and there have been no recurrences. There were no long-term side effects or morbidity from topical 5-FU.

Cautery Ablation

High-grade AIN, by definition, is benign and may take a long time if ever to become malignant. Ablation, particularly in extensive disease, is attractive because it is less morbid than an extensive excision. One disadvantage of ablation is the lack of tissue diagnosis and an invasive carcinoma can be overlooked. Cautery ablation is the most convenient because it is available in every operating room compared to cryosurgery or laser vaporization. It should be performed with the aid of acetic acid painting to visualize the extent of the margins. The cauterization should not be so deep as to cause a chronic unhealed wound. A circumferential involvement of the disease may require a staging ablation about 3 months apart to avoid anal stricture. Another drawback of cautery ablation is the finding that high-grade AIN has also the skin appendage involvement: 57% of hair follicles, 16% of sebaceous glands, and 25% of sweat glands.[50] These structures can be missed by the cautery ablation.

The most recent advancement in the treatment of high-grade AIN is the use of HRA.[27,51] In this way, change in the vascular pattern suggestive of high-grade dysplasia can be identified. The procedure is performed under 3% acetic acid and Lugol's solution painting to delineate the site of the high-grade lesions. The suspicious lesions are biopsied and ablated with electrocautery. Using this technique, Chang and Welton[27] have treated over 400 patients. There were no recurrences among HIV-negative patients after 42 months, but in the HIV-positive patient group, there was a projected 100% recurrence rate by the end of 60 months. The postoperative pain was significant in half of all patients. There was no sphincter dysfunction or anal stenosis.

HRA is slowly gaining popularity in colorectal surgery. Berry et al[51] recommended:

"… the technique is not particularly difficult to learn, but requires a level of clinical experience. It is important to perform HRA on a large number of patients with the disease to learn the clinical pathologic correlations that signify high-grade squamous intraepithelial lesions, and potential areas of invasion. We recommend that interested providers first take an introductory colposcopy course. Providers should become familiar with the basics of colposcopy and be able to recognize and distinguish epithelial and vascular changes that are hallmarks of high-grade squamous intraepithelial lesions. To do HRA well, individuals must be thoroughly trained. It is unlikely that without some training in the basics of colposcopy, one can simply decide to use an operating microscope and recognize the changes that distinguish anal squamous intraepithelial lesions." As good as it appears to be, HRA is not available in all operating rooms and it may not be cost effective if a practice has a low volume of this disease."

A survey of management of perianal Bowen's disease among members of the American Society of Colon and Rectal Surgeons in 2000 showed that 87% of the 663 respondents chose a wide local excision as the treatment of choice for a lesion larger than 3 cm.[52] This approach has now been challenged because of high residual and recurrence rates, even when mapping biopsies have been used. Marchesa et al[40] reported a recurrence rate of 34% in 41 patients who underwent local excision, with a median follow-up of 104 months. Sarmiento et al,[41] in a series of 19 patients, reported a recurrence rate of 31% at 5-year follow-up. Brown et al[32] had histologic evidence of incomplete excision at the initial operation in 56% of 34 patients, and the recurrence rate of 40% with a median follow-up of 41 months. Margenthaler et al,[39] in a series of studies, found that a clear margin was obtained in 23 of the 25 patients (92%), and the recurrence rate was 12% at 3 years' follow-up; they gave credit for this relatively low residual and recurrence rate to aggressive mapping biopsies and wide margin of excision.

Mapping with the application of 3 or 5% acetic acid followed by Lugol's solution may help determine the extent of involvement of the disease more accurately. Even with this, if the skin still harbors the HPV, a recurrence can occur later.

For an extensive involvement of the perianal skin, a circumferential excision should include the anoderm up to the dentate line because of its frequent involvement of the disease especially in HIV-positive patients.[45] In this situation, V–Y island subcutaneous skin flaps can be performed with good results and avoid the use of a split-thickness skin graft.[53]

Evidence now has shown that wide excision of high-grade AIN of perianal area does not preclude a high recurrence rate, even with negative margins. This is partly because it is difficult to accurately determine the margin of the disease, and because the remaining perianal skin may still harbor HPV, especially HPV-16 and HPV-18. Wide excision of perianal skin and anal canal also has high complications, particularly anal stricture, ectropion, and fecal incontinence; some of these patients require a colostomy or a loop ileostomy.[31,53]

In a patient who is found to have a high-grade AIN in a routine hemorrhoidectomy specimen or other anorectal procedures, it is necessary to reexamine the area when the wound has had time to heal. Occasionally, an invasive lesion is underreported and a persistent ulcerated area 2 months after the original procedure should lead to rebiopsy of the area. If the area has healed fully, a thorough inspection of the rest of the anogenital region should identify any remaining severely dysplastic lesions, which should be accordingly treated.[54]

Summary

The management of perianal high-grade AIN or perianal Bowen's disease has changed from the standard, "surgical excision of high-grade AIN remains the treatment of choice"[50] to a more conservative, "close observation with regular biopsy of any suspicious areas to exclude invasive malignancy may be a better treatment option and is the policy currently advocated in this unit."[32] Unless there is an invasive carcinoma, it is reasonable to apply imiquimod[45] or topical 5-FU[46] as an initial treatment. An alternative option may be cautery ablation. Surgical excision, especially an extensive one, should be reserved for patients with symptomatic disease such as untreatable itching, burning, or crusting of the skin.[45] A long-term follow-up is essential because the skin may harbor the virus that perpetuates the disease. Subsequent development of malignancies in other organs should be kept in mind.

Screening for Anal Carcinoma Precursors

Prevention of cervical carcinoma has relied on the identification and treatment of cervical intraepithelial neoplasia before its progression to invasive carcinoma. Typically, women are screened at regular intervals using cervical cytology. Women with abnormal results are referred for colposcopy, to permit visualization of the lesion, and biopsy, to precisely ascertain the level of the disease. Based on the biologic similarity between anal and cervical carcinomas and their respective precursors, similar methods might be used to identify the potential anal carcinoma precursors.[55]

Screening should be considered in the high-risk group: (1) a history of homosexual activity in men and/or a history of receptive anal intercourse; (2) all HIV-positive women, regardless of whether or not they have engaged in anal intercourse; (3) all women with high-grade cervical or vulvar lesions or carcinoma.[35] In homosexual and bisexual men, Goldie et al[56] found that screening every 2 or 3 years for anal squamous intraepithelial lesions with anal cytology would provide life-expectancy benefits comparable to other accepted preventive health measures, and would be cost effective.

Cytology remains the screening test of choice as it is easy to perform and is relatively inexpensive. A Cytette brush (▶ Fig. 10.9) is moistened in saline solution or tap water and is rotated on the perianal skin for 10 to 20 revolutions with firm pressure abrading cells from the area. In the anal canal, very few high-grade squamous intraepithelial lesions (HSIL) occur solely in the transitional zone. The cytological preparation should be taken from the anal verge and lower anal canal only, to avoid fecal contamination in the smears. The brush is then smeared across a glass slide and the smear is fixed for standard fixative for Papanicolaou staining. Another option is to use a wooden spatula. When properly performed, the sensitivity and specificity is over 95% on the presence or absence of abnormal cells.[31]

Abnormal anal cytologic results (LSIL or HSIL) should prompt anoscopic assessment, preferably with magnification and after application of 3 or 5% acetic acid. If one or more well-demarcated lesions are identified (by their white appearance after the application of 3 or 5% acetic acid, and by demonstrating features of vascular punctuation, leukoplakia, papillations, or other topographric irregularities), they should be biopsied if[31,32] there is no contraindication, such as a bleeding disorder.[29,30]

Patients with high-grade AIN should be treated with electrocautery or excisional biopsy. Low-grade AIN should be followed by a repeat screening cytology in 3 to 6 months.[56]

Screening HIV-positive homosexual and bisexual men for anal intraepithelial lesions and squamous cell carcinoma with anal Pap tests offers quality-adjusted life-expectancy benefits at a cost comparable with other accepted clinical preventive interventions.[57]

Human Papilloma Virus Vaccine

Vaccination against HPV types will require universal immunization as opposed to the targeting of "high-risk" persons. Because these are sexually acquired pathogens, immunizing persons before they become sexually experienced will afford the greatest benefit.[58,59] A vaccine against four types of HPV (GARDASIL; Merc & Co, Whitehouse, NJ) is currently available. In girls and young women ages 9 to 26, GARDASIL helps protect against two types of HPV that cause **70% of cervical cancer cases**, and two more types that cause approximately 90% of genital warts cases. In boys and young men ages 9 to 26, GARDASIL helps protect against approximately 90% of genital warts cases. GARDASIL also helps protect girls and young women ages 9 to 26 against about 70% of vaginal cancer cases and up to 50% of vulvar cancer cases. In males and females ages 9 to 26, GARDASIL helps protect against about 80% of anal cancer cases. GARDASIL is not intended to be used for treatment of active genital lesions, AIN, or anal cancers. GARDASIL should be administered intramuscularly as a 0.5-mL dose at the following schedule: 0, 2, and 6 months.[60] It is currently recommended that this vaccine be administered to all persons between the ages of 9 and 26. Future experience will demonstrate the impact on the incidence of HPV-related lesions.

17.6.2 Squamous Cell Carcinoma

General Considerations

Squamous cell carcinomas of the perianal skin resemble those occurring in skin elsewhere in the body. Grossly, they typically have rolled, everted edges with central ulceration (▶ Fig. 17.2). Any chronic unhealed ulcer should be considered a potential squamous cell carcinoma until proven otherwise by biopsy. Squamous cell carcinomas vary in size from as small as < 1 cm to large masses that completely surround and obstruct the anal orifice. The average age of the patient is between 62 and 70 years with a male-to-female ratio approximately equal.[61,62]

Clinical Features

Despite their surface location, squamous cell carcinomas are usually diagnosed late; more than 50% of cases are detected

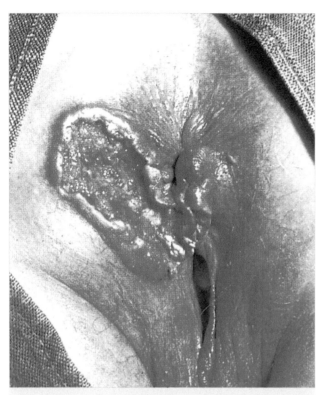

Fig. 17.2 Gross appearance of squamous cell carcinoma with rolled everted edges and central ulceration.

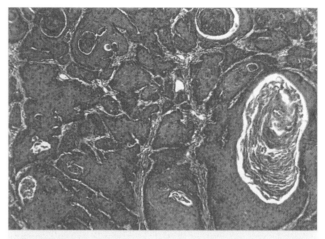

Fig. 17.3 Histologic appearance of squamous cell carcinoma. Note the keratinization.

more than 24 months after the onset of symptoms.[63] The carcinoma is often discovered at a late stage measuring 5 cm or larger in diameter.[62] The usual presentations are a lump, bleeding, pain, discharge, and itching.[61] On rare occasions, squamous cell carcinoma presents as a perianal abscess.[64] Up to 28% of patients with perianal squamous cell carcinoma are misdiagnosed as having hemorrhoids, an anal fissure, an anal fistula, atopic eczema, an anorectal abscess, or a benign neoplasm.[4]

Histologically, these carcinomas are usually well differentiated, with well-developed patterns of keratinization (▸ Fig. 17.3). Local invasion occurs, but the carcinoma is typically slow growing. Lymphatic spread from these carcinomas is directed mainly to the inguinal lymph nodes.

Treatment

Perianal squamous cell carcinoma is five times less common than squamous cell carcinoma of the anal canal.[62] There is limited information in the literature, few authors clearly define the perianal region according to the WHO and the AJCC standards, and the treatment varies widely among different institutions. However, in advanced cases, local excision and abdominoperineal resection (APR) have high failure rates because of local recurrence and inguinal node and distant metastasis.[62,65,66] In properly selected cases, wide local excision remains the cornerstone of the treatment of perianal squamous cell carcinoma. For in situ or microinvasive carcinoma, local excision has a 100% cure rate.[61,67] For superficial well-differentiated or moderately well-differentiated squamous cell carcinoma up to 3 to 4 cm in diameter, Cummings[3] of Princess Margaret Hospital in Toronto has shifted away from radiation therapy toward local excision,

supplemented with a skin graft when necessary, provided that the operation is not anticipated to interfere with anal sphincter function. Cummings reasons, "Although severe damage is infrequent following radiation, chronic irritation of the perianal skin and varying degrees of dysfunction of the anal region are common and can be troublesome."[3] For other less favorable lesions, he recommends chemoradiation. Most authors deliver 40 to 70 Gy.[62,65,66,68] Chemoradiation has also been shown to be superior to radiation alone in nonrandomized studies.[3] Residual or recurrent carcinoma after radiation can be treated with local excision or an APR. Prophylactic radiation to the groin is also recommended, particularly for T2 and T3 lesions.[62,66]

In a series of 54 patients who received radiation with or without chemotherapy, Papillon and Chassard[62] achieved a cancer-specific 5-year survival rate of 80%. The 5- and 10-year cancer-specific survival rates of 86 and 77%, respectively, were reported by Touboul et al[66] in a series of 17 patients. The size of the carcinoma determined the patient's survival. In that study, 5- and 10-year survival rates for T1 lesions were 100 and 100%, respectively, compared to 60 and 40% for T2 lesions, respectively.[4] With proper technique, serious complications from radiation therapy are uncommon. Radionecrosis and fecal incontinence have been claimed to occur only in a few patients.[66]

17.6.3 Perianal Paget's Disease

General Considerations

Perianal Paget's disease is an intraepithelial neoplasm of the perianal skin. In 1874, Sir James Paget first described this disease in relation to the nipple of the female breast.[69] George Thin, in 1881, was the first to describe the cytologic features of Paget's cells, which appeared microscopically as large rounded cells with abundant pale-staining cytoplasm and a large nucleus that is often displaced to the periphery of the cell.[70] The first case of perianal Paget's disease was reported by Darier and Couillaud in 1893.[71] Extramammary Paget's disease may be found in the axilla and the anogenital region (labia majora, penis, scrotum, groin, pubic area, perineum, perianal region, thigh, and buttock).

The histogenesis of perianal Paget's disease is not fully understood, but ultrastructural and immunohistochemical studies have helped to clarify the debate. In contrast to Paget's disease of the nipple, which is invariably associated with an underlying invasive or in situ ductal adenocarcinoma, perianal Paget's disease starts out as a benign neoplasm. It may eventually become invasive and give rise to an adenocarcinoma. The immunohistochemical studies show that, in general, Paget's cells stain positive for apocrine cells and in most cases stain negative for colorectal goblet cells.[72] Unfortunately, many of the markers expressed by perianal Paget's cells are also expressed by signet ring cell carcinoma of the anorectum.[72] However, staining that is negative for all except a marker for anorectal goblet cells almost certainly indicates a spread of Paget's cells from an anorectal mucinous adenocarcinoma. Most authors agree with the concept that Paget's cells are of glandular and probably of apocrine origin.[73,74,75] An alternative hypothesis implicating pluripotential intraepidermal cells cannot be excluded, but the evidence for such a histogenesis is lacking.[73]

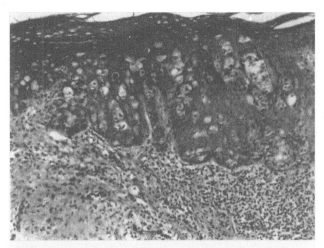

Fig. 17.4 Perianal Paget's disease. Paget's cells are found just above the basal layer.

Clinical Features

Perianal Paget's disease is an uncommon condition that is most commonly found in elderly people with an average age of 66 years. From 1963 to 1995, there have been 194 cases reported in the literature.[76] A PubMed search for publications from 1996 to 2016 found many case reports, a Surveillance Epidemiology and End Results (SEER) registries review, and a few single institution reviews that included patients from previous publications totaling an additional 115 to 215 cases. The lesions appear as a slowly enlarging erythematous, eczematous, and often sharply demarcated perianal skin rash that may ooze or scale and are usually accompanied by pruritus. It is normally located outside the anal canal but may extend up to the level of the dentate line. Because of its similarity to other perianal conditions such as idiopathic pruritus ani, hidradenitis suppurativa, condyloma acuminatum, Crohn's disease, Bowen's disease, and epidermoid carcinoma, the diagnosis of perianal Paget's disease is often delayed because of clinical diagnostic error. In almost one-third of the cases in a series by Jensen et al,[77] the lesion involved the entire circumference of the anus.

Diagnosis

The diagnosis must be confirmed by biopsy and by identification of the characteristic Paget's cells through histologic examination (▶ Fig. 17.4 and ▶ Fig. 17.5). Paget's cells contain a mucoprotein (sialomucin) which stains with periodic acid-Schiff, and cytokeratin (CK) 7, CK20 immunohistochemical staining.[78,79,80] True Paget's disease of the perianal skin must not be confused with the downward intraepidermal spread of a signet ring cell carcinoma of the rectum or with Bowen's disease of the perianal skin. Immunohistochemistry for CK7 and CK20 can differentiate between the true perianal Paget's disease and the downward spread of anorectal adenocarcinoma (pagetoid).[76,77,78] In general, hematoxylin and eosin (H&E) staining is sufficient to diagnose perianal Paget's disease and distinguish it from the grossly similar appearance of perianal Bowen's disease.[79]

A complete large bowel investigation with emphasis on thorough examination of the rectum and anal canal should be performed. The coexistence of visceral carcinomas is well known, with an incidence of about 50%.[76]

Treatment

In the absence of invasive carcinoma, wide excision is the treatment of choice. A small lesion (< 25% of perianal area or anus) can be excised with the wound left open. Larger defects should be closed with a skin flap. Obtaining an adequate microscopically clear margin is important. Because perianal Paget's disease may extend beyond the gross margin of the lesion, mapping the extent of involvement by obtaining multiple biopsies at least 1 cm from the edge of the lesion in all four quadrants, including the dentate line, the anal verge, and the perineum, is essential.[76]

The patient should be prepared with the same bowel preparation and antibiotics administered before a colon resection. The results of a circumferential excision of the perianal skin and the anal canal, with bilateral V–Y island flaps are satisfactory. Of the 15 patients undergoing this technique (not all patients had perianal Paget's disease) reported by Hassan et al,[53] none of them had flap loss or infection. Most complications were minor, including superficial wound separation, flap hematoma, and anal stricture. None of the patients had significant fecal incontinence at the time of follow-up, average 45 months. Perineal wound pain was a problem and 5 of the 15 patients required a diverting ileostomy or colostomy.

Radiation therapy may be an option for perianal Paget's disease. In an extensive review of literature by Brown et al,[81] the authors had difficulty in confirming or refuting the benefit of this mode of treatment. This was due to the rarity of the disease, to the fact that many of the patients were treated for recurrence after a surgical excision, or were medically unfit, and to the lack of standardization in the techniques of radiation therapy. Nevertheless, in a limited cumulative series of nine patients with perianal Paget's disease without invasive carcinoma treated with radiation or chemoradiation, two patients had recurrences at 2 years and 6 years. They believed that radiation therapy could be an alternative treatment for noninvasive Paget's disease that has an involvement extensive enough to require an APR, and for patients who cannot tolerate a general anesthesia. A recurrence after local excision can also be successfully treated with radiation.

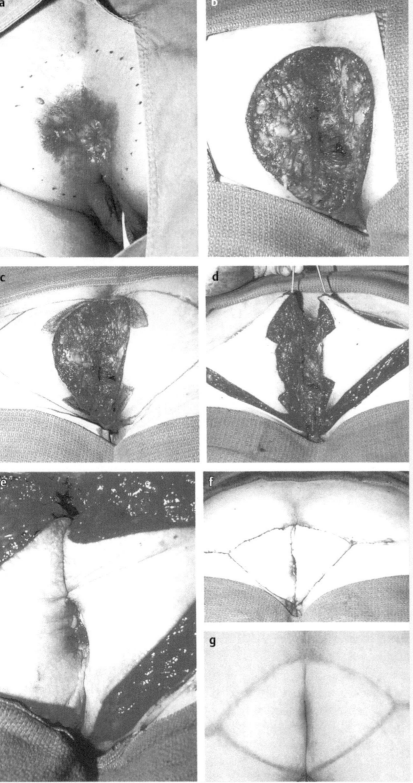

Fig. 17.5 (a) Circumferential perianal Paget's disease. Note the sharply demarcated erythematous and eczematous skin rash. The dotted line marks the extent of the excision. **(b)** Excision deep to subcutaneous fat was made up to the dentate line. **(c)** V flaps were outlined. Shaded areas were tongues of skin to be excised to accommodate the flaps into the anal canal. **(d)** Sliding flaps were deep down to subcutaneous fat. Note the arrowhead shape of the flaps. **(e)** Note accommodation of the flaps into the anal canal. **(f)** The **Y**-shaped flaps at completion. **(g)** Ten months after operation. The patient experienced no fecal incontinence and there had been no recurrence after 8 years of follow-up.

Prognosis

In a patient with noninvasive Paget's disease, the lesion can be cured by wide local excision, although recurrence is high. The recurrence can be reexcised. Long-term follow-up is essential to detect local recurrence and development of invasive Paget's disease or intercurrent invasive carcinoma of the rectum and anal canal.[82,83,84] A patient with invasive perianal Paget's disease has a poor prognosis despite APR, and in most cases, distant metastasis has already occurred at the time of diagnosis.[50] Adjuvant chemoradiation does not seem to help.[81]

17.6.4 Basal Cell Carcinoma

General Considerations

Basal cell carcinomas of the perianal skin are rare. The Mayo Clinic has listed only 20 patients with this type of neoplasm in the 20-year period ending in 1996.[85] This type of carcinoma occurs more frequently in men than in women, usually appearing in the sixth decade. The etiology is unknown but the most consistent factor was an association with basal cell carcinoma on other cutaneous sites (33% of patients) in the series reported by Paterson et al.[85]

Clinical Features

Basal cell carcinomas are usually 1 to 2 cm in diameter and are localized to the perianal skin, although a large lesion may extend into the anal canal. Grossly, they are similar to cutaneous basal cell carcinomas found elsewhere in the body and are characterized by a central ulceration with irregular and raised edges. These carcinomas remain superficial and mobile and rarely metastasize. Histologically, they are similar to basal cell carcinomas of the skin elsewhere (▶ Fig. 17.6). They are of long duration, have a low invasive potential, and must be distinguished from squamous cell carcinomas, which have an entirely different origin and behavior.

In the study by Nielsen and Jensen,[86] almost one-third of patients with basal cell carcinoma of the anal margin were misdiagnosed as having hemorrhoids, an anal fissure, or perianal eczema. The median delay in treatment caused by an erroneous diagnosis was 8 months.

Treatment and Prognosis

Local excision with adequate margins is the treatment of choice for patients with basal cell carcinoma. Local recurrence after local excision is common and accounted for 29% of patients in a series of 27 patients reported on by Nielsen and Jensen[86]; they recommend reexcision as treatment. APR and radiation therapy are reserved for large lesions. The 5-year survival rate in the series by Nielsen and Jensen was 73%, but no patients died as the result of the basal cell carcinoma. In the series reported by Paterson et al,[85] no recurrence or death occurred from perianal

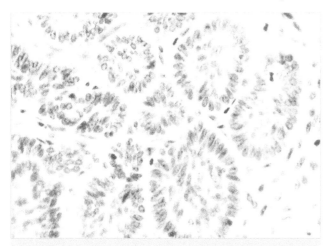

Fig. 17.6 Basal cell carcinoma.

basal cell carcinoma after local excision; however, none of the patients had an invasive carcinoma.

A novel approach is the use of topical imiquimod 5% cream (Aldara, Graceway Pharmaceuticalls, Bristol, TN), an immune response modifier that induces cytokines related to cell-mediated immune response. In the multicenter phase II dose–response open-label trial[87] for small (< 2 cm²) noninvasive basal cell carcinoma of the head, neck, trunk, or limbs, the cream was applied for 6 weeks, followed by an excision for histologic examination. The complete response was achieved in 100, 88, 73, and 70% for the application of twice daily, daily, three times a week, and daily three times a week, respectively.

All of the patients developed local skin reactions with erythema occurring most often and they were dose-related. In the twice-daily group, all the local skin reactions were assessed as severe in two-thirds of the patients, some of whom had vesicles, ulcerations, and excoriations. However, only 1 of the 99 patients who entered the study discontinued because of a medication-related skin reaction at the site of application. Whether this approach can be used for a large or invasive basal cell carcinoma is not known. It is possible to apply it to the basal cell carcinoma of the perianal skin.

17.6.5 Verrucous Carcinoma

Although there is no universal agreement, there is a growing consensus of opinion that the entity that has been termed a "giant condyloma acuminatum" or a "Buschke–Löwenstein tumor" represents a verrucous carcinoma. Similar to anal warts, verrucous carcinoma is associated with HPV-6 and HPV-11. These lesions typically present as large (8 × 8 cm), slow-growing, painful, wartlike growths that are relatively soft and have a cauliflowerlike appearance. The lesions may arise in the perianal skin, anal canal, or distal rectum and are frequently indistinguishable from condylomata acuminata. Although they are histologically benign, their behavior is clinically malignant. The clinical course of these lesions is one of relentless progression and expansion of the neoplasm by extensive erosion and pressure necrosis of surrounding tissues with invasion of the ischioanal fossa, perirectal tissues, and even the pelvic cavity. The invasive nature of these lesions may cause multiple sinuses or fistulous tracts, which may invade fascia, muscle, or the rectum and may cause inflammation, infection, and hemorrhage. The extent of involvement can be precisely determined by CT examination. Microscopically, the lesions bear a marked resemblance to condylomata acuminata with papillary proliferation, keratinization, acanthosis, parakeratosis, and vacuolization of superficial layers. Metastasis from these tumors has not been reported to date.[88,89]

The basic treatment is wide local excision. If the carcinoma involves the anal sphincters, an APR should be performed. At the present time, there have been no reports regarding the use of multimodality therapy in the treatment of verrucous carcinoma, but such consideration may obviate the need for radical extirpative surgery. Squamous cell carcinoma associated with condyloma acuminatum has been effectively treated with chemoradiation. The difference in the two entities may only be one of nomenclature.[88,89]

As an alternative treatment, particularly in unfit patients, Heinzerling et al[90] reported a successful treatment with imiquimod followed by CO₂ laser ablation. In this case, 5% imiquimod was applied to the lesion three times a week and from the second week on once daily. After 6 weeks of treatment, the persisting residual diseases were removed by CO_2 laser under local anesthesia. To prevent recurrences, treatment with imiquimod was continued for 6 weeks after the laser vaporization.

17.7 Neoplasms of the Anal Canal and Anal Canal Intraepithelial Neoplasia

AIN of the anal canal locates in the anal transitional zone as well as the anoderm below the dentate line. AIN of the anal canal has been found in minor surgical specimens such as hemorrhoidectomy, as well as in females with vulvar and cervical neoplasm. There is considerable evidence that AIN of the anal canal is the precursor of anal canal carcinoma, and possibly has a more aggressive behavior than perianal AIN.[30] Similar to perianal AIN, the diagnosis should be confirmed by biopsy, using 3 or 5% acetic acid and Lugol's solution staining as a guide.[32,42] The treatment should be a cautery ablation or local excision. For an extensive involvement of the anoderm, it should be done in stages to avoid anal stricture. AIN of the anal canal found incidentally in hemorrhoidectomy requires no further treatment provided the rest of the anal canal has no high-grade AIN[91]; a periodic follow-up with acetic acid staining is indicated.

Using electrocautery ablation directed by HRA, Chang et al[92] reported 79% recurrence in HIV-positive patients, with a mean recurrence time of 12 months compared with zero recurrence in HIV-negative patients.

17.7.1 Squamous Cell Carcinoma

This general category encompasses a number of different microscopic appearances, including large-cell keratinizing, large-cell nonkeratinizing (transitional), and basaloid (▸ Fig. 17.7).

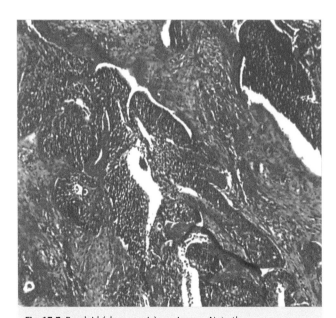

Fig. 17.7 Basaloid (cloacogenic) carcinoma. Note the nonkeratinization.

The term *cloacogenic* carcinoma has been used especially for the basaloid and large-cell nonkeratinizing (transitional) forms of squamous carcinoma. Keratinizing squamous cell carcinomas are rare in the anal canal above the dentate line. Mucoepidermoid carcinoma is extremely rare, if it exists at all in this site. Previously reported examples probably represent squamous cell carcinoma with mucinous microcysts (▸ Fig. 17.8). When carcinomas contain a mixture of cell types, they should be classified according to the appearance that predominates.[1] Because of their similar response to treatment, it is reasonable to group them together as squamous cell carcinoma. To comply with the WHO and the AJCC terminology,[1,2] the term *squamous cell carcinoma* instead of epidermoid carcinoma is used.

Clinical Manifestations

The presentation of squamous cell carcinomas generally follows a long history of minor perianal problems, such as bleeding, which occurs in approximately 50% of the patients.[61,93,94,95] Other signs and symptoms include pruritus, discharge, pain, and an indurated anal mass. Discharge, incontinence, change in bowel habit, pelvic pain, and anovaginal fistula suggest advanced lesions with involvement of the anal sphincter. Almost one-third of the patients in the series study by Stearns and Quan[94] were initially incorrectly diagnosed as having benign or inflammatory disease.

Diagnosis and Workup

The most important part of diagnosis is digital examination of the anal canal. The size, consistency, and fixation of the primary lesion and the presence or absence of pararectal lymph nodes can be determined. Proctoscopy should be done to confirm the digital findings, and the exact location of the neoplasm in relationship to the dentate line should be documented. Biopsy via proctoscope or transanal excision of the neoplasm must be done to determine the histologic type of the carcinoma, thus enabling an appropriate recommendation for treatment. A colonoscopic examination should be done to rule out more proximal associated lesions. Endorectal ultrasonography is useful in evaluating the depth of invasion and detection of lymph node metastasis.

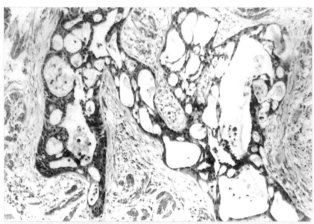

Fig. 17.8 Squamous cell carcinoma of anal canal with mucinous microcysts. This is not a mucoepidermoid carcinoma.[93] (With permission © 1989 Springer-Verlag.)

Both groins must be examined carefully to detect any enlargement of lymph nodes. Enlarged or suspicious lymph nodes in the groin area should be assessed by excision or biopsy because inguinal lymphadenopathy caused by reactive hyperplasia is common.

Character of Squamous Cell Carcinoma of Anal Canal

Even though squamous cell carcinoma of the anal canal is within the easy reach of a finger, the carcinoma is seldom diagnosed early. In a series from the Mayo Clinic, 88% of the carcinomas had already invaded beyond the mucosa before diagnosis.[96] In approximately 50% of the cases, the carcinoma has penetrated the bowel wall or the perianal skin. Invasion of the vaginal septum is more common than involvement of the prostate or urethra. Extensive carcinoma may invade the muscular or bony walls of the pelvis.[97] The anal canal has extensive lymphatic pathways. If the carcinoma is situated above the dentate line, metastases are found along the superior rectal vessels; if the carcinoma is at the dentate line, the lymphatic drainage is toward the internal pudendal, hypogastric, and obturator nodes; and if the carcinoma is below the dentate line, the lymphatic drainage is via the inguinal nodes. A study of lymph node metastasis of carcinoma of the anal canal has been conducted by Wade et al,[98] who used a clearing technique. Their results showed that 44% of the lymph node metastases were found in lymph nodes measuring < 5 mm in diameter. Analysis of maps of lymph nodes allowed these authors to observe that most lymph nodes were located above the peritoneal reflection and were scant in perianal zones. Review articles by Cummings[97] revealed that inguinal metastases are found in 15 to 20% of patients at the time of diagnosis and become apparent later in an additional 10 to 25%. The risk of lymphatic metastases is correlated with the depth of the invasion, the size, and the histologic grade. Nodal metastases are present in 30% of the patients when the smooth muscle is infiltrated and in 58% when the infiltration is beyond the external sphincters. Boman et al[96] found nodal metastases in only 3% of squamous cell carcinomas < 2 cm in diameter but in 25 to 35% of all the larger squamous cell carcinomas. The data from 1973 to 1998 in the SEER cancer registry showed the prevalence by stage was localized in 53%, regional in 38%, and distant in 9%.[12]

Treatment

Local Excision

This therapy should be reserved for early carcinomas or the well-differentiated type that have invaded only the submucosa.

Review of literature reveals that the recurrence rate after local excision is 20 to 78% and the 5-year survival rate is 45 to 85%.[88,98,99] However, properly selected, local excision can be highly successful. 13 of 188 patients with superficially invasive (< 2 cm in diameter) squamous cell carcinoma treated at the Mayo Clinic underwent local excision. Although one required an APR for local recurrence, all were cured at a follow-up of 5 or more years.[96] In the series from St. Mark's Hospital, 8 of 145 patients with squamous cell carcinoma of the anal canal were treated by local excision. The cancer-specific 5-year survival rate was 100%.[8] In general, mobile lesions < 2 cm are suitable for local excision.

Abdominoperineal Resection

In the past, APR with wide excision of perineal tissue formed the basis of treatment.[3] Despite this aggressive approach, the results have been disappointing. The local recurrence rate is 27 to 50% and the 5-year survival rate ranges from 24 to 62%, with a perioperative mortality rate of 2 to 6%.[88] An APR is no longer the primary treatment for invasive squamous cell carcinoma of the anal canal. APR is reserved for those patients who cannot tolerate the chemoradiation and is the primary treatment for failed chemoradiation.

To improve long-term survival and to save some patients from having a colostomy, the use of an APR has been replaced by the use of combined modality therapy for primary treatment.

Chemoradiation Regimen

In 1974, Nigro et al[100] initially attempted giving preoperative 5-FU with mitomycin C (MMC) and radiation in the management of squamous cell carcinoma of the anal canal to enhance the effectiveness of surgery. An APR was performed 4 to 6 weeks after the radiation therapy. Subsequently, they found that most of the surgical specimens contained no residual carcinoma. Nigro[9] then dropped the mandatory APR and instead excised the scar for histologic examination. Patients whose carcinoma grossly disappeared after the chemoradiation treatment required no further operation. Nigro's subsequent regime of the chemoradiation is in Box 17.2.[101] It should be noted that currently the dosage used for radiation varies among different practitioners. Review of the literature via MEDLINE search by Sato et al[102] on the management of carcinoma of the anal canal showed that CHT with 5-FU and MMC was superior in local control, colostomy-free rate, progressive-free survival, and carcinoma-specific survival compared with radiation alone.

Box 17.2 Nigro protocol

Nigro's chemoradiation therapy

External irradiation

- 3,000 rads to the primary carcinoma and pelvic and inguinal nodes; start: day 1 (200 rads/day)

Systemic chemotherapy

- 5-FU 1,000 mg/m^2/24 h as a continuous infusion for 4 days; start: day 1
- Mitomycin C, 15 mg/m^2 as an intravenous bolus; start: day 1 only
- 5-FU, repeat 4-day infusion; start: day 28

There have been questions regarding whether concomitant chemotherapy has the advantage over radiation alone and whether MMC, which is toxic, is necessary. Three well-conducted trials have examined these questions.

The Radiation Therapy Oncology Group and the Eastern Cooperative Oncology Group trial[103] studied the efficacy of MMC added to 5-FU and radiation. Of 291 assessable patients, 145 received 45 to 50.4 Gy pelvic radiation therapy plus 5-FU; 146 received radiation therapy, 5-FU, and MMC. Patients with residual disease on posttreatment biopsy were treated with a salvage regimen that consisted of additional pelvic radiation therapy (9 Gy), 5-FU, and cisplatin.

Posttreatment biopsies were positive in 15% of patients in the 5-FU arm versus 7.7% in MMC arm ($p = 0.135$). At 4 years' follow-up, colostomy rates were lower (9 vs. 22%, $p = 0.002$), colostomy-free survival higher (71 vs. 59%, $p = 0.014$), and disease-free survival higher (75 vs. 51%, $p = 0.0003$) in MMC arm. However, a significant difference in overall survival was not observed at 4 years.

Toxicity was greater in the MMC arm (23 vs. 7%, grade 4 and 5 toxicity, $p < 0.001$). The authors concluded that despite greater toxicity, the use of MMC in a chemoradiation regime for squamous cell carcinoma of the anal canal was justified, particularly in patients with large primary carcinoma. Salvage chemoradiation should be attempted in patients with residual disease following definitive chemoradiation before resorting to radical surgery.

The United Kingdom Coordinating Committee on Cancer Research (UKCCCR) trial[104] was designed to compare combined modality (5-FU, MMC, and radiation) with radiation therapy alone in patients with anal squamous cell carcinoma. In the multicenter trial, 585 patients were randomized to receive 45 Gy RT (290 patients) or RT combined with 5-FU MMC (295 patients). They assessed clinical response 6 weeks after initial treatment: good responders received a boost RT and the poor responders received a salvage surgery. The main end point was local failure rate (26 weeks after initial treatment); secondary end points were overall and cause-specific survival. The results showed that after a median follow-up of 42 months (range, 28–62 months), radiation alone group had a local failure of 59% compared with a 36% rate in the combined modality group. This gave a 46% reduction in the risk of local failure in the patients receiving combined modality (relative risk, 0.54; 95% confidence interval [CI], 0.2–0.69; $p < 0.0001$). The risk of death from anal canal cancer was also reduced in the combined modality therapy arm (relative risk, 0.71; CI, 0.53–0.95; $p = 0.02$). However, there was no overall survival advantage (relative risk, 0.86; CI, 0.67–1.11; $p = 0.25$). Early morbidity was significantly more frequent in the combined modality arm ($p = 0.03$), but late morbidity occurred at similar rates.

The authors concluded that the standard treatment for most patients with anal squamous cell carcinoma should be a combination of RT and infused 5-FU and MMC, with surgery reserved for those who failed this regimen.

The European Organization for Research and Treatment of Cancer Radiotherapy and Gastrointestinal Cooperative Groups conducted a prospective randomized trial to validate the use of concomitant RT and chemotherapy in the treatment of squamous cell carcinoma of the anus.[105]

The study included 103 patients randomized between RT alone ($n = 51$) and a combination of RT and chemotherapy (5-FU continuous infusion plus MMC, $n = 51$). The patients had T3–T4 N0–N3 or T1–T2 N1–N3 squamous cell carcinoma of the anus. The radiation dosage was 45 Gy.

The results showed that at 5-year follow-up, the addition of chemotherapy to radiation therapy resulted in a significant increase in the complete remission rate from 54% for RT alone to 80% for chemoradiation therapy, and from 85 to 96%, respectively, if results are considered after surgical resections. Local recurrence improved by 18%, while colostomy-free rate increased by 32% in the chemoradiation group. Event-free survival, defined as free of local recurrence, no colostomy, and no severe side effects or death, showed significant improvement in favor of the chemoradiation group ($p = 0.03$). The overall survival rates remained similar in both treatment arms. A summary of the three randomized trials is presented in ▶ Table 17.1.

Currently, most investigators recommend combined modality treatment with continuous course radiation (50.4 Gy in 1.8 Gy fractions) plus two cycles of concurrent continuous infusion 5-FU (weeks 1 and 5) plus MMC (days 1 and 29). This regimen is considered by most to be the standard of care. For patients who have T3–T4 disease (primary tumors, greater than 5 cm), it is reasonable to provide a radiation boost with an additional 5.4 to 9.0 Gy.[106] Doses up to 66 to 70 Gy may be needed to treat patients with radiation alone.[107]

The average results of chemoradiation regimen include a complete response rate of 84% (81–87%), a local control rate of 73% (64–86%), and a 5-year survival rate of 77% (66–92%). For patients who have T1–T2 disease, the complete response rates are more than 90%. In patients who have T3–T4 disease, approximately 50% will require salvage APR. If they achieve a complete response following completion of combined modality therapy, only 25% will require a salvage APR.[106,107]

Table 17.1 Summary of randomized controlled trials on squamous cell carcinoma of the anal canal

Study group (year)	Study arms	Statistically significant	Results
Flam et al Intergroup trial[103] (1996)	5-FU + radiation; $n = 145$	Yes: disease-free survival; colostomy-free survival (favoring MMC)	51 vs. 73%, disease-free survival (favoring MMC); follow-up 4 y
	5-FU + MMC + radiation; $n = 146$	No: overall survival	
UKCCCR[104] (1996)	Radiation alone $n = 285$	Yes: local failure; disease-free survival (favoring chemoradiation)	46% reduction local failure; reduction death from cancer (favoring chemoradiation); follow-up 42 mo
	Radiation + 5-FU + MMC; $n = 292$	No: overall survival	
Bartelink et al EORTC[105] (1997)	Radiation alone $n = 52$	Yes: local failure; cancer-free survival (favoring chemoradiation)	80 vs. 54% complete remission; 18% improve in local recurrence; 32% increase in colostomy-free (favoring chemoradiation); follow-up 5 y
	Radiation + 5-FU + MMC; $n = 51$	No: overall survival	

Abbreviations: 5-FU, 5-fluorouracil; MMC, mitomycin C.

An example of chemoradiation treatment of squamous cell carcinoma of the anal canal is illustrated in the study by Myerson et al.[108] During 1975 to 1997, 106 patients with squamous cell carcinoma of the anal canal underwent radiation therapy. The dramatic response to low doses of radiation and concurrent chemotherapy led them to change in policy with most patients receiving chemoradiation, and surgery was reserved for salvage of persistent or recurrent disease. Since 1985, 81 patients have received definitive chemoradiation.

Doses for definitive treatment without chemotherapy were 45 to 50 Gy to the carcinoma and the regional nodes, followed by a boost to a total dose of at least 65 Gy. Substantially lower radiation doses were used with concurrent chemotherapy. A dose of 30 Gy was used for T1/T2, followed by a boost of 10 to 20 Gy (mean 16.19 Gy) and 16 to 30 Gy (mean 23.67 Gy) for T3/T4 lesions. The results of 88 patients that excluded salvage surgery showed: T1-N0 (15 cases, 93 ± 6%); T2-N0 (33 cases, 84 ± 7%); T3-N0 (16 cases, 60 ± 13%); T4-N0 (24 cases, 37 ± 12%) ($p = 0.001$) (▶ Fig. 17.9).

It is important to note the additional malignancies as cited by Myerson et al[108]: 33 additional malignancies in 26 patients. Nineteen of the lesions antedated the squamous carcinoma of the anal canal, and 14 postdated. Types of the malignancies are in ▶ Table 17.2. With exception of the two sarcomas within the radiation portals that occurred 5 and 10 years after radiation without chemotherapy, the additional malignancies were not suggestive of the radiation-induced malignancy.

This information underscores the importance of complete examination in general, in addition to a diligent long-term oncologic screening in patients with squamous cell carcinoma of the anal canal.[109]

Brachytherapy

Brachytherapy is an ideal method to deliver conformal radiation for anal carcinoma while sparing the surrounding healthy structures, such as small intestine and bladder. The primary concern is anal necrosis, and anal necrosis rates reportedly vary from 2% to as high as 76%.[110] Although there are no randomized data, the phase II trials suggest that, even in experienced hands, brachytherapy is associated with higher complication rates than in external beam radiation (EBR) therapy.[106]

Kapp et al,[111] using brachytherapy to boost during a short split between the EBR ± chemotherapy, gave satisfactory results. The rationale of this combination was to improve tolerance of 50 Gy EBR in the pelvis, perineum, and groin. Intestinal or intraluminal brachytherapy was performed using a single high-intensity (^{192}Ir) implant. Dose calculation for needle implants was 6 Gy. EBR was delivered with one dose of 1.8 or 2.0 Gy per day, 5 days a week. After 30 Gy, an interstitial or intraluminal ^{192}Ir high-dose rate (HDR) boost was performed. Depending on the patient's skin reaction, EBR was resumed within 1 to 2 weeks, with an additional 20 Gy. Patients who failed to achieve a complete response received additional brachytherapy.

Follow-up ranged from 3 to 14 months (median, 31 months). The median treatment radiation was 56 days. The 5-year actuarial

Table 17.2 Additional malignancies in patients with squamous cell carcinoma of the anal canal

Type	Number of lesions
Gynecologic	9
Head and neck	6
Lung	5
Colorectal	3
Genitourinary	3
Central nervous system	2
Hematologic	2
Sarcoma	2
Breast	1
Total	33

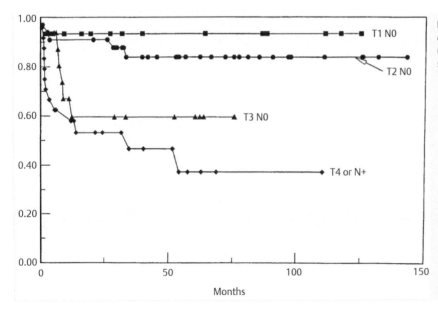

Fig. 17.9 Disease-free survival (Kaplan–Meier) vs. clinical stage. The contribution of surgery (planned or salvage) to the ultimate disease status is included in this figure.

rates of locoregional control (LRC) and disease-specific survival (DSS) were 76 and 76%, respectively. The overall anal preservation was 77 and 97% in patients in whom LRC was achieved. Uncompromised anal function was recorded in 93% of these patients.

Although acute toxicity occurred in 89% in radiochemotherapy group and in 64% of RT alone, predominantly the triad of pronounced skin reaction, diarrhea, and nausea, none of these patients required hospitalization. Late complications that required a temporary colostomy occurred in 7.6% of the patients, for pain relief because of ulceration of the lesions.

The authors concluded that the integration of HDR brachytherapy boost in a split-course EBR regimen ± chemotherapy resulted in excellent sphincter function without an increase of severe complications and with rates of LRC, DSS, and cancer-free survival that compared favorably with those reported in the literature.

Treatment in HIV-Positive Patients

In general, HIV-positive patients have received lower doses of radiation and chemotherapy because of poorer tolerance to therapy and increased complication rate.[106,112,113]

In situ patients with CD-4 counts as low as 105 cells/mL do well with local excision. A low CD-4 count at diagnosis without HAART predicts a poor prognosis because these patients appear to succumb to their HIV status and not the anal disease.[112] Even in the era of HAART and with experienced clinicians, treatment of invasive anal squamous cell carcinoma in HIV-infected patients remains a challenge but the techniques in management will undoubtedly improve in the near future.

At the University of California, San Francisco, HIV-positive patients with invasive anal squamous cell carcinoma and CD-4 counts > 200 cells/mm^3 were treated with chemoradiotherapy in a similar way to patients who were not HIV-infected.[114] Patients with CD-4 counts less than 200 cells/mm^3 were treated using more individualized approaches. In general, the dosage was kept tighter, and prophylactic radiation at nodal areas was not used. These patients had a higher rate of colostomies. Cisplatin was used instead of MMC in some cases. Blazy et al[115] reported their experience of treating anal canal carcinoma in the era of new antiviral drugs, in patients who are HIV-positive. Nine men on highly active antiretroviral therapies with good immune status before CHT received concomitant CHT consisting of 5-FU and cisplatinum, and high-dose RT (60–70 Gy). Six carcinomas were stage I, two were stage II, and one was stage III. CD-4 + cell counts were less than 200/mL for four patients, between 200/mL and 500/mL for four, and more than 500/mL for one. All patients received the planned dose of radiation (260 Gy). The chemotherapy dose was reduced to 25% in six patients. The overall treatment time was 58 days. Grade III hematologic or skin toxicity occurred in four patients. No association was observed between high-grade toxicity and CD-4 + cell count. None of the patients developed opportunistic infections during follow-up. Eight patients were disease-free after a median follow-up of 33 months. Among them, four had no or minor anal function impairment at the last follow-up visit. One patient with T4-N2 disease relapsed locally 1 year after treatment and underwent salvage abdominoperineal excision. The authors concluded that high-dose CHT for anal canal carcinoma is feasible with low toxicity in HIV-positive patients, treated with highly active antiretroviral therapies.

Toxicity of Chemoradiation

Chemoradiation is not to be taken lightly. Reports of complications vary widely in the literature because they are dose and technique dependent. In general, severe complications are increased when the total dose is > 40 Gy. The common complications encountered are dermatitis and mucositis, diarrhea, fecal incontinence, fatigue, bone marrow depression, cystitis, small bowel obstruction, and major arterial stenosis. Death, although very rare, has been reported.[116,117]

Anorectal function was preserved in 88% of patients who underwent chemoradiation, as reported in the series of Cummings et al[116]; the dose was 45 to 55 Gy. Those with severe fecal incontinence required a colostomy. Less severe anorectal dysfunction, such as fecal urgency and occasional fecal incontinence, can be managed satisfactorily with antidiarrheal medications and the adjustment of diet. Complications of chemoradiation can be minimized by split-course radiation.[116] Cisplatin has emerged as a potential replacement for mitomycin in the combination drug regimens. It is a radiation sensitizer and is less myelosuppressive than MMC. However, preliminary results showed the toxicity rate to be similar to MMC regimen.[106,107]

Pattern of Failure and Treatment

The predominant sites of failure after chemoradiation are the pelvis, either the anal area or the regional lymph nodes. In a large series of 190 patients reported by Cummings et al,[116] 41% experienced recurrence at one or more sites. Of those recurrences, 62% were confined to the pelvis, 16% were outside the pelvis, and the rest occurred both inside and outside the pelvis.

Those patients with residual or recurrent carcinoma confined to the pelvis or perianal area should undergo a salvage APR with or without a booster dose of radiation. The outcome is significantly related to the extent of the disease at the time of failure. The series from Memorial Sloan-Kettering Cancer Center showed that T stage did not appear to affect survival after APR ($p = 0.07$).[118] On the other hand, Nguyen et al[119] revealed size to be the only significant factor associated with the need for a stoma ($p = 0.01$), and that node positivity was the only independent predictor of mortality ($p = 0.02$). Inguinal node metastasis at initial presentation, before the chemoradiation, predicted poor outcome after APR for treatment failure. Patients with disease fixed to the pelvic side wall on digital examination at the time of treatment failure fared poorly, with an 8-month median survival and no 5-year survival. Among those with mobile lesions, the median survival is 40 months, with an overall 5-year survival of 47% of those patients.[118] Salvage APR following recurrence can have a long-term survival rate.[117,118,119,120,121,122,123] A dismal result was described in a series by Zelnick et al[122] where there was no 5-year survival.

Inguinal Lymph Nodes

Because of the high morbidity and low yield in the prevention of death from cancer, prophylactic groin dissection is not recommended.[94,95] The simultaneous appearance of inguinal metastasis is an ominous sign. In the series of Gerard et al,[123] of 270 patients with squamous cell carcinoma of the anal canal, synchronous inguinal metastasis occurred in 10%, and metachronous inguinal metastasis in 7.8%. The 5-year overall survival in patients without inguinal lymph node involvement was 73 versus 54% in patients with synchronous lymph node metastasis.

For patients with synchronous lymph node metastasis, the authors recommended a unilateral lymph node dissection immediately followed by a cycle of continuous infusion of 5-FU (day 1–4) and bolus of cisplatinum (day 2–5). Radiation to the involved groin was initiated after completion of the chemotherapy. The dose of the radiation was 45 to 50 Gy over 5 weeks. The results showed local control of the inguinal area in 86%; the 5-year overall survival was 54%.

The initial treatment was inguinal lymph node dissection for patients with a metastatic metachronous inguinal lymph node metastasis. Irradiation started after the wound had healed, delivering 45 to 50 Gy over 5 weeks. No prophylactic irradiation of the contralateral inguinal area was performed. The local control of the inguinal area was observed in 68% of patients so treated and the 5-year overall survival rate was 41%.[123]

Whether prophylactic groin radiation should be performed is controversial. Elective radiation of clinically normal inguinal nodes reduces the risk of late node failure and carries little morbidity. Only 1 of 38 such patients had a late recurrence in the inguinal area after undergoing combination chemotherapy and RT.[124] In series in which the inguinal nodes were not treated electively, the late nodal recurrence rate was 15 to 25%.[96,125,126]

Ulmer et al[127] evaluated the feasibility of the sentinel lymph node technique for groin metastasis of anal squamous cell carcinoma. The lesion in the anal canal was injected submucosally or subdermally with 1-mL Tc^{99m} sulfur colloid in four sites, using a 27-gauge needle and an insulin syringe. Scintigraphy was recorded with a gamma camera. Seventeen hours later, patients with detectable radiocolloid enrichment in the groin underwent lymph node biopsy guided by a handheld gamma probe. Sentinel lymph nodes were detected in 13 of 17 patients (76.5%); metastases were found in the sentinel lymph nodes of 5 of 12 biopsied patients (42%); in two patients the metastases were detected by serial sectioning or immunohistochemical staining after H&E results were negative for carcinoma. Compared with staging using ultrasonography and CT, assessment of the sentinel lymph node provides more reliable staging of inguinal lymph nodes because 44% of all lymph node metastases in anal carcinoma are smaller than 5 mm in diameter.[124] This technique may prove to be a valuable diagnostic workup for anal squamous cell carcinoma. Further studies are warranted.

Drugs for Metastasis

The most frequent sites of visceral metastasis include the liver, lung, bone, and subcutaneous tissues. The prognosis is poor, with a median survival of approximately 9 months. Twenty percent of patients with recurrent carcinoma of the anal canal die from distant metastasis, but most carcinoma-related deaths are secondary to uncontrolled pelvic and perianal disease.[128]

Drugs used to treat metastasis include 5-FU, bleomycin, methyl-CCNU, vincristine, doxorubicin, and cisplatin. Combinations of agents such as bleomycin, vincristine, or methotrexate, plus leucovorin, had also been used. All combinations had resulted in only partial responses.[129] A phase III randomized study is being completed in the United Kingdom for patients who have locally advanced squamous cell carcinoma of the anal canal using different drugs and radiation, including 5-FU/MMC/radiation and 5-FU/cisplatin/radiation.[107]

17.8 Summary

Surgeons must be familiar with the anatomic landmarks of the anal canal and the perianal skin as defined by the WHO and the AJCC, as well as with TNM staging as most current reports and studies use these systems.

Local excision is still the treatment of choice for carcinoma in situ or microscopic invasive carcinoma that has occurred in the anal canal or the perianal area. Unfortunately, only small numbers of the lesions are suitable for this option because most are too large or too advanced at the time of diagnosis. Chemoradiation, which was originally used as the primary treatment of anal canal squamous cell carcinoma, is now also applied to its counterpart in the perianal area. APR is no longer the primary treatment for invasive carcinoma of the anal canal and most perianal carcinomas. Not only does it have a high recurrence, but also local recurrence after APR has a less favorable prognosis. It responds less favorably to chemoradiation than the primary carcinoma, as 52% of patients have persistent disease after the treatment.[130] APR is reserved for local treatment failure of chemoradiation, for anorectal complications of the treatment, especially fecal incontinence, and for those patients who cannot tolerate chemoradiation

17.8.1 Adenocarcinoma

Primary adenocarcinomas of the anus are very rare, constituting 3 to 9% of all anal carcinomas.[131,132,133] The WHO classifies these malignancies into the rectal type, the anal glands, and those within an anorectal fistula.[1]

Rectal Type

This type is the most common adenocarcinoma found in the anal canal. It arises within the upper zone lined by colorectal-type mucosa. Its histology is that of an adenocarcinoma of the large intestine. It is generally difficult or impossible to separate adenocarcinoma of the anal canal from adenocarcinoma of the lower rectum.[1]

Anal Glands

The ducts of the anal glands are lined by squamous epithelium close to their opening in the crypts, by transitional epithelium more deeply, and by mucin-secreting columnar epithelium in the depth of the gland. The histologic picture of these lesions, therefore, may be one of adenocarcinoma or mucoepidermoid carcinoma. It can be differentiated from other types of anal lesions by its haphazardly dispersed, small glands with scant mucin production invading the wall of the anorectal area without an intraluminal component. The glands are positive for CK7.[134,135]

The most characteristic feature of anal duct carcinoma is its extramucosal adenocarcinoma without the involvement of the

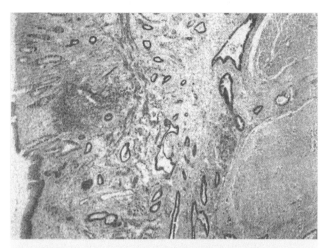

Fig. 17.10 Anal duct carcinoma. Note the intact epithelium.

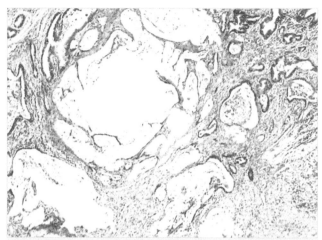

Fig. 17.11 Adenocarcinoma in a fistula-in-ano. Note pools of mucin.

surface epithelium, except when the lesion has become advanced (▸ Fig. 17.10). If there is a break in the surface epithelium, as is often seen clinically, greater perianal involvement or deeper infiltration may provide the only clue to the anal duct origin of these lesions. In a series of 21 patients reported by Jensen et al,[136] nine of the neoplasms were localized in the ischioanal space, seven were in the anal canal, and five were in a fistula-in-ano. Patients usually present with complaints of pain and an extra-anorectal lump, perianal induration, or a perianal abscess. Despite its distal location and its accessibility to digital examination, most anal gland and duct carcinomas are detected late. In the series by Jensen et al,[136] the median duration of symptoms before correct diagnosis was 18 months; the sensation of having a perianal mass, bleeding, pain, soiling, pruritus ani, change in bowel habits, prolapse, and weight loss were common symptoms. Like other malignancies of the anal region, most adenocarcinomas of the anus are diagnosed erroneously by physicians and surgeons, as well as by patients, with a resulting delay in the correct diagnosis. The average size of the carcinoma of the anal canal in the series by Jensen et al[136] was 5 cm and in the perianal area was 10 cm. Sixty-two percent of the patients already had a regional or distant metastasis. Because of the late stage of the carcinoma, 20 of 21 patients died within 18 months after treatment.[136] The primary treatment is an APR, with wide excision of the perineal part.[137] The role of radiation or chemoradiation is unknown.

Anorectal Fistula

Well-differentiated mucinous adenocarcinomas (▸ Fig. 17.11) occasionally develop within an anorectal fistula that may be developmental or acquired.[1] Most often, these carcinomas arise in patients with longstanding perianal disease, especially fistulas.[138,139] Some authors believe that they originate in the anal glands and ducts.[140,141]

Treatment

For a rectal type or a primary adenocarcinoma of anal canal, a wide local excision can be performed for small and well-differentiated carcinomas that have not invaded the muscular wall of the anorectum. In a multicenter study, data collected

Table 17.3 Survival of three modes of treatment of primary anal canal adenocarcinoma

Mode of treatment	Survival	Five year (%)	Ten year (%)
RT/APR	Overall	29	23, $p = 0.02$
RT/CHT	Overall	58	39
APR	Overall	21	21
RT/APR	Disease-free	25	18, $p = 0.038$
RT/CHT	Disease-free	54	20
APR	Disease-free	22	22

Abbreviations: APR, abdominoperineal resection; CHT, chemotherapy; RT, radiotherapy.

for primary adenocarcinoma of the anal canal from patients reported by Belkacémi et al[142] included: 18 T1 (18%), 34 T2 (42%), 22 T3 (27%), and 11 T4 (13%). There were three treatment categories: radiation and surgery, 45 patients; chemoradiation, 31 patients; and APR, 6 patients.

The patients' characteristics were evenly distributed among the three groups. The results showed that recurrence occurred in 37, 36, and 20%, respectively, at 4-year follow-up (not statistically significant). Both the overall and the disease-free 5-year survival were significantly better in the chemoradiation group (▸ Table 17.3). Multivariate analysis revealed four independent prognostic factors for survival: T stage, N stage, histologic grade, and treatment modality.

From this study, it is apparent that from stage T2 onwards, the primary treatment should be chemoradiation and the APR should be reserved for salvage treatment. A small series from Memorial Sloan-Kettering Cancer Center[133] showed that 6 of 13 patients were free of disease after chemoradiation and APR, with a follow-up of 26 months. For adenocarcinomas of the anal gland or an anal fistula, the role of adjuvant therapy is not yet defined due to the uncommon disease.[143] The Nigro chemoradiation regime has been successfully used by Tarazi and Nelson.[144] Of nine patients who used this protocol, six patients were free of disease on follow-up of 2 to 4 years. Papagikos et al[145] recommended a preoperative chemoradiation followed by APR.

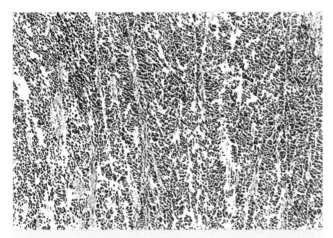

Fig. 17.12 Small cell carcinoma of the large intestine.[93] (With permission © 1989 Springer-Verlag.)

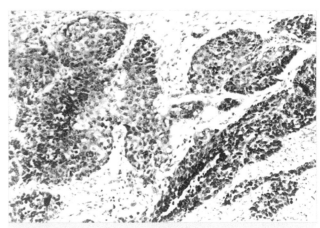

Fig. 17.13 Undifferentiated carcinoma of the large intestine.[93] (With permission © 1989 Springer-Verlag.)

17.8.2 Small Cell Carcinoma

This very rare carcinoma may arise in the anorectal region. It is similar in histology, behavior, and histochemistry to small cell (oat cell) carcinoma of the lung (▶ Fig. 17.12). It is a neuroendocrine carcinoma or a Merkel cell carcinoma. The diagnosis can be confirmed by immunohistochemistry and electron microscopy.[145] This type of lesion has been known to have early and extensive dissemination. The case presented by Paterson et al[146] showed that a 1-cm Merkel cell carcinoma of the anal canal had already metastasized to the liver. Based on Merkel cell carcinoma of other organs, "it is extremely lymphophile; lymph node relapses occur in approximately 80% of the patients with recurrent disease."[147] Merkel cell carcinoma has been known to respond to RT.[147] Whether this mode of treatment is useful for Merkel cell carcinoma of the anal canal is not known.

17.8.3 Undifferentiated Carcinoma

Also very rare, this type of malignant lesion has no glandular structure or other features to indicate definite differentiation (▶ Fig. 17.13). Undifferentiated carcinoma may be distinguished from poorly differentiated carcinoma, small cell carcinoma, lymphoma, or leukemic deposits by the use of mucin stains or immunohistochemical methods.[1] The treatment is the same as for adenocarcinomas. The prognosis can be expected to be poor.

17.8.4 Melanoma

General Considerations

Malignant melanoma is the most depressing of all anorectal malignancies. It is a rare malignant neoplasm of the anorectum that constitutes 1 to 3% of all melanomas. The anal canal is the third most common site, exceeded only by the skin and eyes.[148] The female-to-male ratio is approximately 2:1, and the average age at presentation is approximately 63 years.[149] Evaluation of the NCI SEER data from 1973 to 1992 showed female-to-male ratio as 1.72:1. The mean age was 66 ± 16 years. Mean age by gender was lower for males (57 years) than for females (71 years; p < 0.001). The incidence of anorectal melanoma in young males ages between 25 and 44 years tripled in the San Francisco area when compared with all other locations (14.4 vs. 4.8 per 10 million population; p = 0.06). There was indirect evidence that implicated HIV infection as a risk factor.[150]

Malignant melanoma arises from epithelium of the anal canal, both above and below the dentate line.[151] A few reports describe these lesions as arising from, and being situated in, the rectum.[152,153] Electron microscopy shows that normal melanocytes are present in the rectal mucosa.[152]

Clinical Features

Rectal bleeding, a mass in the anal canal, and anorectal pain are the three most common and most consistent signs and symptoms of malignant melanoma.[149,154] Only 25% of patients have lesions < 1 cm in diameter. The remainder have melanomas as large as 6 cm in diameter, with an average size of 4 cm.[153] Often the mass protrudes through the anus. Weight loss is also a common finding.

Diagnosis

Melanomas are suspected when a pigmented polypoid lesion is noted (▶ Fig. 17.14). Unless an ulceration with raised edges is present, this disease may be confused with a thrombosed hemorrhoid. The majority of melanomas, however, are only lightly pigmented or nonpigmented and are often misdiagnosed as being polyps or other neoplasms of the anal canal. Between 40 and 70% of melanomas of the anal canal are amelanotic and in only 25% of the pigmented lesions is there abundant melanin.[151,155] If melanin is seen on microscopic examination, then the diagnosis is simple. In the amelanotic melanoma, sheets of anaplastic cells may be misinterpreted as undifferentiated squamous cell carcinoma. The most helpful diagnostic feature is the presence of malignant cells in clusters.[155] Endorectal ultrasound is useful to determine the depth of invasion and possible adjacent lymph node metastasis.[156,157]

Mode of Metastasis

Anal canal melanomas have a marked tendency to spread submucosally along the rectum but rarely invade adjacent organs. Review of the literature by Cooper et al[158] showed that 46 of

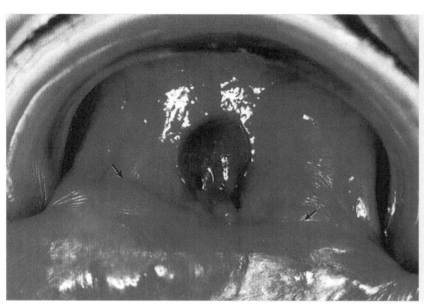

Fig. 17.14 Malignant melanoma of the anal canal. The arrows point at the dentate line.

Table 17.4 Selected series of anal melanoma

Authors	No. of patients	No. of curative WLE and disease-free at 5 years (%)	No. of curative abdominoperineal resection and disease-free at 5 years (%)	Recommended treatment
Pessaux et al 2004[161]	16	11 (29)	4 (0)	WLE
Bullard et al 2003[156]	40	21 (16)	9 (33)	WLE
Thibault et al 1997[149]	50	11 (18)	26 (19)	WLE
Ward et al 1986[162]	21	3 (0)	4 (0)	WLE
Roumen 1996[163]	63	16 (13)	18 (11)	WLE
Brady et al 1995[160]	85	13 (8)	43 (26)	APR
Ross et al 1990[164]	32	12 (8)	14 (0)	WLE
Slingluff et al 1990[165]	24	7 (0)	12 (0)	Multimodality
Goldman et al 1990[166]	49	18 (6)	15 (7)	APR

Abbreviations: APR, abdominoperineal resection; WLE, wide local excision.

120 patients (38%) had metastasis at the time of diagnosis. Perirectal, perianal, and mesenteric lymph nodes were the most common sites of metastasis, followed by inguinal lymph nodes, liver, and lung. Widespread systemic metastases are early and rapid, most commonly to the liver, lung, and bone. Wolff[159] raised a question whether using thickness of the lesion similar to melanoma of the skin can be useful to determine options of treatment and prognosis.

Treatment

There is no survival benefit of adjuvant therapy for melanomas of the anal canal partly because of associated distant metastases in most patients. For the majority of cases, there appears to be no clear-cut choice of surgical treatment between a wide local excision and an APR. Both treatments yield a 5-year survival between 0 and 22%.[149] In the larger series reported by Brady et al[160] of 85 cases and Thibault et al[149] of 50 cases, the 5-year survival rates were 17 and 22%, respectively. Both options of treatment have their proponents (▶ Table 17.4).

Thibault et al[149] reviewed the series from the Mayo Clinic attempting to find predictive factors of survival, including gender, size of the lesion, presence of melanin, depth of penetration, positive perirectal lymph nodes, and wide local excision versus APR, and there was none. This is in contrast to the finding by Brady et al[160] at Memorial Sloan-Kettering Cancer Center that all long-term survivals occurred in women. Indeed, in their study, women with operable disease had a 5-year survival rate of 29%. Although the authors recommend an APR, only one of nine patients who underwent such an operation had positive mesenteric nodes.

It appears that local control of the disease after the operation is not as much a problem as distant metastasis, which is the major cause of death.[156,161,162,163] A reasonable approach is to perform local excision of the lesion, only if this can be accomplished with wide margin and full thickness without causing fecal incontinence. Otherwise, an APR should be performed. Pessaux et al[161] reported 30 patients who underwent APR or wide local excision. Features that showed significantly better results in 5-year survival included: negative inguinal node ($p = 0.031$), duration of symptoms less than 3 months ($p = 0.046$), stage I versus stage II ($p = 0.025$), and nonmelanomic ($p = 0.033$). Tumor size, depth of invasion (in mm), age, gender, and wide local excision versus APR were not statistically different.

References

[1] Fenger C, Frisch M, Marti MC, Parc R. Tumors of the anal canal. In: Hamilton SR, Aaltonen LA, eds. WHO Classification of Tumors. Pathology and Genetics of Tumors of the Digestive System. Lyon: International Agency for Research on Cancer (IARC); 2002:146–155

[2] Green FL, Page DL, Fleming ID, et al. American Joint Committee on Cancer. 6th ed. New York, NY: Springer-Verlag; 2002:139–144, 231–237

[3] Cummings BJ. Editorial. Oncology. 1996; 10:1853–1854

[4] Jensen SL, Hagen K, Shokouh-Amiri MH, Nielsen OV. Does an erroneous diagnosis of squamous-cell carcinoma of the anal canal and anal margin at first physician visit influence prognosis? Dis Colon Rectum. 1987; 30(5):345–351

[5] Williams GR, Talbot IC. Anal carcinoma–a histological review. Histopathology. 1994; 25(6):507–516

[6] Brown DK, Oglesby AB, Scott DH, Dayton MT. Squamous cell carcinoma of the anus: a twenty-five year retrospective. Am Surg. 1988; 54(6):337–342

[7] Greenall MJ, Quan SHQ, Urmacher C, DeCosse JJ. Treatment of epidermoid carcinoma of the anal canal. Surg Gynecol Obstet. 1985; 161(6):509–517

[8] Pintor MP, Northover JMA, Nicholls RJ. Squamous cell carcinoma of the anus at one hospital from 1948 to 1984. Br J Surg. 1989; 76(8):806–810

[9] Nigro ND. Multidisciplinary management of cancer of the anus. World J Surg. 1987; 11(4):446–451

[10] Siegel RL, Miller KD, Jemal A. Cancer statistics, 2015. CA Cancer J Clin. 2015; 65(1):5–29

[11] Deans GT, McAlee JJA, Spence RAJ. Malignant anal tumours. Br J Surg. 1994; 81(4):501–508

[12] Maggard MA, Beanes SR, Ko CY. Anal canal cancer: a population-based reappraisal. Dis Colon Rectum. 2003; 46(11):1517–1523, discussion 1523–1524, author reply 1524

[13] Frisch M. On the etiology of anal squamous carcinoma. Dan Med Bull. 2002; 49(3):194–209

[14] Chang GJ, Sheldon A, Welton ML. Epidemiology and natural history of anal HPV infection and ASIL and cancer in the general population. Semin Colon Rectal Surg. 2004; 15:210–214

[15] Saclarides TJ, Klem D. Genetic alterations and virology of anal cancer. Semin Colon Rectal Surg. 1995; 6:131–134

[16] Palmer JG, Scholefield JH, Coates PJ, et al. Anal cancer and human papillomaviruses. Dis Colon Rectum. 1989; 32(12):1016–1022

[17] Shroyer KR, Kim JG, Manos MM, Greer CE, Pearlman NW, Franklin WA. Papillomavirus found in anorectal squamous carcinoma, not in colon adenocarcinoma. Arch Surg. 1992; 127(6):741–744

[18] Bjørge T, Engeland A, Luostarinen T, et al. Human papillomavirus infection as a risk factor for anal and perianal skin cancer in a prospective study. Br J Cancer. 2002; 87(1):61–64

[19] Frisch M, Glimelius B, van den Brule AJ, et al. Sexually transmitted infection as a cause of anal cancer. N Engl J Med. 1997; 337(19):1350–1358

[20] Welton ML. Etiology of human papilloma virus infections and the development of anal squamous intraepithelial lesions. Semin Colon Rectal Surg. 2004; 15(4):193–195

[21] Mullerat J, Northover J. Human papillomavirus and anal neoplastic lesions in the immunocompromised (transplant) patient. Semin Colon Rectal Surg. 2004; 15(4):215–217

[22] Penn I. Cancers of the anogenital region in renal transplant recipients. Analysis of 65 cases. Cancer. 1986; 58(3):611–616

[23] Gervaz P, Hahnloser D, Wolff BG, et al. Molecular biology of squamous cell carcinoma of the anus: a comparison of HIV-positive and HIV-negative patients. J Gastrointest Surg. 2004; 8(8):1024–1030, discussion 1031

[24] Noffsinger A, Witte D, Fenoglio-Preiser CM. The relationship of human papillomaviruses to anorectal neoplasia. Cancer. 1992; 70(5) Suppl:1276–1287

[25] Cummings BJ. Anal canal carcinoma. In: Hermanek P, Gospodarowicz MK, Henson DE, Hutter RVP, Sobin LH, eds. Prognostic Factors in Cancer. New York, NY: Springer; 1995:80–87

[26] Carter PS. Anal cancer–current perspectives. Dig Dis. 1993; 11(4–5):239–251

[27] Chang GJ, Welton ML. Anal neoplasia. Semin Colon Rectal Surg. 2003; 14:111–118

[28] Bowen JT. Precancerous dermatoses: a study of two cases of chronic atypical epithelial proliferation. J Cutan Dis. 1912; 30:241–255

[29] Fenger C, Nielsen VT. Intraepithelial neoplasia in the anal canal. The appearance and relation to genital neoplasia. Acta Pathol Microbiol Immunol Scand [A]. 1986; 94(5):343–349

[30] Fenger C. Intra-epithelial neoplasia in the anal canal and peri-anal area. Curr Top Pathol. 1990; 81:91–102

[31] Halverson AL. Perianal Bowen's disease then and now: evolution of the treatment for anal high-grade intraepithelial neoplasia. Semin Colon Rectal Surg. 2003; 14(4):213–217

[32] Brown SR, Skinner P, Tidy J, Smith JH, Sharp F, Hosie KB. Outcome after surgical resection for high-grade anal intraepithelial neoplasia (Bowen's disease). Br J Surg. 1999; 86(8):1063–1066

[33] Scholefield JH, Castle MT, Watson NFS. Malignant transformation of high-grade anal intraepithelial neoplasia. Br J Surg. 2005; 92(9):1133–1136

[34] Abbasakoor F, Boulos PB. Anal intraepithelial neoplasia. Br J Surg. 2005; 92(3):277–290

[35] Palefsky JM. Anal squamous intraepithelial lesions in human immunodeficiency virus-positive men and women. Semin Oncol. 2000; 27(4):471–479

[36] Arbesman H, Ransohoff DF. Is Bowen's disease a predictor for the development of internal malignancy? A methodological critique of the literature. JAMA. 1987; 257(4):516–518

[37] Chute CG, Chuang TY, Bergstralh EJ, Su WPD. The subsequent risk of internal cancer with Bowen's disease. A population-based study. JAMA. 1991; 266(6):816–819

[38] Marfing TE, Abel ME, Gallagher DM. Perianal Bowen's disease and associated malignancies. Results of a survey. Dis Colon Rectum. 1987; 30(10):782–785

[39] Margenthaler JA, Dietz DW, Mutch MG, Birnbaum EH, Kodner IJ, Fleshman JW. Outcomes, risk of other malignancies, and need for formal mapping procedures in patients with perianal Bowen's disease. Dis Colon Rectum. 2004; 47(10):1655–1660, discussion 1660–1661

[40] Marchesa P, Fazio VW, Oliart S, Goldblum JR, Lavery IC. Perianal Bowen's disease: a clinicopathologic study of 47 patients. Dis Colon Rectum. 1997; 40(11):1286–1293

[41] Sarmiento JM, Wolff BG, Burgart LJ, Frizelle FA, Ilstrup DM. Perianal Bowen's disease: associated tumors, human papillomavirus, surgery, and other controversies. Dis Colon Rectum. 1997; 40(8):912–918

[42] Scholefield JH, Johnson J, Hitchcock A, et al. Guidelines for anal cytology–to make cytological diagnosis and follow up much more reliable. Cytopathology. 1998; 9(1):15–22

[43] Gupta AK, Browne M, Bluhm R. Imiquimod: a review. J Cutan Med Surg. 2002; 6(6):554–560

[44] Pehoushek J, Smith KJ. Imiquimod and 5% fluorouracil therapy for anal and perianal squamous cell carcinoma in situ in an HIV-1-positive man. Arch Dermatol. 2001; 137(1):14–16

[45] Gottesman L. Editorial. Dis Colon Rectum. 2004; 47:1660–1661

[46] Chang LK, Gottesman L, Breen EL, Bledag R. Anal dysplasia: controversies in management. Semin Colon Rectal Surg. 2004; 15:233–238

[47] Nouri K, O'Connell C, Rivas MP. Imiquimod for the treatment of Bowen's disease and invasive squamous cell carcinoma. J Drugs Dermatol. 2003; 2(6):669–673

[48] Chen K, Shumack S. Treatment of Bowen's disease using a cycle regimen of imiquimod 5% cream. Clin Exp Dermatol. 2003; 28 Suppl 1:10–12

[49] Graham BD, Jetmore AB, Foote JE, Arnold LK. Topical 5-fluorouracil in the management of extensive anal Bowen's disease: a preferred approach. Dis Colon Rectum. 2005; 48(3):444–450

[50] Skinner PP, Ogunbiyi OA, Scholefield JH, et al. Skin appendage involvement in anal intraepithelial neoplasia. Br J Surg. 1997; 84(5):675–678

[51] Berry JM, Jay N, Polefsky JM, Welton ML. State-of-the-art of high-resolution anoscopy as a tool to manage patients at risk for anal cancer. Semin Colon Rectal Surg. 2004; 15(4):218–226

[52] Cleary RK, Schaldenbrand JD, Fowler JJ, Schuler JM, Lampman RM. Treatment options for perianal Bowen's disease: survey of American Society of Colon and Rectal Surgeons members. Am Surg. 2000; 66(7):686–688

[53] Hassan I, Horgan AF, Nivatvongs S. V-Y island flaps for repair of large perianal defects. Am J Surg. 2001; 181(4):363–365

[54] Scholefield JH. Anal intraepithelial neoplasia. Br J Surg. 1999; 86 (11):1363–1364

[55] Welton ML, Winkler B, Darragh TM. Anal-rectal cytology and anal cancer screening. Semin Colon Rectal Surg. 2004; 15:196–200

[56] Goldstone SE, Winkler B, Ufford LJ, Alt E, Palefsky JM. High prevalence of anal squamous intraepithelial lesions and squamous-cell carcinoma in men who have sex with men as seen in a surgical practice. Dis Colon Rectum. 2001; 44(5):690–698

[57] Goldie SJ, Kuntz KM, Weinstein MC, Freedberg KA, Palefsky JM. Cost-effectiveness of screening for anal squamous intraepithelial lesions and anal cancer in human immunodeficiency virus-negative homosexual and bisexual men. Am J Med. 2000; 108(8):634–641

[58] Koutsky LA, Ault KA, Wheeler CM, et al. Proof of Principle Study Investigators. A controlled trial of a human papillomavirus type 16 vaccine. N Engl J Med. 2002; 347(21):1645–1651

[59] Stanberry LR. A human papillomavirus type 16 vaccine. Editorial. N Engl J Med. 2003; 348:1404

[60] http://www.merck.com/product/usa/pi_circulars/g/gardasil/gardasil_pi.pdf. Accessed February 5, 2016

[61] Beahrs OH, Wilson SM. Carcinoma of the anus. Ann Surg. 1976; 184 (4):422–428

[62] Papillon J, Chassard JL. Respective roles of radiotherapy and surgery in the management of epidermoid carcinoma of the anal margin. Series of 57 patients. Dis Colon Rectum. 1992; 35(5):422–429

[63] Möller C, Saksela E. Cancer of the anus and anal canal. Acta Chir Scand. 1970; 136(4):340–348

[64] Nelson RL, Prasad ML, Abcarian H. Anal carcinoma presenting as a perirectal abscess or fistula. Arch Surg. 1985; 120(5):632–635

[65] Fuchshuber PR, Rodriguez-Bigas M, Weber T, Petrelli NJ. Anal canal and perianal epidermoid cancers. J Am Coll Surg. 1997; 185(5):494–505

[66] Touboul E, Schlienger M, Buffat L, et al. Epidermoid carcinoma of the anal margin: 17 cases treated with curative-intent radiation therapy. Radiother Oncol. 1995; 34(3):195–202

[67] Schraut WH, Wang CH, Dawson PJ, Block GE. Depth of invasion, location, and size of cancer of the anus dictate operative treatment. Cancer. 1983; 51 (7):1291–1296

[68] Cummings BJ, Keane TJ, Hawkins NV, O'Sullivan B. Treatment of perianal carcinoma by radiation (RT) or radiation plus chemotherapy (RTCT). Int J Radiat Oncol Biol Phys. 1986; 12:170–173

[69] Paget J. On disease of the mammary areolar preceding cancer of the mammary gland. St. Bartholomew's Hosp Report. 1874; 10:87–89

[70] Tjandra J. Perianal Paget's disease. Report of three cases. Dis Colon Rectum. 1988; 31(6):462–466

[71] Darier J, Couillaud P. Sur un cas de maladie de Paget de la region kerineoanal et scrotale. Ann de Dermatole et de Syph. 1893; 4:25–31

[72] Armitage NC, Jass JR, Richman PI, Thomson JPS, Phillips RKS. Paget's disease of the anus: a clinicopathological study. Br J Surg. 1989; 76(1):60–63

[73] Rosai J. Rosai and Ackerman's Surgical Pathology. 8th ed. St. Louis, MO: CV Mosby; 1996:808–809

[74] Miller LR, McCunniff AJ, Randall ME. An immunohistochemical study of perianal Paget's disease. Possible origins and clinical implications. Cancer. 1992; 69(8):2166–2171

[75] Morson BC, Dawson IMP, Day DW, Jass JR, Price AB, Williams GT. Morson and Dawson's Gastrointestinal Pathology. London: Blackwell Scientific; 1990:673–675

[76] Beck DE. Paget's disease and Bowen's disease of the anus. Semin Colon Rectal Surg. 1995; 6:143–149

[77] Jensen SL, Sjølin KE, Shokouh-Amiri MH, Hagen K, Harling H. Paget's disease of the anal margin. Br J Surg. 1988; 75(11):1089–1092

[78] Park JS, Kerner BA. Perianal Paget's disease. Semin Colon Rectal Surg. 2003; 14:218–221

[79] Ohnishi T, Watanabe S. The use of cytokeratins 7 and 20 in the diagnosis of primary and secondary extramammary Paget's disease. Br J Dermatol. 2000; 142(2):243–247

[80] Goldblum JR, Hart WR. Perianal Paget's disease: a histologic and immunohistochemical study of 11 cases with and without associated rectal adenocarcinoma. Am J Surg Pathol. 1998; 22(2):170–179

[81] Brown RS, Lankester KJ, McCormack M, Power DA, Spittle MF. Radiotherapy for perianal Paget's disease. Clin Oncol. 2002; 14(4):272–284

[82] Sarmiento JM, Wolff BG, Burgart LJ, Frizelle FA, Ilstrup DM. Paget's disease of the perianal region–an aggressive disease? Dis Colon Rectum. 1997; 40 (10):1187–1194

[83] McCarter MD, Quan SH, Busam K, Paty PP, Wong D, Guillem JG. Long-term outcome of perianal Paget's disease. Dis Colon Rectum. 2003; 46 (5):612–616

[84] Marchesa P, Fazio VM, Oliart S, Goldblum JR, Lavery IC, Milsom JW. Long-term outcome of patients with perianal Paget's disease. Am Surg Oncol. 1997; 4:475–480

[85] Paterson CA, Young-Fadok TM, Dozois RR. Basal cell carcinoma of the perianal region: 20-year experience. Dis Colon Rectum. 1999; 42(9):1200–1202

[86] Nielsen OV, Jensen SL. Basal cell carcinoma of the anus—a clinical study of 34 cases. BR J Surg. 1981; 68:856–857

[87] Marks R, Gebauer K, Shumack S, et al. Australasian Multicentre Trial Group. Imiquimod 5% cream in the treatment of superficial basal cell carcinoma: results of a multicenter 6-week dose-response trial. J Am Acad Dermatol. 2001; 44(5):807–813

[88] Gordon PH. Current status–perianal and anal canal neoplasms. Dis Colon Rectum. 1990; 33(9):799–808

[89] Cintron J. Buschke-Lowenstein tumor of the perianal and anorectal region. Semin Colon Rectal Surg. 1995; 6:135–139

[90] Heinzerling LM, Kempf W, Kamarashev J, Hafner J, Nestle FO. Treatment of verrucous carcinoma with imiquimod and CO2 laser ablation. Dermatology. 2003; 207(1):119–122

[91] Foust RL, Dean PJ, Stoler MH, Moinuddin SM. Intraepithelial neoplasia of the anal canal in hemorrhoidal tissue: a study of 19 cases. Hum Pathol. 1991; 22 (6):528–534

[92] Chang GJ, Berry JM, Jay N, Palefsky JM, Welton ML. Surgical treatment of high-grade anal squamous intraepithelial lesions: a prospective study. Dis Colon Rectum. 2002; 45(4):453–458

[93] Jass JR, Sobin LH. Histological Typing of Intestinal Tumors. 2nd ed. Berlin: Springer-Verlag; 1989:90

[94] Stearns MW, Jr, Quan SH. Epidermoid carcinoma of the anorectum. Surg Gynecol Obstet. 1970; 131(5):953–957

[95] Welch JP, Malt RA. Appraisal of the treatment of carcinoma of the anus and anal canal. Surg Gynecol Obstet. 1977; 145(6):837–841

[96] Boman BM, Moertel CG, O'Connell MJ, et al. Carcinoma of the anal canal. A clinical and pathologic study of 188 cases. Cancer. 1984; 54(1):114–125

[97] Cummings BJ. Treatment of primary epidermoid carcinoma of the anal canal. Int J Colorectal Dis. 1987; 2(2):107–112

[98] Wade DS, Herrera L, Castillo NB, Petrelli NJ. Metastases to the lymph nodes in epidermoid carcinoma of the anal canal studied by a clearing technique. Surg Gynecol Obstet. 1989; 169(3):238–242

[99] Jensen SL, Hagen K, Harling H, Shokouh-Amiri MH, Nielsen OV. Long-term prognosis after radical treatment for squamous-cell carcinoma of the anal canal and anal margin. Dis Colon Rectum. 1988; 31(4):273–278

[100] Nigro ND, Vaitkevicius VK, Considine B, Jr. Combined therapy for cancer of the anal canal: a preliminary report. Dis Colon Rectum. 1974; 17(3):354–356

[101] Nigro ND. An evaluation of combined therapy for squamous cell cancer of the anal canal. Dis Colon Rectum. 1984; 27(12):763–766

[102] Sato H, Koh PK, Bartolo DC. Management of anal canal cancer. Dis Colon Rectum. 2005; 48(6):1301–1315

[103] Flam M, John M, Pajak TF, et al. Role of mitomycin in combination with fluorouracil and radiotherapy, and of salvage chemoradiation in the definitive nonsurgical treatment of epidermoid carcinoma of the anal canal: results of a phase III randomized intergroup study. J Clin Oncol. 1996; 14(9):2527–2539

[104] UKCCCR Anal Cancer Trial Working Party. UK Co-ordinating Committee on Cancer Research. Epidermoid anal cancer: results from the UKCCCR randomised trial of radiotherapy alone versus radiotherapy, 5-fluorouracil, and mitomycin. Lancet. 1996; 348(9034):1049–1054

[105] Bartelink H, Roelofsen F, Eschwege F, et al. Concomitant radiotherapy and chemotherapy is superior to radiotherapy alone in the treatment of locally advanced anal cancer: results of a phase III randomized trial of the European Organization for Research and Treatment of Cancer Radiotherapy and Gastrointestinal Cooperative Groups. J Clin Oncol. 1997; 15 (5):2040–2049

[106] Eng C, Abbruzzese J, Minsky BD. Chemotherapy and radiation of anal canal cancer: the first approach. Surg Oncol Clin N Am. 2004; 13(2):309–320, viii

[107] Stafford SL, Martenson JA. Combined radiation and chemotherapy for carcinoma of the anal canal. Oncology (Williston Park). 1998; 12(3):373–377, 381, discussion 382, 384, 38

[108] Myerson RJ, Kong F, Birnbaum EH, et al. Radiation therapy for epidermoid carcinoma of the anal canal, clinical and treatment factors associated with outcome. Radiother Oncol. 2001; 61(1):15–22

[109] Myerson RJ, Shapiro SJ, Lacey D, et al. Carcinoma of the anal canal. Am J Clin Oncol. 1995; 18(1):32–39

[110] Roed H, Engelholm SA, Svendsen LB, Rosendal F, Olsen KJ. Pulsed dose rate (PDR) brachytherapy of anal carcinoma. Radiother Oncol. 1996; 41 (2):131–134

[111] Kapp KS, Geyer E, Gebhart FH, et al. Experience with split-course external beam irradiation +/- chemotherapy and integrated Ir-192 high-dose-rate brachytherapy in the treatment of primary carcinomas of the anal canal. Int J Radiat Oncol Biol Phys. 2001; 49(4):997–1005

[112] Place RJ, Gregorcyk SG, Huber PJ, Simmang CL. Outcome analysis of HIV-positive patients with anal squamous cell carcinoma. Dis Colon Rectum. 2001; 44(4):506–512

[113] Kim JH, Sarani B, Orkin BA, et al. HIV-positive patients with anal carcinoma have poorer treatment tolerance and outcome than HIV-negative patients. Dis Colon Rectum. 2001; 44(10):1496–1502

[114] Berry JM, Palefsky JM, Welton ML. Anal cancer and its precursors in HIV-positive patients: perspectives and management. Surg Oncol Clin N Am. 2004; 13(2):355–373

[115] Blazy A, Hennequin C, Gornet JM, et al. Anal carcinomas in HIV-positive patients: high-dose chemoradiotherapy is feasible in the era of highly active antiretroviral therapy. Dis Colon Rectum. 2005; 48(6):1176–1181

[116] Cummings BJ, Keane TJ, O'Sullivan B, Wong CS, Catton CN. Epidermoid anal cancer: treatment by radiation alone or by radiation and 5-fluorouracil with and without mitomycin C. Int J Radiat Oncol Biol Phys. 1991; 21(5):1115–1125

[117] Tanum G, Tveit KM, Karlsen KO. Chemoradiotherapy of anal carcinoma: tumour response and acute toxicity. Oncology. 1993; 50(1):14–17

[118] Ellenhorn JD, Enker WE, Quan SH. Salvage abdominoperineal resection following combined chemotherapy and radiotherapy for epidermoid carcinoma of the anus. Ann Surg Oncol. 1994; 1(2):105–110

[119] Nguyen WD, Mitchell KM, Beck DE. Risk factors associated with requiring a stoma for the management of anal cancer. Dis Colon Rectum. 2004; 47 (6):843–846

[120] Longo WE, Vernava AM, III, Wade TP, Coplin MA, Virgo KS, Johnson FE. Recurrent squamous cell carcinoma of the anal canal. Predictors of initial treatment failure and results of salvage therapy. Ann Surg. 1994; 220 (1):40–49

[121] Ghouti L, Houvenaeghel G, Moutardier V, et al. Salvage abdominoperineal resection after failure of conservative treatment in anal epidermoid cancer. Dis Colon Rectum. 2005; 48(1):16–22

[122] Zelnick RS, Haas PA, Ajlouni M, Szilagyi E, Fox TA, Jr. Results of abdominoperineal resections for failures after combination chemotherapy and radiation therapy for anal canal cancers. Dis Colon Rectum. 1992; 35(6):574–577, discussion 577–578

[123] Gerard JP, Chapet O, Samiei F, et al. Management of inguinal lymph node metastases in patients with carcinoma of the anal canal: experience in a series of 270 patients treated in Lyon and review of the literature. Cancer. 2001; 92(1):77–84

[124] Cummings BJ, Thomas GM, Keane TJ, Harwood AR, Rider WD. Primary radiation therapy in the treatment of anal canal carcinoma. Dis Colon Rectum. 1982; 25(8):778–782

[125] Papillon J, Montbarbon JF. Epidermoid carcinoma of the anal canal. A series of 276 cases. Dis Colon Rectum. 1987; 30(5):324–333

[126] Stearns MW, Urmacher C, Sternborg SE, Woodruff J, Attiyeh FF. Cancer of the anal canal. Curr Probl Cancer. 1980; 4:1–44

[127] Ulmer C, Bembenek A, Gretschel S, et al. Refined staging by sentinel lymph node biopsy to individualize therapy in anal cancer. Ann Surg Oncol. 2004; 11(3) Suppl:259S–262S

[128] Gupta N, Longo WE, Vernara AM, Wade TP, Johnson FE. Treatment of recurrent epidermoid carcinoma of the anal canal. Semin Colon Rectal Surg. 1995; 6:160–165

[129] Gordon PH. Squamous-cell carcinoma of the anal canal. Surg Clin North Am. 1988; 68(6):1391–1399

[130] Tanum G, Tveit K, Karlsen KO, Hauer-Jensen M. Chemotherapy and radiation therapy for anal carcinoma. Survival and late morbidity. Cancer. 1991; 67 (10):2462–2466

[131] Basik M, Rodriguez-Bigas MA, Penetrante R, Petrelli NJ. Prognosis and recurrence patterns of anal adenocarcinoma. Am J Surg. 1995; 169 (2):233–237

[132] Tarazi R, Nelson R. Adenocarcinoma of the anus. Semin Colon Rectal Surg. 1995; 6:169–173

[133] Beal KP, Wong D, Guillem JG, et al. Primary adenocarcinoma of the anus treated with combined modality therapy. Dis Colon Rectum. 2003; 46 (10):1320–1324

[134] Hobbs CM, Lowry MA, Owen D, Sobin LH. Anal gland carcinoma. Cancer. 2001; 92(8):2045–2049

[135] Morson BC, Sobin LH. Histologic Typing of Intestinal Tumors. Geneva: World Health Organization; 1976

[136] Jensen SL, Shokouh-Amiri MH, Hagen K, Harling H, Nielsen OV. Adenocarcinoma of the anal ducts. A series of 21 cases. Dis Colon Rectum. 1988; 31 (4):268–272

[137] Perkowski PE, Sorrells DL, Evans JT, Nopajaroonsri C, Johnson LW. Anal duct carcinoma: case report and review of the literature. Am Surg. 2000; 66 (12):1149–1152

[138] Fenger C. Anal canal tumors and their precursors. Pathol Annu. 1988; 23(Pt 1):45–66

[139] Schaffzin DM, Stahl TJ, Smith LE. Perianal mucinous adenocarcinoma: unusual case presentations and review of the literature. Am Surg. 2003; 69 (2):166–169

[140] Fenger C, Morson BC. Anal duct carcinoma. [editorial]. Dis Colon Rectum. 1989; 32(4):355–357

[141] Getz SB, Jr, Ough YD, Patterson RB, Kovalcik PJ. Mucinous adenocarcinoma developing in chronic anal fistula: report of two cases and review of the literature. Dis Colon Rectum. 1981; 24(7):562–566

[142] Belkacémi Y, Berger C, Poortmans P, et al. Rare Cancer Network. Management of primary anal canal adenocarcinoma: a large retrospective study from the Rare Cancer Network. Int J Radiat Oncol Biol Phys. 2003; 56 (5):1274–1283

[143] Abel ME, Chiu YS, Russell TR, Volpe PA. Adenocarcinoma of the anal glands. Results of a survey. Dis Colon Rectum. 1993; 36(4):383–387

[144] Tarazi R, Nelson RL. Anal adenocarcinoma: a comprehensive review. Semin Colon Rectal Surg. 1994; 10:235–240

[145] Papagikos M, Crane CH, Skibber J, et al. Chemoradiation for adenocarcinoma of the anus. Int J Radiat Oncol Biol Phys. 2003; 55(3):669–678

[146] Paterson C, Musselman L, Chorneyko K, Reid S, Rawlinson J. Merkel cell (neuroendocrine) carcinoma of the anal canal: report of a case. Dis Colon Rectum. 2003; 46(5):676–678

[147] Coquard R. Merkel cell carcinoma of the anal canal: importance of radiotherapy. [Editorial]. Dis Colon Rectum. 2004; 47(2):256–257, author reply 257

[148] Mason JK, Helwig EB. Ano-rectal melanoma. Cancer. 1966; 19(1):39–50

[149] Thibault C, Sagar P, Nivatvongs S, Ilstrup DM, Wolff BG. Anorectal melanoma—an incurable disease? Dis Colon Rectum. 1997; 40(6):661–668

[150] Cagir B, Whiteford MH, Topham A, Rakinic J, Fry RD. Changing epidemiology of anorectal melanoma. Dis Colon Rectum. 1999; 42 (9):1203–1208

[151] Ward MW, Romano G, Nicholls RJ. The surgical treatment of anorectal malignant melanoma. Br J Surg. 1986; 73(1):68–69

[152] Werdin C, Limas C, Knodell RG. Primary malignant melanoma of the rectum. Evidence for origination from rectal mucosal melanocytes. Cancer. 1988; 61 (7):1364–1370

[153] Quan SHQ. Malignant melanoma of the anorectum. Semin Colon Rectal Surg. 1995; 6:166–168

[154] Antoniuk PM, Tjandra JJ, Webb BW, Petras RE, Milsom JW, Fazio VW. Anorectal malignant melanoma has a poor prognosis. Int J Colorectal Dis. 1993; 8(2):81–86

[155] Chiu YS, Unni KK, Beart RW, Jr. Malignant melanoma of the anorectum. Dis Colon Rectum. 1980; 23(2):122–124

[156] Bullard KM, Tuttle TM, Rothenberger DA, et al. Surgical therapy for anorectal melanoma. J Am Coll Surg. 2003; 196(2):206–211

[157] Malik A, Hull TL, Milsom J. Long-term survivor of anorectal melanoma: report of a case. Dis Colon Rectum. 2002; 45(10):1412–1415, discussion 1415–1417

[158] Cooper PH, Mills SE, Allen MS, Jr. Malignant melanoma of the anus: report of 12 patients and analysis of 255 additional cases. Dis Colon Rectum. 1982; 25 (7):693–703

[159] Wolff BG. Anorectal melanoma. [Editorial]. Dis Colon Rectum. 2002; 45:1415

[160] Brady MS, Kavolius JP, Quan SH. Anorectal melanoma. A 64-year experience at Memorial Sloan-Kettering Cancer Center. Dis Colon Rectum. 1995; 38(2):146–151

[161] Pessaux P, Pocard M, Elias D, et al. Surgical management of primary anorectal melanoma. Br J Surg. 2004; 91(9):1183–1187

[162] Ward MW, Romano G, Nichollo RJ. The surgical treatment of anorectal malignant melanoma. Br J Surg. 1986; 73:68–69

[163] Roumen RM. Anorectal melanoma in The Netherlands: a report of 63 patients. Eur J Surg Oncol. 1996; 22(6):598–601

[164] Ross M, Pezzi C, Pezzi T, Meurer D, Hickey R, Balch C. Patterns of failure in anorectal melanoma. A guide to surgical therapy. Arch Surg. 1990; 125 (3):313–316

[165] Slingluff CL, Jr, Vollmer RT, Seigler HF. Anorectal melanoma: clinical characteristics and results of surgical management in twenty-four patients. Surgery. 1990; 107(1):1–9

[166] Goldman S, Glimelius B, Påhlman L. Anorectal malignant melanoma in Sweden. Report of 49 patients. Dis Colon Rectum. 1990; 33(10):874–877

Part III

Colorectal Disorders

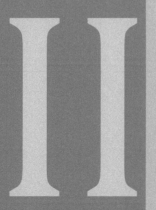

18 Rectal Prolapse

Janice F. Rafferty

Abstract

The term *rectal prolapse* encompasses a spectrum of disorders that result from intussusception or invagination of the rectal wall in a partial-thickness or full-thickness fashion, in varying degrees of protrusion to and through the anal sphincter complex. Surgical treatment is the mainstay of therapy for symptomatic rectal prolapse. Nonoperative therapies have a role for elderly patients with severe comorbidities. For patients with full-thickness prolapse due to straining and constipation, fiber supplements and laxatives can be helpful. Conservative treatments include pelvic floor muscle training and are often recommended as a first step.

Keywords: rectal prolapse, rectal procidentia, operative management, partial thickness, full thickness, classification, fecal leakage, constipation, straining, intussusception

18.1 Introduction

The term *rectal prolapse* encompasses a spectrum of disorders that result from intussusception or invagination of the rectal wall in a partial-thickness or full-thickness fashion, in varying degrees of protrusion to and through the anal sphincter complex. Early authors recognized that the underlying abnormality starts well above the pelvic floor, and described the importance of herniation of the pouch of Douglas[1,2] rather than a disorder of the physiology of the anal sphincter (▶ Fig. 18.1). An anatomic classification of the disorder provided a bit more clarity regarding the differing degrees of prolapse,[3] essentially recognizing the difference between mucosal prolapse (type I), internal intussusception (type II), and full-thickness rectal prolapse (type III). Anatomic abnormalities commonly found in rectal prolapse include diastasis of the levator ani, a deep cul-de-sac, redundant sigmoid colon, patulous anal sphincter, and attenuation of the fibrous attachments between the rectum and the sacrum.[4] No classification system has been universally accepted, and there is no consensus on the relative contribution of various abnormalities such as pelvic floor laxity, prior pregnancy, connective tissue disorders, and chronic constipation to the abnormality that presents as rectal prolapse.

18.2 Symptoms and Risk Factors

The symptoms associated with rectal prolapse can be quite debilitating and have a markedly negative impact on a patient's activities of daily living. Women age 50 and older are six times more likely to present with rectal prolapse than men,[5] with the peak incidence in the seventh decade; multiparity in women is not a prerequisite. Young patients with rectal prolapse are more likely to have a syndrome associated with developmental delay or a psychiatric diagnosis requiring medial therapy.[6] Common patient complaints include fecal incontinence, seepage of mucus, bleeding, discomfort due to protrusion of tissue, and constipation. Fecal incontinence is present in up to 75% of patients with complete rectal prolapse,[7] but the cause of this is unclear. It makes sense that rectal eversion bypassing the anal sphincter would lead to fecal leakage, but other contributing factors likely include continuous stimulation of the rectoanal inhibitory reflex, stretch of the sphincter mechanism, and possibly stretch injury to the pudendal nerve with resultant denervation of the pelvic floor.[8] Patients who complain of "constipation" and the need to strain deserve a closer look, as they may actually have internal intussusception (or occult prolapse) acting as an obstruction to normal defecation.

Risk factors associated with the development of adult prolapse are the same as those that predispose patients to a weak pelvic floor. These include large birth weight of vaginally delivered babies, prior pelvic surgery, increased body mass index, chronic straining, chronic diarrhea, chronic constipation, cystic fibrosis, neurologic diseases that lead to denervation of the pelvic floor (i.e., cauda equina syndrome, spinal cord lesions), connective tissue disorders (i.e., Marfan's syndrome, Ehlers–Danlos syndrome), dementia, and stroke.[9]

18.3 Examination and Evaluation

The diagnosis of circumferential full-thickness rectal prolapse is unmistakable, and must be distinguished from circumferential hemorrhoidal prolapse by the trained observer (▶ Fig. 18.2). However, the seasoned physician must carefully evaluate the understated complaints associated with the spectrum of abnormalities with rectal prolapse. A thorough exam of the abdomen and perineum is indicated.

When examined prone, or in lateral decubitus position, findings commonly include absence of prolapse but a flattened perineum and patulous anus. Despite a wide-open anal canal, many patients can generate a high voluntary squeeze pressure, and this finding should be noted as it can influence the decision of operative approach. Mucus is frequently present on the perianal skin. The prolapse should be visualized directly to make an accurate diagnosis and plan surgical strategy. Asking the patient to sit on the commode and strain can often produce it. Once visualized, the configuration of the mucosal folds, length, and viability of prolapsing segment should be noted, as well as prolapse of other pelvic organs (▶ Fig. 18.3). Mucosal folds should be concentric, as opposed to the radial folds associated with circumferential hemorrhoidal prolapse. With complete prolapse, a sulcus is present between the anus and the protruding mucosa; this finding is not present in a patient with circumferential mucosal or hemorrhoidal prolapse (▶ Fig. 18.4). Proctoscopy will often show a ring of edema and erythema 5 to 6 cm from the anal verge.

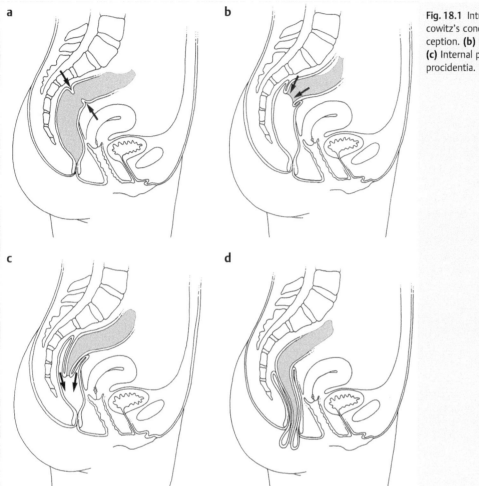

Fig. 18.1 Intussusception analogous to Moschcowitz's concept. **(a)** Starting point of intussusception. **(b)** Early point of intussusception. **(c)** Internal procidentia. **(d)** Complete procidentia.

The patient with *internal intussusception* may complain of "constipation" but on further questioning may admit to a sense of fullness, incomplete evacuation, and passage of bloody mucus. This patient may sit on the toilet for prolonged periods of time attempting to evacuate, with no satisfactory passage of stool. Those with resultant solitary rectal ulcer syndrome may develop deep ulceration of the rectal wall that causes pain and bleeding, and grossly appears similar to neoplastic change, or Crohn's disease. Biopsies, however, will confirm benign disease, showing mucosal and muscular hyperplasia, surface erosion, and mild inflammation—occasionally called colitis cystica profunda. Exam of the perineum may reveal flattening associated with dyssynergia of the pelvic floor, while on digital rectal exam good tone but no mass is found. Straining on the commode often reveals marked perineal descent with opening of the anal orifice revealing mucosa that does not prolapse beyond the anal verge. Proctoscopy will likely reveal a ring of erythema, induration, and possibly ulceration on the anterior rectal wall, 5 to 6 cm from the anal verge.

In addition to physical exam, certain diagnostic tests can be used selectively to refine the diagnosis and expose other associated pathology. Commonly used modalities include defecography or dynamic magnetic resonance imaging (MRI), colonoscopy, and urodynamics. Defecography or dynamic MRI with contrast can clarify the presence and extent of contiguous organ prolapse, such as cystocele, enterocele, sigmoidocele, and vaginal vault. Defecography has altered management strategy in up to 40% of patients presenting with rectal prolapse.[10] The benefit of MRI compared with fluoroscopy is that it is noninvasive, there is no radiation exposure, it provides simultaneous dynamic evaluation of all pelvic organs in multiple planes, and it allows visualization of pelvic floor support structures. Dynamic MRI correlates well with fluoroscopic studies in the identification of pelvic organ prolapse.[11] Depending on patient symptoms, these other organs may require treatment as well.

Colonoscopy rarely changes the management of rectal prolapse, but is important to rule out other abnormalities, especially neoplastic change.[12] Findings visually concerning for neoplasia may be confused with solitary rectal ulcer during endoscopic evaluation. Urodynamics may be indicated to evaluate the patient with concurrent symptoms of a vaginal bulge or urinary incontinence.[13]

The role of pelvic floor physiology testing in the evaluation of rectal prolapse is limited, but may explain the dysfunction in a chronically constipated patient, or define the anatomy of the

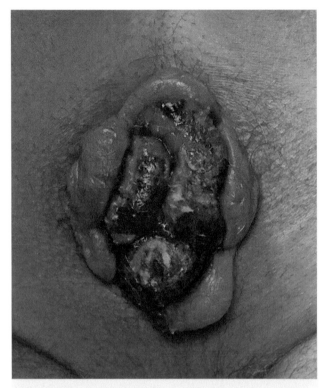

Fig. 18.2 Circumferential prolapsed internal hemorrhoids.

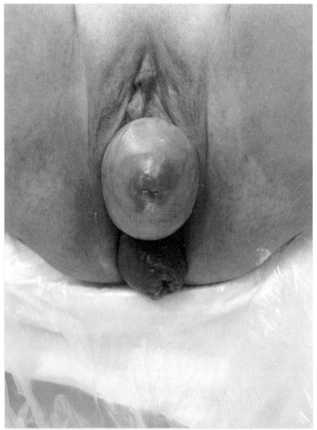

Fig. 18.3 Combined prolapse of the rectum and vagina.

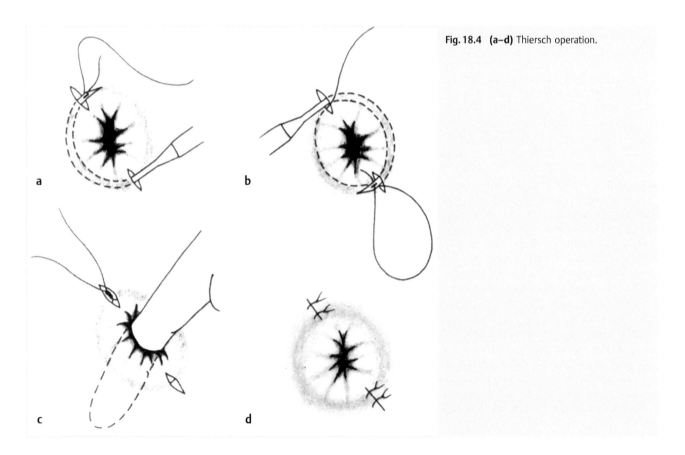

Fig. 18.4 (a–d) Thiersch operation.

anal sphincter in a patient with prior anal surgery who complains of fecal incontinence. Patients who complain of chronic constipation and prolapse should have pelvic floor dyssynergia ruled out with anal manometry and defecography, since they may benefit from pelvic floor physical therapy in the perioperative period. A sitz marker study to rule out colonic inertia may have a role, in addition to a complete metabolic evaluation to rule out one of the myriad causes of slow transit constipation. Delayed pudendal nerve conduction may have prognostic significance for continence, but this is not a reliable predictor of post-op control.[14] In general, patients with fecal incontinence that developed with progressive prolapse will notice improved continence once the prolapse is repaired. Those with questionable sphincter defects and a history of prior anal surgery can have the status of the sphincter complex documented prior to repair using ultrasound technology.

18.4 Treatment

Surgical treatment is the mainstay of therapy for symptomatic rectal prolapse. Nonoperative therapies may have a role in the treatment of elderly patients with severe comorbidities, but are utilized mostly to prevent the frequency and severity of the prolapse, or to assist in reducing the prolapse that is incarcerated.[15] For the patient who produces full-thickness rectal prolapse due to straining and constipation, fiber supplements and laxatives can be helpful in reducing the need to strain. Conservative methods including pelvic floor muscle training are often recommended as a first step, and may lead to an improvement in bowel symptoms.[16]

The anal encirclement procedure was first described in 1891, and has evolved into a procedure that is generally used in the palliative setting. It can be performed under local anesthesia. When combined with a Delorme procedure, outcomes are improved and recurrence rates are decreased.[17] While silver wire was the original implant, other materials have been described such as a monofilament nonabsorbable suture, synthetic mesh, and braided vascular graft. The implant is buried in the ischioanal fat and tied snugly (▶ Fig. 18.4). Bulk-forming agents and laxatives will generally be required following anal encirclement.

Two other approaches, transabdominal and transperineal, are most often considered in the operative repair of rectal prolapse; the range of surgical techniques described to correct the underlying defects reflects the lack of consensus regarding the best operation. A recent review of all randomized controlled trials of surgery to date for managing adult full-thickness rectal prolapse found that the heterogeneity of objectives, interventions, and outcomes makes cogent analysis very difficult. In fact, there were insufficient data across 15 randomized controlled trials involving over 1,000 patients to say which of the abdominal or perineal approaches is most effective.[18]

The recommended surgical approach is therefore patient-specific, and should be dictated by the comorbidities of the patient, the surgeon's preference and experience, and the patient's age and bowel function.[19] Great care should be taken to understand each patient's symptoms, bowel habits, continence, anatomy, and preoperative expectations[20] before choosing the

appropriate surgical technique for a specific patient. Traditionally, for patients who have an acceptable risk profile for abdominal surgery, procedures incorporating transabdominal rectal fixation have been the procedure of choice[13] as they are thought to lead to a lower rate of recurrent prolapse. However, no significant difference has consistently been found in the rate of recurrent prolapse for patients treated with a transabdominal as compared to a transperineal repair.[21] When the patients are appropriately chosen, there is no significant difference in the rate of morbidity and mortality between a perineal or abdominal approach to repair.[22] In addition, no significant difference has been reported in randomized comparisons of perineal procedures and abdominal procedures. All surgical procedures to treat rectal prolapse have been found to result in substantial improvements from baseline in quality of life.[23] The surgical management of external rectal prolapse has evolved, however. More surgeons currently favor an abdominal approach, and the frequency of perineal approach has decreased as evidence mounts that even elderly debilitated patients may tolerate a minimally invasive abdominal procedure. Delorme's operation remains the most popular perineal procedure of choice, but the incidence of the use of Altemeier's procedure has increased.[24]

18.4.1 Transabdominal Rectal Fixation Procedures

The goal of all transabdominal approaches to repair full-thickness rectal prolapse is to draw the prolapsed rectum up out of the pelvis and secure it to the presacral fascia; simple anterior resection without fixation has fallen into disuse as it is associated with a recurrence rate that continues to increase over time.[25] A multitude of procedures have been described for transabdominal fixation, and they differ in their approach (traditional open vs. minimally invasive), extent of rectal mobilization (anterior, posterior, or both), use of mesh (synthetic or biologic), and addition of sigmoid resection. Complete and circumferential mobilization of the rectum down to the level of the pelvic floor for the repair of rectal prolapse has a high rate of postoperative constipation and obstructed defecation,[26] possibly due to division of the autonomic nerves in the lateral stalks,[27] so there is general agreement that limited dissection in the anterior plane, posterior plane, or both, leaving the lateral stalks intact, is preferred. Procedures tend to be performed based on surgeon preference and experience.

Suture Rectopexy

Suture suspension of the rectum to the presacral fascia with nonabsorbable sutures leads to a remarkably low rate of recurrent rectal prolapse (3–9%),[28] whether performed in an open or laparoscopic fashion.[29] Suture fixation was first described in 1959,[30] and prevents redundant bowel from intussuscepting into the distal pelvis. The scarring and fibrosis from not only suture fixation but also complete mobilization of the rectum may play a role in the success of suture rectopexy as well.[31] Of those patients who complain of diarrhea and incontinence in the setting of rectal prolapse, many regain bowel control after this procedure[32,33]; these patients do not

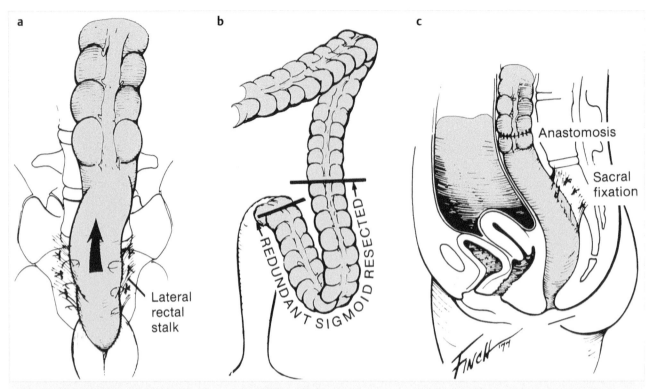

Fig. 18.5 Abdominal proctopexy and sigmoid resection. **(a)** After full mobilization by sharp dissection, the tissues lateral to the rectal wall are swept away laterally. **(b)** Resection of the redundant sigmoid colon. **(c)** Anastomosis completed and rectopexy sutures are placed.

seem predisposed to develop constipation after simple suture rectopexy, whereas approximately 15% of patients experience new constipation following rectopexy. Over half of those who are constipated before surgery are made worse.[34]

The concern over worsening constipation after prolapse repair has led many surgeons to combine suture or mesh rectopexy with sigmoid resection for those patients with preexisting constipation (▶ Fig. 18.5). Adding resection to simple suture suspension seems to improve functional results with minimal increase in morbidity.[29] Segmental resection of the colon appears to reduce the incidence of persistent constipation in a chronically constipated patient,[19] even though segmental resection of the colon for the treatment of constipation, in the absence of prolapse, has not proven to be of benefit. One should consider ruling out colonic inertia before offering a segmental resection to insure the patient does not have dysmotility of the entire colon.

Suture rectopexy, with or without sigmoid colon resection, can also be successfully performed using minimally invasive techniques, with acceptable morbidity and recurrence rates.[35] Patients who undergo laparoscopic rectopexy have been reported to have a shorter length of stay and lower surgical site infection rate than patients who have open abdominal procedures for the repair of a full-thickness rectal prolapse.[36]

Rectopexy Using Mesh

Fixation of the rectum to the sacrum using prosthetic material is thought to decrease the risk of recurrent rectal prolapse. The original mesh fixation described by Ripstein involved mobilization of the rectum, followed by mesh secured to the anterior aspect of the rectum and the presacral fascia bilaterally. While this resulted in acceptable recurrence rates, the incidence of erosion of the mesh on the anterior wall of the rectum was unacceptable. Therefore, the procedure was modified so that mesh was secured to the *lateral* aspect of the rectum and presacral fascia; this resulted in both acceptable recurrence rates and lower complication rates.[37] Still, concerns over complications related to the placement of synthetic mesh in the pelvis—bowel obstruction, ureteral injury, infection—have led many surgeons to abandon its use.

Traditional open surgery for the repair of rectal prolapse has been largely replaced by minimally invasive techniques, which has been well documented to be as effective as traditional open surgery in terms of clinical results, functional results, and recurrence rates. In addition, significant improvements in postoperative pain, length of hospital stay, wound infection rate, and time to recover are widely reported.[38,39] Laparoscopic rectopexy appears to be safe in the older patient as well, and might be a reasonable alternative to perineal repair in selected elderly patients.[40]

The laparoscopic ventral mesh rectopexy (LVMR) has evolved from the Orr–Loygue procedure, which involved anterior and posterior rectal mobilization to the level of the levator ani muscle, with excision of the pouch of Douglas. Two separate pieces of mesh were secured to the anterolateral walls of the rectum and the sacral promontory.[41] This was later modified to a procedure with ventral dissection and mobilization only, without excising the pouch of Douglas, but still incorporating mesh fixation.[42] This appears to reduce the incidence of postoperative constipation, by avoiding posterior lateral mobilization of the rectum. Some authors, however, believe that excision of the abnormally deep pouch of Douglas is an integral part of the procedure that will lead to a lower recurrence rate.[43] LVMR has recurrence rates that are not inferior to traditional open mesh rectopexy (8.2%), with a low rate of mesh-related complications (4.6%).[44] An increased incidence of mesh erosion has been reported when LVMR is combined with perineal surgery, such as posterior colporrhaphy.[45] A recent meta-analysis has failed to show a significant difference between minimally invasive techniques (laparoscopic vs. robotic), although currently there tend to be longer operative times and higher costs with robotic surgery.[46]

The optimal type of mesh used to augment rectal fixation is debatable. Traditionally, synthetic nonabsorbable mesh implants have been used, but have resulted in complications in certain patients including bowel obstruction, erosion into rectum or contiguous organs, and infection. This has led to the occasional use of biologic mesh, and although its safety profile is good, the long-term outcome is not clear.[47] The use of staplers and tackers to fix the mesh to the sacrum, especially in the minimally invasive setting, has been described as faster and easier than the use of sutures, and may be an improvement leading to wider adoption of minimally invasive techniques.[41]

18.4.2 Perineal Procedures

Patients with mucosal prolapse, or a short segment of a full-thickness rectal prolapse, should be considered for a Delorme procedure. In this procedure, the segment of prolapsed rectal mucosa is resected, and the underlying muscle wall is imbricated or plicated. The mucosa is then anastomosed to the top of the anal transition zone (▶ Fig. 18.6). Plication of the muscular wall of the rectum adds bulk above the anal sphincter complex, and may improve continence in select patients with preexisting leakage due to increased rest and squeeze pressures in the anal canal. This procedure is advocated for patients who are considered high risk for general anesthesia or those with preexisting fecal incontinence in the setting of a short segment prolapse.[48] Reported complications are those seen with perineal surgery, including constipation, fecal incontinence, urgency, and tenesmus. In most reports, recurrence rates are higher, but this procedure is easily repeated.

Patients with a longer segment of full-thickness rectal prolapse who are not suitable for general anesthesia, or an abdominal operation, may be best treated with a perineal proctectomy. This procedure was originally described by Dr. William Altemeier at the University of Cincinnati in 1956. It is most commonly recommended for older or debilitated patients with significant comorbidities who have contraindications to abdominal repair. Although recurrence rates may be higher than transabdominal rectal fixation, the complication rate is lower, and length of hospital stay is generally shorter.[49] One of the drawbacks of this approach is resection of the rectal reservoir, which may contribute to defecatory dysfunction after repair of the prolapse. Concurrent posterior levator plication decreases the anorectal angle, and may have a beneficial effect on postoperative continence, however.[50] For this reason, the preference of one of the editors (SDW) is to create a transperineal colonic J pouch and stapled or hand-sewn coloanal anastomosis.[51] Muscle plication is performed with nonabsorbable sutures in the posterior midline prior to performing the handsewn coloanal anastomosis (▶ Fig. 18.7).

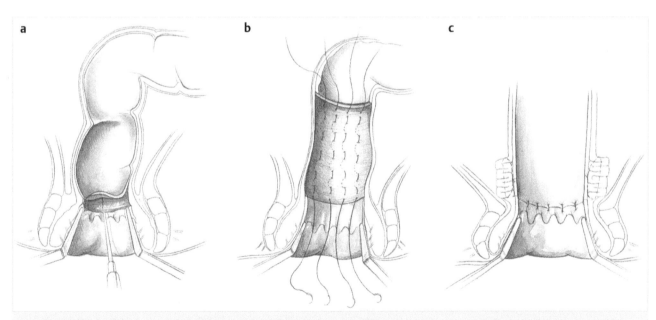

Fig. 18.6 Modified Delorme's technique. **(a)** Endorectal mobilization of mucosa. **(b)** Plication of muscular wall after redundant mucosa excised. **(c)** Completed muscle plication and reanastomosis of mucosal tube.

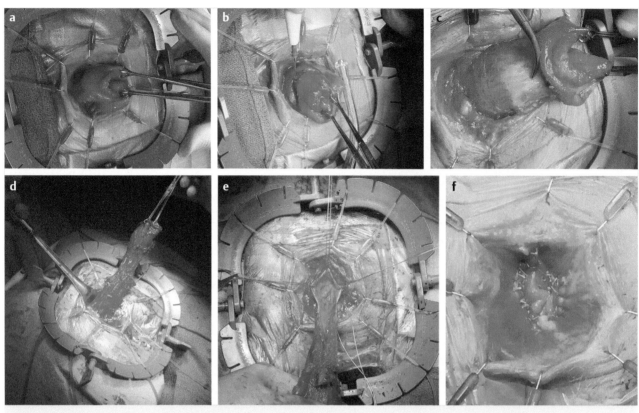

Fig. 18.7 (a–f) Perineal proctectomy.

References

[1] Moscowitz AV. The pathogenesis, anatomy and cure of prolapse of the rectum. Surg Gynecol Obstet. 1912; 15:7–21

[2] Brodén B, Snellman B. Procidentia of the rectum studied with cineradiography. A contribution to the discussion of causative mechanism. Dis Colon Rectum. 1968; 11(5):330–347

[3] Altemeier WA, Culbertson WR, Schowengerdt C, Hunt J. Nineteen years' experience with the one-stage perineal repair of rectal prolapse. Ann Surg. 1971; 173(6):993–1006

[4] Parks AG, Swash M, Urich H. Sphincter denervation in anorectal incontinence and rectal prolapse. Gut. 1977; 18(8):656–665

[5] Kairaluoma MV, Kellokumpu IH. Epidemiologic aspects of complete rectal prolapse. Scand J Surg. 2005; 94(3):207–210

[6] Marceau C, Parc Y, Debroux E, Tiret E, Parc R. Complete rectal prolapse in young patients: psychiatric disease a risk factor of poor outcome. Colorectal Dis. 2005; 7(4):360–365

[7] Kim DS, Tsang CB, Wong WD, Lowry AC, Goldberg SM, Madoff RD. Complete rectal prolapse: evolution of management and results. Dis Colon Rectum. 1999; 42(4):460–466, discussion 466–469

[8] Glasgow SC, Birnbaum EH, Kodner IJ, Fleshman JW, Dietz DW. Preoperative anal manometry predicts continence after perineal proctectomy for rectal prolapse. Dis Colon Rectum. 2006; 49(7):1052–1058

[9] Hatch Q, Steele SR. Rectal prolapse and intussusception. Gastroenterol Clin North Am. 2013; 42(4):837–861

[10] Harvey CJ, Halligan S, Bartram CI, Hollings N, Sahdev A, Kingston K. Evacuation proctography: a prospective study of diagnostic and therapeutic effects. Radiology. 1999; 211(1):223–227

[11] Hetzer FH, Andreisek G, Tsagari C, Sahrbacher U, Weishaupt D. MR defecography in patients with fecal incontinence: imaging findings and their effect on surgical management. Radiology. 2006; 240(2):449–457

[12] Bounovas A, Polychronidis A, Laftsidis P, Simopoulos C. Sigmoid colon cancer presenting as complete rectal prolapse. Colorectal Dis. 2007; 9:665–666

[13] Varma M, Rafferty J, Buie WD, Standards Practice Task Force of American Society of Colon and Rectal Surgeons. Practice parameters for the management of rectal prolapse. Dis Colon Rectum. 2011; 54(11):1339–1346

[14] Felt-Bersma RJ, Tiersma ES, Cuesta MA. Rectal prolapse, rectal intussusception, rectocele, solitary rectal ulcer syndrome, and enterocele. Gastroenterol Clin North Am. 2008; 37(3):645–668, ix

[15] Myers JO, Rothenberger DA. Sugar in the reduction of incarcerated prolapsed bowel. Report of two cases. Dis Colon Rectum. 1991; 34(5):416–418

[16] Hagen S, Stark D. Conservative prevention and management of pelvic organ prolapse in women. Cochrane Database Syst Rev. 2011(12):CD003882

[17] Warwick AM, Zimmermann E, Boorman PA, Smart NJ, Gee AS. Recurrence rate after Delorme's procedure with simultaneous placement of a Thiersch suture. Ann R Coll Surg Engl. 2016; 98(6):419–421

[18] Tou S, Brown SR, Nelson RL. Surgery for complete (full-thickness) rectal prolapse in adults. Cochrane Database Syst Rev. 2015(11):CD001758

[19] Brown AJ, Anderson JH, McKee RF, Finlay IG. Strategy for selection of type of operation for rectal prolapse based on clinical criteria. Dis Colon Rectum. 2004; 47(1):103–107

[20] Bordeianou L, Hicks CW, Kaiser AM, Alavi K, Sudan R, Wise PE. Rectal prolapse: an overview of clinical features, diagnosis, and patient-specific management strategies. J Gastrointest Surg. 2014; 18(5):1059–1069

[21] Ricciardi R, Roberts PL, Read TE, Hall JF, Marcello PW, Schoetz DJ. Which operative repair is associated with a higher likelihood of reoperation after rectal prolapse repair? Am Surg. 2014; 80(11):1128–1131

[22] Mustain WC, Davenport DL, Parcells JP, Vargas HD, Hourigan JS. Abdominal versus perineal approach for treatment of rectal prolapse: comparable safety in a propensity-matched cohort. Am Surg. 2013; 79(7):686–692

[23] Senapati A, Gray RG, Middleton LJ, et al. PROSPER Collaborative Group. PROSPER: a randomised comparison of surgical treatments for rectal prolapse. Colorectal Dis. 2013; 15(7):858–868

[24] Gunner CK, Senapati A, Northover JM, Brown SR. Life after PROSPER. What do people do for external rectal prolapse? Colorectal Dis. 2016; 18(8):811–814

[25] Schlinkert RT, Beart RW, Jr, Wolff BG, Pemberton JH. Anterior resection for complete rectal prolapse. Dis Colon Rectum. 1985; 28(6):409–412

[26] Samaranayake CB, Luo C, Plank AW, Merrie AE, Plank LD, Bissett IP. Systematic review on ventral rectopexy for rectal prolapse and intussusception. Colorectal Dis. 2010; 12(6):504–512

[27] Rutegård J, Sandzén B, Stenling R, Wiig J, Heald RJ. Lateral rectal ligaments contain important nerves. Br J Surg. 1997; 84(11):1544–1545

[28] Graf W, Karlbom U, Påhlman L, Nilsson S, Ejerblad S. Functional results after abdominal suture rectopexy for rectal prolapse or intussusception. Eur J Surg. 1996; 162(11):905–911

[29] Gomes-Ferreira C, Schneider A, Phillippe P, Lacreuse I, Becmeur F. Laparoscopic modified Orr-Loygue mesh rectopexy for rectal prolapse in children. J Ped Surg. 2015; 50(2):353–355

[30] Cutait D. Sacro-promontory fixation of the rectum for complete rectal prolapse. Proc R Soc Med. 1959; 52(Suppl):105

[31] Bishawi M, Foppa C, Tou S, Bergamaschi R, Rectal Prolapse Recurrence Study Group. Recurrence of rectal prolapse following rectopexy: a pooled analysis of 532 patients. Colorectal Dis. 2016; 18(8):779–784

[32] Douard R, Frileux P, Brunel M, Attal E, Tiret E, Parc R. Functional results after the Orr-Loygue transabdominal rectopexy for complete rectal prolapse. Dis Colon Rectum. 2003; 46(8):1089–1096

[33] Foppa C, Martinek L, Arnaud JP, Bergamaschi R. Ten-year follow up after laparoscopic suture rectopexy for full-thickness rectal prolapse. Colorectal Dis. 2014; 16(10):809–814

[34] Aitola PT, Hiltunen KM, Matikainen MJ. Functional results of operative treatment of rectal prolapse over an 11-year period: emphasis on transabdominal approach. Dis Colon Rectum. 1999; 42(5):655–660

[35] Foppa C, Martinek L, Arnaud JP, Bergamaschi R. Ten-year follow up after laparoscopic suture rectopexy for full-thickness rectal prolapse. Colorectal Dis. 2014; 16(10):809–814

[36] Magruder JT, Efron JE, Wick EC, Gearhart SL. Laparoscopic rectopexy for rectal prolapse to reduce surgical-site infections and length of stay. World J Surg. 2013; 37(5):1110–1114

[37] Roberts PL, Schoetz DJ, Jr, Coller JA, Veidenheimer MC. Ripstein procedure. Lahey Clinic experience: 1963–1985. Arch Surg. 1988; 123(5):554–557

[38] Randall J, Smyth E, McCarthy K, Dixon AR. Outcome of laparoscopic ventral mesh rectopexy for external rectal prolapse. Colorectal Dis. 2014; 16(11):914–919

[39] Evans C, Stevenson AR, Sileri P, et al. A Multicenter Collaboration to Assess the Safety of Laparoscopic Ventral Rectopexy. Dis Colon Rectum. 2015; 58 (8):799–807

[40] Dyrberg DL, Nordentoft T, Rosenstock S. Laparoscopic posterior mesh rectopexy for rectal prolapse is a safe procedure in older patients: A prospective follow-up study. Scand J Surg. 2015; 104(4):227–232

[41] Loygue J, Nordlinger B, Cunci O, Malafosse M, Huguet C, Parc R. Rectopexy to the promontory for the treatment of rectal prolapse. Report of 257 cases. Dis Colon Rectum. 1984; 27(6):356–359

[42] D'Hoore A, Cadoni R, Penninckx F. Long-term outcome of laparoscopic ventral rectopexy for total rectal prolapse. Br J Surg. 2004; 91(11):1500–1505

[43] Faucheron JL, Voirin D, Riboud R, Waroquet PA, Noel J. Laparoscopic anterior rectopexy to the promontory for full thickness rectal prolapse in 175 consecutive patients: short- and long-term follow up. Dis Colon Rectum. 2012; 13:561–566

[44] Consten EC, van Iersel JJ, Verheijen PM, Broeders IA, Wolthuis AM, D'Hoore A. Long-term Outcome After Laparoscopic Ventral Mesh Rectopexy: An Observational Study of 919 Consecutive Patients. Ann Surg. 2015; 262(5):742–747, discussion 747–748

[45] van Geluwe B, Wolthuis A, Penninckx F, D'Hoore A. Lessons learned after more than 400 laparoscopic ventral rectopexies. Acta Chir Belg. 2013; 113 (2):103–106

[46] Ramage L, Georgiou P, Tekkis P, Tan E. Is robotic ventral mesh rectopexy better than laparoscopy in the treatment of rectal prolapse and obstructed defecation? A meta-analysis. Tech Coloproctol. 2015; 19 (7):381–389

[47] Smart NJ, Pathak S, Boorman P, Daniels IR. Synthetic or biological mesh use in laparoscopic ventral mesh rectopexy–a systematic review. Colorectal Dis. 2013; 15(6):650–654

[48] Tsunoda A, Yasuda N, Yokoyama N, Kamiyama G, Kusano M. Delorme's procedure for rectal prolapse: clinical and physiological analysis. Dis Colon Rectum. 2003; 46(9):1260–1265

[49] Riansuwan W, Hull TL, Bast J, Hammel JP, Church JM. Comparison of perineal operations with abdominal operations for full-thickness rectal prolapse. World J Surg. 2010; 34(5):1116–1122

[50] Ramanujam PS, Venkatesh KS. Perineal excision of rectal prolapse with posterior levator ani repair in elderly high-risk patients. Dis Colon Rectum. 1988; 31(9):704–706

[51] Baig MK, Galliano D, Larach JA, Weiss EG, Wexner SD, Nogueras JJ. Pouch perineal rectosigmoidectomy: a case report. Surg Innov. 2005; 12 (4):373–375

19 Benign Neoplasms of the Colon and Rectum

David E. Beck

Abstract

The word "polyp" is a nonspecific clinical term that describes any projection from the surface of the intestinal mucosa regardless of its histologic nature. Polyps can be conveniently classified into four categories according to their histologic appearance: neoplastic, hamartomatous, inflammatory, and hyperplastic. This chapter discusses the four classifications of polyps.

Keywords: neoplastic polyps, hamartomatous polyps, inflammatory polyps, lymphoid polyps, hyperplastic polyps, hemangioma, leiomyoma, lipoma, small bowel, large bowel

19.1 Polyps of Colon and Rectum

The word "polyp" is a nonspecific clinical term that describes any projection from the surface of the intestinal mucosa regardless of its histologic nature. Polyps can be conveniently classified into four categories according to their histologic appearance:

1. **Neoplastic**: tubular adenoma, villous adenoma, tubulovillous adenoma, and serrated adenoma.
2. **Hamartomatous**: juvenile polyps, Peutz–Jeghers syndrome (PJS), Cronkhite–Canada syndrome, Cowden's disease.
3. **Inflammatory**: inflammatory polyp or pseudopolyp, benign lymphoid polyp.
4. **Hyperplastic**.

19.1.1 Neoplastic Polyps

Adenomas

A neoplastic polyp is an epithelial growth composed of abnormal glands of the large bowel. A neoplastic polyp has been termed an adenoma and is classified according to the amount of villous component. Those with 0 to 25% villous tissue are classified as tubular adenomas, 25 to 75% as tubulovillous adenomas, and 75 to 100% as villous adenomas.[1] Tubular adenomas (▸ Fig. 19.1) account for 75% of all neoplastic polyps; villous adenomas (▸ Fig. 19.2), 10%; and tubulovillous adenomas (▸ Fig. 19.3), 15%. The villous growth pattern is most prominent in sessile large adenomas, particularly those located distally in the rectum. There remains considerable uncertainty as to the nature of villous growth, whether it is merely a manifestation of continued growth of tubular adenomas or whether it is a distinct phenotype that may reflect an acquired genetic change. In favor of the former is the rarity of small villous adenomas and large purely tubular adenomas.[1]

Dysplasia describes the histologic abnormality of an adenoma according to the degree of atypical cells, categorized as low-grade (mild), moderate, and high (severe). Thus, high-grade dysplasia designates a condition one step away from an invasive carcinoma. The frequency of high-grade dysplasia correlates with the size of the adenoma (▸ Fig. 19.4). The term *carcinoma-in-situ*, or "intramucosal carcinoma," should be avoided, since it implies a biological potential for distant spread, which is unwarranted and could result in overtreatment.[1]

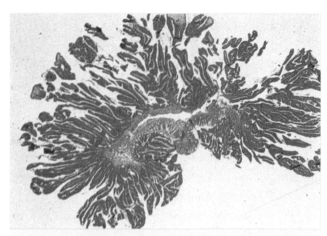

Fig. 19.2 Villous adenoma.

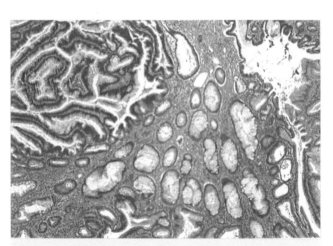

Fig. 19.3 Tubulovillous adenoma; mixture of tubular and villous glands.

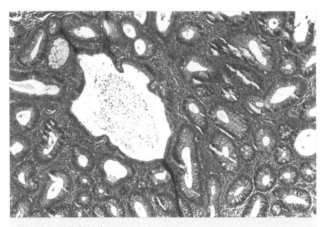

Fig. 19.1 Tubular adenoma.

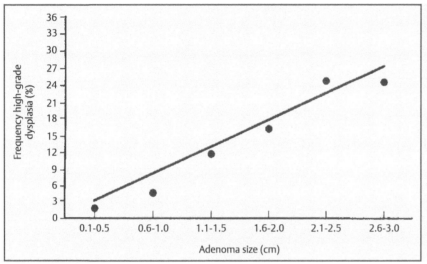

Fig. 19.4 Relationship between adenoma size and frequency of dysplasia.[2] (With permission © 1990 Elsevier.)

Table 19.1 Distribution of colorectal adenomas diagnosed by colonoscopy source[2]

Site	(%)
Cecum	8
Ascending colon	9
Hepatic flexure	4
Transverse colon	10
Splenic flexure descending colon	4
Descending colon	14
Sigmoid colon	43
Rectum	8
Total	100

Table 19.2 Relationship between size of adenoma and carcinoma[7]

Size (cm)	Adenoma (no.)	Invasive carcinoma (%)
< 0.5	5,027	0
0.6–1.5	3,519	2
1.6–2.5	1,052	19
2.6–3.5	510	43
> 3.5	1,080	76

Neoplastic polyps are common. Since data on the clinical recording of adenomas may be biased due to selection of patients and diagnostic methods, most accurate epidemiologic data on adenomas are obtained from autopsy studies. However, data from screening colonoscopy support these data. In autopsy series, adenomas are present in 34 to 52% of males and 29 to 45% of females over 50 years of age. Most adenomas (87–89%) are less than 1 cm in size.[3,4] The number, but not the size, of adenomas, increases with age.[3] Carcinomas are found in 0 to 4%.[3,4,5,6] The National Polyp Study, a multicenter randomized clinical trial in the United States, included 3,371 adenomas in 1,867 patients detected by colonoscopy.[2] This study gives valuable information regarding the natural history and characteristics of polyps: 66.5% of polyps were adenomas, 11.2% were hyperplastic, and 22.3% were classified as "other" (normal mucosa, inflammatory and juvenile polyps, lymphoid hamartomas, submucosal lipomas, carcinoids, and leiomyomas). The majority of the adenomas (69%) were in the left colon (▶ Table 19.1). The sizes of the adenomas were: 0.5 cm, 38%; 0.6 to 1 cm, 37%; and 1 cm, 25%. Colonoscopy studies suggest that the incidence of polyps is greater in males than females.

It is important to note that the size, the extent of villous component, and the increasing age are independent risk factors for high-grade dysplasia. The increased frequency of high-grade dysplasia in adenomas located distal to the splenic flexure is attributable mainly to increased size and villous component rather than to location per se. Multiplicity of adenomas affects the risk of high-grade dysplasia but is dependent on size and villous component and thus is not an independent factor.[2] Invasive carcinomas are uncommon in adenomas < 1 cm, and the incidence increases with an increased size of the adenomas (▶ Table 19.2).[7,8]

Adenoma-Carcinoma Sequence

The Observation

The concept that carcinomas of the colon and rectum derived from benign adenoma was observed by Dukes[9] of St. Mark's Hospital, London, in 1926. Jackman and Mayo[10] coined the term *adenoma-carcinoma sequence* in 1951. After decades of debates and challenges by those who believed that carcinoma of the colon and rectum derived de novo,[11,12] the adenoma-carcinoma sequence has finally become widely accepted and currently is the rationale of the approach to the secondary prevention of colorectal carcinoma by colonoscopic polypectomy.[1,13,14,15,16] Circumstantial evidence supporting the adenoma-carcinoma sequence abounds and explains the high concurrence rate of carcinoma and adenoma and the frequent findings of contiguous benign adenoma in the resected carcinoma.[17] Numerous studies (most of which are retrospective), based on tumor registry reports, hospital records, pathology reports, surgical specimens, and colonoscopy, show a coexistence of adenomas

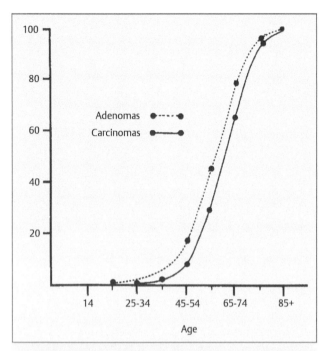

Fig. 19.5 Cumulative incidence of colorectal adenomas and carcinomas recorded in the Norwegian Cancer Registry 1983 to 1985.[19] (With permission © 1991 Springer.)

and adenocarcinomas of the colon and rectum ranging from 13 to 62%.[18] The cumulative incidence curve of adenomas based on data from the Norwegian Cancer Registry precedes the corresponding incidence curve of carcinomas by about 5 years (▶ Fig. 19.5). It should be kept in mind that adenomas are first diagnosed and reported to the cancer registry simultaneously with the diagnosis of colorectal carcinoma, indicating a longer time span between the two types of lesions than the curve indicates. It is manifested also in the natural history of both familial adenomatous polyposis (FAP) and hereditary nonpolyposis colon cancer (HNPCC) syndrome. The latter was originally thought to offer support to the de novo school of thought but several studies have since demonstrated coexisting and contiguous adenomas associated with HNPCC carcinoma with a frequency similar to that observed with sporadic carcinomas.[19] Due to the high prevalence of adenomas and the relatively far less frequent incidence of carcinomas, only a small proportion of adenomas give rise to carcinomas.[20]

Although the adenoma–carcinoma sequence concept has been favored by most authors as the main pathogenesis of colorectal carcinoma, the "de novo" origin of carcinoma developing from normal mucosa has received some attention in recent years as an alternative pathway.[19] In support of this de novo theory, authors[21,22,23] reported early colorectal carcinomas without evidence of adjacent adenomatous cells. In the series reported by Stolte and Bethke[22] of 155 such lesions, 59% of the lesions were polypoid and 34% were flat. However, proponents for the adenoma–carcinoma sequence may argue that these types of lesions are so aggressive that the infiltration destroys the adenomatous remnants. Muto et al[24] thought that all genetic alterations may take place rapidly, one after another, without a chance for morphologic changes to be expressed as seen in the adenoma–carcinoma sequence. They said, "until a specific

responsible gene for de novo carcinoma is detected, de novo carcinoma arising directly from normal mucosa is only an imaginary entity. Until then, the term 'de novo' carcinoma is better avoided and instead de novo-type carcinoma should be used."

Molecular Genetics

Molecular genetic discoveries provide substantial support for the adenoma–carcinoma sequence concept.[25] An adenoma represents an epithelial proliferation derived from a single cell (crypt). Its development occurs as a series of genetic mutations. The progression of colorectal epithelium from normal to adenoma to carcinoma can be simplified as in ▶ Fig. 19.6.

The initial step in colorectal carcinogenesis is the mutation in the *adenomatous polyposis coli (APC)* gene on chromosome 5q. The *APC* gene is inactivated, causing the affected cells to proliferate. These cells are thus primed for subsequent growth-enhancing mutation, which is more likely because of the increased rate of cell division.

Hypomethylation of DNA has been identified as the next factor involved in colorectal carcinogenesis. Loss of methylation of CpG dinucleotides occurs in cells that are already hyperproliferative because of the inactivation of the *APC* gene. These changes produce a growth of the affected cells resulting in adenoma formation. Hypomethylation of DNA may be directly linked to the K-ras (Kirsten rate sarcoma virus) activation that enhances the dysplasia so that the neoplasia can progress.

Because K-ras is an oncogene, mutation of one allele is enough to produce an effect. K-ras mutations can occur in the absence of APC gene mutations but, in this case, are usually limited to aberrant crypt foci (ACF) that do not progress to malignancy. In cells that have already suffered APC mutation (both alleles need two "hits"), K-ras mutation will drive progression. Small adenomas tend to advance to intermediate adenomas.

The transition from intermediate to advanced (or late) adenoma is associated with a distinct genetic alteration on the long arm of chromosome 18. This alteration is correlated with the mutation of a gene that maps to 18q21, named deleted in colon cancer (DCC). Specific DCC mutation has been detected in a number of colorectal carcinomas and carcinomas that have lost the capacity to differentiate into mucus-producing cells that have uniformly lost DCC expression.

The progress from advanced adenoma to carcinoma is frequently accompanied by loss of heterozygosity (i.e., mutation of one of two alleles) on chromosome 17p and mutation of the p53 gene that maps to 17p. These cumulative losses in tumor suppressor gene function accompanied by activation of dominant oncogenes drive the clonal expression of cells from the benign to the malignant site.[25,26] A fuller account of molecular genetics of colon and rectal adenocarcinoma is provided in Chapter 21.

Diagnosis of Large Bowel Adenomas

Clinically, there are two morphologic types of polyps, pedunculated and sessile. The pedunculated polyp has a stem lined with normal mucosa, called a stalk or a pedicle, and has the appearance of a mushroom (▶ Fig. 19.7). A sessile polyp grows flat on the mucosa (▶ Fig. 19.8). A pedunculated polyp rarely is > 4 cm in diameter, whereas a sessile polyp can encompass the entire circumference of the large bowel.

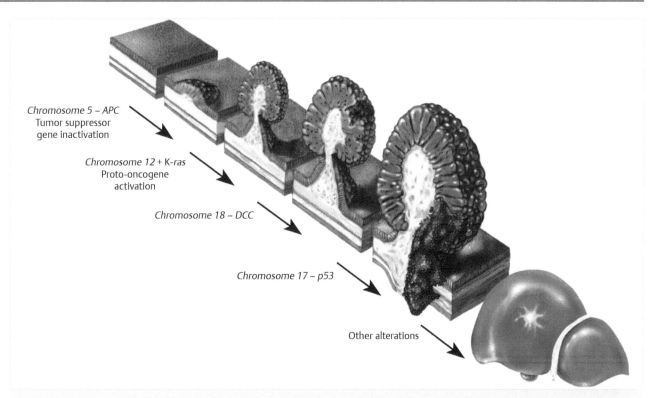

Fig. 19.6 A genetic model for the adenoma-carcinoma sequence. Tumorigenesis proceeds through a series of genetic alterations that accumulate. The histopathologic stages of colorectal tumor development are shown with increasing size and dysplasia until an invasive carcinoma is formed. APC, adenomatous polyposis coli; DCC, deleted in colon cancer. (Reproduced with permission from Nivatvongs and Dorudi.[26])

Chromosome 5 – APC
Tumor suppressor
gene inactivation

Chromosome 12 + K-ras
Proto-oncogene
activation

Chromosome 18 – DCC

Chromosome 17 – p53

Other alterations

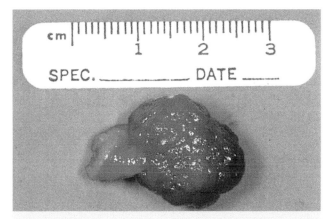

Fig. 19.7 Pedunculated polyp.

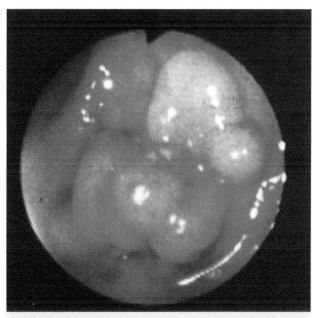

Fig. 19.8 Sessile polyp.

Adenomas of the large bowel are usually asymptomatic and are frequently discovered during routine radiologic studies or endoscopic examinations. Bleeding per rectum is the most common finding if the polyp is situated in the rectum or sigmoid colon. A large pedunculated polyp in the lower part of the rectum may prolapse through the anus. A large villous adenoma may manifest as watery diarrhea; in rare instances, it causes fluid and electrolyte imbalance. Intermittent abdominal pain from recurrent intussusception or spasm may occur with a large colonic polyp but is unusual. Mild anemia may follow chronic bleeding from an ulcerative polyp. With a small polyp, up to 8 mm, biopsy and electrocoagulation can be performed,

preferably using a "hot" biopsy forceps for histopathologic examination. A large polyp should be completely snared or excised and sent for histopathologic examination. A biopsy of a large polyp may not represent the entire lesion and presents difficulty in the interpretation of an invasive carcinoma. Occasionally, biopsy may cause displacement of the gland into the submucosa and can be misinterpreted as an invasive carcinoma.[27] This pseudoadenomatous invasion can also be caused by trauma from hard feces, repeated twisting of the stalk with subsequent ulceration of the surface.[28]

Management of Benign Adenomas

Colonoscopy has revolutionized the management of large bowel polyps. Most polyps throughout the entire colon and rectum can be excised through the colonoscope with minimal morbidity. At the present time, colonic resection or colotomy and polypectomy are reserved for cases in which colonoscopic polypectomy cannot be performed, such as lesions that are too large or too flat, or when the colonoscope cannot be passed to the site of the polyp.

Most pedunculated polyps can be snared in one piece since the pedicles are rarely > 2 cm in diameter. Sessile polyps < 2 cm usually can be snared in one piece. Large sessile polyps may be snared piecemeal and in more than one session or removed with endoscopic mucosal resection or endoscopic submucosal dissection (see Chapter 4). Excised polyps must be prepared properly and sectioned so that all the layers can be examined microscopically and the evidence of invasive carcinoma detected.

Adenomas in the rectum present a unique situation. These lesions can be palpated with finger, suction, or endoscope. If there is no induration, the chance that a lesion is benign is 90%.[29,30] There are a number of ways to remove a large adenoma in the rectum, including proctoscope or a colonoscope, per anal excision, transanal endoscopic microsurgery (TEMS), transanal minimally invasive surgery (TAMIS), and posterior proctotomy.

Patients with a neoplastic polyp have a higher risk of developing another polyp; so follow-up colonoscopy is advised. After the colon and rectum are cleared of polyps, follow-up colonoscopy every 3 to 5 years is recommended. A large sessile polyp, particularly villous type, is prone to recur, and a follow-up check of the polypectomy site should be done every 3 to 6 months the first year, every 6 to 12 months the second year, and every year thereafter to the fifth year. Then colonoscopic examination every 3 to 5 years is appropriate.

The Flat Polyp

In 1985, Muto et al[31] called attention to a separate type of polyp called a "flat" adenoma. This type of polyp is unique in that it is usually small and flat, often with a central depression, and is difficult to detect with colonoscopy or even with the resected colon and rectal specimens. Ninety percent of flat adenomas are < 1 cm and more than half are less than 5 mm.[32] The significance of flat adenomas is the high incidence of carcinomas, which occur in 6% of patients, even when the lesions are as small as 2 to 4 mm, and rapidly rise to 36% when the lesions are 9 to 10 mm. Approximately 10% of the adenomas in the Muto series were flat adenomas. They were most frequently located in the left colon and the rectum. Lynch et al[33] found similar flat adenomas in patients who were members of the same kindred under study for HNPCC. Most of the lesions were in the right colon. The flat adenomas, originally thought to occur mostly among Japanese, have also been found in studies from Australia, Canada, and the United Kingdom.[32]

In a prospective study of 1,000 consecutive patients attending for colonoscopy, flat or depressed lesions were examined by Rembacken et al.[34] Patients were not preselected and the indications were similar to other units in the United Kingdom. A flat adenoma was defined as mucosal elevations with a flat or slightly rounded surface and a height of less than half the diameter of the lesion. In practice, most flat adenomas were less than 2 mm in height and only very broad lesions were 5 mm high. During the examination, they used 0.2% indigo carmine dye, 3 to 6 mL, sprayed directly onto suspicious areas. Magnifying colonoscopy was also used.

The authors identified 321 adenomas; 119 (37%) were flat and 4 (1%) appeared depressed. Fifty-four percent of the flat or depressed lesions were situated between splenic flexure and rectum.

Seventy of the flat lesions (59%) were < 10 mm in size (mean, 5 mm) and 4% had early carcinoma (invasive into submucosa); 49 flat lesions (41%) were > 10 mm (mean, 21 mm), and 29% had early carcinoma. The mean size of the depressed lesions was 9 mm and three of four (75%) had early carcinoma, indicating their aggressiveness compared to other types of lesions.

Rembacken et al[34] suggested, "Western colonoscopists refuse training in the recognition of flat, elevated and depressed lesion in order to detect colorectal neoplasms in their early stages." The readers should note that in this study, all of the patients had indications for colonoscopic examinations and not as a screening examination for low-risk asymptomatic patients. In response to an editorial comment,[35] Rembacken et al wrote,[34] "The use of indigo carmine dye is paramount to the detection of flat and depressed lesions and only takes a few seconds. Without the dye, it is difficult to evaluate non-polypoid lesions because they generally appear to be erythematous patches, easily mistaken for scope trauma. The magnifying colonoscope does not help in the initial recognition of lesions but allows the endoscopists to assess the crypt pattern and predict the histology." Recent molecular analysis of such flat adenomas suggests that they are etiologically distinct from other polypoid adenomas.[36] The mutation rate and the K-ras gene are both significantly reduced (16% in flat adenomas compared to 50% in ordinary colorectal adenomas) and do not occur in the same codons. The management of flat adenomas is the same as for sessile adenomas.

Why Remove a Polyp?

It has generally been accepted that most colorectal carcinomas are derived from benign adenomas through the adenoma-carcinoma sequence. It is estimated that it takes about 5 years from a clean colon to the development of an adenoma and about 10 years from a clean colon to the development of invasive carcinoma.[13] Thus, removal of an adenoma is prophylactic against the development of colorectal carcinoma. Gilbertsen,[37] in a retrospective study, showed that removal of rectal polyps in patients under surveillance with yearly rigid proctosigmoidoscopy results in a lower than expected incidence of rectal carcinoma. This result was confirmed by Selby et al[38] in a case–control study using rigid proctosigmoidoscopy; screening examination produced a 70% reduction in the risk of death from rectal and distal sigmoid carcinoma. The National Polyp Study also showed that colonoscopic polypectomy results in a lower than expected incidence of colorectal carcinoma.[39]

Church studied diminutive (1–5 mm) and small (6–10 mm) adenomas of the colon and rectum, and found that although

Table 19.3 Risk of diminutive and small adenomas. No effect of age, site, or family history[41]

Size (mm)	No.	Severe dysplasia (%)	Invasive carcinoma (%)
1–5 (diminutive)	2,066	44	0.1
6–10 (small)	418	15.6	0.2

the risk of invasive carcinoma was low (0.1 and 0.2%, respectively), the risk of severe dysplasia was significant (4.4 and 15.6%, respectively).[40] He advised a cold excision or a hot snare as appropriate (▶ Table 19.3).

Natural History of Untreated Large Bowel Adenomas

A retrospective review of patients from the precolonoscopic era by Stryker et al[42] analyzed 226 patients who had colonic polyps 210 mm in diameter and in whom periodic radiographic examination of the colon was elected over excision. Twenty-one invasive carcinomas were identified at the site of the index polyp at a mean follow-up of 108 months (range, 24–225 months). The risk of having a polyp ≥ 1 cm in size develop into an invasive carcinoma at 5, 10, and 20 years was 2.5, 8, and 24%, respectively.

Further study of this same group of patients by Otchy et al[43] revealed that the cumulative probability of developing an invasive metachronous carcinoma at a site different from the index polyp was 2% at 5 years, 7% at 10 years, and 12% at 20 years. Over a median duration of polyp surveillance of 4.8 years (range, 1–27 years), 11 (5%) of the index polyps disappeared, 129 (57%) had no growth noted, and 86 demonstrated growth. Forty-two of the 86 polyps (49%) had at least a twofold increase in size. Seventy-one of the 86 polyps were removed, and 24 (34%) were carcinomatous. Fifteen of the 86 polyps that increased in size were not removed, and none of these patients developed a carcinoma. Forty-three of the 129 polyps that did not grow were eventually removed. Five of those polyps had carcinoma and one of these patients also developed a metachronous carcinoma at a later date. In addition, 2 of the 43 patients developed a colon carcinoma in areas distant from the site of the index polyp.

These data further support the recommendation for excision of all colonic polyps ≥ 10 mm in diameter and a periodic examination of the entire colon. Although this study has limitations inherent to any retrospective analysis, comparable prospective data are unlikely to be available in the future because of the widespread availability of colonoscopy and the compelling evidence to recommend the removal of neoplastic polyps.

What Happens to Smaller Adenomas?

Hofstad et al[41] prospectively studied the growth of colorectal polyps. Colonoscopy was performed in 58 subjects. Polyps ≥ 10 mm were removed; polyps < 5 mm and 5 to 9 mm were left behind for a follow-up study. Colonoscopy was followed up by one investigator once a year. On the third year, polyps were removed by snare or hot biopsy. The measurement of the polyps was performed by a measuring probe plus photography. On the third year, 7 of 58 patients had only hyperplastic polyps. Twenty-nine individuals had one adenoma, 17 individuals had two to three

adenomas, and 5 individuals had four to five adenomas. Twenty-five percent of all the adenomas were unchanged in size, whereas 40% displayed growth and 35% showed regression or shrinking in size. Adenomatous polyps < 5 mm showed a tendency to growth, while the adenomas 5 to 9 mm showed a tendency to reduction in size. The hyperplastic polyps showed a similar pattern. There was a tendency to increase growth in the adenomatous polyps in the younger age groups reaching significance from initial examination to the third year and from the first to the second year of re-examination. Moreover, in the patients with four to five adenomas at the initial examination, the polyps showed larger growth than the polyps in patients with only one or two to three adenomas. There were no differences in polyp growth between the sexes. A similar prospective study by Bersentes et al[44] on adenomas of the upper rectum or sigmoid colon, size 3 to 9 mm, showed no regression or consistent linear growth rates with a 2-year follow-up.

In the study by Hofstad et al,[41] 86% of the individuals had at least one new polyp during the 3 years and 75% had at least one new adenoma. The newly discovered polyps were significantly smaller than the average size at initial examination. They were also more frequent in the proximal part of the colon (71%) than the polyps discovered at initial examination (38%). There were more new adenomas among those with more than four to five adenomas at initial examination, than those with one adenoma, reaching significance from initial examination to the first year of examination and from initial examination to third year. There were more new adenomas among patients > 60 years of age than those < 60 years. No differences were found between the sexes.

Adenomas with Invasive Carcinoma

The term *invasive carcinoma* is applied only when the malignant cells have invaded the polyp, either sessile or pedunculated, partially or totally, through the muscularis mucosa into the submucosa. Severely dysplastic cells superficial to the muscularis mucosa do not metastasize and should be classified as atypia (rather than carcinoma in situ or superficial carcinoma).[13] For this type of lesion, complete excision is all that is necessary. Follow-up of these polyps is the same as for benign polyps.

A polyp with invasive carcinoma or a malignant polyp is an early carcinoma. For the TNM classification, it is a T1NxMx. Two classification systems for adenomas with invasive carcinoma have been proposed. In 1985, Haggitt et al[45] proposed a classification for polyps with adenocarcinoma according to the depth of invasion as follows (▶ Fig. 19.9):

- Level 0—Carcinoma in situ or intramucosal carcinoma. These are not invasive.
- Level 1—Carcinoma invading through the muscularis mucosae into the submucosa but limited to the head of the polyp (i.e., above the junction between the adenoma and its stalk).
- Level 2—Carcinoma invading the level of the neck of the adenoma (junction between adenoma and its stalk).
- Level 3—Carcinoma invading any part of the stalk.
- Level 4—Carcinoma invading into the submucosa of the bowel wall below the stalk of the polyp but above the muscularis propria. Although not specifically defined by Haggitt et al, sessile polyps with invasive carcinoma are considered to have level 4 invasion.

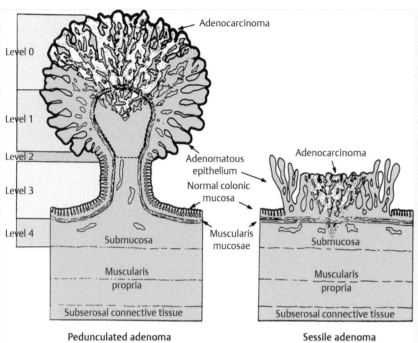

Fig. 19.9 Anatomic landmarks of pedunculated and sessile adenomas.[49] (With permission © 1993 Thieme.)

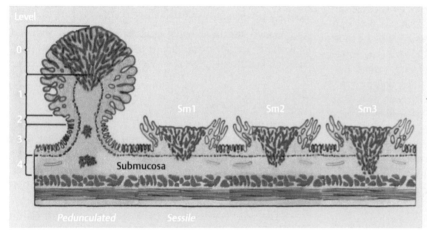

Fig. 19.10 Incorporation of Haggitt classification to Sm system. Sm1, Invasion into upper one-third of submucosa; Sm2, invasion into middle one-third of submucosa; Sm3, invasion into distal one-third of submucosa. Haggitt's pedunculated levels 1, 2, and 3 are all in Sm1; pedunculated level 4 can be Sm1, Sm2, or Sm3. (Source: Mayo Foundation.)

The risk of lymph node metastasis for pedunculated polyp (Haggitt level 1, 2, and 3) is low.[45,46,47,48]

In 1993, Kudo[49] classified the submucosal invasion of the sessile lesions into three levels (▶ Fig. 19.10):

- Sm1—invasion into the upper third of the submucosa.
- Sm2—invasion into the middle third of the submucosa.
- Sm3—invasion into the lower third of the submucosa.

The Sm system appears to be effective and practical and was recommended by a consensus workshop in Paris in 2002.[50] In the series by Nascimbeni et al,[51] the pathologist could evaluate the depth of invasion into Sm1, Sm2, and Sm3 in 97% of the cases. In fact, the Haggitt level for the pedunculated lesion can be incorporated into the Sm system (▶ Fig. 19.10). However, the endoscopists must properly prepare the specimens and the pathologists must properly section them in order to examine the entire layers.

Risk factors for residual cancer or involvement of lymph nodes include: poor differentiation, lymphovascular invasion, depth of invasion in submucosa (e.g., Sm3), and a positive resection margin (< 2 mm from edge of tumor to resected margin).[51,52,53,54]

Patients having lesions with one or more risk factors should undergo an oncologic bowel resection.[52,55,56,57,58] Hagitt level 4 lesions will almost always have a positive margin and will usually require a resection. A malignant lesion that is removed piecemeal also requires further excision or resection. The incidence of residual cancer in the bowel or regional lymph nodes in specimens varies with respect to which risk factors were present but in reported studies has averaged 18% but as high as 50% in some series.[59,60]

For lesions with no risk factors, a complete snaring or a transanal excision is adequate. Close follow-up examination with endoscopy to detect a local recurrence may be performed every 3 to 6 months for the first year. This period can be

Table 19.4 Selected series of local recurrence and survival after transanal excision for T1 carcinoma of the rectum

Institution	No.	LR (%)	5-year survival (%, CSS)	F-U (mo)
University of Minnesota[65]	69	18	95	52
Memorial Sloan Kettering[66]	67	14	74	60
Cleveland Clinic[67]	52	29	75	55
Mayo Clinic[68]	70	7	89	60

Abbreviations: LR, local recurrence; CSS, cancer-specific survival; F-U, follow-up.

extended to every 6 to 12 months in the second year and to every year for the next 2 years. Thereafter, endoscopy every 3 years is adequate.

Rectal polyps merit additional discussion. Those polyps that are early rectal cancers are managed as discussed in Chapter 22.

Transanal excision for a sessile polyp with invasive carcinoma, or a T1 carcinoma of the low rectum has a three- to fivefold higher risk of carcinoma recurrence compared with patients treated by radical resection[61] (▶ Table 19.4). Waiting to perform a radical resection after a local recurrence is a poor choice. In most series, the cancer-free survival for salvage resection in these patients is 50 to 56%.[62,63] On the other hand, an immediate radical resection after local excision (within 1 month) gives a better prognosis, 94% cancer-free survival at 10 years, and is comparable to primary resection in a case–control comparison.[64] In short, local excision for a sessile polyp with invasive carcinoma (T1) of the lower third of rectum has high local recurrence. It appears that the early lesion at this site is a locally disseminated disease. To improve the outcome, the recurrence rate has to be improved: options include doing more radical resection in young and good health patients, finding a better adjuvant therapy, or finding better ways in selection of patients, such as molecular markers in the future.

Serrated Adenoma

This is the term coined by Longacre and Fenoglio-Preiser in 1990[69] to describe a new entity of mixed hyperplastic polyp/adenomatous polyp. In their study of 110 serrated adenomas, compared to 60 traditional adenomas and 40 hyperplastic polyps, they found that these lesions distributed throughout the colon and rectum, with a slight preponderance of large lesions (> 1 cm) occurring in the cecum and appendix.

There are two types of mixed epithelial polyps: one in which adenomatous and hyperplastic glands are mixed (▶ Fig. 19.11a), and one in which the adenoma has a serrated appearance on microscopic examination (▶ Fig. 19.11b). Microscopic examination of the lesions shows goblet cell immaturity, prominent architectural distortion, cytologically atypical nuclei, rare upper zone mitoses, and absence of a thickened collagen table.[66,69]

Grossly, the lesion is flat and smooth; it may look like a plaque or thickened mucosa on colonoscopic examination (▶ Fig. 19.12). This type of lesion can be easily missed on colonoscopy if the colon is overdistended (stretching it flat) or underdistended (causing wrinkle on mucosa to mask it). Unlike

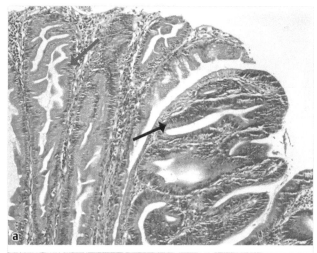

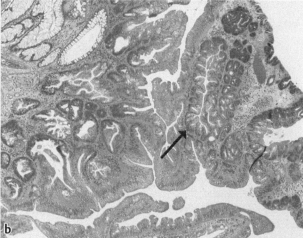

Fig. 19.11 (a) Mixed hyperplastic gland (*red arrow*) and adenomatous gland (*black arrow*). **(b)** Adenomatous gland with serrated appearance (*arrow*). (Courtesy of Thomas C. Smyrk, MD.)

the classic hyperplastic polyps that are small and restricted to the rectum and rectosigmoid colon, serrated adenomas are larger and occur in both proximal and distal colon and rectum.[70] Some of the individuals previously reported as having multiple hyperplastic polyps could instead have had multiple serrated adenomatous polyps.[69]

Based on the observation that 11% of serrated adenomas in the series of Longacre and Fenoglio-Preiser[69] contained foci of intramucosal carcinoma, it was surmised that an individual lesion would carry a significant malignant potential. Nevertheless, the rarity of serrated adenoma (0.6% of colorectal polyps) would minimize their contribution to the overall burden of colorectal malignancy.[65] Torlakovic and Snover[66] reported six patients with serrated adenomatous polyposis. Each patient had at least 50 polyps, ranging from 0.3 to 4.5 cm in size, mostly sessile. Three patients had diffuse polyps, two patients had the polyps in the left colon, and one patient had them in the right colon. Four patients had carcinoma. Serrated adenomas are infrequently observed in endoscopic practice due to underdiagnosis and the potential for rapid evolution to carcinoma. The latter suggestion is supported by the demonstration of DNA microsatellite instability (MSI) in mixed polyps

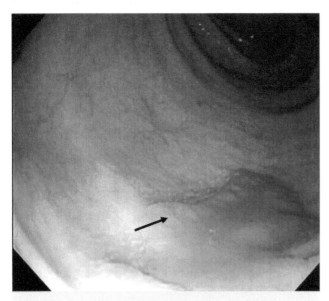

Fig. 19.12 Plaquelike serrated adenoma in transverse colon.

and serrated adenomas and by analogy with the aggressive adenomas in HNPCC.[65]

The known alterations include K-ras mutation, low and occasional high-level MSI, 1pLOH, and methylation of HPP1/TPEF (a putative antiadhesion molecule). Additional genetic alterations may be observed in neoplastic subclones occurring within or adjacent to hyperplastic polyps. These include loss of expression of MGMT or hMLH1.[67]

Sporadic MSI-low (MSI-L) and MSI-high (MSI-H) carcinomas may evolve through the serrated adenoma pathway.[65] The serrated adenoma pathway is likely to show marked molecular heterogeneity, but patterns are beginning to emerge. The view that all, or even most, colorectal carcinomas are initiated by mutation of APC gene and evolve through the classical adenoma-carcinoma sequence may no longer be tenable. This understanding will surely transform our approach to the early detection and prevention of colorectal carcinoma.[65]

The molecular steps that determine growth of ACF into hyperplastic polyp are not known. Colorectal carcinoma is envisioned to arise from hyperplasticlike polyps (or sessile serrated polyps) in which the earliest events might be BRAF mutation synergizing with a methylated and silenced pro-apoptotic gene. Subsequent methylation of hMLH1 or MGMT then predisposes to mutation, dysplastic change, and finally to malignancy that is frequently characterized by MSI-H or MSI-L status. K-ras mutation may substitute for BRAF in methylator pathways culminating in MSI-L and some MSS colorectal carcinomas.[68] Serrated adenomas are neoplastic polyps. The treatment is the same as in adenomatous polyps.

19.1.2 Hamartomatous Polyps

A hamartoma is a malformation or inborn error of tissue development characterized by an abnormal mixture of tissues endogenous to the part, with excess of one or more of these tissues. It may show itself at birth or by extensive growth in the postnatal period.

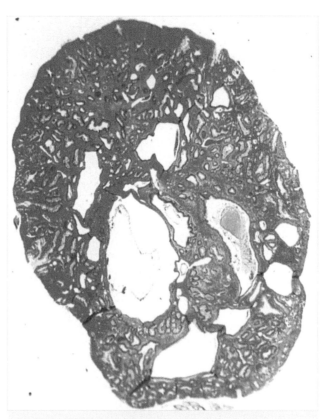

Fig. 19.13 Juvenile or retention polyp. Note the Swiss-cheese appearance from dilated glands.

Juvenile Polyps and Juvenile Polyposis

Juvenile polyps characteristically occur in children, although they may present in adults at any age. This type of polyp is a hamartoma and is not premalignant. Macroscopically, they are pink, smooth, round, and usually pedunculated. The cut section shows a cheeselike appearance from dilated cystic spaces. Microscopic pictures show dilated glands filled with mucus and an abnormality of the lamina propria, which has a mesenchymal appearance (▶ Fig. 19.13). The muscularis mucosa does not participate in the structure of the polyp. Bleeding from the rectum is common. A moderate amount of bleeding can occur if the polyp is autoamputated, a phenomenon not seen in other types of polyps. Intussusception of the colon occasionally occurs if the polyp is large. Treatment is by excision or snaring through a colonoscope or a transanal excision.

Juvenile polyposis is an entity characteristically and biologically distinct from solitary juvenile polyp or other polyposis. The condition was first observed by McColl et al in 1964.[71] The term *juvenile polyposis* rather than juvenile polyposis coli is to be preferred as polyps are also found in the stomach and the small intestine.[72] There are two types of juvenile polyposis: in infancy and in other variable age of onset.[73]

Juvenile polyposis of infancy is a rare form without a family history. The infant presents with diarrhea, either bloody or mucinous, anemia, protein-losing enteropathy, and intussusception; rectal prolapse develops between 8 and 10 months of age and leads to significant morbidity.[73,74] The entire gastrointestinal (GI) tract is usually affected; the prognosis depends on the severity and extent of GI involvement. Death occurs before the age of 2 years in severe cases.[72] Surgery is indicated in cases of intussusception, or polypectomies in cases of rectal prolapse to reduce the leading point of the prolapse. Supportive care to replace fluid and electrolytes or total parenteral nutrition is indicated.[74]

The majority of patients with juvenile polyposis manifest in their first or second decade, but in 15% of patients, the diagnosis is delayed until they are adults. They usually present with rectal bleeding and anemia. Family history of juvenile polyposis is found in 20 to 50% of patients. Various extracolonic abnormalities, described in 11 to 20% of cases, have included digital clubbing, pulmonary arteriovenous fistula, macrocephaly, alopecia, bony swellings, cleft lip, cleft palate, supernumerary teeth, porphyria, arteriovenous malformation affecting the skin, psoriasis, congenital heart disease, malrotation of the gut, abnormalities involving the vitellointestinal duct, double renal pelvis and ureter, acute glomerulonephritis, undescended testes, and bifid uterus and vagina.[72]

Patients with juvenile polyposis usually have 50 to 200 colorectal polyps and a proportion have polyps in the stomach and small intestine. Some patients seem to have relatively few polyps, but these tend to be the parent of the prospectus. It is conceivable that the juvenile polyps are produced only within the first few decades and are subsequently lost through autoamputation. Thus, juvenile polyposis may be diagnosed when a relatively old and asymptomatic parent is screened colonoscopically and the smallest number of polyps found on this basis is 5.[73]

Jass et al[73] proposed a working definition of juvenile polyposis:
- More than five juvenile polyps of the colorectum.
- Juvenile polyps throughout the GI tract.
- Any number of juvenile polyps with a family history of juvenile polyposis.

On the other hand, Giardiello et al[75] suggested that the patients with as few as three juvenile polyps should undergo screening for colorectal neoplasm.

Although there is no evidence that isolated juvenile polyp could be malignant, it is now well established that juvenile polyposis is a precancerous condition.[73,75,76,77,78] The risk of GI malignancy in affected members of juvenile polyposis kindred exceeds 50% in a series of kindred reported by Howe et al.[76]

In a classic paper on juvenile polyposis, Jass et al[73] studied 87 patients with juvenile polyposis recorded in the St. Mark's Polyposis Registry, including 1,032 polyps and 18 patients with colorectal carcinoma. They found that about 20% of juvenile polyps did not conform to the classical description. Grossly, they formed lobular masses (instead of spherical). These atypical juvenile polyps also revealed relatively less lamina propria and more epithelium than that found in the more typical variety and often adopted a villous or papillary configuration. Epithelial dysplasia occurred in both typical and atypical juvenile polyps but more frequently in the latter. Nearly 50% of the atypical juvenile polyps showed some degree of dysplasia similar to adenomas. The 18 patients with colorectal adenocarcinoma had a mean age of 34 years (range, 15–59 years). A high proportion of carcinomas were mucinous and/or poorly differentiated, which was in accord with case reports from other authors.

There is little direct information on the histogenesis of carcinoma in juvenile polyposis. Dysplasia has been shown to occur in two forms: (1) a focus of adenomatous change within a polyp and (2) an adenoma showing no residual juvenile features.[76] On the mechanism of polyp-cancer sequence in juvenile polyposis, Kinzler and Vogelstein[77] postulated,

"an abnormal stroma can affect the development of adjacent epithelial cells is not a new concept. Ulcerative colitis is an autoimmune disease that leads to inflammation and cystic epithelium in the mucosa of the colon. Initially, the imbedded epithelium shows no neoplastic changes, but foci of epithelial neoplasia and progression to cancer eventually develops in many cases. The regeneration that occurs to replace damaged epithelium may increase the probability of somatic mutations in this abnormal microenvironment. The increased risk of cancer in juvenile polyposis syndrome and ulcerative colitis patients, therefore, seems primarily the result of an altered terrain for epithelial cell growth and can be thought of as a landscaper defect."

Juvenile polyposis is an autosomal dominant condition.[76] The germline mutation is in the gene SMAD-4 (also known as DPC-4), located on chromosome 18q21.1.[75,79,80]

There is little information about prophylactic colectomy or proctocolectomy to prevent occurrence of carcinoma. The decision on performing the operation should be dictated by the number and the site of the polyps. Polyps of the colon and rectum that are too numerous for colonoscopy and polypectomies should have an abdominal colectomy with ileorectal anastomosis (IRA) or proctocolectomy with ileal pouch-anal anastomosis (IPAA) or an ileostomy.[72,74,81,82] In a series reported by Oncel et al,[81] 5 of 10 patients who underwent colectomy with IRA for juvenile polyposis required a subsequent proctectomy with a mean follow-up of 9 years (range, 6–34 years). This and other studies suggest that proctocolectomy with ileoanal pouch procedure may be a better option as an initial operation.[81,82]

The proband and relatives of the first degree should be screened, probably starting in the later teen years, by upper and lower GI endoscopy. If this initial screen is negative, a follow-up endoscopy should be performed every 3 years.[83] For patients who have had a colectomy or an ileoanal pouch, surveillance should be performed periodically.[81,82] Howe et al[84] recommended genetic testing as part of the workup. However, given the presumed genetic heterogeneity of this syndrome, failure to show a mutation in SMAD-4 does not support lengthening the surveillance interval to 10 years as they suggested.[81]

Peutz–Jeghers Syndrome

PJS is a rare autosomal dominant disease characterized by GI hamartomatous polyposis and mucocutaneous pigmentation. It was originally described by Peutz in 1921 but was not clearly identified until attention was brought to it by Jeghers et al[85] in 1949. The syndrome comprises melanin spots of buccal mucosa and lips; the face and digits may be involved to a variable extent, but mouth pigmentation is the sine qua non of this portion of the syndrome. The presence of polyps in the small bowel is a constant finding of this syndrome, but the stomach, colon, and rectum also may be involved. The characteristic Peutz–Jeghers polyp has an abnormal muscularis mucosa branching into the lamina propria, giving the appearance of a Christmas tree (▶ Fig. 19.14).

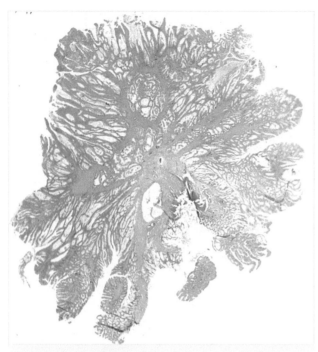

Fig. 19.14 Peutz–Jeghers polyp. Note Christmas-tree appearance from branching of muscularis mucosa.

Diagnosis

Giardiello et al[86] defined a definitive diagnosis of PJS by the presence of histologically confirmed hamartomatous polyps, plus at least two of the following:

- Family history of the syndrome.
- Labial melanin deposits.
- Small bowel polyposis.

The diagnosis is "probable" if two of the three clinical criteria described above are present but without histopathological verification of hamartomatous polyps.[86] Genetic testing may then be used to confirm the diagnosis.[87]

For patients without a family history of PJS, definitive diagnosis depends on the presence of two or more histologically verified Peutz–Jeghers type hamartomatous polyps.[88] For patients with a first-degree relative with PJS, the presence of mucocutaneous hyperpigmentation is sufficient for presumptive diagnosis.[87]

Genetics

To date, the only identifiable mutations causing PJS affect the serine/threonine-protein kinase 11 (STK11, also known as LKB1) gene, located on chromosome 19p13.3. Although PJS is inherited in an autosomal dominant manner, up to 25% of documented cases are not familial. These sporadic cases are felt to be due to de novo mutations in STK11 or low penetrance variance.[87] Genetic testing for STK11 mutations is available but they have variable sensitivity. In familial cases with a known genetic linkage to STK11, testing carries a sensitivity of 70%. In sporadic cases, genetic testing has sensitivity ranging from 30 to 67%. A significant proportion of familial and sporadic Peutz–Jeghers cases may result from mutations in genes other than STK11.[87,88]

High Risk of Cancers

It is a well-known fact that patients with PJS have high risk of developing cancer in many parts of the body. However, the risk varies depending on how the studies are undertaken. Giardiello et al[89] conducted an individual patient meta-analysis to determine the relative risk (RR) of malignancy in patients with PJS compared with general population. The authors used strict criteria for the analysis. Searches of MEDLINE, EMBASE, and referenced articles yielded 94 articles. Only six publications, which consisted of 210 individuals, qualified for the study. The results showed that the RR for all carcinomas was 15.2. A statistically significant increase of RR was noted for: esophagus (57.0), stomach (213.0), small intestine (520.0), colon (84.0), pancreas (132.0), lung (17.0), breast (15.2), uterus (16.0), and ovary (27.0). There was no risk for testicular or cervical malignancy. The cumulative risk for all malignancy was 93% from age 15 to 64 years old.

Carcinoma in Peutz–Jeghers Polyps

Ordinarily, hamartomatous polyps should not degenerate into malignancy. However, there have been reports of invasive adenocarcinoma in Peutz–Jeghers polyps of the small and large intestine, although the risk is not high. Giardiello et al[86] did not detect invasive carcinoma within hamartomatous polyps in any of their patients. The polyps containing hamartomatous, adenomatous, and malignant components have been observed in Peutz–Jeghers polyps of the small and large intestine.[90,91,92,93,94] Spigelman et al[93] surveyed 72 patients registered with PJS at St. Mark's Polyposis Registry. Four patients had nine carcinomas in hamartomatous polyps in stomach, duodenum, jejunum, and colon. This observation suggests that a hamartomatous, adenomatous, and carcinomatous progression may be important in the development of malignancy in Peutz–Jeghers polyps.

Genetic analysis showed that STK11/LKB1 acts as a tumor suppressor gene and may be involved in the early stages of PJS carcinogenesis.[95,96] The results suggest that Peutz–Jeghers-related carcinomas have different molecular genetic alteration compared with those found in sporadic GI carcinomas.[94]

Peutz–Jeghers–Like Mucocutaneous Pigmentation

Characteristic mucocutaneous pigmentation is often the clinical clue that heralds the diagnosis of PJS. The melanotic or lentiginous pigmented macules are dark brown, blue, or blue-brown and located on the vermillion border of the lips (> 90%), buccal mucosa, digits, and occasionally on the periorbital, auricular, perianal, and vulvar skin.[97] The relevance of PJS-like hyperpigmentation in the absence of other features of PJS is not known. Boardman et al[97] coined the term *isolated melanotic mucocutaneous pigmentation* (IMMP). To ascertain the risk of malignancy for patients with IMMP, they identified a group of individuals with mucocutaneous melanotic macules indistinguishable clinically from PJS hyperpigmentation but who did not manifest the other phenotypic characteristics of PJS. To distinguish those patients with possible or definite PJS from those with pigmentation only, the authors applied the diagnostic criteria of Giardiello et al[86] to define definite PJS. Patients who had PJS-like oral hyperpigmentation only and none of the other criteria of

PJS were classified as IMMP. 60 patients with the diagnosis of PJS or PJS-like pigmentation were identified through the patient registry of the Mayo Clinic from 1945 to 1996. Twenty-six unrelated patients were identified with IMMP. There were 16 men and 10 women.

The results showed that 10 individuals developed 12 noncutaneous malignancies including breast (n =1), cervical (n =3), endometrial (n =3), renal (n =1), lung (n =2), colon (n =1), and lymphoma (n =1). The median age of diagnosis of noncutaneous malignancy was 47 years (range, 33–84 years); this compared to a median age of carcinoma in the general population of 68 years. In their previous review of carcinoma risk in PJS patients, the median age at diagnosis of carcinoma was 38 years (range, 16–59 years).[96] The mean interval from the identification of the pigmentation to the development of carcinoma in IMMP patients was 24.2 years, compared to a mean latency period of 19.9 years in PJS patients.[94,95,96,97] Although the magnitude and gender associations of carcinomas in patients with IMMP and PJS are remarkably similar, the authors detected no alterations in the LKB1 among IMMP patients. Is IMMP an entity distinct from PJS? The overlap in the two conditions of phenotypic pigmentary features and the increased risk of malignancy, specifically of the breast and gynecologic tract in women, support the notion that they might share a common genetic origin. Though none of nine individuals with IMMP had mutations in LKB1, 14 to 42% of patients with definite PJS lack LKB1 mutations, suggesting that another yet to be identified gene or genes may be responsible for cases of both PJS and IMMP not caused by LKB1 mutations.[97] Based on the increased RR for gynecologic and breast carcinomas that they detected in their patient population of IMMP, the authors recommend following current screening guidelines for gynecologic and breast carcinoma with thorough evaluation of PJS-like pigmentation. They recommended examination of the GI tract at age 20 years in asymptomatic individuals with PJS-like hyperpigmentation.

Screening

Given the multitude of carcinomas to which these patients are susceptible, aggressive screening protocols are recommended. Upper and lower GI endoscopies are indicated for any adolescent or adult suspected of having PJS. Radiographic studies should also be used to screen for distal small intestinal polyps. Pelvic ultrasound of females and gonadal examination in young men are also recommended.

An at-risk but unaffected relative is a first-degree relative of an individual with PJS who does not meet clinical criteria for PJS. Guidelines for surveillance of affected patients also apply to these at-risk family members. The current guideline for carcinoma screening is summarized in ▶ Table 19.5.

Management of Peutz–Jeghers Polyps

The clinical course of PJS is characterized by asymptomatic periods interspersed with complications such as abdominal pain, intussusception often leading to frank intestinal obstruction, and hemorrhage that is often occult. Small bowel obstruction is the presenting complaint in half of the cases, and exploratory celiotomy due to polyp-induced complications occurs commonly and may do so at quite short intervals.[98] Because this problem is coupled with the significant risk of malignancy in

Table 19.5 Screening recommendations for Peutz–Jeghers syndrome[95]

Organs	Age to begin	Interval (y)	Procedure
Colon	25	2	Colonoscopy
Gastrointestinal tract	10	2	Upper endoscopy
Pancreas	30	1–2	Endoscopic ultrasound; transabdominal ultrasound
Breast	20	2	Mammography
		1	Self-breast exam
Uterus	20	1	Transvaginal ultrasound; endometrial biopsy
Cervix	20	1	Pap smear
Testicular	10	1	Physical exam, ultrasound if clinically indicated

the polyps, the surgical approach is now more aggressive. The current approach is to operate on the patient if the small intestinal polyps are larger than 1.5 cm.[98,99]

Endoscopic resection of Peutz–Jeghers polyps throughout the small intestine at double-balloon enteroscopy without exploratory celiotomy has been reported to be successful.[100] However, in general, an enteroscopy is performed at the time of exploratory celiotomy with polypectomy or resection of the small bowel.[101,102] The indications for surgery included obstructing or intussuscepting polyps, polyps larger than 1.5 cm identified radiologically, or smaller polyps associated with iron deficiency anemia.[102]

In order to achieve more complete polyp clearance, Edwards et al[102] analyzed their experience of using intraoperative enteroscopy in conjunction with exploratory celiotomy. The enteroscope was introduced through an enterotomy at the site of polypectomy for the largest polyps. Depending on the size of the polyps, snare polypectomy, electrocoagulation, or biopsies were performed. In their experience of 25 patients, enteroscopy identified 350 polyps not detected by palpation or transillumination of the bowel by an operating light. All the polyps were removed. There was one early complication of a delayed small bowel perforation at the site of a snare polypectomy that resulted in an urgent reoperation but no long-term sequelae. No patient in this group had required operative polypectomy within 4 years of polyp clearance by intraoperative enteroscopy, compared with registry data of 4 of 23 patients who had more than one exploratory celiotomy within a year. It appears that intraoperative enteroscopy for PJS improves polyp clearance without the need for additional enterotomies and may help to reduce the frequency of exploratory celiotomy.[101]

Cronkhite–Canada Syndrome

Cronkhite–Canada syndrome is characterized by generalized GI polyposis associated with alopecia, cutaneous pigmentation, and atrophy of fingernails and toenails (onychatrophia). It was first deducted in two patients and described by Cronkhite and Canada in 1955.[103] The etiology is unknown. There is no familial inheritance pattern and no associated gene or mutation has been identified.[104]

Diarrhea is a prominent feature of this syndrome, accounting for 46 of 55 patients in the series of Daniel et al.[105] The cause of diarrhea is unknown. Nardone et al[106] reported a case of Cronkhite–Canada syndrome associated with achlorhydria and hypergastrinemia causing direct gastric wall invasion by gram-negative *Campylobacter pylori*. This may explain the diarrhea in those patients. Hair loss was noted in 49 of 55 patients. In most patients, hair loss took place simultaneously from the scalp, eyebrows, face, axillae, pubic areas, and extremities, but in some only loss of scalp hair was described.[105] Nail changes were reported in 51 of 55 patients. In most of them, the nails showed varying degrees of dystrophy, such as thinning and splitting, and partial separation from the nail bed (onycholysis). Complete loss of all fingernails and toenails (onychomadesis), over a period of several weeks, was also noted in some patients.[105]

Hyperpigmentation was present in 45 of 55 patients, ranging from a few millimeters to 10 cm in diameter. The distribution of pigmentary skin changes could be anywhere, including extremities, face, palms, soles, neck, back, chest, scalp, and lips.[105] Other manifestations include nausea, vomiting, weakness, weight loss, abdominal pain, numbness, and tingling of extremities.[105] Electrolyte disturbances are a prominent feature and appear to reflect malabsorption and losses from the GI tract. Total serum protein is also found to be low in most patients due to excessive enteric protein loss.[105]

From radiologic, endoscopic, and autopsy data, the stomach and large intestine were involved in 53 of 55 cases. The actual frequency of small bowel involvement would be inaccurate because the small bowel X-rays and biopsies were not performed in every case, in the series of Daniel et al.[105] From the autopsy data, the number of polyps was greatest in the duodenum, less in the jejunum and proximal ileum, and again increased in the terminal ileum.[105] The polyps consist of cystic dilatation of the epithelial tubules similar to that of juvenile polyps, but the lesions are usually smaller and do not show marked excess of lamina propria.[83,105,106,107,108,109,110,111,112,113,114]

The true incidence of GI carcinoma in Cronkhite–Canada syndrome is unknown. In the review of literature by Daniel et al[105] in 55 cases, they found six cases of carcinoma of the colon and/or rectum, including one case of carcinoma of the stomach. Some of these carcinomas were multiple. Watanabe et al[108] reported a case of Cronkhite–Canada syndrome associated with triple gastric carcinoma. Histopathologic examination revealed that the polyp underwent malignant transformation without an adenoma component.

Management

There has been no specific treatment. The management is symptomatic and the correction of any deficiencies. A complete spontaneous remission has been reported.[109] Resection is reserved for cases in which complications such as carcinoma, bleeding, intussusception, and rectal prolapse develop.[113] Surgery is not usually performed for improvement of protein-losing gastroenteropathy because the protein losing is usually not localized.[110] Hanzawa

et al[110] reported a patient with Cronkhite–Canada syndrome with numerous polyps in the stomach, duodenum, and from cecum to transverse colon. The patient had severe hypoproteinemia and peripheral edema, unresponsive to conservative treatment including elemental diet and hyperalimentation. Scintigraphy with technetium ^{99m}TC-labeled human albumin[111,112] demonstrated a protein-losing region in the ascending colon. An ileo-right colectomy was performed. After the operation, the protein-losing enteropathy stopped; the ectodermal changes improved and other polyps that were a secondary cause to malnutrition regressed.

Cowden's Disease

Cowden's disease is an uncommon familial syndrome of combined ectodermal, endodermal, and mesodermal hamartomas. The disease was named for the propositus by Lloyd and Dennis in 1963.[113] Eighty percent of patients present with dermatologic manifestations, such as keratosis of extremities, the most common being a benign neoplasm of the hair shaft: a trichilemmoma. If a patient is diagnosed with more than one trichilemmoma, consideration should be given to the diagnosis of Cowden's disease. The second most common area of involvement is the central nervous system. Cowden's disease in concert with cerebella gangliocytomatosis is referred to as the Lhermitte–Duclos syndrome. Approximately 40% of affected individuals have macrocephaly as a component of the syndrome. Only 35% of patients who meet the diagnostic criteria for Cowden's disease have GI polyposis.[83]

Polyps in patients with Cowden's disease are small, typically < 5 mm in diameter. Microscopic features are consistent with hamartomas, characterized by disorganization and proliferation of the muscularis mucosa with minimally abnormal overlying mucosa.[114]

Most patients with Cowden's disease have been shown to subsume germline mutations in the PTEN gene located at 10q22.[115] PTEN is a tumor suppressor gene which has been shown to be involved with other forms of carcinoma such as familial thyroid carcinoma, inherited breast carcinoma, prostatic carcinoma, and malignant melanoma.[116,117,118,119,120,121] The majority of patients with Cowden's disease will have some form of benign thyroid or breast disease. In addition, the projected lifetime risk of thyroid malignancy is 10% and of breast malignancy is approximately 30 to 50%.[116,117,118] There has been no reported increased risk of invasive GI malignancy to date.[83]

Screening and surveillance for breast malignancies should include a schedule of monthly breast self-examinations. Clinical examination should be undertaken annually, beginning in the late teen years or as clinically warranted by symptoms. Mammography should be implemented at the age of 25. Although no specific recommendations for thyroid surveillance have been published, annual screening by clinical examination should begin in the late teen years or as symptoms warrant. A thyroid ultrasound may be used in parallel every 1 to 2 years.[83]

GI polyposis should be addressed by endoscopic surveillance. Although no definitive increased risk of colorectal carcinoma has been documented, the syndrome is rare; thus, the true risk may be unrecognized.[83]

Bannayan–Ruvalcaba–Riley Syndrome

This disease encompasses three previously described disorders: Bannayan–Zonana syndrome, Riley–Smith syndrome, and Ruvalcaba–Myhre–Smith syndrome. In 1960, Riley and Smith noted an autosomal dominant condition in which macrocephaly with a slowed cycle motor development, pseudopapilledema, and multiple hemangiomas were observed.[119] In 1971, Bannayan noted the congenital combination of macrocephaly with multiple subcutaneous and visceral lipoma as well as hemangiomas.[120] In 1980, Ruvalcaba described two males with macrocephaly, hamartomatous intestinal polyposis, and pigmentary spotting of the penis.[121] Given the clinical similarities between the conditions and the autosomal dominant pattern of inheritance, geneticists began to accept the notion of combining the disorders into a single entity as Bannayan–Ruvalcaba–Riley syndrome.[87] The syndrome gene is located at chromosome 10q23 133. Intestinal polyposis affects up to 45% of these patients. Usually, multiple hamartomatous polyps are identified with the majority limited to the distal ileum and colon, though they may be seen throughout the GI tract. Histologically, they appear similar to the juvenile polyposis-type polyp.[87]

Bannayan–Ruvalcaba–Riley syndrome is an autosomal dominant condition and, like Cowden's disease, appears to be associated with genetic alterations in the PTEN gene.[122] There has been no increased risk of colorectal carcinoma, other GI malignancies, or extraintestinal malignancy documented in these patients.[83]

19.1.3 Inflammatory and Lymphoid Polyps

Inflammatory polyps, or pseudopolyps, may look grossly like adenomatous polyps. However, microscopic examination shows islands of normal mucosa or mucosa with slight inflammation. They are caused by previous attacks of any form of severe colitis (ulcerative, Crohn's, amebic, ischemic, or schistosomal), resulting in partial loss of mucosa, leaving remnants or islands of relatively normal mucosa.

Radiologically, both the acute and chronic forms appear similar. Distinction can be made with the proctosigmoidoscope, but in the chronic stage a biopsy may be necessary to distinguish the condition from familial polyposis. Inflammatory polyps are not premalignant, and their presence in no way influences the potential malignant status of the patient with ulcerative colitis, a development that remains related to the extent, age of onset, and duration of disease. That these polyps are not premalignant in ulcerative colitis is relative; the potential carcinomatous status of the pseudopolyp in this condition is no more or less than that of the adjacent mucosa.[123]

Benign lymphoid polyps are enlargements of lymphoid follicles commonly seen in the rectum. They may be solitary or diffuse. Their cause is unknown. Lymphoid polyps must not be confused with FAP. The histologic criteria set out by Dawson et al[124] for the diagnosis of benign lymphoid polyps are as follows: the lymphoid tissue must be entirely within the mucosa and submucosa; there must be no invasion of the underlying muscle coat; at least two germinal centers must be present; and if the rectal biopsy fails to include the muscle coat and no germinal centers are seen, the diagnosis is inconclusive.

19.1.4 Hyperplastic Polyps

Hyperplastic polyps, also known as metaplastic polyps, are nonneoplastic polyps commonly found in the rectum as small, pale, and glassy mucosal nodules. Most are 3 to 5 mm, located predominantly in the left colon,[125] although larger ones can be seen in the more proximal part of the colon. Histologic differentiation from neoplastic polyps presents no problem. The characteristic picture is a sawtooth appearance of the lining of epithelial cells, producing a papillary outline (▶ Fig. 19.15). There is no nuclear dysplasia and thus no potential for malignancy.

Despite the colonoscopic findings of more adenomas than hyperplastic polyps, autopsies from Hawaii, Finland, and England demonstrate hyperplastic polyps in excess up to threefold over adenomas, with the great majority of them occurring in the sigmoid colon and rectum. In contrast, adenomas are distributed fairly evenly along the length of the large bowel.[126] The possibility of hyperplastic polyps serving as markers for adenomas has been raised in some colonoscopic data. It is clear, though, that the predictive value of the hyperplastic polyp is low, and the clinical usefulness of the marker must be critically questioned.[126]

Hyperplastic polyposis is a relatively new entity. The following criteria for hyperplastic polyposis have been proposed: (1) at least five histologically diagnosed hyperplastic polyps proximal to the sigmoid colon, of which two are greater than 10 mm in diameter; (2) any number of hyperplastic polyps occurring proximal to the sigmoid in an individual who has a first-degree relative with hyperplastic polyposis; (3) more than 30 hyperplastic polyps of any size, but distributed throughout the colon.[126] Although Williams et al[127] found no association between hyperplastic polyposis and colorectal carcinoma, some of the polyps contained mixture of hyperplastic and adenomatous elements which nowadays would have been classified as serrated adenomas. Subsequent case reports and small series recorded the presentation of colorectal carcinoma in patients with hyperplastic polyposis.[128,129] Colorectal carcinoma complicating hyperplastic polyposis is characterized by

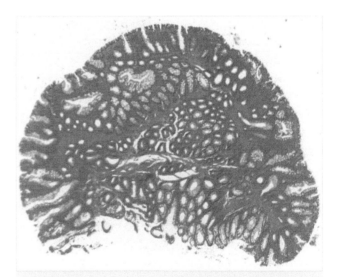

Fig. 19.15 Hyperplastic polyp. Note typical sawtooth appearance of the surface epithelium with a papillary appearance.

early age at onset, multiplicity, frequent location in proximal colon, and greater likelihood of showing the molecular phenotype known as DNA MSI–H.

The association between colorectal carcinoma and hyperplastic polyposis does not prove that carcinomas originate within hyperplastic polyposis. Adenomas might coexist with hyperplastic polyposis and might be the precursors of colorectal carcinomas, or these polyps are in fact serrated adenomas. Little has been reported on the risk of metachronous adenomas in patients with hyperplastic polyps. Bensen et al[130] examined data from two large randomized colorectal chemoprevention trials for possible associations of hyperplastic polyps and adenomatous polyps with subsequent development of these lesions. Of the 1,794 patients randomized in two trials, 1,583 completed two follow-up colonoscopies, and are considered in their analysis. They computed rates of incidence on hyperplastic polyps and adenomas over the 3-year follow-up after the first surveillance examination with polyp status (type and number) at that examination as predictors. During the 3-year follow-up, 320 (20%) had one or more hyperplastic polyps detected, and 564 (36%) had one or more adenomas. Patients with hyperplastic polyps at the first surveillance examination had a higher risk of any hyperplastic polyp recurrence on follow-up than those without hyperplastic polyps (odds ratio, 3.67). Similarly, patients with adenomas at the first surveillance examination had a higher risk of adenoma recurrence than those without adenomas (odds ratio, 2.08). However, the presence of hyperplastic polyps at the first surveillance examination was not significantly associated with adenoma occurrence during follow-up, nor was the presence of adenoma significantly associated with subsequent hyperplastic polyp occurrence.

19.2 Familial Adenomatous Polyposis

FAP is an inherited, non–sex-linked and mendelian-dominant disease characterized by the progressive development of hundreds or thousands of adenomatous polyps throughout the entire large bowel. The clinical diagnosis is based on the histologic confirmation of at least 100 adenomas (▶ Fig. 19.16). However, with the widespread practice of family counseling and the genetic testing, this number of adenomas is no longer rigidly applied. In the absence of a family history of FAP, the number 100 or more is still good to entertain the diagnosis. The important feature of the disease is the fact that one or more of these polyps will eventually develop into an invasive adenocarcinoma unless a prophylactic proctocolectomy is undertaken. The disease has high penetrance, with a 50% chance of development of the disease in the affected family. Approximately 20% of patients with FAP have no family history and their condition represents spontaneous mutation.[131] The term "FAP" is now used to replace the term "familial polyposis coli" because the disease also affects other organs. The older terms Gardner's syndrome, familial polyposis of the GI tract, familial multiple polyposis, and many other names should be avoided.

The incidence of FAP is 1 in 7,000 live births.[132] Although the disease is congenital, there is no evidence that adenomas have ever been present at birth. In his extensive experience with the St. Mark's Hospital, London, Polyposis Registry, Bussey[133] summarized the natural course of FAP in the average untreated patient as follows.

19.2.1 Clinical Manifestations and Diagnosis

Symptoms usually do not develop until there is a full-blown development of polyposis. Bleeding from the rectum and diarrhea are the most common symptoms. The diagnosis is made by endoscopic examination of the colon and rectum or by barium enema studies. It must be confirmed by histologic findings of adenomatous polyps. Only occasionally are tubulovillous adenomas found and villous adenomas are rare. The smallest possible microadenoma consists of only a single crypt, obviously not visible by examination with the naked eye.[134]

The average age at which the disease is diagnosed is 36 years. The adenomas actually appear much earlier, as is seen by comparison with the age of diagnosis in family members called for

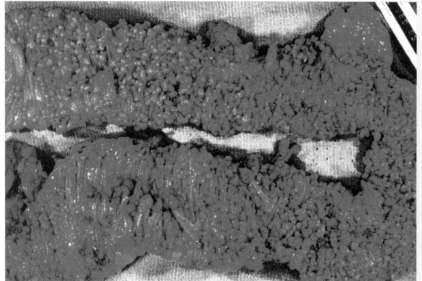

Fig. 19.16 Numerous small adenomatous polyps of the colon and rectum in a patient with familial adenomatous polyposis.

examination. In this group of patients, the average age is 24 years. Nearly two of three patients (65%) who were present because of symptoms already have carcinoma. The average age of colorectal carcinoma in these patients is 39 years, compared with 65 years in the normal population. Since most of the polyps in FAP are small, the best methods of diagnosis are colonoscopy and biopsy. A complete colonic examination has become important since rectal sparing has been reported, even when adenocarcinoma is present in the proximal colon.[135]

Although the rectum is almost invariably involved with polyps, the number of polyps in each segment of the colon and rectum varies from person to person. In general, the left colon has a higher density of polyps than the right colon.[133] In any one patient, the polyps vary in size from barely visible mucosal nodules 1 or 2 mm in diameter, to up to 1 cm or larger. In some patients and families, the adenomas are mostly small, while in others they are large. Most patients with FAP have myriads of polyps, frequently up to 5,000.[136] In a series from Denmark, the risk of developing carcinoma was highest in the rectum, followed by the sigmoid colon (▶ Table 19.6).[136]

19.2.2 Attenuated Familial Adenomatous Polyposis

This is a variant of FAP in which the majority of patients present with between 1 and 50 adenomas, primarily located proximal to the splenic flexure and often morphologically flat.[137,138,139,140,141,142,143,144,145,146] The polyps are diagnosed at the mean age of 44 years, and carcinomas at the mean age of 56 years. Thus, diagnosis of polyps and carcinomas in attenuated familial adenomatous polyposis (AFAP) is generally 10 to 15 years later than in FAP. However, because these data are based on when these lesions are detected and not necessarily on when they arise, the true age of development of polyps and carcinomas in AFAP is unclear. Certainly, lack of recognition of AFAP by patients and by physicians results in fewer patients presenting for voluntary surveillance, perhaps contributing to a delay in diagnosis in these patients.[140]

Patients with AFAP have variability in the number of polyps even within members of the same kindred. Some affected members have few polyps, while others have several hundred. This variability presents difficulties in classifying members of the same kindred as AFAP or FAP. Similar to FAP, colorectal carcinomas in patients with AFAP are generally accompanied by synchronous adenomas.[140] The extracolonic manifestations in AFAP are similar to FAP.

For asymptomatic at-risk individuals belonging to known FAP or AFAP kindreds, genetic testing should be ideally performed between the ages of 10 and 15 years to determine the presence or absence of an APC mutation. A baseline colonoscopy and esophagoduodenoscopy at the time of genetic testing or by the age of 15 years should be performed.[141] In patients with true-negative APC test results (a mutation has been demonstrated in an affected member but not in an at-risk member), a colonoscopy should be performed at the time of genetic testing or by the age of 15. Although the protein truncation test (PTT) is nearly 100% accurate in this setting, endoscopic evaluation serves as confirmation of a negative test. Because polyps occur later in AFAP individuals than in classic FAP, a second colonoscopy at age 20 should be considered to detect late-appearing polyps. If both examinations are negative, no further surveillance is necessary, and the patient may undergo future colorectal carcinoma screening as an average-risk individual.[140]

Patients with AFAP are at increased risk for the development of colorectal carcinoma, but do not have the near certainty of developing colorectal carcinoma that classic FAP patients have. Thus, the indications for prophylactic colectomy differ. In patients with few adenomas, colonoscopic polypectomy is sufficient to clear the affected bowel segments. When multiple polyps are clustered within a single segment of the colon, especially the cecum, resection may be the safest option. When resection is required, a total abdominal colectomy can be performed with an IRA. Because the rectal segment is generally uninvolved in these patients, total proctocolectomy with IPAA does not seem to be required. The rectal segment does need continued surveillance because this mucosa is still at risk. Total abdominal colectomy with IRA may also be required in patients who are difficult to examine fully by colonoscopy and, thus, unable to undergo proper surveillance.[141]

AFAP has two forms: patients with mutations at the five prime of APC are at minimal risk for desmoid disease, whereas patients with mutation in exon 15 are at high risk. This risk of desmoids, often manifest in other relatives who have had an operation, may encourage deferment of surgery. The alternative to colectomy, endoscopic polypectomy with or without chemoprevention, is risky especially when the patient has been shown to carry a germline APC mutation. Colonoscopic surveillance does not prevent carcinoma in all patients with HNPCC; the same can be applied to AFAP; this must be reserved for truly compliant patients who realize the risks.[141]

19.2.3 Molecular Genetics

Using genetic-linkage analysis, it has been determined that FAP is caused by a mutation in the tumor suppressor gene APC located on the long arm of chromosome 5q21–22. The term FAP is not used to describe this gene because familial amyloidotic polyneuropathy takes historical precedence in the genetic literature.[139] The genetic alterations found in the FAP patient's colon and rectal carcinoma are similar to those noted in sporadic carcinoma, except that an APC mutation is already present constitutionally at birth (a germline mutation).

There are correlations between the location of the APC mutation and the clinical phenotype. ▶ Fig. 19.17[143] shows the correlation between the APC genotype and the clinical phenotype. The 15 exons of the APC gene are shown. The locations of germline mutations associated with specific clinical phenotypes are indicated by the dark horizontal lines. Over 34 mutations causing AFAP have

Table 19.6 Distribution of colorectal carcinoma in 109 propositions[137]

	No. of carcinomas	(%)
Right colon	8	6
Transverse colon	6	5
Descending colon	8	6
Sigmoid colon	31	24
Rectum	77	59
Total	130	100

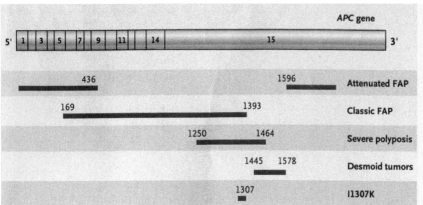

Fig. 19.17 Correlation between the APC genotype and the clinical phenotype.[147]

been reported; these are clustered either at the five prime end (before codon 436) or at the three prime end (after codon 1596) of the APC gene. In contrast, mutations causing classic FAP are located in the central region, and mutations between codons 1250 and 1464 are associated with particularly severe polyposis. Abdominal desmoid tumors are more likely in persons with mutations between codons 1445 and 1578.

The molecular mechanisms that explain why certain APC mutations result in a classic phenotype and others in an attenuated phenotype are currently being elucidated. Most models are predicated on the "two-hit hypothesis"—which states that both alleles of APC must be inactivated in order to initiate tumorigenesis. In ► Fig. 19.18,[143] both copies of chromosome 5 are shown. In classic FAP (panel a), the biallelic inactivation of APC is typically achieved by the combination of an inherited germline mutation in one allele (black X) and a chromosomal deletion of the remaining wild-type allele; this is called loss of heterozygosity. In some cases, the germline APC mutation (red X) can result in the production of a protein that can inhibit the activity of the wild-type protein (white X). This dominant negative effect functionally results in biallelic inactivation.

In AFAP (panel b), the mechanism of APC inactivation is different. Germline mutations involved in AFAP may lead to the formation of alternative APC proteins that are initiated from an internal translation site that is located distal to the truncating mutation. This alternative APC protein does have functional activity. Because of this residual gene activity, an additional "hit" is necessary to fully inactivate APC (panel c). This third "hit" is indicated by the blue X. The second hit is often an intragenic mutation (green X) that inactivates the wild-type APC allele, rather than a large chromosomal deletion as in classic FAP. The red X represents the inherited APC mutation.[143]

19.2.4 Extracolonic Expressions

In 1951, Gardner[144] reported finding osteomatosis, epidermoid cysts, and fibromas of the skin, a triad in FAP known as Gardner's syndrome. The detection of identical mutations in individuals with FAP and Gardner's syndrome helps confirm that at the genetic level they are variants of a common entity.[137] The disease affects the whole body, involving tissues derived from

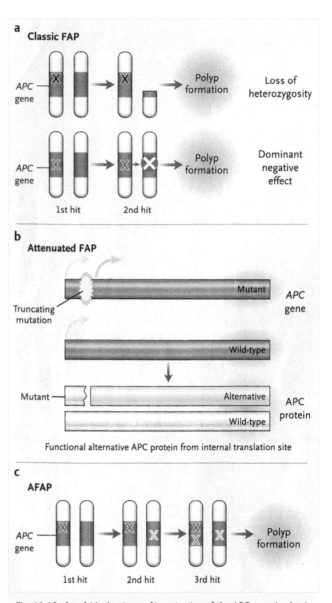

Fig. 19.18 (a–c) Mechanisms of inactivation of the APC gene in classic and attenuated familial adenomatous polyposis (FAP).[147]

all three germ layers.[134] Factors that contribute to the extracolonic manifestations are unresolved. Modifying genetic factors (e.g., other genes or different genetic backgrounds) or environmental variables probably play a role in the final phenotype. Likewise, the role that APC plays in the development of various extracolonic neoplasms and manifestations remains to be defined. There have been some indications that the location of the APC mutation itself may have an effect on the phenotype, although conclusive evidence for this proposal is lacking.[137]

Endodermal Abnormalities

Gastric Polyps

With improved survival rates following colorectal resection, gastric polyps or upper GI lesions have become increasingly important because of the risk of malignant change in duodenal polyps. The introduction of flexible endoscopy has provided more ready access to the upper GI tract, although at present the course of the disease is not precisely known.[145] The prevalence of gastric polyps ranges from 34 to 100%; most of them are hyperplastic type in the fundus of the stomach, and a few adenomatous types have been reported in the antrum.[146,148] When gastric adenomas are present, they seem to be in patients who have duodenogastric reflux in an area exposed to bile.[149]

Duodenal Polyps

In most series, duodenal adenomas occur in more than 90% of FAP patients, particularly in the periampullary region.[147,150,151] The macroscopic appearance of duodenal polyps is very different to that of colonic polyps. The number of the former varies from invisible to over 100. They may present as multiple discrete adenomas (1–10 mm in diameter) or as flat confluent plaques. Sometimes no lesion can be seen and the only clinical abnormality is a prominent ampulla, or the mucosa may appear pale and seem to have a white covering which cannot be removed by rubbing. Biopsy of apparently normal mucosa frequently showed microadenomas.[149] The lifetime risk of adenoma in FAP patients is high. Mutations downstream from codon 1051 seem to be associated with severe periampullary adenomas.[152] Spigelman et al[153] staged the duodenal polyposis according to polyp number, polyp size, and histologic type. The criteria provided a four-stage scoring system (▶ Table 19.7). The classification allows estimation of the severity of duodenal polyposis.

Table 19.7 Staging of duodenal polyposis[154]

Criteria	Grade points		
	1	2	3
Polyp number	1–4	5–20	>20
Polyp size (mm)	1–4	5–10	>10
Histology	Tubular	Tubulovillous	Villous
Dysplasia	Mild	Moderate	Severe

Note: Stage 0, 0 point; stage I, 1–4 points; stage II, 5–6 points; stage III, 7–8 points; stage IV, 9–12 points.

In a prospective study conducted by Domizio et al,[155] over 102 asymptomatic FAP patients were screened with side-viewing video endoscope; duodenal polyps were found to be multiple in two-thirds of patients, with one-third of patients having more than 20. The average size of a duodenal polyp was 9 mm, but they can be much bigger (2 cm). Duodenal polyps were almost always adenomas. Duodenal adenomas were tabular in architecture in about 70% of patients, tubulovillous in 20%, and villous in 10%. Duodenal polyps were not seen in approximately 10% of patients. In just over one-half of these patients, microadenomas were subsequently found. Presumably, if more random biopsies had been taken, more patients with microadenomas would have been found.

Only 10% of patients had stage IV duodenal polyposis, while just under 20% had stage I disease and the remaining, 35% each, had stage II or stage III duodenal polyposis. Those with stage IV disease were older than the rest, implying that duodenal polyposis is a progressive disorder. Advanced duodenal disease might be a marker for the presence of gastric adenomas, as nearly all those with gastric adenomas had stage III or stage IV duodenal polyposis in their series.[155] The risk of duodenal carcinoma in FAP is more than 100 times that of the normal population. Of 222 FAP patients who had a colectomy and IRA at St. Mark's Hospital between 1948 and 1990 (inclusive), duodenal carcinoma accounted for 11 deaths, more than twice the number of deaths attributed to carcinoma of the rectal stump.[156] A retrospective survey based on 10 polyposis registries in the Leeds Castle Polyposis Group showed duodenal and periampullary carcinoma in 30% of 1,225 patients.[154] The major causes of death in a series of 36 FAP patients treated with prophylactic proctocolectomy or colectomy with an IRA at the Cleveland Clinic were desmoid tumor (31%), periampullary carcinoma (22%), and rectal carcinoma (8%).[157] The cause of death from extracolonic diseases is also higher than carcinoma of colon and rectum in recent decades in the series of Belchetz et al.[158]

One of the most difficult problems is the treatment of duodenal adenomas. Bile has been implicated in the pathogenesis of duodenal polyps in patients with FAP. FAP bile has been shown to contain an excess of carcinogens able to form DNA adducts. DNA adducts are chemical modification of DNA, formed by covalent binding of electrophilic carcinogens to DNA, which are implicated in the initiation of carcinogenesis because when they are left unrepaired they can lead to mutations. Modification of the action of these carcinogens may reduce the adduct load to the duodenum and so decrease actual duodenal polyp number. However, in the double-blind randomized placebo-controlled trial conducted by Wallace et al,[159] 26 patients with FAP were randomly assigned to ranitidine, 300 mg daily, or placebo for 6 months after baseline endoscopy. The result showed that acid suppression therapy does not seem to improve duodenal polyposis.

Celecoxib (Celebrex, Pfizer, New York, NY) has been shown to reduce the number of duodenal polyps. Phillips et al[160] conducted a randomized, double-blind, placebo-controlled study of celecoxib, 100 mg twice daily (n = 34), or 400 mg twice daily (n = 32), versus placebo (n = 17), given orally twice daily for 6 months to patients with FAP associated with duodenal polyposis. Efficacy was assessed qualitatively by blinded review of shuffled endoscopy videotapes comparing the extent of duodenal polyposis at entry and at 6 months and quantitatively by measurement of the percentage change in duodenal area covered by discrete and plaquelike adenomas from photographs of high- and low-density polyposis. The results showed a statistically significant effect of 400 mg twice daily celecoxib compared with placebo treatment. Overall, patients taking celecoxib, 400 mg twice daily, showed a 15.5% reduction in involved areas compared with a 1.4% for placebo. The authors suggested that celecoxib might have been indicated in patients with established duodenal disease, particularly when it is severe. However, it is harder to justify its use in patients with lesser duodenal disease, as progression to duodenal carcinoma in these patients with an earlier onset of the disease is unusual.

Some authors successfully eradicated few adenomas of duodenum in FAP patients but the number of these patients had been too small to judge its efficacy.[161,162] In general, endoscopic snaring or thermal contact can be performed only in patients with few small lesions as an initial treatment, or in patients who are not a candidate for major surgery.

The natural history of untreated duodenal and ampullary adenomas in patients with FAP has been studied by Burke et al.[163] A total of 114 FAP patients who had two or more surveillance examinations were followed for a mean of 51 months (range, 10–151 months). Duodenal polyps progressed in size in 26% (25 of 95), number in 32% (34 of 106), and histology in 11% (5 of 45) of patients. Morphology and histology of the main duodenal papilla progressed in 14% (15 of 110) and 11% (12 of 105) of patients, respectively. A minority of FAP patients had progression of endoscopic features and histology of duodenal polyps or the main duodenal papilla when followed over 4 years. An endoscopic surveillance interval of at least 3 years may be appropriate for the majority of untreated patients with FAP.

An operation is indicated if polyps show villous change, severe dysplasia, rapid growth, and induration at endoscopic probing.[147] Duodenectomy or local excision is not preferred because of very high recurrences and complications.[150,164,165,166,167] A pancreatoduodenectomy, particularly duodenectomy with preservation of pancreas, for patients with severe duodenal polyposis or patients who already had carcinoma appears to be the best option.[165,168,169,170] The lifetime risk of duodenal adenomas approaches 100%.[171] Recommendations concerning the age of initiation of upper tract surveillance are not uniform. Some propose that screening for upper GI disease should start at the time of FAP diagnosis. The National Comprehensive Cancer Network, after review of all case reports of duodenal carcinoma in FAP patients, recommended a baseline upper GI endoscopic examination at 25 to 30 years of age. In general, recommendations include: stage 0, every 4 years; stage I, every 2 to 3 years; stage II, every 2 to 3 years; stage III, every 6 to 12 months with consideration for surgery; and stage IV, strongly consider surgery.[171]

Polyps in the Small Bowel

Adenomas have been detected in the ileum following colectomy and IRA and also in Kock's pouch following proctocolectomy. A small number of cases of malignant neoplasms in the small bowel in association with FAP have been recorded; the risk of developing such a lesion appears minimal. Lymphoid polyps have also been noted in FAP, both in the small bowel and colon. Histological confirmation should be undertaken because presentation may mimic FAP.[145]

Mesodermal Abnormalities

Desmoid Tumors

Patients with mutation between codons 1445 and 1578 frequently developed desmoid tumors.[172] Desmoid tumors are benign tumors arising from fibroaponeurotic tissue. It is not known whether they are true neoplasms or the result of a generalized fibroblast abnormality; there is increasing evidence to support the former theory.[173] Although a benign disease, desmoid tumors are focally invasive. They do not metastasize but can be lethal because of aggressive growth with pressure and erosion causing obstruction of the small bowel (▶ Fig. 19.19). A report from the Finnish Polyposis Registry included 202 FAP patients, of whom 169 underwent colectomy. Desmoids were observed in 29 patients (14%): 15 (7%) in the mesentery, 10 (5%) on the abdominal wall, and four (2%) in

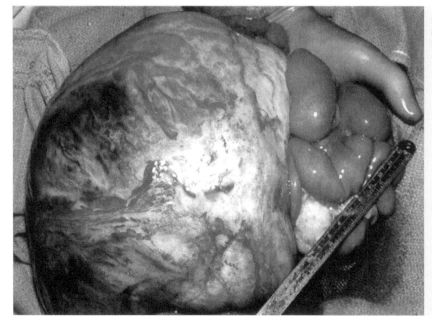

Fig. 19.19 Large desmoid tumor of mesentery causing partial small bowel obstruction. (Courtesy of Roger R. Dozois, MD.)

other sites. The cumulative lifetime risk is 21.0, 1.5, 3.0, 8.9, 16.0, and 18.0% at ages of 10, 20, 30, 40, and 50 years, respectively.[174] Clark et al[175] studied desmoid tumors from St. Mark's Polyposis Registry Database. Eighty-eight patients had 166 desmoids (median age, 32). Eighty-three patients (50%) had the tumor intra-abdominally, with 88% in the small bowel mesentery; 80 patients (48%) had the tumor on the abdominal wall, with 39% in surgical scars; three patients (2%) had the tumor extra-abdominally (chest wall, intrathoracic). All (82%) but 16 patients had already undergone abdominal surgery.

The behavior of desmoids in FAP ranges from rapid growth with symptoms resulting from visceral compression to a more indolent course, or even spontaneous regression. Plaquelike thickening of the small bowel mesentery and the peritoneum that does not amount to a discrete mass has been described as a relatively common finding at celiotomy in patients with FAP undergoing surgery.[176,177]

Hartley et al[176] studied the natural history of these lesions that were incidentally found on celiotomy. A total of 266 patients underwent abdominal surgery for FAP. Incidental intra-abdominal desmoid tumors were identified in 34 patients, 8 at the index surgery and 26 at receliotomy (median 130 months from the index procedure; range, 23–364 months). Intra-abdominal desmoids identified at the time of index surgery influenced the intended procedure in one of eight cases (6-cm mass in mesentery precluded IPAA). Intra-abdominal desmoids identified at second celiotomy influenced the intended surgery procedure in 10 of 26 cases (38%), including one for Kock's pouch, two for IPAA, two difficult pouch reach, two prevented covering stoma, one iliac vein surgery, and two bypass only. Desmoid reaction was found in 1 of the index and 11 of the re-explore celiotomy group. This type of lesion was not an obstacle to the planned surgery. Desmoid reaction or mesenteric fibromatosis is precursor lesion for subsequent desmoid formation. However, the risk for progression in any individual case is likely to be small.[177] Phillips[178] recommended computed tomography (CT) scan of any FAP patients before planned second major surgery, whether for pouch conversion or management of duodenal polyposis.

The most common symptom in patients with intra-abdominal desmoids is a painful abdominal mass (50%). The rest have a painless mass or no palpable mass. The pain is usually caused by bowel obstruction. Other causes of the pain are ureteric obstruction, direct pressure effects of the tumor, or hemorrhage into the tumor.[179] The preferred investigation is the CT scan, which permits serial observation of the tumor.[145,180] Magnetic resonance imaging (MRI) has been shown to provide adequate images of intra-abdominal soft tissue tumors while sparing the patient's exposure to ionizing radiation.[145,181]

Intra-abdominal desmoids are a difficult clinical challenge. Their tendency to recur (65–85%) after removal has encouraged a conservative approach to management.[179] Operation should be preferred for patients in whom life-threatening complications have occurred as a result of local invasion.[145] In many patients, operation is unavoidable. Middleton and Phillips of St. Mark's hospital[182] were forced to remove a large intra-abdominal desmoid tumor from four patients (three patients had FAP). Three had complete excision of their desmoids and all remained well with no recurrence at a median follow-up of 12 (range, 7–14) months. Eight of 22 patients who underwent resection of

their intra-abdominal desmoids at St. Mark's died in the post-operation period.[175] Church[179] cautioned that survey for a large intra-abdominal desmoid is technically extremely difficult, demanding high levels of skill and support. It should only be done in setting of a major medical center. On the other hand, abdominal wall and other superficial desmoids can be often cured by wide excision, especially when the tumor is small. The tumors are extremely resistant to radiotherapy and cytotoxic chemotherapy.[145]

Encouraging reports have appeared following treatment with sulindac, with or without tamoxifen. Church and others[179,183] suggested treatment of intra-abdominal desmoid tumors in FAP with sulindac, 150 mg twice daily. If the tumor continues to grow as shown by clinical observation and CT scan, add tamoxifen, 80 mg/day. If the tumor stabilizes, continue the medications but reduce the tamoxifen dose after 6 months and then gradually discontinue therapy. If the desmoid keeps growing or is still symptomatic, consider chemotherapy. If an intra-abdominal desmoid is discovered during operation and can be resected with a minimum of small bowel and low risk of complications, proceed. If complete excision is impossible, obtain tissue for histologic and estrogen-receptor assays.

Using an antisarcoma regimen consisting of doxorubicin and dacarbazine, Moslein and Dozois[184] used this regimen in nine patients with FAP-related desmoid tumor and it led to complete regression in four patients and partial regression in five patients. Poritz et al[185] treated eight patients with desmoid tumors and FAP who had inoperable GI obstruction and/or uncontrolled pain. The regimen consisted of doxorubicin and dacarbazine followed by carboplatin and dacarbazine. Follow-up at a mean of 42 months in seven patients revealed two patients who achieved complete remission after the therapy. Four patients achieved a partial remission after completing all or some of the chemotherapy regimen; of these, three remained at stable remission, whereas the other was lost to follow-up. There were two recurrences that required further therapy; one of these patients was treated with further chemotherapy, which induced a second remission, and the other was treated with pelvic exenteration and has subsequently died. This cytotoxic regimen should be considered only for patients with fast-growing, life-threatening mesenteric desmoid tumors.

Church et al[186] developed a staging system that can be applied to the management of FAP-related desmoid tumor:

- Stage I: Asymptomatic, not growing. Asymptomatic desmoids are usually small and are found incidentally either during exploratory celiotomy or on CT scan performed for unrelated reasons. Such tumors can be observed, or, at the most, a relatively nontoxic medication such as nonsteroidal anti-inflammatory drugs (NSAIDs) may be prescribed. If a stage I desmoid is found incidentally at surgery and it is easily resectable without the removal of a significant amount of bowel, resection is appropriate.
- Stage II: Symptomatic and 10 cm or less in maximum diameter, not growing. Small desmoids that are causing symptoms (including bowel or ureteral obstruction) need therapy even if they are not obviously growing. If they are resectable with minimal sequelae, then resection is best. If the tumor is unresectable, the addition of tamoxifen or raloxifene to a NSAID offers the possibility of a quicker and more consistent response with low risk of side effects.

- Stage III: Symptomatic and 11 to 20 cm, or asymptomatic and slowly growing desmoids. Larger, symptomatic (including bowel or ureteric obstruction) desmoids, or desmoids that are slowly increasing in size (< 50% increase in diameter in 6 months), need active treatment. Here, the choices include NSAID, tamoxifen, raloxifene, and vinblastine/methotrexate. Antisarcoma chemotherapy can be given if the tumor continues to grow despite less toxic agents.
- Stage IV: Symptomatic, > 20 cm, or rapid growth, or complicated desmoids. These are the worst desmoids: large, or growing rapidly (> 50% increase in diameter within 6 months), these cause life-threatening complications such as sepsis, perforation, or hemorrhage. Here, treatment is an urgent necessity and the possibilities are major exenterative surgery likely to result in significant loss of bowel, antisarcoma therapy, and radiation.

The authors noted that one of the most important uses of the staging system is to allow prospective trials of the various treatment options, some of which are inappropriate for certain stages of tumor.[186] Death from desmoid tumors is caused by either direct effects, such as erosion into a blood vessel or sepsis from an enteric fistula, or secondary effects as the result of desmoid surgery.[179]

Osteomas

Osteomas may occur in any bone but they are most commonly located on the facial skeleton, particularly the mandible. These tumors are benign but may cause symptoms following local growth. They are sometimes identified before the diagnosis of FAP is made.[145]

Teeth

Teeth are derived from both mesoderm and ectoderm. Dental abnormalities, distinct from osteomas of the jaw, have been described in 11 to 80% of individuals with FAP. Although slightly less frequent than osteomas of the jaw, their frequency and the fact that they may appear at an early age are sufficient reasons to make them diagnostically useful. The findings in question are impactions, supernumerary or absent teeth, fused root of first and second molars, and unusually long and tapered roots of posterior teeth.[134]

Ectodermal Abnormalities

Eye Lesions

Although the presence of pigmented lesions of the fundus was noted in a patient with the signs of Gardner's syndrome by Cabot[187] in 1935, it was not until 1980, when Blair and Trempe[188] recorded pigmented lesions in three affected members of a kindred with Gardner's syndrome, that the possibility of using this lesion as a marker for FAP was suggested. The abnormality is considered to be congenital hypertrophy of retinal pigment epithelium (CHRPE). The occurrence of CHRPE is restricted to APC mutation in codons 463 to 1444.[172]

The examination is made by indirect ophthalmoscopy, following instillation of 1% tropicamide for pupil dilatation. It normally appears as a round or oval pigmented lesion with a

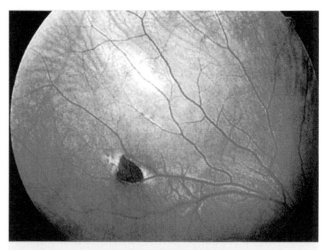

Fig. 19.20 Fundus photograph of the pigmented lesion of the retina (CHRPE). (Courtesy of Helmut Buettmer, MD.)

surrounding pale halo (▶ Fig. 19.20). Microscopic examination shows that CHRPE is a hamartoma. The acronym, while not strictly correct, has become accepted and has continued in use.[153] The incidence of CHRPE in patients with FAP varies widely from 50 to 79%[134,145] compared with 7 and 5% in at-risk groups and in age- and sex-matched individuals, respectively. The sensitivity of CHRPE in FAP is 79% and specificity is 95%.[145]

The presence of CHRPE in a person who is a member of a kindred of a patient manifesting FAP suggests that he or she has inherited the gene. The absence of the lesion does not, however, indicate that the person has not inherited the gene.[145]

Epidermoid Cyst

In patients with FAP, cysts may be found on the limbs, face, and scalp. In the general population, they occur predominantly on the back. Leppard and Bussey[189] found epidermoid cysts in 53% of a series of 74 patients affected by FAP. Perhaps the most significant finding related to epidermoid cysts is their rarity in childhood in any condition other than FAP; skin cysts may be evident before the development of colorectal polyps.[190] Leppard and Bussey[189] recommend that a child with an epidermoid cyst undergo sigmoidoscopy after the age of 14 years but before attaining 30 years of age.

Brain Neoplasms

In 1949, Crail[191] reported a case of synchronous cerebellar medulloblastoma, colonic polyposis (approximately 100 polyps), and papillary carcinoma of the thyroid. This report did not receive widespread recognition at that time.[192] In 1959, Turcot et al[193] described two siblings who presented with colonic polyposis at the ages of 13 and 15 years, respectively. Both patients went on to develop a glioblastoma of the frontal lobe and a medullary medulloblastoma, respectively. The first sibling also had a chromophobe adenoma of the pituitary gland. The authors suggested that these neoplasms might be another extracolonic manifestation of FAP. These associations bear the name Turcot's syndrome.

Hamilton et al[194] studied Turcot's syndrome at the molecular level. Fourteen families with Turcot's syndrome were identified.

Germline mutations in the APC gene characteristic of FAP were evaluated, as well as DNA replication errors and germline mutations in nucleotide mismatch-repair genes characteristic of HNPCC.

Genetic abnormalities were identified in 13 of 14 registry families. Germline APC mutations were detected in 10. The predominant brain tumor in these 10 families was medulloblastoma (11 of 14 patients, or 79%), and the RR of cerebellar medulloblastoma in patients with FAP was 92 times that in the general population. In contrast, the type of brain tumor in the other four families was glioblastoma multiforme. Germline mutations in the mismatch-repair gene hMLH1 or hMMS2 were found in two families.

In the study of the APC gene in 14 families that included at least one affected member, in 12 families classified as having polyposis, mutations were found in 10 (83%). All the mutated genes encoded truncated variance of the APC protein, as is true of the vast majority of patients with FAP. The mutations were heterogeneous in type and location, and there was no association between specific mutations and the development of brain tumors. Two families with polyposis and both families without polyposis had no identifiable germline APC mutations.

Analysis of the hMSH2, hMLH1, hPMS1, and hPMS2 mismatch-repair genes, which are mutated in HNPCC, was carried out in the three patients with neoplasms that contained replication errors. Two had germline alterations: the hPMS2 gene was mutated in one patient and hMLH1 was mutated in another patient. No germline APC mutations were detected in these three patients. The authors concluded that the association between brain neoplasms and multiple colorectal adenomas might result from two distinct types of germline defects: mutation of the APC gene or mutation of the mismatch-repair gene. Molecular diagnosis may contribute to the appropriate care of affected patients.

Review of literature by Matsui et al[195] and Itoh et al[196] revealed that there were 131 documented cases in the medical literature. Of the 35 cases that they considered having true Turcot's syndrome, the average age of death was 20.3 years. Most (76%) died from brain malignancy, 16% died from colorectal carcinoma, and the rest from other causes. Death at young age has made it difficult to determine whether the mode of inheritance is autosomal recessive or autosomal dominant. A more complete list of the extracolonic manifestations of FAP is summarized in ▶ Table 19.8.[192]

19.2.5 Management

Histologic verification of adenomas is essential so that confusion with familial juvenile polyposis, hyperplastic polyposis, pseudopolyposis, and lymphoid polyposis is avoided. Performing total colonoscopy and biopsy is the best choice. Virtually all patients with FAP will develop carcinoma of the colon and rectum by age 40. For this reason, patients with FAP should have prophylactic colectomy. At present, there are several surgical options, and each has advantages and disadvantages.

Proctocolectomy with Ileostomy

This procedure removes all the disease, but an obvious side effect is the creation of a permanent ileostomy, which is not well

Table 19.8 Selected series on risk of rectal carcinoma after colectomy and ileorectal anastomosis

Authors	No. of patients	Year after IRA	Rectal carcinoma rate (%)
Bess et al[208]	143	19	32
Bulow[132]	58	10	13
Sarre et al[212]	133	20	12
De Cosse et al[213]	294	25	13
Nugent and Phillips[210]	224	25	15
Iwama and Mishima[214]	342	15	24
Heiskanen and Järvinen[174]	100	20	25
Jenner and Levitt[215]	55	10	13
Björk et al[197]	195	25	24
Bertario et al[216]	371	20	23
Church et al[200]	62	15	13

Abbreviation: IRA, ileorectal anastomosis.

accepted by most patients, particularly the young ones. With the availability of other alternatives, such as colectomy with IRA and proctocolectomy with an ileoanal pouch procedure (IPAA), proctocolectomy with ileostomy is seldom chosen by patients. However, if there is a carcinoma in the rectum or in patients with a desmoid tumor of the small bowel mesentery, a proctocolectomy should be performed.

Proctocolectomy with Continent Ileostomy

This procedure was a popular option in the 1970s. An ileal reservoir with a nipple valve is created from the terminal ileum and is brought out as an ileostomy. Its advantage over the conventional ileostomy is that an ileostomy bag is not required. The pouch must be evacuated four to six times a day with a catheter. Because of the frequent extrusion of the nipple valve, which results in incontinence, use of the procedure has been limited to a small number of patients. The IPAA now has largely replaced this procedure.

Colectomy with Ileorectal Anastomosis

This procedure minimizes the risk of development of carcinoma up to only the last 12 to 15 cm of the rectum. Patients require lifelong close follow-up, at least once or twice a year, with electrocoagulation of the polyps as indicated. It should be selected for patients in whom the rectum is not carpeted with polyps and who are willing to return for follow-up. The main advantages of this choice are that it is a relatively simple procedure familiar to most surgeons and it has excellent functional results.

Controversy exists about the risk of developing carcinoma in the remaining rectum after colectomy and IRA. The risk varies from series to series, from 0% at the Cleveland Clinic[207] to an overall 32% at the Mayo Clinic.[208] The discrepancy is not clear, but it appears that the risk of developing carcinoma increases with time.[209] The unusually high incidence of carcinoma in the retained rectum in the Mayo Clinic series prompted Bess et al[208] to reanalyze the series 10 years later, with the aim of identifying factors that may contribute to the risks. The following variables do not cause an increase in the risks: male versus female, number of colonic polyps (≥ 100 vs. ≤ 100), family history of polyposis, age at the time of surgery (≥ 40 years vs. ≤ 40 years), and level of ileorectal or ileosigmoid anastomosis (≥ 15 cm vs. ≤ 15 cm). Factors that contribute to an increase in carcinoma risk include the number of preoperative rectal polyps (the risk is increased if there are more than 20 polyps in the remaining rectum) and colonic carcinoma resected at or before colectomy. Of significance is the cumulative risk of carcinoma in the St. Mark's series, increasing from 10% at 20-year follow-up to more than 30% at 35 years.[209]

Risk of Carcinoma in the Retained Rectum

The series from St. Mark's[209] showed that until the age of 50 years, the cumulative risk of carcinoma in the IRA is reasonably low at 10%, increasing sharply to 29% by the age of 60 years. This means that surveillance of the retained rectum in older patients must either be improved or the patients should undergo restorative proctocolectomy in earlier middle age. Nugent and Phillips[210] recommend a flexible videoendoscopy at fixed intervals of 4 months for all patients at risk over the age of 45 years who wish to retain the rectum. A similar age-dependent rectal carcinoma risk is also reported by Heiskanen and Järvinen[211]— 3.9, 12.8, and 25.7% at 40, 50, and 60 years, respectively, and rectal excision rates of 9.5, 26.3, and 44.0%, respectively. The authors also reported a cumulative rectal carcinoma risk of 4.0, 5.6, 7.9, and 25.0% at 5, 10, 15, and 20 years, respectively, after the IRA.

These findings have raised the question of the justification of IRA as the primary treatment of FAP. The planned strategy of two prophylactic operations, first a colectomy with IRA at an earlier age (perhaps 20 years of age), and then a restorative proctectomy at the age of 45 years, doubles the risks of the operations and may also increase the risk of desmoid tumors. Furthermore, a second-stage restorative proctectomy may not result in perfect functional outcome, or is impossible in cases of pelvic fibromatous adhesions or desmoids.[211] The previous recommendation by Bess et al[208] in 1980 is still a good one that the colon and rectum should be removed but the rectum may be retained if there are fewer than 20 polyps in the rectum. Heiskanen and Järvinen[211] now favor proctocolectomy and ileoanal pouch procedure as the primary operation for FAP. A more detailed view of the cumulative rectal carcinoma incidence is shown in ▶ Table 19.9.

Close follow-up of patients with IRA is essential.[197,200,212,213,214,215,216] The retained rectum should be examined, preferably with a flexible sigmoidoscope, once a year or sooner, depending on the number of polyps that should be electrocoagulated. Any time the number of the polyps become too numerous or too large to be safely removed, a proctectomy should be considered. In a series reported by Penna et al[202] of 148 patients with an IRA, 29 required a secondary proctectomy: 16 because the rectal polyps were too numerous, 8 because the patients wished to

Table 19.9 Extracolonic manifestations of familial adenomatous polyposis[210]

Ectodermal origin	Mesodermal origin	Endodermal origin
Epidermoid cyst	Connective tissue	Adenomas
Pilomatrixoma	Fibroma	Stomach
Tumors of central nervous system	Fibrosarcoma	Duodenum
Congenital hypertrophy of the retinal pigment epithelium	Desmoid tumors	Hepatopancreatobiliary system
	Diffuse fibrosis mesenteric retroperitoneum	Small intestine
	Excessive intra-abdominal adhesion	Endocrine tissue
	Lipoma	Adrenal cortex (adenomas)
	Bone	Thyroid gland
	Osteoma	Parathyroid
	Exostosis	Pituitary
	Sclerosis	Pancreatic islets
	Dental	Carcinomas
	Dentigerous cyst	Stomach
	Odontoma	Duodenum
	Supernumerary teeth	Hepatobiliary system
	Unerupted teeth	Small intestine
	Lymphoid	Thyroid gland
	Hyperplasia of ileum	Adrenal gland

discontinue regular surveillance, and 3 because of the discovery of rectal carcinoma (one was Dukes' A 3 years after the IRA, one Dukes' B 14 years after, and one Dukes' C 17 years later). An IPAA was successfully performed in all but three patients who had pelvic desmoid tumors. In a series reported by Nugent and Phillips of 224 patients with IRA, 22 patients developed carcinoma of the rectum. Nine were Dukes' A, four were Dukes' B, and nine were Dukes' C. These carcinomas developed despite a close follow-up; 14 of 22 patients were last examined less than 6 months before. It is essential to realize that despite the close follow-up, surveillance cannot always prevent rectal carcinoma.[198]

Colectomy with IRA has its strong support. Phillips and Spigelman[199] reason that the ileoanal pouch procedure has high morbidity and does not give perfect functional results and that patients can still succumb to other related diseases of FAP.

Bülow et al[201] studied 659 patients undergoing IRA. The data were obtained from the National Polyposis Registries in Denmark, Finland, the Netherlands, and Sweden. They found that chronologic age was the only independent risk factor of developing rectal carcinoma. The risk of secondary proctectomy was higher in patients with mutation in codon 1250 to 1500 than outside this region. None of the 18 patients with

AFAP (mutation in codon 0–200 or greater than 1500) had a secondary proctectomy. Church et al[203] found that the risk of rectal carcinoma after IRA was strongly related to the severity of colorectal polyposis at presentation. Bertario et al[216] found independent predictors of rectal carcinoma after IRA in the FAP with mutation between codon 1250 and 1464 (RR = 4.4).

It is, therefore, reasonable to perform colon resection with IRA in young patients with few adenomas (less than 20 rectal adenomas, less than 1,000 colonic adenomas) and in FAP with mutation in codon 0 to 200 or greater than 1,500.[215,216,217] These patients must understand their responsibility to have a periodic surveillance with an endoscopy, and that they may require a proctectomy in the future.

Regression of Polyps

A temporary spontaneous regression or disappearance of polyps in the rectum after IRA is a common observation. This gives some comfort to clinicians, a hope that perhaps the risk of developing carcinomas can be minimized as well. A study of the effect of colectomy and IRA on rectal mucosal proliferation in FAP showed a significant reduction in rectal mucosal cell proliferation. However, the mechanism is unknown. Sulindac has also been found to markedly reduce epithelial cell proliferation and significant polyp regression, including dysplastic reversion.[205,206] This observation must be guarded, since Spagnesi et al[217] observed the persistence of abnormal rectal mucosal proliferation after sulindac therapy, despite the reduction of number of polyps.

Winde et al[218] conducted a prospective, controlled, non-randomized phase II dose-finding study from sulindac given rectally, and looked at the molecular mechanism by which sulindac worked. The study group (n = 28) and the control group (n = 10) underwent colectomy and IRA, with repeated proctoscopy with endoluminal ultrasound and biopsies every 3 months. The treatment group was given sulindac suppositories, 150 mg twice daily, for 3 months. Visible improvement was followed by a dose reduction to 50 mg daily. Worsening of the polyps required changing to the initial dose level. The results showed that all patients responded to sulindac after 24 weeks (at the latest). Complete reversion was reached with 50 mg/day in 78% of patients. Twenty-two percent had partial reversions of adenomas at latest re-examination and there was no influence on upper GI tract adenomas. There was a permanent antiproliferative effect (Ki-67) of low-dose sulindac, significant blocking of ras mutation activation, and a significant difference of untreated and treated mucosa in mutant p53 content. The follow-up was 4 years. The authors concluded that low-dose antiproliferative sulindac therapy is highly effective in adenoma reversion in FAP patients. Sulindac shows influence on tumor-suppressor genes and on apoptosis markers. All cases with relapse represented by newly developed flat mucosal elevations respond to dose increases.

Giardiello et al[219] conducted a randomized, double-blind, placebo-controlled study looking at whether sulindac can prevent adenoma rather than causing regression of the polyps. The study consisted of 41 young subjects (age range, 8–25 years) who were genotypically affected with familial FAP but phenotypically unaffected. Subjects received either 75 or 150 mg of sulindac orally twice a day or identical-appearing placebo tablets for 48 months. The number and size of new adenomas and the side effects of therapy were evaluated every 4 months for 4 years, and the levels of five major prostaglandins were serially measured in biopsy specimens of normal-appearing colorectal mucosa. The results after 4 years of treatment showed the average rate of compliance exceeded 76% in the sulindac group, and mucosal prostaglandin levels were lower in this group than in the placebo group. During the course of the study, adenomas developed in 9 of 21 subjects (43%) in the sulindac group and 11 of 20 patients in the placebo group (55%). There were no significant differences in the mean number or size of polyps between the groups. The authors concluded that standard doses of sulindac did not prevent the development of adenomas in subjects with FAP. Evidence that sulindac has a short-lived effect on established polyps in patients with FAP has been reported.

The rate of regression of adenomas was greater after 6 months of sulindac treatment than after 9 months and has been reported in some patients who had undergone IRA. Long-term use of sulindac resulted in the development of resistance to this medication.[219] Moreover, colorectal carcinoma has developed in rectal segment in patients with FAP during maintenance therapy with sulindac.[220,221,222]

The lack of efficacy of primary chemoprevention could have been due to resistance to sulindac. Most results do not provide support for the use of NSAIDs such as sulindac for the primary treatment of FAP. Prophylactic colectomy remains the treatment of choice to prevent colorectal carcinoma in patients with this disorder.[219]

Proctocolectomy with Ileal Pouch Procedure

The advantage of the ileal pouch procedure for FAP is its total eradication of the colonic disease. The inconvenience and a small risk of perforation of a long-term or lifetime follow-up of the rectum with proctoscopy or flexible sigmoidoscopy and electrocoagulation in patients who undergo colectomy with IRA thus is eliminated. The argument against its use as the procedure of choice is the fact that it is a more extensive procedure, with high potential for complications, especially sepsis and fecal incontinence. More and more authors and medical centers favor the IPAA as the primary treatment for patients with FAP.[223,224] Although IPAA is a longer, bloodier, and more complex operation with a longer hospital stay than IRA, no significant difference is found between the two groups in terms of complication rate and quality of life in a series of teenagers. IPAA also has few effects on life activities that are especially important at this age.[224,225] The same is true in adult series.[223,226,227] In the series reported by Soravia et al,[228] although IRA had a significantly better functional outcome with regard to nighttime continence and perianal skin irritation, other functional results and the quality of life were similar with IPAA. The authors favored IPAA over IRA because of its lower long-term failure rate.

With concern about the increasing risk of carcinoma in the retained rectum, which is 25% at 20 years after the IRA, Heiskanen and Järvinen[211] favor the IPAA for their patients with FAP as the primary treatment. This approach eliminates the need for a proctectomy, after an IRA.

Proctocolectomy with IPAA for FAP cannot be considered the end of the patient's management. In these patients, adenomas and carcinomas can develop in the ileal pouch, at the anastomosis, or in the anal transitional zone. Church[229] reviewed these problems, searching the MEDLINE database for studies reporting ileoanal pouch adenomas, ileal pouch-anal anastomotic carcinomas, and ileal pouch carcinomas in patients with FAP. Reports of adenomas in Kock's pouches and in Brooke ileostomies in the setting of FAP were also included. The primary end points of the study were the time between pouch (or ileostomy) construction and the diagnosis of neoplasia, the age of the patients at the diagnosis of neoplasia, and the severity of the neoplasia.

The results showed that 18 studies reported pouch neoplasia, 15 with adenomas (98 patients) and 3 with carcinomas (3 patients). Three prospective studies showed that the incidence of the pouch adenomas increases with time of follow-up and that the severity of the polyposis varies. The median time from pouch construction to diagnosis of pouch adenomas was 4.7 years and the range was 0.5 to 12 years.

A prospective review at the Cleveland Clinic showed a rate of 28% for adenomas 3.5 years after stapled IPAA and 14% at 4 years after handsewn IPAA.[230] Similar data had been reported from 97 FAP patients who had an IPAA in a multicenter study by van Duijvendijk et al.[231] At a median follow-up of 78 months (range, 25–137 months), 13 of these patients had adenomas at the anastomosis. The risk for anastomotic adenomas after double-stapled IPAA was 31%, three times that after mucosectomy and handsewn IPAA (10%).[232]

Six studies reported eight patients with carcinoma at the IPAA, who were diagnosed a median of 8 years after pouch construction (range, 3–20 years). One-half of the carcinomas were locally advanced (T4) and one-half were not (T1 or T2). One-half followed stapled anastomosis and one-half were after mucosectomy. There were eight case reports of carcinoma described in an ileostomy in patients with FAP. The median time from ileostomy construction to the ileostomy carcinomas was 25 years (range, 9–40).

Pouch adenomas are difficult to manage endoscopically because of the thin ileal mucosa and the way it is tethered to the submucosa and underlying muscle. Their propensity to occur on suture lines also makes endoscopic treatment difficult. There are no large studies of endoscopic treatment of pouch adenomas, so risks and complication rates are not established. The prospect of coagulating or snaring tens or hundreds of polyps is a concern, however. Pouch excision for uncontrollable polyposis has previously been reported[233] but would be a difficult operation in many patients, usually resulting in an ileostomy and risking complications such as impotence, retrograde ejaculation, ureteric injury, and worsening female fecundity. Chemoprevention of pouch polyposis is, therefore, an attractive alternative. The role of NSAIDs in suppressing colorectal adenomas in FAP is established, and there are anecdotal reports of their use in pouch polyposis. While chemoprevention of colorectal adenomas in FAP using sulindac works only partially and for a limited time, its effectiveness in the ileal pouch has not been systematically studied.[229]

Those caring for patients with FAP need to make sure that endoscopic surveillance is continued after IPAA. The endoscopy has to be accurate and the endoscopists must be aware of the increasing risk of pouch and anastomotic neoplasia. Church[229] recommended pouchoscopy to be done yearly for life, initially to look for anastomotic adenomas and then later to check for pouch adenomas. Once neoplasia is seen, appropriate treatment

needs to be determined. This includes transanal excision of residual, adenoma-bearing anal transitional zone, transanal polypectomy for isolated large (1 cm) pouch adenomas, or sulindac (150 mg twice daily) for multiple (> 10) pouch adenomas.

19.2.6 Genetic Counseling and Testing

The gene responsible for FAP, known as APC, is located on chromosome 5q21. Mutations of the APC gene have been found in patients with FAP. These are often insertions, deletions, and nonsense mutations that lead to frame-shifts and/or premature stop codons in the resulting transcript of the gene. It is not yet clear how the subsequent truncated protein product causes adenomas to form. Capitalizing on the nature of these mutations has led to the development of molecular genetic tests for FAP.[232] It is not carcinoma but the predisposition to carcinoma that is inherited.[233] Genetic testing can capture the opportunity for surgeons to prevent the development of the carcinoma.

Genetic Counseling

Genetic counseling is a dynamic communication process between the patient and the counselor who provides education and support within a multidisciplinary team.[234] Patients and their families must understand the natural history of the disease, the involvement of other blood relatives, and that carcinomas of the large bowel as well as other organs are, in most cases, preventable.

The decision to undergo genetic testing is a personal one based on informed consent. The elements of informed consent include information on the gene being tested and the implications, limitations, and impact of results for the person being tested and two other family members. It should be emphasized that genetic testing is voluntary and the patients need to be aware of alternatives.[234]

The first phase in determining whether genetic testing is appropriate is genetic counseling. This stage educates the patient about the role of inherited causes for developing carcinoma, determines their risk for a malignancy, and provides screening recommendations. The objective is effectively accomplished by understanding the patient's perspective. Education and discussing the benefits and risks of genetic testing through each patient's viewpoint promotes autonomy and lays the foundation for informed consent. An overall general summary of the genetic counseling and testing process is described in ▶ Fig. 19.21.[234]

Genetic Testing

The most important recent development in the management of families of patients with FAP is the use of predictive gene testing. In this context, both children and adults at 50% risk could benefit from genetic testing because of the resultant reduction of uncertainty regardless of test outcome, modifications in screening guidelines for those who do not have the mutant gene, and increased compliance with screening regimens in those who do have the mutant gene.[232]

Because approximately 96% of the mutations in FAP lead to a truncated protein, it has become routine to use the in vitro synthesized-protein assay (IVSP). Sometimes this is called a PTT, for mutation detection. When a truncated protein is identified

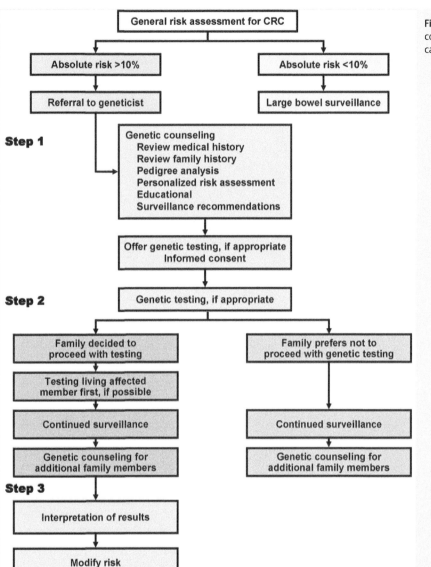

Fig. 19.21 General summary of the genetic counseling and testing process. CRC, colorectal carcinoma.[235]

in the assay, it is possible to localize the mutation to a specific segment of the gene and then use DNA sequencing to determine the mutated nucleotides. However, the use of IVSP as the sole genetic test in FAP misses approximately 20% of APC mutations. Another screening technique is based on analysis of electrophoretic migration of small segments of the wild type and mutant gene (SSCA). The sequential use of two molecular diagnostic tests has become a common practice: a simple and less expensive screening technique (of high sensitivity and moderate specificity) followed by a definitive test of high sensitivity, usually DNA sequencing.[236]

When the mutation in the family is known from one or more affected members previously studied, only one test, usually IVSP, need be performed, as the expression pattern of the mutation is already established for that family. A positive result in such a test is considered a "mutation-positive" result, and the patient can be counseled as recommended. When the mutation in the family is not known, IVSP is performed. In the majority of cases, mutation will be found in the APC gene that can be further characterized by DNA sequencing. Again, a

"mutation-positive" result is obtained leading to the appropriate genetic counseling to the patient. Other options include DNA sequencing and linkage analysis (which tests whether FAP is associated with particular markers in or near APC but requires large families). Even by combining two or more techniques, it is not possible to achieve 100% sensitivity, because the mutations may not be in the coding region of the gene or because a few FAP kindreds do not exhibit linkage to chromosome 5q. Therefore, in such cases, a "no mutation detected" result must not be interpreted as a "negative test" result, with very important considerations for counseling the patient.[236]

Approximately 75% of individuals who carry an APC germline truncating mutation manifest an adenomatous polyp by age 20. These premalignant lesions inevitably evolve to malignancy, and if untreated, the risk for developing colorectal carcinoma is virtually 100% by age 40. Because polyposis often starts before puberty, flexible sigmoidoscopy beginning at puberty is recommended as a screening procedure by most authors.

Mutation carriers require surveillance by gastroduodenoscopy for extracolonic neoplasms in the upper GI tract. Other variant manifestations in FAP include osteomas, cutaneous cysts, and CHRPE. A phenotype-genotype correlation exists. For example, CHRPE is often present if the mutation is located in exon 9–15e of the APC gene. For families who carry mutation in this region, the presence of CHRPE is a diagnostic indication of FAP.

When a mutation has been identified in the family, direct gene testing of relatives who have not yet been clinically assessed will distinguish between those who carry the mutation and those who do not. However, about 30% of FAP cases are caused by new mutations in the APC gene. In these cases, the parents will not carry this mutation and are not at risk of FAP; only descendants of the proband are at 50% risk.

A negative test result is given if the patient does not carry the mutation that is known to exist in their family. In this instance, family members are not at increased risk for developing colorectal carcinoma compared with the general population and should follow guidelines for carcinoma surveillance for that group.

If the patient is affected with FAP and complete coding sequence analysis of the APC gene fails to identify a mutation, this could mean that the APC gene is not responsible for the patient's diagnosis. This is possible because locus heterogeneity has been reported in FAP; not all FAP kindreds are linked to

chromosome 5q. In this case, a "no mutation detected" result, APC gene testing has no predictive value for asymptomatic at-risk relatives. In these families, first-degree relatives should continue colorectal surveillance annually between the ages of 12 and 25 years, every other year between the ages of 25 and 35 years, and every third year between the ages of 35 and 50 years. Family members who have not developed multiple adenomatous polyps on colonoscopic examination by the age of 50 years are assumed to be unaffected by FAP.

Caution should be used in interpreting genetic test results when a mutation is not detected, because these results can be misinterpreted as a negative result. This in turn could lead to controversy in the guidelines in the follow-up care for those with a "no mutation detected" result.

A third scenario with a "no mutation detected" result occurs when an unaffected family member of an APC kindred is tested without testing an affected family member. In such a case, the result does not mean that the unaffected person is not at risk for FAP, because it has not been determined that a mutation in APC is present in the family. It is important that the patient not be falsely reassured, because other mechanisms may inactivate the APC gene, or other genes may be involved. Summary on interpretation of APC genetic testing is in ▶ Fig. 19.22.

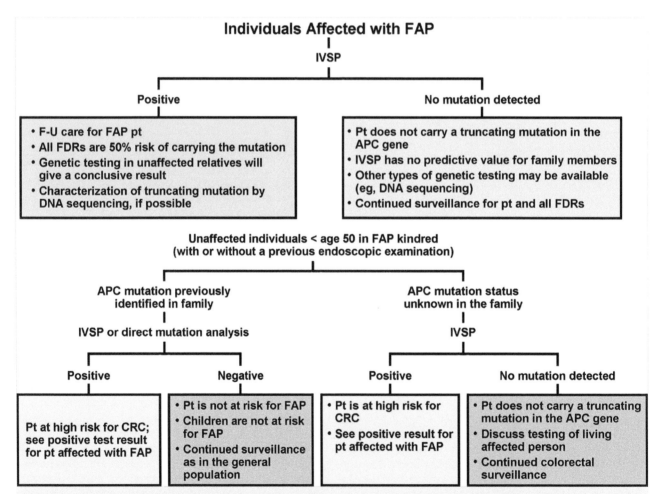

Fig. 19.22 Summary interpretation of APC genetic testing. CRC, colorectal carcinoma; FAP, familial adenomatous polyposis; FDR, first-degree relative; F-U, follow-up; IVSP, in vitro synthesized protein assay (protein truncation test); pt, patient.[235]

19.2.7 When to Screen and When to Operate?

Gene test results can change the risk for FAP from a priori 50% to essentially 0 or 100%. Presymptomatic genetic testing removes the necessity of annual screening of those at-risk individuals who do not have the gene, and probably improves compliance in those who do. No change in conventional screening guidelines for colon polyps is recommended for those whose presymptomatic DNA diagnosis indicates that they have the FAP-causing gene. These individuals should have annual colon and rectal examinations with at least a flexible sigmoidoscopy beginning at approximately 10 or 11 years of age.[232] The age for the start of screening varies from series to series. The St. Mark's series began at 14 years of age or older.[205] Follow-up surveillance for extracolonic neoplasms is also indicated. At this time, the patients should also be counseled to prepare for an eventual prophylactic colectomy and should be given genetic counseling about the risk of FAP for future offspring.

Timing of operation depends on the number of polyps found in the colon and rectum. The natural history of the disease, even though it is highly variable between individual cases, suggests that operation should be performed by 25 years of age, although most of the St. Mark's patients had a colectomy by the age of 20 years. The youngest FAP patient with a carcinoma in the St. Mark's registry is a 17-year-old girl.[205]

For those who have not inherited the APC mutation, colon screening can be significantly reduced to three or fewer time points: at ages 18, 25, and 35 years. These time points are selected to provide the clinician with a management margin that accommodates false negative results from laboratory error and infrequent phenomena, such as tissue mosaicism or de novo mutations. The individual's lifetime risk of colorectal carcinoma becomes the general population's risk of approximately 3%, and colon carcinoma screening should resume again around age 50, according to conventional guidelines. These individuals can also be assured that their offspring will not be at risk for FAP.[232]

19.2.8 Polyposis Registry

The aims of a polyposis registry are to ensure efficient care of patients and their families and to promote and carry out the research that will advance the knowledge of FAP for physicians and surgeons. Data held in a standardized format on computers assist the day-to-day of those in the registry as well as allow for speedy analysis.[233]

A registry deals not only with the patient but also with the patient's family members. Family pedigrees are collected and regularly updated. A counseling team plays an important part in the registry. Early diagnosis, using modern and reliable techniques, timely operation to prevent the onset of carcinoma, and continued surveillance after operation for early detection and treatment of associated carcinomas are key features of a successful registry. The impact of screening on carcinoma incidence in patients with FAP at St. Mark's Registry is shown in ▶ Fig. 19.23. It has a remarkable success in preventing the development of colorectal carcinomas.[233]

The Leed's Castle Polyposis Group in Kent, United Kingdom, was established in June 1985. The aims of this gathering were to discuss the problems facing those who cared for polyposis

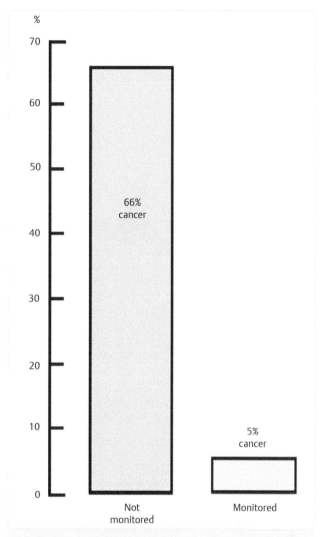

Fig. 19.23 The results of screening by the St. Mark's Polyposis Registry.[237]

patients and to establish an international cooperative organization. In 1992, there were 51 such centers worldwide. The group seeks further knowledge of the etiology, clinical features, prevention, and treatment of FAP in all of its manifestations.[233] As outlined by Church and McGannon,[238] there are three types of FAP registries.

The Countrywide Registry

In this type of registry, cases of FAP from the entire country are collected into one central registry. The registry staff need not undertake direct patient care but must collect and collate data from everywhere. Examples of countrywide registries are those in Denmark, Sweden, Holland, and Singapore.

The Regional Registry

This type fits well with very large or widespread populations or those without a uniform health care system. Regional registries are miniatures of countrywide registries in which families are collected from a defined region, for example, an area health board or a county. Parish, city, and county records contain extensive information with which to flush out family data, and the registry develops lines of communication with hospitals and physicians in its area. Registry staff need not commit to patient care but can offer specialized counseling and testing services. Regional registries are common in the United Kingdom.

The Tertiary Referral Center

This type develops around one or two physicians of repute who work in a tertiary referral medical center and who have a special interest in FAP. Families are accumulated and a patient base is built. Patients may come from all over a country for treatment and return to the registry for surveillance. An example of such a registry is the Cleveland Clinic Foundation. Minnesota Colorectal Cancer Initiative[239] is a community-based Colorectal Cancer Registry run by two physician groups and the University Cancer Center. It is a not-for-profit organization financially supported by health care organizations, pharmaceutical companies, a consulting firm, and other practice groups. It is a model of effective collaboration between an academic tertiary referral center and community health care providers. Enrollment is not limited to individuals with an established diagnosis of a hereditary colorectal cancer syndrome, but is most likely to benefit people who may be at increased risk of developing colorectal or other carcinoma because they have a personal or family history of colorectal carcinoma. Setting up a successful polyposis registry is a large project requiring large sums of funds, space, equipment, and personnel. ▶ Table 19.10 shows the organization of a successful registry.[238]

19.3 Hemangiomas of Large Bowel

Hemangiomas are rare vascular lesions of the large bowel. More than 200 cases have been documented in the literature from 1931 to 1974, with more than 50% involving the rectum.[240] Hemangiomas of the large bowel are congenital, developing from embryonic sequestration of mesodermal tissue. However, whether they represent a simple vascular malformation (hamartoma) or a neoplasm is unsettled.

Capillary hemangiomas consist of a network of fine, newly formed, closely packed capillaries, with a distinct hyperplastic endothelial lining.[241] They are usually encountered at operation and are found mainly in the small intestine, appendix, and perianal skin. This type of hemangioma accounts for 10% of all colon and rectal hemangiomas.[240] Cavernous hemangiomas are large, thin-walled vessels. The stroma has little connective tissue and muscle.

The great majority of patients present early in life with recurrent, painless, and sometimes massive hemorrhage. Nine of 15 cases in the report of Londono-Schimmer et al[242] were first seen at a hospital before the age of 5 years. The age of onset, type, frequency, and severity of bleeding are related to the size, number, and type of vascular malformations. Capillary hemangiomas are characterized by slow, persistent bleeding, producing dark stools and anemia. Cavernous hemangiomas characteristically present early with moderate to severe, painless hemorrhage. The bleeding recurs and increases in severity with each subsequent episode. In severe cases of profuse and unremitting bleeding, an urgent or emergency bowel resection is necessary. This propensity to bleed has been attributed to the lack of muscular and supporting connective tissue in the wall and around the vessels. Anemia is common and accounts for 43% of patients in the series presented by Allred and Spencer.[243] Bowel obstruction accounts for 17% of the cases. Diarrhea, tenesmus, rectal prolapse, and sometimes constipation can occur.

Hemangiomas of the large bowel are often misdiagnosed because of the lack of awareness of the clinical features. They are frequently mistaken for hemorrhoids, inflammatory bowel diseases, polyps, carcinomas, and other entities.[240] At St. Mark's Hospital, 8 of 10 patients had at least one hemorrhoidectomy before the age of 20 years.[237]

Flexible sigmoidoscopy is the most important and most useful part of the workup. The mucosa has a deep blue or dull red color and appears wine or plum colored. The mucosa is usually nodular, with or without dilated veins (▶ Fig. 19.24). Chronic inflammatory changes may mimic proctitis. Usually, there is no mucosal ulceration. Hemorrhoids and ulcerative proctocolitis are the most common misdiagnoses.

Plain abdominal films are useful. Calcification within the venous plexus of the bowel wall represents a sequela of thrombosis

Table 19.10 Staff for a successful registry[238]

Physicians	Administrative	Research
Gastroenterologist	Secretary	Molecular geneticist
Colorectal surgeon	Statistician	Lab technician
Medical geneticist	Computer technician	Research fellows
Pathologist	Financial counselor	Study assistant/ research nurse
	Marketing	

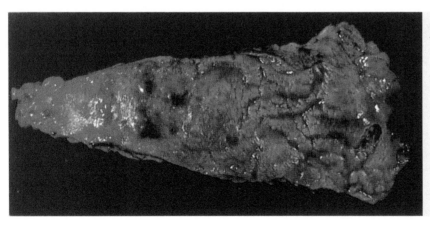

Fig. 19.24 Diffuse hemangioma of rectum. Note thickening and irregular mucosa. (Courtesy of Roger R. Dozois, MD.)

within the neoplasm caused by perivascular inflammation and sluggish blood flow. Phleboliths also accompany hemangiomas at other locations along the GI tract and in venous plexuses of the uterine broad ligament, the urinary bladder, the prostate, and the spleen. Approximately 50% of adults with intestinal hemangiomas are noted to have phlebolith clusters on plain films.[240]

In a patient with an extensive hemangioma, barium enema studies reveal a characteristic scalloped contour of submucosal masses, causing narrowing of the colonic and rectal lumen. It can be differentiated from other neoplastic masses by its compressibility and a longer segment of involvement than polyps or carcinomas. A CT scan of the pelvis may show a large and markedly thickened rectal wall and phleboliths (if present) (▶ Fig. 19.25).

Selective inferior mesenteric arteriography is valuable to assist in determining the extent of the disease, particularly the less extensive hemangiomas in which localization at operation may be difficult. The delayed phase of arteriography may show large venous pooling within the cavernous hemangiomas.[235] Arteriography is also helpful in detecting any abnormal blood vessels in the pelvis.

Hypofibrinogenemia or afibrinogenemia that is caused by a consumptive coagulopathy is occasionally seen in these patients. Isotope studies with ^{51}Cr-labeled platelets suggest sequestration within the hemangiomas. Resection of the hemangiomas has resulted in complete reversal of the coagulopathy.[240]

19.3.1 Treatment

Until 1971, abdominoperineal resection was the only definitive treatment for diffuse hemangiomas of the anorectum. Since then, the St. Mark's group has performed a rectosigmoid resection with preservation of the pelvic floor and sphincter muscles. The entire rectum is mobilized and transected at the level just above the levator ani muscle. The anorectal mucosa and submucosa from the dentate line are stripped from underlying muscle up to the level of the transection. The sigmoid colon or the descending colon is then brought through the denuded anorectum and anastomosed to the dentate line. Londono-Schimmer et al[242] reported success in all 15 patients using this technique and concluded that it is the treatment of

choice. Telander et al[244] successfully performed this operation in four children with rectal hemangiomas associated with Klippel–Trenaunay syndrome, a congenital venous anomaly manifested by extensive hemangiomatous malformation within the pelvis and extremity, hypertrophy of the extremity, and atypical varicosities. Coppa et al,[235] on the other hand, reported that three of eight patients who underwent coloanal sleeve anastomosis had recurrent episodes of rectal bleeding similar to preoperative symptoms, most likely caused by involvement of the anal canal by diffuse cavernous hemangiomas. Ten of those patients who underwent abdominoperineal resection had no recurrent bleeding.

Many other treatments have been reported in literature, all of which are temporary measures. They include colostomy, injection of sclerosing agents, radium implantation, irradiation, ligation of superior rectal arteries, embolization of inferior mesenteric artery, rectal packing, and cryosurgery. The place for the use of the laser in treating diffuse colon and rectal hemangiomas has not been established, but it is doubtful that it would give a permanent cure.

Leiomyomas of the large bowel are rare neoplasms of the smooth muscle of the bowel. In a review of 160 cases of smooth muscle neoplasms of the GI tract by He et al,[245] only four cases involved the rectum, and none was in the colon or the anal canal. A total of 131 patients with benign GI smooth muscle neoplasms were treated at the Massachusetts General Hospital between 1963 and 1987: 8% in the esophagus, 61% in the stomach, 19% in the small intestine, 5% in the colon, and 6% in the rectum.[246] Kusminsky and Bailey[247] reviewed the world literature from 1959 to 1979 and found 79 cases of leiomyoma of the rectum. Leiomyomas are most commonly found in patients 50 to 59 years old and are rare or absent in children.

Miettinen et al[248] studied all the mesenchymal neoplasms involving the rectum and anus coded as leiomyoma, leiomyosarcoma, smooth muscle neoplasm, schwannomas, neurofibromas, nerve sheath, and stromal neoplasm. They used immunohistochemistry. Antibodies to the antigens were: KIT (CD1147), CD34 a-smooth muscle, desmin D33, keratin 18 and 19, neurofilaments, glial fibrillary acidic protein, and S-100 protein. The results showed a total of 133 anorectal GI stromal tumors (GIST). Of these, 50 tumors had been originally diagnosed as

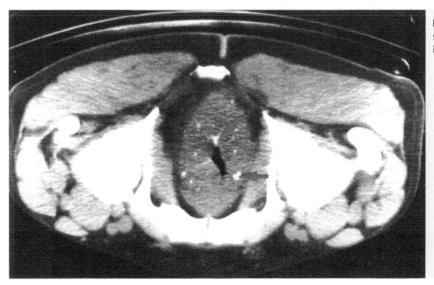

Fig. 19.25 Computed tomography scan of pelvis shows calcification of submucosal vascular plexus in diffuse hemangioma of rectum (*arrows*).

lymphosarcomas, 29 as smooth muscle tumors of uncertain malignant potential, 21 as leiomyomas, and 3 as GIST.

Only three patents were diagnosed as leiomyoma. All three patients were women, age 25, 29, and 38 years. Tumor size was 1.5, 2, and 4 cm in diameter. All tumors were positive for desmin, a-smooth muscle actin, or both. They were negative for CD117 and CD34. One should be cautious to interpret the diagnosis of leiomyomas in the older literature where the study for GIST was not performed.

Leiomyomas of the large bowel usually occur in the rectum and less commonly in the anal canal. The most common finding is the presence of a mass, usually detected as an incidental finding during rectal or proctosigmoidoscopic examination. Most patients with leiomyomas are asymptomatic, but some may present with constipation, bleeding, anorectal pain, and a pressure sensation in the rectum.

Leiomyomas may be pedunculated or sessile, submucosal, extrarectal, or dumbbell shaped to involve both intramural and extramural positions (▶ Fig. 19.26). They may be in the abdomen or may protrude into the retrorectal space. In the anal canal, they may be found submucosally but are most commonly found in the intersphincteric position with a variable relationship to the sphincter muscles.[247] Leiomyomas are firm, rounded, sharply circumscribed neoplasms, but they have no definite capsule microscopically. There are few reliable criteria for separating benign from malignant growths. Most malignant neoplasms are judged by metastases and may not be recognized until months or years later. Some pathologists accept more than two mitoses revealed under high power as evidence of malignancy. Morgan et al[246] concluded that symptomatic gastric and small intestinal leiomyomas with more than two mitoses per 50 high-power field should be suspicious for a malignant potential. Whether this statement can be applied to leiomyomas of the large intestine is unknown. Others do not accept these criteria and do not attempt to differentiate between benign and malignant growths at the time of examination.[249]

Smooth muscle neoplasms of the large bowel may arise from the muscularis mucosa or the muscularis propria. The division into neoplasms arising from the muscularis mucosa of the rectum, muscularis propria, or internal sphincter is based primarily on microscopic appearance to indicate the layer from which the neoplasm appears to arise. Histologically, all neoplasms arising from the muscularis mucosae of the rectum appear totally benign and arid, while the others vary in degree of differentiation. Of the 48 cases at St. Mark's Hospital, 26 arose from muscularis mucosa, 18 from the muscularis propria, and four from the internal sphincter muscle.[249]

19.3.2 Treatment

Since it may not be known which neoplasm is malignant, the key to successful management is complete removal of the lesion. Walsh and Mann[249] reported local excision of 26 neoplasms arising from the muscularis mucosa and four neoplasms arising from the internal sphincter with no recurrence. However, local excision of 18 lesions arising from the muscularis propria resulted in a 60% recurrence rate. Of significance is that the incidence of recurrence after local excision bears no relationship to the degree of histologic differentiation. It appears that for neoplasms arising from the muscularis propria and those > 5 cm in diameter, a radical approach is indicated, that is, bowel resection or even abdominoperineal resection.[247] Vorobyov et al[250] presented their experience of 36 patients with rectal leiomyomas at the Moscow Proctology Institute. The authors recommend electroexcision through the endoscope for a neoplasm < 1 cm in diameter. A transanal excision can be performed for a lesion < 3 cm in diameter. When the lesion is > 5 cm, a resection is advised.

19.4 Lipomas of Large Bowel

Lipomas of the large bowel are uncommon fatty neoplasms. The Mayo Clinic experience reveals 91 cases of large bowel lipomas during the period from 1976 to 1985.[251] Approximately 90% of the large bowel lipomas are in the submucosa and 10% in the subserosa.[251] In order of frequency, the most common sites are the cecum, ascending colon, and sigmoid colon, with one-third to one-half located in the right colon.[251,253] Rare cases of submucosal lipomatous polyps of the colon have been reported.[245,254,255,257,258] In one of

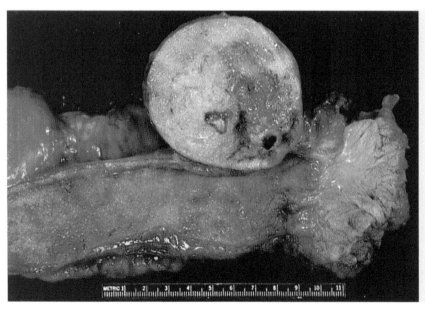

Fig. 19.26 Leiomyoma of the rectum of a patient with ulcerative colitis.

the reports,[258] the number of polyps was between 700 and 1,000 (size 1–9 mm) throughout the entire colon. A subtotal colectomy was performed in this case because of the frequent bowel movement and inability to rule out neoplastic polyps. The specimen did show a combination of tabular adenomas, estimated fewer than 60 in number.

A lipoma < 2 cm rarely causes symptoms. A large lipoma can cause abdominal pain from partial bowel obstruction. Colicky pain may be caused by intermittent intussusception. Lipomas are the most common benign neoplasms that cause intussusception in adults. Bleeding can occur if the mucosa overlying the lipoma is ulcerated, which is usually caused by chronic intussusception.

In the Mayo Clinic series, 46% of the large bowel lipomas were discovered incidentally in the specimens removed for other diseases. Eleven percent of them were resected because of a neoplasm suspected as being a carcinoma.[253]

Barium enema reveals a filling defect in the colon or rectum. A lipoma appears smooth and radiolucent and changes in shape on compression during examination. Despite these characteristics, the correct radiologic diagnosis is not always made. A CT scan is helpful in confirming the presence of fatty tissue in the mass.[256,257] Colonoscopy can confirm the diagnosis in most cases. The lipoma has a characteristic yellowish submucosal soft mass. When pressed with the tip of a biopsy forceps, the lipoma is depressed; this is known as the "cushion sign." A biopsy must include the submucosal layer but seldom is necessary for diagnosis. An ulcerated lipoma can be confused with an adenoma or an adenocarcinoma. Lipomas of the large bowel should not be forgotten in the differential diagnosis of all large bowel neoplasms.

19.4.1 Treatment

Small and asymptomatic lipomas of the large bowel do not require removal. Colonoscopic polypectomy of a large lipoma should be avoided since a tremendous amount of heat is required to cut through the lipoma because of its high water content. The risk of transmural burn, perforation, or bleeding outweighed the benefits in seven lipomas removed by colonoscopic polypectomy by Pfeil et al[258]; three had perforations (size, 4.2 ± 0.7 cm). The authors warned that a lipoma > 2 cm is at the greatest risk for perforation. Symptomatic lipomas should be excised by colotomy or a limited colon resection.[259]

References

[1] O'Brien MJ. Colorectal adenomas: concepts and controversies. Semin Colon Rectal Surg. 1992; 3:195–206
[2] O'Brien MJ, Winawer SJ, Zauber AG, et al. The National Polyp Study. Patient and polyp characteristics associated with high-grade dysplasia in colorectal adenomas. Gastroenterology. 1990; 98(2):371–379
[3] Rickert RR, Auerbach O, Garfinkel L, Hammond EC, Frasca JM. Adenomatous lesions of the large bowel: an autopsy survey. Cancer. 1979; 43(5):1847–1857
[4] Williams AR, Balasooriya BA, Day DW. Polyps and cancer of the large bowel: a necropsy study in Liverpool. Gut. 1982; 23(10):835–842
[5] Vatn MH, Stalsberg H. The prevalence of polyps of the large intestine in Oslo: an autopsy study. Cancer. 1982; 49(4):819–825
[6] Eide TJ, Stalsberg H. Polyps of the large intestine in Northern Norway. Cancer. 1978; 42(6):2839–2848
[7] Nusko G, Mansmann U, Partzsch U, et al. Invasive carcinoma in colorectal adenomas: multivariate analysis of patient and adenoma characteristics. Endoscopy. 1997; 29(7):626–631
[8] Muto T, Bussey HJ, Morson BC. The evolution of cancer of the colon and rectum. Cancer. 1975; 36(6):2251–2270
[9] Dukes C. Simple tumours of the large intestine and their relation to cancer. Br J Surg. 1926; 13(52):720–733
[10] Jackman RJ, Mayo CW. The adenoma-carcinoma sequence in cancer of the colon. Surg Gynecol Obstet. 1951; 93(3):327–330
[11] Castleman B, Krickstein HI. Do adenomatous polyps of the colon become malignant? N Engl J Med. 1962; 267:469–475
[12] Ackerman LV, Spratt JS, Jr, Fischel E. Do adenomatous polyps become cancer? Gastroenterology. 1963; 44:905–908
[13] Morson B. President's address. The polyp-cancer sequence in the large bowel. Proc R Soc Med. 1974; 67(6, Pt 1):451–457
[14] Jass JR. Do all colorectal carcinomas arise in preexisting adenomas? World J Surg. 1989; 13(1):45–51
[15] Nelson RL. Diet and adenomatous polyp risk. Semin Colon Rectal Surg. 1991; 2:262–268
[16] Armitage NC. Intervention studies in adenoma patients. World J Surg. 1991; 15(1):29–34
[17] Kronborg O, Fenger C. Clinical evidence for the adenoma-carcinoma sequence. Eur J Cancer Prev. 1999; 8 Suppl 1:S73–S86
[18] Tierney RP, Ballantyne GH, Modlin IM. The adenoma to carcinoma sequence. Surg Gynecol Obstet. 1990; 171(1):81–94
[19] Eide TJ. Natural history of adenomas. World J Surg. 1991; 15(1):3–6
[20] Eide TJ. Risk of colorectal cancer in adenoma-bearing individuals within a defined population. Int J Cancer. 1986; 38(2):173–176
[21] Shimoda T, Ikegami M, Fujisaki J, Matsui T, Aizawa S, Ishikawa E. Early colorectal carcinoma with special reference to its development de novo. Cancer. 1989; 64(5):1138–1146
[22] Stolte M, Bethke B. Colorectal mini-de novo carcinoma: a reality in Germany too. Endoscopy. 1995; 27(4):286–290
[23] Bedenne L, Faivre J, Boutron MC, Piard F, Cauvin JM, Hillon P. Adenoma–carcinoma sequence or "de novo" carcinogenesis? A study of adenomatous remnants in a population-based series of large bowel cancers. Cancer. 1992; 69(4):883–888
[24] Muto T, Nagawa H, Watanabe T, Masaki T, Sawada T. Colorectal carcinogenesis: historical review. Dis Colon Rectum. 1997; 40(10) Suppl:S80–S85
[25] Church JM, Williams BR, Casey G. Molecular Genetics and Colorectal Neoplasia. A Primer for the Clinician. New York, NY: Igaku-Shoin Medical Publishers; 1996
[26] Nivatvongs S, Dorudi S. Colorectal polyps and their management. In: Williams NS, ed. Colorectal Cancer. London: Churchill Livingstone; 1996:39–54
[27] Dirschmid K, Kiesler J, Mathis G, Beller S, Stoss F, Schobel B. Epithelial misplacement after biopsy of colorectal adenomas. Am J Surg Pathol. 1993; 17(12):1262–1265
[28] Fenoglio-Preiser CM. Colonic polyp histology. Semin Colon Rectal Surg. 1991; 2:234–245
[29] Nivatvongs S, Nicholson JD, Rothenberger DA, et al. Villous adenomas of the rectum: the accuracy of clinical assessment. Surgery. 1980; 87(5):549–551
[30] Galandiuk S, Fazio VW, Jagelman DG, et al. Villous and tubulovillous adenomas of the colon and rectum. A retrospective review, 1964–1985. Am J Surg. 1987; 153(1):41–47
[31] Muto T, Kamiya J, Sawada T, et al. Small "flat adenoma" of the large bowel with special reference to its clinicopathologic features. Dis Colon Rectum. 1985; 28(11):847–851
[32] Muto T, Watanabe T. Flat adenomas and minute carcinomas of the colon and rectum. Perspect Colon Rectal Surg. 1993; 6:117–132
[33] Lynch HT, Smyrk T, Lanspa SJ, et al. Flat adenomas in a colon cancer-prone kindred. J Natl Cancer Inst. 1988; 80(4):278–282
[34] Rembacken BJ, Fujii T, Cairns A, et al. Flat and depressed colonic neoplasms: a prospective study of 1000 colonoscopies in the UK. Lancet. 2000; 355(9211):1211–1214
[35] Radaelli F, Minoli G. Editorial comments. Flat and depressed colonic neoplasms: a prospective study of 1000 colonoscopies in the UK. Gastrointest Endosc. 2001 53:689–691
[36] Minamoto T, Sawaguchi K, Mai M, Yamashita N, Sugimura T, Esumi H. Infrequent K-ras activation in superficial-type (flat) colorectal adenomas and adenocarcinomas. Cancer Res. 1994; 54(11):2841–2844
[37] Gilbertsen VA. Proctosigmoidoscopy and polypectomy in reducing the incidence of rectal cancer. Cancer. 1974; 34(3) suppl:936–939

[38] Selby JV, Friedman GD, Quesenberry CP, Jr, Weiss NS. A case-control study of screening sigmoidoscopy and mortality from colorectal cancer. N Engl J Med. 1992; 326(10):653–657

[39] Winawer SJ, Zauber AG, Ho MN, et al. The National Polyp Study Workgroup. Prevention of colorectal cancer by colonoscopic polypectomy. N Engl J Med. 1993; 329(27):1977–1981

[40] Church JM. Clinical significance of small colorectal polyps. Dis Colon Rectum. 2004; 47(4):481–485

[41] Hofstad B, Vatn MH, Andersen SN, et al. Growth of colorectal polyps: redetection and evaluation of unresected polyps for a period of three years. Gut. 1996; 39(3):449–456

[42] Stryker SJ, Wolff BG, Culp CE, Libbe SD, Ilstrup DM, MacCarty RL. Natural history of untreated colonic polyps. Gastroenterology. 1987; 93(5):1009–1013

[43] Otchy DP, Ransohoff DF, Wolff BG, et al. Metachronous colon cancer in persons who have had a large adenomatous polyp. Am J Gastroenterol. 1996; 91(3):448–454

[44] Bersentes K, Fennerty MB, Sampliner RE, Garewal HS. Lack of spontaneous regression of tubular adenomas in two years of follow-up. Am J Gastroenterol. 1997; 92(7):1117–1120

[45] Haggitt RC, Glotzbach RE, Soffer EE, Wruble LD. Prognostic factors in colorectal carcinomas arising in adenomas: implications for lesions removed by endoscopic polypectomy. Gastroenterology. 1985; 89(2):328–336

[46] Nivatvongs S, Rojanasakul A, Reiman HM, et al. The risk of lymph node metastasis in colorectal polyps with invasive adenocarcinoma. Dis Colon Rectum. 1991; 34(4):323–328

[47] Pollard CW, Nivatvongs S, Rojanasakul A, Reiman HM, Dozois RR. The fate of patients following polypectomy alone for polyps containing invasive carcinoma. Dis Colon Rectum. 1992; 35(10):933–937

[48] Kyzer S, Bégin LR, Gordon PH, Mitmaker B. The care of patients with colorectal polyps that contain invasive adenocarcinoma. Endoscopic polypectomy or colectomy? Cancer. 1992; 70(8):2044–2050

[49] Kudo S. Endoscopic mucosal resection of flat and depressed types of early colorectal cancer. Endoscopy. 1993; 25(7):455–461

[50] The Paris endoscopic classification of superficial neoplastic lesions: esophagus, stomach, and colon: November 30 to December 1, 2002. Gastrointest Endosc. 2003; 58(6) Suppl:S3–S43

[51] Nascimbeni R, Burgart LJ, Nivatvongs S, Larson DR. Risk of lymph node metastasis in T1 carcinoma of the colon and rectum. Dis Colon Rectum. 2002; 45(2):200–206

[52] Muto T, Sawada T, Sugihara K. Treatment of carcinoma in adenomas. World J Surg. 1991; 15(1):35–40

[53] Nivatvongs S. Surgical management of malignant colorectal polyps. Surg Clin North Am. 2002; 82(5):959–966

[54] Kikuchi R, Takano M, Takagi K, et al. Management of early invasive colorectal cancer. Risk of recurrence and clinical guidelines. Dis Colon Rectum. 1995; 38(12):1286–1295

[55] Morson BC, Whiteway JE, Jones EA, Macrae FA, Williams CB. Histopathology and prognosis of malignant colorectal polyps treated by endoscopic polypectomy. Gut. 1984; 25(5):437–444

[56] Richards WO, Webb WA, Morris SJ, et al. Patient management after endoscopic removal of the cancerous colon adenoma. Ann Surg. 1987; 205(6):665–672

[57] Coverlizza S, Risio M, Ferrari A, Fenoglio-Preiser CM, Rossini FP. Colorectal adenomas containing invasive carcinoma. Pathologic assessment of lymph node metastatic potential. Cancer. 1989; 64(9):1937–1947

[58] Cooper HS, Deppisch LM, Gourley WK, et al. Endoscopically removed malignant colorectal polyps: clinicopathologic correlations. Gastroenterology. 1995; 108(6):1657–1665

[59] Robert ME. The malignant colon polyp: diagnosis and therapeutic recommendations. Clin Gastroenterol Hepatol. 2007; 5(6):662–667

[60] Butte JM, Tang P, Gonen M, et al. Rate of residual disease after complete endoscopic resection of malignant colonic polyp. Dis Colon Rectum. 2012; 55(2):122–127

[61] Bentrem DJ, Okabe S, Wong WD, et al. T1 adenocarcinoma of the rectum: transanal excision or radical surgery? Ann Surg. 2005; 242(4):472–477, discussion 477–479

[62] Mellgren A, Sirivongs P, Rothenberger DA, Madoff RD, García-Aguilar J. Is local excision adequate therapy for early rectal cancer? Dis Colon Rectum. 2000; 43(8):1064–1071, discussion 1071–1074

[63] Madbouly KM, Remzi FH, Erkek BA, et al. Recurrence after transanal excision of T1 rectal cancer: should we be concerned? Dis Colon Rectum. 2005; 48(4):711–719, discussion 719–721

[64] Hahnloser D, Wolff BG, Larson DW, Ping J, Nivatvongs S. Immediate radical resection after local excision of rectal cancer: an oncologic compromise? Dis Colon Rectum. 2005; 48(3):429–437

[65] Jass JR. Serrated route to colorectal cancer: back street or super highway? J Pathol. 2001; 193(3):283–285

[66] Torlakovic E, Snover DC. Serrated adenomatous polyposis in humans. Gastroenterology. 1996; 110(3):748–755

[67] Jass JR. Pathogenesis of colorectal cancer. Surg Clin North Am. 2002; 82(5):891–904

[68] Jass JR. Hyperplastic polyps and colorectal cancer: is there a link? Clin Gastroenterol Hepatol. 2004; 2(1):1–8

[69] Longacre TA, Fenoglio-Preiser CM. Mixed hyperplastic adenomatous polyps/serrated adenomas. A distinct form of colorectal neoplasia. Am J Surg Pathol. 1990; 14(6):524–537

[70] Torlakovic E, Skovlund E, Snover DC, Torlakovic G, Nesland JM. Morphologic reappraisal of serrated colorectal polyps. Am J Surg Pathol. 2003; 27(1):65–81

[71] McColl I, Busxey HJ, Veale AM, Morson BC. Juvenile polyposis coli. Proc R Soc Med. 1964; 57:896–897

[72] Desai DC, Neale KF, Talbot IC, Hodgson SV, Phillips RK. Juvenile polyposis. Br J Surg. 1995; 82(1):14–17

[73] Jass JR, Williams CB, Bussey HJ, Morson BC. Juvenile polyposis–a precancerous condition. Histopathology. 1988; 13(6):619–630

[74] Sachatello CR, Hahn IS, Carrington CB. Juvenile gastrointestinal polyposis in a female infant: report of a case and review of the literature of a recently recognized syndrome. Surgery. 1974; 75(1):107–114

[75] Giardiello FM, Hamilton SR, Kern SE, et al. Colorectal neoplasia in juvenile polyposis or juvenile polyps. Arch Dis Child. 1991; 66(8):971–975

[76] Howe JR, Mitros FA, Summers RW. The risk of gastrointestinal carcinoma in familial juvenile polyposis. Ann Surg Oncol. 1998; 5(8):751–756

[77] Kinzler KW, Vogelstein B. Landscaping the cancer terrain. Science. 1998; 280(5366):1036–1037

[78] Järvinen H, Franssila KO. Familial juvenile polyposis coli; increased risk of colorectal cancer. Gut. 1984; 25(7):792–800

[79] Howe JR, Ringold JC, Summers RW, Mitros FA, Nishimura DY, Stone EM. A gene for familial juvenile polyposis maps to chromosome 18q21.1. Am J Hum Genet. 1998; 62(5):1129–1136

[80] Howe JR, Roth S, Ringold JC, et al. Mutations in the SMAD4/DPC4 gene in juvenile polyposis. Science. 1998; 280(5366):1086–1088

[81] Oncel M, Church JM, Remzi FH, Fazio VW. Colonic surgery in patients with juvenile polyposis syndrome: a case series. Dis Colon Rectum. 2005; 48(1):49–55, discussion 55–56

[82] Scott-Conner CE, Hausmann M, Hall TJ, Skelton DS, Anglin BL, Subramony C. Familial juvenile polyposis: patterns of recurrence and implications for surgical management. J Am Coll Surg. 1995; 181(5):407–413

[83] Wirtzfeld DA, Petrelli NJ, Rodriguez-Bigas MA. Hamartomatous polyposis syndromes: molecular genetics, neoplastic risk, and surveillance recommendations. Ann Surg Oncol. 2001; 8(4):319–327

[84] Howe JR, Ringold JC, Hughes JH, Summers RW. Direct genetic testing for Smad4 mutations in patients at risk for juvenile polyposis. Surgery. 1999; 126(2):162–170

[85] Jeghers H, McKusick VA, Katz KH. Generalized intestinal polyposis and melanin spots of the oral mucosa, lips and digits; a syndrome of diagnostic significance. N Engl J Med. 1949; 241(25):993–1005, illust passim

[86] Giardiello FM, Welsh SB, Hamilton SR, et al. Increased risk of cancer in the Peutz-Jeghers syndrome. N Engl J Med. 1987; 316(24):1511–1514

[87] Schreibman IR, Baker M, Amos C, McGarrity TJ. The hamartomatous polyposis syndromes: a clinical and molecular review. Am J Gastroenterol. 2005; 100(2):476–490

[88] Tomlinson IP, Houlston RS. Peutz-Jeghers syndrome. J Med Genet. 1997; 34(12):1007–1011

[89] Giardiello FM, Brensinger JD, Tersmette AC, et al. Very high risk of cancer in familial Peutz-Jeghers syndrome. Gastroenterology. 2000; 119(6):1447–1453

[90] Foley TR, McGarrity TJ, Abt AB. Peutz-Jeghers syndrome: a clinicopathologic survey of the "Harrisburg family" with a 49-year follow-up. Gastroenterology. 1988; 95(6):1535–1540

[91] Narita T, Eto T, Ito T. Peutz-Jeghers syndrome with adenomas and adenocarcinomas in colonic polyps. Am J Surg Pathol. 1987; 11(1):76–81

[92] Perzin KH, Bridge MF. Adenomatous and carcinomatous changes in hamartomatous polyps of the small intestine (Peutz-Jeghers syndrome): report of a case and review of the literature. Cancer. 1982; 49(5):971–983

[93] Spigelman AD, Murday V, Phillips RK. Cancer and the Peutz-Jeghers syndrome. Gut. 1989; 30(11):1588–1590

[94] Boardman LA, Thibodeau SN, Schaid DJ, et al. Increased risk for cancer in patients with the Peutz-Jeghers syndrome. Ann Intern Med. 1998; 128 (11):896–899

[95] Entius MM, Keller JJ, Westerman AM, et al. Molecular genetic alterations in hamartomatous polyps and carcinomas of patients with Peutz-Jeghers syndrome. J Clin Pathol. 2001; 54(2):126–131

[96] Gruber SB, Entius MM, Petersen GM, et al. Pathogenesis of adenocarcinoma in Peutz-Jeghers syndrome. Cancer Res. 1998; 58(23):5267–5270

[97] Boardman LA, Pittelkow MR, Couch FJ, et al. Association of Peutz-Jeghers-like mucocutaneous pigmentation with breast and gynecologic carcinomas in women. Medicine (Baltimore). 2000; 79(5):293–298

[98] Rebsdorf Pedersen I, Hartvigsen A, Fischer Hansen B, Toftgaard C, Konstantin-Hansen K, Büllow S. Management of Peutz-Jeghers syndrome. Experience with patients from the Danish polyposis register. Int J Colorectal Dis. 1994; 9(4):177–179

[99] Spigelman AD, Phillips RK. Peutz-Jeghers syndrome. In: Phillips RK, Spigelman AD, Thomson JP, eds. Familial Adenomatous Polyposis and Other Polyposis Syndromes. London: Edward Arnold; 1994:188–202

[100] Ohmiya N, Taguchi A, Shirai K, et al. Endoscopic resection of Peutz-Jeghers polyps throughout the small intestine at double-balloon enteroscopy without laparotomy. Gastrointest Endosc. 2005; 61(1):140–147

[101] Oncel M, Remzi FH, Church JM, Connor JT, Fazio VW. Benefits of 'clean sweep' in Peutz-Jeghers patients. Colorectal Dis. 2004; 6(5):332–335

[102] Edwards DP, Khosraviani K, Stafferton R, Phillips RK. Long-term results of polyp clearance by intraoperative enteroscopy in the Peutz-Jeghers syndrome. Dis Colon Rectum. 2003; 46(1):48–50

[103] Cronkhite LW, Jr, Canada WJ. Generalized gastrointestinal polyposis; an unusual syndrome of polyposis, pigmentation, alopecia and onychotrophia. N Engl J Med. 1955; 252(24):1011–1015

[104] Hurt S, Mutch MG. The genetic of other polyposis syndromes. Semin Colon Rectal Surg. 2004; 15:158–162

[105] Daniel ES, Ludwig SL, Lewin KJ, Ruprecht RM, Rajacich GM, Schwabe AD. The Cronkhite-Canada Syndrome. An analysis of clinical and pathologic features and therapy in 55 patients. Medicine (Baltimore). 1982; 61(5):293–309

[106] Nardone G, D'Armiento F, Carlomagno P, Budillon G. Cronkhite Canada syndrome: case report with some features not previously described. Gastrointest Endosc. 1990; 36(2):150–152

[107] Rappaport LB, Sperling HV, Stavrides A. Colon cancer in the Cronkhite-Canada syndrome. J Clin Gastroenterol. 1986; 8(2):199–202

[108] Watanabe T, Kudo M, Shirane H, et al. Cronkhite-Canada syndrome associated with triple gastric cancers: a case report. Gastrointest Endosc. 1999; 50 (5):688–691

[109] Russell DM, Bhathal PS, St John DJ. Complete remission in Cronkhite-Canada syndrome. Gastroenterology. 1983; 85(1):180–185

[110] Hanzawa M, Yoshikawa N, Tezuka T, et al. Surgical treatment of Cronkhite-Canada syndrome associated with protein-losing enteropathy: report of a case. Dis Colon Rectum. 1998; 41(7):932–934

[111] Divgi CR, Lisann NM, Yeh SD, Benua RS. Technetium-99 m albumin scintigraphy in the diagnosis of protein-losing enteropathy. J Nucl Med. 1986; 27 (11):1710–1712

[112] Tseng KC, Sheu BS, Lee JC, Tsai HM, Chiu NT, Dai YC. Application of technetium-99m-labeled human serum albumin scan to assist surgical treatment of protein-losing enteropathy in Cronkhite-Canada syndrome: report of a case. Dis Colon Rectum. 2005; 48(4):870–873

[113] Lloyd KM, II, Dennis M. Cowden's disease. A possible new symptom complex with multiple system involvement. Ann Intern Med. 1963; 58:136–142

[114] Carlson GJ, Nivatvongs S, Snover DC. Colorectal polyps in Cowden's disease (multiple hamartoma syndrome). Am J Surg Pathol. 1984; 8(10):763–770

[115] Nelen MR, Padberg GW, Peeters EA, et al. Localization of the gene for Cowden disease to chromosome 10q22–23. Nat Genet. 1996; 13(1):114–116

[116] Hanssen AM, Fryns JP. Cowden syndrome. J Med Genet. 1995; 32 (2):117–119

[117] Starink TM, van der Veen JP, Arwert F, et al. The Cowden syndrome: a clinical and genetic study in 21 patients. Clin Genet. 1986; 29(3):222–233

[118] Longy M, Lacombe D. Cowden disease. Report of a family and review. Ann Genet. 1996; 39(1):35–42

[119] Riley HD, Smith WR. Macrocephaly, pseudopapilledema and multiple hemangioma. Pediatrics. 1960; 26:293–300

[120] Bannayan GA. Lipomatosis, angiomatosis, and macrencephalia. A previously undescribed congenital syndrome. Arch Pathol. 1971; 92(1):1–5

[121] Ruvalcaba RH, Myhre S, Smith DW. Sotos syndrome with intestinal polyposis and pigmentary changes of the genitalia. Clin Genet. 1980; 18(6):413–416

[122] Zigman AF, Lavine JE, Jones MC, Boland CR, Carethers JM. Localization of the Bannayan-Riley-Ruvalcaba syndrome gene to chromosome 10q23. Gastroenterology. 1997; 113(5):1433–1437

[123] Morson BC, Bussey HJ. Predisposing causes of intestinal cancer. Curr Probl Surg. 1970:1–46

[124] Dawson IM, Cornes JS, Morson BC. Primary malignant lymphoid tumours of the intestinal tract. Report of 37 cases with a study of factors influencing prognosis. Br J Surg. 1961; 49:80–89

[125] Khan A, Shrier I, Gordon PH. The changed histologic paradigm of colorectal polyps. Surg Endosc. 2002; 16(3):436–440

[126] Jass JR. Nature and clinical significance of colorectal hyperplastic polyp. Semin Colon Rectal Surg. 1991; 2:246–252

[127] Williams GT, Arthur JF, Bussey HJ, Morson BC. Metaplastic polyps and polyposis of the colorectum. Histopathology. 1980; 4(2):155–170

[128] Hyman NH, Anderson P, Blasyk H. Hyperplastic polyposis and the risk of colorectal cancer. Dis Colon Rectum. 2004; 47(12):2101–2104

[129] Jeevaratnam P, Cottier DS, Browett PJ, Van De Water NS, Pokos V, Jass JR. Familial giant hyperplastic polyposis predisposing to colorectal cancer: a new hereditary bowel cancer syndrome. J Pathol. 1996; 179(1):20–25

[130] Bensen SP, Cole BF, Mott LA, Baron JA, Sandler RS, Halle R. Colorectal hyperplastic polyps and risk of recurrence of adenomas and hyperplastic polyps. Polyps Prevention Study. Lancet. 1999; 354(9193):1873–1874

[131] Rustin RB, Jagelman DG, McGannon E, Fazio VW, Lavery IC, Weakley FL. Spontaneous mutation in familial adenomatous polyposis. Dis Colon Rectum. 1990; 33(1):52–55

[132] Bulow S. The Danish Polyposis Register. Description of the methods of detection and evaluation of completeness. Dis Colon Rectum. 1984; 27 (6):351–355

[133] Bussey HJ. Familial Polyposis Coli. Family Studies, Histopathology, Differential Diagnosis and Results of Treatment. Baltimore, MD: Johns Hopkins University Press; 1975

[134] Talbot IC. Pathology. In: Phillips RK, Spigelman AD, Thomson JP, eds. Familial Adenomatous Polyposis and Other Polyposis Syndromes. London: Edward Arnold; 1994:15–25

[135] Perry RE, Christensen MA, Thorson AG, Williams T. Familial polyposis: colon cancer in the absence of rectal polyps. Br J Surg. 1989; 76(7):744

[136] Bülow S. The risk of developing rectal cancer after colectomy and ileorectal anastomosis in Danish patients with polyposis coli. Dis Colon Rectum. 1984; 27(11):726–729

[137] Powell SM. Clinical applications of molecular genetics in colorectal cancer. Semin Colon Rectal Surg. 1995; 6:2–18

[138] Spirio L, Olschwang S, Groden J, et al. Alleles of the APC gene: an attenuated form of familial polyposis. Cell. 1993; 75(5):951–957

[139] Lynch HT, Smyrk T, McGinn T, et al. Attenuated familial adenomatous polyposis (AFAP). A phenotypically and genotypically distinctive variant of FAP. Cancer. 1995; 76(12):2427–2433

[140] Hernegger GS, Moore HG, Guillem JG. Attenuated familial adenomatous polyposis: an evolving and poorly understood entity. Dis Colon Rectum. 2002; 45(1):127–134, discussion 134–136

[141] Church JM. Editorial. Dis Colon Rectum. 2002; 45:134–135

[142] Hodgson SV, Spigelman AD. Genetics. In: Phillips RK, Spigelman AD, Thomson JP, eds. Familial Adenomatous Polyposis and Other Polyposis Syndromes. London: Edward Arnold; 1994:26–35

[143] Chung DC, Mino M, Shannon KM. Case records of the Massachusetts General Hospital. Weekly clinicopathological exercises. Case 34-2003. A 45-year-old woman with a family history of colonic polyps and cancer. N Engl J Med. 2003; 349(18):1750–1760

[144] Gardner EJ. A genetic and clinical study of intestinal polyposis, a predisposing factor for carcinoma of the colon and rectum. Am J Hum Genet. 1951; 3 (2):167–176

[145] Campbell WJ, Spence RA, Parks TG. Familial adenomatous polyposis. [review]. Br J Surg. 1994; 81(12):1722–1733

[146] Utsunomiya J, Maki T, Iwama T, Matsunaga Y, Ichikawa T. Gastric lesion of familial polyposis coli. Cancer. 1974; 34(3):745–754

[147] Spigelman AD. Familial adenomatous polyposis and the upper gastrointestinal tract. Semin Colon Rectal Surg. 1995; 6:26–28

[148] Marcello PW, Asbun HJ, Veidenheimer MC, et al. Gastroduodenal polyps in familial adenomatous polyposis. Surg Endosc. 1996; 10(4):418–421

[149] Wallace MH, Phillips RK. Upper gastrointestinal disease in patients with familial adenomatous polyposis. Br J Surg. 1998; 85(6):742–750

[150] Bülow S, Alm T, Fausa O, Hultcrantz R, Järvinen H, Vasen H, DAF Project Group. Duodenal adenomatosis in familial adenomatous polyposis. Int J Colorectal Dis. 1995; 10(1):43–46

[151] Church JM, McGannon E, Hull-Boiner S, et al. Gastroduodenal polyps in patients with familial adenomatous polyposis. Dis Colon Rectum. 1992; 35 (12):1170–1173

[152] Björk J, Akerbrant H, Iselius L, et al. Periampullary adenomas and adenocarcinomas in familial adenomatous polyposis: cumulative risks and APC gene mutations. Gastroenterology. 2001; 121(5):1127–1135

[153] Spigelman AD, Williams CB, Talbot IC, Domizio P, Phillips RK. Upper gastrointestinal cancer in patients with familial adenomatous polyposis. Lancet. 1989; 2(8666):783–785

[154] Jagelman DG, DeCosse JJ, Bussey HJ. Upper gastrointestinal cancer in familial adenomatous polyposis. Lancet. 1988; 1(8595):1149–1151

[155] Domizio P, Talbot IC, Spigelman AD, Williams CB, Phillips RK. Upper gastrointestinal pathology in familial adenomatous polyposis: results from a prospective study of 102 patients. J Clin Pathol. 1990; 43(9):738–743

[156] Kashiwagi H, Spigelman AD, Debinski HS, Talbot IC, Phillips RK. Surveillance of ampullary adenomas in familial adenomatous polyposis. [letter]. Lancet. 2003; 344(8936):1582

[157] Arvanitis ML, Jagelman DG, Fazio VW, Lavery IC, McGannon E. Mortality in patients with familial adenomatous polyposis. Dis Colon Rectum. 1990; 33 (8):639–642

[158] Belchetz LA, Berk T, Bapat BV, Cohen Z, Gallinger S. Changing causes of mortality in patients with familial adenomatous polyposis. Dis Colon Rectum. 1996; 39(4):384–387

[159] Wallace MH, Forbes A, Beveridge IG, et al. Randomized, placebo-controlled trial of gastric acid-lowering therapy on duodenal polyposis and relative adduct labeling in familial adenomatous polyposis. Dis Colon Rectum. 2001; 44 (11):1585–1589

[160] Phillips RK, Wallace MH, Lynch PM, et al. FAP Study Group. A randomised, double blind, placebo controlled study of celecoxib, a selective cyclooxygenase 2 inhibitor, on duodenal polyposis in familial adenomatous polyposis. Gut. 2002; 50(6):857–860

[161] Perez A, Saltzman JR, Carr-Locke DL, et al. Benign nonampullary duodenal neoplasms. J Gastrointest Surg. 2003; 7(4):536–541

[162] Alarcon FJ, Burke CA, Church JM, van Stolk RU. Familial adenomatous polyposis: efficacy of endoscopic and surgical treatment for advanced duodenal adenomas. Dis Colon Rectum. 1999; 42(12):1533–1536

[163] Burke CA, Beck GJ, Church JM, van Stolk RU. The natural history of untreated duodenal and ampullary adenomas in patients with familial adenomatous polyposis followed in an endoscopic surveillance program. Gastrointest Endosc. 1999; 49(3, Pt 1):358–364

[164] Soravia C, Berk T, Haber G, Cohen Z, Gallinger S. Management of advanced duodenal polyposis in familial adenomatous polyposis. J Gastrointest Surg. 1997; 1(5):474–478

[165] Penna C, Bataille N, Balladur P, Tiret E, Parc R. Surgical treatment of severe duodenal polyposis in familial adenomatous polyposis. Br J Surg. 1998; 85 (5):665–668

[166] de Vos tot Nederveen Cappel WH, Järvinen HJ, Björk J, Berk T, Griffioen G, Vasen HF. Worldwide survey among polyposis registries of surgical management of severe duodenal adenomatosis in familial adenomatous polyposis. Br J Surg. 2003; 90(6):705–710

[167] Morpurgo E, Vitale GC, Galandiuk S, Kimberling J, Ziegler C, Polk HC, Jr. Clinical characteristics of familial adenomatous polyposis and management of duodenal adenomas. J Gastrointest Surg. 2004; 8(5):559–564

[168] Mackey R, Walsh RM, Chung R, et al. Pancreas-sparing duodenectomy is effective management for familial adenomatous polyposis. J Gastrointest Surg. 2005; 9(8):1088–1093, discussion 1093

[169] Farnell MB, Sakorafas GH, Sarr MG, et al. Villous tumors of the duodenum: reappraisal of local vs. extended resection. J Gastrointest Surg. 2000; 4 (1):13–21, discussion 22–23

[170] Ruo L, Coit DG, Brennan MF, Guillem JG. Long-term follow-up of patients with familial adenomatous polyposis undergoing pancreaticoduodenal surgery. J Gastrointest Surg. 2002; 6(5):671–675

[171] Brosens LA, Keller JJ, Offerhaus GJ, Goggins M, Giardiello FM. Prevention and management of duodenal polyps in familial adenomatous polyposis. Gut. 2005; 54(7):1034–1043

[172] Giardiello FM, Petersen GM, Piantadosi S, et al. APC gene mutations and extraintestinal phenotype of familial adenomatous polyposis. Gut. 1997; 40 (4):521–525

[173] Clark SK, Phillips RK. Desmoids in familial adenomatous polyposis. [review]. Br J Surg. 1996; 83(11):1494–1504

[174] Heiskanen I, Järvinen HJ. Occurrence of desmoid tumours in familial adenomatous polyposis and results of treatment. Int J Colorectal Dis. 1996; 11 (4):157–162

[175] Clark SK, Neale KF, Landgrebe JC, Phillips RK. Desmoid tumours complicating familial adenomatous polyposis. Br J Surg. 1999; 86(9):1185–1189

[176] Hartley JE, Church JM, Gupta S, McGannon E, Fazio VW. Significance of incidental desmoids identified during surgery for familial adenomatous polyposis. Dis Colon Rectum. 2004; 47(3):334–338, discussion 339–340

[177] Lotfi AM, Dozois RR, Gordon H, et al. Mesenteric fibromatosis complicating familial adenomatous polyposis: predisposing factors and results of treatment. Int J Colorectal Dis. 1989; 4(1):30–36

[178] Phillips CV, Goodman KJ, Poole C, the editors of Epidemiologic Perspectives & Innovations. Lead editorial: The need for greater perspective and innovation in epidemiology. Epidemiol Perspect Innov. 2004; 1(1):1

[179] Church JM. Desmoid tumors in patients with familial adenomatous polyposis. Semin Colon Rectal Surg. 1995; 6:29–32

[180] Middleton SB, Clark SK, Matravers P, Katz D, Reznek R, Phillips RK. Stepwise progression of familial adenomatous polyposis-associated desmoid precursor lesions demonstrated by a novel CT scoring system. Dis Colon Rectum. 2003; 46(4):481–485

[181] Healy JC, Reznek RH, Clark SK, Phillips RK, Armstrong P. MR appearances of desmoid tumors in familial adenomatous polyposis. AJR Am J Roentgenol. 1997; 169(2):465–472

[182] Middleton SB, Phillips RK. Surgery for large intra-abdominal desmoid tumors: report of four cases. Dis Colon Rectum. 2000; 43(12):1759–1762, discussion 1762–1763

[183] Bülow S. Sulindac and tamoxifen in the treatment of desmoid tumours in patients with familial adenomatous polyposis. Colorectal Dis. 2001; 3 (4):266–267

[184] Moslein G, Dozois RR. Desmoid tumors associated with familial adenomatous polyposis. Perspect Colon Rectal Surg. 1998; 10:109–126

[185] Poritz LS, Blackstein M, Berk T, Gallinger S, McLeod RS, Cohen Z. Extended follow-up of patients treated with cytotoxic chemotherapy for intra-abdominal desmoid tumors. Dis Colon Rectum. 2001; 44(9):1268–1273

[186] Church J, Berk T, Boman BM, et al. Collaborative Group of the Americas on Inherited Colorectal Cancer. Staging intra-abdominal desmoid tumors in familial adenomatous polyposis: a search for a uniform approach to a troubling disease. Dis Colon Rectum. 2005; 48(8):1528–1534

[187] Cabot RC. Case records of Massachusetts General Hospital: Case 21061. N Engl J Med. 1935; 212:263–267

[188] Blair NP, Trempe CL. Hypertrophy of the retinal pigment epithelium associated with Gardner's syndrome. Am J Ophthalmol. 1980; 90(5):661–667

[189] Leppard B, Bussey HJ. Epidermoid cysts, polyposis coli and Gardner's syndrome. Br J Surg. 1975; 62(5):387–393

[190] Campbell WJ, Spence RA, Parks TG. The role of congenital hypertrophy of the retinal pigment epithelium in screening for familial adenomatous polyposis. Int J Colorectal Dis. 1994; 9(4):191–196

[191] Crail HW. Multiple primary malignancies arising in the rectum, brain, and thyroid; report of a case. U S Nav Med Bull. 1949; 49(1):123–128

[192] Bret MC, Hershman MJ, Glazer G. Other manifestations of familial adenomatous polyposis. In: Phillips RK, Spigelman AD, Thomson JP, eds. Familial Adenomatous Polyposis and Other Polyposis Syndromes. London: Edward Arnold; 1994:143–158

[193] Turcot J, Despres JP, St Pierre F. Malignant tumors of the central nervous system associated with familial polyposis of the colon: report of two cases. Dis Colon Rectum. 1959; 2:465–468

[194] Hamilton SR, Liu B, Parsons RE, et al. The molecular basis of Turcot's syndrome. N Engl J Med. 1995; 332(13):839–847

[195] Matsui T, Hayashi N, Yao K, et al. A father and son with Turcot's syndrome: evidence for autosomal dominant inheritance: report of two cases. Dis Colon Rectum. 1998; 41(6):797–801

[196] Itoh H, Hirata K, Ohsato K. Turcot's syndrome and familial adenomatous polyposis associated with brain tumor: review of related literature. Int J Colorectal Dis. 1993; 8(2):87–94

[197] Björk JA, Akerbrant HI, Iselius LE, Hultcrantz RW. Risk factors for rectal cancer morbidity and mortality in patients with familial adenomatous polyposis after colectomy and ileorectal anastomosis. Dis Colon Rectum. 2000; 43 (12):1719–1725

[198] Heiskanen I, Matikainen M, Hiltunen KM, Laitinen S, Rintala R, Järvinen HJ. Colectomy and ileorectal anastomosis or restorative proctocolectomy for familial adenomatous polyposis. Colorectal Dis. 1999; 1(1):9–14

[199] Phillips RK, Spigelman AD. Can we safely delay or avoid prophylactic colectomy in familial adenomatous polyposis? Br J Surg. 1996; 83(6):769–770

[200] Church J, Burke C, McGannon E, Pastean O, Clark B. Risk of rectal cancer in patients after colectomy and ileorectal anastomosis for familial adenomatous polyposis: a function of available surgical options. Dis Colon Rectum. 2003; 46(9):1175–1181

[201] Bülow C, Vasen H, Järvinen H, Björk J, Bisgaard ML, Bülow S. Ileorectal anastomosis is appropriate for a subset of patients with familial adenomatous polyposis. Gastroenterology. 2000; 119(6):1454–1460

[202] Penna C, Kartheuser A, Parc R, et al. Secondary proctectomy and ileal pouchanal anastomosis after ileorectal anastomosis for familial adenomatous polyposis. Br J Surg. 1993; 80(12):1621–1625

[203] Church J, Burke C, McGannon E, Pastean O, Clark B. Predicting polyposis severity by proctoscopy: how reliable is it? Dis Colon Rectum. 2001; 44 (9):1249–1254

[204] Farmer KC, Phillips RK. Colectomy with ileorectal anastomosis lowers rectal mucosal cell proliferation in familial adenomatous polyposis. Dis Colon Rectum. 1993; 36(2):167–171

[205] Karen P, Nugent MA, Northover J. Total colectomy and ileorectal anastomosis. In: Phillips RK, Spigelman AD, Thomson JP, eds. Familial Adenomatous Polyposis and Other Polyposis Syndromes. London: Edward Arnold; 1994:80–91

[206] Winde G, Schmid KW, Schlegel W, Fischer R, Osswald H, Bünte H. Complete reversion and prevention of rectal adenomas in colectomized patients with familial adenomatous polyposis by rectal low-dose sulindac maintenance treatment. Advantages of a low-dose nonsteroidal anti-inflammatory drug regimen in reversing adenomas exceeding 33 months. Dis Colon Rectum. 1995; 38(8):813–830

[207] Gingold BS, Jagelman D, Turnbull RB. Surgical management of familial polyposis and Gardner's syndrome. Am J Surg. 1979; 137(1):54–56

[208] Bess MA, Adson MA, Elveback LR, Moertel CG. Rectal cancer following colectomy for polyposis. Arch Surg. 1980; 115(4):460–467

[209] Bussey HJ, Eyers AA, Ritchie SM, Thomson JP. The rectum in adenomatous polyposis: the St. Mark's policy. Br J Surg. 1985; 72 Suppl:S29–S31

[210] Nugent KP, Phillips RK. Rectal cancer risk in older patients with familial adenomatous polyposis and an ileorectal anastomosis: a cause for concern. Br J Surg. 1992; 79(11):1204–1206

[211] Heiskanen I, Järvinen HJ. Fate of the rectal stump after colectomy and ileorectal anastomosis for familial adenomatous polyposis. Int J Colorectal Dis. 1997; 12(1):9–13

[212] Sarre RG, Jagelman DG, Beck GJ, et al. Colectomy with ileorectal anastomosis for familial adenomatous polyposis: the risk of rectal cancer. Surgery. 1987; 101(1):20–26

[213] De Cosse JJ, Bülow S, Neale K, et al. The Leeds Castle Polyposis Group. Rectal cancer risk in patients treated for familial adenomatous polyposis. Br J Surg. 1992; 79(12):1372–1375

[214] Iwama T, Mishima Y. Factors affecting the risk of rectal cancer following rectum-preserving surgery in patients with familial adenomatous polyposis. Dis Colon Rectum. 1994; 37(10):1024–1026

[215] Jenner DC, Levitt S. Rectal cancer following colectomy and ileorectal anastomosis for familial adenomatous polyposis. Aust N Z J Surg. 1998; 68(2):136–138

[216] Bertario L, Russo A, Radice P, et al. Genotype and phenotype factors as determinants for rectal stump cancer in patients with familial adenomatous polyposis. Hereditary Colorectal Tumors Registry. Ann Surg. 2000; 231(4):538–543

[217] Spagnesi MT, Tonelli F, Dolara P, et al. Rectal proliferation and polyp occurrence in patients with familial adenomatous polyposis after sulindac treatment. Gastroenterology. 1994; 106(2):362–366

[218] Winde G, Schmid KW, Brandt B, Müller O, Osswald H. Clinical and genomic influence of sulindac on rectal mucosa in familial adenomatous polyposis. Dis Colon Rectum. 1997; 40(10):1156–1168, discussion 1168–1169

[219] Giardiello FM, Yang VW, Hylind LM, et al. Primary chemoprevention of familial adenomatous polyposis with sulindac. N Engl J Med. 2002; 346 (14):1054–1059

[220] Thorson AG, Lynch HT, Smyrk TC. Rectal cancer in FAP patient after sulindac. Lancet. 1994; 343(8890):180

[221] Yang VW, Geiman DE, Hubbard WC, et al. Tissue prostanoids as biomarkers for chemoprevention of colorectal neoplasia: correlation between prostanoid synthesis and clinical response in familial adenomatous polyposis. Prostaglandins Other Lipid Mediat. 2000; 60(1–3):83–96

[222] Niv Y, Fraser GM. Adenocarcinoma in the rectal segment in familial polyposis coli is not prevented by sulindac therapy. Gastroenterology. 1994; 107 (3):854–857

[223] Kartheuser AH, Parc R, Penna CP, et al. Ileal pouch-anal anastomosis as the first choice operation in patients with familial adenomatous polyposis: a ten-year experience. Surgery. 1996; 119(6):615–623

[224] Ziv Y, Church JM, Oakley JR, McGannon E, Fazio VW. Surgery for the teenager with familial adenomatous polyposis: ileo-rectal anastomosis or restorative proctocolectomy? Int J Colorectal Dis. 1995; 10(1):6–9

[225] Parc YR, Moslein G, Dozois RR, Pemberton JH, Wolff BG, King JE. Familial adenomatous polyposis: results after ileal pouch-anal anastomosis in teenagers. Dis Colon Rectum. 2000; 43(7):893–898, discussion 898–902

[226] Ambroze WL, Jr, Dozois RR, Pemberton JH, Beart RW, Jr, Ilstrup DM. Familial adenomatous polyposis: results following ileal pouch-anal anastomosis and ileorectostomy. Dis Colon Rectum. 1992; 35(1):12–15

[227] Setti-Carraro P, Nicholls RJ. Choice of prophylactic surgery for the large bowel component of familial adenomatous polyposis. [review]. Br J Surg. 1996; 83(7):885–892

[228] Soravia C, Klein L, Berk T, O'Connor BI, Cohen Z, McLeod RS. Comparison of ileal pouch-anal anastomosis and ileorectal anastomosis in patients with familial adenomatous polyposis. Dis Colon Rectum. 1999; 42(8):1028–1033, discussion 1033–1034

[229] Church J. Ileoanal pouch neoplasia in familial adenomatous polyposis: an underestimated threat. Dis Colon Rectum. 2005; 48(9):1708–1713

[230] Remzi FH, Church JM, Bast J, et al. Mucosectomy vs. stapled ileal pouch-anal anastomosis in patients with familial adenomatous polyposis: functional outcome and neoplasia control. Dis Colon Rectum. 2001; 44(11):1590–1596

[231] van Duijvendijk P, Vasen HF, Bertario L, et al. Cumulative risk of developing polyps or malignancy at the ileal pouch-anal anastomosis in patients with familial adenomatous polyposis. J Gastrointest Surg. 1999; 3(3):325–330

[232] Petersen GM. Genetic counseling and predictive genetic testing in familial adenomatous polyposis. Semin Colon Rectal Surg. 1995; 6:55–60

[233] Spigelman AD, Thomson JP. Introduction, history and registries. In: Phillips RK, Spigelman AD, Thomson JP, eds. Familial Adenomatous Polyposis and Other Polyposis Syndromes. London: Edward Arnold; 1994:3–14

[234] Wong N, Lasko D, Rabelo R, Pinsky L, Gordon PH, Foulkes W. Genetic counseling and interpretation of genetic tests in familial adenomatous polyposis and hereditary nonpolyposis colorectal cancer. Dis Colon Rectum. 2001; 44 (2):271–279

[235] Coppa GF, Eng K, Localio SA. Surgical management of diffuse cavernous hemangioma of the colon, rectum and anus. Surg Gynecol Obstet. 1984; 159 (1):17–22

[236] Rabelo R, Foulkes W, Gordon PH, et al. Role of molecular diagnostic testing in familial adenomatous polyposis and hereditary nonpolyposis colorectal cancer families. Dis Colon Rectum. 2001; 44(3):437–446

[237] Jeffery PJ, Hawley PR, Parks AG. Colo-anal sleeve anastomosis in the treatment of diffuse cavernous haemangioma involving the rectum. Br J Surg. 1976; 63(9):678–682

[238] Church JM, McGannon E. A polyposis registry: how to set one up and make it work. Semin Colon Rectal Surg. 1995; 6:48–54

[239] Rothenberger DA, Dalberg DL, Leininger A. Minnesota Colorectal Cancer Initiative: successful development and implementation of a community-based colorectal cancer registry. Dis Colon Rectum. 2004; 47(10):1571–1577

[240] Lyon DT, Mantia AG. Large-bowel hemangiomas. Dis Colon Rectum. 1984; 27(6):404–414

[241] Allred HW, Jr. Hemangiomas of the colon, rectum, and anus. Mayo Clin Proc. 1974; 49(10):739–741

[242] Londono-Schimmer EE, Ritchie JK, Hawley PR. Coloanal sleeve anastomosis in the treatment of diffuse cavernous haemangioma of the rectum: long-term results. Br J Surg. 1994; 81(8):1235–1237

[243] Allred HW, Spencer RJ. Hemangiomas of the colon, rectum, and anus. Mayo Clin Proc.. 1974; 49:739–741

[244] Telander RL, Ahlquist D, Blaufuss MC. Rectal mucosectomy: a definitive approach to extensive hemangiomas of the rectum. J Pediatr Surg. 1993; 28 (3):379–381

[245] He LJ, Wang BS, Chen CC. Smooth muscle tumours of the digestive tract: report of 160 cases. Br J Surg. 1988; 75(2):184–186

[246] Morgan BK, Compton C, Talbert M, Gallagher WJ, Wood WC. Benign smooth muscle tumors of the gastrointestinal tract. A 24-year experience. Ann Surg. 1990; 211(1):63–66

[247] Kusminsky RE, Bailey W. Leiomyomas of the rectum and anal canal: report of six cases and review of the literature. Dis Colon Rectum. 1977; 20 (7):580–599

[248] Miettinen M, Furlong M, Sarlomo-Rikala M, Burke A, Sobin LH, Lasota J. Gastrointestinal stromal tumors, intramural leiomyomas, and leiomyosarcomas in the rectum and anus: a clinicopathologic, immunohistochemical, and molecular genetic study of 144 cases. Am J Surg Pathol. 2001; 25(9):1121–1133

[249] Walsh TH, Mann CV. Smooth muscle neoplasms of the rectum and anal canal. Br J Surg. 1984; 71(8):597–599

[250] Vorobyov GI, Odaryuk TS, Kapuller LL, Shelygin YA, Kornyak BS. Surgical treatment of benign, myomatous rectal tumors. Dis Colon Rectum. 1992; 35 (4):328–331

[251] Taylor BA, Wolff BG. Colonic lipomas. Report of two unusual cases and review of the Mayo Clinic experience, 1976–1985. Dis Colon Rectum. 1987; 30 (11):888–893

[252] Gordon RT, Beal JM. Lipoma of the colon. Arch Surg. 1978; 113(7):897–899

[253] Castro EB, Stearns MW. Lipoma of the large intestine: a review of 45 cases. Dis Colon Rectum. 1972; 15(6):441–444

[254] Brouland JP, Poupard B, Nemeth J, Valleur P. Lipomatous polyposis of the colon with multiple lipomas of peritoneal folds and giant diverticulosis: report of a case. Dis Colon Rectum. 2000; 43(12):1767–1769

[255] Santos-Briz A, García JP, González C, Colina F. Lipomatous polyposis of the colon. Histopathology. 2001; 38(1):81–83

[256] Zhang H, Cong JC, Chen CS, Qiao L, Liu EQ. Submucous colon lipoma: a case report and review of the literature. World J Gastroenterol. 2005; 11 (20):3167–3169

[257] Liessi G, Pavanello M, Cesari S, Dell'Antonio C, Avventi P. Large lipomas of the colon: CT and MR findings in three symptomatic cases. Abdom Imaging. 1996; 21(2):150–152

[258] Pfeil SA, Weaver MG, Abdul-Karim FW, Yang P. Colonic lipomas: outcome of endoscopic removal. Gastrointest Endosc. 1990; 36(5):435–438

[259] Chung YF, Ho YH, Nyam DC, Leong AF, Seow-Choen F. Management of colonic lipomas. Aust N Z J Surg. 1998; 68(2):133–135

20 Colorectal Cancer: Screening, Surveillance, and Follow-Up

David E. Beck

Abstract

Despite the plethora of publications on the subject of follow-up strategies for patients who have undergone curative resection for colorectal carcinoma, there is no general agreement on the optimal follow-up program. The efficacy of aggressive and intensive surveillance remains a topic of intense debate. Some data support the contention that surveillance leads to increased rates of early detection and resection of recurrence, but this has not necessarily always translated into improved survival. What constitutes the ideal or even preferred follow-up program remains controversial, and this is clearly reflected by the lack of uniformity among practicing clinicians.

It is important that patients understand the limitations of the postoperative follow-up no matter how minimal or extensive it is. They should actively participate in the decision-making of the follow-up plan. Guidelines from some major societies are helpful on this issue.

Keywords: colorectal cancer, screening, surveillance, follow-up, fecal occult blood test, flexible sigmoidoscopy, colonoscopy, double-contrast barium enema (DCBE), computed tomography colonography (CTC, virtual colonoscopy), fecal DNA testing

20.1 Screening

Screening, which refers primarily to a population approach, has been used interchangeably with early detection. Case finding refers to early detection on an individual basis. These terms refer to the identification of individuals with an increased probability of having colorectal neoplasia. Effective screening tests meet certain criteria. The test should have scientific evidence of effectiveness and identify a significant disease. The benefits should outweigh the harm, and the screened disease should be preventable or treatable when identified. Screening for colorectal cancer meets these criteria.

20.2 Colorectal Carcinoma

In 2018, there were 140,250 estimated new cases of colon and rectal carcinomas in the United States, and of these, 40,500 (29%) were carcinomas of the rectum.[1] Of these, 50,630 (combined colon and rectum) will die, a death rate of 36%.[1] Survival for colon and rectal carcinoma is closely related to the clinical and pathologic stage of the disease at diagnosis. Data from the German Multicenter Study in colorectal carcinoma showed 5-year survival rates in stages I, II, III, and IV as 76, 65, 42, and 16%, respectively (surgical mortality not excluded).[2] More recent National Cancer Institute SEER Cancer Statistics Review for 1975–2013 demonstrated a 5-year survival of 90.1% for localized disease, 71.2% for regional, and 13.5% for distal metastatic disease.[3]

It has become clear that if the disease can be detected at an early stage, the overall prognosis can be improved, with another benefit that some colorectal carcinomas can even be prevented. Most colorectal carcinomas are asymptomatic until a late stage, when some partial obstruction occurs, causing abdominal pain or change in bowel habits. Although carcinoma of the colon and rectum bleeds occasionally and unpredictably, it may be possible to diagnose it in an early stage by examining for occult blood in the stool. Through many observations and studies, including current knowledge of molecular genetics of colorectal carcinoma, the natural history of colorectal carcinoma starts with one crypt. The numerous mutations of genes slowly give rise to a small polyp and this then progresses to an invasive carcinoma that eventually metastasizes. The National Polyp Study (NPS) suggested that it took about 10 years for the development of an invasive carcinoma from a "clean" colon in the majority of patients.[4] This lengthy, stepwise natural history provides a window of opportunity for detecting early carcinoma and removing malignant polyps (▶ Fig. 20.1). Thus, screening strategy can be directed toward detecting early carcinoma to reduce morbidity and mortality as well as removing premalignant polyps to reduce the incidence of colorectal carcinoma.

Various screening tests have been shown to achieve accurate detection of early-stage colorectal carcinomas.[5,6,7,8,9] Evidence from controlled trials and case–control studies suggests varying degrees of persuasiveness that removing adenomatous polyps reduces the incidence of colorectal carcinoma and detecting early-stage carcinomas reduces mortality from the disease. Finally, screening benefits outweigh its harms. The various ways of screening for colorectal carcinoma all have cost-effectiveness ratios comparable to those of other generally accepted screening tests.[10,11] It is important to note that once the screening results are positive, a complete investigation of the entire colon and rectum is mandated to identify colorectal polyps or carcinomas. Screening should be accompanied by efforts to optimize the participation of patients and health care providers, and to

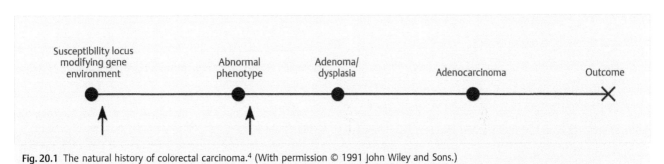

Fig. 20.1 The natural history of colorectal carcinoma.[4] (With permission © 1991 John Wiley and Sons.)

remind patients and providers about the need for rescreening at recommended intervals.[12]

According to the Centers for Disease Control and Prevention (CDC), only two-thirds of eligible patients in the United States have been screened for colorectal carcinoma.[13] A lack of awareness by the respondent of the need for the test and a lack of recommendation by the physician for the test to be performed were found to be the most commonly reported barriers to undergoing the test. Lack of physician recommendation clearly was an important barrier; among persons who reported undergoing no colorectal carcinoma testing or none recently, only 5% reported that a physician had recommended colorectal carcinoma testing.

Approximately 75% of all new cases of colorectal carcinoma occur in people with no known predisposing factors for the disease. Incidence increases with age, beginning around 40 years.[14] People with no predisposing factors are considered to be at average risk for colorectal carcinoma. People with a family history of colorectal carcinoma (i.e., one or more parents, siblings, or children with the disease) but without any apparent defined genetic syndrome account for most of those at high risk (15–20%). Hereditary nonpolyposis colon cancer (HNPCC) accounts for 4 to 7% of all cases and familial adenomatous polyposis (FAP) about 1%. The remainder, about 1%, are attributed to a variety of uncommon conditions: chronic ulcerative colitis, Crohn's colitis, Peutz–Jeghers syndrome, and familial juvenile polyposis, in which the colorectal carcinoma risk is elevated but is not as high as in HNPCC and FAP (▶ Fig. 20.2).[10] Other risk factors that should be kept in mind include older age, a diet high in saturated fats and low in fiber, excessive alcohol consumption, and sedentary lifestyle.[15]

There is no direct evidence as to when screening should stop, but indirect evidence supports stopping screening in people

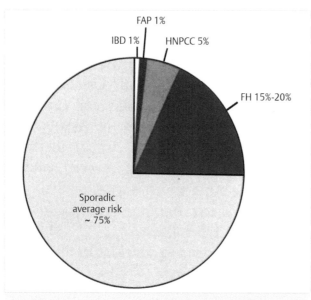

Fig. 20.2 Annual new cases of colorectal carcinoma in men and women: 50 years of age with no special risk factors. FAP, familial adenomatous polyposis; FH, family history; HNPCC, hereditary nonpolyposis colon cancer; IBD, inflammatory bowel disease.[10] (With permission © 1997 Elsevier.)

nearing the end of life. Most polyps take at least 10 years to progress to carcinoma, and screening to detect polyps may not be in the patient's best interest if he or she is not expected to live at least that long. Also, screening and diagnostic tests are, in general, less well tolerated by elderly people. Therefore, there will come a time in most peoples' lives when the rigors of screening and diagnostic evaluation of positive tests are no longer justified by the potential to prolong life. The age at which to stop screening depends on the judgment of the individual patient and his or her clinician, taking into account the lead time between screening and its benefits and the patient's life expectancy.[10]

Screening people at average risk for colorectal carcinoma is different from screening people at high risk. Clinicians should determine an individual patient's risk status well before the earliest potential initiation of screening. The individual's risk status determines when screening should be initiated, and what tests and frequency are appropriate.[12]

Risk stratification can be accomplished by asking several questions aimed at uncovering the risk factors for colorectal cancer.[12] They are as follows:

- Has the patient had colorectal carcinoma or an adenomatous polyp?
- Does the patient have an illness (e.g., inflammatory bowel disease) that predisposes him or her to colorectal carcinoma?
- Has a family member had colorectal carcinoma or an adenomatous polyp? If so, how many? Was it a first-degree relative (parent, sibling, or child), and at what age was the carcinoma or polyp first diagnosed?

A positive response to any of these questions should prompt further efforts to identify and define the specific condition associated with increased risk.

Men and women at average risk should be offered screening with one of the following options beginning at 50 years. A study of a screening colonoscopy in people 40 to 49 years old confirmed that colorectal carcinomas are uncommon in this age group, supporting the recommendation that screening in average risk people begin at age 50 years.[16]

The rationale for presenting multiple options is that no single test has unequivocal superiority, and that giving patients a choice allows them to apply personal preferences and may increase the likelihood that screening will occur. However, the strategies are not equal with regard to evidence of effectiveness, magnitude of effectiveness, risk, or up-front costs. Reviewing the rationale section for each screening test below will provide clinicians with information that they can use in presenting the relative effectiveness of each test to patients. These tests are recommended by the American Gastroenterological Association,[12] the American Cancer Society,[17] and the American Society of Colon and Rectal Surgeons guidelines.

20.3 Colorectal Cancer Screening Tests

A number of tests are available and each has advantages and limitations.[12]

20.3.1 Stool Testing

Fecal Occult Blood Test

This test offers yearly screening with fecal occult blood test (FOBT) using guaiac-based test with dietary restriction (avoidance of red meat for 3 days prior to performing the test). Two samples from each of three consecutive stools should be examined without rehydration. The patients with a positive test on any specimen should be followed up with colonoscopy.[12] The American Gastroenterological Society recommends yearly testing because it is more effective than screening every 2 years. Rehydration is not recommended. Newer guaiac-based tests are available that have improved sensitivity and appear to maintain acceptable specificity. Dietary restrictions during testing are commonly recommended to reduce the false-positive rate for the more sensitive guaiac-based tests but are not necessary for the less sensitive guaiac-based tests.

With longer (18 years) follow-up in the Minnesota trial, FOBT screening every other year was found to reduce colorectal cancer mortality by 21%,[18] a rate consistent with the results of the biennial screening in the two European trials.[7] The incidence of colorectal carcinoma was also reduced in the screened group.[19] A systematic review of three clinical trials[5,6,7,19] has shown that a restricted diet does not reduce the positivity rate for the older, less sensitive guaiac-based tests and that very restricted diets may reduce compliance rates.[20]

Disadvantages of FOBT are that currently available tests for occult blood fail to detect many polyps and some carcinomas. Also, most people who test positive will not have colorectal neoplasia (have a false-positive test result) and, thus, will undergo the discomfort, cost, and risk of colonoscopy without benefit. Colonoscopy is recommended for all those with a positive FOBT because it was a diagnostic procedure used throughout most of the trials and because it is substantially more accurate than double-contrast barium enema (DCBE) for the detection of both small carcinomas and adenomas.[21]

Fecal Immunochemical Test

Fecal immunochemical tests (FITs) are more sensitive at detecting both colorectal carcinomas and adenomas than FOBTs. Many FITs require only one or two stool samples, and none require dietary or medication restrictions, increasing ease of use. In 2008, several U.S. professional societies endorsed the use of FITs to replace FOBTs because of the former's improved performance characteristics and potential for higher participation rates.[22] Countries in Europe and Asia have also adopted widespread colorectal carcinoma screening programs using FITs.[23] However, the diagnostic characteristics of these tests have been difficult to estimate, with reported sensitivities ranging from 25 to 100% for colorectal carcinomas and specificities usually exceeding 90%.[24] A systemic review and meta-analysis of 19 studies found a sensitivity of 79%, a specificity of 95%, and overall accuracy of 96%.[25] Increasing the number of samples did not affect results.

20.3.2 Fecal DNA Testing

Fecal DNA testing is based on the idea that, because carcinoma is a disease of mutations that occur as tissue evolves from normal to adenoma to carcinoma, those mutations should be detectable in stool.[26] Preliminary reports that persons with advanced carcinoma have detectable DNA mutations in stool[27] provided the basis for a large study, using a panel of 21 mutations, in more than 4,000 asymptomatic persons who received screening colonoscopy, fecal DNA testing, and FOBT with Hemoccult II.[28] The DNA marker panel, including mutations in APC, K-ras, and p53, showed a sensitivity of 52% for colorectal carcinoma and specificity of 94%.[29] Such stool-based testing is appealing because it is noninvasive, requires no special colonic preparation, and has the capability of detecting neoplasia throughout the entire length of the colon.[30] Because the DNA alterations in colorectal carcinoma are heterogeneous, assays will need to detect mutations in the number of genes.

The FDA has approved a commercially available test (Cologuard, Exact Sciences, Madison, WI). This is a multitarget stool DNA test consisting of molecular assays for aberrantly methylated *BMP3* and *NDRG4* promoter regions, mutant *KRAS*, and β-actin (a reference gene for human DNA quantity), as well as an immunochemical assay for human hemoglobin. Quantitative measurements of each marker are incorporated into a validated, prespecified, logistic-regression algorithm, with a value of 183 or more for a positive test.[29] A 90-site study of over 12,000 patients comparing a stool DNA test to FIT found that the sensitivity of the DNA test for the detection of both colorectal cancer (92.3%) and advanced precancerous lesions (42.4%) exceeded that of FIT by an absolute difference of nearly 20 percentage points.[29] The future of this test will also depend on factors such as the performance characteristics of alternative tests, testing intervals, complications, costs, patient acceptance, and adherence.[30,31,32]

20.3.3 Flexible Sigmoidoscopy

Screening with flexible sigmoidoscopy is recommended every 5 years. Case-controlled studies have reported that sigmoidoscopy was associated with reduced mortality for colorectal carcinoma.[33,34,35] Colon carcinoma risk in the area beyond the reach of the sigmoidoscope was not reduced. A 5-year interval between screening examinations is a conservative choice. It is supported by the observation that a reduction in colorectal carcinoma deaths related to screening sigmoidoscopy was present up to 10 years from the last screening examination,[33] and that repeat colonoscopy 5 years after a negative colonoscopy found few instances of advanced neoplasia,[36] and follow-up of a cohort of patients after polyp excision showed that development of advanced neoplasia was rare up to 5 years after a negative colonoscopy.[37] The interval is shorter than for colonoscopy because flexible sigmoidoscopy is less sensitive than colonoscopy.

Several studies have shown that the prevalence of proximal advanced adenomas in patients without distal adenomas is in the 2 to 5% range.[38,39,40,41] A flexible sigmoidoscopy followed by colonoscopy if a polyp was found would have identified 70 to 80% of patients with advanced proximal neoplasia.[39] In one randomized controlled trial, screening sigmoidoscopy followed by colonoscopy when polyps were detected was associated with an 80% reduction in colorectal carcinoma incidence.[42]

Yearly FOBT combined with flexible sigmoidoscopy every 5 years in a nonrandomized controlled trial reported a 43% reduction (which was not statistically significant) in colorectal carcinoma deaths in people screened with FOBT and sigmoidoscopy relative to sigmoidoscopy alone.[6] The disadvantage of the FOBT/sigmoidoscopy strategy is that people incur the inconvenience, cost, and complications of both tests with an uncertain gain in effectiveness.

20.3.4 Colonoscopy

Colonoscopy is offered every 10 years. Although there are no studies evaluating whether screening colonoscopy alone reduces the incidence or mortality from colorectal carcinoma in people at average risk, several lines of evidence support the effectiveness of screening colonoscopy.[12] There is direct evidence that screening sigmoidoscopy reduces colorectal carcinoma mortality,[33,34] and colonoscopy allows more of the large bowel to be examined. Colonoscopy has been shown to reduce the incidence of colorectal carcinoma in two cohort studies of people with adenomatous polyps.[37,43] Colonoscopy permits detection and removal of polyps and biopsy of carcinoma throughout the colon. However, colonoscopy involves greater cost, risk, and inconvenience to the patient than other screening tests, and not all examinations visualize the entire colon. The added value of colonoscopy over sigmoidoscopy screening, therefore, involves a tradeoff of incremental benefits and harms.[12]

Choice of a 10-year interval between screening examinations for average-risk people (if the preceding examination is negative) is based on estimates of the sensitivity of colonoscopy and the rate at which advanced adenomas develop. The dwell time from the development of adenomatous polyps to transformation into carcinoma is estimated to be at least 10 years on average.[36,44]

In two large prospective studies of screening colonoscopy, about half of patients with advanced proximal neoplasms had no distal colonic neoplasms.[38,39] Similarly, a prospective study of distal colon findings in a cohort of average-risk persons with carcinoma proximal to the splenic flexure found that 65% had no neoplasm distal to the splenic flexure.[45] A randomized controlled trial of sigmoidoscopy with follow-up colonoscopy for all patients with polyps compared with no screening demonstrated a significant reduction in colorectal carcinoma incidence in the screened patients.[41] A cohort of 154 asymptomatic average-risk persons with negative screening colonoscopies had < 1% incidence of advanced neoplasms at a second colonoscopy 5 years later,[35] lending support to the recommended interval of 10 years. Two colonoscopy studies suggested that flat and depressed adenomas account for 22 and 30% of adenomas,[46,47] and one report suggests that dye spraying is necessary to not miss these lesions.[46] However, the precise prevalence and clinical significance of flat adenomas is uncertain.

By the end of 2000, the U.S. Medicare system had decided to reimburse for colonoscopy screening. Colonoscopy as the best primary screening test began to be discussed and to be advocated by some gastroenterology organizations.[26]

20.3.5 Double-Contrast Barium Enema

This test is recommended every 5 years. The sensitivity of DCBE for large polyps and carcinomas is substantially less than with colonoscopy, the procedure does not permit removal of polyps or biopsy of the carcinomas, and DCBE is more likely than colonoscopy to identify artifacts and other findings (such as stool) as polyps. Patients with an abnormal barium enema need a subsequent colonoscopy.

DCBE is included as an option because it offers an alternative (albeit less sensitive) means to examine the entire colon, it is widely available, and it detects about half of large polyps, which are most likely to be clinically important. Adding flexible sigmoidoscopy to DCBE is not recommended in the screening setting. A 5-year interval between DCBE examinations is recommended because DCBE is less sensitive than colonoscopy in detecting colonic neoplasms.

In a prospective study of DCBE in a surveillance population with a spectrum and prevalence of disease similar to a screened population, DCBE detected 53% of adenomatous polyps 6 to 10 mm in size and 48% of those > 1 cm in size compared with colonoscopy.[31] In a nonrandomized study of 2,193 consecutive colorectal carcinoma cases in community practice, the sensitivity for carcinoma was 85% with DCBE and 95% with colonoscopy.[29]

20.3.6 Computed Tomography Colonography (Virtual Colonoscopy)

Computed tomography colonography (CTC) is not currently an option for mass screening for colorectal carcinoma. It is used as a backup for an incomplete colonoscopy, or for patients who are not suitable for a colonoscopy. However, the advances in technology, techniques, and clinical studies have progressed rapidly. It will be just a matter of time before CTC will become another option for colorectal carcinoma screening (see Chapter 3).

20.4 Screening People at Increased Risk for Colorectal Carcinoma

Screening high-risk people can take several forms. Patients can begin screening at an earlier age if polyps and carcinomas arise at an earlier age, they can be screened more frequently if the evolution from small polyps to carcinoma is more rapid, they can be screened by tests that reach the right colon if the carcinoma occurs more proximally, or they can be screened with more sensitive methods, such as colonoscopy or DCBE rather than FOBT or sigmoidoscopy. Patients already found to have adenomatous polyps are at increased risk for colorectal carcinoma and are candidates for surveillance rather than screening.[10]

20.4.1 Family History of Colorectal Carcinoma or Adenomatous Polyp

This group consists of individuals having one or more first-degree relatives (parent, sibling, or child) with colorectal carcinoma or adenomatous polyps diagnosed at age < 60 years. There is significant evidence that carcinomas arise at an earlier age in these people than in average-risk persons. In effect, the risk of a 40-year-old person with a family history of colorectal carcinoma is comparable to that of an average-risk 50-year-old person.[48] Screening colonoscopy should be started at age 40 years or 10 years younger than the earliest diagnosis in their family, whichever comes first, and repeated every 5 years.[12] Colorectal carcinoma screening recommendations for people with familial or inherited risk are given in ▶ Table 20.1 and ▶ Table 20.2. The lifetime risk of developing colon carcinoma in people with another prior primary cancer is shown in ▶ Table 20.3.

20.4.2 Genetic Syndromes

See Chapter 19 for screening of FAP and Chapter 21 for screening of HNPCC.

20.4.3 Detection of Second Malignancies

Some patients have a higher incidence of a second malignancy than the normal population. Analysis of the Utah Cancer Registry, which documented more than 35,000 carcinomas, revealed that Utah men with one carcinoma have a 1.2 times greater likelihood of developing another carcinoma and Utah women have a 1.5 times greater likelihood than did other persons in the Utah population of the same race, sex, and age who have not had a previous malignancy. In particular, men with primary carcinoma of the colon and rectum have a higher incidence of developing a second carcinoma in the colon, rectum, prostate, or bladder.[49] A complete colonic examination with colonoscopy or flexible

sigmoidoscopy combined with barium enema to check metachronous lesions should be performed every 5 years.

At present, the glycoprotein prostate-specific antigen (PSA) is the most useful marker available for the diagnosis and management of prostate carcinoma. However, PSA is prostate specific but is not sufficiently specific to be used alone as a screening test for prostate carcinoma. PSA is also produced by normal prostatic tissue and can indicate the presence of benign prostatic hyperplasia. The combination of the PSA test and digital rectal examination provides reliable early detection of prostatic carcinoma. These should be performed annually.[50]

Table 20.1 Colon carcinoma screening recommendations for people with familial or inherited risk[12]

Familial risk category	Screening recommendation
First-degree relative with colorectal carcinoma or an adenomatous polyp at age ≥ 60 years, or two second-degree relatives with colorectal carcinoma	Same as average risk but starting at age 40 years
Two or more first-degree relatives[a] with colon carcinoma, or a single first-degree relative with colon carcinoma or adenomatous polyps diagnosed at an age < 60 years	Colonoscopy every 5 years, beginning at age 40 years or 10 years younger than the earliest diagnosis in the family, whichever comes first
One second-degree or any third-degree relative[b,c] with colorectal carcinoma	Same as average risk
Gene carrier or at risk for familial adenomatous polyposis[d]	Sigmoidoscopy annually, beginning at age 10–12 years[e]
Gene carrier or at risk for HNPCC	Colonoscopy, every 1–2 years, beginning at age 20–25 years or 10 years younger than the earliest case in the family, whichever comes first

Abbreviation: HNPCC, hereditary nonpolyposis colon cancer.
[a]First-degree relatives include parents, siblings, and children.
[b]Second-degree relatives include grandparents, aunts, and uncles.
[c]Third-degree relatives include great-grandparents and cousins.
[d]Includes the subcategories of familial adenomatous polyposis, Gardner's syndrome, some Turcot's syndrome families, and attenuated adenomatous polyposis coli (AAPC).
[e]In AAPC, colonoscopy should be used instead of sigmoidoscopy because of the preponderance of proximal colonic adenomas. Colonoscopy screening in AAPC should probably begin in the late teens or early 20 s.

Table 20.2 Familial risk[12]

Familial setting	Approximate lifetime risk of colon carcinoma
General population risk in the United States	6%
One first-degree relative with colon carcinoma[a]	2–3-fold increased
Two first-degree relatives with colon carcinoma[a]	3–4-fold increased
First-degree relative with colon carcinoma diagnosed before age 50	3–4-fold increased
One second- or third-degree relative with colon carcinoma[b,c]	About 1.5-fold increased
Two second-degree relatives with colon carcinoma[b]	About 2–3-fold increased
One first-degree relative with an adenomatous polyp[a]	About 2-fold increased

[a]First-degree relatives include parents, siblings, and children.
[b]Second-degree relatives include grandparents, aunts, and uncles.
[c]Third-degree relatives include great-grandparents and cousins.

Table 20.3 The relative risk of secondary primary malignancy[49]

Site of second malignancy	Sex	Primary lesion of colon (RR)	Primary lesion of rectum (RR)
Stomach	M	1.3	1.0
	F	1.0	1.3
Small intestine (carcinoid, adenocarcinoma)	M	10.2	3.8
	F	5.1	2.0
Kidney	M	1.5	1.2
	F	1.5	1.3
Bladder	M	1.5	1.3
	F	2.0	1.7
Prostate	M	1.3	1.3
Ovary	F	3.0	1.5
Endometrium	F	1.7	1.7
Cervix	F	1.1	1.4
Breast	F	1.3	1.3

Abbreviation: RR, relative risk.

For a 55-year-old man presenting to a physician's office, it is prudent to obtain a serum PSA concentration and perform a digital rectal examination. If both are normal, the patient should be followed with an annual evaluation. If the results of the digital rectal examination are unremarkable but the serum PSA level is mildly elevated (range, 4.1–10.0 mg/L), transrectal ultrasonography should be performed.[51] Cytologic examination of urine for exfoliated cells should be performed annually, if indicated.

In women, a second carcinoma is more likely to occur in the colon, rectum, cervix, uterus, or ovary.[51] Thus, a complete large bowel examination should be performed every 5 years. Mammograpny, pelvic examination, and a Papanicolaou smear test should be performed as part of a routine annual checkup as appropriate.

20.5 Surveillance

Surveillance is the monitoring of people known to have colon or rectal disease.

20.5.1 After Removal of Adenomatous Polyps

The main options for surveillance are colonoscopy and DCBE. The best evidence of the effectiveness of surveillance is from colonoscopy. In the NPS, a cohort of 1,418 patients who had undergone complete colonoscopy and removal of one or more adenomatous polyps from the colon or rectum were followed up for an average of 5.9 years per patient with periodic colonoscopy. After adjusting for age, sex, and polyp size, rates of carcinoma were 76 to 90% lower than expected when compared with three reference groups (from published reports) who had not undergone surveillance. The study used reference groups as controls, with the assumption that patients undergoing polypectomy would have experienced the same incidence of carcinoma as the reference populations who have not undergone polypectomy (▶ Fig. 20.3).

The optional frequency of surveillance was also studied in the NPS. All patients who had undergone prior polypectomy were randomized to undergo surveillance colonoscopy either 1 and 3 years or only 3 years after polypectomy. The two groups showed no difference in the proportion of detected adenomatous polyps with advanced pathology (3% in both groups).[52] This suggests that the first follow-up screening after polypectomy can be deferred for at least 3 years. The study also showed that if the results of the first surveillance colonoscopy are negative, subsequent examinations are highly unlikely to reveal further adenomatous polyps.

Current recommendations for polyp follow-up, developed jointly by the U.S. Multi-Society Task Force on Colorectal Cancer and the American Cancer Society, suggest that patients at increased risk (defined as three or more adenomas, high-grade dysplasia, villous features, or an adenoma 1 cm or larger in size) have a 3-year follow-up colonoscopy. Patients at lower risk (one or two small [<1 cm] tubular adenomas with no high-grade dysplasia) can have a follow-up evaluation in 5 to 10 years. Patients with only hyperplastic polyps should have a 10-year follow-up evaluation, as for average-risk people. There have been recent studies that have reported a significant number of missed cancers by colonoscopy.[53] These recommendations assume high-quality baseline colonoscopy with excellent patient preparation and adequate withdrawal time. An inadequate preparation should alter follow-up recommendations.

There have been no reported studies of surveillance after polypectomy using barium enema and no reported studies comparing surveillance with barium enema versus colonoscopy.[10]

New evidence supports the concept that colonoscopic polypectomy reduces subsequent colorectal carcinoma incidence.[12]

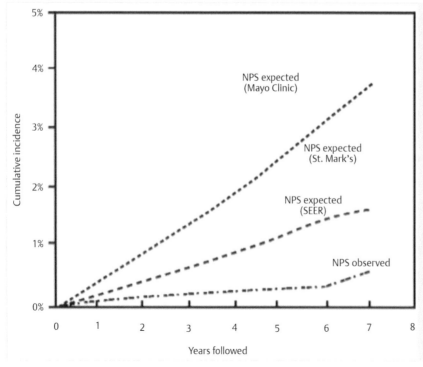

Fig. 20.3 The observed and expected incidences of colorectal carcinoma in a National Polyp Study cohort after having undergone colonoscopic polypectomy. NPS, National Polyp Study; SEER, Surveillance, Epidemiology, and End Results (Program).[26] (With permission © 2005 Elsevier.)

A study of postpolypectomy surveillance demonstrated a 66% reduction in colorectal carcinoma incidence, similar to the previous report of the NPS.[43]

There is no direct evidence related to when to stop surveillance. As with screening, the age at which surveillance should stop depends on the judgment of patients and their clinicians, taking into account the patient's medical history and comorbidity. The characteristics of the polyps removed and the results of follow-up examinations should also be taken into account.

20.5.2 In People with Inflammatory Bowel Disease

The primary goal of surveillance for colorectal carcinoma in patients with inflammatory bowel disease is to detect moderate to severe dysplasia and early carcinoma rather than polyps. Surveillance should be performed in patients with a history of the disease for about 8 years, after which time the risk of carcinoma starts to appear. It is debatable whether surveillance alone is a reliable indicator of prophylactic proctocolectomy (see details in Chapter 23).

20.5.3 Ureterosigmoidostomy

Ureterosigmoidostomy has been replaced for the most part by ileocystoplasty or the ileal conduit and therefore few patients have this condition. Recently, it has been found that patients with ureterocystoplasty or ileal conduit have an equally high risk of developing carcinoma as patients with ureterosigmoidostomy. It takes an average 18 years (range, 5–29 years) for patients with ileocystoplasty or ileal conduit to develop malignancy. Most of the carcinomas or adenomas are at the anastomotic line. At one time in the experimental animal model (rats), it was believed that fecal matter was needed in the urinary stream to develop neoplasia. Later studies disputed this concept and the recent findings of malignancy in ileocystostomy or ileal conduit also confirm that urine alone can cause the malignancy. The pathogenesis is unclear but it appears in animal studies (rats) and the findings in humans that nitrosamines produced by gram-negative bacteria are probably part of the mechanism in carcinogenesis.[27] Patients with ureterosigmoidostomy should have a flexible sigmoidoscopy or colonoscopy. The examinations should begin on the 10th anniversary of the original operation and should be repeated annually.[54] If a polyp is found at the anastomotic line, endoscopic removal is not advisable because most of them are situated at the site of the ureterosigmoidostomy.[55,56] If possible, the patient should have an alternative of urinary diversion.[56,57]

20.5.4 After Curative Resection

Patients with a colorectal carcinoma should have a colonoscopy before the operation to rule out synchronous neoplasms. If the colon is obstructed preoperatively, colonoscopy should be performed approximately 6 months after operation. If this or a complete preoperative examination is normal, subsequent colonoscopy should be offered after 3 years, and then, if normal, every 5 years.[12] The goals of follow-up are to detect local recurrences, distant metastasis, metachronous carcinomas and adenomas, and detection of other primary carcinomas.

The rationale for postoperative follow-up of colorectal carcinoma is based on the assumption that detection of a recurrence in an asymptomatic patient indicates carcinoma at an earlier stage that can be more effectively treated than those detected at a more advanced symptomatic stage.

In general, the investigation includes history and physical examination, endoscopy, carcinoembryonic antigen (CEA), liver function tests, ultrasonography and/or computed tomography (CT) scan, and chest X-ray films.

Approximately 30 to 50% of patients who undergo curative resection for carcinoma of the colon and rectum have a recurrence.[58] In the series by Sugarbaker et al,[59] 85% of patients who develop recurrence do so within 2.5 years, and all sites of recurrence develop at approximately the same period of time, with a median of 17 months. The series by Pihl et al[60] revealed that 50% of liver metastases are clinically obvious within 21 to 22 months of treatment, compared with 22 to 34 months for pulmonary metastases. Recurrences within the abdominal cavity are noted in 84% of all recurrences; 15% have recurrences involving distant metastases only.[59] Approximately 35% of patients have liver metastasis. Of these, the liver is the only site of metastasis in approximately 20%. Between 10 and 22% have pulmonary metastases and approximately 10% of these patients have metastasis isolated to the lungs.[58]

20.6 Recurrences and Metastases

Careful history taking and physical examination provide an effective means of surveillance. Several prospective studies showed that patient symptoms and physical signs can provide the first indication of recurrent carcinoma in 21 to 48% of those with advanced disease.[61,62] In a study by Beart et al,[63] 168 patients who had undergone colorectal resection for cure were followed at least every 15 weeks for up to 4 years. In 41 of 48 patients, symptoms developed before detection by physical examination or biochemical and radiologic investigations. The symptoms included coughing, abdominal and pelvic pain, change in bowel habit, rectal bleeding, and malaise. Physical examination is a frequent indicator of recurrence but is not as sensitive as the presence of symptoms. All patients with positive physical findings were found to have symptoms or a positive CEA test. Recurrent carcinoma that is symptomatic or that can be detected on physical examination is likely to be advanced and not curable.[61]

Alkaline phosphatase seems to be the most sensitive liver function test.[63] However, it also has a high false-positive rate and, therefore, has little predictive value if used alone.[61]

Because chest X-ray films are noninvasive and inexpensive, most clinicians order them annually. Any patient with a questionable or positive lesion should undergo a chest CT scan. A CT scan of the abdomen is not performed routinely, because the results are somewhat unreliable. Its limitation in detecting early pelvic recurrence is compounded by the fact that postoperative artifacts in the pelvis may persist for as long as 2 years. However, a CT scan is invaluable for assessing symptomatic patients and for confirming the clinical impression of recurrences.[58] A CT scan to detect liver metastases is more accurate, with 85 to 90% sensitivity; this is similar to ultrasonography and magnetic resonance imaging (MRI). When CT scan is doubtful, positron emission tomography (PET) can be helpful.[64,65]

A systematic review and meta-analysis of randomized trials suggests a survival benefit associated with performing CT (every 3–12 months).[66] However, others have reported that CT scan did not increase the number of curative hepatectomies.[67] The track record for detecting curable pelvic or local relapse is also disappointing.[68,69,70] When adjuvant radiation therapy is used, related posttreatment changes further complicate the interpretation of such imaging.[71]

CEA is a sensitive marker for identifying recurrence or metastases. CEA level is elevated most commonly in patients with hepatic metastases; 95% of these patients have increased plasma CEA levels. On the other hand, in patients with local abdominal or pelvic recurrences, 17 to 25% have normal CEA levels. Of the 70 patients with recurrences, 89% have elevated plasma CEA levels before the recurrences are detected by any other means. However, CEA does not always detect recurrences or metastases at a resectable stage. In the series reported by Beart et al,[63] 48 patients with elevated CEA were explored and only 1 patient was thought to have a potentially resectable lesion. On the other hand, in another series of 146 asymptomatic patients with elevated CEA, evidence of recurrence was found in 95%, and 58% of these were resectable for potential cure.[72]

In an uncontrolled study by Moertel et al,[73] using a patient population entered into a large National Surgical Adjuvant Trial, the patients were accrued from a variety of settings ranging from small community clinics to large universities and are probably representative of carcinoma in most practices nationwide. Every 12 weeks of the first year, every 4 months for the second year, and every 6 months thereafter, they have evaluations supplemented by hemoglobin and chemical analysis of the blood and chest radiographs. At 24 and 48 weeks and then annually, they underwent either proctoscopy, or colon radiography, or total colonoscopy. Performance of the CEA test was optional, according to the usual practice of the responsible physician. Of a total of 1,216 patients with resected carcinoma of the colon, 1,017 (84%) had CEA monitoring. Among 417 monitored patients with recurrence, 59% had a preceding elevation of CEA concentration. Of 600 patients without recurrence, 16% showed a false-positive result. CEA testing is most sensitive for detecting hepatic or retroperitoneal metastases and relatively insensitive for local, pulmonary, or peritoneal involvement. Surgical explorations were performed in 115 patients with CEA elevations, and 47 recurrences, usually hepatic, were resected with curative intent. On the other hand, 38 patients with normal CEA concentrations and 23 patients not monitored also underwent such resection—usually for a pulmonary or local recurrence. Of all CEA-monitored patients, 2.3% were alive and disease free more than 1 year after the salvage operation (2.9% of those with CEA elevations and 1.9% of those with no elevations). Of patients with no CEA monitoring, 2% were also alive and disease free more than 1 year after the salvage operation. The authors concluded that carcinoma cures attributable to CEA monitoring are, at best, infrequent. It is questionable whether this small gain justifies the substantial cost in dollars and the physical and emotional stress that this intervention may cause patients. Although intensive postoperative follow-up programs, including CEA evaluation, do identify recurrence earlier and thus result in higher resectable rates, they do not translate into a higher survival. Ohlsson et al[68] of Sweden conducted a prospective randomized study investigating the value of intense postoperative follow-up compared with no follow-up in 107 patients followed up from 5.5 to 8.8 years. The study showed no difference in survival. A similar but larger prospective randomized study was conducted by Kjeldsen et al[63] of Denmark. It consisted of 597 patients who also showed no improvement in overall survival or in disease-related survival.

Richard and McLeod[58] critically examined the literature on postoperative follow-up of patients with colorectal carcinoma through a Medline search for articles published from 1966 through February 1996. The report included randomized controlled clinical trials, cohort studies, and descriptive studies. From the findings of their review, the authors believe that there is inconclusive evidence either to support or refute the value of follow-up surveillance programs to detect recurrent colorectal carcinoma. The authors pointed out many flaws in most of the studies, including small sample sizes, patient bias, and variations in follow-up protocols. The authors estimated that even if postoperative surveillance were effective, the survival benefit would not be > 10%. On the other hand, in a meta-analysis of 3,283 patients in seven nonrandomized studies, Bruinvels et al[74] found a 9% better overall survival rate in intensively followed patients, including more asymptomatic recurrences and more operations for recurrence.

Surgeons and patients should understand the limitations of an intensive postoperative follow-up to detect recurrences and metastases. The follow-up regimen should be discussed and individualized to fit each patient's needs.

20.6.1 Metachronous Carcinomas and Polyps

The goal of surveillance after colorectal resection for carcinoma is to clear the adenomas if this has not been done preoperatively and to detect metachronous carcinoma. The incidence of metachronous carcinoma of the large bowel is approximately 2 to 4% within 3 to 20 years.[75,76,77] Periodic examination of the large bowel with colonoscopy every 3 to 5 years provides the most accurate results. An alternative is to use flexible sigmoidoscopy combined with DCBE, possibly CT colography in the near future.

There are no controlled studies of the effectiveness of surveillance strategies in this situation. Available information suggests that the metachronous carcinomas have biological behavior that is not different from initial carcinomas except in increased frequency of occurrence.

20.6.2 Other Primary Malignancies

The detection of other primary carcinomas is not important until the patient has achieved long-term survival. This fact has usually been ignored, unrealized, or forgotten. Enblad et al[49] analyzed the occurrence of a second primary malignant disease in 38,166 patients with carcinoma of the colon and in 23,603 patients with carcinoma of the rectum, as reported to the Swedish Cancer Registry between 1960 and 1981. The overall relative risk (RR) of developing a second primary malignant disease was significantly increased after carcinoma of both the colon (women, RR =1.4; men, RR =1.3) and rectum (women, RR =1.4; men, RR = 1.3). The increased risk of secondary

Table 20.4 Summary of guidelines for colorectal surveillance after primary surgery with curative intent

Procedure or test	ESMO[80]	ASCO[78]	ASCRS[79]
History and physical	Every 3–6 months for first 3 years; then every 6–12 months until year 5	Every 3–6 months for first 3 years; annually thereafter	Every 3–6 months for 2 years. Then every 6 months until year 5
Fecal occult-blood test	Not recommended	No routine testing	Not recommended
Liver function tests	Restricted to patients with suspicious symptoms	No routine testing	No routine testing
CEA	Every 3–6 months for first 3 years; then every 6–12 months until year 5	Every 2–3 months for stage II or III for 2 years or longer. Only in patients who can undergo liver resection	Every 3–6 months for 2 years. Then every 6 months until year 5
Chest X-ray	Restricted to patients with suspicious symptoms	No routine testing. Order when CEA is elevated or symptoms suggestive of pulmonary metastasis	No routine testing
Flexible sigmoidoscopy and endoscopic ultrasound	Every 6 months for 2 years	For patients who have not received pelvic irradiation. Direct imaging of rectum periodically. For patients who have received pelvic irradiation, direct imaging is not suggested	Periodic anastomotic examination in rectal cancer
Colonoscopy	At year 1 and every 3–5 years	Every 3–5 years	Annually for 5 years
CT chest/abdomen/pelvis	Every 6–12 months for the first 3 years in high-risk patients	Not routine	Not routine
Ultrasonography of the abdomen	May be substituted for CT scan	Not addressed	Not addressed

Abbreviations: ASCO; American Society of Clinical Oncology; ASCRS, American Society of Colon and Rectal Surgeons; CEA, carcinoembryonic antigen; CT, computed tomography; ESMO, European Society for Medical Oncology.

primary diseases occurs in the stomach, small intestine, ovary, endometrium, cervix, breast, kidney, bladder, and prostate (▸ Table 20.3).

20.7 Summary

There remains no general agreement on the optimal follow-up program for colorectal cancer. Some data suggest that surveillance leads to increased rates of early detection and resection of recurrence, but this has not necessarily always translated into improved survival. It is important that patients understand the limitations of the postoperative follow-up and they should actively participate in the decision-making of the follow-up plan. Guide-lines from major societies can be helpful in the discussion (see ▸ Table 20.4).[78,79,80]

References

[1] https://seer.cancer.gov/statfacts/html/colorect.html. Accessed June 19, 2018

[2] Hermanek P, Sobin LH. Colorectal carcinoma. In: Hermanek P, Gaspodarowicz MK, Henson DE, Hutter RVP, Sobin LH, eds. Prognostic Factors in Cancer. HCII. International Union against Cancer. Berlin: Springer-Verlag; 1995:64–79. Available at: http://seer.cancer.gov/csr/1975_2013/browse_csr.php?sectionSEL=6&pageSEL=sect_06_table.12.html. Accessed October 30, 2016

[3] Jessup JM, Menck HR, Fremgen A, Winchester DP. Diagnosing colorectal carcinoma: Clinical and molecular approaches. CA Cancer J Clin. 1997; 47:70–92

[4] Winawer SJ, Zauber AG, Stewart E, O'Brien MJ. The natural history of colorectal cancer. Opportunities for intervention. Cancer. 1991; 67(4) Suppl:1143–1149

[5] Mandel JS, Bond JH, Church TR, et al. Reducing mortality from colorectal cancer by screening for fecal occult blood. Minnesota Colon Cancer Control Study. N Engl J Med. 1993; 328(19):1365–1371

[6] Winawer SJ, Flehinger BJ, Schottenfeld D, Miller DG. Screening for colorectal cancer with fecal occult blood testing and sigmoidoscopy. J Natl Cancer Inst. 1993; 85(16):1311–1318

[7] Kronborg O, Fenger C, Olsen J, Jørgensen OD, Søndergaard O. Randomised study of screening for colorectal cancer with faecal-occult-blood test. Lancet. 1996; 348(9040):1467–1471

[8] Hardcastle JD, Chamberlain JO, Robinson MHE, et al. Randomised controlled trial of faecal-occult-blood screening for colorectal cancer. Lancet. 1996; 348 (9040):1472–1477

[9] Kewenter J, Brevinge H, Engarås B, Haglind E, Ahrén C. Results of screening, rescreening, and follow-up in a prospective randomized study for detection of colorectal cancer by fecal occult blood testing. Results for 68,308 subjects. Scand J Gastroenterol. 1994; 29(5):468–473

[10] Winawer SJ, Fletcher RH, Miller L, et al. Colorectal cancer screening: clinical guidelines and rationale. Gastroenterology. 1997; 112(2):594–642

[11] Bond JH. Screening for colorectal cancer: confuting the refuters. Gastrointest Endosc. 1997; 45(1):105–109

[12] Winawer S, Fletcher R, Rex D, et al. Gastrointestinal Consortium Panel. Colorectal cancer screening and surveillance: clinical guidelines and rationale-Update based on new evidence. Gastroenterology. 2003; 124(2):544–560

[13] http://www.cdc.gov/vitalsigns/CancerScreening/ColorectalCancer/index.html Accessed October 30, 2016

[14] Surveillance, Epidemiology and Results (SEER) Program, 1973–1992. Bethesda, MD: National Cancer Institute

[15] Potter JD, Slattery ML, Bostick RM, Gapstur SM. Colon cancer: a review of the epidemiology. Epidemiol Rev. 1993; 15(2):499–545

[16] Imperiale TF, Wagner DR, Lin CY, Larkin GN, Rogge JD, Ransohoff DF. Results of screening colonoscopy among persons 40 to 49 years of age. N Engl J Med. 2002; 346(23):1781–1785

[17] Smith RA, Cokkinides V, Eyre HJ. American Cancer Society Guidelines for the Early Detection of Cancer, 2005. CA Cancer J Clin. 2005; 55(1):31–44, quiz 55–56

[18] Mandel JS, Church TR, Ederer F, Bond JH. Colorectal cancer mortality: effectiveness of biennial screening for fecal occult blood. J Natl Cancer Inst. 1999; 91(5):434–437

[19] Mandel JS, Church TR, Bond JH, et al. The effect of fecal occult-blood screening on the incidence of colorectal cancer. N Engl J Med. 2000; 343(22):1603–1607

[20] Pignone M, Campbell MK, Carr C, Phillips C. Meta-analysis of dietary restriction during fecal occult blood testing. Eff Clin Pract. 2001; 4(4):150–156

[21] Winawer SJ, Stewart ET, Zauber AG, et al. National Polyp Study Work Group. A comparison of colonoscopy and double-contrast barium enema for surveillance after polypectomy. N Engl J Med. 2000; 342(24):1766–1772

[22] Whitlock EP, Lin JS, Liles E, Beil TL, Fu R. Screening for colorectal cancer: a targeted, updated systematic review for the U.S. Preventive Services Task Force. Ann Intern Med. 2008; 149(9):638–658

[23] Chen LS, Yen AM, Chiu SY, Liao CS, Chen HH. Baseline faecal occult blood concentration as a predictor of incident colorectal neoplasia: longitudinal follow-up of a Taiwanese population-based colorectal cancer screening cohort. Lancet Oncol. 2011; 12(6):551–558

[24] Rabeneck L, Rumble RB, Thompson F, et al. Fecal immunochemical tests compared with guaiac fecal occult blood tests for population-based colorectal cancer screening. Can J Gastroenterol. 2012; 26(3):131–147

[25] Lee JK, Liles EG, Bent S, Levin TR, Corley DA. Accuracy of fecal immunochemical tests for colorectal cancer: systematic review and meta-analysis. Ann Intern Med. 2014; 160(3):171–181

[26] Ransohoff DF. Colon cancer screening in 2005: status and challenges. Gastroenterology. 2005; 128(6):1685–1695

[27] Ahlquist DA, Skoletsky JE, Boynton KA, et al. Colorectal cancer screening by detection of altered human DNA in stool: feasibility of a multitarget assay panel. Gastroenterology. 2000; 119(5):1219–1227

[28] Imperiale TF, Ransohoff DF, Itzkowitz SH, Turnbull BA, Ross ME, Colorectal Cancer Study Group. Fecal DNA versus fecal occult blood for colorectal-cancer screening in an average-risk population. N Engl J Med. 2004; 351 (26):2704–2714

[29] Rex DK, Rahmani EY, Haseman JH, Lemmel GT, Kaster S, Buckley JS. Relative sensitivity of colonoscopy and barium enema for detection of colorectal cancer in clinical practice. Gastroenterology. 1997; 112(1):17–23

[30] Walsh JME, Terdiman JP. Colorectal cancer screening: scientific review. JAMA. 2003; 289(10):1288–1296

[31] Zauber AG, Lansdorp-Vogelaar I, Knudsen AB, Wilschut J, van Ballegooijen M, Kuntz KM. Evaluating Test Strategies for Colorectal Cancer Screening — Age to Begin, Age to Stop, and Timing of Screening Intervals: A Decision Analysis of Colorectal Cancer Screening for the U.S. Preventive Services Task Force from the Cancer Intervention and Surveillance Modeling Network (CISNET). Rockville, MD: Agency for Healthcare Research and Quality; March 2009 (AHRQ publication no. 08–05124-EF-2)

[32] Imperiale TF, Ransohoff DF, Itzkowitz SH, et al. Multitarget stool DNA testing for colorectal-cancer screening. N Engl J Med. 2014; 370(14):1287–1297

[33] Selby JV, Friedman GD, Quesenberry CP, Jr, Weiss NS. A case-control study of screening sigmoidoscopy and mortality from colorectal cancer. N Engl J Med. 1992; 326(10):653–657

[34] Newcomb PA, Norfleet RG, Storer BE, Surawicz TS, Marcus PM. Screening sigmoidoscopy and colorectal cancer mortality. J Natl Cancer Inst. 1992; 84 (20):1572–1575

[35] Müller AD, Sonnenberg A. Protection by endoscopy against death from colorectal cancer. A case-control study among veterans. Arch Intern Med. 1995; 155(16):1741–1748

[36] Rex DK, Cummings OW, Helper DJ, et al. 5-year incidence of adenomas after negative colonoscopy in asymptomatic average-risk persons [see comment]. Gastroenterology. 1996; 111(5):1178–1181

[37] Winawer SJ, Zauber AG, Ho MN, et al. The National Polyp Study Workgroup. Prevention of colorectal cancer by colonoscopic polypectomy. N Engl J Med. 1993; 329(27):1977–1981

[38] Levin TR, Palitz A, Grossman S, et al. Predicting advanced proximal colonic neoplasia with screening sigmoidoscopy. JAMA. 1999; 281(17):1611–1617

[39] Lieberman DA, Weiss DG, Bond JH, Ahnen DJ, Garewal H, Chejfec G. Use of colonoscopy to screen asymptomatic adults for colorectal cancer. Veterans Affairs Cooperative Study Group 380. N Engl J Med. 2000; 343(3):162–168

[40] Imperiale TF, Wagner DR, Lin CY, Larkin GN, Rogge JD, Ransohoff DF. Risk of advanced proximal neoplasms in asymptomatic adults according to the distal colorectal findings. N Engl J Med. 2000; 343(3):169–174

[41] Farraye FA, Wallace M. Clinical significance of small polyps found during screening with flexible sigmoidoscopy. Gastrointest Endosc Clin N Am. 2002; 12(1):41–51

[42] Thiis-Evensen E, Hoff GS, Sauar J, Langmark F, Majak BM, Vatn MH. Population-based surveillance by colonoscopy: effect on the incidence of colorectal cancer. Telemark Polyp Study I. Scand J Gastroenterol. 1999; 34(4):414–420

[43] Citarda F, Tomaselli G, Capocaccia R, Barcherini S, Crespi M, Italian Multicentre Study Group. Efficacy in standard clinical practice of colonoscopic polypectomy in reducing colorectal cancer incidence. Gut. 2001; 48(6):812–815

[44] Hofstad B, Vatn M. Growth rate of colon polyps and cancer. Gastrointest Endosc Clin N Am.. 1997; 7:345–363

[45] Rex DK, Chak A, Vasudeva R, et al. Prospective determination of distal colon findings in average-risk patients with proximal colon cancer. Gastrointest Endosc. 1999; 49(6):727–730

[46] Rembacken BJ, Fujii T, Cairns A, et al. Flat and depressed colonic neoplasms: a prospective study of 1000 colonoscopies in the UK. Lancet. 2000; 355 (9211):1211–1214

[47] Saitoh Y, Waxman I, West AB, et al. Prevalence and distinctive biologic features of flat colorectal adenomas in a North American population. Gastroenterology. 2001; 120(7):1657–1665

[48] Fuchs CS, Giovannucci EL, Colditz GA, Hunter DJ, Speizer FE, Willett WC. A prospective study of family history and the risk of colorectal cancer. N Engl J Med. 1994; 331(25):1669–1674

[49] Enblad P, Adami HO, Glimelius B, Krusemo U, Påhlman L. The risk of subsequent primary malignant diseases after cancers of the colon and rectum. A nationwide cohort study. Cancer. 1990; 65(9):2091–2100

[50] Barry MJ. Clinical practice. Prostate-specific-antigen testing for early diagnosis of prostate cancer. N Engl J Med. 2001; 344(18):1373–1377

[51] Oesterling JE. Prostate-specific antigen. Improving its ability to diagnose early prostate cancer. JAMA. 1992; 267(16):2236–2238

[52] Winawer SJ, Zauber AG, O'Brien MJ, et al. The National Polyp Study Workgroup. Randomized comparison of surveillance intervals after colonoscopic removal of newly diagnosed adenomatous polyps. N Engl J Med. 1993; 328 (13):901–906

[53] Winawer SJ, Zauber AG, Fletcher RH, et al. US Multi-Society Task Force on Colorectal Cancer, American Cancer Society. Guidelines for colonoscopy surveillance after polypectomy: a consensus update by the US Multi-Society Task Force on Colorectal Cancer and the American Cancer Society. Gastroenterology. 2006; 130(6):1872–1885

[54] Filmer RB, Spencer JR. Malignancies in bladder augmentations and intestinal conduits. J Urol. 1990; 143(4):671–678

[55] Woodhouse CRJ, British Society for Gastroenterology, Association of Coloproctology for Great Britain and Ireland. Guidelines for monitoring of patients with ureterosigmoidostomy. Gut. 2002; 51 Suppl 5:V15–V16

[56] Hurlstone DP, Wells JM, Bhala N, McAlindon ME. Ureterosigmoid anastomosis: risk of colorectal cancer and implications for colonoscopists. Gastrointest Endosc. 2004; 59(2):248–254

[57] Azimuddin K, Khubchandani IT, Stasik JJ, Rosen L, Riether RD. Neoplasia after ureterosigmoidostomy. Dis Colon Rectum. 1999; 42(12):1632–1638

[58] Richard CS, McLeod RS. Follow-up of patients after resection for colorectal cancer: a position paper of the Canadian Society of Surgical Oncology and the Canadian Society of Colon and Rectal Surgeons. Can J Surg. 1997; 40 (2):90–100

[59] Sugarbaker PH, Gianola FJ, Dwyer A, Neuman NR. A simplified plan for follow-up of patients with colon and rectal cancer supported by prospective studies of laboratory and radiologic test results. Surgery. 1987; 102(1):79–87

[60] Pihl E, Hughes ESR, McDermott FT, Johnson WR, Katrivessis H. Lung recurrence after curative surgery for colorectal cancer. Dis Colon Rectum. 1987; 30 (6):417–419

[61] Kelly CJ, Daly JM. Colorectal cancer. Principles of postoperative follow-up. Cancer. 1992; 70(5) Suppl:1397–1408

[62] Goldberg RM, Fleming TR, Tangen CM, et al. Surgery for recurrent colon cancer: strategies for identifying resectable recurrence and success rates after resection. Eastern Cooperative Oncology Group, the North Central Cancer Treatment Group, and the Southwest Oncology Group. Ann Intern Med. 1998; 129(1):27–35

[63] Beart RW, Jr, Metzger PP, O'Connell MJ, Schutt AJ. Postoperative screening of patients with carcinoma of the colon. Dis Colon Rectum. 1981; 24 (8):585–588

[64] Zheng G, Johnson RJ, Eddleston B, James RD, Schofield PF. Computed tomographic scanning in rectal carcinoma. J R Soc Med. 1984; 77(11):915–920

[65] Tzimas GN, Koumanis DJ, Meterissian S. Positron emission tomography and colorectal carcinoma: an update. J Am Coll Surg. 2004; 198(4):645–652

[66] Renchan AG, Egger M, Saunders MP, O'Dwyer ST. Impact on survival of intensive follow up after curative resection for colorectal cancer: Systematic review and meta-analysis of randomized trials. BMJ. 2002; 384:813–818

[67] Schoemaker D, Black R, Giles L, Toouli J. Yearly colonoscopy, liver CT, and chest radiography do not influence 5-year survival of colorectal cancer patients. Gastroenterology. 1998; 114(1):7–14

[68] Ohlsson B, Breland U, Ekberg H, Graffner H, Tranberg KG. Follow-up after curative surgery for colorectal carcinoma. Randomized comparison with no follow-up. Dis Colon Rectum. 1995; 38(6):619–626

[69] Kjeldsen BJ, Kronborg O, Fenger C, Jørgensen OD. A prospective randomized study of follow-up after radical surgery for colorectal cancer. Br J Surg. 1997; 84(5):666–669

[70] Pietra N, Sarli L, Costi R, Ouchemi C, Grattarola M, Peracchia A. Role of follow-up in management of local recurrences of colorectal cancer: a prospective, randomized study. Dis Colon Rectum. 1998; 41(9):1127–1133

[71] Pfister DG, Benson AB, III, Somerfield MR. Clinical practice. Surveillance strategies after curative treatment of colorectal cancer. N Engl J Med. 2004; 350 (23):2375–2382

[72] Martin EW, Jr, Minton JP, Carey LC. CEA-directed second-look surgery in the asymptomatic patient after primary resection of colorectal carcinoma. Ann Surg. 1985; 202(3):310–317

[73] Moertel CG, Fleming TR, Macdonald JS, Haller DG, Laurie JA, Tangen C. An evaluation of the carcinoembryonic antigen (CEA) test for monitoring patients with resected colon cancer. JAMA. 1993; 270(8):943–947

[74] Bruinvels DJ, Stiggelbout AM, Kievit J, van Houwelingen HC, Habbema JD, van de Velde CJH. Follow-up of patients with colorectal cancer. A meta-analysis. Ann Surg. 1994; 219(2):174–182

[75] Törnqvist A, Ekelund G, Leandoer L. Early diagnosis of metachronous colorectal carcinoma. Aust N Z J Surg. 1981; 51(5):442–445

[76] Luchtefeld MA, Ross DS, Zander JD, Folse JR. Late development of metachronous colorectal cancer. Dis Colon Rectum. 1987; 30(3):180–184

[77] Heald RJ, Bussey HJR. Clinical experiences at St. Mark's Hospital with multiple synchronous cancers of the colon and rectum. Dis Colon Rectum. 1975; 18(1):6–10

[78] Meyerhardt JA, Mangu PB, Flynn PJ, et al. American Society of Clinical Oncology. Follow-up care, surveillance protocol, and secondary prevention measures for survivors of colorectal cancer: American Society of Clinical Oncology clinical practice guideline endorsement. J Clin Oncol. 2013; 31(35):4465–4470

[79] Steele SR, Chang GJ, Hendren S, et al. Clinical Practice Guidelines Committee of the American Society of Colon and Rectal Surgeons. Practice Guideline for the surveillance of patients after curative treatment of colon and rectal cancer. Dis Colon Rectum. 2015; 58(8):713–725

[80] Figueredo A, Rumble RB, Maroun J, et al. Gastrointestinal Cancer Disease Site Group of Cancer Care Ontario's Program in Evidence-based Care. Follow-up of patients with curatively resected colorectal cancer: a practice guideline. BMC Cancer. 2003; 3:26–38

21 Colon Carcinoma: Epidemiology, Etiology, Pathology, and Diagnosis

Philip H. Gordon and David E. Beck

Abstract

Colorectal carcinoma is the third most common internal malignancy, and the second leading cause of carcinoma death.

The incidence and mortality has declined in recent years, most likely due to increased screening. This chapter reviews the incidence, prevalence, epidemiology, etiology, pathology, and diagnosis of malignant colonic neoplasia.

Keywords: malignant neoplasia, colon, incidence, epidemiology, pathology, clinical features, complications, diagnosis, investigations

21.1 Classification

Malignancies of the large intestine assume a major importance because of their frequency in the general population. The types of malignancies and their estimated incidence are listed in ▶ Table 21.1.[1,2]

21.2 Adenocarcinoma

21.2.1 Incidence, Prevalence, and Trends

Colorectal carcinoma is the third most common internal malignancy, and the second leading cause of carcinoma death.[3] It was estimated that in 2017, there would be 95,520 new cases of colon and 39,910 cases of rectal carcinoma in the United States and that 50,260 deaths would result from this disease.[3] The incidence and mortality has declined in recent years most likely due to increased screening. The overall lifetime risk of developing colorectal cancer is 4.7% in men and 4.4% in women.

In the United States, over the past several decades the survival rate has improved for each stage. The current 5-year relative survival for people with stage I colon cancer is about 92%, stage IIA 87%, stage IIB 63%, stage IIIA 89%, stage IIIB 72%, stage IIIC 53%, and stage IV 11%.[3]

Table 21.1 Colon malignancies

Histology	DiSario et al[1] (%)	Kang et al[2] (%)
Adenocarcinoma	94.5	97
Carcinoid	3.3	1.5
Lymphoma	0.3	0.6
Sarcoma	0.1	
Squamous cell carcinoma	0.1	0.3
Plasmacytoma		
Melanoma	0.03	

21.2.2 Epidemiology

An extensive and comprehensive review of the worldwide information on colon carcinoma was collated by Correa and Haenszel.[4] Much of the following information was extracted from their excellent review.

Age

Carcinoma of the large intestine is predominantly a disease of older patients, with the peak incidence being in the seventh decade. However, it must be borne in mind that the disease can occur at virtually any age and may be seen in patients in their 20 s and 30 s.[5] It has been estimated that only 5% of colorectal carcinomas occur in patients who are younger than 40 years of age.[6]

Sex

The incidence of colorectal cancer is slightly higher in men than in women.[3]

Family History

There have been many reports that indicate an increased incidence of colorectal carcinoma in first-order relatives of patients who have suffered from the disease. In a prospective study of 32,085 men and 87,031 women, Fuchs et al[7] found that the age-adjusted relative risk (RR) of colorectal carcinoma for men and women with affected first-degree relatives, when compared with those without a family history of the disease, was 1.72. The RR among study participants with two or more first-degree relatives was 2.75. For participants younger than 45 years, who had one or more affected first-degree relatives, the RR was 5.37.

To compare the risk in relatives of patients with colorectal carcinoma diagnosed at different ages, Hall et al[8] studied two cohorts of patients, 65 diagnosed when they were younger than 45 years of age and 212 patients of all ages. The overall RR of colorectal carcinoma in first-degree relatives was 5.2 in the first group and 2.3 in the second group. The cumulative incidence of colorectal carcinoma for relatives of the young cohort rose steeply from 40 years, reaching 5% at 50 years and 10% at 70 years, compared with the older group, reaching 5% at 70 years and 10% at 80 years.

St John et al[9] conducted a case-control family study of 7,493 first-degree relatives and 1,015 spouses of 523 case-control pairs to determine the RR of developing carcinoma. The authors found an odds ratio (OR) of 1.8 for one and 5.7 for two affected relatives. The risk to parents and siblings was 2.1 times greater, 3.7 for patients diagnosed before 45 years and 1.8 times greater for patients diagnosed at the age of 45 years or older. The cumulative incidence was 11.1, 7.3, and 4.4% among relatives 55 years and older, between 45 and 54 years, and younger than 45 years, respectively. The most recent summary has shown the risk to be increased twofold to fourfold (▶ Table 21.2).[10,11,12,13] Furthermore, people who have a first-degree relative with colorectal carcinoma are estimated to have an average onset of colorectal carcinoma about 10 years earlier than people with sporadic colorectal carcinoma.[9]

Site

The distribution of carcinoma in the various segments of the large bowel has been the subject of several detailed clinical studies. Each of these studies has shown that over the past 50 years there has been a gradual shift in the location of carcinomas from the rectum and left colon toward the right colon. Studies by Mamazza et al[11] and Obrand et al[12] further documented that the left-to-right progression has continued. Reasons for this shift to the right are not entirely clear. A review of patterns in different countries has revealed an increase in the incidence of colon carcinoma with a corresponding decrease in rectal carcinoma.[4] Such findings imply that methods for the early detection and screening of large bowel carcinoma should be directed at the entire colon rather than being limited to the distal 25 cm of the large intestine. Qing et al[13] in a comparison between American and Chinese patients found lesions in 36.3% of white patients versus 26.0% of Asian patients, while carcinomas of the rectum were found in 63.7% of white patients and 74% of Asian patients. The rightward shift has continued in recent decades in the United States[14] and Japan.[15]

Geographic Distribution

There is a wide variation of the incidence of colorectal carcinoma in different countries. In general, countries of the Western world have the highest incidence of colorectal carcinoma, and these include Scotland, Luxembourg, Czechoslovakia, New Zealand, Denmark, and Hungary.

Countries with the lowest incidence include India, El Salvador, Kuwait, Martinique, Poland, and Mexico. The United States and Canada hold an intermediate position.[3,4] In large countries extending over a wide range of latitudes, there may be considerable regional differences that mimic international variations.[4]

It has been suggested that low-risk populations have a relatively increased incidence of right-sided carcinomas, while relatively high-risk communities have an increased risk of left-sided malignancies.[4] There is an increased risk of large bowel carcinoma in urban populations when compared to rural populations. The incidence of colorectal carcinoma in Japanese Americans is higher than in Japanese individuals living in Japan. The children of these immigrants have an incidence approximating that of the general U.S. population. The effects of environmental exposure and food habits can be exemplified by a notable occurrence in Israel. Israelis who were born in Europe or North America run roughly 2.5 times the risk of bowel carcinoma of those born in North Africa or Asia. After their arrival in Israel, the incidence becomes similar.[4]

Race and Religion

Black Americans who once enjoyed a lower incidence of colorectal carcinoma than their white counterparts now suffer a similar incidence of the disease,[4] but the 5-year survival rate for African-Americans is significantly lower than for whites.[16] The risk of large bowel malignancy in American Indians is less than half that for whites in the United States. Individuals of Mexican extraction born in the United States also experience a lower risk for large bowel carcinoma. With respect to religion, Jews in the United States have a higher incidence of colorectal carcinoma, while Mormons and Seventh Day Adventists have a lower rate than the general U.S. population.[4] Ashkenazi Jews have a lifetime colorectal carcinoma risk of 9 to 15%, which differs strikingly from the 5 to 6% colorectal carcinoma risk for non-Ashkenazi members of the general western populations.[17] The lower incidence in Mormons has been attributed to their prohibition of the use of tobacco and alcohol. Self-reported or perceived religiousness has been determined to be a protective factor in the development of colorectal carcinoma (an RR of 0.7).[18]

Occupation

Vobecky et al[19] observed an increased RR of three (i.e., a threefold increase) in the incidence of colorectal carcinoma in individuals working in factories that produce synthetic fibers. In the authors' review of the literature, they found that other workers who were at greater risk of developing large bowel carcinoma included metallurgy workers handling chlorinated oil, manufacturers of transport equipment, weavers, firemen, those working with asbestos or coke by-products, and those working in copper smelters. de Verdier et al[20] found elevated RR of colon carcinoma among male petrol station and/or automobile repair workers (2.3) and men exposed to asbestos (1.8), while elevated RR of rectal carcinoma was found among men exposed to soot (2.2), asbestos (2.2), cutting fluids and/or oils (2.1), and combustion gases from coke, coal, and/or wood (1.9).

A meta-analysis by Homa et al[21] suggested that exposure to amphibole asbestos may be associated with colorectal carcinoma, but exposure to serpentine asbestos is not. Another study failed to find an association between asbestos exposure and

Table 21.2 Estimated relative and absolute risk of developing colorectal carcinoma

Family history	Relative risk	Absolute risk by age 79 y (%)
No family history	1	4[a]
One first-degree relative with colorectal carcinoma	2.3	9[b]
More than one first-degree relative with colorectal carcinoma	4.3	16[b]
One affected first-degree relative diagnosed with colorectal carcinoma before age 45 y	3.9	15[b]
One first-degree relative with colorectal adenoma	2.0	8[b]

[a]Data from SEER database.[10]
[b]The absolute risk of colorectal carcinoma (CRC) for individuals with affected relatives was calculated using the relative risk for CRC and the absolute risk of CRC by age 79 years.

carcinoma of the colon and rectum.[22] Cumulative exposure to organic solvents, dyes, or abrasives also may contribute to an increased risk of colorectal carcinoma.[23,24] Workers involved in the manufacture of polypropylene also exhibit an increased incidence of colorectal carnicoma,[25] but this risk was more recently reported not to exist.[26] Workers with intense exposure to ethyl acrylate and methyl methacrylate for 3 years have an increased risk of colon carcinoma two decades later.[27]

21.2.3 Etiology and Pathogenesis

As with other malignancies, neither the etiology nor the pathogenesis of carcinoma of the colon is known. A number of factors have been considered important in its causation, and certain clinical conditions are considered precursors of carcinoma and will be detailed here.

Polyp–Cancer Sequence

Considerable evidence has accumulated to suggest that most, if not all, carcinomas develop from a precursor polyp, a situation known as the polyp–cancer sequence. This sequence is described in detail in Chapter 19.

Inflammatory Bowel Disease

Although colorectal carcinoma, complicating ulcerative colitis and Crohn's disease, only accounts for 1 to 2% of all cases of colorectal carcinoma in the general population, it is considered a serious complication of the disease and accounts for approximately 15% of all deaths in inflammatory bowel disease patients.

Patients with universal ulcerative colitis, having a more severe inflammation burden and risk of the dysplasia-carcinoma cascade especially those who have had the condition for more than 10 years and those patients who experienced onset in childhood, without doubt are at increased risk of developing carcinoma of the colon or rectum. Lennard-Jones et al[28] reported that the incidence of colorectal carcinoma (in 22 among 401 patients with extensive ulcerative colitis followed over 22 years) was 3, 5, and 13% at 15, 20, and 25 years, respectively. For the 17 patients developing colorectal carcinoma during supervised surveillance (344 patients), Dukes' staging was A or B in 12 patients. In half the carcinoma patients under surveillance, dysplasia signaled the associated carcinoma found only after colectomy in the operative specimens. Others have confirmed the increased risk.[29] Of 3,117 patients with ulcerative colitis followed for up to 60 years through the Swedish Cancer Registry, the RR of colorectal carcinoma was 5.7 (nonsignificant for proctitis), 2.8 for left-sided disease, and 14.8 for pancolitis.[30] Recent figures suggest that the risk of colon carcinoma for people with inflammatory bowel disease increases by 0.5 to 1.0% yearly, 8 to 10 years after diagnosis.[31] Considering the chronic nature of the disease, it is remarkable that there is such a low incidence of colorectal carcinoma in some of the population-based studies, and possible explanations have to be investigated. One possible carcinoma protective factor could be treatment with 5-aminosalicylic acid preparations (5-ASAs).[31]

Adenocarcinoma of the small bowel is extremely rare, compared with adenocarcinoma of the large bowel. Although only few small bowel carcinomas have been reported at sites of involvement with Crohn's disease, the number was significantly increased in relation to the expected number.[31] The incidence of colorectal carcinoma in patients with Crohn's disease has been reported as being 4 to 20 times greater than the general population.[29] In a study of 1,656 patients with Crohn's disease, Ekbom et al[32] indicated RR for colon carcinoma of 3.2 (in Crohn's ileocolitis) to 5.6 (in Crohn's colitis only). With the onset of any Crohn's colitis before the patient was 30 years of age, the RR was 20.9, but only 2.2 when diagnosed after age 30 years.

Genetics

In the last decade and a half, there has been an explosive increase in knowledge about the molecular biology of carcinoma. Publications are legion but often difficult to understand. This notwithstanding, the past decade has been witness to unprecedented progress in the comprehension of the basic mechanisms involved in the genesis of colorectal carcinoma. In his outstanding review of the molecular biology of colorectal carcinoma, Allen[33] attempted to make the subject understandable to the clinician, and the following dissertation draws heavily from that review.

Molecular Biology

The codes that control production of protein enzymes and form the basic information needed for life itself are found within the cell nucleus as long strands of deoxyribonucleic acid (DNA) molecules that are, in turn, composed of four nucleotides: adenine (A), guanine (G), thymine (T), and cytosine (C). Under normal circumstances, adenine only pairs with thymine (A:T), and guanine pairs with cytosine (G:C). As a result of base pairing, cellular DNA forms the familiar stepladder configuration that is twisted into a double helix and supercoiled into microscopically visible structures called chromosomes.

Long DNA sequences are subdivided into smaller segments called genes, each of which contains the information needed for a single protein. Genes are composed of hundreds or thousands of nucleotides. In humans, the entire genetic code, termed the genome, is composed of approximately 3 billion nucleotides organized into approximately 100,000 genes contained within 23 pairs of chromosomes (total, 46). One chromosome in each pair is inherited from the mother and one from the father. Thus, each gene has another similar (but not identical) gene called an allele on the complementary chromosome. Genes can act in a dominant or recessive fashion. For dominant genes, one allele assumes the responsibility for producing the protein and the other allele remains dormant.

The sequence of nucleotides within cellular chromosomes is reproduced faithfully and is passed down from generation to generation during cell division. A "normal" rate of mutation is estimated to be one mistake in every 10 billion base pairs copied. To correct replication errors (RER), a repair mechanism is dependent on genes called mismatch repair genes. Malignant transformation appears to result from the accumulation of mutations within genes that are critical to cell growth and differentiation caused either by an increase in the mutational rate or because the DNA repair process is compromised. A carcinoma is the end result of 4 to 12 genetic changes that convey a growth advantage to the mutated cells. During the initiation phase, there is an increase in the mutational rate of DNA. Mutations in some genes become incorporated into an individual's genome and are passed from generation to generation. These "germline mutations" may occur in genes related to carcinoma and, as a result, cause hereditary carcinoma. Other mutations, termed "somatic," cause a sporadic carcinoma. Knudson[34] proposed that inherited carcinomas arise in individuals with germline mutations of one allele of a recessively acting carcinoma gene, after which only one additional somatic alteration is needed to inactivate the gene and initiate carcinogenesis. Sporadic carcinomas require two somatic mutations (or allelic loss).

Mechanisms of Gene Action

Three major categories of genes have been implicated in carcinoma development: oncogenes,[1] tumor suppressor genes,[2] and mismatch repair genes[3] (▶ Table 21.3). When a proto-oncogene (a normal human growth–related gene) becomes abnormally activated, it drives the cell through the cell cycle facilitating clonal proliferation and is known as an oncogene. Oncogenes act in a dominant fashion because alteration of only one allele is necessary to produce a cellular effect. Oncogenes, however, do not tell the entire story, because only 20% of human carcinomas carry oncogene alterations.

Other genes called tumor suppressor genes can halt the cell cycle even when oncogenes are altered. Tumor suppressor genes act in a recessive manner and promote carcinoma only when they are inactivated by allelic loss or mutations in both alleles. If cells cannot repair DNA damage, tumor suppressor genes such as p53 drive the cell into a suicide mode called apoptosis. A tumor suppressor gene critical to colorectal carcinoma was described on chromosome 5—the adenomatous polyposis coli (APC) gene. It was found to contain an inherited mutation causing truncation of the protein product. Somatic mutations of APC are found early during the neoplastic process in most polyps and carcinomas.

Table 21.3 Genes known to be involved in development of colorectal carcinoma[10,33]

Type	Name	Chromosome
Oncogene	K-ras	12
Tumor suppressor gene	APC	5
	DCC	18
	p53	17
	MCC	5
	TGF-β-RII	3
Mismatch repair gene	hMLH1	3
	hMSH2	2
	hPMS1	2
	hPMS2	7
	hMSH6	2
	hMSH3	5
Others (currently of theoretical importance)	Fat acetylation P450 genes, etc.	Many

The latest genes found to be related to carcinogenesis are called mismatch repair genes, which are needed for cells to repair DNA RER and spontaneous base pair loss. The six DNA mismatch repair genes found in humans to date are hMSH2 (chromosome 2p16), hMLH1 (chromosome 3p21), hPMS1 (chromosome 2q31–33), hPMS2 (chromosome 7q11), hMSH6 (chromosome 2p16), and hMSH3 (chromosome 5q11.2-q13.2). When both copies of these genes are inactivated, DNA mismatch repair is defective, and the cell exhibits an increased frequency of mistakes in DNA replication, thereby accelerating the progression to oncogenesis. The first four genes are regarded to contribute to hereditary non-polyposis colorectal carcinoma (HNPCC) in 31, 33, 2, and 4%, respectively.[35]

The founder mutation MSH2*1906G > C is also considered an important cause of HNPCC in the Ashkenazi Jewish population.[36] This pathogenic mutation accounting for 2 to 3% of colorectal carcinoma in those whose age at diagnosis is less than 60 years is highly penetrant and accounts for approximately one-third of HNPCC in Ashkenazi Jewish families that fulfill the Amsterdam criteria. This founder mutation MSH2*1906 was found in 8% of 1,342 individuals (0.6%) of those of Ashkenazi descent with colorectal carcinoma. A subsequent study[37] sought to characterize the proportion of individuals of Ashkenazi heritage with very early-onset colon carcinoma (diagnosed at age 40 years or younger) that could be attributed to MSH2*1906G > C detected the mutation in 3 of the 41 samples (7.14%) of patients who had colorectal carcinoma diagnosed at age 40 years or younger. The incidence is significantly greater than the 8 in 1,345 (0.6%) observed for cases of colorectal carcinoma in Ashkenazi Jews not selected for age. These results suggest that consideration for testing for the MSH2*1906G > C mutation should be included in the evaluation of Ashkenazi Jewish individuals diagnosed with early onset of colon carcinoma.[38]

hMSH2 and hMLH1 accounted for 63% of kindreds meeting international diagnostic criteria.[38] A recent review by Peltomä-ki[39] cited germline mutations in one of four major HNPCC-associated mismatch repair genes (MLH1, MSH2, MSH6, and PMS2) detected in up to 70 to 80% of such families. More than 400 different predisposing mismatch repair gene mutations are known with approximately 50% effecting MLH1, about 40% MSH2, and about 10% MSH6.[39] The share of PMS2 is less than 5%. The newly identified human mismatch repair gene MLH3 may account for a small percentage of HNPCC. A germline mutation in PMS1 was originally reported in an HNPCC-like family, but there is presently no evidence of PMS1 as an HNPCC predisposition gene. The available data on two additional components of mismatch repair, exonuclease 1 (EXO1) and DNA polymerase, are too limited to allow any reliable assessment of their role in HNPCC predisposition.[39]

Genetic Pathways to Colorectal Carcinoma

Traditionally, carcinoma is seen as a three-step process of initiation, promotion, and progression. Colorectal carcinoma is a genetically heterogeneous disease, and a series of genetic events has been described in the evolution of colorectal carcinoma. The initiation stage (from the beginning to the first mutation) involves a complex (and poorly understood) interplay between environmental factors and host susceptibility (▶ Fig. 21.1). Specific environmental factors are known to modify colorectal carcinoma (▶ Fig. 21.2). For patients with hereditary colorectal carcinoma, the influence of environmental factors is small compared with the power of the underlying genetic mutations. Thus, the risk of initiating colorectal carcinoma is substantially higher in hereditary conditions (100% in patients with polyposis syndromes and approximately 85% in HNPCC).

A number of early reports tried to relate genetic importance to the etiology of colorectal carcinoma. Burt et al[40] examined the inheritance of susceptibility to colonic polyps and carcinomas in a large pedigree with multiple cases of colorectal carcinoma. The authors' analysis suggested that the observed excess of discrete adenomatous polyps and colorectal carcinoma was the result of an inherited autosomal-dominant gene for susceptibility rather than an inherited recessive gene for susceptibility. Solomon et al[41] examined colorectal carcinomas for loss of alleles on chromosome 5. Using a special probe that maps to

chromosome 5q, the authors demonstrated that at least 20% of carcinomas lose one of the alleles present in matched normal tissue. They suggested that becoming recessive for this gene may be a critical step in the progression of a relatively high proportion of colorectal carcinomas. No deletions were found in any other chromosome, which indicates that the loss from chromosome 5 is nonrandom. Law et al[42] reported allelic losses in chromosomes 17 and 18 to be more frequent in colorectal carcinoma than losses on chromosome 5.

It is now believed that the mutation that initiates colonic neoplasia is found in one of two gene loci. The 5q21 loci contain the APC gene, which is altered in more than 70% of all neoplastic lesions. Other polyps and carcinomas demonstrate microsatellite instability (MSI), a hallmark of mismatch repair gene mutations. Depending upon which type of gene has been inactivated, one of two pathways to colorectal carcinoma is followed (▶ Fig. 21.1). In the first pathway, APC gene inactivation leads to a pathway termed loss of heterozygosity (LOH). Approximately 70 to 80% of

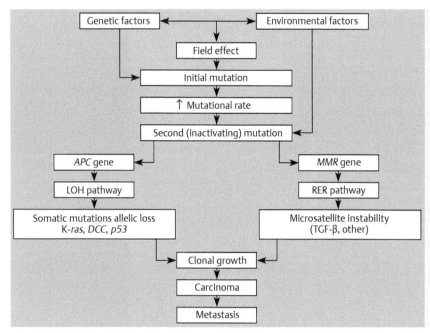

Fig. 21.1 Molecular pathway to colorectal carcinoma. The two arrows associated with the box labeled "genetic factors" illustrate the difference between initiation of a sporadic and hereditary colon carcinoma. The arrow leading from the box labeled "genetic factors" to "initial mutation" illustrates inheritance of a germline mutation capable of initiating neoplasia. APC, adenomatous polyposis coli; LOH, loss of heterozygosity; DCC, deleted in colon carcinoma; MMR, mismatch repair; RER, replication error; TGF-β, transforming growth factor-β.[33]

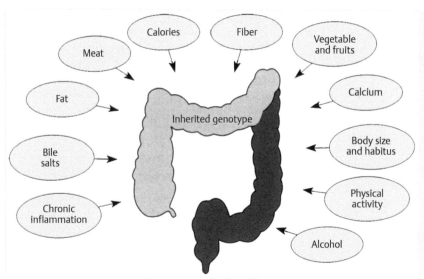

Fig. 21.2 Environmental factors that may contribute to altering colonic mucosa to produce a field effect that precedes initiation of neoplasia. Colonic cells respond to each environmental factor based on the genotype of DNA loci associated with metabolic pathways that relate to the various dietary constituents. Genetic polymorphisms are thought to play a role in determining how individuals respond at a cellular level to various environmental factors.[33]

colorectal carcinoma develops through the LOH pathway following inactivation of the APC gene. The genes involved in the LOH pathway include K-ras, deleted in colon carcinoma (DCC), and p53 in addition to APC (▸ Fig. 21.3). Germline APC mutations initiate the neoplastic process in patients with familial adenomatous polyposis (FAP) and endow all colonic crypt stem cells with a high risk for clonal proliferation.

A large body of evidence supports the concept of a multistep process that typically develops over decades and appears to require at least seven genetic events for completion. But even single altered genes can result in disease (e.g., FAP, HNPCC). In 1990 Fearon and Vogelstein[43] published the now-classic genetic model for colorectal carcinogenesis. The authors proposed a genetic series of events that corresponded to the apparent ordered sequence from a benign to a malignant lesion in histopathologic recognizable stages. They postulated that colorectal carcinoma arises as a result of mutational activation of oncogenes coupled with the mutational inactivation of tumor suppressor genes. Their original suggestion was that there must be mutations in at least four or five genes, but it is now believed to be at least seven for the formation of a carcinoma. Although the genetic alterations often occur according to a preferred sequence, the orderly sequence (▸ Fig. 21.2 and ▸ Fig. 21.3) rarely occurs in any individual carcinoma. It is the total accumulation of genetic alterations rather than their order that is responsible for determining the biologic properties of the carcinoma. The cascade of events described by Fearon and Vogelstein[43] begins with a loss or mutation of the FAP gene on chromosome 5q, resulting in a change from normal epithelium to hyperproliferative epithelium. One of these hyperproliferating cells gives rise to a small

adenoma in which the genome is hypomethylated. The next event involves activation of the K-ras oncogene on the chromosome 12p mutation to form the intermediate adenoma. Unlike oncogenes, tumor suppressor genes are expressed in a recessive manner. Therefore, both allelic copies must be lost or inactivated by point mutations for phenotypic expression to occur. Usually, the DCC gene on chromosome 18q is next to be deactivated or lost, and results in the development of a late adenoma. The final genetic alteration found consistently in colorectal carcinoma is loss and/or mutation of the p53 tumor suppressor gene on chromosome 17p. The p53 gene is altered in 50% of all human carcinomas and in 70% of colorectal carcinomas. Further genetic alterations are required for the development of metastases, subsequently believed to involve the LOH of the Nm23 gene.[44] While there is no obligatory sequence of mutations in the pathway from normal mucosa through adenoma to carcinoma, there is clearly an association of certain types of mutations in specific oncogenes or tumor suppressor genes with early and late states of transformation. This multistep pathway can be observed in sporadic and inherited colorectal carcinoma. Many other genes, such as MCC, TGF-β, Rb, and Myc, have been implicated in the genesis of colorectal carcinoma. Further study of the molecular events will undoubtedly lead to a better understanding of the multistep carcinogenesis and the relative importance of each.

Mismatch repair gene defects initiate an entirely different sequence of events known as the RER pathway. These pathways lead to carcinomas that are biologically quite different. This second pathway to colorectal carcinoma is found in approximately 20% of carcinomas. The RER pathway is similar in both patients with HNPCC and those who develop a spontaneous RER carcinoma. Patients with HNPCC inherit a single defective allele of a mismatch repair gene and require an additional somatic mutation to inactivate the second allele. Spontaneous carcinomas develop after two somatic events inactivate the relevant gene. In either case, inactivation leads to a marked increase in RER. As errors accumulate in microsatellites, malfunction of genes that contain or are near affected microsatellites may occur (▸ Fig. 21.4). Aaltonen et al[45] found the RER-positive phenotype in 77% of colorectal carcinomas from HNPCC patients compared with only 13% of patients with sporadic carcinoma.

How do DNA mismatch repair defects cause carcinoma? The mismatch repair gene defect increases the risk of malignant transformation of the cells, which may ultimately result from the disruption of one or several anticarcinogenic functions of the mismatch repair genes. Peltomäki recently summarized these.[39] First, malfunction of the mismatch repair system is associated with decreased genomic stability, which may manifest itself as highly elevated rates of subtle mutations (MSI) throughout the genome. Second, although mismatch repair–deficient cells typically have a diploid or near-diploid DNA content, loss of heterology-dependent suppression of recombination in these cells may promote gene conversion and expose tumor suppressor genes in analogy to LOH, or allow chromosomal translocations to occur. Furthermore, increased mutational inactivation of genes involved in DNA double-strand break repair may contribute to an elevated degree of chromosomal aberrations in mismatch repair–deficient cells. Third, besides anonymous microsatellite sequences, critical genes may be affected with mutations, conferring a growth advantage on the cells. Typical "target" genes include those involved

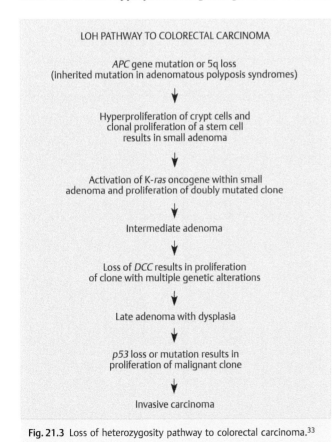

LOH PATHWAY TO COLORECTAL CARCINOMA

APC gene mutation or 5q loss
(inherited mutation in adenomatous polyposis syndromes)

↓

Hyperproliferation of crypt cells and
clonal proliferation of a stem cell
results in small adenoma

↓

Activation of K-*ras* oncogene within small
adenoma and proliferation of doubly mutated clone

↓

Intermediate adenoma

↓

Loss of *DCC* results in proliferation
of clone with multiple genetic alterations

↓

Late adenoma with dysplasia

↓

p53 loss or mutation results in
proliferation of malignant clone

↓

Invasive carcinoma

Fig. 21.3 Loss of heterozygosity pathway to colorectal carcinoma.[33]

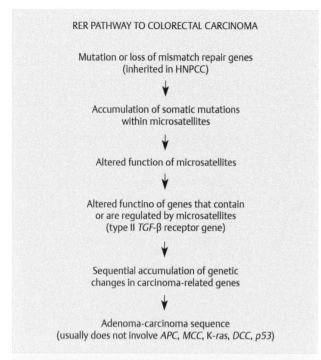

RER PATHWAY TO COLORECTAL CARCINOMA

Mutation or loss of mismatch repair genes
(inherited in HNPCC)

↓

Accumulation of somatic mutations
within microsatellites

↓

Altered function of microsatellites

↓

Altered functino of genes that contain
or are regulated by microsatellites
(type II *TGF-β* receptor gene)

↓

Sequential accumulation of genetic
changes in carcinoma-related genes

↓

Adenoma-carcinoma sequence
(usually does not involve *APC, MCC, K-ras, DCC, p53*)

Fig. 21.4 Genetic alterations often occur according to a preferred sequence.[33]

in growth suppression, apoptosis, or signal transduction. Fourth, there is evidence that failed protection against endogenous or exogenous DNA damage and the ensuing persistence of mutagenic or premutagenic lesions may contribute to genomic instability/MSI in intestinal cells.

There are examples of non-FAP, non-HNPCC hereditary colorectal carcinomas; a family not meeting the Amsterdam criteria with no deficiency of DNA mismatch repair in the malignancy of the proband was found to have a germline mutation of the TGFBR2 gene that encodes the type II TGF-β receptor; loss of the remaining normal allele was observed in the carcinoma.[46] Thus, other biologic mechanisms may underlie non-FAP, non-HNPCC hereditary colorectal carcinoma.

The transition from normal epithelium to adenoma to carcinoma is associated with acquired molecular events. A recent update on the genetic pathway to carcinoma has become available.[13] At least five to seven major molecular alterations may occur when a normal epithelial cell progresses in a colonal fashion to carcinoma. There are at least two major pathways by which these molecular events can lead to colorectal carcinoma. About 85% of colorectal carcinomas are due to events that result in chromosomal instability and the remaining 15% are due to events that result in MSI. Key changes in chromosomal instability carcinomas include widespread alterations in chromosome number (aneuploidy) and detectable losses at the molecular level of portions of chromosome 5q, chromosome 18q, and chromosome 17p; and mutation of the KRAS oncogene. The important genes involved in these chromosome losses are APC (5q), DCC/MADH2/MADH4 (18q), and TP53 (17p), respectively, and chromosome losses are associated with instability at the molecular and chromosomal level. Among the earliest events in the colorectal carcinoma progression pathway is loss of the APC

gene, which appears to be consistent with its important role in predisposing persons with germline mutations to colorectal neoplasms. Acquired or inherited mutations of DNA damage repair genes also play a role in predisposing colorectal epithelial cells to mutations. Not every carcinoma acquires every mutation, nor do mutations always occur in a specific order. The key characteristics of MSI carcinomas are largely intact chromosome complement, but acquisition of defects in DNA repair, such that mutations that may occur in important carcinoma-associated genes are allowed to persist. These types of carcinomas are detectable at the molecular level by alterations in repeating units of DNA that occur normally throughout the genome, known as a DNA microsatellite. Mitotic instability of microsatellites is the hallmark of MSI carcinomas.

MSI, the hallmark of HNPCC, occurs in approximately 15 to 25% of sporadic colorectal carcinomas. According to international criteria, a high degree of MSI (MSI-H) is defined as instability at two or more of five loci or ≥ 30 to 40% of all microsatellite loci studied, whereas instability at fewer loci is referred to as MSI-low (MSI-L). Colorectal carcinomas with MSI-H encompass a group of malignancies with a predilection for the proximal colon, that have diploid DNA content, that are high grade, that are associated with female sex, and have better survival. These features distinguish MSI-H carcinomas from those without widespread MSI, that is, MSI-L or microsatellite-stable (MSS) carcinomas. A majority of MSI-H colon carcinomas are caused by inactivation of MLH1. Whereas the MSI-L subset of colon carcinomas is equally as prevalent as the MSI-H group, immunohistochemical and mutation studies have found no involvement of MLH1, MSH2, MSH6, or MSH3 in the former carcinomas. The clinicopathological features do not seem to distinguish this group from MSS colon carcinomas either.

Clinical Relevance of Basic Genetic Knowledge

An effort by Allen[33] to reclassify the subtypes of colorectal carcinoma based on their molecular pathogenesis and inheritance pattern is depicted in ▶ Table 21.4. Prior to the definition of molecular pathways to colorectal carcinoma, proximal carcinomas were known to have normal cytogenetics, diploid DNA content, slower growth, less frequent metastasis, and a better prognosis compared to distal carcinomas. In addition, the frequency of extracolonic carcinomas had been found to be higher in both patients with colorectal carcinoma and their first-degree relatives when the index colon carcinoma was proximal.

Most carcinomas that arise in the distal colon develop along the LOH pathway, while most proximal carcinomas are RER (▶ Fig. 21.5). Clinical characteristics of LOH carcinomas induce a propensity for left-sided location (80%), aneuploidy, a polyp-to-carcinoma ratio of 20:1, and a total developmental period of 7 to 10 years. The exception to this observation is the rare adenomatous polyposis syndrome variant called hereditary flat adenoma syndrome (HFAS) or attenuated adenomatous polyposis coli (AAPC) syndrome associated with APC mutations. In this syndrome, the inherited point mutation is found upstream from FAP mutations within exons 1 to 4. This subtle difference between FAP and AAPC mutations (sometimes within 10 base pairs of each other) results in dramatically different phenotypes. Patients with AAPC have few polyps (usually fewer than 10); the polyps are diminutive, flat, and located in the proximal

Table 21.4 Classification of colorectal carcinoma based on molecular pathogenesis, genetic pattern, and clinical features[33]

Genetic pattern	Total colorectal carcinoma (%)	Clinical features
LOH		
Sporadic	35	Distal carcinomas (70%), aneuploid DNA, no family history of polyps or colorectal carcinoma, age of colorectal carcinoma older than 60 y
Familial	25	Distal carcinoma, aneuploid, family history of polyps or colorectal carcinoma in several relatives, age of colorectal carcinomas 50–60 y
Inherited (polyposis syndromes)	1–3	More than 100 polyps, early onset of disease (polyps, 10–25 y; colorectal carcinoma, 30–40 y; except HFAS/AAPC)
FAP		Upper gastrointestinal polyps and carcinoma, retinal findings
Gardner's syndrome		Desmoid neoplasms, bone abnormalities
Turcot's syndrome		Medulloblastoma
HFAS/AAPC		Small flat adenomas of proximal colon, usually fewer than 10, late age of onset (50 y or older), gastric fundic polyps
RER		
Sporadic	20	Proximal carcinomas (70%), diploid DNA, better prognosis than LOH carcinomas, age of colorectal carcinoma older than 60 y
Familial	6	Proximal carcinomas, diploid DNA, family history of colorectal carcinoma or polyps, age of colorectal carcinoma of 50–60 y
Inherited (HNPCC)	10	
Lynch syndrome I		Colorectal carcinoma only, proximal carcinomas (70%), diploid, 40% have synchronous or metachronous colorectal carcinoma, age of colorectal carcinoma of 40–45 y
Lynch syndrome II		Lynch I plus carcinoma of endometrium, ovaries, pancreas, stomach, larynx, urinary system, small bowel, bile ducts (vary with families)
Muir–Torre		Lynch syndromes plus skin lesions
Turcot's syndrome		Glioblastomas

Abbreviations: DNA, deoxyribonucleic acid; FAP, familial adenomatous polyposis; HFAS/AAPC, hereditary flat adenoma syndrome/attenuated adenomatous polyposis coli; HNPCC, hereditary nonpolyposis colorectal carcinoma; LOH, loss of heterozygosity; RER, replication error pathway.

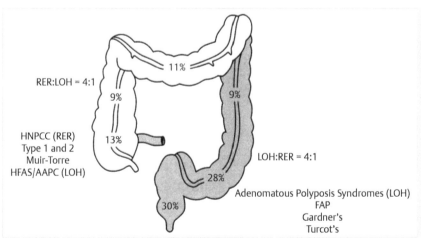

Fig. 21.5 The distribution of neoplastic lesions within the colon is depicted by percentages within the colonic diagram. The ratio of loss of heterozygosity to replication error carcinomas is given for the proximal and distal colon in addition to the locations of most lesions found in various hereditary syndromes.[33]

colon; and a high proportion of polyps progress to carcinomas and they develop late compared with other hereditary neoplasias related to APC mutations. RER carcinomas tend to develop proximal to the splenic flexure (> 70%), have a normal (diploid) DNA content, and carry a better prognosis compared to LOH carcinomas. Molecular analysis of resected carcinomas has led to recognition that LOH carcinomas carry a worse prognosis, stage for stage, than RER carcinomas. To date, the most important molecular marker for prognosis appears to be the DCC gene locus on chromosome 18.

Classification based on genetic patterns and specific syndromes reveals three major forms: sporadic, familial, or inherited. The difference appears to be the method by which the initiating mutation occurs. For sporadic carcinomas, there is a period during which environmental factors influence colon mucosa and eventually alter it so that clonal growth can occur. Familial colorectal carcinoma is defined by patients who have several family members with colon or rectal carcinoma but who do not fit a recognized inherited pattern. Familial colorectal carcinoma may include as many as 30% of patients with colorectal carcinoma when both carcinoma and polyps are included in the pedigree. Explanations for familial clustering could be either shared environment, shared genetics, or both.

Liu et al[47] divided carcinomas with MSI into three classes. The first subset of colorectal carcinomas occurs in patients without a strong family history of colorectal carcinoma (sporadic cases). These account for 12 to 15% of the total colorectal carcinomas in the United States. The second class comprises colon, endometrial, and ovarian carcinomas that develop in patients with a family history of these forms of carcinoma (HNPCC). Virtually all carcinomas that develop in these patients exhibit MSI. The third class of RER carcinomas includes a variable fraction of several types of neoplasms, including those of the lung, breast, and pancreas. The magnitude and prevalence of the microsatellite alterations in this class are generally less pronounced than in RER colorectal carcinomas. The results of Liu et al led to three major conclusions. First, carcinogenesis associated with MMR gene defects usually results from the inactivation of both alleles of the relevant gene. Second, a significant fraction of sporadic RER carcinomas (four of seven in study) arises from mutations in genes other than the four that account for most HNPCC cases. Finally, most sporadic RER carcinomas are not associated with germline mutations of the known match repair genes.

In their review, DeFrancisco and Grady[48] cited the causative genes of HNPCC in decreasing frequency of occurrence to include MLH1, MSH2, MSH6, MLH3, PMS1, PMS2, TGFBR2, and EXO1. Peltomäki summarized the phenotypic features associated with germline mutations manifesting a predisposition to HNPCC.[39] MLH1 is mostly associated with typical HNPCC. Approximately 30% of mutations are of the missense type whose phenotypic manifestations may vary. MSH2 is also mostly associated with typical HNPCC. Extracolonic carcinomas may be more common than in MLH1 mutation carriers. It is a major gene underlying the Muir–Torre syndrome. MSH6 is associated with typical or atypical HNPCC. It is often characterized by late onset, frequent occurrence of endometrial carcinoma, distal location of colorectal carcinomas, and low degree of MSI in carcinomas. PMS2 is also associated with typical or atypical HNPCC. The penetrance of mutations may vary. It is a major gene underlying Turcot's syndrome. MLH3 is seen mostly in atypical HNPCC. It may be characterized by distal location of colorectal carcinomas and variable degrees of MSI in carcinomas. EXO1 is mostly seen in atypical HNPCC. It may be associated with MSI in carcinomas.

Lawes et al[49] reviewed the world literature to determine the clinical importance and prognostic implications of MSI and sporadic carcinoma. In clinical studies, colorectal carcinomas demonstrating MSI respond better to chemotherapy, while in vitro studies using MSI positive cell lines show resistance to radiotherapy and chemotherapy. They concluded MSI may be a useful genetic marker in prognosis and could be an influential factor in deciding treatment options.

Clinical Syndromes

For many years, FAP was considered the only hereditary variety of colon carcinoma. Now, three types of hereditary colorectal carcinomas are recognized: adenomatous polyposis syndromes (Chapter 19), HNPCC, and familial colorectal carcinoma, a group in which families exhibit aggregation of colorectal carcinoma, and/or adenomas, but with no identifiable hereditary syndrome. Approximately 1 to 3% of all colorectal carcinomas are due to hereditary adenomatous polyposis syndromes that include FAP, Gardner's syndrome, Turcot's syndrome, and HFAS/AAPC, all of which begin with germline mutations in the APC gene.

Hereditary Nonpolyposis Colorectal Carcinoma

HNPCC is inherited as an autosomal-dominant pattern with almost complete penetrance. It is estimated that from 0.5 to 6.0% of all colorectal carcinomas can be attributed to HNPCC.[35,50,51,52]

Based on clinical criteria only, Peltomäki[36] noted the estimated incidence of HNPCC varies between 0.5 and 13% of the total colorectal carcinoma burden. Strictly molecular approaches based on the identification of germline mutation carriers among newly diagnosed colorectal patients whose carcinomas showed MSI have arrived at lower estimates—0.3 to 3% of the total colorectal carcinoma burden.

HNPCC has four major subtypes: (1) Lynch type I (site-specific nonpolyposis colorectal carcinoma); (2) Lynch type II (formerly called the carcinoma family syndrome), in which carcinomas occur in the colon and related organs (endometrium, ovaries, stomach, pancreas, and proximal urinary tract, among others); (3) Muir–Torre syndrome, associated with multiple benign and malignant skin neoplasms, sebaceous gland adenomas, carcinomas, and keratoacanthomas[53]; and (4) a variant of Turcot's syndrome (brain neoplasms). HNPCC-related colon carcinomas begin with mutations in the mismatch repair genes and are RER positive.

Clinical criteria were established to confirm the diagnosis of HNPCC at a meeting of the International Collaborative Group on HNPCC in Amsterdam in 1990.[51] The group agreed that minimum criteria should include (1) at least three relatives with histologically verified colorectal carcinoma, one of whom should be a first-degree relative of the other two (those with FAP should be excluded); (2) at least two successive generations should be affected; and (3) in one of the relatives, colorectal carcinoma should have been diagnosed when the patient was younger than 50 years of age.

These criteria have not proved to be comprehensive; therefore, in 1999, the International Collaborative Group developed revised criteria and these are known as Amsterdam-II criteria. They are essentially the same, except that there should be at least three relatives with HNPCC-associated carcinoma (colorectal, endometrial, small bowel, ureter, or renal pelvis). Even this extension of clinical features fails to identify some families with germline mismatch repair gene mutations, so the Bethesda guidelines for testing of colorectal carcinomas for MSI have been developed. They include the following:

1. Individuals with carcinoma in families that meet the Amsterdam criteria.

2. Individuals with two HNPCC-related carcinomas, including synchronous and metachronous colorectal carcinomas or associated extracolonic malignancies (endometrial, ovarian, gastric, hepatobiliary or small bowel carcinoma, or transitional cell carcinoma of the renal pelvis or ureter).

3. Individuals with colorectal carcinoma and a first-degree relative with colorectal carcinoma and/or HNPCC-related extracolonic malignancy and/or a colorectal adenoma; one of the malignancies diagnosed at age younger than 45 years, and the adenoma diagnosed at age younger than 40 years.

4. Individuals with colorectal or endometrial carcinoma diagnosed at age younger than 45 years.

5. Individuals with right-sided colorectal carcinoma with an undifferentiated pattern (solid/cribriform) on histopathology diagnosed at age younger than 45 years. (Note: solid/cribriform defined as poorly differentiated or undifferentiated carcinoma composed of irregular, solid sheets of large eosinophilic cells, and containing small glandlike spaces.)

6. Individuals with signet-ring-cell-type colorectal carcinoma diagnosed at age younger than 45 years. (Note: composed of 50% signet-ring cells.)

7. Individuals with adenomas diagnosed at age younger than 40 years.

In 2002, another workshop was held at the NCI (National Cancer Institute) in Bethesda; the revised guidelines that were created are listed in ▶ Table 21.5.[54] It is estimated that 20 to 25% of population-based cases of colorectal carcinoma meet the Bethesda criteria. It is suggested that for all patients who meet these criteria, a search for MSI is indicated. To establish the most effective and efficient strategy for the detection of MSH2/MLH1 gene carriers in HNPCC, Pinol et al[55] conducted a prospective multicenter nationwide study (the EPICOLON study) in 20 hospitals in the general community in Spain of 1,222 patients with newly diagnosed colorectal carcinoma. MSI testing and MSH2/MLH1 immunostaining were performed in all patients regardless of age, personal or family history, and carcinoma characteristics. Patients whose carcinoma exhibited MSI and/or lack of protein expression underwent MSH2/MLH1 germline testing. The revised Bethesda guidelines were fulfilled by 23.5% of patients and 7.4% had a mismatch repair deficiency, with the carcinoma exhibiting either MSI or loss of protein expression. Germline testing identified mutations in 0.9% in either MSH2 or MLH1 genes. Strategies based on either MSI testing or immunostaining previous selection of patients according to the revised Bethesda guidelines were the most effective (sensitivity, 81.8 and 81.8%; specificity, 98.0 and 98.2%; and positive predictive value, 27.3 and 29.0%, respectively) to identify MSH2/MLH1 gene carriers. They concluded the revised Bethesda guidelines are the most discriminating set of clinical parameters (OR, 33.3).

Table 21.5 The revised Bethesda Guidelines for testing colorectal carcinomas for microsatellite instability (MSI)

Carcinomas from individuals should be tested for MSI in the following situations:

1. Colorectal carcinoma diagnosed in a patient who is younger than 50 y

2. Presence of synchronous, metachronous colorectal, or other HNPCC-associated malignancies[a] regardless of age

3. Colorectal carcinoma with the MSI-H[b] histology[c] diagnosed in a patient who is younger than 60 y[d]

4. Colorectal carcinoma diagnosed in one or more first-degree relatives with an HNPCC-related neoplasm, with one of the neoplasms being diagnosed in a patient younger than 50 y

5. Colorectal carcinoma diagnosed in two or more first- or second-degree relatives with HNPCC-related malignancies regardless of age

[a]HNPCC (hereditary nonpolyposis colorectal carcinoma)-related malignancies include colorectal, endometrial, stomach, ovarian, pancreas, ureter and renal pelvis, biliary tract, and brain (usually glioblastoma as seen in Turcot's syndrome) neoplasms, sebaceous gland adenomas, and keratoacanthomas in Muir–Torre syndrome, and carcinoma of the small bowel.
[b]MSI-H (microsatellite instability-high) in carcinomas refers to changes in two or more of the five National Cancer Institute–recommended panels of microsatellite markers.
[c]Presence of carcinoma infiltrating lymphocytes, Crohn-like lymphocytic reaction, mucinous/signet-ring differentiation, or medullary growth pattern.
[d]There was no consensus among the workshop participants on whether to include the age criteria in guideline 3 above; participants voted to keep younger than 60 years of age in the guidelines.

In conclusion, MSI and immunohistochemistry analysis using antibodies against MLH1, MSH2, PMS2, and MSH6 appeared to be equally effective for the identification of mutation carriers. Despite its name, polyps are a feature of HNPCC, and a review of the literature revealed a polyp incidence in 8 to 17% of first-degree relatives during colonoscopic screening.[38]

Carriers of an MMR defect develop adenomas more frequently than controls. The adenomas identified in carriers are larger, and a significantly higher proportion showed histologic features that are associated with a high risk of malignant degeneration, such as a high degree of dysplasia and the presence of more extensive villous architecture.[56] A relatively high proportion of patients develop colorectal carcinoma within 3 years after a clean colonoscopy and this suggests that the adenoma–carcinoma sequence is accelerated and that the progression from adenoma to carcinoma may take fewer than 3 years.

Genetically speaking, HNPCC syndromes are dominantly inherited with nearly 100% penetrance reported by one group of investigators[50] but only 70 to 80% (i.e., 20–30% of individuals with a predisposing mutation may never develop carcinoma) by others.[57] Asymptomatic gene carriers can pass the causative mutation to their children.[57] The disease is heterogeneous. All first-degree relatives of a patient with HNPCC have a 50% risk of carrying one of the deleterious genes. Adenomas in patients carrying HNPCC gene mutations display MSI, suggesting that mismatch repair defects are important early events in colorectal carcinogenesis. Carcinoma formation requires inactivation of both copies of a given mismatch repair gene, one copy by germline mutation and the other by somatic (acquired) mutation.[57]

Individuals with the Lynch syndrome differ from patients with sporadic colorectal carcinoma in several ways.[35] They show an autosomal-dominant mode of inheritance,[1] a predominance of proximal colonic carcinoma (72% of first colon carcinomas were located in the right colon, and only 25% were found in the sigmoid colon and rectum),[2] an excess of multiple primary colonic carcinomas (18%),[3] an early age of onset (mean, 44 years),[4] a significantly improved survival rate compared with family members with distal colonic and rectal carcinomas when compared with right-sided lesions in an American College of Surgeons series (53% vs. 35% 5-year survivals),[5] and 24% developed metachronous colon carcinoma with a risk for the development of metachronous lesions in 10 years of 40% based on life-table methods.[6] In addition to the above features, Lynch type II syndrome is characterized by a high frequency of other adenocarcinomas and the occasional occurrence of cutaneous manifestations in the form of sebaceous adenomas and carcinomas, epitheliomas, or keratoacanthomas. In a study by Mecklin and Jarvinen,[58] of 40 HNPCC families with 315 affected members, a total of 472 malignancies were identified. They included colorectal (63%), endometrial (8%), gastric (6%), biliopancreatic (4%), and uroepithelial (2%) carcinomas.

The RR of these carcinomas ranges from 3 to 25 times that of the general population.[10] The risk of colorectal carcinoma increases 1.6% per year from age 25 to 75 years in patients with these mutations.[53] In a detailed pedigree analysis of 40 families with HNPCC, Aarnio et al[59] identified 414 patients affected with carcinoma. The risk of any metachronous carcinoma reached 90% after treatment of colorectal carcinoma and 70% after endometrial carcinoma; the second malignancy was most often a new colorectal carcinoma or endometrial carcinoma.[59] Other sites of carcinoma include breast, pancreas, and possible lymphoma and leukemia. The review by DeFrancisco and Grady[48] found the four most common extracolonic carcinomas include (in descending order) endometrial, ovarian, gastric, and transitional cell carcinoma of the uroepithelial tract (bladder, kidney, ureter). Women with HNPCC are at a 10-fold increased risk of endometrial carcinoma, which is usually diagnosed between the ages of 40 and 60 years, that is, 15 years earlier than the general population. The estimated cumulative risk at age 70 years is 40 to 50%. With MSH2 and MLH1 mutations, the risk of colorectal carcinoma or endometrial carcinoma before age 50 years is 20 to 25% compared with 0.2% for the general population.[53] Ovarian carcinoma is less common (incidence approximately 9%). Gastric carcinoma occurs in 5 to 20% of HNPCC families. The RR of gastric carcinoma was 19.3 in MSH2 mutation carriers compared with the general population. Transitional cell carcinoma of the uroepithelial tract occurs in 1% of HNPCC patients. Only the carriers of MSH2 mutations appear to have a significantly increased risk of carcinoma in the urinary tract (RR of 75.3). Overall, the RR of gastric carcinoma, ovarian carcinoma, and carcinoma of the urinary tract has been shown to be higher in patients with mutations in MSH2 as compared to patients with MLH1 mutations. Women with MSH6 mutations appear to be more likely to develop endometrial carcinoma. Other HNPCC-associated extracolonic neoplasms include carcinomas of the small bowel, pancreas, hepatobiliary tree, brain, and skin. The Muir–Torre syndrome, first described in 1967, refers to patients with HNPCC who also develop benign or malignant sebaceous skin neoplasms (sebaceous adenomas, carcinomas, squamous or basal cell), and multiple keratoacanthomas. The syndrome usually arises from mutations in MSH2. The development of glioblastoma multiforme, in association with HNPCC, is called Turcot's syndrome. The Muir–Torre syndrome is also used to describe central nervous system neoplasms occurring in FAP, although these are usually medulloblastomas instead of glioblastomas. Approximately a third of patients with Turcot's syndrome have mutations in one of the mismatch repair genes. HNPCC is associated with a 50% risk of a second carcinoma within 15 years of the initial carcinoma diagnosis[53] compared with 5% in the general population. Information regarding the cumulative risk of developing various HNPCC-associated malignancies has been summarized from several reports and tabulated in
▶ Table 21.6.[10,48,53,59,60]

Plaschke et al[61] analyzed the involvement and phenotypic manifestations of MSH6 germline mutations in families suspected of HNPCC. Patients were preselected among 706 families by MSI, immunohistochemistry, and/or exclusion of MLH1 or MSH2 mutations and were subjected to MSH6 mutation analysis. Clinical and molecular data of MSH6 mutation families were compared with data from families with MLH1 and MSH2 mutations. They identified 27 families with 24 different pathogenic MSH6 germline mutations, representing 3.8% of the total of the families, and 14.7% of all families with DNA mismatch repair gene mutations. The median age of onset of colorectal carcinoma in putative mutation carriers was 10 years higher for MSH6 (54 years) compared with MLH1 and MSH2 (44 years). Relative to other malignancies, colorectal carcinoma was less frequent in MSH6 families compared with MLH1 and MSH2 families. In contrast, the frequency of non–HNPCC-associated neoplasms was increased. Later age of disease onset and lower incidence of colorectal carcinoma may contribute to a lower proportion of identified MSH6 mutations in families suspected of HNPCC. However, in approximately half of these families, at least one patient developed colorectal or endometrial carcinoma in the fourth decade of life. Therefore, a surveillance program as stringent as that for families with MLH1 or MSH2 mutations is recommended.

Table 21.6 Malignancies associated with hereditary nonpolyposis colorectal carcinoma

Malignancy	Median age of onset (y)	Lifetime risk (%)	General population (%)[a]
Colorectal	40–45	78–82	5
Endometrial	45	39–61	1.5
Ovarian	47	9–12	1
Gastric	54	13–19	< 1
Urothelial (bladder, kidney, and ureter)	60	4–10	< 1
Pancreaticobiliary	54	2–18	< 1
Brain	43	1–4	< 1
Small bowel	49	1–4	< 1

[a]Adapted from Boland et al 2001.[53]

Approximately 60% of families that meet the Amsterdam-I criteria (HNPCC) have a hereditary abnormality in a DNA mismatch repair gene. Carcinoma incidence in Amsterdam criteria-I families with mismatch repair gene mutations is reported to be very high, but carcinoma incidence for individuals in Amsterdam criteria-I families with no evidence of a mismatch repair defect is unknown. Lindor et al[62] conducted a study to determine if carcinoma risks in Amsterdam criteria-I families with no apparent deficiency in DNA mismatch repair are different from carcinoma risks in Amsterdam criteria-I families with DNA mismatch repair abnormalities. 161 Amsterdam criteria-I pedigrees from multiple population- and clinic-based sources in North America and Germany were identified and grouped into families with (group A) or without (group B) mismatch repair deficiency by testing. A total of 3,422 relatives were included in the analysis. Group A families from both population- and clinic-based series showed increased incidence of HNPCC-related carcinomas. Group B families showed increased incidence only for colorectal carcinoma (standardized incidence ratio [SIR], 2.3) and to a lesser extent than group A (SIR, 6.1). Families who have fulfilled Amsterdam criteria-I but who have no evidence of DNA mismatch repair defect do not share the same carcinoma incidence as families with HNPCC with mismatch-repair deficiency. Relatives in such families have a lower incidence of colorectal carcinoma than those in families with HNPCC (Lynch syndrome) and incidence may not be increased for other carcinomas. These families should not be described or counseled as having HNPCC. To facilitate distinguishing these entities, the designation of "familial colorectal cancer type X" is suggested to describe this type of familial aggregation of colorectal carcinoma.

Jass[63] dispelled any thoughts that the morphogenetic pathway involved flat adenoma or de novo carcinoma in these cases. In a review of 131 carcinomas, none was small and superficial. Residual adenoma (contiguous with carcinoma) was present in 3 of 3 (100%) in situ carcinomas, 8 of 9 (89%) carcinomas involving only submucosa, 4 of 14 (29%) carcinomas limited to the muscle coat, and 13 of 105 (12%) carcinomas extending beyond the muscle coat. Lynch type II syndrome colon carcinomas show a significant increase in the proportion of mucinous, poorly differentiated carcinomas, and Crohn-like lymphoid reaction around the lesion as well as a higher rate of synchronous and metachronous carcinomas.[35,64]

Other investigators have also studied HNPCC. Sankila et al,[65] compared the survival rates of 175 patients with hMLH1-associated HNPCC with those of 14,000 patients with sporadic colorectal carcinoma diagnosed at less than 65 years. The overall 5-year cumulative relative survival rate was 65% for patients with HNPCC and 44% for patients with sporadic colorectal carcinoma.

In a series of 1,042 Japanese patients who underwent resection for colorectal carcinoma, 3.7% were found to have HNPCC.[66] The characteristic early age of onset, right-sided predominance, and favorable survival were confirmed. Metachronous colorectal carcinoma developed significantly more often in cases with HNPCC (12.8 vs. 1.8%), and metachronous extracolonic malignancies also developed more often (10.2 vs. 3.5%). In cases with HNPCC, the mean interval between initial operation and the diagnosis of the second malignancy was 61 months (range, 12–153 months). These findings stress the importance of long-term follow-up.

Rodríguez-Bigas et al[67] reported the experience from the HNPCC Registry at Roswell Park in Buffalo, New York, which included 301 people in 40 families. In 284 of 301 people, 363 carcinomas were identified. Colorectal carcinomas alone were identified in 64% and in conjunction with extracolonic malignancies in another 11%. Extracolonic malignancies alone were identified in 25%. The median age at diagnosis of colorectal carcinoma was 48 years. Right-sided malignancies predominated (55%), synchronous and metachronous lesions were noted in 33%, and synchronous or metachronous adenomas were documented in 51% of those studied. Generational anticipation was also noted.

Hampel et al[68] assessed the frequency of the mismatch repair genes MLH1, MSH2, MSH6, and PMS2, in patients with a new diagnosis of colorectal carcinoma to identify patients with the Lynch syndrome. Genotyping of the carcinoma for MSI was the primary screening method. Among patients whose screening results were positive for MSI, they searched for germline mutations in the MLH1, MSH2, MSH6, and PMS2 genes with the use of immunohistochemical staining for mismatch repair proteins, genomic sequencing, and deletion studies. Family members of carriers of the mutations were counseled and those found to be at risk were offered mutation testing. Of 1,066 patients enrolled in this study, 19.5% had MSI, and 2.2% of these patients had a mutation causing the Lynch syndrome. Among the 23 probands with the Lynch syndrome, 10 were more than 50 years of age and 5 did not meet the Amsterdam criteria or the Bethesda guidelines for the diagnosis of HNPCC. In the families of 21 of the probands, 117 persons at risk were tested, and of these 52 had Lynch syndrome mutations. They concluded that routine molecular screening of patients with colorectal adenocarcinoma for the Lynch syndrome identified mutations in patients and their family members that otherwise would not have been detected. In most centers, it would not seem feasible to test all patients with colorectal carcinoma.

The characteristics of HNPCC mandate the development of surveillance programs. Screening recommendations have varied, but the recommendation by Lynch et al[69] for gene carriers has been colonoscopy, beginning at age 20 to 25 years or at least 5 years earlier than the earliest age at which colon carcinoma was diagnosed in a particular kindred with the procedure repeated every other year until the patient is 30 years of age and then annually thereafter. The frequency of colonoscopic examination is justified by the finding that HNPCC adenomas have repair deficient cells with rapidly and relentlessly accumulating mutations that support the clinical concept of "aggressive adenomas" and accelerate the adenoma–carcinoma sequence. The authors strongly believe that germline carriers should be offered prophylactic subtotal colectomy.

The importance of screening colonoscopy was underscored by the report of Sankila et al,[65] who compared the colorectal carcinoma death rates of two groups of HNPCC patients—those screened every 3 years and controls who refused screening. The authors' data indicated that one carcinoma was prevented for every 2.8 polypectomies performed. This is in stark contrast to the National Polyp Study data for the general population, which gave a range of 41 to 119 polypectomies per carcinoma prevented.

The importance of screening is further emphasized by the study that compared screened with unscreened (by choice) "controls" evaluated over a 15-year period with 252 relatives at risk for HNPCC, 119 of whom declined screening. In the screened group, 8 of 133 (6%) developed colorectal carcinoma compared to 19 (16%) in the unscreened group.[70] de Vos tot Nederveen Cappel et al[71] examined the stage of the screening detected carcinomas in relation to the surveillance interval and to assess the risk of developing colorectal carcinoma while on the program in 114 families in the Dutch Family Registry. A total of 35 carcinomas were detected while on the program. With intervals between colorectal carcinoma and the preceding surveillance examination of 2 years or less, carcinomas were at Dukes' stage A ($n = 4$), B ($n = 11$), and C ($n = 1$). With intervals of more than 2 years, carcinomas were Dukes' stage A ($n = 3$), B ($n = 10$), and C ($n = 6$). The 10-year cumulative risk of developing colorectal carcinoma was 10.5% in proven mutation carriers, 15.7% after partial colectomy, and 3.4% after subtotal colectomy. There is a substantial risk of developing colorectal carcinoma while on the program. However, all carcinomas but one of subjects who underwent a surveillance examination 2 years or less before detection were at a local stage. They therefore recommend surveillance for HNPCC with an interval of 2 years or less.

For women who are gene carriers, an annual endometrial aspiration curettage should begin at age 30 years. Those patients should be advised of the option of ovarian carcinoma screening with transvaginal ovarian ultrasonography, Doppler color blood flow imagery, and CA-125 evaluation. They should be encouraged to have their children early so they can consider the option of undergoing prophylactic total abdominal hysterectomy and bilateral salpingo-oophorectomy between the ages of 35 and 40 years.

Screening for breast and gastric carcinoma should be initiated earlier in life than might otherwise be considered. If at least one family member is affected, gastroscopy beginning at age 30 to 35 years and every 1 to 2 years is advised.[53] Also, only if at least one family member is affected, ultrasonography of the urinary tract and urine cytology beginning at age 30 to 35 years and every 1 to 2 years is advised.[56]

Mecklin and Jarvinen[72] analyzed 22 Finnish HNPCC families followed up for 7 years. Metachronous neoplasms were diagnosed in 41% of patients treated by segmental resection and 24% of those treated by subtotal colectomy. Extracolonic carcinoma was diagnosed in 30%. The most common malignancy was biliopancreatic carcinoma, which accounted for all five deaths related to carcinoma. The authors concluded that subtotal colectomy is superior to hemicolectomy or segmental resection in patients with HNPCC and that regular follow-up is necessary for surveillance of remaining bowel and extracolonic malignancies.

Itoh et al[73] conducted a study of 130 HNPCC kindreds to determine the risk of death from malignancy in first-degree relatives. The authors found a sevenfold increase in the risk of colon carcinoma in both sexes. In women relatives, the risk of breast carcinoma was increased fivefold, and a lifetime risk of breast carcinoma was 1 in 3.7. From these results, the authors recommended a screening program.

Because clinical premonitory signs such as multiple colonic polyps seen in cases of familial polyposis coli are lacking, the clinician must rely on the clinical findings and a family history typical of HNPCC. Disorders that have been considered in the differential diagnosis of HNPCC have included FAP, attenuated

FAP, juvenile polyposis coli, and Peutz–Jeghers syndrome.[35] Once the diagnosis has been made, the physician is faced with the responsibility of informing the patient that other family members are at risk because the genetic implications for carcinoma expression are profound. Identification of individuals at risk may be aided by inspection of the patient's skin, which may provide clues to the existence of a carcinoma associated with genodermatosis. Criteria providing clues to the diagnosis of Lynch type II syndrome include any patient presenting with an early onset of carcinoma of the colon (particularly of the proximal colon in the absence of multiple polyps), endometrium, or ovaries (particularly when the patient is younger than age 40 years)[1]; any patient with multiple primary carcinomas in which the lesions are integral to Lynch type II syndrome (carcinoma of the colon, endometrium, or ovary and other adenocarcinomas)[2]; and any patient who states that one or more first-degree relatives manifested early onset of the carcinomas integral to Lynch type II syndrome.[3]

It is important to determine whether an HNPCC syndrome is present because the operative procedure of choice for the index carcinoma is subtotal colectomy as opposed to a more limited resection.[35,69] In the case of a woman who has completed her family, the resection may be extended to a prophylactic hysterectomy and bilateral salpingo-oophorectomy because of the patient's inordinately high risk of development of carcinoma of the endometrium and ovaries.

The lifetime risk of endometrial and ovarian carcinomas in HNPCC is up to 60 and 12%, respectively.[74] Watson et al[75] collected data on 80 ovarian carcinoma patients who are members of HNPCC families, including 31 known mutation carriers, 35 presentive carriers (by colorectal/endometrial carcinomas status), and 14 at-risk family members. Among frankly epithelial cases, most carcinomas were well or moderately differentiated. Ovarian carcinoma in HNPCC differs from ovarian in the general population in several clinically important respects. It occurs at a markedly earlier age (42.7 years). It is more likely to be epithelial (95.6%). If it is a frankly invasive epithelial carcinoma, it is more likely to be well or moderately differentiated (85% were International Federation of Obstetrics and Gynecology [FIGO] stage I or II at diagnosis). HNPCC patients with ovarian carcinoma are more likely to have a synchronous endometrial carcinoma (21.5%).

Familial Colorectal Carcinoma

Ten to fifteen percent of patients with colorectal carcinoma and/or colorectal adenomas have other affected family members, but their family histories do not fit the criteria for either FAP or HNPCC and may not appear to follow a recognizable pattern of inheritance, such as autosomal-dominant inheritance. Such families are categorized as having familial colorectal carcinoma. The presence of colorectal carcinoma in more than one family member may be due to genetic factors, shared environmental risk factors or even to chance.[10] With a family history, the risk of colorectal carcinoma is increased earlier in life than later such that at age 45 years the annual incidence is more than three times higher than average-risk people, whereas at age 70, risk is not significantly different. The incidence in a 35- to 40-year-old is about the same as that of an average-risk person at age 50 years. A personal history of adenomatous polyps confers a 15 to 20% risk of subsequently developing polyps. A history of adenomatous polyps in a sibling or parent is also associated with increased risk of colorectal carcinoma. Expert recommendations on screening for such persons are similar to those with a positive family history of colorectal carcinoma. Most experts suggest that screening should begin at age 35 to 40 years when the magnitude of risk is comparable to that of a 50-year-old. Because the risk increases with extent of family history, there is room for clinical judgment in favor of even earlier screening, depending on the details of the family history. A common but unproven clinical practice is to initiate colorectal carcinoma screening 10 years before the age of the youngest colorectal carcinoma case in the family.

Evidence demonstrates that patients in families with breast and colon carcinoma (hereditary breast and colon carcinoma) may have a carcinoma family syndrome caused by CHEK2 1100delC mutations that are present in a subset of the families.[76] The CHEK2 mutation is incompletely penetrant.

Genetic Testing

Genetic testing provides the ability to determine who is and who is not at risk for disease before the onset of symptoms. Such information is becoming essential for proper management of patients and their families. In individuals who inherit mutant genes, simple preventive measures often can reduce morbidity and mortality and allow more thoughtful planning for the future. The benefits of genetic testing are equally important for those families who are found not to carry the relevant mutation; these individuals are spared unnecessary medical procedures and tremendous anxiety. However, genetic testing is not without its problems.

These problems can be broadly divided into psychological or technical in nature. From the societal view, issues related to insurance, employment, discrimination, and privacy have garnered much concern and attention. The technical challenges associated with genetic testing can be just as formidable and are often overlooked. Even when the mutated gene is known, routine genetic testing may fail to identify mutations. As a result of these uncertainties, genetic testing that fails to find the mutation is often inconclusive. Studies have shown that these inconclusive results may be misinterpreted by the patient and physicians and are a source of great anxiety. Because of the complex psychosocial and technical issues, it is clear that genetic testing should never be offered to patients without appropriate genetic counseling.

Prior to embarking upon any genetic testing, it is critically important that the individual at risk of developing carcinoma and the referring physician as well have an understanding of what the testing is designed to do. To this end, genetic counseling is of paramount importance for patients to fully understand the limitations of genetic testing and will aid in the management of patients who are susceptible to colorectal carcinoma. The management of individuals who may be at increased risk for an inherited colorectal carcinoma susceptibility is complex. Knowledge about genetic information can contribute to clinical management at several stages during patient care. Obtaining and interpreting genetic information can be a lengthy process but is essential to avoid harm and to heighten the benefits of genetic testing.

Genetic counseling and interpreting genetic test results can be complex but without knowing the limitations of the methods used and the lifetime probability of developing carcinoma in individuals who carry a gene that predisposes to carcinoma, misinterpretation may lead to false assurance. Wong et al[77] conducted a review of the literature and combined with their clinical and research experience suggested a guide to enable various health care providers to better counsel patients in their quest for advice on prevention, early detection, and surveillance for colorectal carcinoma. Much of the following information was extracted from their review.

Interpretation of genetic tests for colorectal carcinoma is not as straightforward as interpreting a blood sugar test to ascertain whether it is elevated, normal, or lowered. Genetic counseling is a dynamic communication process between the patient and the counselor who provides education and support within a multidisciplinary team. Counseling is targeted toward individuals who are interested in having a personal risk estimate. Those at greatest risk for developing malignancy may benefit by assessing current screening tests, whereas those at lower risk will be reassured that their risk for colorectal carcinoma is not as high as they thought.

Furthermore, survivors of malignancies may want to know their risk of recurrence or of a second primary neoplasm and the risk for their relatives, especially their children. Carcinoma is a genetic disease but is not necessarily inherited. Virtually all neoplasms and certainly all malignant ones result in part from genes that mutate somatically (during one's lifetime). In contrast, a minority of neoplasms arises from an inherited gene that confers susceptibility in development. Genetic counseling is appropriate when the family history is suggestive of a heritable predisposition for malignancy. In general, the counseling process is composed of discrete elements: risk assessment, informative counseling, supportive counseling, and follow-up. Before initiating the process, it is important for the counselor to gain insight into the action of these components from the perspective of the patient. This is initially obtained by contracting. Contracting allows patients to know what to expect from genetic counseling and ensures their needs will be elicited and addressed by the counselor.

The presence or absence of a family history of benign and malignant neoplasms helps determine whether a person has an increased probability of having an inherited susceptibility for malignancy. Other familial traits can be characteristic signs of a genetic syndrome and suggestive that an increased risk for carcinoma may be present in a family. Pedigree analysis is multigenerational and includes details from both sides of the proband's family. Current age or age at death is ascertained for everyone, because early death may explain the absence of a positive family history. Genetic counseling is recommended for individuals with an absolute risk greater than 10% (▶ Table 21.7) for developing carcinoma of the colon and rectum.

Providing risk assessment is only one part of the overall education process in genetic counseling. Explaining what genes are, how they are passed to subsequent generations, and the natural history of the neoplastic disease is an integral part of genetic counseling. Other educational aims include the recommendation or provision of screening modalities for early detection and preventive options. Medical intervention such as prophylactic surgery or chemoprevention, and the possible limitations of these treatments are issues for members of hereditary carcinoma families. Obtaining knowledge may empower the individual and

Table 21.7 Personal and family features that confer a higher than average risk for developing colorectal carcinoma[76]

	Absolute risk to age 70 (%)
Population risk	3–6
Polyps	
Family history	4–7
Personal history	
<1 cm in diameter	3–6
>1 cm in diameter	9–18
Family history of colorectal carcinoma	
1 FDR	
Age <45 y	15–30
Age 45–55 y	6–25
Age >70 y	3–6
1 FDR + 1 SDR	10
2 FDR	15–30
ICG-HNPCC (mutation status unknown)	35–45
Mutation carrier in a gene associated with HNPCC	70–90
FAP (not clinically screened and mutation status unknown)	40–45
APC mutation carrier for FAP	80–90

Abbreviations: APC, adenomatous polyposis coli; FAP, familial adenomatous polyposis; FDR, first-degree relative; ICG-HNPCC, International Collaborative Group on Hereditary Non-Polyposis Colorectal Cancer; SDR, second-degree relative.

family by dispelling the myths about malignancy and by providing guidelines that help in decision making. It also establishes the foundation of informed consent for genetic testing.

Indications

Genetic testing is discussed when the patient's family history of carcinoma falls in the autosomal-dominant mode of inheritance. Appropriate situations include families who carry a mutation in APC, hMLH1, hMSH2, hPMS1, hPMS2, or hMSH6 or families fulfilling the clinical FAP or ICG-HNPCC (International Collaborative Group on Hereditary Non-Polyposis Colorectal Cancer) criteria. The decision to undergo genetic testing is a personal one based on informed consent. The first phase in determining whether genetic testing is appropriate is genetic counseling.

Among FAP families, who are candidates for genetic testing? The diagnosis of FAP is made because of the presence of polyps on examination of the presenting patient (proband or index case). In autosomal-dominant inheritance, on average, 50% of the patient's first-degree relatives (parents, siblings, and offspring) will be at risk. As soon as the FAP diagnosis emerges, either before or after operation, the surgeon should recommend

that all first-degree relatives be examined. If a mutation in APC is identified in the patient's germline DNA, the immediate family and other branches of the family can be encouraged to come forward for genetic counseling and to know their risk status if so desired. If a mutation is not detected, further genetic testing for APC mutations in the family is contraindicated and the clinical decision is to monitor first-degree relatives by colonoscopy at recommended intervals. Depending on the expression of colorectal carcinoma in the proband and the pattern of colorectal carcinoma and other malignancies in the family, genetic testing for HNPCC may be advisable. In every case of FAP, a genetic test to pinpoint the heritable, germline APC mutation is justified, with informed consent of the patient. As far as testing the patient's family is concerned, a common exception (occurring in 30% of probands) is a patient with FAP whose parents are negative on endoscopic examination and who therefore has a "new mutation" in the APC gene. In this instance, the risk for colorectal carcinoma for siblings falls to that of the general population. Nonetheless, children of the patient will require testing (if a mutation was identified in the proband) if so desired, because they are at 50% risk for FAP. The only obvious example in which genetic testing is not recommended would be in an isolated patient with FAP with no living first-degree relatives.

What patients with suspected HNPCC should be referred for genetic counseling and testing? Because HNPCC is not always obvious based on clinical findings, either preoperatively or during resection, the clinical management of a possible HNPCC patient is complex. A detailed family history, with sites of malignancy verified, is critical to determine whether the patient fits the Amsterdam criteria and other associated features of HNPCC. Analysis of neoplastic material would provide assistance in determining whether to test the proband's germline DNA (i.e., a blood sample) for HNPCC mutations (after genetic counseling) and refer the first-degree relatives should a mutation be detected. In the instance of a positive family history, it is ideal for testing to be conducted despite MSI phenotype. The clinical algorithm would be much the same as for FAP, with the exception that the multiple genes might need to be analyzed unless tests on pathogenic samples narrow the search. It is important to point out that at present, detection of a confirmed pathogenic mutation occurs in less than 50% of HNPCC families. In the absence of an identified deleterious mutation, genetic testing is inconclusive, which must be explained to the patient by an individual skilled in genetic counseling. Family members can be given general advice for colorectal carcinoma screening of first-degree relatives of patients with this malignancy.

Techniques

The molecular techniques used in testing for germline mutations in hereditary colorectal carcinoma have been described in detail by Rabelo et al[78] and the following is a synopsis of that work.

Germline DNA can be tested in three ways:

1. With in vitro–synthesized protein (IVSP) assay (also called protein truncation test or in vitro truncation test), specific gene segments are amplified by polymerase chain reaction (PCR) or reversed transcription (RT) PCR, transcribed and translated in vitro, and the protein product is analyzed by gel electrophoresis. If the amplified segment has a mutation that

causes the production of a truncated protein, its smaller size will allow it to be more mobile in the gel.

2. Single-stranded conformation analysis (SSCA) is also a mutation detection technique in which specific gene segments are amplified by PCR or RT-PCR, denatured to separate the stands of the DNA product and analyzed by gel electrophoresis. The mutant DNA often migrates differently under certain conditions, allowing the putative localization of mutation within the segment.

3. DNA sequencing is the criterion standard technique for mutation detection, with up to 99% accuracy. It allows the precise identification of the mutation in the DNA sequence by pinpointing any change in the number or identity of bases.

Pathologic specimens are examined in two ways:

1. A clue to identify colorectal carcinoma caused by HNPCC is by an associated alteration in the length stability of repetitive tract DNA in the carcinoma of an affected individual. This is known as MSI, also called RER-positive phenotype. The presence of MSI + thereby increases the likelihood that direct testing for defects in HNPCC genes will be informative. There are three outcomes of MSI analysis.[56]

   a) If at least two markers tested show instability, the result indicates an increased likelihood that the colorectal carcinoma arose due to an HNPCC-associated mutation (MSI-H).

   b) If no marker shows instability in the absence of a compelling family history, the result is usually interpreted as ruling out HNPCC (MSS stable).

   c) If instability is seen in only one of the markers, the result does not indicate HNPCC. The clinical behavior of MSI-L carcinomas is identical to those with MSS, and does not have the mutational fingerprints of the clinical behavior of MSI-H carcinomas. MSI-L results occur as commonly as do MSI-H results.

2. Immunohistochemistry is a technique for diagnosing a carcinoma that lacks expression of a particular HNPCC gene. It examines either hMLH1 or hMSH2 protein expression in carcinomas by immunostaining using monoclonal antibodies. Formalin-fixed, paraffin-embedded adenocarcinoma tissue is the sample required for testing with a region of normal mucosa adjacent to the carcinoma for comparison. The absence of hMLH1 or hMSH2 immunostaining shows which gene is defective and should be analyzed for the presence of a germline mutation. Studies have shown that the lack of hMLH1 or hMLH2 immunostaining was associated with the presence of MSI +.

Genetic Testing for Familial Adenomatous Polyposis

Presymptomatic genetic diagnosis of FAP in at-risk individuals has been feasible with linkage and direct detection of APC mutations.[10] If one were to use linkage analysis to identify gene carriers, ancillary family members, including more than one affected individual, would need to be studied. With direct detection, fewer family members' blood samples are required than for linkage analysis, but the specific mutation must be identified in at least one affected person by DNA mutation analysis or sequencing. Because approximately 96% of the mutations in FAP lead to a truncated protein, it has become routine to use IVSP assay (sometimes called protein truncation test) for mutation detection. When a truncated protein is identified, it is possible to localize the mutation to a specific segment of the gene and then use DNA sequencing to determine the mutated nucleotide(s). The use of IVSP as the sole genetic test in FAP misses approximately 20% of APC mutations. Another screening technique is based on analysis of electrophoretic migration of small segments of the wild-type mutant gene (SSCA). The sequential use of two molecular diagnostic tests has become a common practice: a simple and less expensive screening technique (of high sensitivity and moderate specificity), followed by a definitive test of high sensitivity, usually DNA sequencing.

These mutation search methods, APC protein truncation testing (from lymphocyte RNA), considerably enhance the feasibility of testing at-risk individuals without requiring DNA from multiple affected family members (as linkage requires). In particular, it is useful for testing in small families or in patients with spontaneous or "de novo" mutations (the first occurrence of FAP in a kindred), which may account for as much as one third of incident cases.[10] Only about 80% of APC mutations can be detected by this method. Therefore, the clinician cannot rule out FAP on the basis of this molecular test alone if other criteria support the FAP diagnosis. When the mutation in a family is known from one or more affected members, one test, usually IVSP, need be performed, as the expression pattern of the mutation is already established for that family. A positive result in such a test is considered a "mutation-positive" result, and the patient can be counseled as recommended. When the mutation in the family is not known, IVSP is performed. In the majority of cases, a mutation will be found in the APC gene that can be further characterized by DNA sequencing. Again, a "mutation-positive" result is obtained leading to the appropriate genetic counseling for the patient. Other options include DNA sequencing and linkage analysis. Even by combining two or more techniques, it is not possible to achieve 100% sensitivity, because the mutations may not be in the coding region of the gene or because a few FAP kindreds do not exhibit linkage to chromosome 5q. In such case, a "no mutation detected" result must not be interpreted as a "negative test" with the very important considerations for counseling the patient.

For at-risk individuals who have been found to be definitively mutation negative by genetic testing, there is no clear consensus on the need for or frequency of colon screening, though it would seem prudent that at least one flexible sigmoidoscopy or colonoscopy examination should be performed in early adulthood (age 18–25 years).[10]

Molecular Genetic Diagnosis of Hereditary Nonpolyposis Colorectal Carcinoma

The HNPCC syndrome is more complex in terms of genetic testing because at least six genes involved in DNA mismatch repair predispose to this syndrome. The two most commonly involved genes are hMSH2 (involved in approximately 45% of cases) and hMLH1 (involved in approximately 49% of cases). Protein truncation is observed in more than 80% of HNPCC cases caused by mutations in hMSH2 and to a lesser degree in hMHL1. Currently, IVSP or SSCA or both are used, followed by DNA sequencing for precise characterization. In the case of a mutation already known in an affected member of the kindred, the same technique used to detect that mutation can be used, and a "mutation-positive" result leads to genetic counseling. If no mutation has been previously described in the kindred, analysis of hMLH1 and hMSH2 in an affected individual by IVSP or SSCA followed by DNA sequencing for confirmation is indicated. If a truncating mutation is found, a causative role can be inferred for the mutation. This "mutation-positive" result allows counseling of the affected individual and further testing of the kindred. If a nontruncating mutation is found, tests such as linkage analysis and functional assays may be required to discriminate between an "inconclusive" and a "mutation-positive" result. It is estimated that approximately 30% of mutations will be missed if IVSP is used as the sole genetic test and that a similar or higher percentage of false negatives may also be expected if SSCA is used instead. Again, even by combining two or more techniques, it is not possible to achieve 100% sensitivity. Other genes may be responsible (locus heterogeneity). A "no mutation detected" result must not be interpreted as a "negative test" result.

Summary

A proposed algorithm for genetic testing of individuals in FAP and HNPCC kindreds is given below. First, use IVSP to locate the mutation, then use DNA sequencing to characterize it precisely in the first affected family member. If the IVSP test is negative, DNA sequencing of the APC gene is warranted. When the mutation is defined for that kindred, the testing of other family members at risk may be accomplished by using IVSP alone. If the mutation in the first affected individual was identified by DNA sequencing, it is logical to continue to use this method for genetic testing of at-risk individuals. Considering the weighty psychological, ethical, and legal implications of the results of genetic tests, the use of two different techniques, one to detect the mutation and the second to identify and confirm it, is recommended in all cases. DNA sequencing, the most sensitive method for mutation detection, should be one of the techniques used. For HNPCC, two techniques are appropriate for initial testing of mutations in these genes, IVSP and SSCA. Screening with IVSP is recommended, but this preference may vary among laboratories. If a mutation is detected by any of these methods, DNA sequencing should be used to identify it precisely in the first affected member of a kindred. If these screening techniques are negative, the sequencing of both hMSH2 and hMLH1 may be warranted. If still negative, in view of the locus heterogeneity seen in HNPCC, the same screening protocol may have to be used for hPMS2, hPMS1, and hMSH6. Again, the use of two different tests in all cases is recommended and DNA sequencing is used and when the pathogenic mutation is defined for that kindred, the testing of other family members at risk may be accomplished with either IVSP or SSCA alone.

When a mutation (a variant gene) is identified by any of the methods, it must be validated as a pathogenic mutation (true-positive result) instead of a polymorphism, a common variant in the protein that does not contribute to the disease phenotype (false positive). When a mutation is not identified ("no mutation detected"), the negative result may be a "true negative" (no predisposing mutations in any relevant genes), or a "false negative" (undetected mutation may exist in known or unknown genes). If the person is affected with colorectal carcinoma, this is either a false negative in a familial colorectal carcinoma syndrome or a sporadic case. This "no mutation detected" result is the one most likely to be misinterpreted, leading to inappropriate genetic counseling. The use of two genetic tests decreases

the rate of false-negative results. DNA sequencing is the most sensitive technique for this purpose and its use is advocated whenever a negative result is obtained by IVSP or SSCP for affected members with a strong family history. Even if the APC gene or all five DNA mismatch repair genes are fully sequenced, there will still be a residue of false-negative results caused by mutations in the noncoding regions of those genes, locus heterogeneity, or in still-unidentified genes.

A "negative test" in patients at risk for FAP or HNPCC will rule out these disorders only if a mutation has been identified in an affected family member. If tests to identify a mutation in an affected family member are negative, a "no mutation detected" result should be considered as noninformative or inconclusive (as if no test had been performed). The correct interpretation of a negative result in mutation analysis of hereditary colorectal carcinoma syndromes is mandatory to avoid adverse outcomes, because a false-negative result may lead to lack of appropriate endoscopic surveillance. Molecular genetic testing must be coupled with appropriate genetic counseling.

Interpretation of Genetic Test Results
Familial Adenomatous Polyposis

A summary for interpreting APC genetic test results is as follows. The implication of a mutation-positive test result is that APC mutation carriers need to be informed that prophylactic colectomy is necessary when adenomatous polyps become evident. Mutation carriers require surveillance by gastroscopy for extracolonic neoplasms in the upper gastrointestinal tract. Other variant manifestations in FAP include osteomas, cutaneous cysts, and congenital hypertrophy of retinal pigment epithelium (CHRPE). When a mutation has been identified in the family, direct gene testing of relatives who have not yet been clinically assessed will distinguish between those who carry the mutation and those who do not. About 30% of FAP cases are caused by new mutations in the APC gene. In these cases, the parents will not carry this mutation and are not at risk of FAP; only descendants of the proband are at 50% risk. What are the implications of a "negative test" result versus "no mutation detected" result? A negative test result is given if the patient does not carry the mutation that is known to exist in their family. In this instance, family members are not at increased risk for developing colorectal carcinoma compared with the general population and should follow guidelines for carcinoma surveillance for that group. If the patient is affected with FAP and complete coding sequence analysis of the APC gene fails to identify a mutation, this could mean that the APC gene is not responsible for the patient's diagnosis. In this case, a "no mutation detected" result, APC gene testing has no predictive value for asymptomatic at-risk relatives. In these families, first-degree relatives should continue colorectal carcinoma surveillance annually between the ages of 12 and 25 years, every other year between the ages of 25 and 35 years, and every third year between 35 and 50 years. Family members who have not developed multiple adenomatous polyps on complete bowel examination by the age of 50 years are assumed to be unaffected by FAP. If a "no mutations detected" result occurs when an unaffected family member from an APC kindred is tested without testing an affected family member, it is important that the patient not be falsely reassured because other mechanisms may inactivate the APC gene or other genes may be involved.

APC I1307K

A mutation in the APC gene termed I1307K was found in about 6% of people of Ashkenazi Jewish descent and about 28% of Ashkenazim with a family history of colorectal carcinoma. It appears to be associated with an approximately twofold increase in colorectal carcinoma risk.[13] This alteration is a transversion of a single base from thymidine to adenine in codon 1307 of the APC gene. Analysis for this mutation is done by allele specific oligonucleotide analysis (extremely sensitive and specific) and consequently delivers a conclusive positive or negative test result. Genetic testing for this alteration is possible, but the clinical utility of such testing is uncertain. The mean age at which colorectal carcinoma occurs in people carrying the I1307K alteration is not known, nor has the natural history of colorectal carcinoma in carriers of I1307K been assessed or compared to sporadic colorectal carcinomas. No screening outcomes have been assessed in carriers of I1307K. Therefore, it is not yet known whether the I1307K carrier state should guide decisions about the age at which screening is initiated, the optimal screening strategy, or the optimal screening interval.[10]

Hereditary Nonpolyposis Colorectal Carcinoma

A summary of interpreting HNPCC genetic testing results is given below. The implication of a positive mutation result is that individuals carrying a mutation in a gene that predisposes to HNPCC should be educated on the risk of colorectal carcinoma as well as carcinoma in other sites: endometrium, stomach, small bowel, biliary tract, ovary, pancreas, renal pelvis, and ureter. The risk to age 70 years for developing any neoplasm may be as high as 90% for males and 70% for females.[79]

For mutation carriers who develop colorectal carcinoma, total abdominal colectomy with ileorectal anastomosis is recommended because the entire colonic mucosa is at risk for malignancy. Proctocolectomy may also be a consideration, because the distal rectum is also a possible site of carcinoma. Prophylactic resection may be an option for mutation carriers unwilling to undergo surveillance or when endoscopic polypectomy is difficult. It should be emphasized that there are no data on whether resection is effective in reducing overall mortality. All first-degree relatives of patients who carry a mutation in one of the mismatch repair genes should be counseled that they have a 50% chance of carrying the same mutation.

What are the implications of a negative test result versus no mutation detected? A patient who tests negative for a known family mutation is not at risk for HNPCC, because it is a conclusive negative test result. Subsequent carcinoma surveillance should be as for the general population. If a mutation in a family with strong circumstantial evidence for HNPCC has not been identified, the interpretation of a "no mutation detected" test result in the HNPCC-associated gene or genes tested is complex. It may be necessary to perform more than one screening test to strengthen the suspicion that a mutation in a mismatch repair gene exists in the family. The difference between a negative test result and a "no mutation detected" result with its subsequent implications is dependent on whether a mutation has been previously identified in the family in HNPCC families. If the person is affected with HNPCC, and no mutation was detected in hMLH1 and hMSH2 with IVSP assay and single-strand conformation polymorphism, other investigations may be offered to determine whether the patient carries a mutation in a mismatch repair gene. For example, testing for MSI in neoplastic tissue may be a worthy investment before sequencing hMLH1 and hMSH2. If no abnormality in hMLH1 and hMSH2 is found by sequencing, analysis of the rarer HNPCC-causing genes is indicated.

Caution should be exercised in providing genetic risk assessment on the basis of currently used germline mutation detection strategies. While screening for hMSH2 gene mutations in HNPCC kindreds, Xia et al[80] observed that using RT-PCR and the protein truncation test, the hMSH2 exon 13 deletion variant was found in more than 90% of individuals. This may lead to a misdiagnosis of HNPCC and has profound implications for counseling and genetic risk assessments of other family members.

Impact of Genetic Testing

Individuals need to know the implications and possible impact of genetic test results before testing. An ambiguous test result may be more distressing than a positive test result. Moreover, genetic testing often yields results that are probabilistic. The psychological burden of knowing that one is at high risk for developing a neoplasm may outweigh the possible benefits from intervention. Results of a study by Keller et al[81] suggest that expressed intention and attitude toward genetic testing do not reliably predict actual uptake of counseling or testing. The actual uptake of genetic testing for HNPCC in a clinical sample of 140 patients fulfilling clinical criteria of HNPCC was 26%. Some 60% of participants experienced pronounced distress related to their potential inheritance of the disorder compared to 35% among nonparticipants. Distress reached a clinically significant level in 28% of participants. Restricted communication within the family was observed frequently. Irrespective of groups, a positive attitude toward obtaining a gene test result predominated. Therefore, the benefits and risks of participating in genetic tests must be described before testing is begun. Undergoing early detection of colorectal carcinoma or prophylactic operation or both can save lives. Surveillance or operation can be targeted to specific sites that are more prone to neoplasia, depending on the identity of the gene. For instance, female members of HNPCC families have a 10-fold increased risk for developing endometrial carcinoma, with an age of onset 10 to 15 years earlier than the same disease in the general population. Options for intervention and early detection and provision of knowledge to other family members are common reasons why individuals seek testing for genes predisposing to carcinoma of the colon and rectum.

Gritz et al[82] examined the impact of HNPCC genetic test results on psychological outcomes among carcinoma-affected and carcinoma-unaffected participants up to 1 year after results disclosure. A total of 155 persons completed study measures before HNPCC genetic testing, and 2 weeks and 6 and 12 months after disclosure of test results. Mean scores on all outcome measures remained stable and within normal limits for carcinoma-affected participants, regardless of mutation status. Among unaffected carriers of HNPCC-predisposing mutations, mean depression, state anxiety, and carcinoma worries scores increased from baseline to 2 weeks post disclosure and decreased from 2 weeks to 6 months post disclosure. Among unaffected noncarriers, mean depression and anxiety scores did not differ, but carcinoma worries scores decreased during the same time period. Affected and unaffected carriers had higher mean test-specific distress scores at 2 weeks post disclosure compared with noncarriers in their respective groups; scores decreased for affected carriers and all unaffected participants from 2 weeks to 12 months post disclosure. Classification of participants into high- versus low-distress clusters using mean scores on baseline psychological measures predicted significantly higher or lower follow-up scores, respectively, on depression, state anxiety, quality of life, and test-specific distress measures, regardless of mutation status. Although HNPCC genetic testing does not result in long-term adverse psychological outcomes, unaffected mutation carriers may experience increased distress during the immediate postdisclosure time period. Furthermore, those with higher levels of baseline mood disturbance, lower quality of life, and lower social support may be at risk for both short- and long-term increased distress.

Examining a person's DNA has the potential for far-reaching consequences beyond the person being tested. Genetic testing can reveal information about relatives with whom we share a common genetic legacy. Despite the possible benefits of testing for susceptibility for malignancy, the uncertainty and limitations of current efforts to lower mortality or morbidity contribute to the psychosocial and ethical complexities. Genetic information must remain confidential. However, breach of confidentiality has been considered permissible if all of the following conditions are met: reasonable effort to encourage disclosure has failed, harm is likely to occur if the information is withheld, the harm is serious and avoidable, and the disease is treatable or preventable.[83] Conflict between issues of privacy and duty to forewarn family members arises because genetic information is, at once, individual and familial. Several key issues may be raised in genetic testing. First, at times genetic test results need to be interpreted in the context of the results of other family members. Second, family members should be independently and autonomously counseled. Third, the decision of each member regarding testing should be followed without coercion by other family members. Fourth, genetic test results have familial implications whether results are disclosed to other family members or not.[84]

To provide information useful in the education and counseling in individuals considering genetic testing, Lerman et al[84] conducted structured interviews with 45 first-degree relatives of colorectal carcinoma patients. Fifty-one percent of respondents indicated that they definitely would want to obtain a genetic test for colon carcinoma susceptibility when it is available. Motivation for genetic testing included the following: to know if more screening tests are needed, to learn if one's children are at risk, and to be reassured. Barriers to testing included concerns about insurance, test accuracy, and how one's family would react emotionally. Most participants anticipated that they would become depressed and anxious if they tested positive for a mutation; many would feel guilty and still worry if they tested negative. These preliminary results underscore the importance of the potential risks, benefits, and limitations of genetic testing with particular emphasis on the possibility of adverse psychological effects and implications for health insurance. Ethical issues of revealing or concealing genetic information will be debated long into the future because the potentially

enormous consequences must be carefully considered. Hadley et al[85] assessed the impact of genetic counseling and testing on the use of endoscopic screening procedures and adherence to recommended endoscopic screening guidelines in 56 symptomatic at-risk individuals in families known to carry an HNPCC mutation. They analyzed data on colonoscopy and flexible sigmoidoscopy screenings collected before genetic counseling and testing and 6 and 12 months postgenetic counseling and testing on 17 mutation-positive and 39 true-negative mutation individuals. Among mutation-negative individuals, use of colonoscopy and flexible sigmoidoscopy decreased significantly between pre- and postgenetic counseling and testing. Among mutation-positive individuals, a nonsignificant increase in use was noted. Age was also associated with use of endoscopic screening after genetic counseling and testing. More mutation-negative individuals strictly adhered to guidelines than did mutation-positive individuals (87 vs. 65%). They concluded genetic counseling and testing for HNPCC significantly influences the use of colonic endoscopy and adherence to recommendations for colon carcinoma screening.

Patients considering genetic testing need to be informed about the potential for genetic discrimination. This is of great concern for asymptomatic family members, because disclosure of a positive mutation result to third parties could be used to limit, raise rates for, or deny access to individual health insurance. However, nondisclosure could nullify a patient's insurance contract.

A survey of medical directors of United States life insurance companies indicated that familial colon or breast carcinoma constituted sufficient grounds to deny insurance (1 of the 27) or charge higher premiums (6 of the 27), despite not having actuarial data to support underwriting (calculating premiums) guidelines pertaining to these carcinomas.

In the United States, several states have safeguards against the potential misuse of genetic information. The potential for misuse of genetic information has led to federal initiatives in the United States to regulate the use of genetic information. In the context of insurance and employment, it is unclear whether the Americans with Disabilities Act of 1990 (ADA) will provide adequate protection to carriers of carcinoma-susceptibility genes, because the Equal Employment Opportunity Commission does not view a person with genetic predisposition for a disease or a carrier of a gene for a late-onset disorder as having a disability. This implies that these persons are not protected under the ADA. Legislation has been introduced to extend the definition of disability to "genetic or medically identified potential of or predisposition toward a physical or mental impairment that substantially limits a major life activity." For now, the ADA has been interpreted to offer protection only to those who develop symptoms.

Health Insurance Portability and Accountability Act (Kennedy–Kassebaum bill) came into effect in the summer of 1997. It defined genetic information as part of an individual's health status. This act was implemented to prohibit employers and insurers from excluding individuals in a group from coverage or charging higher premiums on the basis of health status. Also in 1997, the Genetic Information Nondiscrimination in Health Insurance Act (Slaughter–Snowe bill) called for a ban of the use of "genetic information" in denying or setting rates for group health insurance. In this act, genetic information was defined broadly to include genetic tests as well as information about inherited features. This bill called for a limit on the collection or disclosure of genetic information without the written consent of the individual.

Fourteen states have enacted legislation to provide safeguards and to protect misuse of genetic information by insurers and employers. Other states have followed suit, and amendments are being made to those existing laws in some states, as reviewed by Offit.[86]

In summary, individuals undergoing genetic testing should understand the advantages and disadvantages of receiving and sharing genetic results. Attempting to protect the individual from genetic discrimination by disseminating results to only a few selected medical staff could impede care. So far, there has been no substantial use of genetic information by health insurers, and laws restricting its use have thus far maintained social fairness in the area of health insurance. When integrated with existing testing protocols for colorectal carcinoma and when applied with appropriate caveats particularly regarding interpretation of negative results, genetic testing can result in improved management of patients and families.

Alternate Pathway of Carcinogenesis

An understanding of the mechanisms that explain the initiation and early evolution of colorectal carcinoma should facilitate the development of new approaches to effective prevention and intervention. Jass et al[87] have proposed a model for colorectal neoplasia in which APC mutation is not placed at the point of initiation. Other genes implicated in the regulation of apoptosis and DNA repair may underlie the early development of colorectal carcinoma. Inactivation of these genes may occur not by mutation or loss but through silencing mediated by methylation of the gene's promoter region. hMLH1 and MGMT are examples of DNA repair genes that are silenced by methylation. Loss of expression of hMLH1 and MGMT protein has been demonstrated immunohistochemically in serrated polyps. Multiple lines of evidence point to a "serrated" pathway of neoplasia that is driven by inhibition of apoptosis and the subsequent inactivation of DNA repair genes by promoter methylation. The earliest lesions in this pathway are aberrant crypt foci (ACF). These may develop into hyperplastic polyps or transform while still of microscopic size into admixed polyps, serrated adenomas, or traditional adenomas. Carcinomas developing from these lesions may show high- or low-level MSI (MSI-H and MSI-L, respectively) or may be microsatellite stable (MSS). The suggested clinical model for this alternative pathway is the condition hyperplastic polyposis. Hyperplastic polyposis presents a plausible model for the following reasons:

1. Polyps in this condition may show MSI and silencing of relevant DNA repair genes including hMLH1.

2. Methylation is demonstrated in DNA extracted from hyperplastic polyps in a subset of subjects with hyperplastic polyposis. The finding of methylation is concordant within multiple polyps in such cases, whereas discordant findings occur in subjects with multiple adenomas.

3. The requisite plasticity in methylator pathways is evident in hyperplastic polyposis in which all types of epithelial polyp may occur (hyperplastic, admixed, serrated adenoma, and traditional adenoma), and carcinomas may be MSI-H, MSI-L, or MSS (even within the same subject).

4. The condition hyperplastic polyposis may be familial. Jass et al[87] believe that molecular and morphologic observations have stripped the hyperplastic polyp of its long-presumed innocence. However, the fact that the vast majority of hyperplastic polyps will never progress to carcinoma has not altered. It is impractical to advocate the removal of every minute hyperplastic lesion. On the other hand, more attention might be given to subjects with "high-risk" hyperplastic polyps. High-risk features would include multiplicity (more than 20), size (greater than 10 mm), proximal location, associated polyps with dysplasia, and a family history of colorectal carcinoma. New diagnostic criteria and markers are required to distinguish innocent hyperplastic polyps from their serrated counterparts with a malignant potential that belies their deceptively bland morphology.

21.2.4 Dietary Factors

Dietary factors have been implicated in the etiology of colorectal carcinoma. Prime candidates are dietary fats and fiber-deficient diets. Studies thus far have been inconclusive with respect to which component is most important. Experimental, epidemiological, and clinical evidence shows that diets consumed by Western populations have an important role in the modulation of this disease.[88] The diet contains various mutagens and carcinogens that can be classified into three groups: naturally occurring chemicals that include mycotoxins and plant alkaloids,[1] synthetic compounds exemplified by food additives and pesticides,[2] and compounds produced by cooking,[3] which include polycyclic aromatic hydrocarbons and heterocyclic amines.[89] Since heterocyclic amines are genotoxic compounds, a causal role in some stage of human colon carcinogenesis is plausible.[90]

Fat

Populations with diets high in unsaturated fat and protein, especially if associated with low-fiber ingestion, are associated with a high incidence of colorectal carcinoma. In a Canadian study, patients with colon carcinoma reported a higher intake of total fat, saturated fat, and dietary cholesterol than controls, with the highest RR in saturated fat.[91] In a prospective cohort study of diet and colon carcinoma, Willett et al[92] gathered information on 98,464 nurses. Among the 150 nurses who developed colon carcinoma, the trend for risk with total fat intake ($p < 0.05$) and animal fat ($p < 0.01$) was significant. Animal fat from dairy sources (e.g., butter or ice cream) was not associated with risk. A study by Nigro et al[89] found that animals fed 35% beef fat develop more colon carcinoma than those fed 5% beef fat. Reddy and Maruyana[93] found that a diet containing 20% of either corn or safflower oil increased the incidence of colon carcinoma in animals much more than in those fed 5% of the same fat. Not only is the amount of fat important, but also the type may be equally important. Diets containing high levels of olive oil, coconut oil, or fish oil did not increase the incidence of colon carcinoma more than in animals fed 5% of the same fats. The mechanism of action is believed to be indirect, with the resulting high concentration of fecal bile acids and cholesterol stimulating cell proliferation and acting as promoters of carcinogenesis. However, this seemingly neat hypothesis is not universally accepted. It must be noted that the role of dietary fat is inextricably linked to excretion of bile acids and the ratio of anaerobic to aerobic bacteria.

Meat and Fish

Consumption of red and processed meat has been associated with colorectal carcinoma in many but not all epidemiological studies. Chao et al[94] examined the relationship between recent and long-term meat consumption and the risk of incident colon and rectal carcinoma. A cohort of 148,610 adults aged 50 to 74 years (median, 63 years), residing in 21 states with population-based registries, who provided information on meat consumption in 1982 and again in 1992/1993 were enrolled in the Cancer Prevention Study II Nutrition Cohort. Follow-up identified 1,667 incident colorectal carcinomas. Participants contributed person-years at risk until death or a diagnosis of colon or rectal carcinoma. High intake of red and processed meat reported in 1992/1993 was associated with higher risk of distal colon carcinoma after adjusting for age and energy intake but not after further adjustment for body mass index, cigarette smoking, and other covariates. When long-term consumption was considered, persons in the highest tertile of consumption in both 1982 and 1992/1993 had higher risk of distal colon carcinoma associated with processed meat (RR, 1.50) and ratio of red meat to poultry and fish (RR, 1.53) relative to those persons in the lowest tertile at both time points. Long-term consumption of poultry and fish was inversely associated with risk of both proximal and distal colon carcinoma. High consumption of red meat reported in 1992/1993 was associated with a higher risk of rectal carcinoma (RR, 1.71) as was high consumption reported in both 1982 and 1992/1993 (RR, 1.43). Their results strengthen the evidence that prolonged high consumption of red and processed meat may increase the risk of carcinoma in the distal portion of the large intestine.

Larsson et al[95] prospectively examined whether the association of red meat consumption with carcinoma risk varies by subsite within the large bowel. They analyzed data from 61,433 women aged 40 to 75 years and free from diagnosed carcinoma at baseline. Diet was assessed at baseline using a self-administered food-frequency questionnaire. Over a mean follow-up of 13.9 years, they identified 234 proximal colon carcinomas, 155 distal colon carcinomas, and 230 rectal carcinomas. They observed a significant positive association between red meat consumption and risk of distal colon carcinoma but not of the proximal colon or rectum. The multivariate rate ratio for women who consumed 94 g/d or more of red meat compared to those who consumed less than 50 g/d was 2.22 for the distal colon, 1.03 for proximal colon, and 1.28 for rectum. Although there was no association between consumption of fish and risk of carcinoma at any subsite, poultry consumption was weakly inversely related to risk of total colorectal carcinoma.

Norat et al[96] prospectively followed 478,040 men and women from 10 European countries who were free of carcinoma at enrollment. After a mean follow-up of 4.8 years, 1,329 incident colorectal carcinomas were documented. Colorectal carcinoma risk was positively associated with intake of red and processed meat (highest [> 160 g/d] and lowest [< 20 g/d]; HR = 1.35) and inversely associated with intake of fish (> 80 vs. < 10 g/d, HR = 0.69), but was not related to poultry intake. In this study population, the absolute risk of development of colorectal carcinoma

within 10 years for a study subject aged 50 years was 1.71% for the highest category of red and processed meat intake and 1.28% for the lowest category of intake and was 1.86% for subjects in the lowest category of fish intake and 1.28% for subjects in the highest category of fish intake. Their data confirmed that colorectal carcinoma risk is positively associated with high consumption of red and processed meat and support an inverse association with fish intake.

Fiber

Following his observation of the low incidence of colorectal carcinoma in African natives, Burkitt[97] promoted the idea that their high-fiber intake was responsible for this finding. He further deduced that the Western low-fiber diet along with high carbohydrate and animal fat intake was responsible for the higher incidence of malignancy of the large bowel. Burkitt also noted that when Africans abandon their customary diet, the incidence of carcinoma of the colorectum progressively increases. Diets with a high roughage content result in the production of soft frequent stools. A potential carcinogen in a patient with infrequent stools remains in contact with the colonic and rectal mucosa longer.

Experimental work by Fleiszer et al[98] has supported this thesis in that a high-fiber diet resulted in a diminished incidence of dimethylhydrazine (DMH) induced carcinoma of the colon in rats. Yet the potential protective effect of fiber is controversial. A study by Nigro et al[99] in which a group of rats was given a 30% beef fat and 10% fiber diet, demonstrated no protective effect from wheat bran or cellulose. Animals fed 5% fat and 20 or 30% fiber developed fewer carcinomas than fiber-free controls. This finding suggests that a large quantity of fat can overcome the protective effect of fiber.

From an epidemiologic point of view, Greenwald et al[100] analyzed 55 original reports and found evidence of an inverse association between a high fiber diet and the risk of colon carcinoma. The same group conducted a meta-analysis of 12 methodologically sound and descriptively complete case-control studies and showed protection with an OR of 0.57 (95% confidence interval [CI], 0.50–0.64).[101] Those studies delineating vegetable fiber from total fiber suggested a stronger protective effect from vegetable fiber. Freudenheim et al[103] conducted a case-control study of 850 pairs in which the fiber source was subdivided from grain, fruit, and vegetables and in which the results of consuming soluble versus insoluble fiber were also compared. Fruit and vegetable fiber provided protection against rectal carcinoma in men and women and against colon carcinoma in men. Grain fiber provided protection against colon carcinoma only. Insoluble fractions of grain fiber were more protective in the colon, with both soluble and insoluble fractions from fruit and vegetables protective in the rectum. In a follow-up of 11 years of a German cohort of 1,904 patients, the mortality rate for patients with colon carcinoma was reduced for individuals following a vegetarian lifestyle for over 20 years.[102]

A study with contrary findings was reported. Asano and McLeod[104] conducted a systematic review and meta-analysis to assess the effect of dietary fiber on the incidence or recurrence of colorectal adenomas, the incidence of colorectal carcinoma, and the development of adverse events. Five studies with 4,349 subjects met the inclusion criteria. The interventions were wheat bran fiber, ispaghula husk, or a comprehensive dietary intervention with high fiber whole food sources alone or in combination. When the data were combined there was no difference between the intervention and control groups. The reviewers concluded there is currently no evidence from randomized clinical trials to suggest that increased dietary fiber intake will reduce the incidence or recurrence of adenomatous polyps within a two- to four-year period. Fuchs et al[105] conducted a prospective study of 88,757 women who were 34 to 59 years old and had no history of carcinoma, inflammatory bowel disease, or familial polyposis. During a 16-year follow-up period, 787 cases of colorectal carcinoma were documented. In addition, 1,012 patients with adenomas of the distal colon and rectum were found among 27,530 participants who underwent endoscopy during the follow-up period. After adjustment for age, established risk factors, and total energy intake, they found no association between the intake of dietary fiber and the risk of colorectal carcinoma or colorectal adenoma. The same investigators found no protective effect of fruit or vegetable consumption.[106] Conversely, Terry et al[107] found that total fruit and vegetable consumption was inversely associated with the risk of the development of colorectal carcinoma whereas they observed no association between colorectal carcinoma risk and consumption of cereal fiber. Michels et al[106] prospectively investigated the association between fruit and vegetable consumption and the incidence of colon and rectal carcinoma in two large cohorts: the Nurses' Health Study (88,764 women) and the Health Professionals' Follow-up Study (47,325 men). With a follow-up including 1,743,645 person-years and 937 cases of colon carcinoma, they found little association of colon carcinoma incidence with fruit and vegetable consumption. Although fruit and vegetables may confer protection against some chronic diseases, their frequent consumption did not appear to confer protection from colon and rectal carcinoma in this study. Peters et al[108] used a 137-item food-frequency questionnaire to assess the relation of fiber intake and frequency of colorectal adenoma. The study was done within the prostate, lung, colorectal, ovarian (PLCO) Cancer Screening Trial, a randomized controlled trial designed to investigate methods for early detection of carcinoma. In their analysis, they compared fiber intake of 33,971 participants who were sigmoidoscopy-negative for polyps, with 3,591 cases with at least one histologically verified adenoma in the distal large bowel (i.e., descending colon, sigmoid colon, or rectum). High intakes of dietary fiber were associated with a low risk of colorectal adenoma, after adjustment for potential dietary and nondietary risk factors. Participants in the highest quintile of dietary fiber intake had a 27% lower risk of adenoma than those in the lowest quintile. The inverse association was strongest for fiber from grains and cereals than from fruits. Risks were similar for advanced and nonadvanced adenoma. Risk of rectal adenoma was not significantly associated with fiber intake. Why these two studies reached different results is impossible to answer. The use of different types or sources and amounts of fiber may be one explanation.

In a population-based case-control study, Meyer and White[109] found for both sexes that a higher dietary fiber intake was associated with lower RR for colon carcinoma. Howe et al[110] examined the effects of fiber, vitamin C, and beta-carotene intakes on colorectal carcinoma risk in a combined analysis of data

from 13 case-control studies previously conducted in populations with differing colorectal carcinoma rates and dietary practices. Original data records for 5,287 case subjects with colorectal carcinoma and 10,470 control subjects without disease were combined. Risk decreased as fiber intake increased; RR were 0.79, 0.69, 0.63, and 0.53 for the four highest quintiles of intake compared with the lowest quintile. The inverse association with fiber is seen in 12 of the 13 studies and is similar in magnitude for left- and right-sided colon and rectal carcinomas, for men and for women, and for different age groups. In contrast, after adjustment for fiber intake, only weak inverse associations are seen for the intakes of vitamin C and beta-carotene. This analysis provided substantive evidence that intake of fiber-rich foods is inversely related to risk of carcinomas of both the colon and rectum. If causality is assumed, they estimated that risk of colorectal carcinoma in the United States population could be reduced by 31% (55,000 cases annually) by an average increase in fiber intake from food sources of about 13 g/d, corresponding to an average increase of about 70%. Bingham et al reached the same conclusion. In the biggest study ever published Bingham et al[111] prospectively examined the association between dietary fiber and incidence of colorectal carcinoma in 519,978 individuals aged 25 to 70 years taking part in a study recruited from 10 European countries. Participants completed a dietary questionnaire in 1992 to 1998 and were followed up for the incidence of carcinoma. Follow-up consisted of 1,939,011 person-years, and data for 1,065 reported cases of colorectal carcinoma were included in the analysis. Dietary fiber in foods was inversely related to the incidence of large bowel carcinoma (adjusted RR of 0.75 for the highest vs. lowest quintile of intake), the protective effect being greatest for the left side of the colon, and least for the rectum. After calibration with more detailed dietary data, the adjusted risk for the highest versus lowest quintile of fiber from food intake was 0.58. No food source of fiber was significantly more protective than others, and nonfood supplement sources of fiber were not investigated. They concluded, in populations with low average intake of dietary fiber, an approximate doubling of total fiber intake from foods could reduce the risk of colorectal carcinoma by 40%.

Calcium Deficiency

Slattery et al[112] observed that the dietary intake of calcium decreased the risk of development of colon carcinoma. Calcium can bind intraluminally with bile acids and fatty acids, thus reducing their mitogenic effect.[113] Calcium salts may have antiproliferative effects in the colon of patients who are predisposed to developing large bowel carcinoma.[114] Dietary supplementation with calcium reduces colonic crypt cell production in both normal and hyperplastic mucosa. One of the main pathways used by extracellular calcium to exert its chemopreventive actions is through activation of a calcium-sensing receptor. This results in increased levels of intracellular calcium, inducing a wide range of biological effects, some of which restrain the growth and promote the differentiation of transformed colon cells.[88] Calcium likely reduces lipid damage in the colon by complexing with fat to form mineral-fat complexes or soaps.[115] It has been shown in an increasing number of animal experiments that calcium has the ability to inhibit colon carcinoma. In limited studies in man, the colonic hyperproliferation associated with increased risk of colon carcinoma has been reversed for short periods by the administration of supplemental dietary calcium. In a population-based case-control study, Meyer and White[109] showed that calcium was associated with a decreased risk of colon carcinoma in women only. Baron et al[116] conducted a randomized double-blind trial of the effect of supplementation with calcium carbonate on recurrence of colorectal adenomas. They randomly assigned 930 subjects (mean age, 61 years; 72% men) with a recent history of colorectal adenomas to receive either calcium carbonate (3 g [1,200 mg of elemental calcium] daily) or placebo, with follow-up colonoscopies 1 and 4 years after the qualifying examination. Among the 913 subjects who underwent at least one study colonoscopy, the adjusted risk ratio for any recurrence of adenoma with calcium as compared with placebo was 0.85. At least one adenoma was diagnosed between the first and second follow-up endoscopies in 127 subjects in the calcium group (31%) and 159 subjects in the placebo group (38%). The effect of calcium was independent of initial dietary fat and calcium intake. They concluded calcium supplementation is associated with a significant—though moderate—reduction in the risk of recurrent adenomas. Wu et al[117] examined the association between calcium intake and colon carcinoma risk in two prospective cohorts, the Nurses' Health Study and the Health Professionals Follow-up Study. Their study population included 87,998 women in the former and 47,344 men in the latter. During the follow-up period, 15 years for the Nurses' Health Study cohort, and 10 years for the Health Professionals Follow-up Study, 626 and 399 colon carcinomas were identified in women and men, respectively. In women and men considered together, they found an inverse association between high total calcium intake (>1,250 vs. < 500 mg/day) and distal colon carcinoma (women RR = 0.73, men RR = 0.58, and pooled RR = 0.65). No such association was found for proximal colon carcinoma (women RR = 1.28, men RR = 0.92, and pooled RR = 1.14). The incremental benefit of additional calcium intake beyond approximately 700 mg/d appeared to be minimal.

Wallace et al[118] examined the effect of calcium on the risk of different types of colorectal lesions. They used patients from the Calcium Polyp Prevention Study, a randomized double-blind, placebo-controlled chemoprevention trial among patients with a recent colorectal adenoma in which 930 patients were randomly assigned to calcium carbonate (1,200 mg/d) or placebo. Follow-up colonoscopies were conducted approximately 1 and 4 years after the qualifying examination. The calcium risk ratio for hyperplastic polyps was 0.82, that for tubular adenomas was 0.89, and that for histologically advanced neoplasms was 0.65 compared with patients assigned to placebo. There were no statistically significant differences between the risk ratio for tubular adenomas and that for other types of polyps. The effect of calcium supplementation on adenoma risk was most pronounced among individuals with high dietary intakes of calcium and fiber and with low intake of fat, but the interactions were not statistically significant. Their results suggest that calcium supplementation may have a more pronounced antineoplastic effect on advanced colorectal lesions than on other types of polyps. Taken together, the available evidence suggests that increases in the daily intake of calcium in the diet may provide a means of colorectal carcinoma control.

Although a positive effect has not been proven, it might be prudent for the public to consume diets that contain adequate amounts of calcium.

Magnesium

Larsson et al[119] suggested that a high magnesium intake may reduce the occurrence of colorectal carcinoma in women. In a population-based prospective cohort of 61,433 women aged 40 to 75 years without previous diagnosis of carcinoma at baseline and a mean of 14.8 years (911,042 person-years) of follow-up, 805 incident colorectal carcinoma cases were diagnosed. Compared with women in the lowest quintile of magnesium intake, the multivariate rate ratio was 0.59 for those in the highest quintile. The inverse association was observed for both colon (RR, 0.66) and rectal carcinoma (RR, 0.45).

Micronutrients and Chemical Inhibitors

In geographic regions where the trace element selenium is found to be lacking, there is a higher incidence of colorectal carcinoma, while high selenium areas have low colorectal carcinoma rates.[120] Significantly decreased selenium concentrations in blood samples from patients with colorectal carcinomas and various adenomas have been found when compared to normal controls.[121]

High selenium broccoli decreased the incidence of aberrant crypts in rats with chemically induced colon carcinomas by more than 50% compared with controls.[122] In a case-control study, Nelson et al[123] found that higher levels of selenium produced a protective effect against colon polyps or carcinomas. Jacobs et al[124] conducted a combined analysis of data from three randomized trials—the Wheat Bran Fiber Trial, the Polyp Prevention Trial, and the Polyp Prevention Study, which tested the effects of various nutritional interventions for colorectal adenoma prevention among participants who recently had an adenoma removed during colonoscopy. Selenium concentrations were measured from blood specimens from a total of 1,763 trial participants, and quartiles of baseline selenium were established from pooled data. Analyses of the pooled data showed that individuals whose blood selenium values were in the highest quartile (median = 150 ng/mL) had statistically significantly lower odds of developing a new adenoma compared with those in the lowest quartile (OR = 0.66). They concluded the inverse association between higher blood selenium concentration and adenoma risk supports previous findings indicating that higher selenium status may be related to decreased risk of colorectal carcinoma.

A number of micronutrients and chemicals have been shown to have an inhibitory effect on the development of colorectal carcinoma: phenols, indoles, plant sterols, selenium, calcium, vitamins A, C, and E, and carotenoids.[125] They are present in small amounts in water and in whole grain cereals, fruits, and vegetables. The chemicals in foods that inhibit carcinoma development in laboratory animals have been summarized by Wargovich.[126] They include plant phenols (in grapes, strawberries, and apples), dithiothiones and flavones (in cabbage, broccoli, brussels sprouts, and cauliflower), thioethers (in garlic, onions, and leeks), terpenes (in citrus fruits), and carotenoids (in carrots, yams, and watermelon). Some chemicals not present in the average diet affect the carcinogenic process in animals. Prostaglandin inhibitors and chemicals that influence cell proliferation and differentiation are examples.[127] Some of these agents may be toxic, so the feasibility of administering a combination of agents was studied experimentally by Nigro et al.[128] By the addition of small nontoxic amounts of selenium, 13-cis-retinoic acid, and beta-sitosterol, an additive inhibitory effect resulted in a significant diminution of intestinal carcinoma. Other combinations also have been found effective.[125] Ascorbic acid, diallyl sulfide, and thioether found in garlic and onions also may aid in prevention.[126,129]

Most of the pleiotropic actions of vitamin D are mediated by binding to a nuclear receptor that interacts with specific consensus sites in promoters of specific genes, resulting in downregulation or upregulation of their expression. The actions of vitamin D involve cross-talk with growth factors/cytokines, inhibitory effects on the cell cycle, and stimulation of apoptosis.[88]

Folate lies at the intersection of metabolic pathways involved in DNA methylation and biosynthesis. Three main mechanisms by which decreased levels of folate (and of other dietary one-carbon donors) might increase the risk of carcinoma are alteration of the normal DNA methylation process; imbalance of the steady-state level of DNA precursors, leading to aberrant DNA synthesis and repair; and chromosome and chromatin change.[88]

Alcohol Ingestion

A relationship between alcohol ingestion and development of colorectal carcinoma has been reported (OR, 2.6),[109] specifically the development of rectal carcinoma in association with beer consumption.[4] Daily alcohol drinkers experience a twofold increase in risk of colorectal carcinomas.[130] The positive association had been accounted for primarily by an increased risk of carcinoma in men whose monthly consumption of beer was 15 L or more.[131,132] Beer drinking increases the risk 1.3 to 2.4 times.[132,133,134,135,136,137,138,139,140,141,142,143,144,145,146,147,148,149,150,151,152,153,154,155,156,157,158] In a study of 6,230 Swedish brewery workers, the RR for rectal carcinoma was 1.7, while the risk of colon carcinoma was not significantly increased, supporting the hypothesis that high beer consumption is associated with an increased risk of rectal carcinoma.[136] Newcomb et al[133] found that high levels of alcohol consumption in women (11 or more drinks per week) were associated with an increased risk of large intestinal carcinoma (RR = 1.47).

Maekawa[137] reported that the heavy cumulative intake of alcohol was associated with significantly higher risk of colorectal carcinoma than in nondrinkers (OR = 6.8). The association of alcohol intake with the risk of colorectal carcinoma was not affected by the type of alcoholic beverage. Sharpe et al[138] found the daily consumption of alcohol of any type was associated with increased risks of carcinoma of the distal colon (OR = 2.3), and the rectum (OR = 1.6) but not with an increased risk of a carcinoma of the proximal colon (OR = 1.0).

Smoking

The association of smoking (OR for > 40 pack-years, 3.31) with adenomas (and by implication carcinoma) has been reported.[139] Smoking for 20 years has a strong relation to adenomas, but an induction period of at least 35 years is necessary for colorectal carcinoma.[140,141] Chao[142] examined cigarette smoking in relation to colorectal carcinoma mortality, evaluating smoking duration and intensity, and controlling for potential confounders in the Cancer Prevention Study II. This prospective nationwide mortality study of 1,184,657 adults (age > 30 years) was begun by the American Cancer Society in 1982. After exclusions, their analytic cohort included 312,332 men and 469,019 women, among whom 4,432 colon or rectal carcinoma deaths occurred between 1982 and 1996 among individuals who were carcinoma free in 1982. Multivariate-adjusted colorectal carcinoma mortality rates were highest among current smokers, intermediate among former smokers, and lowest in lifelong nonsmokers. The multivariate-adjusted relative rate for current compared with never smokers was 1.32 among men and 1.41 among women. Increased risk was evident after 20 or more years of smoking for men and women combined as compared with never smokers. Risk among current and former smokers increased with duration of smoking and average number of cigarettes smoked per day; risk in former smokers decreased significantly in years since quitting. If the multivariate-adjusted relative rate estimates in this study do, in fact, reflect causality, then approximately 12% of colorectal carcinoma deaths among both men and women in the general U.S. population in 1997 were attributable to smoking.

Clinical Dietary Studies

A number of case control studies have been reported. Jain et al[143] examined patients with large bowel malignancy and compared them with population and hospital controls. An increased risk was found in persons with an increased intake of saturated fat as well as calories, total protein, total fat, oleic acid, and cholesterol. The strongest effect was that of saturated fat. Potter and McMichael[144] found that dietary protein was the strongest predictor of colon carcinoma with a twofold to threefold RR. In a review, Kritchevsky[145] reported that studies for specific vegetables have been carried out with carrots, broccoli, cabbage, lettuce, potatoes, and legumes. Of a total of 105 studies, 67% have shown no association.

Prospective studies have examined the relationship between diet and subsequent development of colorectal carcinoma. Phillips and Snowdon[146] found a positive association for the risk of colon carcinoma with egg consumption, coffee intake, and weight greater than 125% of ideal weight. No association was noted for use of meat, cheese, milk, or green salad. Garland et al[113] failed to note any association between dietary fat, animal or vegetable protein, ethanol, or energy intake and subsequent colorectal carcinoma. The authors did note a negative association between vitamin D and calcium intake and subsequent colorectal carcinoma. Stemmerman et al[147] studied the relationship between the intake of dietary fat and subsequent colorectal carcinoma during a 15-year follow-up in 7,074 Japanese men and found a negative association between dietary total fat and saturated fat intake and colon carcinoma. The strongest effect was found in the right colon, whereas in contrast a weak positive relationship was found in the rectum. Berry et al,[148] in a study of patients undergoing colonoscopy, analyzed fatty acid and plasma lipid analogs and found that the quality of dietary fat did not influence the development of carcinoma or neoplastic polyps in their population.

The fact that in most high-risk countries there is a positive association between fat or meat intake and risk of large bowel malignancy, but results are inconsistent in low-risk countries, implies that there is perhaps a threshold effect by which a minimal level of fat or meat is necessary to effect the development of colorectal carcinoma. There may be a confounding factor whereby dietary fat or protein increases the risk in persons eating low-fiber diets. In a case-control study of pathologically confirmed, single primary carcinomas of the rectum, the risk of rectal carcinoma increased with an increasing intake of kilocalories, fat, carbohydrate, and iron.[149] The risk decreased with an increasing intake of carotenoids, vitamin C, and dietary fiber from vegetables. Fiber from grains, calcium, retinal, and vitamin E were not associated with risk. Associations of intake with risk were generally stronger for men than for women, except with vitamin C. The associations for carotenoids, vitamin C, and vegetable fiber persisted after stratification on intake of either kilocalories or fat.

Giovannucci et al[150] evaluated the relationship between folate intake and incidence of colon carcinoma in a prospective cohort study of 88,756 women from the Nurses' Health Study. There were 442 with new cases of colon carcinoma. Higher folate intake was related to a lower risk of colon carcinoma (relative ratio 0.69) for intake greater than 400 mg/d compared with intake less than or equal to 200 mg/d after controlling for age; family history of colon carcinoma; aspirin use; smoking; body mass; physical activity; and intake of red meat, alcohol, methionine, and fiber. When intake of vitamins C, D, and E and intake of calcium were also controlled for, results were similar. Women who used multivitamins containing folic acid had no benefit with respect to colon carcinoma after 4 years of use. After15 years of use, risk was markedly lower (relative ratio 0.25) representing 15 instead of 68 new cases of colon carcinoma per 10,000 women of 55 to 69 years of age. Folate from dietary sources alone was related to a modest reduction in risk for colon carcinoma and the benefit of long-term multivitamin use was present across all levels of dietary intakes. In a large study designed to determine the relationship between fish consumption and risk of the development of carcinoma, Fernandez et al[151] noted a consistent pattern of protection against the risk of selected malignancies: colon OR 0.6 and rectum OR 0.5.

21.2.5 Radiation

There have been sporadic reports of carcinoma of the colon and rectum that develops after radiation therapy for a variety of pelvic malignancies.[152,153,154,155,156,157] The average interval between irradiation and the diagnosis of rectal carcinoma is 15.2 years with a range from 14 months to 33 years.[155] There is controversy as to whether the relationship is one of cause and effect or purely coincidental. The characteristics are different from ordinary large bowel carcinoma in that there is a high incidence of mucin-producing carcinoma (53%).[156] Radiation injury was observed in 64% of cases.[156]

Radiation therapy for prostate carcinoma has been associated with an increased rate of pelvic malignancies, particularly bladder carcinoma. Baxter et al[158] conducted a retrospective cohort study using Surveillance, Epidemiology, and End Results (SEER) registry data. They focused on men with prostate carcinoma,

but with no previous history of colorectal carcinoma, treated with either surgery or radiation who survived at least 5 years. They evaluated the effect of radiation on development of carcinoma for three sites: definitely irradiated sites (rectum), potentially irradiated sites (rectosigmoid, sigmoid, and cecum), and nonirradiated sites (the rest of the colon). A total of 30,552 men received radiation, and 55,263 underwent surgery only. Colorectal carcinomas developed in 1,437 patients: 267 in irradiated sites, 686 in potentially irradiated sites, and 484 in nonirradiated sites. Radiation was independently associated with development of carcinoma over time in irradiated sites but not in the remainder of the colon. The adjusted hazards ratio (HR) for development of rectal carcinoma was 1.7 for the radiation group, compared with the surgery only group. Radiation had no effect on development of carcinoma in the remainder of the colon, indicating that the effect is specific to directly irradiated tissue. Hareyama et al[157] described some characteristics of radiation-associated rectal carcinoma. All four of their patients presented with chronic radiation colitis. Radiation-associated rectal carcinoma has a tendency to be diagnosed in the advanced stage and to have a poor prognosis. Since there are no reliable clinical or laboratory indicators of the presence of a curable colorectal carcinoma in the setting of chronic radiation proctocolitis, they recommend surveillance with colonoscopy every 10 years after irradiation in patients with previous pelvic radiotherapy.

21.2.6 Ureteric Implantation

Several reports have documented the development of neoplasia at or near the site of a ureterosigmoidostomy.[159,160,161,162,163,164] The risk of sigmoid carcinoma has been estimated to be anywhere from 8.5 to 10.5 and 80 to 550 times greater in patients with ureterosigmoidostomy than in the normal population.[163,164] Adenomatous polyps at the level of the ureterosigmoidostomy may be precursors of a subsequent carcinoma. The interval between the implantation of ureters and the occurrence of colonic carcinoma varies from 5 to 41 years. Husmann and Spence[165] reviewed the literature to 1990 and found 94 patients who had colonic neoplasia after ureterosigmoidostomy for vesical exstrophy. The average patient age at diagnosis of neoplasia was 33 years with an average latency of 26 years. Blood in the stool and symptoms and signs of ureteral obstruction were cardinal warning signs. Treatment consisted of local extirpation of the lesion with reimplantation of one or both ureters back into the sigmoid in one third of patients. The preferred treatment is either endoscopic destruction of polyps after biopsy or resection of the involved segment with cutaneous loop diversions. If the polyp is located at the mouth of or immediately adjacent to the ureterocolic anastomosis, caution must be exercised to avoid obstruction of the orifice as a result of vigorous electrocautery. Death from carcinoma occurred in 30 of 49 patients. The current trend is away from this type of urinary diversion, but for those individuals who have already had this operation, periodic endoscopic surveillance appears to be in order.

21.2.7 Cholecystectomy

There is considerable epidemiologic evidence to suggest that bile acids play an important role in the development of colorectal malignancy, but their precise action in the initiation or promotion of the neoplastic process remains to be determined.[166] A suggested explanation is that, although before cholecystectomy the bile acid pool circulates two or three times per meal, after cholecystectomy the pool circulates even during fasting. This enhanced circulation results in increased exposure of bile acids to the degrading action of intestinal bacteria, a step in the formation of known carcinogens. Hill[167] has noted a concentration of bile acids in populations of the United States and England that is seven times higher than that in Uganda and India. Populations with a high incidence of colorectal carcinoma have high fecal bile acid concentrations in comparison with those with a low incidence. A high proportion of anaerobic bacteria in these populations caused degradation of bile acids to form known carcinogens. Both deoxycholic and lithocholic acids have been shown to be promoters of colon carcinoma in animal models. These secondary bile acids are the products of bacterial dehydroxylation of the primary bile acids cholic and chenodeoxycholic acid, respectively. The primary bile acids are not promoters of carcinogenesis. Jorgensen and Rafaelsen[168] compared the prevalence of gallstone disease in 145 consecutive patients with colorectal carcinoma with gallstone prevalence in 4,159 subjects randomly selected from a population. The group of patients had a significantly higher prevalence of gallstone disease than the population (OR, 1.59), whereas cholecystectomies occurred with equal frequency in the two groups. There was a nonsignificant trend toward more right-sided carcinomas in patients with gallstones than in patients without gallstones.

Schernhammer et al[169] conducted a prospective study of 85,184 women, 877 of whom developed colorectal carcinoma. They found a significant positive association between cholecystectomy and the risk of colorectal carcinoma (RR = 1.21). The risk was highest for carcinomas of the proximal colon (RR = 1.34) and the rectum (RR = 1.58). Lagergren et al[170] evaluated cholecystectomy and risk of bowel carcinoma with a slightly different result. Cholecystectomized patients identified through the Swedish Inpatient Register were followed up for subsequent carcinoma. In total, 278,460 cholecystectomized patients, contributing 3,519,682 person-years, were followed up for a maximum of 33 years. Cholecystectomized patients had an increased risk of proximal intestinal adenocarcinoma, which gradually declined with increasing distance from the common bile duct. The risk was significantly increased for carcinoma (SIR, 1.77) and carcinoids of the small bowel (SIR, 1.71) and right-sided colon carcinoma (SIR, 1.16). No association was found with more distal bowel carcinoma.

These results, together with available literature, give substantial evidence for an association between gallstones and colorectal carcinoma, an association that is not due to cholecystectomy being a predisposing factor to colorectal carcinoma. Sporadic findings of an association between cholecystectomy and colorectal carcinoma can be explained by the above relationship. Wynder and Reddy[171] were impressed by the correlation between dietary fat intake and colon carcinoma. These authors reasoned that the dietary fat content raised both the concentration of anaerobic bacteria and the amount of bile acid and cholesterol substrates in the gut, thus enhancing the production of bile acid and cholesterol metabolites, which may be the proximate carcinogens.

Considerable attention has been directed to absence of the gallbladder and its possible relationship to the development of colorectal carcinoma. Many studies have been published offering arguments for and against such an association. In their comprehensive review of the controversy, Moorehead and McKelvey[172] found series that suggested an increased RR of developing colorectal carcinoma in the range of 1.59 to 2.27. Higher RR have been reported up to 3.5 for right-sided carcinoma in women, with the highest report being 4.5 for sigmoid lesions.[173,174,175] In a total Icelandic population prospective study of 3,425 individuals who underwent cholecystectomy and were followed up 8 to 33 years, Nielsen et al[176] found an RR of carcinoma in men of 2.73. McFarlane and Welch[177] found an overall OR of 2.78, but it was 6.79 for right-sided lesions. However, this concept is not universally supported. Abrams et al[178] found no relationship between cholecystectomy and the subsequent occurrence of proximal colonic carcinoma. Kune et al[179] and Kaibara et al[180] found no statistical association between previous cholecystectomy and the risk of colorectal carcinoma either in general or in any subsite, age, or sex. Ekbom et al,[181] in a population-based study of 62,615 patients who underwent cholecystectomy, found no overall excess risk of colorectal carcinoma but observed an increased risk among women for right-sided colon carcinoma 15 years or more after operation. In a case-control study conducted by Neugent et al,[182] no significant association was found between cholecystectomy and adenomatous polyps or carcinoma. Even if an association between large bowel neoplasia and biliary tract disease were confirmed, it is possible that there is no direct cause-and-effect relationship. It may be that the diet predisposing to one disease increases the risk of developing the other disease. Resolution of this controversy would be of considerable clinical significance by clearly exposing a readily identifiable at-risk group and offering more intensive screening opportunities to them.

21.2.8 Diverticular Disease

Most surgeons believe that because of the frequency with which both colon carcinoma and diverticular disease exist, it is not uncommon to see both conditions concomitantly without necessarily invoking a cause-and-effect relationship. A study by Boulos et al[183] hinted that patients with diverticular disease might constitute a group at higher risk of developing neoplasia. Morini et al[184] ascertained that adenomas and carcinomas were detected more often in patients with diverticular disease, with an overall OR of 3.0. When examined separately, adenomas maintained their significantly higher frequency, but no difference was observed for carcinomas.

21.2.9 Activity and Exercise

Persky and Andrianopoulos[185] reviewed studies examining the relation between exercise levels and risk of carcinoma. The authors found an RR increase of 1.3 to 2.0 for individuals with sedentary jobs. This association held true only for colon carcinoma, not for rectal carcinoma. Thune and Lund[186] also found a reduced risk for colon carcinoma for men and women who engaged in physical activity at least 4 hours per week. The reduced risk was more marked in the proximal colon. No association between physical activity and rectal carcinoma was observed in men or women. In a case-control study of men with colorectal carcinoma in Japan, physical inactivity based on occupational category increased the risk from the lowest to the highest levels, 1.32 to 1.92 times (rectum and proximal colon, respectively).[133]

In a more recent report contrary results were found by Slattery et al[187]; they conducted a population-based study of 952 incident cases of carcinoma in the rectum and rectosigmoid junction with 1,205 age- and sex-matched controls in Utah and Northern California at the Kaiser Permanente Medical Care Program. Vigorous physical activity was associated with reduced risk of rectal carcinoma in both men and women (OR = 0.60 for men and 0.59 for women). Among men, moderate levels of physical activity were also associated with reduced risk of rectal carcinoma (OR = 0.70). Participation in vigorous activity over the past 20 years conferred the greatest protection for both men and women (OR = 0.55 for men and 0.44 for women). In another case-control study among men, increased physical activity (22 h/wk) was associated with reduced risk for advanced adenomas (OR = 0.4) and for nonadvanced adenomas (OR = 0.8).[188]

Colbert et al[189] examined the association between occupational and leisure physical activity and colorectal carcinoma in a cohort of male smokers. Among the 29,133 men aged 50 to 69 years in the Alpha-Tocopherol, Beta-Carotene Cancer Prevention study, 152 colon and 104 rectal carcinomas were documented during 12 years of follow-up. For colon carcinoma, compared with sedentary workers, men in light occupational activity had an RR of 0.60, whereas those in moderate/heavy activity had an RR of 0.45. For rectal carcinoma, there were risk reductions for those in light (RR, 0.71) and moderate/heavy occupational activity (RR, 0.50). These data provide evidence for a protective role of physical activity in colon and rectal carcinoma. Others support the concept of physical activity as being protective against the development of colon carcinoma.[190,191]

Various mechanisms for this protective effect have been extensively cited. Quadrilatero and Hoffman-Goetz[192] reviewed the published evidence of physical activity and the hypothesized mechanisms. These mechanisms included changes in gastrointestinal transit time, altered immune function and prostaglandin levels, as well as changes in insulin levels, insulinlike growth factors, bile acid secretion, serum cholesterol, and gastrointestinal and pancreatic hormone profiles. There are currently little data to support any of the hypothesized biological mechanisms for the protective effect of exercise on colon carcinoma. It is likely that no one mechanism is responsible for the risk reduction observed in epidemiological and animal studies and therefore, the observed benefits of physical activity in colon carcinoma may be a combination of these and other factors.

21.2.10 Other Factors

A host of seemingly totally unrelated factors have been suggested to play a role in colorectal carcinoma genesis. Many of these are cited below. The risk of colorectal carcinoma is increased following adenocarcinoma of the small bowel.[193]

A factor that has been studied but for which no definitive association has been documented is obesity. With regard to bowel function, a meta-analysis of 14 case-control studies revealed statistically significant risks for colorectal carcinoma associated with both constipation and the use of cathartics (pooled OR, 1.48 and 1.46, respectively).[194]

A meta-analysis of published data revealed that women with a history of breast, endometrial, and ovarian carcinomas have an increased RR of developing colorectal carcinoma of 1.1, 1.4, and 1.6, respectively.[195] Large bowel malignancy correlates with the distribution of endocrine-dependent neoplasms (e.g., breast, endometrium, ovary, or prostate) and arteriosclerotic heart disease. It would be important to know whether there is a protective effect of hormone replacement therapy against colorectal carcinoma. Increased parity was reported to be associated with a decline in the risk of colon carcinoma (OR of 0.44 for women with five children or more relative to nulliparous women), but not for rectal carcinoma.[196] The association with colon carcinoma is restricted to women of 50 years of age or older. A population based case-control study of postmenopausal women revealed that when compared with women who never used hormone replacement therapy, recent users had an RR of 0.54 for colon carcinoma and an RR of 0.91 for rectal carcinoma.[197,198,199,200] Estrogen replacement therapy is associated with a substantially decreased risk in colon carcinoma (RR = 0.71).[201] Users of 1 year or less have an RR of 0.81, while users of 11 years or more have an RR of 0.54. Other investigators found little overall association between colon carcinoma and oral contraceptive use, parity, age at first birth, hysterectomy, oophorectomy status, or age at menopause.[199,200]

In a meta-analysis of 18 epidemiologic studies of postmenopausal hormone therapy and colorectal carcinoma, Grodstein et al[201] found a 20% reduction in risk of colon carcinoma and a 19% decrease in the risk of rectal carcinoma for postmenopausal women who had ever taken hormone therapy compared with women who never used hormones. Much of the apparent reduction in colorectal carcinoma was limited to current hormone users (RR = 0.66). From a case-control study among women, ever use of hormone replacement therapy was more strongly associated with reduced risk of advanced adenomas relative to polyp-free controls (OR = 0.4) than with reduced risk of nonadvanced adenomas (OR = 0.7).[188] Baris et al[202] studied the patterns of carcinoma risk in Sweden and Denmark in 177 patients with acromegaly. Increased risks were found for colon (SIR = 2.6) and rectum (SIR = 2.5). Among other risks, the increased risk for several carcinoma sites among acromegaly patients may be due to the elevated proliferative and antiapoptotic activity associated with increased circulating levels of insulinlike growth factor-1.

Bile acids are suspected from both clinical and experimental studies to have a role in colon carcinogenesis. The twofold increased mortality from colorectal carcinoma is apparent only 15 to 20 years after gastric surgery. It is suggested that the increased mortality from colorectal carcinoma after gastric surgery may be due to altered bile acid metabolism. To determine the relationship between bile acids and increased risk of colorectal neoplasms after truncal vagotomy, Mullen et al[203] conducted a prospective screening study of 100 asymptomatic patients who had undergone truncal vagotomy at least 10 years previously. The patients were investigated by barium enema, colonoscopy, and gallbladder ultrasonography. Control data were obtained from forensic autopsy subjects. The incidence of neoplasms less than 1 cm in the vagotomized group was 14% (11 adenomas and 3 carcinomas) and 3% in controls. The authors found increased proportions of chenodeoxycholic acid and lithocholic acid and decreased proportions of cholic acid in the duodenal bile of vagotomized patients and believe that these abnormalities in bile acid metabolism may help explain the increased risk of colorectal neoplasia 10 years after truncal vagotomy. On the other hand, Fisher et al,[204] in their cohort study of 15,983 males, found no elevation of risk of large bowel carcinoma following gastric surgery for benign disease.

Little et al[205] tested the hypothesis relating bile acids, calcium, and pH to colorectal carcinoma in a large sample of asymptomatic subjects who had participated in fecal occult blood screening. Fecal samples were obtained from 45 cases of carcinoma, 129 subjects with adenoma, 167 fecal occult blood negative controls, and 155 fecal occult blood positive subjects in whom no carcinoma or adenoma was found. No association between colorectal carcinoma and fecal bile acids or pH was observed. Although there was no overall association between colorectal adenomas and fecal bile acids or pH, villous adenomas were associated with increasing concentrations of major bile acids and decreasing concentration of minor bile acids, and there was a suggestion of an inverse association with an acid pH. High levels of fecal calcium were associated with a reduced risk of both colorectal carcinoma and adenoma, but this was not statistically significant. Their study does not support an association between colorectal carcinoma and fecal bile acids. However, there is evidence that increases in major bile acids are associated with villous adenomas.

There is diverse evidence suggesting that intracolonic production of oxygen radicals may play a role in carcinogenesis.[206] The relatively high concentrations of iron in feces, together with the ability of bile pigments to act as iron chelators that support Fenton chemistry, may very well permit efficient hydroxyl radicals generation from superoxide and hydrogen peroxide produced by bacterial metabolism. Such free radical generation in feces could provide a missing link in our understanding of the etiology of colon carcinoma: the oxidation of procarcinogens either by fecal hydroxyl radicals or by secondary peroxyl radicals to form active carcinogens or mitogenic neoplastic promoters. Intracolonic free radical formation may explain the high incidence of carcinoma in the colon and rectum compared with other regions of the gastrointestinal tract, as well as the observed correlation of a higher incidence of colon carcinoma with red meat in the diet, which increases stool iron, and with excessive fat in the diet, which may increase the fecal content of procarcinogens and bile pigments.

Epidemiologic studies and laboratory research have indicated an association between the metabolic activity of the intestinal microflora and carcinoma of the large bowel.[207] It has been suggested that activation of procarcinogens could be mediated enzymatically by intestinal bacteria. The levels of incriminated colonic bacterial enzymes are increased by dietary fat and inhibited by certain dietary fibers. Organic extracts of feces contain a mutagenic substance, presumably derived from bacterial metabolism in the large bowel. Whether this substance or some other organic chemical is the putative proximate carcinogen remains speculative, but the evidence continues to point to intestinal bacteria as the metabolic intermediary in colon carcinoma.

High iron stores may increase the risk of colorectal carcinoma through their contribution to the production of free oxygen radicals. Knekt et al[208] studied serum iron, total iron binding capacity, and transferrin saturation levels in a cohort of 41,276 subjects ranging in age from 20 to 74 years. The authors found an RR of 3.04 for colorectal carcinoma in subjects with transferrin levels exceeding 60%. Asthmatic patients have a reported elevated RR of colon (1.17) and rectum (1.28) carcinoma.[209] The prevalence of colon carcinoma in patients with Barrett's esophagus is 7.6% compared with 1.6% in a control population.[210] Men with esophageal adenocarcinoma may be more likely to be diagnosed with colorectal carcinoma in their lifetime than expected. The opposite association may exist for women.[211] An RR of 3.04 has been calculated for colorectal carcinoma as a result of anthranoid laxative abuse.[212] Younes et al[213] reported that 25% of patients who underwent appendectomy and were found to have mucosal hyperplasia were associated with adenocarcinoma of the colon.

Plasma C-reactive protein concentrations are elevated among persons who subsequently develop colon carcinoma. These data support the hypothesis that inflammation is a risk factor for the development of colon carcinoma in average-risk individuals.[214] Woolcott et al[215] found colon carcinoma risk was inversely associated with coffee. Relative to those drinking fewer than one cup of coffee per day, the OR for those drinking two cups was 0.9, for those drinking three to four cups was 0.8, and for those drinking five or more cups was 0.7. The reduced risk estimates were more pronounced with carcinoma of the proximal colon than the distal colon. Rectal carcinoma risk was not associated with either coffee or tea. In a study of premorbid and personality factors, aggressive hostility was the only variable found to be significant between colon carcinoma patients and controls.[216]

21.2.11 Juvenile versus Adult Carcinoma

To add further confounding information to the matter, two different types of carcinoma may exist. Concerning the wide age range that colorectal carcinoma encompasses, Avni and Feuchtwanger[24] wrote a thought-provoking editorial in which they made a sharp differentiation between "juvenile" and "adult" carcinomas and suggested that a search be made for different etiologies. To support the concept that two different types of colon carcinoma may exist, the authors cited the following observations:

1. In the nonwhite population, the juvenile form occurs up to 16 times more frequently than in the white population, whereas the adult form occurs 10 times more frequently in the white population.
2. Mucinous carcinomas comprise only 5% of all colonic carcinomas, although in the young age group they comprise 76%.
3. In adult patients with colon carcinoma, coexisting polyps can be found in 40 to 50% of patients, whereas in the juvenile group, polyps are exceedingly rare.
4. Alleged nutritional factors in the genesis of colon carcinoma must be present for many years, which cannot be the case in the juvenile group. Moreover, diet in the nonwhite population in whom the juvenile type is more frequent differs from that of the white population.

5. In the adult population with colon carcinoma, a family history of disease is found in 20 to 30%, although this factor is almost nonexistent in the juvenile type.

Only further investigation will resolve this issue.

21.2.12 Prospects for Prevention

Epidemiologic evidence suggests that diet is the principal factor in the cause of colorectal carcinoma. Ingestion of excessive amounts of fat appears to be the major factor. Also noteworthy is the interrelationship between the varying relative amounts of fat and fiber in the diet. For example, in an experimental study on colorectal carcinogenesis by Galloway et al,[217] manipulation of diet resulted in significant differences in alteration of the surface architecture of the colonic mucosa. The high-fat, low-fiber diet was associated with the greatest risk for macroscopic malignant production, and the low-fat, high-fiber diet, with the lowest risk. Furthermore, the sources of fat vary in the degree of their promotional effect.[125] Fiber is considered to inhibit carcinoma, but only the type of fiber found in whole grain cereals, fruits, and vegetables, which contain large amounts of uronic acid, is effective. The exact nature of fat and fiber sources is yet to be delineated.

An effective prevention strategy should be based on an understanding of the pathogenesis of carcinoma, but no such definitive understanding exists. From the available evidence it appears that a high intake of animal fat and protein promotes the formation of colon carcinoma and that certain cruciferous vegetables exert a protective influence. The two-step concept of carcinogenesis includes (1) initiation, about which little is known in human carcinoma, and (2) promotion, which presumably takes a long time to complete. We may well be able to capitalize on the latter fact by the administration of inhibitors during the promotional phase, a concept realized experimentally by Nigro and Bull.[125] Their studies suggested that an appropriate strategy for prevention of carcinoma of the large bowel would be a program aimed at a 10% reduction of fat consumption (i.e., from 40 to 30% of calories) and adoption of a more varied type of fat. The daily addition of 25 to 30 g of dietary fiber, especially grains and vegetables that contain cellulose and uronic acid, may prove effective. A third recommendation is to include in the diet chemical inhibitors such as selenium, retinoids, and plant steroids. Other studies have suggested that other factors, such as calcium and sulfur compounds present in garlic and onions, may be of value in the inhibition of colon carcinoma.[126] Antioxidants such as beta-carotene, vitamin C, vitamin E, and folic acid have been assessed.[218] Individuals with a significant inheritance factor for colon carcinoma may require a supplement to enhance inhibition.

Cassidy et al[219] reported a strong inverse association and suggested a potentially important role for starch in the protection against colorectal carcinoma. This corresponds with the hypothesis that fermentation in the colon is the mechanism for preventing colorectal carcinoma.

Experiments in animals and two epidemiologic studies in humans suggest that aspirin and other nonsteroidal anti-inflammatory drugs (NSAIDs) may be protective against colon carcinoma. Thun et al[220] tested this hypothesis in a prospective mortality study of 662,424 adults who provided information in 1982 on the frequency and duration of their aspirin use. Death rates from colon carcinoma were measured through 1988. The possible influence of other risk factors for colon carcinoma was examined in multivariate analyses for 598 case patients and 3,058 matched control subjects drawn from the cohort. Death rates from colon carcinoma decreased with more frequent aspirin use in both men and women. The RR among persons who used aspirin 16 or more times per month for at least 1 year was 0.60 in men and 0.58 in women. The risk estimates were unaffected when they excluded persons who reported at entry into the study that they had a malignancy, heart disease, stroke, or another condition that might influence both their aspirin use and their mortality. Adjustment for dietary factors, obesity, physical activity, and family history did not alter the findings significantly. No association was found between the use of acetaminophen and the risk of colon carcinoma. The authors concluded that regular aspirin use at low doses may reduce the risk of fatal colon carcinoma.

Rosenberg et al[221] assessed NSAID use in relation to risk of human large bowel carcinoma in a hospital-based case-control study of 1,326 patients with colorectal carcinoma and 4,891 control patients. For regular NSAID use that continued into the year before the interview, the multivariate RR estimate was 0.5. The inverse association was apparent for both colon and rectal carcinoma in men and women and in subjects younger and older than 60 years. Regular NSAID use that had been discontinued at least 1 year previously and nonregular use were not associated with risk. Almost all regular NSAID use was of aspirin-containing drugs. The present data suggest that the sustained use of NSAIDs reduces the incidence of human large bowel carcinoma.

Smalley et al[222] studied how patterns of use (duration, dose, and specific drug) of NSAIDs affected the incidence of colorectal carcinoma. The population-based retrospective cohort study of 104,217 persons aged 65 years or older had at least 5 years of enrollment. Incident histologically confirmed colorectal carcinoma was documented. Users of nonaspirin NSAIDs for at least 48 months of the previous 5 years had an RR of 0.49 for colon carcinoma when compared with those of no use of NSAIDs. Among those with more than 12 months of cumulative use, those using NSAIDs in the past year (recent users) had a relative ratio of 0.61 whereas those with no recent use had a relative ratio of 0.76. No specific NSAID offered a unique protective effect and low dose of NSAIDs appeared to be at least as effective as higher doses. Protection was most pronounced for right-sided lesions. The RR among recent users with more than 12 months of cumulative use was 0.81 for rectal carcinoma, 0.77 for left-sided carcinoma, and 0.48 for right-sided colon carcinoma. In this elderly population, long-term use of nonaspirin NSAIDs nearly halved the risk of colon carcinoma. This study was consistent with previous studies that suggest that duration of use but not daily dose of NSAIDs is an important factor for chemoprevention. Their data also suggest that the protective effect is shared by most NSAIDs, and not confined to a small number of these drugs.

Baron et al[223] performed a randomized double-blind trial of aspirin as a chemopreventive agent against colorectal adenomas. They randomly assigned 1,121 patients with a recent history of histologically documented adenomas to receive placebo (372 patients), 81 mg of aspirin (377 patients), or

325 mg of aspirin (372 patients) daily. Follow-up colonoscopy was performed at least one year after randomization in 97% of patients. The incidence of one or more adenomas was 47% in the placebo group, 38% in the group given 81 mg of aspirin per day, and 45% in the group given 325 mg of aspirin per day. Unadjusted RRs of any adenomas (as compared with the placebo group) were 0.81 in the 81-mg group and 0.96 in the 325-mg group. For advanced neoplasms (adenomas measuring at least 1 cm in diameter or with tubulovillous or villous features, severe dysplasia, or invasive carcinoma), the respective RRs were 0.59 and 0.83. They concluded low-dose aspirin has a moderate chemopreventive effect on adenomas in the large bowel. Since adenoma development can be used as a surrogate marker for the development of carcinoma, the reduction in adenoma development by extrapolation would result in a decrease in the incidence of carcinoma.

In contrast to most observational studies, the randomized Physician's Health Study found no association between aspirin use and colorectal carcinoma after 5 years.[224] In a randomized prospective cohort study, 22,071 healthy male physicians who were 40 to 84 years of age in 1982 were given 325 mg of aspirin every other day. In 1988, the aspirin arm of the randomized trial was stopped early. Participants then chose to receive either aspirin or placebo for the rest of the study. Colorectal carcinoma was diagnosed in 341 patients during the study period. Over 12 years of follow-up, random assignment to aspirin was associated with a RR of colorectal carcinoma of 1.03. The RR for colorectal carcinoma in persons who used aspirin frequently after 1988 was 1.07. In the Physicians Health Study, both randomized and observational analyses indicate that there is no association between the use of aspirin and the incidence of colorectal carcinoma. In their review, Burke et al[225] reported that in population-based observational studies, people had lower rates of colorectal carcinoma if they were taking various agents, including nonsteroidal anti-inflammatory drugs, calcium, and folate. In placebo-controlled trials in patients with FAP and in patients with sporadic colon adenomas, NSAIDs reduced the rates of adenomas, and there is a biologic rationale that they would be effective in reducing colorectal carcinoma as well.

Large-scale chemoprevention trials sponsored by the National Cancer Institute are under way.[226] Agents being evaluated include piroxicam, sulindac, aspirin, acarbose (alpha-glucosidase) inhibitors, and calcium carbonate. Targeted populations include patients with previous adenoma, FAP, history of multiple polyposis, and subjects at risk for colon carcinoma.

21.3 Pathology

21.3.1 Macroscopic Appearance

On gross examination, adenocarcinoma of the colon appears as one of four fairly distinctive types—ulcerative, polypoid, annular, or diffusely infiltrating. The ulcerative carcinoma, the most common type, presents as a roughly circular mass with a raised, irregular, everted edge and a sloughing base. It is confined to one aspect of the bowel wall but may occupy a larger portion of the bowel circumference (▶ Fig. 21.6).

The polypoid, or cauliflower-type, carcinoma presents as a large fungating mass that projects into the lumen and is often of a low-grade malignancy. The ascending colon is a site of predilection (▶ Fig. 21.7).[227] In approximately 10% of cases, the cut surface of the growth may have a gelatinous appearance, due to abundant mucin secretion, and this type has been referred to as a colloid carcinoma.[227]

The annular, or stenosing, carcinoma occupies the entire circumference of the bowel wall. The extent in the long axis is variable. The bowel lumen is usually considerably compromised

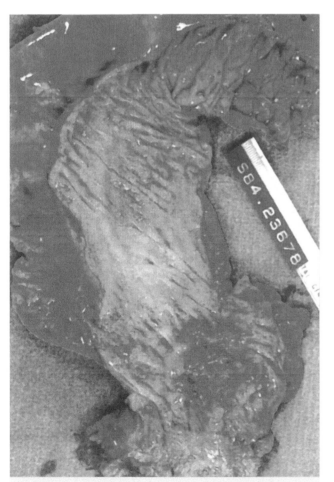

Fig. 21.6 Macroscopic features of an ulcerated adenocarcinoma.

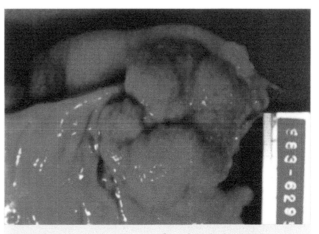

Fig. 21.7 Macroscopic appearance of a polypoid adenocarcinoma.

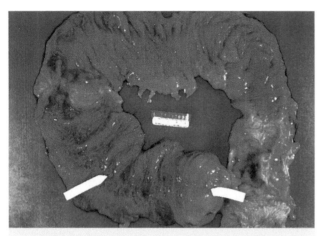

Fig. 21.8 Macroscopic features of an annular carcinoma. Arrows indicate associated adenomas.

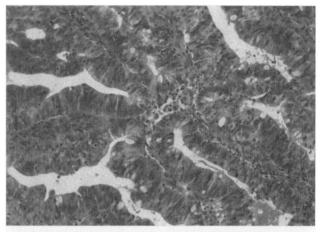

Fig. 21.10 Microscopic appearance of a well-differentiated adenocarcinoma with well-developed glands. (This image is provided courtesy of L.R. Begin, MD.)

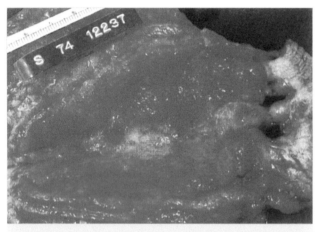

Fig. 21.9 Macroscopic appearance of an infiltrating adenocarcinoma.

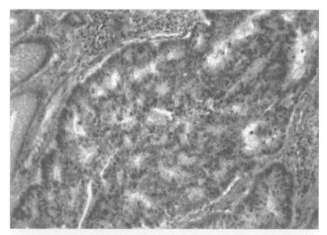

Fig. 21.11 Microscopic appearance of a moderately differentiated adenocarcinoma with gland formation that is less well defined. (This image is provided courtesy of L.R. Begin, MD.)

(▶ Fig. 21.8), and the proximal bowel may demonstrate varying degrees of dilation. Such carcinomas occur with greatest frequency in the transverse and descending colon.[227]

The diffusely infiltrating carcinoma produces a diffuse thickening of the intestinal wall and for the most part is covered with intact mucosa. It is extensively infiltrating, although it preserves the layers of the gastrointestinal wall. It occurs more often in the rectosigmoid, but any portion of the colon may be involved. This variety is similar to linitis plastica of the stomach. It is the type of carcinoma commonly associated with ulcerative colitis (▶ Fig. 21.9). A review of the literature by Papp et al[228] revealed only 85 documented cases of primary linitis plastica of the colon and rectum, characterized by presentation in younger patients and associated with metastatic disease, a higher mortality, and insidious growth, often making detection difficult.

21.3.2 Microscopic Appearance

The histological appearance of carcinoma may vary considerably, with the major importance being related to prognosis. The lesion may be well differentiated (20%; ▶ Fig. 21.10), moderately differentiated (60%; ▶ Fig. 21.11), or poorly differentiated

(20%; ▶ Fig. 21.12).[228] The incidence of lymph node metastases is about 25, 50, and 80% in low-, average-, or high-grade malignancy, respectively. Furthermore, the histologic grade influences survival, with corrected 5-year survival rates of 77, 61, and 29%, for low-, average-, and high-grade rectal malignancies, respectively.[227] Broders[229] popularized a method that divides adenocarcinoma into four grades. In grade 1, 75 to 100% of the cells are differentiated; in grade 2, 50 to 75%; in grade 3, 25 to 50%; and in grade 4, 0 to 25%. The principle of grading by differentiation is based on the biologic law that the higher the degree of differentiation, the less the power of reproduction; therefore, it might be anticipated that well-differentiated carcinomas would proliferate at a slower pace than those that are comparatively undifferentiated. One difficulty in the application of histologic grading is the lack of uniformity in the degree of differentiation throughout the neoplasm. In general, malignant cells are less differentiated at the invading margins than on the surface. Dukes[230] carefully differentiated his classification from that of Broders[229] by noting that the two methods answer different questions. Histologic grade is essentially an

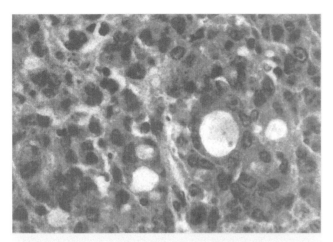

Fig. 21.12 Microscopic features of a poorly differentiated adenocarcinoma with pleomorphic cells and little recognizable gland formation. (This image is provided courtesy of L.R. Begin, MD.)

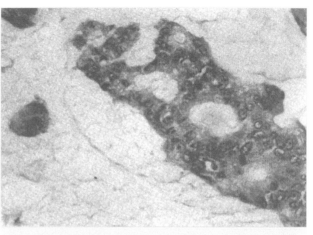

Fig. 21.13 Microscopic features of a mucin-producing adenocarcinoma with abundant extracellular mucin. (This image is provided courtesy of L.R. Begin, MD.)

estimate of the pace of growth, whereas classification into Dukes' A, B, and C cases is a measurement of the boundaries reached. Both methods permit grouping into cases with favorable and unfavorable outcome. Jass et al[231] proposed a grading system that includes the parameters of tubule configuration, advancing margin, and lymphocytic infiltration.

Contrary to what might be expected and what is generally believed, Gibbs[232] reported that rare undifferentiated carcinomas of the large intestine tend to spread circumferentially and do not readily give rise to lymphatic or hematogenous metastases. Affected patients may have a good prognosis.

Colloid, or mucus-producing, lesions may present with varying degrees of differentiation and are said by some to have a poor prognosis (▶ Fig. 21.13). Colloid adenocarcinoma can be classified as extracellular or intracellular, according to the predominant location of the mucin. Most colloid carcinomas are extracellular, with only approximately 2% of all carcinomas of the colon and rectum being the pure signet-ring cell variety. With the latter variety, the patient is unlikely to survive more than 2 years from the time of diagnosis.[227] The largest number of mucinous carcinomas are found in the rectum, but the relative incidence of mucinous carcinoma is higher in the right colon.[233] The primarily intracellular variety of mucinous carcinoma is classified as a signet-ring cell because the mucus pushes the nucleus to the periphery and thereby gives the cells their characteristic appearance. In a review of 426 patients with carcinoma of the rectum and rectosigmoid seen at Memorial Sloan-Kettering Cancer Center, Bonello et al[234] found 4% of the carcinomas to be of the signet-ring cell type, and this accounted for 0.4% of all rectal carcinomas. Umpleby et al[235] compared the clinical and pathologic features of 54 mucinous carcinomas of the large intestine with 576 nonmucinous carcinomas. Lesions were categorized as mucinous if they contained at least 60% mucin by volume. Those with moderate mucin content (60–80%) were indistinguishable in behavior from nonmucinous lesions. By contrast, those with a high mucin content (> 80%) showed several differences from nonmucinous carcinomas. They had a more proximal distribution through the large intestine, they comprised a greater fraction of carcinomas in the under-50 age group (24 vs. 7%), they

were more likely to be Dukes' stage D (58 vs. 31%), and local fixity was more common (70 vs. 37%).

Consequently, the overall resection rate was reduced from 90 to 73%, the curative resection rate from 69 to 42%, and the 5-year survival rate from 37 to 18%. Umpleby et al[235] concluded that colorectal carcinomas of high mucin content require wide excision, tend to recur locally, and carry a poor prognosis. The dramatic difference in this report from others in the literature may be due to this study's strict definition of a mucinous carcinoma as one with greater than 80% mucin content.

In a review of 540 cases of colorectal carcinoma, Okuno et al[236] found that mucinous carcinomas accounted for 6.4% of cases. Such carcinomas were more common in patients of 39 years of age or younger and in women patients. They were most commonly located in the rectum, followed by occurrence in the right colon; however, the relative incidence was higher in the right colon (40.5 vs. 12.5%). These carcinomas were characterized by infiltration of the surrounding tissues (24.3 vs. 7.8%), positive lymph node involvement (75.7 vs. 48.6%), and peritoneal implant (21.6 vs. 4.1%). The cumulative 5- and 10-year survival rates after resection of mucinous carcinoma were 45.5 and 39.8%, respectively; those after curative resection were 77.4 and 63.5%. The authors suggested the need for aggressive lymph node dissection and wide excision of the surrounding tissues for mucinous carcinoma, with special attention paid to local recurrence. This microscopic variety of carcinoma is associated with a higher incidence of metastases and a higher incidence of associated synchronous polyps and carcinoma than nonmucinous carcinomas. The clinical relevance of this association is that it is necessary to perform colonoscopy on patients with mucinous carcinoma.[233]

Anthony et al[237] reported the largest series of signet cell carcinoma of the colon and rectum. There was equal distribution between the right and left colon. Synchronous carcinomas were present in 14%. Nodal or metastatic disease was present in 72% of patients at the time of diagnosis. The 5-year actuarial survival rate was 22%. Patient mortality was due to carcinomatosis in all 22 patients who died. Parenchymal liver involvement occurred in only two patients (9%). Ovarian metastases have been reported in 25 to 60% of patients at time of diagnosis and hence bilateral salpingo-oophorectomy should probably accompany the original resection. Primary linitis plastica of the colon and rectum is an uncommon entity with a poor prognosis. Papp et al[228] found 85 cases reported in the literature. Shirouza et al[238] classified linitis plastica into two types according to histologic growth pattern—the more common scirrhous type and the lymphangiosis type. The scirrhous type is composed mainly of poorly differentiated or signet-ring cells and is accompanied by a severe desmoplastic reaction. The lymphangiosis type is composed mainly of moderately differentiated cells, frequently with glandular formation. The characteristic diffuse tubular thickening and rigidity are the result of fibrotic reaction around infiltrating malignant cells, such as in desmoplasia (see ▶ Fig. 21.9). The microscopic appearance is that of poorly differentiated pleomorphic cells (see ▶ Fig. 21.12).

The pathologist can be instrumental in guiding the surgeon to the appropriate clinical management. Surgeons are often reluctant to recommend major operative procedures for patients with "minimally invasive" carcinoma. Hase et al[239] conducted a study to determine the long-term outcome after curative resection of colorectal carcinomas that extend only into the submucosa. Seventy-nine patients who underwent curative resection were followed for at least 5 years. Formal operation followed attempted endoscopic removal in 25 patients. Lymph node metastases, found in 11 of 79 patients (13.9%), were associated with a worse outcome; 36.4% of node-positive patients developed recurrence versus only 5.9% of node-negative patients. The cumulative survival rate was also worse in node-positive versus node-negative patients: 72.7 versus 91.1% at 5 years and 45.5 versus 65.3% at 10 years. Five histopathologic characteristics were identified as risk factors for lymph node metastases: (1) small clusters of undifferentiated carcinoma cells ahead of the invasive front of the lesion ("tumor budding"), (2) a poorly demarcated invasive front, (3) moderately or poorly differentiated malignant cells in the invasive front, (4) extension of the carcinoma to the middle or deep submucosal layer, and (5) malignant cells in lymphatics. Whereas patients with three or fewer risk factors had no nodal spread, the rate of lymph node involvement with four or more risk factors was 33.3 and 66.7%, respectively. Appropriate bowel resection with lymph node dissection is indicated if a lesion exhibits more than three histologic risk factors for metastasis.

The coexistence of two or more cell types in colonic malignancy has been reported. Novello et al[240] reported cases containing areas with clear adenocarcinomatous and squamous differentiation and morphologic as well as histochemical evidence of neuroendocrine differentiation.

21.3.3 Depressed Carcinoma

A unique macroscopic type of carcinoma rarely recorded in the Western world is the superficial depressed type, which represents de novo growth and is clearly different from that usually seen in the polyp–carcinoma sequence. This type of carcinoma, frequently described in the Japanese population, has a strong tendency to develop into invasive and advanced carcinoma. At our institution, Begin et al[241] described a case of endophytic malignant transformation in a flat adenoma of the colon. The deep component was a well-differentiated adenocarcinoma extending into the serosa and probably was an example of the depressed carcinomas described in the Japanese literature.

Kudo et al[242] published an excellent description of the gross and microscopic features with the subtle nuances of making the diagnosis. The authors reported that the depressed type of invasive carcinoma represented 15.5% of all invasive carcinomas diagnosed on 30,311 endoscopic examinations. The definition of a depressed carcinoma is shown in ▶ Fig. 21.14. To detect the depressed type of carcinoma, it is important to pay special attention to slight changes in the mucosal color during endoscopy—slight redness or, in some cases, pallor (▶ Fig. 21.15). The detection rate was about 1 in 1,000 endoscopic examinations. Indigo carmine spraying of suspicious areas reveals the underlying pathology of the depressed type of carcinoma (▶ Fig. 21.16). Histologic confirmation of such a lesion is seen in ▶ Fig. 21.17. The degree of submucosal extension is depicted in ▶ Fig. 21.18. The management of patients with depressed carcinomas is outlined as an algorithm in ▶ Fig. 21.19. In sm1a and sm1b, extension without vessel invasion, strip biopsy is suitable. For sm1b with vessel invasion, resection is recommended because of the risk of lymph node metastases. For sm2 and sm3 (▶ Fig. 21.18), resection is the preferred treatment. Kubota et al[243] examined 300 surgically resected specimens with a dissecting microscope and found 297 adenomas (240 polypoid, 32 flat, and 25 depressed) along with three nonpolypoid carcinomas. Nonpolypoid adenomas were

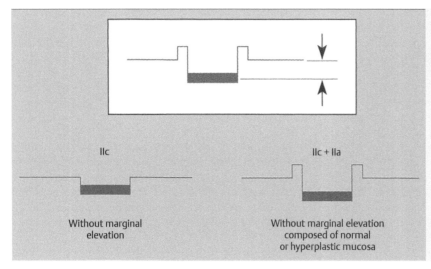

Fig. 21.14 Depressed type of colorectal carcinoma. Definition: carcinoma whose surface is lower than that of neighboring normal mucosa. IIc and IIc + IIa types of carcinoma meet this definition.[242]

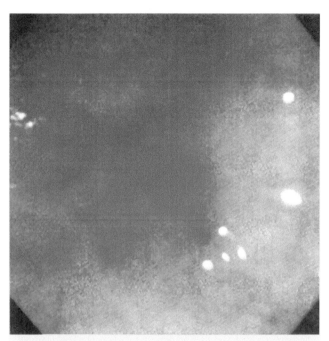

Fig. 21.15 Normal endoscopic image.[242]

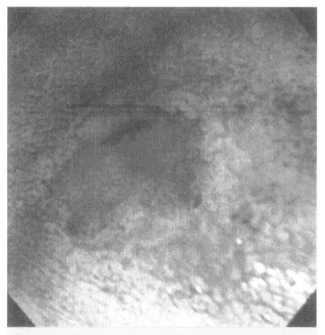

Fig. 21.16 Normal endoscopic image after indigo carmine spraying.[242]

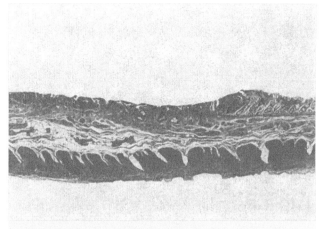

Fig. 21.17 Carcinoma invading the submucosal layer (hematoxylin and eosin stain, original magnification × 10).[242]

The authors found the former to be smaller, more often in the proximal colon, and away from the rectosigmoid area, less frequently well differentiated, with fewer adenomatous remnants, and with more frequent deep invasion and lymphovascular permeation.

Iishi et al[246] reported on a series of 256 early colorectal carcinomas (Dukes' A and B), of which 8% were superficial early carcinomas defined as less than 3 mm in height. These lesions were found scattered throughout the large intestine and were often observed as reddish spots that were easily overlooked without careful observation. Histologically, 90% of these were well differentiated, 24% reached the submucosal layer, and 86% were not associated with adenoma.

Flat lesions are being increasingly recognized with new colonoscopic techniques. Togashi et al[247] reported 10,939 consecutive high-resolution video colonoscopies and indigo carmine spraying to detect flat lesions. All lesions suggesting neoplastic changes were removed by polypectomy or operation. Carcinomas invading beyond the submucosal layer were excluded from this analysis. The gross appearance of flat-type lesions was classified as flat-elevated type or flat-depressed type based on the presence or absence of central depression. A total of 5,408 neoplastic lesions were index lesions, including 5,035 adenomas and 373 carcinomas (124 with submucosal invasion). The prevalence of flat-depressed and flat-elevated lesions were 2.8 and 18.1%, respectively. Submucosal invasion rates were 17.1% in the flat-depressed, 0.8% in the flat-elevated, 1.6% in the sessile, 4.0% in the pedunculated lesions, and 9% in the creeping lesions. The submucosal invasion rate in the flat-depressed lesions was significantly higher than in any others, except for creeping lesions. The percentage of flat-elevated and flat-depressed carcinomas among all carcinomas invading the submucosa was 6.5 and 21.0%, respectively. They concluded that one-quarter of all colorectal carcinomas may be derived from flat lesions. Training in dye spray technique may result in a higher detection rate of flat colonic lesions.

Nivatvongs[248] reviewed the subject of early colorectal carcinoma. Most such carcinomas can be treated by adequate local excision, such as colonoscopic polypectomy and per-anal excision. If there are adverse risk factors, especially poorly

mostly found in the transverse and descending colon. Almost all depressed adenomas were less than 3 mm in dimension (96%), and almost all flat adenomas were less than 3.5 mm in dimension (96.9%). The 3-mm carcinomas ranged in size from 2.4 to 2.9 mm. Minamoto et al[244] suggested that superficial-type adenocarcinomas show rapid growth, aggressive behavior, and may not progress by the adenoma–carcinoma pathway but may rise from a very small superficial-type adenoma.

Tada et al[245] conducted a clinicopathologic study of 62 flat colorectal carcinomas and 80 polypoid colorectal carcinomas.

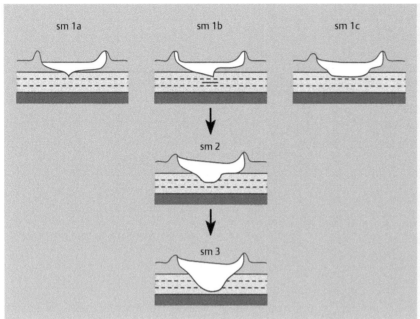

Fig. 21.18 Classification of submucosal invasion of early colorectal carcinoma sm 1, invasion limited to the upper third of the submucosa; sm1a, horizontal invasion limited to less than one quarter of the width of the carcinoma component in the mucosa; sm1b, invasion limited to one quarter to half of the width of the carcinoma component in the mucosa; sm1c, invasion extending to more than half of the width of the carcinoma component in the mucosa; sm2, invasion limited to the middle third of the submucosa; sm3, invasion of the lower third of the submucosa.[242]

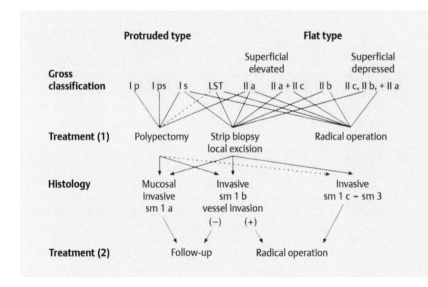

Fig. 21.19 Treatment algorithm for colorectal lesions. p, pedunculated; ps, subpedunculated; s, sessile; LST, laterally spreading type.[242]

differentiated carcinoma, lymphovascular invasion, or incomplete excision, a radical resection is indicated if there is no contraindication. In the case of a low rectal carcinoma, adjuvant chemoradiation should be considered. Recently, a new classification has been developed: sm1 is invasion to the upper one-third of the submucosa, sm2 is invasion to the middle one-third, and sm3 is invasion to the lower one-third. Lesions of sm1 and sm2 have a low risk of local recurrence and lymph node metastasis; local excision is adequate. The sm3 lesions and sm2 flat and depressed types have a high risk of local recurrence and lymph node metastasis; further treatment is indicated.

21.3.4 Sentinel Lymph Node Mapping

Lymph node involvement with metastatic disease has long been recognized as a prognostic discriminant that decreases survival. Ultrastaging by serial sectioning, combined with immunohistochemical techniques, improves detection of lymph node micrometastases. The introduction of sentinel lymph node mapping has provided the potential to facilitate ultrastaging. The impact of staging in the oncologic management of patients may have therapeutic implications. The challenge is to determine the biologic relevance and the prognostic implications. Mulsow et al[249] reviewed the electronic literature (1996–2003) on sentinel node mapping in carcinoma of the colon and rectum. Lymphatic mapping appears to be readily applicable to colorectal carcinomas and identifies those nodes most likely to harbor metastases. Sentinel node mapping carries a false-negative rate of approximately 10% but will also potentially upstage a proportion of patients from node-negative to node-positive following the detection of micro-metastases. The prognostic significance of micrometastases in colorectal carcinoma is required before the staging benefits of sentinel lymph node mapping can be routinely adopted. Bilchik et al[250] proposed a TNM classification for micrometastases and isolated malignant cells.

They studied 120 patients who underwent lymph node mapping before resection of primary colorectal carcinoma. Sentinel nodes were identified using blue dye and/or radiotracer and were examined by hematoxylin and eosin (H&E) staining, cytokeratin immunohistochemistry, and multilevel sectioning. The comparison group comprised 370 patients whose primary colorectal carcinomas were resected without lymph node mapping during the same period. Lymph node mapping was successfully performed in 96% of patients and correctly predicted the status of the nodal basin in 96% of patients. Nodal involvement was identified for 14.3, 30, 74.6, and 83.3% of T1, T2, T3, and T4 carcinomas, respectively, in the study group, and for 6.8, 8.5, 49.3, and 41.8% of T1, T2, T3, and T4 carcinomas, respectively, in the comparison group. The study group had a higher percentage of nodal metastases (53 vs. 36%). They believe lymph node mapping and focused sentinel node analysis should be considered to better stage colorectal carcinoma.

Saha et al[251] used the combination of isosulfan blue (Lymphazurin) 1% and technetium-99 m (^{99m}Tc) sulfur colloid, to test the feasibility and accuracy of lymphatic mapping for colorectal carcinoma. In 57 consecutive patients, mapping was successful in 100% of patients with isosulfan blue and in 89% with sulfur colloid. Lymphatic mapping was accurate in 93% of patients with isosulfan blue versus 92% with sulfur colloid. The combined accuracy was 95%. A total of 709 lymph nodes were found (12.4 per patient): 553 nonsentinel lymph nodes (5.6% nodal positivity) versus 156 sentinel lymph nodes (16.7% nodal positivity). Isosulfan blue detected 152 sentinel lymph nodes, sulfur colloid detected 100, and both modalities detected 96. Of the sentinel lymph nodes detected by isosulfan blue only, 10.7% had nodal metastases, whereas 19.8% of sentinel lymph nodes detected with both modalities had nodal metastases. Nodal disease was detected in 41% of patients with invasive carcinoma. Metastases were detected only in the sentinel lymph nodes in 26% and only by micrometastases in 11% of these patients. The metastatic yield is significantly higher in sentinel lymph nodes identified by both modalities compared with isosulfan blue only. A less encouraging report was published by Bembenek et al.[252] They evaluated the feasibility and utility of lymphatic mapping in 48 patients with rectal carcinoma, 37 of whom had already undergone preoperative radiochemotherapy for locally advanced lesions. An endoscopic injection of sulfur colloid into the submucosa adjacent to the carcinoma was performed 15 to 17 hours before the operation. Ex vivo identification of the nuclide-enriched "sentinel lymph nodes" was performed using a hand-held gamma-probe. The selected sentinel lymph nodes were examined using serial sections and immunohistochemistry. One or more sentinel lymph nodes were found in 46 of the 48 patients. The sentinel lymph node detection rate was 96%. Lymph node metastases were present in 35%. A sensitivity of only 44% and a false-negative rate of 56% were found. Further analysis showed that the method correctly predicted the nodal status only in the small subgroup of patients with early carcinoma without preoperative radiation. They concluded that although lymph node identification shows a relatively high detection rate, the sensitivity in patients with locally advanced irradiated rectal carcinoma is low.

Further studies will be required to determine the ultimate utility of this modality, but even this may not be necessary. The results of the Cancer and Leukemia Group B (CALGB) Protocol 80001, a prospective study conducted in 12 institutions, concluded that sentinel lymph nodes fail to predict nodal status in 52% of cases.[253] Read et al[254] reported that sentinel node mapping would have potentially benefited only 3% and failed to accurately identify nodal metastases in 24% of patients in their study. They concluded the fraction of patients who are benefiting from sentinel lymph node mapping and lymph node ultraprocessing techniques would be 2%. These studies might put the question of sentinel lymph node mapping for colorectal carcinoma to rest. The most recent review of the subject by Stojadinovic et al[255] concluded that there are fundamental questions that remain unanswered: (1) Does sentinel lymph node mapping significantly upstage or increase staging accuracy? (2) Do patients with H&E-negative nodes but nodal metastases have a significantly worse oncologic outcome than those without micrometastases? (3) Does treatment of nodal micrometastases with adjuvant chemotherapy translate into meaningful survival benefit? They believe that until these questions are answered, sentinel lymph node mapping for colorectal carcinoma will likely remain investigational.

Cimmino et al[256] reported that in 267 patients who underwent intraoperative lymphatic mapping with the use of both isosulfan 1% blue dye and radiocolloid injection, five adverse reactions to isosulfan blue were encountered—two cases of anaphylaxis and three cases of "blue hives." The two patients with anaphylaxis experienced cardiovascular collapse, erythema, perioral edema, urticaria, and uvular edema. The blue hives in three patients resolved and transformed to blue patches during the course of the procedures. The incidence of allergic reactions in their series was 2%. Should physicians expand the role of sentinel lymph node mapping, they should consider the use of histamine blockers as prophylaxis and have emergency treatment readily available to treat the life threatening complication of anaphylactic reaction.

21.3.5 Modes of Spread

To produce metastases, malignant cells must succeed in invasion, embolization, survival in the circulation, arrest in a distant capillary bed, and extravasation into and multiplication in organ parenchyma (▶ Fig. 21.20).[257] The outcome of this process depends on the interaction of metastatic cells with multiple host factors. Indeed, the major obstacle to the effective treatment of colon carcinoma metastasis is the biologic heterogeneity of neoplasms. Another challenge to therapy is the finding that different organ environments can modify a metastatic malignant cell's response to systemic therapy. Carcinoma of the colon may spread in one of the following ways: direct continuity, transperitoneal spread, lymphatic spread, hematogenous spread, and implantation.

Direct Continuity

Intramural spread of the carcinoma occurs more rapidly in the transverse than the longitudinal axis of the colon and has been estimated to proceed roughly at the rate of one quarter of the bowel circumference every 6 months. It is unusual for microscopic spread to occur more than 1 cm beyond the grossly visible disease. Radial extension through the bowel wall may result in adherence to abdominal viscera such as the small or large

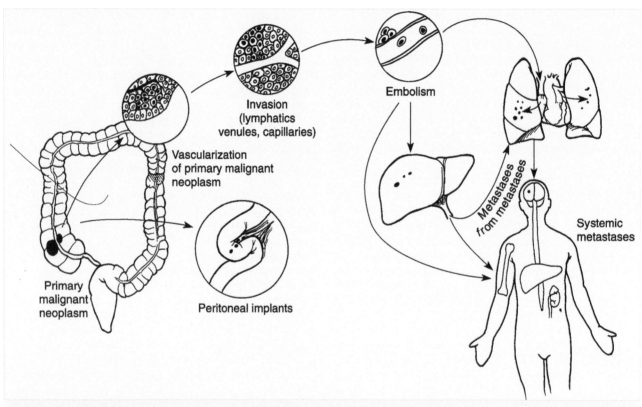

Fig. 21.20 Pathogenesis of metastases from colorectal carcinoma, including metastases from metastases.

gut, stomach, pelvic organs, or abdominal parietes. If the lesion is situated on the retroperitoneal aspect, infiltration of the posterior abdominal wall, duodenum, ureter, perirenal fascia, or iliacus or psoas muscles may occur. Knowledge of the degree of extension is necessary to effect a curative resection. As the carcinoma penetrates the bowel wall, neighboring structures are involved in 10% of patients.[261] Probably one-third to two-thirds of such attached viscera are involved with the neoplastic process. An additional pattern of local spread is perineural invasion, which may reach as far as 10 cm from the primary lesion. Mechanisms involved in invasion of host tissues include (1) mechanical pressure produced by a rapidly proliferating neoplasm may force cords of malignant cells along tissue planes of least resistance, (2) increased cell motility can contribute to malignant cell invasion, and (3) malignant cells may secrete enzymes capable of degrading basement membranes, breaking down barriers between epithelial cells and the stoma.[257]

Transperitoneal Spread

Transmural extension of carcinoma ultimately penetrates the peritoneal surface, following which dissemination may occur in a transcoelomic manner, with implants occurring anywhere on the peritoneal surface or omentum. Approximately 10% of patients with colon carcinoma develop peritoneal deposits.[227]

Lymphatic Spread

The nature of extramural lymphatic spread is of paramount importance in planning the scope of an operation for carcinoma. Indeed, the extent of involvement of the lymphatic system is related to the prognosis of the patient. First metastases usually take place in the paracolic glands nearest the carcinoma and proceed in a stepwise way from gland to gland; however, exceptions to such an orderly progression do occur, and these glands may be missed with the first deposits detected in a more proximal location. Retrograde lymphatic metastases may occur when anterograde blockage is present.

Hematogenous Spread

Blood-borne metastases result in systemic spread of disease, with the liver being the organ most commonly involved. Circulating malignant cells have been found to occur in 28% of patients during induction of anesthesia and in 50% during laparotomy.[258] Surprisingly, follow-up studies of patients with circulating malignant cells during operation have not shown an adverse effect on the ultimate prognosis. Using an experimental melanoma model, it was found that less than 1.0% of cells are viable 24 hours after entry into the circulation and less than 0.1% of these cells eventually produce metastases.[257] Other sites of hematogenous spread include the lung and, less commonly, bone.

Weiss et al[260] analyzed the sequence of events in hematogenous metastasis from colonic carcinoma using 1,541 necropsy reports from 16 centers. The authors' findings were consistent with the cascade hypothesis that metastases develop in discrete steps, first in the liver, next in the lungs, and finally in other sites. There was suggestive evidence in only 216 of 1,194 cases that metastatic patterns (excluding lymph nodes) were causally related to lymph or nonhematogenous pathways. The concept that extrahepatic metastases arise from liver metastases is also supported by Taylor.[261]

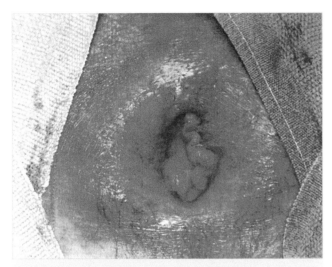

Fig. 21.21 Macroscopic appearance of anal implantation from a proximally located adenocarcinoma of the descending colon.

Implantation

Several reports have been made concerning instances in which exfoliated malignant cells have implanted on raw surfaces, such as with hemorrhoidectomy wounds, fissures-in-ano, fistulas-in-ano, or along the suture line.[259,262,263,264,265,266] Other forms of implantation may relate to an abdominal scar or at the mucocutaneous margin of a colostomy (▶ Fig. 21.21).[257]

21.3.6 Site of Spread

For every 100 patients with intestinal carcinoma, approximately one-half will be cured by operation and 5 will die from lymphatic spread, 10 from local recurrence, and 35 from blood-borne metastases. The organs most frequently involved are the liver (77%), lungs (15%), bones (5%), and brain (5%). The spleen, kidneys, pancreas, adrenals,[267] breast, thyroid, and skin are rarely involved.[227] Even the trachea, tonsils, skeletal muscle, urethra, oral cavity, penis, and nail bed have become involved.[227,268,269,270,271,272]

21.3.7 Staging

It is helpful for the treating physician to be aware of the extent of spread of the disease. By definition, the lesion must penetrate through the muscularis mucosa for it to be considered an invasive carcinoma. Cytologic malignant cells superficial to this layer are considered carcinoma in situ. Dukes[230] originally proposed a classification based on the extent of direct extension along with the presence or absence of regional lymphatic metastases. Dukes' A lesions are those in which growth is confined to the bowel wall, Dukes' B lesions include those in which direct spread has progressed through the full thickness of the wall involving the serosa or fat, and Dukes' C lesions are those in which regional lymph node metastases are present. Dukes' C lesions are further divided into C1, in which lymph nodes are involved near the bowel wall, and C2, in which there is continuous involvement of nodes up to the point of ligature.[273] Not unexpectedly, there is a correlation between histologic grade and the Dukes classification. By common usage, a fourth category, labeled D, has been added. In this group, metastatic disease has advanced beyond the confines of surgical resection, as in the case of a patient with distant metastases or an unresectable local lesion.[274]

Wong et al[275] conducted a study to determine the number of nodes that need to be examined to accurately reflect the histology of the regional lymphatics in colorectal carcinoma. Patients undergoing curative resection for T2 and T3 colorectal carcinomas were reviewed. The number of nodes examined ranged from 0 to 78 (mean, 17 nodes). Node-negative patients had fewer nodes examined (mean, 14 nodes) than node-positive patients (mean, 20 nodes). The entire sample had a node-positive rate of 38.8%. When at least 14 nodes were examined, the percent of patients with at least one positive node was 33.3%. They concluded the examination of at least 14 nodes after resection of T2 or T3 carcinomas of the colon and rectum will accurately stage the lymphatic basin.

The International Union Against Cancer, the American Joint Committee on Cancer, a National Cancer Institute consensus panel, and the College of American Pathologists have all recommended evaluation of at least 12 nodes to ensure adequate sampling.[276,277,278]

The staging of large bowel carcinoma remains a confused topic for most and has been discussed at length.[279] In an effort to better define or categorize patients in order to achieve better prognostication, numerous eponymous modifications have been introduced, but have mostly served only to cloud the issue. Despite the intentions of well-meaning physicians, all in the name of progress, few significant advances have been made. Some of the staging systems proposed are remarkably similar to the Dukes staging system, while others are so detailed that they are cumbersome and unmanageable, difficult to recall and apply, and not practical.[274,279,280,281,282,283,284,285,286,287,288,289] Further confusion has resulted from the fact that the Dukes staging system is frequently misquoted.[287,289]

An ideal staging system would be one that is simple and easy to remember and apply. It should include important prognostic discriminants without becoming too complex. The objectives of a staging system for carcinoma, succinctly enumerated by Davis and Newland,[284] include the following:

1. To aid the physician in planning treatment.
2. To give some indication of prognosis.
3. To assist in the evaluation of treatment results.
4. To facilitate the exchange of information between treatment centers.
5. To contribute to the continuing investigation of human cancer.
6. To provide a method of conveying one group's experience to others without ambiguity.

The most current definitions of the TNM classification are depicted in Box 21.1 and stages in Box 21.2. The completeness of resection designation is seen in Box 21.3.[280] The most commonly used classifications are depicted in ▶ Fig. 21.22.

Box 21.1 TNM (tumor size, node involvement, and metastasis status) classification for colon cancer

Primary tumor (T)

TX	Primary tumor cannot be assessed
T0	No evidence of primary tumor
Tis	Carcinoma in situ: intraepithelial or invasion of lamina propria*
T1	Tumor invades submucosa
T2	Tumor invades muscularis propria
T3	Tumor invades through the muscularis propria into the suberosa, or into nonperitonealized pericolic or perirectal tissues
T4	Tumor directly invades other organs or structures, and/or perforates the visceral peritoneum**,***

* Tis includes cancer cells confined within the glandular basement membrane (intraepithelial) or lamina propria (intramucosal) with no extension through the muscularis mucosae into the submucosa.

** Direct invasion in T4 includes invasion of other segments of the colorectum by way of the serosa; for example, invasion of the sigmoid colon by a carcinoma of the cecum.

*** Tumor that is adherent to other organs or structures, macroscopically, is classified T4. However, if no tumor is present in the adhesion microscopically, the classification should be pT3. The V and L substaging should be used to identify the presence or absence of vascular or lymphatic invasion.

Regional lymph node(s) (N)

NX	Regional lymph nodes cannot be assessed
N0	No regional lymph node metastasis
N1	Metastasis in 1-3 regional lymph nodes
N2	Metastasis in 4 or more regional lymph nodes

A tumor nodule in the pericolorectal adipose tissue of a primary carcinoma without histologic evidence of residual lymph node in the nodule is classified in the pN category as a regional lymph node metastasis if the nodule has the form and smooth contour of a lymph node. If the nodule has an irregular contour, it should be classified in the T category and also coded as V1 (microsopic venous invasion) or as V2 (if it was grossly evident), because there is a strong liklihood that it represents venous invasion.

Distant metastasis (M)

MX	Distant metastasis cannot be assessed
M0	No distant metastasis
M1	Distant metastasis

Source: https://cancerstaging.org/About/news/Pages/Implementation- of-AJCC-8th-Edition-Cancer-Staging-System.aspx. Accessed July 7, 2017.

Box 21.2 Anatomic stage/prognostic groups

Stage grouping

Stage	T	N	M	Dukes*	MAC*
0	Tis	N0	M0	–	–
I	T1	N0	M0	A	A
	T2	N0	M0	A	B1
IIA	T3	N0	M0	B	B2
IIB	T4	N0	M0	B	B3
IIIA	T1-T2	N1	M0	C	C1
IIIB	T3-T4	N1	M0	C	C2/C3
IIIC	Any T	N2	M0	C	C1/C2/C3
IV	Any T	Any N	M1	–	D

* Dukes B is a composite of better (T3, N0, M0) and worse (T4, N0, M0) prognostic groups, as is Dukes C (Any T, N1, M0 and Any T, N2, M0). MAC is the modified Asteler-Coller classification.

Note: The y prefix is to be used for those cancers that are classified after pretreatment, whereas the r prefix is to be used for those cancers that have recurred.

Source: https://cancerstaging.org/About/news/Pages/Implementation- of-AJCC-8th-Edition-Cancer-Staging-System.aspx. Accessed July 7, 2017.

Box 21.3 Completeness of resection designation

- R0: Complete resection, margins histologically negative, no residual tumor left after resection.
- R1: Incomplete resection, margins histologically involved, microscopic tumor remains after resection of gross disease.
- R2: Incomplete resection, margins involved or gross disease remains after resection.

Source: Greene FL, Page DL, Floming ID, et al; American Joint Committee for Cancer. Cancer Staging Handbook. 6th ed. New York, NY: Springer-Verlag; 2002:127–138

21.4 Biology of Growth

The rate of growth of an individual carcinoma is almost certainly the most important prognostic discriminant. Colorectal carcinomas are relatively slow-growing neoplasms, and metastases occur relatively late. In his summary of the results of several series of studies, Spratt,[290] using radiographic measurements, initially calculated a doubling time of 636.5 days in a follow-up of 7.5 years for an unusual case in which a patient was not treated by resection. Similar analysis of 19 other patients revealed a mean doubling time of 620 days, with a 95% range extending from 111 to 3,430 days. Spratt reported the doubling time of pulmonary metastases from colon and rectal carcinoma calculated radiographically

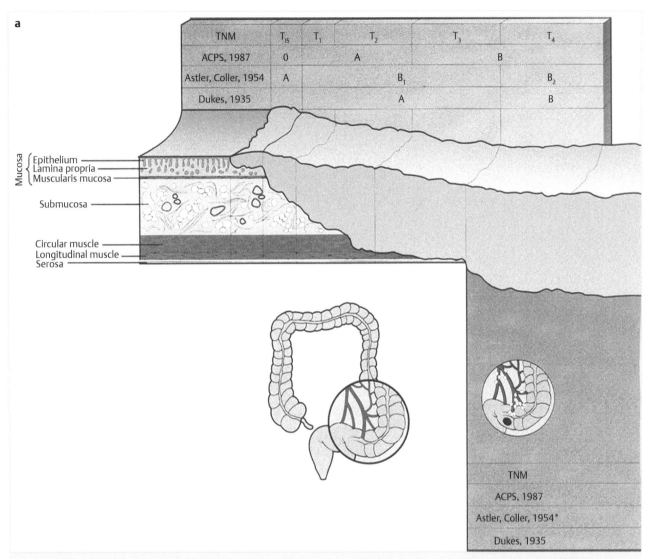

TNM	T_{is}	T_1	T_2	T_3	T_4
ACPS, 1987	0		A		B
Astler, Coller, 1954	A		B_1		B_2
Dukes, 1935			A		B

Mucosa
 Epithelium
 Lamina propria
 Muscularis mucosa
Submucosa
Circular muscle
Longitudinal muscle
Serosa

TNM
ACPS, 1987
Astler, Coller, 1954*
Dukes, 1935

Fig. 21.22 **(a)** Colon wall with anatomic layers and depth of penetration for several proposed staging classifications of colorectal carcinoma. (*Continued*)

to be 109 days, with a 95% range extending from 9 to 1,300 days. He believed that metastatic carcinomas increase their cellular complement six times faster than do primary carcinomas. The doubling time of untreated hepatic metastases has varied between 50 and 95 days.[291,292,293] It has been theorized that the absence of desquamation in the metastatic site accounts for this observed difference. Bolin et al[294] had the opportunity to measure radiographically lesions in 27 patients on two separate occasions, with a median interval of 11 months (4–91 months), and found median doubling time to be 130 days (53–1,570 days). The authors suggested that the high growth rate observed in their investigation was due to the large size of the neoplasm at the time of initial examination. Burnett and Greenbaum[295] believe that although there is little doubt that many colonic carcinomas are slow growing, there is probably a subset of rapidly growing lesions. In a small group of patients, the authors observed doubling times as short as 53 to 150 days. The implication of their report is that

a carcinoma seen on a barium enema study at a given time was not necessarily missed by a negative barium enema study reported, for example, 2 years earlier.

Matsui et al[296] estimated a statistical curve for growth from 31 patients with colorectal carcinoma in which initial lesions were diagnosed as mucosal carcinoma. These lesions were overlooked in the first or second investigations, but were detected later. Initial radiographic features were as follows: 4 pedunculated lesions, 1 semipedunculated lesion, 6 sessile lesions, 9 superficially elevated lesions, and 11 superficially depressed lesions. The diameters of the initial lesions were 12.1 ± 6.1 mm. The final depths of invasion were 6 mucosal carcinomas, 12 submucosal carcinomas, 6 muscularis propria carcinomas, and 7 serosal carcinomas. The observation period between the initial and final examinations was 41.5 ± 25.8 months. Growth speed of early colorectal carcinoma was estimated through a statistically significant growth curve. Estimated doubling time of the volume of early colorectal carcinoma was 26 months.

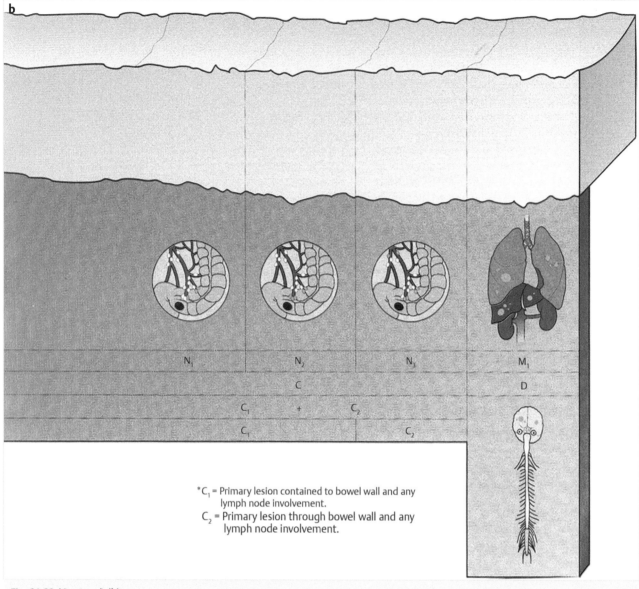

*C_1 = Primary lesion contained to bowel wall and any
lymph node involvement.
C_2 = Primary lesion through bowel wall and any
lymph node involvement.

Fig. 21.22 (*Continued*) **(b)**

21.4.1 Clinical Features and Symptoms

Patients with carcinoma of the large intestine may present in one of three characteristic ways: insidious onset of chronic symptoms, acute intestinal obstruction, or perforation with peritonitis. Aldridge et al[297] reported that those conditions will occur in 77, 16, and 7% of patients, respectively. Mandava et al[298] reported perforated carcinomas in 51 of 1,551 patients (3.3%) with colorectal carcinoma. Localized perforation with abscess formation occurred in 31 patients (61%), and free perforation with generalized peritonitis occurred in 20 patients (39%). Runkel et al,[299] in a review of 923 patients, found the presentation with insidious onset, obstruction, and perforation to occur in 92.0, 6.0, and 2.0% of patients, respectively, with a combination of obstruction and perforation occurring in 0.5% of patients. In a report from Scotland of 750 consecutive patients, an unusually high number (33%) was presented as an emergency.[300]

Depending on the location in the bowel, one or another of the following symptoms may predominate. Bleeding is probably the most common symptom of large bowel malignancy.[301] All too often, the bleeding is attributed by the patient, and regrettably by the physician as well, to hemorrhoids. Despite the fact that the most common cause of rectal bleeding is hemorrhoids, bleeding cannot be dismissed lightly, especially in a middle-aged or older individual. It has been estimated that visible blood per rectum occurs in 10% of the adult population over the age of 30 years.[302] However, Beart et al[301] found that in patients 40 years of age or older with a history of rectal bleeding and known hemorrhoids, 6% had rectal or colon carcinoma and 14% had colon polyps. This underscores the necessity of taking the symptom of bleeding seriously. Bleeding may be occult, as is often the case in right-sided lesions, or overt, being either bright red, dark purple, or even black, depending on the location in the bowel.

The second most common presenting symptom is probably a change in bowel habits, either constipation or diarrhea.[301] The absolute frequency of defecation is not important, but a deviation from what is normal for a given individual may signal the presence of an intestinal neoplasm. Lesions in the proximal colon may not result in a change in bowel symptoms until they are very far advanced. Lesions in the distal colon are more likely to be manifest in symptoms since the stool is more formed in consistency and the bowel lumen is narrower. A progressive narrowing of the caliber of the stool may be reported in the case of a compromised lumen.

Pain may occur with almost equal frequency as the preceding symptom. Abdominal pain may be vague and poorly localized, or it may result from a partially obstructing lesion of the colon. The latter type of pain is generally colicky in nature and may be associated with obstructive symptoms of bloating, nausea, and even vomiting. Rectal pain does not occur with carcinoma unless there is sacral nerve root or sciatic nerve involvement. However, tenesmus may occur with rectal carcinoma. Back pain is a late sign of penetration of retroperitoneal structures.

Other symptoms include mucus discharge, which may coat the stool or be mixed with it. Investigation of weight loss as a solitary complaint only uncommonly yields a large bowel malignancy. However, when associated with a carcinoma, weight loss is usually a sign of advanced disease and bodes a poor prognosis. Nonspecific symptoms of general impairment of health, loss of strength, anemia, and sporadic fever also may be present. Rarely a carcinoma of the cecum obstructs the appendiceal orifice, and the patient presents with the signs and symptoms of acute appendicitis.[303] Bladder involvement may result in urinary frequency, suprapubic pressure, and even pneumaturia if a sigmoidovesical fistula has developed. In the report of the Commission on Cancer,[304] in which 16,527 patients were diagnosed with carcinoma of the colon, the presenting symptoms in order of frequency were abdominal pain (40.5%), change in bowel habits (33.2%), rectal bleeding (28.5%), occult bleeding (34.3%), malaise (16%), bowel obstruction (14.9%), pelvic pain (3.4%), emergency presentation (6.6%), and jaundice (1%).

Iron deficiency anemia is a recognized complication of colorectal carcinoma, especially with right-sided lesions, and failure to investigate the anemia in older patients may lead to a delay in diagnosis. Acher et al[305] conducted a study of all patients presenting with confirmed colorectal carcinoma in a catchment population of 280,000. The criterion for iron deficiency anemia was hemoglobin less than 10.1 g. Of 440 patients with colorectal carcinoma, 38% had iron deficiency anemia at diagnosis and of the latter, 12% were known to have iron deficiency anemia for more than 6 months before diagnosis, and 6% had iron deficiency anemia more than 1 year before diagnosis. Iron deficiency anemia was more common in right-sided carcinomas (65%) than those arising in the left side of the colon and rectum (26%). They concluded the investigation of iron deficiency anemia in older patients is important but in order to detect 26 patients with colorectal carcinoma a year earlier, the investigation of approximately 5,000 patients would be required—a detection rate of less than 1%.

Church and McGannon[306] performed a study to find out how often and how accurately a family history of colorectal carcinoma was recorded in the charts of 100 inpatients on a colorectal surgical floor. The chart review was repeated 4 years later. In the initial review, they found that a family history was recorded in 45 of 100 charts. It was accurate for colorectal carcinoma in 36 charts. Four years later, the rate of family history recording increased to 61 of 96, whereas the accuracy rate did not change. Despite improvement during a 4-year period, there is still room for further improvement.

21.4.2 General and Abdominal Examinations

The general examination may be a guide to the patient's state of nutrition. Any obvious excess weight loss may indicate advanced disease. Pallor may be a sign of anemia. The assessment may help in evaluating the patient's fitness for operation.

Usually, the general abdominal examination fails to reveal significant abnormalities. Occasionally, a mass may be present and may indicate the primary malignancy or possible metastatic disease. The liver may be enlarged, and if it is also umbilicated, this sign would be characteristic of metastatic disease. Ascites may be appreciated. Borborygmi may be present. Abdominal distention may suggest partial obstruction from a constricting lesion. Inguinal and left supraclavicular lymphadenopathy can occur rarely. Peritonitis from a perforated carcinoma may be difficult to differentiate from perforated diverticulitis.

21.4.3 Digital Rectal Examination

Although a digital rectal examination will not identify the presence of a colon carcinoma, it should reveal the presence of a rectal lesion. The examination is described in detail in Chapters 3 and 22. Sometimes a sigmoid carcinoma that hangs down into the cul-de-sac may be palpable.

21.4.4 Extraintestinal Manifestations

Rosato et al[307] noted a number of cutaneous presentations associated with gastrointestinal malignancy. These included acanthosis nigricans, dermatomyositis, and pemphigoid (see Chapter 11). Halak et al[308] reported on the incidence of synchronous colorectal and renal carcinomas and reviewed the literature on that issue. Among 103 patients who underwent colorectal surgery in their series, 5 cases of synchronous colorectal and renal carcinomas were detected (4.9%). A review of the literature suggests the incidence of simultaneous colorectal and renal carcinoma to be 0.04 to 0.5%.

21.4.5 Synchronous Carcinomas

Synchronous carcinomas are not uncommon, and in recent reviews the incidence was found to range from 2 to 8% in colon carcinoma patients.[309,310,311,312] In view of this, it behooves the treating surgeon to evaluate the entire colon, if possible, to determine the presence of other neoplastic lesions. Colonoscopy performed preoperatively in patients undergoing elective resection is the optimal method for assessing the unresected colon for synchronous lesions. In a prospective study of 166 patients, Langevin and Nivatvongs[313] found synchronous carcinomas in

8 patients; 7 of them required resection of more colon than was necessary to treat the index carcinoma. In a study of 320 colorectal patients, Evers et al[310] found synchronous carcinomas in different surgical segments in 6 of 21 patients (38%). Pinol et al[311] conducted a study designed to identify individual and familial characteristics associated with the development of synchronous colorectal neoplasms in patients with colorectal carcinoma. During a 1-year period, 1,522 patients with colorectal carcinoma attended in 25 Spanish hospitals were included. Synchronous colorectal neoplasms were documented in 505 patients (33.2%): adenoma (in 411 patients, 27%); carcinoma (in 27 patients, 1.8%); or both ($n = 67$, 4.4%). Development of these lesions was associated with male gender (OR, 1.94), personal history of colorectal adenoma (OR, 3.39), proximal location of primary carcinoma (OR, 1.4), TNM stage II (OR, 1.31), mucinous carcinoma (OR, 1.89), and family history of gastric carcinoma (OR, 2.03). Based on individual and familial characteristics associated with synchronous colorectal neoplasms, it has been possible to identify a subgroup of patients with colorectal carcinoma prone to multicentricity of neoplasm with potential implications on the delineation of preventive strategies.

If technically and logistically possible, it would be ideal for all patients about to undergo elective resection of carcinoma to have a preoperative colonoscopic examination. If not possible, it is suggested that patients should have postoperative colonoscopy.

21.4.6 Associated Polyps

Neoplastic polyps are frequently associated with carcinoma of the colon, and, indeed, on sigmoidoscopic examination, when a patient is found to have a neoplastic polyp, the entire colon should be assessed to rule out the presence of another associated polyp or an associated malignancy. Approximately 7% of patients with polyps will harbor an associated carcinoma of the colon or rectum.[314] Slater et al[315] studied the relationship between the location of a colorectal carcinoma and the existence of adenomas in 591 patients. The overall incidence of adenomas was 29.7%, with resected specimens of right-sided carcinomas containing adenomas in 47% of cases and left-sided specimens having them in 22%. Thus, the authors suggested that efforts be made to identify polyps preoperatively in patients with colorectal carcinoma. Also, since patients with carcinoma and associated adenomas are at increased risk of developing metachronous carcinoma, the group with right-sided carcinoma should be part of a particularly active surveillance program.

Chu et al[316] retrospectively studied the relationship of colorectal carcinoma with polyps in 1,202 patients. Synchronous polyps were found in 36% of patients. Synchronous carcinoma was found in 4.4% of patients and metachronous carcinoma developed in 3.5% of patients. The incidence of synchronous carcinoma and a metachronous carcinoma increased with synchronous polyps, and varied according to number, size, and histologic features of the polyps. The adjusted 5-year survival rate was improved in patients with synchronous polyps compared with those without synchronous polyps. The pattern of relapse was the same for the synchronous polyp and nonsynchronous polyp groups. The authors even went so far as to recommend subtotal colectomy for colorectal carcinoma and synchronous polyps in good-risk patients.

There is a general trend for the incidence of multiple carcinomas to rise as the number of adenomas increases, whereas in patients in whom there is evidence of only one adenoma being present, the incidence of multiple carcinomas is less than 2%, and the figure for those with more than five adenomas rises to 30%.[231]

21.4.7 Other Associated Malignancies

In a review of 9,329 cases of colorectal carcinoma from the literature, Lee et al[317] found that the incidence of primary malignant neoplasms at sites other than the colon ranged from 3.8 to 7.8%. In a series of 14,235 patients with colon and rectal carcinomas followed for an average of 3.6 years, Tanaka et al[318] observed an elevated risk of second primary malignancies as follows: rectum (observed/expected [O/E], 2.0, men; O/E, 4.3, women), corpus uteri (O/E, 8.2), ovary (O/E, 4.3), and thyroid gland (O/E 4.7, women). These observations were more notable in right-sided colon carcinoma patients than left-sided colon carcinoma and in those younger than 50 years. Schoen et al[319] also found that women with a history of breast, endometrial, or ovarian carcinoma were at a statistically significant increased risk for subsequent colorectal carcinoma (1.1, 1.4, and 1.6, respectively).

21.5 Complications

A number of well-recognized complications of carcinoma of the large bowel may alter its clinical presentation.

21.5.1 Obstruction

Depending on the macroscopic features and location of the malignancy, interference with the passage of intestinal contents may occur. Carcinoma is the most common cause of large bowel obstruction, contributing to 60% of cases in the elderly.[320] Ohman[321] summarized the results of 26 series on colorectal carcinoma reported in the literature. The combined total comprised 23,434 patients of whom 15% presented with obstruction. Incidences ranged from 7 to 29%. In the right colon, carcinomas are usually polypoid, and because of the liquid nature of the intestinal contents, obstruction is unlikely unless it involves the critical ileocecal valve, in which case obstruction may supervene. In the left colon, where the intestinal contents are solid and the nature of the malignancy is more inclined to be annular, occlusion is more likely. Complete obstruction of the colon from carcinoma is often entirely insidious in its onset. The patient often has had progressive difficulty in moving his or her bowels and has taken increasing doses of laxatives until the abdomen has become more distended with pain and eventual obstipation. Nausea and vomiting may supervene. Alternatively, the patient may present with sudden, severe, colicky abdominal pain that persists, and investigation may reveal a complete obstruction. The offending lesion may be surprisingly small, as seen in ▶ Fig. 21.23. On examination, the patient's general condition usually is found to be good, because dehydration and electrolyte depletion are often late phenomena. Examination of the abdomen reveals that it is distended and tympanitic but not

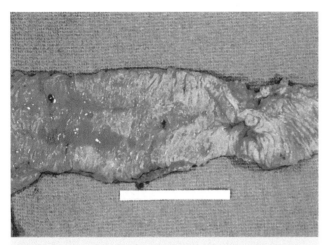

Fig. 21.23 Small adenocarcinoma of splenic flexure in patient who presented with acute colonic obstruction.

tender. Hyperactive peristalsis may be present. It is unlikely that an abdominal mass will be felt in the presence of a distended abdomen. Digital examination may reveal a balloon-type rectum and, in the exceptional case, a palpable carcinoma may be present. A mass in the cul de sac may be appreciated, representing either a sigmoid loop that is hanging down or a cul de sac implant. Sigmoidoscopy may reveal the lower edge of a constricting lesion. The diagnosis is usually suggested from a history of intestinal symptoms and physical findings. Plain X-ray films of the abdomen will reveal the presence of obstruction and indicate its level. The amount of small bowel distention will depend on the competence of the ileocecal valve. The presence of an obstructing carcinoma can be confirmed with an emergency barium enema study.

A nonspecific type of colitis may develop proximal to an obstructing carcinoma of the colon.[322,323] It is reported to occur in 2.0 to 7.5% of cases.[324,325] In most cases, there is a short segment of normal mucosa immediately proximal to the carcinoma, above which the colitic process appears. The etiology of these changes in the colonic mucosa proximal to the obstructed lesion is obscure, although the gross pathology and microscopic features are consistent with those of ischemic colitis in the subacute or chronic phase.[324] The extent of the colitic process varies. It may be unsuspected and discovered only at the time of operation. The extent of resection may be dictated by the length of inflamed bowel. Seow-Choen et al[325] reported that 4 of 204 new cases of colorectal carcinoma seen in a 24-month period were proven to have concomitant proximal ischemic colitis. Ischemic colitis associated with obstructing carcinoma of the colorectum may present dramatically with gangrene or colonic perforation if the acute vascular insufficiency is severe. Less severe degrees of ischemic insult must be recognized intraoperatively because the incorporation of ischemic colon in a colonic anastomosis may result in an anastomotic leak. The National Surgical Adjuvant Breast and Bowel Project (NSABP) trials have suggested that obstructing carcinomas in the right colon carry a more significant risk of recurrence and carcinoma-related mortality than obstructing carcinomas in the left colon.[326] The diminished survival rate in patients presenting with obstructing malignancies does not appear to correlate significantly with annularity of the lesion or the presence of lymph node metastases.

21.5.2 Perforation

The incidence of perforation associated with carcinoma of the colon is in the 6 to 12% range of all hospital admissions for colon carcinoma.[323] A perforation may result in peritonitis, abscess formation, adherence to a neighboring structure, or fistulous communication into a viscus. Perforation is found in conjunction with obstruction in approximately 1% of patients with colorectal carcinoma. In patients with obstruction, concurrent perforation is found in 12 to 19% of patients.[323,327] If acute obstruction supervenes in the middle or distal colon, the cecum may perforate. However, the most common form of perforation is associated with the carcinoma itself. Such perforation may develop suddenly with diffuse peritonitis or more gradually with a localized peritonitis; when it occurs in the cecum, it may resemble appendicitis. Patients with obstruction and a proximal perforation present as desperately ill individuals with generalized peritonitis, dehydration, and electrolyte depletion. Immediate exploratory laparotomy is demanded. Patients without obstruction but with perforation of the carcinoma are also gravely ill and require immediate laparotomy after some correction of dehydration and electrolyte depletion. Patients without obstruction but with perforation of a carcinoma may present with a localized peritonitis. Under these circumstances it may be confused with diverticulitis if the sigmoid colon is involved, or with appendicitis or Crohn's disease if the right colon is involved.

21.5.3 Bleeding

Bleeding is a common symptom of colorectal carcinoma, but massive bleeding is an uncommon presentation.

21.5.4 Unusual Infections Associated with Colorectal Carcinoma

Unusual infections associated with colorectal carcinoma may, in some instances, be the sole clue to the presence of a malignancy. The infections are either related to invasion of tissues or organs in close proximity to the neoplasm or secondary to distant seeding by transient bacteremia arising from necrotic carcinomas. Panwalker[328] identified a series of patients whose clinical presentations included endocarditis (*Streptococcus bovis* bacteremia), meningitis (*S. bovis* bacteremia), nontraumatic gas gangrene (*Escherichia coli*), empyema (*E. coli*, *Bacteroides fragilis*), hepatic abscesses (*Clostridium septicum*), retroperitoneal abscesses (*E. coli*, *B. fragilis*), clostridial sepsis, and colovesical fistulas with urosepsis (*E. coli*). Panwalker also reviewed the English-language literature and identified other infections associated with colon carcinoma, including nontraumatic crepitant cellulitis, suppurative thyroiditis, pericarditis, appendicitis, pulmonary microabscesses, septic arthritis, and fever of unknown origin. Lam et al[329] reported an unusual presentation of colon carcinoma with a purulent pericarditis and cardiac tamponade caused by *B. fragilis.*

443

With or without endocarditis, septicemia caused by *S. bovis* may be associated with an occult colonic malignancy.[330,331] The septicemia also has been described with a variety of gastrointestinal pathologic conditions, such as colonic adenomas, inflammatory bowel disease, and carcinoma of the esophagus. Patients may be entirely asymptomatic, but all patients with endocarditis caused by *S. bovis* should be evaluated for concomitant colon carcinoma.

In a literature review, Panwalker[328] found *S. bovis* bacteremia reported in 467 adults with endocarditis present in 62%, absent in 13%, and of unclear status in the remaining patients. Other organisms associated with endocarditis are *S. salivarius* and enterococcus. An asymptomatic colonic malignancy has been reported in a patient with meningitis caused by *S. salivarius*.[332] *S. bovis* meningitis was reported in 10 adults.[328] Silent colon carcinoma has been reported to present as hepatic abscesses,[333,334] and therefore anaerobic hepatic abscesses might alert the physician to the possibility of a malignancy of the large intestine.

Panwalker[328] found 55 patients with the dramatic clinical presentation of gas gangrene associated with colorectal carcinoma (16 of which were cecal). The gas gangrene was metastatic in 10 patients. Sites included the neck, chest wall, upper extremities, shoulders, and axilla. Kudsk[335] subsequently reported five cases of painful, rapidly spreading gas-producing infection of the lower extremity (three cases), upper extremity (one), and pelvis (one), which represented metastatic *C. septicum* infections in diabetic patients. All had occult carcinomas of the right colon. More recently, Lorimer and Eldus[336] reported three cases of invasive *C. septicum* infection associated with colorectal carcinoma. The authors cited a previous review of 162 cases of nontraumatic *C. septicum* infection, which identified malignant disease in 81%, approximately half of which were colorectal. The carcinoma is typically right sided and always ulcerated, which can occur in three circumstances: occult carcinoma (80%), anastomotic recurrence, or carcinoma that is unresectable or has been bypassed. In summary, gas gangrene associated with colorectal carcinoma is a catastrophic illness that appears to be clostridial, affects diabetic patients disproportionately, and, in almost 50% of cases, is the result of an otherwise silent cecal carcinoma.

21.6 Diagnosis

In a case of carcinoma of the colon the patient's history may not be helpful. Consequently, early diagnosis may depend on screening, which may be directed at the identification of high-risk groups, the use of screening tests, and the investigation of patients with positive screening test results. Early detection is described in Chapter 20. Suffice it to say that a combination of occult blood testing and flexible fiberoptic sigmoidoscopy is the minimum current recommendation.[337] Colonoscopy is ideal and preferable. Atypical dyspepsia and vague abdominal symptoms should be investigated since malignancy may be the cause of otherwise unexplained ill health and anemia. Of course, the symptoms suggestive of the disease, as previously described, should be pursued with the appropriate modalities as described in the discussion of investigations.

For differential diagnosis, a host of conditions may be considered, depending on the predominant symptom complex with which the patient presents. These include inflammatory bowel disease, either of the nonspecific type, such as ulcerative colitis or Crohn's disease, or of the specific type, such as amebiasis, actinomycosis, or tuberculosis. For patients presenting with narrowed bowel, ischemic strictures may be included in the differential diagnosis. Acute abdomen may be confused with conditions such as diverticulitis or appendicitis with abscess, Crohn's disease, foreign body perforation, or even an infarcted appendix epiploica. If marked bleeding is the prominent feature, vascular ectasis, diverticulosis, or acute ischemia are possibilities. With acute obstruction, volvulus, diverticulitis, and Crohn's disease might be considered. Extrinsic pressure from a metastatic carcinoma, endometriosis, or even pancreatitis is possible in appropriate circumstances. Uncommon conditions (e.g., colitis cystica profunda) also can be considered.

21.7 Investigations

21.7.1 Occult Blood Testing

Occult blood determinations are of value in the screening setting; however, for patients who have symptoms that are suggestive of large bowel disease, occult blood testing is inadequate.[337] Certainly patients who relate a history of rectal bleeding do not need occult blood testing to confirm its presence.

21.7.2 Endoscopy

Anoscopy and Sigmoidoscopy

Use of an anoscope to determine the presence of any significant internal hemorrhoids is of value, especially for patients who present with bright-red rectal bleeding.

Sigmoidoscopic examination is an indispensable diagnostic tool in the assessment of rectal carcinoma.[338] The appearance of rectal carcinoma is usually quite distinctive. A protruding mass into the lumen may be seen, but more characteristically a raised everted edge with a central, sometimes necrotic, sloughing base will be noted. The distance from the lower edge of the lesion to the anal verge should be carefully determined because it may be crucial in deciding whether intestinal continuity can be restored. Two points also should be noted: which wall the lesion is located on and whether the lesion is annular. In addition, information can be obtained regarding the mobility of the lesion by placing the end of the sigmoidoscope against the lower margin of the lesion and exerting gentle pressure along the long axis. Mobile carcinomas can be moved and present a quite different sensation from the rigid feel of a fixed carcinoma. The size of the lesion should be recorded, and finally a biopsy should be performed to confirm the diagnosis.

Flexible Fiberoptic Sigmoidoscopy

Flexible fiberoptic sigmoidoscopy has assumed an increasing role in the diagnosis of colon disease.[339,340] Because of its greater length and flexibility than the rigid sigmoidoscope, the flexible sigmoidoscope allows for the detection of a larger number of neoplastic lesions. In addition, equivocal lesions seen on a contrast enema can be elucidated if they are within the reach of the scope. Some surgeons have replaced rigid sigmoidoscopy with flexible sigmoidoscopy, but others, including the authors, believe that the rigid instrument is still superior for the crucial assessment of the distance of a carcinoma from the anal verge and this judgment cannot be made satisfactorily or accurately with a flexible instrument.

Colonoscopy

The role of colonoscopy also has assumed greater importance in the evaluation of colon disease (Chapter 4). In particular, colonoscopy plays a major role in screening for colorectal carcinoma, especially in high-risk patients, as described in Chapter 20. With specific reference to its value in the assessment of patients with large bowel malignancy, colonoscopy has been recommended as a preoperative examination to detect the presence of synchronous neoplastic polyps or carcinomas. Its necessity in the preoperative or at least perioperative setting has been debated, but growing evidence suggests that it plays an important role.[310,341,342] The rationale is that synchronous carcinomas exist in 2 to 7% of cases.[313,343,344] It has been suggested that preoperative colonoscopy alters the operative procedure in one-third of patients.[342] Another group of surgeons, concerned with the potential for implantation of malignant cells, exfoliated by preoperative colonoscopy, has opted for intraoperative palpation to detect synchronous carcinomas and postoperative colonoscopy to clear the colon of polyps.[345]

21.7.3 Radiology

Barium Enema

In the past, the largest number of carcinomas of the colon were diagnosed in the barium enema examination. Currently, colonoscopy is the preferred investigative modality. Various radiologic features may be demonstrated, such as an annular, or "napkin ring," appearance, as is often seen in the left colon (▶ Fig. 21.24). Features distinguishing it from spasm are the irregular, jagged outline and destruction of the mucosa with a typical "apple core" appearance and overhanging edges. A large filling defect representing a bulky neoplasm projecting into the lumen is seen more often in the right colon (▶ Fig. 21.25). A polypoid sessile lesion occupying only one wall of the bowel is demonstrated in ▶ Fig. 21.26. Sometimes a polypoid lesion on a pedicle may be entirely malignant. Occasionally, a complete retrograde obstruction may be present (▶ Fig. 21.27), but this radiologic appearance is not necessarily indicative of a clinically anterograde obstruction.

In an audit of 557 barium enema studies in patients with known carcinomas, a malignant lesion was recorded in 85%.[346] Reviewing cases in which there was failure to perceive a demonstrated lesion or failure to analyze a perceived lesion indicated that 94% of carcinomas should have been reported.

The air-contrast barium enema has been considered superior to the full-column barium enema for detection of small polyps. For detection of large constricting lesions, the single-contrast enema is superior to the double-contrast enema.

In the event of a negative barium enema report, subsequent management will depend on clinical assessment. Should there be a strong degree of clinical suspicion of a carcinoma, colonoscopic evaluation would be in order. If no strong suspicion exists and the barium enema was ordered because of minimal symptoms of constipation, no further investigation may be deemed necessary. If rectal bleeding was the prominent feature and the patient exhibited prominent internal hemorrhoids, hemorrhoid treatment should be performed to eliminate confusion with bleeding of colonic origin. Should bleeding persist after such treatment, colonoscopic examination would be indicated.

Intravenous Pyelography

Previously, there was controversy as to whether an intravenous pyelogram (IVP) is necessary preoperatively. Supporters suggest that it is helpful to know in advance whether the ureters or bladder are involved with the neoplastic process, whether two kidneys are present, or whether additional ureters may be present. Furthermore, in the follow-up of patients who develop urinary tract problems postoperatively, it provides a baseline for differentiating whether these problems are due to a surgical complication or are secondary to pre-existing urologic disease.[347,348] In one study, abnormalities were found in as many as 26% of patients.[348] Adversaries suggest that intravenous pyelography is not cost-effective and is not necessarily reliable in demonstrating the absence of disease

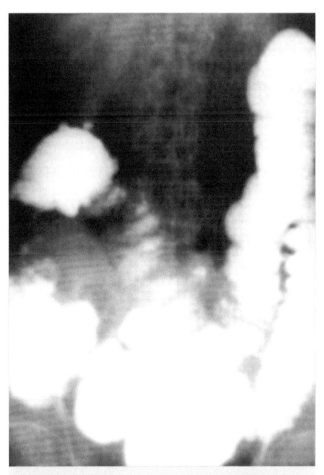

Fig. 21.24 Barium enema study appearance of an annular adenocarcinoma of the colon. (This image is provided courtesy of M. Rosenbloom, MD.)

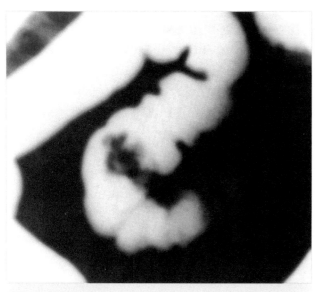

Fig. 21.25 Barium enema study appearance of a polypoid adenocarcinoma of the colon. (This image is provided courtesy of M. Rosenbloom, MD.)

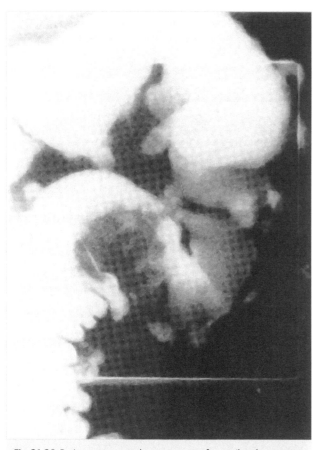

Fig. 21.26 Barium enema study appearance of a sessile adenocarcinoma of the colon. (This image is provided courtesy of M. Rosenbloom, MD.)

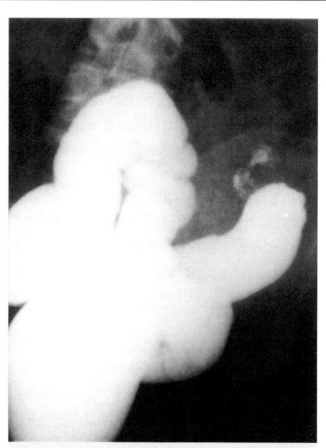

Fig. 21.27 Barium enema study appearance of a complete retrograde obstruction due to adenocarcinoma of the colon. (This image is provided courtesy of M. Rosenbloom, MD.)

Ultrasonography

Sonographic evaluation of colorectal carcinoma can be performed via transcutaneous or intracorporeal approaches. The transcutaneous approach evaluates the liver for metastases and identifies ascites, adenopathy, and an omental cake. Intracorporeal imaging can be performed endoluminally, intraoperatively, or laparoscopically.

Preoperative assessment of the liver by ultrasonography may provide valuable information to consider when recommending the appropriate management of patients with colorectal carcinoma. In a preoperative ultrasonographic study of 195 patients, Grace et al[351] found a false-negative rate of 7.2%.

Both rigid and flexible echoendoscopes are available. Because of the lack of input on the management of the patient with a carcinoma above the peritoneal reflection, endosonography currently finds its role in staging rectal carcinoma. The echo-colonoscope, although available, has not been evaluated extensively. With the advent of laparoscopic colectomy, preoperative endosonography may have an increased role in the future.

Intraoperative liver ultrasonography is currently being touted as the most accurate method for detecting colorectal metastases. It has served to supplement inspection and palpation at the time of laparotomy. The liver can be surveyed by a radiologist or surgeon experienced in intraoperative sonography in 5 to 10 minutes. Although peripheral lesions are easily palpable by

involvement.[349,350] Currently, an abdominal and pelvic (CT) scan, which has become a standard preoperative staging method, provides almost all the information previously sought by the IVP.

the surgeon, deeper lesions may be missed by manual examination. Additional findings may very well alter the course of management, either extending or eliminating the planned procedure. Rafaelsen et al[352] compared diagnostic accuracies of measuring liver enzymes, preoperative ultrasonography, manual palpation, and intraoperative ultrasonography in the detection of liver metastases in 295 consecutive patients with colorectal carcinoma. The presence of metastases was further assessed by ultrasonography 3 months postoperatively. The sensitivity of intraoperative ultrasonography (62 of 64) was significantly superior to that of manual palpation (54 of 64) and preoperative ultrasonography (45 of 64). The lowest sensitivity was presented by the measurement of liver enzymes. The authors concluded that intraoperative ultrasonography reduced the number of patients with liver metastases from being subjected to superfluous or even harmful liver surgery and may increase the number in whom liver surgery will prolong life. They cited six other studies that suggest a higher sensitivity of intraoperative ultrasonography than preoperative ultrasonography in the detection of liver metastases. Meijer et al[353] studied a series of 122 patients who underwent elective resection—34 with suspected liver lesions seen on preoperative CT and ultrasonography and 88 without suspected lesions. Of the 34 patients with suspected lesions, the diagnosis was confirmed with intraoperative ultrasonography in 21 patients, and in the remaining 13 patients, the suspected lesion was shown to be benign. Of the 88 patients with normal preoperative imaging, lesions were detected in five patients. During an 18-month follow-up, 6.5% of patients developed liver metastases not recognized during operation. Machi et al[354] evaluated 189 patients with colorectal carcinoma at the time of operation and revealed that the sensitivity of intraoperative ultrasonography (93.3%) was significantly higher than that of preoperative ultrasonography (41.3%), conventional CT (47.1%), and manual palpation (66.3%). Metastatic liver lesions were detected solely by intraoperative ultrasonography in 9.5% of patients. During the postoperative follow-up period of 18 months or more, liver metastases that were unrecognized during operation appeared in 6.9% of patients. Reevaluation based on these follow-up results indicated that the sensitivity of intraoperative ultrasonography decreased to 82.3%, which was still significantly better than that of other methods. Takeuchi et al[355] reported on a consecutive series of 119 colorectal carcinoma patients who were studied by preoperative extracorporeal ultrasonography, inspection and palpation of the liver at laparotomy, and intraoperative liver ultrasonography. Hepatic metastases were diagnosed in 19 patients—8 by extracorporeal ultrasonography, 7 by palpation, and the last 4 only after intraoperative ultrasonography. Follow-up for a median of 38 months revealed another 8 patients with liver metastases detected at a mean time from operation of 14.7 months. The authors concluded that although intraoperative sonography is a sensitive and useful method in detecting liver metastases, some occult hepatic metastases will remain undetected. Laparoscopic ultrasonography has been used to image the liver and may lead to a less invasive manner of staging the patient and providing pathologic confirmation.

Computed Tomography

CT scanning of the abdomen and pelvis delineates the extent of the disease and excludes metastatic disease in the liver and helps in the preoperative planning of the extent of the operation. Kerner et al[356] used CT of the abdomen and pelvis to augment the preoperative evaluation of 158 consecutive patients with primary, colorectal carcinoma. In 88 patients, findings present on CT were otherwise unknown. Of those, 35% were clinically significant in that they allowed the surgeon to alter the proposed operative procedure or added additional technical information for consideration preoperatively. Findings included liver metastases,[26] atrophic kidney (three), and abdominal wall or contiguous organ invasion.[11] In addition, two other solid organ carcinomas were detected. The authors concluded that CT eliminates the need for a preoperative IVP, improves the preoperative staging of metastatic disease, and provides a baseline for comparison during the postoperative follow-up if recurrence is suspected or adjuvant therapy is planned.

CT has a lower accuracy for identifying early stages of primary colorectal carcinoma, but is useful in examining patients suspected of having extensive disease or recurrent disease with an extrinsic component at an anastomosis.[356,357] Mauchley et al[358] assessed the clinical utility of the practice of routine preoperative CT scanning and determined its cost-effectiveness in 130 colon carcinoma patients. CT scans provided information that was used in treatment planning in 33% of patients and definitively altered the mode of treatment in 16% of patients. The practice saved the institution US$24,018 over 6 years. They concluded routine preoperative CT scanning definitively alters treatment in a small number of cases and is cost-effective.

Magnetic Resonance Imaging

Magnetic resonance imaging (MRI) is a technique that creates images by evaluating nuclei for the absorption or emission of electromagnetic energy in the presence of a stable magnetic field.[359] It has a greater tissue contrast resolution than CT, is multiplanar, and involves no ionizing radiation. The imaging times are longer, the spatial resolution is less than CT, calcifications and bone detail are not as obvious, and the study is more expensive. Certain patients cannot be safely imaged and these include those with cardiac pacemakers, implanted drug infusion pumps, ferromagnetic vascular aneurysm clips, and ocular foreign bodies.

MRI has limitations in assessing depth of penetration of the bowel wall, but this limitation can be partly overcome by larger magnets and newer protocols, which can improve accuracy to 90%. The sensitivity for detecting lymph node metastases ranges from 13 to 40%. Initially, MRI was believed to be better than CT in distinguishing between fibrotic changes and recurrences, but this is probably not so. MRI can be used to assess hepatic metastases. Metastatic lesions to the lungs are better defined by CT. For metastatic lesions involving osseous structures, especially the spine and central nervous system, MRI should be the imaging modality of choice. Zerhouni et al[360] evaluated the accuracy of CT and MRI in staging 478 patients with colorectal carcinoma. CT was more accurate than MRI in the definition of penetration of the muscularis propria by rectal carcinoma (74 vs. 58%). Accuracies were equivalent in depiction of transmural extent of colonic carcinoma. CT and MRI exhibited accuracies of 62 and 64%, respectively, in assessment of lymph node involvement with sensitivities of 48 and 22%, respectively. The accuracy of MRI and CT in the evaluation of liver metastases was equivalent (85%).

447

Positron Emission Tomography

Positron emission tomography (PET) is a method of imaging using a positron-emitting isotope-labeled compound that is incorporated into the biochemical process occurring in organs and tissues of the body. The anatomic and morphologic characteristics are not as well delineated as with other imaging modalities such as CT and MRI, but PET images provide useful information about the nature and physiology of the cellular function of the tissue and have been used to evaluate neoplasms, including colorectal carcinoma. The most widely used isotope is 2-deoxy-2-(^{18}F)fluoro-D-glucose, or fluorodeoxyglucose (FDG). Imaging relies on the premise that there is an enhanced rate of glucose in malignant tissue. PET scanning is more accurate than CT scanning in identifying malignancy. This is especially true in the postoperative follow-up in differentiating recurrent carcinoma from fibrosis. Tempero et al[359] reviewed three studies that compared the results of PET to CT, MRI, and radioimmunoguided scintigraphy (RIGS). In each case, PET sensitivity and specificity were very high and better than the other modalities. The major problems are to clarify the role of PET in clinical management and determine who will be benefitted by this additional expensive, time-consuming study. PET scans may have a role in both the diagnosis of and response to therapy of hepatic metastases.

Several studies have been performed comparing CT scan with PET scan in clinical decision making. Unfortunately, therapeutic decisions are being made based on PET scan data without a clear understanding of how well the diagnostic findings correlate with the clinical findings. Johnson et al[361] conducted a retrospective review of 41 patients with metastatic colorectal carcinoma. All patients had both a CT scan and a PET scan before surgical exploration. PET scan was found to be more sensitive than CT scan when compared with actual operative findings in the liver (100 vs. 69%), extrahepatic region (90 vs. 52%), and abdomen as a whole (87 vs. 61%). Sensitivities to PET scan and CT scan were not significantly different in the pelvic region (87 vs. 61%). It was concluded that PET scanning is more sensitive than CT scanning and more likely to give the correct result when actual metastatic disease is present. The newer option of a PET/CT has resolved many of these issues.

21.7.4 Radioimmunodetection

Radioimmunodetection of carcinoma is usually accomplished by obtaining whole-body gamma scans of patients who have been injected intravenously with an antibody labeled or conjugated with a gamma-emitting radionuclide.[359] In colorectal carcinoma, a variety of antigens have been targeted (e.g., TAG-72 and carcinoembryonic antigen [CEA]). A variety of radionuclides used include iodine-131 (^{131}I), technetium-11 (^{11}Tc), indium-111 (^{111}In), and iodine-125 (^{125}I). Combined results using a variety of antibodies and radionuclides suggest that the sensitivity and detection are high in selected patients; the reports range from a sensitivity of 60% to more than 90%.[359] A number of benefits are attributed to radioimmunodetection. Although it can localize metastases, it is not yet clear whether any changes in management translate into long-term patient benefits. Another goal in monitoring recurrent colorectal carcinoma is to distinguish colorectal carcinoma from benign conditions (e.g., postoperative or radiation changes in the pelvis). False-positive

rates of antibody imaging may be as high as 13%, and it is thus advisable to pursue positive scans with biopsy confirmation.[359] Liver metastases may be diagnosed, but the identification of extrahepatic sites might spare the patient an unnecessary liver resection.

Bertsch et al[362] reported on 32 patients with primary colorectal carcinoma who underwent RIGS after being injected with anti-TAG-72 murine monoclonal antibody CC49 labeled with ^{125}I. Sixteen patients had gross disease and RIGS-positive tissue removed (5 with en bloc resection and 11 with extraregional tissues resected, 2 liver resections, and 25 lymphadenectomies—10 in the gastrohepatic ligament, 5 celiac axis, 6 retroperitoneal, and 4 iliac) and 16 had only traditional extirpation of disease because RIGS-positive tissue was too diffuse. With a median follow-up of 37 months, survival in the former group was 100%, and 14 of 16 patients had no evidence of disease. In the latter group, 14 of 16 patients died and 2 were alive with disease. The same authors reported that for patients with recurrent disease, the addition of RIGS increased the detection rate at operation from 116 sites without RICS to 184 with RIGS (a 57% increase).[363]

Using murine antibody B72.3 labeled with indium-111 (^{111}In-CYT-103, Cytogen), Dominguez et al[364] studied 15 patients with recurrent colorectal carcinoma. It was more accurate than a CT scan, but when the value of the scan was examined with respect to the potential contribution to patient management, it was beneficial in only 13% of patients.

Moffat et al[365] assessed the clinical impact of an anti-carcinoembryonic antigen (anti-CEA) Fab' antibody fragment labeled with ^{99m}Tc pertechnetate in 210 patients with advanced or metastatic colorectal carcinoma. When compared with conventional diagnostic modalities, the CEA scan was superior in the extrahepatic abdomen (55 vs. 32%) and pelvis (69 vs. 48%). Potential clinical benefit was demonstrated in 89 of 210 patients. Corman et al[366] evaluated the role of immunoscintigraphy with ^{111}In satumomab pendetide in 103 patients with colorectal carcinoma. In the 84 patients for whom histopathologic information was available, the sensitivity was 73% and the specificity was 100%, with an overall accuracy of 85% for determining the presence and extent of malignant disease. Investigators judged that the antibody imaging mode was a beneficial contribution in 44% and a negative effect in 2% of case studies. Treatment plans were altered in 17 patients.

The exact role of immunoscintigraphy remains poorly defined. Galandiuk[367] suggested three potentially major roles of immunoscintigraphy in the management of patients who have undergone curative resection: the detection of recurrent disease in patients with an elevated CEA level and either a negative investigation or equivocal findings on CT scan,[1] the exclusion of extra-abdominal disease, prior to planned resection of a presumably isolated recurrence,[2] and earlier detection of recurrence in the follow-up of high-risk patients.[3]

Immunoscintigraphy may allow recurrent disease to be detected at a time when curative resection may still be feasible and result in improved survival and/or effective palliation.

Miscellaneous Investigations

The results of hydrocolonic sonography, a technique of transabdominal sonography following retrograde installation of water into the colon, were compared with conventional transabdominal sonography by Limberg.[368] In a study of 29 patients with carcinoma, the diagnosis was correctly made in 97%, compared with only 31% by conventional sonography. Further studies will be required to determine the utility of this technique. Deranged liver blood flow patterns have been detected in patients with hepatic metastases.[369] The sugar moiety detected from rectal mucus by the galactose oxidase-Schiff (Sham's) test has been studied in screening for colorectal carcinoma. Dian-Yuan et al[370] found a sensitivity of 85.7% for colorectal carcinoma and 47.1% for adenomas in a study of 6,480 subjects older than 40 years of age. This compared favorably to 90.5 and 41.2% for fecal occult blood testing in the same group of individuals. In a study of 330 asymptomatic individuals, Sakamoto et al[371] found an overall specificity of Sham's test of 92.2%.

21.7.5 Cytology

The value of cytology in establishing the diagnosis of carcinoma for the most part has been appreciated only in investigational studies. To date, clinical application has been limited. Brush cytology via the colonoscope has been reported to be 86% accurate in establishing the diagnosis preoperatively, a percentage identical to that of biopsy.[372] A special circumstance in which cell brushings may be of value is when a stricture prevents the colonoscope from reaching the lesion, a situation in which a biopsy cannot be performed. In a study of 33 patients, 15 of whom had proven carcinoma, colonic cytology was positive in 93% of cases, whereas the cytology of control patients was negative.[373] Currently, radiologic-guided fine-needle aspiration has a major role in diagnosing liver lesions and recurrent cancer.

21.7.6 Blood Markers

Liver Function Tests

To determine the presence or absence of anemia, a complete blood count is indicated. Liver function tests often will point to metastatic disease, but a normal liver profile does not rule out hepatic metastases.

Carcinoembryonic Antigen

The initial report of a tumor-specific antigen in human colonic carcinomas by Gold and Freedman[374] heralded a new era in the assessment of the status of patients with colorectal carcinoma. However, CEA evaluation has not fulfilled its promise as a simple blood test that would afford an early diagnosis of carcinoma of the colon. In a comprehensive treatise on the subject, Gold[375] described his life's work on CEA. The following information is drawn from that publication. The CEA molecule is considered an oncodevelopmental human marker of neoplasia initially found in adenocarcinomas of the human digestive system. The molecule has a nominal molecular mass of 180 kDa. The CEA gene family comprises 29 genelike sequences in two defined clusters on chromosome 19.

It is of interest that human colonic carcinoma develops in mucosal tissue that has already undergone multiple steps of genetic change. It has been postulated that these multiple steps create a field effect that is characterized by morphologically normal, but biologically altered, epithelial cells. CEA has been used as a phenotypic marker of this field effect by examining the immunohistochemical expression of CEA on morphologically normal mucosa adjacent to colonic adenocarcinomas. It has been shown very clearly that CEA expression occurs in "normal" mucosa adjacent to a carcinoma and that there is a gradient of CEA expression, falling off at increasing distances from the carcinoma. These data are relevant to both the biology of human colorectal carcinoma and, more practically, the optimal location of surgical resection. Kyzer et al,[376] using statin as a marker, similarly demonstrated that the proliferative rate of mucosa adjacent to a colonic carcinoma is elevated and returns to normal at 5 cm from the carcinoma, even though it is morphologically indistinguishable from its normal counterparts.

The role of CEA in clinical medicine first became a consideration with the development of a radioimmunoassay for circulating CEA. The first series of data, derived from patients with established colonic carcinoma, were most exciting, but more extensive studies revealed the clearly expected false-negative assays, particularly in early-stage bowel carcinoma, and false-positive results in patients with nonenteric carcinoma as well as in others with nonmalignant conditions. Over the years, suggestions for the use of the CEA assay have included detection, diagnosis, monitoring, staging and classification (prognosis), pathology, localization, and therapy.

Normal concentrations of CEA are 2.5 to 5.0 ng/mL, depending on the assay used. CEA concentrations are in general more often elevated in smokers than in nonsmokers, more frequently elevated in men than in women, and more frequently elevated in older subjects than in younger individuals. Racial differences in the frequency of serum elevations of CEA have been suggested but not established. Elevated CEA levels have been described in advanced breast carcinoma, pancreatic carcinoma, lung carcinoma, and other noncolonic adenocarcinomas, but they do not detect early stages of these diseases. Although 80% or more of patients with advanced colonic adenocarcinoma have circulating CEA, the CEA assay should not be used as the sole diagnostic test for suspected carcinoma. CEA levels are not presently useful for distinguishing locally invasive polyps from benign lesions.

Preoperative serum CEA levels in diagnosed colorectal carcinoma are elevated in 40 to 70% of patients. Preoperative serum CEA concentrations correlate inversely with the grade of the carcinoma and directly with the pathologic stage. The CEA is elevated in 95% of patients with well-differentiated lesions, while it is elevated in as few as 30% of those with poorly differentiated adenocarcinomas. The higher the preoperative CEA level, the greater the likelihood of a postoperative recurrence. A significant negative correlation between preoperative elevated plasma CEA levels and patient survival has been observed. Despite disagreement between various groups that have explored the relationship between preoperative CEA levels and prognoses, most studies report that a high preoperative CEA level is indicative of a poor prognosis. This association is often as discriminating as pathologic staging and grading. It is still uncertain which absolute preoperative CEA value reliably discriminates high-risk from low-risk cases for postoperative recurrence.

An increase in the blood CEA concentration in a patient after apparently successful surgical treatment for carcinoma has repeatedly been shown to signal a recurrence of the carcinoma. After apparently complete surgical resection of colorectal carcinoma, the blood CEA concentration, if elevated before operation, decreases to the normal range in nearly all patients. The decrease usually occurs within 1 month but sometimes takes up to 4 months. If levels fail to decrease to the normal range, it is likely that the resection has been incomplete or that the carcinoma has already metastasized. A sustained and progressive rise is strong evidence for recurrence at the primary area or at distant sites. Serial CEA monitoring is currently considered by some authors as the best noninvasive technique for detecting recurrent colorectal carcinoma.

The debate concerning the merit of postoperative determinations of CEA values in monitoring patients with resected colon carcinoma continues. At one extreme are those who feel that the carcinoma cures attributable to CEA monitoring are too infrequent to justify the substantial costs and physical and emotional stress that this intervention may cause for patients. Others believe that intensive follow-up using CEA assays can identify treatable recurrences at a relatively early stage. It has been suggested that when CEA increases more rapidly than an average of 12.6% per month, recurrence should be strongly suspected. Because the overall prognosis for patients with recurrent disease after surgical resection is dismal, serum CEA determination may offer the only chance of a cure for a select group of individuals.

Immunohistochemically, CEA has been identified in carcinomas of the colorectum, breast, lung, uterine cervix, gallbladder, stomach, pancreas, liver, prostate, urinary bladder, and uterus, and in neuroendocrine neoplasms associated with the larynx, lung, and thyroid.[377,378] There are good reasons to regard ulcerative colitis and certain colonic adenomas as premalignant lesions. Immunoperoxidase staining for CEA supports the concept of a polyp–adenoma–carcinoma sequence. Both chronic inflammatory bowel disease and colorectal adenomas show higher tissue CEA concentrations than normal colonic mucosa, suggesting that these situations can be regarded biochemically as premalignant conditions. Results concerning the correlation between positive CEA test results in the carcinoma immunohistochemistry and histologic grade, lymph node involvement, locoregional recurrence, disease-free interval, and patient survival remain controversial.

Initial difficulties have been overcome and several virtually instant and easy-to-use radiolabeling kits for anti-CEA antibodies are available. The reported sensitivities for the detection of liver metastases have ranged from 0 to 94% in different studies, indicating differences largely due to technical ability and knowledge in avoiding pitfalls. The most complete clinical report so far was conducted in Italy. F(ab)2 fragments of the monoclonal antibodies anti-CEA FO23C5, determined to be more suitable than intact immunoglobulin (IgG) or Fab fragments for immunoscintigraphy, were labeled with either ^{131}I or ^{111}In. The variation in results reported by various groups reflects the gamut of potential variables, including the radiolabel used, the route of administration of the conjugate, the size and location of the lesion, the vascularity of the lesion, the patient population studied, the imaging technology used, the unavoidable parameter of subjective interpretation of scans, even in blinded situations, and the type of antibody preparation used. On the basis of the foregoing information, it may, therefore, be concluded that primary lesions with a high CEA content have the best anti-CEA antibody uptake and are most easily imaged and that large fungating carcinomas accumulate a high proportion of the injected labeled antibody in contrast to ulcerating carcinomas with poor vascularity. Hepatic metastases have a high CEA content and a high antibody uptake but may not image well because of the relatively high background uptake of the conjugate by the normal liver.

Adjuvant chemotherapy has had varying success in those patients whose carcinomas have been resected but who are at high risk for recurrence. The ability to detect carcinomas by radioimmunolocalization raises the possibility of treating such lesions by targeting with the same technology.

Other Markers

A host of less well-described markers have been reported to have potential screening value. For example, ornithine decarboxylase activity has been found to be significantly lower in patients with adenomas than in controls, and even lower in patients with carcinoma.[379] Opposite findings were reported by Narisawa et al,[380] who found increased levels in patients with carcinoma. Compared with its activity in control mucosa, urokinase activity has been found to be significantly elevated in adenomas and carcinomas, with levels significantly higher in carcinomas. Tissue plasminogen activator activity is reduced in adenomas and carcinomas, with levels significantly lower in carcinomas.

References

[1] DiSario JA, Burt RW, Kendrick ML, McWhorter WP. Colorectal cancers of rare histologic types compared with adenocarcinomas. Dis Colon Rectum. 1994; 37(12):1277–1280

[2] Kang H, O'Connell JB, Leonardi MJ, Maggard MA, McGory ML, Ko CY. Rare tumors of the colon and rectum: a national review. Int J Colorectal Dis. 2007; 22(2):183–189

[3] American Cancer Society. Key Statistics for Colorectal Cancer: How Common Is Colorectal Cancer? Available at: https://www.cancer.org/cancer/colon-rectal-cancer/about/key-statistics.html. Accessed July 7, 2017

[4] Correa P, Haenszel W. The epidemiology of large-bowel cancer. Adv Cancer Res. 1978; 26:1–141

[5] Corman ML, Veidenheimer MC, Coller JA. Colorectal carcinoma: a decade of experience at the Lahey Clinic. Dis Colon Rectum. 1979; 22(7):477–479

[6] Axtell LM, Cutler SJ, Myers MH, eds. End Results in Cancer, Report No. 4. National Institutes of Health. Publication No. 73. Bethesda, MD: US Department of Health, Education and Welfare, 1972:217–272

[7] Fuchs CS, Giovannucci EL, Colditz GA, Hunter DJ, Speizer FE, Willett WC. A prospective study of family history and the risk of colorectal cancer. N Engl J Med. 1994; 331(25):1669–1674

[8] Hall NR, Bishop DT, Stephenson BM, Finan PJ. Hereditary susceptibility to colorectal cancer. Relatives of early onset cases are particularly at risk. Dis Colon Rectum. 1996; 39(7):739–743

[9] St John DJB, McDermott FT, Hopper JL, Debney EA, Johnson WR, Hughes ES. Cancer risk in relatives of patients with common colorectal cancer. Ann Intern Med. 1993; 118(10):785–790

[10] Genetics of colorectal cancer (PDQR), November 19, 2003. Available at: http://www.cancer.gov/cancerinfo/pdq/genetics/colorectal

[11] Mamazza J, Gordon PH. The changing distribution of large intestinal cancer. Dis Colon Rectum. 1982; 25(6):558–562

[12] Obrand DI, Gordon PH. Continued change in the distribution of colorectal carcinoma. Br J Surg. 1998; 85(2):246–248

[13] Qing SH, Rao KY, Jiang HY, Wexner SD. Racial differences in the anatomical distribution of colorectal cancer: a study of differences between American and Chinese patients. World J Gastroenterol. 2003; 9(4):721–725

[14] Cucino C, Buchner AM, Sonnenberg A. Continued rightward shift of colorectal cancer. Dis Colon Rectum. 2002; 45(8):1035–1040

[15] Takada H, Ohsawa T, Iwamoto S, et al. Changing site distribution of colorectal cancer in Japan. Dis Colon Rectum. 2002; 45(9):1249–1254

[16] Bang KM, White JE, Gause BL, Leffall LD, Jr. Evaluation of recent trends in cancer mortality and incidence among blacks. Cancer. 1988; 61 (6):1255–1261

[17] Lynch HT, Rubinstein WS, Locker GY. Cancer in Jews: introduction and overview. Fam Cancer. 2004; 3(3–4):177–192

[18] Kune GA, Kune S, Watson LF. Perceived religiousness is protective for colorectal cancer: data from the Melbourne Colorectal Cancer Study. J R Soc Med. 1993; 86(11):645–647

[19] Vobecky J, Devroede G, Caro J. Risk of large-bowel cancer in synthetic fiber manufacture. Cancer. 1984; 54(11):2537–2542

[20] de Verdier MG, Plato N, Steineck G, Peters JM. Occupational exposures and cancer of the colon and rectum. Am J Ind Med. 1992; 22(3):291–303

[21] Homa DM, Garabrant DH, Gillespie BW. A meta-analysis of colorectal cancer and asbestos exposure. Am J Epidemiol. 1994; 139(12):1210–1222

[22] Demers RY, Burns PB, Swanson GM. Construction occupations, asbestos exposure, and cancer of the colon and rectum. J Occup Med. 1994; 36 (9):1027–1031

[23] Spiegelman D, Wegman DH. Occupation-related risks for colorectal cancer. J Natl Cancer Inst. 1985; 75(5):813–821

[24] Avni A, Feuchtwanger MM. Juvenile versus adult colonic cancer: distinct different etiologic factors? Dis Colon Rectum. 1984; 27(12):842

[25] Acquavella JF, Douglass TS, Phillips SC. Evaluation of excess colorectal cancer incidence among workers involved in the manufacture of polypropylene. J Occup Med. 1988; 30(5):438–442

[26] Lewis RJ, Schnatter AR, Lerman SE. Colorectal cancer incidence among polypropylene manufacturing workers. An update. J Occup Med. 1994; 36 (6):652–659

[27] Walker AM, Cohen AJ, Loughlin JE, Rothman KJ, DeFonso LR. Mortality from cancer of the colon or rectum among workers exposed to ethyl acrylate and methyl methacrylate. Scand J Work Environ Health. 1991; 17(1):7–19

[28] Lennard-Jones JE, Melville DM, Morson BC, Ritchie JK, Williams CB. Precancer and cancer in extensive ulcerative colitis: findings among 401 patients over 22 years. Gut. 1990; 31(7):800–806

[29] Greenstein AJ, Sachar DB, Smith H, Janowitz HD, Aufses AH, Jr. A comparison of cancer risk in Crohn's disease and ulcerative colitis. Cancer. 1981; 48 (12):2742–2745

[30] Ekbom A, Helmick C, Zack M, Adami HO. Ulcerative colitis and colorectal cancer. A population-based study. N Engl J Med. 1990; 323(18):1228–1233

[31] Munkholm P. Review article: the incidence and prevalence of colorectal cancer in inflammatory bowel disease. Aliment Pharmacol Ther. 2003; 18 Suppl 2:1–5

[32] Ekbom A, Helmick C, Zack M, Adami HO. Increased risk of large-bowel cancer in Crohn's disease with colonic involvement. Lancet. 1990; 336 (8711):357–359

[33] Allen JI. Molecular biology of colorectal cancer: a clinician's view. Perspect Colon Rectal Surg. 1995; 8:181–202

[34] Knudson AG, Jr. Hereditary cancer, oncogenes, and antioncogenes. Cancer Res. 1985; 45(4):1437–1443

[35] Lynch HT, Smyrk T. Hereditary nonpolyposis colorectal cancer (Lynch syndrome). An updated review. Cancer. 1996; 78(6):1149–1167

[36] Foulkes WD, Thiffault I, Gruber SB, et al. The founder mutation MSH2*1906G–>C is an important cause of hereditary nonpolyposis colorectal cancer in the Ashkenazi Jewish population. Am J Hum Genet. 2002; 71 (6):1395–1412

[37] Guillem JG, Rapaport BS, Kirchhoff T, et al. A636P is associated with early-onset colon cancer in Ashkenazi Jews. J Am Coll Surg. 2003; 196(2):222–225

[38] Nyström-Lahti M, Kristo P, Nicolaides NC, et al. Founding mutations and Alu-mediated recombination in hereditary colon cancer. Nat Med. 1995; 1 (11):1203–1206

[39] Peltomäki P. Role of DNA mismatch repair defects in the pathogenesis of human cancer. J Clin Oncol. 2003; 21(6):1174–1179

[40] Burt RW, Bishop DT, Cannon LA, Dowdle MA, Lee RG, Skolnick MH. Dominant inheritance of adenomatous colonic polyps and colorectal cancer. N Engl J Med. 1985; 312(24):1540–1544

[41] Solomon E, Voss R, Hall V, et al. Chromosome 5 allele loss in human colorectal carcinomas. Nature. 1987; 328(6131):616–619

[42] Law DJ, Olschwang S, Monpezat JP, et al. Concerted nonsyntenic allelic loss in human colorectal carcinoma. Science. 1988; 241(4868):961–965

[43] Fearon ER, Vogelstein B. A genetic model for colorectal tumorigenesis. Cell. 1990; 61(5):759–767

[44] Wang L, Patel U, Ghosh L, Chen HC, Banerjee S. Mutation in the nm23 gene is associated with metastasis in colorectal cancer. Cancer Res. 1993; 53 (4):717–720

[45] Aaltonen LA, Peltomäki P, Leach FS, et al. Clues to the pathogenesis of familial colorectal cancer. Science. 1993; 260(5109):812–816

[46] Lu SL, Kawabata M, Imamura T, et al. HNPCC associated with germline mutation in the TGF-beta type II receptor gene. Nat Genet. 1998; 19(1):17–18

[47] Liu B, Nicolaides NC, Markowitz S, et al. Mismatch repair gene defects in sporadic colorectal cancers with microsatellite instability. Nat Genet. 1995; 9(1):48–55

[48] DeFrancisco J, Grady WM. Diagnosis and management of hereditary nonpolyposis colon cancer. Gastrointest Endosc. 2003; 58(3):390–408

[49] Lawes DA, SenGupta S, Boulos PB. The clinical importance and prognostic implications of microsatellite instability in sporadic cancer. Eur J Surg Oncol. 2003; 29(3):201–212

[50] Piepoli A, Santoro R, Cristofaro G, et al. Linkage analysis identifies gene carriers among members of families with hereditary nonpolyposis colorectal cancer. Gastroenterology. 1996; 110(5):1404–1409

[51] Vasen HFA, Mecklin JP, Khan PM, Lynch HT. The International Collaborative Group on Hereditary Non-Polyposis Colorectal Cancer (ICG-HNPCC). Dis Colon Rectum. 1991; 34(5):424–425

[52] Aaltonen LA, Sankila R, Mecklin JP, et al. A novel approach to estimate the proportion of hereditary nonpolyposis colorectal cancer of total colorectal cancer burden. Cancer Detect Prev. 1994; 18(1):57–63

[53] Boland CR, Brown EF, Evans RM, Goldberg A, Short MP. Identifying and Managing Risk for Hereditary Nonpolyposis Colorectal Cancer and Endometrial Cancer (HNPCC). Chicago, IL: American Medical Association and American Gastroenterological Association; 2001:1–21

[54] Umar A, Boland CR, Terdiman JP, et al. Revised Bethesda Guidelines for hereditary nonpolyposis colorectal cancer (Lynch syndrome) and microsatellite instability. J Natl Cancer Inst. 2004; 96(4):261–268

[55] Pinol V, Castells A, Andreu M, et al. Gastrointestinal oncology group of the Spanish gastroenterological association. Accuracy of revised Bethesda guidelines, microsatellite instability, and immunohistochemistry for identification of patients with hereditary non polyposis colorectal cancer. JAMA. 2005; 293(16):1986–1994

[56] De Jong AE, Morreau H, Van Puijenbroek M, et al. The role of mismatch repair gene defects in the development of adenomas in patients with HNPCC. Gastroenterology. 2004; 126(1):42–48

[57] Cunningham C, Dunlop MG. Molecular genetic basis of colorectal cancer susceptibility. Br J Surg. 1996; 83(3):321–329

[58] Mecklin JP, Järvinen HJ. Tumor spectrum in cancer family syndrome (hereditary nonpolyposis colorectal cancer). Cancer. 1991; 68(5):1109–1112

[59] Aarnio M, Mecklin JP, Aaltonen LA, Nyström-Lahti M, Järvinen HJ. Life-time risk of different cancers in hereditary non-polyposis colorectal cancer (HNPCC) syndrome. Int J Cancer. 1995; 64(6):430–433

[60] Brezden-Masley C, Aronson MD, Bapat B, et al. Hereditary nonpolyposis colorectal cancer–molecular basis. Surgery. 2003; 134(1):29–33

[61] Plaschke J, Engel C, Krüger S, et al. Lower incidence of colorectal cancer and later age of disease onset in 27 families with pathogenic MSH6 germline mutations compared with families with MLH1 or MSH2 mutations: the German Hereditary Nonpolyposis Colorectal Cancer Consortium. J Clin Oncol. 2004; 22(22):4486–4494

[62] Lindor NM, Rabe K, Petersen GM, et al. Lower cancer incidence in Amsterdam-I criteria families without mismatch repair deficiency: familial colorectal cancer type X. JAMA. 2005; 293(16):1979–1985

[63] Jass JR. Colorectal adenomas in surgical specimens from subjects with hereditary non-polyposis colorectal cancer. Histopathology. 1995; 27 (3):263–267

[64] Mecklin JP, Sipponen P, Järvinen HJ. Histopathology of colorectal carcinomas and adenomas in cancer family syndrome. Dis Colon Rectum. 1986; 29 (12):849–853

[65] Sankila R, Aaltonen LA, Järvinen HJ, Mecklin JP. Better survival rates in patients with MLH1-associated hereditary colorectal cancer. Gastroenterology. 1996; 110(3):682–687

[66] Tomoda H, Baba H, Oshiro T. Clinical manifestations in patients with hereditary nonpolyposis colorectal cancer. J Surg Oncol. 1996; 61(4):262–266

[67] Rodríguez-Bigas MA, Lee PHV, O'Malley L, et al. Establishment of a hereditary nonpolyposis colorectal cancer registry. Dis Colon Rectum. 1996; 39 (6):649–653

[68] Hampel H, Frankel WL, Martin E, et al. Screening for the Lynch syndrome (hereditary nonpolyposis colorectal cancer). N Engl J Med. 2005; 352 (18):1851–1860

[69] Lynch HT, Smyrk T, Lynch JF. Overview of natural history, pathology, molecular genetics and management of HNPCC (Lynch Syndrome). Int J Cancer. 1996; 69(1):38–43

[70] Järvinen HJ, Aarnio M, Mustonen H, et al. Controlled 15-year trial on screening for colorectal cancer in families with hereditary nonpolyposis colorectal cancer. Gastroenterology. 2000; 118(5):829–834

[71] de Vos tot Nederveen Cappel WH, Nagengast FM, Griffioen G, et al. Surveillance for hereditary nonpolyposis colorectal cancer: a long-term study on 114 families. Dis Colon Rectum. 2002; 45(12):1588–1594

[72] Mecklin JP, Järvinen H. Treatment and follow-up strategies in hereditary nonpolyposis colorectal carcinoma. Dis Colon Rectum. 1993; 36 (10):927–929

[73] Itoh H, Houlston RS, Harocopos C, Slack J. Risk of cancer death in first-degree relatives of patients with hereditary non-polyposis cancer syndrome (Lynch type II): a study of 130 kindreds in the United Kingdom. Br J Surg. 1990; 77 (12):1367–1370

[74] Brown GJ, St John DJ, Macrae FA, Aittomäki K. Cancer risk in young women at risk of hereditary nonpolyposis colorectal cancer: implications for gynecologic surveillance. Gynecol Oncol. 2001; 80(3):346–349

[75] Watson P, Bützow R, Lynch HT, et al. International Collaborative Group on HNPCC. The clinical features of ovarian cancer in hereditary nonpolyposis colorectal cancer. Gynecol Oncol. 2001; 82(2):223–228

[76] Meijers-Heijboer H, Wijnen J, Vasen H, et al. The CHEK2 1100delC mutation identifies families with a hereditary breast and colorectal cancer phenotype. Am J Hum Genet. 2003; 72(5):1308–1314

[77] Wong N, Lasko D, Rabelo R, Pinsky L, Gordon PH, Foulkes W. Genetic counseling and interpretation of genetic tests in familial adenomatous polyposis and hereditary nonpolyposis colorectal cancer. Dis Colon Rectum. 2001; 44 (2):271–279

[78] Rabelo R, Foulkes W, Gordon PH, et al. Role of molecular diagnostic testing in familial adenomatous polyposis and hereditary nonpolyposis colorectal cancer families. Dis Colon Rectum. 2001; 44(3):437–446

[79] Dunlop MG, Farrington SM, Carothers AD, et al. Cancer risk associated with germline DNA mismatch repair gene mutations. Hum Mol Genet. 1997; 6 (1):105–110

[80] Xia L, Shen W, Ritacca F, et al. A truncated hMSH2 transcript occurs as a common variant in the population: implications for genetic diagnosis. Cancer Res. 1996; 56(10):2289–2292

[81] Keller M, Jost R, Kadmon M, et al. Acceptance of and attitude toward genetic testing for hereditary nonpolyposis colorectal cancer: a comparison of participants and nonparticipants in genetic counseling. Dis Colon Rectum. 2004; 47(2):153–162

[82] Gritz ER, Peterson SK, Vernon SW, et al. Psychological impact of genetic testing for hereditary nonpolyposis colorectal cancer. J Clin Oncol. 2005; 23 (9):1902–1910

[83] Statement ASHG, The American Society of Human Genetics Social Issues Subcommittee on Familial Disclosure. ASHG statement. Professional disclosure of familial genetic information. Am J Hum Genet. 1998; 62(2):474–483

[84] Lerman C, Marshall J, Audrain J, Gomez-Caminero A. Genetic testing for colon cancer susceptibility: Anticipated reactions of patients and challenges to providers. Int J Cancer. 1996; 69(1):58–61

[85] Hadley DW, Jenkins JF, Dimond E, de Carvalho M, Kirsch I, Palmer CG. Colon cancer screening practices after genetic counseling and testing for hereditary nonpolyposis colorectal cancer. J Clin Oncol. 2004; 22(1):39–44

[86] Offit K. Clinical Cancer Genetics: Risk Counseling and Management. 1st ed. New York, NY: Wiley-Liss; 1998:301

[87] Jass JR, Whitehall VL, Young J, Leggett BA. Emerging concepts in colorectal neoplasia. Gastroenterology. 2002; 123(3):862–876

[88] Lamprecht SA, Lipkin M. Chemoprevention of colon cancer by calcium, vitamin D and folate: molecular mechanisms. Nat Rev Cancer. 2003; 3(8):601–614

[89] Nigro ND, Singh DV, et al. Effect of dietary beef fat on intestinal cancer formation in rats. J Natl Cancer Inst. 1975; 54:439–442

[90] Nagao M, Sugimura T. Carcinogenic factors in food with relevance to colon cancer development. Mutat Res. 1993; 290(1):43–51

[91] Miller AB, Howe GR, Jain M, Craib KJ, Harrison L. Food items and food groups as risk factors in a case-control study of diet and colo-rectal cancer. Int J Cancer. 1983; 32(2):155–161

[92] Willett WC, Stampfer MJ, Colditz GA, Rosner BA, Speizer FE. Relation of meat, fat, and fiber intake to the risk of colon cancer in a prospective study among women. N Engl J Med. 1990; 323(24):1664–1672

[93] Reddy BS, Maruyana H. Effect of dietary fish oil on colon carcinogenesis in rats. Cancer Res. 1986; 46:3367–3370

[94] Chao A, Thun MJ, Connell CJ, et al. Meat consumption and risk of colorectal cancer. JAMA. 2005; 293(2):172–182

[95] Larsson SC, Rafter J, Holmberg L, Bergkvist L, Wolk A. Red meat consumption and risk of cancers of the proximal colon, distal colon and rectum: the Swedish Mammography Cohort. Int J Cancer. 2005; 113(5):829–834

[96] Norat T, Bingham S, Ferrari P, et al. Meat, fish, and colorectal cancer risk: the European Prospective Investigation into cancer and nutrition. J Natl Cancer Inst. 2005; 97(12):906–916

[97] Burkitt DP. Epidemiology of cancer of the colon and rectum. Cancer. 1971; 28(1):3–13

[98] Fleiszer D, Murray D, MacFarlane J, Brown RA. Protective effect of dietary fibre against chemically induced bowel tumours in rats. Lancet. 1978; 2 (8089):552–553

[99] Nigro ND, Bull AW, Klopfer BA, et al. Effect of dietary fiber on intestinal carcinogenesis in rats. J Natl Cancer Inst. 1979; 62:1097–1102

[100] Greenwald P, Lanza E, Eddy GA. Dietary fiber in the reduction of colon cancer risk. J Am Diet Assoc. 1987; 87(9):1178–1188

[101] Trock B, Lanza E, Greenwald P. Dietary fiber, vegetables, and colon cancer: critical review and meta-analyses of the epidemiologic evidence. J Natl Cancer Inst. 1990; 82(8):650–661

[102] Frentzel-Beyme R, Chang-Claude J. Vegetarian diets and colon cancer: the German experience. Am J Clin Nutr. 1994; 59(5) Suppl:1143S–1152S

[103] Freudenheim JL, Graham S, Horvath PJ, et al. Risks associated with source of fiber and fiber components in cancer of the colon and rectum. Cancer Res. 1990(52):3295–3300

[104] Asano T, McLeod RS. Dietary fibre for the prevention of colorectal adenomas and carcinomas. Cochrane Database Syst Rev. 2002(2):CD003430

[105] Fuchs CS, Giovannucci EL, Colditz GA, et al. Dietary fiber and the risk of colorectal cancer and adenoma in women. N Engl J Med. 1999; 340(3):169–176

[106] Michels KB, Edward Giovannucci, Joshipura KJ, et al. Prospective study of fruit and vegetable consumption and incidence of colon and rectal cancers. J Natl Cancer Inst. 2000; 92(21):1740–1752

[107] Terry P, Giovannucci E, Michels KB, et al. Fruit, vegetables, dietary fiber, and risk of colorectal cancer. J Natl Cancer Inst. 2001; 93(7):525–533

[108] Peters U, Sinha R, Chatterjee N, et al. Prostate, Lung, Colorectal, and Ovarian Cancer Screening Trial Project Team. Dietary fibre and colorectal adenoma in a colorectal cancer early detection programme. Lancet. 2003; 361 (9368):1491–1495

[109] Meyer F, White E. Alcohol and nutrients in relation to colon cancer in middle-aged adults. Am J Epidemiol. 1993; 138(4):225–236

[110] Howe GR, Benito E, Castelleto R, et al. Dietary intake of fiber and decreased risk of cancers of the colon and rectum: evidence from the combined analysis of 13 case-control studies. J Natl Cancer Inst. 1992; 84(24):1887–1896

[111] Bingham SA, Day NE, Luben R, et al. European Prospective Investigation into Cancer and Nutrition. Dietary fibre in food and protection against colorectal cancer in the European Prospective Investigation into Cancer and Nutrition (EPIC): an observational study. Lancet. 2003; 361(9368):1496–1501

[112] Slattery ML, Sorenson AW, Ford MH. Dietary calcium intake as a mitigating factor in colon cancer. Am J Epidemiol. 1988; 128(3):504–514

[113] Garland C, Shekelle RB, Barrett-Connor E, Criqui MH, Rossof AH, Paul O. Dietary vitamin D and calcium and risk of colorectal cancer: a 19-year prospective study in men. Lancet. 1985; 1(8424):307–309

[114] Rozen P, Fireman Z, Wax Y, et al. Oral calcium suppresses colonic mucosal proliferation of persons at risk for colorectal neoplasia. Gastroenterology. 1987; 92:1603

[115] Wargovich MJ, Lynch PM, Levin B. Modulating effects of calcium in animal models of colon carcinogenesis and short-term studies in subjects at increased risk for colon cancer. Am J Clin Nutr. 1991; 54(1) Suppl:202S–205S

[116] Baron JA, Beach M, Mandel JS, et al. Calcium Polyp Prevention Study Group. Calcium supplements for the prevention of colorectal adenomas. N Engl J Med. 1999; 340(2):101–107

[117] Wu K, Willett WC, Fuchs CS, Colditz GA, Giovannucci EL. Calcium intake and risk of colon cancer in women and men. J Natl Cancer Inst. 2002; 94 (6):437–446

[118] Wallace K, Baron JA, Cole BF, et al. Effect of calcium supplementation on the risk of large bowel polyps. J Natl Cancer Inst. 2004; 96(12):921–925

[119] Larsson SC, Bergkvist L, Wolk A. Magnesium intake in relation to risk of colorectal cancer in women. JAMA. 2005; 293(1):86–89

[120] Vernie LN. Selenium in carcinogenesis. Biochim Biophys Acta. 1984; 738 (4):203–217

[121] Rumi G, Imre I, Sülle C, Sarudi I, Kelemen J, Lassú Z. Selenium in the blood of patients with colorectal cancer and neoplastic polyp. Acta Physiol Hung. 1992; 80(1–4):275–279

[122] Finley JW. Reduction of cancer risk by consumption of selenium-enriched plants: enrichment of broccoli with selenium increases the anticarcinogenic properties of broccoli. J Med Food. 2003; 6(1):19–26

[123] Nelson RL, Davis FG, Sutter E, et al. Serum selenium and colonic neoplastic risk. Dis Colon Rectum. 1995; 38(12):1306–1310

[124] Jacobs ET, Jiang R, Alberts DS, et al. Selenium and colorectal adenoma: results of a pooled analysis. J Natl Cancer Inst. 2004; 96(22):1669–1675

[125] Nigro ND, Bull AW. Prospects for the prevention of colorectal cancer. Dis Colon Rectum. 1987; 30(10):751–754

[126] Wargovich MJ. New dietary anticarcinogens and prevention of gastrointestinal cancer. Dis Colon Rectum. 1988; 31(1):72–75

[127] Wattenberg LW. Chemoprevention of cancer. Cancer Res. 1985; 45(1):1–8

[128] Nigro ND, Bull AW, Wilson PS, et al. Combined inhibitors of carcinogenesis or intestinal cancer in rats. J Natl Cancer Inst. 1982; 69:103–107

[129] Colacchio TA, Memoli VA. Chemoprevention of colorectal neoplasms. Ascorbic acid and beta-carotene. Arch Surg. 1986; 121(12):1421–1424

[130] Longnecker MP. A case-control study of alcoholic beverage consumption in relation to risk of cancer of the right colon and rectum in men. Cancer Causes Control. 1990; 1(1):5–14

[131] Pollack ES, Nomura AMY, Heilbrun LK, Stemmermann GN, Green SB. Prospective study of alcohol consumption and cancer. N Engl J Med. 1984; 310 (10):617–621

[132] Newcomb PA, Storer BE, Marcus PM. Cancer of the large bowel in women in relation to alcohol consumption: a case-control study in Wisconsin (United States). Cancer Causes Control. 1993; 4(5):405–411

[133] Kato I, Tominaga S, Ikari A. A case-control study of male colorectal cancer in Aichi Prefecture, Japan: with special reference to occupational activity level, drinking habits and family history. Jpn J Cancer Res. 1990; 81(2):115–121

[134] Riboli E, Cornée J, Macquart-Moulin G, Kaaks R, Casagrande C, Guyader M. Cancer and polyps of the colorectum and lifetime consumption of beer and other alcoholic beverages. Am J Epidemiol. 1991; 134(2):157–166

[135] Serralva MS, Anjos J, Vilaca F. Colorectal carcinoma in patients older than 65 years: prognostic factors. Br J Surg. 1995; 82 suppl 1:35–36

[136] Carstensen JM, Bygren LO, Hatschek T. Cancer incidence among Swedish brewery workers. Int J Cancer. 1990; 45(3):393–396

[137] Maekawa SJ, Aoyama N, Shirasaka D, et al. Excessive alcohol intake enhances the development of synchronous cancerous lesion in colorectal cancer patients. Int J Colorectal Dis. 2004; 19(2):171–175

[138] Sharpe CR, Siemiatycki J, Rachet B. Effects of alcohol consumption on the risk of colorectal cancer among men by anatomical subsite (Canada). Cancer Causes Control. 2002; 13(5):483–491

[139] Kikendall JW, Bowen PE, Burgess MB, Magnetti C, Woodward J, Langenberg P. Cigarettes and alcohol as independent risk factors for colonic adenomas. Gastroenterology. 1989; 97(3):660–664

[140] Giovannucci E, Rimm EB, Stampfer MJ, et al. A prospective study of cigarette smoking and risk of colorectal adenoma and colorectal cancer in U.S. men. J Natl Cancer Inst. 1994; 86(3):183–191

[141] Giovannucci E, Colditz GA, Stampfer MJ, et al. A prospective study of cigarette smoking and risk of colorectal adenoma and colorectal cancer in U.S. women. J Natl Cancer Inst. 1994; 86(3):192–199

[142] Chao A, Thun MJ, Jacobs EJ, Henley SJ, Rodriguez C, Calle EE. Cigarette smoking and colorectal cancer mortality in the cancer prevention study II. J Natl Cancer Inst. 2000; 92(23):1888–1896

[143] Jain M, Cook GM, Davis FG, Grace MG, Howe GR, Miller AB. A case-control study of diet and colo-rectal cancer. Int J Cancer. 1980; 26(6):757–768

[144] Potter JD, McMichael AJ. Diet and cancer of the colon and rectum: a case-control study. J Natl Cancer Inst. 1986; 76(4):557–569

[145] Kritchevsky D. Epidemiology of fibre, resistant starch and colorectal cancer. Eur J Cancer Prev. 1995; 4(5):345–352

[146] Phillips RL, Snowdon DA. Dietary relationships with fatal colorectal cancer among Seventh-Day Adventists. J Natl Cancer Inst. 1985; 74(2):307–317

[147] Stemmermann GN, Nomura AM, Heilbrun LK. Dietary fat and the risk of colorectal cancer. Cancer Res. 1984; 44(10):4633–4637

[148] Berry EM, Zimmerman J, Ligumsky M. The nature of dietary fat and plasma lipids in relation to the development of polyps and carcinoma of the colon. Gastroenterology. 1985; 88:1323

[149] Freudenheim JL, Graham S, Marshall JR, Haughey BP, Wilkinson G. A case-control study of diet and rectal cancer in western New York. Am J Epidemiol. 1990; 131(4):612–624

[150] Giovannucci E, Stampfer MJ, Colditz GA, et al. Multivitamin use, folate, and colon cancer in women in the Nurses' Health Study. Ann Intern Med. 1998; 129(7):517–524

[151] Fernandez E, Chatenoud L, La Vecchia C, Negri E, Franceschi S. Fish consumption and cancer risk. Am J Clin Nutr. 1999; 70(1):85–90

[152] Jao SW, Beart RW, Jr, Reiman HM, Gunderson LL, Ilstrup DM. Colon and anorectal cancer after pelvic irradiation. Dis Colon Rectum. 1987; 30 (12):953–958

[153] Matsuo T, Ito M, Sekine I, Kishikawa M, Taketomi K. Mucosal de novo cancer of the rectum following radiation therapy for uterine cancer. Intern Med. 1993; 32(5):427–429

[154] Tamai O, Nozato E, Miyazato H, et al. Radiation-associated rectal cancer: report of four cases. Dig Surg. 1999; 16(3):238–243

[155] Martins A, Sternberg SS, Attiyeh FF. Radiation-induced carcinoma of the rectum. Dis Colon Rectum. 1980; 23(8):572–575

[156] Shirouzu K, Isomoto H, Morodomi T, Ogata Y, Araki Y, Kakegawa T. Clinicopathologic characteristics of large bowel cancer developing after radiotherapy for uterine cervical cancer. Dis Colon Rectum. 1994; 37(12):1245–1249

[157] Hareyama M, Okubo O, Oouchi A, et al. A case of carcinoma of the rectum after radiotherapy for carcinoma of the cervix. Radiat Med. 1989; 7 (4):197–200

[158] Baxter NN, Tepper JE, Durham SB, Rothenberger DA, Virnig BA. Increased risk of rectal cancer after prostate radiation: a population-based study. Gastroenterology. 2005; 128(4):819–824

[159] Labow SB, Hoexter B, Walrath DC. Colonic adrenocarcinomas in patients with ureterosigmoidostomies. Dis Colon Rectum. 1979; 22(3):157–158

[160] Sheldon CA, McKinley CR, Hartig PR, Gonzalez R. Carcinoma at the site of ureterosigmoidostomy. Dis Colon Rectum. 1983; 26(1):55–58

[161] van Driel MF, Zwiers W, Grond J, Verschueren RC, Mensink HJ. Juvenile polyps at the site of a ureterosigmoidostomy. Report of five cases. Dis Colon Rectum. 1988; 31(7):553–557

[162] Guy RJ, Handa A, Traill Z, Mortensen NJ. Rectosigmoid carcinoma at previous ureterosigmoidostomy site in a renal transplant recipient: report of a case. Dis Colon Rectum. 2001; 44(10):1534–1536

[163] Kälble T, Tricker AR, Friedl P, et al. Ureterosigmoidostomy: long-term results, risk of carcinoma and etiological factors for carcinogenesis. J Urol. 1990; 144 (5):1110–1114

[164] Kliment J, Lupták J, Lofaj M, Horáková M, Beseda A. Carcinoma of the colon after ureterosigmoidostomy and trigonosigmoidostomy for exstrophy of the bladder. Int Urol Nephrol. 1993; 25(4):339–343

[165] Husmann DA, Spence HM. Current status of tumor of the bowel following ureterosigmoidostomy: a review. J Urol. 1990; 144(3):607–610

[166] Zaridze DG. Environmental etiology of large-bowel cancer. J Natl Cancer Inst. 1983; 70(3):389–400

[167] Hill MJ. Mechanism of colorectal carcinogenesis. In: Joosens JV, Hill MJ, Geboers J, eds. Diet and Human Carcinogenesis. Amsterdam: Elsevier Science; 1986:149–164

[168] Jørgensen T, Rafaelsen S. Gallstones and colorectal cancer–there is a relationship, but it is hardly due to cholecystectomy. Dis Colon Rectum. 1992; 35 (1):24–28

[169] Schernhammer ES, Leitzmann MF, Michaud DS, et al. Cholecystectomy and the risk for developing colorectal cancer and distal colorectal adenomas. Br J Cancer. 2003; 88(1):79–83

[170] Lagergren J, Ye W, Ekbom A. Intestinal cancer after cholecystectomy: is bile involved in carcinogenesis? Gastroenterology. 2001; 121(3):542–547

[171] Wynder EL, Reddy BS. Metabolic epidemiology of colorectal cancer. Cancer. 1974; 34(3):801–806

[172] Moorehead RJ, McKelvey STD. Cholecystectomy and colorectal cancer. Br J Surg. 1989; 76(3):250–253

[173] Gafà M, Sarli L, Sansebastiano G, et al. Prevention of colorectal cancer. Role of association between gallstones and colorectal cancer. Dis Colon Rectum. 1987; 30(9):692–696

[174] Hickman MS, Salinas HC, Schwesinger WH. Does cholecystectomy affect colonic tumorigenesis? Arch Surg. 1987; 122(3):334–336

[175] McMichael AJ, Potter JD. Host factors in carcinogenesis: certain bile-acid metabolic profiles that selectively increase the risk of proximal colon cancer. J Natl Cancer Inst. 1985; 75(2):185–191

[176] Nielsen GP, Theodors A, Tulinius H, Sigvaldason H. Cholecystectomy and colorectal carcinoma: a total-population historical prospective study. Am J Gastroenterol. 1991; 86(10):1486–1490

[177] McFarlane MJ, Welch KE. Gallstones, cholecystectomy, and colorectal cancer. Am J Gastroenterol. 1993; 88(12):1994–1999

[178] Abrams JS, Anton JR, Dreyfuss DC. The absence of a relationship between cholecystectomy and the subsequent occurrence of cancer of the proximal colon. Dis Colon Rectum. 1983; 26(3):141–144

[179] Kune GA, Kune S, Watson LF. Large bowel cancer after cholecystectomy. Am J Surg. 1988; 156(5):359–362

[180] Kaibara N, Wakatsuki T, Mizusawa K, Sugesawa A, Kimura O, Koga S. Negative correlation between cholecystectomy and the subsequent development of large bowel carcinoma in a low-risk Japanese population. Dis Colon Rectum. 1986; 29(10):644–646

[181] Ekbom A, Yuen J, Adami HO, et al. Cholecystectomy and colorectal cancer. Gastroenterology. 1993; 105(1):142–147

[182] Neugut AI, Murray TI, Garbowski GC, et al. Cholecystectomy as a risk factor for colorectal adenomatous polyps and carcinoma. Cancer. 1991; 68 (7):1644–1647

[183] Boulos PB, Cowin AP, Karamanolis DG, Clark CG. Diverticula, neoplasia, or both? Early detection of carcinoma in sigmoid diverticular disease. Ann Surg. 1985; 202(5):607–609

[184] Morini S, de Angelis P, Manurita L, Colavolpe V. Association of colonic diverticula with adenomas and carcinomas. A colonoscopic experience. Dis Colon Rectum. 1988; 31(10):793–796

[185] Persky V, Andrianopoulos G. The etiology of cancer of the colon. Is it all in the diet? In: Nelson RL, ed. Problems in Current Surgery. Controversies in Colon Cancer. Philadelphia, PA: JB Lippincott, 1987:11–23

[186] Thune I, Lund E. Physical activity and risk of colorectal cancer in men and women. Br J Cancer. 1996; 73(9):1134–1140

[187] Slattery ML, Edwards S, Curtin K, et al. Physical activity and colorectal cancer. Am J Epidemiol. 2003; 158(3):214–224

[188] Terry MB, Neugut AI, Bostick RM, et al. Risk factors for advanced colorectal adenomas: a pooled analysis. Cancer Epidemiol Biomarkers Prev. 2002; 11 (7):622–629

[189] Colbert LH, Hartman TJ, Malila N, et al. Physical activity in relation to cancer of the colon and rectum in a cohort of male smokers. Cancer Epidemiol Biomarkers Prev. 2001; 10(3):265–268

[190] Longnecker MP, Gerhardsson le Verdier M, Frumkin H, Carpenter C. A case-control study of physical activity in relation to risk of cancer of the right colon and rectum in men. Int J Epidemiol. 1995; 24(1):42–50

[191] White E, Jacobs EJ, Daling JR. Physical activity in relation to colon cancer in middle-aged men and women. Am J Epidemiol. 1996; 144(1):42–50

[192] Quadrilatero J, Hoffman-Goetz L. Physical activity and colon cancer. A systematic review of potential mechanisms. J Sports Med Phys Fitness. 2003; 43(2):121–138

[193] Neugut AI, Santos J. The association between cancers of the small and large bowel. Cancer Epidemiol Biomarkers Prev. 1993; 2(6):551–553

[194] Sonnenberg A, Müller AD. Constipation and cathartics as risk factors of colorectal cancer: a meta-analysis. Pharmacology. 1993; 47 Suppl 1:224–233

[195] Singh S, Morgan MB, Broughton M, Caffarey S, Topham C, Marks CG. A 10-year prospective audit of outcome of surgical treatment for colorectal carcinoma. Br J Surg. 1995; 82(11):1486–1490

[196] Broeders MJ, Lambe M, Baron JA, Leon DA. History of childbearing and colorectal cancer risk in women aged less than 60: an analysis of Swedish routine registry data 1960–1984. Int J Cancer. 1996; 66(2):170–175

[197] Newcomb PA, Storer BE. Postmenopausal hormone use and risk of large-bowel cancer. J Natl Cancer Inst. 1995; 87(14):1067–1071

[198] Calle EE, Miracle-McMahill HL, Thun MJ, Heath CW, Jr. Estrogen replacement therapy and risk of fatal colon cancer in a prospective cohort of postmenopausal women. J Natl Cancer Inst. 1995; 87(7):517–523

[199] Jacobs EJ, White E, Weiss NS. Exogenous hormones, reproductive history, and colon cancer (Seattle, Washington, USA). Cancer Causes Control. 1994; 5 (4):359–366

[200] Marcus PM, Newcomb PA, Young T, Storer BE. The association of reproductive and menstrual characteristics and colon and rectal cancer risk in Wisconsin women. Ann Epidemiol. 1995; 5(4):303–309

[201] Grodstein F, Newcomb PA, Stampfer MJ. Postmenopausal hormone therapy and the risk of colorectal cancer: a review and meta-analysis. Am J Med. 1999; 106(5):574–582

[202] Baris D, Gridley G, Ron E, et al. Acromegaly and cancer risk: a cohort study in Sweden and Denmark. Cancer Causes Control. 2002; 13(5):395–400

[203] Mullan FJ, Wilson HK, Majury CW, et al. Bile acids and the increased risk of colorectal tumours after truncal vagotomy. Br J Surg. 1990; 77(10):1085–1090

[204] Fisher SG, Davis F, Nelson R, Weber L, Haenszel W. Large bowel cancer following gastric surgery for benign disease: a cohort study. Am J Epidemiol. 1994; 139(7):684–692

[205] Little J, Owen RW, Fernandez F, et al. Asymptomatic colorectal neoplasia and fecal characteristics: a case-control study of subjects participating in the nottingham fecal occult blood screening trial. Dis Colon Rectum. 2002; 45 (9):1233–1241

[206] Babbs CF. Free radicals and the etiology of colon cancer. Free Radic Biol Med. 1990; 8(2):191–200

[207] Gorbach SL, Goldin BR. The intestinal microflora and the colon cancer connection. Rev Infect Dis. 1990; 12 Suppl 2:S252–S261

[208] Knekt P, Reunanen A, Takkunen H, Aromaa A, Heliövaara M, Hakulinen T. Body iron stores and risk of cancer. Int J Cancer. 1994; 56(3):379–382

[209] Vesterinen E, Pukkala E, Timonen T, Aromaa A. Cancer incidence among 78,000 asthmatic patients. Int J Epidemiol. 1993; 22(6):976–982

[210] Howden CW, Hornung CA. A systematic review of the association between Barrett's esophagus and colon neoplasms. Am J Gastroenterol. 1995; 90 (10):1814–1819

[211] Vaughan TL, Kiemeney LALM, McKnight B. Colorectal cancer in patients with esophageal adenocarcinoma. Cancer Epidemiol Biomarkers Prev. 1995; 4 (2):93–97

[212] Siegers CP, von Hertzberg-Lottin E, Otte M, Schneider B. Anthranoid laxative abuse–a risk for colorectal cancer? Gut. 1993; 34(8):1099–1101

[213] Younes M, Katikaneni PR, Lechago J. Association between mucosal hyperplasia of the appendix and adenocarcinoma of the colon. Histopathology. 1995; 26(1):33–37

[214] Erlinger TP, Platz EA, Rifai N, Helzlsouer KJ. C-reactive protein and the risk of incident colorectal cancer. JAMA. 2004; 291(5):585–590

[215] Woolcott CG, King WD, Marrett LD. Coffee and tea consumption and cancers of the bladder, colon and rectum. Eur J Cancer Prev. 2002; 11(2):137–145

[216] Kavan MG, Engdahl BE, Kay S. Colon cancer: personality factors predictive of onset and stage of presentation. J Psychosom Res. 1995; 39(8):1031–1039

[217] Galloway DJ, Indran M, Carr K, Jarrett F, George WD. Dietary manipulation during experimental colorectal carcinogenesis: a morphological study in the rat. Int J Colorectal Dis. 1987; 2(4):193–200

[218] Schatzkin A, Kelloff G. Chemo- and dietary prevention of colorectal cancer. Eur J Cancer. 1995; 31A(7–8):1198–1204

[219] Cassidy A, Bingham SA, Cummings JH. Starch intake and colorectal cancer risk: an international comparison. Br J Cancer. 1994; 69(5):937–942

[220] Thun MJ, Namboodiri MM, Heath CW, Jr. Aspirin use and reduced risk of fatal colon cancer. N Engl J Med. 1991; 325(23):1593–1596

[221] Rosenberg L, Palmer JR, Zauber AG, Warshauer ME, Stolley PD, Shapiro S. A hypothesis: nonsteroidal anti-inflammatory drugs reduce the incidence of large-bowel cancer. J Natl Cancer Inst. 1991; 83(5):355–358

[222] Smalley W, Ray WA, Daugherty J, Griffin MR. Use of nonsteroidal anti-inflammatory drugs and incidence of colorectal cancer: a population-based study. Arch Intern Med. 1999; 159(2):161–166

[223] Baron JA, Cole BF, Sandler RS, et al. A randomized trial of aspirin to prevent colorectal adenomas. N Engl J Med. 2003; 348(10):891–899

[224] Stürmer T, Glynn RJ, Lee IM, Manson JE, Buring JE, Hennekens CH. Aspirin use and colorectal cancer: post-trial follow-up data from the Physicians' Health Study. Ann Intern Med. 1998; 128(9):713–720

[225] Burke CA, Bauer WM, Lashner B. Chemoprevention of colorectal cancer: slow, steady progress. Cleve Clin J Med. 2003; 70(4):346–350

[226] Greenwald P, Kelloff G, Burch-Whitman C, Kramer BS. Chemoprevention. CA Cancer J Clin. 1995; 45(1):31–49

[227] Day DW, Jass JR, Price AB, et al, eds. Morson and Dawson's Gastrointestinal Pathology. 4th ed. Malden, MA: Blackwell Science; 2003

[228] Papp JP, Jr, Levine EJ, Thomas FB. Primary linitis plastica carcinoma of the colon and rectum. Am J Gastroenterol. 1995; 90(1):141–145

[229] Broders AC. Grading of carcinoma. Minn Med. 1925; 8:726–730

[230] Dukes CE. The classification of cancer of the rectum. J Pathol Bacteriol. 1932; 35:323–332

[231] Jass JR, Atkin WS, Cuzick J, et al. The grading of rectal cancer: historical perspectives and a multivariate analysis of 447 cases. Histopathology. 1986; 10 (5):437–459

[232] Gibbs NM. Undifferentiated carcinoma of the large intestine. Histopathology. 1977; 1(1):77–84

[233] Sundblad AS, Paz RA. Mucinous carcinomas of the colon and rectum and their relation to polyps. Cancer. 1982; 50(11):2504–2509

[234] Bonello JC, Sternberg SS, Quan SHQ. The significance of the signet-cell variety of adenocarcinoma of the rectum. Dis Colon Rectum. 1980; 23 (3):180–183

[235] Umpleby HC, Ranson DL, Williamson RCN. Peculiarities of mucinous colorectal carcinoma. Br J Surg. 1985; 72(9):715–718

[236] Okuno M, Ikehara T, Nagayama M, Kato Y, Yui S, Umeyama K. Mucinous colorectal carcinoma: clinical pathology and prognosis. Am Surg. 1988; 54 (11):681–685

[237] Anthony T, George R, Rodriguez-Bigas M, Petrelli NJ. Primary signet-ring cell carcinoma of the colon and rectum. Ann Surg Oncol. 1996; 3(4):344–348

[238] Shirouzu K, Isomoto H, Morodomi T, Ogata Y, Akagi Y, Kakegawa T. Primary linitis plastica carcinoma of the colon and rectum. Cancer. 1994; 74 (7):1863–1868

[239] Hase K, Shatney CH, Mochizuki H, et al. Long-term results of curative resection of "minimally invasive" colorectal cancer. Dis Colon Rectum. 1995; 38 (1):19–26

[240] Novello P, Duvillard P, Grandjouan S, et al. Carcinomas of the colon with multidirectional differentiation. Report of two cases and review of the literature. Dig Dis Sci. 1995; 40(1):100–106

[241] Bégin LR, Gordon PH, Alpert LC. Endophytic malignant transformation within flat adenoma of the colon: a potential diagnostic pitfall. Virchows Arch A Pathol Anat Histopathol. 1993; 422(5):415–418

[242] Kudo S, Tamure S, Nakajima T, et al. Depressed type of colorectal cancer. Endoscopy. 1995; 27(1):54–57, discussion 61

[243] Kubota O, Kino I, Kimura T, Harada Y. Nonpolypoid adenomas and adenocarcinomas found in background mucosa of surgically resected colons. Cancer. 1996; 77(4):621–626

[244] Minamoto T, Sawaguchi K, Ohta T, Itoh T, Mai M. Superficial-type adenomas and adenocarcinomas of the colon and rectum: a comparative morphological study. Gastroenterology. 1994; 106(6):1436–1443

[245] Tada S, Yao T, Iida M, Koga H, Hizawa K, Fujishima M. A clinicopathologic study of small flat colorectal carcinoma. Cancer. 1994; 74(9):2430–2435

[246] Iishi H, Kitamura S, Nakaizumi A, et al. Clinicopathological features and endoscopic diagnosis of superficial early adenocarcinomas of the large intestine. Dig Dis Sci. 1993; 38(7):1333–1337

[247] Togashi K, Konishi F, Koinuma K, et al. Flat and depressed lesions of the colon and rectum: Pathogenesis and clinical management. Ann Acad Med Singapore. 2003; 32(2):152–158

[248] Nivatvongs S. Surgical management of early colorectal cancer. World J Surg. 2000; 24(9):1052–1055

[249] Mulsow J, Winter DC, O'Keane JC, O'Connell PR. Sentinel lymph node mapping in colorectal cancer. Br J Surg. 2003; 90(6):659–667

[250] Bilchik AJ, Nora DT, Sobin LH, et al. Effect of lymphatic mapping on the new tumor-node-metastasis classification for colorectal cancer. J Clin Oncol. 2003; 21(4):668–672

[251] Saha S, Dan AG, Berman B, et al. Lymphazurin 1% versus 99mTc sulfur colloid for lymphatic mapping in colorectal tumors: a comparative analysis. Ann Surg Oncol. 2004; 11(1):21–26

[252] Bembenek A, Rau B, Moesta T, et al. Sentinel lymph node biopsy in rectal cancer–not yet ready for routine clinical use. Surgery. 2004; 135(5):498–505, discussion 506–507

[253] Bertagnoli M, Redston M, Miedma B, et al. Sentinel node staging of resectable colon cancer: results of CALG B 80001. Proc Am Soc Clin Oncol. 2004; 22:2465

[254] Read TE, Fleshman JW, Caushaj PF. Sentinel lymph node mapping for adenocarcinoma of the colon does not improve staging accuracy. Dis Colon Rectum. 2005; 48(1):80–85

[255] Stojadinovic A, Allen PJ, Protic M, et al. Colon sentinel lymph node mapping: practical surgical applications. J Am Coll Surg. 2005; 201(2):297–313

[256] Cimmino VM, Brown AC, Szocik JF, et al. Allergic reactions to isosulfan blue during sentinel node biopsy: a common event. Surgery. 2001; 130 (3):439–442

[257] Gutman M, Fidler IJ. Biology of human colon cancer metastasis. World J Surg. 1995; 19(2):226–234

[258] Griffiths JD, McKinna JA, Rowbotham HD, Tsolakidis P, Salsbury AJ. Carcinoma of the colon and rectum: circulating malignant cells and five-year survival. Cancer. 1973; 31(1):226–236

[259] Killingback M, Wilson E, Hughes ESR. Anal metastases from carcinoma of the rectum and colon. Aust N Z J Surg. 1965; 34:178–187

[260] Weiss L, Grundmann E, Torhorst J, et al. Haematogenous metastatic patterns in colonic carcinoma: an analysis of 1541 necropsies. J Pathol. 1986; 150 (3):195–203

[261] Taylor I. Liver metastases from colorectal cancer: lessons from past and present clinical studies. Br J Surg. 1996; 83(4):456–460

[262] Norgren J, Svensson JO. Anal implantation metastasis from carcinoma of the sigmoid colon and rectum–a risk when performing anterior resection with the EEA stapler? Br J Surg. 1985; 72(8):602

[263] Rollinson PD, Dundas SAC. Adenocarcinoma of sigmoid colon seeding into pre-existing fistula in ano. Br J Surg. 1984; 71(9):664–665

[264] Rosenberg IL. The aetiology of colonic suture-line recurrence. Ann R Coll Surg Engl. 1979; 61(4):251–257

[265] Scott NA, Taylor BA, Wolff BG, Lieber MM. Perianal metastasis from a sigmoid carcinoma–objective evidence of a clonal origin. Report of a case. Dis Colon Rectum. 1988; 31(1):68–70

[266] Thomas DJ, Thompson MR. Implantation metastasis from adenocarcinoma of sigmoid colon into fistula in ano. J R Soc Med. 1992; 85(6):361

[267] Murakami S, Terakado M, Hashimoto T, Tsuji Y, Okubo K, Hirayama R. Adrenal metastasis from rectal cancer: report of a case. Surg Today. 2003; 33 (2):126–130

[268] Conti JA, Kemeny N, Klimstra D, Minsky B, Rusch V. Colon carcinoma metastatic to the trachea. Report of a case and a review of the literature. Am J Clin Oncol. 1994; 17(3):227–229

[269] Araki K, Kobayashi M, Ogata T, Takuma K. Colorectal carcinoma metastatic to skeletal muscle. Hepatogastroenterology. 1994; 41(5):405–408

[270] Kupfer HWEM, Theunissen P, Delaere KPJ. Urethral metastasis from a rectal carcinoma. Acta Urol Belg. 1995; 63(4):31–32

[271] Bhutani MS, Pacheco J. Metastatic colon carcinoma to oral soft tissues. Spec Care Dentist. 1992; 12(4):172–173

[272] Vasilevsky CA, Abou-Khalil S, Rochon L, Frenkiel S, Black MJ. Carcinoma of the colon presenting as tonsillar metastasis. J Otolaryngol. 1997; 26(5):325–326

[273] Gabriel WB, Dukes CE, Bussey HJR. Lymphatic spread in cancer of the rectum. Br J Surg. 1935; 23:395–413

[274] Turnbull RB, Jr, Kyle K, Watson FR, Spratt J. Cancer of the colon: the influence of the no-touch isolation technic on survival rates. Ann Surg. 1967; 166 (3):420–427

[275] Wong JH, Severino R, Honnebier MB, Tom P, Namiki TS. Number of nodes examined and staging accuracy in colorectal carcinoma. J Clin Oncol. 1999; 17 (9):2896–2900

[276] Sobin LH, Greene FL. TNM classification: clarification of number of regional lymph nodes for pNo. Cancer. 2001; 92(2):452

[277] Nelson H, Petrelli N, Carlin A, et al. National Cancer Institute Expert Panel. Guidelines 2000 for colon and rectal cancer surgery. J Natl Cancer Inst. 2001; 93(8):583–596

[278] Compton CC, Fielding LP, Burgart LJ, et al. Prognostic factors in colorectal cancer. College of American Pathologists Consensus Statement 1999. Arch Pathol Lab Med. 2000; 124(7):979–994

[279] Chapuis PH, Dixon MF, Fielding LP, et al. Staging of colorectal cancer. Int J Colorectal Dis. 1987; 2(3):123–138

[280] Greene FL, Page DL, Floming ID, et al. American Joint Committee for Cancer. Cancer Staging Handbook. 6th ed. New York, NY: Springer-Verlag, 2002:127–138

[281] Astler VB, Coller FA. The prognostic significance of direct extension of carcinoma of the colon and rectum. Ann Surg. 1954; 139(6):846–852

[282] Chapuis PH, Dent OF, Newland RC, Bokey EL, Pheils MT. An evaluation of the American Joint Committee (pTNM) staging method for cancer of the colon and rectum. Dis Colon Rectum. 1986; 29(1):6–10

[283] Chapuis PH, Dixon MF, Fielding LP, et al. Staging of colorectal cancer. Int J Colorectal Dis. 1987; 2(3):123–138

[284] Davis NC, Newland RC. Terminology and classification of colorectal adenocarcinoma: the Australian clinico-pathological staging system. Aust N Z J Surg. 1983; 53(3):211–221

[285] Gastrointestinal Tumor Study Group. Adjuvant therapy of colon cancer–results of a prospectively randomized trial. N Engl J Med. 1984; 310 (12):737–743

[286] Terrazas JM, Val-Bernal JF, Buelta L. Staging of carcinoma of the colon and rectum. Surg Gynecol Obstet. 1987; 165(3):255–259

[287] Goligher JC. The Dukes' A, B and C categorization of the extent of spread of carcinomas of the rectum. Surg Gynecol Obstet. 1976; 143(5):793–794

[288] Kirklin JW, Dockerty MB, Waugh JM. The role of the peritoneal reflection in the prognosis of carcinoma of the rectum and sigmoid colon. Surg Gynecol Obstet. 1949; 88(3):326–331

[289] Zinkin LD. A critical review of the classifications and staging of colorectal cancer. Dis Colon Rectum. 1983; 26(1):37–43

[290] Newland RC, Chapuis PH, Smyth EJ. The prognostic value of substaging colorectal carcinoma. A prospective study of 1117 cases with standardized pathology. Cancer. 1987; 60(4):852–857

[291] Spratt JS Jr. Gross rates of growth of colonic neoplasms and other variables affecting medical decisions and prognosis. In: Burdette WJ, ed. Carcinoma of the Colon and Antecedent Epithelium. Springfield, IL: Charles C Thomas, 1970:66–77

[292] Finlay IG, Brunton GF, Meek D, et al. Rate of growth of hepatic metastases in colorectal carcinoma. Br J Surg. 1982; 69:689

[293] Havelaar I, Sugarbaker PH. Rate of growth of intraabdominal metastases from colon and rectal cancer followed by serial EOE CT. Cancer. 1984; 54:163–171

[294] Bolin S, Nilsson E, Sjödahl R. Carcinoma of the colon and rectum: growth rate. Ann Surg. 1983; 198(2):151–158

[295] Burnett KR, Greenbaum EI. Rapidly growing carcinoma of the colon. Dis Colon Rectum. 1981; 24(4):282–286

[296] Matsui T, Tsuda S, Yao K, Iwashita A, Sakurai T, Yao T. Natural history of early colorectal cancer: evolution of a growth curve. Dis Colon Rectum. 2000; 43 (10) Suppl:S18–S22

[297] Aldridge MC, Phillips RKS, Hittinger R, Fry JS, Fielding LP. Influence of tumour site on presentation, management and subsequent outcome in large bowel cancer. Br J Surg. 1986; 73(8):663–670

[298] Mandava N, Kumar S, Pizzi WF, Aprile IJ. Perforated colorectal carcinomas. Am J Surg. 1996; 172(3):236–238

[299] Runkel NS, Schlag P, Schwarz V, Herfarth C. Outcome after emergency surgery for cancer of the large intestine. Br J Surg. 1991; 78(2):183–188

[300] The consultant surgeons and pathologists of the Lothian and Borders health boards. Lothian and Borders large bowel cancer project: immediate outcome after surgery. Br J Surg. 1995; 82:888–890

[301] Beart RW, Jr, Melton LJ, III, Maruta M, Dockerty MB, Frydenberg HB, O'Fallon WM. Trends in right and left-sided colon cancer. Dis Colon Rectum. 1983; 26 (6):393–398

[302] Farrands PA, Hardcastle JD. Colorectal screening by a self-completion questionnaire. Gut. 1984; 25(5):445–447

[303] Ramsay JA, Rose TH, Ross T. Colonic carcinoma presenting as an appendiceal abscess in a young woman. Can J Surg. 1996; 39(1):53–56

[304] Beart RW, Steele GD, Jr, Menck HR, Chmiel JS, Ocwieja KE, Winchester DP. Management and survival of patients with adenocarcinoma of the colon and rectum: a national survey of the Commission on Cancer. J Am Coll Surg. 1995; 181(3):225–236

[305] Acher PL, Al-Mishlab T, Rahman M, Bates T. Iron-deficiency anaemia and delay in the diagnosis of colorectal cancer. Colorectal Dis. 2003; 5(2):145–148

[306] Church J, McGannon E. Family history of colorectal cancer: how often and how accurately is it recorded? Dis Colon Rectum. 2000; 43(11):1540–1544

[307] Rosato FE, Shelley WB, Fitts WT, Jr, Miller LD. Nonmetastatic cutaneous manifestations of cancer of the colon. Am J Surg. 1969; 117(2):277–281

[308] Halak M, Hazzan D, Kovacs Z, Shiloni E. Synchronous colorectal and renal carcinomas: a noteworthy clinical entity. Report of five cases. Dis Colon Rectum. 2000; 43(10):1314–1315

[309] Vasilevsky CA, Gordon PH. Colonoscopy in the follow-up of patients with colorectal carcinoma. Can J Surg. 1988; 31(3):188–190

[310] Evers BM, Mullins RJ, Matthews TH, Broghamer WL, Polk HC, Jr. Multiple adenocarcinomas of the colon and rectum. An analysis of incidences and current trends. Dis Colon Rectum. 1988; 31(7):518–522

[311] Piñol V, Andreu M, Castells A, Payá A, Bessa X, Jover R, Gastrointestinal Oncology Group of the Spanish Gastroenterological Association. Synchronous colorectal neoplasms in patients with colorectal cancer: predisposing individual and familial factors. Dis Colon Rectum. 2004; 47(7):1192–1200

[312] Adloff M, Arnaud JP, Bergamaschi R, Schloegel M. Synchronous carcinoma of the colon and rectum: prognostic and therapeutic implications. Am J Surg. 1989; 157(3):299–302

[313] Langevin JM, Nivatvongs S. The true incidence of synchronous cancer of the large bowel. A prospective study. Am J Surg. 1984; 147(3):330–333

[314] Rider JA, Kirsner JB, Moeller HC, Palmer WL. Polyps of the colon and rectum; a four-year to nine-year follow-up study of five hundred thirty-seven patients. J Am Med Assoc. 1959; 170(6):633–638

[315] Slater G, Fleshner P, Aufses AH, Jr. Colorectal cancer location and synchronous adenomas. Am J Gastroenterol. 1988; 83(8):832–836

[316] Chu DZ, Giacco G, Martin RG, Guinee VF. The significance of synchronous carcinoma and polyps in the colon and rectum. Cancer. 1986; 57(3):445–450

[317] Lee TK, Barringer M, Myers RT, Sterchi JM. Multiple primary carcinomas of the colon and associated extracolonic primary malignant tumors. Ann Surg. 1982; 195(4):501–507

[318] Tanaka H, Hiyama T, Hanai A, Fujimoto I. Second primary cancers following colon and rectal cancer in Osaka, Japan. Jpn J Cancer Res. 1991; 82 (12):1356–1365

[319] Schoen RE, Weissfeld JL, Kuller LH. Are women with breast, endometrial, or ovarian cancer at increased risk for colorectal cancer? Am J Gastroenterol. 1994; 89(6):835–842

[320] de Dombal FT, Matharu SS, Staniland JR, et al. Presentation of cancer to hospital as 'acute abdominal pain'. Br J Surg. 1980; 67(6):413–416

[321] Ohman U. Prognosis in patients with obstructing colorectal carcinoma. Am J Surg. 1982; 143(6):742–747

[322] Wolloch Y, Zer M, Lurie M, et al. Ischemic colitis proximal to obstructing carcinoma of the colon. Am J Proctol. 1979; 30:17–22

[323] Saegesser F, Sandblom P. Ischemic lesions of the distended colon: a complication of obstructive colorectal cancer. Am J Surg. 1975; 129(3):309–315

[324] Ueyama T, Yao T, Nakamura K, Enjoji M. Obstructing carcinomas of the colon and rectum: clinicopathologic analysis of 40 cases. Jpn J Clin Oncol. 1991; 21 (2):100–109

[325] Seow-Choen F, Chua TL, Goh HS. Ischaemic colitis and colorectal cancer: some problems and pitfalls. Int J Colorectal Dis. 1993; 8(4):210–212

[326] Wolmark N. NSABP Investigators. The prognostic significance of tumour location and bowel obstruction in Dukes' B and C colorectal cancer. Ann Surg. 1983; 198:743–750

[327] Umpleby HC, Williamson RCN. Survival in acute obstructing colorectal carcinoma. Dis Colon Rectum. 1984; 27(5):299–304

[328] Panwalker AP. Unusual infections associated with colorectal cancer. Rev Infect Dis. 1988; 10(2):347–364

[329] Lam S, Greenberg R, Bank S. An unusual presentation of colon cancer: purulent pericarditis and cardiac tamponade due to Bacteroides fragilis. Am J Gastroenterol. 1995; 90(9):1518–1520

[330] Belinkie SA, Narayanan NC, Russell JC, Becker DR. Splenic abscess associated with Streptococcus bovis septicemia and neoplastic lesions of the colon. Dis Colon Rectum. 1983; 26(12):823–824

[331] Silver SC. Streptococcus bovis endocarditis and its association with colonic carcinoma. Dis Colon Rectum. 1984; 27(9):613–614

[332] Legier JF. Streptococcus salivarius meningitis and colonic carcinoma. South Med J. 1991; 84(8):1058–1059

[333] Lonardo A, Grisendi A, Pulvirenti M, et al. Right colon adenocarcinoma presenting as Bacteroides fragilis liver abscesses. J Clin Gastroenterol. 1992; 14 (4):335–338

[334] Teitz S, Guidetti-Sharon A, Monro H, et al. Pyogenic liver abscess: warning indicator of silent colonic cancer. Dis Colon Rectum. 1995; 58:1220–1223

[335] Kudsk KA. Occult gastrointestinal malignancies producing metastatic Clostridium septicum infections in diabetic patients. Surgery. 1992; 112(4):765–770, discussion 770–772

[336] Lorimer JW, Eidus LB. Invasive Clostridium septicum infection in association with colorectal carcinoma. Can J Surg. 1994; 37(3):245–249

[337] Poleski MH, Gordon PH. Screening for carcinoma of the colon: pitfalls of the hemoccult test. In: Nelson RL, ed. Problems in Current Surgery. Controversies in Colon Cancer. Philadelphia, PA: JB Lippincott, 1987:1–10

[338] Nivatvongs S, Fryd DS. How far does the proctosigmoidoscope reach? A prospective study of 1000 patients. N Engl J Med. 1980; 303(7):380–382

[339] Marks G, Gathright JB, Boggs HW, Ray JE, Castro AF, Salvati E. Guidelines for use of the flexible fiberoptic sigmoidoscope in the management of the surgical patient. Dis Colon Rectum. 1982; 25(3):187–190

[340] Traul DG, Davis CB, Pollock JC, Scudamore HH. Flexible fiberoptic sigmoidoscopy-the Monroe Clinic experience. A prospective study of 5000 examinations. Dis Colon Rectum. 1983; 26(3):161–166

[341] Bernard D, Tassé D, Morgan S, Wassef R. Is preoperative colonoscopy in carcinoma a realistic and valuable proposition? Can J Surg. 1987; 30 (2):87–89

[342] Isler JT, Brown PC, Lewis FG, Billingham RP. The role of preoperative colonoscopy in colorectal cancer. Dis Colon Rectum. 1987; 30(6):435–439

[343] Finan PJ, Ritchie JK, Hawley PR. Synchronous and 'early' metachronous carcinomas of the colon and rectum. Br J Surg. 1987; 74(10):945–947

[344] Reilly JC, Rusin LC, Theuerkauf FJ, Jr. Colonoscopy: its role in cancer of the colon and rectum. Dis Colon Rectum. 1982; 25(6):532–538

[345] Sollenberger LL, Eisenstat TE, Rubin RJ, Salvati EP. Is preoperative colonoscopy necessary in carcinoma of the colon and rectum? Am Surg. 1988; 54 (2):113–115

[346] Thomas RD, Fairhurst JJ, Frost RA. Wessex regional radiology audit: barium enema in colo-rectal carcinoma. Clin Radiol. 1995; 50(9):647–650

[347] Peel AL, Benyon L, Grace RH. The value of routine preoperative urological assessment in patients undergoing elective surgery for diverticular disease or carcinoma of the large bowel. Br J Surg. 1980; 67(1):42–45

[348] Vezeridis MP, Petrelli NJ, Mittelman A. The value of routine preoperative urologic evaluation in patients with colorectal carcinoma. Dis Colon Rectum. 1987; 30(10):758–760

[349] Phillips R, Hittinger R, Saunders V, Blesovsky L, Stewart-Brown S, Fielding P. Preoperative urography in large bowel cancer: a useless investigation? Br J Surg. 1983; 70(7):425–427

[350] Tartter PI, Steinberg BM. The role of preoperative intravenous pyelogram in operations performed for carcinoma of the colon and rectum. Surg Gynecol Obstet. 1986; 163(1):65–69

[351] Grace RH, Hale M, Mackie G, Marks CG, Bloomberg TJ, Walker WJ. Role of ultrasound in the diagnosis of liver metastases before surgery for large bowel cancer. Br J Surg. 1987; 74(6):480–481

[352] Rafaelsen SR, Kronborg O, Larsen C, Fenger C. Intraoperative ultrasonography in detection of hepatic metastases from colorectal cancer. Dis Colon Rectum. 1995; 38(4):355–360

[353] Meijer S, Paul MA, Cuesta MA, Blomjous J. Intra-operative ultrasound in detection of liver metastases. Eur J Cancer. 1995; 31A(7–8):1210–1211

[354] Machi J, Isomoto H, Kurohiji T, et al. Accuracy of intraoperative ultrasonography in diagnosing liver metastasis from colorectal cancer: evaluation with postoperative follow-up results. World J Surg. 1991; 15(4):551–556, discussion 557

[355] Takeuchi N, Ramirez JM, Mortensen NJM, Cobb R, Whittlestone T. Intraoperative ultrasonography in the diagnosis of hepatic metastases during surgery for colorectal cancer. Int J Colorectal Dis. 1996; 11(2):92–95

[356] Kerner BA, Oliver GC, Eisenstat TE, Rubin RJ, Salvati EP. Is preoperative computerized tomography useful in assessing patients with colorectal carcinoma? Dis Colon Rectum. 1993; 36(11):1050–1053

[357] Thoeni RF, Rogalla P. CT for the evaluation of carcinomas in the colon and rectum. Semin Ultrasound CT MR. 1995; 16(2):112–126

[358] Mauchley DC, Lynge DC, Langdale LA, Stelzner MG, Mock CN, Billingsley KG. Clinical utility and cost-effectiveness of routine preoperative computed tomography scanning in patients with colon cancer. Am J Surg. 2005; 189(5):512–517, discussion 517

[359] Tempero M, Brand R, Holdeman K, Matamoros A. New imaging techniques in colorectal cancer. Semin Oncol. 1995; 22(5):448–471

[360] Zerhouni EA, Rutter C, Hamilton SR, et al. CT and MR imaging in the staging of colorectal carcinoma: report of the Radiology Diagnostic Oncology Group II. Radiology. 1996; 200(2):443–451

[361] Johnson K, Bakhsh A, Young D, Martin TE, Jr, Arnold M. Correlating computed tomography and positron emission tomography scan with operative findings in metastatic colorectal cancer. Dis Colon Rectum. 2001; 44(3):354–357

[362] Bertsch DJ, Burak WE, Jr, Young DC, Arnold MW, Martin EW, Jr. Radioimmunoguided surgery for colorectal cancer. Ann Surg Oncol. 1996; 3(3):310–316

[363] Arnold MW, Hitchcock CL, Young DC, Burak WE, Jr, Bertsch DJ, Martin EW, Jr. Intra-abdominal patterns of disease dissemination in colorectal cancer identified using radioimmunoguided surgery. Dis Colon Rectum. 1996; 39(5):509–513

[364] Dominguez JM, Wolff BG, Nelson H, Forstrom LA, Mullan BP. 111 In-CYT-103 scanning in recurrent colorectal cancer–does it affect standard management? Dis Colon Rectum. 1996; 39(5):514–519

[365] Moffat FL, Jr, Pinsky CM, Hammershaimb L, et al. The Immunomedics Study Group. Clinical utility of external immunoscintigraphy with the IMMU-4 technetium-99 m Fab' antibody fragment in patients undergoing surgery for carcinoma of the colon and rectum: results of a pivotal, phase III trial. J Clin Oncol. 1996; 14(8):2295–2305

[366] Corman ML, Galandiuk S, Block GE, et al. Immunoscintigraphy with 111 In-satumomab pendetide in patients with colorectal adenocarcinoma: performance and impact on clinical management. Dis Colon Rectum. 1994; 37(2):129–137

[367] Galandiuk S. Immunoscintigraphy in the surgical management of colorectal cancer. J Nucl Med. 1993; 34(3) Suppl:541–544

[368] Limberg B. Diagnosis and staging of colonic tumors by conventional abdominal sonography as compared with hydrocolonic sonography. N Engl J Med. 1992; 327(2):65–69

[369] Leveson SH, Wiggins PA, Giles GR, Parkin A, Robinson PJ. Deranged liver blood flow patterns in the detection of liver metastases. Br J Surg. 1985; 72(2):128–130

[370] Zhou DY, Feng FC, Zhang YL, et al. Comparison of Shams' test for rectal mucus to an immunological test for fecal occult blood in large intestinal carcinoma screening. Analysis of a check-up of 6480 asymptomatic subjects. Chin Med J (Engl). 1993; 106(10):739–742

[371] Sakamoto K, Muratani M, Ogawa T, Nagamachi Y. Evaluation of a new test for colorectal neoplasms: a prospective study of asymptomatic population. Cancer Biother. 1993; 8(1):49–55

[372] Chen YL. The diagnosis of colorectal cancer with cytologic brushings under direct vision at fiberoptic colonoscopy. A report of 59 cases. Dis Colon Rectum. 1987; 30(5):342–344

[373] Rosman AS, Federman Q, Feinman L. Diagnosis of colon cancer by lavage cytology with an orally administered balanced electrolyte solution. Am J Gastroenterol. 1994; 89(1):51–56

[374] Gold P, Freedman SO. Demonstration of tumor-specific antigens in human colonic cardnomata by immunological tolerance and absorption techniques. J Exp Med. 1965; 121:439–462

[375] Gold P. The carcinoembryonic antigen (CEA): discovery and three decades of study. Perspect Colon Rectal Surg. 1996; 9(2):1–47

[376] Kyzer S, Mitmaker B, Gordon PH, Schipper H, Wang E. Proliferative activity of colonic mucosa at different distances from primary adenocarcinoma as determined by the presence of statin: a nonproliferation-specific nuclear protein. Dis Colon Rectum. 1992; 35(9):879–883

[377] Stein R, Juweid M, Mattes MJ, Goldenberg DM. Carcinoembryonic antigen as a target for radioimmunotherapy of human medullary thyroid carcinoma: antibody processing, targeting, and experimental therapy with 131I and 90Y labeled MAbs. Cancer Biother Radiopharm. 1999; 14(1):37–47

[378] Bockhorn M, Frilling A, Rewerk S, et al. Lack of elevated serum carcinoembryonic antigen and calcitonin in medullary thyroid carcinoma. Thyroid. 2004; 14(6):468–470

[379] Moorehead RJ, Hoper M, McKelvey STD. Assessment of ornithine decarboxylase activity in rectal mucosa as a marker for colorectal adenomas and carcinomas. Br J Surg. 1987; 74(5):364–365

[380] Narisawa T, Takahashi M, Niwa M, et al. Increased mucosal ornithine decarboxylase activity in large bowel with multiple tumors, adenocarcinoma, and adenoma. Cancer. 1989; 63(8):1572–1576

[381] Gelister JSK, Jass JR, Mahmoud M, Gaffney PJ, Boulos PB. Role of urokinase in colorectal neoplasia. Br J Surg. 1987; 74(6):460–463

22 Colon Carcinoma: Treatment

Philip H. Gordon and David E. Beck

Abstract

Operative treatment for carcinoma of the colon has evolved in several stages because of the enormous risk of sepsis. Initially, these stages have included nothing more than a diverting colostomy, subsequent recommendations for exteriorization and double-barrel colostomy, efforts at re-establishing intestinal continuity with various internal stents, resection and anastomosis with proximal diversion, and ultimately resection and primary anastomosis. The acceptance of a one-stage procedure was achieved through the use of mechanical and antimicrobial bowel preparation and improvements in anesthetic and operative techniques.

Keywords: malignancy, colon, carcinoma, anastomosis, curative resection, adjuvant therapy, chemoradiotherapy, complicated carcinomas, obstruction, Hartmann's procedure

22.1 Introduction

Operative treatment for carcinoma of the colon has evolved in several stages because of the enormous risk of sepsis. Initially, these stages have included nothing more than a diverting colostomy, subsequent recommendations for exteriorization and double-barrel colostomy, efforts at re-establishing intestinal continuity with various internal stents, resection and anastomosis with proximal diversion, and ultimately resection and primary anastomosis. The acceptance of a one-stage procedure was achieved through the use of the mechanical and antimicrobial bowel preparation and improvements in anesthetic and operative techniques.

22.2 Curative Resection

22.2.1 Preoperative Evaluation

The general assessment of the patient is discussed in Chapter 5. Fazio et al[1] described a dedicated prognostic index for quantifying operative risk in colorectal carcinoma surgery from data collected from 5,034 consecutive patients undergoing major surgery. Primary end point was 30-day operative mortality. The patients' median age was 66 years. Operative mortality was 2.3% with no significant variability between surgeons or through time. Multivariate analysis identified the following independent risk factors: age (odds ratio [OR] = 1.5 per 10-year increase), American Society of Anesthesiologists (ASA) grade (OR for ASA II, III, IV–V vs. I = 2.6, 4.3, 6.8), tumor/node/metastasis (TNM) staging (OR for stage IV vs. I–III = 2.6), mode of surgery (OR for urgent vs. nonurgent = 2.1), no-carcinoma resection versus carcinoma resection (OR = 4.5), and hematocrit level. The model has implications in everyday practice, because it may be used as an adjunct in the process of informed consent and for monitoring surgical performance through time.[2]

22.2.2 Bowel Preparation

Preoperative bowel preparation has been the subject of considerable controversy. The belief that adequate mechanical preparation and antibiotic preparation are necessary has recently been questioned. As discussed in Chapter 5, most surgeons currently use some form of mechanical cleansing and systemic prophylactic antibiotics. Many are returning to the use of oral antibiotics as well.

22.2.3 Exploration of Abdomen

Before operation, a bladder catheter is routinely inserted into the bladder. A nasogastric tube is not necessary in the vast majority of cases, but an oral gastric tube is placed to decompress the stomach. Incisions should be made in a manner that provides maximum exposure for the planned resection. All operations can be performed through a midline incision and this is the access preferred by most surgeons. For a patient about to undergo a right hemicolectomy, an oblique right-sided abdominal incision is usually adequate and can be extended as needed. For transverse colon lesions, a supraumbilical transverse incision places access immediately in the area of the planned operation, and the incision can be extended in either direction if there is any difficulty encountered in taking down the flexures. For splenic flexure lesions, Rubin et al[3] advocate the use of a left subcostal transverse incision combined with the right lateral position. For left-sided colonic lesions, a subumbilical transverse incision can be used. This permits adequate exposure for even a low anterior resection. For descending colon lesions, an oblique incision may prove very convenient. The use of paramedian incisions appears quite antiquated. For emergency operations, a midline incision seems the access of choice.

When the abdomen has been opened, attention should be directed to ruling out the presence of metastatic disease, with special attention given to the liver and the pelvis. A relatively new technique advocated for the detection of occult hepatic metastases is intraoperative contact ultrasonography.[4] Lesions greater than 1 cm in diameter can be detected in 95% of cases, and those between 0.5 and 1.0 cm in 66% of cases. After assessment of the abdomen, attention is focused on the primary lesion to determine its resectability.

22.2.4 Principles of Resection

Dogma abounds with respect to the technical aspects of operation for colorectal carcinoma. The general principles advocated for all operations for carcinoma include removal of the primary lesion with adequate margin, including the areas of lymphatic drainage. The definition of an adequate margin especially for rectal carcinoma remains controversial. Approximately one-half of the patients seeking operative treatment already have metastatic disease spread to the regional lymph nodes. Controversy exists as to the appropriate extent of lymphatic dissection. Is a segmental resection adequate therapy?

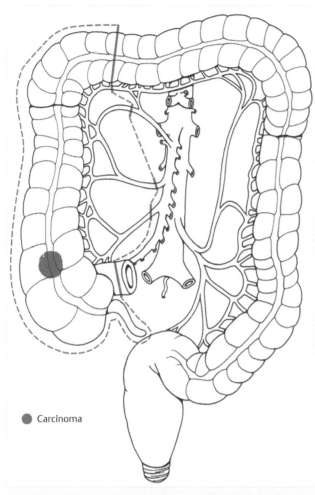

Fig. 22.1 Extent of resection for carcinoma in the cecum or ascending colon.

● Carcinoma

Or with a sigmoid carcinoma, for example, should a formal left hemicolectomy be performed? For the most part, the literature suggests that no survival advantage can be attributed to extended lymph node dissections for left colon and rectal carcinoma.[5,6,7,8] An exception is the isolated report by Enker et al.[9] Without doubt, this operation does result in increased morbidity, with patients often suffering from impotence, bladder difficulties, and potential vascular problems. Any marginal improvement is outweighed by the considerable morbidity. The principle of en bloc resection of involved structures is firmly established. Continued controversy surrounds radical lymph node dissection, luminal ligation, oophorectomy, and the "no-touch technique." What is becoming increasingly evident is that differences in outcome among different surgeons suggest that technique is important. Whether a properly performed lymphadenectomy may produce a therapeutic benefit or whether it is simply a more accurate staging procedure is unknown.

For lesions located in the cecum or the ascending colon, a right hemicolectomy to encompass the bowel served by the ileocolic, right colic, and right branch of the midcolic vessels is recommended (▶ Fig. 22.1). For lesions involving the hepatic flexure, a more extended resection of the transverse colon is indicated (▶ Fig. 22.2). For lesions in the transverse colon, depending on the portion involved, a segment of bowel is removed as shown in ▶ Fig. 22.3. Splenic flexure lesions require removal of the distal half of the transverse colon and the descending colon (▶ Fig. 22.4). Sigmoid lesions are appropriately treated by excision of the sigmoid colon (▶ Fig. 22.5). Some surgeons prefer more radical excisions, but there is no convincing evidence to suggest that prolonged survival or decreased local recurrence will result (▶ Fig. 22.6). Indeed, operative mortality and postoperative complications are reportedly higher.[5] For patients who have synchronous carcinomas in different portions of the colon, a subtotal colectomy seems appropriate (▶ Fig. 22.7). Other suggested indications for subtotal colectomy

Fig. 22.2 Extent of resection for carcinoma in the hepatic flexure.

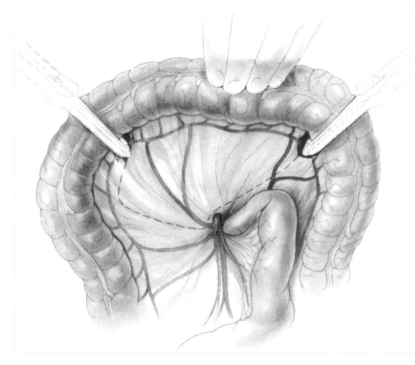

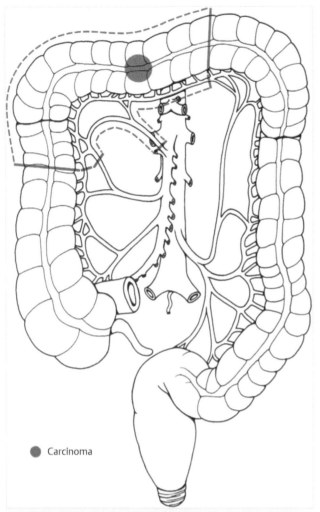

Carcinoma

Fig. 22.3 Extent of resection for carcinoma in the transverse colon.

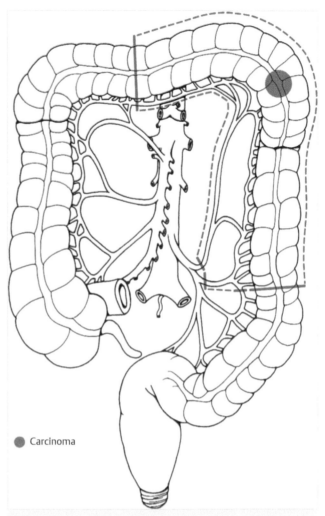

Carcinoma

Fig. 22.4 Extent of resection for carcinoma in the splenic flexure.

include associated polyps (not removed by colonoscopy), acute or subacute obstruction, associated sigmoid diverticulosis (symptomatic), prior transverse colostomy for obstruction, young patient age (< 50 years) with a positive family history, and adherence of the sigmoid colon to a cecal carcinoma.[10]

The techniques described in the following section pertain to good-risk patients. For poor-risk patients or patients undergoing palliative resection, segmental resections are more appropriate. Certain intraoperative precautions have been proposed to eliminate or at least minimize the dissemination of malignant cells. Concern has been expressed that manipulation of the carcinoma results in blood-borne metastases. There is also the risk of exfoliated malignant cells adjacent to the primary lesion becoming implanted at the suture line, in the peritoneal cavity, or in the wound. It has been postulated that handling of the primary lesion early in the operation promotes such dissemination. This thesis was supported by the demonstration of malignant cell in the circulation,[11,12] a finding that led Turnbull et al[13] to popularize the no-touch technique in which lymphovascular channels were ligated prior to any manipulation of the primary lesion. After using this maneuver, they reported improved survival rates for Dukes' C lesions. However,

this was not a controlled trial, and Turnbull's results have not been duplicated. Therefore, the technique has not been adopted by most surgeons as standard therapy. In an effort to avoid implantation of malignant cells shed from the primary carcinoma, Cole et al[12] recommended encirclement of the bowel lumen proximal and distal to the primary lesion. This is a simple addition to the operation and can usually be performed easily. Wound edges can be covered to prevent malignant cell implantation in the wound. In an effort to diminish the risk of implantation of malignant cells distal to the lesion, a host of cytotoxic agents (e.g., Dakin's solution or bichloride of mercury) have been used to irrigate the distal bowel; distilled water has also been used for this purpose. Since none of these cytotoxic agents has been used in a clinical trial setting, their value is in question. As a means of diminishing suture line implantation, iodized catgut was popular for a brief time.[14] Another effort is the intraluminal installation of diluted formalin, in which case local recurrence was reportedly reduced to 2.6 from 14.3% for untreated patients.[15]

None of the techniques tried thus far, including irrigation of the peritoneal cavity or the use of iodized catgut, has been proven of value. However, proximal and distal ligation of the bowel

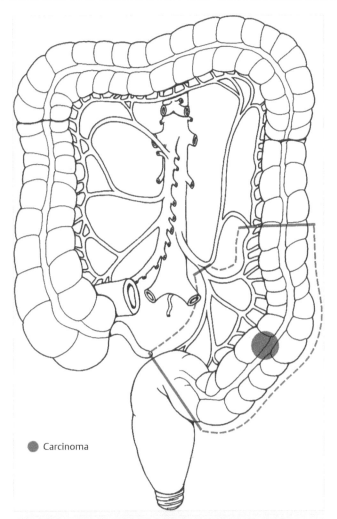

Fig. 22.5 Extent of resection for carcinoma in the sigmoid colon.

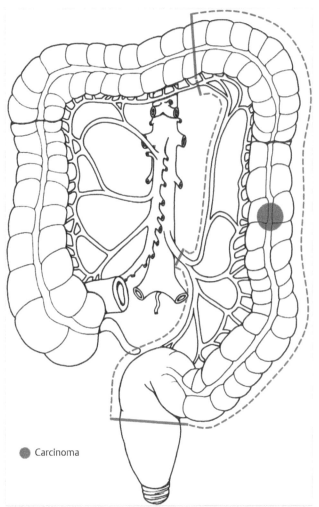

Fig. 22.6 Extended resection preferred by some surgeons for carcinoma in the sigmoid colon.

would appear to be a harmless practice. Adjuvant chemotherapy administered directly into the bowel lumen at the time of operation has been used but not in a trial setting.

Technique

Right Colectomy

With the appropriate retractor in place and the small bowel packed toward the left side of the abdomen, the procedure is begun by incising the parietal peritoneum from just below the terminal ileum toward the hepatic flexure (▶ Fig. 22.8). This can be done with Metzenbaum scissors or preferably by use of diathermy. If feasible, the colon is encircled above and below the carcinoma with umbilical tapes. This procedure is performed as soon as the lesion is appropriately mobile. The right colon is elevated from the retroperitoneum, with care taken not to injure the ureter, gonadal vessels, or inferior vena cava (▶ Fig. 22.9). As dissection is carried toward the hepatic flexure, attention is given to avoiding any injury to the duodenum. Peritoneal division is continued around the hepatic flexure and horizontally along the upper border of the transverse colon, with division of any adhesions to the gallbladder. As dissection continues, the lesser sac is opened by dividing the gastrocolic ligament. Mobilization

is continued for as far as the resection is planned. During this stage of the operation, the second and third portions of the duodenum are exposed, and caution should be exercised to prevent injury to this structure. Next, the greater omentum is transected vertically (▶ Fig. 22.10). The medial aspect of the peritoneum then is incised along the planned area of resection. Mesenteric attachments are divided until the vascular anatomy is clear. The vessels are now displayed, and their trunks are clamped, divided, and the remaining end is ligated (▶ Fig. 22.11). The ileocolic, right colic, and right branches of the middle colic artery are divided in turn. The small vessels adjacent to the small bowel and transverse colon at the level of the proposed transection are divided between clamps, and hemostasis is secured. The two ends of bowel are now ready for division (▶ Fig. 22.12). The technique the surgeon adopts—stapling or suturing—will direct how the bowel is handled.

Surgeons who advocate the no-touch isolation technique ligate the lymphovascular structures as the initial maneuver of the operation. An incision is made in the root of the mesentery, and the trunks of the vessels are identified, divided, and ligated prior to any mobilization. The major concern with this method is the potential need to deal with the ureter, gonadal vessels,

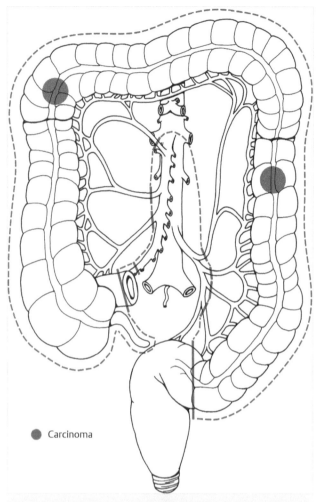

Fig. 22.7 Extent of resection for synchronous carcinomas in different portions of the colon.

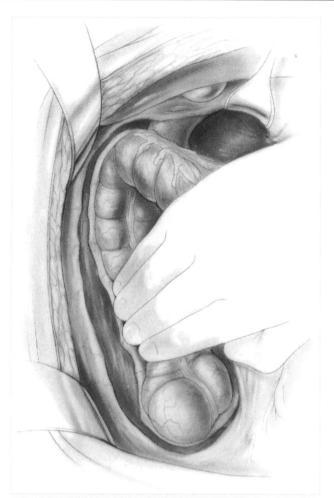

Fig. 22.8 Incision of parietal peritoneum.

and duodenum without the benefit of adequate exposure, which may keep these structures out of harm's way. In terms of long-term survival advantage, the efficacy of this method has not been supported in surgical trials. In a multicenter prospective randomized controlled trial, Wiggers et al[16] compared the no-touch isolation technique to a conventional technique. Both overall and corrected survival data did not differ between the two groups, although there was a tendency toward reduction in the number of occurrences and the length of time to the development of liver metastases with the no-touch technique.

For the re-establishment of intestinal continuity, the authors' preference is to use staplers. A functional end-to-end anastomosis is created in the following way.[17] Once the site of transection has been selected, a small area (less than that necessary for hand-sutured anastomoses) is cleared. Enough fat is cleared from the edge so that when the bowel opening is closed, there is room for the linear stapler to be applied without inclusion of mesenteric fat or appendices epiploicae. Obesity per se is not a contraindication to the use of staplers. In fact, since less clearing is necessary, staplers may have an advantage in such circumstances. The linear cutting instrument (75 mm in length) is applied in the mesenteric–antimesenteric plane (▶ Fig. 22.13a). If the bowel diameter is too large to fit within the jaws of the

instrument, such as with the transverse colon, the instrument is placed so that the tips of the instrument are on the antimesenteric border. Then if the bowel is not completely transected and stapled closed, the open area will occur where an opening would have been made to create the functional end-to-end anastomosis. The advantage of a stapled transection is that little or no devascularization of the bowel is necessary. With manual anastomoses, too little clearing may make anastomotic suturing insecure, and too much may jeopardize the viability of the bowel ends. Caution, however, must be exercised in patients with diverticular disease.

It is often easier to close the mesentery before the anastomosis is constructed, especially with a right hemicolectomy and with patients who are overweight. Completing this step prior to constructing the anastomosis also will diminish the possibility of the error of rotation of the ileum (▶ Fig. 22.13b).

The antimesenteric borders are aligned, and at each corner an amount of tissue just adequate to insert the fork of the anastomosing instrument is excised (▶ Fig. 22.13c). The instrument is inserted to its full length to create a large anastomosis (▶ Fig. 22.13d). The halves of the instrument are joined and the bowel is drawn up, which ensures an anastomosis that is the full length that the instrument is capable of creating (▶ Fig. 22.13e). The anastomosis should be checked to see that it is being created near the antimesenteric border and that no

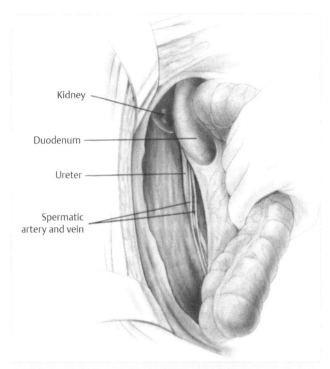

Fig. 22.9 Mobilization of the right colon. Exposure of the duodenum with care taken to avoid injury to retroperitoneal structures.

Labels in figure:
Kidney
Duodenum
Ureter
Spermatic artery and vein

fat, omentum, mesentery, sponge, or viscus is trapped. The halves of the instrument should be gently separated because excessive force may result in disruption of the anastomosis. Some bleeding at the suture line is not uncommon and may be controlled by sponge compression, light cautery, or suture ligature. Excessive cautery may result in a weakened anastomosis and may predispose to leakage. Heavy bleeding should be controlled with fine sutures.

The anastomotic suture lines are held apart in preparation for the application of the linear stapler (▶ Fig. 22.13f). Welter et al[18] showed that with the functional end-to-end anastomosis the area of the anastomosis can be increased by up to one-third of the original bowel lumen if the linear stapler closing staple line is applied so as to hold the anastomosing staple lines in an open V position. There is also the very remote possibility that if the suture lines remain in apposition, unwanted healing may occur from one to the other.

If a stapling instrument is used to close the bowel defect, the staple lines should be slightly staggered when the linear stapler is applied (▶ Fig. 22.13g). This modification was suggested by Chassin et al[19] to avoid too many intersecting staple lines, which may create an ischemic point with potential for a leak. Allis clamps are applied to the tissues being approximated to prevent a portion of the bowel circumference from slipping back as the jaws of the instrument compress the tissue (▶ Fig. 22.13h). The instrument is fired, and the excess tissue is cut away prior to release of the instrument to avoid injury to the anastomosis. A fine ooze of blood is reassuring of a good blood supply to the anastomosis, but more brisk bleeding should be controlled with gentle cautery or a fine suture. Alternatively, the bowel opening can be closed with the application of the linear cutting instrument. This technical variation has

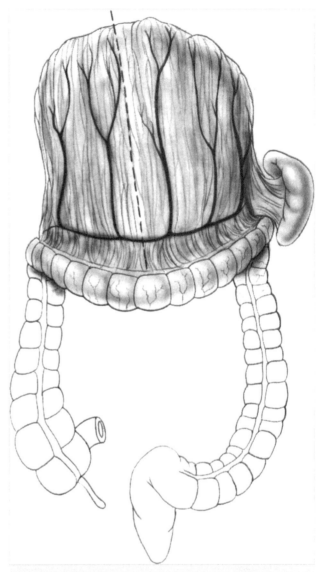

Fig. 22.10 Transection of the greater omentum.

been suggested to reduce the cost of the anastomosis. If adopted, care should be taken to ensure that the instrument application does not compromise the size of the anastomosis. The anastomosis is checked to ensure that it is complete and no leak is present (▶ Fig. 22.13i).

Another option (preferred by DEB) is to close the open defect in layers with two running sutures (polyglactin and polyester). This takes only a little more time, is less expensive than using another stapler, produces an inverted anastomosis, and provides the largest diameter anastomosis (as no bowel tissue is excised.

In a series of 223 anastomoses performed in 205 patients, Kyzer and Gordon reviewed their experience with the use of staples for construction of anastomoses following colonic resection.[20] Indications for operation included malignancy, benign neoplasms, inflammatory bowel disease, and several miscellaneous entities. A functional end-to-end anastomosis using the standard GIA cartridge and the TA 55 instruments was performed. The operative mortality rate was 1.5%, with none of the deaths related to the anastomosis. Intraoperative complications encountered included bleeding, leak (one), tissue fracture (one), instrument failure (four), and technical error (three).

Early postoperative complications related to or potentially related to the anastomosis included bleeding (five), pelvic abscess (one), fistula (one), peritonitis (two), and ischemia of the anastomosis (one). Late complications included five patients with small bowel obstruction, two of whom required operation. Anastomotic recurrences developed in 5.9% of patients. Our experience with stapling instruments has shown them to be a reliable method for performing anastomoses in the colon in a safe and expeditious manner. Complications after functional end-to-end anastomoses reported by other authors are depicted in ▶ Table 22.1.

A variety of commercial instruments are available for the construction of stapled anastomoses (▶ Fig. 22.14).

When a hand-sutured anastomosis is elected, the bowel edges are transected obliquely to ensure adequate blood supply at the bowel edges to be anastomosed. Today most surgeons prefer end-to-end anastomoses. Even where there is a disparity in size of the bowel lumina, as occurs in anastomoses of the ileum to the transverse colon, the discrepancy can be readily overcome by division of the antimesenteric border of the ileum. Considerable controversy has been engendered about whether to use a one-layer or a two-layer anastomosis and the type of suture material to be used. The two-layer technique, which has been used successfully in the past, consists of a posterior row of 4–0 silk or polyglactin (Vicryl, Ethicon) placed on a fine atraumatic needle into the seromuscular layer. An inner layer of 4–0 chromic catgut or polyglactin is placed through the full thickness of the bowel wall, begun on one edge, and continued on the posterior wall in a simple running over-and-over suture but with a change to the Connell suture on the anterior half. The anterior seromuscular layer is then completed with 4–0 silk, polyester, or polyglactin sutures (▶ Fig. 22.15).

A growing number of surgeons have favored a single-layer inverting interrupted technique. A posterior interrupted single layer of a 3–0 or 4–0 absorbable suture has been used. The suture is then continued on the anterior wall (▶ Fig. 22.16). Care must be taken not to invert excessive amounts of tissue, thereby causing narrowing of the lumen, but this is true for any

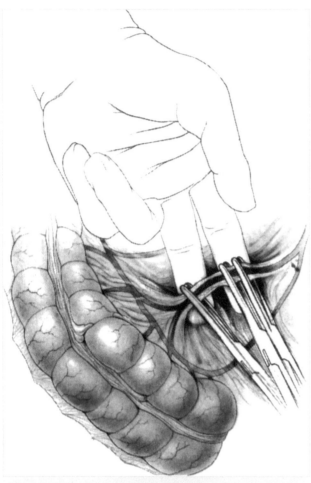

Fig. 22.11 Ligation and division of vessels.

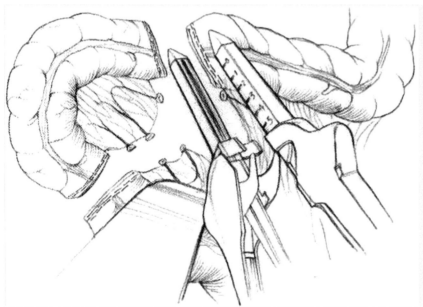

Fig. 22.12 Application of stapler to divide the bowel.

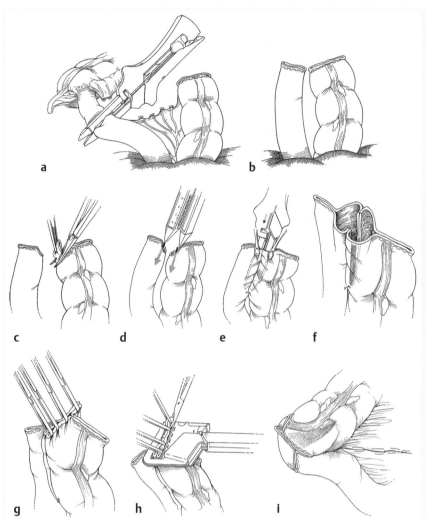

Fig. 22.13 (a) After complete bowel mobilization, the segment of bowel to be resected is transected with the anastomosing stapling instrument. Mesenteric edges are approximated. **(b)** Alignment of proximal and distal resected ends with closure of the mesentery completed. **(c)** Excision of the antimesenteric corner to accommodate the anastomosing stapler. **(d)** Insertion of each limb of the instrument into the bowel ends to be anastomosed. **(e)** With the bowel ends snugly fitted to the neck of the stapler to provide maximum length of anastomosis, the instrument is activated and the anastomosis is accomplished. Suture is placed through antimesenteric border of bowel just beyond the bowel anastomosis. **(f)** Staple line is carefully inspected for proper completion and possible bleeding from the line. **(g)** Approximation of the bowel edges is performed so that the previous staple lines are staggered and the side-to-side anastomosis created is in the open shape of a V. Application of Allis clamps to include the full thickness of the bowel wall and the complete circumference of the bowel. **(h)** Application of the linear stapler with excision of excess tissue. Alternatively, bowel opening can be closed with the anastomosing instrument. **(i)** Completed anastomosis with the staple lines clearly demonstrated.

Table 22.1 Complications after functional end-to-end anastomosis

Author(s)	No. of cases	Bleeding (%)	Fistula or leak (%)	Intraperitoneal abscess (%)	Obstruction or stenosis (%)	Operative mortality (%)
Chassin et al[21]	181	0	1.1	1.7	1.1	0.7
Fortin et al[22]	118	0	5.0	0	0.8	2.5
Brodman and Brodman[23]	88	0	0	2.3	a	0
Reuter[24]	69	0	9.0	a	a	2.9
Scher et al[25]	35		2.9	a		8.6
Steichen and Ravitch[26]	264	0.4	3.4	a	0.8	
Tuchmann et al[27]	51	2.0	6.0	a	a	0.4
Kyzer and Gordon[20]	223	2.2	0.9	0.4	0	1.5
Kracht et al[28]	106	a	2.8	1.9	a	1.9

aNot addressed.

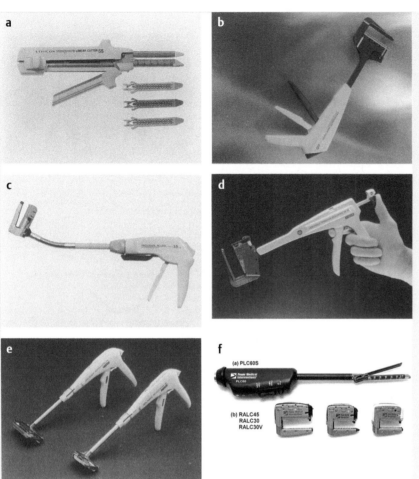

Fig. 22.14 Surgical staplers. **(a)** Proximate reusable 60-mm linear cutter (Ethicon Endosurgery, Inc). **(b)** Proximate right-angle linear stapler 45, 30, and 30 mm vascular (Ethicon Endosurgery Inc). **(c)** Flexible proximate access stapler (Ethicon Endosurgery Inc). **(d)** TA Stapler (Medtronic). **(e)** Roticulator (Covidien). **(f)** Computer-powered linear surgical stapling products (Power Medical Interventions).

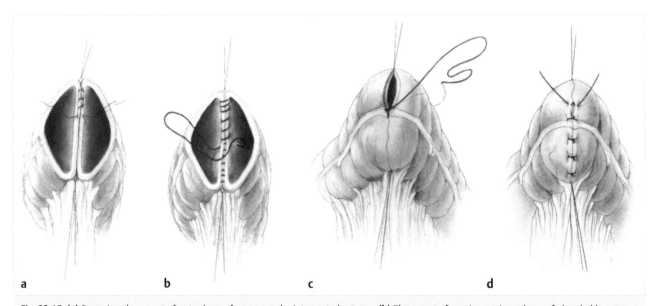

Fig. 22.15 (a) Posterior placement of outer layer of seromuscular interrupted sutures. **(b)** Placement of continuous inner layer of absorbable sutures. **(c)** Continuation of inner layer of sutures anteriorly. **(d)** Completion of anastomosis by anterior placement of layer of interrupted seromuscular sutures.

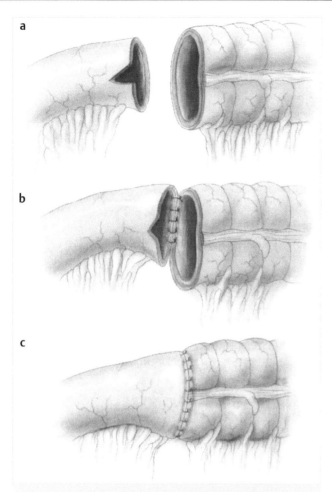

Fig. 22.16 **(a)** When disparity in bowel ends exists, smaller end may be fishmouthed. Alignment of bowel ends for anastomosis. **(b)** Placement of single layer of interrupted sutures in a posterior row. **(c)** Completed anastomosis by placement of anterior row of interrupted sutures.

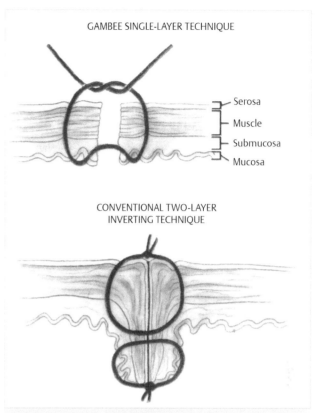

Fig. 22.17 Placement of the Gambee suture is begun with the full-thickness bowel and continued with the mucosa and submucosa on the same side. Suturing is continued on the opposite side with the submucosa and mucosa and then the full-thickness wall. Inverted anastomosis is thus created.

type of hand-sutured anastomosis. Some surgeons prefer to use a Gambee suture for the single-layer anastomosis (▶ Fig. 22.17). Other suture materials such as polypropylene have been used.

Saline irrigation of the abdominal cavity is performed to remove blood, bacteria, and debris. Drains are not necessary. Wounds are closed with continuous absorbable sutures for the fascia, with staples or subcuticular continuous absorbable material used for the skin.

Resection of Transverse Colon

The appropriate operation for a carcinoma of the transverse colon has been a controversial matter. The reason is the desire to fulfill the criteria for resection of the regional lymphatic drainage. Depending on portion of the transverse colon that is involved, drainage may occur through the middle and/or right colic branches and possibly the left colic branches. For a lesion that is located in the midtransverse colon, a transverse colectomy would be in order.

The procedure might begin with division of the greater omentum from the greater curvature of the stomach, either above or below the gastroepiploic arterial arcade, with care taken not to

injure the wall of the stomach (▶ Fig. 22.18). In the event of a very redundant transverse colon, the omentum may be divided vertically on either side at the proposed proximal and distal lines of resection of the colon. For a short transverse colon, the entire omentum may be included in the resected specimen. To avoid tension on the anastomosis, either one or both of the hepatic and splenic flexures will require mobilization. It is often technically easier to resect the right and transverse colon rather than attempt to mobilize both flexures. The technique of mobilization of the hepatic flexure has been described in the discussion of right hemicolectomy.

Mobilization of the splenic flexure is facilitated by incising the lateral peritoneal attachment along the descending colon (▶ Fig. 22.19). As the splenic flexure is approached, great care must be exercised to avoid injury to the spleen. The lienocolic ligament can be accentuated by passage of a finger along the colonic wall from the descending colon side toward the splenic flexure. The ligament then can be clamped and divided, or, alternatively, it can be divided with the use of cautery or other energy sources. Great caution should be exercised in this maneuver since there are frequently numerous adhesions to the splenic capsule. The peritoneum is incised on the mesocolon, and in the process the splenic flexure is mobilized downward and to the right, exposing the retroperitoneum. If the greater omentum becomes a limiting factor, division of the omentum is begun. Varying other posterior attachments

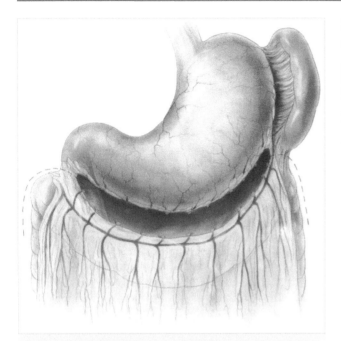

Fig. 22.18 Division of the greater omentum from the greater curvature of the stomach.

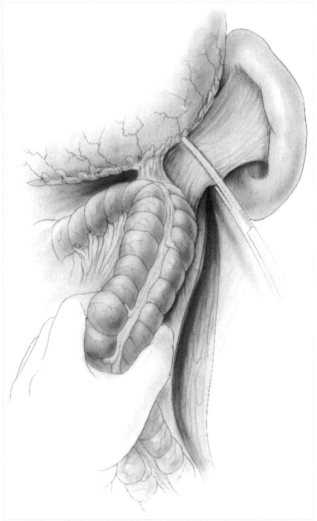

Fig. 22.19 Mobilization of the splenic flexure by division of the lienocolic ligament.

may require division, with care taken not to incite bleeding in this location. The trunk of the middle colic vessel and smaller vessels are secured (▶ Fig. 22.20). It should be noted that the origin of the middle colic vessels is quite proximal on the superior mesenteric vessels and must be pursued with extreme caution to prevent injury to these structures. The bowel is divided and an anastomosis is created as previously described. In reconstituting the mesenteric defect between the ileum and the descending colon, care must be exercised to avoid narrowing of the duodenojejunal junction.

For lesions at or near the hepatic flexure or the ascending colon, a right hemicolectomy is performed. For lesions near the splenic flexure, a partial left colectomy with anastomosis of the transverse colon to the proximal sigmoid is performed (▶ Fig. 22.21). Resection of this type may necessitate division of the left branch of the middle colic and left colic vessels.

Resection of Descending Colon

For lesions of the descending colon, the left branch of the middle colic artery remains intact, but the left colic artery and, depending on the level of the lesion, the first sigmoidal vessels are ligated. The anastomosis is performed between the distal transverse and proximal sigmoid colon. Some surgeons advocate a more formal left hemicolectomy.

Sigmoid Resection

Some controversy exists as to the most appropriate procedure for removal of a sigmoid carcinoma. One school of thought supports the necessity for a radical left hemicolectomy with anastomosis of the transverse colon to the rectum. However, there are a growing number of surgeons who realize that the extended resection has not resulted in increased survival rates. When patients who have lymphatics involved to the root of the

inferior mesenteric artery have these resected, no increased survival rate is noted in comparison with patients who have a less radical procedure.[7] It would, therefore, seem that the extra mobilization, with its potential risks and prolonged operating time, is not justified. The extent of the resection depends on the portion of the sigmoid colon involved. Lesions of the proximal sigmoid would require an anastomosis performed between the descending colon and the distal sigmoid, those of the distal sigmoid would involve an anastomosis between the proximal sigmoid and the upper rectum, and those of the midportion of the sigmoid, depending on the redundancy of the colon, would require an anastomosis between the sigmoid-descending junction and the rectosigmoid. The splenic flexure is not routinely mobilized, but, depending on the location of the lesion and the redundancy of the colon, it may require mobilization to avoid tension on the anastomosis.

The patient may be placed in the supine position, but for more distal lesions it is preferable to have the patient in the modified lithotomy position so that simultaneous access can be obtained through the abdomen and the rectum. This access is

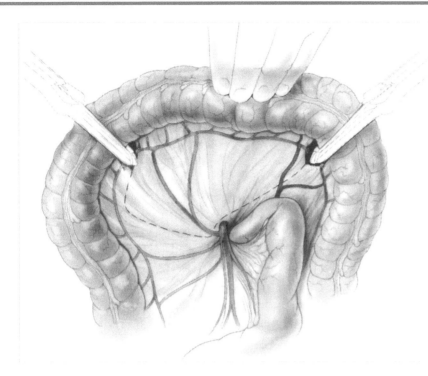

Fig. 22.20 Ligation and division of the middle colic and adjacent smaller vessels.

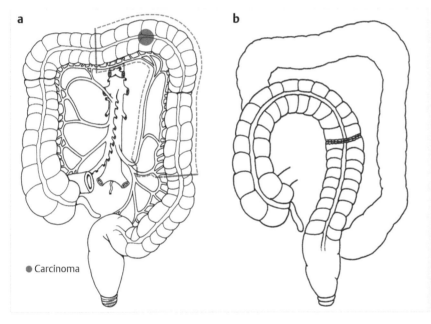

a

b

● Carcinoma

Fig. 22.21 **(a)** Extent of resection for carcinoma near the splenic flexure. **(b)** Result after resection.

necessary to allow use of the circular stapling device or inspection of the anastomosis by proctosigmoidoscopy.

The procedure is initiated by incising the peritoneum along the white line of Toldt in the left paracolic gutter, freeing the distal descending colon and the sigmoid from their developmental attachments from the splenic flexure to the pelvic brim (▶ Fig. 22.22). In the midportion of the sigmoid mesocolon is the intersigmoid fossa, a small depression in the peritoneum that acts as a guide to the underlying ureter (▶ Fig. 22.23). As the sigmoid mesentery is further mobilized, care is taken to displace the mesosigmoid from the left ureter, which is seen coursing over the iliac vessels (▶ Fig. 22.24). The gonadal vessels should be protected in a similar way because injury will result in troublesome bleeding. After lateral mobilization and determination of the

proximal line of resection, the peritoneum over the medial aspect of the mesosigmoid is incised toward the root of the inferior mesenteric artery to the level of the proposed ligation and then downward toward the pelvis. The inferior mesenteric artery, with its left colic and sigmoidal branches, will be identified (▶ Fig. 22.25). The inferior mesenteric artery distal to the left colic branch is then divided and ligated. Smaller vessels leading toward the planned lines of resection are secured, and the bowel is transected proximally and distally. As with the technique for right hemicolectomy, some surgeons advocate ligation and division of the blood supply prior to any other manipulation, but the same general principles pertain. In such a situation, depending on the extent of resection, the inferior mesenteric artery at its origin from the aorta (or distal to the left colic branch) and the inferior mesenteric vein at the level of the duodenum (or more distally for a lesser resection) require ligation and division.[21,22,23, 24,25,26,27,28,29] Abcarian and Pearl[30] have described a simple technique for high ligation of the inferior mesenteric artery and vein. After completion of abdominal exploration, the small bowel is packed away toward the right side of the abdominal cavity to expose the duodenojejunal flexure. The peritoneum overlying the lateral border of the fourth portion of the duodenum is incised,

exposing the inferior mesenteric vein. The vein is mobilized for 2 to 3 cm, ligated in continuity with nonabsorbable suture, and divided. This incision is extended diagonally 5 to 6 cm medially to expose the infrarenal aorta proximal to its bifurcation. The inferior mesenteric artery is easily identified, ligated in continuity, and divided at its origin. The lymph nodes surrounding the takeoff of the inferior mesenteric artery are dissected sharply in a proximal-to-distal manner to allow for their complete excision (▶ Fig. 22.26). Heald[31] recommends division of the inferior mesenteric artery approximately 2 cm from the aorta to preserve the autonomic nerves, which split around its origin.

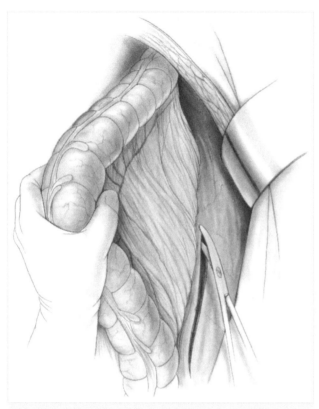

Fig. 22.22 Incision of peritoneum along the white line of Toldt.

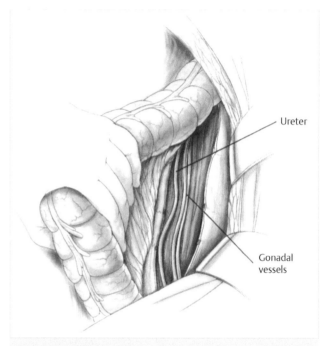

Fig. 22.24 Mobilization of the sigmoid colon with care taken not to injure retroperitoneal structures.

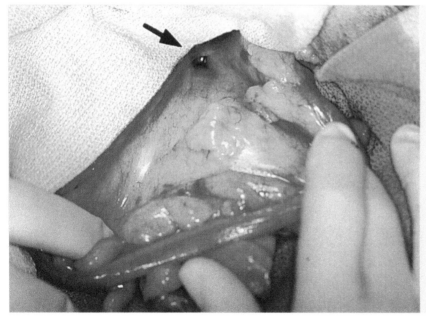

Fig. 22.23 Intersigmoid fossa.

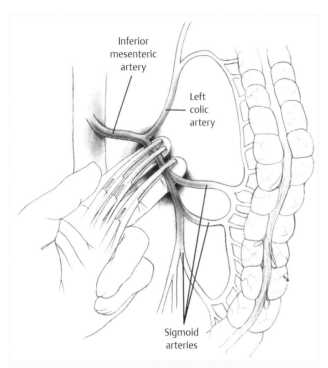

Fig. 22.25 Identification of the inferior mesenteric artery and its left colic and sigmoidal branches.

The anastomosis is then created according to the surgeon's method of choice. However, if the anastomosis is low, the authors' preference is to use the circular stapler as described in detail in this chapter. For surgeons who deem it necessary to perform a radical left hemicolectomy, the operation is conducted in a similar way by combining the mobilization of the sigmoid, the splenic flexure, and the distal transverse colon. The notable difference is the level at which the vessels are secured. To accomplish the radical left hemicolectomy, the posterior parietal peritoneum is incised to expose the inferior mesenteric vessels. The artery is tied flush with the aorta, and the vein is ligated separately at the level of the duodenum (▶ Fig. 22.27).

During the last several years, a variety of individuals including Hohenberger, West, and Quirke have touted the advantages of complete mesocolic excision for the attempted curative treatment of colorectal carcinoma.[32,33,34] While numerous studies have found the technique to confer oncologic benefit, other publications have failed to identify such benefits. Part of the problem may be a confusion between the terms "complete mesocolic excision" and "central venous ligation." Bertelson et al,[35] representing the Dutch Colorectal Cancer Group, were able to echo the results of Hohenberger, West, and Quirke by assessing over 1,000 patients who underwent standard traditional surgery as compared to 364 patients who underwent complete mesocolic excision (CME). The authors identified significant differences in the numbers of lymph nodes retrieved at 10 versus 36, respectively, and also found that 12 nodes were harvested in 89% versus 99%, respectively. Very important was the four-year disease-free survival of 75.9% versus 85.8%, respectively. Other similar differences were identified between the two groups of patients in favor of complete mesocolic excision. Although it is important to perform

complete mesocolic excision, the performance of central venous ligation is more contentious and potentially introduces additional morbidity.

Bilateral Salpingo-Oophorectomy

In a review of their experience and the surgical literature, Birnkrant et al[36] found the incidence of ovarian metastasis from colorectal carcinoma to be approximately 6% with a range of 1.5 to 13.6%. In a prospective controlled study, Graffner et al[37] detected ovarian metastases in 10.3% of patients undergoing operations on all segments of the large bowel. Since bilateral involvement occurs between 50 and 70% of the time, a bilateral oophorectomy is recommended, especially for postmenopausal women.

However, controversy exists about the role of prophylactic oophorectomy during resection of primary colorectal carcinoma. Sielezneff et al[38] attempted to prospectively assess the prognostic impact of simultaneous bilateral oophorectomy in postmenopausal women undergoing curative resection for colorectal carcinoma. Ovarian metastases were detected in 2.4% of the operative specimens. Local recurrence or liver metastases rates were not affected by oophorectomy. Five-year actuarial survival rates were not significantly different whether patients had oophorectomy (81.6%) or not (87.9%). Their results suggested that microscopic synchronous ovarian metastasis is rare at the time of curative resection of a colorectal carcinoma in postmenopausal women and does not modify prognosis. Young-Fadok et al[39] conducted a prospective randomized trial of 152 patients to evaluate the influence of oophorectomy on recurrence and survival in patients with Dukes' B and C stage colorectal carcinomas. In 76 patients randomized to oophorectomy, no incidence of gross or microscopic metastatic disease to the ovary was found. Preliminary survival curves suggest a survival benefit for oophorectomy of 2 to 3 years after operation, but this benefit does not appear to persist at 5 years (▶ Fig. 22.28). There has been no incidence of colorectal carcinoma metastatic to the ovaries in this series of Dukes' B and C stage carcinomas, unlike other nonrandomized studies of all stages, which have reported a 4 to 10% incidence. These authors concluded that the possibility of a survival advantage emphasizes the need to continue this preliminary work.

Concomitant oophorectomy is controversial, and its efficacy in prolonging survival has been questioned since few patients survive 5 years after operation. However, it generally adds little to the operation and will prevent the subsequent development of ovarian carcinoma.[40] Removal of the ovaries at the time of bowel resection will eliminate the need for repeat laparotomy to resect an ovarian mass in approximately 2% of women with large bowel carcinoma.[36] Oophorectomy is often recommended more strongly for patients who have carcinoma of the rectum, but no site in the colon results in a greater proportion of ovarian metastases. The apparent greater proportion from the left colon is probably due to the fact that this portion of the large bowel harbors the largest number of malignancies.

Oophorectomy should be performed in premenopausal women if any gross abnormality of the ovary is detected.[36] Indeed, ovarian metastases of colorectal origin have been reported to occur more commonly in premenopausal women, with rates ranging from 3.8 to 28%.[36,41] This finding might

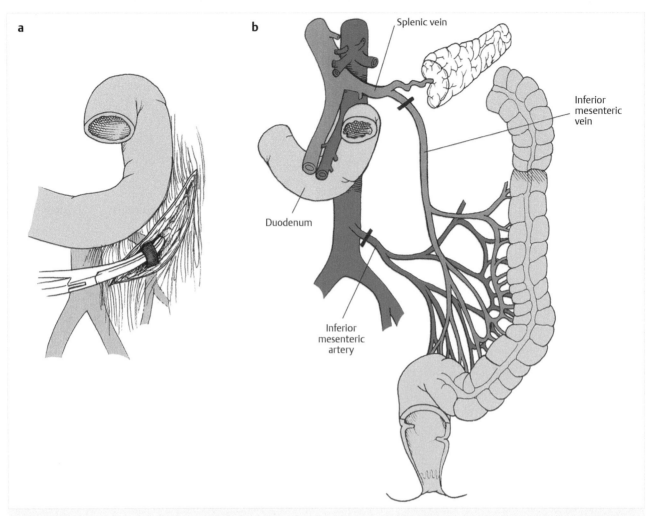

Fig. 22.26 **(a)** High ligation of the inferior mesenteric vein lateral to the fourth portion of the duodenum through a paraduodenal peritoneal incision. **(b)** High ligation of the inferior mesenteric artery at its origin through a diagonal extension of the paraduodenal incision medially to expose the infrarenal aorta.

support the recommendation for prophylactic oophorectomy regardless of patient age.[42] Certainly, contiguous involvement necessitates en bloc resection. Ovarian involvement carries with it a poor prognosis.[43]

22.2.5 Postoperative Care

The postoperative care of the patient is discussed in Chapter 5. It should be noted that it is not necessary to use nasogastric suctioning on a routine basis.

22.3 Adjuvant Therapy

With the advent of new drug combinations, adjuvant chemotherapy has improved survival for colon cancer. Five general principles underlie adjuvant therapy[44]:

1. There may be occult, viable malignant cells in circulation (intravascular, intralymphatic, or intraperitoneal) and/or established, microscopic foci of malignant cells locally, at distant sites, or both.

2. Therapy is most effective when the burden of malignancy is minimal and cell kinetics are optimal.
3. Agents with reported effectiveness against the carcinoma are available.
4. Cytotoxic therapy shows a dose–response relationship and therefore must be administered in maximally tolerated doses, and the duration of therapy must be sufficient to eradicate all malignant cells.
5. The risk-to-benefit ratio for therapy must be favorable to individuals who may remain asymptomatic for their natural life expectancy after resection of their malignancy.

22.3.1 Radiotherapy

Although radiotherapy has been used extensively in various settings for the treatment of rectal carcinoma, it plays a limited role with colon cancer.[45] Exceptions relate to the presence of a carcinoma in a portion of the colorectum fixed to the retroperitoneum (cecum, ascending colon, and descending colon) or pelvis (rectosigmoid or rectum). Indications that have been considered appropriate for postoperative radiotherapy include

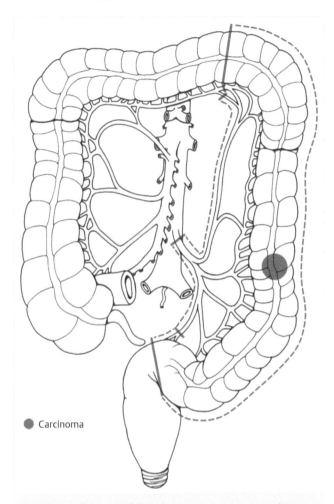

Fig. 22.27 High ligation of the inferior mesenteric artery and vein.

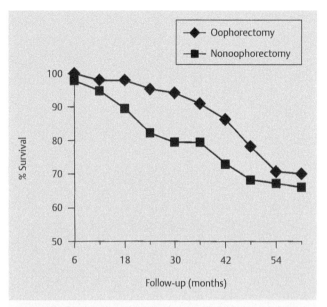

Fig. 22.28 Survival curves for prophylactic oophorectomy during resection for primary colorectal carcinoma.[39] (Reproduced with permission from Wolters Kluwer.)

the following: (1) involvement of lymph nodes; (2) known inadequate margins of resection; (3) adherence to the retroperitoneum, sacrum, or pelvic side walls; (4) transmural penetration to a macroscopic degree; and (5) extensive microscopic penetration with the presence of positive lymph nodes.[46]

A few retrospective, single institution studies have shown that adjuvant radiotherapy improves local control for colon cancer patients at high risk of recurrence after surgery.[47,48,49,50,51,52] Unfortunately, the single randomized prospective trial comparing chemotherapy alone with combined chemotherapy and radiotherapy lacks sufficient power to draw valid conclusions.[53] Current National Comprehensive Cancer Network (NCCN) guidelines recommend that radiotherapy for colon cancer be considered in patients with T4 tumors with penetration to a fixed structure.[54] The radiation field should include the tumor bed as defined by preoperative imaging and the placement of surgical clips at the time of operation. A dose of 45 to 50 Gy in 25 to 28 fractions is recommended and should be delivered with concomitant 5-fluorouracil (5-FU) chemotherapy. Thus, the colorectal surgeon should always be ready to place clips in and around the tumor bed during operations involving the resection of a fixed T4 colon tumor in order to help direct postoperative radiotherapy. Neoadjuvant chemoradiotherapy can be considered for select patients with bulky tumors invading other structures.

22.3.2 Chemotherapy

The use of adjuvant chemotherapy is attractive because it may offer the possibility of identifying patients who are likely to have occult, residual, or disseminated disease at the time of operation. Chemotherapy is most effective when the burden of carcinoma is smallest and the fraction of malignant cells in growth phase is the highest.[55] Currently adjuvant chemotherapy is playing an increasingly important role.[45] For patients with stage III colon cancer, adjuvant chemotherapy has been recommended since 1990.[56] More recently, the National Quality Forum has endorsed metrics related to the administration of chemotherapy in stage III colon cancer patients in order to ensure that patients with stage III colon cancer not only are considered for chemotherapy, but also are given chemotherapy in a timely fashion.[57] For patients with stage I colon cancer, surgery alone is highly successful, and thus no adjuvant therapy is currently recommended. On the other hand, selected patients with stage II colon cancer may benefit from adjuvant treatment and this remains the focus of clinical trials. Finally, stage IV colon cancer patients are usually primarily treated with chemotherapy.

Adjuvant chemotherapy is recommended for all stage III colon cancer patients because it decreases recurrence and increases survival when compared to surgery alone.[58,59] After surgery alone for stage III colon cancer, overall 5-year survival is 40 to 60%.[60,61,62,63,64,65] Current chemotherapeutic regimens improve overall survival to 70 to 80%.[66] Thus, 5-year overall survival of stage III colon cancer patients improves by an absolute 20 to 25% with adjuvant chemotherapy. ▶ Table 22.2 summarizes the results of key clinical trials establishing the efficacy of adjuvant chemotherapy for nonmetastatic colon cancer.[66,67,68,69,70,71] If all patients with stage III colon cancer receive adjuvant chemotherapy, roughly one-third to one-half of disease recurrences would be prevented.

Table 22.2 Key clinical trials establishing the efficacy of adjuvant chemotherapy for colon cancer

Trial	Tumor stage	Comparison	Results	Conclusion
INT 0035 (1990)	Stage III	Surgery alone vs. 5-FU/levamisole	3-y survival 5-FU/levamisole 71% Surgery alone 55%	Post-op adjuvant chemo improves survival for stage III colon cancer
IMPACT 1995[67]	Stage III	Surgery alone vs. 5-FU/leucovorin	3-y survival 5-FU/leucovorin 71% Surgery alone 62%	Post-op adjuvant chemo improves survival for stage III colon cancer
QUASAR 2000[68]	Stage III	5-FU/levamisole vs. 5-FU/folinic acid vs. 5-FU/placebo	Decreased survival and increased recurrence with levamisole compared with placebo	Post-op adjuvant chemo with levamisole inferior to placebo
IMPACT 1999[69]	Stage II	Surgery alone vs. 5-FU/leucovorin	5-y survival = no difference 5-FU/leucovorin 82% Surgery alone 80%	Post-op adjuvant chemo does not improve survival for stage II colon cancer
NSABP (CO-1, CO-2, CO-3, and CO-4) 1999	Stage II	Surgery alone vs. 5-FU + leucovorin and/or levamisole	5-y survival improved with adjuvant treatment 30% mortality reduction with adjuvant treatment	Post-op adjuvant chemo improves survival for stage II colon cancer
MOSAIC 2009[66]	Stages II and III	FOLFOX vs. 5-FU/leucovorin	6-y survival in stage III only FOLFOX 73% 5-FU/leucovorin 68%	FOLFOX superior to 5-FU/LV for stage III colon cancer
XELOXA 2011	Stage III	XELOX vs. 5-FU/leucovorin	3-y disease-free survival XELOX 71% 5-FU/leucovorin 67%	Capecitabine plus oxaliplatin superior to 5-FU/leucovorin

Abbreviation: 5-FU, 5-fluorouracil.

Table 22.3 Current recommended adjuvant chemotherapy regimens for stage III colon cancer

Regimen	Agents and dosage	Frequency
mFOLFOX6	Oxaliplatin 85 mg/m² IV over 2 h, day 1	Every 2 wk
	Leucovorin 400 mg/m² IV over 2 h, day 1	
	5-FU 400 mg/m² IV bolus on day 1, then 1,200 mg/m²/d × 2 d IV continuous infusion	
CapeOx	Oxaliplatin 130 mg/m² IV over 2 h, day 1	Every 3 wk
	Capecitabine 850–1,000 mg/m² oral twice daily for 14 d	

Abbreviations: IV, intravenous; 5-FU, 5-fluorouracil.

Given the significant survival benefit of adjuvant chemotherapy, colon and rectal surgeons need to ensure that their stage III colon cancer patients are evaluated for chemotherapy after surgery. The National Quality Forum has endorsed two metrics regarding the treatment of stage III colon cancer patients.[57] The first metric estimates how many stage III patients are referred or treated with chemotherapy, whereas the second metric looks at the timeliness of the administration of chemotherapy. Specifically, the first metric (measure 0385) determines the percentage of patients ≥ 18 years old who are either referred for adjuvant chemotherapy, prescribed adjuvant chemotherapy, or have previously received adjuvant chemotherapy in the last 12 months. The other metric (measure 0223) determines the percentage of patients younger than 80 years for whom adjuvant chemotherapy is considered or administered within 4 months of the diagnosis. Thus, it is important for colon and rectal surgeons to promptly refer all stage III colon cancer patients for adjuvant chemotherapy.

For patients with stage III colon cancer, the NCCN guidelines recommend adjuvant treatment with folinic acid, fluorouracil and oxaliplatin (FOLFOX) or CapeOx for 6 months.[54] FOLFOX has been found to be superior to 5-FU/leucovorin (LV),[66,72] and CapeOx is superior to bolus 5-FU/LV.[72,73,74] While used frequently in patients with metastatic disease, biologic therapy with antibodies directed at vascular endothelial growth factor A (VEGF-A; bevacizumab) and epidermal growth factor receptor (EGFR) antibody (panitumumab, cetuximab) is not recommended for adjuvant therapy of stage III disease.[75,76,77,78] The current FOLFOX regimen, mFOLFOX6, and the CapeOx regimen are outlined in ▶ Table 22.3. These agents act in different ways on colon cancer cells. 5-Fluorouracil is a pyrimidine analog that incorporates into deoxyribonucleic acid (DNA) to stop DNA synthesis. Capecitabine is an oral 5-FU prolog and thus works in the same way as 5-FU. Folinic acid (LV) is a vitamin B derivative that increases the cytotoxicity of 5-FU. Oxaliplatin inhibits DNA synthesis by forming inter- and intrastrand cross-links in DNA preventing replication and transcription. Using FOLFOX, the survival benefit of adding oxaliplatin to 5-FU does come at a price, the added side effect of peripheral sensory neuropathy (PSN). While 40 to 50% of patients given oxaliplatin will develop PSN, only 10 to 20% of patients will have grade 3 PSN, which is defined as severe symptoms limiting activities of daily living.[79] Fortunately, only 1% of patients will have grade 3 PSN at 12 months after treatment.[66] Since the benefit of the addition of oxaliplatin to 5-FU/LV is unproven in patients over the age of 70 years, capecitabine alone or 5-FU/LV should be considered in elderly patients with stage III colon cancer.[54] Capecitabine-based regimens can be particularly complicated by palmar–plantar erythrodyskinesia (hand–foot syndrome), but this side effect can be limited by symptomatic treatment and resolves after treatment is concluded.[80]

The 5-year overall survival of patients with stage II colon cancer is 65 to 85% with surgery alone.[81] Unlike stage III disease, the role of adjuvant chemotherapy in stage II disease remains controversial, with some studies showing a benefit[70] and others showing no benefit.[82] If there is a benefit to adjuvant chemotherapy in stage II colon cancer patients, the benefit does not improve survival by more than 5% unlike the 25 to 30% improvement for stage III patients receiving adjuvant chemotherapy.[54]

Following surgery for stage II colon cancer, the current NCCN guidelines (February 2015) recommend observation (surgery alone), enrollment in a clinical trial, or adjuvant chemotherapy.[54] To sort out these options, a detailed discussion with the patient is recommended to highlight the potential benefits and risks of chemotherapy. Any high-risk features should be identified and discussed (▶ Table 22.4). Patients with or without high-risk features should consider observation, clinical trial, or chemotherapy with capecitabine or 5-FU/LV. Only those patients with high-risk features should be considered candidates for FOLFOX or CapeOx. It is important to remember that the addition of oxaliplatin has not been shown to improve survival in stage II colon cancer patients.[66] Finally, decision making regarding the use of adjuvant chemotherapy for stage II disease may be aided by performing genetic testing of the tumor after surgical resection. Genetic testing of stage II tumors has been shown to be independently predictive of prognosis. High microsatellite instability (MSI-H) or defective mismatch repair (dMMR) status has been shown to be associated with a lower recurrence rate (11 vs. 26%) after surgical resection alone.[83] In addition, MSI-H tumors do not benefit from 5-FU adjuvant therapy.[75] Thus, MSI/MMR testing is recommended in all patients with stage II disease in order to avoid giving adjuvant chemotherapy in patients who will derive no benefit from it. In addition to MSI/MMR testing, multigene colon cancer assays such as Oncotype Dx, ColoPrint, and ColDx are now available that can also predict prognosis and risk of recurrence. All three of these multigene assays predict recurrence independent from other factors such as TNM stage, MMR status, tumor grade, and nodes.[84,85,86,87,88,89,90] While these assays provide additional information regarding prognosis and recurrence risk, they are not predictive of the potential benefit of chemotherapy, and consequently are, to date, of limited clinical value.

Table 22.4 High-risk factors for recurrence

Poorly differentiated histology (exclusive of those that are MSI-H)

Lymphatic/vascular invasion

Perineural invasion

Close, indeterminate, or positive margins

Bowel obstruction

Localized perforation

Less than 12 lymph nodes examined

Abbreviation: MSI-H, high microsatellite instability.

Bevacizumab (Avastin; Genentech Inc., South San Francisco, CA) is a recombinant humanized anti-VEGF monoclonal antibody that inhibits neoplastic angiogenesis, and has demonstrated survival benefit in patients with previously untreated metastatic colorectal carcinoma when combined with irinotecan/fluorouracil/LV (IFL). Kabbinavar et al[91] combined analysis of data from three randomized clinical studies evaluating bevacizumab in combination with FU/LV alone. The median duration of survival was 17.9 months in 5-FU/LV bevacizumab group compared with 14.6 months in the combined control group, corresponding to a hazard ratio for death of 0.74. The median duration of progression-free survival was 8.8 months in the FU/LV bevacizumab group, compared with 5.6 months in the combined control group, corresponding to a hazard ratio for disease progression of 0.63. The addition of bevacizumab also improved the response rate (34.1 vs. 24.5%).

In a phase III trial, combining bevacizumab with irinotecan, bolus fluorouracil, and LV (IFL) increased survival compared with IFL alone in first-line treatment of patients with metastatic colorectal carcinoma. Hurwitz et al[92] described the efficacy and safety results of the patient cohort who received bevacizumab combined with fluorouracil LV and compared them with results of concurrently enrolled patients who received IFL. Median overall survivals were 18.3 and 15.1 months with fluorouracil LV bevacizumab ($n = 110$) and IFL/placebo ($n = 100$), respectively. Median progression-free survivals were 8.8 and 6.8 months, respectively. Overall response rates were 40 and 37% and median response durations were 8.5 and 7.2 months, respectively. Adverse events consistent with those expected from the fluorouracil LV or IFL-based regimens were seen, as were modest increases in hypertension and bleeding in the bevacizumab arm, which were generally easily managed. They concluded the fluorouracil LV bevacizumab regimen seems as effective as IFL and has an acceptable safety profile. They further concluded that fluorouracil LV bevacizumab is an active alternative treatment regimen for patients with previously untreated metastatic colorectal carcinoma.

While significant progress has been made in defining optimal cytotoxic regimens in the adjuvant treatment of colorectal cancer, several questions remain regarding the optimal duration of chemotherapy treatment, the role of radiotherapy in rectal cancer, the possibility of nonsurgical interventions for rectal cancer, and the emerging role of immunotherapy.

Prior studies have shown no benefit from extending adjuvant therapy beyond 6 months in patients with stage III colon cancer.[93] However, a shorter duration of chemotherapy has not been adequately investigated. CALGB 80702 is currently investigating 6 cycles (3 months) versus 12 cycles (6 months) of FOLFOX chemotherapy in patients with completely resected stage III colon cancer (NCT01150045). This will be one of six ongoing clinical trials evaluating 3 versus 6 months of adjuvant oxaliplatin-based chemotherapy. A meta-analysis of these studies (International Duration Evaluation in Adjuvant Chemotherapy [IDEA] collaboration) will test the noninferiority of a 3-month strategy to a 6-month strategy. In addition to the investigation of the duration of adjuvant treatment in colon cancer, efforts are ongoing to define the role of cyclooxygenase (COX) inhibition on disease recurrence. Analysis of the Nurses' Health Study (NHS) and Health Professional Follow-Up Study (HPFS) has shown a decreased recurrence rate in patients with a diagnosis of colon cancer with regular aspirin intake.[94] The benefit appeared to be limited to patients with COX-2 overexpressing tumors.[95]

These analyses were limited by their retrospective nature and require further support from prospectively conducted trials. CALGB 80702 randomizes all enrolled subjects to celecoxib versus placebo in order to investigate the role of COX-2 inhibition in the adjuvant treatment of colon cancer. Similarly, the A SCOLT clinical trial (NCT00565708) is randomizing patients with stage II or III disease to 3 years of aspirin versus placebo to address the role of aspirin in preventing colorectal cancer recurrence. Finally, several studies are investigating immunotherapy as an adjuvant form of treatment in colon cancer. An ongoing phase III clinical trial is evaluating the role of cytokine-induced killer cell immunotherapy for stage III colon cancer following surgery and completion of adjuvant therapy (NCT02280278).

22.3.3 Immunotherapy

Immunotherapy was believed to have some effect on colon carcinoma, but there is no conclusive evidence to indicate significant improvement in survival.[96] A review of prospective randomized trials by Lise et al,[97] which included an immunotherapy arm, failed to demonstrate any benefit. A report of a controlled randomized trial consisting of a 2-year program of vaccination with bacille Calmette-Guérin (BCG) and neuraminidase-treated autologous carcinoma cells at 5-year follow-up failed to alter either the disease-free interval or the survival of patients.[98] A controlled clinical trial of interferon-a as postoperative surgical adjuvant therapy for patients with colon carcinoma demonstrated significant enhancement of nonspecific immune function but no significant difference in patient survival.[99] A study in which 189 patients with Dukes' C colorectal carcinoma who underwent resection for cure were randomized to observation or postoperative treatment with 17-1A antibody. After a median follow-up of 5 years, antibody treatment was reported to have reduced the overall death rate by 30%.[100] In the future, genetic engineering techniques may allow generation of substances during the immune response, and these may have therapeutic value by modifying the biologic response to malignancy.[101]

22.4 Complicated Carcinomas

Previous studies have reported that emergency presentation of colorectal carcinoma is associated with poor outcome. McArdle

and Hole[102] conducted a study aimed to establish, after adjusting for case mix, the magnitude of the differences in postoperative mortality and survival between patients undergoing elective surgery and those presenting as an emergency. Of 3,200 patients who underwent surgery for colorectal carcinoma, 72.4% of 2,214 elective patients had a potentially curative resection compared with 64.1% of 986 patients who presented as an emergency. Following curative resection, the postoperative mortality rate was 2.8% after elective and 8.2% after emergency operation. Overall survival at 5 years was 57.5% after elective and 39.1% after emergency curative operation; carcinoma-specific survival at 5 years was 70.9 and 52.9%, respectively. The adjusted hazard ratio for overall survival after emergency relative to elective surgery was 1.68 and that for carcinoma-specific survival was 1.90.

Jestin et al[103] identified risk factors in emergency surgery for colonic carcinoma in a large population of 3,259 patients; 806 had an emergency and 2,453 an elective procedure. Patients who had emergency surgery had more advanced carcinomas and a lower survival rate than those who had an elective procedure (5-year survival rate 29.8 vs. 52.4%). There was a stage-specific difference in survival with poorer survival both for patients with stage I and II carcinomas and for those with stage III carcinomas after emergency compared with elective surgery. Emergency surgery was associated with a longer hospital stay (mean 18 vs. 10 days) and higher costs (relative cost 1.5) compared with elective surgery. The duration of hospital stay was the strongest determinant of cost.

22.4.1 Obstruction

When complete obstruction of the colon arises as a result of a carcinoma, the recommended treatment depends on the level of the colon that is obstructed as well as the beliefs and experience of the treating surgeon.[104,105] In their review of 115 obstructing carcinomas, Sjödahl et al[106] found that 37% were right sided (proximal to splenic flexure) and 63% were left sided. Only 4% were Dukes' A, while 15% already had distant metastases.

Interestingly, a study by Nozoe et al[107] found the mean size of the obstructing carcinoma was 3.7 cm, which was significantly smaller than that of nonobstructing carcinomas (5.4 cm). The proportion of lymph node metastases in obstructing carcinomas was 66.9%, which was significantly higher than that in nonobstructing carcinomas (42.4%). The proportion of carcinomas classified into Dukes' C or D in obstructing carcinomas was 84.6% and was significantly higher than that in nonobstructing carcinomas (52.5%).

If the patient's condition can be stabilized and there is evidence of resolution of the occlusion, bowel preparation and elective resection is the ideal solution. This clinical course is unusual, and therefore decisions on how to proceed must be made. For right-sided colonic obstructions, it is generally accepted that the treatment of choice is a resection and primary anastomosis with removal of the right and proximal transverse colon.[108] Even though the bowel is not prepared, the resection usually can be readily accomplished.

When the obstruction is located in the distal transverse colon, the matter of how to proceed is controversial. Some surgeons believe that the patient should have a proximal diversion, followed by a definitive resection. However, under these circumstances a growing number of surgeons have adopted the procedure of an extended right hemicolectomy, followed by a primary ileo-descending colon anastomosis.

Lee et al[109] compared the operative results of 243 patients who had emergency operations for right- and left-sided obstructions from primary colorectal carcinomas. One hundred and seven patients had obstruction at or proximal to the splenic flexure (right-sided lesions) and 136 had lesions distal to the splenic flexure (left-sided lesions). The primary resection rate was 91.8%. Of the 223 patients with primary resection, primary anastomosis was possible in 88% of patients. Among the 101 primary anastomosis patients with left-sided obstruction, segmental resection with on-table lavage was performed in 75 patients and subtotal colectomy was performed in 26 patients. The overall operative mortality rate was 9.4%, although that of the patients with primary resection and anastomosis was 8.1%. The anastomotic leakage rate for those with primary resection and anastomosis was 6.1%. There were no differences in the mortality or leakage rates between patients with right- and left-sided lesions (mortality 7.3 vs. 8.9% and leakage 5.3 vs. 6.9%). Colocolonic anastomosis did not show a significant difference in leakage rate when compared with ileocolonic anastomosis (6.1 vs. 6%).

Three-Stage Procedure

For patients with an obstruction of the left colon, greater controversy exists and a larger number of options are available. Traditionally, these patients have undergone a three-stage operation, with the first stage being a transverse colostomy or possibly a cecostomy, followed by resection and anastomosis, and finally by closure of the colostomy.

In a review of the subject, Deans et al[110] reported that between 70 and 80% of patients having a transverse colostomy undergo resection of their carcinoma during the first hospitalization, with a hospital stay of 30 to 55 days. Overall, 25% of patients do not undergo closure of their colostomy because they are unfit or unwilling to undergo an additional operation. Overall mortality rates range from 2 to 15%, mostly in the 10% range, with morbidity rates ranging from 20 to 37%, often related to stoma complications, ranging from 6 to 14%. Although many reports show that the combined mortality rate of the three-stage procedure is similar to that of primary resection with delayed anastomosis, there is the suggestion that long-term survival is decreased in the three-stage operation.[110] Sjödahl et al[106] found a modest increase in 5-year survival rate of 38% for immediate resection compared with a rate of 29% for a staged resection. Although proximal decompression is still promoted as a simple, safe initial option, the cumulative morbidity and mortality rates, survival disadvantage, prolonged hospital stay, and necessity of repeated operations make the three-stage procedure most unfavored.

Hartmann's Procedure

Some surgeons have advocated an immediate resection without anastomosis (i.e., a proximal colostomy and mucous fistula or closed rectal stump, Hartmann's procedure). The perceived advantages include immediate removal of the carcinoma, avoidance of an anastomosis in less-than-ideal circumstances, and more rapid convalescence and shorter hospital stay. In the event it proves to be permanent, a left-sided colostomy is much less of a burden than a transverse colostomy. The overall operative mortality rate has ranged from 6 to 12%, mostly in the 10% range,[111] with hospital stay ranging from 17 to 30 days. Rates of colostomy closure of 60% or more are common. It must be remembered that significant morbidity can be associated with colostomy closure. In their report on 130 stomas and their subsequent closure, Porter et al[111] experienced a complication rate of 44%. Nevertheless, Hartmann's procedure combines primary resection and relief of the obstruction with acceptable morbidity and mortality rates. It is particularly appropriate for a patient with perforation of the left colon and for the elderly unfit patient.

Subtotal Colectomy

More recently, some surgeons have recommended a subtotal colectomy with primary ileosigmoid anastomosis or even ileorectal anastomosis. Advantages offered by this operation include the following: (1) no stoma problems, (2) a one-stage procedure with a single hospitalization, (3) a shorter hospital stay with financial savings, and (4) removal of synchronous proximal neoplasms and reduced risk of metachronous lesions. Wong et al[112] reported on 35 patients who presented with left-sided obstructing carcinoma. Unsuspected synchronous proximal lesions occurred in 12 patients (32%)—3 carcinomas, 8 adenomas, and 1 with another synchronous carcinoma and polyp. Initial reports stressed the technical demands of this operation, but, with care, good results can be obtained. Operative mortality rates of 3 to 11% have been reported and morbidity rates are low, with a leakage rate of 4% and a hospital stay of 15 to 20 days.[111] Subtotal colectomy carries a risk of diarrhea and/or fecal incontinence, particularly in elderly patients. However, most reported experience has not rated this a significant problem. The overall morbidity rate (6 vs. 44%) and length of hospital stay (17 vs. 34 days) are significantly less than after combined procedures.[113] Perez et al[114] evaluated the results of emergency subtotal colectomy in 35 patients with obstructing carcinoma of the left colon. The postoperative mortality rate was 6%, and complications were significant: wound infection, 28%; ileus, 17%; evisceration, 8%; intestinal obstruction, 8%; and anastomotic leak, 11%. In a series of 35 patients, Lau et al[115] reported a complication rate of 31%, which included an anastomotic leak rate of 3%. Their review of the literature revealed leak rates that ranged from 0 to 4.5% for subtotal colectomy and 0 to 14% for colonic lavage methods.

Chrysos et al[116] reported four patients with obstructing carcinoma of the rectosigmoid junction and upper rectum who underwent a total colectomy, followed by construction of a 10-cm ileal-J pouch that was subsequently anastomosed to the distal rectal stump. One year postoperatively, all patients experienced one to three normal bowel motions daily and no episodes of incontinence. They believe total colectomy with ileal-J-pouch-rectal anastomosis is a reasonable operative alternative in cases with obstructing carcinomas of the rectosigmoid junction, which necessitate removal of the upper rectum.

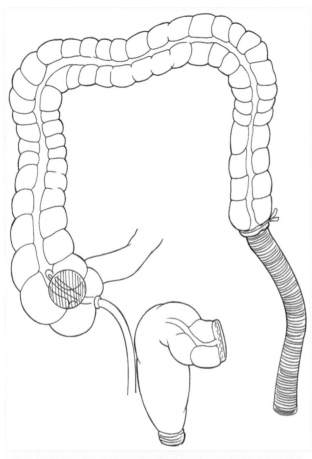

Fig. 22.29 On-table colonic lavage.

On-Table Lavage

Still others have recommended resection of the primary disease combined with on-table lavage and primary anastomosis. A major perceived disadvantage of on-table lavage is that it is time consuming. The operative technique consists of the mobilization of the appropriate segment of colon according to oncologic principles. In most circumstances, both the hepatic and splenic flexures require mobilization. The bowel at an appropriate distance distal to the carcinoma is divided, as is the proximal bowel 5 to 10 cm distal to the proximal site of the anastomosis, thus removing the carcinoma-bearing portion of colon. A no. 22 or 24 bladder catheter is inserted into the cecum through the freshly amputated appendicular stump or through the terminal ileum if the patient has had an appendectomy (▶ Fig. 22.29). The catheter balloon is inflated and held in place by a purse-string suture. A noncrushing clamp is placed across the terminal ileum to prevent reflux of the irrigation fluid. A standard intravenous infusion set is connected to the bladder catheter. The bowel, having been adequately mobilized, permits the distal portion to be placed in a kidney basin and hard fecal scybala can be "milked" into the kidney basin. A sterile corrugated anesthetic scavenger tube, 22 mm in diameter, is then inserted into the distal bowel and secured in place with strong tapes. The free end of this tube is draped over the side of the patient and secured in an appropriate collecting system. The colon is then lavaged with warm isotonic saline solution until the effluent

in the corrugated tube is clear. The volume of lavage solution required is determined by the extent of fecal loading but is usually 3 to 6 L. Lavage time may vary from 20 to 45 minutes. Once the effluent is clear, the bladder catheter is removed, and the appendiceal opening or ileum is closed. A short segment of bowel containing the irrigated tube is resected and an anastomosis created according to the surgeon's preference.

Most series quote an operative mortality rate of approximately 10%.[111] Anastomotic leakage rates following primary anastomosis are low. Tan and Nambiar[117] performed 36 primary resections and anastomoses following intraoperative antegrade colonic lavage for left-sided obstructing carcinoma. There were two deaths (one from anastomotic leak). Other complications included chest infection in 11% and wound infection in 19.4%. Others support this form of management.[114,118,119] Leakage rates are approximately 4%.[111] Wound infection rates remain a problem, with rates of 25 to 60%, and hospital stays of around 20 days.[111]

The Scotia Study Group[120] conducted the first multicenter prospective randomized trial comparing subtotal colectomy with segmental resection and primary anastomosis following intraoperative irrigation for the management of malignant left-sided colonic obstruction. Of the 91 eligible patients recruited by 12 centers, 47 were randomized to subtotal colectomy and 44 to on-table irrigation and segmental colectomy. Hospital mortality and complication rates did not differ significantly, but 4 months after operation, increased bowel frequency (three or more bowel movements per day) was significantly more common in the subtotal colectomy group (14 of 35 vs. 4 of 35). More patients in the subtotal colectomy group reported that they had consulted their general practitioner with bowel problems than those in the segmental resection group (15 of 37 vs. 3 of 35). The authors believe that segmental resection following intraoperative irrigation is the preferred option except when there is cecal perforation or if synchronous neoplasms are present in the colon, when subtotal colectomy is more appropriate.

Chiappa et al[121] reported 39 patients who were treated with intraoperative decompression, on-table lavage, resection, and primary anastomosis. The primary anastomosis was intraperitoneal in 74% and below the peritoneal reflection of the rectum in 26% of patients. Operative mortality was 3% and anastomotic leakage was observed in 6% of patients. Complications included intra-abdominal abscess (3%) and wound infections (8%). Ohman[122] also found a higher operative mortality rate for primary resection (14%) compared with staged resection (5%) and, although there was an early apparent superior survival rate with the staged procedures, it did not persist into the fourth and fifth years. Umpleby and Williamson[123] reported a better 5-year survival rate following resection and anastomosis (48%) than after staged procedures (18%).

Primary Resection

Rather boldly, some surgeons have performed a resection with primary anastomosis in the absence of bowel preparation.[124] An intracolonic bypass has been suggested as treatment.[125] Still others have suggested a primary resection with anastomosis and proximal diversion. In an effort to shed light on the issue, Kronborg[126] conducted a randomized trial in which he compared the results of traditional staged procedures with an initial transverse colostomy, followed by curative resection, and subsequent colostomy closure with immediate resection and end colostomy and mucous fistula with subsequent re-anastomosis. He found no difference in mortality or carcinoma-specific survival rates between the two treatments.

From this constellation of choices, it becomes difficult to select the best one. Ultimately, the selection depends on the surgeon's experience and preference. An informed decision rests on the recognition of the comparable morbidity and mortality rates for the single procedure compared with the combined morbidity and mortality rates of the multiple operations of the staged procedures. Fielding et al[127] recorded an operative mortality rate of 25% for primary resection and 34% for staged resection. This prospective study compared the outcome of primary staged resection in colonic obstruction and failed to show any difference in mortality rates between these options.

The authors' preference is to extend the primary resection for lesions as far as the sigmoid colon. It appears worthwhile to cleanse the bowel distal to the obstruction, and a primary anastomosis then can be constructed between the terminal ileum and the sigmoid colon. The morbidity and mortality rates are lower than those found with the staged approach, and the length of hospitalization is shorter. By eliminating a second or third hospitalization and a temporary colostomy, palliation is better for those patients who ultimately die from recurrent disease. Furthermore, those patients who undergo resection for cure may have increased rates of long-term survival. If the lesion is so distal that there would be little remaining reservoir by resecting all the obstructed colon proximal to the carcinoma, a reasonable alternative would be to cleanse the bowel distal to the carcinoma, perform a primary resection, and use on-table lavage, with a primary anastomosis. In the very debilitated patient, consideration should be given to a right transverse colostomy.

In the exceptional case in which the obstructing lesion is deemed unresectable, a bypass should be performed when possible. For right-sided lesions, an ileotransversostomy can be performed. In other circumstances, a colocolostomy might be deemed appropriate; in any event, this choice would be preferable to a permanent stoma, which would be the last option.

There have been reports on the role of pre-resectional laser recanalization for obstructive carcinomas of the colon and rectum. Eckhauser and Mansour[128] reported on use of the neodymium: yttrium aluminum garnet (Nd:YAG) laser to successfully accomplish decompression and allow for a formal bowel preparation and a definitive one-stage operation. The authors' experience with 29 patients did not involve compromise of patient safety. In several other series, the success rate for recanalization was 80%, with a 2 to 50% procedure-related morbidity and mortality.[111]

22.4.2 Stenting

Intestinal stenting is a procedure that is becoming more widespread. It was first introduced by Dohmoto in 1991[129] as definitive palliative treatment for patients with obstructive disease where resection for cure was not appropriate due to very advanced local disease, metastatic disease, or because of an unacceptably high operative risk. In 1994, Tejero et al[130] proposed stent placement as a "bridge-to-surgery" for emergency relief of colonic obstruction with an aim to subsequent elective resection. The technique can be applied in patients who refused operative treatment. Colostomy can be avoided with an improved quality of life especially in the palliative setting.

Suitable lesions for endoluminal colorectal stenting include obstructing both primary left-sided colorectal carcinomas and extracolonic malignancies such as prostate, bladder, ovarian, or pancreatic. It is also not appropriate for lesions less than 5 cm from the anal verge. The actual length of the lesion is not a theoretical limitation. It is contraindicated in the presence of colonic perforation with peritonitis and would not prove effective with multiple sites of obstruction.

Although it is not mandatory, it is probably best that stents be placed under endoscopic guidance with the aid of fluoroscopy. The administration of prophylactic antibiotics is probably wise. The procedure is conducted under conscious sedation. A catheter over a guide wire is advanced through the lesion. Contrast is injected into the proximal lumen. Once deployed, the stents expand and become incorporated into the surrounding tissue by pressure necrosis, thus anchoring the stent.

Dauphine et al[131] reviewed their experience with 26 self-expanding metal stents as the initial interventional approach in the management of acute malignant large bowel obstruction. In 14 patients, the stents were placed for palliation, whereas in 12, they were placed as a bridge to surgery. In 85%, stent placement was successful on the first occasion. In the remaining four individuals, one was successfully stented at the second occasion, and three required emergency operation. Nine of the 12 patients (75%) in the bridge-to-surgery group underwent elective colon resection. In the palliative group, 29% had reobstruction of the stents and in 9% the stent migrated. In the remaining 62%, the stent was patent until the patient died or until the time of last follow-up. Colonic stents achieved immediate nonoperative decompression and proved to be both safe and effective.

Since first described, there have been numerous publications on the subject. Khot et al[132] conducted a systematic review of the published data on stenting for the treatment of colorectal obstruction. A total of 58 publications were found, of which 29 case series were included in the analysis. Technical and clinical success, complications, and reobstruction, both in palliation and as a "bridge to surgery" were assessed. Pooled results showed that stent insertion was attempted in 598 instances. Technical success was achieved in 92% and clinical success in 88%. Palliation was achieved in 90% of 336 cases, while 85% of 262 insertions succeeded as a "bridge to surgery" (95% had a one-stage operative procedure with a mean time to the operating room of 8.9 days). Technical reasons for failure included inability to place the guide wire, malposition, or perforation. Clinical failures included perforation, persistent obstructive symptoms, or adhesion of colonic wall to the stent. There were three deaths (1%). Perforation occurred 22 times (4%), 1% in balloon dilatation versus 2% in non–balloon dilatation. Stent migration was reported in 10% of 551 technically successful cases. Management included stent removal, stent reinsertion, operation, and no immediate intervention but proceed to planned operation. The rate of stent reobstruction was 10% of the 525, mainly in the palliative group. Reason for obstruction included ingrowth of malignancy, stent migration, and fecal impaction. Bleeding occurred in 5% of patients, the majority requiring no treatment, but three patients received transfusions. Another 5% of patients experienced pain, either abdominal or rectal, and this was controlled with oral analgesics. They concluded that the evidence suggests that colorectal stents offer good palliation and are safe and effective as a "bridge to surgery." Stent usage can avoid the need for a stoma and is associated with low rates of mortality and morbidity. Dilatation of malignant strictures at the time of stent placement appears to be dangerous and should be avoided.

Law et al[133] evaluated the outcomes of self-expanding metallic stents as a palliative treatment for malignant obstruction of the colon and rectum. The insertion of self-expanding metallic stents was attempted for palliation in 52 patients. Successful insertion of the stent was achieved in 50 patients. The median survival of patients was 88 (range, 3–450) days. Complications occurred in 13 patients (25%). These included perforation of the colon ($n = 1$), migration or dislodgement of the stents ($n = 8$), severe tenesmus ($n = 1$), colovesical fistula ($n = 1$), and ingrowth of malignancy ($n = 2$). Insertion of a second stent was required in eight patients. Subsequent operations were performed in nine patients, and stoma creation was required in seven patients.

Saida et al[134] evaluated the long-term prognosis of expandable metallic stent insertion compared with emergency operation without expandable metallic stent. Forty emergency operations and 44 expandable metallic stent insertions were retrospectively compared. Postoperative complications were significantly less frequent in the expandable metallic stent group: wound infection was 14 versus 2%; leakage following anastomosis was 11 versus 3%; 3-year overall survival rate was 50 versus 48%; 5-year survival rate was 44 versus 40% in the emergency operation and expandable metallic stent groups, respectively. They concluded that because preoperative expandable metallic stent insertion for obstructive colorectal carcinoma had good postoperative results and no disadvantages in long-term prognosis, this procedure should be used in preoperative treatments of obstructive colorectal carcinoma.

Martinez-Santos et al[135] evaluated primary anastomosis and morbidity rates obtained with self-expandable stents in comparison with the results of emergency surgical treatment. Patients with left-sided malignant colorectal obstruction were enrolled. Forty-three patients were assigned to preoperative stent and elective operation or palliative stent (emergency surgical treatment). In the stent group, the obstruction was relieved in 95% after the stent placement. Of 26 patients who underwent operative treatment, a primary anastomosis was possible in 84.6 versus 41.4% in the immediate operative group, with lower need for a colostomy (15.4 vs. 58.6%) in the immediate operative group. The anastomotic failure rate was similar and the reintervention rate was lower (0 vs. 17%). The total stay (14.2 vs. 18.5 days), the intensive care unit stay (0.3 vs. 2.9 days), and the number of patients with severe complications (11.6 vs. 41.2%) were significantly lower in the stent group.

Johnson et al[136] studied 36 patients, of whom 18 had obstructing left-sided colon carcinomas relieved by placement of endoluminal stents. These were compared with 18 historical controls with similar clinicopathological features that were treated more conventionally with palliative stoma formation. Both groups of patients gained relief of obstructive symptoms. There were no differences in survival or in-hospital mortality. The median length of palliation was 92 days for stenting and 121 days for palliative stoma formation. Formation of a stoma required a significantly longer stay in the intensive care unit,

but hospital stay was similar. They concluded as an alternative to palliative operation, selected patients benefit from colonic endoluminal stenting with relief of obstructive symptoms and no adverse effect on survival. Patients may be spared the potential problems associated with palliative stoma formation and the morbidity of operation. Stenting can be offered to the very frail patient who would otherwise be managed conservatively.

Meisner et al[137] reported on 104 procedures with self-expanding metal stents performed in 96 patients. The goals of the procedure were either postponement of emergency operation or definitive palliative treatment. Technical success was achieved in 92% and clinical success in 82%. Procedure-related complications included perforation in three patients during stenting and in one instance 6 to 7 hours after. Other technical problems could mainly be overcome by introducing an additional stent. They believe complications seen in the group treated with self-expanding metal stents and subsequent resection (mortality 18% and anastomotic leakage 18%) do not differ from the number of complications usually seen in patients who undergo colorectal resection.

Suzuki et al[138] reviewed 36 patients with malignant obstruction, and 6 patients with benign obstructive disease who underwent placement of self-expandable stents using a combined endoscopic and fluoroscopic technique. Stent placement was successful in 86%. Complication occurred in 44%: migration ($n = 7$), reobstruction ($n = 5$), perforation ($n = 2$), fistula formation ($n = 1$), and stent fracture ($n = 1$). Stent placement was successful in 100% of patients with benign strictures, but post-stent migration was frequent (2/6).

Tomiki et al[139] compared the clinical outcome of 18 patients who had stent placement and 17 patients who underwent only colostomy. The postoperative hospital stay was 22.3 days for stent placement compared with 47.4 days for colostomy. The duration to readmission was 129.2 days for stent placement and 188.4 days for colostomy. The estimated duration of primary stent patency was 106 days. Mean survival period was 134 days in patients with stent placement and 191 days in patients with colostomy. They concluded that stent placement increases the option of palliative treatment and is an effective treatment contributing to improving quality of life.

Sebastian et al[140] systematically reviewed the efficacy and safety of self-expanding metal stents in the setting of malignant colorectal obstruction. Fifty-four studies reported the use of stents in a total of 1,198 patients. The median technical and clinical success rates were 94 and 91%, respectively. The clinical success when used as a bridge to surgery was 71.7%. Major complications related to stent placement included perforation (3.8%), stent migration (11.8%), and reobstruction (7.3%). Stent-related mortality was 0.58%.

Carne et al[141] compared the use of expandable metallic stents as a palliative measure to traditional open surgical management. Patients with left-sided (splenic flexure and distal) colorectal carcinoma and nonresectable metastatic disease (stage IV) were treated with expandable metal stents or open resection or stoma. Twenty-two of 25 patients had colonic stents successfully inserted and 19 patients underwent open operation. The malignancies were primary in 22 stent procedures and 18 open operations. The open operations were laparotomy only ($n = 2$), bypass ($n = 1$), stoma ($n = 7$), resection with anastomosis ($n = 4$), and resection without anastomosis ($n = 5$). The complications after open operation were urinary ($n = 2$), stroke ($n = 1$), cardiac ($n = 2$), respiratory ($n = 2$), deep venous thrombosis ($n = 1$), and anastomotic leak ($n = 1$). There were no stent-related complications. The mean length of stay was significantly shorter in the stent group (4 vs. 10.4 days). There was no difference in survival between the two groups (median survival: stent group, 7.5 months; open operation, 3.9 months). They concluded that patients treated with stents are discharged earlier than after open operation. Stents do not affect survival.

Although stents are expensive, the procedure appears to be cost-effective since emergency operation can be avoided with acute bowel obstruction, and in those with advanced disease no resection of the colon is necessary.

22.4.3 Perforation

Perforation has been reported to occur in 3 to 9% of patients with colorectal carcinomas.[142] Patients who develop a free perforation of the colon associated with a carcinoma present with signs and symptoms of generalized peritonitis. The carcinoma itself may be perforated, or there may be a left-sided carcinoma associated with a right-sided perforation. Each situation is handled differently. In the clinical setting, for treatment of a perforated carcinoma, older reports recommended that the perforation be managed by diversion, with a proximal colostomy or cecostomy performed in association with repair of the perforation. However, this treatment does not relieve the septic process, and the aim of therapy should be to remove the diseased segment. Otherwise, contamination will continue from the level of the stoma to the level of the perforation. On completion of the resection, the question arises as to how to handle the bowel ends. If the patient already has generalized peritonitis, it seems inappropriate to perform a primary anastomosis. In this event, the proximal bowel is brought out as a stoma, and the distal bowel is drawn out as a mucous fistula or closed as a Hartmann pouch. For a right-sided perforation, a similar procedure can be performed. Another option is to resect the perforated diseased bowel and perform a primary anastomosis with a proximal diversionary stoma, either a proximal colostomy or a loop ileostomy. If technically feasible, the two ends of bowel should be brought out adjacent to each other as described for the end loop stoma. The advantage of this technique is that bowel continuity can be established at a later date without the need for a formal laparotomy.

When there is an obstructing lesion of the left colon and a perforation of the right colon, a viable option is a subtotal colectomy encompassing removal of the perforated colon and the malignancy in one operation. Saegesser and Sandblom[143] stressed the fact that simple suture repair of an ischemic colon will not hold and that a temporary colostomy placed in an ischemic or inflamed bowel will pull through. The authors believe that the practice of closure of the perforation and relief of obstruction by colostomy or by exteriorization of the perforated cecum is illogical and inadequate. The surgeon should proceed with resection of the carcinoma and the entire distended part of the ischemic and perforated colon. A subtotal colectomy might even be considered if only a left-sided perforation is present, since this operation would fulfill the criteria of removing the diseased and unprepared bowel. Another option for management of the patient with a perforation remote from the diseased segment is to bring out the perforated segment as a stoma, either by colostomy or cecostomy.

For the patient who presents with localized peritonitis on the right side, the diagnosis may be confused with that of appendicitis. If the diagnosis is definite at the time of laparotomy, it is reasonable to proceed with a right hemicolectomy and primary anastomosis. If the localized peritonitis occurs on the left side, the differential diagnosis will include diverticulitis. Resection of the diseased segment is indicated, and management of the ends involves the same considerations as with the obstructed unprepared bowel.

22.4.4 Bleeding

Massive bleeding from a carcinoma is an unusual complication, but when it arises, it offers the built-in advantage of being a colonic cathartic. Therefore, if bleeding is so profuse that urgent operation is required, a mechanical cleansing is automatically present, and the affected portion of bowel can be resected with a primary anastomosis.

22.4.5 Obstructive Colitis

Obstructive colitis is an ulceroinflammatory condition that occurs in a dilated segment of the colon proximal to an obstructing or partially obstructing lesion. The entity is rarely reported in the literature and the following information was drawn from the review by Tsai et al.[144] Obstructive colitis is only encountered in 0.3 to 3.1% of all colorectal carcinomas and affects both men and women over 50 years of age. Minor degrees of obstructive colitis may be overlooked and its prevalence may be as high as 7% when specifically sought. The left side of the colon, especially the sigmoid colon, is usually involved in obstructive colitis. Patients with obstructive colitis usually complain of bleeding per rectum and abdominal pain as well as nausea and vomiting, all of which are indistinguishable from the symptoms of colorectal carcinoma. Regardless of severity and distribution pattern, a diagnostic feature of obstructive colitis is the presence of an intact mucosal segment of about 2 to 6 cm long between the carcinoma and the colitis. The area of colitis is usually a single confluent area, often with regular geographic margins, which is well demarcated from the surrounding normal mucosa.

Microscopically, focal areas of colitis associated with obstructive colitis show replacement of mucosa by active granulation tissue. Acute and chronic inflammatory cells are moderate in amount and seldom extend beyond sites of granulation. Pseudopolyps of granular tissue or edematous mucosa may occur, and crypt abscesses may involve the mucosa at the ulcer margin. The mucosa in the intervening segment and distal to the obstructing lesion is usually normal. It is differentiated from ulcerative colitis, which is characterized histologically by an intense inflammation of the mucosa and submucosa in addition to the presence of multiple crypt abscesses. The rectum is always involved and the disease extends proximally for varying distances but always with continuity of involvement to the proximal extent of the disease process.

One suggested pathogenic mechanism of obstructive colitis is that of secondary ischemia caused by hypoperfusion. Additional factors, such as preexisting atheroma, anemia, or a past history of pelvic irradiation, may play a role in precipitating the colitis.

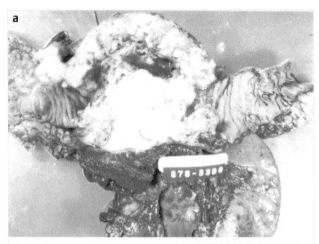

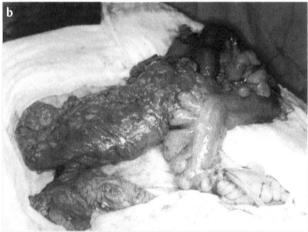

Fig. 22.30 **(a)** Carcinoma of the transverse colon attached to the spleen and greater curvature of the stomach resected en bloc. **(b)** Carcinoma of the transverse colon invading the sigmoid colon.

Obstructive colitis can cause both diagnostic and therapeutic problems. The signs and symptoms arising from obstructive colitis may be attributed to the primary obstructive lesion, which is usually most obvious on radiological and endoscopic studies. Areas of colitis may be a source of septicemia or may perforate and lead to peritonitis. Anastomoses in the unrecognized area of colitis may break down. Up to 25% of cases of obstructive colitis have been associated with anastomotic complications. Their frequently normal appearance at operation may lead to involved segments of colon being used for anastomoses with consequent complications. Because perforation through a colonic carcinoma is a grim prognostic event with negligible 5-year survival, it is important to distinguish this from perforation through the obstructive colitis, which may have a different prognosis. Awareness of the features and incidence of obstructive colitis should help surgeons avoid these diagnostic and therapeutic problems.

22.4.6 Invasion of Adjacent Viscera

Occasionally a carcinoma becomes attached to the abdominal wall or the adjacent viscera, such as the small bowel, urinary bladder, uterus, stomach, spleen, ureter, or duodenum. It is estimated that such attachment occurs in approximately 10% of all patients with colon carcinomas with a reported range of 3.1 to 16.7%.[145] The philosophy of treatment to be followed in these circumstances might best be expressed by the quote attributed to Hippocrates: "To extreme diseases, extreme remedies." In order to perform an adequate curative operation, it sometimes becomes necessary to excise en bloc all or part of the attached viscus (▶ Fig. 22.30). Often, these adhesions are inflammatory in nature and not caused by malignant infiltration, so the prognosis frequently is better than might have been anticipated originally (▶ Table 22.5). With this knowledge, the surgeon should not hesitate to resect attached structures.[146,147,148,149,150,151,152,153,154,155]

Table 22.5 Nature of adhesions between colon and adjacent viscus

Author(s)	No. of patients	Adhesions (%)		5-y survival (%)	Operative mortality (%)
		Carcinomatous	Inflammatory		
Glass et al[146]	69	49	51	70	–
Gall et al[147]	121	55	45	52	12
Hunter et al[148]	28	39	61	61	0
Orkin et al[149]	65	57	43	52	0
Eisenberg et al[150]	58	84	16	0–76[a]	2
Montesani et al[151]	35	71	29	30	0
Curley et al[152]	101	70	30	54	4
Izbicki et al[153]	83	54	46	44 mo (mean)	1
Rowe et al[145]	118	69	31	34–78[b]	4
Carne et al[154]	53	38	62	51	–
Nakafusa et al[155]	53	53	47	77	0

[a]Zero percent survival of those with lymph node metastases; 76% for those without lymph node metastases.
[b]Five-year survival of 78% for those with inflammatory adhesions plus negative lymph nodes; 58% for those with inflammatory adhesions plus positive lymph nodes; 34% for those with invasive adhesions plus positive lymph nodes; 64% for those with invasive adhesions plus negative lymph nodes; 71% for those with negative lymph nodes; 47% for those with positive lymph nodes.

An exception to these recommendations might be when the duodenum or bladder base is extensively involved, in which case the primary lesion is removed and the structures at risk are marked with metal clips. Under these circumstances, the morbidity and mortality rates of the radical operation involving an anterior exenteration or Whipple's procedure would probably exceed any possible benefit derived from a very radical operation. However, Curley et al[156] reported on 12 patients in whom the carcinoma involved the duodenum or pancreatic head and who underwent an en bloc extended right hemicolectomy and pancreaticoduodenectomy. There were no operative deaths, and malignant invasion was confirmed in all patients. At the time of reporting, 8 of the 12 patients were alive at a median of 42 months.

Similarly, Koea et al[157] reported their experience with eight patients with bulky primary carcinomas of the right colon infiltrating the duodenum ($n = 4$) or pancreatic head ($n = 4$) surgically managed at Memorial Sloan Kettering Cancer Center. Six patients presented with anemia, and one patient each with epigastric pain and an abdominal mass. All patients had T4 lesions, whereas five had lymph node metastases at presentation. All patients were resected with clear pathologic margins by either right colectomy and en bloc duodenectomy ($n = 4$) or en bloc pancreaticoduodenectomy ($n = 4$). The 30-day mortality rate was 0. Six patients remained alive and free of disease at a median follow-up of 26 months, and there was one long-term survivor who was alive and free of disease at 84 months after resection.

Talamonti et al[158] reviewed 70 patients who underwent resection of a carcinoma of the colon and rectum with en bloc total cystectomy (36 patients) or partial cystectomy (34 patients). There were three postoperative deaths in the total cystectomy group but none after partial cystectomy. The 5-year actuarial survival rate for the 64 patients with negative resection margins was 52%. In exceptionally good-risk patients, consideration may be given to a total pelvic exenteration.

In a review of 1,918 patients who underwent curative resection for colorectal carcinoma, Gall et al[147] noted that 121 patients had multivisceral organ involvement. Extended multivisceral radical resections resulted in a postoperative mortality rate of 12% (compared to 6% without such resection), with a 5-year survival rate of 54% for patients with inflammatory adherence and 49% for patients with malignant infiltration. In this series, the most frequently used extensions of resection were total hysterectomy (39%), small bowel (21%), urinary bladder (16%), and abdominal wall (4%). It is worth noting that when carcinoma was inadvertently torn or transected during resection, the 5-year survival rate dramatically dropped to 17%. Despite the increased operative mortality with extended resection, the authors of this review believe that the benefit outweighs the disadvantages. Hunter et al[148] reviewed their results of colorectal carcinoma in three treatment groups: standard colectomy, en bloc resection, and colectomy with separation of adherent organs. The 5-year survival rates were 55, 61, and 23%, respectively. No operative mortality occurred with en bloc resection. The 5-year survival rate, recurrence rate, and local recurrence rate for standard colectomy were 55, 33, and 11%, respectively; for en bloc resection, 61, 36, and 18%; and for separation of organs, 23, 77, and 69%. The authors concluded that colorectal carcinoma adherent to adjacent organs must be treated by en bloc resection because separation of organs

results in unacceptably high local recurrence and poor 5-year survival rates. On the other hand, the results of en bloc resection were comparable to those of standard colectomy for non-adherent carcinomas.

Nakafusa et al[155] evaluated the short- or long-term outcome of multivisceral resection relative to that of the standard operation. Of 323 patients, 16.4% received multivisceral resection because of adhesion to other organs. Overall, morbidity rates were 49.1% for multivisceral resection versus 17.8% for the standard operation and postoperative mortality was 0% in both groups. Only multivisceral resection (OR, 2.7) was an independent factor for overall postoperative complications. The survival of patients with multivisceral resection was similar to that after the standard operation (5-year rate, 76.6 vs. 79.5%). Lymph node metastases (hazard ratio, 2.5) and blood transfusion (hazard ratio, 2.4) were independently associated with patient survival.

Kroneman et al[159] evaluated the results of 33 patients who underwent curative en bloc resection. Adherent organs excised included small bowel, urinary bladder, abdominal wall, uterus, duodenum, pancreas, stomach, and kidney. The postoperative morbidity rate was 6%, the mortality was 3%, and the 4-year survival rate was 33%. Poeze et al[160] reported on 1,346 patients with colorectal carcinoma, 144 (11%) of whom underwent multivisceral resections for invasion of adjacent organs. In patients who had disease-free margins, there was no compromise of long-term survival (i.e., local invasion to adjacent organs with or without lymph node involvement was not related to survival). The overall operative mortality rate was 5%. Izbicki et al[153] reported on 83 patients who underwent en bloc resection. Mean survival was 44 months after extended resection. The postoperative mortality, morbidity, and survival rates were comparable to those in patients who underwent nonextended resections.

Landercasper et al[161] reported on 54 of 1,284 patients (4%) who underwent potentially curative resections of right colon lesions found to be adherent to adjacent organs, abdominal wall, or retroperitoneum. Postoperative complications developed in 24% of patients. The mortality rate was 1.9% and the 5-year survival rate was 31%. Only one of nine patients with pancreatic or duodenal adherence treated with limited resection remained disease free. The authors recommend radical en bloc resection if no distant metastases are present. Adjuvant radiation therapy or chemotherapy did not improve survival.

To determine the perioperative mortality and morbidity and the long-term prognosis of patients undergoing extended pelvic resections for localized advanced primary adenocarcinoma of the rectum, Orkin et al[149] reviewed their experience with 65 patients. Local invasion without distant metastases was present in all patients at operation and en bloc resection of all involved organs was performed with intent of cure. Average age at operation was 61 years; 23% were men and 77% were women. Operations included abdominoperineal resection in 57%, low anterior resection in 31%, and Hartmann's procedure in 12%. Additionally, women (81%) with intact uteri underwent en bloc hysterectomy, 77% of women with intact ovaries had oophorectomy, and 50% of women had partial vaginal resection. Twenty-six percent of the 65 patients had a cystectomy, and 2 patients had a portion of small intestine resected in continuity with their carcinoma. Pathologic examination revealed lymph node involvement in 45% and histologic confirmation of adjacent organ extension in 57%. There were no perioperative deaths. Overall 5-year survival was 52% with 65% of deaths attributable to either recurrent carcinoma or a new primary lesion. The cumulative probability of recurrence at 5 years was 39%.

Carne et al[154] reported on multicenter experiences of en bloc bladder resection for colorectal carcinoma adhering to the urinary bladder. Fifty-three patients were identified, of which 45 had en bloc partial cystectomy performed, 4 en bloc total cystectomy, and 4 had the adhesions disrupted and no bladder resection. All patients who did not have a bloc resection developed local recurrence and died from their disease. Mean follow-up was 62 months. The extent of bladder resection did not seem important in determining local recurrence. The decision to perform total rather than partial cystectomy should be based on the anatomic location of the carcinoma.

Rowe et al[145] determined the therapeutic benefit of multivisceral resection in patients with locally advanced colorectal carcinomas. The study population was composed of 118 patients whose resection of the primary lesion included one or more adhesed adjacent secondary organs or structures. Their survival is reported in ▶ Table 22.5, but clinical relevance is that there was no statistically significant difference in the 5-year survival rates when multiple adjacent secondary organs or structures were resected and therefore they believe an aggressive operative approach is warranted.[160,161]

Yamada et al[162] reported 64 patients with locally advanced primary or recurrent rectal carcinoma with abdominoperineal resection with sacral resection performed in 9 patients, anterior pelvic exenteration in 8 patients, total pelvic exenteration in 27 patients, and total pelvic exenteration with sacral resection in 20 patients. Rates of morbidity, reoperation, and mortality were 50, 4.5, and 0% in 22 patients with primary carcinoma, and 60, 2.4, and 2.4% in 42 patients with recurrent disease, respectively. Major complications, such as sepsis, intra-abdominal abscess, and enteric fistula caused one hospital death and reoperation in two patients. In 21 patients who underwent curative resection for primary carcinoma, the overall 5-year survival rates were 74.1% for Dukes' B and 47.4% for Dukes' C although the difference was not statistically significant. Thirty patients with recurrent carcinoma who underwent curative resection had significantly improved survival with a 5-year survival rate of 22.9% compared with 12 patients who underwent palliative resection resulting in a survival rate of 0%.

In an excellent clinical review of the role of extended resection in the initial treatment of locally advanced colorectal carcinoma, Lopez and Monafo[163] collated information on the results of multivisceral resection for colorectal carcinoma. In 11 publications in which 609 patients underwent extended resection for colorectal carcinoma, the operative morbidity rate was 27%, the operative mortality rate was 6%, and lymph node metastases occurred in 39%. The 5-year survival rate was 68% for node-negative status and 23% for node-positive status. If adherence to adjacent viscera was benign, the 5-year survival rate was 68%, but it declined to 40% if the attachment was malignant. Survival in locally advanced colorectal carcinoma is more dependent on lymph node status than on the extent of local invasion.[150] In 23 publications in which 248 patients underwent total pelvic exenteration for rectosigmoid carcinoma, the operative morbidity rate was 60% and the operative mortality rate

was 12%. The 5-year survival rate was 64% for node-negative status and 32% for node-positive status.

In the unique situation in which there is isolated invasion of the prostate by a rectal carcinoma, Campbell et al[164] described the use of radical retropubic prostatectomy in conjunction with restorative proctosigmoidectomy for en bloc excision. This novel technique offers an alternative to total pelvic exenteration, thereby obviating the need for urinary and fecal diversion. The expected 5-year survival of patients subjected to en bloc resection ranged from 30 to 79% (▶ Table 22.5) and thus justifies an aggressive approach.

22.4.7 Urinary Tract Involvement by Colorectal Carcinoma

McNamara et al[165] recently reviewed the literature on urinary tract involvement by colorectal carcinoma with the aim of highlighting technical and oncologic issues that should be considered when dealing with this complex problem. From the relevant literature, they identified three distinct clinical scenarios in which the urinary tract may be affected by colorectal carcinoma: involvement by primary colorectal carcinoma, involvement of recurrent carcinoma, and unexpected intraoperative findings of urinary tract involvement. The following information and guidelines draw heavily from their dissertation.

Primary Involvement of the Urinary Tract

Involvement of the urinary tract system occurs in 5% of patients with primary colorectal carcinoma. Any level of the urinary tract can be affected by direct invasion or be involved with an associated inflammatory mass. Three sites are most commonly affected: the dome of the bladder, the lower ureter, and the base of the bladder. Adherence to or invasion of the dome of the bladder is the most common presentation and most frequently occurs in rectosigmoid malignancies. Locally advanced disease with direct invasion of adjacent organs may result in fistula formation, but half of such patients have no symptoms at presentation. Involvement of the trigone may compromise the intramural ureter. Lower third lesions of the rectum may involve the prostate gland and prostatic urethra. A CT is usually performed as part of the standard investigation of patients with sigmoid or rectal carcinoma but is mandatory in patients with urinary symptoms. In addition to staging, computed tomography (CT) allows localization of the ureters and confirms bilateral renal function, although it tends to overestimate the need for urinary organ resection. CT is more likely to produce a false-positive diagnosis of pelvic floor or piriform muscle invasion than magnetic resonance imaging (MRI) and is less likely to identify sacral bone invasion when it is present. Modern high-resolution MRI (sensitivity 97% and specificity 98%) is superior to CT (sensitivity 70% and specificity 85%) in staging locally advanced primary or recurrent rectal carcinomas, with better detection of penetration of the fascia propria and involvement of the potential circumferential resection margin. Cystoscopy diagnoses the cause of genitourinary symptoms in 79 to 87% of patients with rectal carcinoma. Only 57% of patients with a mucosal abnormality at cystoscopy have bladder invasion at final pathology, yet locating the vesical opening of a malignant rectovesical fistula improves identification of patients who require pelvic exenteration for adequate resection.

Bladder Involvement

If involvement of the dome of the bladder is suspected, en bloc resection of the carcinoma and all adherent bladder should be performed, because of the well-documented difficulty in distinguishing between adherence and invasion macroscopically and the greatly diminished survival experienced by patients in whom the carcinoma is breached during resection. This policy carries the risk that the adjacent organ in the resected specimen may show no evidence of malignant invasion but is justified because no increase in morbidity is reported following multivisceral resection, especially partial cystectomy. No adverse effect on local recurrence or survival has been demonstrated when partial cystectomy is performed instead of total cystectomy for localized malignant involvement, provided the resection is R0.

Involvement of the trigone is less straightforward, and curative resection requires total pelvic exenteration. Total pelvic exenteration is appropriate for direct invasion of the trigone, vesicoureteric junction, or intramural ureter in the absence of distant metastases and has been used in both primary and locally recurrent diseases. Total pelvic exenteration may be combined with sacral resection, especially in patients with local recurrence extending into the presacral space. Bladder reconstruction requires construction of a urinary conduit, of which an ileal conduit is the most common, although cecal or colonic conduits are sometimes used. Supralevator exenteration with double-pouch reconstruction using a colonic J-pouch and a Mainz pouch with sphincter-preserving urethral anastomosis has been described, but long-term results are not available and recurrence in this setting may result in catastrophic complications. Early urologic complications of urinary diversion include ileoureteral anastomotic dehiscence and early hydronephrosis. Late urologic complications include ureteral stenosis and late hydronephrosis. Unsuccessful endoscopic and radiologic management of these complications may lead to the necessity for nephrectomy. Operative mortality rates following total pelvic exenteration ranging between 5 and 33% have been quoted. There is a trend toward increased morbidity in patients who receive preoperative radiotherapy. Review of the literature reveals 3-year survival figures ranging from 30 to 64.5% and 5-year survival figures ranging from 9 to 61%. Some surgeons routinely include intrapelvic dissection of the internal iliac and obturator nodes in their approach to total pelvic exenteration, but no convincing survival advantage has been demonstrated. Total pelvic exenteration has been reported to have a sixfold greater mortality than lesser exenterative procedures.

Ureteric Involvement

Bilateral involvement of the ureters may occur because of compression from extensive nodal disease at the pelvic brim or by invasion of the trigone by the primary carcinoma, but both scenarios usually require total pelvic exenteration if curative resection is desired. In contrast, unilateral ureteric invasion may be approached by en bloc resection of the affected segment, followed by appropriate reconstruction. Ipsilateral ureteroureterostomy over a double-J stent is the simplest form of anastomosis,

but even when combined with use of a vesicopsoas hitch is suitable only for short resections of the distal ureter. Reconstruction following resection of a longer segment may require use of a Boari flap in which a well-vascularized flap of bladder is constructed into a tube to which the proximal ureter may be anastomosed. Cystourethrectomy and ureteric crossover are recommended for unilateral involvement of the ureterovesical junction and may be performed without significantly increasing postoperative morbidity and mortality. Ileal interposition has satisfactory oncologic results and allows resection of a long ureteric segment, but may result in renal damage because of transmission of high intravesical pressures and should only be performed in carefully selected patients. Rarely, nephrectomy may be an acceptable option.

Fistula

Rectourinary fistulation is an uncommon event that rarely occurs in females because of the protective effect afforded by the interposition of the female genital tract. The classic triad of pneumaturia, fecaluria, and recurrent urinary tract infection is unusual, and patients more commonly present with fever, a pelvic mass, or cystitis. Most patients have a urinary tract infection, but pneumaturia is reported by only 10% of patients. Only 21% of fistulas associated with a rectal carcinoma contain malignant cells. The remaining 79% result from interventions (including operation, radiotherapy, and chemotherapy) for rectal carcinoma. The success rates for initial and reoperative surgeries were 21 and 88%, respectively, when malignant cells were identified in the fistula tract as compared with success rates of 44 and 100% for treatment-related fistulas. The decision to administer neoadjuvant chemoradiotherapy must balance the possibility of improved survival and less radical operation against the reported increase in preoperative fistulization and perioperative morbidity and mortality.

Hydronephrosis

In a patient with primary colorectal carcinoma, the most common cause of hydronephrosis is regional nodal disease from a sigmoid or rectal carcinoma at the pelvic brim, but direct extension of a primary carcinoma, local inflammation, and isolated ureteric metastases are possible. Malignant hydronephrosis detected at the time of first diagnosis of colorectal carcinoma is a worrying finding because less than half of such patients have resectable disease.

Radiotherapy

The role of preoperative radiotherapy in rectal carcinoma involving the urinary tract is not yet clear. Downstaging may improve resectability by reducing the extent of operation necessary to obtain negative margins and rendering some inoperable carcinomas resectable.

Unexpected Intraoperative Involvement

A particular difficulty arises when unexpected local extensive disease is identified at operation. Discovery of a rectosigmoid carcinoma adherent to the bladder for which one can envisage a relatively straightforward en bloc resection with primary closure of the bladder clearly differs from a carcinoma likely to require complex reconstruction. Important are issues relating to the quality of the preoperative informed consent, particularly if the proposed resection requires a procedure with the potential for considerably greater morbidity and mortality than anticipated or an unexpected impact on postoperative quality of life such as necessity to create a stoma. In some circumstances, the correct decision is to defer resectional operation in favor of radiotherapy or a subsequent more aggressive one-stage procedure. Fortunately, with current preoperative staging, this occurrence is less common.

Recurrent Colorectal Carcinoma

The finding of hydronephrosis after a previous colorectal resection usually indicates pelvic sidewall disease that precludes resection. It is associated with concomitant metastatic disease in 50% of patients and predicts poor survival, even after salvage operation. Investigation of a patient with suspected recurrence involving the urinary tract should be vigorous to avoid the morbidity and mortality of salvage operation in patients unlikely to benefit. Inoperable metastatic disease should be excluded with spiral CT and MRI or positron emission tomography (PET). Rarely, urinary and/or fecal diversion may be justified in the presence of metastatic disease in patients who are symptomatic but cannot be successfully palliated with less invasive radiologic or endourologic techniques.

Abnormal Renal Function

Patients with abnormal preoperative renal function require optimization of their condition before operation. An elevated preoperative urea level is independently predictive of increased 30-day mortality, while patients who develop acute renal failure postoperatively have a 30-day mortality in excess of 50%. Patients may require preoperative urinary decompression. Early urinary decompression is a priority to prevent or minimize irreversible renal damage. This may take the form of initial retrograde double-J stenting or percutaneous nephrostomy with subsequent endourologic stent insertion.

Palliation

Treatment of unresectable carcinoma involving the urinary tract or potentially resectable local disease in the presence of unresectable metastases should maximize survival without adverse effects on quality of life. Most malignant strictures of the ureter can be treated by an endourologic approach with minimal morbidity, allowing normal micturition without external drainage and with durable results.

22.4.8 Unresectable Carcinoma

In the unusual circumstance in which a lesion is totally unresectable, it usually can be bypassed satisfactorily.

22.4.9 Palliative Resection

One of the most unsatisfying situations facing any surgeon who operates on patients with colon and rectal carcinoma is that of recommending a major abdominal procedure, with its potential complications, to a patient who has definite evidence of incurable disease. The decision regarding operative intervention is usually reached with some trepidation, since many of these patients are in poor physical condition and have a limited life expectancy. However, even for patients with metastatic carcinoma of the large bowel, resection performed to eliminate the symptoms of local disease has been advocated as a worthwhile procedure for avoiding the potential complications of obstruction and massive bleeding and the effects of local invasion of the primary lesion. In general, resections relieve patients of their symptoms and sometimes may even prolong life expectancy.[166] The most common symptoms are pain and bleeding.[167,168]

It has been estimated that 10 to 20% of patients who are seen with primary operable colorectal carcinoma already have associated liver metastases.[166] Unfortunately, not all patients will benefit from resection, and, in fact, some patients will be caused additional morbidity. This morbidity, together with the mortality of the operative procedure, may exceed the benefit of any temporary symptomatic relief. Thus, the role of palliative resection for malignant neoplasms has been questioned from time to time. This is especially true for the decision to perform a palliative abdominoperineal resection, an operation that entails not only an operative procedure of considerable magnitude, but also the establishment of a permanent colostomy in a patient with only a chance of limited survival.

In the presence of metastatic disease, survival will depend on the nature and extent of the metastases. Indeed, some metastatic lesions should be resected in addition to the primary lesion. Survival depends on the pattern of metastatic disease. For example, Joffe and Gordon[167] noted survival with unilobar liver metastases to be 16.9 months, while with bilobar metastases, survival was only 8.5 months. Cady et al[166] noted a survival of 13 months, Takaki et al[169] 12 months, and Goslin et al[170] a similar length of survival. Under such circumstances, the recommendation for resection should be tempered by a consideration of factors such as extensive hepatic replacement or jaundice, marked ascites, or massive peritoneal seeding, in which case life expectancy is very short and no benefit could be accrued from a resection. The prognosis is poor for patients with extensive liver metastases, patients older than 75 years, and patients with a previous history of cardiovascular disease.[167]

Mäkelä et al[171] reviewed 96 patients who underwent palliative operations with an 8% postoperative mortality rate (5% for resections and 17% for nonresection procedures) and a 24% postoperative morbidity rate. Median survival was 10 months (15 months for resections and 7 months for nonresection procedures) and 5% of patients survived longer than 5 years. The median relief of symptoms related to the malignancy was 4 months (4 months after resection and 1 month after nonresection procedures). Twenty-five patients underwent a second palliative operation.

Liu et al[168] studied 68 patients with incurable colon carcinoma to try to identify objective criteria that might help surgeons decide which patients will benefit from palliative operations. The postoperative mortality rate was 10% and the complication rate was 10%. The mean survival after palliative resection was 10.6 months, after bypass was 3.4 months, and after diagnosis in patients not operated on was 2.0 months. Of the variables studied, the only factors affecting survival were poorly differentiated lesions and greater than 50% replacement of liver. The authors concluded that although resection carries with it a relatively high postoperative mortality rate, it is worthwhile as long as hepatic metastases occupy less than 50% of liver volume.

The macroscopic features of the primary disease must be taken into consideration because of the ever-present concern of obstruction. However, endoluminal stenting is an option in dealing with obstructive symptoms.

22.4.10 Synchronous Carcinomas

Recommendations for the appropriate treatment of synchronous carcinomas of the colon are at least in part based on the magnitude of the risk of development of metachronous adenomas and carcinomas after conventional resections. The incidence of synchronous carcinomas has been reported to be 1.5 to 7.6%.[172] In a series of 2,586 patients, an incidence of 1.8% was reported.[172] Bussey et al[173] reported on 3,381 patients who survived conventional resections for carcinoma of the colon and rectum at St. Mark's Hospital in London and found an overall incidence of metachronous carcinoma of 1.5%. The incidence rose to 3% in those cases followed up for at least 20 years. For those patients in whom an associated adenomatous polyp was found in the original operative specimen, the level rose to 5%. In a more recent study, synchronous carcinomas were found in 4.4% of patients.[174] Passman et al[175] reported on an 18-year multi-institutional database of 4,878 patients with colon carcinoma. There were 160 patients (3.3%) with 339 synchronous carcinomas. Eight percent of these patients had more than two lesions at the time of diagnosis. Based on highest stage lesion, 1% of patients were at stage 0, 28% at stage I, 33% at stage II, 25% at stage III, and 11% at stage IV. The disease-specific 5-year survival rate by highest stage was 87% for stage 0 or I, 69% for stage II, 50% for stage III, and 14% for stage IV. These "highest stage" survival rates for patients with synchronous carcinomas were not significantly different from survival of patients with same-stage solitary carcinomas in their database. In light of this, it seems reasonable that if synchronous carcinomas are located in the same anatomic region, a conventional resection should be performed. When the carcinomas are widely separated, a subtotal colectomy is the operation of choice.

22.4.11 Synchronous Polyps and Carcinoma

Recommendation for the treatment of patients with colon carcinoma and associated polyps involves the same considerations as for synchronous carcinomas. However, it also depends on the number, location, and size of these polyps. For example, if the polyps were confined to the region of the index carcinoma, the conventional operation for that portion of the bowel would be indicated. With the availability of colonoscopy, assessment and possible therapy of associated polyps can be accomplished. If the remaining bowel contains only occasional polyps that can be easily excised with the colonoscope, it would appear reasonable to have these polyps excised and to proceed with a conventional resection of the carcinoma. If one of the excised polyps should contain a carcinoma or if the polyps were of a size deemed in excess of colonoscopic polypectomy, a subtotal colectomy would be appropriate.[176] Subtotal colectomy even has

been recommended for colon carcinoma and synchronous polyp in good-risk patients.[174] An individual who has exhibited the propensity for growth of many polyps in the colon, although not in adequate numbers to be considered familial adenomatous polyposis, would still qualify for a subtotal colectomy and ileorectal, or at least ileosigmoid, anastomosis.

22.4.12 Metachronous Carcinoma

Gervaz et al[177] assessed the incidence of metachronous colorectal carcinomas in a population-based study of 500,000 residents. Of this total, 5,006 patients had sporadic carcinoma of the colon or rectum with 34% being located proximal to the splenic flexure. Occurrence of a second primary colorectal carcinoma was observed in 2.4% of this population. The risk for developing a second incidence of primary colorectal carcinoma was higher in patients whose initial carcinoma was located in the proximal colon (3.4 vs. 1.8%; OR, 1.9). The risk for each segment of large bowel was as follows: cecum, 3.4%; right colon, 3%; transverse colon, 3.8%; left colon, 2.8%; sigmoid colon, 1.7%; and rectum, 1.8%. By contrast, the risk for developing a second extracolonic carcinoma did not differ between patients with proximal and distal carcinomas (13.7 vs. 13.4%).

Shitoh et al[178] reported that microsatellite instability can be regarded as an independent marker for predicting the development of metachronous colorectal carcinoma after operation. In a study of 328 colorectal carcinoma patients surveyed by periodic colonoscopy for at least 3 years after operation, 17 metachronous colorectal carcinomas were detected during the follow-up period. The percentage of microsatellite instability–positive cases was 26.4%. Incidences of metachronous colorectal carcinomas in microsatellite instability-positive and microsatellite instability–negative cases were 15.3 and 3%, respectively. The cumulative 5-year incidence of metachronous colorectal carcinomas was significantly higher in microsatellite instability–positive cases than in microsatellite instability–negative cases (12.5 vs. 2.5%).

22.4.13 Treatment of Metastatic Disease

Liver

Metastases to the liver from carcinoma of the colon or rectum are frequent occurrences. Indeed, the liver is the dominant site of treatment failure and the major cause of death in patients with colorectal carcinoma. Studies have demonstrated that up to 30% of patients undergoing apparently curative operation already have hepatic metastases that are not evident to the surgeon at the time of laparotomy.[179,180,181] Furthermore, another 50% have recurrent disease develop within the liver.[182] Some 90% of patients who die from colorectal carcinoma have liver metastases.[183] In a study of doubling times, Finlay et al[184] determined that the mean doubling time for overt metastases was 155 ± 34 days (± standard error of mean [SEM]) compared with 86 ± 12 days for occult metastases. The mean age of the metastases at the time of operation was estimated by extrapolation of the observed growth curve, assuming Gompertzian kinetics, to be 3.7 ± 0.9 years (± SEM) for overt metastases and 2.3 ± 0.4 years for occult metastases.

There is a perception that streamline flow of blood in the portal vein may influence the anatomic distribution of liver metastases, depending on the site of the primary lesion. It has previously been reported that carcinomas arising in the right colon are distributed to the right lobe of the liver 10 times more commonly than to the left lobe, whereas liver metastases from carcinomas arising from the left colon and rectum are believed to be distributed homogenously. Wigmore et al[185] collected data prospectively on the anatomic site of hepatic metastases in 207 patients with colorectal metastases. This study could not find any evidence to support a differential pattern of metastasis within the liver dependent on the location of the primary colorectal carcinoma.

In an effort to accurately detect liver metastases, van Ooijen et al[186] prospectively compared continuous CT angiography to preoperative ultrasonography and conventional CT in 60 patients with primary or secondary colorectal carcinoma. The standard references were palpation of the liver and intraoperative ultrasonography. Continuous CT angiography had a high sensitivity of 94% in contrast to ultrasonography (48%) and conventional CT (52%). However, there was a higher false-positive rate because of variations in the perfusion of normal liver parenchyma. Overall, continuous CT angiography had the highest accuracy (74%) compared with ultrasonography (57%) and CT (57%). The low specificity will hamper its routine application.

Strasberg et al[187] reviewed 43 patients with metastatic colorectal carcinoma referred for hepatic resection after conventional staging with CT. PET scanning was performed on all patients. PET identified additional carcinoma not seen on CT in 10 patients. Operation was contraindicated in 6 of these patients because of the findings on PET. Laparotomy was performed in 37 patients. In all but 2, liver resection was performed. The Kaplan–Meier estimate of overall survival at 3 years was 77%. This figure is higher than the 3-year estimate of survival found in previously published series. They concluded that preoperative PET scan lessens the recurrence rate in patients undergoing hepatic resection for colorectal metastases to the liver by detection of disease not found on conventional imaging. Some patients who will not benefit from operation can thus be spared a laparotomy and major resection.

Liver surgeons usually recommend against biopsy of colorectal liver metastases because of the risk of local dissemination. Rodgers et al[188] conducted a multicenter retrospective review of cases of colorectal liver metastases presenting for operation that had undergone a preoperative biopsy. Of 231 cases of colorectal metastases, 18.6% had undergone a preoperative biopsy. Evidence of dissemination related to the biopsy was 16%. Within the operative period (median 21 months), 3 of the 7 cases with evidence of dissemination and 11 of the 35 without dissemination were alive without disease. They concluded there is a significant risk of local dissemination with biopsy of colorectal liver metastases.

The value of intraoperative hepatic ultrasonography was discussed previously. Fuhrman et al[189] reported on the use of intraoperative ultrasonography in the assessment of porta hepatis lymph nodes and the evaluation of resection margins to determine whether this modality would improve the selection of patients likely to benefit from operation. Of 151 patients undergoing exploration, 30 patients were considered unresectable and 14 (9.2%) demonstrated by intraoperative ultrasonography. The authors concluded that intraoperative ultrasonography did, indeed, improve the selection process.

The question of what to do for patients with these metastases has been a matter of controversy. At one point, any suggestion of an operative approach to metastatic disease was deemed foolish by some. The natural history of untreated hepatic metastases confirms a median survival of 6 to 12 months and of 4.5 months if metastases are synchronous.[190,191,192] If not resected, 3-year survival rates ranged from 3 to 7% and only 1 to 2% of patients will survive for 5 years.[182] Six studies of the natural history of such metastases in a total of 1,151 patients described a 5-year survival rate of 3%. In a study of 484 untreated patients, 6 independent determinants of survival were identified in the following order: (1) percent liver volume replaced by carcinoma, (2) grade of malignancy of the primary lesion, (3) presence of extrahepatic disease, (4) mesenteric lymph node involvement, (5) serum carcinoembryonic antigen (CEA), and (6) patient age.[193] The prognosis is closely related to the extent of liver replacement.

A variety of chemotherapeutic regimens, including systemic chemotherapy and direct intraportal and intra-arterial modes of administration, have been attempted, all with limited and short (if any) benefit, but with the cost of considerable toxicity and anxiety. Systemic chemotherapy has resulted in response rate ranges of 18 to 28%,[194] and the median survival rate ranges of 8 to 14 months.[182] Other efforts have been directed at hepatic artery embolization, hepatic artery ligation, and even irradiation, all without significant worthwhile benefit.

The lack of effective therapeutic alternatives has made hepatic resection the primary treatment consideration. Indeed, worthwhile survival rates in selected patients have been reported (▶ Table 22.6).[195,196,197,198,199,200,201,202,203,204,205,206,207,208, 209,210,211,212,213,214] The timing and extent of operation varies. In the patient who presents with a synchronous lesion, which is amenable to operation, it appears appropriate to excise the lesion at the time of operation. If the lesion requires a major hepatic resection, the combination of partial hepatectomy and colectomy appears to be too great a task for one operation. After the colonic resection, if there is no other evidence of metastases and if a thorough evaluation, including a CT scan, has demonstrated removable disease, proceeding with resection is the treatment of choice. If the patient presents with metastatic disease at a later date, evaluation is necessary to ensure that the metastatic disease is confined; at the same time, evaluation should be performed to rule out the presence of recurrent disease at the area of the index carcinoma. The resection of hepatic metastases in patients with intra-abdominal extrahepatic disease is of no proven benefit.[215] Even with preoperative staging, as many as 26% of patients will have intra-abdominal extrahepatic metastases, most commonly in portal and celiac lymph nodes.[215] It is necessary to rule out evidence of other metastatic disease. Unfortunately, investigation of patients rarely unveils a solitary lesion. Only approximately 10% of patients develop metastases suitable for operation. In their study of the natural history of hepatic metastases from colorectal carcinoma, Wagner et al[216] found that the median survival rate for unresected solitary and multiple unilobar metastases was 21 and 15 months, respectively. Earlier series reported untreated patients to have a median survival of 6 to 12 months. It is understandable why hepatic resection became an attractive option.

Table 22.6 Survival following resection of hepatic metastasis

Author(s)	No. of patients	Survival (%)		Operative mortality (%)	Complication rate (%)
		3 y	5 y		
Hughes et al[195,a]	800		32		
Schlag et al[196]	122	40	30	4	34
Petrelli et al[197]	62		26	8	30
Doci et al[198]	100		30	5	41
Rosen et al[199]	280	47	25	4	
Nakamura et al[200]	31	45	45	3	16
Van Ooijen et al[201]	118		21	8	35
Gayowski et al[202]	204	43	32	1	
Scheele et al[203]	434	45	33	4	22
Fuhrman et al[189,b]	107		44	3	
Hananel et al[204]	26		31	0	66
Rougier et al[205]	123	35	21		
Wade et al[206]	133		26	4	
Wanebo et al[207]	74		24	7	35
Ohlsson et al[208]	111		25	4	
Fong et al[209]	1,001	57	37	3	31
Buell et al[210]	110	54	40	2	21
Elias et al[211]	111	38	20	4	28
Kato et al[212,c]	585		33		
Teh and Ooi[213]	96	71		0	7
Weber et al[214]	62	45	22	0	36

[a]Tumor registry of 24 institutions (24%, 5-year disease-free survival).
[b]Ultimate patient selection with intraoperative ultrasonography.
[c]Postoperative hepatic artery chemotherapy in 33% but no difference in survival noted in those with or without chemotherapy.

Surgical resection of primary colorectal carcinoma in patients with stage IV disease at initial presentation remains controversial. Although bowel resection to manage symptoms such as bleeding, perforation, or obstruction has been advocated, management of asymptomatic patients has not been well defined. Patient-dependent factors (performance status, comorbid disease) and extent of distant metastases are among the considerations that have an impact on the decision to proceed with operative management in asymptomatic stage IV colorectal carcinoma. To ascertain the natural history of a group of untreated patients and to evaluate simultaneously in another group whether or not the administration of systemic chemotherapy modifies this natural history, Luna-Perez et al[218] followed up 77 patients with liver metastases from colorectal carcinoma. Untreated patients consisted of 45 patients; 41 developed extrahepatic metastatic disease and their median survival rate was 13 months. The group who received chemotherapy included 32 patients; 29 developed extrahepatic metastatic disease and their median survival was 15 months. There were no differences in overall survival in both groups. The administration of systemic chemotherapy did not modify the natural course of the disease. Dismal results of this nature mandate a better form of

therapy, namely, operative. Ruo et al[219] reviewed 127 patients who underwent elective resection of their asymptomatic primary colorectal carcinoma. Over the same time period, 103 stage IV patients who did not undergo resection were identified. The resected group could be easily distinguished from the nonresected group by a higher frequency of right colon carcinomas and metastatic disease restricted to the liver or one other site apart from the primary carcinoma. Resected patients had prolonged median (16 vs. 9 months) and 2-year (25 vs. 6%) survival compared with patients who were never resected. Univariate analysis identified three significant prognostic variables (number of distant sites involved, metastases to liver only, and volume of hepatic replacement by malignancy) in the resected group. Volume of hepatic replacement was also a significant predictor of survival. Subsequent to resection of asymptomatic primary colorectal carcinoma, 20% developed postoperative complications. Median hospital stay was 6 days. Two patients (1.6%) died within 30 days of operation. They concluded stage IV patients selected for elective palliative resection of asymptomatic primary colorectal carcinomas had substantial postoperative survival that was significantly better than those never having resection.

A review by Blumgart and Fong[182] revealed an operative mortality of less than 5% in most series, but complications arose in excess of 20% in most series. Myocardial complications were seen in 1%, pleural effusion requiring thoracotomy in 5 to 10%, pneumonia in 5 to 22%, and pulmonary embolism in 1%. Complications specifically related to liver resection included liver failure (3–8%), bile leak and biliary fistula (4%), perihepatic abscess (2–10%), and significant hemorrhage (1–3%). The most common sites for failure were the liver and lung with the liver involved as a site of recurrence in 45 to 75% of patients having liver resection. In light of this, adjuvant systemic chemotherapy seems to be an attractive option, but to date its role is unproven. Because the liver is the most common site of recurrence and may be the sole site in up to 40% of patients, regional hepatic chemotherapy is theoretically attractive, but studies in this arena have also failed to prove the benefit of that therapy. However, some studies are encouraging.

The prognosis of metastatic carcinoma is grave. Kuo et al[220] collected data from 74 patients with stage IV colorectal carcinoma to identify prognostic factors for predicting selection criteria for operative treatment in patients with metastatic disease. Overall survival time was 16.1 months. Survival in the curative resection group was significantly longer than in the noncurative groups (31.9 vs. 12.7 months). The operative mortality and morbidity rates were 5.6 and 21%, respectively. The two most common complications were leakage at the site of anastomosis and urinary tract infection. Based on these results, they concluded that patients older than 65 years with metastases at multiple sites, intestinal obstruction, preoperative CEA level 2,500 ng/mL, lactate dehydrogenase 2,350 units/L, hemoglobin less than 10 mg/dL, or hepatic parenchymal replacement by metastatic disease greater than 25% have poor prognosis for operative intervention. They noted the more aggressively they performed radical resection and metastasectomy in selected patients, the more survival benefits the patients obtained.

Simultaneous Colorectal and Hepatic Resection

Weber et al[214] reported that in selected patients, simultaneous resection of the colorectal primary carcinoma and liver metastases does not increase mortality or morbidity rates compared with delayed resection, even if a left colectomy and/or a major hepatic resection are required. de Santibañes et al[221] reviewed the results of liver resection performed simultaneously with colorectal resection in 71 cases. The median hospital stay was 8 days. Morbidity was 21% and included nine pleural effusions, seven wound abscesses, four instances of hepatic failure, three systemic infections, three intra-abdominal abscesses, and one colonic anastomotic leakage. Operative mortality was 0%. Recurrence rate was 57.7% and progression of disease was detected in 33.8%. Overall and disease-free survivals at 1, 3, and 5 years were 88, 45, and 38% and 67, 17, and 9%, respectively. Prognostic factors with notable influence on patient outcomes were nodal stage as per TNM classification, number of liver metastases, diameter (smaller or larger than 5 cm), liver resection specimen weight (lighter or heavier than 90 g), and liver resection margin (smaller or larger than 1 cm).

Chua et al[222] retrospectively analyzed 96 consecutive patients with synchronously recognized primary carcinoma and hepatic metastases who underwent concurrent (64 patients) or staged

(32 patients) colonic and hepatic resections. No significant differences were observed between concurrent and staged in type of colon resection or hepatic resection, overall operative duration, blood loss, volume of blood products transfused, perioperative morbidity (53 vs. 41%), disease-free survival from date of hepatectomy (median 13 vs. 13 months), or overall survival from date of hepatectomy (median 27 vs. 34 months). There was no operative mortality. Overall duration of hospitalization was significantly shorter for concurrent than for staged resection (mean 11 vs. 22 days). They concluded that concurrent colectomy and hepatectomy is safe and more efficient than staged resection and should be the procedure of choice for selected patients in medical centers with appropriate capacity and experience.

Tocchi et al[223] reviewed the results of 78 patients who underwent resection of primary colorectal carcinoma and hepatic metastases with curative intent. Adverse predictors of the long-term outcome included the number of metastases (> 3), preoperative CEA value greater than 100 ng/mL, resection margin less than 10 mm, and portal nodal status.

Tanaka et al[224] reported on 39 consecutive patients with synchronous colorectal carcinoma metastases to the liver who underwent curative simultaneous "one-stage" hepatectomy and resection of the colorectal primary. Only the volume of the resected liver was selected as a risk factor for postoperative complications (350 g mean resected liver volume in patients with postoperative complications vs. 150 g in those without complications). Patient age of 70 years or older and poorly differentiated mucinous adenocarcinoma as the primary lesion predicted decreased overall survival. They concluded that a one-stage procedure appears desirable for synchronous colorectal hepatic metastases except for patients requiring resection of more than one hepatic section, patients aged 70 years or older, and those with poorly differentiated or mucinous adenocarcinomas as primary lesions.

Currently, there is no consensus as to which factors are important in selecting patients for operation and which factors are important in determining the patient's prognosis. For example, Attiyeh and Wichern[225] found no significant difference in the survival rates of patients with a solitary metastasis and in those with multiple lesions, nor was survival influenced by the size of the metastasis. The survival rate was better in patients whose primary colorectal lesion was Dukes' B compared with those whose lesion was Dukes' C. Adson[226] listed several determinants for a favorable prognosis, including (1) primary colorectal carcinoma of limited locoregional extent (Dukes' A or B), (2) presence of fewer than four liver lesions, (3) metastases that appear a long time after the primary lesion was removed, (4) lesions that can be removed with wide margins, and (5) lack of extrahepatic metastases. Combining their own experience with reports in the literature, Bozzetti et al[227] found that sites of failure after liver resection were hepatic in 16%, extrahepatic in 15%. and both in 14%. Patterns of recurrence in our patients were hepatic in 31%, hepatic and an extrahepatic site in 15%, and lung in 15%.[204] Nagorney[191] reported that the only characteristic associated with prolonged survival was the stage of the primary lesion, with Dukes' B patient survival being greater than Dukes' C. In Nagorney's review, site of origin and degree of differentiation of the primary carcinoma did not correlate with survival rate.

Characteristics of metastatic disease that influenced survival included the number of hepatic metastases (one to three are better than four or more), the interval between diagnosis of the primary lesion and hepatic metastases, the resection margin (a margin > 1 cm is better), and the presence of extrahepatic disease. The size and distribution of lesions within the liver had no association with survival. We were also interested in variables related to survival and reviewed 26 selected patients with liver colorectal metastases who underwent hepatic resection.[204] The patient's age, sex, site of primary lesion, histologic grade, lymph node involvement, location, size, and number of hepatic metastases, type of hepatic resection, and preoperative CEA blood levels were documented. Complete removal with histologically negative resection margins were accomplished in 24 patients. The extent of resection performed was hepatic lobectomy in 12 patients, segmentectomy in 8 patients, and wedge resection in 4 patients. The 5-year survival rate was 30.5%. Patients with metachronous metastases had a better survival rate than those with synchronous lesions (46.6 vs. 13.6%, respectively). None of the other factors studied showed a significant effect on survival. During a median follow-up of 30.9 months, 20 patients developed recurrence of their disease (60% in the liver). There was no perioperative mortality. Morbidity arose in 66% of patients, with a majority of the complications minor. Wanebo et al[207] reported a significant relationship with survival and the number of metastases (three or fewer vs. four or more), the presence of bilobar versus unilobar metastases, and the extent of liver resection (wedge and segmental vs. lobectomy and trisegmentectomy). They believe that resection of bilobar disease or extended resection should generally be avoided, especially in medically compromised patients. Nakamura et al[200] adopted a very aggressive approach for patients suffering from liver metastases. Of 31 patients, 22 underwent lymph node dissection of the hepatic hilus, in the minds of most surgeons, a current contraindication to hepatic resection.

Six of the 22 patients who underwent lymph node dissection had nodes positive for carcinoma. Ten patients underwent removal of recurrent lesions in the liver, lung, adrenal glands, and brain after initial hepatic resection. Based on an overall 5-year survival rate of 45%, the authors concluded that repeat hepatectomy and dissection of hilar lymph nodes improves prognosis in selected patients with hepatic metastases of colorectal carcinoma.

In an analysis of risk factors, Gayowski et al[202] found that gender, Dukes' classification, site of primary colorectal carcinoma, histologic differentiation, size of metastatic lesion, and intraoperative transfusion requirement were not statistically significant prognostic factors. In patients 60 years of age or older, an interval of 24 months or less between colorectal and hepatic resection, four or more metastatic lesions, bilobar involvement, positive resection margins, lymph node involvement, and the direct invasion of adjacent organs were significant poor prognostic factors.

Hughes et al[195] collated information from a registry of 24 participating institutions. Factors that they found to affect prognosis detrimentally were (1) more than four metastatic lesions, (2) a short disease-free interval from initial resection to appearance of metastases (< 1 year), (3) a pathologic margin of less than 1 cm on the liver specimen, and (4) the presence of lymph node metastases at the time of initial resection.

Using a multivariate regression analysis, Scheele et al[203] found that survival was dependent on the presence of satellite metastases, grade of the primary carcinoma, time of the diagnosis of metastases (synchronous vs. metachronous), diameter of the largest metastases (> 5 cm), anatomic versus nonanatomic approach, year of resection, and mesenteric lymph node involvement. Rougier et al[205] studied 544 patients with resected hepatic metastases from colorectal carcinoma to determine prognostic factors. Among the 20 variables assessed, 8 items were singled out. In decreasing order of relative risk, they included performance status (2–4 vs. 0–1), alkaline phosphatase level (greater than normal vs. normal), number of involved segments (24 vs. 3), chemotherapy (no vs. yes), extrahepatic metastases (yes vs. no), primary location (right vs. other), prothrombin time (< 75 vs. > 75%), and resection of the primary carcinoma (no vs. yes). Specific criteria for the selection process are constantly evolving. Adson[226] has offered a thoughtful set of guidelines. Patients whose primary colorectal lesions are well confined, who have one to three evident unilobar hepatic metastases that likely can be removed with wide margins, and who have no evidence of extrahepatic metastases should undergo resection. Patients with extrahepatic metastases, numerous hepatic metastases involving more than one-half of the liver, large lesions that encroach on major hepatic veins, or contralateral hilar ducts or veins or lesions sited so as to preclude resection with free margins have an unfavorable prognosis and should not undergo resection. Unfortunately, many patients do not fall neatly into one of these categories, and the surgeon must exercise considerable judgment in making a definitive recommendation.[227]

The role of neoadjuvant chemotherapy for patients with multiple (five or more) bilobar hepatic metastases irrespective of initial resectability is being considered with increased frequency. Tanaka et al[228] compared the outcome of hepatectomy alone with that of hepatectomy after neoadjuvant chemotherapy for multiple bilobar hepatic metastases from colorectal carcinoma. The outcome of 48 patients treated with neoadjuvant chemotherapy ,followed by hepatectomy was compared with that of 23 patients treated by hepatectomy alone. Patients who received neoadjuvant chemotherapy had better 3- and 5-year survival rates from the time of diagnosis than those who did not (67.0 and 38.9% vs. 51.8 and 20.7%, respectively) and required few extended hepatectomies (four segments or more; 39 of 48 vs. 23 of 23). In patients with bilateral multiple colorectal liver metastases, neoadjuvant chemotherapy before hepatectomy was associated with improved survival and enabled complete resection with fewer extended hepatectomies.

Allen et al[229] compared the treatment and outcome in patients referred for staged resection of synchronous colorectal liver metastases between patients who did not receive neoadjuvant chemotherapy and had exploratory operations after recovery from colon resection and patients who did receive chemotherapy before liver resection. Neoadjuvant chemotherapy was given to 52 patients; in 29 of them, the disease did not progress, but in 17 the disease progressed while they were receiving treatment. Median follow-up was 30 months. Five-year survival was statistically similar between patients who received and did not receive neoadjuvant therapy (43 vs. 35%). Patients within the neoadjuvant group whose disease did not progress while they were receiving chemotherapy experienced significantly improved survival as compared to patients who did not receive chemotherapy (85 vs. 35%). In the setting of synchronous colorectal metastases, the response to neoadjuvant chemotherapy may be a prognostic indicator of survival and may assist in the selection of patients for conventional or experimental adjuvant therapies.

Fong et al[209] reported on 1,001 consecutive patients undergoing liver resection for metastatic colorectal carcinoma. These resections included 237 trisegmentectomies, 394 lobectomies, and 370 resections encompassing less than a lobe. The operative mortality rate was 2.8%. The 5-year survival rate was 37% and the 10-year survival rate was 22%. Seven factors were found to be significant and independent predictors of poor long-term outcome: positive margin, extrahepatic disease, node-positive primary, disease-free interval from primary to metastases less than 12 months, number of hepatic lesions greater than 1 cm, largest hepatic lesion greater than 5 cm, and CEA level greater than 200 ng/mL. When the last five of these criteria were used in a preoperative scoring system, assigning 1 point for each criterion, the total score was highly predictive of outcome. The 5-year actuarial survival for patients with 0 points was 60%, 1 point was 44%, 2 points was 40%, 3 points was 20%, 4 points was 25%, and 5 points was 14%. In fact, no patient with 5 points survived 5 years. Patients with up to two criteria can have a favorable outcome. Patients with three, four, or five criteria should be considered for experimental adjuvant trials.

Iwatsuki et al[230] examined various clinical and pathologic risk factors in 305 consecutive patients who underwent primary hepatic resection for metastatic colorectal carcinoma. Preliminary multivariate analysis revealed that independently significant negative prognosticators were (1) positive surgical margins, (2) extrahepatic carcinoma involvement including the lymph nodes, (3) three or more metastatic lesions, (4) bilobar metastases, and (5) time from treatment of the carcinoma to hepatic recurrence of 30 months or less. Because the survival rates of the 62 patients with positive margins or extrahepatic metastases were uniformly very poor, multivariate analysis was repeated in the remaining 243 patients who did not have these lethal risk factors. The reanalysis revealed that independently significantly poor prognosticators were (1) three or more metastases, (2) metastases size greater than 8 cm, (3) time to hepatic recurrence of 30 months or less, and (4) bilobar metastases. Risk scores (R) for recurrence were divided into five groups: grade 1, no risk factors; grade 2, one risk factor; grade 3, two risk factors; grade 4, three risk factors; and grade 5, four risk factors. Grade 6 consisted of the 62 culled patients with positive margins or extrahepatic metastases. Estimated 5-year survival rates of grade 1 to 6 patients were 48.3, 36.6, 19.9, 11.9, 0, and 0%, respectively. The proposed risk-score grading predicted the survival differences.

Smith et al[231] found that in patients who are undergoing curative resection of hepatic colorectal metastases, an elevated expression of the biomarkers hTERT and Ki-67 are better predictors of poor long-term survival than is a score based on clinical features. Kato et al[212] reported on 585 patients who underwent hepatectomy at 18 institutions. The 5-year survival rate for those treated by hepatectomy was significantly higher (32.9%) than for those not undergoing hepatectomy (3.4%). After hepatectomy for hepatic metastases, the most prevalent form of recurrence was in the remnant liver (41.4%), followed by recurrence of pulmonary metastases (19.2%), and other

(7.2%). Factors of the primary carcinoma that adversely affect prognosis included poorly differentiated adenocarcinoma or mucinous carcinoma, depth of invasion, lymph node metastases of stage n3 and n4 by the Japanese classification of colorectal carcinoma, number of metastatic lymph nodes of more than four, and Dukes' stage D. Factors at the time of hepatectomy adversely affecting prognosis after operation for hepatic metastases included residual carcinoma, extrahepatic metastases, hepatic metastases of degree H3 stipulated by the Japanese classification of colorectal carcinoma, number of metastases of four or more, pathology of hepatic metastases of poorly differentiated carcinoma, resection margin of less than 10 mm, and CEA value higher than normal preoperative and 1-month postoperative.

Indications for hepatectomy in patients with four or more hepatic colorectal metastases remain controversial. Imamura et al[232] reviewed data from 131 patients who underwent a total of 198 hepatectomies. Patients were grouped according to the number of metastases. The 5-year survival rate of patients with 1 to 3, 4 to 9, and 10 or more metastases were 51, 46, and 25%, respectively. They concluded hepatic resection for patients with four to nine metastases clearly is warranted. On the other hand, in high volume centers at which the operative mortality rate is nearly zero, the presence of 10 or more nodules may not be an absolute contraindication to surgical therapy.

In the review by Jaeck[233] the 5-year survival rate for resection of colorectal liver metastases ranged from 20 to 54%. However, the resectability rate of colorectal liver metastases is reported to be less than 20%. This limitation is mainly due to insufficient remnant liver and to extrahepatic disease. Among extrahepatic locations, lymph node metastases are often considered indications of a very poor prognosis and a contraindication to resection. He found that the presence of hepatic pedicle lymph node metastases ranged from 10 to 20%. When located near the hilum and along the hepatic pedicle, they should not be considered an absolute contraindication to resection, and extended lymphadenectomy should be performed. However, when they reach the celiac trunk, there is no survival benefit after resection of colorectal liver metastases.

Elias et al[234] reported the long-term outcome and prognostic factors of 75 patients who underwent a complete R0 resection of extrahepatic disease simultaneously with hepatectomy for colorectal liver metastases. Extrahepatic disease localization included peritoneal carcinomatosis (limited), hilar lymph nodes, local recurrences, retroperitoneal nodes, lung, ovary, and abdominal wall. The mortality rate was 2.7% and morbidity was 25%. After a median follow-up of 4.9 years, the overall 3- and 5-year survival rates were 45 and 28%, respectively. They concluded extrahepatic disease in colorectal carcinoma patients with liver metastases should no longer be considered as a contraindication to hepatectomy. However, there must be an intended R0 resection, and it is inappropriate for patients with multiple extrahepatic disease sites or more than five liver metastases.

The optimal operative strategy for the treatment of synchronous resectable colorectal liver metastases has not been defined. Martin et al[235] reviewed their experience with 240 patients who were treated surgically for primary adenocarcinoma of the large bowel and synchronous hepatic metastasis. One hundred thirty-four patients underwent simultaneous resection of a colorectal primary and hepatic metastases in a single operation (group 1), and 106 patients underwent staged operations (group 2). Simultaneous resections tend to be performed for right colon primaries, smaller, and fewer liver metastases, and less extensive liver resection. Complications were less common in the simultaneous resection group, with 49% sustaining 142 complications compared with 67% sustaining 197 complications for both hospitalizations in the staged resection group. Patients having simultaneous resection required fewer days in hospital (median 10 vs. 18 days). Perioperative mortality was similar (3 each in simultaneous and staged). They believe simultaneous resection should be considered a safe option in selected patients with resectable synchronous colorectal metastases.

Nelson and Freels[236] assessed the effect of posthepatic resection with hepatic artery chemotherapy on overall survival. Trials were sought in Medline, the Cochrane Controlled Trial Register, the Cochrane Hepatobiliary Group Trials Register, and through contact of trial authors and reference lists using key words. Overall survival at 5 years in the hepatic artery group was 45 and 40% in the control group. No significant advantage was found in the meta-analysis for hepatic artery and chemotherapy measuring overall survival. Adverse events related to hepatic artery therapy were common including five therapy-related deaths. They concluded that this added intervention for the treatment of metastatic colorectal carcinoma cannot be recommended at this time.

Clancy et al[237] conducted a meta-analysis of prospective clinical trials to determine if adjuvant hepatic arterial infusion confers a survival benefit to treat residual microscopic disease after curative hepatic resection for colorectal carcinoma metastases. Prospective clinical trials comparing hepatic arterial chemotherapy after curative hepatic resection for colorectal carcinoma metastases against a control arm were included. The outcome measure was survival difference at 1 and 2 years after operation. Seven studies met the inclusion criteria, and all except one were randomized trials. The survival difference in months was not statistically significant at 2 years. Based on these findings, they concluded routine adjuvant hepatic artery infusion after curative resection for colorectal carcinoma of the liver cannot be recommended.

Bines et al[238] reported on a review of 131 patients who underwent hepatic resection for metastatic colorectal carcinoma. There were 31 recurrences and, of those, 13 underwent re-resection with a morbidity rate of 23%, a mortality rate of 8%, and a 5-year survival rate of 23%. The authors concluded that in properly selected patients, repeat resection yields results similar to those after initial resection. Wanebo et al[207] reported that 12% of their patients had repeated resection of metastases, with an overall 5-year survival rate of 43% after the first resection and 22% after the second resection. In their review of 10 reports, Blumgart and Fong[182] noted that between 15 and 40% of patients who undergo resection for hepatic metastases have the liver as the sole site of recurrence, and approximately one-third will be candidates for further resection. In the 146 patients collated, the operative mortality rate was 3%, and the complications encountered were similar to those that developed after initial resection. These results were in highly selected patients. The median survival was greater than 30 months when calculated from the time of second liver resection and greater than

47 months when calculated from the time of the first resection. However, there were only four 5-year survivors. Although resection is feasible, only approximately 5% of all patients undergoing further resection will come to a second resection.[182] Wanebo et al[239] reported recurrence rates in 65 to 85% of patients after initial hepatectomy for metastases for colorectal carcinoma. Approximately one-half of these have liver metastases and in 20 to 30% only the liver is involved. The opportunity for resection is frequently limited because of diffuse liver disease or extrahepatic extension, and only approximately 10 to 25% of these patients have conditions amenable to resection. The authors' comprehensive review of the 28 series showed that the mean interval between the first and second liver resections varied from 9 to 33 months and was approximately 17.5 months in the two largest series. The median survival in the series reporting 10 or more patients was 19 months (mean, 24 months), which is comparable to data in the single resection series. In the large French Association series containing 1,626 patients with single resections and 144 patients with two resections, the 5-year survival rates were 25 and 16%, respectively. The recurrence rate after repeat resection was high (> 60%), and half of the recurrences were in the liver. The prognostic factors favoring repeat resection are variable, but they include absence of an extrahepatic extension of carcinoma and a complete resection of liver metastases. The authors concluded that repeat hepatic liver resection for metastatic colorectal carcinoma in carefully selected patients appears warranted. From their own experience and review of the literature, Pinson et al[240] came to the same conclusion. For patients collected from the literature, the authors constructed a survival curve (▶ Fig. 22.31). Fernández-Trigo et al[241] were also encouraged to perform repeat hepatic resections for colorectal metastases because it remains the only curative treatment. Others concur with this course of management.[242]

Takahashi et al[243] reviewed clinical data of patients undergoing repeat hepatectomy for metastatic colorectal carcinoma compared with those of initial hepatectomy to determine criteria for

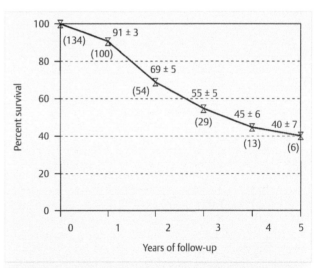

Fig. 22.31 Survival curve for 134 patients undergoing second hepatic operations for colorectal metastasis (collected from 15 reports in the literature).[240] (Reproduced with permission from Wolters Kluwer.)

repeat hepatectomy. For 22 patients who underwent repeat hepatectomy, no mortality and an 18% morbidity rate were observed. The 3-year survival rate after hepatectomy was 49%. The only poor prognostic factor after repeat hepatectomy was a serum CEA level greater than 50 ng/mL before initial hepatectomy. Suzuki et al[244] assessed the risks and clinical benefits of repeat hepatectomy for those patients who underwent hepatectomy for colorectal metastases. There was no operative mortality after repeat hepatectomy in 26 patients. Operative bleeding was significantly increased in the second hepatectomy, but operating time, duration of hospital stay, and performance status after the second hepatectomy were comparable with those of the initial hepatectomy. The median survival time from the second hepatectomy was 31 months and the 3- and 5-year survival rates were 62 and 32%, respectively. A short disease-free interval (6 months or less) between the initial hepatectomy and diagnosis of hepatic recurrence in the remnant liver was significantly associated with poor survival after the second hepatectomy. Oshowo et al[245] conducted a study aimed to compare outcome in patients with solitary colorectal liver metastases treated by operation ($n = 20$) or by radiofrequency ablation. Most patients in both groups also received systemic chemotherapy. Median survival after liver resection was 41 months with a 3-year survival of 55.4%. There was one postoperative death and morbidity was minimal. Median survival after radiofrequency ablation was 37 months with a 3-year survival of 52.6%. In this study, survival after resection or radiofrequency ablation of solitary colorectal liver metastases was comparable. The latter is less invasive and requires either an overnight stay or day-case facilities only.

Berber et al[246] determined the predictors of survival at the time of laparoscopic radiofrequency thermal ablation in 135 patients with colorectal liver metastases who were not candidates for resection. The median survival for all patients was 28.9 months. Patients with a CEA less than 200 ng/mL had improved survival compared to those with a CEA more than 200 ng/mL (34 vs. 16 months). Patients with the dominant lesion less than 3 cm in diameter had a median survival of 38 versus 34 months for lesions 3 to 5 cm, and 21 months for lesions greater than 5 cm. Survival approached significance for patients with one to three metastases versus more than three metastases (29 vs. 22 months). The presence of extrahepatic disease did not affect survival. Only the largest liver metastases more than 5 cm was found to be a significant predictor of mortality with a 2.5-fold increased risk of death versus the largest liver metastases less than 3 cm in size.

Ueno et al[247] collected data from 68 patients who underwent resection of colorectal liver metastases who might benefit from prophylactic regional chemotherapy. The extrahepatic recurrence rate at 3 years after hepatectomy was 57.8%. Three variables were independently associated with extrahepatic recurrence including raised serum level of CEA after hepatectomy (relative risk 5.4), venous invasion of the primary carcinoma (relative risk 4.0), and high-grade budding of the primary carcinoma (relative risk 3.1). Patients with none of these risk factors had a 3-year extrahepatic recurrence rate of 7.1% compared with 61.6% for those with one risk factor and 100% for those with two or three risk factors. This system might be used on an individual basis to select patients with colorectal liver metastases for regional chemotherapy or systemic chemotherapy after operative intervention. The value of postoperative chemotherapy following resection of hepatic metastases was reviewed by Cohen and Kemeny.[248] Two studies compared hepatic artery infusion with no treatment and no overall survival benefit was reported. In one study, there was a modest 2-year survival improvement from 72 to 86%. Drugs used included floxuridine (FUDR), and 5-FU/LV, and in light of newer drugs used for systemic chemotherapy, this improvement may not be relevant. For patients with unresectable liver metastases, Gray et al[249] reported on the use of embolization of yttrium-90-containing microspheres into the liver via a catheter inserted into the hepatic artery at laparotomy. In 29 patients, the CEA levels fell in the 26 patients in whom this therapy was tested, and there was CT evidence of reduction in 48% of the 22 patients re-examined. Some patients also received continuous chemotherapy infusion to potentiate the radiation effect. Although this is an important first step, there is no evidence that reduction of disease is translated to either improved survival or quality of life. Stubbs et al[250] treated 50 patients with advanced nonresectable colorectal liver metastases with selective internal radiation therapy. Estimated liver involvement was less than 25% in 30 patients, 25 to 50% in 13 patients, and greater than 50% in 7 patients. A single dose of between 2.0 and 3.0 GBq of 90-yttrium microspheres was injected into the hepatic artery via a subcutaneous port and followed at 4-week intervals by regional chemotherapy with 5-FU. Treatment-related morbidity did occur including a 12% incidence of duodenal ulceration. Median survival for patients with extrahepatic disease was 6.9 months. For patients with no extrahepatic disease, median survival was 17.5 months. Substantial destruction of liver metastases can be achieved in more than 90% of patients with a single treatment. Lang and Brown[251] recommended the selective embolization of doxorubicin and ethiodized oil for unresectable hepatic metastases. In his review, Stuart[252] found that chemoembolization for patients with metastatic colorectal carcinoma appears to be a reasonable alternative for many who are not operative candidates. Response rates of approximately 50% have been reported, with survival longer than would be expected in studies of systemic therapy among patients who had failed standard chemotherapy. Survival may be especially enhanced in treated patients who have no extrahepatic metastases.

Cryoablation has also been used in this clinical setting but has not yet been proven to improve outcome.[182] For patients with unresectable hepatic metastases, Weaver et al[253] reported the use of hepatic cryosurgery with or without resection in 140 patients, 119 of whom had carcinomas that were colorectal in origin. The median number of lesions treated was three. The operative mortality rate was 4%, and complications included coagulopathy, hypothermia, myoglobinuria, pleural effusion, acute tubular necrosis, and infection. The median survival rate was 27 months. Ruers et al[254] reported on the long-term efficacy of cryosurgery as an adjunct to hepatic resection in patients with colorectal liver metastases not amenable to resection alone. Thirty patients met the following inclusion criteria: metastases confined to the liver and judged unresectable, 10 or fewer metastases, cryosurgery alone or in combination with hepatic resection allowed disease clearance. Median follow-up was 26 months. Overall, 1- and 2-year survival rates were 76 and 71%, respectively. Median survival was 32 months.

Disease-free survival rates at 1 and 2 years were 35% and 7%, respectively. Six patients developed recurrence at the site of cryosurgery; given that the total number of cryosurgery-treated lesions was 69, the local recurrence rate was 9%.

Lung

Pulmonary metastases occur in approximately 10% of all patients with adenocarcinoma of the colon and rectum, and the majority of these are only one facet of a generalized spread of disease. About 10% of these patients, that is, 1% of the total, will develop solitary pulmonary metastases. The criteria for determining resectability of pulmonary metastases are similar to those applied to resection of hepatic metastases:

- Ideally, the pulmonary metastasis should be solitary. If more than one is involved, the lesions should be confined to one lung; if bilateral, the lesion in each lung must be solitary.
- The primary colorectal carcinoma should be controlled locally.
- There should be no other evidence of metastases.
- The patient's medical condition should allow for thoracotomy and pulmonary resection.

A number of prognostic discriminants, including disease-free interval, number of metastases, grade, stage, and location of the primary carcinoma, age and sex of the patient, location of the pulmonary metastases, and type of pulmonary resection, have been examined. None is uniformly reliable in the management of a particular patient, and there is no agreement on the importance of each individual factor. The predictive value of the route of venous drainage on prognosis was investigated in a consecutive series of 44 patients who underwent curative resection of pulmonary metastases from colorectal carcinoma.[255] The primary lesion was located in the colon in 14 patients and in the upper third of the rectum in 11 patients, thus indicating blood drainage directed toward the portal vein (group I). In 10 and 9 cases, respectively, the initial growth was in the middle and lower third of the rectum with the venous outflow at least partially directed into the vena cava (group II). There was no obvious difference in the two groups regarding the initial site of carcinoma recurrence. The liver was involved in 4 of 15 patients failing in group I as opposed to 4 of 13 patients with hematogenous relapse in group II. Median survival and disease-free survival times were significantly longer in patients in group I (58.4 and 50.2 months, respectively) than in patients in group II (30.9 and 16.8 months, respectively), and even more pronounced in colon carcinoma patients (75.4 and 60.2 months, respectively) when compared with rectal carcinoma patients (31.0 and 17.9 months, respectively). In contrast, survival curves did not differ significantly when the two groups with different routes of drainage (5-year survival rate, 53 vs. 38%; 5-year disease-free survival rate, 43 vs. 37%), or carcinomas of the colon and rectum (5-year survival rate, 67 vs. 38%; 5-year disease-free survival rate, 60 vs. 32%), were compared using the log-rank test. The primary carcinoma site therefore does not become a major criterion in selecting patients for surgical resection.

Saclarides et al[256] reported on 23 patients who underwent 35 thoracotomies for metastatic colorectal carcinoma. The pulmonary disease was diagnosed within an interval of 0 to 105 months (average, 33.4 months) after colon resection. Fifteen patients underwent a single thoracotomy (12 patients had solitary lesions and 3 patients had multiple nodules). Eight patients underwent multiple thoracotomies. The median survival following thoracotomy was 28 months, the 3-year survival rate was 45%, and the 5-year survival rate was 16%. Factors that had no significant bearing on survival included the origin and stage of the primary carcinoma and the patient's age and sex. An interval before thoracotomy of 3 years had an impact on survival. Patients who underwent multiple thoracotomies had a significantly prolonged survival. Patients who underwent a single thoracotomy for a solitary lesion had a significantly prolonged survival compared with patients who underwent a single thoracotomy for multiple metastases. After thoracotomy, 14 patients eventually developed recurrent disease, which was confined to the lung in only 4 patients. Of these 14 patients, 11 subsequently died of carcinoma. The authors concluded that thoracotomy for metastatic disease should be considered when the primary carcinoma is controlled, the lungs are the only site of metastatic disease, and there is adequate lung reserve to withstand surgery.

In a review of 12 series of patients, including their own, Brister et al[257] summarized the results of 335 patients who underwent pulmonary resection. The authors found overall 2- and 5-year survival rates of 70 and 30%, respectively. In their series, the only factor significant in determining survival was a long disease-free interval. It seems logical that a longer disease-free interval reflects a slower growing malignancy and would in turn be associated with a longer post-thoracotomy survival. In a series of 76 pulmonary resections, Wade et al[206] found a projected 5-year survival rate of 36%, a mean survival rate of 38 months, and a 3% operative mortality rate.

Kanemitsu et al[258] studied factors that might be helpful in predicting survival in 313 patients (the largest number) with pulmonary metastases from colorectal carcinoma who were candidates for thoracotomy. Pulmonary resections included 137 lobectomies, 132 partial resections, 38 segmentectomies, and 6 pneumonectomies. Overall survival rates were 90.4% in 1 year, 53% at 3 years, and 38.3% at 5 years. The 1-, 3-, and 5-year survival rates of patients with pulmonary metastases from colorectal carcinoma who did not undergo thoracotomy were 58.6, 8.5, and 1.9%, respectively. They identified five variables as independent predictors of 3-year survival: prethoracotomy CEA level, number of pulmonary lesions, presence of hilar or mediastinal infiltrated lymph nodes, histology of the primary carcinoma, and presence of extrathoracic disease. Their model has moderate predictive ability to discriminate between patients who are likely to survive after thoracotomy for pulmonary metastases from colorectal carcinoma.

Watanabe et al[259] also reviewed 49 patients to identify prognostic factors for overall survival and risk factors for further intrapulmonary recurrence after resection of pulmonary metastases from colorectal carcinoma. Survival after resection of pulmonary metastases was 78% at 3 years and 56% at 5 years. Solitary pulmonary metastases were significantly correlated with survival. The pathological features of the primary colorectal carcinoma had no impact on survival. Histologically, incomplete resection of pulmonary metastasis significantly correlated with pulmonary re-recurrence.

Negri et al[260] reported on the development of a preoperative chemotherapy strategy for patients selected to undergo pulmonary metastasectomy from colorectal carcinoma in 31 patients.

The median age at operation was 61 years. Twenty (65%) proceeded directly to operation and 5 of these patients received postoperative chemotherapy. Eleven (35%) received preoperative chemotherapy, which consisted of fluoropyrimidine in combination with either oxaliplatin or mitomycin C, except for 1 patient who received single agent CPT-11; 82% had a partial response and 18% had stable disease. In total, 39 thoracic operations (6 bilateral and 1 incomplete) were undertaken. There were no postoperative deaths. Twenty percent who had initial operation had postoperative complications compared to 18% of the preoperative chemotherapy group. Overall 3- and 5-year survival rates after the first thoracic operation were 65.2 and 26.1%, respectively. Disease-free interval, number of pulmonary metastases, previous resection of hepatic metastases, prethoracotomy CEA, and preoperative chemotherapy were not found to be significant prognostic factors for survival. They concluded resection of lung metastases has a low morbidity and mortality and results in long-term survival for 20 to 30% of patients. Furthermore, in this clinical setting, preoperative chemotherapy produced a high response rate with no patients experiencing disease progression prior to operation.

King et al[261] assessed the safety and efficacy of imaging-guided percutaneous radiofrequency ablation for local control of lung metastases from colorectal carcinoma. Forty-four metastatic lesions in 19 patients were treated successfully at 25 treatment sessions. Five of 19 patients were retreated for new lesions. There were 13 pneumothoraces following the 25 treatments, and 6 patients required drainage. Six months after treatment, CT demonstrated that 3 lesions had progressed, 25 metastases were stable or smaller, and 11 were no longer visible. At 12 months, 5 metastases had progressed, 11 were smaller or stable, and 9 were not visible.

Retreatment for recurrence or new metastases is feasible and occurred in five patients in this series. Some patients also received concomitant chemotherapy. Improving long-term survival is not the only goal of treatment. Relief of symptoms such as cough, hemoptysis, and pain is also beneficial. Furthermore, survival benefit has been shown for repeat pulmonary metastasectomy.

Ike et al[262] evaluated results of their strategy for intensive follow-up after resection of colorectal carcinoma and aggressive resection of lung metastases. The follow-up program for lung metastases includes a serum CEA assay every 2 months and chest X-ray every 6 months. Operative resection of lung metastases was performed if the primary and any nonpulmonary metastases had been controlled, lung metastases numbered four or fewer, and pulmonary functional reserve was adequate. Standard operation for lung metastases was lobectomy and lymph node dissection was added in cases where the metastases were over 3 cm in size. Forty-two patients underwent 50 lung resections for metastatic colorectal carcinoma. Overall 5-year survival rate after resection of lung metastases from colorectal carcinoma was 63.7%. Patients with well-differentiated primary carcinoma, a solitary metastatic nodule, and disease-free interval of at least 2 years after initial operation are likely to be long-term survivors.

Ishikawa et al[263] reviewed retrospectively the clinical course of 37 patients who underwent operative resection of primary colorectal carcinoma and metastatic lung disease. Multivariate analysis indicated that the existence of an extranodal malignant deposit in the primary lesion (hazard ratio = 4.55) and three or more lung metastases (hazard ratio = 2.9) were significant indicators for poor prognosis. They divided the patients into two groups; group A (n = 12) had neither of these two parameters and group B (n = 25) comprised all other patients. Survival rate at 3 and 5 years were 90.9 and 90.9% in group A and 16.1 and 8.1% in group B, respectively; and disease-free survival after thoracotomy was as follows: 3- and 5-year disease-free survival rate, 52.9 and 39.7% in group A; 5.3 and 5.3% in group B. They identified an extranodal malignant deposit at the primary carcinoma site as a new significant prognostic factor after resection of pulmonary metastases from colorectal carcinoma. Resection of pulmonary metastases is expected to be very useful for patients without extranodal deposits and fewer than three pulmonary metastases.

Zink et al[264] reviewed medical records of 110 patients operated on for pulmonary metastases of colorectal origin. The median time interval between diagnosis of the primary carcinoma and thoracotomy was 35 months. After resection of the pulmonary metastases, the 3- and 5-year post-thoracotomy survival measured 57 and 32.6%, respectively. The overall survival was significantly correlated with the disease-free interval and the number of intrapulmonary metastases. Treatment, stage, and grade of the primary carcinoma, occurrence of liver metastases and local recurrences, mode of treatment of metastases, and postoperative residual stage had no significant correlation with either total or post-thoracotomy survival.

Irshad et al[265] reviewed 49 patients treated operatively for pulmonary metastases from colorectal carcinoma. The perioperative death rate was 4%. Overall 5- and 10-year survival rates were 55 and 40%, respectively. The mean interval between the initial colonic resection and resection of pulmonary metastases was 36 months. Variables that carried a poor prognosis included more than one pulmonary lesion, a disease-free interval less than 2 years, and moderately or poorly differentiated colorectal carcinoma. The 16 patients who received chemotherapy after their thoracotomy had a 5-year survival rate of 51% compared with 54% for the 33 patients who did not receive chemotherapy, demonstrating postoperative chemotherapy has no survival benefit.

Vogelsang et al[266] evaluated clinically relevant prognostic factors to define a subgroup of patients who would most benefit from resection of lung metastases from colorectal carcinoma. There were 75 patients with pulmonary metastases from colorectal carcinoma who underwent 104 R0 lung resections. Patients who had no evidence of recurrent extrathoracic disease, no more than three metastases on either side, lobectomy as the maximum operative procedure, and adequate cardiorespiratory function were eligible for operation. Overall median survival was 33 months with 3- and 5-year survival rates of 47 and 27%, respectively. Prognostic groups included patients with a maximum metastasis size of 3.75 cm or less with a disease-free interval of more than 10 months and patients with larger metastases and a shorter disease-free interval. Median survival and 5-year survival were 45 months and 39% in the former group and 24 months and less than 11% in the latter.

When a solitary pulmonary shadow occurs synchronously with a large bowel carcinoma, the dual problems of the nature of the pulmonary lesion and the priority of management arise. Based on the principles of management of metastatic lesions, this clinical situation should not be a dilemma. The large bowel malignancy should be handled without regard for the pulmonary lesion. If the surgeon achieves a curative resection, thus fulfilling the criterion of control of local disease, and there is no other evidence of metastatic disease, attention can be directed toward the pulmonary lesion, usually 2 or 3 months later. The pulmonary lesion may, in fact, prove to be a primary lung carcinoma.

Assessment of the contribution of surgery to the treatment of pulmonary metastases from carcinoma of the colorectum demonstrated that it is a valid treatment option with survival benefit. An aggressive operative policy directed toward metastatic carcinoma confined to the lung has resulted in a rewarding rate of disease-free survivals and appreciable palliative benefit for appropriately selected patients. Even multiple metastases may be successfully managed as long as the cardinal principles of patient selection are observed. Pulmonary resection is attended with little risk (operative mortality rates ranging from 0 to 4% and major complication rates from 0 to 12%); the survival results justify an aggressive operative approach.[256] Accordingly, patient follow-up should include regular chest X-ray examinations to detect subsequent metastases amenable to operative therapy.

Liver and Lung

Although simple lung or liver metastasectomy from colorectal carcinoma has proved effective in selected patients, the subject of simultaneous biorgan metastasectomies is seldom addressed. Mineo et al[267] reported on 29 patients who presented simultaneous ($n = 12$) or sequential liver before lung ($n = 10$) and lung before liver ($n = 7$) metastases. All metastases were successfully resected in a total of 56 separate procedures. In 35 thoracic procedures, 45 metastases were removed by wedge resection ($n = 36$) or lobectomy ($n = 9$). In addition, 47 liver metastases were resected with wedge ($n = 24$), segmentectomy ($n = 13$), or lobectomy ($n = 10$). There were no perioperative deaths and the morbidity rate was 10.7%. All patients were followed for a minimum of 3 years. Median survival from the second metastasectomy was 41 months, with a 5-year survival rate of 51.3%. Risk-factor distribution among the three metastatic pattern groups was insignificant. Premetastasectomy elevated levels of both CEA and CA19–9, and mediastinal or celiac lymph node status, were significantly associated with survival, although number of metastasectomies, disease-free interval, and simultaneous versus sequential diagnosis were not. In the multivariate analysis, only elevated CEA plus CA19–9 was significantly associated with survival. They concluded that either simultaneous or sequential lung and liver metastasectomy can be successfully treated by operation.

Ike et al[268] retrospectively analyzed 48 patients who underwent pulmonary resection for metastatic colorectal carcinoma, 27 of whom had lung metastases alone and 15 had previous partial hepatectomy, and 6 had previous resection of local or lymph node recurrence. Five-year survival rates after resection of lung metastases were 73% in patients without preceding recurrence, 50% following previous partial hepatectomy, and 0% after resection of previous local recurrence. There was no significant difference in survival after lung resection between patients who had sequential liver and lung resection versus those who had lung resection alone.

Nagakura et al[269] analyzed retrospectively a total of 136 patients who underwent resection of hepatic or pulmonary metastases of colorectal origin. Eighty-four patients underwent hepatectomy alone, 25 underwent pulmonary resection alone, and 27 underwent both hepatic and pulmonary resection. The 27 patients undergoing hepatic and pulmonary resections were divided into two groups: 17 patients with sequentially detected hepatic and pulmonary metastases and 10 patients with simultaneously detected metastases. Patient survival after hepatic and pulmonary resection was comparable with that after hepatic alone and that after pulmonary resection alone. Among the 27 patients undergoing hepatic and pulmonary resection, the outcomes after resection were significantly better in patients with sequentially detected metastases (cumulative 5-year survival of 44%) than in those with simultaneously detected ones (cumulative 5-year survival of 0%). They concluded patients with sequentially detected hepatic and pulmonary metastases from a colorectal primary are good candidates for aggressive metastasectomy, but simultaneous detection of these metastases does not warrant resection.

Ovary

The mechanism of spread of large bowel carcinoma to ovary is not clear. Postulated methods include implantation from intraperitoneal spread, hematogenous spread, and lymphatic dissemination. Immunostaining for cytokeratin 7 (CK7; positive in ovarian carcinoma) and cytokeratin 20 (positive in colorectal carcinoma) is a useful technique for making the distinction between the organs of origin.[270] The development of ovarian metastases was discussed in the section on treatment. Colon carcinoma may present as metastatic disease to the ovaries in a Krukenberg-like pattern.[271] Treatment consists of bilateral salpingo-oophorectomy (▶ Fig. 22.32). In a study of a series of patients who presented with what appeared to be primary ovarian neoplasms but actually were ovarian metastases from a colonic origin, Herrera-Ornelas et al[272] found that survival was similar to that of patients who were primarily diagnosed as having large bowel carcinoma and subsequently developed ovarian metastases. Average life expectancy after diagnosis was 16.5 months. In their review of 63 patients with metachronous ovarian metastases, Morrow and Enker[273] found that such disease was part of diffuse intra-abdominal disease in 55% of patients. The mean survival rate following operation was 16.6 months. Ability to remove all gross disease at the time of oophorectomy was the major determinant of survival. Patients rendered disease free had a mean survival of 48 months compared with 9.6 months in patients with unresectable disease. Morrow and Enker believe that bilateral oophorectomy is warranted as part of the palliative treatment of women with metastatic disease to prevent the development of large symptomatic metastases that require further therapy.

Huang et al[274] reviewed the impact of elective and therapeutic oophorectomy on the natural history of colorectal carcinoma. A total of 155 patients were studied. Synchronous ovarian metastases occurred in 90 patients (58.1%); metachronous ovarian metastases occurred in 41.9%. Estimated 5-year survival for patients with synchronous ovarian metastases was 9 versus 20% for metachronous ovarian metastases. Resection of metastatic disease was associated with an improved 5-year survival

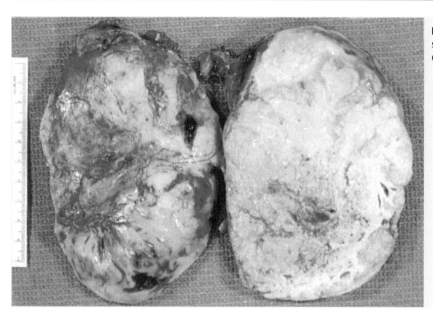

Fig. 22.32 Example of bilateral ovarian metastases in a patient presenting with acute colonic obstruction.

for synchronous ovarian metastases (15 vs. 0%) and metachronous ovarian metastases (24 vs. 0%) if patients were disease free postoperatively. Other clinical characteristics including age, menopausal status, stage, and location of primary carcinoma had no significant impact on survival. Thus, ovarian metastases from colorectal carcinoma are associated with a poor outcome. Although there is no survival advantage associated with resection of occult microscopic disease, long-term survival is possible if patients are rendered surgically disease free.

Bone

Metastases to the bone are usually associated with widely disseminated disease. Besbeas and Stearns[275] reported osseous involvement in 6.9% of patients, 5.1% as part of widespread metastases and 1.8% with skeletal metastases only. Sites of metastatic disease included the skull, scapula, clavicle, ribs, vertebrae, pelvic bones, humerus, and femur. The interval from initial diagnosis to manifestation of osseous metastases ranged from 10 months to 6 years and 11 months in that report. Bonnheim et al[276] reported a 4% incidence of osseous metastases. Scuderi et al[277] reported a case of sternal metastases as the initial presentation of an unknown rectal carcinoma. They stated osseous metastases occur in 3.8 to 10.5% of cases of rectal carcinoma. Isolated bony metastases are very rare and usually represent a late manifestation, being part of diffuse metastatic disease. Operation is an option in cases of solitary sternal localization but must be reserved for patients in good general condition. Treatment is directed toward pain control, and this is often achieved through radiotherapy. The mean period from onset of osseous metastases to death was 10 to 13.2 months.[275,276]

Brain

Wong and Berkenblit[278] reviewed therapeutic options and expected outcomes for patients with brain metastases. They reported that the median survival with no treatment was 1 to 2 months; with steroids 2 to 3 months; with whole-brain radiotherapy 3 to 6 months; with operation and whole-brain radiotherapy 10 to 16 months; with radiosurgery and whole-brain radiotherapy 6 to 15 months; and with chemotherapy 8 to 12 months. Because the majority of cytotoxic agents seem to be unable to penetrate the blood–brain barrier, the role of chemotherapy in the treatment of brain metastases remains controversial. A few of the newly developed cytotoxic agents can cross the blood–brain barrier and may have a role in the treatment of patients with brain metastases. They noted studies that demonstrated the antineoplastic activity of topotecan against brain metastases, with objective response rates ranging from 33 to 63% in patients with various solid malignancies mostly of lung origin. This result may be explained by the lack of exposure of brain metastases to previous cytotoxic agents, suggesting a role for topotecan in patients with brain metastases. Early studies have also suggested that topotecan, an apparent radiosensitizer, may be particularly effective in combination with radiotherapy, the current standard of care for patients with brain metastases. Alden et al[279] reviewed their experience with brain metastases from colorectal carcinoma. The authors identified 19 of their own patients and collected information from other reports. Fifty-eight percent of the patients had disseminated disease at initial diagnosis. The mean interval between treatment of the primary lesion and the diagnosis of brain metastases was 32.1 months. The brain was the sole site of metastatic disease in 21% of patients. Lesions were solitary in 63%, exclusively cerebral in 53%, cerebellar in 32%, or both in 15%. Presenting complaints ranged from ataxia (63%), headaches (21%), dizziness (26%), and weakness (32%) to seizures (16%), dysphasia (21%), and mental status changes (21%).

Diagnosis is established by CT scanning (▶ Fig. 22.33) or MRI. Treatment consists of steroids to decrease intracranial swelling and radiation or craniotomy in special circumstances. Survival is dismal with no 1-year survivors in the series of 19 patients reviewed by Alden et al.[279] The median survival rate following craniotomy was 4.9 months and following radiation was 2.6 months. Survival was not affected by the number or location of metastatic lesions or whether the brain was the sole site of metastatic disease. Because of the dismal survival rate, the authors believe that craniotomy is rarely indicated, except in the rare patient who has minimal neurologic impairment, a long

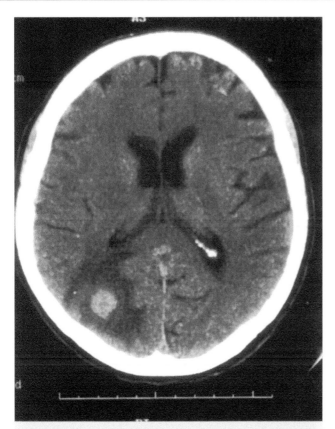

Fig. 22.33 CT scan demonstrating metastasis to brain. The hyperdense thick-walled lesion is surrounded by a "halo"-vasogenic (white matter) edema.

Peritoneal Carcinomatosis

Intraperitoneal carcinomatosis accounts for 25 to 35% of recurrences of colorectal carcinoma.[282] Studies demonstrate that peritoneal carcinomatosis is not necessarily a terminal condition with no options for treatment for cure. The combination of aggressive, cytoreductive surgery and intra-abdominal hyperthermia chemotherapy improves long-term overall survival in selected patients but is a time-consuming procedure and entails high mortality (5%) and morbidity (35%).[282] Most commonly used drugs are mitomycin C and platinum compounds, which have synergistic toxic effects on malignant cells when hyperthermia is applied. The three principal studies dedicated to the natural history of peritoneal carcinomatosis from colorectal carcinoma consistently showed median survival ranging between 6 and 8 months. Glehen et al[283] conducted a retrospective multicenter study to evaluate the international experience with cytoreductive surgery and perioperative intraperitoneal chemotherapy and to identify the principal prognostic indicators. The study included 506 patients from 28 institutions. The median age was 51 years. The median follow-up was 53 months. The morbidity and mortality rates were 22.9 and 4%, respectively. The overall median survival was 19.2 months. Patients in whom cytoreductive surgery was complete had a median survival of 32.4 months, compared with 8.4 months for patients in whom complete cytoreductive surgery was not possible. Positive independent prognostic indicators by multivariate analysis were complete cytoreduction, treatment by a second procedure, limited extent of peritoneal carcinomatosis, age less than 65 years, and use of adjuvant chemotherapy. The use of neoadjuvant chemotherapy, lymph node involvement, presence of liver metastases, and poor histologic differentiation were negative independent prognostic indicators.

Culliford et al[284] reported aggressive treatment of peritoneal metastases from colon carcinoma by surgical cytoreduction and infusional intraperitoneal chemotherapy may benefit select patients. There were 64 patients having surgical debulking and intraperitoneal (FUDR) plus LV for peritoneal metastases. Primary carcinoma sites were 47 in the colon and 17 in the appendix. Peritoneal metastases were synchronous in 48 patients and metachronous in 16 patients. Patients received intraperitoneal FUDR (1,000 mg/m^2 daily for 3 days) and intraperitoneal LV (240 mg/m^2) with a median cycle number of 4. The median number of complications was 1 with no treatment-related mortality. Only 9% required termination of intraperitoneal chemotherapy because of complications. The median follow-up was 17 months. The median survival was 34 months; 5-year survival was 28%. The 5-year survival was 54% for complete and 16% for incomplete resection.

Occasionally, a few discrete nodules on the peritoneum are present at the time of colonic resection and it would seem appropriate to excise these. Verwaal et al[285] conducted a randomized trial of cytoreduction and hyperthermia intraperitoneal chemotherapy versus systemic chemotherapy and palliative surgery in patients with peritoneal carcinomatosis of colorectal carcinoma. Of the 105 patients randomly assigned with a median follow-up of 21.6 months, the median 5-year survival was 12.6 months in the standard therapy arm and 22.3 months in the experimental therapy arm. The treatment-related mortality

disease-free interval, a solitary metastasis, and no extracranial disease. The authors believe that for most patients, radiation is the treatment of choice.

Hammoud et al[280] reported on 100 patients with brain metastases secondary to colorectal carcinoma. Of these patients, 36 underwent operation, 57 underwent radiotherapy alone, and the remaining 7 received steroids. The median interval between the diagnosis of the primary carcinoma and the diagnosis of brain metastasis was 26 months. The median survival time was 1 month for patients who received only steroids, 3 months for those who received radiotherapy, and 9 months for those who underwent operation. The early onset of brain metastases was associated with a poor prognosis.

Farnell et al[281] reported that brain metastases occur in 25 to 35% of all patients with malignancies, with colorectal carcinoma accounting for approximately 8% of these. Of 150 patients with brain metastases, 82% had concomitant extracerebral metastases, especially in the lungs. Only 16% of patients survived more than 1 year. The median survival rates for all patients receiving operation and radiotherapy,[43] operation alone,[11] radiotherapy alone,[82] and supportive care[17] were 42, 45, 16, and 8 weeks, respectively. Of the patients treated with radiotherapy, 30% showed regression and three had complete regression. Given the similar results in patients treated with operation plus radiotherapy and those treated with operation alone, the authors believe that consideration should be given to withholding radiotherapy to obviate its side effects.

in the aggressive therapy group was 8%. In their review of the literature of 11 other reports on similar therapy, median reported survival ranged from 6 to 39 months mostly in the 15-month rage, but the best series reported a 30% 5-year survival. Verwaal et al[286] reported updated data on 117 patients treated by cytoreduction and hyperthermic intraperitoneal chemotherapy. The median survival was 21.8 months. The 1-, 3-, and 5-year survival rates were 75, 28, and 19%, respectively. In 59 patients, a complete cytoreduction was achieved, and in 41 patients there was minimal residual disease. The median survival of these patient groups was 42.9 and 17.4 months, respectively. When gross macroscopic disease was left behind, as was the case in 17 patients, the median survival was 5 months. Involvement of the small bowel before cytoreduction was associated with poor outcome.

In patients with widespread peritoneal deposits, such an approach seems excessively aggressive. Improved outcomes for selected patients with peritoneal spread have been reported. Shen et al[287] reviewed their experience of cytoreductive surgery and intraperitoneal hyperthermic chemotherapy with mitomycin C in 77 patients. Peritoneal carcinomatosis was synchronous and metachronous in 27 and 73% of patients, respectively. Seventy-five percent of patients had received chemotherapy prior to intraperitoneal hyperthermic chemotherapy. Complete resection of all gross disease was accomplished in 48% of patients. Overall survival at 1, 3, and 5 years was 56, 25, and 17%, respectively. With a median follow-up of 15 months, the median overall survival was 16 months. Perioperative morbidity and mortality were 30 and 12%, respectively.

Hematologic toxicity occurred in 19%. Poor performance status, bowel obstruction, malignant ascites, and incomplete resection of gross disease were independent predictors of decreased survival. Patients with complete resection of all gross disease had a 5-year overall survival of 34% with a median overall survival of 28 months.

Elias et al[288] conducted a two-center prospective randomized trial comparing postoperative peritoneal chemotherapy plus systemic chemotherapy versus systemic chemotherapy alone, after complete cytoreduction surgery of colorectal peritoneal carcinomatosis. Analysis of 35 patients showed that complete resection of peritoneal carcinomatosis resulted in a 2-year survival of 60%, far above the classic 10% survival rate among patients with colorectal peritoneal carcinomatosis treated with systemic chemotherapy and symptomatic surgery. In this small series, postoperative intraperitoneal chemotherapy did not demonstrate any advantage for survival.

Other Metastatic Disease

Metastatic carcinoma that involves the spleen is usually a manifestation of widely disseminated disease, but solitary splenic metastases have been reported.[289] Cutaneous metastasis of rectal adenocarcinoma is a rare event occurring in fewer than 4% of all patients with rectal carcinoma.[290,291] When present, it typically signifies disseminated disease with a poor prognosis.[292] Metastatic colonic carcinoma may present in an old operative scar. Metastases to the glans penis,[293] pancreas,[294] and vagina (not contiguous disease)[295] have been reported. Metastatic colon carcinoma has even presented as a testicular hydrocele[296] or to the testis.[297]

22.4.14 Carcinoma in Young Patients

It has been reported that carcinoma of the colon occurring under the age of 40 years carries with it a poor prognosis. It has been suggested that this is due to the fact that patients present at a later stage in their development because the diagnosis had not been suspected. In a depressing report by Radhakrishnan and Bruce,[298] eight children with primary carcinoma of the colon presented with the common symptom being right iliac fossa pain. All children had poorly differentiated, highly aggressive lesions. In spite of operation and adjuvant therapy, all the children died within 1 year of presentation.

22.5 Postoperative Complications

The complications that may be encountered following colonic surgery are discussed in detail in Chapter 33. Nevertheless, one very detailed and extraordinarily carefully studied series of cases should be cited. Killingback et al[299] reviewed 1,418 elective resections with anastomoses by a single colorectal surgeon. Postoperative mortality was 1.6%. Significant adverse events, which were potentially avoidable, occurred in 45.5% of the patients who died. The morbidity rate was (41.6%). Clinical anastomotic leaks occurred more frequently in extraperitoneal anastomoses (4.7%) than in intraperitoneal anastomoses (0.2%). Anastomotic leak caused the death of two patients (0.14%). Routine prophylactic anticoagulation did not decrease the incidence of pulmonary embolism. Significant thrombophlebitis at the intravenous cannula site occurred in 3.8%, wound infection in 2.1%, and postural peripheral nerve injury in the upper limbs occurred in 0.8%. Unscheduled operations were required in 2.7% of patients. A classification of anastomotic leak is suggested to assist in comparisons of this complication, which remains a significant concern following extraperitoneal anastomoses.

22.6 Results

In an effort to determine the survival rate following operations for colon carcinoma, review of the plethora of reports makes the reader quickly realize that the literature consists of a maze of information. In attempting to compare the results from various institutions, it rapidly becomes apparent that a host of reporting methods have been used. For example, some authors present overall survival rates of all patients who present with colon carcinoma. Others present data only for those who underwent an operation, while still others present data only for those who presumably had a curative operation. Some authors present survival data for subsets of patients according to the Dukes classification, while others state that they are using the Dukes classification but, in fact, are using some variation of it, and therefore survival data are not comparable. Some reports use actuarial methods correcting the data for the age of the patients, thereby attempting to give a more accurate survival statistic. Some authors have used corrected 5-year survival rates by means of life tables to exclude deaths not due to carcinoma but caused by intercurrent disease. Presumably, this method is being used to increase the precision of reporting rather than making the survival statistics look better because, by definition, the corrected survival rate is always higher than the crude survival rate.

Estimates of survival are commonly used in the literature to describe outcomes in patients treated for carcinoma. Terms such as carcinoma-specific and carcinoma-free survival are frequently quoted although often without clear definitions. Platell and Semmens[300] compared survival estimates on the same population of patients but using different definitions of what constitutes an event. This was to highlight some of the variation that can occur when different techniques are used to perform these calculations. The study included 497 patients with a mean age of 68 years, and a male-to-female ratio of 1.3: 1. They were followed for a mean of 2.2 years. The various survivals at 5 years were as follows: (1) overall survival, 55.6%; (2) carcinoma-specific survival, 67%; (3) carcinoma-free survival, 49.9%; (4) recurrence-free survival, 43.5%; and (5) relative survival, 73.4%. The 5-year survival calculations for this group of patients with colorectal carcinoma varied by as much as 30% depending on how the data were censored. This highlights that there needs to be a clear and accountable definition on how survival curves are calculated and presented in the literature to allow for meaningful interpretation and comparisons.

It is not unreasonable to assume that figures quoted from major surgical centers would offer better survival rates because a higher standard of care is assumed. However, these figures may not be representative of the majority of regional hospitals.

Statistics from tumor registries may be more representative. The crude 5-year survival rates reported from cancer registries have been less impressive, partly because a proportion of these patients almost certainly had only palliative excisions and partly because statistics for those patients who are alive 5 years after operation are expressed as a percentage of those submitted to surgical treatment and not of those surviving that treatment. Thus, operative deaths would be included among the nonsurvivors, making the number of 5-year survivors correspondingly less.

A more useful measure of surgical treatment is the overall or absolute survival rate, which expresses the number of patients alive and well after 5 years as a percentage of the total number of patients presenting to hospital with carcinoma of the colon in the first instance, not as a percentage of the immediate survivors of operation. The absolute survival rate automatically takes into account the resectability and operative mortality rates as well as the success of the operation in eradicating the carcinoma.

Despite this confusing information and with full recognition of the limitations of the exercise, an effort has been made to extract a number of representative series of reasonable size, and these are presented in ▶ Table 22.6 and ▶ Table 22.7.[301,302,303,304,305,306,307,308,309,310,311,312,314,315,316,317] In a review of 22 series, Devesa et al[318] determined that the corrected 5-year survival rates for patients with large bowel carcinoma operated on for cure varies from 44 to 68%.

Table 22.7 Results of curative operation for colon carcinoma

Author(s)	No. of patients	Resectability rates (%)	Operative mortality (%)	5-y survival (%)	
				Crude	Corrected
Corman[433]	1,008	95	4		
Pihl et al[301]	434		7		76
Stefanini et al[302]	436	81	3		
Zhou et al[303]	302	71	2	73	
Umpleby et al[304]	439		13	27	59
Isbister and Fraser[305]	1,505			43	
Wied et al[306]	442			47	
Glass et al[146]	413		3		82
Davis et al[307]	405		3	38	52
Moreaux and Catala[308]	646		1	78	
Brown et al[309]	550	85	7		
Enblad et al[310]	38,166		3		46
Jatzko et al[311]	223	98	2	81	
Clemmesen and Sprechler[312]	212			47	
Singh et al[313]	304	99	3		59 (10 y)
Carraro et al[314]	256	–	4	60	
Read et al[315]	316		2	84	

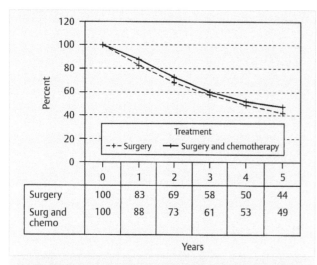

Fig. 22.34 Relative survival for 1985 to 1988 colon carcinoma cases (combined American Joint Committee on Cancer [AJCC] stage group III) by treatment modality.[318] (Reproduced with permission from Wolters Kluwer.)

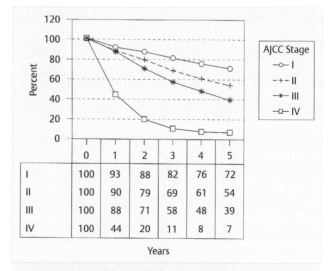

Fig. 22.36 Relative 5-year survival rate for carcinoma of rectum by combined pathologic and clinical AJCC staging. Percent survival by stage is shown in boxes below graph.[308] (Reproduced with permission from John Wiley and Sons.)

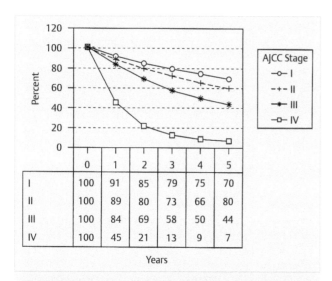

Fig. 22.35 Relative survival for 1985 to 1988 colon carcinoma cases by combined AJCC stage group.[318] (Reproduced with permission from Wolters Kluwer.)

The Commission on Cancer Data from the National Cancer Data Base reports time trends in stage of disease, treatment patterns, and survival for patients with selected carcinomas. The 1993 data for patients with colon carcinoma are described.[319] Five calls for data yielded 3,700,000 cases of carcinoma for the years 1985 through 1993 from hospital cancer registries across the United States, including 36,937 cases of colon carcinoma from 1988 and 44,812 from 1993. Interesting trends are as follows: (1) the elderly patients (> 80 years) present with earlier stage disease than do younger patients; (2) the National Cancer Institute recognized that cancer centers have more patients with advanced disease than do other types of hospitals; (3) all ethnic groups have generally similar stages of disease at presentation except for African-Americans, who have a slightly higher incidence of stage IV disease; (4) the proximal migration of the primary carcinoma continues; 54.7% of primary colon carcinoma arose in the right colon in 1993 compared with 50.9% in 1988; (5) an interaction between grade and stage of carcinoma seems present, and patients with stage III colon carcinoma who received adjuvant chemotherapy had a 5% improvement in 5-year relative survival (▶ Fig. 22.34); (6) the data suggest an important biologic role for grade of carcinoma. They also suggest that African-Americans and other ethnic groups have the same outcome as non-Hispanic whites but that access to medical care may still be less. Finally, the use of adjuvant therapy for stage III colon carcinoma may just be beginning to be appreciated. The relative 5-year survival rates for patients with colon carcinoma are depicted in ▶ Fig. 22.35. Comparable data for those with rectal carcinoma are shown in ▶ Fig. 22.36.

Survival rates for patients presenting with obstructing and perforating carcinomas are considerably more dismal. Representative reports are shown in ▶ Table 22.8, ▶ Table 22.9, and ▶ Table 22.10.[320,321,322,323,324,325,327,328,329,330,331,332,333,334,335,336, 337,338,339,340,341] The factors primarily contributing to this distressingly poor outlook are the low curability and survival rates for patients with large bowel obstruction secondary to colorectal carcinoma because of advanced disease at the time of diagnosis and treatment. Serpell et al[325] reported a reduction in curative resection rate from 71% in patients without obstruction to 50% in those with obstruction. A review of the literature by Smithers et al[108] revealed an operative mortality of 9 to 35% for emergency right hemicolectomy. Indeed, emergency operations of all kinds carry a higher operative mortality rate than do elective operations. Goodall and Park[124] reported on 40 patients with an obstructed left colon who underwent primary resection and anastomosis with a 5% mortality rate and a 40% complication rate.

Table 22.8 Five-year survival according to Dukes' staging following curative resection

| Author(s) | Dukes' A | | | Dukes' B | | | Dukes' C | | |
| | No. of patients | Survival (%) | | No. of patients | Survival (%) | | No. of patients | Survival (%) | |
		Crude	Corrected		Crude	Corrected		Crude	Corrected
Corman et al[433]	225	81	95	332	62	90	204	35	55
Pihl et al[301]	109		88	208		78	90		60
Eisenberg et al[316]	101		75–87[a]	274		64–85[a]	501		39–43[a]
Isbister and Fraser[305]	172	64		427	58		354	32	
Davis et al[307]	24	71	96	125	65	87	85	36	52
Read et al[315]	73	99		151	87		92	72	
Staib et al[317]	184	82		388	74		246	49	

[a]Range depending on portion of colon affected.

Table 22.9 Overall 5-year survival for patients with obstructing carcinoma

| Author(s) | No. of patients | Operative mortality (%) | Survival (%) | |
			Crude	Corrected
Kelley et al[320]	156	18	18	
Ohman[122]	148	9	16	
Brief et al[321]	41	2	78	
Crooms and Kovalcik[322]	37	3	33	
Umpleby and Williamson[123]	124	20	18	
Phillips et al[323]	713	23		25
Willett et al[324]	77		31	
Serpell et al[325]	148	9		
Ueyama et al[326]	40	0	52	
Mulcahy et al[327]	115	17		
Sjödahl et al[106]	92	12	36	
Chen et al[328]	120	5	33	
Carraro et al[314]	177	10	46	

Mandava et al[343] reported that in their series of 51 patients with perforated colorectal carcinoma, if the patients with metastatic disease and operative mortalities were excluded, there was a 58% 5-year survival rate in the remaining 32 patients. Scott et al[344] reported on risk factors in patients presenting in an emergency with colorectal carcinoma. Of 905 patients with colorectal carcinoma admitted to a single hospital, 272 (30%) were admitted as emergencies. Emergency patients had more advanced lesions (Dukes' B and C, 96 vs. 88% of those admitted electively), a shorter history (median, 3 vs. 11 weeks), were less likely to be fully ambulatory (44 vs. 80%), and more likely to have abdominal pain (74 vs. 51%) and vomiting (40 vs. 10%). More emergency patients were given stomas (56 vs. 35%) and died in hospital (19 vs. 8%). Of those who survived to be discharged, patients admitted as an emergency spent longer in hospital (median stay, 16 vs. 13 days) and had a poor overall 5-year survival rate (29 vs. 39%). Emergency patients were significantly older (median, 74 vs. 72 years) and were much more likely to be widowed (41 vs. 27%) than those admitted for elective surgery. The authors concluded that if the personal and resource disaster of emergency colorectal carcinoma admission is to be reduced, screening strategies targeted by demographic characteristics require investigation.

Anderson et al[345] conducted a prospective study of 570 patients presenting with colorectal carcinoma over a 6-year period. Of these, 363 were admitted electively and 207 presented as emergencies. In the elective group, the proportion of resected lesions was greater (77 vs. 64%), the operative mortality rate was lower (9 vs. 19%), and the 5-year disease-related survival rate was higher (37 vs. 19%). These differences may relate to the greater resection rates in the elective situation. Clemmesen and Sprechler[312] reported on the results of 803 patients with colorectal carcinoma, 273 of whom required emergency admission. Immediate operation was performed on 76 of these patients, 37 for obstruction, 15 for perforation, and 24 for other indications. The operative mortality rate for this group was 25%.

Other factors to consider are advanced disease and high-risk elderly patients. Fitzgerald et al[346] reviewed the perioperative mortality and long-term survival in elderly and high-risk patients with colorectal neoplasia. Elderly high-risk patients with localized disease were compared with those with advanced disease. Over a 5-year period, 82 high-risk (at least one major organ system disease) or elderly (age ≥ 70 years) patients underwent an operation for colorectal neoplasia. Overall, 43 of 82 patients (52%) had advanced disease (obstruction, perforation, hemorrhage, or metastatic disease), while 39 of 82 patients (48%) had localized disease. Preoperative comorbid diseases included coronary atherosclerosis, 59 (72%); previous myocardial infarction,

Table 22.10 Results of immediate resection and primary anastomosis for obstructing carcinoma of the left colon

Authors	Procedure	No. of patients	Operative mortality (%)	Complication rate (%)
Amsterdam and Krispin[104]	Segmental resection	25	12	60
Hughes et al[329]	TAC or STC	52	12	
Morgan et al[330]	TAC or STC	16	13	
White and Macfie[105]	LHC or sigmoid resection	35	9	29
Feng et al[331]	STC or segmental resection	15	7	27
Halevy et al[332]	STC	22	5	36
Slors et al[333]	TAC and IRA	10	10	30
Stephenson et al[113]	STC	31	3	6
Runkel et al[142]	STC, LHC	21	14	46
Antal et al[334]	STC	40	0	25
Brief et al[321]	STC	23	4	29
Tan et al[335]	Segmental resection	23	9	43
Murray et al[336]	Segmental resection	21	0	60
Sjödahl et al[106]	Not stated	18	6	17
Stewart et al[118]	Segmental resection	60	7	
Arnaud and Bergamaschi[337]	STC	44	7	7
Lau et al[115]	STC or segmental resection	35	6	31
Carraro et al[314]	Segmental or STC	107	10	–

Abbreviations: IRA, ileorectal anastomosis; LHC, left hemicolectomy; STC, subtotal colectomy; TAC, total abdominal colectomy.

17 (21%); previous arrhythmia, 10 (12%); emphysema, 32 (39%); renal failure, 6 (7%); and cirrhosis, 3 (4%). At the time of operation, 26 patients (32%) had metastatic disease. Six patients (7%) died in the perioperative period. There was no difference in major morbidity between patients operated on for localized and for advanced disease. The mean actuarial 18-month survival rate was less for patients with advanced disease. Sixty-eight patients (83%) were alive at a follow-up of 17.7±29 months postoperatively. The morbidity and mortality rates associated with resection of colorectal neoplasia in high-risk elderly patients are acceptable even in the presence of advanced disease. In select patients, resection offers the best palliation and may improve the quality of remaining life.

Colorectal carcinoma in cirrhotic patients is different from that in patients without the liver disease. Gervaz et al[347] retrospectively analyzed 72 patients operated on for colorectal adenocarcinoma with confirmed liver cirrhosis at the time of abdominal exploration. There were 43% Child A, 42% Child B, and 15% Child C. The median age was 70 years, and the mean duration of follow-up was 46 months. Postoperative death was 13%. The risk factors were an elevated bilirubin and prolonged prothrombin time. Liver metastases developed in 10%. For the whole group, 1-, 3-, and 5-year survival rates were 69, 49, and 35%, respectively. Child A patients had a significantly better survival rate than the combined group of Child B and C patients. The risks for long-term survival were decreased albumin and prolonged prothrombin time. The Child classification, and not the TNM stage of the carcinoma, predicts the risk of postoperative death and long-term

survival. Kotake et al[348] examined trends of colorectal carcinoma in relation to age, gender, site, and survival during a 20-year period. The multi-institutional registry of the Japanese Society for Cancer of the Colon and Rectum offered 87,695 surgical cases with invasive adenocarcinoma. The number of cases showed a 2.5-fold increase with consistent male predominance confined to the distal colon and rectum. Colon carcinoma in the last 5-year period was more likely right sided for females (OR, 1.26) and males (OR, 1.16) compared with the first period. Carcinomas in younger patients were more likely at stage III to IV in the late 1990s if the carcinomas were in the distal colon, the rectum (for both genders), or the proximal colon (for females). Survival was improved except for cases with proximal colon carcinoma of stage IV. In the multivariate analysis, hazard ratios for death in the postoperative 5 years were 0.77, 0.59, and 0.66 for proximal colon, distal colon, and rectal carcinomas, respectively, in the last period as compared with those in the first period. Reduced hazard ratio for females was the largest for proximal colon carcinoma with stages I and II. Although surgical outcome was largely improved, delayed presentation or diagnosis in younger patients remained a problem.

Wang et al[349] investigated the clinical features, diagnosis, treatment, and prognosis of 37 patients with multiple primary carcinomas. The incidence of multiple primary colorectal carcinomas was 2.7% in patients with primary colorectal carcinomas, 15 cases were patients with synchronous carcinomas, and 22 cases were diagnosed as metachronous carcinomas. Most carcinomas were located in the right colon and rectum. Fifty-five percent of metachronous carcinomas were diagnosed within 3 years after resection of the initial lesion and 41% of metachronous carcinomas occurred after 8 years. Radical resections were performed in all patients except for one case. The 5-year survival rate of synchronous carcinomas was 72.7% and those of metachronous carcinomas after the first carcinoma and second carcinoma were 71.4 and 38.9%, respectively. Their results indicate the importance of complete preoperative examination and careful intraoperative exploration and periodic postoperative surveillance.

Immunosuppression used in transplantation is associated with an increased incidence of various carcinomas. Papaconstantinou et al[350] defined the characteristics and survival patterns of transplant patients developing de novo colorectal carcinomas. A total of 150 transplant patients with de novo colorectal carcinoma were identified: 93 kidney, 29 heart, 27 liver, and 1 lung. Mean age of transplantation was 53 years. Age of transplantation of colorectal carcinoma diagnosis was not significant for gender, race, or stage of disease. Compared to National Cancer Institute Surveillance Epidemiology and End Results database, transplantation patients had a younger mean age of colorectal carcinoma diagnosis (58 vs. 70 years) and a worse 5-year survival (overall 44 vs. 62%, Dukes' A and B 74 vs. 90%, Dukes' C 20 vs. 66%, and Dukes' D 0 vs. 9%). Their data suggest that chronic immunosuppression results in a more aggressive biology. Frequent post-transplantation colorectal screening program may be warranted.

22.7 Prognostic Discriminants

Over the years, many factors that might influence survival rates have been studied, and different authors have placed varying degrees of confidence on certain ones. For example, in a large prospective analysis of 2,524 patients who had undergone curable resection, the prognostic factors in order of importance were (1) lymph node status, (2) mobility of the carcinoma, (3) number of positive lymph nodes, (4) presence of bowel obstruction, and (5) depth of penetration of the primary lesions.[351]

In a review of the literature and combined with his experience, Jass[352] summarized the important variables as follows. The pathologist should provide the staging, completeness of excision (resection lines), extent of spread through the bowel wall, lymph node or satellite nodule involvement, especially involvement of nodes at the apex of the vascular pedicle, and the number of nodes. Other variables should be considered. For completeness of documentation, carcinoma of the large bowel should be typed as adenocarcinoma, mucinous adenocarcinoma, signet-ring cell carcinoma, undifferentiated carcinoma, or other. In addition, the grade of differentiation, well, moderate, or poor, should be stated. However, type and grade of carcinoma have little or no independent prognostic value.

Classification of carcinoma as expanding or diffusely infiltrating has been shown to be of prognostic importance in a number of multivariate studies. Most large bowel carcinomas are relatively well circumscribed. Approximately 25% show an irregular margin of growth with tongues of neoplastic cells dissecting between the normal structures of the bowel wall, making it difficult to define a clear border of the carcinoma. The term "diffuse infiltration" does not imply massive intramural spread, a type of spread very rarely seen in the large bowel.

The presence of venous invasion by carcinoma should be recorded because this may have a bearing on the documentation of extent of spread. The presence of venous invasion is strongly correlated with distant spread. When cases with distant spread are excluded, the prognostic value of venous spread is greatly diminished and is absent in some multivariate studies. The presence of perineural and lymphatic spread influences prognosis adversely, but these factors were not found to be independent when Jass[352] examined 500 specimens from the prospectively collected Australian series. A conspicuous lymphocytic infiltrate, either within an inflammatory mantle at the growing edge of the carcinoma or arranged within nodular collections around small serosal vessels, confers a favorable prognosis that has been shown to be independent.

The following discussion, although not totally comprehensive, elaborates on the factors that most often have been considered relevant.[353,354]

22.7.1 Clinical Features

Age

Survival rates of patients younger than 40 years of age are frequently believed to be lower than overall survival rates. The 5-year survival rates in this group of patients range from 16 to 43%.[355,356,357,358,359,360] The poor prognosis in young patients has been attributed to the larger portion of poorly differentiated lesions, a larger number of mucinous lesions, and a lower potential for curative resection.[355,356] Not all authors believe that young patients have a less favorable prognosis.[361,362] Svendson et al[363] reported that patients who are between 40 and 60 years of age at the time of diagnosis have a worse prognosis than both younger and older patients.

Cusack et al[359] conducted a retrospective review of 186 patients younger than 40 years of age. Regional lymph node metastases, distant metastases, or both were seen on first examination in 66% of young patients. The authors identified three biologic indicators of aggressive and potentially metastatic biology: signet-ring cell carcinoma (11.1%), infiltrating edge of the carcinoma (69%), and aggressive (poorly differentiated) grade (41%). Vascular invasion in stage II disease was also a significant negative prognostic variable. These histologic measures of more aggressive disease in part account for the higher rate of advanced disease at presentation in patients younger than 40 years of age.

Liang et al[364] compared 138 consecutive patients with colorectal carcinoma aged younger than 40 years with 339 patients aged 60 years or older. The younger patients with colorectal carcinoma had more mucin-producing (14.5 vs. 4.7%) and poorly differentiated (7.2 vs. 3.3%) carcinomas, a higher incidence of synchronous (5.8 vs. 1.2%) and metachronous (4.0 vs. 0.6%) colorectal carcinomas, and more advanced stage than older patients. The operative mortality rate was lower (0.7 vs. 5.0%), and carcinoma-specific survival was similar (in stage I, II, and III disease) or better (in stage IV disease). There was a higher percentage of normal p53 expression (61.1 vs. 46.8%) and high frequency of microsatellite instability (29.4 vs. 6.3%) and a similar family history of carcinoma (17.5 vs. 14.2%), compared with older patients.

O'Connell et al[366] performed the most comprehensive systematic review focusing on colorectal carcinoma in the young aiming to (1) characterize the disease in the young population and (2) determine how colorectal carcinoma in this population should be further addressed regarding detection and treatment. A Medline literature search chose 55 studies that examined 6,425 patients younger than 40 years. Approximately 7% of all colorectal carcinomas consisted of patients younger than 40 years. They found that colorectal carcinoma in the young population appears to be more aggressive, to present with later stage (66% of patients younger than 40 years presented with Dukes' C and D lesions compared with 32 to 49% reported for patients older than 40 years), and to have poorer pathologic findings (higher prevalence of mucinous or poorly differentiated lesions including signet-ring cell carcinoma—one of the main distinctions between the disease in older versus younger patients). Mucinous lesions constituted an average of 21% of carcinoma in younger patients compared with an average of 10–15% of patients of all ages with colorectal carcinoma. The average percentage of lesions found to be poorly differentiated was 27% for the young group compared with 2–29% of patients older than 40. The average overall 5-year survival for young patients was 33% compared with 61% overall 5-year survival reflecting presentation with later stage disease, thus appearing to have a poorer prognosis. However, if detected early, young patients with Dukes' stage A or B lesions have better overall 5-year survival rates. Average-adjusted 5-year survival for Dukes' A, B, and C lesions are as follows: 94%, 77%, and 39%. A crucial issue is that close attention must be paid to young patients who present with common symptoms of colorectal carcinoma. O'Connell et al[367] used a national-level, population-based cancer registry to compare rectal carcinoma outcomes between young versus older populations. All patients with rectal carcinoma in the Surveillance Epidemiology and End Results Cancer database from 1991 to 1999 were evaluated. Young (range 20–40 years; $n = 466$) and older groups (range 60–80 years; $n = 11,312$) were compared for patient and carcinoma characteristics, treatment patterns, and 5-year overall and stage-specific survival. Mean ages for the groups were 34.1 and 70 years. The young group was comprised of more Black and Hispanic patients compared with the older group. Young patients were more likely to present with late stage disease (young vs. older: stage III, 27 vs. 20% and stage IV, 17.4 vs. 13.6%, respectively). The younger group also had worse grade (poorly differentiated 24.3 vs. 14%, respectively). Although the majority of both groups received surgery (85% for each), significantly more young patients received radiation. Importantly, overall and stage-specific, 5-year survival rates were similar for both groups.

From a group of 2,495 patients with malignancies of the colon and rectum, Turkiewicz et al[368] identified 61 patients with colorectal carcinoma who were younger than 40 years at presentation. Their clinical data were then compared with the larger group of older patients. A positive family history was the most consistent risk factor, present in 34% of patients. Despite this, only 1 patient out of 61 had been diagnosed as a result of a screening program. The overall 5-year survival among younger patients was 53%. The 5-year survival rates in younger patients were better than for older patients for the Australian Clinicopathological Staging A and B reaching statistical significance for both of these stages. Their results indicate that young patients with colorectal carcinoma have the potential to do just as well as older ones.

For the prognosis of elderly patients, conflicting reports are found. A common notion is that aged patients have less biologically aggressive neoplasms. Newland et al[369] found that in patients over 75 years of age, the hazard ratio for survival was 1.98. Coburn et al[370] compared 177 cases of colorectal carcinoma in patients older than 80 years to 623 in patients younger than 80 years. There was no difference in operative mortality between the two groups. Octogenarians and nonagenarians more often displayed obstruction or perforation, elevated preoperative CEA levels, right-sided lesions, and solitary hepatic metastases. The actuarial 5-year survival rate was 32% in the older patients and 48% in the younger group. Others report that the prognosis for the elderly is not different from that of younger patients.[371,372,373]

Sex

Some authors have reported a slightly higher incidence of carcinoma of the colon in women than in men, but the 5-year survival rates are slightly higher in women.[3] However, others have reported poorer survival rates in women.[374] The hazard ratio for the male gender has been estimated at 1.27.[369]

History

As might be expected, patients who are asymptomatic have better survival rates than symptomatic patients do.[375,376,377] Patients who have rectal bleeding as a presenting symptom have a better prognosis than do those presenting with other symptoms of colonic carcinoma.[376] The number of symptoms is also a prognostic discriminant since patients with more than two symptoms have a poorer prognosis.[374]

There appears to be no correlation between the duration of symptoms and survival. In a study of 152 patients, Goodman and Irvin[375] found no difference in the survival rate for patients in whom the diagnosis was delayed greater than 12 weeks from the onset of symptoms compared with those who presented early. They did find that patients with anemia and no abdominal symptoms had a significantly higher survival rate than those presenting with abdominal symptoms. Patients who ignore their symptoms tend to have biologically more favorable lesions. Ironically, in patients with a longer history of symptoms, there appears to be either no effect on survival or a better survival rate.[376,377,378] Wiggers et al[379] found that patients who had symptoms for a very short time (< 1 week) or a very long time (> 6 months) had a poorer survival rate than those in the intermediate range, but this was not statistically significant. This apparent paradox may be explained by the fact that patients with aggressive lesions (i.e., annular, constricting, or poorly differentiated) are compelled to seek help early. Patients with less acute symptoms often exhibit lesions of average grade and may ultimately prove to have a better prognosis.

Obstruction

The incidence of intestinal obstruction has been reported to be between 7 and 29% of all patients with colon and rectal cancer.[380] The occurrence of acute obstruction diminishes the ultimate survival rate and increases the immediate hazard to the patient.[376,380,382,383,384] In a review of 12 reports, Sugarbaker et al[46] found a median overall survival rate of 20% and a 5-year survival rate of

40% with curative surgery. The authors attributed this dismal prognosis to the fact that only about one-half of the patients had potentially curative operations and that the operations were accompanied by high morbidity and mortality rates, with a median hospital mortality rate of 18% and complications occurring in one-third to one-half of the patients.

Wang et al[380] conducted a study to assess the long-term prognosis of patients with obstructing carcinoma of the right colon. The 256 patients who were status post curative resection of right colon adenocarcinoma were classified as obstruction group ($n = 35$) or nonobstruction group ($n = 221$). The overall (49 vs. 22%), distant (40 vs. 18%), and local (14 vs. 5%) recurrence rates were significantly higher in obstructive patients than in nonobstructive patients. Long-term crude (36 vs. 77%) and carcinoma-specific survival rates (46 vs. 83%) were significantly lower in obstructed patients. Multivariate analysis demonstrated that obstruction and stage were both independent prognostic factors.

Carraro et al[314] reported on a series of 528 patients with colonic carcinoma, 34% of whom presented with obstruction. One-stage primary resection and anastomosis as curative treatment were performed in 107 obstructed and 256 nonobstructed patients. Three hundred and thirty-six potentially cured survivors (94 in the former group and 242 in the latter) were followed for a median of 55 months. During follow-up, local recurrence occurred in 37 patients (12 obstructed [12.8%] and 25 nonobstructed [10.4%]), and metastatic disease in obstructed (27.6%) and nonobstructed (17.8%). Multivariate analysis of survival showed that over 70 years of age Dukes' stage, histologic grade, and recurrence were the only prognostic factors. After one-stage emergency curative treatment, patients presenting with obstructing carcinomas of the colon have a smaller survival probability than that of patients with nonobstructing lesions.

Chen et al[328] reviewed the medical records of 1,950 patients with colorectal carcinoma. Patients were grouped as follows: group 1, complete colonic obstruction without perforation ($n = 120$); group 2, complete obstruction with perforation at the site of the carcinoma ($n = 35$); group 3, complete obstruction with perforation proximal to the carcinoma ($n = 13$); and group 4, nonobstructing, nonperforated carcinomas ($n = 1,682$). When compared with group 4, group 1 had a more advanced Dukes' stage, older age, greater incidence of colonic versus rectal carcinomas, and a poorer carcinoma-free survival. Groups 2 and 3 had a greater incidence of colonic versus rectal carcinomas, and group 3 had a greater operative mortality. No significant differences were found between groups 1, 2, and 3. Independent factors favorable to carcinoma-free survival were female gender, well-differentiated pathology, uncomplicated cases, colon versus rectal location, and early stage. The perioperative mortality rate for perforated colorectal carcinoma at the site of the carcinoma was 9%; for obstructive colorectal carcinoma, it was 5%. Perioperative mortality was much greater for perforations of the colon and rectum occurring proximal to the carcinoma (31%). Survival was worse for patients with obstruction (33%), or perforation proximal to the carcinoma (33%).

Perforation

In comparison with obstruction, perforation has an even greater detrimental effect on the ultimate outcome for the patient. In a review of four reports, Sugarbaker et al[46] found a median overall 5-year survival rate of only 9% and a 5-year survival rate of 33% with curative surgery. The median curative operative rate was 55%, with a hospital mortality rate of 30%. For patients with a free perforation into the peritoneal cavity, the 5-year survival rate was a dismal 7.3%, whereas for a localized perforation, the 5-year survival rate was 41.4%. Another report shows an even higher postoperative mortality of 52%.[123]

Khan et al[341] reviewed 48 patients presenting with acute colonic perforation associated with colorectal carcinoma. Thirty-six had perforation of the carcinoma, 11 proximal to the carcinoma, and 1 distal to the primary carcinoma. Patients who perforated proximal to the carcinoma were older (74.5 vs. 64.7 years) and had a longer length of stay (46.8 vs. 11.6 days). Fourteen patients had stage II disease, 19 stage III, and 15 stage IV. Thirty-day mortality was 14%. Of the 30-day survivors, 60% had curative resection (21 with local perforation and 9 with proximal perforation). Thirty-three percent had either unresectable or metastatic disease on exploration. One-year survival was 55%. Five-year disease-free survival was 14%. There were no long-term survivors after perforation proximal to the carcinoma although disease stage was comparable in both groups.

Adjacent Organ Involvement

Direct invasion of adjacent viscera does not preclude the possibility of a curative resection, and every effort must be made to perform a resection if technically possible. A review of 25 reports in the literature by Sugarbaker et al[46] noted a median adjacent organ involvement in 9%, an operative mortality rate of 8%, and a salvage rate of 30% to 50%. This includes fistulization into an adjacent viscus such as the urinary bladder. Although adjacent organ involvement represents more advanced disease, curative resection may still be possible. However, extensive operation is associated with a higher morbidity and mortality.

Presence of Metastatic Disease

It is axiomatic that patients with metastatic disease bear a poorer prognosis than those who are free of disseminated disease. The rare exception is the situation in which the metastatic disease can be resected for cure.

Systemic Manifestations

Patients who develop symptoms of weight loss, anorexia, weakness, or anemia frequently do so in the presence of advanced disease, which does not bode well for the patient.

Obesity

To determine the relationship between body mass index and rates of sphincter preserving operations, overall survival, recurrence, and treatment-related toxicities, Meyerhardt et al[381] evaluated a nested cohort of 1,688 patients with stage II and III rectal carcinoma participating in a randomized trial of postoperative fluorouracil-based chemotherapy and radiation therapy. Obese patients were more likely to undergo an abdominoperineal resection than normal-weight patients (OR, 1.77). Increasing adiposity in men was a strong predictor of having an abdominoperineal resection. Obese men with rectal carcinoma were also more likely than normal-weight men to have a local recurrence (hazard ratio, 1.61). In contrast, obesity was not predictive of carcinoma recurrence in women nor was body mass index predictive of overall mortality in either men or women. Underweight patients had an increased risk of death (hazard ratio, 1.43) compared with normal-weight patients but no increase in carcinoma recurrences. Among all study participants, obese patients had a significantly lower rate of grade 3 to 4 leukopenia, neutropenia, and stomatitis and a lower rate of any grade 3 or worse toxicity when compared with normal-weight individuals.

Technique of Resection

Various efforts have been made to diminish the risk of dissemination of malignant cells during the operation, but for the most part the results have not been conclusive. In their large multicenter trial, Phillips et al[382] reported considerable surgeon-related variation with respect to local recurrence. The patients of surgeons with considerable experience had fewer recurrences of disease. Possible causes cited for local recurrence include inadequate resection, suture implantation of malignant cells, and development of a second primary carcinoma at the anastomosis site. The authors state that surgeons should be aware that a small group of our colleagues are obtaining results substantially better than those of the majority, and they conclude that these good results have been achieved by meticulous attention to detail.

In a comprehensive review of the literature, Sugarbaker and Corlew[383] analyzed available data and concluded that there was no survival benefit with the use of radical left hemicolectomy instead of segmental resection, the use of the no-touch technique instead of conventional techniques, or the adoption of control of intraluminal spread of malignant cells. En bloc resection of an attached structure did seem important. The inadvertent intraoperative perforation of the bowel during a curative resection has a decidedly detrimental effect, in terms of both survival and local recurrence.[384] The 5-year survival rate with bowel disruption was 23%, and the rate fell as low as 14% when the carcinoma itself was disrupted. Local recurrence rose to 67% in Dukes' B cases with spillage and as high as 87% when Dukes' C carcinomas were perforated at the time of operation.[384] Other authors have reported that spillage of malignant cells at the time of operation reduces 5-year survival after resection for cure from 70 to 44%.[385]

Akyol et al[386] examined anastomotic leaks as a risk factor for recurrence. At a mean follow-up of 25 months, 46.9% of patients with leaks developed a recurrence compared with 18.5% for those without a leak. Cancer-specific mortality rates at 24 months were higher for patients with leaks (36.9 vs. 12.6%). Fujita et al[387] also found that for patients with anastomotic leakage, the incidence of local recurrence was higher (21.2 vs. 2.4%) and the disease-free survival rate was lower in Dukes' A and B patients (55 vs. 80% at 5 years), but not in Dukes' C patients than in patients with no leakage.

In a study of 403 patients, Bell et al[388] found that after adjustment for lymph node metastases, the distal resection margin of resection, non-total anatomical dissection of the rectum, and the level of the anastomosis identified a significant association between anastomotic leakage and local recurrence (hazard ratio 3.8). They concluded that leakage following a colorectal anastomosis after potentially curative resection for carcinoma of the rectum is an independent predictor of local recurrence.

Rouffet et al[389] reviewed 270 consecutive patients randomly allotted to undergo either left hemicolectomy or left segmental colectomy. Left hemicolectomy removed the entire left colon along with the origin of the inferior mesenteric artery and the dependent lymphatic territory. Left segmental colectomy removed a more restrictive segment of the colon and left the origin of the inferior mesenteric artery unmolested. Both groups were similar with regard to preoperative risk factors. The number of early postoperative abdominal and extra-abdominal complications was similar in both groups. Overall, early postoperative mortality was 4% higher, in left hemicolectomy (6%) than in the left segmental colectomy (2%). Median survival was 10 years, and nearly equivalent in both groups. The two actuarial survival curves were similar. Bowel movement frequency was significantly increased after left hemicolectomy during the first postoperative year. Their results suggest that survival after left segmental colectomy is equivalent to that of left hemicolectomy. Inadvertent perforation of the bowel during curative resection for colon carcinoma has a definite adverse effect. Slanetz[384] reported a drop in 5-year survival rates from 29 to 14% when disruption occurred during dissection. Local recurrence developed in 75% of cases involving spillage of malignant cells.

Colorectal Specialization and Surgical Volume

In an audit from a Scottish series of 646 anastomoses, the overall anastomotic leak rate was 4.8% (3.2% for colonic carcinoma and 8.9% after resection for rectal carcinoma).[390] Intersurgeon variation was scrutinized. When the anastomosis was performed by 5 of the 28 surgeons responsible for 50% of the patients, the leak rate was 4.2 vs. 14.3% for the others. The authors support the concept of specialized units.

The impact of the variability in surgical skill among surgeons has also been reported in a multicenter study by Reinbach et al.[391] There was a significant difference between colorectal surgeons with regard to postoperative mortality rates, which varied from 8 to 30%, anastomotic leakage rates, which ranged from 0 to 25%, wound sepsis rates, which ranged from 6 to 35%, and local recurrence rates, which ranged from 0 to 29%. The 10-year survival rate varied from 0 to 63%. There are many studies that now stress the point that we cannot ignore the fact that there exists a variability of skill among surgeons.

Volume

Meyerhardt et al[392] studied a nested cohort of 1,330 patients with stage II and stage III rectal carcinoma participating in a multicenter adjuvant chemotherapy trial. They analyzed differences in rates of sphincter-preserving operations, overall survival, and carcinoma recurrence by hospital surgical volume. They observed a significant difference in the rates of abdominoperineal resections across tertiles of hospital procedure volume (46.3% for patients resected at low-volume, 41.3% at medium-volume, and 31.8% at high-volume hospitals). This higher rate of sphincter-sparing operation at high-volume centers was not accompanied by any increase in recurrence rates. Hospital surgical volume did not predict overall disease-free, or local recurrence-free survival. Patients who did not complete the planned adjuvant chemotherapy, as well as those who underwent operation at low-volume hospitals, had a significant increase in carcinoma recurrence (hazard ratio 1.94) and a nonsignificant trend toward increased overall mortality and local recurrence. In contrast, no significant volume–outcome relation was noted among patients who did complete postoperative therapy.

Schrag et al[393] conducted a retrospective population-based cohort study utilizing the Surveillance, Epidemiology and End Results-Medicare linked database that identified 2,815 rectal carcinoma patients aged 65 years and older. They found surgeon volume was better than hospital procedure volume at predicting long-term survival and can have a significant impact on survival for patients with rectal carcinoma. From the same database, Schrag et al[394] identified 24,166 colon carcinoma patients aged 65 years and older. As opposed to their findings with rectal carcinoma, high hospital procedure volume remained a strong predictor of low postoperative mortality rates for each outcome with and without adjustment for surgeon procedure volume. Surgeon-specific procedure volume was also an important predictor of surgical outcomes for 30-day mortality, and for 2-year mortality, although this effect was attenuated after adjusting for hospital volume. Hospital volume and surgeon volume were each an important predictor of the ostomy rate. Among high-volume institutions and surgeons, individual providers with unusually high ostomy rates could be identified. Both hospital- and surgeon-specific procedure volumes predict outcomes following colon carcinoma resection, but hospital volume may exert a stronger effect. In an analysis of 600 patients undergoing resections for rectal carcinoma, Hermanek and Hohenberger[395] reported that the patients of low-volume surgeons experienced an increased risk of local recurrence.

Borowski et al[396] examined surgeon volume and specialization as defined as membership of the Association of Coloproctology of Great Britain and Ireland (ACPGBI) as independent prognostic factors for operative morbidity and mortality for patients undergoing operations for colorectal carcinoma. A total of 5,948 patients in a regional center in the United Kingdom underwent operations with an operative mortality of 7.9%. Mortality risk was significantly reduced for surgeons who performed more than 20 operations per year, while ACPGBI membership was not significant. Although membership demonstrated an interest, it did not necessarily represent specialty training. Surgeons with a high case volume or specialized interest were more likely to achieve bowel continuity than low-volume surgeons and nonspecialists following rectal resection. There was no significant difference in anastomotic leak rate (5.1%).

Martling et al[397] compared outcomes in patients being operated upon by high-volume surgeons (> 12 operations per year) with low-volume surgeons (12 operations or fewer per year). Forty-six surgeons operated on 652 patients. Five high-volume surgeons operated on 48% of the patients. In these, outcome was significantly better than in patients treated by low-volume surgeons (local recurrence rate 4 vs. 10%; rate of rectal carcinoma death 11 vs. 18%).

Wibe[398] examined the influence of caseload on long-term outcome following standardization of rectal carcinoma surgery at a national level. Data relating to all 3,388 Norwegian patients with rectal carcinoma treated for cure were recorded in a national database. Treating hospitals were divided into four groups according to their annual caseload: hospitals in group 1 carried out 30 or more procedures, those in group 2 performed

20 to 29 procedures, group 3 10 to 19 procedures, and group 4 fewer than 10 procedures. The 5-year local recurrence rates were 9.2, 14.7, 12.5, and 17.5%, and 5-year overall survival rates were 64.4, 64.0, 60.8, and 57.8%, respectively, in the four hospital caseload groups. An annual hospital caseload of fewer than 10 procedures increased the risk of local recurrence compared with that in hospitals where 30 or more procedures were performed each year (hazard ratio, 1.9). Overall survival was lower for patients treated at hospitals with an annual caseload of fewer than 10 versus hospitals with 30 or more (hazard ratio, 1.2).

Colorectal Specialization

Callahan et al[399] examined the relationship of surgeon subspecialty training and interests to in-hospital mortality while controlling for both hospital and surgeon volume. A large Statewide Planning and Research Cooperative System was used to identify 48,582 patients who underwent colectomy. Surgical subspecialty training and interests was defined as surgeons who were members of the Society of Surgical Oncology (training/interest; $n = 68$) or the American Society of Colon and Rectal Surgeons (training/interest; $n = 61$). Overall mortality for colectomy patients was 4.6%; the adjusted mortality rate for subspecialty versus non–specialty-trained surgeons was 2.4 versus 4.8%, respectively. For colectomies, risk-adjusted mortality is substantially lower when performed by subspecialty interested and trained surgeons, even after accounting for hospital and surgeon volume and patient characteristics. These findings may have implications for surgical training programs and for regionalization of complex surgical procedures.

Rosen et al[400] examined variations in operative mortality among surgical specialists who perform colorectal surgery. Mortality rates were compared between 6 board-certified colorectal surgeons and 33 other institutional surgeons using comparable colorectal procedure codes and a validated database indicating patient severity of illness. Thirty-five ICD-9-CM procedure codes were used to identify 2,805 patients who underwent colorectal surgery. Atlas, a state-legislated outcome database, was used by the hospital's Quality Assurance Department to rank the Admission Severity Group (ASG) of 1,753 patients (higher ASG, 0–4, indicates increasing medical instability). Colorectal surgeons had an 8-year mean in-hospital mortality rate of 1.4% compared with 7.3% by other institutional surgeons. There was a significantly lower mortality rate for colorectal surgeons compared with other institutional surgeons in ASG2 (0.8 vs. 3.8%, respectively) and ASG3 (5.7 and 16.4%, respectively). Board-certified colorectal surgeons had a lower in-hospital mortality rate than other institutional surgeons as patients' severity of illness increased.

Platell et al[401] reviewed patients with colorectal carcinoma managed in general surgery units versus a colorectal unit. These results were compared to a historical control group treated within general surgical units at the same hospital. There were 974 patients involved in the study with no significant differences in the demographic details for the three groups. Patients in the colorectal group were more likely to have rectal carcinoma and stage I carcinomas and less likely to have stage II carcinomas. Patients treated in the colorectal group had a significantly higher overall 5-year survival when compared with the general surgical group and the historical control group (56 vs. 45 vs. 40%, respectively). Survival regression analysis identified age, ASA scores, disease stage, adjuvant chemotherapy, and treatment in a colorectal unit (hazards ratio 0.67) as significant independent predictors of survival. The results suggest that there may be a survival advantage for patients with colon and rectal carcinoma being treated within a specialist colorectal unit.

Read et al[402] determined the effect of surgeon specialty on disease-free survival and local control in patients with carcinoma of the rectum. The records of 384 consecutive patients treated by colorectal surgeons (n = 251) and noncolorectal surgeons (n = 133) were reviewed independently by physicians in the Division of Radiation Oncology. Local recurrence was defined as pelvic recurrence occurring in the presence or absence of distant metastatic disease. Actuarial disease-free survival and local control rates at 5 years were 77 and 99% for colorectal surgeons versus 68 and 84% for noncolorectal surgeons. Multivariate analysis revealed that pathologic stage and background of the surgeon were the only independent predictors of disease-free survival and that pathologic stage, background of the surgeon, and proximal location of the carcinoma were independent predictors of local control. Sphincter preservation was more common by colorectal surgeons (52%) than noncolorectal surgeons (30%). They concluded good outcome for patients with carcinoma of the rectum is associated with subspecialty training in colon and rectal surgery.

Dorrance et al[403] examined the effect of the surgeon's specialty on patient outcome after potentially curative colorectal carcinoma surgery to identify factors that may help explain differences in outcome among specialty groups. In a large teaching hospital, 378 patients underwent potentially curative operation for colorectal carcinoma by surgeons with specialty interests, vascular or transplant, general, and colorectal surgeons. At a median follow-up of 45 months, the only factors associated with a significant reduced local recurrence rate were the length of the resection specimen (OR, 0.56) and colorectal specialty. Patients operated on by a general surgeon were 3.42 times more likely to develop a local recurrence than those operated on by a colorectal surgeon. For overall recurrence, early-stage disease, absence of vascular invasion, and colorectal specialty were the only factors associated with significantly improved outcome at multivariate analysis. These data show that surgeons with an interest in colorectal carcinoma achieve lower local and overall recurrence rates compared with vascular, transplant, or general surgeons.

Martling et al[404] evaluated the effects of an initiative to teach the TME technique on outcomes at 5 years after surgery. The study population comprised all 447 patients who underwent abdominal operations for rectal carcinoma in Stockholm County. Outcomes were compared with those in the Stockholm I (790 patients) and Stockholm II (542 patients) radiotherapy trials. The permanent stoma rate was reduced from 60.3 and 55.3% in the Stockholm I and II trials, respectively, to 26.5% in the TME project. Five-year local recurrence rates decreased from 21.9 and 19.1% to 8.2%, respectively. Five-year carcinoma-specific survival rates increased from 66.0 and 65.7% in the Stockholm trials to 77.3% in the TME project (hazard ratio, 0.62). They concluded that a surgical teaching program had a major impact on rectal carcinoma outcome.

McArdle and Hole[405] conducted a study to determine whether differences in survival following surgery for colorectal carcinoma were due to differences in caseload or degree of specialization. The outcome in 3,200 patients who underwent resection for colorectal carcinoma was analyzed on the basis of caseload and degree of specialization of individual surgeons.

Carcinoma-specific survival at 5 years following curative resection varied among surgeons from 53.4 to 84.6%; the adjusted hazard ratios varied from 0.48 to 1.55. Carcinoma-specific survival rate at 5 years following curative resection was 70.2, 62.0, and 65.9% for surgeons with a high, medium, and low case volume, respectively. There were no consistent differences in the adjusted hazard ratios by volume. Carcinoma-specific survival rate at 5 years following curative resection was 72.7% for those treated by specialists and 63.8% for those treated by nonspecialists; the adjusted hazard ratio for nonspecialists was 1.35. They concluded the differences in outcome following apparently curative resection for colorectal carcinoma among surgeons appear to reflect the degree of specialization rather than case volume. It is likely that increased specialization will lead to further improvements in survival.

Perioperative Blood Transfusion

Clinical and experimental studies indicate that transfusion of blood has immunomodulating properties and that the behavior of some neoplasms may be influenced by the immune system of the host. It has been suggested that blood transfusion in the perioperative period adversely affects the rate of carcinoma recurrence and is even associated with increased mortality.[406,407] Leite et al[408] noted a 5-year survival rate of 37% for patients who were transfused compared with 60% for nontransfused patients. Furthermore, it has been suggested that the number of units of blood transfused perioperatively in patients operated on for colon carcinoma has a progressively strong negative influence on survival.[409] It has been reported that the incidence of recurrence is higher in those patients who receive transfusion during the operation than in those who receive transfusion either before or after operation; however, the study indicated that factors influencing the need for blood transfusion during the operation had a greater bearing on prognosis than the receipt of the blood per se.[410] As with other prognosis discriminants, various authors have presented conflicting views.[411,412] To resolve some of the controversy over the degree of immunomodulation by perioperative blood transfusion and its effect on oncologic surgery, Chung et al[411] reviewed all studies published between 1982 and 1990 using the statistical method of Mantel–Haenszel–Peto to determine a cumulative estimate of the direction and magnitude of this association. Some 20 articles were included in the analysis, representing 5,236 patients. The cumulative OR (95% confidence interval) of disease recurrence, death from carcinoma, and death from any cause were 1.80 (1.30–2.51), 1.76 (1.15–2.66), and 1.63 (1.12–2.38), respectively. These results support the hypothesis that perioperative blood transfusion is associated with an increased risk of recurrence of colorectal carcinoma and death from this malignancy.

Splenectomy has been considered a possible factor in the survival of patients operated on for colorectal carcinoma.[412] The mechanism responsible for this adverse impact is undefined, but it may fall into the category of modulation of the immune response—others disagree.[413]

Previous Appendectomy

Armstrong et al[414] studied a series of 519 patients presenting with carcinoma of the cecum in relation to a history with or without previous appendectomy. Previous appendectomy was associated with a higher incidence of local fixity, invasion of the abdominal wall, metastatic spread, and poor differentiation. These differences were reflected in a significantly lower resection rate for carcinomas in patients who had undergone appendectomy. The survival of patients who had previously had appendectomy was significantly reduced. Local recurrence was more common and often was noted to be in the old appendectomy wound itself. In this study, appendectomy did not increase the risk of carcinogenesis in the cecum but worsened the prognosis for patients who subsequently developed carcinoma of the cecum.

22.7.2 Pathologic Features

Numerous pathologic features have been studied in an effort to define and refine the prognosis of a given patient. In a very meticulous and thorough study, Newland et al[369] analyzed data from 579 patients collected prospectively during a follow-up ranging between 6 months and 21.5 years. Six variables showed significant independent effects on survival on multivariate analysis. In diminishing potency, these variables were apical lymph node involvement, spread involving a free serosal surface, invasion beyond the muscularis propria, location in the rectum, venous invasion, and high-grade malignancy. Significant independent effects also were shown for patient age and gender. The number of involved lymph nodes added no significant independent prognostic information. The authors recommend that all six independent variables be included in any future protocol for stratifying this prognostically diverse group of patients. Many of the individual discriminants are discussed below.

Location

Most reports suggest that rectal carcinoma has a poorer prognosis than colon carcinoma.[369,373,383] In the report by Polissar et al[374] colon carcinoma resulted in a significantly worse prognosis than rectal carcinoma. Newland et al[369] reported a hazard ratio of 1.53. In contrast, the study by Martin et al[415] found no difference in 5-year survival rates on the basis of site of the carcinoma. In patients with colon carcinoma, opinion has differed as to whether a right-sided lesion has a better prognosis,[383] a left-sided lesion has a better prognosis,[304] or the prognoses are equal. Several authors believe that right-sided lesions carry a poorer prognosis.[416]

Size

In contrast to other malignancies, it has been reported that the size of a carcinoma of the colon bears little relationship to prognosis.[417,418] Other authors have expressed the opposite opinion.[416,419]

Configuration

The macroscopic features of a colon carcinoma appear to reflect its biologic activity. Polypoid lesions tend not to deeply invade the bowel wall, whereas ulcerating lesions more often penetrate the wall and are associated with a poorer prognosis.

Lumen encirclement is a strong prognostic discriminant.[373] Rate of survival with full circumferential involvement was found to be 29.7% at 5 years, whereas when less than half of the lumen was involved, the 5-year survival rate was 53.9%.[383]

Survival and local recurrence are significantly better for patients with exophytic (polypoid and sessile) carcinomas than for those with nonexophytic (ulcerated and flat raised lesions).[420] Exophytic lesions include significantly more stage T1 and fewer T2 and T3 carcinomas, and a significantly smaller proportion of carcinomas that show venous and lymphatic invasion than the nonexophytic lesions.

Microscopy

Although histologic grading is valuable in assessing prognosis, no uniform system of grading exists. Broders' grade 1 carries a relatively good prognosis, while grades 3 and 4 have a poor prognosis. Approximately one-half of patients fall into the grade 2 category, which makes this grading system of limited help. Furthermore, there is frequently a discrepancy between the preoperative and postoperative assessments. In their review, Sugarbaker et al[46] summarized the findings of many studies and concluded that malignancies of higher grades have less chance for cure than those of lower grades. Other microscopic features associated with a diminished chance for cure include more advanced primary lesions, cases involving increased frequency of venous invasion, increased frequency of distant metastases, increased frequency of perineural invasion, and increased frequency of metastases to lymph nodes. Preoperative biopsy is of limited prognostic value unless a poorly differentiated lesion is present, in which case the likelihood of lymphatic metastases is greater. Newland et al[369] estimated that the hazard ratio for survival for patients with a high-grade carcinoma was 1.48.

Carcinomas that secrete large amounts of mucus are associated with reduced survival. Yamamoto et al[421] compared the clinicopathologic features of patients with a mucinous carcinoma (6.6% of their patients) to a nonmucinous carcinoma. They found that mucinous carcinomas were more likely to invade adjacent viscera (29 vs. 10%), show lymph node involvement beyond the pericolic region (50 vs. 26%), have a reduced rate of curative resection (34 vs. 69%), have a higher recurrence rate (27 vs. 19%), and result in a poorer 5-year survival rate (33 vs. 53%). Green et al[422] found that stage for stage, the 5-year overall survival rate was the same for mucinous and nonmucinous carcinomas. However, the 5-year survival rate for mucinous carcinoma of the rectum was decidedly worse than nonmucinous carcinoma (11 vs. 57%). In a review of 352 patients with colorectal carcinoma, followed for a minimum of 5 years, Secco et al[423] found that mucinous adenocarcinomas represented 11.1% and signet-ring cell carcinomas represented 1.1% of cases. Mucinous carcinomas were most frequently located in the rectum (61.5%) and in the sigmoid colon (15.3%). Patients presented with Dukes' C and metastatic disease in 41 and 15% of cases, respectively. Disease recurrence was more frequently observed in patients with mucinous (51.7%) or signet-ring lesions (100%) compared with adenocarcinomas. Five-year survival rates were 45, 28, and 0% in patients with adenocarcinoma, mucinous adenocarcinoma, or signet-ring cell carcinomas, respectively.

Signet-ring cell adenocarcinomas (i.e., cells with abundant intracellular mucus) have a particularly poor prognosis. Chen et al[424] identified 61 signet-ring cell carcinoma patients and compared their clinical data and outcomes to those of 144 consecutive patients with non-signet–ring cell mucinous rectal carcinomas and 2,414 consecutive patients with nonmucinous rectal carcinomas. The incidence of signet-ring cell carcinomas was 1.39% of rectal carcinomas. Mean patient age at onset of signet-ring cell carcinomas (48.1 years) was significantly lower than that for non-signet–ring cell mucinous carcinomas (57.4 years) and nonmucinous carcinomas (62.6 years). The proportion of late stage (TNM III and IV) carcinomas was significantly higher in signet-ring cell carcinomas (90%) than in non-signet–ring cell mucinous carcinomas (69%) and nonmucinous carcinomas (48%). There were more carcinomas located in the lower rectum in signet-ring cell carcinomas (46%) than in non-signet–ring mucinous carcinomas (34%) and nonmucinous carcinomas (29%). Signet-ring cell carcinomas were significantly larger (5.7 cm) than non-signet–ring cell mucinous carcinoma (4.3 cm) and nonmucinous lesions (3.8 cm). A higher percentage of patients with signet-ring cell carcinoma (42.6%) received abdominoperineal resection for treatment. In carcinomas with TNM stage IV, the rate of spread via hematogenous route was significantly lower in signet-ring cell carcinomas (18.5%) than in non-signet–ring cell mucinous (43.5%) and in nonmucinous carcinomas (69%). The rate of spread via seeding to the peritoneum was lower in signet-ring cell carcinomas (22.2%) than in non-signet–ring cell mucinous carcinomas (43.5%) but higher than in nonmucinous carcinomas (2.7%). The rate of spread via the lymphatic route was higher in signet-ring cell carcinoma (44.4%) than in non-signet–ring cell mucinous carcinoma (26.1%) and significantly higher than in nonmucinous carcinomas (12.3%). The 1-, 2-, and 5-year overall signet-ring cell carcinoma survival rates were 73.9, 36.3, and 23.3%, respectively, which were significantly poorer than those of non-signet–ring cell mucinous carcinomas and nonmucinous carcinomas. For the signet-ring cell carcinomas, the 1-, 2-, and 5-year disease-free survival rates were 84, 44.2, and 30.3%, respectively, which are comparable with general data of stage III rectal carcinoma in the world. They concluded that diffuse infiltration of signet-ring cells enhanced the tendency of mucinous carcinomas of the rectum to express local extension and lymphatic involvement but not peritoneal seeding.

Nissan et al[425] compared 46 patients with signet-ring cell carcinomas with 3,371 patients with primary non-signet–ring cell carcinomas. Lymphatic and peritoneal spread was more common among the signet-ring cell carcinoma group. Approximately one-third of signet-ring cell carcinoma patients presented with metastatic disease. Mean survival time of signet-ring cell carcinoma group was 45.4 months compared with 78.5 months for the control patients group. The cumulative survival curve of patients with signet-ring cell carcinoma resembles that of patients with poorly differentiated rectal carcinomas.

The pathologic diagnosis of scirrhous carcinoma of the large bowel carries a very poor prognosis. Extent of penetration of the bowel wall is associated with a reduced prognosis. Greater extramural spread is associated with an increased incidence of nodal involvement.[418] Hase et al[426] examined 663 specimens from patients who underwent curative resection for colorectal carcinoma and identified small clusters of undifferentiated malignant cells ahead of the invasive front of the lesion, which they labeled "tumor budding." The presence of this feature resulted in a diminished 5-year survival rate (22 vs. 71%). In a study of 138 patients, Tanaka et al[427] reported recurrence in 48% of patients with "tumor budding" compared with 4.5% without this histologic feature. Cumulative disease-specific survivals at 5 years were 74 and 98%, respectively. In a review of 196 resected stage II and III colon carcinomas, Okuyama et al[428] found budding detected significantly more frequently in lesions with lymph node metastases (stage III) than in lesions without it. Patients with budding-positive lesions had worse outcome than those with budding-negative lesions with 50.6% with budding-positive lesions and 8.1% with budding-negative lesions developing recurrence. Patients with budding-positive lesions had a worse prognosis than patients without it. Moreover, no significant difference in survival curves was observed between patients with budding-positive stage II lesions and those with stage III lesions.

An additional histologic feature that may correlate with prognosis is the presence or absence of an inflammatory infiltrate. For patients whose resected specimens demonstrated infiltration of lymphocytes around blood vessels, together with hyperplasia of paracortical regions in lymph nodes, Pihl et al[301] found a 5-year recurrence-free interval of 85%, while patients who lacked these characteristics exhibited a survival rate of 69%.

Gagliardi et al[429] studied the relationship between acinar growth patterns in 138 patients with rectal carcinoma and survival. Lesions were classified according to size, 28 microacinar and 110 macroacinar. Patients with microacinar (small regular tubules) had a significantly reduced 5-year survival rate compared with those with macroacinar (large irregular tubules) lesions (43 vs. 68%).

Residual Disease

Local residual disease predicts poor patient survival after resection for colorectal carcinoma. Chan et al[430] determined the prevalence of residual carcinoma in a line of resection in a large prospective series and identified other pathology variables that may influence survival in the absence of distant metastases. The overall prevalence of residual carcinoma in a line of resection was 5.9%. Of 12 pathology variables examined, only high-grade and apical node metastases were independently associated with survival in the subset of 120 patients with residual disease in a line of resection but without distant metastases. The 2-year survival rate for patients with neither of these adverse features was 46.4% as compared with only 7.7% in those who had both.

Dukes' Staging

The numerous eponymous modifications of the Dukes classification have not allowed any meaningful comparison to be made from one report to another. However, within each of these modifications a more advanced stage represents a poorer prognosis. If a staging system of local, regional, and distant categories were adopted, it might permit comparison and agreement on survival of a given category of patient.

Histologic activity offers a means of estimating biologic behavior, and this association has been reflected in the Dukes classification. The effect of Dukes' staging on survivorship was reported from the Lahey Clinic in Boston in a study of 344 patients treated for colorectal carcinoma. The uncorrected 5-year survivorship for Dukes' A, B, and C patients was 85, 65, and 46%, respectively, while the corresponding corrected values were 100, 78, and 54%.[383]

Newland et al[369] conducted a multivariate survival analysis on the depth of invasion. For spread beyond the muscularis propria, the authors found a hazard ratio of 1.68, and for spread involving the free serosal surface, the hazard ratio was 1.71. In another report, the same authors found that the survival rates of patients with clinicopathologic stage A or B closely matched their expected survival as predicted from the general population.[417] Males with stage B carcinomas were the only exception and their reduced survival rates were due to four clinical variables (cardiovascular complications, permanent stoma, urgent operation, or respiratory complications) and one pathologic variable (direct spread involving a free serosal surface).

Greene et al[431] proposed a new TNM staging strategy for node-positive colon and rectal carcinoma because the current stage III designation of colon carcinoma excludes prognostic subgroups stratified for mural penetration (T1–T4) or nodal involvement (N1 vs. N2). They analyzed 50,042 patients with stage III colon carcinoma reported to the National Cancer Data Base. Three distinct subcategories with a traditional stage III cohort of colon carcinoma were identified—IIIA: T1/T2, N1; IIIB: T3/T4, N1; and IIIC: any T, N2. Five-year observed survival rates for these three subcategories were 59.8%, IIIA; 42.0%, IIIB; and 27.3%, IIIC. Analysis of this large dataset supports stratification into three subsets, confirming the benefit of adjuvant chemotherapy in each subgroup. They subsequently analyzed data entered in the National Cancer Data Base for 5,987 stage III patients with rectal carcinoma.[432] Five-year observed survival rates for stage III subcategories were 55.3% in IIIA; 35.3% in IIIB; and 24.5% in IIIC. Stratifying for treatment outcome, stage IIIA patients having operation alone had poorer observed 5-year survival (39%) than patients treated with operation and adjuvant chemotherapy or radiation therapy (60%). Similar outcomes occurred in IIIB (operation alone 21.7% and chemo/radiotherapy 40.9%) and in IIIC (operation alone 12.2% and chemo/radiotherapy 28.9%). The effect of postoperative adjuvant therapy was beneficial in all subsets.

Lymph Node Status

The most important prognostic variable in colon carcinoma is the presence or absence of lymph node metastases. Patients with colorectal carcinoma found to have regional lymph node metastases after curative resection form a large and prognostically diverse group. In studies focusing on the level of lymph node involvement and the number of affected lymph nodes, the number of lymph nodes involved correlates with survival in some reports. In a report by Corman et al,[433] if more than three lymph nodes were positive, the overall survival rate was 18%, but with one to three nodes involved, the survival rate was 45 to 50%. An analysis of the National Surgical Adjuvant Breast and Bowel Project (NSABP) clinical trials by Wolmark et al[434] revealed a relative risk of death of 1.9 and 3.4 for patients with one to four and five to nine positive lymph nodes, respectively. Gardner et al[435] also found that prognosis worsened with an increased number of involved lymph nodes. Patients who had six

or more involved nodes were 4.6 times as likely to die from the disease as patients with only one involved node. Cohen et al[436] reported that when one to three nodes were involved, the 5-year survival rate was 66%, but was reduced to 37% when four or more nodes were positive. Similarly, Tang et al[437] found that the number of lymph nodes involved had an impact on survival. In a retrospective study of 538 patients, the 5-year survival rate for patients with one to three positive nodes was 69%, 44% for those with four to nine positive nodes, and 29% for those with 10 or more positive nodes. Conversely, Newland et al[369] reported that the number of involved lymph nodes added no significant independent prognostic information. Most potent in their analysis was apical node involvement, which they calculated to have a hazard ratio of 1.79 in their multivariate survival analysis. Such involvement was present in 9% of their node-positive patients. Malassagne et al[438] found that both the number of lymph nodes involved and apical node involvement were prognosticators. The 5-year survival rates were 17 and 45% for patients with and without apical lymph node involvement, respectively, and 44 and 6% for those with four or fewer nodes involved compared with those with more than four positive nodes, respectively.

Swanson et al[439] examined data from the National Cancer Data Base to determine whether the number of examined lymph nodes is prognostic for T3N0 colon carcinoma. A total of 35,787 prospectively collected cases of T3N0 colon carcinomas that were surgically treated and pathologically reported as T3N0M0 were analyzed. The 5-year relative survival rate for T3N0M0 colon carcinoma varied from 64% if one or two lymph nodes were examined to 86% if more than 25 lymph nodes were examined. Three strata of lymph nodes[1,2,3,4,5,6,7,8,9,10,11,12,216] distinguished significantly different observed 5-year survival rates. These results demonstrate that the prognosis of T3N0 colon carcinoma is dependent on the number of lymph nodes examined. The authors felt that a minimum of 13 lymph nodes should be examined to label a T3 colon carcinoma as node negative.

Fisher et al[440] examined the presumably negative nodes of a larger cohort of patients for what they designated nodal mini-micrometastases on parameters of survival. Mini-micrometastases were detected by immunohistochemical staining of the original lymph node sections with anticytokeratin A1/A3 in a total of 241 Dukes' A and B patients with rectal and 158 with colonic carcinoma. Nodal mini-micrometastases were detected in 18% of patients in this cohort, but this additional finding failed to exhibit any significant relationship to overall recurrence free survival. Other reports have recorded mini-micrometastases in 19 to 39% of cases and this probably relates to the number of sections taken at the time of study. Sakuragi et al[441] sought predictive markers of lymph node metastases to assist in management of 278 T1 colorectal carcinomas. Depth of submucosal invasion and lymphatic channel invasion were accurate predictive factors for lymph node metastases. The authors believe these two factors could be used in selecting appropriate cases for operation after endoscopic resection.

Tepper et al[442] analyzed data from 1,664 patients with T3, T4, or node-positive rectal carcinoma treated in a national intergroup trial of adjuvant therapy with chemotherapy and radiation therapy to assess the association between the number of lymph nodes found by the pathologist in the surgical specimen and the time to relapse and survival outcomes. No significant differences were found by quartiles among patients determined to be node positive. Approximately 14 nodes needed to be studied to define nodal status accurately. Examining greater number of nodes increased the likelihood of proper staging.

Venous Invasion

In a personal study of more than 1,000 operative specimens, Morson and Dawson[443] found regional venous involvement in 35% of cases. Submucosal venous spread occurred in 10%, and in 25% there was evidence of permeation of extramural vessels. In the former cases, there was little or no effect on prognosis, but extramural venous involvement reduced 5-year survival rates from 55 to approximately 30%. In the report by Corman et al,[433] patients with Dukes' C lesions and blood vessel invasion had a 31% 5-year survival rate compared with 43% without blood vessel invasion. Comparable figures for Dukes' B lesions were 55 and 70%, respectively. The former percent is not significant, but the latter reached statistical significance. A subsequent report from the Lahey Clinic found a difference with and without blood vessel invasion.[383] Minsky et al[444] reviewed a series of 168 patients who underwent potentially curative resection. The authors found that patients who had extramural blood vessel invasion had a significantly decreased 5-year survival rate compared with patients who had intramural blood vessel invasion or no vascular invasion at all. When extramural and intramural invasion were combined, the difference disappeared. Krasna et al[445] found that the 3-year survival rate decreased from 62.2% in patients without vascular invasion to 29.7% in patients demonstrating vascular invasion. In 128 operative specimens, Horn et al[446] identified venous invasion in 22%. The 5-year survival rate in those with venous invasion was 32.9 vs. 84.3% for those without venous invasion. Newland et al[369] identified venous invasion in 28.8% of their series, and in 81% of those patients extramural veins were involved. The authors calculated a hazard ratio of 1.49 in the multivariate survival analysis.

In a very thorough study, Sternberg et al[447] investigated venous invasion as a predictor of prognosis in colorectal carcinoma. The reported incidence of venous invasion in colorectal carcinoma specimens varies between 10 and 89.9%, mainly as a result of the interobserver variability and differences in specimen processing. Their study goal was to assess and compare the incidence of venous invasion diagnosed on hematoxylin and eosin (H&E) stained tissue versus tissue stained with both H&E and an elastic fiber stain. Venous invasion was assessed on sections from 81 colorectal carcinomas resected from patients with synchronous distant metastases. Only stage IV carcinomas were studied for the following reasons: (1) it can be assumed that in all patients with distant hematogenous metastases venous invasion had occurred, thus enabling the false negative rate to be calculated; (2) there can be no dispute about the clinical relevance of the various characteristics of venous invasion identified in the carcinomas of patients with synchronous distant hematogenous metastases; and[3] to eliminate the effect of variance in carcinoma staging on the incidence of venous invasion. Initially, H&E-stained sections were studied for venous invasion. Sections that were negative or questionable with regard to venous invasion were then stained with an elastic fiber stain and a second final search for venous invasion was carried out. Venous invasion was identified in 51.9% on H&E-stained sections. The addition of the elastic fiber stain enabled the diagnosis of venous invasion in 38.5% of the remaining specimens, increasing the overall incidence to 70.4%. Of the 57 positive specimens, venous invasion was minimal in 47.4%, intermediate in 8.8%, and massive in 43.9%. Only intramural veins were involved in 31.6%, only extramural veins in 45.6%, and both intramural and extramural veins in 22.8% of the positive specimens. The filling type of venous invasion was found in 71.9%, the floating type in 49.1%, and the infiltrating type in 10.5% of the positive specimens. There was no significant difference between the incidence of venous invasion in the colon (70%) versus rectal and rectosigmoid carcinomas (71.4%) nor in the incidence of venous invasion in patients with hepatic (70%) versus nonhepatic (72.7%) metastases. Only minimal venous invasion is required for the seeding of clinically relevant hematogenous metastases, which emphasizes the careful dedicated search for venous invasion that is required from the pathologist. Although extramural venous invasion was predominant in stage IV colorectal carcinomas, in a third of lesions only intramural venous invasion was found. This suggests that intramural venous invasion may also seed clinically relevant hematogenous metastases, and should therefore also be considered as an indicator of poor prognosis.

Perineural Invasion

Perineural invasion has been shown to have a detrimental effect on prognosis. Its presence may be part of the overall penetration of the bowel wall. The association of disseminated disease has been reported.[448] Krasna et al[445] found that the 3-year survival rate decreased from 57.7% in patients without neural invasion to 29.6% in patients with neural invasion. Of 128 operative specimens examined by Horn et al[446] neural invasion was demonstrated in 32%. The 5-year survival rate in patients with neural invasion was 64.3% compared with 81.1% when neural invasion was not demonstrated.

Ueno et al[449] investigated perineural invasion in 364 patients who underwent curative resection for rectal carcinoma penetrating the muscular layer. A grading system was established based on the "intensity" (number of perineural invasion foci in a 20-power field) and "depth" (distance from the muscularis propria). Perinural invasion (PNI) zero was defined as without perineural invasion, PNI-1 as intensity of less than five foci and depth less than 10 mm, and PNI-2 as five or more foci or 10 mm or greater depth of invasion. Perineural invasion was observed in 14% and strongly correlated with pathological lymph node metastases. Five-year survival was related to the perineural invasion (74% in PNI-0, 50% in PNI-1, and 22% in PNI-2). The rate of local recurrence was also related to PNI stage: 43% in PNI-2 and 9% in PNI-0 and PNI-1. The PNI grading system may be useful in prognosis and may allow case selection for intensive postoperative adjuvant therapy.

22.7.3 Biochemical and Special Investigations

Preoperative Carcinoembryonic Antigen Levels

An analysis of data from 945 patients entered into the NSABP revealed a strong correlation between preoperative CEA levels and the Dukes' classes.[448] The mean CEA level progressively increased with each Dukes' category, and the mean value for each of the four classes was significantly different. Mean values (±SE) for Dukes' A, B, C, and D (metastatic or contiguous disease) were 3.9±0.6, 9.3±1.4, 32.1±8.9, and 251±84, respectively. The prognostic function was independent of the number of positive histologic lymph nodes and unrelated to the presence or absence of obstruction. Preoperative levels correlated with the degree of lumen encirclement by the carcinoma, with lesions involving more than one-half the circumference being associated with significantly lower preoperative CEA levels. The relative risk of developing a treatment failure was associated with preoperative CEA in both Dukes' B and C patients. For patients with Dukes' B lesions, those with a CEA of 2.5 to 10 had 1.2 times the likelihood of developing a recurrence as those with less than 2.5, while those with a CEA level greater than 10 had 3.24 times the likelihood. For patients with Dukes' C lesions, the respective risks were 1.77 and 1.76. Although some authors have come to the same conclusion,[437] others have found the correlation true only for patients with Dukes' C lesions.[450] An important caveat to note is that poorly differentiated carcinomas produce little CEA, and therefore a normal preoperative CEA in a patient with a poorly differentiated carcinoma does not suggest a favorable prognosis.[451] Several authors have found CEA determinations to be of little prognostic significance.[452] However, a clearer relationship has been demonstrated between persistently elevated levels of CEA in the postoperative period and early recurrence.[453]

Liver Function Tests

Abnormal results of liver function tests have been associated with a poor prognosis,[454] but not uniformly so.[379]

Other Blood Tests

Low serum protein levels have been reported to be associated with a poor prognosis. Factors found to have no effect on prognosis include hemoglobin level, white blood count, and erythrocyte sedimentation rate.[379]

DNA Distribution

Several studies have reported that patients who exhibit an abnormal DNA pattern, that is, other than the normal diploid pattern, suffer a higher recurrence rate.[455,456,457,458] Giaretti et al[459] found DNA aneuploidy present in 31% of adenomas and 74% of adenocarcinomas. DNA ploidy correlated with the size and the degree of dysplasia but not with histologic type. From the same center, it was determined that fresh-frozen material gave a higher incidence of DNA aneuploidy than paraffin-embedded material (79 vs. 41%).[460] Armitage et al[456] found that 55% of their patients had cells with abnormal DNA (aneuploid). Of this group, only 19% of patients survived 5 years, compared with 43% of patients with diploid neoplasms. In contrast, Jones et al[460] found that after the surgeon's assessment of operability, the pathologic classification, and the patient's age were considered, the DNA ploidy status conferred no independent survival value. Halvorsen and Johannesen[461] reported a significant survival advantage in patients with diploid lesions compared to those with nondiploid lesions but no difference between carcinoma of the rectum and colon. The authors concluded that

ploidy does not contribute to the explanation of why patients with rectal carcinoma had a poorer prognosis than those with colon carcinoma. Venkatesh et al[455] compared two parameters in DNA analysis and found that the odds of survival were 3.7 times greater in patients with aneuploidy rather than aneuploidy plus an S-phase fraction greater than 20%.

Genetic Alteration

Among the most recent factors considered in the galaxy of prognostic discriminants are molecular genetic alterations.[462] Fractional allelic loss, a measure of allelic deletions, has provided independent prognostic information. Distant metastases were significantly associated with high fractional allelic loss and with deletions of 17p and 18q. Further associations were found between allelic losses and a family history of carcinoma, left-sided location of a carcinoma, and absence of extracellular mucin.

Jen et al[463] reported that patients with stage II disease have a 5-year survival rate of 93% when the carcinoma has no evidence of allelic loss of chromosome 18q, but only 54% when there was an allelic loss. In patients with stage III disease, 5-year survival is 52% without allelic loss and 38% with loss. An overall hazard ratio for death in patients with allelic loss of chromosome 18q is 2.83. It has also been reported that patients with CD44 v6-positive carcinomas have a poorer prognosis than those with negative lesions.[464] Overexpression of ras p21 was reportedly associated with an increased incidence of lymphatic invasion, depth of invasion, incidence of liver metastases, and decreased operative curability and long-term survival.[465]

Overall expression of p53 has been found to be an independent predictor of recurrence in Dukes' B and C carcinomas by some authors[466,467] and not a predictor by others.[468] Auvinen et al[467] reported patients with p53 overexpression had a corrected 5-year survival rate of 37% compared with that of 58% in patients with normal expression. Corresponding 10-year rates were 34 and 54%, respectively. TP53 gene mutations (topographic genotyping) have been associated with decreased survival.[469]

Shibata et al[470] found that in patients with stage II disease whose carcinoma expressed DCC, the 5-year survival rate was 94.3%, whereas in patients with DCC-negative lesions, the survival rate was 61.6%. In patients with stage III disease, the survival rates were 59.3 and 33.2%, respectively.

Wang et al[471] used DNA chip technology to systematically identify new prognostic markers for relapse in Dukes' B carcinoma patients. Gene expression profiling identified a 23-gene signature that predicts recurrence in Dukes' B patients. The overall performance accuracy was 78%. Thirteen of 18 relapse patients and 15 of 18 disease-free patients were predicted correctly, giving an OR of 13. The clinical value of these markers is that the patients at a high predictive risk of relapse (13-fold risk) could be upstaged to receive adjuvant therapy, similar to Dukes' C patients.

Lim et al[472] analyzed the association between MSI status and clinicopathological features and prognosis in 248 sporadic colorectal carcinoma patients of which 9.3% had MSI carcinomas. MSI sporadic colorectal carcinomas were found predominantly in the proximal colon and were associated with poor differentiation, a lower preoperative serum CEA level, and less frequent systemic metastases than MSI carcinomas. Low grade, low T-stage, no lymph node metastases, no systemic metastases, adjuvant chemotherapy, and MSI status were independent favorable prognostic factors for survival in sporadic colorectal carcinoma patients.

Kohonen-Corish et al[473] undertook a detailed analysis of the prognostic significance of MSI-L and loss of methyltransferase (MGMT) protein expression in colon carcinoma in 183 patients with clinicopathologic stage C colon carcinoma who had not received adjuvant therapy. They showed that MSI-L defines a group of patients with poorer survival than microsatellite stable (MSS) patients and that MSI-L was an independent prognostic indicator in stage III colon carcinoma. Loss of MGMT protein expression was associated with the MSI-L phenotype but was not a prognostic factor for overall survival in colon carcinoma. p-16 methylation was significantly less frequent in MSI-L than in MSI-H and MSS carcinomas and was not associated with survival.

To derive a more precise estimate of the prognostic significance of MSI, Popat et al[474] reviewed and pooled data from 32 eligible studies that reported survival in a total of 7,642 cases, including 1,277 with MSI. There was no evidence of publication bias. The combined hazard ratio estimate for overall survival associated with MSI was 0.65. This benefit was maintained restricting analyses to clinical trial patients (HR = 0.69) and patients with locally advanced colorectal carcinoma (HR = 0.67).

Sialomucin Staining

Oncogenic transformation of colonic epithelium is accompanied by increased secretion of sialomucin at the expense of the normally predominant sulfomucins. For patients who exhibit a sialomucin-predominant pattern, there is an increased incidence for local recurrence and a predicted diminution of 5-year survival.[475]

Nuclear Morphometry

In search of a reliable prognostic discriminant, Mitmaker et al[476] used nuclear morphometry to assess 100 cases of colorectal carcinoma in which patients who underwent curative resection were followed for at least 5 years. Each case was staged according to the Dukes classification and graded histologically. The nuclear shape factor was defined as the degree of circularity of the nucleus, with a perfect circle recorded as 1.0. A nuclear shape factor greater than 0.84 was associated with a poor outcome. This variable proved to be a highly significant predictor of survival and independent of the variables of sex, age, histologic grade, and Dukes' classification.

Plasminogen Activity

Studies of tissue plasminogen activity have revealed that overall survival curves are related to the ratio of urokinase-type plasminogen activators to tissue-type plasminogen activators.[477] A ratio greater than 0.22 in normal mucosa of patients with Dukes' B and C carcinoma has a decreased probability of survival with a Cox's hazard ratio of 2.8.

Sialyl Lewis^x Antigen Expression

Based on data of 114 patients who underwent curative resections, sialyl Lewis^x antigen–positive patients had a higher incidence of recurrence in distant organs, especially in the liver, than that of sialyl Lewis^x–negative patients.[478] The 5-year disease-free survival rates of sialyl Lewis^x–positive and –negative patients were 57.7 and 89.1%, respectively.

Proliferating Cell Nuclear Antigen Labeling Findings

Proliferating cell nuclear antigen expressions of the invasive margin of a carcinoma were shown to be significantly higher in patients who were noted to have venous invasions, a higher potential for metastases to lymph nodes and liver, and less differentiated lesions.[479]

22.8 Recurrent Disease

22.8.1 Follow-up

The most appropriate follow-up for patients who have been operated on for carcinoma of the colon has not been determined. Any follow-up program should focus on the detection of resectable anastomotic and locoregional failure, liver and lung metastases, and metachronous lesions. In a retrospective analysis of 5,476 patients with colon or rectal carcinoma, Cali et al[480] calculated the annual incidence for metachronous carcinomas to be 0.35%. Current recommendations for follow-up are described in Chapter 20. However, the wisdom of any type of follow-up has been questioned. The rationale for such a stance is the belief that little effective therapy is available when recurrences develop. Opponents argue that intensive follow-up is not worth the effort and expense, since as many as 62% of new lesions are detected when the patient presents with symptoms between scheduled follow-up sessions.[217,453,481,482] Proponents of intensive follow-up state that if a recurrent or metachronous lesion is detected when a patient is asymptomatic, the probability of cure by repeat resection will be increased, since the newly detected lesion will be at a more favorable stage than if the patient were symptomatic.[483,484] In support of the latter argument, Bühler et al[483] reported on a series in which patients with asymptomatic anastomotic recurrence had a re-resection rate of 66%, with a survival rate of 12 to 72 months, whereas none of the patients who were symptomatic had a resection for cure and the survival rate in this group was 1 to 24 months. In a report in which 1,293 patients were rigorously followed, 299 recurrences were detected in 168 patients (local recurrence, 40%; liver metastases, 29%; and other, 31%).[484] Of these patients, 51% with local recurrence and 47% with liver metastases were asymptomatic. Radical operation was performed in 50% of those with local recurrences and in 26% of those with liver metastases. The 3-year survival rate after reoperation was 35% in those with local recurrence and 33% in those with liver metastases. The 5-year survival rates were 23 and 15%, respectively. These results demonstrate the benefit of aggressive follow-up. Yamamoto et al[485] reported the results of 974 patients who underwent a curative resection. Recurrence developed locally in 7.2%; liver, 4.8%; and lung, 3.6%. The percentages of patients who underwent reoperation or curative resection were 77 and 24% of those with local recurrence, 34 and 38% of those with liver metastases, and 17 and 100% of those with pulmonary metastases, respectively. The 3-and 5-year survival rates were 13 and

9% after reoperation for local recurrence, 14 and 0% for liver metastases, and 53 and 53% after reoperation for pulmonary metastases, respectively.

In an extensive review by Wade et al[206] of 22,715 patients who underwent colectomy for carcinoma, 12,150 presented with metastatic disease. The estimated surveillance costs averaged $1.3 million per life saved by resection, or $203,000 per year of added life. Despite the apparent high price tag for postoperative studies, the authors believe that surveillance should continue. The costs of eliminating surveillance after curative colectomy would be paid every year by the patients who would die annually with recurrent carcinoma of the colon and rectum, by those who would lose 20 to 28 months of added life gained on average with resection of their isolated colorectal metastases, and by the patients whose cure would be sacrificed. There is a need to determine which tests and regimens can best identify metastatic disease at an early enough stage to allow curative treatment for those who will benefit from it.

22.8.2 Incidence

In an excellent review, Devesa et al[318] found that the incidence of recurrence varied because of multiple biases of classification and treatment, different methods of determining recurrence, and statistical manipulation. From their study, it was noted that all series quote the incidence of recurrence by Dukes' staging or by some modification of Dukes' staging (e.g., Dukes' A from 0 to 13%, Dukes' B from 11 to 61%, and Dukes' C from 32 to 88%). Although anastomotic recurrences are not uncommon with low anterior resection, such a development following a right hemicolectomy or intraperitoneal anastomosis is considered a rare entity.

22.8.3 Contributing Factors

Sugarbaker et al[46] have suggested several possible reasons that "curative" resections fail: (1) metastases in the lymphatic channels or nodes may result in unrecognized residual carcinoma, (2) malignant cells may be exfoliated from the primary lesion into veins prior to or during the operation, (3) malignant cells may persist at the circumferential margins of resection, and (4) malignant cells may be disseminated at the time of resection. Implantation is more likely to result in the development of early recurrence at the suture line, whereas metachronous carcinogenesis provides a likely explanation for the development of late recurrences.[486] Indeed, all four mechanisms may play a role to a lesser or greater extent.

22.8.4 Patterns

Depending on the location of the original resection, patterns of recurrence vary with respect to the development of local, anastomotic, regional, or distant failure as well as the time to recurrence.[487,488] The definition of local recurrence generally includes recurrence in areas contiguous to the bed of the primary resection or recurrence at the site of anastomosis. Distant spread represents metastases to sites beyond the location of resection. Local pelvic failure is common in rectal carcinoma because of narrow radial margins defined by the anatomic limits of dissection. Colon carcinoma tends to fail in the peritoneal cavity, the liver, or distant sites, with a relatively small component of isolated local failure. This pattern explains the emphasis on radiotherapy as adjuvant therapy for rectal carcinoma and systemic chemotherapy for colonic carcinoma. In a review of several series, Devesa et al[318] found that 30 to 50% of patients with recurrence of colon carcinoma manifested locoregional failure. Distant metastases are present in up to 80% of patients with recurrence. The liver is most often involved in 50 to 80% of autopsy studies, followed by lung, bone, and other sites. In a follow-up of 487 patients for a median of 48 months (range, 15–132 months), Böhm et al[489] documented recurrence in 31%. Of those, distant metastases were found in 51%, only local recurrence in 31%, and both local and distant metastases in 18%. In the review by Obrand and Gordon[490] the reported recurrence rates after curative resection of large bowel adenocarcinoma varied widely from 3 to 50%.

The patterns of recurrence from several selected series are presented in ▶ Table 22.11. It is often difficult to separate series of colon carcinoma from those of rectal carcinoma because the reports often are combined. Rodriguez-Bigas et al[491] conducted a retrospective analysis of the prognostic significance of anastomotic recurrence in 50 patients with colorectal carcinoma. All carcinomas were located above 10 cm from the anal verge. Forty anastomotic recurrences (80%) followed resection of sigmoid or proximal rectal lesions. The overall disease-free interval was 13 months, with 90% of recurrences diagnosed within 24 months of the primary resection. Forty-five recurrences (90%) were associated with synchronous or metachronous metastases. The overall median survival rate following the recurrence was 16 months (37 months if the anastomosis was the only recurrence site). Of five patients alive without evidence of disease, all were asymptomatic, and recurrence was confined to the anastomosis. The authors concluded that anastomotic recurrence following resection of colorectal carcinoma frequently heralds disseminated disease but can be potentially resected for cure if it is the only site in an otherwise asymptomatic patient. Willett et al[324] reported that in patients with obstructing lesions, local failure developed in 42%, approximately one-third of whom had local failure only. In patients with perforated carcinoma, 44% developed local failure. The incidence of local failure and distant metastases in their control group was 14 and 21%, respectively.

With respect to the time frame, Ekman et al[217] found that 70% of all recurrences of colon carcinoma were detected within 2 years of operation and 90% were detected within 4 years. A review of the literature by Devesa et al[318] noted that 60 to 84% of recurrences became apparent within 2 years of the initial operation and 90% within 4 years (median, 22 months).[493,494,495] With respect to location, Malcolm et al[492] found overall recurrence rates of 24, 10, 11.5, and 34%, respectively, for carcinoma of the right, transverse, left, and sigmoid colon.

In a study to determine the incidence and patterns of recurrence after curative resection of colorectal carcinoma, Obrand and Gordon[490] conducted a retrospective review of 524 patients, 448 operated on with curative intent. The overall recurrence rate was 27.9%. The anastomotic recurrence rate was 11.7%. Locoregional recurrence rates, including anastomotic recurrences, were higher in patients with rectal lesions than colon lesions (20.3 vs. 6.2%). Distant metastases developed in 14.4% of patients (13.9% for colon carcinoma and 15.5% for rectal carcinoma).

Table 22.11 Patterns of recurrence following curative resection for colon carcinoma

Authors	No. of patients	Duration of follow-up (y)	Recurrence (%)			Total	Time to recurrence (mo)	5-y survival (%)
			Local	Distal	Local and distant			
Olson et al[481]	214	5.0	7		16	23		49
Malcolm et al[492]	191	5.0	1	22	5	28	1–102	21
Boey et al[493]	146		10	15	10	35	4–40	
Russell et al[487]	550	4.0	5	19	10	34	2–102	
Umpleby et al[304]	329	5.0	18	22	7	47		27
Willett et al[494]	533	5.0	6	12	13	31		63
Gunderson et al[495]	91		19	20	39			
Galandiuk et al[496,a]	818	2.0–11.5	5	34	4	43	0.5–98 (median, 17)	
Obrand and Gordon[490,a]	448	1–15 (median, 70 mo)	13	13	2	28	2–100 (median, 17)	47[b]

[a]Includes colon and rectal carcinoma.
[b]Forty-seven percent alive at average of 80 months.

The average time to recurrence was 21.3 months (median, 17 months; range, 2–100 months). The average time for anastomotic recurrence was 16.2 versus 22.9 months for distant disease and 18.9 months for regional recurrence. Colon recurrences occurred at a median of 16 versus 17 months for rectal recurrences. Patients with Dukes' A lesions had a 17.6% recurrence rate, those with Dukes' B had a 23.4% rate, and those with Dukes' C had 43.7%. Patients who did not undergo any intervention after diagnosis of recurrence survived an average of 28 months. Those who received palliative treatment survived an average of 39 months. Of those patients who underwent reoperation, 24% had re-resection for cure. Anastomotic re-resections accounted for 20 of 30 resections. A majority of recurrences (69.4%) occurred within 24 months of the original operation and 95% recurred by 48 months. For those who received adjuvant therapy, the mean and median times to recurrence were 25.4 and 22.0 months, respectively. For those patients who did not receive any adjuvant treatment, the mean and median times to recurrence were 19.8 and 16.0 months, respectively. Neither of these reached statistical significance on multivariate analysis. Forty-seven percent of these patients were alive at a mean of 8 months. Those who died of their disease did so at an average of 53 months. Positive predictive factors for recurrence included the site of the lesion (rectum vs. colon), stage, invasion of contiguous organs, and presence of perforation. Age, sex, degree of differentiation, mucin secretion, and gross morphology were not found to be predictive factors.

Risk factors previously associated with increased recurrence rates include patient's sex, age, Dukes' stage, site of primary carcinoma (colon vs. rectum), infiltration of adjacent organs, perforation, and histology and size of the carcinoma, among others. Adverse prognostic factors reported by Galandiuk et al[496] include males doing worse than females, rectum worse than colon, Dukes' C worse than B, grades 3 and 4 worse than 1 and 2, adhesions and/or invasion worse than none, perforation worse than none, and nondiploid worse than diploid.

The clinical relevance of seeking factors capable of predicting recurrence is to permit the physician to focus on subsets of patients who might most appropriately be targeted for aggressive adjuvant therapy and postoperative surveillance programs that will expedite the diagnosis of recurrent disease at a time when potentially curative therapy can be instituted. This is true even for patients who develop metastatic disease such as liver or lung metastases where curative resections are still favorable in selected circumstances.

Disease recurrence in the abdominal wall from primary colorectal carcinoma has received renewed attention after the recognition of port site metastases in patients undergoing laparoscopic colorectal resections. Koea et al[497] reviewed 31 patients presenting to Memorial Sloan Kettering Cancer Center with recurrent disease in the abdominal wall between 7 and 183 months after operation. Primary carcinomas were located in the right colon in 17 patients, left colon in 2 patients, sigmoid colon in 7 patients, and rectum in 3 patients. Nineteen percent of primary carcinomas were perforated, 45% were poorly differentiated, 92% were transmural (T3 or T4), and 51% had lymph node metastases at presentation. Twenty-two patients presented with a symptomatic abdominal wall mass, whereas recurrence in the abdominal wall was found incidentally in nine patients undergoing laparotomy. Four patients had isolated abdominal wall disease, whereas the remaining 27 were found to have associated intra-abdominal disease. Six patients who were left with residual intra-abdominal carcinoma after abdominal wall resection had a median survival of 4 months. Twenty-five patients underwent a histologically complete resection of recurrence restricted to the abdominal wall alone ($n = 4$; median survival time, 18 months), abdominal wall and in continuity resection of adherent viscera ($n = 15$; median survival time, 12.5 months), or resection of abdominal wall and intra-abdominal recurrence at a distant site ($n = 6$, median survival time, 22 months, although only one patient remained alive with disease). The actual 2- and 5-year survival rates were 16 and 3%, respectively. They concluded abdominal wall metastases are often indicators of recurrent intra-abdominal disease; aggressive resection in patients with disease restricted to the abdominal wall and associated adherent viscera can result in local disease control.

22.8.5 Clinical Features

The first suspicion of recurrence may be the insidious failure of general health signaled by malaise, weight loss, and anorexia. Vague discomfort as well as occasional bowel symptoms may be present. General physical examination is usually unrewarding, but as the disease progresses, a mass in the abdominal wall or within the abdominal cavity as well as ascites may be present.

22.8.6 Investigations

In the detection of local recurrence or peritoneal seeding, physical examination and radiologic tests are not sensitive. Barium enema examination may reveal the recurrence, but sometimes minor changes have been interpreted as a surgical tailoring defect and anastomotic recurrences are not likely to be detected early. Colonoscopy will more directly detect anastomotic recurrences, but mucosal disruption caused by locoregional recurrence is reported to occur in less than 3% of patients.[443]

Barillari et al[498] evaluated the effectiveness of routine colonoscopy in 481 patients who underwent curative resection. Approximately 10% of patients developed intraluminal recurrences, with more than half arising in the first 24 months. CT is not a reliable diagnostic test for low-volume masses on peritoneal surfaces. Jacquet et al[499] found an overall sensitivity of 79%. Sensitivity was 90% for nodules greater than 0.5 cm but only 28% for nodules less than 0.5 cm. Sensitivity was lowest in the pelvis (60%). The newest technology available to detect recurrent disease is fluorodeoxyglucose (FDG) PET. Delbeke et al[500] assessed the accuracy of [18]FDG-PET in patients with recurrent colorectal carcinoma in detecting liver metastases compared with CT and CT portography, detecting extrahepatic metastases compared with CT and evaluating the impact on patient management. Fifty-two patients previously treated for colorectal carcinoma presented on 61 occasions with suspected recurrence and underwent PET of the entire body. The final diagnosis was obtained by pathology ($n = 44$) or clinical and radiological follow-up ($n = 17$). A total of 166 suspicious lesions were identified. Of the 127 intrahepatic lesions, 104 were malignant and of the 39 extrahepatic lesions, 34 were malignant. PET was more accurate (92%) than CT and CT portography (78 and 80%, respectively) in detecting liver metastases and more accurate than CT for extrahepatic metastases (92 and 71%, respectively). PET detected unsuspected metastases in 17 patients and altered surgical management in 28% of patients. They concluded PET is the most accurate noninvasive method for staging patients for recurrent metastatic colorectal carcinoma and plays an important role in management decisions in this setting.

Libutti et al[342] evaluated the PET scan and CEA scan as a means of localizing recurrent colorectal carcinoma. In 28 patients explored, disease was found at operation in 94%. Ten had

unresectable disease. PET scan predicted unresectable disease in 90% of patients. CEA scans failed to predict unresectable disease in any patient. In 16 patients found to have resectable disease or disease that could be treated with regional therapy, PET scan predicted this in 81% and CEA scan in 13%.

Desai et al[501] determined the effect of PET on surgical decision making in patients with metastatic or recurrent colorectal carcinoma. A total of 114 patients with advanced colorectal carcinoma were imaged with CT and PET scans. Forty-two of the 114 patients deemed to have resectable disease on the basis of CT, PET altered therapy in 40% on the basis of extrahepatic disease, bilobar involvement, thoracic involvement, retroperitoneal lymphadenopathy, bone involvement, and supraclavicular disease. In 25 patients with liver metastases, only PET found additional disease in 72%, extrahepatic disease, chest disease, retroperitoneal lymphadenopathy, and bone disease. Both scans underestimated small-volume peritoneal metastases discovered at laparotomy.

Whiteford et al[502] evaluated the records of 105 patients who underwent 101 CT and 109 PET scans for suspected metastatic colorectal carcinoma. Clinical correlation was confirmed at time of operation, histologically, or by clinical course. The overall sensitivity and specificity of PET scan in detection of clinically relevant carcinoma were higher (87 and 68%) than for CT plus other conventional diagnostic studies (66 and 59%). The sensitivity of PET scan in detecting mucinous carcinoma was lower (58%) than for nonmucinous carcinoma (92%). The sensitivity of PET scanning in detecting locoregional recurrence was higher than for CT plus colonoscopy (90 vs. 71%, respectively). The sensitivity of PET in detecting hepatic metastases was higher than for CT (89 vs. 71%). The sensitivity of PET scanning in detecting extrahepatic metastases exclusive of locoregional recurrence was higher for CT plus other conventional diagnostic studies (94 vs. 67%). PET scanning altered clinical management in a beneficiary manner in 26% of cases when compared with evaluation of CT plus other conventional diagnostic studies.

Johnson et al[503] compared CT scan with PET scan in clinical decision making. A retrospective review of 41 patients with metastatic colorectal carcinoma who had both CT and PET scans before operative exploration was performed. All patients underwent re-exploration. Findings were divided into hepatic, extrahepatic, and pelvic regions of the abdomen. PET scan was found to be more sensitive than CT scan when compared with operative findings in the liver (100 vs. 69%), extrahepatic region (90 vs. 52%), and abdomen as a whole (87 vs. 61%). Sensitivities of PET scan and CT scan were not significantly different in the pelvic region (87 vs. 61%). In each case, specificity was not significantly different between the two examinations. However, PET scanning is more sensitive than CT scanning and more likely to give the correct result when actual metastatic disease is present.

22.8.7 Role of Carcinoembryonic Antigen

One area in which CEA may be of value is in the early detection of recurrence. However, this is not always the case, and when the CEA level is elevated, there is often other evidence of recurrence. In their review of the literature, Devesa et al[318] found higher than normal blood CEA levels in less than 50% of patients with early or localized failure and in approximately 75% of patients with widely disseminated disease nearly always involving the liver. The percentage of patients with lung metastases or peritoneal seeding who show elevated CEA levels is very low. False-positive results are found in 6 to 25% of cases. Transient elevations of CEA have been reported to occur in 7 to 36% of patients without demonstrable recurrent carcinoma.

In a remarkable series reported by Minton et al[504] in which a CEA-directed second-look procedure was practiced on asymptomatic patients, approximately half of the patients were found to have a recurrence amenable to resection for cure. The 5-year survival rate for this group was 30%. In those patients with recurrences after a second-look procedure, a small select group was slated to undergo a third-look (and possibly a fourth-look) procedure in an attempt to make them disease-free. The authors justify this aggressive approach because of the unresponsiveness of colorectal carcinoma to other treatment modalities.

Careful preoperative assessment must be performed to exclude those patients with unresectable metastatic disease. The surgeon must be aware that CEA levels may be elevated in non-malignant conditions. Several authors have reported the benefit of a CEA-directed second-look operation.[493,505,506] However, most surgeons have not encountered such uniformly encouraging results. In a selected review of four series comprising 203 patients, Wanebo and Stevens[450] found 80% with recurrent carcinoma. Disease was localized in 46%, and 54% had distant metastases. CEA levels at exploration ranged from 6.5 ng/mL (Ohio State University) to 25 ng/mL (Memorial Sloan Kettering Cancer Center); 36% of the entire group underwent resection for cure, but the range was 7% (Roswell Park Memorial Institute) to 72% (Ohio State University).

Hida et al[506] reported on the usefulness of postoperative CEA monitoring for second-look operations. Seven hundred and fifty-six patients with Dukes' B and C, who had undergone curative resection, were monitored postoperatively using CEA and imaging techniques. A second-look operation was performed on any patient with a potentially resectable recurrence and, in addition, a second-look operation was performed when a persistently rising CEA value was detected. Recurrence developed in 18.8% of patients and 90.8% of the recurrences were detected within the first 3 years following curative resection. When comparing carcinomas of the colon with those of the rectum, the former were associated with significantly more hepatic and intra-abdominal recurrences, whereas the latter had significantly more locoregional and pulmonary recurrences. Seventy-two patients underwent a second-look operation. Of those patients, 54.2% had all of their disease resected and 1.4% had no detectable disease at the second look. Among the 142 patients with recurrence, 50% of patients underwent a second-look operation. The resectable group carried a significantly better survival than the unresectable recurrence group (41.3 vs. 5.2%). The authors concluded that complete removal of colorectal carcinoma recurrences by second-look operations, on the basis of postoperative, follow-up CEA, and imaging technique findings, results in improved survival.

22.8.8 Treatment

Operative Treatment

Reluctance on the part of many surgeons to engage in the close follow-up of patients who previously have undergone resection for carcinoma of the colon and rectum lies in the pessimistic reports of the limited prospect for patients being amenable to re-excisional surgery. Böhm et al[489] reported that 24% of patients could undergo further curative resection but only 25% of those (6% of all recurrences) were free of disease for more than 2 years. Nevertheless, some reports have been encouraging and it is well worthwhile to operate on some of these individuals.[507] Follow-up is important for several reasons: (1) a second primary large bowel malignancy may be detected at an early stage of development, (2) patients who have had a colorectal carcinoma are at a higher risk of developing a primary malignancy in another organ (e.g., the breast or endometrium), and (3) recurrent disease may be diagnosed when it is localized and thus be amenable to curative therapy. Gwin et al[508] reviewed 28 patients with nonhepatic intra-abdominal recurrence of carcinoma of the colon and were able to report 15 patients who had a median actuarial survival of 25.5 months. Disease-free survival was prolonged for these patients when the time to recurrence was greater than 16 months. Patients who underwent palliative resection did better than those who had a bypass. Using CEA-directed second-look operations, Minton et al[504] reported a re-resection for cure in 60% of patients with a 5-year survival of 30%. In a review of several series published in the 1980s, Herfarth et al[509] found reoperation rates ranging from 18 to 60%, with an average of 31%.

The value of operation for patients with incurable colorectal carcinoma is controversial. Law et al[510] evaluated the outcomes of 180 patients undergoing operation for incurable colorectal carcinoma. Seventeen patients died in the postoperative period. Operative mortality was significantly higher in patients with nonresection procedures. Median survival of patients with resection was significantly longer than in those without resection (30 vs. 17 weeks). Other independent factors that were significantly associated with poor survival were the presence of ascites, presence of bilobar liver metastases, and absence of chemotherapy and/or radiation therapy. In the presence of these factors, the balance between the benefit and risk of operation should be carefully considered before decision for operative treatment.

Bowne et al[511] reported their experience with surgical resection for patients with locoregional recurrent colon carcinoma. A total of 744 patients with recurrent colon carcinoma were identified and 100 (13.4%) underwent exploration with curative intent for potentially resectable locoregional recurrence: 75 with isolated locoregional recurrence, and 25 with locoregional recurrence and resectable distant disease. The median follow-up for survivors was 27 months. Locoregional recurrence was classified into four categories: anastomotic, mesenteric/nodal, retroperitoneal, and peritoneal. Median survival for all patients was 30 months. Fifty-six patients had an R0 resection (including distant sites). Factors associated with prolonged disease-specific survival included R0 resection; age younger than 60 years; early stage of primary disease; and no associated distant disease. Poor prognostic factors included more than one site of recurrence and involvement of the mesenteric/nodal basin. The ability to obtain an R0 resection was the strongest predictor of outcome, and these patients had a median survival of 66 months.

Intraoperative Radiotherapy

Because of the inadequacy of operation or radiation therapy alone to treat recurrent locally advanced disease, a multimodality approach of intraoperative electron beam radiotherapy (IORT) combined with operation has been advocated.[512] Willett et al[512] reported that 5-year actuarial local control and disease-free survival rates for 30 patients undergoing this treatment program were 26 and 19%, respectively.

Taylor et al[513] reported on 100 colonic carcinoma patients treated with combination therapy including surgical resection, chemotherapy, and external plus intraoperative radiotherapy. The 5-year survival was 24.7%. The 38 patients with recurrent disease whose disease was completely resected had a 37.4% 5-year survival.

Endoscopic Laser Therapy

For the recurrent lesion that is unresectable, relief of obstruction and control of bleeding or secretions may be obtained by the use of endoscopic laser therapy.[514] This therapy offers no relief of pain nor would there be any expected improvement in survival. However, an important advantage of this mode of therapy is that it can be performed with little or no sedation, thus avoiding the risks of general anesthesia and major surgery. In addition, it can be performed on an outpatient basis in most cases and can be applied on a repetitive schedule because there is no limiting cumulative dose for laser energy. Finally, systemic side effects are few, and thus patient acceptance is good.[515] The symptoms of obstruction or bleeding can be controlled in 80 to 90% of patients with a complication rate of less than 10% and a mortality rate of approximately 1%.[128,516,517,518,519,520,521,522,523] Not all reports support the palliative virtues of lasers. In one report, two-thirds of patients with large lesions showed little improvement and required alternative operative management.[524] Courtney et al[525] reported their experience with high-powered diode laser to palliate 57 patients with inoperable colorectal carcinoma with neodymium:yttrium aluminum garnet (Nd:YAG). The median number of treatments received by each patient was 3 (range, 1–16 treatments), with a median interval between treatments of 9.5 (range, 1–25) weeks. Lifelong palliation of symptoms occurred in 89% of patients. Major complications were two perforations and one hemorrhage, giving an overall complication rate of 5.3%. One of the patients who experienced perforation died, giving an overall mortality rate of 1.8% for the procedure. The median survival by laser therapy was 8.5 months with a probability of survival at 24 months of 15%. The role of metallic stenting has been described previously. For the individual in whom laser therapy or stenting is unsuitable or unsuccessful and who ultimately presents with an obstruction secondary to recurrence, a stoma may be the last desperate effort at palliation.

Cytoreductive Surgery and Hyperthermic Intraperitoneal Chemotherapy

Hyperthermic intraoperative intraperitoneal chemotherapy has been proposed to treat peritoneal carcinomatosis arising from colon carcinoma, which is usually regarded as a lethal clinical entity. Pilati et al[526] reviewed 46 patients treated for peritoneal carcinomatosis from colorectal carcinoma. Thirty-four patients were treated with complete cytoreductive surgery, immediately followed by intraoperative hyperthermic intraperitoneal chemotherapy with mitomycin C and cisplatin. No operative deaths were reported. The postoperative morbidity rate was 35%. No severe locoregional or systemic toxicity was observed. The 2-year overall survival was 31% and the median survival time and the median time to local disease progression were 18 and 13 months, respectively. Survival and local disease control in patients with well and moderately differentiated colon carcinoma were significantly better than in those with poorly differentiated lesions. Considering the dismal prognosis of this condition, hyperthermic intraoperative intraperitoneal chemotherapy seems to achieve encouraging results in a selected group of patients affected with resectable peritoneal carcinomatosis arising from colon carcinoma.

Verwaal et al[527] evaluated the outcome after the treatment of peritoneal carcinomatosis of colorectal carcinoma by cytoreduction and hyperthermic intraperitoneal chemotherapy. Recurrence within the study period of 7.5 years was 65%. For patients who had undergone a gross incomplete initial cytoreduction, the median duration of survival after recurrence was 3.7 months. If a complete cytoreduction had been accomplished initially, the median duration of survival after recurrence was 11.1 months. After effective initial treatment, a second surgical debulking for recurrent disease resulted in median survival duration of 10.3 months and after treatment with chemotherapy it was 8.5 months. The survival was 11.2 months for patients who received radiotherapy for recurrent disease. Patients who did not receive further therapy survived 1.9 months. They concluded treatment of recurrence after cytoreduction and hyperthermic intraperitoneal chemotherapy is often feasible and seems worthwhile in selected patients.

Management of Malignant Ureteral Obstruction

The patient who develops a malignant ureteral obstruction poses a special and difficult problem in the decision-making process. A thoughtful and reasoned approach to the subject was outlined by Smith and Bruera,[528] from whom much of the following information has been obtained. The patient presents with an upper urinary tract obstruction with clinical manifestations including flank pain, hematuria, fever, sepsis, and pyuria. In cases of high-grade obstruction, oliguria, anuria, or uremia may be presenting features. The diagnosis may be suspected based on retroperitoneal lymphadenopathy seen on abdominal pelvic CT or hydronephrosis seen on abdominal ultrasonography. The imaging method of choice for proving ureteral obstruction is excretory urography.

It is in the management of these patients that the decision-making process is difficult. An important consideration in the decision to treat these patients is their performance status. Some patients are already bedridden, severely symptomatic, and may not require treatment of their obstruction. Other patients may still be active with expressed, clearly defined personal goals that they can achieve with a few more months of life. For those patients deemed appropriate for aggressive therapy, both pharmacologic and urologic interventions may prove beneficial. It has clearly been shown that resection is contraindicated.[196]

Pharmacologic treatments include the use of agents with antineoplastic activity or agents capable of reducing edema. In the latter category, patients with acute or chronic renal failure are treated with intravenous rehydration and a trial of high-dose corticosteroids (intravenous dexamethasone, 10 mg every 6 hours for 48 hours).

The role of urologic intervention in the management of malignant ureteral obstruction in advanced disease is not well defined. Some authors contend that active intervention is unwarranted with long-term progression of an underlying malignancy. Keidan et al[529] reviewed 20 patients with advanced pelvic malignancy and concluded that before recommending percutaneous nephrostomy, the factors of in-hospital mortality (35% never left the hospital), limited survival (an additional 35% spent < 6 weeks at home before they died), significant morbidity (55% required multiple tube changes), and poor quality of life should be considered. Others argue that decision making should be guided by clinical indications and contraindications. Published indications for urinary diversion in malignant ureteral obstruction include bilateral hydronephrosis, unilateral ureteral obstruction with renal insufficiency, and unilateral pyelonephritis. Contraindications include the evidence of rapid progression of underlying disease for which no further antineoplastic treatment is planned, other life-threatening medical problems for which no further treatment is planned, and asymptomatic unilateral malignant ureteral obstruction with normal stable renal function in patients whose previous ureteral stenting has failed. Endoscopic retrograde placement of double J (double pig-tail) type ureteral stents is generally considered the first-line urinary diversion procedure. Failing this, percutaneous nephrostomy tubes can be placed successfully in nearly all cases. Open nephrostomy, with its significant mortality and complication rates associated with prolonged hospitalization, makes this a less attractive option. Anterograde and bidirectional stenting, subcutaneous stenting, and cutaneous ureterostomy have a limited role. In the final analysis, the decision regarding the management of ureteral obstruction needs to be highly personalized and follow a careful discussion with the patient and/or his or her family.

Nonoperative Treatment

For the most part, radiotherapy has not been used in the treatment of recurrent carcinoma of the colon because of the effects of radiation on the remaining abdominal viscera. However, specific localized areas of known recurrence can be treated by radiotherapy.

Chemotherapy in the form of various drugs, dosage scheduling, and routes of administration has been used for the treatment of colon carcinoma. The most frequently used drug has been 5-FU, which offered response rates in the 15% range. Addition of other drugs as described previously has improved response rates.

Pain Management

For patients in whom no active treatment is available, it is imperative that the treating physician ensure that the patient is relieved of pain by the prescription of progressively strong analgesics as necessary. Chronic severe carcinoma pain often is not well controlled because of an inadequate understanding of the nature of pain. Common causes of chronic pain in patients with carcinoma include the following[530]:

- Peripheral neuropathies due to radiation, chemotherapy (typically platinum, paclitaxel, and vincristine), erosion by the malignancy.
- Radiation fibrosis.
- Chronic postsurgical incisional pain.
- Phantom pain.
- Arthropathies and musculoskeletal pain due to changes in posture or mobility.
- Visceral pain due to damage to viscera or blockage due to the malignancy.

Most chronic pain in patients with carcinoma is neuropathic pain. Physicians often unnecessarily limit the dosage of analgesia because they have the ill-founded fear that the patient will become addicted to the drug. The basis of rational management is an appropriate analgesic given regularly in dosages adequate to suppress pain continuously. The stable of drugs might include traditional analgesics such as acetylsalicylic acid, acetaminophen, and pentazocine; anti-inflammatory agents such as acetylsalicylic acid, indomethacin, and phenylbutazone, valuable in the management of painful bony metastases; psychotropic analgesics such as tricyclic antidepressants (e.g., amitriptyline) and phenothiazine tranquilizers; and, ultimately, narcotics such as meperidine, methadone, codeine, and morphine. Drug selection climbs the "analgesic ladder" from nonopioid for mild pain to opioid with or without adjuvant medication for severe pain from carcinoma (▶ Fig. 22.37).[531] A combination of agents is often useful. Since many of the narcotics result in constipation, patients should be prescribed laxatives at the same time (see Chapter 31). For patients in whom pain cannot be controlled by traditional oral and parenteral methods, Waterman et al[532] have used epidural and intrathecal infusion with morphine. Excellent or good relief of pain was obtained in 70% of patients. It is a method of delivery that can be used in an outpatient setting. For patients in whom the pain is still not controlled, regional therapies should be considered, such as celiac plexus block or sympathetic blockade. Failing this, a neuroablative procedure should be offered, such as rhizotomy, neurolysis of primary afferent nerves or their ganglia, or cordotomy.[531,532]

An often-neglected aspect of the care of patients with advanced carcinoma is the anorexia and associated weight loss suffered by these terminally ill patients. Foltz et al[533] determined that nutritional counseling produced a significant increase in caloric intake. The augmented regimen included a target caloric intake with 25% of total calories derived from protein sources as well as zinc and magnesium supplementation. Increases in intake were not associated with significant weight gain or increased percent protein intake, but they had some effect on minimizing weight loss or stabilizing weight, even in patients with advanced disease who were undergoing systemic chemotherapy.

22.8.9 Results of Reoperation

The virtue of re-resection of local recurrence for cure has been questioned, but it is undeniable that some patients with local

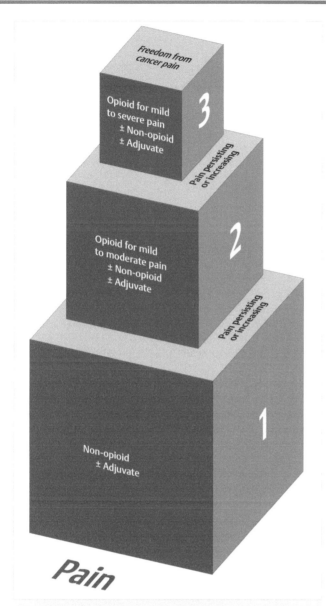

Fig. 22.37 "Analgesic ladder" of pain control.

recurrence are amenable to cure. Reports of success for the re-section of local recurrence for cure have varied widely, but 5-year survivals in the 30% range have been recorded.[504] Since many reports have documented that most recurrences occur within the first 2 years after resection of the primary lesion,[481] it seems reasonable to concentrate follow-up efforts during that period. Those opposed to intensive follow-up state that the poor reoperation rate for cure, ranging from 7 to 20%, negates the cost and effort applied.[217,443,481,482] However, Bühler et al[483] noted that repeat resections for cure were possible in 66% of patients who were asymptomatic at the time that the recurrent lesion was detected, whereas in symptomatic patients, the lesion was usually unresectable. In a series of 30 patients with anastomotic recurrence, Vassilopoulos et al[534] found that the majority of patients were diagnosed within 2 years of initial operation, but in this series the diagnosis was usually based on persistent signs and symptoms. Nevertheless, resection for cure was still feasible in 50% of the cases, with a 5-year survival rate

of 49% and only a 3% operative mortality rate. In the report by Pihl et al,[535] an anastomotic recurrence rate of 2.7% was detected with a re-resection rate of 40%. Other authors also believe that re-resection offers the best outlook with regard to survival.[536] Barillari et al[498] detected a 10% intraluminal recurrence rate in a series of 481 patients. Of the 29 patients who underwent a second operation, 17 had a radical procedure and, in this group, the 5-year survival rate was 70.6%. The authors concluded that asymptomatic patients more frequently underwent another operation for cure and thus had a better survival rate.[532]

22.8.10 Intestinal Obstruction Due to Recurrent Carcinoma

A very difficult situation that challenges the clinical judgment of even the most experienced surgeon is the management of patients presenting with bowel obstruction after treatment of the primary malignancy when the feared cause is metastatic disease. Inappropriate operation does not improve outcome. Stellato and Shenk[537] reviewed the literature on this subject and concluded that patients should be treated as any other patient manifesting intestinal obstruction, the rationale being that 26 to 38% of the bowel obstructions in patients with a history of malignancy are not secondary to recurrent or metastatic disease and that operative mortality rates for patients with carcinoma are comparable (9–15%) with those of patients presenting with obstruction without a history of malignancy. While 10 to 30% of patients obtain relief of obstruction by nasogastric decompression (two-thirds within 3 days), 40% require operation. More than 35% of those with obstruction due to recurrent carcinoma obtain relief of their symptoms with operation. Predictors of poor outcome include the presence of shock, ascites, or an abdominal mass, with mortality rates of 100, 70, and 54%, respectively. Known carcinomatosis has a 40% 30-day mortality rate. van Ooijen et al[538] reviewed the management of 59 patients with intestinal obstruction (38 patients with advanced carcinoma of the ovary and 21 patients with peritoneal carcinomatosis of other organs). The authors concluded that operative therapy for the relief of intestinal obstruction should only be considered in patients who do not present with manifest ascites or palpable masses and in patients with carcinoma of the ovary for whom effective chemotherapy is available. The rationale is simply that patients with masses or ascites had a median postoperative survival of only 36 days. Percutaneous gastrostomy should be the method of choice for other patients.

Although the overall prognosis is poor in patients with malignant obstruction, the median survival being 6 months, operation still offers the best hope for palliation.[537] Lau and Lorentz[539] believe that a more aggressive approach is appropriate. In a review of 30 patients with unresectable intra-abdominal disease, 63% had bowel function restored. Obstruction recurred after a mean symptom-free interval of 120 days in 8 of 19 patients initially relieved. Another operation was performed in 3 of these patients. The authors believe that their results, with a median survival of 192 days for those who benefitted from operation, justify a more positive approach toward this problem and when conservatism fails, laparotomy should be undertaken in patients who are not terminally ill.

Butler et al[540] also believe in an aggressive approach. The authors reviewed 54 patients with small bowel obstruction who had a previous diagnosis of carcinoma. Forty patients were initially treated nonoperatively, and 28% of those resolved after a mean 7 days of nasogastric suction. Five developed recurrent small bowel obstruction. Thirty-seven patients underwent laparotomy, at which time 68% were found to have obstruction due to recurrent carcinoma, with a mean survival of 5 months. Major postoperative complications occurred in 49% of patients, the most common being failure of resolution of the obstruction. The 30-day and in-hospital mortality rates of the 25 surgically treated patients were 24 and 28%, respectively. The authors concluded that (1) patients should be given an initial trial of nonoperative therapy, (2) patients with no known recurrence or a long interval to development of small bowel obstruction should be aggressively treated with early operation if nonoperative treatment fails, and (3) for patients with known abdominal recurrence in whom nonoperative therapy fails, the results of operative palliation are grim.

Miller et al[541] conducted a study to determine the efficacy and long-term prognosis for operative versus nonoperative treatment of small bowel obstruction secondary to malignant disease. There were 32 patients accounting for 74 admissions. Colorectal neoplasm was the principal primary malignant disease that led to small bowel obstruction. The median time between diagnosis of the malignant disease and small bowel obstruction was 1.1 years. At their initial presentation, 80% of patients were treated by operation, but 47% of these patients had an initial trial of nonoperative treatment. Reobstruction occurred in 57% of patients who were operated on compared with 72% of patients who were not. The median time to reobstruction was 17 months for patients who underwent operation compared with 2.5 months for patients who did not. Also, 71% of patients were alive and symptom free 30 days after discharge from the operative treatment compared with 52% after nonoperative treatment. Postoperative morbidity was 67%. Mortality was 13%, and 94% of patients eventually died from complications of their primary disease. They concluded that small bowel obstruction secondary to malignant disease usually indicates a grim prognosis. Operative treatment has better outcome than nonoperative management in terms of symptom-free interval and reobstruction rates. However, it is marked by high postoperative morbidity. They recommend that after a short trial of nasogastric decompression, patients with obstruction secondary to malignant disease be operated on if clinical factors indicate they will survive the operation.

For patients with malignant large bowel obstruction, stent placement may successfully relieve obstruction and this subject has been described previously. Other methods to relieve malignant large bowel obstruction include Nd:YAG laser or balloon dilatation. Krouse et al in their excellent review of palliative care of the patient with malignant obstruction detailed the wide range of possible pharmacologic management.[542] It may include opioids for pain control, metoclopramide for nausea and vomiting, and other antiemetics (prochlorperazine, promethazine, and haloperidol, to mention a few). Treatment of dehydration and nutritional depletion is controversial. Octreotide will be effective in the relief of symptoms of malignant bowel obstruction. Corticosteroids have been used in the hope of reducing edema around the malignancy.

August et al[543] reported on the use of home parenteral nutrition in patients with inoperable malignant bowel obstruction. In a review of 17 patients so treated, most patients and families (82%) perceived therapy as beneficial, with a median survival of 90 days. In most circumstances, members of the nutritional support team agreed in that home parenteral nutrition facilitates compassionate home care for carefully selected patients. Despite their encouraging report, one should be circumspect about embarking on such a program.

At times, because of diffuse involvement of the intestine by carcinomatosis, a percutaneous endoscopic gastroscopy may avoid the need for celiotomy. When used selectively, it can improve the quality of life of the carcinoma patient by relieving intractable vomiting and by providing an avenue for nutrition in a partially functioning gastrointestinal tract.

Parker and Baines[544] questioned the philosophy of the compulsion to operate on the assumption that obstruction always demands operative intervention. The authors point out a mortality rate of 13% with a median survival of 10 months, but in malnourished patients the mortality rate can climb to 72%. Emergency operation increases the mortality rate threefold and, although survival may be increased by a few months, the relief of symptoms lasts only 2 months overall. To counteract these depressing data, good prognostic factors include an early-stage or low-grade initial lesion, a long interval from first operation, a well-nourished patient, and the fact that in one-third of patients with previous carcinoma, the obstruction is caused by benign disease. The decision to operate must be made with as much information as possible. Barium studies, CT, MRI, ultrasonography, or endoscopic evaluation may be beneficial. When the decision is made not to operate, adequate analgesia, antiemetics, and antisecretagogues should be administered.

22.9 Colorectal Carcinoma Complicating Pregnancy

Colorectal carcinoma in pregnancy is a rare condition and has been estimated to occur in 0.001 to 0.100% of pregnancies.[545] As of 1993, 205 cases were reported in the literature. Colorectal carcinoma that presents in pregnancy usually does so at an advanced stage because the individuals are young and the diagnosis is usually not entertained, while any symptoms that do arise are often attributed to the pregnancy.[546] The most common presenting complaint is abdominal pain, followed by nausea and vomiting, constipation, abdominal distention, rectal bleeding, fever, and backache.

To better characterize the disease under this circumstance, Bernstein et al[545] surveyed the membership of the American Society of Colon and Rectal Surgeons and identified 41 cases of large bowel carcinoma who presented during pregnancy or the immediate postpartum period. The mean age at presentation was 31 years (range, 16–41 years). Spatial distribution within the large bowel was as follows: right colon, 3; transverse colon, 2; left colon, 2; sigmoid colon, 8; and rectum, 26. Staging at presentation was Dukes' A, 0; B, 16; C, 17; and metastatic, 6. Two patients were unstaged. The average follow-up was 41 months. The stage-for-stage survival was similar to patients with colorectal carcinoma in the general population. For those with rectal lesions, the 5-year survival rate for Dukes' B was 83% and Dukes' C, 27%, and for the colon, 75 and 33%, respectively. Noteworthy was the distal distribution, with 64% in their series and 86% in the literature located in the rectum, in contradistinction to the changing distribution in the general population where a migration to the right has been documented. Also, patients presented at an advanced stage (60% had Dukes' C or metastatic) and this probably accounts for the poor prognosis generally attributed to patients who develop colorectal carcinoma during pregnancy. A delay in diagnosis may in part account for the advanced stage of these lesions. It has been suggested that elevated levels of circulating estrogen and progesterone may stimulate growth of the carcinomas. The poor prognosis may in part be a reflection of the patient's age, as many believe that patients younger than 40 years of age are destined to a poor outcome.

Operative excision is the treatment of choice but, in pregnancy, operability, period of gestation, religious belief, and the patient's desire for children might be considered. In the first two trimesters, the appropriate operation should be recommended, leaving the pregnancy intact.[546] Total abdominal hysterectomy has been recommended if the uterus is found to be involved.[547] If the lesion is unresectable or is obstructing, a colostomy or "hidden" colostomy should be performed to help provide time for the fetus to reach viability. In the third trimester, it has been suggested that treatment be delayed until fetal pulmonary maturity is demonstrated. At that time, labor may be induced or a cesarean section performed, often without the lesion being removed. Simultaneous removal is not usually recommended because of increased vascularity in the pelvis. The definitive operation can be delayed for a few weeks after vaginal delivery. In the event the lesion is inoperable, the pregnancy can be allowed to proceed until viability is ensured, following which palliative measures can be undertaken.

Colorectal carcinoma coupled with pregnancy is a devastating combination yielding a poor prognosis. Whether this apparent poor prognosis reflects a delay in diagnosis, a biologically aggressive carcinoma in young women, or a hormonally driven carcinoma remains to be determined.[545]

22.9.1 Ovarian Carcinoma Involving the Colon

Involvement of the colon by advanced ovarian carcinoma is not uncommon. In these circumstances, the question arises as to the propriety of large bowel resection. Hertel et al[548] reported on 100 patients with International Federation of Gynecology and Obstetrics (FIGO) stage IIIc ovarian carcinoma who underwent pelvic en bloc resection with excision of the rectosigmoid colon as part of the primary or secondary cytoreductive operation. Malignant involvement of the rectum was confirmed histopathologically: infiltration of the serosa in 28% of patients, infiltration of the muscularis in 31% of patients, and infiltration of the mucosa in 14% of patients. Histopathologically confirmed pelvic R0 resection was achieved in 85% of patients. Pelvic recurrence occurred in 4.7% of 85 optimally debulked patients compared to 60% of 15 patients with suboptimal pelvic resection status. End colostomy could be prevented in 94% of patients. They concluded pelvic en bloc surgery with rectosigmoid resection was justified by histopathological outcome since deperitonealization with preservation of the rectosigmoid would

have left malignancy in situ in 73% of patients with suspected cul-de-sac involvement. This recommendation of course can only be made if there is no other evidence of metastatic disease as is the usual situation with ovarian carcinoma.

22.9.2 Malakoplakia and Colorectal Carcinoma

Malakoplakia is a characteristic inflammatory condition that is usually seen in the urogenital tract. Gastrointestinal malakoplakia is seen in association with a variety of conditions such as ulcerative colitis, diverticular disease, adenomatous polyps, and carcinoma. Pillay and Chetty[549] reported four cases of colorectal carcinoma associated with malakoplakia. Three of the cases were encountered in males and the patients ranged in age from 55 to 64 years. One case each occurred in the cecum/ascending colon and descending colon, while the remaining two were located in the rectum. All four cases were Dukes' stage B carcinoma. Furthermore, all four cases had spread to pericolonic fat and two had perforated. Microscopic examination showed the malakoplakia to be present at the infiltrating edge of the carcinoma. The draining lymph nodes were involved by malakoplakia to varying degrees in all cases. From their series and the literature review, malakoplakia associated with colorectal carcinoma tends to occur in elderly males in the rectum. The malakoplakia is found at the infiltrating front of the carcinoma and is not admixed with the neoplastic glands. Although lymph node involvement by malakoplakia has been reported only once previously, all four cases in this series showed evidence of involvement. The association does not appear to have any prognostic significance.

References

[1] Fazio VW, Tekkis PP, Remzi F, Lavery IC. Assessment of operative risk in colorectal cancer surgery: the Cleveland Clinic Foundation colorectal cancer model. Dis Colon Rectum. 2004; 47(12):2015–2024

[2] Portnoy J, Kagan E, Gordon PH, Mendelson J. Prophylactic antibiotics in elective colorectal surgery. Dis Colon Rectum. 1983; 26(5):310–313

[3] Rubin RJ, White RA, Eisenstat TE, et al. Left subcostal transverse incision combined with the right lateral position for excising the splenic flexure: a reintroduction. Perspect Colon Rectal Surg. 1988; l(2):41–47

[4] Thomas WM, Morris DL, Hardcastle JD. Contact ultrasonography in the detection of liver metastases from colorectal cancer: an in vitro study. Br J Surg. 1987; 74(10):955–956

[5] Busuttil RW, Foglia RP, Longmire WP, Jr. Treatment of carcinoma of the sigmoid colon and upper rectum. A comparison of local segmental resection and left hemicolectomy. Arch Surg. 1977; 112(8):920–923

[6] Dwight RW, Higgins GA, Keehn RJ. Factors influencing survival after resection in cancer of the colon and rectum. Am J Surg. 1969; 117(4):512–522

[7] Grinnell RS. Results of ligation of inferior mesenteric artery at the aorta in resections of carcinoma of the descending and sigmoid colon and rectum. Surg Gynecol Obstet. 1965; 120:1031–1036

[8] Pezim ME, Nicholls RJ. Survival after high or low ligation of the inferior mesenteric artery during curative surgery for rectal cancer. Ann Surg. 1984; 200 (6):729–733

[9] Enker WE, Laffer UT, Block GE. Enhanced survival of patients with colon and rectal cancer is based upon wide anatomic resection. Ann Surg. 1979; 190 (3):350–360

[10] Brief DK, Brener BJ, Goldenkranz R, et al. Defining the role of subtotal colectomy in the treatment of carcinoma of the colon. Ann Surg. 1991; 213 (3):248–252

[11] Fisher ER, Turnbull RB, Jr. The cytologic demonstration and significance of tumor cells in the mesenteric venous blood in patients with colorectal carcinoma. Surg Gynecol Obstet. 1955; 100(1):102–108

[12] Cole WH, Packard D, Southwick HW. Carcinoma of the colon with special reference to prevention of recurrence. J Am Med Assoc. 1954; 155 (18):1549–1553

[13] Turnbull RB, Jr, Kyle K, Watson FR, Spratt J. Cancer of the colon: the influence of the no-touch isolation technic on survival rates. Ann Surg. 1967; 166 (3):420–427

[14] Cohn I, Jr, Floyd CE, Atik M. Control of tumor implantation during operations on the colon. Ann Surg. 1963; 157:825–838

[15] Long RTL, Edwards RH. Implantation metastasis as a cause of local recurrence of colorectal carcinoma. Am J Surg. 1989; 157(2):194–201

[16] Wiggers T, Jeekel J, Arends JW, et al. No-touch isolation technique in colon cancer: a controlled prospective trial. Br J Surg. 1988; 75(5):409–415

[17] Gordon PH, Dalrymple S. The use of staples for reconstruction after colonic and rectal surgery. In: Ravitch MM, Steichen FM, eds. Principles and Practice of Surgical Stapling. Chicago, IL: Year Book Medical Publishers, 1987:402–431

[18] Welter R, Charlier A, Psalmon F. Personal communication. In: Steichen FM, Ravitch MM, eds. Stapling in Surgery. Chicago: Year Book Medical Publishers, 1988:271

[19] Chassin JL, Rifkind KM, Turner JW. Errors and pitfalls in stapling gastrointestinal tract anastomoses. Surg Clin North Am. 1984; 64(3):441–459

[20] Kyzer S, Gordon PH. The stapled functional end-to-end anastomosis following colonic resection. Int J Colorectal Dis. 1992; 7(3):125–131

[21] Chassin JL, Rifkind KM, Sussman B, et al. The stapled gastrointestinal tract anastomosis: incidence of postoperative complications compared with the sutured anastomosis. Ann Surg. 1978; 188(5):689–696

[22] Fortin CL, Poulin EC, Leclerc Y. Evaluation de l'utilisation des appareils d'autosuture en chirurgie digestive. Can J Surg. 1979; 22(6):580–582

[23] Brodman RF, Brodman HR. Staple suturing of the colon above the peritoneal reflection. Arch Surg. 1981; 116(2):191–192

[24] Reuter MJP. Les sutures mécaniques en chirurgie digestive et pulmonaire. Thesis. Université Louis Pasteur, Faculté de Médecine de Strasbourg, France, 1982

[25] Scher KS, Scott-Conner C, Jones CW, Leach M. A comparison of stapled and sutured anastomoses in colonic operations. Surg Gynecol Obstet. 1982; 155 (4):489–493

[26] Steichen FM, Ravitch MM. Stapling in Surgery. Chicago, IL: Year Book Medical Publishers, 1984:271

[27] Tuchmann A, Dinstl K, Strasser K, Armbruster C. Stapling devices in gastrointestinal surgery. Int Surg. 1985; 70(1):23–27

[28] Kracht M, Hay JM, Fagniez PL, Fingerhut A. Ileocolonic anastomosis after right hemicolectomy for carcinoma: stapled or hand-sewn? A prospective, multicenter, randomized trial. Int J Colorectal Dis. 1993; 8(1):29–33

[29] Corman ML. Colon and Rectal Surgery. 2nd ed. Philadelphia, PA: JB Lippincott, 1989:417

[30] Abcarian H, Pearl RK. Simple technique for high ligation of the inferior mesenteric artery and vein. Dis Colon Rectum. 1991; 34(12):1138

[31] Heald RJ. Anterior resection of the rectum. In: Fielding LP, Goldberg SM, eds. Rob and Smith's Operative Surgery. Surgery of the Colon, Rectum, and Anus. 5th ed. London: Butterworth-Heinemann Ltd, 1993:456–471

[32] West NP, Morris EJ, Rotimi O, Cairns A, Finan PJ, Quirke P. Pathology grading of colon cancer surgical resection and its association with survival: a retrospective observational study. Lancet Oncol. 2008; 9:857–865

[33] West NP, Hohenberger W, Weber K, Perrakis A, Finan PJ, Quirke P. Complete mesocolic excision with central vascular ligation produces an oncologically superior specimen compared with standard surgery for carcinoma of the colon. J Clin Oncol. 2010; 28:272–278

[34] Hohenberger W, Weber K, Matzel KE, Papadopoulos T, Merkel S. Standardized surgery for colonic cancer: complete mesocolic excision and central ligation–technical notes and outcome. Colorectal Dis. 2009; 11:354–364

[35] [35] Bertelsen CA, Neuenschwander AU, Jansen JE, et al; Danish Colorectal Cancer Group. Disease-free survival after complete mesocolic excision compared with conventional colon cancer surgery: a retrospective, population-based study. Lancet Oncol. 2015;16(2):161-168. Epub 2014 Dec 31.

[36] Birnkrant A, Sampson J, Sugarbaker PH. Ovarian metastasis from colorectal cancer. Dis Colon Rectum. 1986; 29(11):767–771

[37] Graffner HOL, Alm PO, Oscarson JEA. Prophylactic oophorectomy in colorectal carcinoma. Am J Surg. 1983; 146(2):233–235

[38] Sielezneff I, Salle E, Antoine K, Thirion X, Brunet C, Sastre B. Simultaneous bilateral oophorectomy does not improve prognosis of postmenopausal women undergoing colorectal resection for cancer. Dis Colon Rectum. 1997; 40(11):1299–1302

[39] Young-Fadok TM, Wolff BG, Nivatvongs S, Metzger PP, Ilstrup DM. Prophylactic oophorectomy in colorectal carcinoma: preliminary results of a randomized, prospective trial. Dis Colon Rectum. 1998; 41(3):277–283, discussion 283–285

[40] Cutait R, Lesser ML, Enker WE. Prophylactic oophorectomy in surgery for large-bowel cancer. Dis Colon Rectum. 1983; 26(1):6–11

[41] O'Brien PH, Newton BB, Metcalf JS, Rittenbury MS. Oophorectomy in women with carcinoma of the colon and rectum. Surg Gynecol Obstet. 1981; 153 (6):827–830

[42] MacKeigan JM, Ferguson JA. Prophylactic oophorectomy and colorectal cancer in premenopausal patients. Dis Colon Rectum. 1979; 22(6):401–405

[43] Blamey S, McDermott F, Pihl E, Price AB, Milne BJ, Hughes E. Ovarian involvement in adenocarcinoma of the colon and rectum. Surg Gynecol Obstet. 1981; 153(1):42–44

[44] Steele G, Augenlicht L, Begg C, et al. National Institutes of Health consensus development conference statement: adjuvant therapy for patients with colon and rectal cancer. JAMA. 1990; 264:1444

[45] Sentovich SM, Fakih M. Colorectal cancer: postoperative adjuvant therapy. In: Steele SR, Hull TL, Read TE, Saclarides TJ, Senagore AJ, Whitlow CB, eds. The ASCRS Textbook of Colon and Rectal Surgery. New York, NY: Springer; 2016:547–554

[46] Sugarbaker PH, Gunderson LL, Wittes RE. Colorectal cancer. In: DeVita VT Jr., Hellman S, Rosenberg SA, eds. Cancer Principles and Practices of Oncology. 2nd ed. Philadelphia, PA: JB Lippincott, 1985:795–884

[47] Willett CG, Fung CY, Kaufman DS, Efird J, Shellito PC. Postoperative radiation therapy for high-risk colon carcinoma. J Clin Oncol. 1993; 11(6):1112–1117

[48] Schild SE, Gunderson LL, Haddock MG, Wong WW, Nelson H. The treatment of locally advanced colon cancer. Int J Radiat Oncol Biol Phys. 1997; 37 (1):51–58

[49] Amos EH, Mendenhall WM, McCarty PJ, et al. Postoperative radiotherapy for locally advanced colon cancer. Ann Surg Oncol. 1996; 3(5):431–436

[50] Duttenhaver JR, Hoskins RB, Gunderson LL, Tepper JE. Adjuvant postoperative radiation therapy in the management of adenocarcinoma of the colon. Cancer. 1986; 57(5):955–963

[51] Ghossein NA, Samala EC, Alpert S, et al. Elective postoperative radiotherapy after incomplete resection of colorectal cancer. Dis Colon Rectum. 1981; 24 (4):252–256

[52] Wong CS, Harwood AR, Cummings BJ, Keane TJ, Thomas GM, Rider WD. Postoperative local abdominal irradiation for cancer of the colon above the peritoneal reflection. Int J Radiat Oncol Biol Phys. 1985; 11(12):2067–2071

[53] Martenson JA, Jr, Willett CG, Sargent DJ, et al. Phase III study of adjuvant chemotherapy and radiation therapy compared with chemotherapy alone in the surgical adjuvant treatment of colon cancer: results of intergroup protocol 0130. J Clin Oncol. 2004; 22(16):3277–3283

[54] National Comprehensive Cancer Network. Colon Cancer version 2. 2015. Available at: http://www.nccn.org

[55] Schabel FM, Jr. Rationale for perioperative anticancer treatment. Recent Results Cancer Res. 1985; 98:1–10

[56] Conference NC. NIH consensus conference. Adjuvant therapy for patients with colon and rectal cancer. JAMA. 1990; 264(11):1444–1450

[57] National Quality Forum. Endorsement summary: cancer measures. 2012. Available at: http://www.qualityforum.org

[58] Laurie JA, Moertel CG, Fleming TR, et al. The North Central Cancer Treatment Group and the Mayo Clinic. Surgical adjuvant therapy of large-bowel carcinoma: an evaluation of levamisole and the combination of levamisole and fluorouracil. J Clin Oncol. 1989; 7(10):1447–1456

[59] Moertel CG, Fleming TR, Macdonald JS, et al. Levamisole and fluorouracil for adjuvant therapy of resected colon carcinoma. N Engl J Med. 1990; 322 (6):352–358

[60] Gastrointestinal Tumor Study Group. Adjuvant therapy of colon cancer–results of a prospectively randomized trial. N Engl J Med. 1984; 310 (12):737–743

[61] Gilbert JM, Hellmann K, Evans M, et al. Randomized trial of oral adjuvant razoxane (ICRF 159) in resectable colorectal cancer: five-year follow-up. Br J Surg. 1986; 73(6):446–450

[62] Grage TB, Moss SE. Adjuvant chemotherapy in cancer of the colon and rectum: demonstration of effectiveness of prolonged 5-FU chemotherapy in a prospectively controlled, randomized trial. Surg Clin North Am. 1981; 61 (6):1321–1329

[63] Higgins GA, Jr, Amadeo JH, McElhinney J, McCaughan JJ, Keehn RJ. Efficacy of prolonged intermittent therapy with combined 5-fluorouracil and methyl-CCNU following resection for carcinoma of the large bowel. A Veterans Administration Surgical Oncology Group report. Cancer. 1984; 53(1):1–8

[64] Laurie J, Moertel C, Fleming T, et al. Surgical adjuvant therapy of poor prognostic colorectal cancer with levamisole alone or combined levamisole and 5fluorouracil. A North Central Cancer Treatment Group and Mayo Clinic study. Proc Am Soc Clin Oncol. 1986; 5:316

[65] Jemal A, Siegel R, Ward E, et al. Cancer statistics, 2006. CA Cancer J Clin. 2006; 56(2):106–130

[66] André T, Boni C, Navarro M, et al. Improved overall survival with oxaliplatin, fluorouracil, and leucovorin as adjuvant treatment in stage II or III colon cancer in the MOSAIC trial. J Clin Oncol. 2009; 27(19):3109–3116

[67] Efficacy of adjuvant fluorouracil and folinic acid in colon cancer. International Multicentre Pooled Analysis of Colon Cancer Trials (IMPACT) investigators. Lancet. 1995; 345(8955):939–944

[68] QUASAR Collaborative Group. Comparison of fluorouracil with additional levamisole, higher-dose folinic acid, or both, as adjuvant chemotherapy for colorectal cancer: a randomised trial. Lancet. 2000; 355(9215):1588–1596

[69] Efficacy of adjuvant fluorouracil and folinic acid in B2 colon cancer. International Multicentre Pooled Analysis of B2 Colon Cancer Trials (IMPACT B2) investigators. J Clin Oncol. 1999; 17(5):1356–1363

[70] Mamounas E, Wieand S, Wolmark N, et al. Comparative efficacy of adjuvant chemotherapy in patients with Dukes' B versus Dukes' C colon cancer: results from four National Surgical Adjuvant Breast and Bowel Project adjuvant studies (C-01, C-02, C-03, and C-04). J Clin Oncol. 1999; 17(5):1349–1355

[71] Haller DG, Tabernero J, Maroun J, et al. Capecitabine plus oxaliplatin compared with fluorouracil and folinic acid as adjuvant therapy for stage III colon cancer. J Clin Oncol. 2011; 29(11):1465–1471

[72] André T, Boni C, Mounedji-Boudiaf L, et al. Multicenter International Study of Oxaliplatin/5-Fluorouracil/Leucovorin in the Adjuvant Treatment of Colon Cancer (MOSAIC) Investigators. Oxaliplatin, fluorouracil, and leucovorin as adjuvant treatment for colon cancer. N Engl J Med. 2004; 350(23):2343–2351

[73] Kuebler JP, Wieand HS, O'Connell MJ, et al. Oxaliplatin combined with weekly bolus fluorouracil and leucovorin as surgical adjuvant chemotherapy for stage II and III colon cancer: results from NSABP C-07. J Clin Oncol. 2007; 25(16):2198–2204

[74] Twelves C, Wong A, Nowacki MP, et al. Capecitabine as adjuvant treatment for stage III colon cancer. N Engl J Med. 2005; 352(26):2696–2704

[75] Alberts SR, Sargent DJ, Nair S, et al. Effect of oxaliplatin, fluorouracil, and leucovorin with or without cetuximab on survival among patients with resected stage III colon cancer: a randomized trial. JAMA. 2012; 307(13):1383–1393

[76] Taieb J, Tabernero J, Mini E, et al. PETACC-8 Study Investigators. Oxaliplatin, fluorouracil, and leucovorin with or without cetuximab in patients with resected stage III colon cancer (PETACC-8): an open-label, randomised phase 3 trial. Lancet Oncol. 2014; 15(8):862–873

[77] Allegra CJ, Yothers G, O'Connell MJ, et al. Bevacizumab in stage II-III colon cancer: 5-year update of the National Surgical Adjuvant Breast and Bowel Project C-08 trial. J Clin Oncol. 2013; 31(3):359–364

[78] de Gramont A, Van Cutsem E, Schmoll HJ, et al. Bevacizumab plus oxaliplatin-based chemotherapy as adjuvant treatment for colon cancer (AVANT): a phase 3 randomised controlled trial. Lancet Oncol. 2012; 13(12):1225–1233

[79] Zedan AH, Hansen TF, Fex Svenningsen A, Vilholm OJ. Oxaliplatin-induced neuropathy in colorectal cancer: many questions with few answers. Clin Colorectal Cancer. 2014; 13(2):73–80

[80] Nagore E, Insa A, Sanmartín O. Antineoplastic therapy-induced palmar plantar erythrodysesthesia ("hand-foot") syndrome. Incidence, recognition and management. Am J Clin Dermatol. 2000; 1(4):225–234

[81] Parkin DM, Bray F, Ferlay J, Pisani P. Global cancer statistics, 2002. CA Cancer J Clin. 2005; 55(2):74–108

[82] Schrag D, Gelfand S, Bach P, et al. Adjuvant chemotherapy for stage II Colon cancer: insight from a SEER-Medicare cohort. Proc Am Soc Clin Oncol. 2001; 20:488

[83] Sargent DJ, Marsoni S, Monges G, et al. Defective mismatch repair as a predictive marker for lack of efficacy of fluorouracil-based adjuvant therapy in colon cancer. J Clin Oncol. 2010; 28(20):3219–3226

[84] O'Connell MJ, Lavery I, Yothers G, et al. Relationship between tumor gene expression and recurrence in four independent studies of patients with stage II/III colon cancer treated with surgery alone or surgery plus adjuvant fluorouracil plus leucovorin. J Clin Oncol. 2010; 28(25):3937–3944

[85] Gray RG, Quirke P, Handley K, et al. Validation study of a quantitative multigene reverse transcriptase-polymerase chain reaction assay for assessment of recurrence risk in patients with stage II colon cancer. J Clin Oncol. 2011; 29(35):4611–4619

[86] Venook AP, Niedzwiecki D, Lopatin M, Ye X, Lee M, Friedman PN, et al. Biologic determinants of tumor recurrence in stage II Colon cancer: validation study of the 12-gene recurrence score in cancer and leukemia group B (CALGB) 9581. J Clin Oncol. 2013; 31(14):1775–1781

[87] Yothers G, O'Connell MJ, Lee M, et al. Validation of the 12-gene colon cancer recurrence score in NSABP C-07 as a predictor of recurrence in patients with stage II and III colon cancer treated with fluorouracil and leucovorin (FU/LV) and FU/LV plus oxaliplatin. J Clin Oncol. 2013; 31(36):4512–4519

[88] Salazar R, Roepman P, Capella G, et al. Gene expression signature to improve prognosis prediction of stage II and III colorectal cancer. J Clin Oncol. 2011; 29(1):17–24

[89] Kopetz S, Tabernero J, Rosenberg R, et al. Genomic classifier ColoPrint predicts recurrence in stage II colorectal cancer patients more accurately than clinical factors. Oncologist. 2015; 20(2):127–133

[90] Kennedy RD, Bylesjo M, Kerr P, et al. Development and independent validation of a prognostic assay for stage II colon cancer using formalin-fixed paraffin-embedded tissue. J Clin Oncol. 2011; 29(35):4620–4626

[91] Kabbinavar FF, Hambleton J, Mass RD, Hurwitz HI, Bergsland E, Sarkar S. Combined analysis of efficacy: the addition of bevacizumab to fluorouracil/leucovorin improves survival for patients with metastatic colorectal cancer. J Clin Oncol. 2005; 23(16):3706–3712

[92] Hurwitz HI, Fehrenbacher L, Hainsworth JD, et al. Bevacizumab in combination with fluorouracil and leucovorin: an active regimen for first-line metastatic colorectal cancer. J Clin Oncol. 2005; 23(15):3502–3508

[93] Haller DG, Catalano PJ, Macdonald JS, et al. Phase III study of fluorouracil, leucovorin, and levamisole in high-risk stage II and III colon cancer: final report of Intergroup 0089. J Clin Oncol. 2005; 23(34):8671–8678

[94] Chan AT, Ogino S, Fuchs CS. Aspirin and the risk of colorectal cancer in relation to the expression of COX-2. N Engl J Med. 2007; 356(21):2131–2142

[95] Chan AT, Ogino S, Fuchs CS. Aspirin use and survival after diagnosis of colorectal cancer. JAMA. 2009; 302(6):649–658

[96] Wolmark N, Fisher B, Rockette H, et al. Postoperative adjuvant chemotherapy or BCG for colon cancer: results from NSABP protocol C-01. J Natl Cancer Inst. 1988; 80(1):30–36

[97] Lise M, Gerard A, Nitti D, et al. Adjuvant therapy for colorectal cancer. The EORTC experience and a review of the literature. Dis Colon Rectum. 1987; 30(11):847–854

[98] Gray BN, Walker C, Andrewartha L, Freeman S, Bennett RC. Melbourne trial of adjuvant immunotherapy in operable large bowel cancer. Aust N Z J Surg. 1988; 58(1):43–46

[99] Wiesenfeld M, O'Connell MJ, Wieand HS, et al. Controlled clinical trial of interferon-gamma as postoperative surgical adjuvant therapy for colon cancer. J Clin Oncol. 1995; 13(9):2324–2329

[100] Reithmuller G, Schnieder-Godicke E, Schlimok G, et al. Randomized trial of monoclonal antibody for adjuvant therapy of resected Dukes' C colorectal carcinoma. Lancet. 1994; 343:1177–1183

[101] Guillou PJ. Potential impact of immunobiotechnology on cancer therapy. Br J Surg. 1987; 74(8):705–710

[102] McArdle CS, Hole DJ. Emergency presentation of colorectal cancer is associated with poor 5-year survival. Br J Surg. 2004; 91(5):605–609

[103] Jestin P, Nilsson J, Heurgren M, Påhlman L, Glimelius B, Gunnarsson U. Emergency surgery for colonic cancer in a defined population. Br J Surg. 2005; 92(1):94–100

[104] Amsterdam E, Krispin M. Primary resection with colocolostomy for obstructive carcinoma of the left side of the colon. Am J Surg. 1985; 150(5):558–560

[105] White CM, Macfie J. Immediate colectomy and primary anastomosis for acute obstruction due to carcinoma of the left colon and rectum. Dis Colon Rectum. 1985; 28(3):155–157

[106] Sjödahl R, Franzén T, Nyström PO. Primary versus staged resection for acute obstructing colorectal carcinoma. Br J Surg. 1992; 79(7):685–688

[107] Nozoe T, Yasuda M, Honda M, Inutsuka S, Korenaga D. Obstructing carcinomas of the colon and rectum have a smaller size compared with those of non-obstructing carcinomas. Oncol Rep. 2001; 8(6):1313–1315

[108] Smithers BM, Theile DE, Cohen JR, Evans EB, Davis NC. Emergency right hemicolectomy in colon carcinoma: a prospective study. Aust N Z J Surg. 1986; 56(10):749–752

[109] Lee YM, Law WL, Chu KW, Poon RT. Emergency surgery for obstructing colorectal cancers: a comparison between right-sided and left-sided lesions. J Am Coll Surg. 2001; 192(6):719–725

[110] Deans GT, Krukowski ZH, Irwin ST. Malignant obstruction of the left colon. Br J Surg. 1994; 81(9):1270–1276

[111] Porter JA, Salvati EP, Rubin RJ, Eisenstat TE. Complications of colostomies. Dis Colon Rectum. 1989; 32(4):299–303

[112] Wong SK, Eu KW, Lim SL, et al. Total colectomy removes undetected proximal synchronous lesions in acute left-sided colonic obstruction. Tech Coloproctol. 1996; 4:87–88

[113] Stephenson BM, Shandall AA, Farouk R, Griffith G. Malignant left-sided large bowel obstruction managed by subtotal/total colectomy. Br J Surg. 1990; 77 (10):1098–1102

[114] Perez MD, de Fuenmayor ML, Calvo N, et al. Morbidity of emergency subtotal colectomy in obstructing carcinoma of the left colon. Br J Surg. 1995; 82 Suppl:33

[115] Lau PW, Lo CY, Law WL. The role of one-stage surgery in acute left-sided colonic obstruction. Am J Surg. 1995; 169(4):406–409

[116] Chrysos E, Athanasakis E, Vassilakis JS, Zoras O, Xynos E. Total colectomy and J-pouch ileorectal anastomosis for obstructed tumours of the rectosigmoid junction. ANZ J Surg. 2002; 72(2):92–94

[117] Tan SG, Nambiar R. Resection and anastomosis of obstructed left colonic cancer: primary or staged? Aust N Z J Surg. 1995; 65(10):728–731

[118] Stewart J, Diament RH, Brennan TG. Management of obstructing lesions of the left colon by resection, on-table lavage, and primary anastomosis. Surgery. 1993; 114(3):502–505

[119] Kressner U, Antonsson J, Ejerblad S, Gerdin B, Påhlman L. Intraoperative colonic lavage and primary anastomosis–an alternative to Hartmann procedure in emergency surgery of the left colon. Eur J Surg. 1994; 160(5):287–292

[120] Scotia Study Group. Single-stage treatment for malignant left-sided colonic obstruction: a prospective randomized clinical trial comparing subtotal colectomy with segmental resection following intraoperative irrigation. The SCOTIA Study Group. Subtotal Colectomy versus On-table Irrigation and Anastomosis. Br J Surg. 1995; 82(12):1622–1627

[121] Chiappa A, Zbar A, Biella F, Staudacher C. One-stage resection and primary anastomosis following acute obstruction of the left colon for cancer. Am Surg. 2000; 66(7):619–622

[122] Ohman U. Prognosis in patients with obstructing colorectal carcinoma. Am J Surg. 1982; 143(6):742–747

[123] Umpleby HC, Williamson RCN. Survival in acute obstructing colorectal carcinoma. Dis Colon Rectum. 1984; 27(5):299–304

[124] Goodall RG, Park M. Primary resection and anastomosis of lesions obstructing the left colon. Can J Surg. 1988; 31(3):167–168

[125] Ravo B. Colorectal anastomotic healing and intracolonic bypass procedure. Surg Clin North Am. 1988; 68(6):1267–1294

[126] Kronborg O. The missing randomized trial of two surgical treatments for acute obstruction due to carcinoma of the left colon and rectum. An interim report. Int J Colorectal Dis. 1986; 1(3):162–166

[127] Fielding LP, Stewart-Brown S, Blesovsky L. Large-bowel obstruction caused by cancer: a prospective study. BMJ. 1979; 2(6189):515–517

[128] Eckhauser ML, Mansour EG. Endoscopic laser therapy for obstructing and/or bleeding colorectal carcinoma. Am Surg. 1992; 58(6):358–363

[129] Dohmoto M. New method-endoscopic implantation of rectal stent in palliative treatment of malignant stenosis. Digestiva. 1991; 3:1507–1512

[130] Tejero E, Mainar A, Fernández L, Tobío R, De Gregorio MA. New procedure for the treatment of colorectal neoplastic obstructions. Dis Colon Rectum. 1994; 37(11):1158–1159

[131] Dauphine CE, Tan P, Beart RW, Jr, Vukasin P, Cohen H, Corman ML. Placement of self-expanding metal stents for acute malignant large-bowel obstruction: a collective review. Ann Surg Oncol. 2002; 9(6):574–579

[132] Khot UP, Lang AW, Murali K, Parker MC. Systematic review of the efficacy and safety of colorectal stents. Br J Surg. 2002; 89(9):1096–1102

[133] Law WL, Choi HK, Lee YM, Chu KW. Palliation for advanced malignant colorectal obstruction by self-expanding metallic stents: prospective evaluation of outcomes. Dis Colon Rectum. 2004; 47(1):39–43

[134] Saida Y, Sumiyama Y, Nagao J, Uramatsu M. Long-term prognosis of preoperative "bridge to surgery" expandable metallic stent insertion for obstructive colorectal cancer: comparison with emergency operation. Dis Colon Rectum. 2003; 46(10) Suppl:S44–S49

[135] Martinez-Santos C, Lobato RF, Fradejas JM, Pinto I, Ortega-Deballón P, Moreno-Azcoita M. Self-expandable stent before elective surgery vs. emergency surgery for the treatment of malignant colorectal obstructions: comparison of primary anastomosis and morbidity rates. Dis Colon Rectum. 2002; 45 (3):401–406

[136] Johnson R, Marsh R, Corson J, Seymour K. A comparison of two methods of palliation of large bowel obstruction due to irremovable colon cancer. Ann R Coll Surg Engl. 2004; 86(2):99–103

[137] Meisner S, Hensler M, Knop FK, West F, Wille-Jørgensen P. Self-expanding metal stents for colonic obstruction: experiences from 104 procedures in a single center. Dis Colon Rectum. 2004; 47(4):444–450

[138] Suzuki N, Saunders BP, Thomas-Gibson S, Akle C, Marshall M, Halligan S. Colorectal stenting for malignant and benign disease: outcomes in colorectal stenting. Dis Colon Rectum. 2004; 47(7):1201–1207

[139] Tomiki Y, Watanabe T, Ishibiki Y, et al. Comparison of stent placement and colostomy as palliative treatment for inoperable malignant colorectal obstruction. Surg Endosc. 2004; 18(11):1572–1577

[140] Sebastian S, Johnston S, Geoghegan T, Torreggiani W, Buckley M. Pooled analysis of the efficacy and safety of self-expanding metal stenting in malignant colorectal obstruction. Am J Gastroenterol. 2004; 99(10):2051–2057

[141] Carne PW, Frye JN, Robertson GM, Frizelle FA. Stents or open operation for palliation of colorectal cancer: a retrospective, cohort study of perioperative outcome and long-term survival. Dis Colon Rectum. 2004; 47(9):1455–1461

[142] Runkel NS, Schlag P, Schwarz V, Herfarth C. Outcome after emergency surgery for cancer of the large intestine. Br J Surg. 1991; 78(2):183–188

[143] Saegesser F, Sandblom P. Ischemic lesions of the distended colon: a complication of obstructive colorectal cancer. Am J Surg. 1975; 129(3):309–315

[144] Tsai MH, Yang YC, Leu FJ. Obstructive colitis proximal to partially obstructive colonic carcinoma: a case report and review of the literature. Int J Colorectal Dis. 2004; 19(3):268–272

[145] Rowe VL, Frost DB, Huang S. Extended resection for locally advanced colorectal carcinoma. Ann Surg Oncol. 1997; 4(2):131–136

[146] Glass RE, Fazio VW, Jagelman DG, Lavery IC, Weakley FL, Forsythe SR. The results of surgical treatment of cancer of the colon at the Cleveland Clinic from 1965–1975: classification of the spread of colon cancer and long-term survival. Int J Colorectal Dis. 1986; 1(1):33–39

[147] Gall FP, Tonak J, Altendorf A. Multivisceral resections in colorectal cancer. Dis Colon Rectum. 1987; 30(5):337–341

[148] Hunter JA, Ryan JA, Jr, Schultz P. En bloc resection of colon cancer adherent to other organs. Am J Surg. 1987; 154(1):67–71

[149] Orkin BA, Dozois RR, Beart RW, Jr, Patterson DE, Gunderson LL, Ilstrup DM. Extended resection for locally advanced primary adenocarcinoma of the rectum. Dis Colon Rectum. 1989; 32(4):286–292

[150] Eisenberg SB, Kraybill WG, Lopez MJ. Long-term results of surgical resection of locally advanced colorectal carcinoma. Surgery. 1990; 108(4):779–785, discussion 785–786

[151] Montesani C, Ribotta G, De Milito R, et al. Extended resection in the treatment of colorectal cancer. Int J Colorectal Dis. 1991; 6(3):161–164

[152] Curley SA, Carlson GW, Shumate CR, Wishnow KI, Ames FC. Extended resection for locally advanced colorectal carcinoma. Am J Surg. 1992; 163(6):553–559

[153] Izbicki JR, Hosch SB, Knoefel WT, Passlick B, Bloechle C, Broelsch CE. Extended resections are beneficial for patients with locally advanced colorectal cancer. Dis Colon Rectum. 1995; 38(12):1251–1256

[154] Carne PW, Frye JN, Kennedy-Smith A, et al. Local invasion of the bladder with colorectal cancers: surgical management and patterns of local recurrence. Dis Colon Rectum. 2004; 47(1):44–47

[155] Nakafusa Y, Tanaka T, Tanaka M, Kitajima Y, Sato S, Miyazaki K. Comparison of multivisceral resection and standard operation for locally advanced colorectal cancer: analysis of prognostic factors for short-term and long-term outcome. Dis Colon Rectum. 2004; 47(12):2055–2063

[156] Curley SA, Evans DB, Ames FC. Resection for cure of carcinoma of the colon directly invading the duodenum or pancreatic head. J Am Coll Surg. 1994; 179(5):587–592

[157] Koea JB, Conlon K, Paty PB, Guillem JG, Cohen AM. Pancreatic or duodenal resection or both for advanced carcinoma of the right colon: is it justified? Dis Colon Rectum. 2000; 43(4):460–465

[158] Talamonti MS, Shumate CR, Carlson GW, Curley SA. Locally advanced carcinoma of the colon and rectum involving the urinary bladder. Surg Gynecol Obstet. 1993; 177(5):481–487

[159] Kroneman H, Castelein A, Jeekel J. En bloc resection of colon carcinoma adherent to other organs: an efficacious treatment? Dis Colon Rectum. 1991; 34(9):780–783

[160] Poeze M, Houbiers JGA, van de Velde CJH, Wobbes T, von Meyenfeldt MF. Radical resection of locally advanced colorectal cancer. Br J Surg. 1995; 82 (10):1386–1390

[161] Landercasper J, Stolee RT, Steenlage E, Strutt PJ, Cogbill TH. Treatment and outcome of right colon cancers adherent to adjacent organs or the abdominal wall. Arch Surg. 1992; 127(7):841–845, discussion 845–846

[162] Yamada K, Ishizawa T, Niwa K, Chuman Y, Aikou T. Pelvic exenteration and sacral resection for locally advanced primary and recurrent rectal cancer. Dis Colon Rectum. 2002; 45(8):1078–1084

[163] Lopez MJ, Monafo WW. Role of extended resection in the initial treatment of locally advanced colorectal carcinoma. Surgery. 1993; 113(4):365–372

[164] Campbell SC, Church JM, Fazio VW, Klein EA, Pontes JE. Combined radical retropubic prostatectomy and proctosigmoidectomy for en bloc removal of locally invasive carcinoma of the rectum. Surg Gynecol Obstet. 1993; 176 (6):605–608

[165] McNamara DA, Fitzpatrick JM, O'Connell PR. Urinary tract involvement by colorectal cancer. Dis Colon Rectum. 2003; 46(9):1266–1276

[166] Cady B, Monson DO, Swinton NW, Sr. Survival of patients after colonic resection for carcinoma with simultaneous liver metastases. Surg Gynecol Obstet. 1970; 131(4):697–700

[167] Joffe J, Gordon PH. Palliative resection for colorectal carcinoma. Dis Colon Rectum. 1981; 24(5):355–360

[168] Liu SK, Church JM, Lavery IC, Fazio VW. Operation in patients with incurable colon cancer: is it worthwhile? Dis Colon Rectum. 1997; 40(1):11–14

[169] Takaki HS, Ujiki GT, Shields TS. Palliative resections in the treatment of primary colorectal cancer. Am J Surg. 1977; 133(5):548–550

[170] Goslin R, Steele G, Jr, Zamcheck N, Mayer R, MacIntyre J. Factors influencing survival in patients with hepatic metastases from adenocarcinoma of the colon or rectum. Dis Colon Rectum. 1982; 25(8):749–754

[171] Mäkelä J, Haukipuro K, Laitinen S, Kairaluoma MI. Palliative operations for colorectal cancer. Dis Colon Rectum. 1990; 33(10):846–850

[172] Fegiz G, Ramacciato G, Indinnimeo M, et al. Synchronous large bowel cancer: a series of 47 cases. Ital J Surg Sci. 1989; 19(1):23–28

[173] Bussey HJR, Wallace MH, Morson BC. Metachronous carcinoma of the large intestine and intestinal polyps. Proc R Soc Med. 1967; 60(3):208–210

[174] Chu DZJ, Giacco G, Martin RG, Guinee VF. The significance of synchronous carcinoma and polyps in the colon and rectum. Cancer. 1986; 57(3):445–450

[175] Passman MA, Pommier RF, Vetto JT. Synchronous colon primaries have the same prognosis as solitary colon cancers. Dis Colon Rectum. 1996; 39(3):329–334

[176] Fogler R, Weiner E. Multiple foci of colorectal carcinoma; argument for subtotal colectomy. N Y State J Med. 1980; 80(1):47–51

[177] Gervaz P, Bucher P, Neyroud-Caspar I, Soravia C, Morel P. Proximal location of colon cancer is a risk factor for development of metachronous colorectal cancer: a population-based study. Dis Colon Rectum. 2005; 48(2):227–232

[178] Shitoh K, Konishi F, Miyakura Y, Togashi K, Okamoto T, Nagai H. Microsatellite instability as a marker in predicting metachronous multiple colorectal carcinomas after surgery: a cohort-like study. Dis Colon Rectum. 2002; 45(3):329–333

[179] Leveson SH, Wiggins PA, Giles GR, Parkin A, Robinson PJ. Deranged liver blood flow patterns in the detection of liver metastases. Br J Surg. 1985; 72(2):128–130

[180] Finlay IG, McArdle CS. Occult hepatic metastases in colorectal carcinoma. Br J Surg. 1986; 73(9):732–735

[181] Machi J, Isomoto H, Kurohiji T, et al. Detection of unrecognized liver metastases from colorectal cancers by routine use of operative ultrasonography. Dis Colon Rectum. 1986; 29(6):405–409

[182] Blumgart LH, Fong Y. Surgical options in the treatment of hepatic metastasis from colorectal cancer. Curr Probl Surg. 1995; 32(5):333–421

[183] Rosenberg IL. The aetiology of colonic suture-line recurrence. Ann R Coll Surg Engl. 1979; 61(4):251–257

[184] Finlay IG, Meek D, Brunton F, McArdle CS. Growth rate of hepatic metastases in colorectal carcinoma. Br J Surg. 1988; 75(7):641–644

[185] Wigmore SJ, Madhavan K, Redhead DN, Currie EJ, Garden OJ. Distribution of colorectal liver metastases in patients referred for hepatic resection. Cancer. 2000; 89(2):285–287

[186] van Ooijen B, Oudkerk M, Schmitz PIM, Wiggers T. Detection of liver metastases from colorectal carcinoma: is there a place for routine computed tomography arteriography? Surgery. 1996; 119(5):511–516

[187] Strasberg SM, Dehdashti F, Siegel BA, Drebin JA, Linehan D. Survival of patients evaluated by FDG-PET before hepatic resection for metastatic colorectal carcinoma: a prospective database study. Ann Surg. 2001; 233(3):293–299

[188] Rodgers MS, Collinson R, Desai S, Stubbs RS, McCall JL. Risk of dissemination with biopsy of colorectal liver metastases. Dis Colon Rectum. 2003; 46(4):454–458, discussion 458–459

[189] Fuhrman GM, Curley SA, Hohn DC, Roh MS. Improved survival after resection of colorectal liver metastases. Ann Surg Oncol. 1995; 2(6):537–541

[190] Bengtsson G, Carlsson G, Hafström L, Jönsson PE. Natural history of patients with untreated liver metastases from colorectal cancer. Am J Surg. 1981; 141(5):586–589

[191] Nagorney DM. Hepatic resection for metastases from colorectal cancer. In: Nelson RL, ed. Problems in Current Surgery. Controversies in Colon Cancer. Philadelphia, PA: JB Lippincott; 1987:83–92

[192] Palmer M, Petrelli NJ, Herrera L. No treatment option for liver metastases from colorectal adenocarcinoma. Dis Colon Rectum. 1989; 32(8):698–701

[193] Stangl R, Altendorf-Hofmann A, Charnley RM, Scheele J. Factors influencing the natural history of colorectal liver metastases. Lancet. 1994; 343(8910):1405–1410

[194] Vauthey JN, Marsh RdeW, Cendan JC, Chu NM, Copeland EM. Arterial therapy of hepatic colorectal metastases. Br J Surg. 1996; 83(4):447–455

[195] Hughes K, Scheele J, Sugarbaker PH. Surgery for colorectal cancer metastatic to the liver. Optimizing the results of treatment. Surg Clin North Am. 1989; 69(2):339–359

[196] Schlag P, Hohenberger P, Herfarth C. Resection of liver metastases in colorectal cancer–competitive analysis of treatment results in synchronous versus metachronous metastases. Eur J Surg Oncol. 1990; 16(4):360–365

[197] Petrelli N, Gupta B, Piedmonte M, Herrera L. Morbidity and survival of liver resection for colorectal adenocarcinoma. Dis Colon Rectum. 1991; 34(10):899–904

[198] Doci R, Gennari L, Bignami P, Montalto F, Morabito A, Bozzetti F. One hundred patients with hepatic metastases from colorectal cancer treated by resection: analysis of prognostic determinants. Br J Surg. 1991; 78(7):797–801

[199] Rosen CB, Nagorney DM, Taswell HF, et al. Perioperative blood transfusion and determinants of survival after liver resection for metastatic colorectal carcinoma. Ann Surg. 1992; 216(4):493–504, discussion 504–505

[200] Nakamura S, Yokoi Y, Suzuki S, Baba S, Muro H. Results of extensive surgery for liver metastases in colorectal carcinoma. Br J Surg. 1992; 79(1):35–38

[201] van Ooijen B, Wiggers T, Meijer S, et al. Hepatic resections for colorectal metastases in The Netherlands. A multi-institutional 10-year study. Cancer. 1992; 70(1):28–34

[202] Gayowski TJ, Iwatsuki S, Madariaga JR, et al. Experience in hepatic resection for metastatic colorectal cancer: analysis of clinical and pathologic risk factors. Surgery. 1994; 116(4):703–710, discussion 710–711

[203] Scheele J, Stang R, Altendorf-Hofmann A, Paul M. Resection of colorectal liver metastases. World J Surg. 1995; 19(1):59–71

[204] Hananel N, Garzon J, Gordon PH. Hepatic resection for colorectal liver metastases. Am Surg. 1995; 61(5):444–447

[205] Rougier PH, Milan C, Lazorthes F, et al. Prospective study of prognostic factors in patients with unresected hepatic metastases from colorectal cancer. Br J Surg. 1995; 82:1397–1400

[206] Wade TP, Virgo KS, Li MJ, Callander PW, Longo WE, Johnson FE. Outcomes after detection of metastatic carcinoma of the colon and rectum in a national hospital system. J Am Coll Surg. 1996; 182(4):353–361

[207] Wanebo HJ, Chu QD, Vezeridis MP, Soderberg C. Patient selection for hepatic resection of colorectal metastases. Arch Surg. 1996; 131(3):322–329

[208] Ohlsson B, Stenram U, Tranberg KG. Resection of colorectal liver metastases: 25-year experience. World J Surg. 1998; 22(3):268–276, discussion 276–277

[209] Fong Y, Fortner J, Sun RL, Brennan MF, Blumgart LH. Clinical score for predicting recurrence after hepatic resection for metastatic colorectal cancer: analysis of 1001 consecutive cases. Ann Surg. 1999; 230(3):309–318, discussion 318–321

[210] Buell JF, Rosen S, Yoshida A, et al. Hepatic resection: effective treatment for primary and secondary tumors. Surgery. 2000; 128(4):686–693

[211] Elias D, Ouellet JF, Bellon N, Pignon JP, Pocard M, Lasser P. Extrahepatic disease does not contraindicate hepatectomy for colorectal liver metastases. Br J Surg. 2003; 90(5):567–574

[212] Kato T, Yasui K, Hirai T, et al. Therapeutic results for hepatic metastasis of colorectal cancer with special reference to effectiveness of hepatectomy: analysis of prognostic factors for 763 cases recorded at 18 institutions. Dis Colon Rectum. 2003; 46(10) Suppl:S22–S31

[213] Teh CS, Ooi LL. Hepatic resection for colorectal metastases to the liver: The National Cancer Centre/Singapore General Hospital experience. Ann Acad Med Singapore. 2003; 32(2):196–204

[214] Weber JC, Bachellier P, Oussoultzoglou E, Jaeck D. Simultaneous resection of colorectal primary tumour and synchronous liver metastases. Br J Surg. 2003; 90(8):956–962

[215] Lefor AT, Hughes KS, Shiloni E, et al. Intra-abdominal extrahepatic disease in patients with colorectal hepatic metastases. Dis Colon Rectum. 1988; 31(2):100–103

[216] Wagner JS, Adson MA, Van Heerden JA, Adson MH, Ilstrup DM. The natural history of hepatic metastases from colorectal cancer. A comparison with resective treatment. Ann Surg. 1984; 199(5):502–508

[217] Ekman CA, Gustavson J, Henning A. Value of a follow-up study of recurrent carcinoma of the colon and rectum. Surg Gynecol Obstet. 1977; 145(6):895–897

[218] Luna-Perez P, Rodriguez-Coria DF, Arroyo B, Gonzalez-Macouzet J. The natural history of liver metastases from colorectal cancer. Arch Med Res. 1998; 29(4):319–324

[219] Ruo L, Gougoutas C, Paty PB, Guillem JG, Cohen AM, Wong WD. Elective bowel resection for incurable stage IV colorectal cancer: prognostic variables for asymptomatic patients. J Am Coll Surg. 2003; 196(5):722–728

[220] Kuo LJ, Leu SY, Liu MC, Jian JJM, Hongiun Cheng S, Chen CM. How aggressive should we be in patients with stage IV colorectal cancer? Dis Colon Rectum. 2003; 46(12):1646–1652

[221] de Santibañes E, Lassalle FB, McCormack L, et al. Simultaneous colorectal and hepatic resections for colorectal cancer: postoperative and long term outcomes. J Am Coll Surg. 2002; 195(2):196–202

[222] Chua HK, Sondenaa K, Tsiotos GG, Larson DR, Wolff BG, Nagorney DM. Concurrent vs. staged colectomy and hepatectomy for primary colorectal cancer with synchronous hepatic metastases. Dis Colon Rectum. 2004; 47 (8):1310–1316

[223] Tocchi A, Mazzoni G, Brozzetti S, Miccini M, Cassini D, Bettelli E. Hepatic resection in stage IV colorectal cancer: prognostic predictors of outcome. Int J Colorectal Dis. 2004; 19(6):580–585

[224] Tanaka K, Shimada H, Matsuo K, et al. Outcome after simultaneous colorectal and hepatic resection for colorectal cancer with synchronous metastases. Surgery. 2004; 136(3):650–659

[225] Attiyeh FF, Wichern WA, Jr. Hepatic resection for primary and metastatic tumors. Am J Surg. 1988; 156(5):368–373

[226] Adson MA. Resection of liver metastases–when is it worthwhile? World J Surg. 1987; 11(4):511–520

[227] Bozzetti F, Doci R, Bignami P, Morabito A, Gennari L. Patterns of failure following surgical resection of colorectal cancer liver metastases. Rationale for a multimodal approach. Ann Surg. 1987; 205(3):264–270

[228] Tanaka K, Adam R, Shimada H, Azoulay D, Lévi F, Bismuth H. Role of neoadjuvant chemotherapy in the treatment of multiple colorectal metastases to the liver. Br J Surg. 2003; 90(8):963–969

[229] Allen PJ, Kemeny N, Jarnagin W, DeMatteo R, Blumgart L, Fong Y. Importance of response to neoadjuvant chemotherapy in patients undergoing resection of synchronous colorectal liver metastases. J Gastrointest Surg. 2003; 7 (1):109–115, discussion 116–117

[230] Iwatsuki S, Dvorchik I, Madariaga JR, et al. Hepatic resection for metastatic colorectal adenocarcinoma: a proposal of a prognostic scoring system. J Am Coll Surg. 1999; 189(3):291–299

[231] Smith DL, Soria JC, Morat L, et al. Human telomerase reverse transcriptase (hTERT) and Ki-67 are better predictors of survival than established clinical indicators in patients undergoing curative hepatic resection for colorectal metastases. Ann Surg Oncol. 2004; 11(1):45–51

[232] Imamura H, Seyama Y, Kokudo N, et al. Single and multiple resections of multiple hepatic metastases of colorectal origin. Surgery. 2004; 135(5):508–517

[233] Jaeck D. The significance of hepatic pedicle lymph nodes metastases in surgical management of colorectal liver metastases and of other liver malignancies. Ann Surg Oncol. 2003; 10(9):1007–1011

[234] Elias D, Sideris L, Pocard M, et al. Results of R0 resection for colorectal liver metastases associated with extrahepatic disease. Ann Surg Oncol. 2004; 11:274–280

[235] Martin R, Paty P, Fong Y, et al. Simultaneous liver and colorectal resections are safe for synchronous colorectal liver metastasis. J Am Coll Surg. 2003; 197(2):233–241, discussion 241–242

[236] Nelson RL, Freels S. A systematic review of hepatic artery chemotherapy after hepatic resection of colorectal cancer metastatic to the liver. Dis Colon Rectum. 2004; 47(5):739–745

[237] Clancy TE, Dixon E, Perlis R, Sutherland FR, Zinner MJ. Hepatic arterial infusion after curative resection of colorectal cancer metastases: a meta-analysis of prospective clinical trials. J Gastrointest Surg. 2005; 9(2):198–206

[238] Bines SD, Doolas A, Jenkins L, Millikan K, Roseman DL. Survival after repeat hepatic resection for recurrent colorectal hepatic metastases. Surgery. 1996; 120(4):591–596

[239] Wanebo HJ, Chu QD, Avradopoulos KA, Vezeridis MP. Current perspectives on repeat hepatic resection for colorectal carcinoma: a review. Surgery. 1996; 119(4):361–371

[240] Pinson CW, Wright JK, Chapman WC, Garrard CL, Blair TK, Sawyers JL. Repeat hepatic surgery for colorectal cancer metastasis to the liver. Ann Surg. 1996; 223(6):765–773, discussion 773–776

[241] Fernández-Trigo V, Shamsa F, Sugarbaker PH. Repeat liver resections from colorectal metastasis. Repeat Hepatic Metastases Registry. Surgery. 1995; 117(3):296–304

[242] Que FG, Nagorney DM. Resection of "recurrent" colorectal metastases to the liver. Br J Surg. 1994; 81(2):255–258

[243] Takahashi S, Inoue K, Konishi M, Nakagouri T, Kinoshita T. Prognostic factors for poor survival after repeat hepatectomy in patients with colorectal liver metastases. Surgery. 2003; 133(6):627–634

[244] Suzuki S, Sakaguchi T, Yokoi Y, et al. Impact of repeat hepatectomy on recurrent colorectal liver metastases. Surgery. 2001; 129(4):421–428

[245] Oshowo A, Gillams A, Harrison E, Lees WR, Taylor I. Comparison of resection and radiofrequency ablation for treatment of solitary colorectal liver metastases. Br J Surg. 2003; 90(10):1240–1243

[246] Berber E, Pelley R, Siperstein AE. Predictors of survival after radiofrequency thermal ablation of colorectal cancer metastases to the liver: a prospective study. J Clin Oncol. 2005; 23(7):1358–1364

[247] Ueno H, Mochizuki H, Hashiguchi Y, Hatsuse K, Fujimoto H, Hase K. Predictors of extrahepatic recurrence after resection of colorectal liver metastases. Br J Surg. 2004; 91(3):327–333

[248] Cohen AD, Kemeny NE. An update on hepatic arterial infusion chemotherapy for colorectal cancer. Oncologist. 2003; 8(6):553–566

[249] Gray BN, Anderson JE, Burton MA, et al. Regression of liver metastases following treatment with yttrium-90 microspheres. Aust N Z J Surg. 1992; 62 (2):105–110

[250] Stubbs RS, Cannan RJ, Mitchell AW. Selective internal radiation therapy with 90yttrium microspheres for extensive colorectal liver metastases. J Gastrointest Surg. 2001; 5(3):294–302

[251] Lang EK, Brown CL, Jr. Colorectal metastases to the liver: selective chemoembolization. Radiology. 1993; 189(2):417–422

[252] Stuart K. Chemoembolization in the management of liver tumors. Oncologist. 2003; 8(5):425–437

[253] Weaver ML, Atkinson D, Zemel R. Hepatic cryosurgery in the treatment of unresectable metastases. Surg Oncol. 1995; 4(5):231–236

[254] Ruers TJ, Joosten J, Jager GJ, Wobbes T. Long-term results of treating hepatic colorectal metastases with cryosurgery. Br J Surg. 2001; 88(6):844–849

[255] Scheele J, Altendorf-Hofmann A, Stangl R, Gall FP. Pulmonary resection for metastatic colon and upper rectum cancer. Is it useful? Dis Colon Rectum. 1990; 33(9):745–752

[256] Saclarides TJ, Krueger BL, Szeluga DJ, Warren WH, Faber LP, Economou SG. Thoracotomy for colon and rectal cancer metastases. Dis Colon Rectum. 1993; 36(5):425–429

[257] Brister SJ, de Varennes B, Gordon PH, Sheiner NM, Pym J. Contemporary operative management of pulmonary metastases of colorectal origin. Dis Colon Rectum. 1988; 31(10):786–792

[258] Kanemitsu Y, Kato T, Hirai T, Yasui K. Preoperative probability model for predicting overall survival after resection of pulmonary metastases from colorectal cancer. Br J Surg. 2004; 91(1):112–120

[259] Watanabe I, Arai T, Ono M, et al. Prognostic factors in resection of pulmonary metastasis from colorectal cancer. Br J Surg. 2003; 90(11):1436–1440

[260] Negri F, Musolino A, Normon AR, et al. The development for preoperative chemotherapy strategy for patients selected to undergo pulmonary metastectomy from colorectal cancer. J Clin Oncol. 2004; 145:202S

[261] King J, Glenn D, Clark W, et al. Percutaneous radiofrequency ablation of pulmonary metastases in patients with colorectal cancer. Br J Surg. 2004; 91 (2):217–223

[262] Ike H, Shimada H, Ohki S, Togo S, Yamaguchi S, Ichikawa Y. Results of aggressive resection of lung metastases from colorectal carcinoma detected by intensive follow-up. Dis Colon Rectum. 2002; 45(4):468–473, discussion 473–475

[263] Ishikawa K, Hashiguchi Y, Mochizuki H, Ozeki Y, Ueno H. Extranodal cancer deposit at the primary tumor site and the number of pulmonary lesions are useful prognostic factors after surgery for colorectal lung metastases. Dis Colon Rectum. 2003; 46(5):629–636

[264] Zink S, Kayser G, Gabius HJ, Kayser K. Survival, disease-free interval, and associated tumor features in patients with colon/rectal carcinomas and their resected intra-pulmonary metastases. Eur J Cardiothorac Surg. 2001; 19 (6):908–913

[265] Irshad K, Ahmad F, Morin JE, Mulder DS. Pulmonary metastases from colorectal cancer: 25 years of experience. Can J Surg. 2001; 44(3):217–221

[266] Vogelsang H, Haas S, Hierholzer C, Berger U, Siewert JR, Präuer H. Factors influencing survival after resection of pulmonary metastases from colorectal cancer. Br J Surg. 2004; 91(8):1066–1071

[267] Mineo TC, Ambrogi V, Tonini G, et al. Long-term results after resection of simultaneous and sequential lung and liver metastases from colorectal carcinoma. J Am Coll Surg. 2003; 197(3):386–391

[268] Ike H, Shimada H, Togo S, Yamaguchi S, Ichikawa Y, Tanaka K. Sequential resection of lung metastasis following partial hepatectomy for colorectal cancer. Br J Surg. 2002; 89(9):1164–1168

[269] Nagakura S, Shirai Y, Yamato Y, Yokoyama N, Suda T, Hatakeyama K. Simultaneous detection of colorectal carcinoma liver and lung metastases does not warrant resection. J Am Coll Surg. 2001; 193(2):153–160

[270] Jass JR, Atkin WS, Cuzick J, et al. The grading of rectal cancer: historical perspectives and a multivariate analysis of 447 cases. Histopathology. 1986; 10 (5):437–459

[271] Traina TA, Leonard GD, Tang L, Paty PB, Maki RG. Metastatic colon cancer to the ovaries in a Krukenberg-like pattern. J Clin Oncol. 2005; 23 (22):5255–5256

[272] Herrera-Ornelas L, Natarajan N, Tsukada Y, et al. Adenocarcinoma of the colon masquerading as primary ovarian neoplasia. An analysis of ten cases. Dis Colon Rectum. 1983; 26(6):377–380

[273] Morrow M, Enker WE. Late ovarian metastases in carcinoma of the colon and rectum. Arch Surg. 1984; 119(12):1385–1388

[274] Huang PP, Weber TK, Mendoza C, Rodriguez-Bigas MA, Petrelli NJ. Long-term survival in patients with ovarian metastases from colorectal carcinoma. Ann Surg Oncol. 1998; 5(8):695–698

[275] Besbeas S, Stearns MW, Jr. Osseous metastases from carcinomas of the colon and rectum. Dis Colon Rectum. 1978; 21(4):266–268

[276] Bonnheim DC, Petrelli NJ, Herrera L, Walsh D, Mittelman A. Osseous metastases from colorectal carcinoma. Am J Surg. 1986; 151(4):457–459

[277] Scuderi G, Macrì A, Sfuncia G, et al. Sternal metastasis as initial presentation of a unknown rectal cancer. Int J Colorectal Dis. 2004; 19(3):292–293

[278] Wong ET, Berkenblit A. The role of topotecan in the treatment of brain metastases. Oncologist. 2004; 9(1):68–79

[279] Alden TD, Gianino JW, Saclarides TJ. Brain metastases from colorectal cancer. Dis Colon Rectum. 1996; 39(5):541–545

[280] Hammoud MA, McCutcheon IE, Elsouki R, Schoppa D, Patt YZ. Colorectal carcinoma and brain metastasis: distribution, treatment, and survival. Ann Surg Oncol. 1996; 3(5):453–463

[281] Farnell GF, Buckner JC, Cascino TL, O'Connell MJ, Schomberg PJ, Suman V. Brain metastases from colorectal carcinoma. The long term survivors. Cancer. 1996; 78(4):711–716

[282] Knorr C, Reingruber B, Meyer T, Hohenberger W, Stremmel C. Peritoneal carcinomatosis of colorectal cancer: incidence, prognosis, and treatment modalities. Int J Colorectal Dis. 2004; 19(3):181–187

[283] Glehen O, Kwiatkowski F, Sugarbaker PH, et al. Cytoreductive surgery combined with perioperative intraperitoneal chemotherapy for the management of peritoneal carcinomatosis from colorectal cancer: a multi-institutional study. J Clin Oncol. 2004; 22(16):3284–3292

[284] Culliford AT, IV, Brooks AD, Sharma S, et al. Surgical debulking and intraperitoneal chemotherapy for established peritoneal metastases from colon and appendix cancer. Ann Surg Oncol. 2001; 8(10):787–795

[285] Verwaal VJ, van Ruth S, de Bree E, et al. Randomized trial of cytoreduction and hyperthermic intraperitoneal chemotherapy versus systemic chemotherapy and palliative surgery in patients with peritoneal carcinomatosis of colorectal cancer. J Clin Oncol. 2003; 21(20):3737–3743

[286] Verwaal VJ, van Ruth S, Witkamp A, Boot H, van Slooten G, Zoetmulder FA. Long-term survival of peritoneal carcinomatosis of colorectal origin. Ann Surg Oncol. 2005; 12(1):65–71

[287] Shen P, Hawksworth J, Lovato J, et al. Cytoreductive surgery and intraperitoneal hyperthermic chemotherapy with mitomycin C for peritoneal carcinomatosis from nonappendiceal colorectal cancer. Ann Surg Oncol. 2004; 11(2):178–186

[288] Elias D, Delperro JR, Sideris L, et al. Treatment of peritoneal carcinomatosis from colorectal cancer: impact of complete cytoreductive surgery and difficulties in conducting randomized trials. Ann Surg Oncol. 2004; 11(5):518–521

[289] Mainprize KS, Berry AR. Solitary splenic metastasis from colorectal carcinoma. Br J Surg. 1997; 84(1):70

[290] Rendi MH, Dhar AD. Cutaneous metastasis of rectal adenocarcinoma. Dermatol Nurs. 2003; 15(2):131–132

[291] Tsai HL, Huang YS, Hsieh JS, Huang TJ, Tsai KB. Signet-ring cell carcinoma of the rectum with diffuse and multiple skin metastases–a case report. Kaohsiung J Med Sci. 2002; 18(7):359–362

[292] Gabriele R, Borghese M, Conte M, Basso L. Sister Mary Joseph's nodule as a first sign of cancer of the cecum: report of a case. Dis Colon Rectum. 2004; 47(1):115–117

[293] Tan BK, Nyam DC, Ho YH. Carcinoma of the rectum with a single penile metastasis. Singapore Med J. 2002; 43(1):39–40

[294] Tutton MG, George M, Hill ME, Abulafi AM. Solitary pancreatic metastasis from a primary colonic tumor detected by PET scan: report of a case. Dis Colon Rectum. 2001; 44(2):288–290

[295] Chagpar A, Kanthan SC. Vaginal metastasis of colon cancer. Am Surg. 2001; 67(2):171–172

[296] Charles W, Joseph G, Hunis B, Rankin L. Metastatic colon cancer to the testicle presenting as testicular hydrocele. J Clin Oncol. 2005; 23(22):5256–5257

[297] Tiong HY, Kew CY, Tan KB, Salto-Tellez M, Leong AF. Metastatic testicular carcinoma from the colon with clinical, immunophenotypical, and molecular characterization: report of a case. Dis Colon Rectum. 2005; 48(3):582–585

[298] Radhakrishnan CN, Bruce J. Colorectal cancers in children without any predisposing factors. A report of eight cases and review of the literature. Eur J Pediatr Surg. 2003; 13(1):66–68

[299] Killingback M, Barron P, Dent O. Elective resection and anastomosis for colorectal cancer: a prospective audit of mortality and morbidity 1976–1998. ANZ J Surg. 2002; 72(10):689–698

[300] Platell CF, Semmens JB. Review of survival curves for colorectal cancer. Dis Colon Rectum. 2004; 47(12):2070–2075

[301] Pihl E, Hughes ESR, McDermott FT, Milne BJ, Korner JM, Price AB. Carcinoma of the colon. Cancer specific long-term survival. A series of 615 patients treated by one surgeon. Ann Surg. 1980; 192(1):114–117

[302] Stefanini P, Castrini G, Pappalardo G. Surgical treatment of cancer of the colon. Int Surg. 1981; 66(2):125–131

[303] Zhou XG, Yu BM, Shen YX. Surgical treatment and late results in 1226 cases of colorectal cancer. Dis Colon Rectum. 1983; 26(4):250–256

[304] Umpleby HC, Bristol JB, Rainey JB, Williamson RC. Survival of 727 patients with single carcinomas of the large bowel. Dis Colon Rectum. 1984; 27 (12):803–810

[305] Isbister WH, Fraser J. Survival following resection for colorectal cancer. A New Zealand national study. Dis Colon Rectum. 1985; 28(10):725–727

[306] Wied U, Nilsson T, Knudsen JB, Sprechler M, Johansen A. Postoperative survival of patients with potentially curable cancer of the colon. Dis Colon Rectum. 1985; 28(5):333–335

[307] Davis NC, Evans EB, Cohen JR, Theile DE, Job DM. Colorectal cancer: a large unselected Australian series. Aust N Z J Surg. 1987; 57(3):153–159

[308] Moreaux J, Catala M. Carcinoma of the colon: long-term survival and prognosis after surgical treatment in a series of 798 patients. World J Surg. 1987; 11(6):804–809

[309] Brown SC, Walsh S, Sykes PA. Operative mortality rate and surgery for colorectal cancer. Br J Surg. 1988; 75(7):645–647

[310] Enblad P, Adami HO, Bergström R, Glimelius B, Krusemo U, Påhlman L. Improved survival of patients with cancers of the colon and rectum? J Natl Cancer Inst. 1988; 80(8):586–591

[311] Jatzko G, Lisborg P, Wette V. Improving survival rates for patients with colorectal cancer. Br J Surg. 1992; 79(6):588–591

[312] Clemmesen T, Sprechler M. Recording of patients with colorectal cancer on a database: results and advantages. Eur J Surg. 1994; 160(3):175–178

[313] Singh S, Morgan BF, Broughton M, et al. A 10 year prospective audit of outcome of surgical treatment for colorectal carcinoma. Br J Surg. 1995; 82:1486–1490

[314] Carraro PG, Segala M, Cesana BM, Tiberio G. Obstructing colonic cancer: failure and survival patterns over a ten-year follow-up after one-stage curative surgery. Dis Colon Rectum. 2001; 44(2):243–250

[315] Read TE, Mutch MG, Chang BW, et al. Locoregional recurrence and survival after curative resection of adenocarcinoma of the colon. J Am Coll Surg. 2002; 195(1):33–40

[316] Eisenberg B, Decosse JJ, Harford F, Michalek J. Carcinoma of the colon and rectum: the natural history reviewed in 1704 patients. Cancer. 1982; 49 (6):1131–1134

[317] Staib L, Link KH, Blatz A, Beger HG. Surgery of colorectal cancer: surgical morbidity and five- and ten-year results in 2400 patients: monoinstitutional experience. World J Surg. 2002; 26(1):59–66

[318] Devesa JM, Morales V, Enriquez JM, et al. Colorectal cancer. The bases for a comprehensive follow-up. Dis Colon Rectum. 1988; 31(8):636–652

[319] American College of Surgeons. The National Cancer Data Base Report on colon cancer, Nov 23, 2004. Available at: www.facs.org

[320] Kelley WE, Jr, Brown PW, Lawrence W, Jr, Terz JJ. Penetrating, obstructing, and perforating carcinomas of the colon and rectum. Arch Surg. 1981; 116 (4):381–384

[321] Brief DK, Brener BJ, Goldenkranz R, Alpert J, Yalof I, Parsonnet V. An argument for increased use of subtotal colectomy in the management of carcinoma of the colon. Am Surg. 1983; 49(2):66–72

[322] Crooms JW, Kovalcik PJ. Obstructing left-sided colon carcinoma. Appraisal of surgical options. Am Surg. 1984; 50(1):15–19

[323] Phillips RKS, Hittinger R, Fry JS, Fielding LP. Malignant large bowel obstruction. Br J Surg. 1985; 72(4):296–302

[324] Willett C, Tepper JE, Cohen A, Orlow E, Welch C. Obstructive and perforative colonic carcinoma: patterns of failure. J Clin Oncol. 1985; 3(3):379–384

[325] Serpell JW, McDermott FT, Katrivessis H, Hughes ES. Obstructing carcinomas of the colon. Br J Surg. 1989; 76(9):965–969

[326] Ueyama T, Yao T, Nakamura K, et al. Obstructing carcinoma of the colon and rectum: clinicopathologic analysis of 40 cases. Jpn J Clin Oncol. 1991; 21:100–109

[327] Mulcahy HE, Skelly MM, Husain A, O'Donoghue DP. Long-term outcome following curative surgery for malignant large bowel obstruction. Br J Surg. 1996; 83(1):46–50

[328] Chen HS, Sheen-Chen SM. Obstruction and perforation in colorectal adenocarcinoma: an analysis of prognosis and current trends. Surgery. 2000; 127 (4):370–376

[329] Hughes ESR, McDermott FT, Polglase AL, Nottle P. Total and subtotal colectomy for colonic obstruction. Dis Colon Rectum. 1985; 28(3):162–163

[330] Morgan WP, Jenkins N, Lewis P, Aubrey DA. Management of obstructing carcinoma of the left colon by extended right hemicolectomy. Am J Surg. 1985; 149(3):327–329

[331] Feng YS, Hsu H, Chen SS. One-stage operation for obstructing carcinomas of the left colon and rectum. Dis Colon Rectum. 1987; 30(1):29–32

[332] Halevy A, Levi J, Orda R. Emergency subtotal colectomy. A new trend for treatment of obstructing carcinoma of the left colon. Ann Surg. 1989; 210 (2):220–223

[333] Slors JF, Taat CW, Mallonga ET, Brummelkamp WH. One-stage colectomy and ileorectal anastomosis for complete left-sided obstruction of the colon. Neth J Surg. 1989; 41(1):1–4

[334] Antal SC, Kovacs ZG, Feigenbaum V, Engelberg M. Obstructing carcinoma of the left colon: treatment by extended right hemicolectomy. Int Surg. 1991; 76(3):161–163

[335] Tan SG, Nambiar R, Rauff A, Ngoi SS, Goh HS. Primary resection and anastomosis in obstructed descending colon due to cancer. Arch Surg. 1991; 126 (6):748–751

[336] Murray JJ, Schoetz DJ, Jr, Coller JA, Roberts PL, Veidenheimer MC. Intraoperative colonic lavage and primary anastomosis in nonelective colon resection. Dis Colon Rectum. 1991; 34(7):527–531

[337] Arnaud JP, Bergamaschi R. Emergency subtotal/total colectomy with anastomosis for acutely obstructed carcinoma of the left colon. Dis Colon Rectum. 1994; 37(7):685–688

[338] Michowitz M, Avnieli D, Lazarovici I, Solowiejczyk M. Perforation complicating carcinoma of colon. J Surg Oncol. 1982; 19(1):18–21

[339] Badía JM, Sitges-Serra A, Pla J, Ragué JM, Roqueta F, Sitges-Creus A. Perforation of colonic neoplasms. A review of 36 cases. Int J Colorectal Dis. 1987; 2 (4):187–189

[340] Carraro PG, Segala M, Orlotti C, Tiberio G. Outcome of large-bowel perforation in patients with colorectal cancer. Dis Colon Rectum. 1998; 41 (11):1421–1426

[341] Khan S, Pawlak SE, Eggenberger JC, Lee CS, Szilagy EJ, Margolin DA. Acute colonic perforation associated with colorectal cancer. Am Surg. 2001; 67 (3):261–264

[342] Libutti SK, Alexander HR, Jr, Choyke P, et al. A prospective study of 2-[18F] fluoro-2-deoxy-D-glucose/positron emission tomography scan, 99mTc-labeled arcitumomab (CEA-scan), and blind second-look laparotomy for detecting colon cancer recurrence in patients with increasing carcinoembryonic antigen levels. Ann Surg Oncol. 2001; 8(10):779–786

[343] Mandava N, Kumar S, Pizzi WF, Aprile IJ. Perforated colorectal carcinomas. Am J Surg. 1996; 172(3):236–238

[344] Scott NA, Jeacock J, Kingston RD. Risk factors in patients presenting as an emergency with colorectal cancer. Br J Surg. 1995; 82(3):321–323

[345] Anderson JH, Hole D, McArdle CS. Elective versus emergency surgery for patients with colorectal cancer. Br J Surg. 1992; 79(7):706–709

[346] Fitzgerald SD, Longo WE, Daniel GL, Vernava AM, III. Advanced colorectal neoplasia in the high-risk elderly patient: is surgical resection justified? Dis Colon Rectum. 1993; 36(2):161–166

[347] Gervaz P, Pak-art R, Nivatvongs S, Wolff BG, Larson D, Ringel S. Colorectal adenocarcinoma in cirrhotic patients. J Am Coll Surg. 2003; 196(6):874–879

[348] Kotake K, Honjo S, Sugihara K, et al. Changes in colorectal cancer during a 20-year period: an extended report from the multi-institutional registry of large bowel cancer, Japan. Dis Colon Rectum. 2003; 46(10) Suppl:S32–S43

[349] Wang HZ, Huang XF, Wang Y, Ji JF, Gu J. Clinical features, diagnosis, treatment and prognosis of multiple primary colorectal carcinoma. World J Gastroenterol. 2004; 10(14):2136–2139

[350] Papaconstantinou HT, Sklow B, Hanaway MJ, et al. Characteristics and survival patterns of solid organ transplant patients developing de novo colon and rectal cancer. Dis Colon Rectum. 2004; 47(11):1898–1903

[351] Phillips RKS, Hittinger R, Blesovsky L, Fry JS, Fielding LP. Large bowel cancer: surgical pathology and its relationship to survival. Br J Surg. 1984; 71 (8):604–610

[352] Jass JR. Pathologists' perspective on colorectal cancer. Perspect Colon Rectal Surg. 1991; 4:327–332

[353] Adkins RB, Jr, DeLozier JB, McKnight WG, Waterhouse G. Carcinoma of the colon in patients 35 years of age and younger. Am Surg. 1987; 53 (3):141–145

[354] Behbehani A, Sakwa M, Ehrlichman R, et al. Colorectal carcinoma in patients under age 40. Ann Surg. 1985; 202(5):610–614

[355] Koh SJ, Johnson WW. Cancer of the large bowel in children. South Med J. 1986; 79(8):931–935

[356] Rao BN, Pratt CB, Fleming ID, Dilawari RA, Green AA, Austin BA. Colon carcinoma in children and adolescents. A review of 30 cases. Cancer. 1985; 55 (6):1322–1326

[357] Okuno M, Ikehara T, Nagayama M, Sakamoto K, Kato Y, Umeyama K. Colorectal carcinoma in young adults. Am J Surg. 1987; 154(3):264–268

[358] Chapuis PH, Dent OF, Fisher R, et al. A multivariate analysis of clinical and pathological variables in prognosis after resection of large bowel cancer. Br J Surg. 1985; 72(9):698–702

[359] Cusack JC, Giacco GG, Cleary K, et al. Survival factors in 186 patients younger than 40 years old with colorectal adenocarcinoma. J Am Coll Surg. 1996; 183 (2):105–112

[360] Palmer ML, Herrera L, Petrelli NJ. Colorectal adenocarcinoma in patients less than 40 years of age. Dis Colon Rectum. 1991; 34(4):343–346

[361] Adloff M, Arnaud JP, Schloegel M, Thibaud D, Bergamaschi R. Colorectal cancer in patients under 40 years of age. Dis Colon Rectum. 1986; 29 (5):322–325

[362] Enblad G, Enblad P, Adami HO, Glimelius B, Krusemo U, Påhlman L. Relationship between age and survival in cancer of the colon and rectum with special reference to patients less than 40 years of age. Br J Surg. 1990; 77 (6):611–616

[363] Svendson LB, Sorensen C, Kjersgaard P, et al. The influence of age upon the survival of curative operation for colorectal cancer. Int J Colorectal Dis. 1989; 4:123–127

[364] Liang JT, Huang KC, Cheng AL, Jeng YM, Wu MS, Wang SM. Clinicopathological and molecular biological features of colorectal cancer in patients less than 40 years of age. Br J Surg. 2003; 90:205–214

[365] de Mello J, Struthers L, Turner R, Cooper EH, Giles GR. Multivariate analyses as aids to diagnosis and assessment of prognosis in gastrointestinal cancer. Br J Cancer. 1983; 48(3):341–348

[366] O'Connell JB, Maggard MA, Livingston EH, Yo CK. Colorectal cancer in the young. Am J Surg. 2004; 187(3):343–348

[367] O'Connell JB, Maggard MA, Liu JH, Etzioni DA, Ko CY. Are survival rates different for young and older patients with rectal cancer? Dis Colon Rectum. 2004; 47(12):2064–2069

[368] Turkiewicz D, Miller B, Schache D, Cohen J, Theile D. Young patients with colorectal cancer: how do they fare? ANZ J Surg. 2001; 71(12):707–710

[369] Newland RC, Dent OF, Lyttle MN, Chapuis PH, Bokey EL. Pathologic determinants of survival associated with colorectal cancer with lymph node metastases. A multivariate analysis of 579 patients. Cancer. 1994; 73(8):2076–2082

[370] Coburn MC, Pricolo VE, Soderberg CH. Factors affecting prognosis and management of carcinoma of the colon and rectum in patients more than eighty years of age. J Am Coll Surg. 1994; 179(1):65–69

[371] Irvin TT. Prognosis of colorectal cancer in the elderly. Br J Surg. 1988; 75 (5):419–421

[372] Arnaud JP, Schloegel M, Ollier JC, Adloff M. Colorectal cancer in patients over 80 years of age. Dis Colon Rectum. 1991; 34(10):896–898

[373] Mulcahy HE, Patchett SE, Daly L, O'Donoghue DP. Prognosis of elderly patients with large bowel cancer. Br J Surg. 1994; 81(5):736–738

[374] Polissar L, Sim D, Francis A. Survival of colorectal cancer patients in relation to duration of symptoms and other prognostic factors. Dis Colon Rectum. 1981; 24(5):364–369

[375] Goodman D, Irvin TT. Delay in the diagnosis and prognosis of carcinoma of the right colon. Br J Surg. 1993; 80(10):1327–1329

[376] Pescatori M, Maria G, Beltrani B, Mattana C. Site, emergency, and duration of symptoms in the prognosis of colorectal cancer. Dis Colon Rectum. 1982; 25 (1):33–40

[377] Sanfelippo PM, Beahrs OH. Factors in the prognosis of adenocarcinoma of the colon and rectum. Arch Surg. 1972; 104(4):401–406

[378] Nilsson E, Bolin S, Sjödahl R. Carcinoma of the colon and rectum. Delay in diagnosis. Acta Chir Scand. 1982; 148(7):617–622

[379] Wiggers T, Arends JW, Volovics A. Regression analysis of prognostic factors in colorectal cancer after curative resections. Dis Colon Rectum. 1988; 31 (1):33–41

[380] Wang HS, Lin JK, Mou CY, et al. Long-term prognosis of patients with obstructing carcinoma of the right colon. Am J Surg. 2004; 187(4):497–500

[381] Meyerhardt JA, Tepper JE, Niedzwieki D, et al. Impact of body mass index on outcomes and treatment-related toxicity in patients with stage II and III rectal cancer: findings from Intergroup Trial 0114. J Clin Oncol. 2004; 22:648–657

[382] Phillips RK, Hittinger R, Blesovsky L, Fry JS, Fielding LP. Local recurrence following "curative" surgery for large bowel cancer: I. The overall picture. Br J Surg. 1984; 71(1):12–16

[383] Sugarbaker PH, Corlew S. Influence of surgical techniques on survival in patients with colorectal cancer. Dis Colon Rectum. 1982; 25(6):545–557

[384] Slanetz CA, Jr. The effect of inadvertent intraoperative perforation on survival and recurrence in colorectal cancer. Dis Colon Rectum. 1984; 27(12):792–797

[385] Zirngibl H, Husemann B, Hermanek P. Intraoperative spillage of tumor cells in surgery for rectal cancer. Dis Colon Rectum. 1990; 33(7):610–614

[386] Akyol AM, McGregor JR, Galloway DJ, Murray GD, George WD. Anastomotic leaks in colorectal cancer surgery: a risk factor for recurrence? Int J Colorectal Dis. 1991; 6(4):179–183

[387] Fujita S, Teramoto T, Watanabe M, Kodaira S, Kitajima M. Anastomotic leakage after colorectal cancer surgery: a risk factor for recurrence and poor prognosis. Jpn J Clin Oncol. 1993; 23(5):299–302

[388] Bell SW, Walker KG, Rickard MJ, et al. Anastomotic leakage after curative anterior resection results in a higher prevalence of local recurrence. Br J Surg. 2003; 90(10):1261–1266

[389] Rouffet F, Hay JM, Vacher B, et al. French Association for Surgical Research. Curative resection for left colonic carcinoma: hemicolectomy vs. segmental colectomy. A prospective, controlled, multicenter trial. Dis Colon Rectum. 1994; 37(7):651–659

[390] The consultant surgeons and pathologists of the Lothian and Borders health boards. Lothian and Borders large bowel cancer project: immediate outcome after surgery. Br J Surg. 1995; 82:888–890

[391] Reinbach DH, McGregor JR, Murray GD, O'Dwyer PJ. Effect of the surgeon's specialty interest on the type of resection performed for colorectal cancer. Dis Colon Rectum. 1994; 37(10):1020–1023

[392] Meyerhardt JA, Tepper JE, Niedzwiecki D, et al. Impact of hospital procedure volume on surgical operation and long-term outcomes in high-risk curatively resected rectal cancer: findings from the Intergroup 0114 Study. J Clin Oncol. 2004; 22(1):166–174

[393] Schrag D, Panageas KS, Riedel E, et al. Hospital and surgeon procedure volume as predictors of outcome following rectal cancer resection. Ann Surg. 2002; 236(5):583–592

[394] Schrag D, Panageas KS, Riedel E, et al. Surgeon volume compared to hospital volume as a predictor of outcome following primary colon cancer resection. J Surg Oncol. 2003; 83(2):68–78, discussion 78–79

[395] Hermanek P, Hohenberger W. The importance of volume in colorectal cancer surgery. Eur J Surg Oncol. 1996; 22(3):213–215

[396] Borowski DW, Kelly SB, Ratcliffe AA, et al. Small caseload in colorectal cancer surgery is associated with adverse outcome. Br J Surg. 2004; 91 Suppl 1:73

[397] Martling A, Cedermark B, Johansson H, Rutqvist LE, Holm T. The surgeon as a prognostic factor after the introduction of total mesorectal excision in the treatment of rectal cancer. Br J Surg. 2002; 89(8):1008–1013

[398] Wibe A, Eriksen MT, Syse A, Tretli S, Myrvold HE, Søreide O, Norwegian Rectal Cancer Group. Effect of hospital caseload on long-term outcome after standardization of rectal cancer surgery at a national level. Br J Surg. 2005; 92(2):217–224

[399] Callahan MA, Christos PJ, Gold HT, Mushlin AI, Daly JM. Influence of surgical subspecialty training on in-hospital mortality for gastrectomy and colectomy patients. Ann Surg. 2003; 238(4):629–636, discussion 636–639

[400] Rosen L, Stasik JJ, Jr, Reed JF, III, Olenwine JA, Aronoff JS, Sherman D. Variations in colon and rectal surgical mortality. Comparison of specialties with a state-legislated database. Dis Colon Rectum. 1996; 39(2):129–135

[401] Platell C, Lim D, Tajudeen N, Tan JL, Wong K. Dose surgical sub-specialization influence survival in patients with colorectal cancer? World J Gastroenterol. 2003; 9(5):961–964

[402] Read TE, Myerson RJ, Fleshman JW, et al. Surgeon specialty is associated with outcome in rectal cancer treatment. Dis Colon Rectum. 2002; 45(7):904–914

[403] Dorrance HR, Docherty GM, O'Dwyer PJ. Effect of surgeon specialty interest on patient outcome after potentially curative colorectal cancer surgery. Dis Colon Rectum. 2000; 43(4):492–498

[404] Martling A, Holm T, Rutqvist LE, et al. Impact of a surgical training programme on rectal cancer outcomes in Stockholm. Br J Surg. 2005; 92(2):225–229

[405] McArdle CS, Hole DJ. Influence of volume and specialization on survival following surgery for colorectal cancer. Br J Surg. 2004; 91(5):610–617

[406] Parrott NR, Lennard TWJ, Taylor RMR, Proud G, Shenton BK, Johnston ID. Effect of perioperative blood transfusion on recurrence of colorectal cancer. Br J Surg. 1986; 73(12):970–973

[407] Wobbes T, Joosen KH, Kuypers HH, Beerthuizen GI, Theeuwes GM. The effect of packed cells and whole blood transfusions on survival after curative resection for colorectal carcinoma. Dis Colon Rectum. 1989; 32(9):743–748

[408] Leite JF, Granjo ME, Martins MI, Reis RC, Monteiro JC, Castro-Sousa F. Effect of perioperative blood transfusions on survival of patients after radical surgery for colorectal cancer. Int J Colorectal Dis. 1993; 8(3):129–133

[409] Arnoux R, Corman J, Péloquin A, Smeesters C, St-Louis G. Adverse effect of blood transfusions on patient survival after resection of rectal cancer. Can J Surg. 1988; 31(2):121–126

[410] Francis DMA, Judson RT. Blood transfusion and recurrence of cancer of the colon and rectum. Br J Surg. 1987; 74(1):26–30

[411] Chung M, Steinmetz OK, Gordon PH. Perioperative blood transfusion and outcome after resection for colorectal carcinoma. Br J Surg. 1993; 80(4):427–432

[412] Davis CJ, Ilstrup DM, Pemberton JH. Influence of splenectomy on survival rate of patients with colorectal cancer. Am J Surg. 1988; 155(1):173–179

[413] Varty PP, Linehan IP, Boulos PB. Does concurrent splenectomy at colorectal cancer resection influence survival? Dis Colon Rectum. 1993; 36(6):602–606

[414] Armstrong CP, Ahsan Z, Hinchley G, Prothero DL, Brodribb AJ. Appendicectomy and carcinoma of the caecum. Br J Surg. 1989; 76(10):1049–1053

[415] Martin MB, Fontrier T, Jarman W, Sterchi JM. Colon and rectal carcinoma. Forty years and 1400 cases. Am Surg. 1987; 53(3):146–148

[416] Alley PG, McNee RK. Age and sex differences in right colon cancer. Dis Colon Rectum. 1986; 29(4):227–229

[417] Newland RC, Dent OF, Chapuis PH, Bokey L. Survival after curative resection of lymph node negative colorectal carcinoma. A prospective study of 910 patients. Cancer. 1995; 76(4):564–571

[418] Wolmark N, Fisher ER, Wieand HS, Fisher B. The relationship of depth of penetration and tumor size to the number of positive nodes in Dukes C colorectal cancer. Cancer. 1984; 53(12):2707–2712

[419] Bjerkeset T, Morild I, Mørk S, Søreide O. Tumor characteristics in colorectal cancer and their relationship to treatment and prognosis. Dis Colon Rectum. 1987; 30(12):934–938

[420] Chambers WM, Khan U, Gagliano A, Smith RD, Sheffield J, Nicholls RJ. Tumour morphology as a predictor of outcome after local excision of rectal cancer. Br J Surg. 2004; 91(4):457–459

[421] Yamamoto S, Mochizuki H, Hase K, et al. Assessment of clinicopathologic features of colorectal mucinous adenocarcinoma. Am J Surg. 1993; 166(3):257–261

[422] Green JB, Timmcke AE, Mitchell WT, Hicks TC, Gathright JB, Jr, Ray JE. Mucinous carcinoma: just another colon cancer? Dis Colon Rectum. 1993; 36(1):49–54

[423] Secco GB, Fardelli R, Campora E, et al. Primary mucinous adenocarcinomas and signet-ring cell carcinomas of colon and rectum. Oncology. 1994; 51(1):30–34

[424] Chen JS, Hsieh PS, Hung SY, et al. Clinical significance of signet ring cell rectal carcinoma. Int J Colorectal Dis. 2004; 19(2):102–107

[425] Nissan A, Guillem JG, Paty PB, Wong WD, Cohen AM. Signet-ring cell carcinoma of the colon and rectum: a matched control study. Dis Colon Rectum. 1999; 42(9):1176–1180

[426] Hase K, Shatney C, Johnson D, Trollope M, Vierra M. Prognostic value of tumor "budding" in patients with colorectal cancer. Dis Colon Rectum. 1993; 36(7):627–635

[427] Tanaka M, Hashiguchi Y, Ueno H, Hase K, Mochizuki H. Tumor budding at the invasive margin can predict patients at high risk of recurrence after curative surgery for stage II, T3 colon cancer. Dis Colon Rectum. 2003; 46(8):1054–1059

[428] Okuyama T, Nakamura T, Yamaguchi M. Budding is useful to select high-risk patients in stage II well-differentiated or moderately differentiated colon adenocarcinoma. Dis Colon Rectum. 2003; 46(10):1400–1406

[429] Gagliardi G, Stepniewska KA, Hershman MJ, Hawley PR, Talbot IC. New grade-related prognostic variable for rectal cancer. Br J Surg. 1995; 82(5):599–602

[430] Chan CL, Chafai N, Rickard MJ, Dent OF, Chapuis PH, Bokey EL. What pathologic features influence survival in patients with local residual tumor after resection of colorectal cancer? J Am Coll Surg. 2004; 199(5):680–686

[431] Greene FL, Stewart AK, Norton HJ. A new TNM staging strategy for node-positive (stage III) colon cancer: an analysis of 50,042 patients. Ann Surg. 2002; 236(4):416–421, discussion 421

[432] Greene FL, Stewart AK, Norton HJ. New tumor-node-metastasis staging strategy for node-positive (stage III) rectal cancer: an analysis. J Clin Oncol. 2004; 22(10):1778–1784

[433] Corman ML, Veidenheimer MC, Coller JA. Colorectal carcinoma: a decade of experience at the Lahey Clinic. Dis Colon Rectum. 1979; 22(7):477–479

[434] Wolmark N, Fisher B, Wieand HS. The prognostic value of the modifications of the Dukes' C class of colorectal cancer. An analysis of the NSABP clinical trials. Ann Surg. 1986; 203(2):115–122

[435] Gardner B, Feldman J, Spivak Y, et al. Investigations of factors influencing the prognosis of colon cancer. Am J Surg. 1987; 153(6):541–544

[436] Cohen AM, Tremiterra S, Candela F, Thaler HT, Sigurdson ER. Prognosis of node-positive colon cancer. Cancer. 1991; 67(7):1859–1861

[437] Tang R, Wang JY, Chen JS, et al. Survival impact of lymph node metastasis in TNM stage III carcinoma of the colon and rectum. J Am Coll Surg. 1995; 180(6):705–712

[438] Malassagne B, Valleur P, Serra J, et al. Relationship of apical lymph node involvement to survival in resected colon carcinoma. Dis Colon Rectum. 1993; 36(7):645–653

[439] Swanson RS, Compton CC, Stewart AK, Bland KI. The prognosis of T3N0 colon cancer is dependent on the number of lymph nodes examined. Ann Surg Oncol. 2003; 10(1):65–71

[440] Fisher ER, Colangelo L, Wieand S, Fisher B, Wolmark N. Lack of influence of cytokeratin-positive mini micrometastases in "Negative Node" patients with colorectal cancer: findings from the national surgical adjuvant breast and bowel projects protocols R-01 and C-01. Dis Colon Rectum. 2003; 46(8):1021–1025, discussion 1025–1026

[441] Sakuragi M, Togashi K, Konishi F, et al. Predictive factors for lymph node metastasis in T1 stage colorectal carcinomas. Dis Colon Rectum. 2003; 46(12):1626–1632

[442] Tepper JE, O'Connell MJ, Niedzwiecki D, et al. Impact of number of nodes retrieved on outcome in patients with rectal cancer. J Clin Oncol. 2001; 19(1):157–163

[443] Day DW, Jass JR, Price AB, et al., eds. Morson and Dawson's Gastrointestinal Pathology. 4th ed. Malden, MA: Blackwell Science; 2008

[444] Minsky BD, Mies C, Rich TA, Recht A, Chaffey JT. Potentially curative surgery of colon cancer: the influence of blood vessel invasion. J Clin Oncol.. 1988; 6(1):119–127

[445] Krasna MJ, Flancbaum L, Cody RP, Shneibaum S, Ben Ari G. Vascular and neural invasion in colorectal carcinoma. Incidence and prognostic significance. Cancer. 1988; 61(5):1018–1023

[446] Horn A, Dahl O, Morild I. Venous and neural invasion as predictors of recurrence in rectal adenocarcinoma. Dis Colon Rectum. 1991; 34(9):798–804

[447] Sternberg A, Amar M, Alfici R, Groisman G. Conclusions from a study of venous invasion in stage IV colorectal adenocarcinoma. J Clin Pathol. 2002; 55(1):17–21

[448] Martin EW, Jr, Joyce S, Lucas J, Clausen K, Cooperman M. Colorectal carcinoma in patients less than 40 years of age: pathology and prognosis. Dis Colon Rectum. 1981; 24(1):25–28

[449] Ueno H, Hase K, Mochizuki H. Criteria for extramural perineural invasion as a prognostic factor in rectal cancer. Br J Surg. 2001; 88:994–1000

[450] Wanebo HJ, Stevens W. Surgical treatment of locally recurrent colorectal cancer. In: Nelson RL, ed. Problems in Current Surgery. Controversies in Colon Cancer. Philadelphia, PA: JB Lippincott; 1987:115–129

[451] Steele G, Jr, Zamcheck N. The use of carcinoembryonic antigen in the clinical management of patients with colorectal cancer. Cancer Detect Prev. 1985; 8(3):421–427

[452] Moertel CG, O'Fallon JR, Go VL, O'Connell MJ, Thynne GS. The preoperative carcinoembryonic antigen test in the diagnosis, staging, and prognosis of colorectal cancer. Cancer. 1986; 58(3):603–610

[453] Beart RW, Jr, O'Connell MJ. Postoperative follow-up of patients with carcinoma of the colon. Mayo Clin Proc. 1983; 58(6):361–363

[454] Lahr CJ, Soong SJ, Cloud G, Smith JW, Urist MM, Balch CM. A multifactorial analysis of prognostic factors in patients with liver metastases from colorectal carcinoma. J Clin Oncol. 1983; 1(11):720–726

[455] Venkatesh KS, Weingart DJ, Ramanujam PJ. Comparison of double and single parameters in DNA analysis for staging and as a prognostic indicator in patients with colon and rectal carcinoma. Dis Colon Rectum. 1994; 37(11):1142–1147

[456] Armitage NC, Robins RA, Evans DF, Turner DR, Baldwin RW, Hardcastle JD. The influence of tumour cell DNA abnormalities on survival in colorectal cancer. Br J Surg. 1985; 72(10):828–830

[457] Kokal W, Sheibani K, Terz J, Harada JR. Tumor DNA content in the prognosis of colorectal carcinoma. JAMA. 1986; 255(22):3123–3127

[458] Araki Y, Isomoto H, Morodomi T, Shirouzu K, Kakegawa T. Survival of rectal carcinoma patients studied with flow cytometric DNA analysis. Kurume Med J. 1990; 37(4):277–283

[459] Giaretti W, Sciallero S, Bruno S, Geido E, Aste H, Di Vinci A. DNA flow cytometry of endoscopically examined colorectal adenomas and adenocarcinomas. Cytometry. 1988; 9(3):238–244

[460] Jones DJ, Moore M, Schofield PF. Prognostic significance of DNA ploidy in colorectal cancer: a prospective flow cytometric study. Br J Surg. 1988; 75(1):28–33

[461] Halvorsen TB, Johannesen E. DNA ploidy, tumour site, and prognosis in colorectal cancer. A flow cytometric study of paraffin-embedded tissue. Scand J Gastroenterol. 1990; 25(2):141–148

[462] Kern SE, Fearon ER, Tersmette KW, et al. Clinical and pathological associations with allelic loss in colorectal carcinoma [corrected]. JAMA. 1989; 261(21):3099–3103

[463] Jen J, Kim H, Piantadosi S, et al. Allelic loss of chromosome 18q and prognosis in colorectal cancer. N Engl J Med. 1994; 331(4):213–221

[464] Herrlich P, Pals S, Ponta H. CD44 in colon cancer. Eur J Cancer. 1995; 31A(7–8):1110–1112

[465] Miyahara M, Saito T, Kaketani K, et al. Clinical significance of ras p21 overexpression for patients with an advanced colorectal cancer. Dis Colon Rectum. 1991; 34(12):1097–1102

[466] Diez M, Gonzalez A, Enriquez JM, et al. Prediction of recurrence in B-C stages of colorectal cancer by p-53 expression. Br J Surg. 1995; 82(26) (Suppl 1)

[467] Auvinen A, Isola J, Visakorpi T, Koivula T, Virtanen S, Hakama M. Overexpression of p53 and long-term survival in colon carcinoma. Br J Cancer. 1994; 70(2):293–296

[468] Grewal H, Guillem JG, Klimstra DS, Cohen AM. p53 nuclear overexpression may not be an independent prognostic marker in early colorectal cancer. Dis Colon Rectum. 1995; 38(11):1176–1181

[469] Pricolo VE, Finkelstein SD, Wu TT, et al. Prognostic value of TP53 and K-ras-2 mutational analysis in stage III carcinoma of the colon. Am J Surg. 1996; 171(1):41–46

[470] Shibata D, Reale MA, Lavin P, et al. The DCC protein and prognosis in colorectal cancer. N Engl J Med. 1996; 335(23):1727–1732

[471] Wang Y, Jatkoe T, Zhang Y, et al. Gene expression profiles and molecular markers to predict recurrence of Dukes' B colon cancer. J Clin Oncol. 2004; 22(9):1564–1571

[472] Lim SB, Jeong SY, Lee MR, et al. Prognostic significance of microsatellite instability in sporadic colorectal cancer. Int J Colorectal Dis. 2004; 19(6):533–537

[473] Kohonen-Corish MR, Daniel JJ, Chan C, et al. Low microsatellite instability is associated with poor prognosis in stage C colon cancer. J Clin Oncol. 2005; 23(10):2318–2324

[474] Popat S, Hubner R, Houlston RS. Systematic review of microsatellite instability and colorectal cancer prognosis. J Clin Oncol. 2005; 23(3):609–618

[475] Habib NA, Dawson PM, Bradfield JWB, Williamson RC, Wood CB. Sialomucins at resection margin and likelihood of recurrence in colorectal carcinoma. Br Med J (Clin Res Ed). 1986; 293(6546):521–523

[476] Mitmaker B, Begin LR, Gordon PH. Nuclear shape as a prognostic discriminant in colorectal carcinoma. Dis Colon Rectum. 1991; 34(3):249–259

[477] Verspaget HW, Sier CF, Ganesh S, Griffioen G, Lamers CB. Prognostic value of plasminogen activators and their inhibitors in colorectal cancer. Eur J Cancer. 1995; 31A(7–8):1105–1109

[478] Nakamori S, Kameyama M, Imaoka S, et al. Increased expression of sialyl Lewisx antigen correlates with poor survival in patients with colorectal carcinoma: clinicopathological and immunohistochemical study. Cancer Res. 1993; 53(15):3632–3637

[479] Teixeira CR, Tanaka S, Haruma K, Yoshihara M, Sumii K, Kajiyama G. Proliferating cell nuclear antigen expression at the invasive tumor margin predicts malignant potential of colorectal carcinomas. Cancer. 1994; 73(3):575–579

[480] Cali RL, Pitsch RM, Thorson AG, et al. Cumulative incidence of metachronous colorectal cancer. Dis Colon Rectum. 1993; 36(4):388–393

[481] Olson RM, Perencevich NP, Malcolm AW, Chaffey JT, Wilson RE. Patterns of recurrence following curative resection of adenocarcinoma of the colon and rectum. Cancer. 1980; 45(12):2969–2974

[482] Cochrane JP, Williams JT, Faber RG, Slack WW. Value of outpatient follow-up after curative surgery for carcinoma of the large bowel. BMJ. 1980; 280(6214):593–595

[483] Bühler H, Seefeld U, Deyhle P, Buchmann P, Metzger U, Ammann R. Endoscopic follow-up after colorectal cancer surgery. Early detection of local recurrence? Cancer. 1984; 54(5):791–793

[484] Wenzl E, Wunderlich M, Herbst F, et al. Results of a rigorous follow-up system in colorectal cancer. Int J Colorectal Dis. 1988; 3(3):176–180

[485] Yamamoto Y, Imai H, Iwamoto S, Kasai Y, Tsunoda T. Surgical treatment for the recurrence of colorectal cancer. Surg Today. 1996; 26(3):164–168

[486] Umpleby HC, Williamson RC. Anastomotic recurrence in large bowel cancer. Br J Surg. 1987; 74(10):873–878

[487] Russell AH, Tong D, Dawson LE, Wisbeck W. Adenocarcinoma of the proximal colon. Sites of initial dissemination and patterns of recurrence following surgery alone. Cancer. 1984; 53(2):360–367

[488] Gunderson LL, Tepper JE, Dosoretz DE, et al. Patterns of failure after treatment of gastrointestinal cancer. In: Cox JD, ed. Proceedings of CROS-NCI Conference on Patterns of Failure after Treatment of Cancer. Vol. 2. Cancer Treatment Symposium; 1983

[489] Böhm B, Schwenk W, Hucke HP, Stock W. Does methodic long-term follow-up affect survival after curative resection of colorectal carcinoma? Dis Colon Rectum. 1993; 36(3):280–286

[490] Obrand DI, Gordon PH. Incidence and patterns of recurrence following curative resection for colorectal carcinoma. Dis Colon Rectum. 1997; 40(1):15–24

[491] Rodriguez-Bigas MA, Stulc JP, Davidson B, Petrelli NJ. Prognostic significance of anastomotic recurrence from colorectal adenocarcinoma. Dis Colon Rectum. 1992; 35(9):838–842

[492] Malcolm AW, Perencevich NP, Olson RM, Hanley JA, Chaffey JT, Wilson RE. Analysis of recurrence patterns following curative resection for carcinoma of the colon and rectum. Surg Gynecol Obstet. 1981; 152(2):131–136

[493] Boey J, Cheung HC, Lai CK, Wong J. A prospective evaluation of serum carcinoembryonic antigen (CEA) levels in the management of colorectal carcinoma. World J Surg. 1984; 8(3):279–286

[494] Willett CG, Tepper JE, Cohen AM, Orlow E, Welch CE. Failure patterns following curative resection of colonic carcinoma. Ann Surg. 1984; 200(6):685–690

[495] Gunderson LL, Sosin H, Levitt S. Extrapelvic colon: areas of failure in a reoperation series: implications for adjuvant therapy. Int J Radiat Oncol Biol Phys. 1985; 11(4):731–741

[496] Galandiuk S, Wieand HS, Moertel CG, et al. Patterns of recurrence after curative resection of carcinoma of the colon and rectum. Surg Gynecol Obstet. 1992; 174(1):27–32

[497] Koea JB, Lanouette N, Paty PB, Guillem JG, Cohen AM. Abdominal wall recurrence after colorectal resection for cancer. Dis Colon Rectum. 2000; 43(5):628–632

[498] Barillari P, Ramacciato G, Manetti G, Bovino A, Sammartino P, Stipa V. Surveillance of colorectal cancer: effectiveness of early detection of intraluminal recurrences on prognosis and survival of patients treated for cure. Dis Colon Rectum. 1996; 39(4):388–393

[499] Jacquet P, Jelinek JS, Steves MA, Sugarbaker PH. Evaluation of computed tomography in patients with peritoneal carcinomatosis. Cancer. 1993; 72(5):1631–1636

[500] Delbeke D, Vitola JV, Sandler MP, et al. Staging recurrent metastatic colorectal carcinoma with PET. J Nucl Med. 1997; 38(8):1196–1201

[501] Desai DC, Zervos EE, Arnold MW, Burak WE, Jr, Mantil J, Martin EW, Jr. Positron emission tomography affects surgical management in recurrent colorectal cancer patients. Ann Surg Oncol. 2003; 10(1):59–64

[502] Whiteford MH, Whiteford HM, Yee LF, et al. Usefulness of FDG-PET scan in the assessment of suspected metastatic or recurrent adenocarcinoma of the colon and rectum. Dis Colon Rectum. 2000; 43(6):759–767, discussion 767–770

[503] Johnson K, Bakhsh A, Young D, Martin TE, Jr, Arnold M. Correlating computed tomography and positron emission tomography scan with operative findings in metastatic colorectal cancer. Dis Colon Rectum. 2001; 44(3):354–357

[504] Minton JP, Hoehn JL, Gerber DM, et al. Results of a 400-patient carcinoembryonic antigen second-look colorectal cancer study. Cancer. 1985; 55(6):1284–1290

[505] Staab HJ, Anderer FA, Stumpf E, Hornung A, Fischer R, Kieninger G. Eighty-four potential second-look operations based on sequential carcinoembryonic antigen determinations and clinical investigations in patients with recurrent gastrointestinal cancer. Am J Surg. 1985; 149(2):198–204

[506] Hida J, Yasutomi M, Shindoh K, et al. Second-look operation for recurrent colorectal cancer based on carcinoembryonic antigen and imaging techniques. Dis Colon Rectum. 1996; 39(1):74–79

[507] Waldron RP, Donovan IA. Clinical follow-up and treatment of locally recurrent colorectal cancer. Dis Colon Rectum. 1987; 30(6):428–430

[508] Gwin JL, Hoffman JP, Eisenberg BL. Surgical management of nonhepatic intra-abdominal recurrence of carcinoma of the colon. Dis Colon Rectum. 1993; 36(6):540–544

[509] Herfarth C, Schlag P, Hohenberger P. Surgical strategies in locoregional recurrences of gastrointestinal carcinoma. World J Surg. 1987; 11(4):504–510

[510] Law WL, Chan WF, Lee YM, Chu KW. Non-curative surgery for colorectal cancer: critical appraisal of outcomes. Int J Colorectal Dis. 2004; 19(3):197–202

[511] Bowne WB, Lee B, Wong WD, et al. Operative salvage for locoregional recurrent colon cancer after curative resection: an analysis of 100 cases. Dis Colon Rectum. 2005; 48(5):897–909

[512] Willett CG, Shellito PC, Tepper JE, Eliseo R, Convery K, Wood WC. Intraoperative electron beam radiation therapy for recurrent locally advanced rectal or rectosigmoid carcinoma. Cancer. 1991; 67(6):1504–1508

[513] Taylor WE, Donohue JH, Gunderson LL, et al. The Mayo Clinic experience with multimodality treatment of locally advanced or recurrent colon cancer. Ann Surg Oncol. 2002; 9(2):177–185

[514] Wodnicki H, Goldberg R, Kaplan S, Yahr WZ, Kreiger B, Russin D. The laser: an alternative for palliative treatment of obstructing intraluminal lesions. Am Surg. 1988; 54(4):227–230

[515] Buchi KN. Endoscopic laser surgery in the colon and rectum. Dis Colon Rectum. 1988; 31(9):739–745

[516] Bown SG, Barr H, Matthewson K, et al. Endoscopic treatment of inoperable colorectal cancers with the Nd YAG laser. Br J Surg. 1986; 73(12):949–952

[517] Faintuch JS. Endoscopic laser therapy in colorectal carcinoma. Hematol Oncol Clin North Am. 1989; 3(1):155–170

[518] Krasner N. Lasers in the treatment of colorectal disease. Symposium. Int J Colorectal Dis. 1989; 4:1–29

[519] Tan CC, Iftikhar SY, Allan A, Freeman JG. Local effects of colorectal cancer are well palliated by endoscopic laser therapy. Eur J Surg Oncol. 1995; 21(6):648–652

[520] Mandava N, Petrelli N, Herrera L, Nava H. Laser palliation for colorectal carcinoma. Am J Surg. 1991; 162(3):212–214, discussion 215

[521] Chia YW, Ngoi SS, Goh PMY. Endoscopic Nd:YAG laser in the palliative treatment of advanced low rectal carcinoma in Singapore. Dis Colon Rectum. 1991; 34(12):1093–1096

[522] Arrigoni A, Pennazio M, Spandre M, Rossini FP. Emergency endoscopy: recanalization of intestinal obstruction caused by colorectal cancer. Gastrointest Endosc. 1994; 40(5):576–580

[523] Dittrich K, Armbruster C, Hoffer F, Tuchmann A, Dinstl K. Nd:YAG laser treatment of colorectal malignancies: an experience of 4 1/2 years. Lasers Surg Med. 1992; 12(2):199–203

[524] Bright N, Hale P, Mason R. Poor palliation of colorectal malignancy with the neodymium yttrium-aluminium-garnet laser. Br J Surg. 1992; 79(4):308–309

[525] Courtney ED, Raja A, Leicester RJ. Eight years experience of high-powered endoscopic diode laser therapy for palliation of colorectal carcinoma. Dis Colon Rectum. 2005; 48(4):845–850

[526] Pilati P, Mocellin S, Rossi CR, et al. Cytoreductive surgery combined with hyperthermic intraperitoneal intraoperative chemotherapy for peritoneal carcinomatosis arising from colon adenocarcinoma. Ann Surg Oncol. 2003; 10(5):508–513

[527] Verwaal VJ, Boot H, Aleman BM, van Tinteren H, Zoetmulder FA. Recurrences after peritoneal carcinomatosis of colorectal origin treated by cytoreduction and hyperthermic intraperitoneal chemotherapy: location, treatment, and outcome. Ann Surg Oncol. 2004; 11(4):375–379

[528] Smith P, Bruera E. Management of malignant ureteral obstruction in the palliative care setting. J Pain Symptom Manage. 1995; 10(6):481–486

[529] Keidan RD, Greenberg RE, Hoffman JP, Weese JL. Is percutaneous nephrostomy for hydronephrosis appropriate in patients with advanced cancer? Am J Surg. 1988; 156(3, Pt 1):206–208

[530] Ballantyne JC. Chronic pain following treatment for cancer: the role of opioids. Oncologist. 2003; 8(6):567–575

[531] Cherny NI, Portenoy RK. The management of cancer pain. CA Cancer J Clin. 1994; 44(5):263–303

[532] Waterman NG, Hughes S, Foster WS. Control of cancer pain by epidural infusion of morphine. Surgery. 1991; 110(4):612–614, discussion 614–616

[533] Foltz A, Besser P, Ellenberg S, et al. Effectiveness of nutritional counseling on caloric intake, weight change and percent protein intake in patients with advanced colorectal and lung cancer. Nutrition. 1987; 3:263–271

[534] Vassilopoulos PP, Yoon JM, Ledesma EJ, Mittelman A. Treatment of recurrence of adenocarcinoma of the colon and rectum at the anastomotic site. Surg Gynecol Obstet. 1981; 152(6):777–780

[535] Pihl E, Hughes ESR, McDermott FT, Price AB. Recurrence of carcinoma of the colon and rectum at the anastomotic suture line. Surg Gynecol Obstet. 1981; 153(4):495–496

[536] Mäkelä J, Kairaluoma MI. Reoperation for colorectal cancer. Acta Chir Scand. 1986; 152:151–155

[537] Stellato TA, Shenk RR. Gastrointestinal emergencies in the oncology patient. Semin Oncol. 1989; 16(6):521–531

[538] van Ooijen B, van der Burg ME, Planting AS, Siersema PD, Wiggers T. Surgical treatment or gastric drainage only for intestinal obstruction in patients with carcinoma of the ovary or peritoneal carcinomatosis of other origin. Surg Gynecol Obstet. 1993; 176(5):469–474

[539] Lau PWK, Lorentz TG. Results of surgery for malignant bowel obstruction in advanced, unresectable, recurrent colorectal cancer. Dis Colon Rectum. 1993; 36(1):61–64

[540] Butler JA, Cameron BL, Morrow M, Kahng K, Tom J. Small bowel obstruction in patients with a prior history of cancer. Am J Surg. 1991; 162(6):624–628

[541] Miller G, Boman J, Shrier I, Gordon PH. Small-bowel obstruction secondary to malignant disease: an 11-year audit. Can J Surg. 2000; 43(5):353–358

[542] Krouse RS, McCahill LE, Easson AM, Dunn GP. When the sun can set on an unoperated bowel obstruction: management of malignant bowel obstruction. J Am Coll Surg. 2002; 195(1):117–128

[543] August DA, Thorn D, Fisher RL, Welchek CM. Home parenteral nutrition for patients with inoperable malignant bowel obstruction. JPEN J Parenter Enteral Nutr. 1991; 15(3):323–327

[544] Parker MC, Baines MJ. Intestinal obstruction in patients with advanced malignant disease. Br J Surg. 1996; 83(1):1–2

[545] Bernstein MA, Madoff RD, Caushaj PF. Colon and rectal cancer in pregnancy. Dis Colon Rectum. 1993; 36(2):172–178

[546] Van Voorhis B, Cruikshank DP. Colon carcinoma complicating pregnancy. A report of two cases. J Reprod Med. 1989; 34(11):923–927

[547] Nesbitt JC, Moise KJ, Sawyers JL. Colorectal carcinoma in pregnancy. Arch Surg. 1985; 120(5):636–640

[548] Hertel H, Diebolder H, Herrmann J, et al. Is the decision for colorectal resection justified by histopathologic findings: a prospective study of 100 patients with advanced ovarian cancer. Gynecol Oncol. 2001; 83(3):481–484

[549] Pillay K, Chetty R. Malakoplakia in association with colorectal carcinoma: a series of four cases. Pathology. 2002; 34(4):332–335

23 Other Malignant Lesions of the Colon and Rectum

Philip H. Gordon and David E. Beck

Abstract

This chapter discusses a number of uncommon malignant lesions of the colon and rectum, including their incidence, clinical features, imaging procedures, chemical activity, and treatment.

Keywords: malignant lesions, carcinoid, lymphoma, sarcoma, squamous cell carcinoma, adenosquamous carcinoma, plasmacytoma, melanoma, schwannoma, angiosarcoma

23.1 Carcinoid

The carcinoid neoplasm is one member of a collection of neoplasms grouped together because of a common biochemical function. These neoplasms all incorporate and store large amounts of amine precursor (5-hydroxytryptophan) and have the ability to decarboxylate this substrate, leading to the production of several biologically active amines; thus, the acronym APUD (amine precursor uptake and decarboxylation) is derived.[1]

23.1.1 Incidence

Carcinoids arise from neuroectodermal derivatives. The gastrointestinal tract is the most common site and in decreasing order of frequency, the locations of carcinoids are the appendix, ileum, rectum, colon, and stomach.[2] Approximately 5% of all carcinoids are located in the colon.[2,3] In the Connecticut Registry with 54 colonic carcinoids, 48% were in the cecum, 16% in the ascending colon, 6% in the transverse colon, 11% in the descending colon, 13% in the sigmoid colon, and 6% were not assigned.[4] The incidence of rectal carcinoids was 1.3% of noncarcinoid neoplasms of the rectum; for the colon, the incidence was 0.3% of noncarcinoid neoplasms of the colon.[5] In the Connecticut Registry, the age-adjusted incidence was 0.31 cases per 100,000 population/y.[4] Colonic involvement accounted for only 2.5% of all gastrointestinal carcinoids and 2.8% of all carcinoids.[6] Rectal carcinoids accounted for 12 to 15% of all carcinoids, and carcinoids of the remainder of the colon accounted for 7% of all carcinoids.[7]

23.1.2 Clinical Features

Carcinoids most commonly occur in the seventh and eighth decades of life, with a female preponderance of 2:1.[1,6] Colonic carcinoids may present as a simple polyp or as a gross malignancy that is indistinguishable from carcinoma radiologically and has an "apple core" appearance. These carcinoids may be entirely asymptomatic, found in 0.014% of rectal examinations, or they may produce symptoms indistinguishable from those of carcinoma. Colonic carcinoids are usually symptomatic.[6] Once they have been diagnosed, a search for other neoplasms should be made because the incidence of synchronous and metachronous neoplasms has been reported as high as 42%.[6] Gastrointestinal carcinoid is associated with a high incidence of second primary malignancy. Gerstle et al[8] reviewed their experience with 69 patients with carcinoids of the gastrointestinal tract and found that 42% had second synchronous neoplasms and 4% had a metachronous neoplasm. The gastrointestinal tract was the site of 43% of these additional neoplasms with half of these being carcinomas of the colon and rectum. Tichansky et al[9] conducted a search of the National Cancer Institute Surveillance, Epidemiology, and End Results database from 1973 to 1996 and found 2,086 patients with colorectal carcinoids. Patients with colorectal carcinoids had an increased rate of carcinoma in the colon and rectum, small bowel, esophagus/stomach, lung/bronchus, urinary tract, and prostate, when compared with the control population. Most of the gastrointestinal carcinomas were synchronous carcinomas, whereas lesions outside the gastrointestinal tract were mostly metachronous neoplasms. After the diagnosis of colorectal carcinoid neoplasms, patients should undergo appropriate screening and surveillance for carcinoma at these other sites.

Most gastrointestinal carcinoids are incidentally discovered at laparotomy or autopsy. The discovery of an asymptomatic gastrointestinal carcinoid during the operative treatment of another malignancy will usually only require resection and has little effect on the prognosis of the individual. Carcinoids may be associated with multiple endocrine neoplasia, (especially of the parathyroid,) but most of these are associated with carcinoids of foregut origin.[10] Carcinoids of midgut and hindgut origin occur more frequently and produce significant endocrine relationships other than serotonin production. The diagnosis may be established by demonstrating elevated blood levels of serotonin or elevated urinary levels of 5-hydroxyindoleacetic acid.

In the series reported by Rosenberg and Welch,[6] 44% of patients had signs of local spread, while 38% of patients had distant metastases. The liver was involved in 35.5% of the patients and the lung in 8%. In a review by Berardi,[11] 57% of patients with colonic carcinoids already had metastases, and of these, 42% had distant metastases. In the series reported by Gerstle et al,[8] the overall incidence of metastatic carcinoid at presentation was 32%. The most common sites of metastatic disease were lymph nodes in 82%, liver in 68%, satellite lesions to adjacent small bowel in 32%, peritoneum in 27%, and omentum in 18%. Only 1 of 18 appendiceal carcinoids metastasized and that only to the local lymph nodes. Four of nine colorectal carcinoids metastasized to the lymph nodes and liver. Other sites of metastatic disease included bone.[12]

23.1.3 Pathology

Macroscopically, carcinoids may vary in appearance from nodular thickening in the mucosa and submucosa to a sessile or pedunculated polypoid lesion, and they may have a yellowish tinge. Larger lesions may ulcerate and become annular, or they may obstruct and metastasize to regional lymph nodes or the liver (▶ Fig. 23.1). The malignant character of these lesions correlates with size, location, and tissue invasion. Carcinoids of the appendix and rectum rarely metastasize.[7] Lesions less than 2 cm rarely metastasize, whereas 80% of lesions greater than

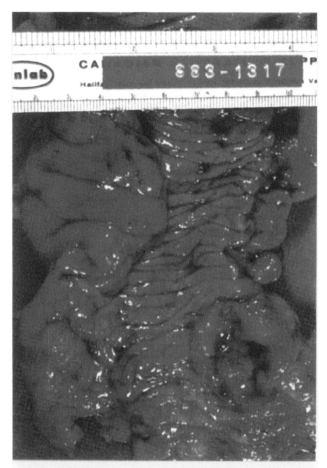

Fig. 23.1 Macroscopic features of a carcinoid of the large bowel. Lesion appears as a yellowish-tinged protruding mass.

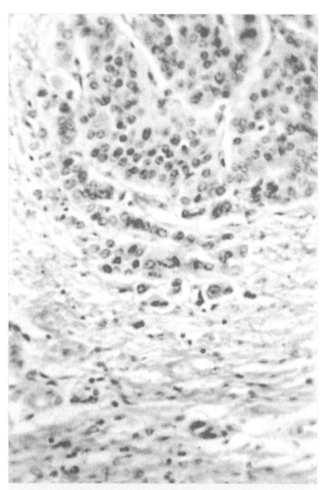

Fig. 23.2 Microscopic features of a carcinoid with uniform small cells in a trabecular anastomotic pattern. Although the lesion is not cytologically malignant, invasion into the muscle is evident. (This image is provided courtesy of H. Srolovitz, MD.)

2 cm in diameter do metastasize. Superficially invasive lesions have a better prognosis than do deeply penetrating ones. In his review, Berardi[11] found multiple carcinoids in 4.2% of patients with colonic carcinoids as compared with 30% of patients with ileal carcinoids. Associated malignancy of the colon was found in 2.5% of patients with colonic carcinoids as compared with 30 to 53% of patients with ileal carcinoids.

Microscopically, carcinoids consist of uniform, small, round, or polygonal cells with prominent round nuclei and eosinophilic cytoplasmic granules (▶ Fig. 23.2). They usually demonstrate one of five histologic patterns: insular, trabecular, glandular, undifferentiated, or mixed. In decreasing order of median survival time in years, the growth patterns are ranked as follows: mixed insular plus glandular, 4.4; insular, 2.9; trabecular, 2.5; mixed insular plus trabecular 2.3; mixed growth pattern, 1.4; glandular, 0.9; and undifferentiated, 0.5.[13]

23.1.4 Imaging Procedures

The hypervascular nature of carcinoids and their metastases allows an aggressive role by the radiologist in diagnosis and interventional management.[14] Double-contrast studies still best define the primary neoplasms. The "spoke wheel" configuration of the desmoplastic mesenteric masses and lymph node metastases are best seen by CT, whereas hepatic metastases can be demonstrated by CT, CT angioportography, ultrasonography,

MRI, and octreotide scintigraphy. Superior mesenteric angiography of the small bowel and cecum is useful when scanning procedures are not revealing. Percutaneous needle biopsy with radiologic guidance may confirm the diagnosis.

Octreotide scintigraphy may have a fourfold impact on patient management.[15] It may detect resectable lesions that would be unrecognized with conventional imaging techniques, it may prevent operation in patients whose lesions have metastasized to a greater extent than can be detected with conventional imaging, it may direct the choice of therapy in patients with inoperable carcinoids, and, in the future, it may be used to select patients for radionuclide therapy.

23.1.5 Chemical Activity

Carcinoids secrete serotonin, a substance with pronounced pharmacologic effects, including flushing of the face, neck, anterior chest wall, and hands; increased peristalsis leading to diarrhea; constriction of bronchi presenting as wheezing; and cardiac valvular lesions with right-sided heart failure (pulmonary stenosis). Other components of the syndrome include a rise in pulmonary arterial pressure, hypotension, edema, pellagralike skin lesions, peptic ulcers, arthralgia, and weight loss.[16]

This constellation of symptoms, known as the carcinoid syndrome, usually occurs with metastases to the liver. Other products such as bradykinin, histamine, vasoactive intestinal peptide, adrenocorticotropic hormone (ACTH), 5-hydroxytryptophan, and prostaglandins produce part of the syndrome complex. The syndrome occurs primarily with carcinoids of the small bowel but not with those of the colon or rectum.

Foregut carcinoids, which are argentaffin negative and argyrophil positive, produce the serotonin precursor 5-hydroxytryptophan. Midgut carcinoids are usually both argyrophil positive and argentaffin positive, are frequently multicentric in origin, and may be associated with the carcinoid syndrome. Hindgut carcinoids are rarely argyrophil positive or argentaffin positive, are usually unicentric, and are not usually associated with the carcinoid syndrome (▶ Fig. 23.3). The carcinoid syndrome is a rare clinical entity that occurs with a prevalence of 1.6% in patients with carcinoids and almost only if liver metastases are present.[17] Berardi[11] estimated that less than 5% of colonic carcinoids cause the carcinoid syndrome. In a series by Rosenberg and Welch,[6] 4.2% of patients had either symptoms suggestive of the syndrome or elevated 5-hydroxyindoleacetic acid levels.

23.1.6 Treatment

Appendiceal carcinoids less than 1 cm in diameter can be treated adequately by appendectomy, but if they are greater than 2 cm in diameter, a right hemicolectomy should be performed.[2] The rationale for the latter recommendation is that the average rate of metastases is 30%.[2] For lesions between 1 and 2 cm, in which the risk of metastases is between 0 and 1%, the decision-making process is more difficult. Appendectomy is probably sufficient but additional criteria may be considered, such as extension to the mesoappendix or subserosal lymphatic invasion.[18] A more aggressive approach may be advised for younger patients.[2] Gouzi et al[19] recommended that other than having a size greater than 2 cm and base location, the presence of mucin production is a further indication for secondary right hemicolectomy.

The recommended treatment for small bowel carcinoids is wide segmental resection. Because the average lymph node involvement is 44%,[2] relevant lymph node drainage should be included. Meticulous intraoperative examination is indicated because 20 to 40% of small bowel carcinoids are multicentric and simultaneous adenocarcinomas of other parts of the gastrointestinal tract occur at a rate of 8 to 29%.[2] For colonic carcinoids, the standard operation for adenocarcinoma should be performed.

Metastatic disease occurs more frequently with carcinoids of the colon. If there is distant disease, resection of the primary lesion is still recommended to alleviate symptoms (because a long survival period is possible).[7] Partial hepatectomy should be considered if technically feasible.[16,20] Beaton et al[21] have shown the value of aggressive operative debulking in reducing and sometimes obliterating the manifestations of the syndrome. For patients with unresectable metastatic carcinoids to the liver, combining either operative hepatic dearterialization or hepatic intra-arterial embolization with chemotherapy has reportedly been effective in inducing regression of the liver metastases.[14,20,22]

Chemotherapeutic agents used have included 5-fluorouracil (5-FU), streptozotocin delivered via hepatic artery or portal vein catheters, or floxuridine (FUDR) and doxorubicin administered systemically.[23,24,25] A number of other pharmacologic and cytotoxic agents have been used to control the carcinoid syndrome.[26] Each is aimed at neutralizing one of the pharmacologically active products released by the carcinoid. Vinik and Moattari[23] have reported the successful use of somatostatin analog in the management of the carcinoid syndrome. The symptoms of diarrhea, flushing, and wheezing can be dramatically reduced or even abolished. Ahlman et al[20] pursued an aggressive policy in the management of patients with midgut carcinoid syndrome and bilobar disease. After primary operation to relieve symptoms of intestine obstruction and ischemia, the authors performed successful embolizations of hepatic arteries. Patients with remedial disease were treated by octreotide. In a series of 64 patients, the authors obtained a 70% 5-year survival rate.

23.1.7 Results

Five-year survival rates for patients with colonic carcinoids are reported to be 52%.[15] Survival rates reported by Rosenberg and Welch[6] were 51, 25, and 10% at 2, 5, and 10 years, respectively. In the Connecticut Registry, 2- and 5-year survival rates were 56 and 33%, respectively. The 5-year survival by Dukes' staging was as follows: A, 83%; B, 43%; C, 35%; and metastatic, 21%. In a 25-year population-based study of 36 colonic carcinoids, Spread et al[3] found a perioperative mortality of 22%. Actuarial survival rates at 2 and 5 years were 34 and 26%, respectively. In the authors' review, the size of the lesion and invasion into muscularis propria, the two major histopathologic prognostic factors for carcinoids, were not found to influence survival significantly. Stage, histologic pattern, differentiation, nuclear grade, and mitotic rate (> 20 mitosis/10 high power fields [hpf])

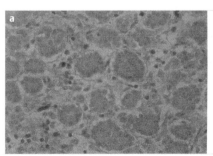
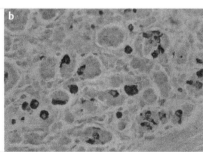

Fig. 23.3 (a) Microscopic appearance of a carcinoid with demonstration of argyrophilic granules by Fontana's stain. **(b)** Microscopic appearance of a carcinoid demonstrating argentaffin tissue. (The images are provided courtesy of L.R. Begin, MD.)

proved to be prognostic factors. The 5-year survival rate in patients with appendiceal carcinoids was 90 to 100%.[2] The overall 5-year survival rate for small bowel carcinoids was 50 to 60%.[2] The 5-year survival rate decreases from 75% for local disease to 59% for patients with positive nodes to 20 to 35% if liver metastases are present.

23.2 Lymphoma

23.2.1 Incidence

Lymphoma may occur as a primary lesion or as part of a generalized malignant process involving the gastrointestinal tract. As a primary lesion, it constitutes only 0.5% of all cases of neoplastic disease of the colon, and yet it is the second most common malignant disease of the colon. Lymphoma comprises 6 to 20% of cases of primary gastrointestinal lymphoma[7,24,25,26,27] and accounts for 5 to 10% of all non-Hodgkin's lymphoma.[25] It most commonly involves the cecum (70%), with the rectum and ascending colon next in order of frequency.[25,27] A more recent publication cited distribution sites of primary large bowel lymphoma as cecum 37.5%, descending colon 25%, ascending colon 25%, and rectum 12.5%.[26] It can occur at any age from 3 to 81 years, but the average age is 50 years. Men are affected twice as often as women, but a recent publication cited the reverse.[26]

23.2.2 Pathology

Lymphomas represent a diverse group of neoplasms. At least six major classifications of non-Hodgkin's lymphoma are in use, but there is no consensus among them. Three macroscopic types are seen.[28] Annular or plaquelike thickenings are the most common type, followed by bulky protuberant growths, and, rarely, thickened and aneurysmal dilatations of the bowel wall. The cut surface has a uniform fleshy appearance (▶ Fig. 23.4). Regional lymph nodes are involved in one-half of all cases, but such involvement is not related to prognosis. Multiple primary foci are quite common. Malignant lymphomas may present as multiple polypoid protrusions of the entire colon and may mimic adenomatosis coli. Roentgenographically, 86% of colonic lymphomas are single lesions, 8% are multiple discrete lesions,

and 6% show a diffuse colonic involvement.[17] Dawson et al[29] presented these criteria for a primary lymphoma of the gastrointestinal tract: (1) no palpable peripheral lymphadenopathy, (2) normal roentgenographic findings except at the primary site, (3) normal white blood cell count and differential, (4) tract lesion with only regional lymph node involvement, and (5) no involvement of the liver or spleen.

The large series of large bowel lymphomas reported by Jinnai et al[25] were classified histologically in order of frequency as follows: histiocytic, lymphocytic, mixed, and Hodgkin's disease. The incidence of each variety varies from series to series, but in the combined series it was as follows: histiocytic type, 43%; lymphocytic type, 29%; mixed type, 14%; and Hodgkin's disease, 3.5% (▶ Fig. 23.5).[24] In one series of 15 patients, histologically 40% were classified as high-grade and 60% as intermediate-grade non-Hodgkin's lymphoma. The neoplasms usually presented at an advanced stage: in 87%, the lymphoma had spread to the adjacent mesentery, the regional lymph nodes, or both when first diagnosed.[27]

23.2.3 Clinical Features

Lymphomas of the colon are characterized by abdominal pain in more than 90% of patients. Otherwise, the symptoms may be indistinguishable from those of carcinoma, with changes in bowel habits such as diarrhea or constipation, bleeding, weight loss, weakness, and possibly fever. Tender abdominal masses are present in 80% of patients on initial examination.[24] If ulceration supervenes, bleeding may be more prominent. Obstruction occurs in 20 to 25% of patients, but perforation is infrequent.[24] Multiple lesions constitute 8% of cases.[30]

The radiologic signs observed during barium enema studies for non-Hodgkin's lymphoma are as follows: a small nodular pattern frequently with multiple lesions (45.7%), a diffuse or infiltrating pattern (25.4%), a filling defect (22.9%), endoluminal and exoluminal images (17.8%), ulcerating patterns (3.4%), and a pure mesenteric form (0.8%).[31,32] Lymphomas of the colon may produce the same radiologic appearance as carcinomas and similarly may be indistinguishable from carcinomas at laparotomy. The colonoscopic appearance of a follicular lymphoma

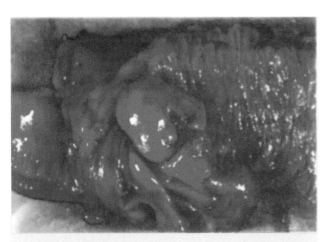

Fig. 23.4 Grayish fish-flesh appearance of a lymphoma of the large bowel. Note that the mucosa is intact.

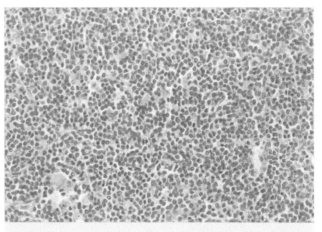

Fig. 23.5 Microscopic features of a poorly differentiated lymphoma of the colon demonstrating a somewhat nodular pattern, pleomorphism, and a degree of cellular necrosis. (This image is provided courtesy of L. R. Begin, MD.)

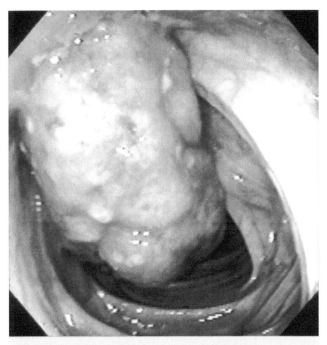

Fig. 23.6 Colonoscopic appearance of a colonic lymphoma.

is seen in ▸ Fig. 23.6. Biopsy will clarify the diagnosis, but diagnosis still may be difficult because of the superficial nature of the biopsy.

Once the diagnosis is made, staging should be performed through an adequate history, physical examination, barium enema, complete blood count, liver function tests, chest X-ray films, bone marrow assay, CT scan of the abdomen, and lymphangiography.[7]

23.2.4 Treatment

The treatment of primary lymphoma of the colon is resection. At laparotomy, appropriate staging with liver biopsy, lymph node biopsy, and splenectomy has been recommended.[7] Only one-third of lymphomas are confined to the bowel wall at laparotomy.[31] For unresectable lesions, radiation is beneficial. Chemotherapy is recommended for systemic disease.

23.2.5 Results

The overall 5-year survival rate is approximately 40% (range, 20–55%).[24,28] When regional lymph nodes are involved, 5-year survivals fall to 12%. There is a marked difference in survival rate between patients who undergo resection only and those who receive supplementary radiotherapy, 83 versus 16%.[31]

In a series of 130 cases of primary lymphoma of the large intestine, Jinnai et al[25] reported a resection rate for cure of 55%, with most operations being abdominoperineal resections and others low anterior resections or hemicolectomies. Survival rates at 5 and 10 years were 39.8 and 33.2%, respectively. Corresponding survival rates after curative resection were 44.2 and 40%. Prognosis was better when the lesion was 5 cm in diameter, intraluminal, and without lymph node metastases. When lymphomas were analyzed according to histologic type, 5- and 10-year survival rates of curative resection were both 38.9% for histiocytic type, both 43% for lymphocytic type, 43.8 and 21.9% for the mixed type, and both 100% for Hodgkin's disease. Overall 5-year survival rates were 25.4, 33.2, 35.4, and 40%, respectively. The growth pattern for the lesions was intraluminal for about 50%, extramural in 15%, intramural in 25%, and unknown in the remainder. Corresponding 5-year survival rates were 47, 20, and 12%. The 10-year survival rates were the same for intraluminal and extramural lesions, but no patients in the intramural group survived more than 7 years. The 5- and 10-year survival rates were 18.5% for patients with lymph node metastases, and 45.4 and 37.1%, respectively, for patients without metastases.

Doolabh et al[33] reported their experience with seven cases of primary colonic lymphoma, which represented 1.4% of all non-Hodgkin's lymphoma, 14% of gastrointestinal non-Hodgkin's lymphoma, and 0.9% of all colonic malignancies diagnosed during the period of their study. The most common presentation was nonspecific abdominal pain. The lack of specific symptoms delayed diagnoses from 1 to 12 months. All patients underwent laparotomy with resection. The most common location of the lymphoma was the cecum (71%). Regional lymph nodes were affected in all but one patient. All lymphomas were B-cell lymphomas (five small noncleaved cells and two large cells). Six of seven patients received adjuvant chemotherapy. Of the six patients available for follow-up, four remained alive (12, 19, 23, and 25 months after diagnosis). In both patients who died, the disease recurred diffusely.

Fan et al[34] identified 37 cases of primary colorectal lymphoma that comprised 0.48% of all cases of colon malignancies. The most common presenting sign and symptoms were abdominal pain (62%), abdominal mass (54%), and weight loss (43%). The most frequent site of involvement was the cecum (45%). Histologically, 78% were classified as high-grade lymphoma and 22% as intermediate-grade to low-grade lymphoma. Fifty-seven percent of cases received adjuvant chemotherapy. The 5-year survival was 33% for all patients and 39% for patients treated with combination chemotherapy.

23.3 Sarcoma

There are a large variety of very uncommon neoplasms arising from mesenchymal tissues. Malignancies that fit into this category are classified as sarcomas and include leiomyosarcoma, liposarcoma, hemangiosarcoma, fibrosarcoma, fibrous histiocytoma, neurofibrosarcoma, lymphangiosarcoma, and Kaposi's sarcoma.

Leiomyosarcoma of the colon is a rare pathologic entity, with only 58 recorded cases at the time of review of the literature by Suzuki et al.[35] This type of sarcoma occurs two to six times more commonly in the rectum than in the colon in both sexes and most commonly appears in the fifth and sixth decades of life.[36] The lesion arises from the smooth muscle of the bowel. Macroscopically, it may range from a small nodule to a large mass, which is covered by mucosa in its early stages but eventually may become ulcerated (▸ Fig. 23.7). The lesion may be intramural, endoenteric, exoenteric, or dumbbell shaped (endoenteric and exoenteric) in position. It is usually a low-grade malignancy, and histologically it may be very difficult to differentiate from a benign leiomyoma (▸ Fig. 23.8). Hematogenous spread results in

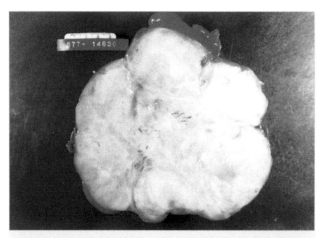

Fig. 23.7 Macroscopic appearance of a transected leiomyosarcoma of the descending colon.

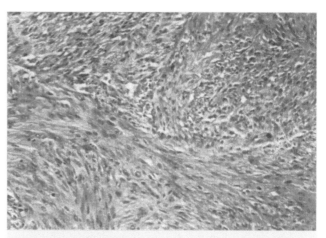

Fig. 23.8 Microscopic features of the leiomyosarcoma shown in ▸ Fig. 23.7. Relatively well-differentiated cells may be difficult to distinguish from those of a benign leiomyoma. (This image is provided courtesy of L.R. Bégin, MD, Montreal, Canada.)

metastases to the liver and the lung.[37] Regional lymph nodes are rarely involved. Early diagnosis is seldom accomplished before complications such as bleeding or obstruction occur.[37] Symptoms are similar to those of carcinoma: changes in bowel habit, rectal bleeding, passage of mucus, and, in the more advanced stage, weight loss. If the lesion is causing obstructive symptoms, abdominal pain may occur either as an ache or cramping. Rarely will an abdominal mass be palpable. Barium enema reveals a polypoid or constricting lesion that is usually indistinguishable from carcinoma. Colonoscopy and biopsy may be helpful if they are performed preoperatively. The treatment is resection as performed for carcinoma, and, in fact, the diagnosis will probably be made only after histologic examination of the resected specimen. Curative resection has been reported in 45% of patients.[38] The 5-year survival rates are meaningless because of the paucity of cases. Pulmonary and hepatic metastases may occur many years later. The prognosis depends on the Broders grade, with grades 1 and 2 representing better prognoses than grades 3 and 4.[39,40] Shiu et al[36] noted that endoenteric lesions carried a good prognosis and that exoenteric neoplasms invaded adjacent structures or perforated into the peritoneal cavity. Three clinicopathologic factors adversely affect prognosis: (1) lesions > 5 cm in diameter, (2) extraintestinal invasion or perforation, and (3) high histopathologic grade of malignancy. Patients rarely survive 5 years after operation and almost two-thirds die within 1 year.[39] Radiation or chemotherapy, alone or in combination, have not been found to be effective.[40]

For the most part, the other sarcomas in this group are pathologic curiosities, and their symptomatology and management are similar to those of leiomyosarcoma. For example, a primary osteosarcoma arising in the colon has been reported.[41] The ultimate diagnosis of these conditions is probably also made from the resected specimen.[42]

23.4 Squamous Cell Carcinoma

Primary squamous cell carcinoma of the large intestine is another exceedingly uncommon neoplasm. It is estimated that adenosquamous and squamous cell carcinoma of the large intestine comprise 0.05 to 0.10% of all large bowel malignancies.[43] Only 72

cases had been reported in the English-language literature until 1992.[43] Subsequently, DiSario et al[44] reported another 75 cases. In their review of the literature, Michelassi et al[45] found synchronous squamous cell carcinoma of the colon present in 3.2% of the collected cases; 10% had either antecedent, synchronous, or metachronous adenocarcinoma of the colon. The reported age range was 32 to 91 years. Mixed adenosquamous cell carcinoma occurs in men and women with equal frequency, but there are twice as many men in the squamous cell group. It has been suggested that a number of criteria must be satisfied before a diagnosis of primary squamous cell carcinoma of the large bowel is entertained[46]: (1) there must be no evidence in any other organ of a squamous cell carcinoma that might spread directly into the lower bowel or provide a source of intestinal metastases, (2) the affected bowel should not be involved in a fistulous tract lined with squamous cells (colocutaneous fistulas have been described in association with squamous cell carcinoma), and (3) when squamous cell carcinoma occurs in the rectum, care must be taken to exclude origin from the anal canal (i.e., there should be a lack of continuity between the lesion and the anal canal epithelium).

Several mechanisms that have been proposed for the pathogenesis of this entity were reviewed by Vezeridis et al.[47] They include (1) proliferation of uncommitted reserve or basal cells following mucosal injury, (2) squamous metaplasia of glandular epithelium, resulting from chronic irritation, (3) origin from embryonal nests of committed or uncommitted ectodermal cells remaining in an ectopic site after embryogenesis, (4) squamous metaplasia of an established colorectal adenocarcinoma, and (5) squamous differentiation arising in an adenoma. Associated conditions that have been described include ulcerative colitis, irradiated bowel, chronic colocutaneous fistulas, schistosomiasis, and colonic duplication.[45] Symptoms, investigations, and assessment are similar to those of colon carcinoma. Lesions are distributed throughout the large bowel with 25 to 50% of all reported cases located in the rectum.[43] Coexistent disease has been reported—schistosomiasis, ulcerative colitis, colonic duplication, amebiasis, ovarian carcinoma previously treated with radiation, prostatic carcinoma, and ovarian teratoma. Macroscopic features may not be dissimilar

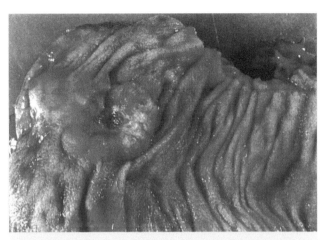

Fig. 23.9 Example of a squamous cell carcinoma of the large bowel, showing features similar to those of an adenocarcinoma.

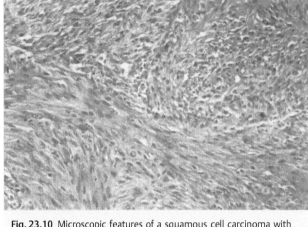

Fig. 23.10 Microscopic features of a squamous cell carcinoma with clusters of squamous cells in the stroma.

to those of adenocarcinoma (▶ Fig. 23.9). Microscopic features are demonstrated in ▶ Fig. 23.10. Of the cases in the literature, approximately half were pure squamous cell carcinoma, and the other half were mixed adenosquamous cell carcinoma. Treatment consists of resection of the affected segment. For rectal lesions, it has been suggested that multimodality therapy, as described by Nigro, be the first line of treatment and that only when this therapy fails should extensive operative procedures be used.[46] Conversely, the Nigro protocol may be used as adjuvant therapy. The 5-year survival rate was 50% for patients with Dukes' B lesions and 33% for those with Dukes' C lesions; no patients with metastatic disease survived.[45,47,48]

23.5 Adenosquamous Carcinoma

This malignancy contains both adenocarcinomatous and squamous carcinomatous elements that are separate although contiguous, thus making a distinction from the common squamous metaplasia in an adenocarcinoma. It may be found in all parts of the large bowel but mostly in the right colon and rectum. They are very aggressive neoplasms that may have a worse prognosis than the more common form of colonic adenocarcinoma. Furthermore, the squamous component, in particular, may have a greater potential for metastasizing and can do so as an undifferentiated-appearing carcinoma.[49] Frizelle et al[50] searched the Mayo Clinic Tissue Registry for all primary cases of squamous and adenosquamous carcinoma of the colon and rectum. Cases were divided into pure squamous cell carcinoma ($n = 11$), mixed adenosquamous carcinoma ($n = 31$), and adenocarcinoma with benign-appearing squamous metaplasia (adenoacanthoma; $n = 2$). Right-sided lesions were the most common (43%). Metastatic disease was evident at presentation in 49% of patients, the most common sites in order being liver, peritoneal, and lung. The 5-year overall survival was 34%, stage I to III disease had a 65% 5-year survival rate, and stage IV mean survival time was 8.5 months. For node-positive and node-negative diseases, 23 and 85%, respectively, survived 5 years.

23.6 Plasmacytoma

Primary plasmacytoma involving the colon is an exceedingly rare lesion.[30,51] Presenting symptoms are nonspecific for gastrointestinal disease and may include abdominal pain, rectal bleeding, weight loss, nausea, vomiting, and anorexia. The lesion may be single or multiple and consists of polypoid or nodular protrusions. In the presence of intestinal involvement, appropriate scans and bone marrow biopsy should be obtained to rule out bone and marrow involvement. Microscopically, the plasmacytoma lesion is composed of many plasma cells. In most cases, treatment has consisted of resection of the involved colon. An 80% 10-year survival can be expected.[7] However, if the diagnosis can be made by colonoscopic biopsy, treatment options include chemotherapy and radiotherapy.[52]

23.7 Melanoma

Primary melanoma of the colon is a distinctly uncommon entity. Indeed, since melanoblasts are necessary for the development of melanoma and since they are found in tissues of ectodermal origin (not in the large intestine above the mucocutaneous junction), it is questionable whether primary intestinal melanoma occurs at all. When the colon is involved, the disease is usually metastatic in origin.

Tessier et al[53] conducted a review of the literature in which they identified 88 cases of metastatic melanoma to the colon to which they added 24 patients. The mean age of their patients was 63.9 years. The interval time between diagnosis of the primary and metastatic disease to the colon was 7.5 years. Presenting symptoms included bleeding (51%), obstruction (29%), pain (20%), weight loss (11%), and perforation (7%). The frequency of these symptoms is comparable to those in the literature. Colonoscopy was the most commonly used diagnostic test (58%), followed by exploratory laparotomy (25%), autopsy (8%), and barium enema (8%). Resection was performed in 61% of patients with 39% having positive lymph nodes. The 1-year survival rate was 60% and the 5-year survival rate was 33%.

Much of the following information has been obtained from the review by Tessier et al.[53] Radiologic studies of the gastrointestinal tract have shown a wide variation of abnormalities with the small intestine having the most diverse findings. A "bull's eye" or "target" sign on barium studies is a well-described finding in the small intestine, stomach, and duodenum. Findings of colonic involvement on barium studies may include multiple submucosal nodules, intussusception, large ulcerative lesions, and extrinsic masses compressing the colon. Macroscopically, the lesions are characteristically mucosal or submucosal, may be polypoid or infiltrative, single or multiple, and melanotic or amelanotic.

On endoscopic examination, these lesions may appear amelanotic but may have enough pigmentation to be easily recognizable on gross or microscopic examination. Intussusception of the colon, multiple colonic polyps, and fungating masses resembling colon carcinoma have been described on endoscopy. Colonoscopy not only is the most reliable study, but also offers the benefit of obtaining tissue for diagnosis. Special stains such as nuclear S100 and cytoplasmic HMB-45 may be necessary to secure the diagnosis.

There has been much debate as to the benefit of operation in patients with metastatic disease to the gastrointestinal tract from malignancy. Resection was performed in 75% of patients in the series of Tessier et al[53] and in 61% of patients from historic data. The average time until death after operation was 27.5 months. Nonoperative candidates died within 7.8 months after diagnosis. Patients with negative nodes had an average survival of 34.7 months, whereas those with positive nodes lived an average of 20.4 months. In their group, 87.5% of patients had another organ involved at the time of presentation, highlighting the rarity of isolated colonic metastases. From the literature review, the long-term survival for isolated colonic metastases was 58.7 months. It would appear, therefore, that resection of isolated metastases to the colon is beneficial and negative nodal status is indicative of a favorable prognosis. Over 90% of patients who underwent operative resection of gastrointestinal metastases have also reported improvement in their symptoms, further supporting a role for operative intervention in symptomatic patients. In the series of Tessier et al,[53] patients presenting with obstruction or perforation had a dismal prognosis with no patient surviving longer than 10 months.

23.8 Leukemic Infiltration

Although a solid neoplasm is not involved in leukemia of the colon, it might be appropriate to include this disease in this section. The following account draws heavily from the work of Moir et al.[54] The underlying pathology of leukemia of the colon is a neutropenic enterocolitis with primarily cecal involvement (typhlitis). The edema and hemorrhagic infarction may be seen elsewhere in the gastrointestinal tract. Neutropenic enterocolitis occurs particularly in patients with acute myelogenous leukemia undergoing high-dose cytosine arabinoside chemotherapy, but it is also seen in patients with other hematologic disorders.[55]

Four pathophysiologic mechanisms have been proposed: (1) enteric vascular ischemia caused by stasis or shock contributes to mucosal ulceration and subsequent invasion by pathogens, (2) mucosal necrosis caused by intramural neoplastic infiltrate alone or in combination with necrosis induced by chemotherapy allows entry of organisms into the bowel wall, (3) bleeding into the mucosa or submucosa secondary to thrombocytopenia causes mucosal disruption and subsequent invasion by colonic flora, and (4) focal fecal ulceration provides entry for pathogens.[56]

The clinical triad is comprised of neutropenia, sepsis, and abdominal pain.[57] The onset, which is heralded by prodromal fever, watery or bloody diarrhea, and abdominal distention, occurs during the phase of severe neutropenia. Symptoms may localize in the right lower quadrant with an associated increase in systemic toxicity. The diagnosis can be confirmed by several re-examinations, abdominal radiographs (showing partial small bowel obstruction, thickened and irregular mucosal folds, and air within the bowel wall), ultrasonography, or radionucleotide scans (gallium- or indium-labeled white blood cells). CT findings include an edematous cecum and/or right colon, spiculation, and inflammation of the pericolic fat, and pneumatosis—all thought to be pathognomonic for neutropenic typhlitis.[57]

The mainstay of management is complete bowel rest with total parenteral nutrition, nasogastric suction, broad-spectrum antibiotics, and avoidance of laxatives or antidiarrheal agents. Granulocyte support may be helpful. Patients with a history of typhlitis should have prophylactic bowel rest and total parenteral nutrition instituted at the beginning of further chemotherapy. Patients with ongoing severe systemic sepsis who do not respond to chemotherapy and those with overt perforation, obstruction, massive hemorrhage, or abscess formation will require operative intervention. All necrotic material must be resected, usually by right hemicolectomy, ileostomy, and mucous fistula. Depending on the extent of bowel involvement, a more extensive resection may be required. Anastomosis is not advised. To prevent recurrence, elective right hemicolectomy has been suggested if additional courses of chemotherapy are required.[57]

23.9 Neuroendocrine Lesions of the Colorectum

In their review of the subject, Vilor et al[58] noted that neuroendocrine proliferations have been classified into three types: benign (glicentin, PP- or peptide YY-producing carcinoid), low-grade malignant (serotonin-producing carcinoid), and high-grade malignant (neuroendocrine carcinoma). Neuroendocrine carcinomas have further been subdivided into the oat cell type and intermediate cell type. The incidence of neuroendocrine carcinomas is less than 0.1% of all malignancies at this site. Thomas and Sobin[59] noted that only 38 of 108,303 colonic and 18 of 46,618 rectal malignancies were small cell carcinomas. The preferred sites of occurrence are the cecum and rectum.[60] Microscopically, neuroendocrine neoplasms are recognized by their characteristically cytologic appearance with lack of tubule formation and submucosal growth pattern. They are argyrophilic and diffusely immunoreactive for neuron-specific enolase and synaptophysin. Most reported cases show metastases to the lymph nodes or distant organs at the time of diagnosis. Only approximately 10% of patients survive 1 year.

Bernick et al[61] identified 38 patients with neuroendocrine carcinomas from a database comprising 6,495 patients (0.6%). These endocrine carcinomas did not include carcinoids. Average patient age was 57 years: 44.7% males and 55.3% females. Locations of the carcinomas were as follows: 17 colon, 14 rectum, 6 anal canal, and

1 appendix. Pathology was reviewed and carcinomas were categorized as small cell carcinomas ($n = 22$) or large cell neuroendocrine carcinoma ($n = 16$). Eighty percent stained positive by means of immunohistochemistry for neuroendocrine markers, including chromogranin, synaptophysin, and/or neuron-specific enolase. Metastatic disease was detected at the time of diagnosis in 69.4% of patients. As a group, these carcinomas had a poor prognosis with a mean survival of 10.4 months. One-, 2-, and 3-year survivals were 46, 26, and 13%, respectively. There was no significant difference in survival based on pathological subtypes. Median follow-up time was 9.4 months.

23.10 Medullary Carcinoma of the Colon

Wick et al[62] studied 68 sporadic colorectal carcinomas with medullary features and compared them with 35 poorly differentiated purely "enteric" colorectal carcinomas and 15 purely neuroendocrine carcinomas of grades II and III, all in patients lacking a family history of colorectal carcinoma. Medullary carcinomas were significantly more common in the ascending colon than were enteric carcinomas, but there was no significant dissimilarity to neuroendocrine carcinomas. Purely enteric carcinomas occurred more often in the rectosigmoid than medullary carcinomas or neuroendocrine carcinomas. Medullary carcinomas arose in older patients, and a marked sex difference also was noted. Despite an infiltrative growth pattern, medullary carcinoma was less likely than enteric carcinomas to manifest with stage III or IV disease, but there was no stage-related difference from neuroendocrine carcinomas. Although the histologic images of medullary carcinomas were evocative of neuroendocrine differentiation, chromogranin positivity and synaptophysin reactivity in that group did not differ meaningfully from enteric colorectal carcinomas but was dissimilar to the 100% labeling of neuroendocrine carcinomas. p53 immunolabeling was similar in the three groups of carcinomas. Follow-up data in the study cases showed that 5-year mortality was 40% for medullary carcinomas, 59% for enteric carcinomas, and 93% for neuroendocrine carcinomas. Medullary colorectal carcinoma seems to be a distinct clinicopathologic variant of colorectal carcinoma, which does not have a neuroendocrine lineage. The biologic behavior of medullary carcinoma was better than that for enteric carcinomas or neuroendocrine carcinomas.

23.11 Carcinosarcoma

A unique case of carcinosarcoma of the colon has been reported.[63] It invaded the bowel wall deeply, metastasized widely, resisted multi-agent chemotherapy, and caused the patient's death 4 years later. It was composed of adenosquamous carcinoma admixed with sarcoma showing osseous, cartilaginous, and nonspecific spindle-cell differentiation.

23.12 Schwannoma

Schwannomas of the colon and rectum are uncommon. Miettinen et al[64] identified 20 colorectal schwannomas from the files of the Armed Forces Institute of Pathology. The schwannomas occurred equally in men and women in a wide age range (18–87 years). The most common location was cecum, followed by sigmoid and rectosigmoid, transverse colon, descending colon, and rectum. The lesions commonly presented as polypoid intraluminal protrusions often with mucosal ulceration. Rectal bleeding, colonic obstruction, and abdominal pain were the most common presenting symptoms. The most common histologic variant ($n = 15$) was a spindle-cell schwannoma with a trabecular pattern and vague or no Verocay bodies. These neoplasms ranged from 0.5 to 5.5 cm in diameter. A lymphoid cuff with germinal centers typically surrounded these lesions and focal nuclear atypia was often present, but mitotic activity never exceeded 5 per 50 HPF. All lesions were strongly positive for S100 protein and negative for CD117 (KIT), neurofilament proteins, smooth muscle actin, and desmin. Colorectal schwannomas behaved in a benign fashion with no evidence of aggressive behavior or connection with neurofibromatosis 1 or 2, based on follow-up information on 18 patients.

23.13 Angiosarcoma

Colorectal sarcomas are rare, accounting for less than 0.001% of all colorectal malignancies. Brown et al[65] recently reviewed the literature on the subject and the following information has been extracted from that review. Thirteen cases of colonic angiosarcoma have been reported in the literature. The majority (61%) of the patients were females. The locations of the sarcoma were as follows: sigmoid ($n = 5$), cecum ($n = 4$), rectum ($n = 2$), descending colon ($n = 1$), and multiple colonic sites ($n = 1$). Most patients presented with rectal bleeding ($n = 7$), abdominal pain ($n = 6$), abdominal mass ($n = 5$), and/or weight loss ($n = 3$). Although chronic lymphedema, radiation, thorium dioxide (Thorotrast) exposure, and a number of syndromes have been cited as risk factors for angiosarcoma, none of these were noted in the cases of colonic angiosarcoma reported in the literature. The presence of a foreign body, a predisposing factor noted in other cases of angiosarcoma, was seen in only one patient with colonic angiosarcoma who had a surgical sponge left in the abdomen after previous operation.

The histomorphology revealed dissecting, atypical vascular channels with plump and layered endothelial cells and areas of solid and spindled cells with an infiltrative and destructive growth pattern typical of angiosarcoma. The differential diagnosis would include sarcomatoid carcinoma, metastatic melanoma, and other sarcomas. Size has been shown to be an independent prognostic factor in angiosarcoma. In this series, five of six patients with a colonic angiosarcoma less than 5 cm in largest diameter were alive at last follow-up (13–24 months postoperatively). Conversely, only one of six patients with a colonic angiosarcoma sized 25 cm was alive at last follow-up.

Patient age ranged from 16 to 77 years. Six of seven patients older than age 60 years had rapid progression of their disease leading to death, whereas four of six patients younger than 60 years were still alive at the last reported follow-up (13–36 months postoperatively).

A review of the literature on colorectal angiosarcoma revealed that surgical excision is the only management shown to result in long-term survival. All survivors had surgical resection of the lesion and none received adjuvant radiotherapy or chemotherapy for the primary lesion. The patient with the longest recorded survival is a 16-year-old female who had multiple peritoneal metastases at the time of her original operation. Despite incomplete resection of the lesion and no adjuvant therapy, the patient was alive and well at 36 months follow-up. These early findings suggest that the patient's age at the time of diagnosis may influence the prognosis of the disease.

With so few reported cases of angiosarcoma of the colon and rectum, the role of adjuvant therapy is unclear. Generally, there seems to be little or no survival benefit with adjuvant chemotherapy in the treatment of sarcoma, and limited experience in angiosarcoma has shown similarly disappointing results. However, doxorubicin-based regimens have shown response rates of 25% in subset analysis of a randomized controlled trial of chemotherapy in sarcoma. The role of adjuvant radiotherapy is unclear.

23.14 Choriocarcinoma

Primary choriocarcinoma of the colon is a very rare neoplasm with only seven reported cases in the world literature, all but two of which were associated with an adjacent adenocarcinoma.[66] This has led to the suggestion that colonic choriocarcinomas may arise from the more typical adenocarcinoma, a process of further dedifferentiation. The overall poor prognosis may reflect the late diagnosis and the high volume of metastatic disease.

23.14.1 Metastases from Other Sources

Patients who present with a suspected colonic neoplasm and a past history of another malignancy should be considered to have possible metastatic disease, especially if the constriction appears extramucosal and the lesion is at the splenic flexure. If the colonic lesion is a squamous carcinoma, an extracolonic source should be sought because primary squamous cell carcinoma of the colon is extremely rare. Metastases from carcinoma of the lung[67] or breast[68,69] presenting as primary colonic neoplasms have been reported. In a review of the literature, Washington and McDonagh[70] found the most common sources of metastases to the colon and rectum to be melanoma, lung, and breast. From their own series of surgical autopsy specimens, the authors added gynecologic, bladder, prostate, and pancreas. Survival after the development of gastrointestinal involvement is generally poor, with most patients surviving less than 1 year. However, long-term palliation may be achieved in a small subset of patients, chiefly with single small bowel deposits of melanoma or those with breast carcinoma responsive to tamoxifen.

For patients with locally advanced ovarian carcinoma with contiguous extension to or encasement of the reproductive organs, pelvic peritoneum, cul de sac, and sigmoid colon, Bristow et al[71,72] reported on 31 consecutive patients undergoing radical oophorectomy and en bloc rectosigmoid colectomy with primary stapled anastomosis. All patients had advanced stage epithelial ovarian carcinoma: International Federation of Gynecology and Obstetrics (FIGO) stage III B (6.5%), stage III C (64.5%), and stage IV (29%). There was one anastomotic breakdown requiring reoperation and colostomy. Complete clearance of macroscopic pelvic disease was achieved in all cases. Overall, 87.1% of patients were left with optimal (≤ 1 cm) residual disease and 61.3% were visibly disease free. There were no postoperative deaths, but major and minor postoperative morbidity occurred in 12.9 and 35.5% of patients, respectively. They concluded that resection of locally advanced ovarian carcinoma significantly contributes to a maximal cytoreductive effort.

References

[1] Nakano PH, Bloom RR, Brown BC, Gray SW, Skandalakis JE, Kibbe JM. Apudomas. Am Surg. 1987; 53(9):505–509

[2] Stinner B, Kisker O, Zielke A, Rothmund M. Surgical management for carcinoid tumors of small bowel, appendix, colon, and rectum. World J Surg. 1996; 20(2):183–188

[3] Spread C, Berkel H, Jewell L, Jenkins H, Yakimets W. Colon carcinoid tumors. A population-based study. Dis Colon Rectum. 1994; 37(5):482–491

[4] Ballantyne GH, Savoca PE, Flannery JT, Ahlman MH, Modlin IM. Incidence and mortality of carcinoids of the colon. Data from the Connecticut Tumor Registry. Cancer. 1992; 69(10):2400–2405

[5] Godwin JD, II. Carcinoid tumors. An analysis of 2,837 cases. Cancer. 1975; 36 (2):560–569

[6] Rosenberg JM, Welch JP. Carcinoid tumors of the colon. A study of 72 patients. Am J Surg. 1985; 149(6):775–779

[7] Walker MJ. Rare tumours of the colon and rectum. In: Nelson RL, ed. Problems in Current Surgery: Controversies in Colon Cancer. Philadelphia, PA: JB Lippincott; 1987:141–153

[8] Gerstle JT, Kauffman GL, Jr, Koltun WA. The incidence, management, and outcome of patients with gastrointestinal carcinoids and second primary malignancies. J Am Coll Surg. 1995; 180(4):427–432

[9] Tichansky DS, Cagir B, Borrazzo E, et al. Risk of second cancers in patients with colorectal carcinoids. Dis Colon Rectum. 2002; 45(1):91–97

[10] Duh QY, Hybarger CP, Geist R, et al. Carcinoids associated with multiple endocrine neoplasia syndromes. Am J Surg. 1987; 154(1):142–148

[11] Berardi RS. Carcinoid tumors of the colon (exclusive of the rectum): review of the literature. Dis Colon Rectum. 1972; 15(5):383–391

[12] Jolles PR. Rectal carcinoid metastatic to the skeleton. Scintigraphic and radiographic correlation. Clin Nucl Med. 1994; 19(2):108–111

[13] Johnson LA, Lavin P, Moertel CG, et al. Carcinoids: the association of histologic growth pattern and survival. Cancer. 1983; 51(5):882–889

[14] Wallace S, Ajani JA, Charnsangavej C, et al. Carcinoid tumors: imaging procedures and interventional radiology. World J Surg. 1996; 20(2):147–156

[15] Kwekkeboom DJ, Krenning EP. Somatostatin receptor scintigraphy in patients with carcinoid tumors. World J Surg. 1996; 20(2):157–161

[16] Woods HF, Bax NDS, Smith JAR. Small bowel carcinoid tumors. World J Surg. 1985; 9(6):921–929

[17] Creutzfeldt W. Carcinoid tumors: development of our knowledge. World J Surg. 1996; 20(2):126–131

[18] Bowman GA, Rosenthal D. Carcinoid tumors of the appendix. Am J Surg. 1983; 146(6):700–703

[19] Gouzi JL, Laigneau P, Delalande JP, et al. The French Associations for Surgical Research. Indications for right hemicolectomy in carcinoid tumors of the appendix. Surg Gynecol Obstet. 1993; 176(6):543–547

[20] Ahlman H, Westberg G, Wängberg B, et al. Treatment of liver metastases of carcinoid tumors. World J Surg. 1996; 20(2):196–202

[21] Beaton H, Homan W, Dineen P. Gastrointestinal carcinoids and the malignant carcinoid syndrome. Surg Gynecol Obstet. 1981; 152(3):268–272

[22] Azizkhan RG, Tegtmeyer CJ, Wanebo HJ. Malignant rectal carcinoid: a sequential multidisciplinary approach for successful treatment of hepatic metastases. Am J Surg. 1985; 149(2):210–214

[23] Vinik A, Moattari AR. Use of somatostatin analog in management of carcinoid syndrome. Dig Dis Sci. 1989; 34(3) Suppl:14S–27S

[24] Henry CA, Berry RE. Primary lymphoma of the large intestine. Am Surg. 1988; 54(5):262–266

[25] Jinnai D, Iwasa Z, Watanuki T. Malignant lymphoma of the large intestine-operative results in Japan. Jpn J Surg. 1983; 13(4):331–336

[26] Pandey M, Kothari KC, Wadhwa MK, Patel HP, Patel SM, Patel DD. Primary malignant large bowel lymphoma. Am Surg. 2002; 68(2):121–126

[27] Zighelboim J, Larson MV. Primary colonic lymphoma. Clinical presentation, histopathologic features, and outcome with combination chemotherapy. J Clin Gastroenterol. 1994; 18(4):291–297

[28] Zinzani PL, Magagnoli M, Pagliani G, et al. Primary intestinal lymphoma: clinical and therapeutic features of 32 patients. Haematologica. 1997; 82(3):305–308

[29] Dawson IMP, Cornes JS, Morson BC. Primary malignant lymphoid tumours of the intestinal tract. Report of 37 cases with a study of factors influencing prognosis. Br J Surg. 1961; 49:80–89

[30] Sidani MS, Campos MM, Joseph JI. Primary plasmacytomas of the colon. Dis Colon Rectum. 1983; 26(3):182–187

[31] Contreary K, Nance FC, Becker WF. Primary lymphoma of the gastrointestinal tract. Ann Surg. 1980; 191(5):593–598

[32] Bruneton JN, Thyss A, Bourry J, Bidoli R, Schneider M. Colonic and rectal lymphomas. A report of six cases and review of the literature. RoFo Fortschr Geb Rontgenstr Nuklearmed. 1983; 138(3):283–287

[33] Doolabh N, Anthony T, Simmang C, et al. Primary colonic lymphoma. J Surg Oncol. 2000; 74(4):257–262

[34] Fan CW, Changchien CR, Wang JY, et al. Primary colorectal lymphoma. Dis Colon Rectum. 2000; 43(9):1277–1282

[35] Suzuki A, Fukuda S, Tomita S, et al. An unusual case of colonic leiomyosarcoma presenting with fever–significant uptake of radioactivity of gallium-67 in the tumor. Gastroenterol Jpn. 1984; 19(5):486–492

[36] Shiu MH, Farr GH, Egeli RA, Quan SH, Hajdu SI. Myosarcomas of the small and large intestine: a clinicopathologic study. J Surg Oncol. 1983; 24(1):67–72

[37] Stavorovsky M, Jaffa AJ, Papo J, Baratz M. Leiomyosarcoma of the colon and rectum. Dis Colon Rectum. 1980; 23(4):249–254

[38] Akwari OE, Dozois RR, Weiland LH, Beahrs OH. Leiomyosarcoma of the small and large bowel. Cancer. 1978; 42(3):1375–1384

[39] Berkley KM. Leiomyosarcoma of the large intestine, excluding the rectum. Int Surg. 1981; 66(2):177–179

[40] Nuessle WR, Magill TR, III. Leiomyosarcoma of the transverse colon. Report of a case with discussion. Dis Colon Rectum. 1990; 33(4):323–326

[41] Shimazu K, Funata N, Yamamoto Y, Mori T. Primary osteosarcoma arising in the colon: report of a case. Dis Colon Rectum. 2001; 44(9):1367–1370

[42] Smith JA, Bhathal PS, Cuthbertson AM. Angiosarcoma of the colon. Report of a case with long-term survival. Dis Colon Rectum. 1990; 33(4):330–333

[43] Schneider TA, II, Birkett DH, Vernava AM, III. Primary adenosquamous and squamous cell carcinoma of the colon and rectum. Int J Colorectal Dis. 1992; 7(3):144–147

[44] DiSario JA, Burt RW, Kendrick ML, McWhorter WP. Colorectal cancers of rare histologic types compared with adenocarcinomas. Dis Colon Rectum. 1994; 37(12):1277–1280

[45] Michelassi F, Mishlove LA, Stipa F, Block GE. Squamous-cell carcinoma of the colon. Experience at the University of Chicago, review of the literature, report of two cases. Dis Colon Rectum. 1988; 31(3):228–235

[46] Lafreniere R, Ketcham AS. Primary squamous carcinoma of the rectum. Report of a case and review of the literature. Dis Colon Rectum. 1985; 28(12):967–972

[47] Vezeridis MP, Herrera LO, Lopez GE, Ledesma EJ, Mittleman A. Squamous-cell carcinoma of the colon and rectum. Dis Colon Rectum. 1983; 26(3):188–191

[48] Juturi JV, Francis B, Koontz PW, Wilkes JD. Squamous-cell carcinoma of the colon responsive to chemotherapy. Dis Colon Rectum. 1999; 42:102–109

[49] Cerezo L, Alvarez M, Edwards O, Price G. Adenosquamous carcinoma of the colon. Dis Colon Rectum. 1985; 28(8):597–603

[50] Frizelle FA, Hobday KS, Batts KP, Nelson H. Adenosquamous and squamous carcinoma of the colon and upper rectum: a clinical and histopathologic study. Dis Colon Rectum. 2001; 44(3):341–346

[51] Lattuneddu A, Farneti F, Lucci E, Garcea D, Ronconi S, Saragoni L. A case of primary extramedullary plasmacytoma of the colon. Int J Colorectal Dis. 2004; 19(3):289–291

[52] Sperling RI, Fromowitz FB, Castellano TJ. Anaplastic solitary extramedullary plasmacytoma of the cecum. Report of a case confirmed by immunoperoxidase staining. Dis Colon Rectum. 1987; 30(11):894–898

[53] Tessier DJ, McConnell EJ, Young-Fadok T, Wolff BG. Melanoma metastatic to the colon: case series and review of the literature with outcome analysis. Dis Colon Rectum. 2003; 46(4):441–447

[54] Moir CR, Scudamore CH, Benny WB. Typhlitis: selective surgical management. Am J Surg. 1986; 151(5):563–566

[55] Taylor AJ, Dodds WJ, Gonyo JE, Komorowski RA. Typhlitis in adults. Gastrointest Radiol. 1985; 10(4):363–369

[56] McClenathan JH. Metastatic melanoma involving the colon. Report of a case. Dis Colon Rectum. 1989; 32(1):70–72

[57] Keidan RD, Fanning J, Gatenby RA, Weese JL. Recurrent typhlitis. A disease resulting from aggressive chemotherapy. Dis Colon Rectum. 1989; 32(3):206–209

[58] Vilor M, Tsutsumi Y, Osamura RY, et al. Small cell neuroendocrine carcinoma of the rectum. Pathol Int. 1995; 45(8):605–609

[59] Thomas RM, Sobin LH. Gastrointestinal cancer. Cancer. 1995; 75(1) Suppl:154–170

[60] Saclarides TJ, Szeluga D, Staren ED. Neuroendocrine cancers of the colon and rectum. Results of a ten-year experience. Dis Colon Rectum. 1994; 37(7):635–642

[61] Bernick PE, Klimstra DS, Shia J, et al. Neuroendocrine carcinomas of the colon and rectum. Dis Colon Rectum. 2004; 47(2):163–169

[62] Wick MR, Vitsky JL, Ritter JH, Swanson PE, Mills SE. Sporadic medullary carcinoma of the colon: a clinicopathologic comparison with nonhereditary poorly differentiated enteric-type adenocarcinoma and neuroendocrine colorectal carcinoma. Am J Clin Pathol. 2005; 123(1):56–65

[63] Weidner N, Zekan P. Carcinosarcoma of the colon. Report of a unique case with light and immunohistochemical studies. Cancer. 1986; 58(5):1126–1130

[64] Miettinen M, Shekitka KM, Sobin LH. Schwannomas in the colon and rectum: a clinicopathologic and immunohistochemical study of 20 cases. Am J Surg Pathol. 2001; 25(7):846–855

[65] Brown CJ, Falck VG, MacLean A. Angiosarcoma of the colon and rectum: report of a case and review of the literature. Dis Colon Rectum. 2004; 47(12):2202–2207

[66] Le DT, Austin RC, Payne SN, Dworkin MJ, Chappell ME. Choriocarcinoma of the colon: report of a case and review of the literature. Dis Colon Rectum. 2003; 46(2):264–266

[67] Carr CS, Boulos PB. Two cases of solitary metastases from carcinoma of the lung presenting as primary colonic tumours. Br J Surg. 1996; 83(5):647

[68] Voravud N, el-Naggar AK, Balch CM, Theriault RL. Metastatic lobular breast carcinoma simulating primary colon cancer. Am J Clin Oncol. 1992; 15(4):365–369

[69] Law WL, Chu KW. Scirrhous colonic metastasis from ductal carcinoma of the breast: report of a case. Dis Colon Rectum. 2003; 46(10):1424–1427

[70] Washington K, McDonagh D. Secondary tumors of the gastrointestinal tract: surgical pathologic findings and comparison with autopsy survey. Mod Pathol. 1995; 8(4):427–433

[71] Bristow RE, del Carmen MG, Kaufman HS, Montz FJ. Radical oophorectomy with primary stapled colorectal anastomosis for resection of locally advanced epithelial ovarian cancer. J Am Coll Surg. 2003; 197(4):565–574

[72] Olson RM, Perencevich NP, Malcolm AW, Chaffey JT, Wilson RE. Patterns of recurrence following curative resection of adenocarcinoma of the colon and rectum. Cancer. 1980; 45(12):2969–2974

24 Rectal Adenocarcinoma

John R.T. Monson, Lawrence Lee, and Steven D. Wexner

Abstract

Modern care of the patient with rectal carcinoma is multidisciplinary and requires close cooperation of surgery, medical and radiation oncology, radiology, and pathology specialties. Accurate locoregional staging will influence the decision to administer neoadjuvant therapies. Preoperative chemoradiation will decrease the local recurrence rates for locally advanced rectal cancer by 50%. High-quality surgery according to total mesorectal excision principles remains essential for curative resection, as is specialized pathologic evaluation of the surgical specimen. Newer organ-preserving modalities further contribute to the treatment armamentarium. Adjuvant therapy is controversial but remains the standard of care. Patients should further be followed after definitive management according to established surveillance protocols to identify local and distant recurrences. Optimization of outcomes for patients with rectal carcinoma is dependent on adherence to these principles of high-quality evidence-based care.

Keywords: rectal cancer, total mesorectal excision, adjuvant therapy, surveillance, local recurrence, distal recurrence, evidence-based care, multidisciplinary care, locoregional staging

24.1 Introduction

Cancers arising in the rectum (i.e., the distal 15 cm of the large bowel) share many of the same genetic and pathologic characteristics of cancer originating in the more proximal colon, but the anatomic constraints of the bony pelvis along with the proximity to other urogenital structures, anal sphincters, and autonomic nerves create significant issues for surgical access. As a result, rectal cancer outcomes have been historically worse than those of colon cancers. Rectal cancer surgery has evolved from perineal (Jacques Lisfranc)[1] and posterior (Paul Kraske)[2] approaches in the 1800s to the introduction of the abdominoperineal excision by Sir Ernest Miles in 1908[3] and the sphincter-preserving anterior resection by Dixon in 1948.[4] However, local recurrence rates and survival remained poor until the introduction of the total mesorectal excision (TME) concept, which emphasizes dissection along the avascular "holy plane" and en bloc removal of the rectum and its encompassing mesorectum, by R.J. Heald in 1982.[5] Local recurrence rates further improved when the benefits of neoadjuvant (chemo)radiation were demonstrated by the German Rectal Cancer Study[6] and the Swedish Rectal Cancer Trial.[7] The introduction of minimally invasive techniques and organ preservation has further added to the treatment armamentarium. The management of rectal cancer has become truly multidisciplinary with optimal management dependent on medical and radiation oncologists, radiologists, pathologists, and surgeons.

24.2 Epidemiology and Presentation

Colorectal cancer is common, with an estimated 1.4 million new cases worldwide including 693,900 deaths.[8] Incidence rates are highest in North America, Europe, Oceania, and Japan, but are increasing in many countries in which rates are historically low.[9] The reasons for this increase in countries in Latin America, Asia, and Eastern Europe are thought to be changing dietary and activity patterns, and increase in smoking prevalence.[10,11,12] In the United States, it is estimated that 134,500 new colorectal cancer cases are diagnosed annually, including 39,220 rectal cancers.[13] While still among the highest in the world, the incidence rate in the United States and Western Europe is starting to decrease, likely as a result of screening and removal of precancerous lesions.[14,15] However, the incidence of colorectal cancer in patients younger than 50 years is increasing at a rate of 2.1% per year from 1992 to 2012, for whom average-risk screening is not recommended. Young-onset colorectal cancer is more likely to be left sided or rectal, poorly differentiated, have mucinous or signet-ring cell histology, and present at advanced stages.[16,17] The large majority of these patients were symptomatic with rectal bleeding (50–60%), abdominal pain (30–60%), or change in bowel habits (20–70%),[16,17,18] which likely prompted further evaluation given that screening of asymptomatic average-risk individuals in this age group is not standard of care. However, stage-specific survival in young-onset colorectal cancer is similar to cancers occurring in older individuals.[19] The molecular genetics of colorectal cancer are covered in detail elsewhere and will not be discussed in this chapter.

Patients with colorectal cancer can present in three ways: asymptomatic individuals in whom the tumor is detected on routine screening; evaluation after worrisome symptoms; or emergently with perforation, obstruction, or life-threatening bleeding. However, 80 to 90% of colorectal cancers are detected after evaluation for symptoms—most commonly rectal bleeding, abdominal pain, and change in bowel habits.[20,21] In contrast, emergent presentation occurs in approximately 5 to 10% of patients, usually as a result of obstruction.[22] Despite the increase in screening programs, 20 to 30% of patients with newly diagnosed colorectal cancer will not have previously undergone a screening colonoscopy.[20,21,22] Furthermore, approximately 20% of patients will have stage IV disease at presentation, most commonly to the liver, lungs, or peritoneum as a result of hematogenous spread. The liver is usually the initial site of metastasis due to the portal venous drainage of the large bowel. However, tumors in the distal rectum often develop pulmonary metastases first because the inferior rectal vein drains directly into the vena cava instead of the portal vein.

24.3 Preoperative Evaluation

Once the diagnosis of rectal cancer is made, the patient must undergo complete evaluation prior to initiation of any treatment (▶ Table 24.1).[23] A comprehensive history and physical examination should be performed to assess for associated signs and symptoms. The history should include any current comorbidities that might affect perioperative management, previous surgical history, and complete family history. Concerning cancer-specific history may include significant weight loss, extensive bleeding per rectum, tenesmus, pain with defecation, and obstructive symptoms. The presence of any of these symptoms should alert the clinician to more advanced disease. In particular, tenesmus, the sensation of incomplete evacuation or constant feeling of needing to evacuate, is suggestive of a large and potentially fixed tumor. Pain with defecation may suggest lower tumors with possible sphincter involvement, as rectal cancer above the anorectal junction is typically painless unless there is invasion of surrounding structures. Pretreatment history should also include sphincter and urinary function, as well as sexual function in males, as these may be affected by neoadjuvant and/or surgical therapy. Perioperative cardiac risk assessment should be performed according to the American College of Cardiology/American Heart Association guidelines.[24] The patient should also be specifically questioned about functional capacity by determining if they can climb two flights of stairs without shortness of breath. This activity represents a functional capacity of at least four metabolic equivalents (METs). Physical examination should assess for any previous abdominal incisions that might affect potential surgical approach. A digital rectal examination (DRE) must be performed to assess for sphincter involvement. Palpable low rectal tumors should also be evaluated if they are mobile and soft, or hard and fixed. For lesions that are not palpable, the surgeon should also perform a rigid proctoscopy to determine the distal extent of the tumor. Patients should undergo a full colonoscopy if not already done to rule out synchronous lesions, which are found in approximately 3 to 5% of patients from population-based studies.[25,26]

Table 24.1 Full preoperative evaluation for patients with rectal adenocarcinoma

Baseline

- History and physical examination including digital rectal examination
- Colonoscopy to rule out synchronous lesions
- Rigid proctoscopy to assess tumor height and location within bowel lumen
- Carcinoembryonic antigen
  - Other routine laboratory tests are not indicated

Imaging

- Computed tomography (CT) scans of the chest, abdomen, and pelvis
- Pelvic MRI
- Endorectal ultrasound
  - Positron emission tomography CT is not routinely indicated

Preoperative planning

- Presentation at multidisciplinary tumor board for consideration of neoadjuvant therapy
  - Pathology review
  - Radiology review

A carcinoembryonic antigen (CEA) level should be obtained for every patient before surgery. It must be noted that the purpose of the CEA is not for screening or diagnosis. A meta-analysis of the diagnostic characteristics of CEA for colorectal cancer reported a pooled sensitivity of 46% (95% confidence interval [CI]: 0.45–0.47) and specificity of 89% (95% CI: 0.88–0.92).[27,28] Other etiologies for an elevated CEA include gastritis, peptic ulcer disease, diverticulitis, liver disease, chronic obstructive pulmonary disease, diabetes, and other acute inflammatory states. CEA may also be falsely elevated in smokers.[29] Several surgical and medical oncology societies have recommended against the use of tumor markers, including CEA, as a screening or diagnostic test.[30,31] CEA does have utility as a prognostic tool, as well as for surgical planning and posttreatment surveillance, and therefore a baseline measurement should be obtained prior to any treatment. Patients with preoperative serum CEA ≥ 5 ng/mL have worse prognosis, stage for stage, than patients with serum CEA < 5 ng/mL.[31,32,33,34] Furthermore, normalization of CEA in patients with an elevated serum CEA who are undergoing neoadjuvant therapy is a strong predictor of complete pathologic response.[35,36,37] Elevated CEA levels that do not normalize after curative resection should raise the suspicion of residual disease and should prompt further evaluation. Likewise, patients with rising CEA levels after curative resection should undergo systemic imaging to rule out local and/or distant recurrence. Routine laboratory tests other than a CEA are not necessary. Transaminases are neither sensitive nor specific for liver metastases.

Staging is performed according to the American Joint Commission on Cancer 7th edition TNM classification (▶ Table 24.2 and ▶ Table 24.3). Computed tomography (CT) scans of the

Table 24.2 Staging groups (AJCC 7th edition)

Primary tumor (T)

TX: tumor cannot be assessed
T0: no evidence of primary tumor
Tis: carcinoma in situ (intramucosal)
T1: invasion into submucosa
T2: invasion into muscularis propria
T3: invasion through muscularis propria into pericolorectal tissues
T4a: tumor penetrates to the surface of the visceral peritoneum
T4b: tumor directly invades or is adherent to other organs or structures

Regional lymph nodes (N)

NX: regional lymph nodes cannot be assessed
N0: no regional lymph node metastases
N1: metastases in 1–3 regional lymph nodes
N1a: metastasis in 1 regional lymph node
N1b: metastases in 2–3 regional lymph nodes
N1c: tumor deposits in the subserosa, mesentery, or nonperitonealized pericolic or perirectal tissues without regional lymph node metastases
N2: metastases in 4 or more regional lymph nodes
N2a: metastases in 4–6 regional lymph nodes
N2b: metastases in 7 or more regional lymph nodes

Distant metastasis (M)

M0: no distant metastasis
M1: distant metastasis
M1a: metastasis confined to 1 organ or site (e.g., lung, liver, or nonregional lymph node)
M1b: metastases to more than 1 organ and/or peritoneum

Source: © 2010 American Joint Committee on Cancer

Table 24.3 AJCC 7th edition staging groups

Stage	T	N	M
0	Tis	N0	M0
I	T1	N0	M0
	T2	N0	M0
IIa	T3	N0	M0
IIb	T4a	N0	M0
IIc	T4b	N0	M0
IIIa	T1–T2	N1/N1c	M0
	T1	N2a	M0
IIIb	T3–T4a	N1/N1c	M0
	T2–T3	N2a	M0
	T1–T2	N2b	M0
IIIc	T4a	N2a	M0
	T3–T4a	N2b	M0
	T4b	N1–N2	M0
IVa	Any T	Any N	M1a
IVb	Any T	Any N	M1b

Source: © 2010 American Joint Committee on Cancer

chest, abdomen, and pelvis are required to rule out concurrent distant metastases. CT scans of the abdomen and pelvis may show tumor-related complications such as perforation, obstruction, or clear invasion into surrounding organs, or distant metastases or lymphatic involvement. It must be noted that CT scan has limited sensitivity for low-volume lesions (especially under 0.5–1.0 cm). According to one study, only 11% of nodules less than 0.5 cm were seen on CT scan, and only 37% of lesions between 0.5 and 1.0 cm were seen.[38,39] An extremely elevated CEA in the absence of metastatic disease apparent on CT imaging should alert the clinician about the possibility of peritoneal carcinomatosis. In these cases, a positron emission tomography (PET) scan may be useful.[27,28] Even if the PET scan is normal, visual and/or manual inspection of the peritoneal cavity at the beginning of a curative-intent procedure is imperative to rule out synchronous metastatic disease prior to undergoing proctectomy. Routine CT imaging of the chest is controversial, as the incidence of indeterminate lesions is high, but these nodules are often benign; however, numerous groups include this as the optimal imaging choice; for example, in the United States both National Comprehensive Cancer Network (NCCN) and the American College of Surgeons Commission on Cancer (ACS CoC) National Accreditation program for Rectal Cancer (NAPRC) recommend CT rather than plain chest X-ray.

In theory, venous drainage of lower rectal cancers directly enters into the vena cava circulation, and bypassing the liver, through the hemorrhoidal veins. In one systematic review of 12 studies including 5,873 patients, 9% had indeterminate pulmonary nodules on preoperative chest CT, but only 11% of these lesions (~1% of the total population) declared themselves to be colorectal metastases during surveillance.[40] Given the low incidence of malignancy in these indeterminate pulmonary nodules, further preoperative evaluation can be avoided, and these lesions can be followed during surveillance. If equivocal suspicious findings on CT scan are found, the patient should undergo more specific testing, such as liver magnetic resonance imaging

(MRI). The additional imaging techniques should be not routinely performed in the absence of other findings on CT scan as they are not generally useful and add unnecessary costs and burden for the patient.

A PET scan need not be routinely ordered if the patient has no evidence of metastatic disease on staging CT scans. A PET scan may be useful in the setting of resectable liver metastases to detect any extrahepatic disease that may render the patient not a candidate for curative resection, or in the situations with an elevated CEA but no metastatic disease on CT imaging.

24.3.1 Local Staging

The two imaging modalities that are the most useful for local staging of rectal adenocarcinoma are transrectal ultrasound (TRUS) and MRI. Both modalities are more accurate than CT for assessing the depth of tumor invasion, nodal staging, and assessment of the circumferential resection margin (CRM). CT of the pelvis can define tumor invasion into surrounding structures for larger tumors, but does not adequately assess depth of invasion for smaller tumors.[41,42,43,44] CT also does not accurately diagnose malignant perirectal adenopathy, with a sensitivity of only 49%.[45] The utility of preoperative CT is to detect tumor-related complications such as perforation, malignant fistula, or obstruction.

Transrectal Ultrasound

TRUS can differentiate between the specific layers of the rectal wall and other surrounding anatomic structures, especially those situated anteriorly, based on their different acoustic impedances (▶ Fig. 24.1). The 10-mHz crystal is most commonly used for rectal cancer staging, and has a resolution of 0.4 mm and focal range of 1.5 to 4 cm. The anal sphincter complex is especially well visualized on TRUS, but the distal most length of rectum at the anorectal junction is difficult to assess by TRUS. The optimal image requires that the transducer probe be situated in the middle of the rectum with good opposition of the rectal wall with the water-filled balloon. Tumors appear as extensions of the first hypoechoic wall. Ultrasound T-staging is based on tumor disruption of the different echographic layers of the rectal wall. The entire length of the tumor needs to be imaged as the depth of invasion is not uniform. This may cause the patient significant discomfort for tumors that are large, bulky, or near obstructing. Metastatic lymph nodes appear as hypoechoic deposits usually at the level of or proximal to the tumor, are round rather than oval, and have ill-defined borders. However, small tumor deposits may not sufficiently alter the echogenic profile of the lymph node to be detected by TRUS. As such, TRUS is technically difficult and operator dependent.

Prior to the widespread use of MRI, TRUS was considered the gold standard for locoregional staging of rectal cancer. Early studies found high diagnostic accuracy for TRUS. In a systematic review of studies published before 1993, the overall accuracy of endorectal ultrasound (ERUS) for T-staging was 84%, with 97% sensitivity and 87% specificity.[46] In particular, ERUS was highly accurate in differentiating between T1/T2 and T3 and greater, which had important management implications as T3 and above tumors should undergo neoadjuvant chemotherapy, whereas T1/T2 tumors can undergo upfront resection (in the

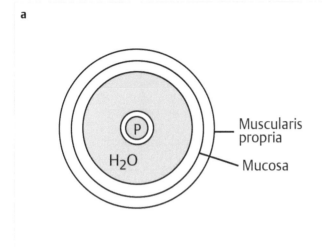
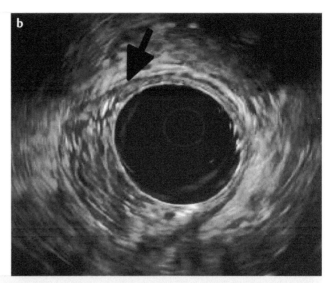

Fig. 24.1 **(a)** Five ultrasonographic layers of rectum. Layers of rectal wall are seen as rings, which represent interfaces between tissues of different density. Critical ring is outer dark ring, which represents muscularis propria. Penetration of this ring by carcinoma denotes cT3 and above. **(b)** EUS appearance of a cT3 tumor. The black arrow points to the muscularis propria, which is breached by the tumor and is not readily apparent where the tumor is located. EUS, endorectal ultrasound.

absence of nodal metastases). However, later studies have shown TRUS to be less accurate than previously reported. In one of the largest studies on the use of TRUS for locoregional rectal cancer staging, 7,096 patients underwent TRUS followed by surgical resection without neoadjuvant therapy.[47] The overall concordance between clinical stage as reported by TRUS and final pathologic staging was only 64.7% (95% CI: 63.6–65.8). Tumors were overstaged in 17.3%, and understaged in 18%. The accuracy of TRUS varied significantly based on T-stage, with highest clinical–pathological concordance for TRUS-staged T1 tumors (kappa = 0.591) and lowest for T4 tumors (kappa = 0.321). Hospitals that performed over 30 TRUS per year had the highest diagnostic accuracy (73.1%; 95% CI: 69.4–76.5), whereas hospitals with less than 10 TRUS per year reported a diagnostic accuracy of only 63.2% (95% CI: 61.5–64.9). Another study of 545 patients reported the overall accuracy of TRUS for T-staging to be 69%, and 64% for N-staging.[48] Tumors were more often overstaged (18%) than understaged (13%). Other more recent studies report that TRUS is less reliable in differentiating between early T3 with minimal extramural spread and more advanced T3 tumors, as well as differentiating between T2 and early T3.[48,49] This disadvantage is particularly relevant as it may over- or undertreat a significant proportion of patients with rectal cancer under evaluation for neoadjuvant therapies. These results suggest that TRUS may be an accurate diagnostic modality to diagnose earlier stage tumors if local expertise is available.

The diagnostic accuracy of TRUS for nodal staging (70–75%) is similar to that of CT (55–65%) and MRI (60–65%).[50,51] A meta-analysis of 35 studies including 2,732 patients reported the pooled sensitivity and specificity of TRUS for nodal staging to be 73.2% (95% CI: 70.6–75.6) and 75.8% (95% CI: 73.5–78.0), respectively.[52] The additional value of fine-needle aspiration (FNA) to TRUS for the evaluation of nodal status is equivocal.[53] Perirectal nodes are typically too small to be visualized by TRUS unless they contain metastatic deposits, at which point they can be detected by visual morphology alone and do not require

FNA biopsy confirmation. However, assessment of lymph nodes outside of the focal range of the TRUS probe, such as the lateral pelvic nodes, is lacking.

TRUS is also limited for the assessment of the mesorectal fascia, which has therapeutic and prognostic importance. Anteriorly, TRUS can detect CRM involvement at the level of the seminal vesicles, prostate, and vagina based on the close proximity of these structures to the rectal wall. Posteriorly, TRUS cannot assess the CRM based on the lack of adjacent structures. In these cases, MRI offers a clear advantage over TRUS.

Magnetic Resonance Imaging

Pelvic or rectal MRI has replaced EUS as the local staging modality. MRI offers excellent resolution and assessment of the tissues and anatomic structures of the pelvis and has replaced ERUS as the imaging modality of choice for most expert groups and authorities (▶ Fig. 24.2). Its specific advantage over other imaging options includes the ability to predict involvement of the CRM and to visualize extramural vascular invasion (EMVI).

Rectal MRI is typically performed on a 1.5- or 3-T MRI scanner. Endorectal surface coils can be used, but are very uncomfortable for the patient, and the development of high-resolution surface coils has also led to the reduction in their use. Specific rectal cancer protocols with multiplanar T2-weighted images including axial, coronal, sagittal, oblique axial, and oblique coronal view with or without multiaxial diffusion-weighted imaging should be used. The examination is performed with the patient supine. The rectum should be cleansed with enemas to decrease image misinterpretation caused by stool. Several different rectal solutions can be administered to provide a negative contrast against the rectal wall. The radiologist should be provided with tumor-specific information such as the estimated height and dimensions of the tumor, as well as any previous pelvic surgeries.

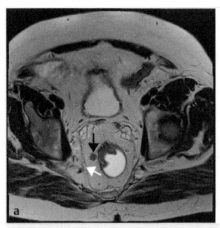 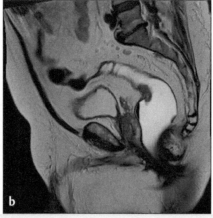 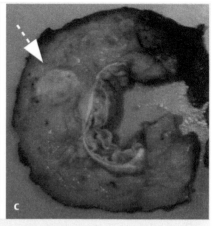

Fig. 24.2 MRI scan of a cT3N1 tumor. **(a)** Axial image with black arrow showing an enlarged lymph node in the mesorectum, and the white arrow the mesorectal fascia, which is not threated by the tumor. **(b)** Sagittal image of a cT3N1 tumor located in the midrectum. **(c)** Gross pathology of the resected specimen. White dotted arrow points to the lymph node seen on MRI in **(a)**. MRI, magnetic resonance imaging.

MRI may have difficulty in differentiating between the mucosa and the submucosa, as they appear as a single inner hyperintense layer on T2-weighted imaging. The muscularis propria is an intermediate hypointense layer, and the mesorectal fat appears hyperintense. The mesorectal fascia can also be clearly seen as a thin hypointense layer surrounding the mesorectal fat. Rectal tumors appear as intermediate signal intensity lesions between the high signal intensity of fat and low intensity of muscle on T2-weighted imaging and demonstrate enhancement after contrast administration. MRI has difficulty in distinguishing between early T1/T2 tumors and they are often combined together as tumors confined to the bowel wall. Invasion into the perirectal fat can be clearly seen on thin section MRIs and is crucial in differentiating between T2 and T3 tumors. The extent of extramural spread measured by MRI is highly accurate when measured against final pathology, and can be used to determine the need for neoadjuvant therapies for select T3 tumors.[54] Metastatic nodes appear as nodular structures in the mesorectum at the level of or slightly proximal to the tumor. They can also be seen along the internal iliac or superior rectal vessels. Nodes smaller than 3 mm are not well visualized on MRI, but can still harbor malignancy.[55] Lymph nodes are considered metastatic if they are larger than 5 mm in shortest axis, those with spiculated or irregular borders, or have a mottled appearance.[56,57] Enlarged nodes in the mesorectum in the context of rectal cancer are usually considered malignant, but nodes can be reactive to rectal manipulation such as biopsy and tattooing during endoscopy. Administration of newer contrast agents[58,59] or diffusion weighted imaging[60] can also be used to diagnose metastatic nodes, but these techniques are still considered experimental and are not yet widely used. MRI can also detect extramural vascular invasion, which appears as tumor deposits spreading directly off the tumor along lateral rectal vessels, which also has prognostic implications.[61,62]

The accuracy of MRI for locoregional staging has been addressed in a meta-analysis of 21 studies that used histopathologic analysis as the reference.[63] In this study, the sensitivity and specificity of MRI to detect T3/T4 over T1/T2 was 87% (95% CI: 81–92) and 75% (95% CI: 65–80), nodal metastases 77% (95% CI: 69–84) and 71% (95% CI: 59–81), and involved CRM 77%

(95% CI: 57–90) and 94% (95% CI: 88–97), respectively. However, the authors noted that there was significant heterogeneity among the studies in terms of the definition of a positive lymph node or an involved CRM.

The role of MRI in the locoregional staging of rectal cancer has evolved significantly over the past decade. The Magnetic Resonance Imaging in Rectal Cancer European Equivalence (MERCURY) study group has contributed important data that have shifted the modality of choice from TRUS to MRI. There are several major advantages of MRI over TRUS that make it the preferred imaging modality for the locoregional staging of rectal cancer, especially when neoadjuvant therapy is under consideration. While sensitivity and specificity of the two modalities for T- and nodal-staging are roughly equal, MRI can accurately predict involvement of the CRM as well as the depth of extramural invasion for cT3 tumors. These two findings will subsequently dictate further neoadjuvant management. Improvements in technology will allow for better resolution and enhanced accuracy of MRI staging.

Several studies have shown that depth of extramural invasion has important prognostic implications. Patients with invasion greater than 5 mm have worse cancer-specific survival compared to patients with less than 5 mm invasion (54 vs. 85% at 5 years; p < 0.001).[64,65] Increased depth of invasion is also associated with an increased risk of nodal metastases.[66] These findings suggest that the importance of distinguishing between T1/T2 and T3 tumors is less essential than identifying T3 tumors with greater than 5-mm invasion into the perirectal fat. The MERCURY study group showed that thin-slice MRI can reliably identify the depth of invasion for patients with T3 tumors within 0.5 mm of the final histopathological result.[54] MRI can also identify patients with high risk for positive CRM in which a part of the tumor of a metastatic deposit or lymph node is less than 1 mm from mesorectal fascia before neoadjuvant therapy[67] after surgical resection with 94% accuracy.[68] MRI-involved CRM also predicted local recurrence, disease-free, and overall survival.[69] The utility of MRI assessment of extramural depth of invasion, CRM status, and extramural vascular invasion was demonstrated in a study in which patients were divided into "good prognosis" and "bad prognosis." Patients with "good prognosis" tumors had T1/T2 or T3 disease with safe CRM (tumor > 1 mm from mesorectal fascia), no evidence of extramural vascular invasion, and extramural depth of invasion less than 5 mm on preoperative MRI. None of these patients received pre- or postoperative radiotherapy and all underwent TME proctectomy. Local recurrence rate for these patients was 3% with 85% disease-free and 68% overall survival at 5 years. These findings suggest that MRI can be used to detect tumors that would traditionally undergo neoadjuvant chemoradiation that could undergo upfront resection with good outcomes. However, this approach is not yet standard of care.

Imaging after Neoadjuvant Chemoradiation

Certain patients may benefit from restaging after completion of neoadjuvant chemoradiation. MRI and TRUS can be used to assess response to neoadjuvant therapy, but their accuracy is poor as both have difficulty in differentiating between residual tumor and radiation-induced edema, inflammation, or fibrosis. Restaging will be discussed later in this chapter. A systematic review of 30 studies reporting on the accuracy of restaging MRI and TRUS after neoadjuvant chemoradiation published up to 2011 demonstrated that both modalities have poor accuracy for T-stage (65%, 95% CI: 56–72 for TRUS; 52%, 95% CI: 44–59% for MRI) and N-stage (both modalities had 72% accuracy).[70] MRI was able to accurately predict CRM involvement after neoadjuvant therapy. Given these data, restaging with MRI and TRUS remains difficult, and neither of these studies should be used as the sole method to assess tumor (complete) response. Newer MRI technologies such as diffusion-weighted imaging or dynamic contrast-enhanced MRI may potentially increase the ability to accurately assess tumor response by directly measuring local microcirculation and cellular environment.[71] These techniques are still limited to large specialty centers and have not been disseminated into smaller practices. PET scan may also be able to detect pathologic response, although the data are conflicting.[72,73]

24.3.2 Multidisciplinary Tumor Board

All patients with rectal cancer should be discussed upon presentation to the institution at a multidisciplinary tumor board conference.[74] These conferences should consist of a panel of surgeons, radiologists, pathologists, medical oncologists, and radiation oncologists that are specialized in the care of patients with rectal cancer. Management decisions to proceed with neoadjuvant therapy, upfront surgery, or other strategies are decided on using a consensus multidisciplinary team approach. Previous studies have demonstrated that the multidisciplinary approach improves decision making, clinical, outcomes, and patient experience for patients with a variety of cancers.[75,76,77,78] Specifically for rectal cancer, the implementation of multidisciplinary tumor boards was associated with lower incidences of permanent stoma and local recurrence, improved delivery of evidence-based care, and, most importantly, better overall survival.[79,80] The importance of the multidisciplinary tumor board in the management of patients with rectal cancer is such that it is included among the core components of the American College of Surgeons (ACS) Commission on Cancer (CoC) National Accreditation Program for Rectal Cancer (NAPRC).[81,82]

It is the goal of the NAPRC to provide standards for multidisciplinary management to improve the quality and delivery of care for patients with rectal adenocarcinoma.[81] Outcomes in the United States are highly variable. While it is difficult to study variability in more exact measures of outcome such as local recurrence rates and survival, colostomy rates are felt to be an appropriate metric of decreased surgical quality in rectal cancer.[83] As of 2007, 60% of patients undergoing proctectomy for rectal cancer received a permanent colostomy.[84] Two studies by Ricciardi et al[84,85] demonstrate that rates of permanent colostomy are highly variable and excessive. County-level data from 21 U.S. states revealed that 40% of surgeons performed only abdominoperineal resection (APR) for their patients with rectal cancer,[85] while a study of greater than 7,500 proctectomies from 11 states found that half of all patients received a permanent colostomy.[86] A recent study of over 47,000 patients using data from the Nationwide Inpatient Sample found that colostomy rates had decreased in the United States from 65% in 1988 to 40% in 2006. However, there was marked variability between high- and low-volume hospitals (colostomy rates 44 vs. 57%, respectively) and even the lowest colostomy rate reported was still far in excess of what would be considered acceptable in European countries where quality improvement programs have been successfully implemented.[83]

This variability between high- and low-volume centers also extends to delivery of neoadjuvant care, as well as other surgical quality measures. Analysis of the National Cancer Database (NCDB) demonstrated that a higher proportion of rectal cancer patients received evidence-based neoadjuvant therapy in high-volume (more than 30 rectal resections per year) compared to low-volume centers.[87] The inverse relationship was also true, in that patients were more likely to receive adjuvant chemoradiotherapy at low-volume centers. Hodgson et al[88] also reported that low-volume hospitals had higher permanent colostomy and 30-day mortality and lower 2-year survival compared to hospitals in the higher quartiles of volume, using the California Cancer Registry. These and other studies were included in a Cochrane meta-analysis, which demonstrated that higher hospital volume was significantly associated with improved 5-year survival.[89]

24.4 Neoadjuvant Therapy

24.4.1 Indications

The use of neoadjuvant therapy has led to a significant reduction in local recurrence rates for patients with resectable adenocarcinoma of the rectum. Traditionally, patients underwent upfront surgical resection, followed by chemoradiotherapy in the adjuvant setting for patients with advanced tumors, positive margins, and/or node-positive disease. The treatment paradigm has drastically changed since the late 1990s and early 2000s when several seminal trials demonstrated significantly improved outcomes for preoperative treatment. At present, the current standard of care for neoadjuvant therapy includes long-course chemoradiation, usually with 50.4 Gy delivered in 28 fractions with concurrent fluoropyrimidine-based radio-sensitizing chemotherapy and surgery after 6 to 8 weeks, or short-course preoperative radiotherapy delivered as 25 Gy in 5 fractions over 1 week, followed by surgery within a week of completion of therapy. The current accepted indications for neoadjuvant chemoradiotherapy are provided in ▶ Table 24.4.

24.4.2 Overview of Neoadjuvant Strategies

The best regimen for neoadjuvant therapy has not been determined, with significant variability internationally. In the United States, long-course chemoradiation is the favored approach for any patient with an indication for neoadjuvant therapy, whereas in Europe, short-course radiotherapy is preferred. What is clear from the data is that both neoadjuvant long-course chemoradiation and short-course radiotherapy reduce the risk of local recurrence by approximately 50% without major differences in disease-free and overall survival, especially in patients undergoing proctectomy according to TME principles. One potential benefit of long-course chemoradiation is the potential for significant tumor regression with 10 to 15% incidence of complete pathologic response, which may favorably impact prognosis. An overview of the seminal randomized controlled trials that have influenced current neoadjuvant management will be reviewed below.

Preoperative versus Postoperative Chemoradiotherapy

Several randomized trials have compared the use of chemoradiation in the preoperative versus postoperative setting and

Table 24.4 Indications for neoadjuvant chemoradiotherapy in patients with rectal cancer

Standard of care indications for neoadjuvant radiation with or without concomitant chemotherapy

- T3–T4, any N (short-course radiotherapy is not recommended for T4b tumors)
- Any T, N1–N2
- Tumors in the lower third of the rectum in which sphincter-saving surgery may not be possible without tumor regression
- Tumor invasion into sphincter complex (long-course chemoradiation recommended)
- Threatened (within 1–2 mm) or involved mesorectal fascia

have generally demonstrated a 50% risk reduction in local recurrence in favor of preoperative therapy (▶ Table 24.5). Long-course chemoradiation has been largely based on a study by the German Rectal Cancer Study Group in which 823 patients with clinical T3/T4 or node-positive tumors were randomized to either neoadjuvant or adjuvant chemoradiation.[6] The preoperative group received 50.4 Gy delivered in 28 fractions over 5 weeks with a 5-day continuous infusion of fluorouracil (5-FU) during the first and fifth weeks, followed by surgery with TME technique 6 weeks after completion of chemoradiation. The postoperative group received the same regimen in the adjuvant setting with an additional 5.4-Gy boost to the tumor bed. Both groups received additional four cycles of bolus 5-FU (4 weeks after surgery in the preoperative group, and 4 weeks after completion of chemoradiation in the postoperative group). The 5-year local recurrence rate was 6% in the preoperative group versus 13% in the postoperative group ($p = 0.006$), but no difference in 5-year disease-free (68 vs. 65%) or overall survival (76 vs. 74%). Long-term follow-up data from this trial demonstrated a persistent benefit in the reduction of local recurrence (7 vs. 10%; $p = 0.048$) but again with no differences in disease-free (70 vs. 70%) or overall (60 vs. 60%) survival.[90] Preoperative therapy did improve sphincter preservation in the subset of patients thought to require APR ($n = 194$) before treatment (39 vs. 20%; $p = 0.004$). Complete clinical response was seen in 8% overall in the preoperative group. There were no differences in postoperative morbidity between the two groups.

The National Surgical Adjuvant Breast and Bowel Project (NSABP) R-03 trial randomly assigned 267 patients with clinical T3/T4 or node-positive tumors to a similar protocol as the German Rectal Cancer Study Group, but without mandatory TME surgery.[91] In this study, there were no differences in 5-year local recurrence rates (11% in both arms) and overall survival (75 vs. 66%; $p = 0.065$) between preoperative and postoperative groups despite a 16.5% incidence of complete pathologic response in patients receiving preoperative chemoradiation. However, an improvement in disease-free survival was seen in the preoperative

Table 24.5 Randomized controlled trials comparing preoperative and postoperative chemoradiation for rectal cancer

	German trial[6]		NSABP R-03[91]		Korean trial[92]	
	Preoperative	Postoperative	Preoperative	Postoperative	Preoperative	Postoperative
Regimen	CRT 50.4 Gy[a]	CRT 55.8 Gy[a]	CRT 50.4 Gy[a]	CRT 50.4 Gy[a]	CRT 50 Gy[b]	CRT 50 Gy[b]
Number of patients	421	402	130	137	107	113
TME surgery	Yes		No		Yes	
Sphincter-saving resection	69%	71%	48%	39%	68%	42%
Postoperative morbidity	36%	34%	25%	23%	–	–
pCR	8%	0%	15%	0%	17%	0%
5-y local recurrence	6%	13%	11%	11%	5%	6%
5-y DFS	68%	65%	65%	53%	73%	74%
5-y OS	76%	74%	75%	66%	83%	85%

Abbreviations: CRT, chemoradiotherapy; DFS, disease-free survival; OS, overall survival; TME, total mesorectal excision.
[a]Concomitant chemotherapy with infusional 5-FU.
[b]Concomitant chemotherapy with capecitabine.

group (65 vs. 53%; $p = 0.011$). The discrepancy in results between the NSABP R-03 and the German Rectal Cancer Study Group trials may be the lack of uniform TME surgery in the NSABP R-03 study.

A third trial conducted in Korea compared pre- and postoperative chemoradiation with capecitabine as the chemosensitizing agent with pelvic radiotherapy along with surgery according to TME principles for patients with clinical T3/T4 or node-positive tumors.[92] This trial could not demonstrate the benefit of preoperative chemoradiation as the 5-year rates of local recurrence, disease-free, and overall survival were similar between the two groups. Pathologic complete response was seen in 17%. One benefit of neoadjuvant chemoradiation in this study was a higher incidence of sphincter preservation in low-lying tumors (68 vs. 42%).

Preoperative Radiotherapy with or without Concurrent Chemotherapy

Several randomized trials have shown that the addition of concurrent chemotherapy as a radiosensitizing agent decreases local recurrence rates by 50% compared to preoperative radiotherapy alone. The largest study, the European Organization for Research and Treatment of Cancer (EORTC) 22921 trial, used a 2 × 2 factorial design to randomly assign patients with clinical T3/T4 tumors into four groups: preoperative radiotherapy alone (45 Gy over 5 weeks), preoperative chemoradiation (bolus 5-FU/leucovorin [LV] on weeks 1 and 5 of radiotherapy), preoperative radiotherapy and postoperative chemotherapy, and preoperative chemoradiation and postoperative chemotherapy. TME surgery was performed in only 37% of all procedures. Local recurrence was lower in all groups receiving chemotherapy regardless of the timing of administration compared to preoperative radiotherapy alone (17% for preoperative radiotherapy alone, 8.7% for preoperative chemoradiation, 9.6% for preoperative radiotherapy and postoperative chemotherapy, and 7.6% for preoperative chemoradiation and postoperative chemotherapy; $p = 0.002$). However, no survival benefit at 5 years was found between any of the four groups. These results persisted at 10-year follow-up.[93]

The French Fédération Francophone de Canérologie Digestive (FFCD) 9203 trial randomly assigned 742 patients with clinical T3/T4 to a preoperative radiotherapy regimen 45 Gy in 25 fractions with 5-FU/LV during the first and fifth weeks versus radiotherapy alone.[94] Surgery was performed within 3 and 10 weeks after completion of radiotherapy. TME was recommended but not required. Both arms received adjuvant chemotherapy. Local recurrence at 5 years was lower in patients who received chemoradiation (8.1 vs. 16.5%; $p = 0.004$).

Preoperative Short-Course Radiotherapy versus Surgery Alone

The role of preoperative short-course radiotherapy versus surgery alone has been investigated in three randomized trials (▶ Table 24.6). The three trials are consistent in reporting a decrease in local recurrence for patients receiving preoperative radiotherapy versus surgery alone, with a significant effect even in patients undergoing TME surgery. The Swedish Rectal Cancer Trial randomized 1,168 patients with resectable rectal adenocarcinoma to preoperative short-course radiotherapy regimen consisting of 25 Gy delivered in 5 fractions over a 1-week period followed by surgery within 1 week versus surgery alone with no additional radiotherapy.[7] Importantly, surgery was not performed according to TME principles in this trial, and approximately one-third of the included patients were stage I tumors. Patients receiving preoperative radiotherapy experienced a significantly lower local recurrence (11 vs. 27%; $p < 0.001$) and higher overall survival (58 vs. 48%; $p = 0.002$) at 5 years compared to patients in the surgery-only arm. Long-term follow-up data reported the persistent benefits in local control and overall survival after a median of 13-year follow-up.[95] However, this trial must be interpreted with caution, as the surgical technique did not adhere to TME principles, which may explain the 27% local recurrence rate in the surgery-only arm, which is more than double that of the surgery-only arms in the Dutch Colorectal Cancer Group and MRC-CR07 trials that included TME-guided surgery. The 16% difference in local recurrence between the two arms may also explain the survival advantage in the preoperative therapy arm, which again was not seen in the two other trials.

The Dutch Colorectal Cancer Group trial investigated the role of short-course radiotherapy in patients undergoing proctectomy according to TME principles. This trial enrolled 1,861 patients

Table 24.6 Randomized controlled trials comparing preoperative short-course radiotherapy + surgery versus surgery alone

	Swedish trial		Dutch trial		MRC CR-07	
	Preoperative 5 × 5 Gy	Surgery	Preoperative 5 × 5 Gy	Surgery	Preoperative 5 × 5 Gy	Surgery + selective postoperative RTX
Number of patients	583	585	924	937	674	676
TME surgery	No		Yes		Yes	
CRM positive	–	–	16%	16%	10%	12%
Perineal wound complications	20%	10%[a]	26%	18%	35%	22%
5-year local recurrence	11%	27%[a]	5.6%	10.9%[a]	4.7%	11.5%[a]
5-year OS	58%	48%[a]	64.2%	63.5%	70.3%	67.9%

Abbreviations: CRM, circumferential resection margin; OS, overall survival; RTX, radiotherapy; TME, total mesorectal excision.
[a]$p < 0.05$.

to Swedish-style preoperative short-course 5 × 5 Gy radiotherapy and then surgery versus surgery alone. Postoperative therapy was administered to patients with intraoperative tumor spillage or positive margins. Five-year local recurrence was lower in the preoperative therapy arm (5.6 vs. 10.9%; $p < 0.001$), but no differences in overall survival (64.2 vs. 63.5%; $p = 0.902$). Long-term follow-up of this trial demonstrated the improvement in local recurrence rates for the preoperative radiotherapy arm persisted at 10 years (5 vs. 11%; $p < 0.001$). Overall survival was similar between the two arms (48 vs. 49%; $p = 0.20$). Importantly, local recurrence rates were still lower after preoperative radiotherapy in patients with a negative circumferential margin (3 vs. 9%; $p < 0.001$).

The Medical Research Council CR-07/National Cancer Institute of Canada (NCIC) Clinical Trials Group C016 randomly assigned 1,350 patients with operable rectal cancer to preoperative 5 × 5 Gy radiotherapy followed by surgery versus surgery and selective postoperative chemoradiation (45 Gy in 25 fractions with concurrent infusional 5-FU) for positive CRM on pathology. Both groups were administered adjuvant chemotherapy if they had positive CRM and/or positive nodes. There were no differences in the incidence of CRM positivity after surgery between the two arms, but 5-year local recurrence rates were lower in the preoperative radiotherapy arm (4.7 vs. 11.5%; $p < 0.001$). The preoperative radiotherapy arm also had improved disease-free (73.6 vs. 66.7%; $p = 0.013$), but not overall survival (70.3 vs. 67.9%; $p = 0.91$).

Preoperative Short-Course Radiotherapy versus Long-Course Chemoradiation

Several trials have directly compared preoperative short-course radiotherapy to long-course chemoradiation and have not demonstrated an improvement in local recurrence or sphincter preservation for either approach. The Polish Colorectal Study Group randomly assigned 312 patients with clinically accessible T3/T4 tumors to conventional chemoradiation with 50.4 Gy in 28 fractions with bolus 5-FU/LV or short-course radiotherapy with 5 × 5 Gy and surgery within 1 week.[96] All patients underwent TME surgery. This study was powered to detect a 15% difference in sphincter preservation between the two arms, with the decision to perform sphincter preservation at the time of surgery. Compliance was higher and there was less early radiation toxicity in the short-course radiotherapy arm. The incidence of complete response was 16% in the chemoradiation arm compared to 1% in the short-course radiotherapy arm ($p < 0.001$). There were also higher rates of positive CRM in the short-course radiotherapy arm (12.9 vs. 4.4%; $p = 0.017$), but these findings did not translate into higher sphincter preservation (58 vs. 61%; $p = 0.57$), 4-year local recurrence (9 vs. 14%; $p = 0.170$), disease-free survival (55.6 vs. 58.4%; $p = 0.820$), or overall survival (66.2 vs. 67.2%; $p = 0.960$) in the chemoradiation arm.

The Trans-Tasman Radiation Oncology Group 01.04 trial also compared conventional long-course chemoradiation with 50.4 Gy with infusional 5-FU versus short-course radiotherapy with 5 × 5 Gy in a randomized trial of 326 patients with cT3N0–2M0 rectal adenocarcinoma.[97] Similarly to the Polish Colorectal Study Group trial, complete pathologic response was higher in the chemoradiation arm (15 vs. 1%), but there was no difference in the proportion of patients undergoing APR for tumors less than 5 cm from the anal verge (short-course 79 vs. long-course

77%) or margin positivity (5 vs. 4%). At 5-year follow-up, local recurrence rates were similar (5.7 vs. 7.5%; $p = 0.51$), as were disease-free and overall survival, and late complications.

Short-course radiotherapy is generally not recommended for patients with clinical T4 or large bulky tumors since it is not used to induce downsizing or downstaging. However, there have been some data to support the use of consolidation chemotherapy after short-course radiotherapy. One trial randomly assigned 541 patients with clinical T4 or fixed T3 tumors to preoperative short-course radiotherapy followed by 6 cycles of FOLFOX4 (folinic acid, fluorouracil, and oxaliplatin) followed by surgery versus long-course chemoradiation but with the addition of oxaliplatin to bolus 5-FU/LV.[98] In this study, toxicity was lower in the short-course radiotherapy arm but there were similar rates of R0 resection and complete pathologic response. At 3-year follow-up, overall survival was higher in the short-course group. While these results appear promising, the control arm of this study used oxaliplatin along with 5-FU/LV, which has been shown to increase treatment toxicity without any improvement in outcomes compared to conventional 5-FU-based chemotherapy.

Timing of Surgery after Neoadjuvant Therapy

The optimal timing of surgery after completion of neoadjuvant therapy has not yet been determined. Traditionally, this interval was 6 weeks based on the protocol used by the German Rectal Cancer Study Group.[6] However, tumor response to radiotherapy takes time—one study reported that a tumor size of 54 cm³ would require an interval of 20 weeks to regress to less than 0.1 cm³.[99] Pooled results of 13 observational studies including 3,584 patients show that delaying surgery beyond 8 weeks increased the incidence of pathologic complete response by 6% without increasing complications, but with no difference in R0 resections or disease-free or overall survival.[100] Similarly, an analysis of the National Cancer Database reported that an interval greater than 8 weeks was associated with increased pCR (odds ratio [OR]: 1.12; 95% CI: 1.01–1.25) and tumor downstaging (OR: 1.11; 95% CI: 1.02–1.25) compared to 6- to 8-week interval.[101] There have been two randomized trials investigating the timing of surgery after neoadjuvant radiation. The Lyon R90–01 trial compared 2 weeks versus 6 to 8 weeks after long-course radiotherapy and reported a higher pathologic complete response in the longer duration (26 vs. 10%), but with no differences in overall survival.[102] However, this trial used preoperative long-course radiotherapy with 39 Gy in 13 fractions without concurrent chemotherapy rather than conventional chemoradiation, thus limiting the generalizability of these results to standard practice.

The French Research Group of Rectal Cancer Surgery 6 (GREC-CAR-6) trial randomly assigned 265 patients with clinical T3/T4 or node-positive tumors of the mid and low rectum who received conventional neoadjuvant long-course chemoradiation to surgery 7 versus 11 weeks after completion of neoadjuvant therapy.[103] The longer 11-week interval to surgery did not increase the incidence of pathologic complete response (17 vs. 15%; $p = 0.60$), which was the primary endpoint of the study, or sphincter preservation (90 vs. 89%). The 11-week arm also experienced higher postoperative morbidity (44.5 vs. 32%; $p = 0.040$) through higher medical complications (32.8 vs. 19.2%; $p = 0.014$), but similar rates of anastomotic leakage and a trend toward more perineal wound problems after APR and conversion to open surgery. The quality of mesorectal excision was also worse in the 11-week arm (complete mesorectum 78.7 vs. 90%; $p = 0.016$). The authors concluded that waiting 11 weeks for surgical resection after completion of chemoradiation did not confer any benefit over a 7-week interval and increased postoperative morbidity. Many surgeons now wait 10 to 12 weeks following the completion of neoadjuvant chemoradiotherapy.

Alternative Chemotherapeutic Agents during Neoadjuvant Radiotherapy

At the present time, current standard of care for patients undergoing long-course chemoradiation is to deliver infusional 5-FU during neoadjuvant radiotherapy, with capecitabine as an oral alternative for 5-FU. Two trials have compared capecitabine to infusional 5-FU as the radiosensitizing agent during radiotherapy.[104,105] In both trials, locoregional control and overall survival were similar between the two agents, but with different toxicity profiles. These data suggest the equivalency of oral capecitabine and infusional 5-FU during radiotherapy for neoadjuvant therapy.

Oxaliplatin has also been investigated as an addition to 5-FU-based chemotherapy during neoadjuvant radiotherapy in multiple randomized trials with mixed results.[105,106,107,108,109] In all trials, the toxicity profile of oxaliplatin was higher than that of traditional 5-FU-based chemotherapy. Only two trials demonstrated benefit in terms of improved pathologic complete response rates[108,109] and disease-free survival.[108] Given its greater toxicity profile and unclear effectiveness, oxaliplatin should not be routinely administered as part of neoadjuvant chemotherapy during radiotherapy. Irinotecan has also been investigated in the neoadjuvant setting, but its efficacy was not demonstrated in a small trial of 106 patients,[110] although some benefit has been reported in nonrandomized trials.[111,112,113] The addition of bevacizumab or epidermal growth factor inhibitors to traditional 5-FU-based chemoradiotherapy does not have any level I evidence for or against the inclusion of these agents.

Initial Neoadjuvant Chemotherapy Instead of Chemoradiation

While the previously mentioned studies have investigated the addition of different agents to chemotherapy during neoadjuvant radiotherapy, the use of neoadjuvant chemotherapy rather than chemoradiotherapy is under active investigation. As the MERCURY study group has shown, select tumors with favorable characteristics that would otherwise undergo neoadjuvant (chemo)radiotherapy can undergo upfront resection without increased risk of local recurrence or worse survival.[114] Furthermore, modern chemotherapy regimens are effective against rectal cancer and are better tolerated in the preoperative versus postoperative setting. This approach may allow for more selective use of radiotherapy, which would spare the patient from the short- and long-term effects of radiation. A pilot study of 32 patients from Memorial Sloan Kettering Cancer Center prospectively enrolled patients with stage II or III rectal cancer to a preoperative regimen of six cycles of FOLFOX (including four cycles of bevacizumab) followed by restaging. Patients with T4 lesions,

CRM involvement on preoperative MRI, and/or bulky nodal disease were excluded. Patients who demonstrated stable or responsive disease underwent surgery, while those demonstrating progression underwent conventional long-course chemoradiation. All patients in this study were able to achieve R0 resection, including 25% with complete pathologic response. After a median follow-up of 54 months, there were no locoregional recurrences and 4-year disease-free and overall survival were 92 (95% CI: 82.1–100) and 91.6% (84.0–100), respectively. This study formed the basis of the ongoing multi-institutional PROSPECT trial that should further define management for patients with favorable stage II or III tumors. Initial results of the FOWARC trial, which randomly assigned 495 patients with clinical stage II or III rectal cancer to conventional preoperative chemoradiation, preoperative long-course radiotherapy with concurrent FOLFOX, or FOLFOX alone, show that the chemotherapy arm had equal tumor downsizing to the conventional chemoradiation arm but with less toxicity and postoperative complications.[109] Long-term results are still pending. Despite these promising data, patients with T3N0 or T1–3N1 disease should still undergo conventional neoadjuvant chemoradiation unless they cannot or are unwilling to receive pelvic radiation, unless they are part of a clinical trial.

Induction chemotherapy prior to chemoradiation should be considered for patients with locally invasive tumors (T4) or those with bulky nodal disease, At present, current standard of care indicates that patients undergoing neoadjuvant chemoradiation with curative intent should receive adjuvant chemotherapy, but a multicenter study of specialty cancer centers reported that a sizable minority of these patients do not receive adjuvant chemotherapy.[115] Administering systemic therapy in the neoadjuvant setting may lead to higher rates of resectability and pathologic complete response. In addition, neoadjuvant chemotherapy addresses potential systemic disease earlier and in a more effective manner. FOLFOX is generally better tolerated in the neoadjuvant setting and more patients complete the proposed therapy. While there are no randomized trials, several phase II trials report promising results. A study from the United Kingdom prospectively enrolled patients with high-risk criteria on MRI (tumors within 1 mm of the mesorectal fascia, at or below the levators, extending ≥ 5 mm into the perirectal fat, T4, or T1–2N2) into a treatment regimen consisting of 12 weeks of neoadjuvant capecitabine and oxaliplatin, followed by conventional long-course chemoradiation and TME surgery.[116] Radiologic response was seen in 74% after completion of chemotherapy and 89% after chemotherapy and chemoradiation, while 96% of patients who underwent surgery had R0 resection. Disease-free and overall survival at 3 years were 68 and 83%, respectively. A Spanish study randomly assigned 108 patients to induction versus adjuvant chemotherapy with capecitabine/oxaliplatin for patients undergoing preoperative chemoradiation and TME surgery for T3/T4 or node-positive tumors.[117] Patients in the induction arm were better able to tolerate systemic chemotherapy, but no differences in short-term outcomes were found. Despite the lack of randomized data supporting its effectiveness, induction chemotherapy is recognized as an acceptable option according to the NCCN guidelines for patients with an indication for neoadjuvant (chemo)radiation, although it is generally reserved for patients with high-risk tumors in which there is concern of a positive margin, or with bulky nodal disease.

24.4.3 Morbidity of Neoadjuvant Therapy

The benefits of an approximate 50% reduction in local recurrence for both neoadjuvant long-course chemoradiation or short-course radiotherapy and the 10 to 15% pathologic complete response is associated with significant adverse events that result from these therapies.

The EORTC 22921 study demonstrated that the addition of concurrent chemotherapy to a long-course dose of radiotherapy increases the incidence of grade 3 or higher toxicity during neoadjuvant treatment by almost 50% (7.4% for radiotherapy alone vs. 13.9% for chemoradiation; $p < 0.001$).[118] In the Polish Colorectal Study Group trial, patients undergoing long-course chemoradiation had a much higher incidence of grade 3/4 toxicity compared to the short-course radiotherapy arm (18.2 vs. 3.2%; $p < 0.001$),[96] although this was not replicated in the Trans-Tasman trial.[97] The German Rectal Cancer Study Group trial showed no difference in toxicity between pre- and postoperative long-course chemoradiation, although the incidence of anastomotic stenosis was higher in patients receiving postoperative chemoradiation.[6] Because of the lower toxicity profile, compliance is higher for short-course radiotherapy.

However, short-course radiotherapy may have a significant negative impact on postoperative morbidity. In all three trials comparing preoperative short-course radiotherapy versus upfront surgery, the preoperative radiotherapy arm had higher perineal wound complications.[7,119,120] The Stockholm III randomized trial compared preoperative 5 × 5 short-course radiotherapy with a short (1-week) and long (4- to 8-week) interval to surgery and long-course radiotherapy with a long interval to surgery.[121] The incidence of postoperative complications was highest in patients who underwent preoperative 5 × 5 radiotherapy but had surgery 11 to 17 days after radiotherapy (65%). There were no complications between short- and long-course radiotherapy, although the long-course arm did not receive concurrent chemotherapy. The Polish Colorectal Study Group also reported no differences in quality of life as measured by the EORTC QLQ-C30 or sexual dysfunction between long-course chemoradiation and short-course radiotherapy.[122] Preoperative radiotherapy is also associated with significant impairments in anorectal function. Analyses of long-term data from the Swedish Rectal Cancer trial and the Dutch trial reported higher rates of fecal and urinary incontinence and small bowel obstructions in patients who received preoperative radiotherapy versus upfront surgery.[123,124,125] These impairments are likely a result of radiotherapy rather than the mode of delivery (i.e., same long-term effects regardless or short- or long-course regimens).[126] Preoperative radiotherapy does not appear to increase the risk of secondary malignancy.[127] These data underline the importance of accurate staging to avoid overtreatment.

Assessment of Tumor Response after Neoadjuvant Therapy

The benefit of repeating the staging investigations after completion of neoadjuvant therapy and prior to surgery is not clear. Several studies have reported a change in management in up to 15% of patients based on repeat CT, PET, or MRI, mostly based on the interval development of metastatic disease.[128,129,130,131,132] Restaging may also demonstrate significant tumor regression, which has important prognostic implications.[133] The MERCURY study reported that tumor regression grade was significantly associated with both disease-free and overall survival. Those with a good tumor regression grade had better 5-year overall survival compared to those with poor response (72 vs. 27%; $p = 0.001$).[134] The German CAO/ARO/AIO-94 trial also showed that patients with a complete response had a 10-year disease-free survival of 89.5% compared to 73.6% for moderate regression and 63% for poor regression.[135] A retrospective review of 725 patients reported similar findings.[136] While the GREC-CAR-6 study did not demonstrate a difference in pathologic complete response after 11- versus 6-week interval between completion of chemoradiation and surgery, other studies have shown a higher incidence of tumor regression or pathologic complete response with longer interval to surgery.[137,138,139,140] Given these data, it is reasonable to perform repeat DRE, CEA, endoscopy, and MRI to assess tumor response between 4 and 6 weeks after completion of neoadjuvant chemoradiation. Patients who demonstrate evidence of significant tumor regression on repeat staging and who are asymptomatic should be considered for a longer interval to surgery to induce further response, although this should be balanced against the potentially increased risk of postoperative complications.[103,137,140] Patients with minimal to no response should undergo surgery within the usual 6- to 8-week intervals.

24.4.4 Summary of the Decision-Making Process for Preoperative Therapy

Patients with clinical stage I tumors (cT1–2, cN0) have a very low rate of local recurrence if high-quality TME is performed; thus, these patients do not usually require neoadjuvant chemoradiation. Subgroup analyses of the Dutch trial reported a 1.7% 5-year local recurrence for stage I tumors, with no statistically significant reduction in local recurrence with the addition of preoperative short-course radiotherapy. In comparison, 5-year local recurrence for stage I tumors decreased from 15% for surgery alone to 5% for the short-course radiotherapy arm in the original Swedish trial, but this may be reflective of the radiotherapy making up for suboptimal surgery (no TME performed) in this study. However, neoadjuvant therapy should be considered for stage I tumors if the preoperative MRI demonstrates a threatened CRM. This is mainly relevant for low rectal tumors as the mesorectum is significantly thinner at this level. The Norwegian Colorectal Cancer Group demonstrated that T2 tumors with a CRM ≤ 2 mm after resection were at much higher risk of local recurrence versus those with a CRM greater than 2 mm (hazard ratio [HR[: 2.76; 95% CI: 1.05–7.38).[141] Neoadjuvant therapy should also be considered in cases where the tumor encroaches on the sphincter complex. In these cases, neoadjuvant chemoradiation may result in tumor downsizing or also downstaging and allow for a sphincter-preserving procedure where an APR would have been otherwise required.

Neoadjuvant chemoradiation has been traditionally recommended for patients with clinical stage II tumors (cT3–4, N0). Pooled analysis from rectal cancer adjuvant trials (before the

TME era) demonstrates an 84% 5-year overall survival for T3N0 tumors, with a local recurrence rate ranging from 5 to 11% based on the postoperative regimen used.[142] The addition of preoperative radiotherapy was shown to decrease local recurrence in the Swedish[7,95] and CR07[120] trials, but not in the Dutch trial.[119,143] While the results of the Swedish trial may not be generalizable in the TME era, the difference in local recurrence rates in the Dutch and CR07 trials may be attributable to the inclusion of adjuvant chemotherapy in the CR07 trial. However, there is emerging evidence to suggest that not all cT3 tumors require preoperative treatment. Patients with T3N0 tumors with less than 5 mm of extramural spread or with a clear CRM greater than 2 mm have acceptable rates of local recurrence (in the 5–10% range depending on the plane of dissection).[64,144] One of the issues has been inaccurate local staging techniques, but the MERCURY study group has shown that high-resolution MRI can predict a pathologically negative CRM as well as accurately assess extramural spread within 0.5 mm of final histopathological measurement.[54,68,69] Furthermore, high-resolution MRI can identify good prognosis cT3 tumors with a clear CRM greater than 1 mm, extramural extension less than 5 mm, and absence of lymphovascular invasion that can undergo proctectomy and TME without need for neoadjuvant therapy with local recurrence rates of less than 5%.[114] However, this approach is not yet standard of care in North America, and these patients should be discussed at a multidisciplinary rectal cancer tumor board to discuss the possible management strategies. Patients with cT4 tumors are at high risk of local recurrence and distant metastasis up to 20 and 60%, respectively.[145] Therefore, these patients should undergo long-course chemoradiation to improve local control and minimize distant recurrence.

Patients with stage III disease (i.e., any cT, cN1–2) should be considered for neoadjuvant therapy with long-course chemoradiation or short-course preoperative radiotherapy. Long-course chemoradiation is standard of care in North America for patients with stage III disease compared to the European approach where short-course Swedish-style radiotherapy is more common. Regardless, it is clear from the available data that patients with N + disease have a significantly higher risk of local recurrence and potentially worse survival outcomes in the absence of neoadjuvant treatment. Long-term follow-up of the Swedish trial showed 23% local recurrence rate for patients treated with preoperative short-course radiotherapy followed by surgery compared to 46% for patients treated with surgery alone ($p < 0.001$) at a median follow-up of 13 years. No differences in cancer-specific or overall survival were found between the two groups. Again it must be noted that the higher rates of local recurrence in the Swedish trial are reflective of the non-TME surgical technique. Similarly, 12-year follow-up of the Dutch rectal cancer trial showed a significant decrease in local recurrence from 19% in the surgery-alone group compared to 9% in the preoperative short-course radiotherapy + surgery group ($p < 0.001$). Just like in the Swedish trial, no difference in overall survival was found between the two groups. The MRC CR07 trial also demonstrated a significantly lower local recurrence rate at 3 years for stage III rectal cancer patients treated with preoperative radiotherapy (HR: 0.46; 95% CI: 0.28–0.76).

Finally, patients who present with synchronous stage IV distant metastases in the setting of rectal cancer (i.e., stage IV disease) should be managed based on burden of disease and symptoms arising from the primary rectal tumor. Preoperative systemic therapy should be strongly considered based on the EORTC Intergroup trial 40983 in patients with resectable hepatic disease, which is randomizing patients to six cycles of FOLFOX4 before and after liver resection vs. surgery alone, of which 46% were rectal cancers.[146] The 3-year progression-free survival increased from 28.1% in the surgery-only arm to 36.2% in the perioperative chemotherapy arm ($p = 0.041$). A liver-first strategy should be adopted as cancer survival is related to burden of systemic disease rather than the primary tumor.[147] The optimal strategy with regard to the timing and type of radiotherapy has not yet been determined. One potential strategy is the administration of perioperative oxaliplatin-based systemic therapy with liver surgery, followed by short-course radiotherapy and then proctectomy. Short-course radiotherapy may be more tolerable in this setting compared to long-course chemoradiation, and shortens time to proctectomy if patients are symptomatic. While preoperative chemoradiation does not affect overall survival, decreasing the risk of local recurrence in patients with resectable disease is still a valid goal given the morbidity of a pelvic recurrence. In cases with unresectable distant metastases, systemic therapy should be initiated with interval restaging to assess for conversion to resectability. The management of the primary tumor is controversial. Patients with obstructive symptoms should be considered for a diverting ostomy prior to starting systemic therapy. However, even patients with a near-obstructing lesion are likely to be able to avoid surgery with palliative radiotherapy and chemotherapy. In one study, only 23% of patients with a near-obstructing lesion required palliative stoma creation with 5×5 Gy irradiation, followed by oxaliplatin-based chemotherapy.[148] In patients with limited remaining lifespan, or those who are unable to tolerate surgery, systemic therapy, and/or radiation, colonic stenting should be considered.

24.5 Principles of Rectal Cancer Surgery

24.5.1 Local Excision

Select patients with early rectal cancer can be managed by local excision instead of radical surgery. Early rectal cancer is defined as well to moderately differentiated clinical T1 tumors with absence of lymphovascular and perineural invasion. These patients are at the lowest risk of lymph node metastasis and local recurrence and therefore are amenable for local excision with curative intent. The main controversy surrounding management of early rectal cancer is trade-off between the excellent oncologic outcomes associated with radical surgery for T1 tumors (with 5-year survival approaching 90%)[149,150,151] and the lower perioperative and long-term morbidity associated with local excision, as radical surgery is associated with significant perioperative complications and long-term functional impairments.[152,153] The indications according to the most recent NCCN and American Society of Colon and Rectal Surgeons (ASCRS) guidelines for local excision are reported in ▶ Table 24.7. The main limitation of local excision is the inability to pathologically assess the draining nodal basins; therefore, careful selection of patients is necessary. Locoregional recurrence after local excision for T1 tumors can be as high as 20%,[154] although it is

Table 24.7 Indications for curative intent local excision for early rectal cancer

NCCN guidelines[162]	ASCRS practice parameters[23]
Less than 30% of the bowel Less than 3 cm in size Mobile T1 only Absence of lymphovascular (LVI) and perineural (PNI) invasion Well or moderately differentiated No evidence of lymphadenopathy on preoperative staging investigations	T1 only without high-risk features Well to moderately differentiated No LVI or PNI Less than 3 cm in diameter

more commonly quoted in the 10 to 15% range.[150,155,156,157] Furthermore, tumor biology of the rectum is different than that of the colon.[158] The incidence of nodal involvement for T1 tumors of the rectum can be high as 18%, whereas it is 3 to 8% in the colon.[149,158,159] Kikuchi et al[160] showed that the risk of lymph node involvement was associated with the depth of invasion into the submucosa. None of the patients with tumors that invaded into the first third of the submucosa (sm1) had nodal involvement or local recurrence compared to 8% of patients with invasion into the middle third (sm2) and 20% of patients with invasion into the deepest third (sm3). An analysis of T1 tumors undergoing radical excision from the Surveillance, Epidemiology, and End Results database reported that the overall incidence of nodal involvement was 16.3%.[159] Tumors that were sized over 1.5 cm and poorly differentiated were at significantly higher risk. Similarly, a meta-analysis of 23 studies including 4,510 patients reported that T1 tumors with greater than 1 mm invasion into the submucosa (OR: 3.87; 95% CI: 1.50–10.00), lymphovascular invasion (OR: 4.81; 95% CI: 3.14–7.37), and poor differentiation (OR: 5.60; 95% CI: 2.90–10.82) were independent risk factors for lymph node metastasis.[161] Similarly, larger tumors, depth of invasion beyond sm1, and lymphovascular invasion were found to be independent predictors of local recurrence after local excision of rectal cancer in an Association of Coloproctology of Great Britain and Ireland Transanal Endoscopic Microsurgery Collaborative study.[155] Patients with any of these risk factors should not undergo curative local excision, or if these features are found on final pathology after local excision, radical surgery should be recommended.

Local excision can be performed via traditional transanal excision (TAE) or through an advanced transanal endoscopic surgery (TES) operating platform such as transanal endoscopic microsurgery (TEMS), transanal endoscopic operation (TEO), or transanal minimally invasive surgery (TAMIS). While traditional local excision was limited to tumors situated in the low rectum due to the lack of access of mid- and high-rectal lesions using Parks retractors, newer platforms have been developed which offer better visualization of and access to the lesion, allowing for an improved resection quality. TEMS was first reported by Dr. Gerard Buess in 1984,[163] which used a rigid operating platform with stereoscopic views (resectoscope) to gain endoluminal access. TEO was introduced as an alternative to TEMS. Subsequently, TAMIS was described by Atallah et al in 2010 as a less expensive alternative to TES.[164] Endoluminal access is obtained using a soft single-incision operating port and standard laparoscopic equipment. The SILSPort (Covidien, New Haven, CT) was first used, but since then specialized operating ports developed specifically for TAMIS have been developed, such as the GelPOINT Path (Applied Medical, Rancho Santa Margarita, CA). There are no in vivo comparative data between the different operating platforms, and the choice will be dictated by surgeon preference and equipment availability.[165] However, TEMS has been compared to traditional TAE using Parks retractors and has been shown to be superior in terms of resection quality. A meta-analysis showed that TES was associated with a lower incidence of lesion fragmentation (OR: 0.10; 95% CI: 0.04–0.21), positive margins (OR: 0.19; 95% CI: 0.11–0.31), and local recurrence (OR: 0.25; 95% CI: 0.15–0.40) with no difference in complications (OR: 1.02; 95% CI: 0.66–1.58).[166] It must be noted that tumors excised by TAE were located almost solely in the distal rectum, which have a worse prognosis compared to lesions in the upper two-thirds, and these results may be due to selection bias. Nevertheless, the poor outcomes associated with TAE are even more reason to use an advanced operating platform (TES) to approach these lesions.

In cases with diagnostic uncertainty, local excision can act as an "excisional biopsy" and further management dictated by final pathologic results. Given the limitations of the current locoregional staging modalities, there will be a not insignificant proportion of patients who will be understaged or will have risk factors for lymph node metastasis or local recurrences that were not apparent on the preoperative biopsy. These patients should undergo salvage radical excision within 30 days of the initial local excision. Perioperative outcomes appear to be similar between salvage TME after local excision and upfront TME[167,168]; however, one study reported a higher APR rate.[168] The authors hypothesized that the inflammatory process post-TES made a low colorectal or coloanal anastomosis (CAA) not feasible. Several studies have shown that salvage surgery in these cases does not compromise oncologic outcomes.[169,170] Patients who refuse radical surgery or are too medically unfit can be considered for adjuvant chemoradiotherapy, although level I data to support such an approach are lacking. Case series from MD Anderson and Memorial Sloan Kettering Cancer Centers show that adjuvant radiotherapy without concomitant chemotherapy may provide adequate local control,[171,172] although recurrence rate are still high and survival may still be inferior compared to radical resection. Long-term follow-up of the Cancer and Leukemia Group B (CALGB) 8984 trial demonstrated that 10-year local recurrence rates for T2 lesions treated with local excision and postoperative chemoradiation was 18% compared to 8% for T1 lesions treated with local excision alone.[173] Disease-free and overall survival was also lower in the T2 lesions despite chemoradiotherapy.

TES requires establishing pneumorectum through the transanal operating port when rigid platforms are employed. For TEMS, the dedicated system using a continuous flow model that prevents billowing is a key component of the technology. Standard laparoscopic insufflators and equipment can be used when flexible platforms are utilized, although newer insufflation technologies such as the high-flow CO_2 (AirSeal, ConMed, Utica, NY) reduce the amount of luminal bellowing and greatly facilitate the procedure. Regardless of the operating platform that is used, a full-thickness excision into the mesorectal fat with at least 1 cm surrounding should be performed for malignant lesions

(▶ Fig. 24.3), as a submucosal resection is at high risk of residual disease (OR: 6.47; 95% CI: 3.00–13.97 compared to full-thickness excision).[155] Lesions as high as 15 cm from the anal verge can be resected via TEO, although the risk of intraperitoneal perforation is highest for anterior lesions located 7 cm and above from the anal verge. The resulting full-thickness defect can either be closed or left open, as the data are equivocal. There may be fewer complications if the defect is closed,[174] but this theory has not been definitively proven.[175] Clearly if peritoneal perforation occurs, the resulting defect must be closed. This can be performed via the transanal approach, or a transabdominal approach if the resulting loss of pneumorectum precludes endoluminal closure. There are no data to suggest that oncologic outcomes are compromised if peritoneal perforation occurs. These cases are usually done as outpatient surgery, unless there is concern about peritoneal violation or bleeding. The most common immediate postoperative complications include pain, urinary retention, and

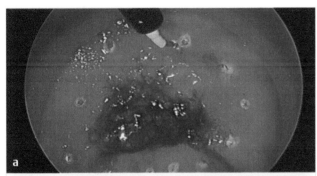

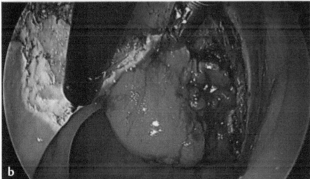

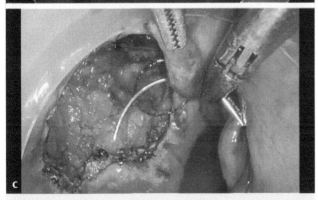

Fig. 24.3 Local excision of an early rectal cancer using the transanal minimally invasive surgery platform. **(a)** Marking 1-cm margin around the lesion. **(b)** Full-thickness excision into the perirectal fat. **(c)** Final defect and closure.

bleeding. Anorectal function impairment can occur, but usually resolves within 6 months.[176,177,178]

Several studies have shown less postoperative morbidity and comparable long-term outcomes between local excision and radical resection for T1 rectal adenocarcinoma. Winde et al[179] randomly assigned 52 patients with well to moderately differentiated T1 tumors to TAE versus anterior resection. There were fewer early complications and equal survival outcomes, although this study was underpowered to detect any real differences in these outcomes. Meta-analyses have reported significantly lower perioperative complications (8.2 vs. 47.2%; $p = 0.01$) and mortality (0 vs. 3.7%; $p = 0.01$) for local excision by TES compared to radical surgery.[180] However, TES local excision was associated with a higher incidence of local recurrence compared to radical resection, but without any differences in disease-free or overall survival.[180,181] If only "low-risk" T1 cancers are considered (well to moderate differentiation, absence of lymphovascular invasion), recurrence rate after TES was similar to that of radical surgery (4 vs. 3%), whereas for "high-risk" T1 tumors (poor differentiation or presence of lymphovascular invasion), TES had significantly higher rates of local recurrence (33 vs. 18%). Local excision is also associated with improved quality of life compared to radical surgery for early rectal cancer. Lezoche et al[182] demonstrated that quality-of-life impairments as measured by the EORTC QLQ–C30 and QLQ–CR38 lasted only 1 month after TES local excision, whereas these impairments persisted up to 6 months after laparoscopic TME. At 1 year, neither TES nor the laparoscopic TME had any changes from baseline. Long-term data show that local excision by TES and laparoscopic TME has similar quality of life (EORTC QLQ–C30 and EQ-5D), but there was a higher incidence of defecation problems in patients undergoing radical surgery.[183]

The cost of rigid TES platforms is approximately US$80,000, whereas the main equipment costs of TAMIS are related to the disposable transanal port, which costs approximately US$600 to 800.[184] However, a cost analysis comparing local excision by TES versus open surgery for early rectal cancer reported that only 12 TES cases were required to recoup the capital costs of the equipment.[185] Furthermore, the improved resection quality offered over traditional TAE should offset the increased equipment costs by minimizing recurrences and associated high treatment costs.

Surveillance after local excision of early rectal cancer should follow NCCN guidelines and include history, physical examination, and CEA every 3 to 6 months for the first 2 years, then every 6 months thereafter for a total of 5 years. Given the risk of local recurrence, close endoscopic and radiologic follow-up should also be considered as part of the surveillance strategy. Flexible sigmoidoscopy (to detect mucosal recurrence) and MRI of the rectum (to detect mural recurrences that may not be apparent by endoscopy) every 3 to 6 months for the first 2 years is reasonable.

If recurrence is detected, a complete staging workup should be performed to assess whether the recurrence is locoregional or if there are distant metastases. Early studies that reported outcomes of local recurrence after TAE for T1 and T2 tumors reported that locoregional recurrences were often advanced and required multivisceral resection in a significant proportion of patients.[186,187,188] An R0 resection was achieved in 79 to 94% of patients undergoing surgical salvage. Survival was poor in these patients and was not equivalent to those undergoing upfront radical resection. More recent studies reporting on outcomes for local recurrences after TEMS report that 61 to 88% of patients with recurrent disease were eligible for curative salvage surgery, and that this may not negatively impact survival as compared to upfront surgery.[189,190] However, these data are heterogeneous in terms of the surveillance strategy and available technologies over the study periods. Better present imaging modalities allow for more accurate clinical staging, which may improve patient selection for local excision. Nevertheless, these data underscore the importance of proper patient selection for these procedures.

Local Excision after Chemoradiation

Unlike T1 tumors, T2 lesions have a much higher failure rate after local excision alone. Locoregional recurrence for T2 tumors is at least double that of T1 tumors, ranging from 13 to 30%,[156,162,191,192] which may be in part due to the 30 to 40% incidence of occult nodal involvement.[192] Despite this, a significant proportion of patients with T2 tumors are treated with local excision alone.[193] This has led to the application of neoadjuvant chemoradiation prior to local excision in order to reduce local recurrence rate and avoid the morbidity of radical oncologic surgery. There are some data to support this approach. Lezoche et al[182] randomly assigned 100 patients with T2N0M0 tumors less than 3 cm within 6 cm of the anal verge to local excision by TES versus laparoscopic TME after long-course neoadjuvant chemoradiation with 50.4 Gy and concomitant infusional 5-FU. Tumors were downstaged in 51% of cases, with 28% in the TEMS and 26% in the surgery arm achieving ypT0. No patients in the surgery arm had positive lymph nodes on final pathology. After a median follow-up of 9.6 years, the local recurrence rate was similar for both arms (TES 12 vs. surgery 10%; $p = 0.686$), as was cancer-related (89 vs. 94%; $p = 0.687$) and overall (72 vs. 80%; $p = 0.609$) survival. Similarly, the ACOSOG Z6041 phase II trial investigated a preoperative chemoradiation regimen consisting of capecitabine, oxaliplatin, and 54-Gy radiotherapy, followed by local excision for patients with clinical T2N0 tumors.[194] Of the 77 patients who completed the preoperative regimen and underwent local excision, 64% experienced tumor downstaging with 44% overall achieving a pathologic complete response.[195] Three-year disease-free and overall survival was 88.2 and 94.8%, respectively.

Despite these promising data, the success of this approach appears to be dependent on the tumor response to neoadjuvant therapy. In a systematic review of 20 studies including 1,068 patients, Hallam et al demonstrated that the rate of local recurrence was high if a pathologic complete response was not obtained.[196] After a median follow-up of 54 months, local recurrence occurred in 4.0% (95% CI: 1.9–6.9) of patients with ypT0, 12.1% (95% CI: 6.3–19.4) for ypT1, 23.6% (95% CI: 13.0–36.1) for ypT2, and 59.6% (95% CI: 32.6–83.8) for ypT3. The pooled local recurrence rate for tumors ≥ ypT1 was 21.9% (95% CI: 15.9–28.5). Similarly, the rate of distant metastasis was 2.8% (95% CI: 0.8–6.1) for ypT0 and 20.9% (95% CI: 14.7–27.9) for tumors ≥ ypT1. The significantly higher failure rate for tumors ≥ ypT1 may be explained by the fact that more than 20% of ypT1/T2 tumors had residual lymph node metastases after radical surgery, as was shown in the German CAO/ARO/AIO-94 trial.[197] Perez et al[198] also showed that patients with cT2–4N0M0 that do not demonstrate complete clinical response (cCR)

after chemoradiation have a high incidence of unfavorable histology (ypT2 or 3 in at least 66%). These data suggest that local excision alone after neoadjuvant chemotherapy in patients without apparent complete clinical or pathologic response would result in understaging and undertreatment in a significant proportion of patients.

Another consideration is that perioperative morbidity after local excision post-neoadjuvant chemoradiation is high. Several studies have reported that a significant proportion of patients experienced a rectal wound complication after local excision. Marks et al[199] showed that 33% of patients receiving neoadjuvant therapy had a complication versus 5% in patients who did not ($p < 0.05$). Rectal wound complications were also higher (25 vs. 0%; $p = 0.015$). Perez et al[200] also showed that patients undergoing local excision after neoadjuvant therapy had significantly more rectal wound dehiscence (70 vs. 23%; $p = 0.03$), and pain requiring readmission (43 vs. 7%; $p = 0.02$).[200] Anorectal function also appears to be significantly impaired in these patients. Gornicki et al[201] showed that anorectal function and quality of life was similar between local excision and radical surgery after neoadjuvant chemoradiation, suggesting that the benefits of local excision in terms of preserved function were lost with neoadjuvant treatment. Similarly, Habr-Gama et al[202] demonstrated that local excision after chemoradiation was associated with significantly worse anorectal function, as measured by manometry and the Fecal Incontinence Index and Quality of Life assessment, compared to patients who underwent observation. Given the equivocal results from the current data, local excision after neoadjuvant chemoradiation for cT2N0 tumors should not be routinely offered unless patients are unwilling or unable to undergo radical resection. Two multicenter randomized trials are currently underway to investigate this approach: ChemorAdiation therapy for rectal cancer in the distal Rectum followed by organ-sparing Transanal endoscopic microSurgery (CARTS) and Transanal endoscopic microsurgery and Radiotherapy in Early rectal Cancer (TREC).[203,204] Until the results of these trials are available, this approach should only be performed as part of a clinical trial.

24.5.2 Watch and Wait

Oncologic TME surgery for patients who are medically operable remains the standard of care for patients regardless of clinical response to neoadjuvant therapy. The incidence of complete pathologic response (pCR) after long-course chemoradiation ranges from 10 to 44%, with improved oncologic outcomes in these patients compared to those without pCR.[205,206,207] Maas et al performed an individual patient data meta-analysis including 3,105 patients who received neoadjuvant chemoradiation and TME.[207] The overall pCR rate was 16%, with patients achieving pCR having improved local control (HR: 0.41; 95% CI: 0.21–0.81) disease-free (HR: 0.54; 95% CI: 0.40–0.73) and overall (HR: 0.65; 95% CI: 0.47–0.89) survival compared to patients with residual disease. Given the improved outcomes with pCR and the significant short- and long-term morbidity and mortality associated with radical surgery, there has been interest in identifying patients for which surgery can be avoided ("watch-and-wait" approach).[208]

Habr-Gama et al[209] were the first to report outcomes for the watch-and-wait approach. In their study, 29% of patients who underwent long-course chemoradiation were deemed to have cCR at 8 weeks using a combination of endoscopic and radiologic (CT with or without TRUS) findings. Patients with apparent cCR underwent intensive surveillance for possible recurrence with monthly follow-ups for repeat DRE, proctoscopy, and serum CEA levels, and CT scan every 6 months. These 79 patients were compared to 22 patients who had pCR on surgical pathology. After a median follow-up of 57 months, 2 patients in the observation group experienced a local recurrence that was successfully salvaged and 3 developed metastatic disease. There were no differences in disease-specific (92 vs. 83%) or overall survival (100 vs. 88%) between the observation and surgery groups. A later follow-up study on 183 patients, of which 90 (49%) had cCR (the increase in cCR was due to a change in the definition of a cCR), reported that local recurrence developed in 28 patients (31%).[210] Of these, 17 had recurred within 12 months of observation and 11 afterward. Salvage was possible in 93% with R0 resections in 89%. Overall survival at 5 years was 91%.

A Dutch study showed that only 1 patient out of 21 with cCR had a local recurrence after a mean follow-up of 25 months, which was managed by local excision.[211] No patients undergoing observation in this study had distant metastases. The endoscopic, radiologic MRI, and clinical criteria to identify patients with cCR were more stringent than Brazilian study, as was the surveillance protocol. There was no difference in disease-free or overall survival when compared to patients who underwent resection and had pCR, with better bowel function in the observation group. Similarly, the experience from Memorial Sloan Kettering Cancer Center reported 6 recurrences out of 32 patients managed by observation alone after median follow-up of 28 months.[212] All of the local recurrences were salvageable. There were no differences in 2-year disease-free (88 vs. 98%; $p = 0.27$) and overall (96 vs. 100%; $p = 0.56$) survival between observation and patients who were resected with a pCR.

The Oncologic Outcomes after Clinical Complete Response in Patients with Rectal Cancer (OnCoRe) study[213] performed a propensity-score-matched analysis of patients undergoing induction chemoradiotherapy managed by watch-and-wait or surgical resection from four United Kingdom cancer centers. Primary outcome in this study was non-regrowth disease-free survival. A total of 129 patients were observed after cCR, of which 34% had experienced local regrowth. Salvage therapy was feasible in 88% of these patients. After one-to-one matching with patients undergoing surgical resection, there were no differences in 3-year non-regrowth disease-free (88 vs. 78%) or overall (96 vs. 87%) survival between watch-and-wait and resected patients. These combined data suggest that observation after cCR may not need surgery, although prospective randomized trials are lacking. At the present time, surgical resection is recommended for patients who are medically operable and willing to undergo surgery.

One of the significant barriers to the watch-and-wait approach is the ascertainment of cCR of the primary tumor as well as nodal status. Lymph nodes may contain residual tumor in up to 10% of patients with ypT0.[214,215] A combination of physical examination with endoscopic and radiologic evaluation should be used, as the diagnostic accuracy of each of these modalities is low. Assessment by DRE and proctoscopy was only able to correctly predict pathologic complete response in 25% of cases.[216] Endoscopic findings of complete response include whitening of the mucosa, telangiectasia

without mucosal ulcerations, and subtle loss of pliability of the rectal wall (▶ Fig. 24.4). Residual disease should be highly suspected in the presence of a palpable nodule, ulceration, or irregularity. However, up to 61 to 74% of patients with a pCR may still have mucosal abnormalities suggestive of an incomplete clinical response.[217,218] Similarly, 27% of patients with endoscopic findings suggestive of cCR had residual disease.[217] Complete response is similarly problematic to accurately predict on radiologic imaging. MRI has difficulty distinguishing between residual tumor and radiation-induced edema or fibrosis. In cases of complete response, a scar replaces the site of the tumor, which is represented as an area of low signal intensity on T2-weighted imaging.[219] Newer MRI techniques such as diffusion-weight imaging may improve diagnostic accuracy for assessment of tumor response.[71] PET/CT shows promise since complete response should eliminate metabolic activity of the tumor. A systematic review of 34

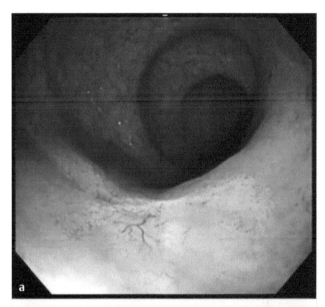

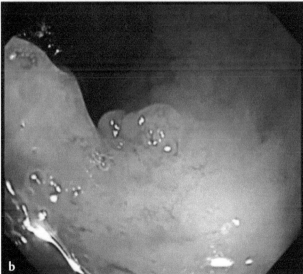

Fig. 24.4 Endoscopic appearance after neoadjuvant chemoradiation. **(a)** Complete clinical response demonstrating whitening of the mucosa and telangiectasia with no mucosal abnormalities. **(b)** Incomplete clinical response with residual mucosal abnormality.

studies including 1,526 patients reported a 71% sensitivity of PET/CT for the detection of complete response.[72] A prospective study by Perez et al[220] reported that clinical evaluation alone accurately detected residual cancer in 91% of cases, and PET/CT increased overall accuracy to 96%. Normalization of CEA after neoadjuvant therapy is also reflective of tumor response.[35,221] Finally, local excision of the tumor scar may confirm mural sterility, but is associated with significant pain and wound complications.[199,222]

It is not clear when to perform this assessment, as studies have ranged between 4 and 10 weeks.[209,211,212] Perez et al[223] performed PET/CT at 6 and 12 weeks after completion of neoadjuvant chemoradiation and reported that patients in whom the SUVmax increased during this interval were unlikely to develop cCR or significant tumor regression. However, not all patients should wait 12 weeks for definitive management, be it resection or observation. The GRECCAR-6 trial did not demonstrate any difference in pCR between patients randomized to 7- versus 11-week interval to surgery (15.0 vs. 17.4%; $p = 0.598$), but the patients in the 11-week arm experienced increased postoperative morbidity (44.5 vs. 32.0%; $p = 0.040$).[103] It is reasonable to assess tumor response at a minimum of 6 weeks after completion of neoadjuvant chemotherapy. Patients who demonstrate significant or complete mucosal response based on DRE/proctoscopy may be considered for further evaluation of complete response, whereas patients with moderate to poor response should undergo resection within 6 to 8 weeks after completion of neoadjuvant therapy as per current guidelines.

Patients who exhibit evidence of cCR should be willing and able to undergo a strict surveillance protocol, especially during the first year as this is when the majority of recurrences occur. Based on the approach of Habr-Gama et al,[209] patients should undergo monthly follow-up with DRE or proctoscopy for the first 3 months, then every 2 to 3 months for the remainder of the first year. CEA is checked every 2 months. Radiologic evaluation using CT or MRI should be done at the time of initial tumor assessment, and then every 6 months. Follow-up visits should continue every 3 months after the first year. Suspicious findings on clinical assessment or imaging should prompt further evaluation or radical surgery.

24.6 Surgical Resection

24.6.1 Total Mesorectal Excision

The introduction of the concept of the total mesorectal excision (TME) by Professor R.J. Heald in the 1980s revolutionized rectal cancer surgery.[5,224,225] Heald described dissection in the avascular "holy plane" between the visceral and parietal layers of the endopelvic fascia ensuring en bloc removal of the primary tumor and associated mesentery, lymphatics, vascular, and perineural tumor deposits, as well as preserving autonomic nerve and reducing bleeding.[5,224] The operative steps of a TME are reported in ▶ Table 24.8. Local recurrence rate in Heald's TME series of 115 curative-intent rectal cancer resections was 2.7% after a mean follow-up of 4.2 years.[225] Prior to TME, rectal mobilization by blunt dissection, which leaves much of the mesorectum behind, was associated with local recurrence rates as high as 30 to 40% (▶ Table 24.9).[226,227,228] Many other series have reported a significant improvement in oncologic outcomes after

the introduction of TME.[229,230,231,232] Arbman et al[232] demonstrated that the rate of local recurrence decreased from 11 to 3% after the TME technique was introduced.[232] Köckerling et al reported a decrease in local recurrence rates from 39.4 to 9.8% and an improvement in 5-year overall survival from 50 to 71% after adoption of TME in a retrospective series of 1,581 consecutive patients undergoing R0 resection for rectal cancer.[230] The introduction of TME in the Netherlands decreased local recurrence from 16% for conventional blunt dissection techniques to 9% in patients undergoing TME surgery without preoperative radiotherapy in the Dutch TME trial.[231] Comparatively, local recurrence rate in patients undergoing non-TME surgery and without preoperative radiotherapy in the Swedish Rectal Cancer trial was 27%.[7]

Obtaining a negative CRM is crucial in local control. Quirke et al were among the first to realize the importance of the CRM.[66] A microscopic positive margin or tumor ≤ 1 mm from the inked surface is predictive of poor oncologic outcomes.[66,236,237,238,239] A review by Nagtegaal and Quirke[239] including over 17,500 patients reported that patients with a negative CRM had lower risk of local recurrence (HR: 0.37; 95% CI: 0.23–0.58), fewer distant metastases (HR: 0.36; 95% CI: 0.23–0.54), and improved overall survival (HR: 1.7; 95% CI: 1.3–2.3). The effect of a positive CRM was even more pronounced in the setting of surgery after neoadjuvant therapy. In the Dutch TME trial, patients with a positive CRM after neoadjuvant therapy were much more likely to develop local recurrence (HR: 10.0; 95% CI: 6.7–25.0)

Table 24.8 Operative steps of a total mesorectal excision

1. Ligation of the inferior mesenteric artery at its origin
2. Complete mobilization of the splenic flexure
3. Transection of the proximal left colon
4. Sharp dissection in the avascular plane into the pelvis anterior to the presacral (Waldeyer's) fascia and outside the fascia propria or enveloping visceral fascia
5. Division of lymphatics and middle hemorrhoidal vessels anterolaterally at the level of the pelvic floor
6. Inclusion of all pelvic fat and lymphatic material to the level of the anorectal ring or at least 2 cm below the level of the distal margin

Table 24.9 Incidence of local recurrence after curative proctectomy in the pre-total mesorectal excision era

Study	N	Follow-up	Local recurrence
Wilson and Beahrs[233]	345	Minimum 5 y	13%
Cass et al[234]	280	Minimum 1 y	28%
Rao et al[235]	204	Minimum 5 y	22%
Påhlman and Glimelius[226]	197	Minimum 5 y	38%
Pilipshen et al[227]	412	Minimum 5 y	25%
Arbman et al[232]	142	2 y	13%
Kapiteijn et al[231]	269	Median 78 mo	16%
Folkesson et al[95]	454 (surgery alone)	Median 13 y	26%

compared to patients with a positive CRM without neoadjuvant therapy (HR: 3.8; 95% CI: 3.3–5.6).[238,240] This effect is likely due to tumor biology, as tumors not responding to radiotherapy is a poor prognostic sign in and of itself.[134,135]

Pretreatment CRM involvement is more likely as the T and N stage increases.[66,239] CRM involvement can be from direct or discontinuous spread from the primary tumor, lymphatic or perineural invasion, or positive lymph nodes. However, the importance of a positive CRM due to tumor within a lymph node is not clear. Nagtegaal et al[238] reported that the incidence of local recurrence was 22.1% for patients with a positive CRM due to direct tumor extension compared to 12.4% for patients with an involved CRM due to nodal disease. Similarly, Birbeck et al reported that local recurrence in patients with CRM involvement due to tumor within a lymph node (10.5%) was not significantly different compared to patients with a negative CRM (10.0%).[241] All other modes of CRM involvement had significantly higher rates of local recurrence.

The proper plane of dissection during TME will decrease CRM involvement. The CRM is also more likely to be involved in a muscularis propria (19–29%) compared to the mesorectal (1.6–14.6%) plane of dissection.[242] The grade of mesorectum is determined macroscopically after resection and can be graded as complete (mesorectal plane of dissection), nearly complete (intramesorectal plane), or incomplete (muscularis propria plane; ▶ Table 24.10 and ▶ Fig. 24.5, ▶ Fig. 24.6, ▶ Fig. 24.7). In an analysis of the surgical specimens of the surgery-only arm of the Dutch TME trial, Nagtegaal et al reported that the patients with a complete or a nearly complete mesorectum had fewer recurrences compared to patients with an incomplete TME (21.5 vs. 35.6%; $p = 0.01$) but with no difference in overall survival.[243] This effect remained significant even for patients with a negative CRM (> 1 mm), as patients with a complete or nearly complete TME had fewer recurrences (14.9 vs. 28.6%; $p = 0.03$) and better overall survival (90.5 vs. 76.9%; $p < 0.05$), suggesting that the quality of the TME has important prognostic value beyond decreasing CRM positivity. Similarly, Quirke et al[244] graded the mesorectal specimens for 1,157 patients included in the CR07 trial and reported that the rates of CRM positivity were 9% for

the mesorectal, 12% for the intramesorectal, and 19% for the muscularis propria plane. CRM involvement was associated with worse 3-year local recurrence and disease-free survival for all planes of surgery. In patients with a negative CRM, the incidence of local recurrence was 4% for mesorectal and 13% for muscularis propria plane (log rank $p = 0.0039$). Overall, patients receiving preoperative radiotherapy and a complete mesorectum had a local recurrence rate of only 1%. However, 11.1 to 56.4% of patients with a positive CRM had a mesorectal plane of dissection, suggesting that CRM involvement may also be a marker of poor tumor biology in addition to surgical technique.[239] Hall et al[245] demonstrated that CRM involvement in the setting of a complete mesorectum was associated with worse 5-year disease-free and overall survival but not local recurrence. The plane of TME dissection and subsequent mesorectal grade therefore has important implications for both oncologic outcomes and quality of care.

Level of Inferior Artery Ligation and Splenic Flexure Mobilization

Metastatic lymphovascular spread follows the lymphatic chains along the inferior mesenteric artery (IMA) and vein. There is no consensus regarding the level of ligation along the IMA. The IMA can be ligated at the origin of the superior rectal artery, just distal to the takeoff of the left colic artery (low tie), or at its origin from the aorta (high tie). A low tie results in preservation of the left colic artery and supposed improved blood supply to the descending and sigmoid colon, but may not provide enough length to perform a tension-free anastomosis for low colorectal anastomoses, especially if the sigmoid is resected. Conversely, a high tie will result in the vascular supply of the colonic conduit relying on the middle colic and marginal arteries. As long as the marginal artery is not compromised, high tie should not result in devascularization and will allow more length to perform a low anastomosis.[246]

There are no oncologic advantages in low versus high ligation of the IMA. High tie may yield a greater lymph node harvest and improve staging, but the available data have not been able to demonstrate a survival advantage for high tie versus low tie.[247,248] High tie does include the apical nodes at the root of the IMA, which may have prognostic value.[249,250] Kim et al[250] reported that patients with apical nodal involvement had a significantly worse survival than patients without for stage III/IV colorectal cancer (38 vs. 58%, HR: 2.58; 95% CI: 1.59–4.18). In the absence of clear data, high ligation of the IMA does not have to be routinely performed. The decision of the level of vessel ligation depends on the amount of mobilization required to form a tension-free anastomosis and whether there are any suspicious nodes at the origin of the IMA.

The decision to perform a splenic flexure mobilization should be individualized to each patient depending on anatomy and tumor characteristics. Patients who require a low colorectal or a coloanal anastomosis are more likely to require splenic flexure mobilization to obtain enough length to perform a tension-free anastomosis.[251] In order to obtain maximum length in these patients, the splenic flexure should be mobilized completely, the omentum separated from the transverse colon, and the IMV ligated at the inferior edge

Table 24.10 Pathologic macroscopic grading of the mesorectum

Grade of mesorectum	
Mesorectal plane (complete)	• Intact mesorectum with only minor irregularities • No defects deeper than 5 mm • No coning toward the distal margin of the resection specimen • Smooth CRM on transverse sections
Intramesorectal plane (nearly complete)	• Moderate bulk to the mesorectum • One or more defects deeper than 5 mm • Moderate coning • No visible muscularis propria • Irregular CRM on transverse sections
Muscularis propria plane (incomplete)	• Exposed muscularis propria • Moderate to marked coning • Irregular CRM on transverse sections

Abbreviation: CRM, circumferential resection margin.

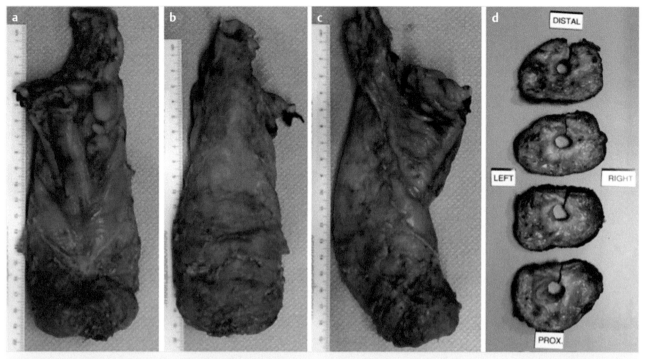

Fig. 24.5 (a–d) Macroscopic appearance of a complete mesorectum (mesorectal plane).

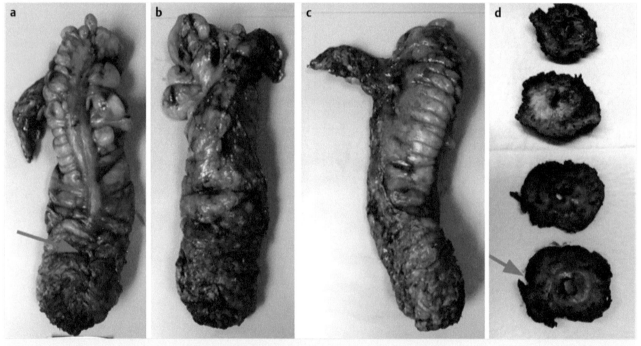

Fig. 24.6 (a–d) Macroscopic appearance of a nearly complete mesorectum (intramesorectal plane). The red arrow marks a small (<5 mm) defect in the mesorectum, demonstrated on the anterior and cross-sectional views.

of the pancreas and the IMA at its origin from the aorta. The additional length that the splenic flexure takedown provides can also allow for removal of the sigmoid colon so that the anastomosis is fashioned using the descending colon. Karanjia et al[252] reported that use of the sigmoid colon was an independent predictor for anastomotic leak. However, there does not appear to be any difference in anastomotic complications if the splenic flexure is not mobilized for cancers of the upper rectum and rectosigmoid as long as the principles of a tension-free anastomosis are followed.

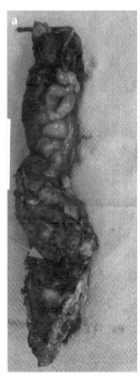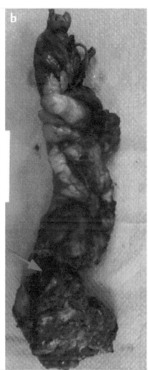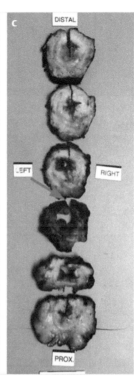

Fig. 24.7 Macroscopic appearance of an incomplete mesorectum (muscularis propria plane). The red arrow marks the full-thickness defect in the rectal wall, demonstrated on the **(a)** anterior, **(b)** posterior, and **(c)** cross-sectional views.

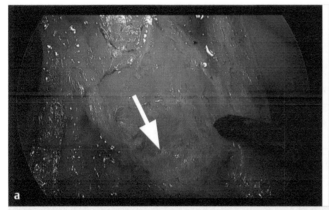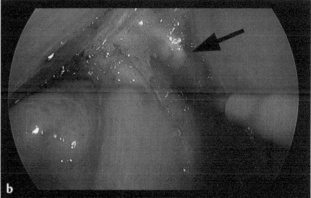

Fig. 24.8 Images from a laparoscopic total mesorectal excision (TME). **(a)** Posterior dissection. The white arrow denotes the avascular TME plane. **(b)** Anterior dissection. The black arrow demonstrates the right seminal vesicle. The tumor in this case was anterior so the dissection included Denonvillier's fascia.

Pelvic Dissection

Sharp dissection in the avascular areolar plane that represents the fusion between the visceral and parietal layers of the endopelvic fascia begins in the posterior midline and proceeds posteriorly until the desired level of distal margin. Once the posterior mobilization is completed, the dissection proceeds laterally in the same areolar plane until it is completed circumferentially (▶ Fig. 24.8). Dissection in the correct plane avoids injury to the presacral plexus with potentially major hemorrhage, as well as minimizes sexual dysfunction due to inadvertent nervous injury. The autonomic nerves of the inferior hypogastric plexus lie superficial to the endopelvic fascia and are at highest risk of injury during the posterolateral pelvic mobilization. These nerves should be identified and carefully dissected away from the mesorectum on both sides. Middle rectal arteries are present in approximately 20% of patients and may be encountered laterally during deep pelvic dissection—these vessels can easily be taken using electrocautery or an energy device. The anterior dissection should proceed along Denonvillier's fascia down to the pelvic floor or the desired distal margin. Denonvillier's fascia should be included for tumors that are located anteriorly, which puts the neurovascular bundles of Walsh and seminal vesicles at risk for injury. Posterior tumors do not require Denonvillier's fascia to be included in the resection specimen. Once the mesorectum is completely mobilized, the distal margin should be verified by DRE or endoscopy prior to transection, and a stapled colorectal or handsewn CAA created.

Dissection in the proper TME plane results in less sexual and urinary dysfunction compared to conventional blunt dissection. Maurer et al compared the incidence of autonomic pelvic nerve function in patients undergoing TME versus non-TME surgery.[253] Urinary function between the two groups was similar, but higher proportion of patients undergoing TME surgery preserved their ability to achieve orgasm and ejaculate, even when preexisting poor genital functions were excluded from the analysis. Furthermore, more patients undergoing non-TME surgery reported significant deterioration from baseline sexual function compared to TME surgery patients. Nevertheless, the incidence of sexual and urinary dysfunction is high even after TME, and patients should be counseled appropriately. Nerve injury and pelvic scarring may cause damage to the superior and inferior hypogastric plexuses, manifesting in disorders of ejaculation and impotence, respectively.[254] The prevalence is surprisingly high, as a cross-sectional study in rectal cancer survivors reported that 43% of sexually active men and 39% of sexually active women reported sexual dysfunction.[255] This effect appears to improve with time, as Stamopoulos et al reported that 66% of males reported sexual dysfunction at 3 months, which improved to only 14% by 6 months.[256] Similarly, the incidence of urinary dysfunction is also high. Among patients who were continent before treatment, urinary incontinence persisted in 27% of patients and difficulty voiding in 20% at 5 years in the Dutch TME trial.[257] Incontinence arises from sympathetic injury at the superior hypogastric plexus, whereas retention symptoms result from parasympathetic injury at the inferior hypogastric plexus. Urinary dysfunction is usually temporary and often resolves within 3 to 6 months after surgery, but persistence of symptoms at 1 year is usually permanent.[258] Laparoscopic or robotic approaches may reduce these risks, although data are conflicting. Data from two earlier randomized trials comparing laparoscopic versus open TME reported higher rates of sexual, but not bladder, impairments in patients undergoing laparoscopic surgery.[259,260] Patient-reported outcomes from the COlorectal cancer Laparoscopic or Open Resection II (COLOR II) trial showed no differences between the two approaches[261]; however, nonrandomized studies demonstrate significant benefit for the laparoscopic approach.[262,263,264]

Tumor-Specific Mesorectal Excision

A TME is not oncologically necessary for tumors of the rectosigmoid and upper rectum. A TME by definition requires removal of the entire mesorectal envelope down to the levators and subsequent low pelvic anastomosis. However, low anastomoses are associated with increased risk of anastomotic leak,[252] as well as worse intestinal functional outcomes.[265] Furthermore, distal mesorectal metastatic nodal deposits are rarely found beyond 5 cm.[5,266,267] Consequently, tumors in the upper rectum can be managed by a tumor-specific mesorectal excision (TSME). The ASCRS practice parameters recommended mesorectal excision no less than 5 cm beyond the lowest extent of the tumor.[23] In particular, the mesorectum should be transected perpendicular to the bowel wall at least 5 cm from lower edge of the tumor to avoid "coning" and leaving residual mesorectum that may contain metastatic deposits. TSME has been shown to result in equal oncologic outcomes with decreased perioperative morbidity as compared to a TME for upper rectal cancers. Data from

the Cleveland Clinic showed that upper rectal cancers treated with TSME had similar oncologic outcomes as sigmoid cancer.[268] Upper rectal cancers had lower 5-year local recurrence (2.8 vs. 8.6%; $p = 0.003$) and cancer-specific death (12.7 vs. 25.6%; $p < 0.001$) than rectal cancers in the mid- and low rectum treated with TME, with a trend toward higher anastomotic leak rates for low-rectal cancers. Similarly, a series of 514 patients with rectal cancer treated with surgery alone at the Mayo Clinic reported 5-year local recurrence and disease-free survival of 7 and 78% for anterior resection and TSME for upper third of the rectum compared to 6 and 83% for LAR with CAA and TME for tumors in the middle and lower third of the rectum.[269]

Distal Margin

Distal intramural tumor spread is uncommon and is found beyond 1 cm from the primary tumor in less than 10% of cases.[270] A 2-cm distal mural margin will remove all microscopic tumor in the majority of cases and is recommended in the most recent ASCRS practice parameters for rectal cancer.[23] Old surgical dogma necessitated a 5-cm distal margin, but early work in the pre-TME era from Williams et al[270] and Pollet and Nicholls[271] showed that there was no difference in local recurrence between patients with a 2- versus 5-cm distal margin. Vernava et al[272] further showed that a 1-cm distal margin was adequate if TME was performed. An analysis from the NSABP R-01 trial showed no difference in treatment failure and survival between patients undergoing sphincter-saving procedures with distal resection margins (DRM) of less than 2, 2 to 2.9, and ≥ 3 cm.[273] However, a smaller margin is also likely to be adequate especially in the setting of TME and neoadjuvant chemoradiotherapy.[274,275] Guillem et al[274] showed that only 2 out of 109 patients demonstrated intramural tumor extension beyond the gross mucosal edge of the residual tumor after long-course chemoradiation, with maximum spread of 0.95 mm. Distal resection margins are ≤ 1 cm[275] and ≤ 5 mm[276] and have been shown to be oncologically safe after preoperative chemoradiation. A systematic review of 17 studies reported no difference in local recurrence rates between DRM ≤ 5 mm, less than 1 cm, and greater than 1 cm.[276] The ability to obtain a smaller DRM without compromising oncologic outcomes is especially useful for distal tumors for which 2 cm may not be possible in the setting of sphincter preservation. However, 2-cm distal margins should be obtained if feasible.

24.6.2 Laparoscopic Total Mesorectal Excision

An analysis of the National Inpatient Sample from 2009 to 2011 reported that only 16% of patients underwent minimally invasive techniques for rectal cancer surgery.[277] Most of the laparoscopic resections (72% overall) were done at high-volume centers (25 + cases per year) and the use of laparoscopy increased over the study period in high-volume centers only. A similar analysis of the National Cancer Database showed that 42% of resections were done laparoscopically in American College of Surgeons' Commission on Cancer accredited centers from 2010 to 2012.[278] The data suggest that the majority of rectal cancer resections are still performed via the open approach except in specialist high-volume centers. The ASCRS clinical practice guidelines suggest that laparoscopic TME be performed with similar oncologic outcomes as open TME as long as the technical expertise is available.[23]

Current evidence suggests that laparoscopic TME is superior to open surgery in terms of postoperative recovery and perioperative morbidity. A Cochrane review in 2014 including 14 randomized trials with 3,528 patients reported that laparoscopic TME resulted in shorter hospitalization (weighted mean difference: –2.16 days; 95% CI: –3.22 to –1.10), faster postoperative recovery (time to normal diet, time to first defecation, analgesia use, and pain), and similar overall morbidity (OR: 0.94; 95% CI: 0.80–1.10). Wound infections (OR: 0.68; 95% CI: 0.50–0.93) and bleeding complications (OR: 0.30; 95% CI: 0.10–0.93) were fewer in the TME group. Patients in the laparoscopic TME group also had fewer small bowel obstructions (OR: 0.30; 95% CI: 0.12–0.75) over the long term. Operating time was higher in the laparoscopic group (weighted mean difference: 37.5 min; 95% CI: 27.8–47.2), but there were no differences in intraoperative complications (OR: 0.86; 95% CI: 0.62–1.18). Direct medical costs were also higher for the laparoscopic group.

Several studies have also demonstrated equivalence of oncologic outcomes between laparoscopic and open TME. The Cochrane review did not find a difference in the lymph node harvest (weighted mean difference: –0.43 lymph nodes; 95% CI: –1.13–0.26) or CRM involvement (OR: 0.99; 95% CI: 0.71–1.40). Five-year local recurrence (OR: 0.94; 95% CI: 0.49–1.81), and disease-free (OR: 1.02; 95% CI: 0.76–1.38) and overall (OR: 1.00; 95% CI: 0.70–1.42) survival were also similar between the two approaches. A summary of study characteristics and perioperative and oncologic outcomes for the larger trials (> 100 patients per arm) comparing laparoscopic and open TME are shown in ▶ Table 24.11 and ▶ Table 24.12. The Cochrane review did not include long-term outcomes of the COLOR II and the Comparison of Open versus laparoscopic surgery for mid or low REctal cancer After Neoadjuvant chemoradiotherapy (COREAN) trials, but these trials did not demonstrate differences between the two arms and are unlikely to influence the overall null effect. Two recent randomized trials, the American College of Surgeons Oncology Group (ACOSOG) Z6051 and Australasian Laparoscopic Cancer of the Rectum Trial (ALaCaRT), were also not included in the Cochrane review. Both of these trials were designed as noninferiority trials with a composite measure including quality of the mesorectum, CRM, and DRM as the primary outcome. The ACOSOG Z6051 trial randomly assigned 462 patients with stage II/III rectal cancer less than 12 cm from the anal verge to laparoscopic or open TME.[279] Almost all patients in this study underwent neoadjuvant chemoradiation. The trial was powered using a one-sided noninferiority margin of –6% using composite measure of a complete or nearly complete mesorectum, negative CRM, and negative DRM. There were no statistically significant differences in any of the individual outcomes, and the trial did not demonstrate noninferiority in the primary composite outcome for the laparoscopic arm (81.7 vs. 86.9%; difference: –5.3%; one-sided 95% CI: –10.8% to ∞). Long-term oncologic outcomes are not yet available, but the authors concluded that based on short-term pathologic outcomes the results of the trial did not support the use of laparoscopic TME.

The ALaCaRT study randomized 475 patients with rectal cancer less than 15 cm from the anal verge to laparoscopic versus open TME.[287] Patients with T4 lesions or an involved CRM were excluded in this trial, and 50% of patients in each arm underwent neoadjuvant radiotherapy. The primary outcome in this trial was also a composite measure of complete mesorectum (nearly complete grades were considered failure), negative CRM, and DRM. This trial was powered based on a one-sided noninferiority margin of –8% for the primary composite measure. Noninferiority could also not be established based on the trial results, as the difference in the primary composite measure was –7.0% (95% CI: –12.4 to ∞), with 82% successful resection in the laparoscopic arm and 89% in the open arm. Subgroup analysis demonstrates significant benefits for the open approach for T3 lesions and patients receiving neoadjuvant radiotherapy. Oncologic outcomes for this trial are also not available at present.

Table 24.11 Characteristics and short-term outcomes of the large randomized trials comparing laparoscopic and open total mesorectal excision

Trial	N	RTX	Tumor height	Sphincter saving	Conversion	30-d complications	Length of stay
Lujan et al[280]	O: 103 L: 101	O: 77% L: 73%	O: 6.2 cm L: 5.5 cm	O: 79% L: 76%	8%	O: 33% L: 34%	O: 9.9 d (6.8) L: 8.2 d (7.3)
CLASICC[281,282]	O: 128 L: 253	–	–	O: 73% L: 75%	34%	O: 37% L: 40%	O: 13 d (9–18) L: 11 d (9–15)
COLOR II[283,284]	O: 345 L: 699	O: 58% L: 59%	O: 66% < 10 cm L: 68% < 10 cm	–	17%	O: 37% L: 40%	O: 9 d (7–14) L: 8 d (6–13)
COREAN[285,286]	O: 170 L: 170	100%	O: 5.6 cm L: 5.3 cm	O: 86% L: 89%	1%	O: 23.5% L: 21.2%	O: 9 d (8–12) L: 8 d (7–12)
ACOSOG Z6051[279]	O: 239 L: 242	O: 97% L: 98%	O: 6.3 cm L: 6.1 cm	O: 76% L: 77%	11.3%	O: 58.1% L: 57.1%	O: 7.0 d (3.4) L: 7.3 d (5.4)
ALaCaRT[287]	O: 235 L: 238	O: 50% L: 50%	O: 79% < 10 cm L: 78% < 10 cm	O: 93% L: 92%	8.8%	No difference	O: 8 d (6–12) L: 8 d (6–12)

Abbreviations: L, laparoscopic; O, open; RTX, radiotherapy.

Table 24.12 Pathologic and long-term oncologic outcomes of the large randomized trials comparing laparoscopic and open total mesorectal excision

	+ CRM	Complete TME	–DRM	LR	DFS	OS
Lujan et al[280]	O: 3% L: 4%	–	O: 0% L: 0%	(5 y) O: 5.3% L: 4.8%	(5 y) O: 81% L: 85%	(5 y) O: 75% L: 72%
CLASICC[281,282]	O: 14% L: 16%	–	–	(5 y) O: 7.6% L: 9.4%	(5 y) O: 52.1% L: 53.2%	(5 y) O: 52.9% L: 60.3%
COLOR II[283,284]	O: 10% L: 10%	O: 92% L: 88%	O: 3 cm [1.8–5][a] L: 3 cm [2–4.8][a]	(3 y) O: 5% L: 5%	(3 y) O: 70.8% L: 74.8%	(3 y) O: 83.6% L: 86.7%
COREAN[285,286]	O: 4.1% L: 2.9%	O: 74.7% L: 72.4%	O: 2 cm [1–3.5][a] L: 2 cm [1–3.5][a]	(3 y) O: 4.9% L: 2.6%	(3 y) O: 72.5% L: 79.2%	(3 y) O: 90.4% L: 91.7%
ACOSOG Z6051[279]	O: 7.7% L: 12.1%	O: 81.5% L: 72.9%	O: 98.2% L: 98.3%	–	–	–
ALaCaRT[287]	O: 3% L: 7%	O: 92% L: 87%	O: 99% L: 99%	–	–	–

[a]Quantity of cm represents the mean, value in brackets represents the range.

Abbreviations: CRM, circumferential resection margin; DFS, disease free survival; DRM, distal resection margin; L, laparoscopic; LR, local recurrence; O, open; OS, overall survival; TME, total mesorectal excision.

The results of the ACOSOG Z6051 and the ALaCaRT trials were unexpected and run counter to the previous evidence. However, oncologic outcomes for these trials are not yet available, and until strong evidence to the contrary can be provided, it is likely that laparoscopic TME is oncologically equivalent to open TME, but with significant short-term advantages.

24.6.3 Robotic Total Mesorectal Excision

The robotic surgical system (da Vinci Surgical System; Intuitive Surgical, Inc., Sunnyvale, CA) has been proposed as an alternative to laparoscopy to provide many of the advantages of the minimally invasive approach for TME but with improved optics and angle of dissection with increased range of motion. Proponents of the robotic platform suggest that the three-dimensional 10-fold magnification, and instrument stability, and improved surgeon ergonomics may result in better dissection quality and preservation of the autonomic nerves.[280,281,282,283,284,285,286,287,288,289,290] The largest series to date originated from Korea in which 370 patients underwent robotically assisted tumor-specific TME.[291] Mean operative time was 363 minutes with 0.8% conversion rate. CRM involvement was seen in 5.7% of cases and 3.6% of patients experienced a local recurrence with a mean overall follow-up of 26.5 months. Pigazzi et al[292] reported a multi-institutional series with 143 patients with similar results as the Korean study, except with less CRM involvement (0.7%). Compared to open TME, retrospective observational studies have reported equal histopathological outcomes but with increased operative duration for robotic TME.[293,294] The improved visualization offered by the robotic surgery platform is also advocated to minimize pelvic autonomic nerve injury. Luca et al[295] described sexual and urinary function after robotic and laparoscopic TME. Patients in the robotic group experienced less sexual dysfunction at 1 month after surgery than the laparoscopic group, although the two groups were similar at 1 year. Urinary function was similar between the groups throughout the follow-up period. Kim et al[264] also reported that robotic TME was associated with quicker recovery of erectile function compared to laparoscopy.

Robotic TME has been described in two ways: a hybrid approach where mobilization of the left colon and splenic flexure, and vessel ligation is performed laparoscopically and the pelvic dissection is performed robotically; or where the entire procedure is performed via the robotic approach. A single pilot randomized trial including 36 patients (18 robotic and 18 laparoscopic TME) did not demonstrate any differences in perioperative and pathologic outcomes, except for a shorter hospital stay in the robotic arm (6.9 days [standard deviation (SD): 1.3] vs. 8.7 days [SD: 1.3]; $p < 0.001$).[296] A systematic review comparing laparoscopic and robotic TME identified 8 studies including 554 robotic cases and 675 laparoscopic cases.[297] In the pooled analysis, robotic TME was associated with less conversion to open surgery (OR: 0.23; 95% CI: 0.10–0.52), less CRM involvement (OR: 0.44; 95% CI: 0.20–0.96), and less erectile dysfunction (HR: 0.09; 95% CI: 0.02–0.42) compared to laparoscopic TME. Other outcomes, including operative duration, lymph node harvest, postoperative morbidity, and recovery of gastrointestinal (GI) function, were similar between the two techniques. Baik et al[296] reported that a complete mesorectum was obtained in 92.8% of robotic TME compared to 75.4% of laparoscopic TME ($p = 0.033$). Costs for robotic TME are significantly higher than for laparoscopic surgery. Kim and Kang reported that the mean total hospital costs were $14,080 for robotic TME, $9,120 for laparoscopic TME, and $8,386 for open TME in Korea.[298] Similarly, Leong et al[299] reported that the direct costs for robotic TME were at least three times higher than that of laparoscopic TME due to the capital costs of the robotic system and disposable instruments. These observational results suggest that robotic TME is feasible and is likely to have equal outcomes as laparoscopic TME, but at significantly higher costs.

Several large randomized trials comparing robotic and laparoscopic TME are currently underway, including the Robotic versus Laparoscopic Resection for Rectal cancer (ROLARR)[300] and several others from South Korea.[301,302] The results of these trials will help define the effectiveness of the robotic TME.

Initial results of the ROLARR trial have been presented at the ASCRS (Boston, MA) and EAES (Bucharest, Hungary) meetings in 2015 and subsequently published[303]. A total of 471 patients were randomized, including 234 laparoscopic and 237 robotic TMEs. The primary outcome in this trial was conversion to open surgery. The overall conversion rate was 10.1%, and no difference was found between the two approaches (laparoscopic 12.2 vs. robotic 8.1%; *p* =0.158). In the a priori defined subgroup analyses, the robotic approach demonstrated lower conversion rates in male patients (OR: 0.46 95% CI: 0.21–0.99), but did not reach statistical significance for low tumors or for obese patients. Notably, the main reason for conversion in both arms was for the completion of the rectal dissection. Important secondary endpoints of this trial included CRM involvement (laparoscopic 6.3 vs. robotic 5.1%), intraoperative complications (14.8 vs. 15.3%), and 30-day morbidity (31.7 vs. 33.1%). These results suggest that robotic TME conferred no clear benefit compared to laparoscopy for conversion, CRM involvement, and postoperative morbidity. Final results of this trial will include other endpoints such as technical, functional, and oncologic outcomes, quality of life, and cost.

24.6.4 Transanal Total Mesorectal Excision

Despite advances in surgical technique and neoadjuvant therapy, obtaining a negative CRM resection with intact TME had remained challenging, particularly for patients with tumors in the distal rectum.[304] More recently, transanal TME (TA-TME) has emerged as a new technique for performing TME for rectal cancer with curative intent.[305] In the TA-TME approach, an advanced endoscopic platform is introduced transanally, and a rectum is purse-stringed closed distal to the tumor. A circumferential full-thickness proctotomy is performed, and the TME is carried out distal to proximal (▶ Fig. 24.9). Splenic flexure takedown, ligation of the IMA, and the proximal rectal dissection are performed transabdominally. Proponents of the TA-TME argue the technique offers excellent access to the distal rectum, allows for establishment of a distal negative resection margin, and has advantages in dealing with difficult pelvic anatomy.[306] The "bottom-up" technique has been proposed as a way to overcome a narrow pelvis and perform sphincter-preserving surgery for cancers of the distal rectum.

Experience with this technique is limited to case series from a few specialized centers. An international registry from 66 surgical units in 23 countries reported short-term and pathologic outcomes of the first 720 cases (of which 634 were cancer

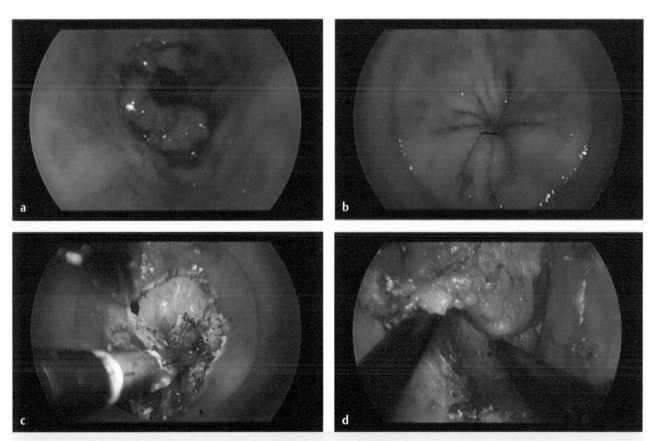

Fig. 24.9 Images from a transanal total mesorectal excision (TME). **(a)** Tumor in situ. **(b)** Purse-string closure of the rectal lumen at least 1 cm below the tumor, ensuring a negative distal margin. **(c)** Full-thickness proctotomy and entry into the TME plane anteriorly. **(d)** Posterior dissection during transanal TME. Note the avascular space denoting the TME plane.

cases).[307] Most participating surgical units had fewer than 10 cases (68%), whereas only 13 centers (20%) had done more than 20 cases. The mean tumor height was 6.0 cm, and 56% received neoadjuvant (chemo)radiotherapy. Pathologic outcomes were excellent, as 96% of cancer cases had complete or nearly complete mesorectum, and 4% had CRM involvement. A poor-quality resection, defined by an incomplete mesorectum or R1 resection, occurred in 7.4% of cases. Morbidity within 30 days was 32.6%, which is comparable to contemporary laparoscopic TME studies. However, long-term oncologic outcomes are not yet available, and the learning curve has not yet been defined. A randomized clinical trial comparing TA-TME and laparoscopic TME is currently enrolling patients.[308] Until these data are available, TA-TME should remain investigational.

24.6.5 Abdominoperineal Excision

Since the introduction of proctectomy according to TME principles, sphincter preservation, urogenital function, and local recurrence have improved.[309] Yet, oncologic outcomes for patients undergoing abdominoperineal excision (APE) for low-rectal cancer in the TME era are still inferior to those undergoing low anterior resection (LAR).[310] Data from the Norwegian Rectal Cancer Project demonstrated that the 5-year overall survival was worse after APE compared to LAR (HR: 1.3; 95% CI: 1–1.6).[311] Analysis of pooled data from five European rectal cancer trials showed that APE compared to LAR was an independent risk factor for CRM involvement (OR: 2.52; 95% CI: 1.69–3.76), local recurrence (HR: 1.36; 95% CI: 1.07–1.72), cancer-specific (1.17; 95% CI: 1.02–1.34), and overall survival (HR: 1.31; 95% CI: 1.11–1.56).[312] These differences in oncologic outcomes may be explained by tumor-related and surgical technique–related factors. While there is significant emphasis on the technique of pelvic dissection along TME planes, there is little standardization of the perineal portion of the APE. TME principles dictate meticulous sharp dissection in the areolar tissue enveloping the mesorectal fascia to the top of the anorectal ring, at which point the mesorectum is separated off of the levator muscles. The perineal portion of the APE follows the external sphincter until the top of the anal canal, at which point the levators are divided close to the rectal wall. This approach typically results in a "waist" at this level, which is often where the tumor is situated and where the mesorectum is the thinnest. The waisting effect increases the risk of bowel perforation and CRM involvement, since the sphincter muscles form the CRM below the level of the levators. Nagtegaal et al analyzed 373 APE specimens as part of the Dutch TME trial and reported that the plane of dissection was intrasphincteric/submucosal or perforated in 36% of cases, and the remainder was sphincteric. The majority of patients who had perforation during dissection were during APE (13.7% of APE specimens vs. 2.5% of anterior resections; $p < 0.001$).[313] Involvement of the CRM during APE was associated with significantly worse local recurrence and overall survival.[314] A Norwegian population-based cohort study also showed that the risk of perforation was significantly higher during APE (OR: 5.6; 95% CI: 3.5–8.8), with worse 5-year local recurrence rates (28.8 vs. 9.9%; $p < 0.001$) and overall survival (41.5 vs. 67.1%; $p < 0.001$) after perforation.[315] Patients undergoing APE also have higher T stages and lower tumors,[311] which are both poor prognostic factors.

While there is much emphasis on sphincter preservation for patients with low rectal cancer, there will be certain scenarios in which an APE is necessary (▶ Table 24.13). Tumors that involve the distal mesorectal fascia, levator muscle, or sphincter complex may require an APE to obtain a clear radial or distal margin. However, there is much variability in the APE rate between surgeons and institutions. A nested cohort study within the Intergroup 0114 trial reported that the APE rate was 46% for low-volume (0–8 cases per year), 41% for medium-volume (8–16 cases per year), and 32% for high-volume (17 + cases per year) hospitals.[316] Similarly, a UK population-based analysis reported that the APE rate varied from 8.5 to 52.6% across different hospitals.[317] Given this variability along with the high rates of CRM involvement, and inadvertent bowel perforation with subsequent poor oncologic outcomes associated with an APE, there have been attempts to provide a standardized approach for APE.[318] Three types of APE can be defined based on patient- and tumor-related factors: intersphincteric APE, extralevator

Table 24.13 Indications for abdominoperineal excision (APE) for rectal cancer

Intersphincteric APE: total mesorectal excision (TME) along mesorectal fascia until the top of the anal canal. Perineal dissection between internal and external sphincter muscles. Dissection planes meet at level of puborectalis

- Tumor not involving the levators or sphincter complex but restoration of intestinal continuity not wanted or not advisable due to:
  - History of fecal incontinence
  - Highly comorbid patient that would not tolerate an anastomotic complication
  - High risk of anastomotic leak
  - Patient preference

Extralevator (ELAPE): TME along mesorectal fascia until the top of levator muscles (i.e., lateral attachments of the levator muscles). Perineal dissection just lateral to the external sphincter and along levator muscle fascia. Dissection planes meet at the lateral origins of the levator muscles at the obturator internus muscle.

- Tumor involving the sphincter complex (T2–T4)
- Low tumor (< 5 cm from the anal verge) threatening the circumferential resection margin

Ischioanal APE: TME along mesorectal fascia until the top of levator muscles (i.e., lateral attachments of the levator muscles). Perineal dissection begins with a skin incision depending on the extent of tumor involvement and directed toward the ischial tuberosities. Dissection proceeds upward along the obturator internus muscle to remove the ischioanal fat en bloc.

- Locally advanced rectal cancer that involves the levator muscles, ischioanal fat, or perianal skin
- Tumor perforation into ischioanal space

APE (ELAPE), and ischioanal APE (▶ Table 24.13 and ▶ Fig. 24.10). For all three types, the abdominal portion is identical. Pathologic macroscopic grading of the resected sphincter complex (valid for ELAPE and ischioanal APE only) is performed in similar manner graded as the mesorectum and is divided into three categories: extralevator, sphincteric, and intrasphincteric/submucosal planes (▶ Table 24.14 and ▶ Fig. 24.11).[239]

The concept of ELAPE was first introduced by Holm et al[320] in 2007 in which the authors described 28 cases in which the perineal dissection was performed in the prone position and the levators were resected en bloc with the sphincter complex and rectum with gluteus flap reconstruction. This resulted in a more "cylindrical" APE specimen without a waist effect at the level of the anorectal ring. In this initial report, perforation occurred in 1 of the 28 (4%) and CRM involvement in 2 of 28 (7%) cases. A subsequent study by West et al[321] compared 176 ELAPE with 124 standard APE specimens and reported that ELAPE removed more tissue outside of the smooth muscle, resulting in less CRM involvement (20.3 vs. 49.6%; $p < 0.001$) and intraoperative perforation (8.2 vs. 28.2%; $p < 0.001$). However, perineal wound complications were higher in the ELAPE group (38 vs. 20%; $p = 0.019$). Similarly, a systematic review of 14 studies comparing 1,097 patients undergoing ELAPE and 4,147 patients undergoing standard APE reported lower rates of CRM involvement (9.6 vs.

15.4%; $p = 0.022$), inadvertent bowel perforation (4.1 vs. 10.4%; $p = 0.004$), and local recurrence (6.6 vs. 11.9%; $p < 0.001$) after ELAPE.[322] However, a different review did not find any significant differences in CRM involvement or inadvertent bowel perforation between the two techniques.[323] However, one of the criticisms of these studies is the lack of a consistent definition of a "standard APE," which biases the effect toward the null.[319]

Holm et al's[319] initial description of the ELAPE technique positioned the patient in the prone jackknife position, instead of the traditional supine lithotomy position, for the perineal dissection.[320] The authors suggested that the prone positioning offered better exposure during the difficult perineal dissection. However, intraoperative changes in patient positioning may increase operative time and expose the patients to the risk of accidental extubation during transfer. There are also conflicting reports on whether the prone position results in better perineal dissection. de Campos-Lobato et al compared 168 patients undergoing APE (81 prone and 87 lithotomy) and reported similar rates of CRM involvement, bowel perforation, perioperative morbidity, and survival between the two groups.[324] Martijnse et al[325] also reported excellent outcomes for ELAPE in the supine lithotomy positioning compared to conventional APE. There is no clear evidence for the superiority of one position

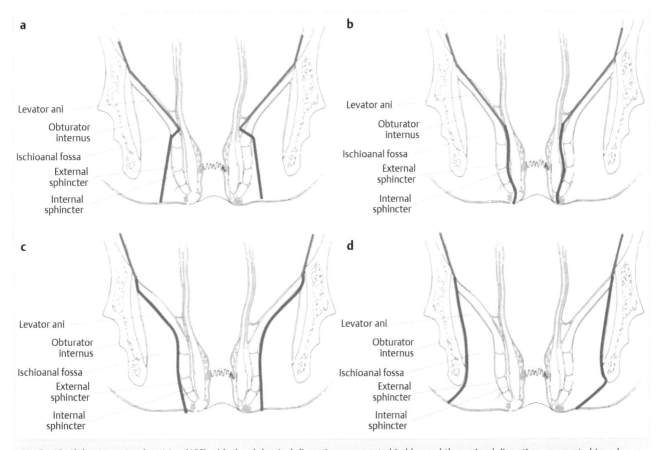

Fig. 24.10 Abdominoperineal excision (APE) with the abdominal dissection represented in blue and the perineal dissection represented in red. **(a)** Traditional APE that comes in at the junction between the distal-most aspect of the TME and the top of the sphincter complex, resulting in a "waist" potentially at the level of the tumor. **(b)** Intersphincteric APE where the perineal dissection is performed between the internal and external sphincter muscles. **(c)** Extralevator APE where the perineal dissection removes the entire sphincter complex and the levators to their lateral origins at the obturator internus. **(d)** Ischioanal APE where the perineal dissection removes the ischioanal fat en bloc for tumors that invade into this space (the skin incision is dependent on the extent of tumor involvement). (Adapted from Holm 2014.[319])

Table 24.14 Pathologic macroscopic grading of the sphincter complex

Grade of sphincter complex	
Extralevator	• Cylindrical specimen without waisting • Levators removed en bloc
Sphincteric plane	• Slight waist effect • No significant defects or perforations
Intrasphincteric/sub- mucosal plane	• Significant waist effect • Perforation or missing areas of muscularis propria

over another, and the choice should be left to the surgeon's discretion. The prone position may allow for better exposure and facilitate teaching, but with no difference in resection quality.

Closure of the perineal wound after APE is also problematic. The incidence of perineal complications can be as high as 50%, especially if patients have received preoperative radiotherapy.[326] ELAPE and ischioanal APE may also increase the risk of wound complications given the larger perineal defect.[321] There are multiple options for perineal wound closure, including primary closure, omental pedicle and musculocutaneous rotational flaps, and biologic mesh repair. The rectus abdominis, gluteus maximus, and gracilis muscles can be used as musculocutaneous flaps, with varying success.[327,328] Reconstruction of the perineum using biologic mesh is a promising option with similar results as flap repair but with less morbidity.[329] At present, there is no standardized approach for perineal wound closure, and the choice should be made based on anatomic factors and available expertise. Primary closure can be safely performed for intersphincteric APE and possibly ELAPE, but with a higher risk of perineal wound dehiscence. Patients undergoing ELAPE or ischioanal APE should be evaluated by a plastic surgeon in the preoperative setting to determine advanced reconstructive options.

Low-Lying Tumors: Restorative Proctectomy with Intersphincteric Dissection versus Abdominoperineal Excision

In the era of multidisciplinary management for rectal cancer and the increased concentration within high-volume specialty institutions, the proportion of patients undergoing sphincter-preserving surgery has been used as a measure of quality. It is therefore tempting to perform a restorative proctectomy with a low colorectal or CAA with or without an intersphincteric resection (ISR) for all patients with a low-lying rectal tumor in the absence of sphincter involvement. The classification of low-lying rectal tumors was best described by Rullier et al[330] (▶ Fig. 24.12), who classified tumors into four types based on location in relation to the anorectal ring and sphincters, as well as the surgical technique required for complete extirpation. Type I lesions (> 1 cm above the anorectal ring) can be treated by TME and CAA. Type II lesions (within 1 cm from the top of the anorectal ring) require a partial ISR. Type III lesions are located within the anal canal but only involve the internal anal sphincter, but require a complete ISR. Finally, type IV lesions invade into the external anal sphincter and require an APE (extent depends on the depth of invasion). In their series of 404 patients, Rullier et al reported no difference in 5-year local recurrence (6, 5, 9, and 17% for types I,

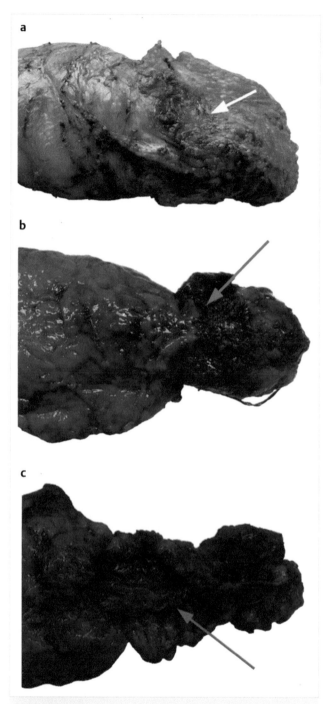

Fig. 24.11 Macroscopic appearance of **(a)** extralevator plane of dissection. The white arrow demonstrates the cut edge of the levators enveloping a cylindrical specimen with no defects in the sphincter muscles or levators. **(b)** Sphincteric plane of dissection. The red arrow demonstrates the "waist" effect by coning at the level of the puborectalis. **(c)** Intrasphincteric/submucosal plane of dissection. The gray arrow demonstrates where the sphincter complex has been entered and the rectal tube has been perforated.

II, III, and IV, respectively; $p = 0.186$) between the four tumor types. However, type IV lesions (i.e., invading into external sphincter and requiring APE) had higher risk of distant recurrence, and worse overall and disease-free survival, which is reflective of other published data. Postoperative morbidity was

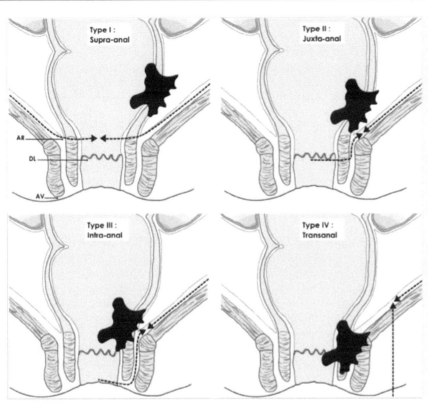

Fig. 24.12 Rullier's classification of low rectal tumors. (Adapted from Rullier et al 2013.[330])

also similar between the four groups. However, functional outcomes were not described in this study.

In these cases, high-resolution MRI is useful as the MERCURY study group demonstrated that intersphincteric plane involvement can be accurately predicted on pretreatment imaging and can help define the feasibility of an ISR or need for an abdominoperineal excision (APE).[331] Neoadjuvant chemoradiation can also downsize the tumor to allow for sphincter preservation, although tumors that do not respond to preoperative therapy should proceed with APE.[332] APE has also been associated with poor quality of life on the basis of the permanent stoma and high perineal wound morbidity. However, there may be patients in whom an APE may be desirable over a low anastomosis. Patients with preexisting poor sphincter function should be counseled against a restorative procedure, as function after a low colorectal or CAA will be worse compared to higher anastomoses,[333] especially in the setting of an ISR and preoperative radiotherapy. Up to 75 to 85% of patients complain of some degree of fecal incontinence after low restorative procedures.[334,335] Parc et al[336] demonstrated that patients with an ultralow LAR or a CAA undergoing preoperative radiation reported more daily bowel movements (4.2 [SD: 3.5] vs. 3.5 [SD: 2.6]; $p = 0.032$) and more urgency (85 vs. 67%; $p = 0.002$) than nonradiated patients. A CAA with an ISR may also have worse anorectal function, as Bretagnol et al showed that patients with an ISR had more fecal incontinence (Wexner score: 10.8 vs. 6.9; $p < 0.001$) and used more antidiarrheals (60 vs. 35%; $p = 0.04$) than patients undergoing a CAA without ISR.[337] However, the degree of incontinence is related to the amount of internal sphincter that is removed.[338] Low anastomoses are also at higher risk of anastomotic leak and proximal diversion should be performed routinely in these patients.

APE may not have as great of an impact on patient-reported outcomes as is generally thought. An analysis of patient-reported outcomes in the NSABP R-04 study administered the FACT-C and EORTC CR38 quality-of-life questionnaires preoperatively and at 1 year to patients undergoing sphincter preservation versus APE. No differences in global quality of life were found between the two groups at 1 year, although APR patients reported less sexual enjoyment, worse micturition symptoms, and body image compared to baseline, whereas patients undergoing sphincter preservation had worse GI function.[339] Multiple other studies have also reported similar global quality of life between APE and low colorectal/coloanal anastomoses with worse sexual function after APE and worse GI function after low restorative procedures.[334,335,340,341] APE may also be associated with better cognitive and social function subscale scores, and less pain and sleep disturbance symptoms.[340] These findings should be used in the decision-making process when deciding between a low restorative procedure and APE.

Lateral Lymph Node Dissection

Nodal involvement of the lateral lymph nodes along the obturator and iliac vessels occurs in approximately 10 to 25% of patients.[342] Lateral lymph node metastases are associated with higher rates of local recurrence and decreased survival.[342,343,344] In the current TNM staging system, involvement of the lateral lymph node chain is considered M1 disease. However, Japanese surgeons routinely perform lateral lymph node dissection, especially for patients with locally advanced rectal cancer or tumors below the peritoneal reflection. Proponents of this approach cite improved local control and improved outcomes.[345,346] Indeed, the lateral compartment is frequently involved in recurrent disease.[347,348] A meta-analysis comparing lateral lymph node dissection with conventional surgery did not find any improvement in 5-year local recurrence rates, disease-free or overall survival between the two groups, but male urinary and sexual dysfunction was higher in the extended lymphadenectomy group.[349] A comparison between patients undergoing TME and adjuvant chemoradiotherapy and those undergoing TME and lateral lymph node dissection did not report any difference in survival between the two groups, but higher rates of locoregional recurrence in patients who did not receive adjuvant chemoradiotherapy were reported.[350] Another study that compared outcomes between the Dutch TME trial and patients undergoing TME and lateral lymph node dissection at the Japanese National Cancer Hospital reported local recurrence rates of 6.9% for patients with extended resection, 5.8% for preoperative short-course radiotherapy + TME, and 12.1% for TME alone. Recurrence in the lateral pelvis was lowest in the radiotherapy + TME group (0.8%) compared to extended resection (2.2%) and TME alone (2.7%).[348] These data suggest that lateral lymph node dissection should not be routinely performed, as the weight of evidence does not support its oncologic benefit. In the case of recurrent disease, however, the lateral compartment should be cleared if clinically involved, as this has been associated with improved outcomes.[351]

24.6.6 Anastomotic Technique

Hand-Sewn versus Stapled

A colorectal anastomosis can be fashioned using a circular stapler or a handsewn anastomosis, with the exception of low anastomosis around the anal canal, in which a handsewn CAA is usually necessary. The invention of circular staplers in the 1970s allowed for more patients to undergo sphincter-preserving surgery, despite early concern of increased local recurrence, which ultimately was not borne out.[352,353,354] A stapled anastomosis can be created using the double-purse string technique or double-stapled technique. There have been few direct comparisons between the two techniques,[355,356] and both appear to be associated with low rates of anastomotic leak. A double-purse-string technique avoids crossing staple lines and the "dog-ears" of the residual transverse staple line, but it requires meticulous application of the distal purse string, which may not always be possible for a low infraperitoneal rectal stump.[357]

There are also no data to support the superiority of a stapled versus a handsewn anastomosis. However, there is much variability in the technical details of handsewn anastomoses in the type of suture used, spacing of bites, continuous versus interrupted, etc., which make comparisons difficult. A Cochrane systematic review and meta-analysis identified nine randomized trials comparing stapled and handsewn anastomoses including a total of 1,233 patients, although all trials were published prior to 1995.[358] The incidence of anastomotic leak was similar between the two groups (OR: 0.80; 95% CI: 0.51–1.24) regardless of supra- or infraperitoneal location. There was some evidence to suggest that stapled anastomosis had a higher incidence of hemorrhage for supraperitoneal location (OR: 6.82; 95% CI: 1.15, 40.41) although this was based on a single trial. There was also a higher incidence of stricture (OR: 3.99; 95% CI: 2.00, 7.96) based on four studies, but duration of follow-up and definition of

stricture differed greatly among these studies. Stapled anastomosis was 7.6 minutes faster on average (95% CI: 2.3, 12.9) to create than the handsewn technique. Other secondary outcomes such as reoperation, length of stay, wound infection, and mortality were equal. These data suggest that the choice of anastomotic technique should be decided based on surgeon comfort and technical ability. However, the decision may be predicated on the location of the anastomosis and therefore familiarity with both techniques is necessary.

Compression

Compression anastomosis represents a third option for colorectal anastomotic creation. Several devices are currently available on market that create a sutureless anastomosis by entrapping the ischemic ends of the divided bowel together with eventual sloughing and release of the compression rings to be excreted with feces. Most of these devices involve a nitinol adaptive compression clip (Compress Anastomosis Clip; CAC, NiTi Surgical Solutions, Netanya, Israel) or ring (Compression Anastomosis Ring, ColonRing or CAR, NiTi Surgical Solutions, Netanya, Israel) depending on the thickness of the bowel. In a review of 1,180 patients undergoing end-to-end anastomosis, the leak rate was 3.2% with the compression ring, with only 4 patients having a technical failure requiring redoing anastomosis.[359] Another postmarketing evaluation with 266 patients reported similar results with 5.3% incidence of anastomotic leak, with 3.1% incidence for low anastomoses.[360] However, when the CAR was directly compared with conventional stapled or handsewn anastomosis, the incidence of anastomotic leak was similar (2.2% for CAR and 3% for conventional).[361] Another meta-analysis comparing all compression anastomosis regardless of device to conventional anastomoses reported similar incidence of anastomotic leak, but earlier return to bowel function and shorter length of stay.[362] However, compression anastomosis was associated with higher incidence of bowel obstruction. It is also commerically available.

Reconstructive Techniques

Several different options are available for reconstruction after LAR. In cases where a significant portion of the rectum remains, functional outcomes are likely to be minimally affected. Lewis et al[363] reported that native rectum has much better function than a neorectum created using a colonic reservoir, with higher capacity, resting anal pressure, and volume required for maximal sphincter inhibition. Similarly, Montesani et al[364] showed that important functional deficits and manometric findings appeared in patients once anastomoses were created in the lower third of the rectum. Therefore, in patients undergoing partial TME and in whom a colorectal anastomosis can be performed in a supraperitoneal location, there does not appear to be any benefit for additional reconstructive techniques beyond a straight end-to-end colorectal anastomosis.

However, in patients undergoing complete TME and in whom a low anastomosis is required, attention must be paid to the method of restoration of intestinal continuity to avoid significant problems with urgency, frequency, and incontinence. It is clear that there is some degree of dysfunctional physiologic response of the anal sphincter in relation to the neorectum. Williamson et al[365] reported that patients undergoing LAR did not recover resting anal pressure or the volume required to elicit maximum rectoanal inhibitory reflex by 1 year after surgery, and these manometric findings correlated with significant deteriorations in urgency and leakage. Fürst et al[366] also demonstrated that neorectal reservoir volume was not the main determinant in functional outcomes after reconstruction post-LAR.

▶ Fig. 24.13 shows the different options that are available for neorectal reconstruction, which include straight coloanal anastomosis (CAA), side-to-end CAA, transverse coloplasty, and colonic J-pouch. Transverse coloplasty was first described by Z'graggen et al[367] in which an 8-cm longitudinal colostomy is made 2 cm proximal to the anvil in the cut edge of the colon. The colostomy is then closed transversely in two layers to create an increased rectal reservoir. At 2 months after surgery, mean stool frequency was reported to be 3.4 in 24 hours, which decreased to 2.1 per 24 hours at 8 months, with no reports of incomplete evacuation. The colonic J-pouch was described in 1986 by Parc et al[368] and Lazorthes et al[369] in which a colonic

reservoir is created in J-configuration with a common channel of at least 6 to 8 cm. Studies have shown that the maximal benefit of the colonic J-pouch is within the first year, but by 2 to 3 years after surgery the functional outcomes between a straight CAA and a colonic J-pouch were less profound but still evident.[370,371] Hüttner et al[372] performed a systematic review and meta-analysis of all randomized trials comparing the different reconstructive options. The colonic J-pouch had better continence, less frequency, and less use of antidiarrheal medications when compared to straight CAA in the early (< 8 months) and intermediate (8–18 months) postoperative periods, although the differences between the two techniques were less pronounced in the later periods. Transverse coloplasty and side-to-end CAA had similar functional outcomes compared to colonic J-pouch. Importantly, however, both transverse coloplasty (OR: 2.45; 95% CI: 1.00–5.22) and straight coloanal anastomosis (OR: 2.49; 95% CI: 1.03–5.17) were at higher risk of anastomotic leak compared to colonic J-pouch, whereas side-to-end CAA showed no difference (OR: 1.03; 95% CI: 0.38–2.25). These data suggest that the formation of a colonic J-pouch or a side-to-end CAA is the preferred method of neorectum reconstruction after LAR, as

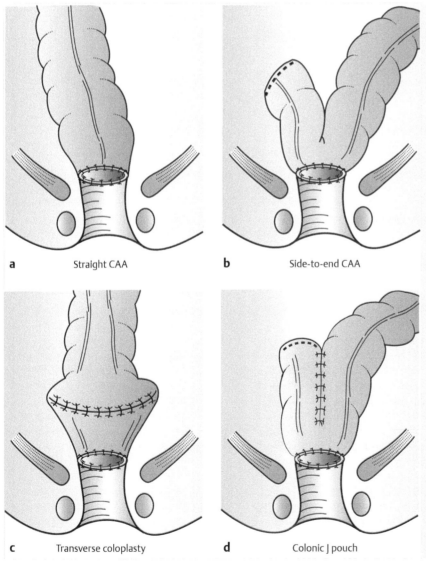

Fig. 24.13 Reconstructive options after low anterior resection. **(a)** Straight coloanal anastomosis. **(b)** Side-to-end coloanal anastomosis. **(c)** Transverse coloplasty. **(d)** Colonic J-pouch. (Adapted from Hüttner et al 2015.[372])

a   Straight CAA

b   Side-to-end CAA

c   Transverse coloplasty

d   Colonic J pouch

long as there is enough length on the mobilized colon and the pelvis is large enough to admit the reservoir.

Defunctioning Stoma

The decision to form a protective stoma has been a matter of debate for many years. Proximal diversion may reduce the impact of anastomotic leak and pelvic sepsis, but it requires a second operation and is associated with high morbidity. Analysis of the data suggests that a defunctioning stoma should be selectively used in patients undergoing restorative proctectomy. A meta-analysis of 4 randomized trials and 21 nonrandomized studies that included 11,429 patients reported a lower clinical anastomotic leak rate (relative risk [RR]: 0.39; 95% CI: 0.23–0.66) and lower reoperation rate (RR: 0.29; 95% CI: 0.16–0.53) for patients who underwent a diverting stoma.[373] These effect estimates were similar in the nonrandomized studies. Another recent meta-analysis that included more recent studies reported similar conclusions.[374] It is recommended to routinely create a diverting loop ileostomy after primary anastomosis for patients with a low pelvic anastomosis after neoadjuvant radiotherapy, intraoperative anastomotic complications, and those with risk factors for poor wound healing. It should be strongly considered for patients who may not tolerate the physiologic sequelae of an anastomotic leak or those in whom the potential impact of delaying adjuvant systemic therapy outweighs the potential morbidity of a stoma. If proximal diversion is undertaken, a loop ileostomy is preferred over a loop colostomy due to less stoma prolapse and ease of closure.[373] However, loop ileostomies are associated with an important risk of dehydration and subsequent readmission. Messaris et al reported that 16.1% of patients with a loop ileostomy were readmitted within 60 days, of which the indication for readmission was dehydration in 43%.[375] Another study reported that patients with a diverting ileostomy were at significantly higher risk of a postoperative hospital-based acute encounter compared to patients without (OR: 2.28; 95% CI: 2.15–2.42), mostly due to infection, renal failure, or dehydration.[376] Patient education for stoma management is especially important and may improve stoma proficiency and quality of life, and decrease length of stay, readmissions, and costs.[377,378,379] Patients should also be counseled about the risk of stoma nonclosure, which occurs in 10 to 24% of cases.[380,381] Risk factors for permanent stoma after "temporary" loop ileostomy include development of metastatic disease, postoperative complications, and comorbid status.[380,381,382]

All patients in whom a temporary or permanent stoma may be requred should be preoperatively marked to ensure optimal placement. Complications after stoma are common, occurring in approximately one-third of patients, and poor stoma placement can cause significant problems such as skin irritation, poor appliance fitting, and pain.[383,384] Preoperative evaluation by an enterostomal therapist to determine optimal stoma site and provide education reduces adverse outcomes and improves patients' satisfaction and quality of life related to their ostomy.[385,386] Furthermore, intensive preoperative stoma teaching has been shown in a randomized trial to improve time to stoma proficiency, decrease complications, hospital stay, unplanned stoma-relative interventions, and costs.[387] Detailed guidelines have been jointly published by the ASCRS and the Wound Ostomy Continence Nurses Society.[388]

Pelvic Drainage

The use of prophylactic closed-suction pelvic drains has been the subject of much controversy. Advocates for their use suggest that it allows for early detection of anastomotic complications before deterioration of physiologic status and may avoid the need for operative intervention by controlling sepsis, whereas opponents argue that they cause additional complications and delay discharge. Multiple randomized trials have investigated the question of drainage versus no drainage, and meta-analyses of these trials have failed to demonstrate a benefit, although often intra- and extraperitoneal colorectal anastomoses were combined.[389] No difference was found in the incidence of anastomotic leakage when randomized trials of drain placement after extraperitoneal anastomoses only were meta-analyzed, although there was a benefit when observational studies were included.[390] The largest trial was performed by the French Research Group of Rectal Cancer Surgery (GRECCAR) in which 494 patients with infraperitoneal anastomosis after proctectomy for rectal cancer were randomly assigned to drainage versus no drainage.[391] The incidence of protective stoma and neoadjuvant radiotherapy was similar between the two groups. The main results of this trial reported no difference in the incidence of pelvic sepsis (16.1% drain vs. 18.0% no drain; $p = 0.58$), along with no difference in the time to diagnosis of pelvic sepsis. Secondary endpoints were also similar, which included reintervention, postoperative morbidity and mortality, and length of stay after surgery. Based on these data, there does not appear to be any clinically important benefit for pelvic drainage; however, the data also suggest that they do not appear to cause harm.

Fluorescence Angiography

Fluorescence angiography is a newer method to assess the vascular supply of the conduit. Sterile indocyanine green (ICG), which is a hydrophilic molecule that binds mainly to plasma proteins and remains intravascular for 2 to 5 minutes, is injected and then excited using polarized infrared light (in the 800-nm spectrum). The infrared light can be a stand-alone system such as the PINPOINT or SPY Elite or integrated within the laparoscopic camera (1588 AIM, Stryker, La Jolla, CA). Selective excitation of the plasma protein-bound ICG is thus a surrogate for blood flow, and is used to assess the microcirculation of the cut edge of the colon to be used for anastomosis (► Fig. 24.14). Noncomparative studies report that the use of ICG may affect surgical technique and result in a low rate of anastomotic leak. Watanabe et al demonstrated that 20% of patients had minimal or no perfusion of the rectosigmoid junction once the sigmoid branch of the IMA was divided (i.e., flow only through the marginal artery) using ICG; however, there was no difference in anastomotic leak rates based on perfusion pattern.[392] Gröne et al[393] reported a change in surgical decision making in 28% of cases of low rectal or CAA with ICG assessment. The Perfusion Assessment in Laparoscopic Left-Sided/Anterior Resection (PILLAR) II multi-institutional study reported that perfusion assessment altered the surgical plan in 11 of 139 patients, including 9 patients in whom the proximal transection margin was changed and 1 patient in whom the anastomosis was refashioned due to poor blood supply. Overall, the anastomotic leak

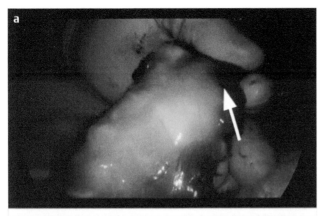

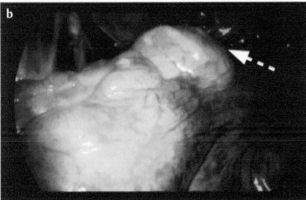

Fig. 24.14 Intraoperative assessment of microcirculation of the colonic conduit using fluorescence angiography with indocyanine green. **(a)** The white arrow demonstrates the demarcation where the marginal artery has been divided. **(b)** The dashed white arrow demonstrates the verification of the vascular supply up to the anvil.

rate was 1.4% (2/139), with none occurring in the 11 patients whose surgical plan was altered with perfusion assessment.[394] A randomized trial, PILLAR III, is currently ongoing.[395]

Until the results of PILLAR III are published, there is no level I evidence for immunofluorescence perfusion assessment. There have been few comparative studies, which have reported equivocal results. Kim et al[396] compared 123 patients undergoing robotic LAR with ICG versus 313 without. There were 13 patients in the ICG group that required a change in surgical decision making due to ICG, and a composite outcome of leak, abscess, and stricture was lower in the ICG group (0.8 vs. 5.3%; p = 0.031). Kudszus et al[397] showed a trend toward fewer reoperations secondary to anastomotic leak in patients undergoing colorectal surgery that underwent ICG perfusion assessment (2.5 vs. 7.5%; p = 0.079), although the difference was not statistically significant, and it is unclear how many of the patients underwent a low colorectal anastomosis. Finally, Kin et al[398] matched 173 patients undergoing left-sided or rectal resections based on age, gender, level of anastomosis, neoadjuvant pelvic radiotherapy, and proximal diversion. In this study, 4.6% of patients in the ICG group underwent additional colon resection based on the appearance on immunofluorescence perfusion assessment, but fluorescence angiography did not significantly affect the anastomotic leak rate (OR: 1.3; 95% CI: 0.5–3.2). The conclusions that can be made based on these data are limited,

and the utility of immunofluorescence angiography has yet to be clearly defined.

Endoluminal Stenting for Obstructing Tumors

Patients who present with tumor-related emergencies have increased mortality and worse prognosis.[399,400] In the absence of life-threatening bleeding or perforation, patients who present with obstructing lesions may be considered for an endoluminal stent either as a bridge to surgery or for palliation. Theoretically, endoluminal stent placement allows for colonic decompression with subsequent one-stage resection and primary anastomosis. Much of the available data combined left-sided colonic and rectal obstructions. The Dutch Stent-In 2 trial randomly assigned 98 patients with obstructing left-sided colorectal cancer to receive colonic stenting as a bridge to surgery or emergency surgery.[401] The trial had to be prematurely terminated before the targeted sample size of 120 patients due to the increase in morbidity in the colonic stenting arm. The success rate of stenting (defined as successful stent placement and resolution of obstruction) was 70%, with 12.7% of patients experiencing a procedure- or stent-related perforation. At final analysis, there were no differences in morbidity or mortality, and stoma rates in the two arms were similar (stent 57.4 vs. surgery 66.6%; p = 0.35). There was no difference in quality-of-life outcomes between the two arms at 6 months. The authors concluded that stenting offered no clinical advantage over emergency surgery. Further analysis of the 58 patients with malignant obstructions in the Stent-In 2 trial (26 stent, 32 surgery) demonstrated a higher risk of recurrence for patients in the stent arm, with worse 4-year disease-free survival in the stent arm (30 vs. 49%; p = 0.007), although there was no difference in disease-specific survival (66 vs. 87%; p = 0.099). In particular, patients with tumor perforation as a result of stenting had significantly worse outcomes. While this analysis was limited by the small sample size, these data are concerning for oncologic outcomes for stented patients.[402] A Cochrane meta-analysis of five randomized trials including 208 patients reported an overall incidence of successful stent insertion of 86.02%, but a higher incidence of clinical relief of obstruction in the emergency surgery group compared to stenting (OR: 0.06; 95% CI: 0.01–0.32).[403] Overall morbidity showed no difference between the two groups (OR: 0.79; 95% CI: 0.47–1.34).

The decision to perform endoluminal stenting versus emergency surgery in patients with obstructing rectal cancer is dependent on the patient's physiologic status, location of the tumor, presence of distant metastases, and whether the tumor is resectable upfront. Low rectal tumors may not be appropriate for stenting as impingement of the stent onto the anal sphincter complex can cause significant tenesmus and pain. Furthermore, the length of bowel wall that is involved by the endoluminal stent often needs to be resected, which may preclude sphincter preservation if an adequate distal cuff cannot be preserved. Patients with malignant rectal obstructions often have locally advanced tumors, which should be ideally treated with multimodal neoadjuvant therapy as outlined earlier. There are little to no data to support the use of neoadjuvant therapy in the setting of a stented lesion. A diverting loop ostomy is likely to be a more appropriate treatment option in these cases. The improved survival of patients with metastatic disease may also play an important role in deciding whether to perform an upfront diversion, as stent migration rates are high.

24.7 Adjuvant Therapy

24.7.1 Postoperative Chemotherapy

The administration of postoperative adjuvant chemotherapy in patients who received neoadjuvant chemoradiation is controversial. NCCN guidelines recommends adjuvant therapy for all patients with stage II and III rectal cancer following neoadjuvant chemoradiation and surgery if they did not receive neoadjuvant chemotherapy regardless of the final pathologic results. A Cochrane review of 21 randomized trials comparing adjuvant fluoropyrimidine-based chemotherapy versus observation after potentially curative rectal cancer surgery reported significant benefit for disease-free (HR: 0.75; 95% CI: 0.68–0.83) and overall (HR: 0.83; 95% CI: 0.76–0.91) survival in patients treated with adjuvant therapy.[404] However, no modern agents were studied, and only one of the included trials included routine preoperative chemoradiation. Accordingly, the majority of patients in the United States receive adjuvant chemotherapy after neoadjuvant chemoradiation.[115] However, data to support this approach in the era of neoadjuvant therapy are lacking, as none of the four randomized trials[118,405,406,407] that have directly investigated this issue were able to demonstrate a statistically significant benefit for adjuvant chemotherapy.[408]

The EORTC 22921 trial (described earlier) did not demonstrate a difference in disease-free or overall survival at 5 or 10 years in patients who received additional four cycles of 5-FU/LV versus observation alone after preoperative radiation with or without concurrent chemotherapy.[93,118] A subgroup analysis of patients in this trial that had R0 resection showed that 5-year disease-free and overall survival was improved for patients who were downstaged to ypT0–2 compared to those with ypT3–4,[409] although this effect was no longer significant at 10-year follow-up.[93] Only 43% of patients in this trial assigned to the adjuvant therapy arms completed the full course. Another study from 10 Korean institutions did not demonstrate an improvement in relapse-free survival for adjuvant chemotherapy patients with ypT0–2N0, although there was a significant interaction with tumor regression grade.[410] It is unclear from these data whether tumor response is predictive of response to adjuvant chemotherapy or merely a prognostic indicator.[411]

The Italian I-CNR-RT trial randomly assigned 655 patients with locally advanced rectal cancer (T3–4, any N) treated with neoadjuvant chemoradiation and surgery to 6 cycles of 5-FU/LV or observation.[405] There were no differences in disease-free and overall (69 vs. 70%) survival between the two arms, although 28% of patients assigned to the adjuvant chemotherapy arm did not receive the intervention. A subgroup analysis of patients with persistent node-positive disease also did not demonstrate any difference in overall survival (52 vs. 51%).

The United Kingdom Chronicle trial compared 18 weeks of adjuvant capecitabine/oxaliplatin versus observation in patients undergoing long-course chemoradiation and curative resection.[407] The trial was closed prematurely due to poor accrual, as only 113 were randomly assigned to one of the two groups out of a planned 390 for each arm. This trial did not demonstrate any difference in disease-free or overall survival due to the limited sample size, but compliance was poor. While 98% in the treatment arm started adjuvant chemotherapy, 39% had to have dose reductions and only 48% completed all six cycles.

The PROCTOR-SCRIPT trial randomly assigned 437 patients with stage II/III rectal cancer who underwent preoperative radiotherapy or chemoradiotherapy and TME to either adjuvant therapy with 5-FU/LV (PROCTOR) or capecitabine (SCRIPT).[406] Overall survival at 5 years did not demonstrate any advantage for patients in the adjuvant chemotherapy arm (80 vs. 79%), nor was there any difference in effect of adjuvant chemotherapy after preoperative short-course radiotherapy or long-course chemoradiation. This trial did close early because of poor accrual.

An individual patient data meta-analysis of these four trials that included 1,196 patients with stage II or III rectal cancer that underwent R0 resection showed no significant difference in disease-free (HR: 0.91; 95% CI: 0.77–1.07) or overall (HR: 0.97; 95% CI: 0.81–1.17) survival between patients who received adjuvant chemotherapy versus observation alone.[412] Subgroup analysis did demonstrate a disease-free survival advantage for patients undergoing adjuvant therapy with tumors 10 to 15 cm from the anal verge (HR: 0.59; 95% CI: 0.40–0.85) due to fewer distant metastases (HR: 0.61; 95% CI: 0.40–0.94). No differences were reported in the other subgroups, including stage II vs. III, LAR vs. APR, or short-course radiotherapy vs. long-course (chemo)radiation. Another meta-analysis that also included nonrandomized studies reported an improvement in 5-year disease-free (OR: 0.71; 95% CI: 0.60–0.83) and overall (OR: 0.64; 95% CI: 0.46–0.88) survival for patients receiving adjuvant therapy.[413] However, the effect magnitude was much stronger in the nonrandomized data. Data from randomized data only did not demonstrate a difference for overall survival (OR: 0.93; 95% CI: 0.64–1.34), but disease-free survival was higher (OR: 0.81; 95% CI: 0.66–0.99). As such, this meta-analysis should be interpreted with caution. Finally, an analysis of the National Cancer Database showed that adjuvant therapy was associated with improved overall survival in patients undergoing adjuvant chemotherapy after neoadjuvant therapy and curative resection for both node-negative and node-positive rectal cancer.[414]

The addition of newer chemotherapeutic agents in adjuvant therapy regimens may provide a benefit over fluoropyrimidine-based regimens alone. The advanced rectal cancer after preoperative chemoradiotherapy (ADORE) trial randomized 321 patients who underwent neoadjuvant therapy and surgery to adjuvant FOLFOX or 5-FU/LV. Three-year disease-free survival was higher in the FOLFOX arm (71.6 vs. 62.9%; $p = 0.047$), with no difference in toxicity between the two arms.[415] The German CAO/ARO/AIO-04 trial also found an improvement in 3-year disease-free survival when oxaliplatin was added to conventional preoperative fluoropyrimidine-based chemoradiation and adjuvant chemotherapy (75.9 vs. 71.2%; $p = 0.03$), also with no difference in chemotherapy-related toxicity.[416]

Despite equivocal data, adjuvant chemotherapy for patients who received neoadjuvant (chemo)radiation remains the standard of care. Current NCCN guidelines recommend FOLFOX or capecitabine/oxaliplatin as first-line therapy, although 5-FU/LV or capecitabine alone may be appropriate if a good response with neoadjuvant therapy with these agents were obtained. A 4-month course with adjuvant FOLFOX is adequate if long-course neoadjuvant chemoradiation was given. If induction chemotherapy was given, adjuvant therapy can be omitted. Patients undergoing upfront surgery who are upstaged to node-positive disease or have high-risk features on final surgical pathology should be considered for adjuvant chemoradiation or a full 6-month course of adjuvant chemotherapy. Adjuvant therapy should begin as soon as the patient is medically able to derive maximum benefit. A large systematic review and meta-analysis including over 15,000 patients reported that each 4-week delay in adjuvant therapy results in a 14% decrease in overall survival.[417]

Postoperative Chemoradiation

Radiotherapy delivered in the neoadjuvant setting has several major advantages. As described earlier, two seminal randomized trials have demonstrated the superiority of neoadjuvant versus adjuvant chemoradiation for stage II/III rectal cancer in terms of local control and disease-free survival.[6,91] Neoadjuvant radiotherapy may also downstage or downsize the tumor to facilitate sphincter preservation. Surgery-naïve tissues are also more sensitive to radiotherapy due to improved tissue vascularization and oxygenation. Finally, preoperative therapy lowers the risk of potential radiation-induced injury to the small bowel that often falls into the pelvis after surgery, as well as avoids radiation to the neorectum with its subsequent functional impairments. These advantages are weighed against the possibility of overtreatment of tumors that are clinically overstaged. Improvements in locoregional staging have lowered, but not eliminated, this risk.

However, adjuvant chemoradiation has a role for select patients. Patients with clinical stage I tumors who undergo upfront surgery and are upstaged to stage II or III, or patients who undergo upfront surgery for preoperative low-risk T3N0 tumors who have a positive CRM, incomplete TME, or residual disease after surgery should be considered for postoperative chemoradiation to reduce the risk of locoregional recurrence and distant metastasis. Two early trials established the benefits of adjuvant therapy over observation alone after curative resection of rectal cancer. The Gastrointestinal Tumor Study Group (GTSG) 7175 trial randomly assigned 227 patients with Dukes' B2 and C rectal cancer to observation, postoperative radiotherapy only, postoperative chemotherapy only, or postoperative chemoradiation.[418,419] Relapse-free and overall survival after a median 46-month follow-up was significantly higher in the chemoradiotherapy group compared to surgery alone. This study utilized older chemotherapy agents that are no longer in use, but still established the benefits of fluoropyrimidine-based chemoradiation. The NSABP R-01 randomly assigned 555 patients with Dukes' B and C rectal cancer to surgery alone, surgery + chemotherapy, or surgery + radiotherapy.[420] Disease-free survival was higher in the adjuvant chemotherapy group, but local recurrence was lowest in the radiotherapy arm. Overall survival was equal in all three arms. Modern therapy delivered in the adjuvant setting usually consists of fluoropyrimidine-based sandwich therapy (chemotherapy, then chemoradiation, and then chemotherapy).[421,422,423]

There may be certain tumors with favorable characteristics for which adjuvant chemoradiotherapy may not be necessary. There are data to suggest that patients with T3N0 may benefit from adjuvant chemotherapy alone instead of adjuvant chemoradiation if neoadjuvant therapy was not given. A pooled analysis of 3,791 patients by Gunderson et al[142] from five randomized trials comparing different adjuvant chemotherapy regimens (without neoadjuvant therapy) showed that patients with T3N0 disease undergoing surgery and adjuvant chemotherapy alone had favorable 5-year overall survival rates compared to patients undergoing adjuvant chemoradiation (84 vs. 74% and 76% for the INT 0114 and NCCTG/NSABP data). For T1–2N1, the magnitude of effects was also similar in the two groups (84 vs. 82% and 83%). For patients in the moderately high-risk (T1–2N2, T3N1, T4N0) and high-risk (T3N2, T4N1, T4N2) groups, overall and disease-free survival was inferior in the surgery + chemotherapy compared to the surgery + chemoradiation arms. However, these trials mostly used chemotherapeutic agents that are no longer in use and did not employ surgery according to TME principles. The Dutch TME trial showed that 12-year local recurrence rate for the surgery-only arm was 8% for patients with T3–4N0 tumors with TME surgery, compared to 9 to 13% for patients with T3–4N0 in the pooled analysis without TME surgery (which includes adjuvant chemotherapy or chemoradiation).[142,143] Furthermore, the MERCURY study group demonstrated that tumors with good prognostic features on preoperative MRI can forego radiotherapy both pre- and postoperatively. Patients with CRM greater than 1 mm, T1–3b (< 5 mm of extramural depth of invasion for T3 tumors), absence of extramural vascular invasion, and any N stage can undergo upfront surgery (with selective adjuvant chemotherapy for node-positive tumors on final pathology) without adjuvant chemoradiation with a 2.3% local recurrence rate, and 5-year disease-free and overall survival of 76 to 95% and 65 to 81%, respectively. These results compare more than favorably to the Gunderson et al pooled analysis,[142] Dutch TME trial,[119,143] and CR07[120] data. These data suggest that adjuvant chemoradiation can be safely omitted in patients with favorable low-risk tumors who did not receive neoadjuvant therapy, but this approach should only be performed in the context of a multidisciplinary tumor board discussion and close surveillance and/or a clinical trial.

Adjuvant chemoradiation may also be difficult for patients to tolerate and is also associated with important functional impairments. Chemoradiation delivered in the neoadjuvant setting is associated with fewer adverse events and better compliance compared to the adjuvant setting.[424] Radiating the neorectum may also worsen anorectal function. Data from 10-year median follow-up study of patients receiving adjuvant (chemo)radiation showed that 39% had poor functional outcomes, including urgency (36%), increased frequency (26%), and incontinence (25% needing to wear a pad).[425] Kollmorgen et al[426] compared patients who received adjuvant chemoradiation after anterior resection for rectal cancer versus those with surgery only with a minimum of 2-year follow-up. Patients undergoing adjuvant chemoradiotherapy had more bowel movements per day (median 7 vs. 2; p < 0.001), clustering, nighttime movements, urgency, and incontinence (41 vs. 10% wore a pad; p < 0.001) compared to the patients who did not receive radiotherapy. Adjuvant chemoradiation has also been shown to have a larger impact on bowel function compared to neoadjuvant therapy. Frykholm et al[427] reported data on functional outcomes in a randomized trial comparing preoperative short-course ($n = 255$) versus postoperative long-course ($n = 127$) radiotherapy after rectal cancer resection with a minimum follow-up of 5 years. Patients in the adjuvant radiotherapy arm had a significantly higher incidence of small bowel obstruction (11 vs. 5%; $p = 0.05$) and overall chronic radiation-induced complications (41 vs. 20%; $p = 0.017$). The German Rectal Cancer Study Group also showed that postoperative chemoradiotherapy had more long-term grade 3 or 4 adverse events (24 vs. 14%; $p = 0.01$), including a higher incidence of anastomotic strictures (12 vs. 4%; $p = 0.003$).[6] The use of a colonic J-pouch may improve function after radiation.[428] Adjuvant radiotherapy carries a significant risk of radiation-induced injury to the small bowel, as they tend to fall into the pelvis postsurgery and be exposed to the radiation fields. One study showed that the probability of developing treatment-induced bowel injury at 5 years was 19%.[429] However, radiation delivered in the neoadjuvant setting is also associated with significant risk of chronic bowel injury as per long-term follow-up data of the Swedish and Dutch trials.[124,125,430] Sexual function can also be significantly affected postradiation, although the maximal negative effect was seen at 8 months and improved thereafter.[431] Patients must be informed of both the acute and chronic adverse events associated with radiotherapy, especially given the more recent data questioning its use in the adjuvant setting.

Changes in the Delivery of Perioperative Therapy

The perioperative delivery of (chemo)radiation has undergone a dramatic paradigm shift since the 1990s. Traditionally, chemoradiation was administered in the adjuvant setting, which has the advantage of treatment according to final pathologic staging and the avoidance of overtreatment, but at the significant cost of irradiating the neorectum with its subsequent consequences on anorectal function. The Swedish Rectal Cancer Trial was the first to definitively demonstrate the superiority of neoadjuvant delivery of radiotherapy, despite the low proportion of patients undergoing TME surgery in this study.[7] The subsequent Dutch TME trial and MRC CR07 provided evidence of the superiority of preoperative radiotherapy even with TME surgery.[119,120] The German Rectal Cancer Study Group and NSABP R-03 further demonstrated the superiority of neoadjuvant administration of long-course chemoradiation over adjuvant delivery.[6,91] These seminal studies have shifted delivery of (chemo)radiotherapy from the adjuvant to the neoadjuvant setting, although the debate regarding preoperative short-course radiotherapy versus long-course chemoradiation has yet to be resolved. While these therapies have all consistently demonstrated a 50% decrease in local recurrence rates over the control intervention, this benefit comes with the cost of significant short- and long-term adverse events due to chemo- and radiotherapy toxicity. There are also a certain proportion of patients who will be overtreated based on preoperative staging, but advances

in imaging modalities, especially MRI, will more accurately define patients who will benefit from neoadjuvant therapy. Data from the MERCURY study group have shown that MRI characteristics can help identify patients in whom radiotherapy may not be required, regardless of timing of delivery.[54,69,331] As these technologies continue to refine and more data become available, the indications for radiotherapy will become more selective, thus minimizing the number of patients exposed to unnecessary harm and maximizing delivery to those who will benefit the most. Genetic markers that predict response to neoadjuvant chemoradiation will further allow the clinician to deliver individualized treatment plans to reduce morbidity and optimize outcomes.[432,433,434]

24.7.2 Measuring Quality

Even in the era of multidisciplinary rectal cancer care, good surgical technique remains paramount to ensure optimal oncologic outcomes. As discussed earlier, surgeons should strive for a TME specimen that has no breaches in the mesorectal fascia (complete mesorectum grade), negative circumferential, and DRM. Pathologic processing of the surgical specimen plays a key role in quality assessment. Pathology reports should include all factors of prognostic importance, including macroscopic evaluation of the mesorectum quality, status of the circumferential margin, lymph node harvest, tumor regression (in cases where neoadjuvant therapy was delivered), histological classification, lymphovascular and perineural invasion, and tumor staging. This report should be reviewed and discussed at the multidisciplinary tumor board to determine optimal adjuvant treatment and measure the quality of surgery. These data may also be used to assess the quality of locoregional staging modalities. For example, the accuracy of nodal involvement on preoperative MRI can be compared to final pathology. Training programs or quality improvement programs can be targeted at centers or individuals based on these pathologic data. Standardization of locoregional staging, surgery, and pathologic assessment has been shown to improve cancer outcomes. The Norwegian Rectal Cancer Project was launched in 1993 as a national training program for surgeons and pathologists on surgery according to TME principles and pathologic reporting in order to improve rectal cancer outcomes.[435] This initiative was established as a multidisciplinary effort from the onset—data on surgical quality and reporting were continuously fed back to the clinicians and institutions. As a result, the rate of TME surgery increased and local recurrence decreased from 12 to 6%. Similar national programs were established in Sweden, Denmark, and the United Kingdom with similar results.[408,436,437] A comparable program does not exist in the United States, despite a wide variability in the care delivery and outcomes.[74,87,304] ACS CoC NAPRC was designed to fill this void and improve outcomes in the USA.

24.8 Surveillance

The goal of posttreatment surveillance is to detect locoregional or metastatic recurrences that may be resectable for cure, as well as detect metachronous neoplasms. The surveillance recommendations from the NCCN and the American Society of

Clinical Oncology (ASCO) and Cancer Care Ontario (CCO)[438] are shown in ► Table 24.15. Both guidelines recommend intensive surveillance strategies for the first 5 years. An analysis of 20,898 patients from 18 randomized trials on adjuvant therapy demonstrated that the risk of treatment failure was highest between years 1 and 3 during surveillance.[439] This risk continued to risk until year 4 for patients with stage III disease, after which time the risk of recurrence was similar to that of stage II patients. After 5 years, the recurrence rate per year did not exceed 1.5%, regardless of disease stage. In another study involving 4,023 patients, only 4.3% of the recurrences occurred after 5 years.[440] Hepatic or pulmonary metastases were equally common in patients with rectal cancer.

Intensive surveillance strategies include a combination of history and physical examination, serum CEA levels, endoscopy, and imaging studies. Multiple randomized trials have shown that an intensive surveillance strategy detects more recurrences that can be treated with curative intent, but with little to no difference in overall or cancer-specific survival. The Follow-up After Colorectal Surgery (FACS) trial randomly assigned 1,202 patients to four groups: CEA only, CT only, CEA+CT, or minimum follow-up.[441] The absolute difference in the intensive follow-up groups compared to minimum follow-up ranged from 4.3 to 5.7% (overall $p = 0.02$), but with no difference in number of deaths from any cause (difference between intensive and minimum follow-up: 2.3%; 95% CI: –2.6, 7.1) or disease-specific colorectal cancer deaths (difference 1.1%; 95% CI: –2.7, 5.0). The CEAwatch trial from the Netherlands randomized 3,223 patients to an intensive surveillance program including serum CEA levels every 2 months with imaging in cases of two consecutive CEA rises versus standard care consisting of history and physical, liver ultrasound, chest X-ray, and serum CEA every 6 months for the first 3 years, then annually thereafter.[442] Similar to the FACS study, the proportion of patients who recurred that underwent curative intent therapy was higher in the intensive surveillance group (OR: 2.84; 95% CI: 1.38–5.86), as was the time to diagnosis of recurrence (HR: 1.45; 95% CI: 1.08–1.95). Survival outcomes were not reported in this trial. These results were mirrored in a Cochrane meta-analysis of 15 studies including 5,403 patients, which demonstrated a higher incidence of salvage surgery with curative intent (RR: 1.98; 95% CI: 1.53–2.56)

and fewer symptomatic recurrences (RR: 0.59; 95% CI: 0.41–0.86) for intensive surveillance, but no difference in overall (HR: 0.90; 95% CI: 0.78–1.02) or relapse-free (HR: 1.03; 95% CI: 0.90–1.18) survival.[443] Furthermore, an intensive surveillance strategy should only be considered for patients who may be candidates for further treatment in case of a locoregional recurrence or distant metastasis. Patients who are unwilling or medically unable to tolerate therapy can undergo symptomatic surveillance.

The purpose of surveillance colonoscopy is to detect metachronous lesions, rather than detecting local recurrence. Patients with a history of colorectal cancer have an increased risk of developing second cancers, especially in the first 2 years following treatment.[444] The proximal colon is at highest risk of metachronous cancers.[445] The value of routine proctoscopy to evaluate for anastomotic recurrence is unclear. Pelvic recurrences can usually be felt by DRE and true anastomotic recurrence is uncommon,[446] thus limiting the value of endoluminal evaluation of the anastomosis.[447] The 2015 update to the NCCN rectal cancer guidelines has removed routine surveillance proctoscopy, except for patients who have undergone transanal local excision. However, other society guidelines continue to recommend proctoscopy.

In the case of alarming symptoms or an increasing serum CEA, a complete history and physical, imaging studies, and endoscopic evaluation should be performed. Both the trend and the absolute serum CEA value should be considered, as well as the preoperative value. When CEA levels rise after initial normalization following primary curative treatment, this should be considered an ominous sign and worthy of urgent investigation. However, not all tumors produce CEA and it should not be the only modality used during surveillance. A Cochrane meta-analysis reported that the sensitivity of a CEA cutoff of 2.5 μg/L had a pooled sensitivity of 82% (95% CI: 78–86) and specificity of 80% (95% CI: 59–92).[448] A threshold of 10 μg/L had a pooled sensitivity of 68% (95% CI: 53–79) and specificity of 97% (95% CI: 90–99). A lower CEA threshold will improve sensitivity at the expense of a high number of false positives. However, levels above 15 to 35 μ/L almost always represent true positives.[449] Treatment should not be initiated in the setting of an elevated CEA without documented evidence of disease. A PET/CT in this setting may be useful, as a systematic review of the utility of PET/CT for elevated CEA reported a pooled sensitivity of 94.1%

Table 24.15 Surveillance strategies after curative resection of rectal cancer

The National Comprehensive Cancer Network (NCCN) guidelines[a]	American Society of Clinical Oncology (ASCO) and Cancer Care Ontario (CCO)[438]
• History and physical examination every 3–6 mo for 2 y, then every 6 mo for a total of 5 y • CEA every 3–6 mo for 2 y, then every 6 mo for a total of 5 y • Proctoscopy (with EUS or MRI) every 3–6 mo for the first 2 y, then every 6 mo for a total of 5 y; patients with transanal excision only • Chest and abdominal/pelvic CT every 3–6 mo for 2 y, then every 6–12 mo for a total of 5 y • Complete colonoscopy at 1 y except if no preoperative colonoscopy due to obstructing lesion, colonoscopy in 3–6 mo • If advanced adenoma, repeat in 1 y • If no advanced adenoma, repeat in 3 y, then every 5 y • PET scan not routinely recommended	• History, physical examination, and CEA every 3–6 mo for 5 y • Rectosigmoidoscopy every 6 mo for 2–5 y for patients who did not receive pelvic radiation • Chest and abdominal/pelvic CT annually for 3 y. Consider imaging every 6–12 mo for the first 3 y for high-risk patients. • Complete colonoscopy 1 y after initial surgery. If a complete colonoscopy was not performed prior to surgery, it should be done after completion of adjuvant therapy. If normal, repeat at 5 y. • Any new or persistent symptoms suggestive of a recurrence • PET scan not routinely recommended

[a]Source: http://www.nccn.org
Abbreviations: CEA, carcinoembryonic antigen; CT, computed tomography; EUS, endorectal ultrasound; MRI, magnetic resonance imaging; PET, positron emission tomography.

(95% CI: 89.4–97.1) and specificity of 77.2% (95% CI: 66.4–85.9).[450] However, its role in the setting of negative high-quality CT imaging is unclear. PET/CT also cannot differentiate between hypermetabolic activity due to inflammation in the setting of a chronic pelvic sepsis versus disease recurrence. Therefore, PET/CT can be considered for patients with an elevated CEA but with an otherwise negative workup.

24.9 Pelvic Recurrence

Patients with locoregional recurrence or metastatic lesions should undergo a full evaluation as outlined previously, and presentation at multidisciplinary tumor board conference for discussion of therapeutic options. For patients who are found to have metastatic disease at initial presentation or during surveillance, perioperative chemotherapy and restaging to assess tumor response prior to curative resection should be considered. A hepatobiliary or thoracic surgeon should be present at the multidisciplinary tumor board conference to evaluate the resectability of hepatic and pulmonary metastases. A full discussion of the management strategies for metastatic disease is beyond the scope of this chapter and will be addressed in another chapter.

In the case of suspected locoregional recurrence, a complete history and physical examination, repeat imaging with pelvic MRI and CT scan of the chest, abdomen, and pelvis, as well as full endoscopic evaluation to rule out synchronous lesions in the colon, are required. Symptoms such as significant pelvic or sciatic pain and/or neuropathy are concerning for tumor invasion into the pelvic sidewall. Every effort should be made to obtain tissue biopsy as imaging modalities may have difficulty in distinguishing between true tumor recurrence and scar tissue. These patients should be presented at a multidisciplinary tumor board conference to determine resectability based on MRI, and consideration of perioperative (chemo)radiotherapy. There are several different classification systems for pelvic recurrences, but in general tumors should be classified based on involvement of surrounding structures. Anterior resections involve the neorectum and urogynecologic structures, posterior resections include the sacrum, and lateral resections include the iliac vessels and other structures in the lumbosacral plexus. Multiple points of tumor fixation decrease the ability to achieve an R0 resection.[451] Patients who require an anterior compartment resection only have the best outcomes since the probability of achieving an R0 resection is the highest.[451,452] Lateral invasion into the pelvic sidewall is at significantly higher risk of an incomplete resection.[453] Unresectable disease includes recurrences that invade major vascular structures, sacral involvement above S2, and extensive sidewall disease. Certain specialized centers have expanded their indications and are pursuing more extensive resections as there are some data to suggest improved oncologic outcomes.[453,454,455] The ultimate decision regarding resectability should be dependent on the ability to achieve an R0 resection and the available technical expertise. Certainly these patients should be referred to a high-volume institution given the complexities of management. Even in these centers, R0 resection is achieved in only 50 to 60% of patients.[456,457] In cases of residual disease or an area concerning for microscopically positive margins, intraoperative radiotherapy can be delivered.[457]

The most important prognostic factor for locally recurrent rectal cancer is the ability to achieve a complete resection with microscopically negative margins. Local recurrence rates are usually reported to be in the range of 15 to 25% for R0 resections, and are significantly higher for patients with R1–R2 disease.[456,457,458,459] Median survival times in the published literature vary from 8 to 38 months, and are also highly dependent on the radicality of the resection.[460] Harris et al[456] showed that 5-year cancer-specific survival was 44% with clear margins, compared to 26 and 10% for patients with R1 and R2 diseases, respectively. Most patients recurred with systemic disease, rather than local re-recurrence. Pelvic exenteration can be performed with minimal mortality and acceptable morbidity rates at specialized centers. In a review of 23 studies, complication rates ranged from 37 to 100% (median 57%) and mortality 0 to 25% (median 2.2%).[460] Involvement of other surgical specialties such as urology, orthopaedics/neurosurgery, and reconstructive surgery is often required, especially in the setting of multivisceral resections. Most, if not all, patients will require a permanent end colostomy. The perineal wound is often a source of considerable morbidity. Available data suggest that the use of myocutaneous flaps such as gracilis or rectus abdominis may decrease the incidence of major perineal wound complications compared to primary closure.[461]

Ideally, all patients with recurrent rectal carcinoma should be treated with preoperative (chemo)radiation, but in the era of multimodal therapy, a significant proportion of patients will have already received radiation to the pelvis as part of their initial primary tumor treatment. The value of reirradiation is unclear. The risks of further irradiating surrounding tissues that may have already reached their maximum radiation tolerance during primary treatment need to be balanced with the potential of improving R0 resectability. Acute toxicity during irradiation occurs in 5 to 20% of patients and up to a third of patients will require a break or termination.[462] Late toxicity can also occur in up to a third of patients. A systematic review of nine studies including 474 patients with locally recurrent rectal carcinoma that had been previously irradiated reported that reirradiation with external beam radiotherapy with or without intraoperative radiotherapy was associated with improved R0 resection rates, local control, and overall survival.[463] The most important factor in determining prognosis was R0 resection, regardless of whether reirradiation was given. Radiation toxicity and perioperative morbidity and mortality were acceptable. Harris et al analyzed the outcomes of 533 patients with locally recurrent rectal cancer from five high-volume institutions and reported that preoperative chemoradiotherapy was the only modality to improve 5-year overall survival when an R0 resection was obtained.[456] Perioperative chemotherapy or radiotherapy alone improved survival for patients with R2 resections.

24.10 Conclusion

The management of rectal cancer has evolved significantly since the initial description of the Miles operation in 1908. Modern care of the patient with rectal carcinoma is multidisciplinary and requires close cooperation of surgery, medical and radiation oncology, radiology, and pathology specialties. This is a true example of personalized medicine with bespoke treatment strategies for individual patients. Accurate locoregional staging will influence the decision to administer neoadjuvant therapies. Preoperative chemoradiation will decrease the local recurrence rates for locally advanced rectal cancer by 50%. High-quality surgery according to TME principles remains essential for curative resection, as is specialized pathologic evaluation of the surgical specimen. Newer organ-preserving modalities further contribute to the treatment armamentarium. Adjuvant therapy is controversial but remains the standard of care. Patients should further be followed after definitive management according to established surveillance protocols to identify local and distant recurrences. Optimization of outcomes for patients with rectal carcinoma is dependent on adherence to these principles of high-quality evidence-based care.

References

[1] Lisfranc J. Mémoire sur l'éxcision de la partie inférieure du rectum devenue carcinomateuse. Mém Acad R Chir. 1833; 3:291–302

[2] Kraske P. Zur Exstirpation Hochsitzender Mast Darm Krebse. Verh Deutsch Ges Chir. 1885; 14:464–474

[3] Miles WE. A method of performing abdominoperineal excision for carcinoma of the rectum and of the terminal portion of the pelvic colon. Lancet. 1908; 2:1812–1813

[4] Dixon CF. Anterior resection for malignant lesions of the upper part of the rectum and lower part of the sigmoid. Ann Surg. 1948; 128(3):425–442

[5] Heald RJ, Husband EM, Ryall RD. The mesorectum in rectal cancer surgery: the clue to pelvic recurrence? Br J Surg. 1982; 69(10):613–616

[6] Sauer R, Becker H, Hohenberger W, et al. Preoperative versus postoperative chemoradiotherapy for rectal cancer. N Engl J Med. 2004:1731–1740

[7] Cedermark B, Dahlberg M, Glimelius B, Påhlman L, Rutqvist LE, Wilking N, Swedish Rectal Cancer Trial. Improved survival with preoperative radiotherapy in resectable rectal cancer. N Engl J Med. 1997; 336(14):980–987

[8] Ferlay J, Soerjomataram I, Ervik M, et al. GLOBOCAN 2012 v1.0, Cancer Incidence and Mortality Worldwide: IARC Cancer Base No. 11. Lyon, France: International Agency for Research on Cancer; 2013

[9] Torre LA, Siegel RL, Ward EM, Jemal A. Global cancer incidence and mortality rates and trends: an update. Cancer Epidemiol Biomarkers Prev. 2016; 25 (1):16–27

[10] Zhang J, Dhakal IB, Zhao Z, Li L. Trends in mortality from cancers of the breast, colon, prostate, esophagus, and stomach in East Asia: role of nutrition transition. Eur J Cancer Prev. 2012; 21(5):480–489

[11] Arnold M, Karim-Kos HE, Coebergh JW, et al. Recent trends in incidence of five common cancers in 26 European countries since 1988: analysis of the European Cancer Observatory. Eur J Cancer. 2015; 51(9):1164–1187

[12] Chatenoud L, Bertuccio P, Bosetti C, et al. Trends in mortality from major cancers in the Americas: 1980–2010. Ann Oncol. 2014; 25(9):1843–1853

[13] Siegel RL, Miller KD, Jemal A. Cancer statistics, 2016. CA Cancer J Clin. 2016; 66(1):7–30

[14] Bosetti C, Bertuccio P, Malvezzi M, et al. Cancer mortality in Europe, 2005–2009, and an overview of trends since 1980. Ann Oncol. 2013; 24 (10):2657–2671

[15] Ryerson AB, Eheman CR, Altekruse SF, et al. Annual Report to the Nation on the Status of Cancer, 1975–2012, featuring the increasing incidence of liver cancer. Cancer. 2016; 122(9):1312–1337

[16] Dozois EJ, Boardman LA, Suwanthanma W, et al. Young-onset colorectal cancer in patients with no known genetic predisposition: can we increase early recognition and improve outcome? Medicine (Baltimore). 2008; 87(5):259–263

[17] Myers EA, Feingold DL, Forde KA, Arnell T, Jang JH, Whelan RL. Colorectal cancer in patients under 50 years of age: a retrospective analysis of two institutions' experience. World J Gastroenterol. 2013; 19(34):5651–5657

[18] Taggarshe D, Rehil N, Sharma S, Flynn JC, Damadi A. Colorectal cancer: are the "young" being overlooked? Am J Surg. 2013; 205(3):312–316, discussion 316

[19] Ahnen DJ, Wade SW, Jones WF, et al. The increasing incidence of young-onset colorectal cancer: a call to action. Mayo Clin Proc. 2014; 89(2):216–224

[20] Hatch QM, Kniery KR, Johnson EK, et al. Screening or symptoms? How do we detect colorectal cancer in an equal access health care system? J Gastrointest Surg. 2016; 20(2):431–438

[21] Neugut AI, Garbowski GC, Waye JD, et al. Diagnostic yield of colorectal neoplasia with colonoscopy for abdominal pain, change in bowel habits, and rectal bleeding. Am J Gastroenterol. 1993; 88(8):1179–1183

[22] Moreno CC, Mittal PK, Sullivan PS, et al. Colorectal cancer initial diagnosis: screening colonoscopy, diagnostic colonoscopy, or emergent surgery, and tumor stage and size at initial presentation. Clin Colorectal Cancer. 2016; 15 (1):67–73

[23] Monson JR, Weiser MR, Buie WD, et al. Standards Practice Task Force of the American Society of Colon and Rectal Surgeons. Practice parameters for the management of rectal cancer (revised). Dis Colon Rectum. 2013; 56(5):535–550

[24] Fleisher LA, Fleischmann KE, Auerbach AD, et al. American College of Cardiology, American Heart Association. 2014 ACC/AHA guideline on perioperative cardiovascular evaluation and management of patients undergoing noncardiac surgery: a report of the American College of Cardiology/American Heart Association Task Force on practice guidelines. J Am Coll Cardiol. 2014; 64(22):e77–e137

[25] Mulder SA, Kranse R, Damhuis RA, et al. Prevalence and prognosis of synchronous colorectal cancer: a Dutch population-based study. Cancer Epidemiol. 2011; 35(5):442–447

[26] Latournerie M, Jooste V, Cottet V, Lepage C, Faivre J, Bouvier AM. Epidemiology and prognosis of synchronous colorectal cancers. Br J Surg. 2008; 95 (12):1528–1533

[27] Flamen P, Hoekstra OS, Homans F, et al. Unexplained rising carcinoembryonic antigen (CEA) in the postoperative surveillance of colorectal cancer: the utility of positron emission tomography (PET). Eur J Cancer. 2001; 37 (7):862–869

[28] Whiteford MH, Whiteford HM, Yee LF, et al. Usefulness of FDG-PET scan in the assessment of suspected metastatic or recurrent adenocarcinoma of the colon and rectum. Dis Colon Rectum. 2000; 43(6):759–767, discussion 767–770

[29] Alexander JC, Silverman NA, Chretien PB. Effect of age and cigarette smoking on carcinoembryonic antigen levels. JAMA. 1976; 235(18):1975–1979

[30] Locker GY, Hamilton S, Harris J, et al. ASCO. ASCO 2006 update of recommendations for the use of tumor markers in gastrointestinal cancer. J Clin Oncol. 2006; 24(33):5313–5327

[31] Duffy MJ, van Dalen A, Haglund C, et al. Clinical utility of biochemical markers in colorectal cancer: European Group on Tumour Markers (EGTM) guidelines. Eur J Cancer. 2003; 39(6):718–727

[32] Wolmark N, Fisher B, Wieand HS, et al. The prognostic significance of preoperative carcinoembryonic antigen levels in colorectal cancer. Results from NSABP (National Surgical Adjuvant Breast and Bowel Project) clinical trials. Ann Surg. 1984; 199(4):375–382

[33] Lindmark G, Bergström R, Påhlman L, Glimelius B. The association of preoperative serum tumour markers with Dukes' stage and survival in colorectal cancer. Br J Cancer. 1995; 71(5):1090–1094

[34] Park IJ, Choi GS, Lim KH, Kang BM, Jun SH. Serum carcinoembryonic antigen monitoring after curative resection for colorectal cancer: clinical significance of the preoperative level. Ann Surg Oncol. 2009; 16(11):3087–3093

[35] Kleiman A, Al-Khamis A, Farsi A, et al. Normalization of CEA levels post-neoadjuvant therapy is a strong predictor of pathologic complete response in rectal cancer. J Gastrointest Surg. 2015; 19(6):1106–1112

[36] Wallin U, Rothenberger D, Lowry A, Luepker R, Mellgren A. CEA: a predictor for pathologic complete response after neoadjuvant therapy for rectal cancer. Dis Colon Rectum. 2013; 56(7):859–868

[37] Probst CP, Becerra AZ, Aquina CT, et al. Watch and wait?: elevated pretreatment CEA is associated with decreased pathological complete response in rectal cancer. J Gastrointest Surg. 2016; 20(1):43–52, discussion 52

[38] Jacquet P, Jelinek JS, Steves MA, Sugarbaker PH. Evaluation of computed tomography in patients with peritoneal carcinomatosis. Cancer. 1993; 72 (5):1631–1636

[39] Koh JL, Yan TD, Glenn D, Morris DL. Evaluation of preoperative computed tomography in estimating peritoneal cancer index in colorectal peritoneal carcinomatosis. Ann Surg Oncol. 2009; 16(2):327–333

[40] Nordholm-Carstensen A, Wille-Jørgensen PA, Jorgensen LN, Harling H. Indeterminate pulmonary nodules at colorectal cancer staging: a systematic review of predictive parameters for malignancy. Ann Surg Oncol. 2013; 20 (12):4022–4030

[41] Kim NK, Kim MJ, Yun SH, Sohn SK, Min JS. Comparative study of transrectal ultrasonography, pelvic computerized tomography, and magnetic resonance imaging in preoperative staging of rectal cancer. Dis Colon Rectum. 1999; 42 (6):770–775

[42] Zerhouni EA, Rutter C, Hamilton SR, et al. CT and MR imaging in the staging of colorectal carcinoma: report of the Radiology Diagnostic Oncology Group II. Radiology. 1996; 200(2):443–451

[43] Rifkin MD, Ehrlich SM, Marks G. Staging of rectal carcinoma: prospective comparison of endorectal US and CT. Radiology. 1989; 170(2):319–322

[44] Butch RJ, Stark DD, Wittenberg J, et al. Staging rectal cancer by MR and CT. AJR Am J Roentgenol. 1986; 146(6):1155–1160

[45] Kobayashi H, Kikuchi A, Okazaki S, et al. Diagnostic performance of multidetector row computed tomography for assessment of lymph node metastasis in patients with distal rectal cancer. Ann Surg Oncol. 2015; 22(1):203–208

[46] Solomon MJ, McLeod RS. Endoluminal transrectal ultrasonography: accuracy, reliability, and validity. Dis Colon Rectum. 1993; 36(2):200–205

[47] Marusch F, Ptok H, Sahm M, et al. Endorectal ultrasound in rectal carcinoma: do the literature results really correspond to the realities of routine clinical care? Endoscopy. 2011; 43(5):425–431

[48] Garcia-Aguilar J, Pollack J, Lee SH, et al. Accuracy of endorectal ultrasonography in preoperative staging of rectal tumors. Dis Colon Rectum. 2002; 45(1):10–15

[49] Jürgensen C, Teubner A, Habeck JO, Diener F, Scherübl H, Stölzel U. Staging of rectal cancer by EUS: depth of infiltration in T3 cancers is important. Gastrointest Endosc. 2011; 73(2):325–328

[50] Badger SA, Devlin PB, Neilly PJ, Gilliland R. Preoperative staging of rectal carcinoma by endorectal ultrasound: is there a learning curve? Int J Colorectal Dis. 2007; 22(10):1261–1268

[51] Lahaye MJ, Engelen SM, Nelemans PJ, et al. Imaging for predicting the risk factors—the circumferential resection margin and nodal disease—of local recurrence in rectal cancer: a meta-analysis. Semin Ultrasound CT MR. 2005; 26(4):259–268

[52] Puli SR, Reddy JB, Bechtold ML, Choudhary A, Antillon MR, Brugge WR. Accuracy of endoscopic ultrasound to diagnose nodal invasion by rectal cancers: a meta-analysis and systematic review. Ann Surg Oncol. 2009; 16(5):1255–1265

[53] Harewood GC, Wiersema MJ, Nelson H, et al. A prospective, blinded assessment of the impact of preoperative staging on the management of rectal cancer. Gastroenterology. 2002; 123(1):24–32

[54] MERCURY Study Group. Extramural depth of tumor invasion at thin-section MR in patients with rectal cancer: results of the MERCURY study. Radiology. 2007; 243(1):132–139

[55] Kono Y, Togashi K, Utano K, et al. Lymph node size alone is not an accurate predictor of metastases in rectal cancer: a node-for-node comparative study of specimens and histology. Am Surg. 2015; 81(12):1263–1271

[56] Kim JH, Beets GL, Kim MJ, Kessels AG, Beets-Tan RG. High-resolution MR imaging for nodal staging in rectal cancer: are there any criteria in addition to the size? Eur J Radiol. 2004; 52(1):78–83

[57] Brown G, Richards CJ, Bourne MW, et al. Morphologic predictors of lymph node status in rectal cancer with use of high-spatial-resolution MR imaging with histopathologic comparison. Radiology. 2003; 227(2):371–377

[58] Lambregts DM, Beets GL, Maas M, et al. Accuracy of gadofosveset-enhanced MRI for nodal staging and restaging in rectal cancer. Ann Surg. 2011; 253(3):539–545

[59] Heijnen LA, Lambregts DM, Martens MH, et al. Performance of gadofosveset-enhanced MRI for staging rectal cancer nodes: can the initial promising results be reproduced? Eur Radiol. 2014; 24(2):371–379

[60] Yu XP, Wen L, Hou J, et al. Discrimination between Metastatic and Nonmetastatic Mesorectal Lymph Nodes in Rectal Cancer Using Intravoxel Incoherent Motion Diffusion-weighted Magnetic Resonance Imaging. Acad Radiol. 2016; 23(4):479–485

[61] Smith NJ, Barbachano Y, Norman AR, Swift RI, Abulafi AM, Brown G. Prognostic significance of magnetic resonance imaging-detected extramural vascular invasion in rectal cancer. Br J Surg. 2008; 95(2):229–236

[62] Brown G, Radcliffe AG, Newcombe RG, Dallimore NS, Bourne MW, Williams GT. Preoperative assessment of prognostic factors in rectal cancer using high-resolution magnetic resonance imaging. Br J Surg. 2003; 90(3):355–364

[63] Al-Sukhni E, Milot L, Fruitman M, et al. Diagnostic accuracy of MRI for assessment of T category, lymph node metastases, and circumferential resection margin involvement in patients with rectal cancer: a systematic review and meta-analysis. Ann Surg Oncol. 2012; 19(7):2212–2223

[64] Merkel S, Mansmann U, Siassi M, Papadopoulos T, Hohenberger W, Hermanek P. The prognostic inhomogeneity in pT3 rectal carcinomas. Int J Colorectal Dis. 2001; 16(5):298–304

[65] Shin R, Jeong SY, Yoo HY, et al. Depth of mesorectal extension has prognostic significance in patients with T3 rectal cancer. Dis Colon Rectum. 2012; 55(12):1220–1228

[66] Quirke P, Durdey P, Dixon MF, Williams NS. Local recurrence of rectal adenocarcinoma due to inadequate surgical resection. Histopathological study of lateral tumour spread and surgical excision. Lancet. 1986; 2(8514):996–999

[67] Taylor FG, Quirke P, Heald RJ, et al. MERCURY Study Group. One millimetre is the safe cut-off for magnetic resonance imaging prediction of surgical margin status in rectal cancer. Br J Surg. 2011; 98(6):872–879

[68] MERCURY Study Group. Diagnostic accuracy of preoperative magnetic resonance imaging in predicting curative resection of rectal cancer: prospective observational study. BMJ. 2006; 333(7572):779

[69] Taylor FG, Quirke P, Heald RJ, et al. Magnetic Resonance Imaging in Rectal Cancer European Equivalence Study Group. Preoperative magnetic resonance imaging assessment of circumferential resection margin predicts disease-free survival and local recurrence: 5-year follow-up results of the MERCURY study. J Clin Oncol. 2014; 32(1):34–43

[70] Memon S, Lynch AC, Bressel M, Wise AG, Heriot AG. Systematic review and meta-analysis of the accuracy of MRI and endorectal ultrasound in the restaging and response assessment of rectal cancer following neoadjuvant therapy. Colorectal Dis. 2015; 17(9):748–761

[71] Hötker AM, Garcia-Aguilar J, Gollub MJ. Multiparametric MRI of rectal cancer in the assessment of response to therapy: a systematic review. Dis Colon Rectum. 2014; 57(6):790–799

[72] Maffione AM, Marzola MC, Capirci C, Colletti PM, Rubello D. Value of (18)F-FDG PET for predicting response to neoadjuvant therapy in rectal cancer: systematic review and meta-analysis. AJR Am J Roentgenol. 2015; 204(6):1261–1268

[73] Guillem JG, Ruby JA, Leibold T, et al. Neither FDG-PET Nor CT can distinguish between a pathological complete response and an incomplete response after neoadjuvant chemoradiation in locally advanced rectal cancer: a prospective study. Ann Surg. 2013; 258(2):289–295

[74] Dietz DW, Consortium for Optimizing Surgical Treatment of Rectal Cancer (OSTRiCh). Multidisciplinary management of rectal cancer: the OSTRICH. J Gastrointest Surg. 2013; 17(10):1863–1868

[75] Gabel M, Hilton NE, Nathanson SD. Multidisciplinary breast cancer clinics. Do they work? Cancer. 1997; 79(12):2380–2384

[76] Stephens MR, Lewis WG, Brewster AE, et al. Multidisciplinary team management is associated with improved outcomes after surgery for esophageal cancer. Dis Esophagus. 2006; 19(3):164–171

[77] Birchall M, Bailey D, King P, South West Cancer Intelligence Service Head and Neck Tumour Panel. Effect of process standards on survival of patients with head and neck cancer in the south and west of England. Br J Cancer. 2004; 91(8):1477–1481

[78] Coory M, Gkolia P, Yang IA, Bowman RV, Fong KM. Systematic review of multidisciplinary teams in the management of lung cancer. Lung Cancer. 2008; 60(1):14–21

[79] Morris E, Haward RA, Gilthorpe MS, Craigs C, Forman D. The impact of the Calman-Hine report on the processes and outcomes of care for Yorkshire's colorectal cancer patients. Br J Cancer. 2006; 95(8):979–985

[80] Burton S, Brown G, Daniels IR, Norman AR, Mason B, Cunningham D, Royal Marsden Hospital, Colorectal Cancer Network. MRI directed multidisciplinary team preoperative treatment strategy: the way to eliminate positive circumferential margins? Br J Cancer. 2006; 94(3):351–357

[81] Wexner SD, Berho ME. The rationale for and reality of the new national accreditation program for rectal cancer. Dis Colon Rectum. 2017; 60(6):595–602

[82] Berho M, Narang R, Van Koughnett JA, Wexner SD. Modern multidisciplinary perioperative management of rectal cancer. JAMA Surg. 2015; 150(3):260–266

[83] Paquette IM, Kemp JA, Finlayson SR. Patient and hospital factors associated with use of sphincter-sparing surgery for rectal cancer. Dis Colon Rectum. 2010; 53(2):115–120

[84] Ricciardi R, Virnig BA, Madoff RD, Rothenberger DA, Baxter NN. The status of radical proctectomy and sphincter-sparing surgery in the United States. Dis Colon Rectum. 2007; 50(8):1119–1127, discussion 1126–1127

[85] Ricciardi R, Roberts PL, Read TE, Marcello PW, Schoetz DJ, Baxter NN. Variability in reconstructive procedures following rectal cancer surgery in the United States. Dis Colon Rectum. 2010; 53(6):874–880

[86] Ricciardi R, Roberts PL, Read TE, Baxter NN, Marcello PW, Schoetz DJ. Who performs proctectomy for rectal cancer in the United States? Dis Colon Rectum. 2011; 54(10):1210–1215

[87] Monson JR, Probst CP, Wexner SD, et al. Consortium for Optimizing the Treatment of Rectal Cancer (OSTRiCh). Failure of evidence-based cancer care in the United States: the association between rectal cancer treatment, cancer center volume, and geography. Ann Surg. 2014; 260(4):625–631, discussion 631–632

[88] Hodgson DC, Zhang W, Zaslavsky AM, Fuchs CS, Wright WE, Ayanian JZ. Relation of hospital volume to colostomy rates and survival for patients with rectal cancer. J Natl Cancer Inst. 2003; 95(10):708–716

[89] Archampong D, Borowski D, Wille-Jørgensen P, Iversen LH. Workload and surgeon's specialty for outcome after colorectal cancer surgery. Cochrane Database Syst Rev. 2012;(3):CD005391

[90] Sauer R, Liersch T, Merkel S, et al. Preoperative versus postoperative chemoradiotherapy for locally advanced rectal cancer: results of the German CAO/ARO/AIO-94 randomized phase III trial after a median follow-up of 11 years. J Clin Oncol. 2012; 30(16):1926–1933

[91] Roh MS, Colangelo LH, O'Connell MJ, et al. Preoperative multimodality therapy improves disease-free survival in patients with carcinoma of the rectum: NSABP R-03. J Clin Oncol. 2009; 27(31):5124–5130

[92] Park JH, Yoon SM, Yu CS, Kim JH, Kim TW, Kim JC. Randomized phase 3 trial comparing preoperative and postoperative chemoradiotherapy with capecitabine for locally advanced rectal cancer. Cancer. 2011; 117(16):3703–3712

[93] Bosset JF, Calais G, Mineur L, et al. EORTC Radiation Oncology Group. Fluorouracil-based adjuvant chemotherapy after preoperative chemoradiotherapy in rectal cancer: long-term results of the EORTC 22921 randomised study. Lancet Oncol. 2014; 15(2):184–190

[94] Gérard JP, Conroy T, Bonnetain F, et al. Preoperative radiotherapy with or without concurrent fluorouracil and leucovorin in T3–4 rectal cancers: results of FFCD 9203. J Clin Oncol. 2006; 24(28):4620–4625

[95] Folkesson J, Birgisson H, Pahlman L, Cedermark B, Glimelius B, Gunnarsson U. Swedish Rectal Cancer Trial: long lasting benefits from radiotherapy on survival and local recurrence rate. J Clin Oncol. 2005; 23(24):5644–5650

[96] Bujko K, Nowacki MP, Nasierowska-Guttmejer A, Michalski W, Bebenek M, Kryj M. Long-term results of a randomized trial comparing preoperative short-course radiotherapy with preoperative conventionally fractionated chemoradiation for rectal cancer. Br J Surg. 2006; 93(10):1215–1223

[97] Ngan SY, Burmeister B, Fisher RJ, et al. Randomized trial of short-course radiotherapy versus long-course chemoradiation comparing rates of local recurrence in patients with T3 rectal cancer: Trans-Tasman Radiation Oncology Group trial 01.04. J Clin Oncol. 2012; 30(31):3827–3833

[98] Bujko K, Wyrwicz L, Rutkowski A, et al. Polish Colorectal Study Group. Long-course oxaliplatin-based preoperative chemoradiation versus 5 × 5 Gy and consolidation chemotherapy for cT4 or fixed cT3 rectal cancer: results of a randomized phase III study. Ann Oncol. 2016; 27(5):834–842

[99] Dhadda AS, Zaitoun AM, Bessell EM. Regression of rectal cancer with radiotherapy with or without concurrent capecitabine: optimising the timing of surgical resection. Clin Oncol (R Coll Radiol). 2009; 21(1):23–31

[100] Petrelli F, Sgroi G, Sarti E, Barni S. Increasing the interval between neoadjuvant chemoradiotherapy and surgery in rectal cancer: a meta-analysis of published studies. Ann Surg. 2016; 263(3):458–464

[101] Probst CP, Becerra AZ, Aquina CT, et al. Consortium for Optimizing the Surgical Treatment of Rectal Cancer (OSTRiCh). Extended intervals after neoadjuvant therapy in locally advanced rectal cancer: the key to improved tumor response and potential organ preservation. J Am Coll Surg. 2015; 221(2):430–440

[102] Francois Y, Nemoz CJ, Baulieux J, et al. Influence of the interval between preoperative radiation therapy and surgery on downstaging and on the rate of sphincter-sparing surgery for rectal cancer: the Lyon R90–01 randomized trial. J Clin Oncol. 1999; 17(8):2396

[103] Lefevre JH, Mineur L, Kotti S, et al. Effect of interval (7 or 11 weeks) between neoadjuvant radiochemotherapy and surgery on complete pathologic response in rectal cancer: a multicenter, randomized, controlled trial (GRECCAR-6). J Clin Oncol. 2016; 34(31):3773–3780

[104] Hofheinz RD, Wenz F, Post S, et al. Chemoradiotherapy with capecitabine versus fluorouracil for locally advanced rectal cancer: a randomised, multicentre, non-inferiority, phase 3 trial. Lancet Oncol. 2012; 13(6):579–588

[105] Allegra CJ, Yothers G, O'Connell MJ, et al. Neoadjuvant 5-FU or capecitabine plus radiation with or without oxaliplatin in rectal cancer patients: a phase III randomized clinical trial. J Natl Cancer Inst. 2015; 107(11):djv248

[106] Gérard JP, Azria D, Gourgou-Bourgade S, et al. Comparison of two neoadjuvant chemoradiotherapy regimens for locally advanced rectal cancer: results of the phase III trial ACCORD 12/0405-Prodige 2. J Clin Oncol. 2010; 28(10):1638–1644

[107] Corazzelli G, Capobianco G, Arcamone M, et al. Long-term results of gemcitabine plus oxaliplatin with and without rituximab as salvage treatment for transplant-ineligible patients with refractory/relapsing B-cell lymphoma. Cancer Chemother Pharmacol. 2009; 64(5):907–916

[108] Rödel C, Liersch T, Becker H, et al. German Rectal Cancer Study Group. Preoperative chemoradiotherapy and postoperative chemotherapy with fluorouracil and oxaliplatin versus fluorouracil alone in locally advanced rectal cancer: initial results of the German CAO/ARO/AIO-04 randomised phase 3 trial. Lancet Oncol. 2012; 13(7):679–687

[109] Deng Y, Chi P, Lan P, et al. Modified FOLFOX6 with or without radiation versus fluorouracil and leucovorin with radiation in neoadjuvant treatment of locally advanced rectal cancer: initial results of the Chinese FOWARC multicenter, open-label, randomized three-arm phase III trial. J Clin Oncol. 2016; 34(27):3300–3307

[110] Mohiuddin M, Paulus R, Mitchell E, et al. Neoadjuvant chemoradiation for distal rectal cancer: 5-year updated results of a randomized phase 2 study of neoadjuvant combined modality chemoradiation for distal rectal cancer. Int J Radiat Oncol Biol Phys. 2013; 86(3):523–528

[111] Navarro M, Dotor E, Rivera F, et al. A phase II study of preoperative radiotherapy and concomitant weekly irinotecan in combination with protracted venous infusion 5-fluorouracil, for resectable locally advanced rectal cancer. Int J Radiat Oncol Biol Phys. 2006; 66(1):201–205

[112] Willeke F, Horisberger K, Kraus-Tiefenbacher U, et al. A phase II study of capecitabine and irinotecan in combination with concurrent pelvic radiotherapy (CapIri-RT) as neoadjuvant treatment of locally advanced rectal cancer. Br J Cancer. 2007; 96(6):912–917

[113] Gollins S, Sun Myint A, Haylock B, et al. Preoperative chemoradiotherapy using concurrent capecitabine and irinotecan in magnetic resonance imaging-defined locally advanced rectal cancer: impact on long-term clinical outcomes. J Clin Oncol. 2011; 29(8):1042–1049

[114] Taylor FG, Quirke P, Heald RJ, et al. MERCURY Study Group. Preoperative high-resolution magnetic resonance imaging can identify good prognosis stage I, II, and III rectal cancer best managed by surgery alone: a prospective, multicenter, European study. Ann Surg. 2011; 253(4):711–719

[115] Khrizman P, Niland JC, ter Veer A, et al. Postoperative adjuvant chemotherapy use in patients with stage II/III rectal cancer treated with neoadjuvant therapy: a national comprehensive cancer network analysis. J Clin Oncol. 2013; 31(1):30–38

[116] Chua YJ, Barbachano Y, Cunningham D, et al. Neoadjuvant capecitabine and oxaliplatin before chemoradiotherapy and total mesorectal excision in MRI-defined poor-risk rectal cancer: a phase 2 trial. Lancet Oncol. 2010; 11(3):241–248

[117] Fernández-Martos C, Pericay C, Aparicio J, et al. Phase II, randomized study of concomitant chemoradiotherapy followed by surgery and adjuvant capecitabine plus oxaliplatin (CAPOX) compared with induction CAPOX followed by concomitant chemoradiotherapy and surgery in magnetic resonance imaging-defined, locally advanced rectal cancer: Grupo cancer de recto 3 study. J Clin Oncol. 2010; 28(5):859–865

[118] Bosset JF, Collette L, Calais G, et al. EORTC Radiotherapy Group Trial 22921. Chemotherapy with preoperative radiotherapy in rectal cancer. N Engl J Med. 2006; 355(11):1114–1123

[119] Kapiteijn E, Marijnen CA, Nagtegaal ID, et al. Dutch Colorectal Cancer Group. Preoperative radiotherapy combined with total mesorectal excision for resectable rectal cancer. N Engl J Med. 2001; 345(9):638–646

[120] Sebag-Montefiore D, Stephens RJ, Steele R, et al. Preoperative radiotherapy versus selective postoperative chemoradiotherapy in patients with rectal cancer (MRC CR07 and NCIC-CTG C016): a multicentre, randomised, trial. Lancet. 2009; 373(9666):811–820

[121] Pettersson D, Cedermark B, Holm T, et al. Interim analysis of the Stockholm III trial of preoperative radiotherapy regimens for rectal cancer. Br J Surg. 2010; 97(4):580–587

[122] Pietrzak L, Bujko K, Nowacki MP, et al. Polish Colorectal Study Group. Quality of life, anorectal and sexual functions after preoperative radiotherapy for rectal cancer: report of a randomised trial. Radiother Oncol. 2007; 84(3):217–225

[123] Peeters KC, van de Velde CJ, Leer JW, et al. Late side effects of short-course preoperative radiotherapy combined with total mesorectal excision for rectal cancer: increased bowel dysfunction in irradiated patients: a Dutch colorectal cancer group study. J Clin Oncol. 2005; 23(25):6199–6206

[124] Pollack J, Holm T, Cedermark B, et al. Late adverse effects of short-course preoperative radiotherapy in rectal cancer. Br J Surg. 2006; 93(12):1519–1525

[125] Birgisson H, Påhlman L, Gunnarsson U, Glimelius B. Late gastrointestinal disorders after rectal cancer surgery with and without preoperative radiation therapy. Br J Surg. 2008; 95(2):206–213

[126] Loos M, Quentmeier P, Schuster T, et al. Effect of preoperative radio(chemo)therapy on long-term functional outcome in rectal cancer patients: a systematic review and meta-analysis. Ann Surg Oncol. 2013; 20(6):1816–1828

[127] Martling A, Smedby KE, Birgisson H, et al. Risk of second primary cancer in patients treated with radiotherapy for rectal cancer. Br J Surg. 2017; 104(3):278–287

[128] McBrearty A, McCallion K, Moorehead RJ, et al. Re-staging following long-course chemoradiotherapy for rectal cancer: does it influence management? Ulster Med J. 2016; 85(3):178–181

[129] Schneider DA, Akhurst TJ, Ngan SY, et al. Relative value of restaging MRI, CT, and FDG-PET scan after preoperative chemoradiation for rectal cancer. Dis Colon Rectum. 2016; 59(3):179–186

[130] Bisschop C, Tjalma JJ, Hospers GA, et al. Consequence of restaging after neoadjuvant treatment for locally advanced rectal cancer. Ann Surg Oncol. 2015; 22(2):552–556

[131] Davids JS, Alavi K, Andres Cervera-Servin J, et al. Routine preoperative restaging CTs after neoadjuvant chemoradiation for locally advanced rectal cancer are low yield: a retrospective case study. Int J Surg. 2014; 12(12):1295–1299

[132] Ayez N, Alberda WJ, Burger JW, et al. Is restaging with chest and abdominal CT scan after neoadjuvant chemoradiotherapy for locally advanced rectal cancer necessary? Ann Surg Oncol. 2013; 20(1):155–160

[133] Rödel C, Martus P, Papadoupolos T, et al. Prognostic significance of tumor regression after preoperative chemoradiotherapy for rectal cancer. J Clin Oncol. 2005; 23(34):8688–8696

[134] Patel UB, Taylor F, Blomqvist L, et al. Magnetic resonance imaging-detected tumor response for locally advanced rectal cancer predicts survival outcomes: MERCURY experience. J Clin Oncol. 2011; 29(28):3753–3760

[135] Fokas E, Liersch T, Fietkau R, et al. Tumor regression grading after preoperative chemoradiotherapy for locally advanced rectal carcinoma revisited: updated results of the CAO/ARO/AIO-94 trial. J Clin Oncol. 2014; 32(15):1554–1562

[136] Park IJ, You YN, Agarwal A, et al. Neoadjuvant treatment response as an early response indicator for patients with rectal cancer. J Clin Oncol. 2012; 30(15):1770–1776

[137] Foster JD, Jones EL, Falk S, Cooper EJ, Francis NK. Timing of surgery after long-course neoadjuvant chemoradiotherapy for rectal cancer: a systematic review of the literature. Dis Colon Rectum. 2013; 56(7):921–930

[138] Sloothaak DA, Geijsen DE, van Leersum NJ, et al. Dutch Surgical Colorectal Audit. Optimal time interval between neoadjuvant chemoradiotherapy and surgery for rectal cancer. Br J Surg. 2013; 100(7):933–939

[139] Kalady MF, de Campos-Lobato LF, Stocchi L, et al. Predictive factors of pathologic complete response after neoadjuvant chemoradiation for rectal cancer. Ann Surg. 2009; 250(4):582–589

[140] Garcia-Aguilar J, Smith DD, Avila K, Bergsland EK, Chu P, Krieg RM, Timing of Rectal Cancer Response to Chemoradiation Consortium. Optimal timing of surgery after chemoradiation for advanced rectal cancer: preliminary results of a multicenter, nonrandomized phase II prospective trial. Ann Surg. 2011; 254(1):97–102

[141] Bernstein TE, Endreseth BH, Romundstad P, Wibe A, Norwegian Colorectal Cancer Group. Circumferential resection margin as a prognostic factor in rectal cancer. Br J Surg. 2009; 96(11):1348–1357

[142] Gunderson LL, Sargent DJ, Tepper JE, et al. Impact of T and N stage and treatment on survival and relapse in adjuvant rectal cancer: a pooled analysis. J Clin Oncol. 2004; 22(10):1785–1796

[143] van Gijn W, Marijnen CA, Nagtegaal ID, et al. Dutch Colorectal Cancer Group. Preoperative radiotherapy combined with total mesorectal excision for resectable rectal cancer: 12-year follow-up of the multicentre, randomised controlled TME trial. Lancet Oncol. 2011; 12(6):575–582

[144] Eriksen MT, Wibe A, Haffner J, Wiig JN, Norwegian Rectal Cancer Group. Prognostic groups in 1,676 patients with T3 rectal cancer treated without preoperative radiotherapy. Dis Colon Rectum. 2007; 50(2):156–167

[145] Braendengen M, Tveit KM, Berglund A, et al. Randomized phase III study comparing preoperative radiotherapy with chemoradiotherapy in nonresectable rectal cancer. J Clin Oncol. 2008; 26(22):3687–3694

[146] Nordlinger B, Sorbye H, Glimelius B, et al. EORTC Gastro-Intestinal Tract Cancer Group, Cancer Research UK, Arbeitsgruppe Lebermetastasen und -tumoren in der Chirurgischen Arbeitsgemeinschaft Onkologie (ALM-CAO), Australasian Gastro-Intestinal Trials Group (AGITG), Fédération Francophone de Cancérologie Digestive, (FFCD). Perioperative chemotherapy with FOLFOX4 and surgery versus surgery alone for resectable liver metastases from colorectal cancer (EORTC Intergroup trial 40983): a randomised controlled trial. Lancet. 2008; 371(9617):1007–1016

[147] Lam VW, Laurence JM, Pang T, et al. A systematic review of a liver-first approach in patients with colorectal cancer and synchronous colorectal liver metastases. HPB. 2014; 16(2):101–108

[148] Tyc-Szczepaniak D, Wyrwicz L, Kepka L, et al. Palliative radiotherapy and chemotherapy instead of surgery in symptomatic rectal cancer with synchronous unresectable metastases: a phase II study. Ann Oncol. 2013; 24(11):2829–2834

[149] Bentrem DJ, Okabe S, Wong WD, et al. T1 adenocarcinoma of the rectum: transanal excision or radical surgery? Ann Surg. 2005; 242(4):472–477, discussion 477–479

[150] Endreseth BH, Myrvold HE, Romundstad P, Hestvik UE, Bjerkeset T, Wibe A, Norwegian Rectal Cancer Group. Transanal excision vs. major surgery for T1 rectal cancer. Dis Colon Rectum. 2005; 48(7):1380–1388

[151] Peng J, Chen W, Sheng W, et al. Oncological outcome of T1 rectal cancer undergoing standard resection and local excision. Colorectal Dis. 2011; 13(2):e14–e19

[152] Scheele J, Lemke J, Meier M, Sander S, Henne-Bruns D, Kornmann M. Quality of life after sphincter-preserving rectal cancer resection. Clin Colorectal Cancer. 2015; 14(4):e33–e40

[153] Ridolfi TJ, Berger N, Ludwig KA. Low anterior resection syndrome: current management and future directions. Clin Colon Rectal Surg. 2016; 29(3):239–245

[154] Mellgren A, Sirivongs P, Rothenberger DA, Madoff RD, García-Aguilar J. Is local excision adequate therapy for early rectal cancer? Dis Colon Rectum. 2000; 43(8):1064–1071, discussion 1071–1074

[155] Bach SP, Hill J, Monson JR, et al. Association of Coloproctology of Great Britain and Ireland Transanal Endoscopic Microsurgery (TEM) Collaboration. A predictive model for local recurrence after transanal endoscopic microsurgery for rectal cancer. Br J Surg. 2009; 96(3):280–290

[156] You YN, Baxter NN, Stewart A, Nelson H. Is the increasing rate of local excision for stage I rectal cancer in the United States justified?: a nationwide cohort study from the National Cancer Database. Ann Surg. 2007; 245(5):726–733

[157] Ptok H, Marusch F, Meyer F, et al. Colon/Rectal Cancer (Primary Tumor) Study Group. Oncological outcome of local vs radical resection of low-risk pT1 rectal cancer. Arch Surg. 2007; 142(7):649–655, discussion 656

[158] Nascimbeni R, Burgart LJ, Nivatvongs S, Larson DR. Risk of lymph node metastasis in T1 carcinoma of the colon and rectum. Dis Colon Rectum. 2002; 45(2):200–206

[159] Brunner W, Widmann B, Marti L, Tarantino I, Schmied BM, Warschkow R. Predictors for regional lymph node metastasis in T1 rectal cancer: a population-based SEER analysis. Surg Endosc. 2016; 30(10):4405–4415

[160] Kikuchi R, Takano M, Takagi K, et al. Management of early invasive colorectal cancer. Risk of recurrence and clinical guidelines. Dis Colon Rectum. 1995; 38(12):1286–1295

[161] Beaton C, Twine CP, Williams GL, Radcliffe AG. Systematic review and metaanalysis of histopathological factors influencing the risk of lymph node metastasis in early colorectal cancer. Colorectal Dis. 2013; 15(7):788–797

[162] National Comprehensive Cancer Network. NCCN Clinical Practice Guidelines in Oncology (NCCN Guidelines). Rectal Cancer. Version 2.2016. Fort Washington, PA: NCCN; 2016

[163] Buess G, Theiss R, Günther M, Hutterer F, Pichlmaier H. Endoscopic surgery in the rectum. Endoscopy. 1985; 17(1):31–35

[164] Atallah S, Albert M, Larach S. Transanal minimally invasive surgery: a giant leap forward. Surg Endosc. 2010; 24(9):2200–2205

[165] Rimonda R, Arezzo A, Arolfo S, Salvai A, Morino M. TransAnal Minimally Invasive Surgery (TAMIS) with SILS™ port versus Transanal Endoscopic Microsurgery (TEM): a comparative experimental study. Surg Endosc. 2013; 27(10):3762–3768

[166] Clancy C, Burke JP, Albert MR, O'Connell PR, Winter DC. Transanal endoscopic microsurgery versus standard transanal excision for the removal of rectal neoplasms: a systematic review and meta-analysis. Dis Colon Rectum. 2015; 58(2):254–261

[167] Levic K, Bulut O, Hesselfeldt P, Bülow S. The outcome of rectal cancer after early salvage TME following TEM compared with primary TME: a case-matched study. Tech Coloproctol. 2013; 17(4):397–403

[168] Morino M, Allaix ME, Arolfo S, Arezzo A. Previous transanal endoscopic microsurgery for rectal cancer represents a risk factor for an increased abdominoperineal resection rate. Surg Endosc. 2013; 27(9):3315–3321

[169] Hahnloser D, Wolff BG, Larson DW, Ping J, Nivatvongs S. Immediate radical resection after local excision of rectal cancer: an oncologic compromise? Dis Colon Rectum. 2005; 48(3):429–437

[170] Borschitz T, Heintz A, Junginger T. The influence of histopathologic criteria on the long-term prognosis of locally excised pT1 rectal carcinomas: results of local excision (transanal endoscopic microsurgery) and immediate reoperation. Dis Colon Rectum. 2006; 49(10):1492–1506, discussion 1500–1505

[171] Bouvet M, Milas M, Giacco GG, Cleary KR, Janjan NA, Skibber JM. Predictors of recurrence after local excision and postoperative chemoradiation therapy of adenocarcinoma of the rectum. Ann Surg Oncol. 1999; 6(1):26–32

[172] Wagman R, Minsky BD, Cohen AM, Saltz L, Paty PB, Guillem JG. Conservative management of rectal cancer with local excision and postoperative adjuvant therapy. Int J Radiat Oncol Biol Phys. 1999; 44(4):841–846

[173] Greenberg JA, Shibata D, Herndon JE, II, Steele GD, Jr, Mayer R, Bleday R. Local excision of distal rectal cancer: an update of cancer and leukemia group B 8984. Dis Colon Rectum. 2008; 51(8):1185–1191, discussion 1191–1194

[174] Brown C, Raval MJ, Phang PT, Karimuddin AA. The surgical defect after transanal endoscopic microsurgery: open versus closed management. Surg Endosc. 2016; 31(3):1078–1082

[175] Hahnloser D, Cantero R, Salgado G, Dindo D, Rega D, Delrio P. Transanal minimal invasive surgery for rectal lesions: should the defect be closed? Colorectal Dis. 2015; 17(5):397–402

[176] Barendse RM, Oors JM, de Graaf EJ, et al. The effect of endoscopic mucosal resection and transanal endoscopic microsurgery on anorectal function. Colorectal Dis. 2013; 15(9):e534–e541

[177] Herman RM, Richter P, Walega P, Popiela T. Anorectal sphincter function and rectal barostat study in patients following transanal endoscopic microsurgery. Int J Colorectal Dis. 2001; 16(6):370–376

[178] Allaix ME, Rebecchi F, Giaccone C, Mistrangelo M, Morino M. Long-term functional results and quality of life after transanal endoscopic microsurgery. Br J Surg. 2011; 98(11):1635–1643

[179] Winde G, Nottberg H, Keller R, Schmid KW, Bünte H. Surgical cure for early rectal carcinomas (T1). Transanal endoscopic microsurgery vs. anterior resection. Dis Colon Rectum. 1996; 39(9):969–976

[180] Wu Y, Wu YY, Li S, et al. TEM and conventional rectal surgery for T1 rectal cancer: a meta-analysis. Hepatogastroenterology. 2011; 58(106):364–368

[181] Lu JY, Lin GL, Qiu HZ, Xiao Y, Wu B, Zhou JL. Comparison of transanal endoscopic microsurgery and total mesorectal excision in the treatment of T1 rectal cancer: a meta-analysis. PLoS One. 2015; 10(10):e0141427

[182] Lezoche E, Paganini AM, Fabiani B, et al. Quality-of-life impairment after endoluminal locoregional resection and laparoscopic total mesorectal excision. Surg Endosc. 2014; 28(1):227–234

[183] Doornebosch PG, Tollenaar RA, Gosselink MP, et al. Quality of life after transanal endoscopic microsurgery and total mesorectal excision in early rectal cancer. Colorectal Dis. 2007; 9(6):553–558

[184] McLemore EC, Weston LA, Coker AM, et al. Transanal minimally invasive surgery for benign and malignant rectal neoplasia. Am J Surg. 2014; 208(3):372–381

[185] Maslekar S, Pillinger SH, Sharma A, Taylor A, Monson JR. Cost analysis of transanal endoscopic microsurgery for rectal tumours. Colorectal Dis. 2007; 9(3):229–234

[186] Weiser MR, Landmann RG, Wong WD, et al. Surgical salvage of recurrent rectal cancer after transanal excision. Dis Colon Rectum. 2005; 48(6):1169–1175

[187] Friel CM, Cromwell JW, Marra C, Madoff RD, Rothenberger DA, Garcia-Aguílar J. Salvage radical surgery after failed local excision for early rectal cancer. Dis Colon Rectum. 2002; 45(7):875–879

[188] Madbouly KM, Remzi FH, Erkek BA, et al. Recurrence after transanal excision of T1 rectal cancer: should we be concerned? Dis Colon Rectum. 2005; 48(4):711–719, discussion 719–721

[189] Stipa F, Giaccaglia V, Burza A. Management and outcome of local recurrence following transanal endoscopic microsurgery for rectal cancer. Dis Colon Rectum. 2012; 55(3):262–269

[190] Doornebosch PG, Ferenschild FT, de Wilt JH, Dawson I, Tetteroo GW, de Graaf EJ. Treatment of recurrence after transanal endoscopic microsurgery (TEM) for T1 rectal cancer. Dis Colon Rectum. 2010; 53(9):1234–1239

[191] Garcia-Aguilar J, Mellgren A, Sirivongs P, Buie D, Madoff RD, Rothenberger DA. Local excision of rectal cancer without adjuvant therapy: a word of caution. Ann Surg. 2000; 231(3):345–351

[192] Paty PB, Nash GM, Baron P, et al. Long-term results of local excision for rectal cancer. Ann Surg. 2002; 236(4):522–529, discussion 529–530

[193] Gopaul D, Belliveau P, Vuong T, et al. Outcome of local excision of rectal carcinoma. Dis Colon Rectum. 2004; 47(11):1780–1788

[194] Garcia-Aguilar J, Renfro LA, Chow OS, et al. Organ preservation for clinical T2N0 distal rectal cancer using neoadjuvant chemoradiotherapy and local excision (ACOSOG Z6041): results of an open-label, single-arm, multi-institutional, phase 2 trial. Lancet Oncol. 2015; 16(15):1537–1546

[195] Garcia-Aguilar J, Shi Q, Thomas CR, Jr, et al. A phase II trial of neoadjuvant chemoradiation and local excision for T2N0 rectal cancer: preliminary results of the ACOSOG Z6041 trial. Ann Surg Oncol. 2012; 19(2):384–391

[196] Hallam S, Messenger DE, Thomas MG. A systematic review of local excision after neoadjuvant therapy for rectal cancer: are ypT0 tumors the limit? Dis Colon Rectum. 2016; 59(10):984–997

[197] Sprenger T, Rothe H, Conradi LC, et al. Stage-dependent frequency of lymph node metastases in patients with rectal carcinoma after preoperative chemoradiation: results from the CAO/ARO/AIO-94 trial and from a comparative prospective evaluation with extensive pathological workup. Dis Colon Rectum. 2016; 59(5):377–385

[198] Perez RO, Habr-Gama A, São Julião GP, et al. Transanal local excision for distal rectal cancer and incomplete response to neoadjuvant chemoradiation: does baseline staging matter? Dis Colon Rectum. 2014; 57(11):1253–1259

[199] Marks JH, Valsdottir EB, DeNittis A, et al. Transanal endoscopic microsurgery for the treatment of rectal cancer: comparison of wound complication rates with and without neoadjuvant radiation therapy. Surg Endosc. 2009; 23(5):1081–1087

[200] Perez RO, Habr-Gama A, São Julião GP, Proscurshim I, Scanavini Neto A, Gama-Rodrigues J. Transanal endoscopic microsurgery for residual rectal cancer after neoadjuvant chemoradiation therapy is associated with significant immediate pain and hospital readmission rates. Dis Colon Rectum. 2011; 54(5):545–551

[201] Gornicki A, Richter P, Polkowski W, et al. Anorectal and sexual functions after preoperative radiotherapy and full-thickness local excision of rectal cancer. Eur J Surg Oncol. 2014; 40(6):723–730

[202] Habr-Gama A, Lynn PB, Jorge JM, et al. Impact of organ-preserving strategies on anorectal function in patients with distal rectal cancer following neoadjuvant chemoradiation. Dis Colon Rectum. 2016; 59(4):264–269

[203] Verseveld M, de Graaf EJ, Verhoef C, et al. CARTS Study Group. Chemoradiation therapy for rectal cancer in the distal rectum followed by organ-sparing transanal endoscopic microsurgery (CARTS study). Br J Surg. 2015; 102(7):853–860

[204] ISRCTN Register. Transanal endoscopic microsurgery (TEM) and radiotherapy in early rectal Cancer: a randomised phase II feasibility study. Available at: http://www.isrctn.com/ISRCTN14422743?q=Transanal. Accessed November 25, 2016

[205] Stipa F, Chessin DB, Shia J, et al. A pathologic complete response of rectal cancer to preoperative combined-modality therapy results in improved oncological outcome compared with those who achieve no downstaging on the basis of preoperative endorectal ultrasonography. Ann Surg Oncol. 2006; 13(8):1047–1053

[206] Valentini V, Coco C, Picciocchi A, et al. Does downstaging predict improved outcome after preoperative chemoradiation for extraperitoneal locally advanced rectal cancer? A long-term analysis of 165 patients. Int J Radiat Oncol Biol Phys. 2002; 53(3):664–674

[207] Maas M, Nelemans PJ, Valentini V, et al. Long-term outcome in patients with a pathological complete response after chemoradiation for rectal cancer: a pooled analysis of individual patient data. Lancet Oncol. 2010; 11(9):835–844

[208] Monson JRT, Arsalanizadeh R. Surgery for patients with rectal cancer-time to listen to the patients and recognize reality. JAMA Oncol. 2017; 3(7):887–888

[209] Habr-Gama A, Perez RO, Nadalin W, et al. Operative versus nonoperative treatment for stage 0 distal rectal cancer following chemoradiation therapy: long-term results. Ann Surg. 2004; 240(4):711–717, discussion 717–718

[210] Habr-Gama A, Gama-Rodrigues J, São Julião GP, et al. Local recurrence after complete clinical response and watch and wait in rectal cancer after neoadjuvant chemoradiation: impact of salvage therapy on local disease control. Int J Radiat Oncol Biol Phys. 2014; 88(4):822–828

[211] Maas M, Beets-Tan RG, Lambregts DM, et al. Wait-and-see policy for clinical complete responders after chemoradiation for rectal cancer. J Clin Oncol. 2011; 29(35):4633–4640

[212] Smith JD, Ruby JA, Goodman KA, et al. Nonoperative management of rectal cancer with complete clinical response after neoadjuvant therapy. Ann Surg. 2012; 256(6):965–972

[213] Renehan AG, Malcomson L, Emsley R, et al. Watch-and-wait approach versus surgical resection after chemoradiotherapy for patients with rectal cancer (the OnCoRe project): a propensity-score matched cohort analysis. Lancet Oncol. 2016; 17(2):174–183

[214] Park IJ, You YN, Skibber JM, et al. Comparative analysis of lymph node metastases in patients with ypT0–2 rectal cancers after neoadjuvant chemoradiotherapy. Dis Colon Rectum. 2013; 56(2):135–141

[215] Perez RO, Habr-Gama A, Nishida Arazawa ST, et al. Lymph node micrometastasis in stage II distal rectal cancer following neoadjuvant chemoradiation therapy. Int J Colorectal Dis. 2005; 20(5):434–439

[216] Hiotis SP, Weber SM, Cohen AM, et al. Assessing the predictive value of clinical complete response to neoadjuvant therapy for rectal cancer: an analysis of 488 patients. J Am Coll Surg. 2002; 194(2):131–135, discussion 135–136

[217] Smith FM, Wiland H, Mace A, Pai RK, Kalady MF. Clinical criteria underestimate complete pathological response in rectal cancer treated with neoadjuvant chemoradiotherapy. Dis Colon Rectum. 2014; 57(3):311–315

[218] Smith FM, Chang KH, Sheahan K, Hyland J, O'Connell PR, Winter DC. The surgical significance of residual mucosal abnormalities in rectal cancer following neoadjuvant chemoradiotherapy. Br J Surg. 2012; 99(7):993–1001

[219] O'Neill BD, Brown G, Heald RJ, Cunningham D, Tait DM. Non-operative treatment after neoadjuvant chemoradiotherapy for rectal cancer. Lancet Oncol. 2007; 8(7):625–633

[220] Perez RO, Habr-Gama A, Gama-Rodrigues J, et al. Accuracy of positron emission tomography/computed tomography and clinical assessment in the detection of complete rectal tumor regression after neoadjuvant chemoradiation: long-term results of a prospective trial (National Clinical Trial 00254683). Cancer. 2012; 118(14):3501–3511

[221] Jang NY, Kang SB, Kim DW, et al. The role of carcinoembryonic antigen after neoadjuvant chemoradiotherapy in patients with rectal cancer. Dis Colon Rectum. 2011; 54(2):245–252

[222] Habr-Gama A, São Julião GP, Perez RO. Pitfalls of transanal endoscopic microsurgery for rectal cancer following neoadjuvant chemoradiation therapy. Minim Invasive Ther Allied Technol. 2014; 23(2):63–69

[223] Perez RO, Habr-Gama A, São Julião GP, et al. Optimal timing for assessment of tumor response to neoadjuvant chemoradiation in patients with rectal cancer: do all patients benefit from waiting longer than 6 weeks? Int J Radiat Oncol Biol Phys. 2012; 84(5):1159–1165

[224] Heald RJ. A new approach to rectal cancer. Br J Hosp Med. 1979; 22 (3):277–281

[225] Heald RJ, Ryall RD. Recurrence and survival after total mesorectal excision for rectal cancer. Lancet. 1986; 1(8496):1479–1482

[226] Påhlman L, Glimelius B. Local recurrences after surgical treatment for rectal carcinoma. Acta Chir Scand. 1984; 150(4):331–335

[227] Pilipshen SJ, Heilweil M, Quan SH, Sternberg SS, Enker WE. Patterns of pelvic recurrence following definitive resections of rectal cancer. Cancer. 1984; 53 (6):1354–1362

[228] Hurst PA, Prout WG, Kelly JM, Bannister JJ, Walker RT. Local recurrence after low anterior resection using the staple gun. Br J Surg. 1982; 69(5):275–276

[229] Maurer CA, Renzulli P, Kull C, et al. The impact of the introduction of total mesorectal excision on local recurrence rate and survival in rectal cancer: long-term results. Ann Surg Oncol. 2011; 18(7):1899–1906

[230] Köckerling F, Reymond MA, Altendorf-Hofmann A, Dworak O, Hohenberger W. Influence of surgery on metachronous distant metastases and survival in rectal cancer. J Clin Oncol. 1998; 16(1):324–329

[231] Kapiteijn E, Putter H, van de Velde CJ, Cooperative Investigators of the Dutch ColoRectal Cancer Group. Impact of the introduction and training of total mesorectal excision on recurrence and survival in rectal cancer in The Netherlands. Br J Surg. 2002; 89(9):1142–1149

[232] Arbman G, Nilsson E, Hallböök O, Sjödahl R. Local recurrence following total mesorectal excision for rectal cancer. Br J Surg. 1996; 83(3):375–379

[233] Wilson SM, Beahrs OH. The curative treatment of carcinoma of the sigmoid, rectosigmoid, and rectum. Ann Surg. 1976; 183(5):556–565

[234] Cass AW, Million RR, Pfaff WW. Patterns of recurrence following surgery alone for adenocarcinoma of the colon and rectum. Cancer. 1976; 37 (6):2861–2865

[235] Rao AR, Kagan AR, Chan PM, Gilbert HA, Nussbaum H, Hintz BL. Patterns of recurrence following curative resection alone for adenocarcinoma of the rectum and sigmoid colon. Cancer. 1981; 48(6):1492–1495

[236] de Haas-Kock DF, Baeten CG, Jager JJ, et al. Prognostic significance of radial margins of clearance in rectal cancer. Br J Surg. 1996; 83(6):781–785

[237] Adam IJ, Mohamdee MO, Martin IG, et al. Role of circumferential margin involvement in the local recurrence of rectal cancer. Lancet. 1994; 344 (8924):707–711

[238] Nagtegaal ID, Marijnen CA, Kranenbarg EK, van de Velde CJ, van Krieken JH, Pathology Review Committee, Cooperative Clinical Investigators. Circumferential margin involvement is still an important predictor of local recurrence in rectal carcinoma: not one millimeter but two millimeters is the limit. Am J Surg Pathol. 2002; 26(3):350–357

[239] Nagtegaal ID, Quirke P. What is the role for the circumferential margin in the modern treatment of rectal cancer? J Clin Oncol. 2008; 26(2):303–312

[240] Marijnen CA, Nagtegaal ID, Kapiteijn E, et al. Cooperative Investigators of the Dutch Colorectal Cancer Group. Radiotherapy does not compensate for positive resection margins in rectal cancer patients: report of a multicenter randomized trial. Int J Radiat Oncol Biol Phys. 2003; 55(5):1311–1320

[241] Birbeck KF, Macklin CP, Tiffin NJ, et al. Rates of circumferential resection margin involvement vary between surgeons and predict outcomes in rectal cancer surgery. Ann Surg. 2002; 235(4):449–457

[242] Bosch SL, Nagtegaal ID. The importance of the pathologist's role in assessment of the quality of the mesorectum. Curr Colorectal Cancer Rep. 2012; 8 (2):90–98

[243] Nagtegaal ID, van de Velde CJ, van der Worp E, Kapiteijn E, Quirke P, van Krieken JH, Cooperative Clinical Investigators of the Dutch Colorectal Cancer Group. Macroscopic evaluation of rectal cancer resection specimen: clinical significance of the pathologist in quality control. J Clin Oncol. 2002; 20 (7):1729–1734

[244] Quirke P, Steele R, Monson J, et al. MRC CR07/NCIC-CTG CO16 Trial Investigators, NCRI Colorectal Cancer Study Group. Effect of the plane of surgery achieved on local recurrence in patients with operable rectal cancer: a prospective study using data from the MRC CR07 and NCIC-CTG CO16 randomised clinical trial. Lancet. 2009; 373(9666):821–828

[245] Hall NR, Finan PJ, al-Jaberi T, et al. Circumferential margin involvement after mesorectal excision of rectal cancer with curative intent. Predictor of survival but not local recurrence? Dis Colon Rectum. 1998; 41(8):979–983

[246] Bonnet S, Berger A, Hentati N, et al. High tie versus low tie vascular ligation of the inferior mesenteric artery in colorectal cancer surgery: impact on the gain in colon length and implications on the feasibility of anastomoses. Dis Colon Rectum. 2012; 55(5):515–521

[247] Titu LV, Tweedle E, Rooney PS. High tie of the inferior mesenteric artery in curative surgery for left colonic and rectal cancers: a systematic review. Dig Surg. 2008; 25(2):148–157

[248] Lange MM, Buunen M, van de Velde CJ, Lange JF. Level of arterial ligation in rectal cancer surgery: low tie preferred over high tie. A review. Dis Colon Rectum. 2008; 51(9):1139–1145

[249] Malassagne B, Valleur P, Serra J, et al. Relationship of apical lymph node involvement to survival in resected colon carcinoma. Dis Colon Rectum. 1993; 36(7):645–653

[250] Kim JC, Lee KH, Yu CS, et al. The clinicopathological significance of inferior mesenteric lymph node metastasis in colorectal cancer. Eur J Surg Oncol. 2004; 30(3):271–279

[251] Marsden MR, Conti JA, Zeidan S, et al. The selective use of splenic flexure mobilization is safe in both laparoscopic and open anterior resections. Colorectal Dis. 2012; 14(10):1255–1261

[252] Karanjia ND, Corder AP, Bearn P, Heald RJ. Leakage from stapled low anastomosis after total mesorectal excision for carcinoma of the rectum. Br J Surg. 1994; 81(8):1224–1226

[253] Maurer CA, Z'Graggen K, Renzulli P, Schilling MK, Netzer P, Büchler MW. Total mesorectal excision preserves male genital function compared with conventional rectal cancer surgery. Br J Surg. 2001; 88(11):1501–1505

[254] Maas CP, Moriya Y, Steup WH, Klein Kranenbarg E, van de Velde CJ. A prospective study on radical and nerve-preserving surgery for rectal cancer in the Netherlands. Eur J Surg Oncol. 2000; 26(8):751–757

[255] Hendren SK, O'Connor BI, Liu M, et al. Prevalence of male and female sexual dysfunction is high following surgery for rectal cancer. Ann Surg. 2005; 242 (2):212–223

[256] Stamopoulos P, Theodoropoulos GE, Papailiou J, et al. Prospective evaluation of sexual function after open and laparoscopic surgery for rectal cancer. Surg Endosc. 2009; 23(12):2665–2674

[257] Lange MM, Maas CP, Marijnen CA, et al. Cooperative Clinical Investigators of the Dutch Total Mesorectal Excision Trial. Urinary dysfunction after rectal cancer treatment is mainly caused by surgery. Br J Surg. 2008; 95 (8):1020–1028

[258] Lange MM, van de Velde CJ. Urinary and sexual dysfunction after rectal cancer treatment. Nat Rev Urol. 2011; 8(1):51–57

[259] Quah HM, Jayne DG, Eu KW, Seow-Choen F. Bladder and sexual dysfunction following laparoscopically assisted and conventional open mesorectal resection for cancer. Br J Surg. 2002; 89(12):1551–1556

[260] Jayne DG, Brown JM, Thorpe H, Walker J, Quirke P, Guillou PJ. Bladder and sexual function following resection for rectal cancer in a randomized clinical trial of laparoscopic versus open technique. Br J Surg. 2005; 92(9):1124–1132

[261] Andersson J, Abis G, Gellerstedt M, et al. Patient-reported genitourinary dysfunction after laparoscopic and open rectal cancer surgery in a randomized trial (COLOR II). Br J Surg. 2014; 101(10):1272–1279

[262] Asoglu O, Matlim T, Karanlik H, et al. Impact of laparoscopic surgery on bladder and sexual function after total mesorectal excision for rectal cancer. Surg Endosc. 2009; 23(2):296–303

[263] Yang L, Yu YY, Zhou ZG, et al. Quality of life outcomes following laparoscopic total mesorectal excision for low rectal cancers: a clinical control study. Eur J Surg Oncol. 2007; 33(5):575–579

[264] Kim JY, Kim NK, Lee KY, Hur H, Min BS, Kim JH. A comparative study of voiding and sexual function after total mesorectal excision with autonomic nerve preservation for rectal cancer: laparoscopic versus robotic surgery. Ann Surg Oncol. 2012; 19(8):2485–2493

[265] Brown CJ, Fenech DS, McLeod RS. Reconstructive techniques after rectal resection for rectal cancer. Cochrane Database Syst Rev. 2008(2):CD006040

[266] Hida J, Yasutomi M, Maruyama T, Fujimoto K, Uchida T, Okuno K. Lymph node metastases detected in the mesorectum distal to carcinoma of the rectum by the clearing method: justification of total mesorectal excision. J Am Coll Surg. 1997; 184(6):584–588

[267] Scott N, Jackson P, al-Jaberi T, Dixon MF, Quirke P, Finan PJ. Total mesorectal excision and local recurrence: a study of tumour spread in the mesorectum distal to rectal cancer. Br J Surg. 1995; 82(8):1031–1033

[268] Lopez-Kostner F, Lavery IC, Hool GR, Rybicki LA, Fazio VW. Total mesorectal excision is not necessary for cancers of the upper rectum. Surgery. 1998; 124(4):612–617, discussion 617–618

[269] Zaheer S, Pemberton JH, Farouk R, Dozois RR, Wolff BG, Ilstrup D. Surgical treatment of adenocarcinoma of the rectum. Ann Surg. 1998; 227(6):800–811

[270] Williams NS, Dixon MF, Johnston D. Reappraisal of the 5 centimetre rule of distal excision for carcinoma of the rectum: a study of distal intramural spread and of patients' survival. Br J Surg. 1983; 70(3):150–154

[271] Pollett WG, Nicholls RJ. The relationship between the extent of distal clearance and survival and local recurrence rates after curative anterior resection for carcinoma of the rectum. Ann Surg. 1983; 198(2):159–163

[272] Vernava AM, III, Moran M, Rothenberger DA, Wong WD. A prospective evaluation of distal margins in carcinoma of the rectum. Surg Gynecol Obstet. 1992; 175(4):333–336

[273] Wolmark N, Fisher B, National Surgical Adjuvant Breast and Bowel Project. An analysis of survival and treatment failure following abdominoperineal and sphincter-saving resection in Dukes' B and C rectal carcinoma. A report of the NSABP clinical trials. Ann Surg. 1986; 204(4):480–489

[274] Guillem JG, Chessin DB, Shia J, et al. A prospective pathologic analysis using whole-mount sections of rectal cancer following preoperative combined modality therapy: implications for sphincter preservation. Ann Surg. 2007; 245(1):88–93

[275] Kuvshinoff B, Maghfoor I, Miedema B, et al. Distal margin requirements after preoperative chemoradiotherapy for distal rectal carcinomas: are < or = 1 cm distal margins sufficient? Ann Surg Oncol. 2001; 8(2):163–169

[276] Rutkowski A, Nowacki MP, Chwalinski M, et al. Acceptance of a 5-mm distal bowel resection margin for rectal cancer: is it safe? Colorectal Dis. 2012; 14 (1):71–78

[277] Yeo HL, Abelson JS, Mao J, Cheerharan M, Milsom J, Sedrakyan A. Minimally invasive surgery and sphincter preservation in rectal cancer. J Surg Res. 2016; 202(2):299–307

[278] Sun Z, Kim J, Adam MA, et al. Minimally invasive versus open low anterior resection: equivalent survival in a national analysis of 14,033 patients with rectal cancer. Ann Surg. 2016; 263(6):1152–1158

[279] Fleshman J, Branda M, Sargent DJ, et al. Effect of laparoscopic-assisted resection vs open resection of stage II or III rectal cancer on pathologic outcomes: the ACOSOG Z6051 randomized clinical trial. JAMA. 2015; 314(13):1346–1355

[280] Lujan J, Valero G, Hernandez Q, Sanchez A, Frutos MD, Parrilla P. Randomized clinical trial comparing laparoscopic and open surgery in patients with rectal cancer. Br J Surg. 2009; 96(9):982–989

[281] Guillou PJ, Quirke P, Thorpe H, et al. MRC CLASICC trial group. Short-term endpoints of conventional versus laparoscopic-assisted surgery in patients with colorectal cancer (MRC CLASICC trial): multicentre, randomised controlled trial. Lancet. 2005; 365(9472):1718–1726

[282] Jayne DG, Thorpe HC, Copeland J, Quirke P, Brown JM, Guillou PJ. Five-year follow-up of the Medical Research Council CLASICC trial of laparoscopically assisted versus open surgery for colorectal cancer. Br J Surg. 2010; 97 (11):1638–1645

[283] Bonjer HJ, Deijen CL, Abis GA, et al. COLOR II Study Group. A randomized trial of laparoscopic versus open surgery for rectal cancer. N Engl J Med. 2015; 372(14):1324–1332

[284] van der Pas MH, Haglind E, Cuesta MA, et al. COlorectal cancer Laparoscopic or Open Resection II (COLOR II) Study Group. Laparoscopic versus open surgery for rectal cancer (COLOR II): short-term outcomes of a randomised, phase 3 trial. Lancet Oncol. 2013; 14(3):210–218

[285] Kang SB, Park JW, Jeong SY, et al. Open versus laparoscopic surgery for mid or low rectal cancer after neoadjuvant chemoradiotherapy (COREAN trial): short-term outcomes of an open-label randomised controlled trial. Lancet Oncol. 2010; 11(7):637–645

[286] Jeong SY, Park JW, Nam BH, et al. Open versus laparoscopic surgery for mid-rectal or low-rectal cancer after neoadjuvant chemoradiotherapy (COREAN trial): survival outcomes of an open-label, non-inferiority, randomised controlled trial. Lancet Oncol. 2014; 15(7):767–774

[287] Stevenson AR, Solomon MJ, Lumley JW, et al. ALaCaRT Investigators. Effect of laparoscopic-assisted resection vs open resection on pathological outcomes in rectal cancer: the ALaCaRT randomized clinical trial. JAMA. 2015; 314 (13):1356–1363

[288] Ballantyne GH, Moll F. The da Vinci telerobotic surgical system: the virtual operative field and telepresence surgery. Surg Clin North Am. 2003; 83 (6):1293–1304, vii

[289] Lanfranco AR, Castellanos AE, Desai JP, Meyers WC. Robotic surgery: a current perspective. Ann Surg. 2004; 239(1):14–21

[290] Baik SH. Robotic colorectal surgery. Yonsei Med J. 2008; 49(6):891–896

[291] Baik SH, Kim NK, Lim DR, Hur H, Min BS, Lee KY. Oncologic outcomes and perioperative clinicopathologic results after robot-assisted tumor-specific mesorectal excision for rectal cancer. Ann Surg Oncol. 2013; 20(8):2625–2632

[292] Pigazzi A, Luca F, Patriti A, et al. Multicentric study on robotic tumor-specific mesorectal excision for the treatment of rectal cancer. Ann Surg Oncol. 2010; 17(6):1614–1620

[293] Ghezzi TL, Luca F, Valvo M, et al. Robotic versus open total mesorectal excision for rectal cancer: comparative study of short and long-term outcomes. Eur J Surg Oncol. 2014; 40(9):1072–1079

[294] deSouza AL, Prasad LM, Ricci J, et al. A comparison of open and robotic total mesorectal excision for rectal adenocarcinoma. Dis Colon Rectum. 2011; 54 (3):275–282

[295] Luca F, Valvo M, Ghezzi TL, et al. Impact of robotic surgery on sexual and urinary functions after fully robotic nerve-sparing total mesorectal excision for rectal cancer. Ann Surg. 2013; 257(4):672–678

[296] Baik SH, Ko YT, Kang CM, et al. Robotic tumor-specific mesorectal excision of rectal cancer: short-term outcome of a pilot randomized trial. Surg Endosc. 2008; 22(7):1601–1608

[297] Wang Y, Zhao GH, Yang H, Lin J. A pooled analysis of robotic versus laparoscopic surgery for total mesorectal excision for rectal cancer. Surg Laparosc Endosc Percutan Tech. 2016; 26(3):259–264

[298] Kim NK, Kang J. Optimal total mesorectal excision for rectal cancer: the role of robotic surgery from an expert's view. J Korean Soc Coloproctol. 2010; 26 (6):377–387

[299] Leong QM, Son DN, Cho JS, et al. Robot-assisted intersphincteric resection for low rectal cancer: technique and short-term outcome for 29 consecutive patients. Surg Endosc. 2011; 25(9):2987–2992

[300] Collinson FJ, Jayne DG, Pigazzi A, et al. An international, multicentre, prospective, randomised, controlled, unblinded, parallel-group trial of robotic-assisted versus standard laparoscopic surgery for the curative treatment of rectal cancer. Int J Colorectal Dis. 2012; 27(2):233–241

[301] Choi CS. A Trial to Assess Robot-assisted Surgery and Laparoscopy-assisted Surgery in Patients with Mid or Low Rectal Cancer (COLRAR). NCT01423214. 2016. Available at: http://clinicaltrials.gov/ct2/show/NCT01423214

[302] Park JW. Clinical assessment of laparoscopic and robotic surgery for rectal cancer-randomized phase II trial. NCT01591798. 2016. Available at: http://clinicaltrials.gov/ct2/show/NCT01591798

[303] Jayne D, Pigazzi A, Marshall H, et al. Effect of Robotic-Assisted vs. Conventional Laparascopic Surgery on Risk of Conversion to Open Laparotomy Among Patients Undergoing Resection for the Rectal Cancer: The ROLARR Randomized Clinical Trial. JAMA. 2017; 318(16):1569–1580

[304] Rickles AS, Dietz DW, Chang GJ, et al. Consortium for Optimizing the Treatment of Rectal Cancer (OSTRiCh). High rate of positive circumferential resection margins following rectal cancer surgery: a call to action. Ann Surg. 2015; 262(6):891–898

[305] Heald RJ. A new solution to some old problems: transanal TME. Tech Coloproctol. 2013; 17(3):257–258

[306] Atallah S, Martin-Perez B, Albert M, et al. Transanal minimally invasive surgery for total mesorectal excision (TAMIS-TME): results and experience with the first 20 patients undergoing curative-intent rectal cancer surgery at a single institution. Tech Coloproctol. 2014; 18(5):473–480

[307] Penna M, Hompes R, Arnold S, et al. Transanal total mesorectal excision: international registry results of the first 720 cases. Ann Surg. 2017; 266(1):111–117

[308] Deijen CL, Velthuis S, Tsai A, et al. COLOR III: a multicentre randomised clinical trial comparing transanal TME versus laparoscopic TME for mid and low rectal cancer. Surg Endosc. 2016; 30(8):3210–3215

[309] Martling AL, Holm T, Rutqvist LE, Moran BJ, Heald RJ, Cedermark B. Effect of a surgical training programme on outcome of rectal cancer in the County of Stockholm. Stockholm Colorectal Cancer Study Group, Basingstoke Bowel Cancer Research Project. Lancet. 2000; 356(9224):93–96

[310] Marr R, Birbeck K, Garvican J, et al. The modern abdominoperineal excision: the next challenge after total mesorectal excision. Ann Surg. 2005; 242(1):74–82

[311] Wibe A, Syse A, Andersen E, Tretli S, Myrvold HE, Søreide O, Norwegian Rectal Cancer Group. Oncological outcomes after total mesorectal excision for cure for cancer of the lower rectum: anterior vs. abdominoperineal resection. Dis Colon Rectum. 2004; 47(1):48–58

[312] den Dulk M, Putter H, Collette L, et al. The abdominoperineal resection itself is associated with an adverse outcome: the European experience based on a pooled analysis of five European randomised clinical trials on rectal cancer. Eur J Cancer. 2009; 45(7):1175–1183

[313] Nagtegaal ID, van de Velde CJ, Marijnen CA, van Krieken JH, Quirke P, Dutch Colorectal Cancer Group, Pathology Review Committee. Low rectal cancer: a call for a change of approach in abdominoperineal resection. J Clin Oncol. 2005; 23(36):9257–9264

[314] den Dulk M, Marijnen CA, Putter H, et al. Risk factors for adverse outcome in patients with rectal cancer treated with an abdominoperineal resection in the total mesorectal excision trial. Ann Surg. 2007; 246(1):83–90

[315] Eriksen MT, Wibe A, Syse A, Haffner J, Wiig JN, Norwegian Rectal Cancer Group, Norwegian Gastrointestinal Cancer Group. Inadvertent perforation during rectal cancer resection in Norway. Br J Surg. 2004; 91(2):210–216

[316] Meyerhardt JA, Tepper JE, Niedzwiecki D, et al. Impact of hospital procedure volume on surgical operation and long-term outcomes in high-risk curatively resected rectal cancer: findings from the Intergroup 0114 Study. J Clin Oncol. 2004; 22(1):166–174

[317] Morris E, Quirke P, Thomas JD, Fairley L, Cottier B, Forman D. Unacceptable variation in abdominoperineal excision rates for rectal cancer: time to intervene? Gut. 2008; 57(12):1690–1697

[318] Moore TJ, Moran BJ. Precision surgery, precision terminology: the origins and meaning of ELAPE. Colorectal Dis. 2012; 14(10):1173–1174

[319] Holm T. Controversies in abdominoperineal excision. Surg Oncol Clin N Am. 2014; 23(1):93–111

[320] Holm T, Ljung A, Häggmark T, Jurell G, Lagergren J. Extended abdominoperineal resection with gluteus maximus flap reconstruction of the pelvic floor for rectal cancer. Br J Surg. 2007; 94(2):232–238

[321] West NP, Anderin C, Smith KJ, Holm T, Quirke P, European Extralevator Abdominoperineal Excision Study Group. Multicentre experience with extralevator abdominoperineal excision for low rectal cancer. Br J Surg. 2010; 97 (4):588–599

[322] Stelzner S, Koehler C, Stelzer J, Sims A, Witzigmann H. Extended abdominoperineal excision vs. standard abdominoperineal excision in rectal cancer: a systematic overview. Int J Colorectal Dis. 2011; 26(10):1227–1240

[323] Krishna A, Rickard MJ, Keshava A, Dent OF, Chapuis PH. A comparison of published rates of resection margin involvement and intra-operative perforation between standard and 'cylindrical' abdominoperineal excision for low rectal cancer. Colorectal Dis. 2013; 15(1):57–65

[324] de Campos-Lobato LF, Stocchi L, Dietz DW, Lavery IC, Fazio VW, Kalady MF. Prone or lithotomy positioning during an abdominoperineal resection for rectal cancer results in comparable oncologic outcomes. Dis Colon Rectum. 2011; 54(8):939–946

[325] Martijnse IS, Dudink RL, West NP, et al. Focus on extralevator perineal dissection in supine position for low rectal cancer has led to better quality of surgery and oncological outcome. Ann Surg Oncol. 2012; 19(3):786–793

[326] Bullard KM, Trudel JL, Baxter NN, Rothenberger DA. Primary perineal wound closure after preoperative radiotherapy and abdominoperineal resection has a high incidence of wound failure. Dis Colon Rectum. 2005; 48(3):438–443

[327] Nisar PJ, Scott HJ. Myocutaneous flap reconstruction of the pelvis after abdominoperineal excision. Colorectal Dis. 2009; 11(8):806–816

[328] Khoo AK, Skibber JM, Nabawi AS, et al. Indications for immediate tissue transfer for soft tissue reconstruction in visceral pelvic surgery. Surgery. 2001; 130(3):463–469

[329] Foster JD, Pathak S, Smart NJ, et al. Reconstruction of the perineum following extralevator abdominoperineal excision for carcinoma of the lower rectum: a systematic review. Colorectal Dis. 2012; 14(9):1052–1059

[330] Rullier E, Denost Q, Vendrely V, Rullier A, Laurent C. Low rectal cancer: classification and standardization of surgery. Dis Colon Rectum. 2013; 56 (5):560–567

[331] Battersby NJ, How P, Moran B, et al. MERCURY II Study Group. Prospective validation of a low rectal cancer magnetic resonance imaging staging system and development of a local recurrence risk stratification model: the MERCURY II study. Ann Surg. 2016; 263(4):751–760

[332] Weiser MR, Quah HM, Shia J, et al. Sphincter preservation in low rectal cancer is facilitated by preoperative chemoradiation and intersphincteric dissection. Ann Surg. 2009; 249(2):236–242

[333] Guren MG, Eriksen MT, Wiig JN, et al. Norwegian Rectal Cancer Group. Quality of life and functional outcome following anterior or abdominoperineal resection for rectal cancer. Eur J Surg Oncol. 2005; 31(7):735–742

[334] Digennaro R, Tondo M, Cuccia F, et al. Coloanal anastomosis or abdominoperineal resection for very low rectal cancer: what will benefit, the surgeon's pride or the patient's quality of life? Int J Colorectal Dis. 2013; 28 (7):949–957

[335] Konanz J, Herrle F, Weiss C, Post S, Kienle P. Quality of life of patients after low anterior, intersphincteric, and abdominoperineal resection for rectal cancer–a matched-pair analysis. Int J Colorectal Dis. 2013; 28(5):679–688

[336] Parc Y, Zutshi M, Zalinski S, Ruppert R, Fürst A, Fazio VW. Preoperative radiotherapy is associated with worse functional results after coloanal anastomosis for rectal cancer. Dis Colon Rectum. 2009; 52(12):2004–2014

[337] Bretagnol F, Rullier E, Laurent C, Zerbib F, Gontier R, Saric J. Comparison of functional results and quality of life between intersphincteric resection and conventional coloanal anastomosis for low rectal cancer. Dis Colon Rectum. 2004; 47(6):832–838

[338] Barisic G, Markovic V, Popovic M, Dimitrijevic I, Gavrilovic P, Krivokapic Z. Function after intersphincteric resection for low rectal cancer and its influence on quality of life. Colorectal Dis. 2011; 13(6):638–643

[339] Russell MM, Ganz PA, Lopa S, et al. Comparative effectiveness of sphincter-sparing surgery versus abdominoperineal resection in rectal cancer: patient-reported outcomes in National Surgical Adjuvant Breast and Bowel Project randomized trial R-04. Ann Surg. 2015; 261(1):144–148

[340] How P, Stelzner S, Branagan G, et al. Comparative quality of life in patients following abdominoperineal excision and low anterior resection for low rectal cancer. Dis Colon Rectum. 2012; 55(4):400–406

[341] Kasparek MS, Hassan I, Cima RR, Larson DR, Gullerud RE, Wolff BG. Quality of life after coloanal anastomosis and abdominoperineal resection for distal rectal cancers: sphincter preservation vs quality of life. Colorectal Dis. 2011; 13(8):872–877

[342] Hida J, Yasutomi M, Fujimoto K, Maruyama T, Okuno K, Shindo K. Does lateral lymph node dissection improve survival in rectal carcinoma? Examination of node metastases by the clearing method. J Am Coll Surg. 1997; 184 (5):475–480

[343] Steup WH, Moriya Y, van de Velde CJ. Patterns of lymphatic spread in rectal cancer. A topographical analysis on lymph node metastases. Eur J Cancer. 2002; 38(7):911–918

[344] Ueno H, Mochizuki H, Hashiguchi Y, Hase K. Prognostic determinants of patients with lateral nodal involvement by rectal cancer. Ann Surg. 2001; 234 (2):190–197

[345] Fujita S, Yamamoto S, Akasu T, Moriya Y. Lateral pelvic lymph node dissection for advanced lower rectal cancer. Br J Surg. 2003; 90(12):1580–1585

[346] Hojo K, Sawada T, Moriya Y. An analysis of survival and voiding, sexual function after wide iliopelvic lymphadenectomy in patients with carcinoma of the rectum, compared with conventional lymphadenectomy. Dis Colon Rectum. 1989; 32(2):128–133

[347] Kusters M, Marijnen CA, van de Velde CJ, et al. Patterns of local recurrence in rectal cancer; a study of the Dutch TME trial. Eur J Surg Oncol. 2010; 36 (5):470–476

[348] Kusters M, Beets GL, van de Velde CJ, et al. A comparison between the treatment of low rectal cancer in Japan and the Netherlands, focusing on the patterns of local recurrence. Ann Surg. 2009; 249(2):229–235

[349] Georgiou P, Tan E, Gouvas N, et al. Extended lymphadenectomy versus conventional surgery for rectal cancer: a meta-analysis. Lancet Oncol. 2009; 10 (11):1053–1062

[350] Kim JC, Takahashi K, Yu CS, et al. Comparative outcome between chemoradiotherapy and lateral pelvic lymph node dissection following total mesorectal excision in rectal cancer. Ann Surg. 2007; 246(5):754–762

[351] Heriot AG, Byrne CM, Lee P, et al. Extended radical resection: the choice for locally recurrent rectal cancer. Dis Colon Rectum. 2008; 51(3):284–291

[352] Bokey EL, Chapuis PH, Hughes WJ, Koorey SG, Dunn D. Local recurrence following anterior resection for carcinoma of the rectum with a stapled anastomosis. Acta Chir Scand. 1984; 150(8):683–686

[353] Colombo PL, Foglieni CL, Morone C. Analysis of recurrence following curative low anterior resection and stapled anastomoses for carcinoma of the middle third and lower rectum. Dis Colon Rectum. 1987; 30(6):457–464

[354] Bisgaard C, Svanholm H, Jensen AS. Recurrent carcinoma after low anterior resection of the rectum using the EEA staple gun. Acta Chir Scand. 1986; 152:157–160

[355] Chiarugi M, Buccianti P, Sidoti F, Franceschi M, Goletti O, Cavina E. Single and double stapled anastomoses in rectal cancer surgery; a retrospective study on the safety of the technique and its indication. Acta Chir Belg. 1996; 96 (1):31–36

[356] Moore JW, Chapuis PH, Bokey EL. Morbidity and mortality after single- and double-stapled colorectal anastomoses in patients with carcinoma of the rectum. Aust N Z J Surg. 1996; 66(12):820–823

[357] Marecik SJ, Chaudhry V, Pearl R, Park JJ, Prasad LM. Single-stapled double-pursestring anastomosis after anterior resection of the rectum. Am J Surg. 2007; 193(3):395–399

[358] Neutzling CB, Lustosa SA, Proenca IM, da Silva EM, Matos D. Stapled versus handsewn methods for colorectal anastomosis surgery. Cochrane Database Syst Rev. 2012(2):CD003144

[359] Masoomi H, Luo R, Mills S, Carmichael JC, Senagore AJ, Stamos MJ. Compression anastomosis ring device in colorectal anastomosis: a review of 1,180 patients. Am J Surg. 2013; 205(4):447–451

[360] D'Hoore A, Albert MR, Cohen SM, et al. COMPRES collaborative study group. COMPRES: a prospective postmarketing evaluation of the compression anastomosis ring CAR 27(™) /ColonRing(™). Colorectal Dis. 2015; 17 (6):522–529

[361] Tabola R, Cirocchi R, Fingerhut A, et al. A systematic analysis of controlled clinical trials using the NiTi CAR™ compression ring in colorectal anastomoses. Tech Coloproctol. 2017; 21(3):177–184

[362] Slesser AA, Pellino G, Shariq O, et al. Compression versus hand-sewn and stapled anastomosis in colorectal surgery: a systematic review and meta-analysis of randomized controlled trials. Tech Coloproctol. 2016; 20 (10):667–676

[363] Lewis WG, Holdsworth PJ, Stephenson BM, Finan PJ, Johnston D. Role of the rectum in the physiological and clinical results of coloanal and colorectal anastomosis after anterior resection for rectal carcinoma. Br J Surg. 1992; 79 (10):1082–1086

[364] Montesani C, Pronio A, Santella S, et al. Rectal cancer surgery with sphincter preservation: functional results related to the level of anastomosis. Clinical and instrumental study. Hepatogastroenterology. 2004; 51(57):718–721

[365] Williamson ME, Lewis WG, Finan PJ, Miller AS, Holdsworth PJ, Johnston D. Recovery of physiologic and clinical function after low anterior resection of the rectum for carcinoma: myth or reality? Dis Colon Rectum. 1995; 38 (4):411–418

[366] Fürst A, Burghofer K, Hutzel L, Jauch KW. Neorectal reservoir is not the functional principle of the colonic J-pouch: the volume of a short colonic J-pouch does not differ from a straight coloanal anastomosis. Dis Colon Rectum. 2002; 45(5):660–667

[367] Z'graggen K, Maurer CA, Birrer S, Giachino D, Kern B, Büchler MW. A new surgical concept for rectal replacement after low anterior resection: the transverse coloplasty pouch. Ann Surg. 2001; 234(6):780–785, discussion 785–787

[368] Parc R, Tiret E, Frileux P, Moszkowski E, Loygue J. Resection and colo-anal anastomosis with colonic reservoir for rectal carcinoma. Br J Surg. 1986; 73 (2):139–141

[369] Lazorthes F, Fages P, Chiotasso P, Lemozy J, Bloom E. Resection of the rectum with construction of a colonic reservoir and colo-anal anastomosis for carcinoma of the rectum. Br J Surg. 1986; 73(2):136–138

[370] Joo JS, Latulippe JF, Alabaz O, Weiss EG, Nogueras JJ, Wexner SD. Long-term functional evaluation of straight coloanal anastomosis and colonic J-pouch: is the functional superiority of colonic J-pouch sustained? Dis Colon Rectum. 1998; 41(6):740–746

[371] Dehni N, Tiret E, Singland JD, et al. Long-term functional outcome after low anterior resection: comparison of low colorectal anastomosis and colonic J-pouch-anal anastomosis. Dis Colon Rectum. 1998; 41(7):817–822, discussion 822–823

[372] Hüttner FJ, Tenckhoff S, Jensen K, et al. Meta-analysis of reconstruction techniques after low anterior resection for rectal cancer. Br J Surg. 2015; 102 (7):735–745

[373] Tan WS, Tang CL, Shi L, Eu KW. Meta-analysis of defunctioning stomas in low anterior resection for rectal cancer. Br J Surg. 2009; 96(5):462–472

[374] Gu WL, Wu SW. Meta-analysis of defunctioning stoma in low anterior resection with total mesorectal excision for rectal cancer: evidence based on thirteen studies. World J Surg Oncol. 2015; 13:9

[375] Messaris E, Sehgal R, Deiling S, et al. Dehydration is the most common indication for readmission after diverting ileostomy creation. Dis Colon Rectum. 2012; 55(2):175–180

[376] Tyler JA, Fox JP, Dharmarajan S, et al. Acute health care resource utilization for ileostomy patients is higher than expected. Dis Colon Rectum. 2014; 57 (12):1412–1420

[377] Danielsen AK, Burcharth J, Rosenberg J. Patient education has a positive effect in patients with a stoma: a systematic review. Colorectal Dis. 2013; 15 (6):e276–e283

[378] Nagle D, Pare T, Keenan E, Marcet K, Tizio S, Poylin V. Ileostomy pathway virtually eliminates readmissions for dehydration in new ostomates. Dis Colon Rectum. 2012; 55(12):1266–1272

[379] Hardiman KM, Reames CD, McLeod MC, Regenbogen SE. Patient autonomy-centered self-care checklist reduces hospital readmissions after ileostomy creation. Surgery. 2016; 160(5):1302–1308

[380] Pan HD, Peng YF, Wang L, et al. Risk factors for nonclosure of a temporary defunctioning ileostomy following anterior resection of rectal cancer. Dis Colon Rectum. 2016; 59(2):94–100

[381] Kim MJ, Kim YS, Park SC, et al. Risk factors for permanent stoma after rectal cancer surgery with temporary ileostomy. Surgery. 2016; 159(3):721–727

[382] Chun LJ, Haigh PI, Tam MS, Abbas MA. Defunctioning loop ileostomy for pelvic anastomoses: predictors of morbidity and nonclosure. Dis Colon Rectum. 2012; 55(2):167–174

[383] Park JJ, Del Pino A, Orsay CP, et al. Stoma complications: the Cook County Hospital experience. Dis Colon Rectum. 1999; 42(12):1575–1580

[384] Crooks S. Foresight that leads to improved outcome: stoma care nurses' role in siting stomas. Prof Nurse. 1994; 10(2):89–92

[385] Person B, Ifargan R, Lachter J, Duek SD, Kluger Y, Assalia A. The impact of preoperative stoma site marking on the incidence of complications, quality of life, and patient's independence. Dis Colon Rectum. 2012; 55(7):783–787

[386] Bass EM, Del Pino A, Tan A, Pearl RK, Orsay CP, Abcarian H. Does preoperative stoma marking and education by the enterostomal therapist affect outcome? Dis Colon Rectum. 1997; 40(4):440–442

[387] Chaudhri S, Brown L, Hassan I, Horgan AF. Preoperative intensive, community-based vs. traditional stoma education: a randomized, controlled trial. Dis Colon Rectum. 2005; 48(3):504–509

[388] American Society of Colon and Rectal Surgeons Committee Members, Wound Ostomy Continence Nurses Society Committee Members. ASCRS and WOCN joint position statement on the value of preoperative stoma marking for patients undergoing fecal ostomy surgery. J Wound Ostomy Continence Nurs. 2007; 34(6):627–628

[389] Zhang HY, Zhao CL, Xie J, et al. To drain or not to drain in colorectal anastomosis: a meta-analysis. Int J Colorectal Dis. 2016; 31(5):951–960

[390] Rondelli F, Bugiantella W, Vedovati MC, et al. To drain or not to drain extraperitoneal colorectal anastomosis? A systematic review and meta-analysis. Colorectal Dis. 2014; 16(2):O35–O42

[391] Denost Q, Rouanet P, Faucheron JL, et al. French Research Group of Rectal Cancer Surgery (GRECCAR). To drain or not to drain infraperitoneal anastomosis after rectal excision for cancer: the GRECCAR 5 randomized trial. Ann Surg. 2017; 265(3):474–480

[392] Watanabe J, Ota M, Suwa Y, et al. Evaluation of the intestinal blood flow near the rectosigmoid junction using the indocyanine green fluorescence method in a colorectal cancer surgery. Int J Colorectal Dis. 2015; 30 (3):329–335

[393] Gröne J, Koch D, Kreis ME. Impact of intraoperative microperfusion assessment with Pinpoint Perfusion Imaging on surgical management of laparoscopic low rectal and anorectal anastomoses. Colorectal Dis. 2015; 17 Suppl 3:22–28

[394] Jafari MD, Wexner SD, Martz JE, et al. Perfusion assessment in laparoscopic left-sided/anterior resection (PILLAR II): a multi-institutional study. J Am Coll Surg. 2015; 220(1):82–92.e1

[395] A study assessing perfusion outcomes with PINPOINT® near infrared fluorescence imaging in low anterior resection (PILLAR III). https://clinicaltrials.gov/ct2/show/NCT02205307. Accessed December 1, 2016

[396] Kim JC, Lee JL, Yoon YS, Alotaibi AM, Kim J. Utility of indocyanine-green fluorescent imaging during robot-assisted sphincter-saving surgery on rectal cancer patients. Int J Med Robot. 2016; 12(4):710–717

[397] Kudszus S, Roesel C, Schachtrupp A, Höer JJ. Intraoperative laser fluorescence angiography in colorectal surgery: a noninvasive analysis to reduce the rate of anastomotic leakage. Langenbecks Arch Surg. 2010; 395 (8):1025–1030

[398] Kin C, Vo H, Welton L, Welton M. Equivocal effect of intraoperative fluorescence angiography on colorectal anastomotic leaks. Dis Colon Rectum. 2015; 58(6):582–587

[399] Diggs JC, Xu F, Diaz M, Cooper GS, Koroukian SM. Failure to screen: predictors and burden of emergency colorectal cancer resection. Am J Manag Care. 2007; 13(3):157–164

[400] McArdle CS, Hole DJ. Emergency presentation of colorectal cancer is associated with poor 5-year survival. Br J Surg. 2004; 91(5):605–609

[401] van Hooft JE, Bemelman WA, Oldenburg B, et al. collaborative Dutch Stent-In study group. Colonic stenting versus emergency surgery for acute left-sided malignant colonic obstruction: a multicentre randomised trial. Lancet Oncol. 2011; 12(4):344–352

[402] Sloothaak DA, van den Berg MW, Dijkgraaf MG, et al. collaborative Dutch Stent-In study group. Oncological outcome of malignant colonic obstruction in the Dutch Stent-In 2 trial. Br J Surg. 2014; 101(13):1751–1757

[403] Sagar J. Colorectal stents for the management of malignant colonic obstructions. Cochrane Database Syst Rev. 2011(11):CD007378

[404] Petersen SH, Harling H, Kirkeby LT, Wille-Jørgensen P, Mocellin S. Postoperative adjuvant chemotherapy in rectal cancer operated for cure. Cochrane Database Syst Rev. 2012(3):CD004078

[405] Sainato A, Cernusco Luna Nunzia V, Valentini V, et al. No benefit of adjuvant Fluorouracil Leucovorin chemotherapy after neoadjuvant chemoradiotherapy in locally advanced cancer of the rectum (LARC): Long term results of a randomized trial (I-CNR-RT). Radiother Oncol. 2014; 113(2):223–229

[406] Breugom AJ, van Gijn W, Muller EW, et al. Cooperative Investigators of Dutch Colorectal Cancer Group and Nordic Gastrointestinal Tumour Adjuvant Therapy Group. Adjuvant chemotherapy for rectal cancer patients treated with preoperative (chemo)radiotherapy and total mesorectal excision: a Dutch Colorectal Cancer Group (DCCG) randomized phase III trial. Ann Oncol. 2015; 26(4):696–701

[407] Glynne-Jones R, Counsell N, Quirke P, et al. Chronicle: results of a randomised phase III trial in locally advanced rectal cancer after neoadjuvant chemoradiation randomising postoperative adjuvant capecitabine plus oxaliplatin (XELOX) versus control. Ann Oncol. 2014; 25(7):1356–1362

[408] Bujko K, Glynne-Jones R, Bujko M. Does adjuvant fluoropyrimidine-based chemotherapy provide a benefit for patients with resected rectal cancer who have already received neoadjuvant radiochemotherapy? A systematic review of randomised trials. Ann Oncol. 2010; 21(9):1743–1750

[409] Collette L, Bosset JF, den Dulk M, et al. European Organisation for Research and Treatment of Cancer Radiation Oncology Group. Patients with curative resection of cT3–4 rectal cancer after preoperative radiotherapy or radiochemotherapy: does anybody benefit from adjuvant fluorouracil-based chemotherapy? A trial of the European Organisation for Research and Treatment of Cancer Radiation Oncology Group. J Clin Oncol. 2007; 25(28):4379–4386

[410] Park IJ, Kim DY, Kim HC, et al. Role of adjuvant chemotherapy in ypt0–2n0 patients treated with preoperative chemoradiation therapy and radical resection for rectal cancer. Int J Radiat Oncol Biol Phys. 2015; 92(3):540–547

[411] Chan AK, Wong A, Jenken D, Heine J, Buie D, Johnson D. Posttreatment TNM staging is a prognostic indicator of survival and recurrence in tethered or fixed rectal carcinoma after preoperative chemotherapy and radiotherapy. Int J Radiat Oncol Biol Phys. 2005; 61(3):665–677

[412] Breugom AJ, Swets M, Bosset JF, et al. Adjuvant chemotherapy after preoperative (chemo)radiotherapy and surgery for patients with rectal cancer: a systematic review and meta-analysis of individual patient data. Lancet Oncol. 2015; 16(2):200–207

[413] Petrelli F, Coinu A, Lonati V, Barni S. A systematic review and meta-analysis of adjuvant chemotherapy after neoadjuvant treatment and surgery for rectal cancer. Int J Colorectal Dis. 2015; 30(4):447–457

[414] Kulaylat AS, Hollenbeak CS, Stewart DB, Sr. Adjuvant chemotherapy improves overall survival of rectal cancer patients treated with neoadjuvant chemoradiotherapy regardless of pathologic nodal status. Ann Surg Oncol. 2017; 24(5):1281–1288

[415] Hong YS, Nam BH, Kim KP, et al. Oxaliplatin, fluorouracil, and leucovorin versus fluorouracil and leucovorin as adjuvant chemotherapy for locally advanced rectal cancer after preoperative chemoradiotherapy (ADORE): an open-label, multicentre, phase 2, randomised controlled trial. Lancet Oncol. 2014; 15(11):1245–1253

[416] Rödel C, Graeven U, Fietkau R, et al. German Rectal Cancer Study Group. Oxaliplatin added to fluorouracil-based preoperative chemoradiotherapy and postoperative chemotherapy of locally advanced rectal cancer (the German CAO/ARO/AIO-04 study): final results of the multicentre, open-label, randomised, phase 3 trial. Lancet Oncol. 2015; 16(8):979–989

[417] Biagi JJ, Raphael MJ, Mackillop WJ, Kong W, King WD, Booth CM. Association between time to initiation of adjuvant chemotherapy and survival in colorectal cancer: a systematic review and meta-analysis. JAMA. 2011; 305(22):2335–2342

[418] Gastrointestinal Tumor Study Group. Prolongation of the disease-free interval in surgically treated rectal carcinoma. N Engl J Med. 1985; 312(23):1465–1472

[419] Douglass HO, Jr, Moertel CG, Mayer RJ, et al. Gastrointestinal Tumor Study Group. Survival after postoperative combination treatment of rectal cancer. N Engl J Med. 1986; 315(20):1294–1295

[420] Fisher B, Wolmark N, Rockette H, et al. Postoperative adjuvant chemotherapy or radiation therapy for rectal cancer: results from NSABP protocol R-01. J Natl Cancer Inst. 1988; 80(1):21–29

[421] Smalley SR, Benedetti JK, Williamson SK, et al. Phase III trial of fluorouracil-based chemotherapy regimens plus radiotherapy in postoperative adjuvant rectal cancer: GI INT 0144. J Clin Oncol. 2006; 24(22):3542–3547

[422] O'Connell MJ, Martenson JA, Wieand HS, et al. Improving adjuvant therapy for rectal cancer by combining protracted-infusion fluorouracil with radiation therapy after curative surgery. N Engl J Med. 1994; 331(8):502–507

[423] Tepper JE, O'Connell M, Niedzwiecki D, et al. Adjuvant therapy in rectal cancer: analysis of stage, sex, and local control: final report of intergroup 0114. J Clin Oncol. 2002; 20(7):1744–1750

[424] Minsky BD, Cohen AM, Kemeny N, et al. Combined modality therapy of rectal cancer: decreased acute toxicity with the preoperative approach. J Clin Oncol. 1992; 10(8):1218–1224

[425] Lupattelli M, Mascioni F, Bellavita R, et al. Long-term anorectal function after postoperative chemoradiotherapy in high-risk rectal cancer patients. Tumori. 2010; 96(1):34–41

[426] Kollmorgen CF, Meagher AP, Wolff BG, Pemberton JH, Martenson JA, Illstrup DM. The long-term effect of adjuvant postoperative chemoradiotherapy for rectal carcinoma on bowel function. Ann Surg. 1994; 220(5):676–682

[427] Frykholm GJ, Glimelius B, Påhlman L. Preoperative or postoperative irradiation in adenocarcinoma of the rectum: final treatment results of a randomized trial and an evaluation of late secondary effects. Dis Colon Rectum. 1993; 36(6):564–572

[428] Dehni N, McNamara DA, Schlegel RD, Guiguet M, Tiret E, Parc R. Clinical effects of preoperative radiation therapy on anorectal function after proctectomy and colonic J-pouch-anal anastomosis. Dis Colon Rectum. 2002; 45(12):1635–1640

[429] Miller AR, Martenson JA, Nelson H, et al. The incidence and clinical consequences of treatment-related bowel injury. Int J Radiat Oncol Biol Phys. 1999; 43(4):817–825

[430] Peeters KC, Marijnen CA, Nagtegaal ID, et al. Dutch Colorectal Cancer Group. The TME trial after a median follow-up of 6 years: increased local control but no survival benefit in irradiated patients with resectable rectal carcinoma. Ann Surg. 2007; 246(5):693–701

[431] Heriot AG, Tekkis PP, Fazio VW, Neary P, Lavery IC. Adjuvant radiotherapy is associated with increased sexual dysfunction in male patients undergoing resection for rectal cancer: a predictive model. Ann Surg. 2005; 242(4):502–510, discussion 510–511

[432] Maring ED, Tawadros PS, Steer CJ, Lee JT. Systematic review of candidate single-nucleotide polymorphisms as biomarkers for responsiveness to neoadjuvant chemoradiation for rectal cancer. Anticancer Res. 2015; 35(7):3761–3766

[433] Nelson B, Carter JV, Eichenberger MR, Netz U, Galandiuk S. Genetic polymorphisms in 5-Fluorouracil-related enzymes predict pathologic response after neoadjuvant chemoradiation for rectal cancer. Surgery. 2016; 160(5):1326–1332

[434] Villafranca E, Okruzhnov Y, Dominguez MA, et al. Polymorphisms of the repeated sequences in the enhancer region of the thymidylate synthase gene promoter may predict downstaging after preoperative chemoradiation in rectal cancer. J Clin Oncol. 2001; 19(6):1779–1786

[435] Wibe A, Møller B, Norstein J, et al. Norwegian Rectal Cancer Group. A national strategic change in treatment policy for rectal cancer: implementation of total mesorectal excision as routine treatment in Norway. A national audit. Dis Colon Rectum. 2002; 45(7):857–866

[436] Khani MH, Smedh K. Centralization of rectal cancer surgery improves long-term survival. Colorectal Dis. 2010; 12(9):874–879

[437] Bulow S, Harling H, Iversen LH, Ladelund S, Danish Colorectal Cancer Group. Survival after rectal cancer has improved considerably in Denmark–secondary publication. Ugeskr Laeger. 2009; 171(38):2735–2738

[438] Meyerhardt JA, Mangu PB, Flynn PJ, et al. American Society of Clinical Oncology. Follow-up care, surveillance protocol, and secondary prevention measures for survivors of colorectal cancer: American Society of Clinical Oncology clinical practice guideline endorsement. J Clin Oncol. 2013; 31(35):4465–4470

[439] Sargent D, Sobrero A, Grothey A, et al. Evidence for cure by adjuvant therapy in colon cancer: observations based on individual patient data from 20,898 patients on 18 randomized trials. J Clin Oncol. 2009; 27(6):872–877

[440] Seo SI, Lim SB, Yoon YS, et al. Comparison of recurrence patterns between ≤ 5 years and > 5 years after curative operations in colorectal cancer patients. J Surg Oncol. 2013; 108(1):9–13

[441] Primrose JN, Perera R, Gray A, et al. FACS Trial Investigators. Effect of 3 to 5 years of scheduled CEA and CT follow-up to detect recurrence of colorectal cancer: the FACS randomized clinical trial. JAMA. 2014; 311(3):263–270

[442] Verberne CJ, Zhan Z, van den Heuvel E, et al. Intensified follow-up in colorectal cancer patients using frequent carcino-embryonic antigen (CEA) measurements and CEA-triggered imaging: results of the randomized "CEAwatch" trial. Eur J Surg Oncol. 2015; 41(9):1188–1196

[443] Jeffery M, Hickey BE, Hider PN, See AM. Follow-up strategies for patients treated for non-metastatic colorectal cancer. Cochrane Database Syst Rev. 2016; 11:CD002200

[444] Green RJ, Metlay JP, Propert K, et al. Surveillance for second primary colorectal cancer after adjuvant chemotherapy: an analysis of Intergroup 0089. Ann Intern Med. 2002; 136(4):261–269

[445] Liu L, Lemmens VE, De Hingh IH, et al. Second primary cancers in subsites of colon and rectum in patients with previous colorectal cancer. Dis Colon Rectum. 2013; 56(2):158–168

[446] Wiig JN, Wolff PA, Tveit KM, Giercksky KE. Location of pelvic recurrence after "curative" low anterior resection for rectal cancer. Eur J Surg Oncol. 1999; 25 (6):590–594

[447] Martin LA, Gross ME, Mone MC, et al. Routine endoscopic surveillance for local recurrence of rectal cancer is futile. Am J Surg. 2015; 210(6):996–1001, discussion 1001–1002

[448] Nicholson BD, Shinkins B, Pathiraja I, et al. Blood CEA levels for detecting recurrent colorectal cancer. Cochrane Database Syst Rev. 2015(12):CD011134

[449] Litvak A, Cercek A, Segal N, et al. False-positive elevations of carcinoembryonic antigen in patients with a history of resected colorectal cancer. J Natl Compr Canc Netw. 2014; 12(6):907–913

[450] Lu YY, Chen JH, Chien CR, et al. Use of FDG-PET or PET/CT to detect recurrent colorectal cancer in patients with elevated CEA: a systematic review and meta-analysis. Int J Colorectal Dis. 2013; 28(8):1039–1047

[451] Hahnloser D, Nelson H, Gunderson LL, et al. Curative potential of multimodality therapy for locally recurrent rectal cancer. Ann Surg. 2003; 237 (4):502–508

[452] Suzuki K, Dozois RR, Devine RM, et al. Curative reoperations for locally recurrent rectal cancer. Dis Colon Rectum. 1996; 39(7):730–736

[453] Dozois EJ, Privitera A, Holubar SD, et al. High sacrectomy for locally recurrent rectal cancer: can long-term survival be achieved? J Surg Oncol. 2011; 103(2):105–109

[454] Milne T, Solomon MJ, Lee P, et al. Sacral resection with pelvic exenteration for advanced primary and recurrent pelvic cancer: a single-institution experience of 100 sacrectomies. Dis Colon Rectum. 2014; 57(10):1153–1161

[455] Abdelsattar ZM, Mathis KL, Colibaseanu DT, et al. Surgery for locally advanced recurrent colorectal cancer involving the aortoiliac axis: can we achieve R0 resection and long-term survival? Dis Colon Rectum. 2013; 56 (6):711–716

[456] Harris CA, Solomon MJ, Heriot AG, et al. The outcomes and patterns of treatment failure after surgery for locally recurrent rectal cancer. Ann Surg. 2016; 264(2):323–329

[457] Holman FA, Bosman SJ, Haddock MG, et al. Results of a pooled analysis of IOERT containing multimodality treatment for locally recurrent rectal cancer: results of 565 patients of two major treatment centres. Eur J Surg Oncol. 2017; 43(1):107–117

[458] Bhangu A, Ali SM, Brown G, Nicholls RJ, Tekkis P. Indications and outcome of pelvic exenteration for locally advanced primary and recurrent rectal cancer. Ann Surg. 2014; 259(2):315–322

[459] Dresen RC, Gosens MJ, Martijn H, et al. Radical resection after IORT-containing multimodality treatment is the most important determinant for outcome in patients treated for locally recurrent rectal cancer. Ann Surg Oncol. 2008; 15(7):1937–1947

[460] Yang TX, Morris DL, Chua TC. Pelvic exenteration for rectal cancer: a systematic review. Dis Colon Rectum. 2013; 56(4):519–531

[461] Devulapalli C, Jia Wei AT, DiBiagio JR, et al. Primary versus flap closure of perineal defects following oncologic resection: a systematic review and meta-analysis. Plast Reconstr Surg. 2016; 137(5):1602–1613

[462] Guren MG, Undseth C, Rekstad BL, et al. Reirradiation of locally recurrent rectal cancer: a systematic review. Radiother Oncol. 2014; 113(2):151–157

[463] van der Meij W, Rombouts AJ, Rütten H, Bremers AJ, de Wilt JH. Treatment of locally recurrent rectal carcinoma in previously (chemo)irradiated patients: a review. Dis Colon Rectum. 2016; 59(2):148–156

25 Ulcerative Colitis

Quinton Hatch, Scott R. Steele, and Steven D. Wexner

Abstract

Ulcerative colitis is a potentially complex and crippling disease process, challenging for the provider and cruel to the patient. While many patients are successfully managed with minimal medical intervention, a significant number will progress to severe, debilitating, and intractable disease, ultimately necessitating a high-risk surgery. Multidisciplinary discussion and formation of a solid therapeutic alliance are critical parts of the treatment process, particularly in refractory cases. It should be kept in mind that chronic ulcerative colitis patients often have an innate understanding of their own disease process that far outweighs clinical data. The risk of any intervention is not insignificant, and ultimately it is the patient who has to live with the outcome. Individualized medical and surgical care should therefore be the standard. In practice, this principle is not easy to follow, as it necessitates thorough and often lengthy counseling. However, the ability to provide a potentially curative surgery to a patient who has been experiencing the pain and humiliation of ulcerative colitis is a privilege worthy of additional effort.

Keywords: ulcerative colitis, inflammatory bowel disease, colectomy, pouch

25.1 Introduction

Inflammatory bowel disease (IBD) has been described in various forms and terms since Roman times. It is simultaneously fascinating and exasperating that after two millennia this disease spectrum continues to perplex patients and physicians alike. Certainly the aptly named Soranus (AD 117) could not have imagined that the noncontagious diarrhea he described would remain a mysterious phenomenon in an era where living organs can be grown from stem cells.[1]

It was not until 1859 that Sir Samuel Wilks coined the term "ulcerative colitis" (UC).[2] The term itself is a bit of a misnomer, as the inflammation generally emanates from the rectum, and ulceration is not a "sine qua non" of the disease. Knowledge of the gross and histologic manifestations of UC became further refined over the course of the next century, and an increasing interest in defining UC as a unique disease process separate from Crohn's disease (CD) and ischemic colitis developed. A number of etiologic theories were described, including infection,[3] colonic "mucinases,"[4] allergy,[5] psychological factors,[6] and autoimmunity.[7,8] Most physicians currently favor the autoimmune theory, which has shaped the modern framework of how we manage UC. Nevertheless, the debate rages on, as immune-modulating medications have variable and inconsistent impacts on the natural history of the disease. Furthermore, the multiple phenotypic variants in and of themselves likely favor a multifactorial mechanism. It could easily be argued that, despite advances in modern medicine and extensive research in the field of IBD, the most accurate definition to this day was spelled out by F.T. De Dombal in 1968, who described UC as follows[9]:

"An inflammatory disease of unknown origin, characterized clinically by recurrent attacks of bloody diarrhea, and pathologically by a diffuse inflammation of the wall of the large bowel. The inflammatory changes spread proximally from the rectum; and are confined to (or most severe in) the colonic and rectal mucosa".

These qualities help distinguish UC from CD, which is generally characterized by full-thickness inflammation impacting any portion of the gastrointestinal tract. Confinement to the colonic and rectal mucosa adds surgical options to the armamentarium against UC, with proctocolectomy offering hope of a surgical "cure." In practice, however, the distinction between the two disease processes is somewhat blurred, and many initially thought to have UC turn out to have CD (and vice versa). Physicians and patients must therefore accept some degree of uncertainty when implying one diagnosis over the other.

The impact of IBD on patient lifestyle and psyche cannot be overstated. Many of these patients have lived for years with chronic pain, debilitating anxiety, and routine humiliation due to fecal incontinence. As such, a therapeutic alliance must be established early, ideally in a multidisciplinary setting. Of utmost importance to this alliance is an upfront and thorough explanation of the natural history of the disease, diagnostic limitations, the role of both medications and surgery, and establishment of realistic therapeutic goals that fit with the patient's life plan.

25.2 Epidemiology

The global incidence of UC ranges from 0.6 to 24.3 cases per 100,000 life years.[10,11] While regional variations exist, it seems clear that UC diagnosis rates have increased across the globe over the last 50 years.[10] Molodecky et al[10] recently performed a systematic review of global IBD epidemiologic data between 1930 and 2008. Sixty percent of UC studies reporting at least 10 years of data showed a statistically significant increasing incidence, with increases ranging from 2.4 to 18.1%. Interestingly, only 23% of UC studies performed after 1980 showed a significant increase, suggesting either a true leveling off or simply the calm after a flurry of new diagnoses secondary to increased disease awareness. Corroborating data presented in previous large series, the study found that Europe and North America had the highest disease incidences, reported at 24.3 and 19.2 per 100,000 person-years, respectively. Asia and the Middle East followed similar trends toward increasing incidence; however, their rates were significantly lower at 6.3 per 100,000 person-years.

The prevalence of UC in the 1980s and 1990s ranged from 6 to 246 cases per 100,000 persons, with the largest populations not surprisingly located in North America (37.5–246 cases per 100,000 persons) and Europe (21.4–243 cases per 100,000 persons). Health insurance data suggest there are approximately 512,000 UC patients in the United States alone,[12] with an extrapolated annual treatment cost of $2.1 billion dollars.

Thorough analysis of global trends reveals that UC rates may be more heavily influenced by industrialization than by regional genotypic tendencies. Central to this argument is the parallel between UC rates and the level of industrialization. Developing countries have exceedingly low rates of UC, but as societies become industrialized higher rates of UC emerge. CD rates tend to lag behind UC in this setting, although the trend is the same. Whether these increased rates of IBD are due to improved health care and diagnostic awareness or some inherent gastrointestinal assault associated with the "Western lifestyle" has yet to be determined.[11]

UC is usually diagnosed in the third to fourth decade of life, with the mean age of diagnosis 5 to 10 years later than what is seen with CD.[10,13,14,15] Although it has classically been thought of as having a bimodal age distribution with a second, smaller peak in the sixth to seventh decade, recent epidemiologic studies have not supported this pattern.[11] Pediatric IBD accounts for 7 to 10% of all IBD cases, although UC accounts for a much smaller percentage of this population with an incidence of only 0.8 per 100,000 person-years (compared to 5.2 per 100,000 person-years for pediatric CD).[16,17,18]

While the data are mixed, large regional series have suggested a slight (60%) male predominance in UC.[15,19,20] Undoubtedly contributing to this is an increasing incidence of UC in males in recent years (with a corresponding decrease in females).[15] Interestingly, the pediatric population seems to exhibit the opposite gender profile in UC, with females carrying the bulk of the disease burden. The shift in differential gender balance, if one exists, seems to occur between the ages of 14 and 17 years.[16]

There seem to be variations in IBD incidence and prevalence based on race and ethnicity. People of Jewish descent have higher rates of IBD, and tend to have higher rates than other ethnicities regardless of the geographic location. African Americans were once thought to be at lower risk when compared to whites; however, more recent data suggest similar rates of disease.[21] Conversely, Asian-Americans, Hispanic-Americans, and Native Americans are much less likely to develop IBD.[22,23] As with geographic differences, it is unclear how much of an impact culture and lifestyle have on these differential disease patterns. Studies of migrant populations suggest that disease patterns may have more to do with the environment than was previously thought. Evidence of this is seen in South Asians, traditionally with low rates of IBD, who migrate to the United Kingdom and develop an increased risk for IBD when compared to whites.[24,25,26] Age at migration seems to impact this risk, with the highest disease rates seen in those who move before the age of 15 years.[26]

25.3 Etiology

The increased incidence of IBD in "Western," industrialized countries coupled with 8- to 10-fold higher rates of IBD among first-degree relatives of IBD probands suggests a multifactorial etiology, with contributions from both the environment and the genome.[27,28] Specific etiologic theories include aberrant immune regulation, defective mucosal barrier function, defective microbial clearance, persistent specific infection, and dysbiosis (abnormal ratio of beneficial and detrimental commensal microbial agents; ▶ Fig. 25.1).[29]

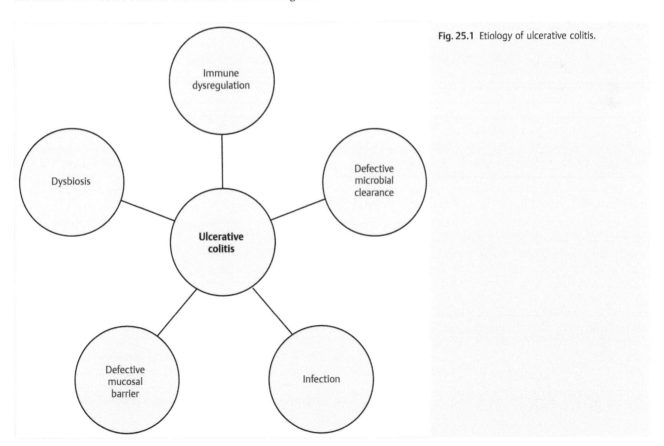

Fig. 25.1 Etiology of ulcerative colitis.

Genetic correlates have come to light in recent years, in large part due to the completion of the Human Genome Project in 2003. A thorough understanding of the genetics of IBD will undoubtedly contribute to the understanding of the various etiologic theories, and will hopefully provide new targets for therapeutic intervention. At this point, however, the relative contributions of associated genes, the environment, the gut microbiome, infection, and any as yet unknown elements to the IBD phenotype are uncertain.

Human single nucleotide polymorphism and candidate gene studies together with studies using mouse models of experimental colitis have identified 200 gene loci, and approximately 300 gene candidates, associated with IBD.[30,31,32] At least 23 of these loci are specifically associated with UC, although the vast majority is associated with both CD and UC. Most, if not all, of these genes are involved in immunoregulation, mucosal barrier integrity and microbial clearance, and/or homeostasis.[29]

25.3.1 Aberrant Immune Regulation

A direct link between IBD-associated genetic abnormalities and the phenotypic expression of altered immunity has not been firmly established. What seems clear, however, is that patients with IBD have activated innate and acquired immune systems, with loss of tolerance to resident enteric bacteria.[33,34]

Under normal circumstances, intestinal macrophages and epithelial cells have the ability to reside in areas of high bacterial loads without causing inflammation. This is due to the downregulation of bacterial recognition receptors (such as Toll-like receptor [TLR] and cluster of differentiation 14 [CD14]) on these cells.[35] When activated by bacterial recognition, TLR molecules on the surface of innate immune effector cells bind microbial adjuvants and initiate the nuclear factor κ-light-chain-enhancer of activated B cells (NF-κB) pathway.[36] Induction of this pathway ultimately results in an increase in proinflammatory cytokines, which have been directly implicated in the pathogenesis of both forms of IBD.[29] Interleukin-1 beta (IL-1β), tumor necrosis factor-α (TNF-α), IL-6, and IL-18 have all been found to be increased in patients with active UC. A similar pattern is found in CD, although IL-12, IL-23, and IL-27 are also increased.[29] Inhibition of these cytokines attenuates experimental colitis, and represents the foundation for anti-TNF-α therapy.

The reason for the upregulation of the innate immune response including activated macrophages and dendritic cells and the presumed resultant loss of tolerance to commensal gut flora is the subject of considerable debate. Recent studies have suggested that loss-of-function mutations in the IL-10 R anti-inflammatory gene may play a role in the exaggerated immune reaction. While the limited studies have linked this mutation to a severe form of early-onset CD, it has been found to be associated with UC as well.[37,38] Certainly it makes intuitive sense for a defect in an anti-inflammatory cytokine to result in exaggerated immunogenicity. Abnormal expression of TLR molecules may be another causative factor, a theory that has gained recent popularity.[39]

Adaptive immunity is also altered in IBD, generally through dysregulation of T-helper cell type 1 (Th1) and Th2 pathways. Alterations of Th1 responses have been associated with CD in animal models, while UC is generally thought to be related to abnormalities in the Th2 response. This atypical Th2 response in UC has not been elucidated; however, it is felt to be mediated by natural killer T cells that secrete IL-13 upon activation by antigen-presenting cells.[29]

25.3.2 Defective Mucosal Barrier Function

Compromise of the gut mucosal barrier layer has also been theorized to play a role in the pathogenesis of IBD. This mechanism has been postulated to be secondary to an intrinsic defect in patients with IBD, which would allow either primary poor functioning of the barrier or defective barrier repair after insults such as ulcerogenic medications or infections. The theory is at least indirectly supported by genetic studies, with MDR1 (UC) and NOD2 (CD) genes presumably playing a role in maintenance of the intestinal mucosal barrier. MDR1 mediates excretion of xenobiotic molecules, and possibly bacteria, from epithelial cells, while NOD2 potentially plays a role in bacterial clearance and production of antimicrobial α-defensins by Paneth's cells.[29,40,41]

25.3.3 Defective Microbial Clearance

Some studies have noted the persistence of bacteria in the gut tissue and lymph nodes of CD patients,[29] which is the basis for the defective microbial clearance theory of IBD. Other studies showing significant increases in the number of mucosally adherent enteric bacteria in active UC and CD lend additional support to this theory.[42] It is believed by many that this increase in the adherent bacterial load is secondary to aberrant innate immunity resulting in defective killing of bacteria.[43]

It seems counterintuitive that there would be increases in the numbers of adherent gut bacteria in IBD given the previously described intolerance to normal commensal organisms; however, these are not mutually exclusive theories. It may be that intolerance of normal bacteria due to alterations in TLRs and the NF-κB pathway coupled with defective bacterial killing results in the dysfunctional and self-perpetuating nonspecific inflammation we see in IBD. One can easily see how a defective mucosal barrier along with the presence of more virulent commensal organisms would further exacerbate this problem. This complex interplay likely explains the difficulty understanding, much less treating, CD and UC.

A number of IBD-associated genes have functional roles in these pathways, and may in part explain the genetic foundation for the phenotypic variants. NOD2, which is associated with CD rather than UC, is heavily involved in NF-κB activation as well as autophagy and localization of bacteria in autophagolysosomes.[44] IRGM (UC and CD) and ATG16L1 (CD) are also thought to be involved with autophagy, and therefore the ability to clear bacteria.[31] Another gene thought to be associated with bacterial clearance is IL23R. Interestingly, a mutation in the IL23R gene has been found to be protective against both CD and UC.[27,28,45] While it is unclear what impact these genetic variants have on the development and course of IBD, the correlations are striking and seem to corroborate prevailing pathogenic theories.[29]

25.3.4 Persistent Specific Infection

Gastrointestinal infection can break the mucosal barrier, initiate inflammation, and stimulate innate immunity. Despite these insults, most people who develop an infection ultimately clear the infection without adverse sequelae. Nevertheless, there are several chronic infectious processes that have been associated with CD and, to a lesser extent, UC.

The first of these potential culprits is *Mycobacterium avium* subspecies *paratuberculosis* (MAP), which causes a granulomatous infection of the gastrointestinal tract in ruminants that is similar to the granulomatous inflammation of CD.[46] MAP may be encountered in contaminated drinking water, and has been implicated in IBD due to series reporting 55 and 22% incidences of MAP-positive blood cultures in CD and UC, respectively.[47] Additional credence to this theory was added after a series demonstrated that 52% of resected CD specimens contained MAP DNA.[48] In that study, MAP was present in approximately 2% of UC and 5% of control specimens, which argues against a link between MAP and UC. These results are similar to other series suggesting a much stronger link between MAP and CD than MAP and UC.

The other bacterial infection that has been associated with IBD is enteroadherent and invasive *Escherichia coli*, which has been recovered from 22% of mucosal biopsies from CD patients (compared to just 6% of controls).[49] Interestingly, CD patients with *NOD2* polymorphisms and infection with this *E. coli* strain have decreased expression of TNF and IL-10, a phenotype consistent with ulceration, fistulas, and defective clearance of intracellular infections.[40,42,50,51] No studies have shown a link between *E. coli* and UC.

Another infection historically linked to IBD, albeit not UC specifically, was measles. This inference was based on post-World War II data from Sweden showing a higher incidence of IBD in people born within 3 months of a measles epidemic.[52,53] This finding has not been replicated in subsequent studies, and concern for IBD risk with live measles virus vaccines is unfounded based on available literature.[11]

25.3.5 Dysbiosis

Alterations in the homeostasis of the gut microbiome can lead to a relative overgrowth of certain commensal organisms. *E. coli*, *Bacteroides* spp., *Enterococcus*, *Klebsiella*, and *Clostridia* have all been implicated in the inflammation of experimental colitis and IBD through this phenomenon, often referred to as dysbiosis. The process may be further exacerbated by the acquisition of virulence factors by these normal resident bacteria.[49,54]

Diet is often felt to play a role in dysbiosis, and a dietary link could help explain the increased risk of IBD in Western societies.[11] While the validity of this theory remains open for debate, dietary components can certainly alter the macro- and microenvironment of the gut, potentially impacting the composition and virulence of commensal microorganisms. In fact, studies have shown that dietary iron potentiates the growth and virulence of intracellular organisms, while dietary aluminum stimulates the inflammatory response.[55,56,57] Furthermore, a paucity of colonic short chain fatty acids from a relative scarcity of *Lactobacillus* or *Bifidobacteria* may have detrimental effects on maintenance of an effective mucosal barrier.[58]

Another potential contributor to dysbiosis is the so-called "hygiene hypothesis," which suggests that protective immunity is stimulated by early exposure to pathogens and parasites.[29] Whether aware of this theory by name or not, parents who routinely allow their children to eat dirt and/or food off the floor with the thought that it will improve their immune system subscribe to this principle. The thought is that early development of protective immunity against low-virulence organisms prevents a later, more aggressive immunologic response due to a mature, robust immune system at first exposure. Some have suggested that dysbiosis caused by a lack of early pathogen exposure may be a contributing factor to increased rates of IBD in developed countries. The experimental improvement in symptoms with the delivery of pig whipworms to the gut in active UC and CD patients argues in support of this theory.[59,60]

25.4 Modifiable Risk Factors

Given the high financial, psychological, and physiologic cost and chronicity of IBD, it is important to have a thorough understanding of modifiable risk factors so that we might mitigate the severity of illness. Cigarette smoking, oral contraceptives, and diet have all been theorized to impact the natural history and even development of IBD in the first place.

25.4.1 Smoking

In contrast to CD in which smoking is a risk factor for surgery and recurrence, paradoxically active smoking may impart some benefit in UC.[61,62,63,64] While controversial, given the widely publicized adverse effects of smoking on other body systems, smoking has consistently been linked with a decreased risk of UC. A 1989 meta-analysis concluded that smokers were 40% less likely to develop active UC as opposed to nonsmokers.[62] There have also been reports that smokers with UC are less likely to be hospitalized and have a colectomy when compared to nonsmokers.[61] The reasons for this protective effect are unclear, but are theorized to be related to the impact of nicotine on rectal blood flow, colonic mucus, cytokines, and eicosanoids.[65,66] Unfortunately, the beneficial impacts of smoking on UC are not long lasting and patients who smoke and subsequently quit tend to have more active disease, more hospitalizations, and an increased dependence on corticosteroids and immune modulators.[67] Furthermore, former smokers are 70% more likely to develop UC than those who never smoked.[62]

25.4.2 Oral Contraceptives

Oral contraceptives have been studied in relation to IBD. While the data are not entirely clear, the bulk of the literature does seem to support an increased risk of developing either CD or UC in women who used oral contraceptives.[68,69,70] Whether the use of oral contraceptives has an impact on preexisting IBD remains unclear.

25.4.3 Diet

Perhaps the most studied dietary association with IBD is sugar; however, the results of the studies are mixed, with some series showing a relationship but others not.[71,72,73,74] Limited studies attempting to link fiber and fat intake to IBD have also yielded inconsistent results.[74,75,76,77,78] Given these varied results, it is not surprising that most studies regarding the impact of dietary modifications on IBD have been disappointing.[79] Recent studies out of Seattle Children's, however, have yielded some promising results with the utilization of the "specific carbohydrate diet" (SCD) for treatment of CD and UC within the pediatric population.[80] While further studies are needed, their early results suggest that the dietary association is stronger than once thought, and may be utilized to improve symptoms if not induce remission.

25.4.4 Appendectomy

There are numerous other proposed risk factors for UC; however, one that has garnered considerable attention is appendectomy. Early retrospective data, to include a meta-analysis incorporating almost 3,600 cases and 4,600 controls, suggested a significant inverse association between appendectomy and UC, with a 69% decreased risk of UC in those who had previously undergone appendectomy.[81] Subsequent cohort studies have tempered these findings somewhat, although appendectomy for appendicitis does seem to confer a protective effect against the development of UC. This statistic is especially true in patients who undergo appendectomy before the age of 20 years.[82]

25.5 Pathology

The most common manifestation of UC is circumferential confluent mucosal inflammation starting in the rectum and extending proximally, with the most substantial disease burden generally seen in the rectum. There may be an element of terminal ileitis in continuity with cecal inflammation, referred to as "backwash ileitis." Patchy inflammation with "skip lesions" is not the norm, and the presence of this pattern should bias the clinician in favor of CD. Nevertheless, some degree of heterogeneity may be expected, especially in treated UC patients as the mucosa heals. A common finding in patients actively undergoing treatment for UC is an appearance of "rectal sparing."[83,84,85,86] Kim et al[86] looked at sequential endoscopies in UC patients undergoing therapy and found that 59% of patients had patchy disease, rectal sparing, or both at some point during treatment. The specific pattern of heterogeneity was not associated with the type of therapy (including steroid use and rectal therapy). It is important to be cognizant of this healing pattern lest we mistakenly label all healing UC patients with CD. It is for this reason that the first colonoscopic evaluation for IBD is generally the most accurate for ascertaining UC versus CD.

The colorectal mucosa in early UC may grossly appear edematous, with confluent erythema and a loss of vascular markings. As the disease progresses, the mucosa will develop granularity with micropurulence and bleeding. Advanced UC will be marked by the characteristic pseudopolyp formation, deep (even full-thickness) ulcerations, gross purulence, mucosal bridging, and varied mucosal thickness (▶ Table 25.1).[87,88]

There are no pathognomonic histopathological features of UC, which makes definitive diagnosis difficult even after the colon and rectum are excised. The diagnosis generally rests on the gross morphology combined with the absence of histopathologic findings more consistent with CD including noncaseating

Table 25.1 Endoscopic and histopathologic findings in ulcerative colitis

	Endoscopy	Histopathology
Early	Confluent erythema	Vascular congestion
	Loss of vascular markings	Crypt distortion, branching
	Edema	Mucosal inflammation
		Goblet cell mucin depletion
Intermediate	Bleeding	Lamina propria neutrophils
	Micropurulence	Loss of mucosa with retention of crypts
	Granularity	Uniform crypt abscesses
Advanced/late	Ulceration	Deeper submucosal inflammation
	Purulence	Pseudopolyps
	Pseudopolyps	Mucosal bridging
	Mucosal bridging	Crypt destruction
	Variable mucosal thickness	Dysplasia

Source: Koltun 2011.[89]

granulomas, vasculitis, and neuronal hyperplasia. Even the thickness of inflammation can be misleading, as severe cases of UC may have full-thickness inflammation. Despite these caveats, routine UC has a fairly predictable microscopic profile. Early disease is generally characterized by mucosal inflammation, crypt distortion, goblet cell mucin depletion, and vascular congestion. Neutrophil infiltration of the lamina propria in intermediate disease is associated with crypt abscesses and loss of mucosa with preservation of the crypts themselves. Crypt destruction, pseudopolyps, and deeper invasion of inflammation are the hallmarks of advanced disease.[88] It is in late disease where we tend to identify dysplasia; however, it can only be interpreted when identified in noninflamed bowel, as many dysplastic features are similar to inflammation (▶ Table 25.1).[89]

It should be noted here that there is a population of colitis patients who do not classically fall in line with the routine presentation of either UC or CD. These patients may have rectal sparing disease with confluent colonic inflammation or confluent inflammation of the rectum and descending colon with nonspecific ulcerations elsewhere. Stated differently, these patients may have gross characteristics of both CD and UC. In the absence of pathognomonic histopathologic findings, it is exceedingly difficult to resolve the diagnosis. Rates of this indeterminate colitis are cited at 10 to 15%; however, it is likely even higher, as 4 to 10% of patients who undergo ileal pouch anal anastomosis (IPAA) "develop" CD in the pouch.[89,90] As such, all patients with a diagnosis of UC who are considering pouch reconstruction must be counseled with a reasonable degree of uncertainty, especially in cases that are not straightforward.

25.6 Clinical Manifestations

Signs and symptoms of a UC flare depend largely on the severity and location of disease. The most common findings are blood and mucus in the stools. Tenesmus, urgency, increased stool frequency, fecal incontinence, and pain with defecation are common, as the majority of the disease burden is generally in the rectum. Fecal incontinence is certainly the most distressing and anxiety-producing element of the disease, and as with tenesmus and urgency, is due to noncompliance of the rectum and loss of receptive relaxation. While diarrhea is common, up to 25% of patients may complain of constipation with a sense of incomplete evacuation.[89] Left lower quadrant abdominal pain, followed by flank and back pain is the norm as the disease progresses to involve the sigmoid and descending colon, respectively. Abdominal distention may also be present.

The severity of pain generally signifies severity of inflammation, and as the colonic lumen narrows with edema, the intensity of peristaltic pain increases. Nausea is extremely common, and likely reflects either downstream effects of circulating inflammatory mediators or inflammation of the stomach secondary to direct apposition with inflamed colon as opposed to frank obstruction. Weight loss is also common with chronic UC, which is likely a multifactorial phenomenon dependent on protein loss via the inflamed mucosa, avoidance of oral intake, and the metabolic demand of constant inflammation.

Some patients may smolder with advanced disease for some time before manifesting systemic signs of illness such as fevers and tachycardia. Others, however, may manifest these symptoms earlier in the process, possibly indicating a more severe disease phenotype. Regardless, development of these clinical features may be a harbinger of progression to life-threatening colitis, and warrants close attention and aggressive medical therapy. Certainly any further progression to peritonitis or evidence of severe colonic dilation is of grave concern, generally mandating urgent total abdominal colectomy.

Acute complications of UC include progression to life-threatening colitis, severe bleeding, and perforation, each of which is a manifestation of severe disease rather than an indicator of disease chronicity. The term toxic megacolon has largely been replaced, at least in concept if not the vernacular, by life-threatening colitis. This shift simply accounts for the fact that "toxic" patients need not have colonic dilatation. It likely reflects a severe UC phenotype, as 60% of patients who ultimately develop toxic colitis do so in the first 3 years, with half of those occurring in the first year. Severe bleeding may occur in up to 10% of patients over the course of their disease, with approximately 3% developing life-threatening hemorrhage necessitating colectomy. Acute perforation is another dire consequence of acute UC, with a mortality risk of up to 50%.[91] It may occur either with or without the presence of fulminant colitis. Perforation in the absence of fulminant disease generally occurs very early in the disease process, before the colon becomes scarred and resistant to perforation.

It should be noted that immune suppression might mask peritonitis. Furthermore, IBD patients are at risk for developing a superseding infectious colitis, usually *Clostridium difficile*, which may be the underlying etiology of the presumed disease exacerbation.[92,93] These two points must be at the forefront of the clinician's thought process when evaluating and managing a patient with new-onset severe signs and symptoms.

25.7 Extraintestinal Manifestations

Both UC and Crohn's disease are marked by a variety of extraintestinal manifestations, the severity of which generally parallels the severity of colonic inflammation. Population-based studies report the overall incidence of extraintestinal disease at up to 40%, with 10% of patients having extraintestinal manifestations at the time of IBD diagnosis (▶ Table 25.2).[94,95,96] These numbers likely underestimate the true incidence, as patients may or may not link their extraintestinal symptoms with their disease, and as such may not report them.

25.7.1 Musculoskeletal

Arthropathies are a common finding in IBD, occurring in approximately 30% of patients. Peripheral arthropathy constitutes the vast majority of these; however, approximately 5% of IBD patients develop axial arthritis (ankylosing spondylitis). The joint pain can be debilitating, and seems to reflect the severity of colorectal inflammation. The importance of this correlation is significant, as a patient with severe urgency, frequent stooling, and difficulty moving due to substantial joint pain will almost undoubtedly become a prisoner of IBD due to fecal incontinence. In addition to arthropathy, IBD patients

Table 25.2 Extraintestinal manifestations of ulcerative colitis

	Extraintestinal manifestation
Musculoskeletal	Peripheral arthropathy
	Axial arthropathy (ankylosing spondylitis)
	Osteopenia
	Osteoporosis
Ophthalmologic	Episcleritis
	Scleritis
	Uveitis
Cutaneous	Erythema nodosum
	Pyoderma gangrenosum
	Sweet's syndrome
	Aseptic abscess syndrome
	Bowel-associated dermatosis–arthritis syndrome
	Cutaneous vasculitides
	Malignant melanoma
Hepatobiliary	Primary sclerosing cholangitis
Hematologic	Deep venous thrombosis
	Pulmonary embolism
	Mesenteric venous thrombosis (postoperative)

frequently develop osteopenia and osteoporosis. It is unknown if a primary link between IBD and bone loss exists, as chronic corticosteroid use and deconditioning are both substantial risk factors for bone disease. Regardless, bone disease represents a significant morbidity, and likely explains the 40% increased risk of bone fractures in IBD.[94]

25.7.2 Ophthalmologic

Episcleritis, scleritis, and uveitis impact approximately 2 to 5% of patients with UC. Episcleritis manifests as "red eye" and generally does not cause pain or visual disturbance. Unlike other ophthalmologic complications, inflammation of the episclera generally parallels colorectal inflammation. Episcleritis lies in stark contrast to scleritis, which causes severe pain and visual impairment. Uveitis is more common in women with IBD, is associated with arthritis, and causes pain and redness. Neither scleritis nor uveitis appear to reflect the degree of colorectal inflammation, and in fact may be present even in the absence of gastrointestinal symptoms.[97,98]

25.7.3 Cutaneous

IBD patients are predisposed to a variety of skin conditions. It is important to document these, as many of the medications used to treat IBD can themselves have dermatologic complications and therefore confound the treatment algorithm. Erythema nodosum is the most common inflammatory skin condition associated with IBD; it occurs in 3 to 10% of UC patients. These lesions tend to occur on the extensor surfaces of extremities, especially the anterior tibia, and consist of 1- to 5-mm raised, tender, red or violet subcutaneous nodules.[99] Pyoderma gangrenosum is the second most common skin manifestation in IBD, although it is still a rare condition occurring in only 0.75% of patients. These lesions most commonly occur on the legs but may occur anywhere and have been found adjacent to ileostomies and wounds.[99,100] They appear as single or multiple erythematous papules or pustules, which are often preceded by trauma to the skin. Dermal necrosis then leads to deep ulcerations containing sterile purulence. Up to 50% of patients who present with pyoderma gangrenosum have IBD.[101] Erythema nodosum generally parallels gut inflammation, while pyoderma gangrenosum does not. Neutrophilic dermatoses such as Sweet's syndrome, aseptic abscess syndrome, and bowel-associated dermatosis–arthritis syndrome, and cutaneous vasculitides may also occur in IBD, although they are quite rare. IBD may also be a risk factor for malignant melanoma.[102]

25.7.4 Hepatobiliary

Both UC and CD are associated with primary sclerosing cholangitis (PSC), fatty liver, and autoimmune liver disease.[89] PSC occurs in approximately 3% of UC patients, although UC may be present in up to 73% of PSC cases.[103] The risk of both colorectal and hepatobiliary malignancies is thought to be increased in UC patients with PSC.[104]

25.7.5 Hematologic

Patients with IBD have a twofold to threefold increased risk of deep venous thrombosis (DVT) and pulmonary embolism (PE)

when compared to the general population.[105] The incidence of DVT within this population is 30.7 per 10,000 person-years and is similar between UC and CD (30.0 for UC and 31.4 for CD). Risk of PE is higher in UC than in CD, with incidences of 19.8 and 10.3 per 10,000 person-years, respectively.[106] Patients younger than 40 years suffering from active inflammation and more extensive colonic disease have the highest baseline risk within this group.[106,107] The phenomenon cannot be explained by surgery or inflammation alone, as the risk in IBD exceeds that in non-IBD surgery (other than oncologic), rheumatoid arthritis, or celiac disease (other inflammatory conditions).[108] The entire etiology for the unique intrinsic coagulopathy in IBD has not been established; however, the inflammation associated with IBD can certainly shift the hematologic homeostasis toward a prothrombotic state. Implicated in this process are increased plasma levels of thrombotic factors, several of which are acute-phase reactants; decreased levels of natural anticoagulants; reduced fibrinolytic activity; endothelial damage and dysfunction leading to downregulation of the anticoagulant thrombomodulin and endothelial protein C receptor, ultimately affecting the conversion of protein C into its activated form; and an inherent thrombophilia.[109] These factors likely contribute to the 3 to 5% risk of mesenteric venous thrombosis, a feared complication of colectomy in IBD. Initial reports of this complication were associated with mortality as high as 50%; however, heightened awareness in recent years has led to more frequent diagnosis, earlier intervention with anticoagulation, and lower overall morbidity and mortality.[89,110,111]

25.8 Classification

The most utilized clinical assessment tool for UC was described by Truelove and Witts in 1954 (▶ Table 25.3).[112] They described disease as either mild or severe based on bowel frequency, blood in the stool, fever, heart rate, hemoglobin, and erythrocyte sedimentation rate (ESR). Initially used to monitor the impact of cortisone on disease, the simplicity and relevance of the model have allowed some variation of it to be used in nearly all modern grading systems. Modern variations of this system such as the Montreal and Mayo classifications include "moderate" categories as well as colonoscopic appearance, but otherwise use similar clinical criteria.[113,114] The Montreal Working Party also felt it necessary to include a parallel classification system stratifying UC by extent of disease, with separate categories for isolated proctitis, left-sided disease, and pancolitis.[113]

Table 25.3 Truelove and Witts' ulcerative colitis activity index

	Mild	Severe
Fever	Absent	>37.5
Heart rate	<90	>90
Blood in stool	+	+++
Stool frequency	<4	>6
Erythrocyte sedimentation rate	<30	>30
Hemoglobin	>75% normal	<75% normal

Source: Koltun 2011.[89]

25.9 Natural History

The most common manifestations of UC are blood and mucus in the stool, although other signs and symptoms may be present depending on the location and severity of inflammation. As previously discussed, the involvement of the rectum generally leads to frequent bowel movements, tenesmus, urgency, a sensation of inadequate evacuation, and fecal incontinence. The latter is generally a progressive problem, worsening as the rectum scars and loses capacitance. Abdominal and back pain may be present as well, depending on the presence and severity of inflammation in the intra-abdominal and retroperitoneal colon.

In order to understand the typical disease progression, we must understand the historical context, to include patient outcomes prior to the development of adequate therapies. The "natural history" of UC was altered dramatically by the widespread use of corticosteroids for UC, which was spawned by the landmark work of Truelove and Witts in 1954.[112] Prior to this time, patients were at the whim of their disease process, as few treatment options were available. In fact, limited series from the early 1930s suggested that as many as 75% of patients died within 1 year of an acute presentation.[115] A larger subsequent series by Edwards and Truelove clearly identified a dichotomy between outcomes of UC flares before and after 1954. That study reported outcomes in 624 patients treated for acute UC exacerbations between 1938 and 1962, and identified an overall mortality rate of 14% prior to 1953 versus 4% thereafter. This included a 34% mortality rate among those referred for severe colitis, which was significant in that 19% of patients had severe disease at the initial attack, and 18% of patients would have a severe attack at some point.[116] The 1954 pivotal study itself compared mortality rates in patients with severe UC who received either cortisone or placebo, and found a significant mortality reduction from 24% in the placebo group to 7% among patients who received cortisone.[112] Despite similar rates of steroid responsiveness in the decades since the initial studies, mortality rates have continued to downtrend and currently reside at approximately 1%.[117] These improved outcomes are presumably due to additional rescue therapies, improved supportive care, and recognition of the importance of surgical intervention in medication-refractory cases.[102]

Modern epidemiologic data suggest that the first presentation of UC is usually for an attack of mild severity (73%), although more than one in four patients will initially manifest moderate (27%) or severe disease (1%).[18,118,119] Duration of an UC "flare" is highly variable, ranging from several weeks to several months, with a small contingent developing intractable disease. This range is independent of treatment, as patients have varying response profiles to the therapeutic options.

Langholz et al[119] published a series of 1,161 UC patients managed from 1962 to 1987 who were followed from diagnosis up to 25 years. They found that the probability of progression to a relapsing course was approximately 90%. Active disease in any given year was predicted by active disease in the preceding year, indicating that sick patients tend to stay sick. In years 3 to 7 after diagnosis, 25% of patients were in remission, 18% had active disease in all years, and 57% had intermittent relapses. Twenty-four percent of patients had a colectomy within the first 10 years. While this study is outdated, and even at the time included patients from several generations of medical therapy, it shows a baseline natural history in patients largely managed by steroid pulses alone.[18]

A more recent population-based study by Solberg et al[120] followed 423 UC patients for 10 years (1990–1994 to 2000–2004). Similar to the Langholz study, Solberg et al[120] found that a large percentage of patients develop relapsing disease (83%), although approximately half the patients were relapse free over the last 5 years of the study. The most notable finding in this study was a significantly decreased 10-year rate of colectomy. The 9.8% colectomy rate in the 1990s marked a 58% decrease in colectomy when compared to the years between 1962 and 1987. This change likely reflects advancements in medical management, most notably the widespread use of aminosalicylates and immune-modulating medications. The study was cut off in the year infliximab was approved for use in UC, so biologic therapy likely did not impact the results of this study.

A number of patient and environmental factors have been associated with relapse. Among these are younger age at diagnosis, female gender, and more extensive disease at presentation. Additionally, frequent relapses tend to beget more relapses, again emphasizing that healthy patients stay healthy and sick patients stay sick. Stress has also been linked to relapses, which can lead to a vicious cycle of worsening disease with stress causing relapses, and relapses inducing more relapses. As previously discussed, active smoking and potentially appendectomy confer some degree of protection from relapse. Interestingly, systemic symptoms such as fever and weight loss are associated with fewer relapses, although this is presumably due to a higher likelihood of early colectomy.[14,67,118,120,121,122,123,124,125]

As UC is a dynamic disease, it is important to consider not only the relapse itself, but also the progression of disease extent over time. Gower-Rousseau et al observed a series of pediatric patients with UC and found that 28% of patients have isolated proctitis, 35% left-sided colitis, and 37% extensive colitis at initial presentation. In this cohort, the disease course was characterized by extension of inflammation in 49% of patients.[126] This is not dissimilar to other studies identifying 20 to 53% proximal extension rates, depending on the initial segment involved.[119,120,127] Patients with proctitis have a ~ 50% chance of extension, and those with disease proximal to the sigmoid colon have a 9% chance of progression to pancolitis. Interestingly, regression may also be observed when the disease is followed over time. In fact, the probability of regression has been reported as high as 76.8% for substantial colitis and 75.7% for pancolitis after 25 years.[119,120,127]

Stricture and neoplasia are feared sequelae of chronic UC inflammation. In 1966, De Dombal et al[9] reviewed their 10-year UC data and found that 11% of UC patients had a stricture within the study period. The majority of these strictures were located in the rectum, which was not surprising as the majority of the patients had rectal disease. Stricture rates in those with panproctocolitis were over 17%, while those with left-sided and isolated rectal disease had 7.5 and 3.6% stricture rates, respectively. Interestingly, the stricture rate did not seem to correlate with duration of disease, as a number of patients had strictures on initial presentation.[9] Stricture rates since the De Dombal study have been reported from 3 to 11%.[128,129,130] The underlying issue is not, however, the stricture per se, but rather the underlying dysplasia or neoplasia.[129,130] While a minority of strictures will have malignant cells on endoscopic biopsy, approximately 40% will return with carcinoma in the resected specimen and an additional 33% will have high-grade dysplasia.[131]

Meta-analysis of premillennial UC data suggested that the risk of colorectal carcinoma among UC patients is approximately 3.7%, with pancolitis conferring an even higher risk of 5.4%. The same study found the cumulative risk of colorectal carcinoma by decade was 2% at 10 years, 8% at 20 years, and 18% at 30 years.[132] These findings underlie the recommendation for endoscopic surveillance starting after 8 years of disease duration in pancolitis. More recent studies, however, suggest much lower probabilities, with cumulative risks in the new millennium being reported at 1, 2, and 5% after 10, 20, and more than 20 years of disease duration, respectively.[133] The decreased risk in recent studies likely reflects either the benefits of rigorous endoscopic surveillance or overall improved disease management rather than a shift in disease phenotype.[134,135]

Whether or not the most recent therapeutic advancements are impacting the natural history of UC remains unknown. Infliximab was the first biologic agent added to the UC armamentarium in 2004. Since then, several relatively small, randomized controlled trials have shown a decrease in early colectomy rates among UC patients started on infliximab.[136,137] Despite these favorable trends, any beneficial effect in chronic, refractory UC has been called into question.[138] Unfortunately, no significant long-term epidemiological studies are available to address the impacts of the most modern iteration of medical management.

25.10 Diagnosis

25.10.1 Clinical History

Prior to strategizing a diagnostic approach to any patient complaining of abdominal pain and altered bowel habits, it is important to have a thorough understanding of the differential diagnosis. Thinking in terms of the larger picture will prevent "tunnel vision" with regard to medical and surgical decision making.

CD impacting the colon may present in similar fashion to UC. In fact, it may be difficult to distinguish the two disease processes. While the medical management does not differ significantly, differentiation between the forms of IBD is critical for management of patient expectations and surgical planning. Crohn's colitis constitutes approximately 30% of CD cases, and most commonly presents with diarrhea and bleeding similar to UC. Patchy "skip" lesions and rectal sparing are commonly found in CD, and may help differentiate the processes; however, treated UC may present with a heterogeneous appearance as the mucosa heals in a disorganized fashion.[86] While "backwash ileitis" may be present in UC patients with pancolitis, any other evidence of small bowel disease, intestinal fistulas, perianal disease, or hallmark histopathologic findings of CD point to a diagnosis of CD. Determining a definitive diagnosis is exceedingly difficult in the absence of these tell-tale findings, and patients should be counseled regarding the degree of uncertainty.

Infectious colitis or proctitis must be excluded prior to immunosuppressive treatment for a UC flare. Not only can these infections present in similar fashion to UC, but they may also occur more frequently in IBD due to recurrent hospitalizations, administration of immunomodulatory and antimicrobial agents that disturb the intestinal flora, and a decreased

nutritional status. These risk factors are especially important for *C. difficile* infections, which are present in 5 to 19% of patients admitted with an IBD exacerbation.[92,93] Other bacteria that may cause inflammatory diarrhea include *Shigella* spp., enterohemorrhagic or enteroinvasive *E. coli*, *Campylobacter jejuni*, *Salmonella* spp., *Yersinia enterocolitica*, *M. tuberculosis*, *Vibrio parahaemolyticus*, and *Chlamydia trachomatis*. Parasitic infections may also mimic a UC flare, and include *Entamoeba histolytica*, *Schistosoma* spp., *Balantidium coli*, and *Trichinella spiralis*. Cytomegalovirus (CMV) is a fairly ubiquitous pathogenic virus with low virulence. In the immune suppressed, however, it may produce "CMV colitis," which can worsen rapidly and sometimes necessitate urgent colectomy. Different pathogens are responsible for isolated proctitis. These include sexually transmitted diseases such as *Neisseria gonorrhoeae*, Herpes simplex virus, and *C. trachomatis*. Other proctitis causing organisms are *Treponema pallidum* and CMV.[139] A thorough review of infectious diarrhea is outside the scope of this chapter; however, the importance of ruling out such an infection before starting pulse immunosuppression cannot be overstated. At a minimum, all patients with an inflammatory or infectious colitis require laboratory evaluation of the stool to include stool culture, fecal leukocytes, fecal ova, and parasites, and the presence of *C. difficile* toxin. In patients who are immune suppressed, it is prudent to take colonic mucosal biopsies to rule out CMV colitis.

A number of other conditions can mimic the clinical profile of UC. These include lymphoma, chronic mesenteric ischemia, radiation colitis, diversion colitis, solitary rectal ulcer syndrome, graft versus host disease, diverticular colitis, and medication-associated colitis. In addition to clinical history, the diagnosis of UC requires direct visualization of the colon via endoscopy, radiographic imaging studies, and evaluation for serologic markers specific to IBD or UC.

25.10.2 Endoscopy

Endoscopy is the gold standard for diagnosis of UC, as the entire extent of the disease process can effectively be surveyed. Additional imaging modalities only need be utilized if the clinical history is such that additional diagnoses, such as CD, need to be entertained. Colonoscopy allows for tissue biopsy as well as assessment of the gross appearance and specific pattern of inflammation. Complications of IBD such as strictures, fistulas, bleeding, or neoplasm may be readily identified. Colonoscopic examination alone is generally enough to diagnose UC in the right clinical setting, especially if tissue biopsies return without sarcoid-type giant cell granulomas, which would indicate CD. Colonoscopic findings consistent with mild UC include edema, confluent erythema, and loss of vascular markings, generally starting in the rectum. Moderate disease is marked by mucosal granularity, bleeding, and micropurulence, and may show further proximal extension of disease. Severe disease may be noted by ulcerations with deep penetration into the bowel wall, pseudopolyp formation, frank purulence, variable thinning and thickening of the mucosa, strictures, and mucosal bridging.[88,89] Deep ulceration at colonoscopy predicts worse outcomes and higher risk of surgery.[140] The findings in severe disease may have significant overlap with CD, which makes definitive diagnosis difficult. Another caveat to the "classic" findings is that the confluent erythema emanating from the rectum may be absent in a UC patient with healing disease. As previously discussed, a significant number of UC patients on treatment will appear to have rectal-sparing and/or patchy disease.[83,86]

The decision to perform endoscopy in the setting of severe disease should not be taken lightly. Despite studies reporting its safety, the general feeling is that the risk of perforation is increased. Nevertheless, patients with intractable, severe, disease will require tissue biopsies and stool samples to exclude concurrent infection. Rigid or flexible proctoscopy is generally undertaken in these situations, with biopsies taken below the peritoneal reflection.[89]

25.10.3 Imaging

Plain Film X-Rays

X-rays still play a role when considering the patient who presents acutely with abdominal pain. Upright abdominal films will reveal the presence of free air or "toxic megacolon," a term that has all but fallen out of favor due to the fact that patients can be "toxic" without having "megacolon." Nevertheless, colonic dilatation ≥ 6 cm or cecal diameter greater than 9 cm in the setting of fever, tachycardia, and abdominal pain is a grave concern that mandates urgent surgical intervention.[141,142] More subtle findings on plain films include nodularity of the mucosa suggesting the presence of pseudopolyps, mucosal edema ("thumbprinting"), and an ahaustral, "lead-pipe" colon, which is suggestive of chronic disease.

Contrast Enema

Double-contrast barium enema is not required for the diagnosis of CD; however, it is useful to help exclude CD when there is any question of small bowel involvement. The specific benefit of rectal contrast over small bowel follow-through is that it more clearly delineates the terminal ileum as there is less interference from proximal intestinal loops.

Enteroclysis

Enteroclysis is preferred over small bowel follow-through for detailed assessment of the small intestine. In fact, this technique is more sensitive than computed tomography (CT) for the detection of small bowel fistulas and early mucosal abnormalities.[143] Nevertheless, this study is not widely utilized as it is labor intensive and requires nasointestinal tube placement, which is never desirable for the patient. The study entails placement of a post-pyloric nasal tube, followed by repetitive small boluses of barium contrast, which will coat the bowel wall. Each bolus is followed by insufflation of air to distend the small bowel, and a spot film is taken. The additional detail offered by this technique is not generally worth the added time and labor. As such, if a contrast study is obtained to evaluate the small bowel, it is generally either standard small bowel follow-through or CT.

Computed Tomography

CT of the abdomen and pelvis is the most commonly obtained radiographic study in the acute evaluation of IBD. As with plain films, the role of CT in UC is negligible when the diagnosis of UC is secure. The benefit of CT is twofold: first, it has the ability to evaluate all intra-abdominal organs simultaneously and, second, it can evaluate the thickness of the entire intestinal wall. It must be emphasized here that a CT scan to evaluate the bowel wall specifically is severely limited if intraluminal contrast is not used. We therefore recommend a full oral contrast load with consideration of rectal contrast if a CT scan is to be performed for any diagnostic study in IBD. In UC specifically, signs that may be identified on CT include increased perirectal and presacral fat, heterogeneous colonic thickening, target or "double-halo" sign of the colon, and strictures.[144]

Magnetic Resonance

The role of magnetic resonance imaging (MRI) in IBD is still evolving. While less efficient and more costly than CT for an abdominal survey,[143] its ability to objectively quantify severity of inflammation in the bowel and mesentery may hold promise for monitoring response to medical therapy.[145,146] It may also have a unique role in characterizing perianal fistulas in CD, although this technology would have limited use in UC unless the diagnosis is in question. In addition, the lack of radiation exposure is appealing.

Ultrasound

Ultrasonography may be used as an adjunctive measure to assess response to therapy in IBD patients. A transabdominal wall ultrasound (TABS) can assess for strictures or other bowel wall thickening. Some functional data can be obtained as well, as peristalsis can be observed.[147] The technique is obviously operator dependent, and the data obtained are nonspecific, which may account for the lack of enthusiasm for TABS in the United States.

Nuclear Medicine

Nuclear imaging techniques have shown some promise in distinguishing CD from UC, and may be utilized to assess response to therapy as well. These studies rely on injection of the patient's own radionuclide-labeled white blood cells, and have been shown to accurately delineate the anatomic extent of inflammation. Newer techniques use Technetium-99 m haxamethyl-propylamine-oxime (HMPAO), which has improved sensitivity over older, Indium-111 labeling. While the specificity is inadequate to differentiate infectious versus idiopathic or autoimmune inflammation, studies have shown 93 to 98% accuracy in differentiating CD from UC.[89,148,149] These findings are based on the differential anatomic patterns of inflammation between CD and UC, so it may be that nuclear imaging provides little if any information that is not readily obtained by more traditional techniques. Given its high sensitivity for identifying inflammation, nuclear medicine may have a future role in assessing response to therapy. Whether this methodology offers any benefit beyond standard MRI has yet to be determined.

25.10.4 Capsule Endoscopy

Wireless capsule endoscopy is an additional imaging modality used in IBD. The primary benefit of this technique is that it allows visualization of the small bowel when CD is suspected.[150]

There is no role for this technology in classic cases of UC, although it provides additional diagnostic information in indeterminate cases.

25.10.5 Serologic Testing

A number of serum tests may be obtained in IBD in order to assess the degree of inflammation and aid in diagnosis. C-reactive protein (CRP) and ESR are the only two widely used tests for assessing general systemic inflammation. Neither measurement is sensitive or specific for IBD, but they may give an idea as to the level of inflammation in an IBD flare if other causes of inflammation are ruled out. ESR is felt to correlate more with colitis than small bowel disease irrespective of CD versus UC. The results of ESR and CRP may be misleading, as elevation can indicate anything from a perirectal abscess to pneumonia. A normal level can also be somewhat misleading, as the degree of inflammation may not correlate with a patient's symptoms. Such a scenario could involve a symptomatic stricture without significant active inflammation.[151]

An ever-increasing number of IBD-associated serologic markers have been identified. Among these are antineutrophil cytoplasmic antibodies (pANCA) and anti-Saccharomyces cerevisiae antibodies (ASCA), which were the first two widely used markers. It is felt that the presence or absence of these markers may help differentiate CD from UC in cases that are clinically in question. pANCA is more frequently identified in UC patients (50–70% of UC vs. 20–30% of CD) and may indicate a more medically refractory phenotype.[152] ASCA is more frequently associated with CD, although it may be present in 10 to 15% of UC patients as well. Other serologic markers such as anti-outer membrane porin C (anti-OmpC), anti-CBir1, anti-A4-Fla2, and anti-Fla-X have since been associated with IBD and are in clinical use; however, their utility in diagnosis is not as well established. In addition to aiding in diagnosis of IBD, both pANCA and antiCBir1 have been found to predict the risk of pouch complications after IPAA.[153]

25.10.6 Genetic Studies

A number of genetic markers have been identified that may help differentiate CD from UC. Out of 200 known DNA loci associated with IBD, at least 23 are associated with UC alone.[30,32] *ATG16L1*, *ECM1*, *NKX2-3*, and *STAT3* are currently in clinical use, although of those only *ECM1* is UC specific. There is a test on the market that combines these four genetic markers with several associated serologic and inflammatory markers. Reliance on such technology is variable, and at this point it is unclear what additional diagnostic benefit is gained from such testing. However, it likely has a future role in tailoring not only medication therapy, but also the decision to proceed with proctocolectomy with IPAA versus end ileostomy in medically refractory UC patients.

25.11 Medical Management

As with CD, UC is a chronic and debilitating disease with no definitive curative nonsurgical options. This realization alone is both humbling for the provider and terrifying for patients. As such, it is preferable to hold discussions with UC patients in a multidisciplinary setting, where the gastroenterologist and surgeon can establish cohesive therapeutic goals with specific input from a well-counseled patient.

The medical management of UC is predicated on a combination of disease distribution, disease severity, and clinical response to treatment (▶ Table 25.4). Unpredictable responses to individual medication classes mean that management is a dynamic process, constantly being tailored to a patient's disease phenotype. In addition to the fluidity built into treatment algorithms themselves, there are different philosophies with regard to upfront, aggressive management with biologic agents ("top-down" approach) versus a "step-up" approach for severe UC. Unfortunately, despite all algorithms and best intentions, it may appear that we are pursuing trial-and-error medicine in patients who ultimately have medically refractory UC, which is not far from the truth. With each intervention requiring 6 to 17 weeks to be deemed a failure, this approach may be particularly costly to the patient's lifestyle and trust in the medical community. It is therefore imperative that a therapeutic relationship be developed early on, with a thorough explanation of the potential limitations of medical management.

25.11.1 Induction of Remission

Proctitis

Mild to moderate UC confined to the rectum is generally treated by topical therapy alone, although oral adjuncts may be used as well. Mesalamine (5-ASA) and steroids are the mainstays of therapy; both indications are available in a variety of formulations. Suppositories are the preferred method of delivery for isolated proctitis as they are easier to administer, leak less, and have been shown to target the site of inflammation more effectively than liquid or foam enemas.[154,155] Randomized controlled trials suggest that topical mesalamine is more effective than monotherapy with topical steroids, oral mesalamine, or placebo at inducing remission, with 63 to 94% of patients experiencing a clinical response within 4 to 6 weeks.[102,156,157,158,159,160] The dosage administered should be 1 to 2 g daily, although there is no increased dose response above 1 g. Divided daily doses are no more effective than once daily.[161,162]

Topical steroids are four to five times more likely to induce remission than placebo,[163] although they are considered second-line therapy due to randomized controlled trials showing inferiority to topical mesalamine.[156,157,158,159,160] Nevertheless, topical steroids continue to play a role in those who do not tolerate mesalamine or in patients who are refractory to topical mesalamine monotherapy. Formulations and dosing are variable in the studies, which may account for the wide-ranging response rate of 35 to 70% at 4 weeks.[156,157,158]

If patients are not responsive to topical monotherapy, combination therapy with topical mesalamine and budesonide may be more efficacious than either therapy alone. A randomized controlled trial comparing topical mesalamine (2 g/d) plus topical budesonide (3 g/d) to either therapy alone noted clinical, endoscopic, and histologic improvement at 4 weeks in 100, 76, and 71% for combination therapy, mesalamine, and budesonide, respectively. Endoscopic remission followed a similar trend favoring combination therapy, with 37, 30, and 10% of patients showing complete endoscopic healing at 4 weeks.[156]

Table 25.4 Medical management of ulcerative colitis

Disease category	Segment	Treatment options depending on responsiveness and side effects
Induction		
Mild to moderate	Rectum	Topical mesalamine
		Topical steroids
		Topical mesalamine plus topical steroids
		Oral mesalamine plus topical mesalamine and topical steroids
		Oral mesalamine plus oral steroids plus topical mesalamine plus topical steroids
	Left sided	Oral mesalamine plus topical mesalamine
		Oral mesalamine plus topical steroids
		Oral mesalamine plus topical mesalamine and topical steroids
		Oral mesalamine plus oral steroids plus topical mesalamine plus topical steroids
	Extended	Oral mesalamine plus topical mesalamine
		Oral mesalamine plus topical steroids
		Oral mesalamine plus oral steroids plus topical mesalamine plus topical steroids
Severe	Any	Intravenous methylprednisolone or hydrocortisone
		Intravenous calcineurin inhibitor
		Tumor necrosis factor-α (TNF-α) inhibitor
Relapsing	Any	Add a thiopurine to baseline management
		Biologic agent
Steroid dependent	Any	Add a thiopurine to baseline management
		Biologic agent
Steroid refractory	Any	Add a thiopurine to baseline management
		Biologic agent
Maintenance		
In remission	Any	Oral mesalamine
		Oral mesalamine plus topical mesalamine
		Oral mesalamine plus topical mesalamine and topical steroids
Steroid dependent	Any	Add a thiopurine or methotrexate to baseline management
		Biologic agent
Steroid refractory	Any	Add a thiopurine or methotrexate to baseline management
		Biologic agent

While not as effective as topical mesalamine, oral mesalamine may be utilized as monotherapy or in combination with other agents for distal UC. When used as monotherapy, a 4-g daily dose of pH-dependent release oral mesalamine is more effective than placebo or lower doses.[154,164,165,166] The combination of oral (2.4 g/d) and topical mesalamine, however, was found to be more efficacious than either application alone in patients with disease progression halting within 50 cm of the anal verge.[167,168]

Ultimately, patients with mild to moderate ulcerative proctitis should be started on mesalamine suppositories. Combination therapies with topical steroid and/or oral mesalamine should be considered in refractory patients. If inflammation is ongoing, systemic therapy with oral steroids is indicated in order to induce remission. It is this final group of patients that may go on to require immune modulation, biologic therapy, or surgery if the rectal inflammation cannot be controlled.[102]

Left-Sided Colitis

The treatment algorithm for mild to moderate left-sided UC is similar to that for ulcerative proctitis, with several minor distinctions. First-line therapy consists of combination therapy with oral (2–4 g/d) and topical mesalamine, which was found to have improved disease activity indices (–5.2 for combination therapy; –4.4 for topical mesalamine; –3.9 for oral mesalamine) and clinical improvement at 8 weeks (86% for combination therapy vs. 68% for monotherapy) for left-sided disease.[102,168,169] Remission rates at 8 weeks were similarly improved by combination therapy, with 64% remission in those on combination therapy versus 43% of those on oral mesalamine only.[169] The argument for this combination is strengthened when data from the treatment of more extensive UC are extrapolated to left-sided UC.[170]

The bulk of the literature suggests the superiority of topical 5-ASA over topical steroids for left-sided UC, although the data are not as strong as they are for isolated proctitis.[163,171,172] Topical steroids are therefore a reasonable second line, especially in the case of 5-ASA hypersensitivity (bleeding and urgency 3–5 days after starting therapy; resolves in 72 hours with discontinuation of 5-ASA). Additionally, combining steroid and mesalamine topical therapy with oral mesalamine in cases refractory to oral and topical mesalamine alone may result in clinical improvement. While no comparative studies of this triple therapy exist, there is evidence to suggest that dual topical therapy results in improved remission rates when compared to either therapy alone.[156] Regardless of whether mesalamine or steroids are being used, topical agents should be delivered via enema (foam or liquid) as opposed to suppository form.[102] Neither foam nor liquid enemas have shown superiority over the other.[173] Low- and high-volume doses also show equivalent efficacy, although the low-volume dose is better tolerated.[174]

Although oral mesalamine alone is better tolerated than is oral sulfasalazine, it is no more effective.[175] As described earlier, a single daily 2- to 4-g dose of pH-dependent release oral mesalamine is more effective than placebo when used as monotherapy for left-sided colitis.[164,166] While the literature is somewhat mixed, most agree that any dose-dependent effect is negligible at doses over 2 g/d.[154,165,166] Combined analysis of the studies limited to pH-dependent release oral mesalamine has shown 8-week remission rates of approximately 40%, which marks a 100% increase in efficacy over earlier formulations.[166] Once daily dosing with 3-g oral mesalamine has been associated with improved remission rates when compared to 3-g divided daily dosing (86 vs. 73%).[176] Once-daily oral mesalamine dosing has not been comparatively evaluated as part of combined modality therapy.

While most patients with left-sided UC will experience symptomatic improvement within 2 weeks, it may take up to 16 weeks for mesalamine responders to achieve remission.[177, 178,179,180,181,182] Within this time frame, the patient will have ongoing symptoms to some degree, and may not respond at all. As such, a discussion regarding the timing for escalation of therapy often takes place prior to declaration of failure of first-line treatments. Oral steroids are the next line of therapy, and induce remission in the majority of patients.[102,183,184] Unfortunately they are not without complications, and an extensive discussion should be undertaken in which the patient is thoroughly counseled regarding the desired time-to-response versus steroid-induced side effects. Regardless, oral corticosteroids are likely needed in cases of clinical deterioration, continued rectal bleeding beyond 14 days, and inability to achieve remission after 40 days of appropriate mesalamine and/or topical steroid therapy.[102]

Extensive Ulcerative Colitis

Extensive UC, also referred to as pancolitis, refers to inflammation extending proximal to the splenic flexure. This disease pattern requires oral therapy as the proximal extent of the inflammation cannot effectively be reached by topical agents. It should be noted that the data driving the treatment of both left-sided colitis and extensive colitis are largely drawn from the same studies, which include a heterogeneous patient population. As such, much of the treatment of mild-to-moderate extensive colitis has already been reviewed.

First-line therapy is a single daily dose of 2- to 4-g oral mesalamine in addition to a 1-g mesalamine enema. This combined therapy effectively targets both the proximal and distal extents of the disease, and results in an 8-week remission rate of 63%.[102,168,169,175,180,185] Topical steroids are therefore a reasonable alternative to topical mesalamine, especially in the case of 5-ASA hypersensitivity.

Patients who do not respond to first-line therapy, or who have a relapse of disease while on maintenance therapy, require oral steroids. Truelove and Witts initially reported the benefit of cortisone for the treatment of UC in 1954.[112] A follow-up study used a regimen of a 20-mg divided daily dose of prednisolone in addition to topical hydrocortisone. The remission rate in this group of patients was 76%, which represented a significant improvement over the 52% seen with sulfasalazine alone.[184] The oral steroid regimen for induction of remission is 40 to 60 mg of prednisone or prednisolone daily. These dosages are based largely on a 1962 study by Baron et al, which showed a 50% revision rate for patients with pancolitis regardless of whether they received 60- or 40-mg daily prednisone doses.[186] Most prefer a 40-mg dose, as the side-effect profile worsens with little or no additional therapeutic benefit above this dose.[186]

Given the considerable side-effect profile, steroids are not intended as maintenance therapy. As such, a reasonable taper must be implemented such that steroid dependence is recognized early, but not at the cost of early relapse. Steroid courses less than 3 weeks in duration have been associated with early relapses. As such, an 8-week course starting with 40-mg prednisolone per day for 1 week and reducing by 5 mg/d every week is recommended by the most recent European consensus.[102]

Budesonide is an alternative oral steroid with limited systemic effects due to first pass metabolism. While attractive in concept due to the lack of side effects, numerous studies have failed to identify any benefit of budesonide over mesalamine. A newer formulation with a colonic release mechanism (budesonide multimatrix [MMX]) has improved remission rates over placebo (15 vs. 7%), and is most effective in left-sided patients who are mesalamine responsive. Nevertheless, a recent Cochrane review found no definitive data to suggest a benefit of budesonide MMX over standard budesonide, much less over mesalamine.[187]

Severe Ulcerative Colitis

Severe UC is defined as at least six bloody stools daily, abdominal tenderness with signs of systemic toxicity including fever (> 37.5 °C), tachycardia (> 90 bpm), anemia (hgb < 75% normal), and increased ESR (> 30 mm/h).[188] Historically, these cases carried a high mortality burden, with up to 75% of patients dying within the first year of a severe flare. The era of corticosteroid salvage was ushered in by the landmark study of Truelove and Witts in 1954; outcomes have improved dramatically since that time. Nevertheless, a significant number of severely inflamed patients progress to fulminant, life-threatening colitis.

While the clinical urgency of a toxic patient with presumed fulminant UC must be acknowledged, uninformed decision making can be potentially catastrophic. In the moment, it is of dire importance that intestinal infection be ruled out or at least treated empirically before starting immune suppression. Patients with inflammatory bowel disease (IBD) are at increased risk for *C. difficile* and CMV infections for a variety of reasons, and failure to address these as potential confounders, if not primary etiologies, could mean the difference between life and death.[92,93,189,190,191,192,193,194] Clostridial infection may easily be determined by stool studies, which should be performed on admission for any UC flare. Biopsies are needed to effectively rule out CMV colitis. As such, an unprepared, limited flexible sigmoidoscopy with biopsies should be undertaken in truly refractory cases that do not require urgent surgical intervention. While the decision to perform endoscopy in the face of acute inflammation is never taken lightly, the information obtained could be of vital importance. Infected patients should be treated with appropriate antimicrobials, and consideration should be given to withholding immunosuppression (when able).[194,195] In addition to excluding or treating infection, a number of other measures should be undertaken to ensure the patient is medically "optimized"[102]:

- Liberal fluid resuscitation and correction of electrolytes should be undertaken, as hypokalemia and hypomagnesemia can promote toxic colonic dilation.[91]
- DVT chemoprophylaxis should be administered, as patients with IBD are at increased risk for venous thromboembolism compared to controls. The risk further increases during an acute flare independent of other risk factors.[196,197]
- Nutritional support should be undertaken, particularly in patients who suffer from malnutrition at baseline. Enteral feeding is preferable to parenteral, as bowel rest with intravenous

(IV) nutrition has not shown any benefit and is associated with significantly more complications (35 vs. 9%).[198,199]

- Narcotics, anticholinergics, antidiarrheals, and nonsteroidal anti-inflammatories should be limited as they may increase the risk of progression to toxic colonic dilatation.[91,200,201]
- Topical mesalamine or corticosteroids may be given if tolerated; however, there are no comparative studies to suggest a benefit in this setting.[184,202]
- Appropriate antibiotics should be given empirically if infection is suspected. There is no therapeutic advantage to antibiotics in the absence of infection.[203,204,205]

Patients admitted for severe UC should be given IV steroids; both methylprednisolone 60 mg/24 h and hydrocortisone 100 mg every 4 hours are effective. Higher dosages, continuous infusions, and prolonged courses beyond 7 to 10 days do not confer added benefit.[102,117,206,207] Approximately 67% of patients will respond to IV steroids, although 29% of patients will ultimately stall or deteriorate, necessitating a colectomy.[117]

Cyclosporine may be an alternative to IV steroids in this setting, although it is less studied. A small, randomized controlled trial comparing cyclosporine 4 mg/kg/d to methylprednisolone 40 mg/d in 30 patients with severe acute UC resulted in equivalent (if not improved) efficacy in obtaining a clinical response in the cyclosporine group (67% for cyclosporine vs. 53% for methylprednisolone). It should be emphasized here that this is not the standard of care, and should only be considered in patients in whom steroids should be avoided (history of steroid psychosis, osteoporosis, poorly controlled diabetes).

Clinical response should be continuously assessed, and decision making should be undertaken in a multidisciplinary setting with a surgeon and a gastroenterologist, with input from the patient. Steroid-refractory patients must be identified early and projected to either rescue therapy or surgery, as delayed colectomy is associated with high morbidity.[208,209]

Intravenous Steroid Refractory Ulcerative Colitis

If declaration of success or failure has not already been made, the third day of treatment marks a critical junction in decision making. Continued administration of ineffective high-dose IV steroids in this setting risks progression of disease, delayed colectomy, and increased morbidity.[208,209] Any discussion regarding salvage attempts using cyclosporine, infliximab, or tacrolimus should be framed such that expectations are appropriately managed. Ideally, the patient has already met with the surgical team and enterostomal therapist, as it is important to have already established a foundation of trust should the patient deteriorate. Certainly if significant clinical improvement is not seen by day 3, a surgical consultation must be sought even as salvage therapy is undertaken. Colectomy is indicated if improvement is not seen after 4 to 7 days of salvage therapy.[102]

A number of clinical, biochemical, and radiologic/endoscopic markers have been used to predict the likelihood of steroid failure and progression to urgent colectomy. Fever, tachycardia, and elevation of inflammatory markers such as ESR and CRP are all associated with increased colectomy rates despite aggressive steroids. ESR greater than 75 mm/h and fever greater than 38 °C at the time of admission confers a 4.6- and 8.8-fold increased

risk of colectomy on that admission.[210] Days 2 to 5 are critical for repeat assessment of risk for steroid nonresponse. Greater than 12 bowel movements in 24 hours on day 2 of steroids is associated with colectomy in 55% of patients.[211] Greater than eight bowel movements, three to eight bowel movements in addition to a CRP > 45 mg/L, or the product of number of stools multiplied by 0.14 CRP equaling ≥ 8 on day 3 of steroids is suggestive of a 75 to 85% chance of acute progression to colectomy.[212,213] If the result is less than a 40% reduction in the bowel movements on day 5, the conclusion is that the patient did not respond to steroids.[210] Colonic dilatation greater than 5.5 cm, mucosal islands, and/or small bowel ileus noted on radiography each predict a 73 to 75% chance of same-admission colectomy.[211,214] The presence of severe ulceration noted on endoscopy predicts progression to colectomy in 93% of patients.[215] These dire numbers should be used to set the stage for the patient's decision regarding salvage therapy versus procession directly to surgery.

Refractory Proctitis and Distal Colitis

A category of disease that warrants separate discussion is refractory proctitis and distal colitis. By definition, these patients have failed topical mesalamine and/or topical steroids as well as oral mesalamine and steroids. These patients suffer from the most distressing symptoms (urgency, tenesmus, incontinence), but may not progress to fulminant disease or even develop the dangerous signs of fevers and abdominal pain and distention.[102] As such, the decision to proceed with surgery is never forced and the patient is left in limbo, suffering from disease, medication side effects, and the tormenting decision regarding whether or not to proceed with "elective" surgery.

In these situations, it is important to exclude medication noncompliance, alternative diagnoses, and proximal constipation/dysmotility (which may decrease the concentration of medication delivered to the site of inflammation). If these alternative explanations are not identified, additional treatments may be considered. Remaining therapeutic options include oral and/or rectal calcineurin inhibitors and biologics.[216,217,218,219] The overall efficacy of these salvage therapies specifically for isolated distal disease has not been established; however, they are not likely any more efficacious than in more extensive colitis. A considerable number of these patients will therefore fail salvage therapy.

Alternative therapies are not validated; however, small trials have suggested some conferred benefit with fatty acid enemas, lidocaine enemas, acetarsol suppositories, epidermal growth factor (EGF) enemas, and transdermal nicotine patches.[220,221,222,223,224,225] Cohort studies also suggest that up to 90% of patients with ulcerative proctitis may have significant improvement in disease activity after appendectomy, suggesting a possible etiologic link if not a potential therapeutic intervention.[226]

Salvage Therapy

Cyclosporine has shown efficacy as salvage monotherapy in steroid-refractory severe acute UC, with 76 to 85% of patients avoiding colectomy on that admission. Median time to improvement in pooled series is approximately 4 days, which allows for timely colectomy in those who do not respond.[102,227,228,229,230,231]

Response rates are no different between 2 and 4 mg/kg/d,[102, 227,228,229,230,231] and considering the narrow therapeutic index, significant side effect profile, and 3 to 4% risk of death with cyclosporine, the 2 mg/kg/d dosing has become the most commonly used regimen.[102] Responders should be transitioned to oral cyclosporine at a dose of 5 mg/kg/d divided twice daily. This regimen is generally continued for 3 to 4 months, and is given in conjunction with a standard maintenance therapy for steroid-refractory patients such as azathioprine (see section on maintenance therapy).[232]

While relatively effective for avoidance of colectomy in the short term, the long-term impact of cyclosporine on colon salvage is questionable. Follow-up data suggest that between 58 and 88% of patients who required cyclosporine rescue underwent a colectomy within 7 years.[230,233] Patients who were able to maintain some degree of remission on a thiopurine, or who were thiopurine naïve at baseline, were much more likely to avoid colectomy over the long term after cyclosporine salvage.[230,234,235]

Tacrolimus has a similar mechanism of action as cyclosporine (calcineurin inhibitor) but binds a different receptor. Both have multiple downstream immunologic effects, with inhibition of IL-2 likely the most significant. Several trials have shown a benefit in terms of induction of remission, symptomatic improvement, and decreased steroid requirements. Ogata et al performed a randomized controlled trial to identify dose efficacy of oral tacrolimus for salvage therapy. Results of treatment with high trough concentrations (10–15 ng/mL), low trough concentrations (5–10 ng/mL), and placebo were compared at 2 weeks. Sixty-eight percent of patients in the high-trough group experienced symptomatic improvement, with 20% entering clinical remission and 79% showing evidence of mucosal healing. These marked a substantial improvement over placebo (10% improvement) and low trough (18% improvement), although the study was underpowered to show a significant difference between the high- and low-trough strategies. An open label extension of that study showed the majority of patients who were improved at week 2 remained improved over an extended period, with 55% of patients demonstrating an improvement in disease activity index at week 10. Prednisolone doses were weaned from 19.7 mg/d at study entry to 7.8 mg/d at week 10.[236] A more recent prospective observational study showed clinical remission at 4 weeks in 76% of steroid refractory patients treated with tacrolimus.[237] The results of this latter study, while encouraging, are likely confounded by the inclusion of patients with moderate disease. Other case series have shown mixed outcomes, with clinical improvement rates ranging from 47 to 90%.[238,239,240] Long-term colectomy-free survival has been reported as 57% at 44 months; however, this included patients with both moderate and severe diseases.[238]

Infliximab has demonstrated efficacy for rescue therapy in patients with steroid-refractory severe acute UC. Case series report 20 to 75% colectomy rates in steroid refractory severe colitis treated with infliximab.[241,242,243,244,245] Järnerot et al[136] performed a randomized controlled trial comparing colectomy rates in patients with steroid-refractory severe and moderately severe UC who received a 5 mg/kg dose of infliximab versus those who received placebo. Colectomy rates at 3 months and 3 years were significantly lower in those who received infliximab (29 vs. 67%; $p = 0.017$ and 50% vs. 76%; $p = 0.02$, respectively).[246]

The Active Ulcerative Colitis Trial 1 (ACT-1) and ACT-2 randomized controlled trials evaluated infliximab induction and maintenance therapy in ambulatory patients with moderate to severe active UC. Clinical remission occurred significantly more in the infliximab group relative to placebo (≥ 30 vs. 15%). The studies also identified significantly decreased rates of colectomy at 54 weeks in the infliximab group (10 vs. 17%; $p = 0.02$).[137] It should be noted that the ACT studies looked at ambulatory patients specifically and were not evaluating true salvage therapy per se, which likely explains the lower overall colectomy rate in its population when compared to inpatient studies.

The decision to proceed with a calcineurin inhibitor versus infliximab in acute, steroid refractory colitis is not straightforward. Pooling of available nonrandomized data suggests superiority of infliximab over cyclosporine, with therapeutic response rates of 75 and 55%, respectively. Similarly, nonrandomized 3- and 12-month colectomy rates were lower in patients treated with infliximab (24 vs. 43% and 21 vs. 37%, respectively), although the difference at 3 months was not statistically significant.[247] However, recent randomized controlled trials have refuted the superiority of infliximab, and meta-analysis of the three studies suggests similar clinical response rates of 43.8% for infliximab and 41.7% for cyclosporine. The 3- and 12-month colectomy rates of 26.5 versus 26.4 and 34 versus 43%, respectively, were also similar.[247,248,249,250]

In the absence of definitive data showing superiority of one rescue therapy over another, the treatment decided upon should be patient-centric. With the widespread use of infliximab for maintenance therapy, the decision regarding salvage therapy is often made by default, as the inflammation is already refractory to infliximab. Cyclosporine is therefore preferable in these patients if an attempt at rescue therapy is desired. Another theoretical benefit of cyclosporine over infliximab is the shorter half-life (8 hours vs. 8–10 days, respectively), which may be a factor for those who believe that infliximab imparts an increased risk for postoperative infections. Infliximab, however, has the desirable feature of being able to be continued for maintenance therapy in responders. In patients who are naïve to both therapies and do not have a contraindication to either, there is some evidence to suggest the safety of sequential therapy if one fails.[251] Nevertheless, current recommendations discourage this strategy in favor of early colectomy based on prior studies suggesting an adverse risk-to-benefit ratio.[102,252,253]

An area of ongoing research is the ability to predict response to infliximab. Jürgens et al[254] correlated inflammatory markers and IBD-associated genetic variations to infliximab response in patients with moderate to severe UC. High CRP levels, ANCA seronegativity, and homozygosity for IBD-associated variants of the *IL23R* gene were associated with improved clinical responses. In the future, such predictive models will hopefully be able to guide our decision making as it pertains to escalation of medical care, timing of surgery, and even the recommendation for pouch reconstruction versus stoma.

Management in the Ambulatory Setting

Patients who respond to initial management may stratify into a number of disease courses. These categories include relapsing disease, steroid dependence, refractory, and long-term remission.

The ultimate goal of medical management is long-term, steroid-free remission. Achievement of that goal depends on a symbiosis between disease phenotype, patient compliance, and selection of the appropriate therapeutic agent.

Relapsing Disease

Early relapsing disease (< 3 months) should be treated with induction therapy as before, depending on the severity and extent of disease. Additionally, azathioprine or mercaptopurine should be started in order to minimize the risk of ongoing relapses or smoldering disease. Repeat endoscopy is unnecessary unless it will change management (i.e., proximal extension necessitating the addition of oral mesalamine). Relapses greater than 3 months apart should be treated as they were previously, without the addition of immune modulators.[102]

Steroid Dependence

Steroid dependence is defined as the inability to taper glucocorticoids to less than 10 mg/d within 3 months of starting steroids without recurrent disease.[255] Steroids should not be indefinitely continued due to the substantial side effect profile. Ardizzone et al[256] compared azathioprine with mesalamine for induction and maintenance of steroid-free remission. Patients on 40 mg/d of prednisolone were randomized to receive azathioprine 2 mg/kg/d or oral mesalamine 3.2 g/d. After 6 months, 53% of patients in the azathioprine group were in steroid-free remission compared to 21% in the mesalamine group (odds ratio [OR], 4.78; 95% confidence interval [CI], 1.6–14.5). Longer-term follow-up in an uncontrolled study looking at steroid-dependent patients suggested a similar benefit of azathioprine, with 12-, 24-, and 36-month steroid-free remission rates of 55, 45, and 42%, respectively.[257] As such, azathioprine should be the mainstay therapy in all steroid-dependent ambulatory patients without a contraindication.

Oral Steroid Refractory

Ambulatory patients with UC refractory to oral steroids already stratify into a challenging disease phenotype. This group is the subject of intense pharmacologic research, and really is the target population for the use of "biologic" therapy. While these medications have generated the majority of publicity in recent years, there may be a role for thiopurines and calcineurin inhibitors as well.

Biologic Therapy

The drive behind ongoing research on biologic therapies in autoimmunity is based on the inadequacy of disease control with the use of conventional therapies. Currently, there are six biologic agents used in UC: infliximab, adalimumab, golimumab, vedolizumab, etrolizumab, and tofacitinib, all of which are superior to placebo for both induction and maintenance of remission.[258] While no direct comparative studies have been performed, a recent meta-analysis including available randomized controlled data indirectly compared infliximab to adalimumab, and found that infliximab is more likely to induce a clinical response (OR, 2.36; 95% CI, 1.22–4.63) and mucosal healing (OR, 2.02; 95% CI, 1.13–3.59).

Tumor Necrosis Factor-α Inhibitors

Infliximab: The approval of infliximab for UC in 2004 opened new avenues and offered medically refractory patients hope for remission. The ACT-1 and ACT-2 randomized controlled trials evaluated the efficacy of infliximab (TNF-α inhibitor) for induction of remission in such patients. A 5-mg dose was as effective as was a 10-mg dose at inducing remission, which was observed in 21% of patients at 30 weeks (compared to 7% of controls/placebo). The studies also identified significantly decreased rates of colectomy at 54 weeks in the infliximab group (10 vs. 17%; *p* = 0.02).[137] A more recent placebo-controlled trial looking at immune-modulator-naïve patients with steroid-refractory UC suggests that the combination of infliximab and azathioprine has an additive, if not synergistic, effect on remission induction. Sixteen-week steroid-free remission was achieved in 24, 22, and 40% of patients taking azathioprine monotherapy, infliximab monotherapy, and combination therapy, respectively.[259] It is therefore recommended that infliximab be administered in combination with azathioprine.

Adalimumab: Another TNF-α inhibitor that has shown promise in induction and maintenance of remission is adalimumab. The recommended initial dose of adalimumab is 160 mg, followed by a second dose 2 weeks later of 80 mg, and a maintenance dose of 40 mg every other week, thereafter. A randomized controlled trial comparing adalimumab to placebo in steroid refractory, moderately severe UC showed improved 8-week steroid-free remission rates in the adalimumab group (18.5 vs. 9.2%). At 8 weeks, there was no substantial difference in remission rates between the subgroup who was on steroid therapy at the time of adalimumab induction and those who were not (16.9 vs. 9%).[260] In contrast, another randomized controlled trial looking at the efficacy of adalimumab for long-term steroid-free remission suggested that patients who were on steroids when adalimumab was started had significantly higher 54-week steroid-free remission rates than those who were not (13.3 vs. 5.7%).[261] This likely indicates improved efficacy for adalimumab in steroid dependency as opposed to steroid refractory, although it had a benefit in both groups. Interestingly, this study included patients who had previously been on infliximab, suggesting that failure of one TNF-α inhibitor may not translate to a failure of all.

Golimumab: Golimumab is another recently investigated TNF-α inhibitor in refractory moderate to severe UC. While the same volume of data do not exist, it appears from randomized controlled trials that its efficacy for inducing and maintaining remission is similar to infliximab and adalimumab. Sandborn et al studied 6-week clinical response rates for two different induction doses of golimumab (200 mg and then 100 mg, or 400 mg and then 200 mg, 2 weeks apart) and found 51 and 55% responses for 200/100 mg and 400/200 mg doses, respectively. These were in comparison to a 30% improvement rate for patients randomized to placebo. Fifty-four-week follow-up using maintenance doses of golimumab found a persistent clinical response rate of 47% for patients receiving a 50-mg dose every 4 weeks and 50% of patients receiving a 100-mg dose every 4 weeks. Remission and mucosal healing rates were higher among patients receiving the 100-mg maintenance dose (27.8 and 42.4%) than those receiving the 50-mg maintenance dose (23.2 and 41.7%) or placebo (15.6 and

26.6%; $p < 0.004$).[262] Impact of maintenance therapy was only analyzed in patients who had a response to the induction dose.

Sequential TNF-α Inhibitors

Recent studies have looked at the impact of sequential TNF-α inhibitor use in ambulatory refractory UC.[263] Contrary to intuition, the data seem to suggest that failure of two consecutive TNF-α inhibitors does not predict a nonresponse to a third. De Silva et al[263] found that over 50% of patients trialing a third anti-TNF agent after failure of two previous anti-TNF therapies were able to remain on the third agent for over a year. Three year follow-up data are less encouraging, with only 25% remaining on the same therapy by that time. Prior primary nonresponders to the first anti-TNF agent and persistent disease activity at 3 months after commencement of a third anti-TNF predicted poorer response.

Other Biologic Therapies

Vedolizumab: Vedolizumab imparts its effect through a different mechanism than the TNF-α inhibitors. Specifically, it is a recombinant humanized, anti-alpha-4-beta-7 integrin monoclonal antibody. As integrins regulate migration of leukocytes to the gut, it is hoped that this medication will more selectively target the area of inflammation in IBD. Furthermore, the mere fact that it is different mechanistically offers hope for patients who are either intolerant of or refractory to TNF-α inhibitors. Randomized controlled trials have suggested the efficacy of vedolizumab for induction and maintenance of remission in moderate to severe UC that has failed conventional management.[264, 265,266] In one such randomized trial, a 300-mg dose induced a 6-week clinical response rate of 47%, compared to 22% in patients who were given placebo. Clinical remission and mucosal healing were also improved at the 6-week mark compared to placebo (17 vs. 5% and 41 vs. 25%, respectively); 52-week remission rates were significantly higher in patients who received vedolizumab at either 8-week (42%) or 4-week (45%) intervals when compared to placebo (29%). Similar to golimumab studies, the impact of maintenance therapy was only analyzed in patients who had a response to the induction dose.[265,266]

Etrolizumab: The newest biologic agent to be used in ulcerative colitis (UC) is the monoclonal antibody etrolizumab. As with vedolizumab, it functions via a gut selective mechanism and is designed to interrupt the immune cell trafficking into the intestine via binding of α4β77 and 8 and αEβ79 integrin heterodimers. A recent randomized controlled trial suggested a 21% clinical remission rate at week 10 in patients receiving 100-mg etrolizumab every 4 weeks. This was in comparison to the 0% remission rate in the placebo group. Post hoc analysis suggested a relationship between *ITGAE* gene expression in the baseline colonoscopic biopsy sample and the achievement of clinical remission, with higher rates of gene expression correlating to higher rates of remission.[267] The role of etrolizumab in UC is still being determined.

Tofacitinib: Tyrosine kinases such as Janus kinase 1 (JAK1) and JAK3 are intracellular molecules that help regulate the signal transmission of interleukins, and may play a role in the pathogenesis of UC. Tofacitinib (CP-690, 550) is an oral inhibitor of JAK1, JAK2, and JAK3. Inhibition of these Janus kinases ultimately results in blockage of signaling of a number of cytokines presumably implicated in IBD. These include gamma-chain, containing cytokines such as IL-2, IL-4, IL-7, IL-9, IL-15, and IL-21. A recent randomized, placebo-controlled trial for tofacitinib in moderate to severe UC identified a 15-mg twice-daily dose as the most efficacious regimen, with 8-week clinical remission rate of 41 vs. 10% with placebo.[268]

Thiopurines

While not considered induction agents per se, thiopurines have been shown to induce remission in a significant number of patients, and should be started in all steroid-dependent and steroid-refractory cases.[102] A 30-year cohort study from the Oxford IBD clinic suggested an overall remission rate of 58% for UC patients treated with azathioprine, which increased to 87% of patients who received treatment for 6 months.[269] Unfortunately, these results were confounded by the lack of a control group. Furthermore, the high rate of remission in those treated for 6 months ignored the patients who ultimately failed thiopurine therapy and proceeded to either colectomy or another treatment modality. Nevertheless, recent randomized controlled trials corroborate the efficacy of azathioprine for induction of remission. As previously discussed, azathioprine is as effective as infliximab for induction of remission in steroid-refractory ambulatory patients with moderate to severe UC (24 vs. 22%). Nevertheless, it is the additive effect of the infliximab/azathioprine combination that provides the best patient outcomes (44% remission at 16 weeks) in this patient population.[259] An additional role for azathioprine in induction therapy is as an adjunct to, and ultimately a replacement for, IV cyclosporine in salvage therapy. The transition to azathioprine or 6-mercaptopurine after cyclosporine rescue was associated with much lower long-term colectomy rates when compared to those who remained on 20 weeks of cyclosporine alone (20 vs. 45%, respectively).[270]

Calcineurin Inhibitors

Aside from their role in rescue therapy for IV steroid-refractory UC, calcineurin inhibitors may be considered for remission induction in moderate to severe steroid-refractory disease. Given the IV dosing and narrow toxicity profile, use of cyclosporine has predominantly been relegated to rescue therapy. Tacrolimus, on the other hand, has shown that it may have a place in the armamentarium against moderate to severe ambulatory UC. A placebo-controlled trial has been performed in this patient population. While some of the patients were hospitalized, and while 25% were receiving at least 30-mg prednisolone, these patients did not meet criteria for severe disease mandating rescue therapy. While no patients were in remission after 2 weeks, 68% of those who received tacrolimus adjusted to a trough level of 10 to 15 ng/mL experienced a partial response. This was in comparison to the placebo group and a trough level of 5 to 10 ng/mL group, which experienced partial response rates of 10 and 38%, respectively. The mean dose of prednisolone was also decreased from 19.7 to 7.8 mg/d by week 10.[236] A retrospective series looking at the impact of tacrolimus in moderate to severe steroid-refractory UC demonstrated remission rates of 72% at 12 weeks. Concomitant administration of a thiopurine resulted in significant improvement in remission rate (85 vs. 61%), which adds credence to the prior assertion that all steroid-dependent and steroid-refractory patients should be started on a thiopurine.[271] Most recently, an observational series investigating the use of tacrolimus in moderate to severe UC patients who were not on concurrent steroids suggested early remission rates as high as 90%, with 73% remaining in remission at 10 months.[272]

Methotrexate

The data regarding methotrexate use in UC are limited. The few prospective studies are small, use different doses, and have variable results. The only randomized controlled trial to address methotrexate use (12.5-mg oral dose, weekly) in this population identified 46.7 and 48.6% remission rates in the methotrexate and control groups, respectively.[273] A randomized comparison of 6-mercaptopurine (1.5 mg/kg/d), 5-ASA (3 g/d), and methotrexate (15 mg/wk) in a mixed group of steroid-dependent CD and UC patients found 30-week remission rates of 79, 25, and 58%, respectively.[274] A recent Cochrane review found that there was no evidence to support its use in UC.[275]

25.11.2 Maintenance

Critical analysis of the data regarding maintenance is challenging, as remission is defined differently across studies. It may be defined clinically as the absence of a relapse within 6 to 12 months, which is not only somewhat subjective, but also depends on a universal definition of relapse, which also is not well established. Certainly an increase in stool frequency and recurrence of rectal bleeding confirmed endoscopically is an accurate definition of relapse; however, it cannot be stated that the mere absence of these symptoms indicates remission unless the patient is also off corticosteroids. Additionally, not all studies use endoscopy when evaluating for persistent remission, and even in those that do, the disease activity index scales themselves are subjective in that mucosal friability is in the eye of the beholder.

The goal of maintenance therapy is to maintain steroid-free remission. As more than half of UC patients relapse within a year after an acute flare, it is recommended that continuous maintenance therapy be delivered. A number of risk factors for relapsing disease have been identified. The most consistent across studies is the frequency of prior relapses, suggesting that flares beget more flares. Certainly histopathologic analysis suggesting persistent polymorphonuclear leukocytes in the rectal mucosa has been shown to confer up to a twofold increased risk of relapse. Other factors include the presence of extraintestinal manifestations, younger age, and low fiber diet.[121,122,125,276,277,278,279,280] Stress and being single have also been associated with relapse, and on multivariable analysis have been shown to be stronger predictors of relapse than nonsteroidal anti-inflammatory drugs (NSAIDs), antibiotics, or infection.[281] The strongest correlation with relapsing disease, however, is adherence to medical therapy. A greater than fivefold increased risk of relapse was seen among patients who filled less than 80% of their prescriptions.[282]

After remission, the choice of how to stay in remission is of critical importance. The decision is predicated on the severity of disease, extent of disease, response to previous therapies (especially the regimen that precipitated remission), previous failures, long-term safety profile, and cancer prevention.[102]

Aminosalicylates

For steroid-responsive patients and those who are in remission with aminosalicylates, oral mesalamine is the first-line maintenance treatment. A recent Cochrane review found that mesalamine and other 5-ASA therapies are inversely associated with failure of remission when compared with placebo (OR, 0.47; 95% CI, 0.36–0.62).[172] Topical mesalamine is also helpful, with series showing a 12-month failure of remission rate of 20 to 48% compared to 47 to 89% with placebo.[167,204,283,284,285] Meta-analysis comparing topical mesalamine to placebo for 12-month remission maintenance identified a 16-fold increased chance of remission maintenance with topical mesalamine.[172] Combination of oral and topical mesalamine is slightly more efficacious than oral mesalamine alone and may be administered indefinitely.[102,286] However, a significant number of patients prefer oral treatment alone for maintenance with topical therapy as needed for relapses.[287]

There is no clear dose-response effect for 5-ASA drugs over 0.8 g/d when used for maintenance therapy.[102] Nevertheless, doses as high as 3 g/d are in use, and there is some literature to support these higher maintenance doses. While relapse rates may be similar at 12 months, it appears that patients receiving higher doses (i.e., 2.5–3 g/d) may be in remission for longer periods before recurrence within that year. This finding is especially true for patients with extensive or frequently relapsing disease.[288,289] As with induction therapy, once-daily dosing is as effective as, and preferable to, divided daily dosing.[180,185,290,291] In contrast to induction therapy, pH-dependent release formulations of 5-ASA are not associated with improved outcomes. Any of the oral 5-ASA products may therefore be used for maintenance therapy.[164,292]

Thiopurines

All patients with steroid-dependent UC, steroid-refractory UC, or those who were given a calcineurin inhibitor to induce remission should be started on a thiopurine such as azathioprine or 6-mercaptopurine. Other patients that derive benefit from starting these medications are those with mild to moderate disease with early or frequent relapses despite optimized 5-ASA therapy.[102] A number of small, randomized controlled trials have evaluated the impact of thiopurines on remission maintenance.[274,293,294,295,296,297] A Cochrane review of these studies found that azathioprine had superior outcomes when compared to placebo for failure of remission maintenance (OR, 0.41; 95% CI, 0.24–0.70).[298] A larger randomized controlled trial comparing azathioprine to mesalamine as maintenance therapy for steroid-dependent UC has since been undertaken. This study found that a 2 mg/kg/d dose of azathioprine had improved steroid-free, clinical, and endoscopic remission rates when compared to 3.2 g/d of mesalamine (53 vs. 21%).[256] Long-term data from observational studies suggest 5-year remission rates as high as 62% for azathioprine maintenance therapy.[269]

Thiopurines have a unique role as first-line maintenance therapy for patients in whom remission was induced via calcineurin inhibitors. Unlike biologic agents started for remission, calcineurin inhibitors cannot be continued indefinitely as maintenance drugs due to the significant side-effect profile and unacceptably high risk. In light of this fact, an alternate maintenance therapy is necessary. The rationale for starting with a thiopurine, even in patients who are aminosalicylate naïve, is the high 12-month colectomy rate in patients salvaged with cyclosporine (36–69%).[214,227,230,299] One series reporting long-term outcomes suggests that patients who were successfully converted to either azathioprine or mercaptopurine after calcineurin-inhibitor rescue therapy have substantially lower 5-year colectomy rates than those who were not (20 vs. 45%). This was corroborated in another study looking at 1- and 7-year colectomy-free rates after cyclosporine salvage, which showed a significant discordance between those who received thiopurine maintenance (80 and 60%, respectively) versus those who did not (47 and 15%, respectively).[299]

Methotrexate

The efficacy of methotrexate for maintenance of remission has not been thoroughly studied. One placebo-controlled trial looked at a weekly 12.5-mg dose of methotrexate for remission and maintenance in refractory UC. Patients were followed for 9 months, at which point there was no difference between methotrexate and placebo for either remission or maintenance thereof.[273] These findings may be the result of subtherapeutic dosing rather than a true lack of efficacy. A likely more representative study was an open-label comparison of mercaptopurine (1 mg/kg), methotrexate (15 mg/week), and 5-ASA (3 g/d) in steroid-dependent, active UC. Thirty-week remission rates were highest in mercaptopurine, although there was no statistically significant difference between mercaptopurine (79%) and methotrexate (58%). Patients who achieved clinical remission at 30 weeks were then followed for 72 weeks to determine the efficacy of maintenance therapy. Methotrexate appeared to be inferior to mercaptopurine for this use, as long-term maintenance of remission was achieved in 64, 14, and 0% of patients on mercaptopurine, methotrexate, and placebo, respectively.[274] Retrospective studies looking at the efficacy of 20 to 25 mg of IV methotrexate for remission in this population have identified 30 to 80% remission rates,[300] which may suggest a role for high-dose methotrexate in either remission or maintenance in patients who cannot tolerate or have failed thiopurines. Long-term prospective data evaluating these larger doses of methotrexate in UC do not exist at this time.

Biologic Agents

Tumor necrosis alpha inhibitors have shown efficacy in treating moderate to severe UC refractory to corticosteroids and/or immune modulators. Specific comparative data regarding maintenance regimens in this difficult patient population are lacking. However, it is generally recommended that patients who initially respond to TNF-α inhibitors be maintained on that agent over the long term. The addition or continuation of thiopurines as maintenance therapy in this setting is the subject of some debate.

Infliximab

The ACT-1 randomized, placebo-controlled trial found a 35% remission rate at week 54 in medically refractory UC patients treated with 5 mg/kg dosing of infliximab. This was in comparison to a 54-week remission rate of 17% in the placebo group. Fifty-four-week steroid-free remission rates were 24 and 10%, respectively, and sustained remission over the entirety of 54 weeks was 20 and 7%, respectively. Data from the ACT-2 study followed the same trends, although follow-up only went as far as 30 weeks. ACT-2 saw sustained remission rates of 15% in patients on 5 mg/kg infliximab as compared to 2% with placebo.[301] While clinical response rates were substantially higher than actual remission rates, the relatively low rates of both short- and long-term remission are somewhat daunting.

An observational series with long-term observational follow-up suggested that 68% of patients who had an initial response to infliximab would achieve a sustained clinical response on maintenance doses of the same. Seventeen percent of those who initially responded to infliximab regressed to the point of needing a colectomy over a median follow-up of 33 months. Independent predictors of colectomy included a lack of short-term response to infliximab, a baseline CRP ≥ 5 mg/L, and previous treatment with IV steroids or cyclosporine.[241] The mechanism by which circulating antibodies to infliximab might impact long-term maintenance therapy is not well understood. ACT-1 and ACT-2 patients in the infliximab group had at least 14 and 12% antibody development, respectively. Unfortunately, the tests were inconclusive the majority of the time, so the actual rate of antibody formation could not be ascertained. Interestingly, patients with higher circulating antibodies had improved long-term responses compared to those without. This seemed counterintuitive, and was theorized to be due to low serum concentration levels of the drug in those who did not develop antibodies.[301] Regardless, the addition of an immune-modulating agent to the regimen appears to improve remission rates, perhaps in part due to inhibition of antibody development.[253] Panaccione et al conducted a placebo-controlled trial looking at immune-modulator-naïve patients with steroid-refractory UC, and found that the combination of infliximab and azathioprine has an additive, if not synergistic, effect on remission induction. Sixteen-week steroid-free remission was achieved in 24, 22, and 40% of patients taking azathioprine monotherapy, infliximab monotherapy, and combination therapy, respectively. Antibodies to infliximab were reported in 17% of patients treated with infliximab monotherapy and 3% of patients treated with combination therapy. Unfortunately, antibody testing was inaccurate as only 38% of patients had evaluable samples, and 60% of those were inconclusive.[259] Based on the Panaccione study, it is recommended that infliximab be administered in combination with azathioprine. It seems that antibodies to infliximab develop early, and studies of combined therapy in CD have suggested that the thiopurine may be discontinued after 6 months with no loss of response to infliximab over 2 years.[302]

Adalimumab

Several randomized placebo-controlled trials have reported the efficacy of adalimumab for remission and maintenance therapy in patients with medically refractory moderate to severe UC.[260,261]

The Ulcerative Colitis Long-Term Remission and Maintenance with Adalimumab (ULTRA) trial found a clinical remission rate of 16.5% at 8 weeks in patients receiving 160-/80-mg adalimumab. This was in comparison to the placebo group, which had a 9.3% remission rate. Corresponding values at week 52 were 17.3 and 8.5%, respectively. These numbers were improved in patients who had not previously been on an anti-TNF-α agent. Such patients had 21.3 and 22% 8- and 52-week remission rates, respectively. Patients who had previously been on a TNF-α inhibitor fared worse, with 9.2 and 10.2% remission rates at 8 and 52 weeks.[260,261] Four-year follow-up data have now been released, and suggest that one-third of patients randomized to the adalimumab group remained on adalimumab at week 208. Corticosteroid discontinuation was reported in 59% of these patients, and remission confirmed by mucosal healing was observed in 28% of patients.[303] Indirect comparative data suggest the inferiority of adalimumab when compared to infliximab in anti-TNF-α inhibitor-naïve patients.[258] As such, the role of adalimumab is likely as a sequential therapy for those who have failed or not tolerated infliximab. Unfortunately, it is this group that has the least robust response.

Golimumab

Fifty-four-week follow-up of moderate to severe UC patients who were induced and maintained with golimumab found a persistent clinical response rate of 47% for patients receiving a 50-mg dose every 4 weeks and 50% of patients receiving a 100-mg dose every 4 weeks. Remission and mucosal healing rates were higher among patients receiving the 100-mg maintenance dose (27.8 and 42.4%) than those receiving the 50-mg maintenance dose (23.2 and 41.7%) or placebo (15.6 and 26.6%; $p < 0.004$).[262] It should be noted that the impact of maintenance therapy was only analyzed in patients who had a response to the induction dose.

Vedolizumab

Randomized controlled trials have suggested the efficacy of vedolizumab for induction and maintenance of remission in moderate to severe UC that has failed conventional management.[264,265,266] While no direct comparison studies have been undertaken, a network meta-analysis suggested that vedolizumab is as efficacious as TNF-α inhibitors for induction and maintenance of remission; however, its adverse event profile is lower.[258] Follow-up of randomized controlled data indicated that 52-week remission rates were significantly higher in patients who received vedolizumab at either 8-week (42%) or 4-week (45%) intervals when compared to placebo (29%). Similar to golimumab studies, the impact of maintenance therapy has only been analyzed in patients who had a response to the induction dose.[266] Long-term follow-up studies addressing maintenance therapy with etrolizumab or tofacitinib are lacking.

25.11.3 Primary Nonresponse to Tumor Necrosis Factor-α Inhibitors

Primary nonresponse is defined as a lack of improvement of clinical signs and symptoms with induction therapy.[304] A declaration of nonresponse should not be made before 14 weeks for infliximab or 12 weeks with adalimumab.[305,306] It occurs in 10 to 30% of patients, and is predicted by disease duration greater than 2 years, active smoking, and elevation of CRP.[305,307] Recent studies have also sought to determine genetic markers that may have prognostic significance with regard to response to therapeutics. Genetic mutations in the apoptosis pathway such as FASL and caspace-9 have been associated with primary nonresponse to TNF-α inhibitors.[308] Management of primary nonresponse is contingent on several objective criteria. The presence of high serum drug levels and no anti-TNF antibodies suggests a true primary nonresponse.[309] Two options exist in this case, with limited data backing. Conversion to a second TNF-α inhibitor has been shown in limited series to be safe, with response efficacy in the range of 50 to 65%.[310] An alternative strategy is to switch biologic class and start with a gut-selective agent such as vedolizumab, which has been shown to induce remission in approximately 26% of patients that have previously failed anti-TNF therapy.[311] The presence of low serum drug levels and no anti-TNF antibodies does not indicate nonresponse to therapy, but rather subtherapeutic dosing. Pharmacokinetic profiling, therapeutic drug monitoring, and calculated dose escalation are appropriate in this scenario.[304] Post hoc analysis of the ACT-1 and ACT-2 trials suggests the presumed efficacy of this strategy, as the presence of infliximab levels approximately 41 µ/mL at 8 weeks had a positive predictive value of 80% for clinical response.[301,312] Therapeutic drug monitoring may be especially important in severe UC, as the massive inflammation is associated with increased clearance of infliximab and resultant primary nonresponse.[313]

Secondary loss of response, or simply loss of response, occurs when patients have an initial clinical response but subsequently lose responsiveness during maintenance.[304] Specific data regarding loss of response to TNF-α inhibitors in UC is lacking. Nevertheless, ACT-1 and ACT-2 data suggest its occurrence, as remission rates at 30 weeks were significantly higher than those at 54 weeks (74 vs. 66%).[301] Systematic review of the CD literature suggests a 20% loss of response per patient-year, with 24% requiring dose escalation per patient-year.[314] If loss of response is verified, therapeutic drug monitoring is in order.

Loss of response is associated with formation of anti-TNF antibodies, which either interfere with TNF binding or enhance clearance of the drug through the reticuloendothelial system.[315] Anti-TNF antibodies develop in at least 12 to 17% of patients on infliximab monotherapy.[259,301] Dose escalation is generally not advised in these patients, as the clinical response is unlikely and the risk of infusion reaction is significantly increased.[316,317] Conversion to another TNF-α inhibitor is well tolerated and is associated with a complete or partial response in 92% of patients.[316] Small studies have even shown efficacy for a third sequential TNF-α inhibitor if options such as surgery or other drug classes are not desirable.[263,318] An alternative is to start an immune modulator such as azathioprine, mercaptopurine, or methotrexate either as prevention from initial induction or at the time of loss of response. The evidence for starting immune modulation upfront is more robust. Two small case series demonstrated decreased antibody levels and increased drug trough levels with use of immune modulation, which led to improved clinical response.[319,320,321,322,323]

Primary prevention of loss of response may be undertaken by starting an immune modulator upfront, using therapeutic drug monitoring to achieve infliximab troughs between 4 and 7 µ/mL, pretreating with corticosteroids, and ensuring that patients adhere to scheduled delivery of the TNF-α inhibitor rather than relying on episodic dosing.[305,321,324,325,326,327,328,329,330,331]

25.11.4 Medication Side Effects and Tolerance

Mesalamine

Mesalamine's effect is imparted by topical interaction only. As such, its side effects cannot be analyzed by pharmacokinetic comparisons, although absorption may influence adverse events. Mesalamine is not tolerated in up to 15% of patients, and as many as 3% of patients will have acute intolerance resembling a colitis flare.[102] Specific symptoms include diarrhea, headache, nausea, rash, and exceedingly rare (< 1%) thrombocytopenia. Nevertheless, systematic review has identified mesalamine as safe, with adverse event rates similar to those of placebo.[332]

Calcineurin Inhibitors

Hypertension, paresthesias, tremors, and headaches are the most common side effects of cyclosporine and tacrolimus, although hypomagnesemia, renal impairment, and gastrointestinal upset impact approximately half of all patients. Cyclosporine-related neurological side effects are increased in cases of hypomagnesemia and low cholesterol, and should be avoided in these groups. Tacrolimus may induce diabetes.[102,236] Opportunistic infection is a significant concern in these patients as well. A study of long-term outcomes of severe UC patients treated with IV cyclosporine found that 3.5% of these patients died of either *Pneumocystis jiroveci* or *Aspergillus fumigatus* pneumonia.[333]

Thiopurines

A recent study evaluated the long-term outcomes of nearly 4,000 IBD patients who were on thiopurine maintenance therapy for a median of 44 months. The cumulative incidence of adverse events was 26%, with an annual risk of 7% per patient-year of treatment. The most frequent adverse events were nausea (8%), hepatotoxicity (4%), myelotoxicity (4%), and pancreatitis (4%). Four patients developed lymphoma. Crohn's disease (CD) patients had higher rates of nausea, hepatotoxicity, and pancreatitis when compared to UC. Overall, 17% of patients discontinued thiopurine treatment due to adverse events. Thirty-seven percent of these patients started thiopurines again and 40% of them had adverse events again.[334]

TNF-α Inhibitors

In placebo-controlled trials in moderate to severe UC, serious adverse events occurred less frequently in the infliximab groups than they did with placebo (10.7–21.5% with 5-mg dosing, 9.2–23.8% with 10-mg dosing, and 19.5–25.6% with placebo). Infectious complications were the most common adverse events, occurring in 27 to 43% of patients treated with 5-mg infliximab versus 24 to 39% with placebo. Serious infections occurred much less frequently in both groups (1.7–2.5% with 5-mg infliximab vs.

0.8–4.1% with placebo). Infusion reactions occurred in 10% of infliximab patients, although this increased to 35.7% of patients who developed infliximab antibodies. Basal cell carcinoma, colorectal dysplasia, CMV infection, and demyelinating disease were reported in less than 0.1% of patients.[301] Placebo-controlled trials regarding adalimumab had similarly low rates of serious infections (2.2% with adalimumab vs. 6.5% with placebo). Injection site reactions were more frequent with adalimumab than with placebo (46.9 vs. 16.4%). Long-term follow-up of patients receiving maintenance therapy with adalimumab saw the emergence of rare side effects such as lymphoma (0.1%), demyelinating disease (0.1%), congestive heart failure (0.2%), CMV infection (0.2%), liver injury (0.5%), and death (0.1%).[303]

Vedolizumab

The adverse event profile for vedolizumab is actually quite favorable based on randomized controlled trials and a separate meta-analysis. Rates of serious adverse effects (12.4 vs. 13.5%), serious infections (1.9 vs. 29%), and development of cancer (0.2 vs. 1.1%) are all similar to, if not lower than, that seen with placebo.[266]

Etrolizumab

Rates of overall and serious adverse events are not significantly different between etrolizumab and placebo, ranging from 48 to 61% and 5 to 12%, respectively. Influenzalike illness, rash, and arthralgias were more frequently encountered in patients receiving 100 mg of etrolizumab when compared to placebo (7 vs. 2%, 7 vs. 2%, and 15 vs. 9%, respectively).[267]

Tofacitinib

Adverse event rates appear to be similar between patients on placebo and on tofacitinib, although serious infectious complications, although rare (1.3% of all tofacitinib patients), may occur more frequently in higher dosages (6% of patients receiving 10-mg dose). There also seems to be a dose-dependent increase in high-density lipoprotein (HDL) and low-density lipoprotein (LDL) levels at 8 weeks. These metabolic derangements spontaneously correct after discontinuation of the drug. Perhaps the most concerning adverse event observed in patients receiving tofacitinib was a neutropenia, with absolute neutrophil counts less than 1,500 cells/mm^3, as occurred in approximately 2% of patients who received tofacitinib.[268]

25.11.5 Alternative Therapies

Helminths

The hygiene hypothesis, which suggests that protective immunity is stimulated by early exposure to pathogens and parasites, backed by experimental evidence suggesting that some helminths moderate immune-mediated colitis, led to a randomized, placebo-controlled trial of *Trichuris suis* ova in mild to moderate UC. The experimental group was given 2,500 ova every 2 weeks for 12 weeks. Forty-three percent of patients in the treatment group experienced clinical improvement at 12 weeks versus 17% with placebo.[59,60] A recent meta-analysis of helminthic therapy for IBD found insufficient evidence to draw any conclusions about the efficacy or safety of the treatment.[335]

Leucocytapheresis

Leucocytapheresis is a technique involving extracorporeal removal of leucocytes via a series of filters. The therapy removes up to 100% of neutrophils and monocytes and 20 to 60% of lymphocytes. A number of limited studies have suggested benefit; however, the only well-designed randomized controlled trial failed to show any clinical improvement using the technique.[336,337,338,339,340,341,342] While the practice is relatively common in Japan, better quality randomized controlled trials will need to be undertaken before this procedure gains more widespread popularity.

Several alternative therapies aim to treat UC by addressing the "dysbiosis" theory of IBD, in which self-perpetuating inflammation is in part due to alterations in the colonic bacterial and nutritional homeostasis. Antibiotics, probiotics, fecal transplant, and restrictive diets are among the proposed therapies.

Antibiotics

Antibiotics may be useful as an adjunct to steroids for induction of remission in active UC. Unfortunately, the data are conflicting and difficult to interpret. However, meta-analysis of nine randomized controlled trials using an assortment of antibiotic regimens in active UC suggested that antibiotics are associated with an improved clinical response (OR, 2.17; 95% CI, 1.54–3.05).[343] Randomized, placebo-controlled trials have used a regimen of amoxicillin 1,500 mg/d, tetracycline 1,500 mg/d, and metronidazole 750 mg/d for 2 weeks and found significantly higher rates of remission at 3 months with antibiotics (44.8 vs. 22.8%).[344] There has been speculation that the benefit is a result of alterations in the bacterial homeostasis of the gut rather than a direct effect of antibiotics. Bench studies have confirmed that this combination of antibiotics induces long-term alterations in the gut flora, which would corroborate this theory.[345] Additional studies evaluating the possible benefit of long-term antibiotics for maintenance of remission have been undertaken. While both ciprofloxacin and metronidazole have shown promising results in terms of long-term remission when added to standard therapies, the data are inadequate to make formal recommendations.[346,347,348]

Probiotics

Limited data exist regarding the use of probiotics for the treatment of UC. Only one trial has identified an improved clinical response in active mild to moderate UC treated with probiotics. Miele et al[349] randomized newly diagnosed UC patients to receive either standard therapy with mesalamine and steroids plus placebo or mesalamine and steroids with concomitant VSL#3. The authors found a 93% clinical response rate in the VSL#3 plus standard therapy group in comparison with a 36% response with standard therapy alone. Follow-up over 1 year suggested improved long-term remission in the VSL#3 group, with only 21% of these patients suffering a relapse compared to 73% with placebo. The E. coli strain Nissle 1917 is another probiotic that has shown benefit as a maintenance therapy. An equivalence study for long-term maintenance therapy using either standard 5-ASA or E. coli Nissle 1917 for 12 months was undertaken. Relapse rates of 45 and 36% were seen in the probiotic and the 5-ASA groups, respectively. Because these rates were not statistically different, it was concluded that E. coli Nissle 1917 is noninferior to standard 5-ASA for maintenance therapy.[350]

Restrictive Diets

A number of studies have previously evaluated restrictive diets for the treatment of IBD, with mixed and largely disappointing results. Recently, however, the implementation of a "specific carbohydrate diet" (SCD) in IBD has proven to be reassuring, particularly in the pediatric population.[80,351,352,353] While the case series are small, it seems that disease activity indices decrease in conjunction with induction of dietary carbohydrate restrictions. Obih et al[80] evaluated the impact of SCD on 26 children with either CD or UC, and found that UC disease index scores decreased from 28 to 18 over 6 months following SCD implementation. Another small series used SCD as primary therapy for IBD in children, and noted 100% resolution of symptoms by 3 months.[353] A case series in adults who utilized SCD in conjunction with, and sometimes as a replacement for, standard therapy reported 66% symptom resolution within 10 months with a mean time to improvement of 29 days. Patient surveys rated SCD as greater than 90% effective at controlling acute flares and maintaining remission.[351] Kakodkar et al[352] suggest that the altered nutrients entering the colon with SCD result in a shift in the microbiome, which may influence the course of inflammation. While prospective, controlled studies are needed, these small case series may represent a turning point in the way we view and manage IBD.

Fecal Transplant

With the emergence of fecal transplantation as the definitive therapy for recurrent C. difficile colitis,[354] the technique has gained widespread interest for its potential efficacy in the treatment of other gastrointestinal maladies. Certainly the potential benefits in UC, a disease characterized at least in part by a dysfunctional microbial homeostasis, are astounding. The first randomized controlled trial to look at fecal transplant in UC was recently undertaken. Clinical response and remission rates at 7 months were significantly improved in the fecal transplant group in comparison to placebo (39 and 24%, respectively, vs. 24 and 5%, respectively).[355] This study is the first solid evidence supporting a primary role for alteration of the microbiome in the treatment of UC.

25.12 Surgical Management

It is understandable, although perhaps unfortunate, that the flow of any medical text proceeds from the simplest algorithm to the most complex, often ending with a surgical procedure and its potential complications. In reality, the "surgical" UC patient may be quite young with no clear antecedent history of gastrointestinal symptoms. In such a case, the majority of the medical algorithm is bypassed. Other patients are at the opposite extreme of the spectrum, languishing for years with intractable fecal incontinence, excruciating pain, and a keen sense of the limitations of modern medicine to help. This latter patient suffers through the entire algorithm many times over, awaiting approval of the next medication, awaiting some sort of relief, awaiting something definitive, awaiting the end of the chapter. The timing of elective surgery is often dictated by the degree of lifestyle compromise and morbidity from the disease and/or its medical treatments. The adverse side effects of the medical regimens may be worse than the symptoms of the disease.

The distinction between CD and UC needs to be the fulcrum on which every operative decision in IBD rests, as the gastrointestinal manifestations of UC are obliterated with resection of the colon and rectum, while no such palliation exists for CD. Patient counseling to this point is exceedingly important, as is the recognition that we are not infrequently wrong. Given the uncertainty of diagnosis and potential morbidity of any colorectal operation, the approach to the IBD patient should be to maximally educate, establish realistic expectations, and ultimately relinquish to patient autonomy.

The operative management of UC has undergone a remarkable evolution in the century since surgery was introduced as a therapeutic option. In 1893, Mayo-Robson[356] of Leeds performed the first documented UC surgery when he created a colostomy in order to irrigate the diseased colon. This concept was subsequently refined and formalized, and by 1909 cecostomy and appendicostomy were the surgical procedures of choice for primary colonic inflammation.[357,358] These interventions had the distinct advantage of relatively low output compared to ileostomy, which was a desirable component as no formal stoma appliances had been invented. Furthermore, the goal of the fistula was not to divert the fecal stream but to provide access for the infusion of various solutions.

Fecal diversion was not part of the collective thinking early in the 20th century. It was not until 1913 that Brown of St. Louis espoused the benefits of physiologic rest of the inflamed colon by fecal diversion.[359] Ensuing years saw a philosophical divide among surgeons who subscribed to the principle of either colonic irrigation with an appendicostomy or fecal diversion with an ileostomy. Unfortunately, the limitations of enterostomal therapy at the time fated the ileostomy to be a highly morbid procedure, generally reserved for only the sickest patients.

The development of the first stoma appliance in 1944 ushered in the modern era of UC surgery.[360] This new technology, coupled with the Brian Brooke's ("Brooke") ileostomy developed 8 years later,[361] dramatically improved the quality of life with an ileostomy and made it a much more palatable procedure. The ability to have a tolerable end ileostomy allowed for definitive surgery, and the single-stage proctocolectomy championed by Brooke became the gold standard.[361,362] Nevertheless, the patient's desire to avoid an ileostomy often superseded the tolerability of fecal diversion. The remaining evolution of UC surgery has therefore not been driven by improvement in disease control, but rather refinements in techniques to either restore gastrointestinal continuity or mitigate the impact of life with an ileostomy.

25.12.1 Emergent Indications

Life-Threatening Severe Colitis

Life-threatening UC, often referred to as fulminant colitis, presents with rapid-onset abdominal pain, abdominal distention, persistent bloody diarrhea, and signs of toxicity such as fevers and tachycardia (▶ Table 25.5). Many will have anemia and/or a profound leukocytosis.[363] These patients must be treated aggressively with fluid resuscitation, electrolyte replacement, and high-dose IV steroids. It is important to rule out infectious etiologies before starting corticosteroids. A nasogastric tube may be placed, although this is unlikely to decompress a colon with a competent ileocecal valve. If the etiology is in question, as it is in the 10% of patients presenting for the first time with fulminant colitis,[364] the diagnosis should be confirmed with flexible sigmoidoscopy. If the patient remains stable but without substantial improvement over the next 24 to 48 hours, rescue therapy with a calcineurin inhibitor or an anti-TNF-α agent may be considered. Short-term results of rescue therapy in this population are encouraging, with 76 to 85% of patients avoiding colectomy on that admission. Long-term patient expectations should be tempered, however, as follow-up data suggest that between 58 and 88% of patients who required cyclosporine rescue underwent a colectomy within 7 years.[230,233]

So-called "toxic megacolon" is an extreme variant of fulminant colitis in which all or a segment of the transverse or left colon is dilated to more than 5.5 cm. It occurs in up to 2.5% of those with UC, and, as with fulminant colitis, may be the initial presentation.[91,364] The medical algorithm is unchanged from

Table 25.5 Surgical indications and recommended procedures in ulcerative colitis

	Indication	Treatment
Emergent	Life-threatening colitis	Total abdominal colectomy with end ileostomy ± mucus fistula
		Turnbull-"blowhole" colostomy
	Massive hemorrhage	Total abdominal colectomy with end ileostomy
		Total proctocolectomy with end ileostomy if rectal bleeding
	Perforation	Total abdominal colectomy with end ileostomy
		Turnbull-"blowhole" colostomy
	Obstruction	Total abdominal colectomy with end ileostomy ± mucus fistula
		Turnbull-"blowhole" colostomy
Nonemergent	Intractable disease	Restorative proctocolectomy
		Total proctocolectomy with end ileostomy or continent ileostomy
		Total abdominal colectomy with end ileostomy ± mucus fistula[a]
	Dysplasia or malignancy	Individualized, see ▶ Table 25.6
	Extraintestinal manifestations	Restorative proctocolectomy
		Total proctocolectomy with end ileostomy or continent ileostomy

[a]Patients who are acutely ill and unresponsive to medications or who have been on at least 20 mg of prednisone per day for 6 weeks first undergo subtotal colectomy with end ileostomy.[102]

Table 25.6 Surgical management of colorectal dysplasia in the setting of ulcerative colitis

Lesion appearance	Dysplasia grade	Treatment
Flat	Low grade	Individualized
	High grade	Colectomy/with end ileostomy, possible interval completion proctectomy and ileal pouch anal anastomosis (IPAA) if no recurrence
Raised: adenomatous	Low grade	Endoscopic polypectomy ok if margin is clear of dysplasia and inflammation
	High grade	Colectomy/with end ileostomy, possible interval completion proctectomy and IPAA if no recurrence
Raised: nonadenomatous	Low grade	Colectomy/with end ileostomy, possible interval completion proctectomy and IPAA if no recurrence
	High grade	Colectomy/with end ileostomy, possible interval completion proctectomy and IPAA if no recurrence

that of fulminant colitis, although broad-spectrum antibiotics should be administered in conjunction with high-dose steroids.[91] Early surgical consultation is an absolute necessity, as a delay in operative management risks perforation and 30% mortality.[364] A lack of response within 24 to 48 hours necessitates either operative intervention or rescue therapy. Rescue therapy, even when successful in the short term, should be viewed as a bridge to a more "elective" surgery, as at least 35% of these patients will require a proctocolectomy within a year and up to 88% by 7 years.[230]

Massive Hemorrhage

Hemorrhage to the point of hemodynamic instability is a rare occurrence in UC (~1%), although it does account for approximately 10% of urgent colectomies for UC.[365] These patients should be initially managed as any other gastrointestinal bleed with resuscitation, localization, and hemorrhage control. Upper gastrointestinal sources should be ruled out and high-dose IV steroids should be administered. A stable patient may be monitored for 24 to 72 hours for improvement on steroids; however, the majority of patients will require surgery. The bleeding is usually from a diffuse mucosal injury and is therefore not amenable to colonoscopic or endovascular hemorrhage control techniques. Massive hemorrhage from both the colon and rectum is likely the one and only indication for an emergent proctocolectomy. If possible, it is preferred to leave the rectum in situ in the acute setting to facilitate a staged completion proctectomy with an ileal pouch anastomosis. In approximately 12% of cases, the rectal stump will continue to bleed despite steroids and diversion; however, it is usually relatively minor bleeding that can be conservatively managed.

Perforation

Colonic perforation is related to extent and severity of disease, occurring in as many as 20% of UC patients presenting with fulminant pancolitis. The patients are acutely ill upon presentation, and mortality rate is approximately 50%.[366] Observation with immune suppression therefore has no role in any patient with a full-thickness perforation. Abdominal colectomy with ileostomy and Hartmann closure of the rectum or construction of an either open or closed mucous fistula is the procedure of choice.

Obstruction

Strictures are present in 3 to 17% of patients with UC, with approximately one in three located in the rectum.[9,128,130] Stricturing disease may ultimately result in a large bowel obstruction, which necessitates surgical excision due to both the risk of perforation and the potential for malignant cells within the stricture.[128] It has been suggested that approximately 40% of resected strictures will return with carcinoma in the resected specimen and an additional 33% will have high-grade dysplasia.[131]

25.12.2 Nonemergent Indications

Intractable Disease

Intractable colorectal inflammation is the most common indication for nonemergent surgery in UC (▶ Table 25.5).[365] These patients are either unable to tolerate a steroid taper without recurrence of symptoms, intolerant of medical therapy due to severe side effects, or have persistent symptoms despite maximal medical therapy.[128] The gold-standard surgery is a total proctocolectomy with or without pouch reconstruction. Excision of the entire colon and rectum, regardless of the extent of the disease at the time of surgery, will remove the entirety of the primary disease process and correct several extraintestinal manifestations. The difficulty in these cases is that maximal medical therapy is a fluid definition depending on available medications and the person prescribing them. With new biologic therapies in the pipeline, recent studies reporting some success with trialing a third sequential TNF-α inhibitor, and some clinicians supporting the off-label use of unproven biologics in UC, it is easy to imagine a situation where a smoldering patient is eternally strung along in hopes of a medical "cure." The lack of a clear-cut line in the sand is one of the more frustrating aspects of UC for both patients and surgeons alike, and highlights the necessity for multidisciplinary collaboration.

Dysplasia, Malignancy of the Colon or Rectum, or Cancer Prophylaxis

UC is associated with a 0.5 to 1% increased risk per year after 10 years, regardless of severity of disease activity.[366] This equates to a 20% risk at 20 years and a greater than 30% risk at 35 years.[367] It stands to reason that patients who are younger at diagnosis are at higher risk for subsequent development of colorectal cancer. Cancer risk is also correlated with extent of disease, as an increase in inflamed surface area imposes a higher mathematical probability of developing inflammation-related cancer.[368] Furthermore, the mere presence of low-grade dysplasia in one portion of the colon suggests that the entirety of the diseased colon and rectum is at risk for synchronous malignancy.[369] As such, patients with colorectal malignancy, high-grade dysplasia, dysplasia-associated lesion or mass (DALM), or low-grade dysplasia are candidates for colectomy or proctocolectomy (▶ Table 25.6).[369,370] Ileal pouch anal anastomosis (IPAA) is not contraindicated in the setting of malignancy, and the decision to proceed with pouch reconstruction is based on tumor location and patient preference rather than a specific algorithm.[365] Caution should be exercised, however, in the setting of more advanced (T3) lesions, as these may represent an aggressive phenotype predisposing to metastases. A conservative approach consisting of abdominal colectomy and end ileostomy, followed by IPAA after an observation period of at least 12 months is recommended in these patients.[371] Patients with low or middle rectal cancer should be advised against IPAA, as they are at increased risk for subsequent radiation therapy (close margins, local recurrence), which renders a pouch poorly functional at best.

The management of colorectal dysplasia in the setting of UC is a controversial subject, and current recommendations are based on the macroscopic pattern and microscopic characteristics of the lesion.[129,130,370,371,372] Microscopic patterns of dysplasia include high and low grade, either of which should be verified by a second pathologist given the degree of variability in the findings.[372,373,374] Macroscopic patterns include "flat" and "raised" lesions. Flat lesions are endoscopically undetectable and are generally discovered on random biopsies or on pathological evaluation of a resected specimen.[129,130,370] Flat lesions containing high-grade dysplasia are associated with exceedingly high rates of occult malignancy, ranging from 42 to 67%.[375,376,377] Colectomy is therefore recommended in any UC patient with a flat lesion and high-grade dysplasia.[378] Flat lesions with low-grade dysplasia have a dramatically different natural history, with a positive predictive value for progression to high-grade dysplasia or cancer of only 14.6%.[379] Long-term follow-up studies have found rates of progression to malignancy to be exceedingly low, approaching the malignancy rates seen in the age-matched general public.[380,381] As such, it is unclear if upfront colectomy is indicated in these patients. An individualized, patient-centric approach may therefore be taken in such cases.[378] Moreover, re-review of all biopsies by an expert colorectal pathologist is essential.

Raised lesions are described as adenomatous or nonadenomatous. Adenomalike lesions appear as a normal polyp not associated with inflammatory bowel disease (IBD). They are generally well circumscribed, non-necrotic, and pedunculated or sessile. These lesions may be treated as any other adenomatous polyp, with endoscopic polypectomy. This recommendation is based on long-term follow-up data suggesting exceedingly low rates of adenocarcinoma development after polypectomy.[382,383,384] Nonadenomatous raised lesions include velvety patches, plaques, irregular nodules, abnormal thickening, strictures, and broad-based masses.[129,130,385,386,387] There is a strong association between nonadenomatous UC-related polyps and synchronous and metachronous gastrointestinal malignancies, ranging from 38 to 83%.[370] It is therefore necessary to proceed with full oncologic resection, which in the typical case of UC consists of a total proctocolectomy.

Extraintestinal Manifestations

While UC-related joint, eye, and skin manifestations are often improved following proctocolectomy, surgery is rarely indicated for extraintestinal manifestations alone. The reason for this is twofold. First, appropriate medical management of colorectal inflammation generally controls the extraintestinal manifestations that are improved with proctocolectomy. Second, these manifestations are rarely severe enough to justify the potential morbidity of resection of the entire colon and rectum. Additionally, the most concerning extraintestinal manifestations such as ankylosing spondylitis, PSC, and liver dysfunction are not impacted by excision of the primary offending organ. Nevertheless, there are several instances where secondary gains justify colectomy or proctocolectomy. Extreme growth and developmental delays in children with UC can be reversed with removal of the colon. This is likely the most common indication for colectomy to treat an extraintestinal manifestation. Another, less common indication for colectomy or proctocolectomy is refractory pyoderma gangrenosum, which resolves after colectomy in approximately 50% of patients. A rare extraintestinal manifestation of UC is severe hemolytic anemia, which may require urgent colectomy with splenectomy if refractory to immune suppression.[365]

25.12.3 Surgical Options and Outcomes

The ultimate goal of surgical therapy for UC is removal of the entire intestinal disease burden. Total proctocolectomy is therefore the procedure of choice, and offers the chance for a surgical "cure." Nevertheless, there are alternative strategies that may play roles in select situations. In all, there are six available surgical options for the UC patient, depending on the clinical scenario. These include subtotal colectomy with end ileostomy, transverse loop ("blow-hole") colostomy of Turnbull, total proctocolectomy with end (Brooke) ileostomy, total proctocolectomy with continent (Koch) ileostomy, abdominal colectomy with ileorectal anastomosis, and total proctocolectomy with IPAA.

The transition of a UC patient from the medical to the surgical domain carries with it a number of implications that complicate surgical decision making. With the enlarging medication armamentarium for UC, the period of time before surgical consultation for "failed medical management" is ever increasing. Thus, the first contact the surgeon has with the UC patient is often in the setting of fulminant colitis or long-standing steroid-dependent or steroid-refractory disease. Neither of these scenarios necessarily indicates a medically "optimized" patient, and all increase the patient's risk for developing postoperative complications such as anastomotic leak. Thus, the fear of postoperative complications as justification for delay of elective surgery becomes a self-fulfilling prophecy. It is for the sake of these patients that a staged approach to restorative proctocolectomy is undertaken. Consensus guidelines suggest that patients who are acutely ill and unresponsive to medications or who have been on at least 20 mg of prednisone per day for 6 weeks first undergo subtotal colectomy with end ileostomy.[102] It should be noted at this point that having been on biologic or immune-modulating medications other than steroids does not, in and of itself, necessitate a staged approach.

25.12.4 Subtotal Colectomy with End Ileostomy

In 1951, Crile and Thomas[388] advocated for total abdominal colectomy with end ileostomy to control severe colitis. Adoption of this management strategy reduced the mortality rate of toxic megacolon from 63% (with ileostomy alone) to only 14%. More recent series suggest a mortality rate less than 10%, with pelvic sepsis rates approximately 10%, and overall morbidity rates greater than 30%.[389,390] The procedure is not definitive. Rather, it is a temporizing measure to control the bulk of the disease burden and ensure colonic decompression while allowing the patient time to wean from steroids and optimize nutrition prior to endeavoring upon a high-risk IPAA. The hidden benefit in this strategy is that it allows for a more accurate pathologic diagnosis, thereby minimizing the risk of a CD "recurrence" in the pouch. There is no urgency to definitive surgery after subtotal colectomy with end ileostomy, as long as the rectal stump is appropriately surveyed for malignancy.

Procedure

Whether by laparotomy or laparoscopy, upon entry the abdomen is explored to evaluate for CD or malignancy. Attention is then turned to the right colon, which is mobilized by either lateral-to-medial or medial-to-lateral dissection. With the former, the cecum is retracted medially and the peritoneum is incised along white line of Toldt. Using broad sweeps with a blunt instrument, the right colon is swept medially in the retroperitoneal avascular plane and the peritoneal reflection is serially incised as the mobilization continues cephalad to the level of the hepatic flexure and the duodenal sweep. Staying in the appropriate plane will allow for a bloodless dissection in which Gerota's fascia, the right ureter, and the duodenum are maintained in their posterior retroperitoneal position.

At this point, the hepatic flexure must be mobilized. To do so, the greater omentum is retracted anteriorly and the lesser sac is entered by incising the gastrocolic ligament in an avascular plan adjacent to the wall of the transverse colon. This plane is then developed by gentle sweeping of the transverse colon inferiorly, further exposing the avascular plane of the gastrocolic ligament. The line of dissection is thus carried toward the hepatic flexure. The dissection plane between the omentum and posterior wall of the lesser sac becomes fused as the hepatocolic ligament is approached. It is important at this point that substantial attention is given to discerning the omentum, which is to be incised from the transverse colon mesentery. The hepatic flexure of the colon is then retracted inferiorly and remaining retroperitoneal attachments are incised. This maneuver should expose the second portion of the duodenum and connect the two dissection planes.

The orientation of the working instruments should then be reversed and the omentum dissected off the transverse colon proceeding toward the splenic flexure. This dissection should be continued until further mobilization of the splenic flexure becomes difficult. Attention should then be turned to the descending colon, which must be mobilized from the retroperitoneum before splenic flexure mobilization can be completed. The sigmoid colon is retracted medially and the peritoneum incised along the white line of Toldt, exposing the avascular

retroperitoneal plane. Similar to the right colon mobilization, the avascular plane is further developed by broad sweeping of the sigmoid and descending colon medially. As it is exposed, the peritoneum is incised. It is important to stay close to the colon wall lest the dissection continue posterior to Gerota's fascia. The dissection is continued superiorly to the splenic flexure of the colon, which is then retracted medially to allow for the division of any remaining lienocolic or retroperitoneal attachments.

Medial-to-lateral dissection of the ascending and descending colon is an alternative strategy often used with laparoscopic, hand-assisted, or robotic-assisted surgery. Medial-to-lateral dissection of the right colon starts with anterior retraction on the cecum to "tent" the ileocolic artery. The peritoneum is then scored immediately adjacent to the artery and the avascular retroperitoneal plane is developed from the pelvic brim to the duodenum using gentle blunt dissection. The hepatic flexure is then taken down as previously described and the white line of Toldt is divided, completing the mobilization. Medial-to-lateral dissection of the left colon proceeds in similar fashion. The sigmoid colon is grasped and retracted anteriorly such that the superior hemorrhoidal vessel "tents." The peritoneum adjacent to the artery is then scored and the avascular plane is identified and gently developed. The left ureter should be identified and kept down with the retroperitoneal structures. The medial dissection plane should extend from the pelvic brim to the superior mesenteric vein. Once mobilized medially, the white line of Toldt is incised and the mobilization of the splenic flexure completed.

With the entire colon mobilized, the right colic (if present) and middle colic vascular pedicles should be ligated. The ileocolic and inferior mesenteric pedicles should remain undisturbed, with the mesenteric dissection being carried out immediately adjacent to the bowel wall. The terminal ileum is then divided and the distal resection point is identified. The entire rectum should be left in situ to facilitate later completion proctectomy. Many will leave a small amount of sigmoid colon as well, which allows even greater ease in establishing the dissection plane at the time of completion proctectomy. The entire mobilized specimen is then brought out of the incision and passed off the table.

Management of the Rectal Stump

The fate of the rectal stump is of great concern, as "blowout" of the staple line may occur in up to 12% of patients.[391,392,393] This complication is incredibly morbid, and options for management of the stump are designed to mitigate this risk. The stump may be converted into a mucus fistula or left in situ with a temporary decompression tube in place. A third option is to bring the proximal stapled end of the rectosigmoid into the subcutaneous fat and secure it there. When managed in this fashion, a rectal stump leak will in essence become a mucus fistula to the anterior abdominal wall.[391,394] Finally, the ileostomy is matured and the abdomen is closed.

25.12.5 Turnbull-Blowhole Colostomy

Despite improvements in severe UC outcomes with the use of abdominal colectomy and end ileostomy, Turnbull proposed a skin-level loop colostomy in addition to loop ileostomy in cases of toxic megacolon. The rationale for this maneuver was two-fold: first, it avoided iatrogenic injury secondary to handling of the friable, diseased colon. Second, it avoided the problems associated with management of the difficult rectal stump.[395] The procedure is largely of historical interest, as most do not find that it imparts a benefit over abdominal colectomy in the era of modern medicine. Nevertheless, it continues to have a role in the most unstable patients and in pregnant women in whom colonic dissection around the gravid uterus is undesirable. Another benefit of Turnbull's procedure in pregnant women is that it avoids the need for bringing the rectosigmoid stump out as mucus fistula, which may not be feasible in the presence of a gravid uterus.[396]

Procedure

An upper midline incision is made and the abdomen is explored. The terminal ileum is identified and a loop is brought out through the abdominal wall in the right lower quadrant using a muscle-splitting technique. The exteriorized loop is secured at the skin level using a stoma rod placed through a mesenteric window immediately adjacent to the bowel wall. The midpoint of the transverse colon is then identified through either the same incision or a second, 5-cm, epigastric incision. The fascia and skin are then closed from inferior to superior, ending at the bulging colon edge. If a separate incision was used to find the transverse colon, then the entirety of the original midline wound may be closed. The loop ileostomy is then matured.

Attention is then turned toward creation of the blowhole colostomy. The omentum and seromuscular layers of the transverse colon are secured to the peritoneum and fascia using interrupted or running 3–0 absorbable (chromic cat gut) suture. A second row of sutures is created to secure the seromuscular layers of the colon to the subcutaneous fat. At this point, the colon is opened transversely. The decompression that ensues allows the colon to rise to skin level within the wound. The colon edge is then secured to the skin with interrupted 3–0 absorbable sutures.

25.12.6 Total Proctocolectomy and End Ileostomy

Total proctocolectomy and Brooke's ileostomy was the gold standard for UC surgery prior to the refinement of pouch reconstruction in 1978.[397] The procedure provides outstanding disease control and eliminates any future chance of colorectal cancer. It is also less technically demanding than reconstructive procedures and is routinely performed in a single stage in the nonemergent setting. Reluctance on the patient's behalf to undergo this procedure as opposed to restorative proctocolectomy is because of the presence of a permanent abdominal stoma. While some individual quality-of-life studies report that ileostomates have a life quality similar to an age-matched cohort of the general population, almost 25% of these patients are restricted in their social and recreational activities, and 15% would consider conversion to pouch reconstruction.[398] Additionally, the idea of an uncontrollable fecal stream necessitating the continuous wear of a containment device is unappealing to many.

Procedure

Any combination of open laparoscopic, hand-assisted open, or robotic platforms may be utilized for this operation. The abdominal colectomy portion of the procedure is undertaken in the manner as was previously described (subtotal colectomy with end ileostomy). With the entire colon mobilized, the right colic (if present), middle colic, and inferior mesenteric vascular pedicles should be ligated. The ileocolic pedicle should remain undisturbed for the time being. Ligation of the vascular pedicles at their roots ("high ligation") need not be performed in the absence of dysplasia or cancer. Care must be taken when ligating and dividing the inferior mesenteric vessels, as the sympathetic nerve complex controlling ejaculation in males and bladder emptying in females resides at the root of the inferior mesenteric artery. This is also the point at which ureteral injuries may occur if the ureter has not been identified and protected. The terminal ileum is then divided and the entire mobilized specimen brought out of the incision (if open).

The small bowel and omentum are then packed into the upper abdomen and the table is placed in slight reversed Trendelenburg to gain exposure to the pelvis. Attention is turned to the pelvic dissection. The high anterior rectum is grasped and elevated anteriorly to place the mesorectum on stretch. The avascular presacral plane is identified at the sacral promontory and the peritoneum is scored. This incision is carried inferiorly along the right rectum. The presacral plane is then developed, ensuring that the pelvic hypogastric nerves and the ureters are not injured in the process. The left and right lateral rectal attachments are divided while holding countertraction. If present, the middle rectal artery will be encountered during this portion of the dissection and should be ligated and divided.

The anterior rectal dissection differs somewhat between male and female patients. In males, the rectovesical fold is exposed with anterior displacement of the bladder and posterior displacement of the rectum. The left and right peritoneal incisions are then connected through the fold. This maneuver helps avoid injury to the prostatic plexus and nervi erigentes by remaining posterior to Denonvillier's fascia. In females, the uterus is retracted anteriorly and the uterosacral ligaments arching around the rectum are identified. The rectouterine peritoneal fold is then grasped between these ligaments and incised. The areolar plane is entered and the vagina is dissected away from the rectum. The dissection is complete when the anorectal ring is reached.

The perineal portion of the procedure is then undertaken. An intersphincteric dissection plane is preferred for IBD in the absence of rectal malignancy (the entire sphincter complex must be removed in the case of rectal cancer). Leaving the external sphincter muscle in place allows for a healthy, well-vascularized perineal closure. To start, a circumferential incision is made just outside the anal verge and the intersphincteric plane is entered. The intersphincteric plane is then developed circumferentially to the level of the anorectal ring, where the previous dissection plane should be encountered after incising the muscularis propria posteriorly. The muscularis propria is then divided circumferentially at the level of the anorectal ring. The entire specimen is then delivered through the perineal incision.

If rectal cancer is present, an intersphincteric perineal incision is inappropriate. In this case, the perineal skin is incised circumferentially 2 cm outside the anal verge. The incision is then deepened into the ischiorectal fat to the level of the levator muscles. The muscularis propria is then incised in the posterior midline, allowing entry into the pelvic cavity. To ensure an appropriate incision point, it is important to palpate the coccyx and anococcygeal ligament. Once the incision is made, an index finger is inserted and the levators are finger-hooked and divided with cautery. The specimen is then brought out through the perineal incision. In the absence of rectal cancer, it is preferable to proceed with an intersphincteric perineal dissection, as it minimizes the risk of perineal wound complications.[399] An omental pedicle flap may also be placed into the pelvis as a buttress. This technique has been found to protect against wound complications.[400]

The pelvis should then be thoroughly irrigated. No closed-suction drain is necessary, although many surgeons will elect to leave a pelvic drain as part of their practice. Attention is then turned to creation of the end ileostomy. Ideally, the patient was evaluated and marked for stoma placement by an enterostomal therapist preoperatively. A 2-cm circular piece of skin is excised at the marked site. This is carried down to the level of the anterior fascia. The fascia is incised and the rectus muscle is split, allowing access to the posterior fascia, which is also incised. The aperture should be large enough to accommodate two fingers. An atraumatic grasper is then inserted through the aperture and the staple line of the terminal ileum is grasped. The terminal ileum is then pulled through the abdominal wall, ensuring that the ileum is sufficiently mobilized from the mesentery to allow 5 to 6 cm of protrusion. The staple line is then excised and the stoma is matured. A budding, everted ileostomy is ideal, and is best achieved with the use of "three-bite" sutures. This technique involves a full-thickness "bite" of the cut edge of the bowel, a seromuscular bite of the bowel approximately two finger breadths below the cut edge, and a dermal bite of the skin. Care must be taken not to include the epidermis, as mucosal cells can be implanted and cause issues with appliance fit. When placed in the four cardinal directions around the stoma, these sutures evert the mucosa, thereby creating a spout that allows appropriate positioning of the stoma appliance and protection of the serosa against infection.

Outcomes

In addition to any psychosocial disadvantages to proctocolectomy and end ileostomy, there exist several drawbacks to the ileostomy itself. Stomal complications will almost invariably arise, with rates as high as 76% at 20 years for UC-associated ileostomies. Skin problems are the most common individual complication, occurring in 34% of patients. Twenty-eight percent of UC ileostomies will necessitate revision over time, generally for stomal retraction (occurring in 17%) or parastomal herniation (occurring in 16%).[401] The frequency with which these complications arise is the primary argument for IPAA in a patient who is not abjectly opposed to ileostomy on psychosocial grounds. In such a patient, the risk of stoma complications must be carefully weighed against the risk of IPAA complications in the context of that patient's lifestyle. Ultimately, over 90% of ileostomates are happy with their lifestyle and recognize it as a part of their salvation from chronic illness.

Other complications of this operation are not unique to proctocolectomy and Brooke's ileostomy, but are simply consistent with major abdominal surgery, pelvic dissection, and closure of a perineal wound. The overall morbidity rate is 20% in the non-emergent setting, with the primary risks being hemorrhage, contamination, sepsis, small bowel obstruction, and neural injury. Bladder and sexual dysfunctions are more commonly seen in women and are associated with parasympathetic nerve injury and perineal scarring. Impotence is reported to occur in up to 5% of males, while almost 30% of females describe dyspareunia after proctectomy.[365,402]

Perineal wound complications may occur in up to 25% of these patients,[403,404] which is one of the main reasons to stage the proctocolectomy in patients who present acutely or after prolonged steroid courses. Intersphincteric perineal dissection with closure of the dead space has been shown to decrease the rate of perineal wound complications, and is the preferred approach in the absence of rectal cancer.[399] The buttressing of the perineal repair with an omental pedicle flap has also been found to improve wound healing.[400] Wound breakdown is generally managed with local wound care, although the most severe cases may require flap reconstruction, often with gracilis muscle.[405,406]

25.12.7 Kock Continent Ileostomy

The Kock continent ileostomy was developed as a way to mitigate some of the adverse aspects of an end ileostomy, namely, persistent drainage of the gastrointestinal tract and constant need for a fecal containment system. It is rarely performed in the modern era given the technical complexity in combination with the relatively high complication rate. Nevertheless, the procedure may have a role in select patients who have difficulties with the wear of an appliance. It may also be utilized for those who have either failed a Brooke ileostomy or who cannot undergo IPAA due to perianal disease, low rectal cancer, or poor sphincter function. CD is an absolute contraindication to continent ileostomy, as recurrence in the pouch necessitating excision results in the loss of at least 45 cm of terminal ileum. Relative contraindications include obesity and age over 40 years, as they are associated with an increased risk of pouch dysfunction.[407,408] A thorough workup and frank discussion with the patient must therefore be undertaken before deciding to proceed with a Kock pouch.

Procedure

A continent ileostomy may be undertaken as part of the index total proctocolectomy or as a revision of a previously placed end ileostomy. In either case, it is essential that the entirety of the small bowel be inspected for evidence of CD prior to proceeding. In the classic description by Kock, two 15-cm limbs are secured together to form an isoperistaltic pouch. The adjacent limbs should be created such that an additional 15 cm of terminal ileum remain as an efferent limb. The antimesenteric border of the adjacent limbs is then incised and the edges of the back wall of the pouch are further secured with continuous absorbable suture. A valve is then created from the efferent 15 cm of terminal ileum. To create the valve, the proximal portion of the efferent limb is scarified and 5 cm of corresponding mesentery is divided. The efferent limb is then intussuscepted into the pouch where it is secured in place with a noncutting staple load or absorbable suture. The intussuscipiens is further secured to the sidewall of the pouch with an additional noncutting staple load or absorbable suture. It is important to tailor the length of the intussuscipiens and the efferent limb such that the entirety of the pouch will sit posterior to the fascia while allowing adequate length to secure the efferent limb to the skin without tension or redundancy. The efferent limb is then brought through the abdominal wall in the preoperatively defined stoma location and is sutured flush to the skin. The pouch is then firmly anchored to the posterior rectus sheath using absorbable suture. The ileostomy is then cannulated by a wide plastic tube with large fenestrations to facilitate gravity drainage. The tube is left in place for the first 10 postoperative days, at which point the tube is occluded for progressively longer periods. The catheter may be removed when it can be occluded for 8 hours without patient discomfort. The patient may then self-catheterize three times a day at his or her convenience. It is not uncommon for the process of expanding and "functionalizing" the pouch to take 6 weeks.

Outcomes

Postoperative complications are not uncommon after continent ileostomy, which is in large part why they are not routinely performed. One survey study looking at long-term outcomes reported a 36% pouch excision rate at a mean of 15 years. Reasons for excision were nipple valve slippage (42%), fistulas (26%), refractory pouchitis (23%), and CD (6%).[409] Valve slippage tends to occur due to telescopic movement of the intussuscipiens, which can be improved by a mesh wrap. Unfortunately, this modification results in unacceptably high rates of fistula formation, and a reliable alternative has not been described. Lepistö et al[410] identified slightly improved long-term success rates (71% at 29 years); however, it was noted on Kaplan–Meier analysis to be far inferior to IPAA. Furthermore, 59% of patients in the study required a re-reconstruction and 98% of patients required a surgical intervention on the pouch within 29 years. Nevertheless, it remains an option for select patients managed in centers with adequate experience.

25.12.8 Total Abdominal Colectomy and Ileorectal Anastomosis

Removal of the diseased colon with ileoproctostomy has been used in various forms since 1943.[411] The benefits of this procedure include preservation of gastrointestinal continuity in addition to avoidance of pelvic dissection, thereby mitigating the risk of impotence, bladder dysfunction, and infertility. Of equal importance is the fact that it leaves other options available should the primary surgery fail. While controversial, it remains an option in UC for select patients with a pliable, distensible rectum and no perianal disease. In the modern era, it is primarily reserved for patients with indeterminate colitis or high-risk patients who are not good candidates for IPAA. It also warrants consideration in teenagers for whom an expeditious return to school is desirable and young women who would like to preserve fertility, but not at the cost of an ileostomy.[412] Clearly, these discussions must be taken on a case-by-case basis, and must include extensive counseling as to the risks and benefits of leaving rectal disease behind. Functional results depend on the level of the anastomosis, the state of the rectum, and the natural history of the individual patient's UC phenotype (which cannot be accurately predicted). Contraindications to ileorectal

anastomosis include a severely diseased and nondistensible rectum, rectal dysplasia or cancer, perianal disease, or a poorly functioning anal sphincter complex.[408]

Procedure

The steps of total abdominal colectomy have previously been reviewed, especially including preservation of the ileocolic and inferior mesenteric vascular pedicles. The tenets are unchanged in cases where an ileorectal anastomosis is to be performed, with the caveat that the patient should be positioned in lithotomy position.

Once the specimen has been removed, gastrointestinal continuity is restored via either an end-to-end or side-to-end ileorectal anastomosis. As with any anastomosis, the ileorectal connection must have healthy proximal and distal conduit, good blood supply, and be tension free and technically perfect. The decision to hand sew or use staples is left to the surgeon's discretion, although most prefer a circular stapled anastomosis using a double-stapling technique.

The staple line of the terminal ileum is removed sharply. The significant size discrepancy between the terminal ileum and the rectum is mitigated by using a 28-, 29-, 31-, or 33-mm stapler, the anvil of which is inserted into the opened end of the ileum and secured with a purse-string suture (the authors use 2–0 Prolene). Fat and blood vessels are cleared from the anvil post so that a flush circular staple line is achieved. An assistant then inserts the stapler into the anus. Under direct visualization, and with constant communication between surgeon and assistant, the stapler spike is exposed and placed through the rectum near the midportion of the rectal staple line. The anvil is then brought onto the spike while ensuring that the small bowel mesentery is not twisted, that no bowel is trapped under the internal hernia defect, and that the vagina is reflected anteriorly and inferiorly out of the staple line. The stapler is then fired, completing the anastomosis. The donuts are inspected for integrity and an air leak test is performed. If a leak is noted, it should be directly repaired or the anastomosis redone. Well vascularized distal sigmoid colon has been left in situ with the rectum. Another potential problem is that the stapler may fracture rather than seal the rectum or sigmoid. Should this problem occur, a more distal transection is employed. Should the situation recur, ultimately suture of the stump with pelvic and transrectal drainage may be required. A proximal diversion may be created if there is any question about the quality of, or the patient's ability to heal, the anastomosis.

Outcomes

In appropriately selected patients, outcomes from total abdominal colectomy and ileorectal anastomosis for UC are generally favorable. Morbidity rates range from 8 to 28% with anastomotic leak rates of 2 to 9%, and 0 to 4% mortality rates. Sexual and bladder functions are preserved, and anastomotic leaks are a fairly rare occurrence, with rates of 2 to 9%.[409] Most patients have four to five bowel movements per day and one at night, although the reported ranges are quite variable. Fecal incontinence is rare. The most recent data regarding long-term (20-year) outcomes of ileorectal anastomosis for UC come from a study by da Luz Moreira et al[413] in 2010. This study reported an average of six bowel movements a day, with nighttime seepage in 5%, and urgency in 68%. These data conflict somewhat with a previous 20-year follow-up study by Leijonmarck et al, who reported an average of four bowel movements a day, none at night, and 100% fecal continence.[414] Pastore et al[415] identified a median of six daily and one nocturnal bowel movement, with 53% of patients requiring routine antidiarrheal medication and 31% requiring either systemic or topical steroids.

The major concerns with this procedure revolve around the leaving of diseased rectum in situ. While patients with minimal rectal inflammation at the time of surgery tend to have an excellent prognosis, the rectum may go on to be the source of intractable or recurrent inflammation in 8 to 45% of patients.[416] This manifests as severe diarrhea, bleeding, tenesmus, urgency, and incontinence. One in four subsequently require proctectomy with either an end ileostomy or IPAA, although extended follow-up to 20 years suggests the rectal excision rate may be as high as 53%.[413,416] da Luz Moreira[413] found cumulative probabilities of having a functional ileoproctostomy at 5, 10, 15, and 20 years of 81, 74, 56, and 46%, respectively. Aside from a lack of rectal inflammation preoperatively, no studies have identified specific risk factors for ileoproctostomy failure. Turnbull, however, was of the opinion that an anastomosis 6 cm or less above the peritoneal reflection improved inflammation in the first perioperative months and ultimately reduced the incidence of ileoproctostomy failure.[417] Regardless, the potential for intractable inflammation and possible need for future proctectomy must be explained to any patient considering an ileorectal anastomosis in this setting.

The other major concern in these patients is the cancer risk in the retained rectum. The 20-year follow-up study by da Luz Moreira[413] in 2010 found dysplasia rates of 7, 9, 20, and 25% at 5, 10, 15, and 20 years, respectively. When followed over time, 42% of patients with rectal dysplasia after ileorectal anastomosis will progress to adenocarcinoma within 9 years.[418] Overall rectal cancer rates after ileorectal anastomosis for UC range from 0 to 18% depending on the series, with the majority of these cancers appearing after 15 to 20 years.[416] The da Luz Moreira[413] study identified rectal cancer rates of 0, 2, 5, and 14% at 5, 10, 15, and 20 years, respectively.

Of particular concern is the relative frequency of advanced stage (*t*umor size, *n*ode involvement, and *m*etastasis status [TNM] stages III–IV) rectal cancers among patients who undergo ileoproctostomy for UC. Baker et al identified a 62% 3-year mortality after a rectal cancer diagnosis in this population.[419] A subsequent study by Johnson et al reported nodal or distant metastatic disease in 8 out of 10 rectal cancers identified after ileoproctostomy for UC.[418] Whether this is due to more aggressive tumor biology or inadequate endoscopic surveillance is unknown. Regardless, it is imperative that patients be placed into standard UC surveillance programs (once or twice yearly flexible proctoscopy with multiple biopsies). This necessity should be discussed with the patient preoperatively, particularly young patients who will need lifelong surveillance. The presence of dysplasia or local malignancy in the retained rectum should be managed as any other rectal cancer, with the definitive procedure being oncologic resection. Ileal pouch reconstruction may be considered if the tumor is high, small, node negative, and adjuvant chemotherapy is not predicted.

25.12.9 Total Proctocolectomy and Ileal Pouch Anal Anastomosis

The earliest ileoanal anastomosis was described by Vignolo in 1912 when he used the distal ileum as an interposition graft between the sigmoid colon and anus to avoid mandatory colostomy after proctectomy.[420] This maneuver, when coupled with his previous description of mucosal proctectomy, set the stage for the anal ileostomy refined by Ravitch and Sabiston in 1947.[421] The pioneering efforts of Champeau in 1950 and Goligher in 1951 subsequently identified the potential benefits of the ileal J pouch and the temporary loop ileostomy, respectively.[422,423] These concepts mark the foundations of the modern-day restorative proctocolectomy described by Parks in 1978, which has become the gold-standard surgical procedure for UC.[397]

The allure of a well-functioning IPAA seems obvious in that it avoids a permanent abdominal stoma without compromising quality of life. Nevertheless, the decision between proctocolectomy with Brooke ileostomy and IPAA must not be taken lightly, as complications associated with IPAA can be substantial. At a minimum, the decision to proceed with IPAA subjects the patient to a longer recovery with greater uncertainty. Therefore, IPAA should not be a foregone conclusion in all candidate patients, as some will elect a permanent ileostomy when appropriately counseled.

All UC patients with preserved anal sphincter function, no evidence of small bowel or perineal CD, and without the need for pelvic radiation are technically candidates for restorative proctocolectomy. Relative contraindications include advanced age, desired future pregnancy, a history of perianal suppurative disease, obesity, and the presence of isolated CD. Each of these findings warrants some concern and should prompt careful consideration prior to proceeding with pouch reconstruction.

Procedure

The conduct of the proctocolectomy portion of restorative proctocolectomy has previously been discussed, although in contrast to the patient receiving a planned end ileostomy, the IPAA patient must be positioned in lithotomy to enable access to the perineum. Additionally, the mesentery of the right colon must be taken close to the bowel wall in order to preserve the ileocolic vascular pedicle, which supplies the future pouch. Another caveat is that rectal dissection to the pelvic floor may conclude in one of two ways depending on surgeon preference. For the double-circular stapled technique, the dissection is carried to the top of the anal canal at which point the rectum is divided. However, if a mucosectomy and hand-sewn ileoanal anastomosis are to be carried out, the distal rectum may be clamped and sharply divided to permit perineal mucosectomy to about 4 cm proximal to the dentate line, thereby allowing for a protective muscular cuff around the high-risk pouch anastomosis.

Mucosal stripping begins after rectal division by positioning the patient in the high lithotomy position. A Lone Star (Lone Star Medical Products, Stafford, TX) retractor is positioned such that the dentate line is clearly exposed. A dilute epinephrine solution (1:200,000) is injected circumferentially in the submucosal plane from the dentate line to the levators. A 360-degree incision is then made in the mucosa at the level of the dentate line. Sharp dissection is then used to circumferentially develop a plane between the mucosa and the internal sphincter to a level approximately 4 cm proximal to the dentate line. The excised mucosa and remaining proximal rectum are then removed, leaving a distal muscular cuff of rectum.

The terminal ileum is then exteriorized either through the midline or Pfannenstiel incision (depending on whether the proctocolectomy was performed open or with laparoscopic assistance) and the pouch is constructed. The most commonly used pouch configuration is the J pouch, which will be described here. The terminal ileum is aligned in a J configuration with each limb approximately 15 to 25 cm in length and the mesentery oriented posteriorly. The pouch must then be assessed for tension by pulling it inferiorly. The proposed apex of the pouch must reach 4 to 5 cm below the superior border of the symphysis pubis in order to reach the anal canal without undue tension. If additional length is needed, a series of procedures may be undertaken. First, complete mobilization of the mesentery to the level of the duodenum should be carried out. The anterior peritoneum can then be scored every 1 to 2 cm over the course of the primary vessel supplying the pouch. This maneuver will allow for another 1 to 2 cm of length. A limited Kocher maneuver may also be performed. If the length is still not adequate, then division of small vessels between major restrictive blood vessels may be undertaken to create mesenteric windows. Finally, if tension is still present, division of a restraining vessel is necessary. To avoid pouch ischemia, a bulldog clamp is placed across the proposed vessel to be divided. The end of the ileum should then be inspected for any evidence of ischemia, and if present this vessel should not be divided. These steps may then be repeated on another restricting vessel. Once adequate length is achieved, stay sutures are used to secure the afferent and efferent limbs in this position in the "J" configuration with the mesentery oriented posteriorly. An enterotomy is then made at the antimesenteric apex of the pouch. The common wall of the two limbs is then divided using two consecutive firings of a 100-mm linear stapler. The pouch is then pulled into the pelvis through the muscular cuff and the anastomosis between the pouch apex and the dentate line is carried out. Four anchoring sutures incorporating the full thickness of the pouch and a generous amount of internal sphincter are then placed in at right angles to secure the pouch in position. The anastomosis is then completed by placing additional sutures between each anchoring stitch.

If a double circular stapled anastomosis is to be undertaken, the rectum is divided approximately 2 cm proximal to the dentate line using a right-angled linear stapler. The pouch is then created as previously described, and the anvil of a mid-sized circular stapler is placed through the apical enterotomy and secured. An air-leak test is then performed on the rectal stump. Any leaks should be immediately oversewn. The stapler is then passed through the anus and the spike is advanced near the midpoint of the staple line. Ensuring there is no twisting of the pouch mesentery, the pouch is brought into the pelvis and the anvil is secured on the spike. The stapler is then closed and fired, completing the anastomosis. Whether or not to provide a proximal diversion is up to surgeon discretion. When elected, a standard loop ileostomy in the most tension-free loop of ileum is preferred.

Falk et al[424] in 1993 and Schmitt et al[425] in 1994 described the first laparoscopic pouch operations. Since that time, laparoscopic pouch surgery has become the preferred approach and is now successfully achieved in the majority of patients undergoing pouch surgery.[426,427] A variety of laparoscopic approaches have been described including standard laparoscopy, single-port laparoscopy, hand-assisted surgery, and robotic pouch surgery. Pouch construction has been described through the umbilicus, through the anus, and even transanally. Laparoscopic pouch procedures have also been combined with transanal surgery as a dual-access minimal access platform procedure.

Technical Points

Type of Anastomosis

One technical factor that has been shown to impact both complication rates and functional outcomes is the type of ileoanal anastomosis. Kirat et al directly compared outcomes between hand-sewn and stapled IPAA in over 3,100 patients who received an IPAA. The groups were similar in terms of demographics and nutrition. The study found that double circular stapled anastomoses were associated with significantly decreased rates of septic complications (17 vs. 21%), anastomotic stricture (16 vs. 22%), and pouch failure (4 vs. 11%) when compared to hand-sewn anastomoses. Functional outcomes were similarly improved when a stapled anastomosis was performed. Specifically, fecal incontinence (2 vs. 6%), daytime seepage (20 vs. 35%), nighttime seepage (35 vs. 61%), dietary restrictions (27 vs. 34%), social restrictions (14 vs. 20%), quality-of-life score (8.2 vs. 8.0), and quality-of-health score (8.1 vs. 7.9) all favored a stapled anastomosis over hand-sewn anastomoses ($p < 0.02$).[428] Despite the apparent superiority of the stapled anastomosis, the ability to perform a hand-sewn ileoanal anastomosis is a critical tool, as an intraoperative problem with a stapled anastomosis cannot be remedied with a second stapler fire.

Pouch Configuration

A number of pouches have been proposed since Parks' original description of the triple-loop S pouch.[397] These include the double-loop J pouch, quadruple-loop W pouch, and the lateral isoperistaltic H pouch.[429,430,431] As with most procedures that have multiple variations, no one pouch is perfect. General issues that have plagued pouches are evacuation problems, pouch distention resulting in stasis and pouchitis, and obstructive defecation. Early S pouches were especially problematic, as the 5-cm outlet tract caused evacuation problems requiring pouch catheterization.[397] For obvious reasons, this construction led to high rates of stasis and pouchitis. H pouches had similar difficulties due to the long efferent tract.[432] The W pouch offers the largest capacity and a short outlet, both of which allow for good functionality.[430] Two randomized controlled studies comparing W and J pouch outcomes at 1 year found conflicting results. Johnston et al[433] identified equivalent stooling frequency, nocturnal stooling, seepage, and fecal incontinence rates, while Selvaggi et al[434] found significantly improved frequency of defecation and nighttime defecation in W pouch patients when compared to J pouch patients (three vs. five bowel movements in 24 hours and 17 vs. 50% nocturnal defecation, respectively). Despite the initial troubles with S pouches, refinement of the technique with a shortening of the exit conduit to 2 cm provided improved functionality.[408] Furthermore, the S pouch provides an additional 2 to 4 cm of length, so it is a reasonable option for patients in whom length is an issue. A recent study comparing outcomes of hand-sewn J pouches to S pouches (which must be hand sewn given their construction) found lower rates of pouch fistulas, pelvic sepsis, and pouch-related hospitalizations among S pouch patients. At 12-month follow-up S pouch patients had fewer bowel movements ($p < 0.001$), less frequent pad use ($p = 0.001$), and a lower fecal incontinence severity index score ($p = 0.015$).[435]

Diversion

The debate regarding proximal diversion of the fecal stream after pouch surgery is centered around fear of pelvic sepsis and the resulting pouch dysfunction. The data are mixed regarding the overall impact of fecal diversion on IPAA outcomes. Meta-analysis by Westin–Petrides in 2008 identified a significant correlation between no-diversion and anastomotic leak (OR, 2.37; $p = 0.002$). Such data suggest a protective role for proximal diversion, and consensus recommendations call for a protective ileostomy in the majority of cases.[102] Nevertheless, large series and recent meta-analyses exist in which similar leak rates are identified regardless of the presence of a protective stoma, suggesting there is a population of patients in whom diversion may be safely deferred.[436,437] The largest such study suggested that ileostomy may be avoided without increased morbidity in patients who receive a technically sound, tension-free, stapled anastomosis in the absence of malnutrition, toxicity, anemia, or prolonged steroid use.[437] This scenario is rare, as the majority of UC patients who come to surgery do so only after failure of prolonged medical management or when systemically ill.

Outcomes

While IPAA is a relatively safe procedure in terms of mortality (0.1%), the potential for early and late morbidity is quite high (34 and 29%, respectively).[438] Meta-analysis of all relevant case series since 2000 found that outright pouch failure is rarely seen (4.7%), although the additive rates of anastomotic stricture (16.5%), pelvic sepsis (7.5%), pouch fistula (4.5%), and sexual dysfunction (3.0%) suggest the potential for a considerable impact both acutely and in the long term.[416] Furthermore, greater than 25% of patients will develop nonspecific inflammation of the ileal pouch (pouchitis), which may necessitate resumption of steroid enemas, mesalamine, or even pouch excision in severe, refractory cases.[438,439,440,441,442,443]

Functional outcomes have not changed substantially over the last several decades,[416] and depend almost exclusively on patient selection, technical precision, proper healing of the pelvic pouch, and type of pouch and anastomosis. The average frequency of bowel movements is 6 per day, with one to two overnight stools. Mild and severe fecal incontinences occur in 14 and 6% of patients, respectively.[436] Despite these difficulties, most patients are highly satisfied with their pouch function after the year-long initial adjustment. Quality of life and social functioning, it would appear from the literature, are comparable to a healthy, age-matched cohort.[444,445] These reassuring long-term results are predicated on appropriate patient selection, technically and fundamentally sound surgery, and the establishment of realistic expectations by the surgeon before any procedure is undertaken.

Specific Complications

Pelvic Sepsis

Pelvic abscess is one of the most feared complications after IPAA, as the largest series to date found a significant association

between pelvic sepsis and pouch failure (hazard ratio [HR], 3.3; 95% CI, 2.2–4.8; $p < 0.001$).[438] Sepsis is generally due to anastomotic dehiscence or infected pelvic hematoma. Early leaks occur in approximately 5% of patients and account for the majority of cases, although late leaks (seen in 2% of patients) may contribute as well.[438] Rates of pelvic sepsis after IPAA have improved since 2000, with meta-analyses suggesting a 21% decrease in the new millennium (6.3 from 9.5%).[416,438] The reasons for the decreased rates in recent years are not clear, although increased familiarity and experience combined with more frequent use of the stapled anastomosis undoubtedly contribute. Acute manifestations include fevers, tenesmus, frequency, or bleeding and purulence from the pouch. Subacute or smoldering abscesses may present later as a perineal fistula. Regardless of the timing of symptoms, CT or MRI should be obtained for diagnosis. IV broad-spectrum antibiotics should be started and fluid collections should be drained. Percutaneous drainage is preferred, although endoanal drainage is a good option, particularly if percutaneous access does not adequately clear the septic source. If the endoanal approach is utilized, it is important to establish wide drainage into the pouch and curette the cavity. Open drainage via laparotomy may be entertained, although this should be considered a last resort after multiple attempts at local control. If a subclinical leak is detected on endoscopy or imaging before ileostomy reversal, local procedures should be undertaken, with direct repair of any leaks and endoanal drainage of any fluid collection. The loop ileostomy should remain in place until complete healing is documented.

Anastomotic Stricture

Stricture is a fairly common complication after IPAA. The literature reports rates ranging from 5 to 38%, depending on follow-up, technique, and series size.[438,440,441,442,443] Some variability may be accounted for by differential definitions of stricture, with some defining it as any narrowing requiring dilations and others defining it as a narrowing causing mechanical outlet obstruction. Fazio et al studied the outcomes of over 3,700 pouches, and using the former definition found a 5% chance of early stricture, which increased to 11% in long-term follow-up.[438] The underlying etiology for stricture formation is believed to be anastomotic tension predisposing to leakage and infection. Poor blood supply is likely another contributing factor, particularly in cases where mesenteric vessels need to be taken to obtain adequate length on the pouch. Most commonly the stricture is weblike, fracturing easily with gentle finger dilation. Nevertheless, fibrotic strictures can occur and often require multiple dilations in the operating room. Fifty percent of these patients will retain adequate pouch function, although some may require transanal anastomotic resection with pouch advancement.[440,443,446,447]

Fistulas

Fistulas occur in 1 to 16% of pouches, and are attributed to pelvic sepsis and anastomotic leak.[438,447,448,449,450,451] They may also indicate CD as the underlying disease; however, Fazio et al found low rates of fistula formation in both UC and CD patients undergoing IPAA (1.3%). Pouch-vaginal fistulas are particularly problematic as they are quite distressing to patients, may be difficult to resolve, and are associated with pouch failure (HR,

4.5; 95% CI, 3.1–6.6; p < 0.001).[438] They occur in 3 to 16% of women who undergo an IPAA, and as with other pouch fistulas are associated with pelvic sepsis.[448,449,450,451] Iatrogenic vaginal injury during low rectal dissection and/or ileoanal anastomosis is another causative factor, although it is unknown how often this occurs. The management of perineal or vaginal fistulas depends on the degree and severity of fistulization and symptoms. There is no role for medical management unless it is determined that CD is the etiology. In such cases, infliximab may be beneficial.[452] Certainly source control must be obtained in cases where a drainable fluid collection is identified. Observation or seton drainage may be all that is needed in patients with minimally symptomatic fistulas.[450] Fecal diversion may be undertaken and is a reasonable option, particularly in those who suffer from incontinence. This alone will not promote fistula healing; however, the diversion should improve the outcome of definitive repair in these patients. An abdominal or perineal approach may be taken for repair, depending on the height of the anastomosis. A pouch-vaginal fistula from a high (above the anorectal ring) anastomosis generally should be approached through the abdomen, with pouch mobilization, repair of the vaginal wall, and creation of a new anastomosis.[408] An omental buttress should be placed in the cul de sac if possible. This approach results in fistula healing rates of approximately 80%.[446,453,454,455] A low anastomosis is amenable to a perineal approach. A pouch-vaginal fistula in the anal canal may be addressed via an endoanal ileal advancement flap[448,451,456,457] transvaginal repair, or a gracilis interposition.[458] In contrast to rectovaginal fistulas, neither side of an anovaginal fistula is in a high-pressure zone, which likely explains the equivalent results in limited series. In fact, many would argue that the transvaginal approach is preferable, as the risk of sphincter damage is mitigated.[408] Gracilis muscle interposition flaps have also been used in especially high-risk repairs.[451]

Pouchitis

Pouchitis is the most common complication after IPAA, and may be divided into acute (< 4 weeks in duration) and chronic (> 4 weeks in duration) disease states. Thirty-nine percent of UC patients with an IPAA develop at least one episode in 25 years, while 17% suffer from chronic inflammation of the pouch.[438] Fifty percent of patients who resolve an episode of pouchitis will eventually recur.[459,460,461] Patients present with abdominal cramping, fevers, pelvic pain, and increased stool frequency.[408,461,462] Extraintestinal manifestations may also develop secondary to pouch inflammation.[378] These symptoms are nonspecific, and may represent alternative diagnoses such as CD of the pouch, cuffitis, or an irritable pouch.[463,464,465,466] Adverse sequelae from pouchitis include abscesses, fistulas, pouch anal stenosis, and pouch failure.[438,460]

Given the broad differential, diagnosis of pouchitis must be confirmed by pouchoscopy. Endoscopic findings consistent with true pouchitis include diffuse, patchy erythema, edema, granularity, and friability. Staple line erosions do not necessarily indicate pouchitis. Interestingly, pouches undergo colonic metaplasia, which tends to correlate with the time of pouchitis onset and may explain why patients who develop pouchitis generally do so in the first 3 years. Histology is otherwise relatively ineffective for diagnosing pouchitis, as nonspecific mucosal inflammation is generally all that is seen.

While many believe the inflammation is due to bacterial overgrowth, the etiology is not entirely understood. As with other inflammatory bowel conditions, it likely represents a common manifestation of different multifactorial etiologies. This could explain the discordant responses to therapy between acute and chronic pouchitis, with acute pouchitis generally responding quickly to antibiotics, while chronic pouchitis requires long-term antibiotics, anti-inflammatories, and ultimately pouch excision in refractory cases. Active smoking is a risk factor for acute pouchitis, while smoking may have a protective effect against the development of chronic pouchitis. Other risk factors include colorectal dysplasia, the lack of prior use of anxiolytics, and preoperative steroid use. The presence of serologic markers such as pANCA and CBir1 before colectomy is predictive of both acute and chronic pouchitis.

The differential diagnosis for pouchitis includes CD, cuffitis, and irritable pouch, all of which may be mistakenly identified as pouchitis. Crohn's disease (CD) of the pouch occurs in approximately 4% of IPAA patients, and may be unmasked by smoking. Cuffitis is simply inflammation of the narrow cuff of mucosa that is left in place with a stapled anastomosis. These patients often present with bleeding and arthralgias. Irritable pouch syndrome is a diagnosis of exclusion, and is likely under-recognized. It is a functional disorder that manifests as pouchitis, but occurs in the setting of a structurally normal pouch. It is felt to be due to a visceral hypersensitivity analogous to irritable bowel syndrome, and may have an association with anxiolytic use.

Various scoring models for pouchitis have been developed. The pouchitis disease activity index (PDAI) proposed by Sandborn et al is a thorough evaluation of disease severity, and includes symptomatology, endoscopic findings, and histologic examination.[462] Given the necessity for endoscopy and biopsies, it has largely been used in research protocols rather than clinical practice. Nevertheless, a modified version excluding histologic examination has shown promising correlation, and may be used more readily in the clinical setting.[467] Other scores such as the Moskowitz index and an index from Heidelberg may be used as well, although these tests are not directly comparable.

No large, randomized controlled trials regarding the management of pouchitis have been conducted; however, placebo-controlled trials and small, randomized controlled trials have suggested the efficacy of metronidazole and ciprofloxacin as first-line therapy for acute pouchitis. Comparative studies and a Cochrane review found ciprofloxacin to be superior to metronidazole in terms of PDAI, symptom score, and endoscopic score. Budesonide enemas are likely as efficacious as metronidazole.[459,468,469,470,471] Probiotic therapy may be of benefit for maintenance therapy after resolution of an acute flair, which lends credence to the bacterial overgrowth theory.[471,472] For refractory cases, infectious etiologies such as *C. difficile* and CMV should be ruled out. Furthermore, alternative diagnoses such as CD, cuffitis, fistulas, and irritable pouch should be considered. When unresponsive pouchitis is confirmed, combination therapy using ciprofloxacin and flagyl, steroid enemas, and mesalamine may be considered. Each of these second-line treatments showed a benefit in underpowered studies.[473,474,475] Immune modulators and biologic therapies may be utilized as third-line medications. While all studies regarding these alternative medications are lacking in terms of methodology, they have demonstrated the efficacy of cyclosporine enemas, infliximab, and adalimumab in treating intractable pouchitis.[241,476,477,478,479]

Infertility

Rectal excision with pouch reconstruction is associated with a 30 to 70% reduction in female fecundity.[480,481,482,483] The etiology is presumably pelvic adhesions, although this has not been proven. Given the significant risk of infertility, along with the fact that many women with UC are in their child-bearing years, ileorectal anastomosis or even end ileostomy may be preferred to total proctocolectomy with end ileostomy.

25.13 Other Debates

25.13.1 Obesity

Several authors have described the adverse effects of obesity on pouch construction (▶ Table 25.7).[484,485,486] Most recently, the group at the Mayo Clinic have calculated a specific risk as related to increasing BMI.[486] The problems of obesity include difficulty in gaining sufficient length to create a pouch anal anastomosis and secondly in creating a satisfactorily distal proximal loop ileostomy. The ability to laparoscopically complete the procedure as well as the rate of pelvic sepsis and other postoperative complications all increase with increasing body mass index.

If a pouch does not reach the anus, a variety of lengthening maneuvers may be undertaken including scoring the peritoneum, making full-thickness incisions between vessels in the peritoneum and mesentery, or dividing intermediate vessels to gain length. It may be safest to divide these intermediate vessels by transiently applying bulldog clamps while observing the pouch. Indocyanine green fluorescence imaging is a useful adjunct to more objectively assess blood supply after bulldog clamp application. If after satisfactory time has elapsed and pouch viability is evident ideally by indocyanine green imaging, then the vessels may be carefully divided. If a pouch still does not reach, then it should not be constructed, but instead an end ileostomy should be created. Ideally these maneuvers should be undertaken prior to rectal mobilization. It is much more beneficial to perform an end ileostomy and leave the rectum or rectosigmoid as a Hartmann stump rather than leaving only the anus to ideally facilitate a more safe subsequent pelvic dissection and pouch construction without nerve sacrifice. These instances tend to occur in obese patients. After significant weight loss, pouch construction and pouch anal anastomosis may be possible. It is ideal to avoid near total proctocolectomy leaving the anus in place and pouch construction to then discover that a pouch does not reach. Therefore, a trial reach is generally attempted after full mobilization of small bowel to the level of the superior mesenteric artery and vein as well as the head of the pancreas and prior to rectal mobilization and then again after distal transection. Only after adequate reach has been demonstrated is the pouch constructed. Because of the possibility of a pouch not reaching the consent form should always include both subtotal colectomy and permanent ileostomy.

25.13.2 Age

When pouches were first described, surgeons were cautioned against performing these operations in patients older than 50 years. The indications for pouch surgery have broadened and numerous series have clearly documented satisfactory results in patients in their 60s and 70s, and occasionally even older. Success rates for IPAA surgery in patients with indeterminate colitis are somewhere between the success rates for patients with CD and the success rates for patients with UC. The most important decision-making variable is a history of or the contemporaneous presence of perianal sepsis. Patients with perianal sepsis have higher failure rates presumably because of the actual diagnosis of CD. Accordingly, the decision to perform IPAA in a patient with indeterminate colitis is heavily weighted

Table 25.7 Outcomes of ileal pouch anal anastomosis in obese patients

Author and year	Study design	N	Mean BMI (kg/m²)	Outcomes
Efron et al 2001[484]	Case matched	Obese = 31 Nonobese = 31	33.7	• Longer operative time (229 vs. 196 min; $p = 0.02$) • Higher perioperative morbidity (32 vs. 9.6%; $p = 0.058$) • More stomal complications (10 vs. 0%) • More incisional hernias (13 vs. 3%; $p = NS$) • Significantly higher rate of pelvic sepsis (16 vs. 0%; $p < 0.05$) • Similar hospital length of stay (9.7 vs. 7.7 d; $p = 0.13$) • Comparable functional outcome
Canedo et al 2010[485]	Case matched	Obese = 65 Nonobese = 65	34	• Higher incidence of cardiorespiratory comorbidities ($p = 0.044$) • Longer operative time ($p = 0.001$) • Longer hospital stay ($p = 0.009$) • Higher incidence of incisional hernia ($p = 0.01$)
Klos et al 2014[486]	Case matched	Obese = 75 Nonobese = 103	35	• Increased rate of overall complications (80 vs. 64%; $p = 0.03$) • Increased pouch-related complications (61 vs. 26%; $p < 0.01$) • Anastomotic/pouch strictures (27 vs. 6%; $p < 0.01$) • Inflammatory pouch complications (17 vs. 4%; $p < 0.01$) • Pouch fistulas (12 vs. 3%; $p = 0.03$)

Table 25.8 Outcomes of ileal pouch anal anastomosis in elderly patients

Author and year	Patients	Bowel frequency	Continence	Manometry	Morbidity and mortality
Reissman et al 1996[487]	14 (>60) 126 (<60)	Higher>60 (night)	Same	Same	Same
Dayton et al 1996[488]	32 (>55) 423 (<55)	Higher>55	Higher>55	–	Dehydration Higher>55
Tan et al 1997[489]	28 (>50) 43 (<50)	Same	Same	–	Same
Takao et al 1998[490]	17 (>60) 105 (<60)	Same	Same	Same	–
Delaney et al 2003[491]	154 (56–65) 42 (>65)	Higher>65 (night)	Decline with time	–	–
Pinto et al 2011[492]	33 (>65) 126 (<65)	Same	Same	Same	Dehydration Higher>65
Ramage et al 2016[493]	Systematic review: • Safe in older patients • Increased risk of dehydration • Worse postoperative function but seems to level out with time • Does not appear to significantly impact on overall quality of life and patient satisfaction				

by the reason for the diagnosis of indeterminate colitis. In the patient who had a subtotal colectomy for acute toxic colitis, full-thickness disease may be present, but the finding of skip areas and granulomas would certainly tilt the decision away from UC toward CD. Accordingly, each patient must be individually counseled. Furthermore, it is important to remember that the diagnosis of indeterminate colitis can only be made after the colon has been removed. It is not a diagnosis made by either endoscopy or histopathologic review of endoscopic biopsies (▶ Table 25.8).[487,488,489,490,491,492,493]

25.13.3 Reoperative Pouch Surgery

The longer IPAA has been performed and the more patients upon whom it has been performed, the more reoperative IPAA operations have been performed. These reoperations are generally done because of sepsis or poor function. Within the former category are included pouch perineal and pouch anal fistulas as well as a variety of leaks from any of the staple lines. Contingent upon suspicion for CD consideration may be given to either pouch excision or pouch revision. If pouch revision is considered, all patients must understand that the original pouch may not be salvageable and may require excision. If excision is undertaken and length is sufficient, a second pouch may be created, but ultimately a permanent ileostomy may result. Some of the larger series have suggested that roughly two-thirds of patients in whom reoperative pouch surgery is attempted can ultimately maintain a functioning pouch. However, reoperative pouch surgery usually entails a mucosectomy and virtually always includes construction of loop ileostomy unless the reoperative surgery is some type of minor perianal procedure such as placement of a seton. The definitive operations are generally performed as a combination of intra-abdominal and transperineal procedures. There are some exceptions to this statement including patients in whom the efferent limb has fistulized sometimes to the prior ileostomy site. The limb can often be successfully stapled across and shortened. The second reason

for reoperative pouch surgery includes poor function, which might be incontinence or severe chronic pouchitis. In either of these instances, pouch excision with construction of a permanent stoma may be preferable to reconstructing a new J pouch. It may also be feasible to perform these repeat pouch operations whether revisions, reconstructions, or excisions in a laparoscopic manner. Regardless of whether such an operation is undertaken by laparoscopy or through a laparotomy, bilateral ureteric catheters may be helpful to facilitate ureteric identification and, should it occur, identify ureteric injury.

25.14 Postoperative Considerations

25.14.1 Dysplasia and Malignancy

Patients with lower or middle third rectal cancers with threatened circumferential margins should undergo neoadjuvant therapy prior to surgery as postoperative radiation therapy renders a pouch poorly functional or even ischemic. Severe adverse sequelae such as a necrotic pouch are even possible.[494]

IPAA mitigates the risk of rectal cancer, and should be considered almost mandatory when dysplasia is identified in the colon or rectum.[416] Nevertheless, the risk is not eliminated entirely, presumably due to the inevitable retention of mucosal remnants in the anal transition zone. These mucosal remnants have been a point of contention, particularly as they pertain to the argument over perineal proctectomy and hand-sewn ileoanal anastomosis versus a double circular stapled anastomosis. A rim of the anal transition zone is left in place out of necessity with the stapled anastomosis, which may account for the improved functional outcomes with this technique. Opponents of the stapled anastomosis felt that this could represent a cancer risk to the patient in the same way that ileoproctostomy does; however, the literature has not borne this out. Follow-up series of stapled pouch anastomoses have found exceedingly low rates of dysplasia in the anal transition zone after at least 10 years, with rates ranging from 0 to 4%. None of these series identified a cancer; and dysplasia, when it did occur, was found in the first 2 to 3 years after surgery.[495,496,497]

The largest single study to take on this issue not only confirmed that dysplasia is rare in these patients, but also found that the type of anastomosis does not appear to make a difference in terms of the risk. The study looked at 25-year follow-up data from over 3,200 patients who underwent IPAA at the Cleveland Clinic between 1984 and 2009. Twenty-three patients (0.72%) developed dysplasia and 11 (0.36%) developed adenocarcinoma of the pouch or anal transition zone. Rates of overall neoplasia were 0.9, 1.3, 1.9, 4.2, and 5.1% at 5, 10, 15, 20, and 25 years, respectively. Multivariable analysis identified preoperative cancer and dysplasia as the only independent risk factors for postoperative neoplasia. Neither mucosectomy nor stapled anastomosis was associated with the development of neoplasia. In fact, rates of pouch cancer were actually higher in patients who had a mucosectomy compared to those who underwent a stapled anastomosis (1.3 vs. 0.3%).[498]

Another group of IPAA patients who may be at risk for dysplasia are those who suffer from chronic pouchitis. Banasiewicz et al[499] reviewed their series of 276 UC patients treated with an IPAA and found that 24% had chronic pouchitis, 1.8% had low-grade dysplasia, and 1.1% had high-grade dysplasia. Logistic regression identified pouchitis as a predictor of dysplasia (OR, 13.48; $p < 0.02$). Given the increased risk of dysplasia in the setting of chronic pouchitis or preoperative dysplasia, some have called for surveillance endoscopy in these higher risk populations.[499,500,501]

25.14.2 Pregnancy

In the event a pouch patient becomes pregnant, a common concern is the mode of delivery. Standard vaginal delivery can cause pudendal nerve terminal motor latency through stretch, which generally does not result in adverse sequelae with regard to fecal continence. In pouch patients, however, there is an over-reliance on a functioning sphincter mechanism to maintain continence. This is in large part due to the absence of solid stools and abnormal rectal sensation and anorectal inhibition. The fear among surgeons is that pudendal nerve stretch or significant perineal trauma will result in long-standing fecal incontinence; however, this fear is unfounded based on the limited literature. Remzi et al[502] looked at the impact of childbirth on anal sphincter function and integrity after restorative proctocolectomy. The study found that pudendal nerve motor latency was normal after vaginal delivery. Sphincter defects were detected on ultrasound in approximately 50% of pouch patients after vaginal delivery. This was in contrast to the 30% sphincter disruption rate seen in standard vaginal deliveries in the population and the 13% rate identified in pouch patients who underwent caesarian section. These injuries, while distressing to the patient, did not have any clinical impact on the functioning of the pouch. Another, smaller study by Gearhart et al[503] has corroborated the benign nature of these sphincter defects in pouch patients. Despite the apparent safety of vaginal delivery after IPAA, many surgeons continue to recommend caesarian section for pregnant pouch patients, with series suggesting caesarian section rates of 38 to 76%.[504]

25.15 Conclusion

UC is a potentially complex and crippling disease process, challenging for the provider and cruel to the patient. While many patients are successfully managed with minimal medical intervention, a significant number will progress to severe, debilitating, and intractable disease, ultimately necessitating a high-risk surgery. Multidisciplinary discussion and formation of a solid therapeutic alliance are critical parts of the treatment process, particularly in refractory cases. It should be kept in mind that chronic UC patients often have an innate understanding of their own disease process that far outweighs clinical data. The risk of any intervention is not insignificant, and ultimately it is the patient who has to live with the outcome. Individualized medical and surgical care should therefore be the standard. In practice, this principle is not easy to follow, as it necessitates thorough and often lengthy counseling. However, the ability to provide a potentially curative surgery to a patient who has been experiencing the pain and humiliation of UC is a privilege worthy of additional effort.

References

[1] Soranus of Ephesus (c. 117 AD). Quoted by Mettler CC. History of Medicine. Philadelphia, PA: Blakiston; 1947

[2] Wilks S, Moxon W. Lectures on Pathological Anatomy. 2nd ed. London: J&A Churchill; 1875

[3] Bargen J. Experimental studies on etiology of chronic ulcerative colitis. J Am Med Assoc. 1924; 83:332

[4] Meyer K, Gellhorn A, Prudden J. Lysozyme in chronic ulcerative colitis. Proc Soc Exp Biol Med. 1947; 65(2):221

[5] Rosenberg EW, Fischer RW. DNCB allergy in the guinea pig colon. Arch Dermatol. 1964; 89:99–103

[6] Grace W, Wolf S, Wolff H. The Human Colon. New York, NY: Hoeber; 1951

[7] Cornelis W. Quoted by Kraft, Bregman, and Kirsner (1962); 1958

[8] Broberger O, Perlmann P. Autoantibodies in human ulcerative colitis. J Exp Med. 1959; 110:657–674

[9] De Dombal FT, Watts JM, Watkinson G, Goligher JC. Local complications of ulcerative colitis: stricture, pseudopolyposis, and carcinoma of colon and rectum. BMJ. 1966; 1(5501):1442–1447

[10] Molodecky NA, Soon IS, Rabi DM, et al. Increasing incidence and prevalence of the inflammatory bowel diseases with time, based on systematic review. Gastroenterology. 2012; 142(1):46–54.e42, quiz e30

[11] Loftus EV, Jr. Clinical epidemiology of inflammatory bowel disease: Incidence, prevalence, and environmental influences. Gastroenterology. 2004; 126(6):1504–1517

[12] Kappelman MD, Rifas-Shiman SL, Kleinman K, et al. The prevalence and geographic distribution of Crohn's disease and ulcerative colitis in the United States. Clin Gastroenterol Hepatol. 2007; 5(12):1424–1429

[13] Björnsson S, Jóhannsson JH. Inflammatory bowel disease in Iceland, 1990–1994: a prospective, nationwide, epidemiological study. Eur J Gastroenterol Hepatol. 2000; 12(1):31–38

[14] Cosnes J, Carbonnel F, Beaugerie L, Blain A, Reijasse D, Gendre JP. Effects of appendicectomy on the course of ulcerative colitis. Gut. 2002; 51(6):803–807

[15] Loftus EV, Jr, Silverstein MD, Sandborn WJ, Tremaine WJ, Harmsen WS, Zinsmeister AR. Ulcerative colitis in Olmsted County, Minnesota, 1940–1993: incidence, prevalence, and survival. Gut. 2000; 46(3):336–343

[16] Auvin S, Molinié F, Gower-Rousseau C, et al. Incidence, clinical presentation and location at diagnosis of pediatric inflammatory bowel disease: a prospective population-based study in northern France (1988–1999). J Pediatr Gastroenterol Nutr. 2005; 41(1):49–55

[17] Kelsen J, Baldassano RN. Inflammatory bowel disease: the difference between children and adults. Inflamm Bowel Dis. 2008; 14 Suppl 2:S9–S11

[18] Langholz E, Munkholm P, Nielsen OH, Kreiner S, Binder V. Incidence and prevalence of ulcerative colitis in Copenhagen county from 1962 to 1987. Scand J Gastroenterol. 1991; 26(12):1247–1256

[19] Bernstein CN, Wajda A, Svenson LW, et al. The epidemiology of inflammatory bowel disease in Canada: a population-based study. Am J Gastroenterol. 2006; 101(7):1559–1568

[20] Cosnes J, Gower-Rousseau C, Seksik P, Cortot A. Epidemiology and natural history of inflammatory bowel diseases. Gastroenterology. 2011; 140 (6):1785–1794

[21] Sawczenko A, Sandhu BK, Logan RF, et al. Prospective survey of childhood inflammatory bowel disease in the British Isles. Lancet. 2001; 357 (9262):1093–1094

[22] Blanchard JF, Bernstein CN, Wajda A, Rawsthorne P. Small-area variations and sociodemographic correlates for the incidence of Crohn's disease and ulcerative colitis. Am J Epidemiol. 2001; 154(4):328–335

[23] Sonnenberg A, McCarty DJ, Jacobsen SJ. Geographic variation of inflammatory bowel disease within the United States. Gastroenterology. 1991; 100 (1):143–149

[24] Carr I, Mayberry JF. The effects of migration on ulcerative colitis: a three-year prospective study among Europeans and first- and second- generation South Asians in Leicester (1991–1994). Am J Gastroenterol. 1999; 94 (10):2918–2922

[25] Montgomery SM, Morris DL, Pounder RE, Wakefield AJ. Asian ethnic origin and the risk of inflammatory bowel disease. Eur J Gastroenterol Hepatol. 1999; 11(5):543–546

[26] Probert CS, Jayanthi V, Pinder D, Wicks AC, Mayberry JF. Epidemiological study of ulcerative proctocolitis in Indian migrants and the indigenous population of Leicestershire. Gut. 1992; 33(5):687–693

[27] Cho JH. The genetics and immunopathogenesis of inflammatory bowel disease. Nat Rev Immunol. 2008; 8(6):458–466

[28] Cho JH, Brant SR. Recent insights into the genetics of inflammatory bowel disease. Gastroenterology. 2011; 140(6):1704–1712

[29] Sartor RB. Mechanisms of disease: pathogenesis of Crohn's disease and ulcerative colitis. Nat Clin Pract Gastroenterol Hepatol. 2006; 3(7):390–407

[30] Liu JZ, van Sommeren S, Huang H, et al. International Multiple Sclerosis Genetics Consortium, International IBD Genetics Consortium. Association analyses identify 38 susceptibility loci for inflammatory bowel disease and highlight shared genetic risk across populations. Nat Genet. 2015; 47(9):979–986

[31] Loddo I, Romano C. Inflammatory bowel disease: genetics, epigenetics, and pathogenesis. Front Immunol. 2015; 6:551

[32] McGovern DP, Kugathasan S, Cho JH. Genetics of inflammatory bowel diseases. Gastroenterology. 2015; 149(5):1163–1176.e2

[33] Duchmann R, Kaiser I, Hermann E, Mayet W, Ewe K, Meyer zum Büschenfelde KH. Tolerance exists towards resident intestinal flora but is broken in active inflammatory bowel disease (IBD). Clin Exp Immunol. 1995; 102 (3):448–455

[34] Mow WS, Vasiliauskas EA, Lin YC, et al. Association of antibody responses to microbial antigens and complications of small bowel Crohn's disease. Gastroenterology. 2004; 126(2):414–424

[35] Smythies LE, Sellers M, Clements RH, et al. Human intestinal macrophages display profound inflammatory anergy despite avid phagocytic and bacteriocidal activity. J Clin Invest. 2005; 115(1):66–75

[36] Iwasaki A, Medzhitov R. Toll-like receptor control of the adaptive immune responses. Nat Immunol. 2004; 5(10):987–995

[37] Uhlig HH, Schwerd T, Koletzko S, et al. COLORS in IBD Study Group and NEOPICS. The diagnostic approach to monogenic very early onset inflammatory bowel disease. Gastroenterology. 2014; 147(5):990–1007.e3

[38] Glocker EO, Frede N, Perro M, et al. Infant colitis: it's in the genes. Lancet. 2010; 376(9748):1272

[39] Østvik AE, Granlund AV, Torp SH, et al. Expression of Toll-like receptor-3 is enhanced in active inflammatory bowel disease and mediates the excessive release of lipocalin 2. Clin Exp Immunol. 2013; 173(3):502–511

[40] Hisamatsu T, Suzuki M, Reinecker HC, Nadeau WJ, McCormick BA, Podolsky DK. CARD15/NOD2 functions as an antibacterial factor in human intestinal epithelial cells. Gastroenterology. 2003; 124(4):993–1000

[41] Kobayashi KS, Chamaillard M, Ogura Y, et al. Nod2-dependent regulation of innate and adaptive immunity in the intestinal tract. Science. 2005; 307 (5710):731–734

[42] Swidsinski A, Ladhoff A, Pernthaler A, et al. Mucosal flora in inflammatory bowel disease. Gastroenterology. 2002; 122(1):44–54

[43] Korzenik JR, Dieckgraefe BK. Is Crohn's disease an immunodeficiency? A hypothesis suggesting possible early events in the pathogenesis of Crohn's disease. Dig Dis Sci. 2000; 45(6):1121–1129

[44] Cooney R, Baker J, Brain O, et al. NOD2 stimulation induces autophagy in dendritic cells influencing bacterial handling and antigen presentation. Nat Med. 2010; 16(1):90–97

[45] Duerr RH, Taylor KD, Brant SR, et al. A genome-wide association study identifies IL23R as an inflammatory bowel disease gene. Science. 2006; 314 (5804):1461–1463

[46] Sartor RB. Does Mycobacterium avium subspecies paratuberculosis cause Crohn's disease? Gut. 2005; 54(7):896–898

[47] Naser SA, Ghobrial G, Romero C, Valentine JF. Culture of mycobacterium avium subspecies paratuberculosis from the blood of patients with Crohn's disease. Lancet. 2004; 364(9439):1039–1044

[48] Autschbach F, Eisold S, Hinz U, et al. High prevalence of mycobacterium avium subspecies paratuberculosis IS900 DNA in gut tissues from individuals with Crohn's disease. Gut. 2005; 54(7):944–949

[49] Darfeuille-Michaud A, Boudeau J, Bulois P, et al. High prevalence of adherent-invasive Escherichia coli associated with ileal mucosa in Crohn's disease. Gastroenterology. 2004; 127(2):412–421

[50] Liu Y, van Kruiningen HJ, West AB, Cartun RW, Cortot A, Colombel JF. Immunocytochemical evidence of Listeria, Escherichia coli, and Streptococcus antigens in Crohn's disease. Gastroenterology. 1995; 108(5):1396–1404

[51] Peeters H, Bogaert S, Laukens D, et al. CARD15 variants determine a disturbed early response of monocytes to adherent-invasive Escherichia coli strain LF82 in Crohn's disease. Int J Immunogenet. 2007; 34(3):181–191

[52] Ekbom A, Wakefield AJ, Zack M, Adami HO. Perinatal measles infection and subsequent Crohn's disease. Lancet. 1994; 344(8921):508–510

[53] Wakefield AJ, Ekbom A, Dhillon AP, Pittilo RM, Pounder RE. Crohn's disease: pathogenesis and persistent measles virus infection. Gastroenterology. 1995; 108(3):911–916

[54] Lodes MJ, Cong Y, Elson CO, et al. Bacterial flagellin is a dominant antigen in Crohn disease. J Clin Invest. 2004; 113(9):1296–1306

[55] Erichsen K, Milde AM, Arslan G, et al. Low-dose oral ferrous fumarate aggravated intestinal inflammation in rats with DSS-induced colitis. Inflamm Bowel Dis. 2005; 11(8):744–748

[56] Lerner A. Aluminum as an adjuvant in Crohn's disease induction. Lupus. 2012; 21(2):231–238

[57] Perl DP, Fogarty U, Harpaz N, Sachar DB. Bacterial-metal interactions: the potential role of aluminum and other trace elements in the etiology of Crohn's disease. Inflamm Bowel Dis. 2004; 10(6):881–883

[58] Sartor RB. Therapeutic manipulation of the enteric microflora in inflammatory bowel diseases: antibiotics, probiotics, and prebiotics. Gastroenterology. 2004; 126(6):1620–1633

[59] Summers RW, Elliott DE, Urban JF, Jr, Thompson RA, Weinstock JV. Trichuris suis therapy for active ulcerative colitis: a randomized controlled trial. Gastroenterology. 2005; 128(4):825–832

[60] Summers RW, Elliott DE, Urban JF, Jr, Thompson R, Weinstock JV. Trichuris suis therapy in Crohn's disease. Gut. 2005; 54(1):87–90

[61] Boyko EJ, Perera DR, Koepsell TD, Keane EM, Inui TS. Effects of cigarette smoking on the clinical course of ulcerative colitis. Scand J Gastroenterol. 1988; 23(9):1147–1152

[62] Calkins BM. A meta-analysis of the role of smoking in inflammatory bowel disease. Dig Dis Sci. 1989; 34(12):1841–1854

[63] Pullan RD, Rhodes J, Ganesh S, et al. Transdermal nicotine for active ulcerative colitis. N Engl J Med. 1994; 330(12):811–815

[64] Sandborn WJ, Tremaine WJ, Offord KP, et al. Transdermal nicotine for mildly to moderately active ulcerative colitis. A randomized, double-blind, placebo-controlled trial. Ann Intern Med. 1997; 126(5):364–371

[65] Agarwal A, Rhodes J. Smoking and IBD. IBD Monitor. 2003; 4:114–119

[66] Rubin DT, Hanauer SB. Smoking and inflammatory bowel disease. Eur J Gastroenterol Hepatol. 2000; 12(8):855–862

[67] Beaugerie L, Massot N, Carbonnel F, Cattan S, Gendre JP, Cosnes J. Impact of cessation of smoking on the course of ulcerative colitis. Am J Gastroenterol. 2001; 96(7):2113–2116

[68] Boyko EJ, Theis MK, Vaughan TL, Nicol-Blades B. Increased risk of inflammatory bowel disease associated with oral contraceptive use. Am J Epidemiol. 1994; 140(3):268–278

[69] Corrao G, Tragnone A, Caprilli R, et al. Cooperative Investigators of the Italian Group for the Study of the Colon and the Rectum (GISC). Risk of inflammatory bowel disease attributable to smoking, oral contraception and breastfeeding in Italy: a nationwide case-control study. Int J Epidemiol. 1998; 27(3):397–404

[70] Godet PG, May GR, Sutherland LR. Meta-analysis of the role of oral contraceptive agents in inflammatory bowel disease. Gut. 1995; 37(5):668–673

[71] Järnerot G, Järnmark I, Nilsson K. Consumption of refined sugar by patients with Crohn's disease, ulcerative colitis, or irritable bowel syndrome. Scand J Gastroenterol. 1983; 18(8):999–1002

[72] Mayberry JF, Rhodes J, Allan R, et al. Diet in Crohn's disease two studies of current and previous habits in newly diagnosed patients. Dig Dis Sci. 1981; 26(5):444–448

[73] Reif S, Klein I, Lubin F, Farbstein M, Hallak A, Gilat T. Pre-illness dietary factors in inflammatory bowel disease. Gut. 1997; 40(6):754–760

[74] Tragnone A, Valpiani D, Miglio F, et al. Dietary habits as risk factors for inflammatory bowel disease. Eur J Gastroenterol Hepatol. 1995; 7(1):47–51

[75] Geerling BJ, Dagnelie PC, Badart-Smook A, Russel MG, Stockbrügger RW, Brummer RJ. Diet as a risk factor for the development of ulcerative colitis. Am J Gastroenterol. 2000; 95(4):1008–1013

[76] Persson PG, Ahlbom A, Hellers G. Diet and inflammatory bowel disease: a case-control study. Epidemiology. 1992; 3(1):47–52

[77] Russel MG, Engels LG, Muris JW, et al. Modern life' in the epidemiology of inflammatory bowel disease: a case-control study with special emphasis on nutritional factors. Eur J Gastroenterol Hepatol. 1998; 10(3):243–249

[78] Shoda R, Matsueda K, Yamato S, Umeda N. Epidemiologic analysis of Crohn disease in Japan: increased dietary intake of n-6 polyunsaturated fatty acids and animal protein relates to the increased incidence of Crohn disease in Japan. Am J Clin Nutr. 1996; 63(5):741–745

[79] Riordan AM, Ruxton CH, Hunter JO. A review of associations between Crohn's disease and consumption of sugars. Eur J Clin Nutr. 1998; 52 (4):229–238

[80] Obih C, Wahbeh G, Lee D, et al. Specific carbohydrate diet for pediatric inflammatory bowel disease in clinical practice within an academic IBD center. Nutrition. 2016; 32(4):418–425

[81] Koutroubakis IE, Vlachonikolis IG, Kouroumalis EA. Role of appendicitis and appendectomy in the pathogenesis of ulcerative colitis: a critical review. Inflamm Bowel Dis. 2002; 8(4):277–286

[82] Andersson RE, Olaison G, Tysk C, Ekbom A. Appendectomy and protection against ulcerative colitis. N Engl J Med. 2001; 344(11):808–814

[83] Bernstein CN, Shanahan F, Anton PA, Weinstein WM. Patchiness of mucosal inflammation in treated ulcerative colitis: a prospective study. Gastrointest Endosc. 1995; 42(3):232–237

[84] Park SH, Yang SK, Park SK, et al. Atypical distribution of inflammation in newly diagnosed ulcerative colitis is not rare. Can J Gastroenterol Hepatol. 2014; 28(3):125–130

[85] Joo M, Odze RD. Rectal sparing and skip lesions in ulcerative colitis: a comparative study of endoscopic and histologic findings in patients who underwent proctocolectomy. Am J Surg Pathol. 2010; 34(5):689–696

[86] Kim B, Barnett JL, Kleer CG, Appelman HD. Endoscopic and histological patchiness in treated ulcerative colitis. Am J Gastroenterol. 1999; 94 (11):3258–3262

[87] Chutkan RK, Scherl E, Waye JD. Colonoscopy in inflammatory bowel disease. Gastrointest Endosc Clin N Am. 2002; 12(3):463–483, viii

[88] Waye JD. The role of colonoscopy in the differential diagnosis of inflammatory bowel disease. Gastrointest Endosc. 1977; 23(3):150–154

[89] Koltun W. IBD: diagnosis and evaluation. In: Beck D, Roberts P, Saclarides T, et al., eds. The ASCRS Textbook of Colon and Rectal Surgery. 2nd ed. New York, NY: Springer; 2011:449–462

[90] Price AB. Overlap in the spectrum of non-specific inflammatory bowel disease: "colitis indeterminate". J Clin Pathol. 1978; 31(6):567–577

[91] Gan SI, Beck PL. A new look at toxic megacolon: an update and review of incidence, etiology, pathogenesis, and management. Am J Gastroenterol. 2003; 98(11):2363–2371

[92] Issa M, Ananthakrishnan AN, Binion DG. Clostridium difficile and inflammatory bowel disease. Inflamm Bowel Dis. 2008; 14(10):1432–1442

[93] Issa M, Vijayapal A, Graham MB, et al. Impact of clostridium difficile on inflammatory bowel disease. Clin Gastroenterol Hepatol. 2007; 5(3):345–351

[94] Bernstein CN, Blanchard JF, Rawsthorne P, Yu N. The prevalence of extraintestinal diseases in inflammatory bowel disease: a population-based study. Am J Gastroenterol. 2001; 96(4):1116–1122

[95] Monsén U, Sorstad J, Hellers G, Johansson C. Extracolonic diagnoses in ulcerative colitis: an epidemiological study. Am J Gastroenterol. 1990; 85 (6):711–716

[96] Ricart E, Panaccione R, Loftus EV, Jr, et al. Autoimmune disorders and extraintestinal manifestations in first-degree familial and sporadic inflammatory bowel disease: a case-control study. Inflamm Bowel Dis. 2004; 10 (3):207–214

[97] Lyons JL, Rosenbaum JT. Uveitis associated with inflammatory bowel disease compared with uveitis associated with spondyloarthropathy. Arch Ophthalmol. 1997; 115(1):61–64

[98] Petrelli EA, McKinley M, Troncale FJ. Ocular manifestations of inflammatory bowel disease. Ann Ophthalmol. 1982; 14(4):356–360

[99] Farhi D, Cosnes J, Zizi N, et al. Significance of erythema nodosum and pyoderma gangrenosum in inflammatory bowel diseases: a cohort study of 2402 patients. Medicine (Baltimore). 2008; 87(5):281–293

[100] Keltz M, Lebwohl M, Bishop S. Peristomal pyoderma gangrenosum. J Am Acad Dermatol. 1992; 27(2)(Pt 2):360–364

[101] Powell FC, Schroeter AL, Su WP, Perry HO. Pyoderma gangrenosum: a review of 86 patients. Q J Med. 1985; 55(217):173–186

[102] Dignass A, Lindsay JO, Sturm A, et al. Second European evidence-based consensus on the diagnosis and management of ulcerative colitis part 2: current management. J Crohn's Colitis. 2012; 6(10):991–1030

[103] Bambha K, Kim WR, Talwalkar J, et al. Incidence, clinical spectrum, and outcomes of primary sclerosing cholangitis in a United States community. Gastroenterology. 2003; 125(5):1364–1369

[104] Poritz LS, Koltun WA. Surgical management of ulcerative colitis in the presence of primary sclerosing cholangitis. Dis Colon Rectum. 2003; 46(2):173–178

[105] Yuhara H, Steinmaus C, Corley D, et al. Meta-analysis: the risk of venous thromboembolism in patients with inflammatory bowel disease. Aliment Pharmacol Ther. 2013; 37(10):953–962

[106] Bernstein CN, Blanchard JF, Houston DS, Wajda A. The incidence of deep venous thrombosis and pulmonary embolism among patients with inflammatory bowel disease: a population-based cohort study. Thromb Haemost. 2001; 85(3):430–434

[107] Papa A, Gerardi V, Marzo M, Felice C, Rapaccini GL, Gasbarrini A. Venous thromboembolism in patients with inflammatory bowel disease: focus on prevention and treatment. World J Gastroenterol. 2014; 20(12):3173–3179

[108] Miehsler W, Reinisch W, Valic E, et al. Is inflammatory bowel disease an independent and disease specific risk factor for thromboembolism? Gut. 2004; 53(4):542–548

[109] Danese S, Papa A, Saibeni S, Repici A, Malesci A, Vecchi M. Inflammation and coagulation in inflammatory bowel disease: the clot thickens. Am J Gastroenterol. 2007; 102(1):174–186

[110] Fichera A, Cicchiello LA, Mendelson DS, Greenstein AJ, Heimann TM. Superior mesenteric vein thrombosis after colectomy for inflammatory bowel disease: a not uncommon cause of postoperative acute abdominal pain. Dis Colon Rectum. 2003; 46(5):643–648

[111] James AW, Rabl C, Westphalen AC, Fogarty PF, Posselt AM, Campos GM. Portomesenteric venous thrombosis after laparoscopic surgery: a systematic literature review. Arch Surg. 2009; 144(6):520–526

[112] Truelove SC, Witts LJ. Cortisone in ulcerative colitis; preliminary report on a therapeutic trial. BMJ. 1954; 2(4884):375–378

[113] Satsangi J, Silverberg MS, Vermeire S, Colombel JF. The Montreal classification of inflammatory bowel disease: controversies, consensus, and implications. Gut. 2006; 55(6):749–753

[114] Schroeder KW, Tremaine WJ, Ilstrup DM. Coated oral 5-aminosalicylic acid therapy for mildly to moderately active ulcerative colitis. A randomized study. N Engl J Med. 1987; 317(26):1625–1629

[115] Hardy TL, Bulmer E. Ulcerative colitis: a survey of ninety-five cases. BMJ. 1933; 2(3800):812–815

[116] Edwards FC, Truelove SC. The course and prognosis of ulcerative colitis. Gut. 1963; 4:299–315

[117] Turner D, Walsh CM, Steinhart AH, Griffiths AM. Response to corticosteroids in severe ulcerative colitis: a systematic review of the literature and a meta-regression. Clin Gastroenterol Hepatol. 2007; 5(1):103–110

[118] Langholz E, Munkholm P, Davidsen M, Binder V. Course of ulcerative colitis: analysis of changes in disease activity over years. Gastroenterology. 1994; 107(1):3–11

[119] Langholz E, Munkholm P, Davidsen M, Nielsen OH, Binder V. Changes in extent of ulcerative colitis: a study on the course and prognostic factors. Scand J Gastroenterol. 1996; 31(3):260–266

[120] Solberg IC, Lygren I, Jahnsen J, et al. IBSEN Study Group. Clinical course during the first 10 years of ulcerative colitis: results from a population-based inception cohort (IBSEN Study). Scand J Gastroenterol. 2009; 44(4):431–440

[121] Bitton A, Peppercorn MA, Antonioli DA, et al. Clinical, biological, and histologic parameters as predictors of relapse in ulcerative colitis. Gastroenterology. 2001; 120(1):13–20

[122] Bitton A, Sewitch MJ, Peppercorn MA, et al. Psychosocial determinants of relapse in ulcerative colitis: a longitudinal study. Am J Gastroenterol. 2003; 98 (10):2203–2208

[123] Henriksen M, Jahnsen J, Lygren I, et al. Ibsen Study Group. Clinical course in Crohn's disease: results of a five-year population-based follow-up study (the IBSEN study). Scand J Gastroenterol. 2007; 42(5):602–610

[124] Hoie O, Wolters FL, Riis L, et al. European Collaborative Study Group of Inflammatory Bowel Disease. Low colectomy rates in ulcerative colitis in an unselected European cohort followed for 10 years. Gastroenterology. 2007; 132(2):507–515

[125] Levenstein S, Prantera C, Varvo V, et al. Stress and exacerbation in ulcerative colitis: a prospective study of patients enrolled in remission. Am J Gastroenterol. 2000; 95(5):1213–1220

[126] Gower-Rousseau C, Dauchet L, Vernier-Massouille G, et al. The natural history of pediatric ulcerative colitis: a population-based cohort study. Am J Gastroenterol. 2009; 104(8):2080–2088

[127] Ayres RC, Gillen CD, Walmsley RS, Allan RN. Progression of ulcerative proctosigmoiditis: incidence and factors influencing progression. Eur J Gastroenterol Hepatol. 1996; 8(6):555–558

[128] Cima RR, Pemberton JH. Surgical indications and procedures in ulcerative colitis. Curr Treat Options Gastroenterol. 2004; 7(3):181–190

[129] Rutter MD, Saunders BP, Wilkinson KH, et al. Cancer surveillance in long-standing ulcerative colitis: endoscopic appearances help predict cancer risk. Gut. 2004; 53(12):1813–1816

[130] Rutter MD, Saunders BP, Wilkinson KH, Kamm MA, Williams CB, Forbes A. Most dysplasia in ulcerative colitis is visible at colonoscopy. Gastrointest Endosc. 2004; 60(3):334–339

[131] Lashner BA, Turner BC, Bostwick DG, Frank PH, Hanauer SB. Dysplasia and cancer complicating strictures in ulcerative colitis. Dig Dis Sci. 1990; 35(3):349–352

[132] Eaden JA, Abrams KR, Mayberry JF. The risk of colorectal cancer in ulcerative colitis: a meta-analysis. Gut. 2001; 48(4):526–535

[133] Lutgens MW, van Oijen MG, van der Heijden GJ, Vleggaar FP, Siersema PD, Oldenburg B. Declining risk of colorectal cancer in inflammatory bowel disease: an updated meta-analysis of population-based cohort studies. Inflamm Bowel Dis. 2013; 19(4):789–799

[134] Eaden J, Abrams K, Ekbom A, Jackson E, Mayberry J. Colorectal cancer prevention in ulcerative colitis: a case-control study. Aliment Pharmacol Ther. 2000; 14(2):145–153

[135] Karlén P, Kornfeld D, Broström O, Löfberg R, Persson PG, Ekbom A. Is colonoscopic surveillance reducing colorectal cancer mortality in ulcerative colitis? A population based case control study. Gut. 1998; 42(5):711–714

[136] Järnerot G, Hertervig E, Friis-Liby I, et al. Infliximab as rescue therapy in severe to moderately severe ulcerative colitis: a randomized, placebo-controlled study. Gastroenterology. 2005; 128(7):1805–1811

[137] Sandborn WJ, Rutgeerts P, Feagan BG, et al. Colectomy rate comparison after treatment of ulcerative colitis with placebo or infliximab. Gastroenterology. 2009; 137(4):1250–1260, quiz 1520

[138] Rizzo G, Pugliese D, Armuzzi A, Coco C. Anti-TNF alpha in the treatment of ulcerative colitis: a valid approach for organ-sparing or an expensive option to delay surgery? World J Gastroenterol. 2014; 20(17):4839–4845

[139] Guerrant R, Lima A. Inflammtory enteritides. In: Mandell G, Bennett J, Dolin R, eds. Principles and Practice of Infectious Diseases, 5th ed. Philadelphia, PA: Churchill Livingstone; 2000

[140] Carbonnel F, Lavergne A, Lémann M, et al. Colonoscopy of acute colitis. A safe and reliable tool for assessment of severity. Dig Dis Sci. 1994; 39(7):1550–1557

[141] Fazio VW. Toxic megacolon in ulcerative colitis and Crohn's colitis. Clin Gastroenterol. 1980; 9(2):389–407

[142] Jalan KN, Sircus W, Card WI, et al. An experience of ulcerative colitis. I. Toxic dilation in 55 cases. Gastroenterology. 1969; 57(1):68–82

[143] Mowat C, Cole A, Windsor A, et al. IBD Section of the British Society of Gastroenterology. Guidelines for the management of inflammatory bowel disease in adults. Gut. 2011; 60(5):571–607

[144] Carucci LR, Levine MS. Radiographic imaging of inflammatory bowel disease. Gastroenterol Clin North Am. 2002; 31(1):93–117, ix

[145] Maccioni F, Viscido A, Broglia L, et al. Evaluation of Crohn disease activity with magnetic resonance imaging. Abdom Imaging. 2000; 25(3):219–228

[146] Schreyer AG, Gölder S, Seitz J, Herfarth H. New diagnostic avenues in inflammatory bowel diseases. Capsule endoscopy, magnetic resonance imaging and virtual enteroscopy. Dig Dis. 2003; 21(2):129–137

[147] Gasche C, Moser G, Turetschek K, Schober E, Moeschl P, Oberhuber G. Transabdominal bowel sonography for the detection of intestinal complications in Crohn's disease. Gut. 1999; 44(1):112–117

[148] Annese V, Lombardi G, Perri F, et al. Variants of CARD15 are associated with an aggressive clinical course of Crohn's disease: an IG-IBD study. Am J Gastroenterol. 2005; 100(1):84–92

[149] Li DJ, Freeman A, Miles KA, Wraight EP. Can 99Tcm HMPAO leucocyte scintigraphy distinguish between Crohn's disease and ulcerative colitis? Br J Radiol. 1994; 67(797):472–477

[150] Lopes S, Figueiredo P, Portela F, et al. Capsule endoscopy in inflammatory bowel disease type unclassified and indeterminate colitis serologically negative. Inflamm Bowel Dis. 2010; 16(10):1663–1668

[151] Camilleri M, Proano M. Advances in the assessment of disease activity in inflammatory bowel disease. Mayo Clin Proc. 1989; 64(7):800–807

[152] Cambridge G, Rampton DS, Stevens TR, McCarthy DA, Kamm M, Leaker B. Anti-neutrophil antibodies in inflammatory bowel disease: prevalence and diagnostic role. Gut. 1992; 33(5):668–674

[153] Coukos JA, Howard LA, Weinberg JM, Becker JM, Stucchi AF, Farraye FA. ASCA IgG and CBir antibodies are associated with the development of Crohn's disease and fistulae following ileal pouch-anal anastomosis. Dig Dis Sci. 2012; 57(6):1544–1553

[154] Gionchetti P, Rizzello F, Venturi A, et al. Comparison of oral with rectal mesalazine in the treatment of ulcerative proctitis. Dis Colon Rectum. 1998; 41(1):93–97

[155] van Bodegraven AA, Boer RO, Lourens J, Tuynman HA, Sindram JW. Distribution of mesalazine enemas in active and quiescent ulcerative colitis. Aliment Pharmacol Ther. 1996; 10(3):327–332

[156] Mulder CJ, Fockens P, Meijer JW, van der Heide H, Wiltink EH, Tytgat GN. Beclomethasone dipropionate (3 mg) versus 5-aminosalicylic acid (2 g) versus the combination of both (3 mg/2 g) as retention enemas in active ulcerative proctitis. Eur J Gastroenterol Hepatol. 1996; 8(6):549–553

[157] Lémann M, Galian A, Rutgeerts P, et al. Comparison of budesonide and 5-aminosalicylic acid enemas in active distal ulcerative colitis. Aliment Pharmacol Ther. 1995; 9(5):557–562

[158] Farup PG, Hovde O, Halvorsen FA, Raknerud N, Brodin U. Mesalazine suppositories versus hydrocortisone foam in patients with distal ulcerative colitis. A comparison of the efficacy and practicality of two topical treatment regimens. Scand J Gastroenterol. 1995; 30(2):164–170

[159] Lucidarme D, Marteau P, Foucault M, Vautrin B, Filoche B. Efficacy and tolerance of mesalazine suppositories vs. hydrocortisone foam in proctitis. Aliment Pharmacol Ther. 1997; 11(2):335–340

[160] Gionchetti P, D'Arienzo A, Rizzello F, et al. Italian BDP Study Group. Topical treatment of distal active ulcerative colitis with beclomethasone dipropionate or mesalamine: a single-blind randomized controlled trial. J Clin Gastroenterol. 2005; 39(4):291–297

[161] Andus T, Kocjan A, Müser M, et al. International Salofalk Suppository OD Study Group. Clinical trial: a novel high-dose 1 g mesalamine suppository (Salofalk) once daily is as efficacious as a 500-mg suppository thrice daily in active ulcerative proctitis. Inflamm Bowel Dis. 2010; 16(11):1947–1956

[162] Lamet M. A multicenter, randomized study to evaluate the efficacy and safety of mesalamine suppositories 1 g at bedtime and 500 mg twice daily in patients with active mild-to-moderate ulcerative proctitis. Dig Dis Sci. 2011; 56(2):513–522

[163] Marshall JK, Irvine EJ. Rectal corticosteroids versus alternative treatments in ulcerative colitis: a meta-analysis. Gut. 1997; 40(6):775–781

[164] Ito H, Iida M, Matsumoto T, et al. Direct comparison of two different mesalamine formulations for the induction of remission in patients with ulcerative colitis: a double-blind, randomized study. Inflamm Bowel Dis. 2010; 16(9):1567–1574

[165] Kam L, Cohen H, Dooley C, Rubin P, Orchard J. A comparison of mesalamine suspension enema and oral sulfasalazine for treatment of active distal ulcerative colitis in adults. Am J Gastroenterol. 1996; 91(7):1338–1342

[166] Sandborn WJ, Kamm MA, Lichtenstein GR, Lyne A, Butler T, Joseph RE. MMX Multi Matrix System mesalazine for the induction of remission in patients with mild-to-moderate ulcerative colitis: a combined analysis of two randomized, double-blind, placebo-controlled trials. Aliment Pharmacol Ther. 2007; 26(2):205–215

[167] Marteau P, Crand J, Foucault M, Rambaud JC. Use of mesalazine slow release suppositories 1 g three times per week to maintain remission of ulcerative proctitis: a randomised double blind placebo controlled multicentre study. Gut. 1998; 42(2):195–199

[168] Safdi M, DeMicco M, Sninsky C, et al. A double-blind comparison of oral versus rectal mesalamine versus combination therapy in the treatment of distal ulcerative colitis. Am J Gastroenterol. 1997; 92(10):1867–1871

[169] Marteau P, Probert CS, Lindgren S, et al. Combined oral and enema treatment with Pentasa (mesalazine) is superior to oral therapy alone in patients with extensive mild/moderate active ulcerative colitis: a randomised, double blind, placebo controlled study. Gut. 2005; 54(7):960–965

[170] Ford AC, Achkar JP, Khan KJ, et al. Efficacy of 5-aminosalicylates in ulcerative colitis: systematic review and meta-analysis. Am J Gastroenterol. 2011; 106(4):601–616

[171] Manguso F, Balzano A. Meta-analysis: the efficacy of rectal beclomethasone dipropionate vs. 5-aminosalicylic acid in mild to moderate distal ulcerative colitis. Aliment Pharmacol Ther. 2007; 26(1):21–29

[172] Marshall JK, Thabane M, Steinhart AH, Newman JR, Anand A, Irvine EJ. Rectal 5-aminosalicylic acid for induction of remission in ulcerative colitis. Cochrane Database Syst Rev. 2010; 20(1):CD004115

[173] Cortot A, Maetz D, Degoutte E, et al. Mesalamine foam enema versus mesalamine liquid enema in active left-sided ulcerative colitis. Am J Gastroenterol. 2008; 103(12):3106–3114

[174] Eliakim R, Tulassay Z, Kupcinskas L, et al. International Salofalk Foam Study Group. Clinical trial: randomized-controlled clinical study comparing the efficacy and safety of a low-volume vs. a high-volume mesalazine foam in active distal ulcerative colitis. Aliment Pharmacol Ther. 2007; 26 (9):1237–1249

[175] Sutherland L, Macdonald J. Oral 5-aminosalicylic acid for induction of remission in ulcerative colitis. Cochrane Database Syst Rev 2006:CD000543

[176] Kruis W, Kiudelis G, Rácz I, et al. International Salofalk OD Study Group. Once daily versus three times daily mesalazine granules in active ulcerative colitis: a double-blind, double-dummy, randomised, non-inferiority trial. Gut. 2009; 58(2):233–240

[177] Hanauer SB, Sandborn WJ, Kornbluth A, et al. Delayed-release oral mesalamine at 4.8 g/day (800 mg tablet) for the treatment of moderately active ulcerative colitis: the ASCEND II trial. Am J Gastroenterol. 2005; 100 (11):2478–2485

[178] Hanauer S, Schwartz J, Robinson M, et al. Mesalamine capsule for treatment of active ulcerative colitis: results of a controlled trial: Pentasa Study Group. Am J Gastroenterol. 1993; 88:1188–1197

[179] Kamm MA, Lichtenstein GR, Sandborn WJ, et al. Randomised trial of once- or twice-daily MMX mesalazine for maintenance of remission in ulcerative colitis. Gut. 2008; 57(7):893–902

[180] Kamm MA, Sandborn WJ, Gassull M, et al. Once-daily, high-concentration MMX mesalamine in active ulcerative colitis. Gastroenterology. 2007; 132 (1):66–75, quiz 432–433

[181] Lichtenstein GR, Kamm MA, Boddu P, et al. Effect of once- or twice-daily MMX mesalamine (SPD476) for the induction of remission of mild to moderately active ulcerative colitis. Clin Gastroenterol Hepatol. 2007; 5(1):95–102

[182] Lichtenstein GR, Ramsey D, Rubin DT. Randomised clinical trial: delayed-release oral mesalazine 4.8 g/day vs. 2.4 g/day in endoscopic mucosal healing: ASCEND I and II combined analysis. Aliment Pharmacol Ther. 2011; 33 (6):672–678

[183] Lennard-Jones JE, Longmore AJ, Newell AC, Wilson CW, Jones FA. An assessment of prednisone, salazopyrin, and topical hydrocortisone hemisuccinate used as out-patient treatment for ulcerative colitis. Gut. 1960; 1:217–222

[184] Truelove SC, Watkinson G, Draper G. Comparison of corticosteroid and sulphasalazine therapy in ulcerative colitis. BMJ. 1962; 2(5321):1708–1711

[185] Kruis W, Jonaitis L, Pokrotnieks J, et al. International Salofalk OD Study Group. Randomised clinical trial: a comparative dose-finding study of three arms of dual release mesalazine for maintaining remission in ulcerative colitis. Aliment Pharmacol Ther. 2011; 33(3):313–322

[186] Baron JH, Connell AM, Kanaghinis TG, Lennard-Jones JE, Jones AF. Out-patient treatment of ulcerative colitis. Comparison between three doses of oral prednisone. BMJ. 1962; 2(5302):441–443

[187] Sherlock ME, MacDonald JK, Griffiths AM, Steinhart AH, Seow CH. Oral budesonide for induction of remission in ulcerative colitis. Cochrane Database Syst Rev. 2015(10):CD007698

[188] Sands BE. Fulminant colitis. J Gastrointest Surg. 2008; 12(12):2157–2159

[189] Domènech E, Vega R, Ojanguren I, et al. Cytomegalovirus infection in ulcerative colitis: a prospective, comparative study on prevalence and diagnostic strategy. Inflamm Bowel Dis. 2008; 14(10):1373–1379

[190] Jen MH, Saxena S, Bottle A, Aylin P, Pollok RC. Increased health burden associated with clostridium difficile diarrhoea in patients with inflammatory bowel disease. Aliment Pharmacol Ther. 2011; 33(12):1322–1331

[191] Kishore J, Ghoshal U, Ghoshal UC, et al. Infection with cytomegalovirus in patients with inflammatory bowel disease: prevalence, clinical significance and outcome. J Med Microbiol. 2004; 53(Pt 11):1155–1160

[192] Nguyen GC, Kaplan GG, Harris ML, Brant SR. A national survey of the prevalence and impact of clostridium difficile infection among hospitalized inflammatory bowel disease patients. Am J Gastroenterol. 2008; 103(6):1443–1450

[193] Papadakis KA, Tung JK, Binder SW, et al. Outcome of cytomegalovirus infections in patients with inflammatory bowel disease. Am J Gastroenterol. 2001; 96(7):2137–2142

[194] Rahier JF, Ben-Horin S, Chowers Y, et al. European Crohn's and Colitis Organisation (ECCO). European evidence-based consensus on the prevention, diagnosis and management of opportunistic infections in inflammatory bowel disease. J Crohn's Colitis. 2009; 3(2):47–91

[195] Ben-Horin S, Margalit M, Bossuyt P, et al. European Crohn's and Colitis Organization (ECCO). Combination immunomodulator and antibiotic treatment in patients with inflammatory bowel disease and clostridium difficile infection. Clin Gastroenterol Hepatol. 2009; 7(9):981–987

[196] Grainge MJ, West J, Card TR. Venous thromboembolism during active disease and remission in inflammatory bowel disease: a cohort study. Lancet. 2010; 375(9715):657–663

[197] Kappelman MD, Horvath-Puho E, Sandler RS, et al. Thromboembolic risk among Danish children and adults with inflammatory bowel diseases: a population-based nationwide study. Gut. 2011; 60(7):937–943

[198] González-Huix F, Fernández-Bañares F, Esteve-Comas M, et al. Enteral versus parenteral nutrition as adjunct therapy in acute ulcerative colitis. Am J Gastroenterol. 1993; 88(2):227–232

[199] McIntyre PB, Powell-Tuck J, Wood SR, et al. Controlled trial of bowel rest in the treatment of severe acute colitis. Gut. 1986; 27(5):481–485

[200] Kefalakes H, Stylianides TJ, Amanakis G, Kolios G. Exacerbation of inflammatory bowel diseases associated with the use of nonsteroidal anti-inflammatory drugs: myth or reality? Eur J Clin Pharmacol. 2009; 65(10):963–970

[201] Takeuchi K, Smale S, Premchand P, et al. Prevalence and mechanism of nonsteroidal anti-inflammatory drug-induced clinical relapse in patients with inflammatory bowel disease. Clin Gastroenterol Hepatol. 2006; 4 (2):196–202

[202] Rice-Oxley J, Truelove S. Ulcerative colitis course and prognosis. Lancet. 1950; 255:663–666

[203] Chapman RW, Selby WS, Jewell DP. Controlled trial of intravenous metronidazole as an adjunct to corticosteroids in severe ulcerative colitis. Gut. 1986; 27(10):1210–1212

[204] Mantzaris GJ, Hatzis A, Petraki K, Spiliadi C, Triantaphyllou G. Intermittent therapy with high-dose 5-aminosalicylic acid enemas maintains remission in ulcerative proctitis and proctosigmoiditis. Dis Colon Rectum. 1994; 37 (1):58–62

[205] Mantzaris GJ, Petraki K, Archavlis E, et al. A prospective randomized controlled trial of intravenous ciprofloxacin as an adjunct to corticosteroids in acute, severe ulcerative colitis. Scand J Gastroenterol. 2001; 36(9):971–974

[206] Bossa F, Fiorella S, Caruso N, et al. Continuous infusion versus bolus administration of steroids in severe attacks of ulcerative colitis: a randomized, double-blind trial. Am J Gastroenterol. 2007; 102(3):601–608

[207] Rosenberg W, Ireland A, Jewell DP. High-dose methylprednisolone in the treatment of active ulcerative colitis. J Clin Gastroenterol. 1990; 12(1):40–41

[208] Randall J, Singh B, Warren BF, Travis SP, Mortensen NJ, George BD. Delayed surgery for acute severe colitis is associated with increased risk of postoperative complications. Br J Surg. 2010; 97(3):404–409

[209] Roberts SE, Williams JG, Yeates D, Goldacre MJ. Mortality in patients with and without colectomy admitted to hospital for ulcerative colitis and Crohn's disease: record linkage studies. BMJ. 2007; 335(7628):1033–1036

[210] Benazzato L, D'Incà R, Grigoletto F, et al. Prognosis of severe attacks in ulcerative colitis: effect of intensive medical treatment. Dig Liver Dis. 2004; 36 (7):461–466

[211] Lennard-Jones JE, Ritchie JK, Hilder W, Spicer CC. Assessment of severity in colitis: a preliminary study. Gut. 1975; 16(8):579–584

[212] Lindgren SC, Flood LM, Kilander AF, Löfberg R, Persson TB, Sjödahl RI. Early predictors of glucocorticosteroid treatment failure in severe and moderately severe attacks of ulcerative colitis. Eur J Gastroenterol Hepatol. 1998; 10 (10):831–835

[213] Travis SP, Farrant JM, Ricketts C, et al. Predicting outcome in severe ulcerative colitis. Gut. 1996; 38(6):905–910

[214] Chew CN, Nolan DJ, Jewell DP. Small bowel gas in severe ulcerative colitis. Gut. 1991; 32(12):1535–1537

[215] Carbonnel F, Boruchowicz A, Duclos B, et al. Intravenous cyclosporine in attacks of ulcerative colitis: short-term and long-term responses. Dig Dis Sci. 1996; 41(12):2471–2476

[216] Bouguen G, Roblin X, Bourreille A, et al. Infliximab for refractory ulcerative proctitis. Aliment Pharmacol Ther. 2010; 31(11):1178–1185

[217] Lawrance IC, Copeland TS. Rectal tacrolimus in the treatment of resistant ulcerative proctitis. Aliment Pharmacol Ther. 2008; 28(10):1214–1220

[218] Sandborn WJ, Tremaine WJ, Schroeder KW, et al. A placebo-controlled trial of cyclosporine enemas for mildly to moderately active left-sided ulcerative colitis. Gastroenterology. 1994; 106(6):1429–1435

[219] van Dieren JM, van Bodegraven AA, Kuipers EJ, et al. Local application of tacrolimus in distal colitis: feasible and safe. Inflamm Bowel Dis. 2009; 15 (2):193–198

[220] Breuer RI, Soergel KH, Lashner BA, et al. Short chain fatty acid rectal irrigation for left-sided ulcerative colitis: a randomised, placebo controlled trial. Gut. 1997; 40(4):485–491

[221] Forbes A, Britton TC, House IM, Gazzard BG. Safety and efficacy of acetarsol suppositories in unresponsive proctitis. Aliment Pharmacol Ther. 1989; 3 (6):553–556

[222] Guslandi M, Frego R, Viale E, Testoni PA. Distal ulcerative colitis refractory to rectal mesalamine: role of transdermal nicotine versus oral mesalamine. Can J Gastroenterol. 2002; 16(5):293–296

[223] Saibil F. Lidocaine enemas for intractable distal ulcerative colitis: Efficacy and safety. Gastroenterology. 1998; 114:A1073

[224] Scheppach W, German-Austrian SCFA Study Group. Treatment of distal ulcerative colitis with short-chain fatty acid enemas. A placebo-controlled trial. Dig Dis Sci. 1996; 41(11):2254–2259

[225] Sinha A, Nightingale J, West KP, Berlanga-Acosta J, Playford RJ. Epidermal growth factor enemas with oral mesalamine for mild-to-moderate left-sided ulcerative colitis or proctitis. N Engl J Med. 2003; 349(4):350–357

[226] Bolin TD, Wong S, Crouch R, Engelman JL, Riordan SM. Appendicectomy as a therapy for ulcerative proctitis. Am J Gastroenterol. 2009; 104 (10):2476–2482

[227] Cohen RD, Stein R, Hanauer SB. Intravenous cyclosporin in ulcerative colitis: a five-year experience. Am J Gastroenterol. 1999; 94(6):1587–1592

[228] D'Haens G, Lemmens L, Geboes K, et al. Intravenous cyclosporine versus intravenous corticosteroids as single therapy for severe attacks of ulcerative colitis. Gastroenterology. 2001; 120(6):1323–1329

[229] Lichtiger S, Present DH, Kornbluth A, et al. Cyclosporine in severe ulcerative colitis refractory to steroid therapy. N Engl J Med. 1994; 330(26):1841–1845

[230] Moskovitz DN, Van Assche G, Maenhout B, et al. Incidence of colectomy during long-term follow-up after cyclosporine-induced remission of severe ulcerative colitis. Clin Gastroenterol Hepatol. 2006; 4(6):760–765

[231] Van Assche G, D'Haens G, Noman M, et al. Randomized, double-blind comparison of 4 mg/kg versus 2 mg/kg intravenous cyclosporine in severe ulcerative colitis. Gastroenterology. 2003; 125(4):1025–1031

[232] Sands B. IBD: medical management. In: Beck D, Roberts P, Saclarides T, et al., eds. The ASCRS Textbook of Colon and Rectal Surgery. New York, NY: Springer; 2011:463–478

[233] Campbell S, Travis S, Jewell D. Ciclosporin use in acute ulcerative colitis: a long-term experience. Eur J Gastroenterol Hepatol. 2005; 17(1):79–84

[234] Bamba S, Tsujikawa T, Inatomi O, et al. Factors affecting the efficacy of cyclosporin A therapy for refractory ulcerative colitis. J Gastroenterol Hepatol. 2010; 25(3):494–498

[235] Walch A, Meshkat M, Vogelsang H, et al. Long-term outcome in patients with ulcerative colitis treated with intravenous cyclosporine A is determined by previous exposure to thiopurines. J Crohn's Colitis. 2010; 4(4):398–404

[236] Ogata H, Matsui T, Nakamura M, et al. A randomised dose finding study of oral tacrolimus (FK506) therapy in refractory ulcerative colitis. Gut. 2006; 55(9):1255–1262

[237] Kawakami K, Inoue T, Murano M, et al. Effects of oral tacrolimus as a rapid induction therapy in ulcerative colitis. World J Gastroenterol. 2015; 21 (6):1880–1886

[238] Baumgart DC, Wiedenmann B, Dignass AU. Rescue therapy with tacrolimus is effective in patients with severe and refractory inflammatory bowel disease. Aliment Pharmacol Ther. 2003; 17(10):1273–1281

[239] Fellermann K, Tanko Z, Herrlinger KR, et al. Response of refractory colitis to intravenous or oral tacrolimus (FK506). Inflamm Bowel Dis. 2002; 8 (5):317–324

[240] Högenauer C, Wenzl HH, Hinterleitner TA, Petritsch W. Effect of oral tacrolimus (FK 506) on steroid-refractory moderate/severe ulcerative colitis. Aliment Pharmacol Ther. 2003; 18(4):415–423

[241] Ferrante M, D'Haens G, Dewit O, et al. Belgian IBD Research Group. Efficacy of infliximab in refractory pouchitis and Crohn's disease-related complications of the pouch: a Belgian case series. Inflamm Bowel Dis. 2010; 16 (2):243–249

[242] Ferrante M, Vermeire S, Katsanos KH, et al. Predictors of early response to infliximab in patients with ulcerative colitis. Inflamm Bowel Dis. 2007; 13 (2):123–128

[243] Jakobovits SL, Jewell DP, Travis SP. Infliximab for the treatment of ulcerative colitis: outcomes in Oxford from 2000 to 2006. Aliment Pharmacol Ther. 2007; 25(9):1055–1060

[244] Lees CW, Heys D, Ho GT, et al. Scottish Society of Gastroenterology Infliximab Group. A retrospective analysis of the efficacy and safety of infliximab as rescue therapy in acute severe ulcerative colitis. Aliment Pharmacol Ther. 2007; 26(3):411–419

[245] Regueiro M, Curtis J, Plevy S. Infliximab for hospitalized patients with severe ulcerative colitis. J Clin Gastroenterol. 2006; 40(6):476–481

[246] Gustavsson A, Järnerot G, Hertervig E, et al. Clinical trial: colectomy after rescue therapy in ulcerative colitis—3-year follow-up of the Swedish-Danish controlled infliximab study. Aliment Pharmacol Ther. 2010; 32 (8):984–989

[247] Narula N, Marshall JK, Colombel JF, et al. Systematic review and meta-analysis: infliximab or cyclosporine as rescue therapy in patients with severe ulcerative colitis refractory to steroids. Am J Gastroenterol. 2016; 111(4):477–491

[248] Laharie D, Bourreille A, Branche J, et al. Groupe d'Etudes Thérapeutiques des Affections Inflammatoires Digestives. Ciclosporin versus infliximab in patients with severe ulcerative colitis refractory to intravenous steroids: a parallel, open-label randomised controlled trial. Lancet. 2012; 380(9857):1909–1915

[249] Scimeca D, Bossa F, Annese V, et al. Infliximab vs oral cyclosporin in patients with severe ulcerative colitis refractory to intravenous steroids. A controlled, randomized study. Paper presented at the United European Gastroenterology Week 2012, Amsterdam, The Netherlands, 2012

[250] Williams J, Alam M, Alrubaiy L, et al. Comparative clinical effectiveness of infliximab and ciclosporin for acute severe ulcerative colitis: early results from the CONSTRUCT trial. Paper presented at the United European Gastroenterology Week 2014, Vienna, Austria, 2014

[251] Narula N, Fine M, Colombel JF, Marshall JK, Reinisch W. Systematic review: sequential rescue therapy in severe ulcerative colitis: do the benefits outweigh the risks? Inflamm Bowel Dis. 2015; 21(7):1683–1694

[252] Leblanc S, Allez M, Seksik P, et al. GETAID. Successive treatment with cyclosporine and infliximab in steroid-refractory ulcerative colitis. Am J Gastroenterol. 2011; 106(4):771–777

[253] Maser EA, Villela R, Silverberg MS, Greenberg GR. Association of trough serum infliximab to clinical outcome after scheduled maintenance treatment for Crohn's disease. Clin Gastroenterol Hepatol. 2006; 4(10):1248–1254

[254] Jürgens M, Laubender RP, Hartl F, et al. Disease activity, ANCA, and IL23 R genotype status determine early response to infliximab in patients with ulcerative colitis. Am J Gastroenterol. 2010; 105(8):1811–1819

[255] Dignass A, Eliakim R, Magro F, et al. Second European evidence-based consensus on the diagnosis and management of ulcerative colitis part 1: definitions and diagnosis. J Crohn's Colitis. 2012; 6(10):965–990

[256] Ardizzone S, Maconi G, Russo A, Imbesi V, Colombo E, Bianchi Porro G. Randomised controlled trial of azathioprine and 5-aminosalicylic acid for treatment of steroid dependent ulcerative colitis. Gut. 2006; 55(1):47–53

[257] Chebli LA, Chaves LD, Pimentel FF, et al. Azathioprine maintains long-term steroid-free remission through 3 years in patients with steroid-dependent ulcerative colitis. Inflamm Bowel Dis. 2010; 16(4):613–619

[258] Danese S, Fiorino G, Peyrin-Biroulet L, et al. Biological agents for moderately to severely active ulcerative colitis: a systematic review and network meta-analysis. Ann Intern Med. 2014; 160(10):704–711

[259] Panaccione R, Ghosh S, Middleton S, et al. Combination therapy with infliximab and azathioprine is superior to monotherapy with either agent in ulcerative colitis. Gastroenterology. 2014; 146(2):392–400.e3

[260] Reinisch W, Sandborn WJ, Hommes DW, et al. Adalimumab for induction of clinical remission in moderately to severely active ulcerative colitis: results of a randomised controlled trial. Gut. 2011; 60(6):780–787

[261] Sandborn WJ, van Assche G, Reinisch W, et al. Adalimumab induces and maintains clinical remission in patients with moderate-to-severe ulcerative colitis. Gastroenterology. 2012; 142(2):257–265.e1, 3

[262] Sandborn WJ, Feagan BG, Marano C, et al. PURSUIT-SC Study Group. Subcutaneous golimumab induces clinical response and remission in patients with moderate-to-severe ulcerative colitis. Gastroenterology. 2014; 146(1):85–95, quiz e14–e15

[263] de Silva PS, Nguyen DD, Sauk J, Korzenik J, Yajnik V, Ananthakrishnan AN. Long-term outcome of a third anti-TNF monoclonal antibody after the failure of two prior anti-TNFs in inflammatory bowel disease. Aliment Pharmacol Ther. 2012; 36(5):459–466

[264] Bickston SJ, Behm BW, Tsoulis DJ, et al. Vedolizumab for induction and maintenance of remission in ulcerative colitis. Cochrane Database Syst Rev. 2014 (8):CD007571

[265] Feagan BG, Greenberg GR, Wild G, et al. Treatment of ulcerative colitis with a humanized antibody to the alpha4beta7 integrin. N Engl J Med. 2005; 352 (24):2499–2507

[266] Feagan BG, Rutgeerts P, Sands BE, et al. GEMINI 1 Study Group. Vedolizumab as induction and maintenance therapy for ulcerative colitis. N Engl J Med. 2013; 369(8):699–710

[267] Vermeire S, O'Byrne S, Keir M, et al. Etrolizumab as induction therapy for ulcerative colitis: a randomised, controlled, phase 2 trial. Lancet. 2014; 384 (9940):309–318

[268] Sandborn WJ, Ghosh S, Panes J, et al. Study A3921063 Investigators. Tofacitinib, an oral Janus kinase inhibitor, in active ulcerative colitis. N Engl J Med. 2012; 367(7):616–624

[269] Fraser AG, Orchard TR, Jewell DP. The efficacy of azathioprine for the treatment of inflammatory bowel disease: a 30 year review. Gut. 2002; 50 (4):485–489

[270] Cohen RD, Woseth DM, Thisted RA, Hanauer SB. A meta-analysis and overview of the literature on treatment options for left-sided ulcerative colitis and ulcerative proctitis. Am J Gastroenterol. 2000; 95(5):1263–1276

[271] Schmidt KJ, Herrlinger KR, Emmrich J, et al. Short-term efficacy of tacrolimus in steroid-refractory ulcerative colitis: experience in 130 patients. Aliment Pharmacol Ther. 2013; 37(1):129–136

[272] Inoue T, Murano M, Narabayashi K, et al. The efficacy of oral tacrolimus in patients with moderate/severe ulcerative colitis not receiving concomitant corticosteroid therapy. Intern Med. 2013; 52(1):15–20

[273] Oren R, Arber N, Odes S, et al. Methotrexate in chronic active ulcerative colitis: a double-blind, randomized, Israeli multicenter trial. Gastroenterology. 1996; 110(5):1416–1421

[274] Maté-Jiménez J, Hermida C, Cantero-Perona J, Moreno-Otero R. 6-mercaptopurine or methotrexate added to prednisone induces and maintains remission in steroid-dependent inflammatory bowel disease. Eur J Gastroenterol Hepatol. 2000; 12(11):1227–1233

[275] Wang Y, MacDonald JK, Vandermeer B, Griffiths AM, El-Matary W. Methotrexate for maintenance of remission in ulcerative colitis. Cochrane Database Syst Rev. 2015(8):CD007560

[276] Leo S, Leandro G, Di Matteo G, Caruso ML, Lorusso D. Ulcerative colitis in remission: it is possible to predict the risk of relapse? Digestion. 1989; 44 (4):217–221

[277] Riley SA, Mani V, Goodman MJ, Dutt S, Herd ME. Microscopic activity in ulcerative colitis: what does it mean? Gut. 1991; 32(2):174–178

[278] Riley SA, Mani V, Goodman MJ, Lucas S. Why do patients with ulcerative colitis relapse? Gut. 1990; 31(2):179–183

[279] Vidal A, Gómez-Gil E, Sans M, et al. Life events and inflammatory bowel disease relapse: a prospective study of patients enrolled in remission. Am J Gastroenterol. 2006; 101(4):775–781

[280] Wright R, Truelove SR. Serial rectal biopsy in ulcerative colitis during the course of a controlled therapeutic trial of various diets. Am J Dig Dis. 1966; 11(11):847–857

[281] Bernstein CN, Singh S, Graff LA, Walker JR, Miller N, Cheang M. A prospective population-based study of triggers of symptomatic flares in IBD. Am J Gastroenterol. 2010; 105(9):1994–2002

[282] Kane S, Huo D, Aikens J, Hanauer S. Medication nonadherence and the outcomes of patients with quiescent ulcerative colitis. Am J Med. 2003; 114 (1):39–43

[283] d'Albasio G, Pacini F, Camarri E, et al. Combined therapy with 5-aminosalicylic acid tablets and enemas for maintaining remission in ulcerative colitis: a randomized double-blind study. Am J Gastroenterol. 1997; 92(7):1143–1147

[284] d'Albasio G, Trallori G, Ghetti A, et al. Intermittent therapy with high-dose 5-aminosalicylic acid enemas for maintaining remission in ulcerative proctosigmoiditis. Dis Colon Rectum. 1990; 33(5):394–397

[285] Miner P, Daly R, Nester T, et al. The effect of varying dose intervals of mesalamine enemas for the prevention of relapse in distal ulcerative colitis. Gastroenterology. 1994; 106:A736

[286] Casellas F, Vaquero E, Armengol JR, Malagelada JR. Practicality of 5-aminosalicylic suppositories for long-term treatment of inactive distal ulcerative colitis. Hepatogastroenterology. 1999; 46(28):2343–2346

[287] Moody GA, Eaden JA, Helyes Z, Mayberry JF. Oral or rectal administration of drugs in IBD? Aliment Pharmacol Ther. 1997; 11(5):999–1000

[288] Fockens P, Mulder CJ, Tytgat GN, et al. Dutch Pentasa Study Group. Comparison of the efficacy and safety of 1.5 compared with 3.0 g oral slow-release mesalazine (Pentasa) in the maintenance treatment of ulcerative colitis. Eur J Gastroenterol Hepatol. 1995; 7(11):1025–1030

[289] Paoluzi OA, Iacopini F, Pica R, et al. Comparison of two different daily dosages (2.4 vs. 1.2 g) of oral mesalazine in maintenance of remission in ulcerative colitis patients: 1-year follow-up study. Aliment Pharmacol Ther. 2005; 21(9):1111–1119

[290] Dignass AU, Bokemeyer B, Adamek H, et al. Mesalamine once daily is more effective than twice daily in patients with quiescent ulcerative colitis. Clin Gastroenterol Hepatol. 2009; 7(7):762–769

[291] Sandborn WJ, Korzenik J, Lashner B, et al. Once-daily dosing of delayed-release oral mesalamine (400-mg tablet) is as effective as twice-daily dosing for maintenance of remission of ulcerative colitis. Gastroenterology. 2010; 138(4):1286–1296, 1296.e1–1296.e3

[292] Prantera C, Kohn A, Campieri M, et al. Clinical trial: ulcerative colitis maintenance treatment with 5-ASA: a 1-year, randomized multicentre study comparing MMX with Asacol. Aliment Pharmacol Ther. 2009; 30(9):908–918

[293] Cassinotti A, Actis GC, Duca P, et al. Maintenance treatment with azathioprine in ulcerative colitis: outcome and predictive factors after drug withdrawal. Am J Gastroenterol. 2009; 104(11):2760–2767

[294] Hawthorne AB, Logan RF, Hawkey CJ, et al. Randomised controlled trial of azathioprine withdrawal in ulcerative colitis. BMJ. 1992; 305(6844):20–22

[295] Jewell DP, Truelove SC. Azathioprine in ulcerative colitis: final report on controlled therapeutic trial. BMJ. 1974; 4(5945):627–630

[296] Sood A, Kaushal V, Midha V, Bhatia KL, Sood N, Malhotra V. The beneficial effect of azathioprine on maintenance of remission in severe ulcerative colitis. J Gastroenterol. 2002; 37(4):270–274

[297] Sood A, Midha V, Sood N, Avasthi G. Azathioprine versus sulfasalazine in maintenance of remission in severe ulcerative colitis. Indian J Gastroenterol. 2003; 22(3):79–81

[298] Timmer A, McDonald JW, Macdonald JK. Azathioprine and 6-mercaptopurine for maintenance of remission in ulcerative colitis. Cochrane Database Syst Rev. 2007(1):CD000478

[299] Actis GC, Fadda M, David E, Sapino A. Colectomy rate in steroid-refractory colitis initially responsive to cyclosporin: a long-term retrospective cohort study. BMC Gastroenterol. 2007; 7:13

[300] Wahed M, Louis-Auguste JR, Baxter LM, et al. Efficacy of methotrexate in Crohn's disease and ulcerative colitis patients unresponsive or intolerant to azathioprine/mercaptopurine. Aliment Pharmacol Ther. 2009; 30 (6):614–620

[301] Rutgeerts P, Sandborn WJ, Feagan BG, et al. Infliximab for induction and maintenance therapy for ulcerative colitis. N Engl J Med. 2005; 353 (23):2462–2476

[302] Van Assche G, Magdelaine-Beuzelin C, D'Haens G, et al. Withdrawal of immunosuppression in Crohn's disease treated with scheduled infliximab maintenance: a randomized trial. Gastroenterology. 2008; 134 (7):1861–1868

[303] Colombel JF, Sandborn WJ, Ghosh S, et al. Four-year maintenance treatment with adalimumab in patients with moderately to severely active ulcerative colitis: Data from ULTRA 1, 2, and 3. Am J Gastroenterol. 2014; 109 (11):1771–1780

[304] Roda G, Jharap B, Neeraj N, Colombel JF. Loss of response to anti-TNFs: definition, epidemiology, and management. Clin Transl Gastroenterol. 2016; 7:e135

[305] Hanauer S, Feagan B, Lichtenstein G, et al. ACCENT I Study Group. Maintenance infliximab for Crohn's disease: the ACCENT I randomized trial. Lancet. 2002; 59:1541–1549

[306] Sands BE, Anderson FH, Bernstein CN, et al. Infliximab maintenance therapy for fistulizing Crohn's disease. N Engl J Med. 2004; 350(9):876–885

[307] Sprakes MB, Ford AC, Warren L, Greer D, Hamlin J. Efficacy, tolerability, and predictors of response to infliximab therapy for Crohn's disease: a large single centre experience. J Crohn's Colitis. 2012; 6(2):143–153

[308] Ben-Horin S, Kopylov U, Chowers Y. Optimizing anti-TNF treatments in inflammatory bowel disease. Autoimmun Rev. 2014; 13(1):24–30

[309] Ainsworth MA, Bendtzen K, Brynskov J. Tumor necrosis factor-alpha binding capacity and anti-infliximab antibodies measured by fluid-phase radioimmunoassays as predictors of clinical efficacy of infliximab in Crohn's disease. Am J Gastroenterol. 2008; 103(4):944–948

[310] Allez M, Karmiris K, Louis E, et al. Report of the ECCO pathogenesis workshop on anti-TNF therapy failures in inflammatory bowel diseases: definitions, frequency and pharmacological aspects. J Crohn's Colitis. 2010; 4 (4):355–366

[311] Sands BE, Feagan BG, Rutgeerts P, et al. Effects of vedolizumab induction therapy for patients with Crohn's disease in whom tumor necrosis factor antagonist treatment failed. Gastroenterology. 2014; 147(3):618–627.e3

[312] Adedokun OJ, Sandborn WJ, Feagan BG, et al. Association between serum concentration of infliximab and efficacy in adult patients with ulcerative colitis. Gastroenterology. 2014; 147(6):1296–1307.e5

[313] Fausel R, Afzali A. Biologics in the management of ulcerative colitis: comparative safety and efficacy of TNF-α antagonists. Ther Clin Risk Manag. 2015; 11:63–73

[314] Colombel JF, Sandborn WJ, Rutgeerts P, et al. Adalimumab for maintenance of clinical response and remission in patients with Crohn's disease: the CHARM trial. Gastroenterology. 2007; 132(1):52–65

[315] Rojas JR, Taylor RP, Cunningham MR, et al. Formation, distribution, and elimination of infliximab and anti-infliximab immune complexes in cynomolgus monkeys. J Pharmacol Exp Ther. 2005; 313(2):578–585

[316] Afif W, Loftus EV, Jr, Faubion WA, et al. Clinical utility of measuring infliximab and human anti-chimeric antibody concentrations in patients with inflammatory bowel disease. Am J Gastroenterol. 2010; 105(5):1133–1139

[317] Vande Casteele N, Gils A, Singh S, et al. Antibody response to infliximab and its impact on pharmacokinetics can be transient. Am J Gastroenterol. 2013; 108(6):962–971

[318] Gisbert JP, Chaparro M. Use of a third anti-TNF after failure of two previous anti-TNFs in patients with inflammatory bowel disease: is it worth it? Scand J Gastroenterol. 2015; 50(4):379–386

[319] Baert F, Noman M, Vermeire S, et al. Influence of immunogenicity on the long-term efficacy of infliximab in Crohn's disease. N Engl J Med. 2003; 348 (7):601–608

[320] Ben-Horin S, Waterman M, Kopylov U, et al. Addition of an immunomodulator to infliximab therapy eliminates antidrug antibodies in serum and restores clinical response of patients with inflammatory bowel disease. Clin Gastroenterol Hepatol. 2013; 11(4):444–447

[321] Hanauer SB, Wagner CL, Bala M, et al. Incidence and importance of antibody responses to infliximab after maintenance or episodic treatment in Crohn's disease. Clin Gastroenterol Hepatol. 2004; 2(7):542–553

[322] Ong DE, Kamm MA, Hartono JL, Lust M. Addition of thiopurines can recapture response in patients with Crohn's disease who have lost response to anti-tumor necrosis factor monotherapy. J Gastroenterol Hepatol. 2013; 28 (10):1595–1599

[323] Sandborn WJ, Hanauer SB, Rutgeerts P, et al. Adalimumab for maintenance treatment of Crohn's disease: results of the CLASSIC II trial. Gut. 2007; 56 (9):1232–1239

[324] Colombel JF, Feagan BG, Sandborn WJ, Van Assche G, Robinson AM. Therapeutic drug monitoring of biologics for inflammatory bowel disease. Inflamm Bowel Dis. 2012; 18(2):349–358

[325] Farrell RJ, Alsahli M, Jeen YT, Falchuk KR, Peppercorn MA, Michetti P. Intravenous hydrocortisone premedication reduces antibodies to infliximab in Crohn's disease: a randomized controlled trial. Gastroenterology. 2003; 124 (4):917–924

[326] Grell M, Douni E, Wajant H, et al. The transmembrane form of tumor necrosis factor is the prime activating ligand of the 80 kDa tumor necrosis factor receptor. Cell. 1995; 83(5):793–802

[327] Grell M, Zimmermann G, Gottfried E, et al. Induction of cell death by tumour necrosis factor (TNF) receptor 2, CD40 and CD30: a role for TNF-R1 activation by endogenous membrane-anchored TNF. EMBO J. 1999; 18 (11):3034–3043

[328] Haridas V, Darnay BG, Natarajan K, Heller R, Aggarwal BB. Overexpression of the p80 TNF receptor leads to TNF-dependent apoptosis, nuclear factor-kappa B activation, and c-Jun kinase activation. J Immunol. 1998; 160(7):3152–3162

[329] Rutgeerts P, Van Assche G, Vermeire S. Optimizing anti-TNF treatment in inflammatory bowel disease. Gastroenterology. 2004; 126(6):1593–1610

[330] Tartaglia LA, Pennica D, Goeddel DV. Ligand passing: the 75-kDa tumor necrosis factor (TNF) receptor recruits TNF for signaling by the 55-kDa TNF receptor. J Biol Chem. 1993; 268(25):18542–18548

[331] Vande Casteele N, Gils A. Preemptive dose optimization using therapeutic drug monitoring for biologic therapy of Crohn's disease: avoiding failure while lowering costs? Dig Dis Sci. 2015; 60(9):2571–2573

[332] Loftus EV, Jr, Kane SV, Bjorkman D. Systematic review: short-term adverse effects of 5-aminosalicylic acid agents in the treatment of ulcerative colitis. Aliment Pharmacol Ther. 2004; 19(2):179–189

[333] Arts J, D'Haens G, Zeegers M, et al. Long-term outcome of treatment with intravenous cyclosporin in patients with severe ulcerative colitis. Inflamm Bowel Dis. 2004; 10(2):73–78

[334] Chaparro M, Ordás I, Cabré E, et al. Safety of thiopurine therapy in inflammatory bowel disease: long-term follow-up study of 3931 patients. Inflamm Bowel Dis. 2013; 19(7):1404–1410

[335] Garg SK, Croft AM, Bager P. Helminth therapy (worms) for induction of remission in inflammatory bowel disease. Cochrane Database Syst Rev. 2014 (1):CD009400

[336] Dignass AU, Eriksson A, Kilander A, Pukitis A, Rhodes JM, Vavricka S. Clinical trial: five or ten cycles of granulocyte-monocyte apheresis show equivalent efficacy and safety in ulcerative colitis. Aliment Pharmacol Ther. 2010; 31 (12):1286–1295

[337] Kruis W, Dignass A, Steinhagen-Thiessen E, et al. Open label trial of granulocyte apheresis suggests therapeutic efficacy in chronically active steroid refractory ulcerative colitis. World J Gastroenterol. 2005; 11(44):7001–7006

[338] Oxelmark L, Hillerås P, Dignass A, et al. Quality of life in patients with active ulcerative colitis treated with selective leukocyte apheresis. Scand J Gastroenterol. 2007; 42(3):406–407

[339] Sandborn WJ. Preliminary data on the use of apheresis in inflammatory bowel disease. Inflamm Bowel Dis. 2006; 12 Suppl 1:S15–S21

[340] Sands BE, Sandborn WJ, Feagan B, et al. Adacolumn Study Group. A randomized, double-blind, sham-controlled study of granulocyte/monocyte apheresis for active ulcerative colitis. Gastroenterology. 2008; 135(2):400–409

[341] Sawada K, Kusugami K, Suzuki Y, et al. Leukocytapheresis in ulcerative colitis: results of a multicenter double-blind prospective case-control study with sham apheresis as placebo treatment. Am J Gastroenterol. 2005; 100 (6):1362–1369

[342] Yamamoto T, Umegae S, Kitagawa T, et al. Granulocyte and monocyte adsorptive apheresis in the treatment of active distal ulcerative colitis: a prospective, pilot study. Aliment Pharmacol Ther. 2004; 20(7):783–792

[343] Wang SL, Wang ZR, Yang CQ. Meta-analysis of broad-spectrum antibiotic therapy in patients with active inflammatory bowel disease. Exp Ther Med. 2012; 4(6):1051–1056

[344] Ohkusa T, Kato K, Terao S, et al. Japan UC Antibiotic Therapy Study Group. Newly developed antibiotic combination therapy for ulcerative colitis: a double-blind placebo-controlled multicenter trial. Am J Gastroenterol. 2010; 105(8):1820–1829

[345] Koido S, Ohkusa T, Kajiura T, et al. Long-term alteration of intestinal microbiota in patients with ulcerative colitis by antibiotic combination therapy. PLoS One. 2014; 9(1):e86702

[346] Gilat T, Leichtman G, Delpre G, Eshchar J, Bar Meir S, Fireman Z. A comparison of metronidazole and sulfasalazine in the maintenance of remission in patients with ulcerative colitis. J Clin Gastroenterol. 1989; 11(4):392–395

[347] Present DH. Ciprofloxacin as a treatment for ulcerative colitis-not yet. Gastroenterology. 1998; 115(5):1289–1291

[348] Turunen UM, Färkkilä MA, Hakala K, et al. Long-term treatment of ulcerative colitis with ciprofloxacin: a prospective, double-blind, placebo-controlled study. Gastroenterology. 1998; 115(5):1072–1078

[349] Miele E, Pascarella F, Giannetti E, Quaglietta L, Baldassano RN, Staiano A. Effect of a probiotic preparation (VSL#3) on induction and maintenance of remission in children with ulcerative colitis. Am J Gastroenterol. 2009; 104 (2):437–443

[350] Kruis W, Fric P, Pokrotnieks J, et al. Maintaining remission of ulcerative colitis with the probiotic Escherichia coli Nissle 1917 is as effective as with standard mesalazine. Gut. 2004; 53(11):1617–1623

[351] Kakodkar S, Farooqui AJ, Mikolaitis SL, Mutlu EA. The specific carbohydrate diet for inflammatory bowel disease: a case series. J Acad Nutr Diet. 2015; 115(8):1226–1232

[352] Kakodkar S, Mikolaitis S, Engen P, et al. The bacterial microbiome of inflammatory bowel disease patients on the specific carbohydrate diet (SCD). Gastroenterology. 2013; 144 Suppl:S552

[353] Suskind DL, Wahbeh G, Gregory N, Vendettuoli H, Christie D. Nutritional therapy in pediatric Crohn disease: the specific carbohydrate diet. J Pediatr Gastroenterol Nutr. 2014; 58(1):87–91

[354] Ramsauer B. Duodenal infusion of feces for recurrent clostridium difficile. N Engl J Med. 2013; 368(22):2144

[355] Moayyedi P, Surette MG, Kim PT, et al. Fecal microbiota transplantation induces remission in patients with active ulcerative colitis in a randomized controlled trial. Gastroenterology. 2015; 149(1):102–109.e6

[356] Mayo-Robson A. Case of colitis with ulcerative colitis treated by inguinal colostomy. Trans Clin Soc London.. 1893; 26:213–215

[357] Keetle. Quoted by: Brooke BN. Ulcerative Colitis and Its Surgical Treatment. Edinburgh: E&S Livingston; 1954

[358] Weir R. A new use for the useless appendix in surgical treatment of obstinate colitis. Med Rec. 1902; 62:201

[359] Brown J. The value of complete physiological rest of the large bowel in the treatment of certain ulcerative and obstructive lesions of this organ. Surg Gynecol Obstet. 1913; 16:610–613

[360] Strauss A, Strauss S. Surgical treatment of ulcerative colitis. Surg Clin North Am. 1944; 24:211–224

[361] Brooke BN. The management of an ileostomy, including its complications. Lancet. 1952; 2(6725):102–104

[362] Parc YR, Radice E, Dozois RR. Surgery for ulcerative colitis: historical perspective. A century of surgical innovations and refinements. Dis Colon Rectum. 1999; 42(3):299–306

[363] Kornbluth A, Sachar DB, Practice Parameters Committee of the American College of Gastroenterology. Ulcerative colitis practice guidelines in adults: American College Of Gastroenterology, Practice Parameters Committee. Am J Gastroenterol. 2010; 105(3):501–523, quiz 524

[364] Becker JM. Surgical therapy for ulcerative colitis and Crohn's disease. Gastroenterol Clin North Am. 1999; 28(2):371–390, viii–ix

[365] Parray FQ, Wani ML, Malik AA, et al. Ulcerative colitis: a challenge to surgeons. Int J Prev Med. 2012; 3(11):749–763

[366] Danovitch SH. Fulminant colitis and toxic megacolon. Gastroenterol Clin North Am. 1989; 18(1):73–82

[367] Munkholm P. Review article: the incidence and prevalence of colorectal cancer in inflammatory bowel disease. Aliment Pharmacol Ther. 2003; 18 Suppl 2:1–5

[368] Sharan R, Schoen RE. Cancer in inflammatory bowel disease. An evidence-based analysis and guide for physicians and patients. Gastroenterol Clin North Am. 2002; 31(1):237–254

[369] Gorfine SR, Bauer JJ, Harris MT, Kreel I. Dysplasia complicating chronic ulcerative colitis: is immediate colectomy warranted? Dis Colon Rectum. 2000; 43(11):1575–1581

[370] Odze RD. Adenomas and adenoma-like DALMs in chronic ulcerative colitis: a clinical, pathological, and molecular review. Am J Gastroenterol. 1999; 94 (7):1746–1750

[371] Wiltz O, Hashmi HF, Schoetz DJ, Jr, et al. Carcinoma and the ileal pouch-anal anastomosis. Dis Colon Rectum. 1991; 34(9):805–809

[372] Riddell RH, Goldman H, Ransohoff DF, et al. Dysplasia in inflammatory bowel disease: standardized classification with provisional clinical applications. Hum Pathol. 1983; 14(11):931–968

[373] Eaden J, Abrams K, McKay H, Denley H, Mayberry J. Inter-observer variation between general and specialist gastrointestinal pathologists when grading dysplasia in ulcerative colitis. J Pathol. 2001; 194(2):152–157

[374] Odze RD, Goldblum J, Noffsinger A, Alsaigh N, Rybicki LA, Fogt F. Interobserver variability in the diagnosis of ulcerative colitis-associated dysplasia by telepathology. Mod Pathol. 2002; 15(4):379–386

[375] Bernstein CN, Shanahan F, Weinstein WM. Are we telling patients the truth about surveillance colonoscopy in ulcerative colitis? Lancet. 1994; 343 (8889):71–74

[376] Connell WR, Lennard-Jones JE, Williams CB, Talbot IC, Price AB, Wilkinson KH. Factors affecting the outcome of endoscopic surveillance for cancer in ulcerative colitis. Gastroenterology. 1994; 107(4):934–944

[377] Hata K, Watanabe T, Kazama S, et al. Earlier surveillance colonoscopy programme improves survival in patients with ulcerative colitis associated colorectal cancer: results of a 23-year surveillance programme in the Japanese population. Br J Cancer. 2003; 89(7):1232–1236

[378] Van Assche G, Dignass A, Bokemeyer B, et al. European Crohn's and Colitis Organisation. Second European evidence-based consensus on the diagnosis and management of ulcerative colitis part 3: special situations. J Crohn's Colitis. 2013; 7(1):1–33

[379] Thomas T, Abrams KA, Robinson RJ, Mayberry JF. Meta-analysis: cancer risk of low-grade dysplasia in chronic ulcerative colitis. Aliment Pharmacol Ther. 2007; 25(6):657–668

[380] Befrits R, Ljung T, Jaramillo E, Rubio C. Low-grade dysplasia in extensive, long-standing inflammatory bowel disease: a follow-up study. Dis Colon Rectum. 2002; 45(5):615–620

[381] Lim CH, Dixon MF, Vail A, Forman D, Lynch DA, Axon AT. Ten year follow up of ulcerative colitis patients with and without low grade dysplasia. Gut. 2003; 52(8):1127–1132

[382] Cairns SR, Scholefield JH, Steele RJ, et al. British Society of Gastroenterology, Association of Coloproctology for Great Britain and Ireland. Guidelines for colorectal cancer screening and surveillance in moderate and high risk groups (update from 2002). Gut. 2010; 59(5):666–689

[383] Farraye FA, Odze RD, Eaden J, Itzkowitz SH. AGA technical review on the diagnosis and management of colorectal neoplasia in inflammatory bowel disease. Gastroenterology. 2010; 138(2):746–774, 774.e1–774.e4, quiz e12–e13

[384] Vieth M, Behrens H, Stolte M. Sporadic adenoma in ulcerative colitis: endoscopic resection is an adequate treatment. Gut. 2006; 55(8):1151–1155

[385] Blackstone MO, Riddell RH, Rogers BH, Levin B. Dysplasia-associated lesion or mass (DALM) detected by colonoscopy in long-standing ulcerative colitis: an indication for colectomy. Gastroenterology. 1981; 80 (2):366–374

[386] Butt JH, Konishi F, Morson BC, Lennard-Jones JE, Ritchie JK. Macroscopic lesions in dysplasia and carcinoma complicating ulcerative colitis. Dig Dis Sci. 1983; 28(1):18–26

[387] Lennard-Jones JE, Melville DM, Morson BC, Ritchie JK, Williams CB. Precancer and cancer in extensive ulcerative colitis: findings among 401 patients over 22 years. Gut. 1990; 31(7):800–806

[388] Crile G, Jr, Thomas CY, Jr. The treatment of acute toxic ulcerative colitis by ileostomy and simultaneous colectomy. Gastroenterology. 1951; 19 (1):58–68

[389] Alves A, Panis Y, Bouhnik Y, Maylin V, Lavergne-Slove A, Valleur P. Subtotal colectomy for severe acute colitis: a 20-year experience of a tertiary care center with an aggressive and early surgical policy. J Am Coll Surg. 2003; 197(3):379–385

[390] Patel SC, Stone RM. Toxic megacolon: results of emergency colectomy. Can J Surg. 1977; 20(1):36–38

[391] Carter FM, McLeod RS, Cohen Z. Subtotal colectomy for ulcerative colitis: complications related to the rectal remnant. Dis Colon Rectum. 1991; 34 (11):1005–1009

[392] Ozuner G, Strong SA, Fazio VW. Effect of rectosigmoid stump length on restorative proctocolectomy after subtotal colectomy. Dis Colon Rectum. 1995; 38(10):1039–1042

[393] Wøjdemann M, Wettergren A, Hartvigsen A, Myrhøj T, Svendsen LB, Bülow S. Closure of rectal stump after colectomy for acute colitis. Int J Colorectal Dis. 1995; 10(4):197–199

[394] McKee RF, Keenan RA, Munro A. Colectomy for acute colitis: is it safe to close the rectal stump? Int J Colorectal Dis. 1995; 10(4):222–224

[395] Turnbull RB, Jr. Surgical treatment of ulcerative colitis: early results after colectomy and low ileorectal anastomosis. Dis Colon Rectum. 1959; 2(3):260–263

[396] Ooi BS, Remzi FH, Fazio VW. Turnbull-blowhole colostomy for toxic ulcerative colitis in pregnancy: report of two cases. Dis Colon Rectum. 2003; 46 (1):111–115

[397] Parks AG, Nicholls RJ. Proctocolectomy without ileostomy for ulcerative colitis. BMJ. 1978; 2(6130):85–88

[398] Camilleri-Brennan J, Steele RJ. Objective assessment of quality of life following panproctocolectomy and ileostomy for ulcerative colitis. Ann R Coll Surg Engl. 2001; 83(5):321–324

[399] Berry AR, de Campos R, Lee EC. Perineal and pelvic morbidity following perimuscular excision of the rectum for inflammatory bowel disease. Br J Surg. 1986; 73(8):675–677

[400] Killeen S, Devaney A, Mannion M, Martin ST, Winter DC. Omental pedicle flaps following proctectomy: a systematic review. Colorectal Dis. 2013; 15 (11):e634–e645

[401] Leong AP, Londono-Schimmer EE, Phillips RK. Life-table analysis of stomal complications following ileostomy. Br J Surg. 1994; 81(5):727–729

[402] Wikland M, Jansson I, Asztély M, et al. Gynaecological problems related to anatomical changes after conventional proctocolectomy and ileostomy. Int J Colorectal Dis. 1990; 5(1):49–52

[403] Baudot P, Keighley MR, Alexander-Williams J. Perineal wound healing after proctectomy for carcinoma and inflammatory disease. Br J Surg. 1980; 67 (4):275–276

[404] Lubbers EJ. Healing of the perineal wound after proctectomy for nonmalignant conditions. Dis Colon Rectum. 1982; 25(4):351–357

[405] Hurst RD, Gottlieb LJ, Crucitti P, Melis M, Rubin M, Michelassi F. Primary closure of complicated perineal wounds with myocutaneous and fasciocutaneous flaps after proctectomy for Crohn's disease. Surgery. 2001; 130(4):767–772, discussion 772–773

[406] Rius J, Nessim A, Nogueras JJ, Wexner SD. Gracilis transposition in complicated perianal fistula and unhealed perineal wounds in Crohn's disease. Eur J Surg. 2000; 166(3):218–222

[407] Kock NG, Darle N, Hultén L, Kewenter J, Myrvold H, Philipson B. Ileostomy. Curr Probl Surg. 1977; 14(8):1–52

[408] Murrell Z, Fleshner P. Ulcerative colitis: surgical management. In: Beck D, Roberts P, Saclarides T, et al., eds. The ASCRS Textbook of Colon and Rectal Surgery. New York, NY: Springer; 2011:479–497

[409] Litle VR, Barbour S, Schrock TR, Welton ML. The continent ileostomy: long-term durability and patient satisfaction. J Gastrointest Surg. 1999; 3(6):625–632

[410] Lepistö AH, Järvinen HJ. Durability of Kock continent ileostomy. Dis Colon Rectum. 2003; 46(7):925–928

[411] Devine H. Method of colectomy for desperate cases of ulcerative colitis. Surg Gynecol Obstet. 1943; 76:136

[412] Mortier PE, Gambiez L, Karoui M, et al. Colectomy with ileorectal anastomosis preserves female fertility in ulcerative colitis. Gastroenterol Clin Biol. 2006; 30(4):594–597

[413] da Luz Moreira A, Kiran RP, Lavery I. Clinical outcomes of ileorectal anastomosis for ulcerative colitis. Br J Surg. 2010; 97(1):65–69

[414] Leijonmarck CE, Löfberg R, Ost A, Hellers G. Long-term results of ileorectal anastomosis in ulcerative colitis in Stockholm County. Dis Colon Rectum. 1990; 33(3):195–200

[415] Pastore RL, Wolff BG, Hodge D. Total abdominal colectomy and ileorectal anastomosis for inflammatory bowel disease. Dis Colon Rectum. 1997; 40 (12):1455–1464

[416] Scoglio D, Ahmed Ali U, Fichera A. Surgical treatment of ulcerative colitis: ileorectal vs ileal pouch-anal anastomosis. World J Gastroenterol. 2014; 20 (37):13211–13218

[417] Turnbull RB, Jr, Hawk WA, Weakley FL. Surgical treatment of toxic megacolon. Ileostomy and colostomy to prepare patients for colectomy. Am J Surg. 1971; 122(3):325–331

[418] Johnson WR, McDermott FT, Hughes ES, Pihl EA, Milne BJ, Price AB. The risk of rectal carcinoma following colectomy in ulcerative colitis. Dis Colon Rectum. 1983; 26(1):44–46

[419] Baker WN, Glass RE, Ritchie JK, Aylett SO. Cancer of the rectum following colectomy and ileorectal anastomosis for ulcerative colitis. Br J Surg. 1978; 65 (12):862–868

[420] Vignolo Q. Nouveau procede operatoire pour retablir la continuite intestinale dans les resections rectosigmoidiennes etendues. Arch Gen Chir. 1912; 6:621–643

[421] Ravitch MM, Sabiston DC, Jr. Anal ileostomy with preservation of the sphincter; a proposed operation in patients requiring total colectomy for benign lesions. Surg Gynecol Obstet. 1947; 84(6):1095–1099

[422] Champeau. In: Delannoy E, Martinot M, eds.: Traitement chirugical de la rectocolite ulcero-hemorrhagique. Paris: Masson et Compagnie; 1957:86–88

[423] Goligher JC. The functional results after sphincter-saving resections of the rectum. Ann R Coll Surg Engl. 1951; 8(6):421–438

[424] Falk PM, Beart RW, Jr, Wexner SD, et al. Laparoscopic colectomy: a critical appraisal. Dis Colon Rectum. 1993; 36(1):28–34

[425] Schmitt SL, Cohen SM, Wexner SD, Nogueras JJ, Jagelman DG. Does laparoscopic-assisted ileal pouch anal anastomosis reduce the length of hospitalization? Int J Colorectal Dis. 1994; 9(3):134–137

[426] Fleming FJ, Francone TD, Kim MJ, Gunzler D, Messing S, Monson JR. A laparoscopic approach does reduce short-term complications in patients undergoing ileal pouch-anal anastomosis. Dis Colon Rectum. 2011; 54(2):176–182

[427] Causey MW, Stoddard D, Johnson EK, et al. Laparoscopy impacts outcomes favorably following colectomy for ulcerative colitis: a critical analysis of the ACS-NSQIP database. Surg Endosc. 2013; 27(2):603–609

[428] Kirat HT, Remzi FH, Kiran RP, Fazio VW. Comparison of outcomes after handsewn versus stapled ileal pouch-anal anastomosis in 3,109 patients. Surgery. 2009; 146(4):723–729, discussion 729–730

[429] Fonkalsrud EW. Total colectomy and endorectal ileal pull-through with internal ileal reservoir for ulcerative colitis. Surg Gynecol Obstet. 1980; 150 (1):1–8

[430] Nicholls RJ, Lubowski DZ. Restorative proctocolectomy: the four loop (W) reservoir. Br J Surg. 1987; 74(7):564–566

[431] Utsunomiya J, Iwama T, Imajo M, et al. Total colectomy, mucosal proctectomy, and ileoanal anastomosis. Dis Colon Rectum. 1980; 23(7):459–466

[432] Stone MM, Lewin K, Fonkalsrud EW. Late obstruction of the lateral ileal reservoir after colectomy and endorectal ileal pullthrough procedures. Surg Gynecol Obstet. 1986; 162(5):411–417

[433] Johnston D, Williamson ME, Lewis WG, Miller AS, Sagar PM, Holdsworth PJ. Prospective controlled trial of duplicated (J) versus quadruplicated (W) pelvic ileal reservoirs in restorative proctocolectomy for ulcerative colitis. Gut. 1996; 39(2):242–247

[434] Selvaggi F, Giuliani A, Gallo C, Signoriello G, Riegler G, Canonico S. Randomized, controlled trial to compare the J-pouch and W-pouch configurations for ulcerative colitis in the maturation period. Dis Colon Rectum. 2000; 43 (5):615–620

[435] Wu XR, Kirat HT, Kalady MF, Church JM. Restorative proctocolectomy with a handsewn IPAA: S-pouch or J-pouch? Dis Colon Rectum. 2015; 58(2):205–213

[436] de Zeeuw S, Ahmed Ali U, Donders RA, Hueting WE, Keus F, van Laarhoven CJ. Update of complications and functional outcome of the ileo-pouch anal anastomosis: overview of evidence and meta-analysis of 96 observational studies. Int J Colorectal Dis. 2012; 27(7):843–853

[437] Remzi FH, Fazio VW, Gorgun E, et al. The outcome after restorative proctocolectomy with or without defunctioning ileostomy. Dis Colon Rectum. 2006; 49(4):470–477

[438] Fazio VW, Kiran RP, Remzi FH, et al. Ileal pouch anal anastomosis: analysis of outcome and quality of life in 3707 patients. Ann Surg. 2013; 257(4):679–685

[439] Hueting WE, Buskens E, van der Tweel I, Gooszen HG, van Laarhoven CJ. Results and complications after ileal pouch anal anastomosis: a meta-analysis of 43 observational studies comprising 9,317 patients. Dig Surg. 2005; 22(1–2):69–79

[440] Lewis WG, Kuzu A, Sagar PM, Holdsworth PJ, Johnston D. Stricture at the pouch-anal anastomosis after restorative proctocolectomy. Dis Colon Rectum. 1994; 37(2):120–125

[441] Marcello PW, Roberts PL, Schoetz DJ, Jr, Coller JA, Murray JJ, Veidenheimer MC. Long-term results of the ileoanal pouch procedure. Arch Surg. 1993; 128(5):500–503, discussion 503–504

[442] Prudhomme M, Dozois RR, Godlewski G, Mathison S, Fabbro-Peray P. Anal canal strictures after ileal pouch-anal anastomosis. Dis Colon Rectum. 2003; 46(1):20–23

[443] Senapati A, Tibbs CJ, Ritchie JK, Nicholls RJ, Hawley PR. Stenosis of the pouch anal anastomosis following restorative proctocolectomy. Int J Colorectal Dis. 1996; 11(2):57–59

[444] Heikens JT, de Vries J, van Laarhoven CJ. Quality of life, health-related quality of life and health status in patients having restorative proctocolectomy with ileal pouch-anal anastomosis for ulcerative colitis: a systematic review. Colorectal Dis. 2012; 14(5):536–544

[445] Carmon E, Keidar A, Ravid A, Goldman G, Rabau M. The correlation between quality of life and functional outcome in ulcerative colitis patients after proctocolectomy ileal pouch anal anastomosis. Colorectal Dis. 2003; 5 (3):228–232

[446] Fazio VW, Tjandra JJ. Pouch advancement and neoileoanal anastomosis for anastomotic stricture and anovaginal fistula complicating restorative proctocolectomy. Br J Surg. 1992; 79(7):694–696

[447] Galandiuk S, Scott NA, Dozois RR, et al. Ileal pouch-anal anastomosis. Reoperation for pouch-related complications. Ann Surg. 1990; 212(4):446–452, discussion 452–454

[448] Groom JS, Nicholls RJ, Hawley PR, Phillips RK. Pouch-vaginal fistula. Br J Surg. 1993; 80(7):936–940

[449] Johnson PM, O'Connor BI, Cohen Z, McLeod RS. Pouch-vaginal fistula after ileal pouch-anal anastomosis: treatment and outcomes. Dis Colon Rectum. 2005; 48(6):1249–1253

[450] Keighley MR, Grobler SP. Fistula complicating restorative proctocolectomy. Br J Surg. 1993; 80(8):1065–1067

[451] Wexner SD, Rothenberger DA, Jensen L, et al. Ileal pouch vaginal fistulas: incidence, etiology, and management. Dis Colon Rectum. 1989; 32(6):460–465

[452] Colombel JF, Ricart E, Loftus EV, Jr, et al. Management of Crohn's disease of the ileoanal pouch with infliximab. Am J Gastroenterol. 2003; 98(10):2239–2244

[453] Cohen Z, Smith D, McLeod R. Reconstructive surgery for pelvic pouches. World J Surg. 1998; 22(3):342–346

[454] Paye F, Penna C, Chiche L, Tiret E, Frileux P, Parc R. Pouch-related fistula following restorative proctocolectomy. Br J Surg. 1996; 83(11):1574–1577

[455] Zinicola R, Wilkinson KH, Nicholls RJ. Ileal pouch-vaginal fistula treated by abdominoanal advancement of the ileal pouch. Br J Surg. 2003; 90 (11):1434–1435

[456] Lee PY, Fazio VW, Church JM, Hull TL, Eu KW, Lavery IC. Vaginal fistula following restorative proctocolectomy. Dis Colon Rectum. 1997; 40(7):752–759

[457] Ozuner G, Hull T, Lee P, Fazio VW. What happens to a pelvic pouch when a fistula develops? Dis Colon Rectum. 1997; 40(5):543–547

[458] Burke D, van Laarhoven CJ, Herbst F, Nicholls RJ. Transvaginal repair of pouch-vaginal fistula. Br J Surg. 2001; 88(2):241–245

[459] Hurst RD, Molinari M, Chung TP, Rubin M, Michelassi F. Prospective study of the incidence, timing and treatment of pouchitis in 104 consecutive patients after restorative proctocolectomy. Arch Surg. 1996; 131(5):497–500, discussion 501–502

[460] Shen B, Fazio VW, Remzi FH, Lashner BA. Clinical approach to diseases of ileal pouch-anal anastomosis. Am J Gastroenterol. 2005; 100(12):2796–2807

[461] Shen B, Achkar JP, Lashner BA, et al. Endoscopic and histologic evaluation together with symptom assessment are required to diagnose pouchitis. Gastroenterology. 2001; 121(2):261–267

[462] Sandborn WJ, Tremaine WJ, Batts KP, Pemberton JH, Phillips SF. Pouchitis after ileal pouch-anal anastomosis: a Pouchitis Disease Activity Index. Mayo Clin Proc. 1994; 69(5):409–415

[463] Pemberton JH. The problem with pouchitis. Gastroenterology. 1993; 104 (4):1209–1211

[464] Shen B, Achkar JP, Lashner BA, et al. Irritable pouch syndrome: a new category of diagnosis for symptomatic patients with ileal pouch-anal anastomosis. Am J Gastroenterol. 2002; 97(4):972–977

[465] Shen B, Lashner BA, Bennett AE, et al. Treatment of rectal cuff inflammation (cuffitis) in patients with ulcerative colitis following restorative proctocolectomy and ileal pouch-anal anastomosis. Am J Gastroenterol. 2004; 99 (8):1527–1531

[466] Shepherd NA, Hultén L, Tytgat GN, et al. Pouchitis. Int J Colorectal Dis. 1989; 4(4):205–229

[467] Shen B, Achkar JP, Connor JT, et al. Modified pouchitis disease activity index: a simplified approach to the diagnosis of pouchitis. Dis Colon Rectum. 2003; 46(6):748–753

[468] Holubar SD, Cima RR, Sandborn WJ, Pardi DS. Treatment and prevention of pouchitis after ileal pouch-anal anastomosis for chronic ulcerative colitis. Cochrane Database Syst Rev. 2010(6):CD001176

[469] Madden MV, McIntyre AS, Nicholls RJ. Double-blind crossover trial of metronidazole versus placebo in chronic unremitting pouchitis. Dig Dis Sci. 1994; 39(6):1193–1196

[470] Shen B, Achkar JP, Lashner BA, et al. A randomized clinical trial of ciprofloxacin and metronidazole to treat acute pouchitis. Inflamm Bowel Dis. 2001; 7 (4):301–305

[471] Singh S, Stroud AM, Holubar SD, Sandborn WJ, Pardi DS. Treatment and prevention of pouchitis after ileal pouch-anal anastomosis for chronic ulcerative colitis. Cochrane Database Syst Rev. 2015(11):CD001176

[472] Gionchetti P, Rizzello F, Venturi A, et al. Oral bacteriotherapy as maintenance treatment in patients with chronic pouchitis: a double-blind, placebo-controlled trial. Gastroenterology. 2000; 119(2):305–309

[473] Gionchetti P, Rizzello F, Poggioli G, et al. Oral budesonide in the treatment of chronic refractory pouchitis. Aliment Pharmacol Ther. 2007; 25 (10):1231–1236

[474] Gionchetti P, Rizzello F, Venturi A, et al. Antibiotic combination therapy in patients with chronic, treatment-resistant pouchitis. Aliment Pharmacol Ther. 1999; 13(6):713–718

[475] Mimura T, Rizzello F, Helwig U, et al. Four-week open-label trial of metronidazole and ciprofloxacin for the treatment of recurrent or refractory pouchitis. Aliment Pharmacol Ther. 2002; 16(5):909–917

[476] Barreiro-de Acosta M, García-Bosch O, Gordillo J, et al. Grupo Joven GETECCU. Efficacy of adalimumab rescue therapy in patients with chronic refractory pouchitis previously treated with infliximab: a case series. Eur J Gastroenterol Hepatol. 2012; 24(7):756–758

[477] Barreiro-de Acosta M, García-Bosch O, Souto R, et al. Grupo joven GETECCU. Efficacy of infliximab rescue therapy in patients with chronic refractory pouchitis: a multicenter study. Inflamm Bowel Dis. 2012; 18(5):812–817

[478] Calabrese C, Gionchetti P, Rizzello F, et al. Short-term treatment with infliximab in chronic refractory pouchitis and ileitis. Aliment Pharmacol Ther. 2008; 27(9):759–764

[479] Winter TA, Dalton HR, Merrett MN, Campbell A, Jewell DP. Cyclosporin A retention enemas in refractory distal ulcerative colitis and "pouchitis". Scand J Gastroenterol. 1993; 28(8):701–704

[480] Gorgun E, Remzi FH, Goldberg JM, et al. Fertility is reduced after restorative proctocolectomy with ileal pouch anal anastomosis: a study of 300 patients. Surgery. 2004; 136(4):795–803

[481] Johnson P, Richard C, Ravid A, et al. Female infertility after ileal pouch-anal anastomosis for ulcerative colitis. Dis Colon Rectum. 2004; 47(7):1119–1126

[482] Olsen KO, Joelsson M, Laurberg S, Oresland T. Fertility after ileal pouch-anal anastomosis in women with ulcerative colitis. Br J Surg. 1999; 86 (4):493–495

[483] Ørding Olsen K, Juul S, Berndtsson I, Oresland T, Laurberg S. Ulcerative colitis: female fecundity before diagnosis, during disease, and after surgery compared with a population sample. Gastroenterology. 2002; 122(1):15–19

[484] Efron JE, Uriburu JP, Wexner SD, et al. Restorative proctocolectomy with ileal pouch anal anastomosis in obese patients. Obes Surg. 2001; 11(3):246–251

[485] Canedo JA, Pinto RA, McLemore EC, Rosen L, Wexner SD. Restorative proctectomy with ileal pouch-anal anastomosis in obese patients. Dis Colon Rectum. 2010; 53(7):1030–1034

[486] Klos CL, Safar B, Jamal N, et al. Obesity increases risk for pouch-related complications following restorative proctocolectomy with ileal pouch-anal anastomosis (IPAA). J Gastrointest Surg. 2014; 18(3):573–579

[487] Reissman P, Teoh TA, Weiss EG, Nogueras JJ, Wexner SD. Functional outcome of the double stapled ileoanal reservoir in patients more than 60 years of age. Am Surg. 1996; 62(3):178–183

[488] Dayton MT, Larsen KR. Should older patients undergo ileal pouch-anal anastomosis? Am J Surg. 1996; 172(5):444–447, discussion 447–448

[489] Tan HT, Connolly AB, Morton D, Keighley MR. Results of restorative proctocolectomy in the elderly. Int J Colorectal Dis. 1997; 12(6):319–322

[490] Takao Y, Gilliland R, Nogueras JJ, Weiss EG, Wexner SD. Is age relevant to functional outcome after restorative proctocolectomy for ulcerative colitis?: prospective assessment of 122 cases. Ann Surg. 1998; 227(2):187–194

[491] Delaney CP, Fazio VW, Remzi FH, et al. Prospective, age-related analysis of surgical results, functional outcome, and quality of life after ileal pouch-anal anastomosis. Ann Surg. 2003; 238(2):221–228

[492] Pinto RA, Canedo J, Murad-Regadas S, Regadas SF, Weiss EG, Wexner SD. Ileal pouch-anal anastomosis in elderly patients: is there a difference in morbidity compared with younger patients? Colorectal Dis. 2011; 13(2):177–183

[493] Ramage L, Qiu S, Georgiou P, Tekkis P, Tan E. Functional outcomes following ileal pouch-anal anastomosis (IPAA) in older patients: a systematic review. Int J Colorectal Dis. 2016; 31(3):481–492

[494] Wu XR, Kiran RP, Mukewar S, Remzi FH, Shen B, Shen B. Diagnosis and management of pouch outlet obstruction caused by common anatomical problems after restorative proctocolectomy. J Crohn's Colitis. 2014; 8(4):270–275

[495] Coull DB, Lee FD, Henderson AP, Anderson JH, McKee RF, Finlay IG. Risk of dysplasia in the columnar cuff after stapled restorative proctocolectomy. Br J Surg. 2003; 90(1):72–75

[496] O'Riordain MG, Fazio VW, Lavery IC, et al. Incidence and natural history of dysplasia of the anal transitional zone after ileal pouch-anal anastomosis: results of a five-year to ten-year follow-up. Dis Colon Rectum. 2000; 43 (12):1660–1665

[497] Remzi FH, Fazio VW, Delaney CP, et al. Dysplasia of the anal transitional zone after ileal pouch-anal anastomosis: results of prospective evaluation after a minimum of ten years. Dis Colon Rectum. 2003; 46(1):6–13

[498] Kariv R, Remzi FH, Lian L, et al. Preoperative colorectal neoplasia increases risk for pouch neoplasia in patients with restorative proctocolectomy. Gastroenterology. 2010; 139(3):806–812, 812.e1–812.e2

[499] Banasiewicz T, Marciniak R, Paszkowski J, et al. Pouchitis may increase the risk of dysplasia after restorative proctocolectomy in patients with ulcerative colitis. Colorectal Dis. 2012; 14(1):92–97

[500] Duff SE, O'Dwyer ST, Hultén L, Willén R, Haboubi NY. Dysplasia in the ileoanal pouch. Colorectal Dis. 2002; 4(6):420–429

[501] Hurlstone DP, Shorthouse AJ, Cross SS, Brown S, Sanders DS, Lobo AJ. High-magnification chromoscopic pouchoscopy: a novel in vivo technique for surveillance of the anal transition zone and columnar cuff following ileal pouch-anal anastomosis. Tech Coloproctol. 2004; 8(3):173–178, discussion 178

[502] Remzi FH, Gorgun E, Bast J, et al. Vaginal delivery after ileal pouch-anal anastomosis: a word of caution. Dis Colon Rectum. 2005; 48(9):1691–1699

[503] Gearhart SL, Hull TL, Schroeder T, Church J, Floruta C. Sphincter defects are not associated with long-term incontinence following ileal pouch-anal anastomosis. Dis Colon Rectum. 2005; 48(7):1410–1415

[504] Cornish JA, Tan E, Teare J, et al. The effect of restorative proctocolectomy on sexual function, urinary function, fertility, pregnancy and delivery: a systematic review. Dis Colon Rectum. 2007; 50(8):1128–1138

26 Crohn's Disease

Scott R. Steele and Steven D. Wexner

Abstract

Crohn's disease remains a complex disease process with many different manifestations. Although advances in medical therapy continue to evolve and significantly alter the way patients are managed, surgeons still play a large role in both the medical and surgical therapy of the disease. Due to its recurring nature, surgeons must adhere to the principles of preventing and managing disease complications versus aiming for cure. By focusing on the maximization of functional outcomes, surgeons can optimize outcomes through a multimodality approach and minimize additional complications. All providers caring for Crohn's disease must be cognizant of the wide array of presentations and inherent difficulties in managing this disease. Medical management remains the mainstay of therapy, although the majority of patients will require surgery at some point in their life due to complications associated with the disease. Adherence to principles of surgery and a thorough understanding of the recurring nature of the disease will aid in allowing patients to have the best outcomes.

Keywords: Crohn's disease, fistula, fissure, colitis, anorectal, inflammatory bowel disease

26.1 Introduction

Despite being a relatively common inflammatory disorder, Crohn's disease (CD) remains an enigma, with the spectrum of disease widely variable, the pathogenesis still unknown, and the treatment strategies continuing to evolve. Early reports in the latter half of the 1800s of CD-like inflammation surfaced that included mostly obstructive symptoms, and were more attributed to ulcerative colitis or intrinsic strictures. Interestingly, the vast majority of pathological findings were located in the colon.[1] When it finally was described, this disorder may have just as easily been referred to by another eponym had the authors decided against going with the alphabetized listing of its authors (Crohn, Ginzburg, and Oppenheimer) in the 1932 JAMA publication "Regional ileitis: a pathological and clinical entity."[2] In this publication, the authors were able to successfully characterize the inflammatory condition that led to strictures and multiple fistulas; however, they incorrectly felt it was localized to the terminal ileum. Had the authorship proceeded with a more prosurgical angle, the entity may have been named Berg's disease, as it was the idea of Dr. A.A. Berg, a surgeon, to evaluate the original 52 specimens who were also his patients.[3] Moreover, some readers may not realize that one of the initial descriptions of the condition was actually first made in 1769 by the Italian physician Giovanni Battista Morgagni—the same physician who named anal columns, the aortic sinus, and the space for certain types of congenital diaphragmatic hernias.[4] Over time, our understanding of this condition, its epidemiology, and pathogenesis has improved. From Lockhart-Mummery and Morson's accurate description of CD in the large intestine in 1960[5,6] to the identification of the NOD2 genetic abnormality associated with a susceptibility to CD in 2001,[7] our knowledge

regarding a broad array of aspects of this idiopathic, ulcerogenic, inflammatory condition of the gastrointestinal (GI) tract continues to evolve.

To date, CD remains a predominately medically treated condition, with several new classes of medical therapy available for both primary and recalcitrant disease. Yet, somewhat hidden in this fact is that three-quarters or more of all patients will require at least one operation during their lifetime.[6] Furthermore, the waxing and waning of symptoms, propensity for recurrence, and varying intervals between flares result in a lack of a "one-size-fits-all" treatment approach. All physicians, regardless of specialty, must therefore be cognizant of the impact of treatment decisions, as not only must the problem at hand be addressed, but also the patient's future function must be carefully weighed when considering the proper therapeutic endeavor. Surgeons need to be exceedingly aware of the indications, surgical options, and expected outcomes for patients with CD, as well as have a thorough understanding of the principles guiding both medical and surgical care to maximize outcomes. While operative intervention may be required to address complications of the disease or in the setting of failed medical management, these overriding doctrines need to be balanced with avoiding an overaggressive surgical approach that can dramatically impact the patient's future course.

26.2 Epidemiology

The true incidence and prevalence of CD is unknown. In part, this data void is secondary to the wide variety of presentations of the disease, for which a patient's symptoms may be inaccurately attributed to another diagnosis. Yet with improved diagnostic methods and a higher degree of awareness and focus on the disease itself, CD has seen an increase in incidence during the last 50 years.[8] Traditionally, CD is described as having a bimodal distribution relative to age of onset, initially between 15 and 30 years, followed by a later, albeit smaller, peak in the sixth to ninth decades.[7] More recently, systematic reviews have found an annual incidence of CD ranging from 20.2 per 100,000 person-years in North America and 12.7 per 100,000 person-years in Europe to 5.0 per 100,000 person-years in Asia and the Middle East.[9] Looking longitudinally, the mean age at diagnosis has slowly shifted from late teens to late 20 s to early 30 s, although this finding may be more of an indicator that more patients are living longer and being diagnosed later in life—artificially pushing the mean to the right.[10] Even within regions, variations exist—the incidence in western Europe is almost twice that of eastern Europe, whereas the highest incidence of inflammatory bowel disease (IBD) in the world is in the Faroe Islands. Within England, Hindus and Sikhs have a lower risk than does the general population. While data in developing countries remain relatively sparse, both the incidence and prevalence of CD are increasing in the United States and around the world, including more recently in Asia. There is also an association with latitude, with increased incidences in higher latitude areas (including Canada, Scandinavia, and Australia) compared to regions closer to the equator. Gender has a yet undefined role, with some reports stating a 20 to 30% increased risk of CD in women, and other demonstrating males and females to be equally affected. Ethnicity has a much more established pattern, with whites and certain ethnic groups such as those of Ashkenazi Jewish descent having higher overall rates.[11] In general, Native American Indian and Black populations are affected at much lower rates.

Although CD is not inherited through traditional Mendelian genetics, it appears to have a familial predisposition that leads to higher rates within families. A family history in patients with CD occurs in 2 to 14% of patients.[12] This statistic translates to 15- to 35-fold increase among family members above the general population. Even closer examination reveals an approximate 5% age-adjusted lifetime risk of a first-degree relative of a CD proband developing IBD (up to 8% for those of Jewish ancestry).[13] The concordance rate for monozygotic twins ranges from 20 to 50%,[14] suggesting that genetics do play a role and that the disease is not entirely dependent on environmental and/or acquired factors. Furthermore, there does not appear to be a genetic concordance with the phenotypical manifestations of fibrostenotic, fistulizing, phlegmonous, or extent of disease among relatives. This risk does not seem to affect second-degree relatives, as they do not appear to have an increased risk association.

26.3 Etiology and Pathogenesis

Despite tremendous progress in the overall understanding of the disease and advancements in the comprehension of the various phenotypical manifestations, the exact etiology of CD remains unknown. Most hypotheses include interplay among the genetic composition of the individual along with environmental, bacteriological, immunological, and epidemiological factors that contribute to its development. Leading theories suggest that CD involves one or more of the following: (1) an antigen or infectious source, (2) a weakened host defense that allows for greater exposure to that source, or (3) an abnormal host response (▶ Table 26.1).[15] Efforts in each of these areas continue in attempt to determine which are causative factors versus those that are simply associations.

Current theories revolve around the host–microbiome interaction, and the variable response that occurs along several pathways that may ultimately lead to the chronic inflammatory state seen in CD.[16] In this model, intestinal microorganisms initiate an inappropriately regulated host immune response that results in a cascade of events ranging from altered permeability of the intestinal lumen to autoimmune "attacks" on several host organ systems.[17] This defective mucosal barrier allows exposure

Table 26.1 Possible etiological factors associated with Crohn's disease

Source	Associative factors
I. Genetics	Positive family history, IBD genes, ethnicity
II. Immune	Mucosal abnormalities/barrier, adaptive immunity (B- and T-cell response), pathogen recognition, microbiome
III. Infectious	Bacterial pathogens (*Mycobacterium avium paratuberculosis*), viral (paramyxovirus, measles)
IV. Environmental	Smoking, NSAIDs, location

Abbreviations: IBD, inflammatory bowel disease; NSAID, nonsteroidal anti-inflammatory drugs.

to luminal antigens as well as creates a microenvironment where continuous stimulation of underlying cells upregulates an inflammatory cascade leading to an out-of-proportion and inappropriate proinflammatory response. As such, the fecal and intestinal mucosal bacterial composition is known to be altered in CD patients; however, it is unknown if this occurs as a result of the inflammatory process, or is itself a contributing factor to disease development.[18] Furthermore, this alteration in mucosal permeability has been demonstrated to be present in up to 10 to 15% of CD family members that do not display any characteristics of the disease. Whether the permeability is a primary causative factor or the end result of another process remains undetermined. What seems more clear through proteomic and metagenomic evaluation of commensal and altered GI microbiota in CD patients is that there is an inappropriate pattern recognition with the microbiota serving as the driver of the disease pathogenesis.[19]

Beginning in 1996, linkage studies of the human genome have helped with the discovery of several IBD genes that signify patients who are susceptible to CD development.[20] Most attention has revolved around the NOD2 (formerly CARD15) gene on chromosome 16, a region felt to be involved in host interactions with bacterial lipopolysaccharide.[21] Genetic differences in the pattern-recognition proteins for which NOD2 codes may lead to an impaired sensing and handling of bacteria by the immune system, disrupting the tenuous balance of normal tolerance versus initiating an incorrect immune response. Since then, genome-wide association studies have provided insight that polymorphisms in genes such as ATG16L1 and IRGM play a role in autophagy in patients with CD. This process involves the regulation of cell development and differentiation, senescence, and ultimately the inflammatory system response to what the body deems is normal and abnormal.[22] In addition, other genes such as TLR4, HLA, and IRF5 are involved in the innate and adaptive immune system response seen in CD patients. Other causative immune factors have included overexpression and dysregulation of tumor necrosis factor (TNF), an imbalance between proinflammatory and anti-inflammatory cytokines, and an impaired mucosal susceptibility in sampling gut antigens.[23] Combined, all these contribute to regulatory mechanisms that may be altered and play a role in CD pathogenesis.

Infectious theories also persist,[24] with specific organisms including *Mycobacterium avium* subspecies *paratuberculosis* (i.e., Johne's disease), *Campylobacter concisus*, adherent-invasive *Escherichia coli* (AIEC), and non–*H. pylori Helicobacter* species among the most common agents cited. Although the beneficial effects of antibiotics in the treatment of CD provide indirect evidence for a bacterial etiology, no distinct organism has been identified to date. Similarly, several viruses have been postulated to have an association with CD, the most common being Epstein–Barr virus (EBV), cytomegalovirus (CMV), and measles. However, systematic reviews have found little evidence to support this notion.[25] Additionally, environmental factors are felt to play a role, highlighted by the well-established link to smoking with both an increased susceptibility and worsened clinical course. Smokers have been shown to have an odds ratio over threefold for the development of the disease, as well as more flares, worse clinical and endoscopic disease severity, higher rate of recurrent disease, and much more apt to undergo resection when compared to nonsmokers.[8,26,27] Food also appears to play a role. While patients with CD frequently have concomitant food intolerances, the role of dietary habits remains debatable.[28] Previously, dietary factors ranging from refined sugar, starches, dietary fats, and low fiber have been described as having an association with the development of CD. However, the dietary theory has not been proven; rather than a causative effect, it is felt that the microbiome in the human GI tract is heavily influenced by dietary intake, leading to a local environment ripe to foster susceptibility to CD. Finally, oral contraceptive use has been shown to increase the risk anywhere from 1.4-fold to fivefold, with higher rates with prolonged use,[27,29] and something that may be diminished in part or altogether following discontinuation. The mechanism for this association remains unknown.

26.4 Pathology

26.4.1 Microscopic Examination

Classically, the presence of noncaseating granulomas on pathological examination is pathognomonic of CD. However, in reality they are only found in 25 to 42% of patients, and may simply be a marker of more virulent disease.[30] In addition, occasional granulomas may be found in patients with chronic mucosal ulcerative colitis (MUC).[31] Furthermore, granulomas may be present but are not typically demonstrated on the specimens that are taken with routine depth endoscopic biopsies, rather only visible on resected full-thickness specimens. Other histological evidence of CD includes architectural distortion of the size, shape, and symmetry of the crypts, ulcerations, pseudopolyps, and skip areas—some of which may also be found in ulcerative colitis.

26.4.2 Gross Examination

Discriminating features of CD include the potential for full-thickness involvement of the bowel wall due to transmural inflammation. This disease manifestation results in coalescing of the aphthous ulcerations and formation of a cobblestone mucosal appearance. The inflammation is demonstrated in the mucosa and submucosa when viewed endoscopically. Externally, the presence of "creeping fat," where the mesenteric fat extends over the serosal surface of the bowel wall, results in the characteristic fat "creeping" over the normally distinct mesenteric/bowel wall interface. Gross pathological examination of CD specimens may range from acutely inflamed, edematous, hyperemic bowel to thickened, fibrotic, or "woody." Finally, the mesentery is classically thickened, with marked edema and friability, and is generally hypervascular in nature. This translates into a foreshortened mesentery in active and even chronic disease. The bowel will have areas of dilation proximal to a stricture(s), which are also interspersed by segments of normal-appearing bowel. Finally, in contrast to ulcerative colitis, the disease may occur anywhere along the GI tract from mouth to anus.

26.5 Diagnosis

The diagnosis of CD relies upon a combination of clinical, radiological, endoscopic, and laboratory findings. Simple well-known CD facts such as the absence of a "curative" surgery, and a disease hallmarked by lifelong periods of flares and quiescent disease provide some insight but are not enough to make the definitive diagnosis. CD falls under the umbrella of IBD along with ulcerative colitis, as well as indeterminate colitis. In both CD and ulcerative colitis, there is no specific test at present to permit a definitive diagnosis; rather this combination of history and physical examination, laboratory, radiographic, and endoscopic findings is crucial. Unfortunately, approximately 5 to 15% of patients with ulcerative colitis will eventually be diagnosed with CD, and this fact may have widespread ramifications if they have undergone a restorative proctocolectomy. In addition, certain patients are labeled as having indeterminate colitis, due to their expression of manifestations of both diseases.[32,33]

26.5.1 Laboratory Analysis

No single laboratory examination will provide a definitive diagnosis of CD; yet, there are tests available to help discriminate between CD and other disease processes. Routine serum profiles such as perinuclear antineutrophil cytoplasmic antibodies (p-ANCA) and anti-*Saccharomyces cerevisiae* antibodies (ASCA) have traditionally been used to help differentiate CD from ulcerative colitis. The former is a known marker associated with ulcerative colitis, whereas elevated levels of ASCA are associated with CD. Unfortunately, only 30 to 50% of CD patients will test positive for ASCA, and up to 10% of healthy individuals will also have elevated serum levels.[34]

C-reactive protein is a nonspecific marker for inflammation that has been useful in tracking disease activity and response to treatment. More recently, fecal biomarkers such as fecal calprotectin,[35] lactoferrin, and neopterin[36] are used to monitor intestinal inflammation, and have been shown to reliably correlate with disease activity and mucosal healing as measured endoscopically.[37] In addition, they may play a role in helping make a distinction between IBD and functional bowel disorders, with reported sensitivities and specificities of approximately 80 to 85%.[38] While nonspecific, persistent elevations in fecal biomarkers have been shown also to correlate with higher levels of recurrence following surgical resection.[39]

Serologic and Genetic Markers

Despite all efforts, certain IBD patients may be unclear as to which underlying disorder afflicts them: CD, ulcerative colitis, or indeterminate colitis. In these situations, serum testing with the Prometheus (San Diego, CA) antigen testing panel is a useful diagnostic aid. This panel uses two 2-mL (serum and whole blood) specimens to test for various serogenetic markers such as ASCA, OmpC, CBir1, pANCA, and single nucleotide polymorphism (SNP) 8, SNP12, and SNP13. This CD prognostic test combines the serologic markers with the genetic mutations with the goal of identifying the risk of developing disease complications and determining optimal treatment options. While disease progression is the primary focus of the CD prognostic test, other Prometheus testing is most helpful in excluding IBD, but may also have a role in differentiating between MUC and indeterminate colitis and CD.[6,40] At present, these biomarkers may be found in up to 80% of patients with IBD (not just CD), while these will be absent in approximately 15 to 20% with IBD. Unfortunately, to date the panel still lacks the specificity to reliably determine the definitive diagnosis. Hopefully as additional antigens and markers are added to the panel, these types of tests will become more clinically useful.

26.5.2 Radiology

Radiological evaluation of patients with CD is an invaluable part of the assessment. In addition to providing information on the acuity of the process, diagnostic imaging is used to determine the extent of disease, any associated fistula or abscess, and enable periodic review of disease status during treatment.

Plain Films

A radiological evaluation with plain films is often a routine part of the diagnostic evaluation of these patients, though the degree to which it is helpful is debatable. An abdominal flat plate and upright film can aid in simple things such as in the setting of a possible bowel obstruction, to exclude toxic megacolon, or to evaluate for pneumoperitoneum. While these studies are quick and easy to obtain and provide focused information in light of the clinical scenario, they lack specificity.

Fluoroscopic Imaging

Historically, contrast studies such as a barium enema helped diagnose CD by identifying longitudinal and transverse linear ulcerations that create cobblestone and nodular patterns, skip lesions, fistulas, and strictures.[41] A small bowel follow-through had also been a long-standing modality utilized to evaluate for strictures, active disease (highlighted by ulceration, mucosal granularity, and loss of villous morphology), and fistulas. Yet, with newer studies such as computed tomography (CT) and magnetic resonance (MR) enterography, traditional barium studies are becoming more infrequent. Although these studies may be performed only with single-contrast techniques, double-contrast techniques with radio-opaque contrast media followed by X-ray-negative distended contrast media or air may be utilized. Negative aspects include the manpower and time it takes to complete, along with the radiation exposure to the patient.

Computed Tomography

In many centers, CT has now largely replaced the barium enema and small bowel follow-through, with the added ability to identify the extent of the disease and involvement of surrounding structures, manifested by segmental bowel thickening, mesenteric fat stranding, and intra-abdominal fluid.[42] Additionally, CT is useful to identify secondarily involved organs or provide information that may be pertinent to preoperative planning, such as bladder or vaginal air indicating presence of a fistula, an adjacent psoas abscess in ileocecal disease, or ureteral obstruction that may require stenting. CT and MR enterography provide improved detail of the mucosal surface and are especially useful in depicting fistulas and strictures, along with the added benefit of lower levels of radiation exposure. The latter benefit is especially relevant considering the generally younger patient population, body habitus, and potential need for lifelong repeat imaging associated with CD.

Magnetic Resonance Imaging

MR enterography in particular has been shown to be over 85% accurate in predicting stenosis, abscess, and fistula in preoperative planning, as well as changing the surgical strategy/approach in up to 10% of CD patients.[43] Furthermore, its sensitivity (85–90%), specificity (100%), and negative predictive value (77%) have made it ideal for detecting recurrent disease after surgery.[44,45]

Magnetic resonance imaging (MRI) has also been particularly useful in the evaluation of complex perianal fistulas seen in CD patients, identifying secondary "hidden" tracts and occult abscesses that lend to higher failure rates if not addressed.[46] More recently, diffusion-weighted imaging and magnetization transfer imaging sequences have allowed bowel resolution previously not achievable to help identify disease, depict disease activity, and target interventions.[47]

Positron Emission Tomography Scan

Another modality typically not associated with IBD, fluorine-18 fluorodeoxyglucose (F^{18}-FDG) positron emission tomography (PET) has been used for the assessment of CD largely in academic and research centers to date.[48] While cost seems to be somewhat prohibitive, this emerging indication has the potential to (1) determine disease activity in a noninvasive manner, (2) provide information regarding subclinical disease, (3) deliver a qualitative measure of response to treatment, and (4) indicate disease activity that would otherwise be unobtainable by traditional methods.

Video Capsule Endoscopy

Finally, video capsule endoscopy uses wireless technology to capture continuous images of the upper GI tract mucosa. As up to 30% of patients will have disease limited to the small bowel, capsule endoscopy plays a unique role to determine disease presence and activity that are outside the reach of endoscopy and the limitations of traditional small bowel imaging. While the diagnostic yield may not be as high, it has been shown to be comparable to ileocolonoscopy and better than small bowel follow-through for the detection of small bowel inflammation.[49] Furthermore, negative predictive values range from 96 to 100%, essentially ruling out the diagnosis of CD when the results are normal.[50] It is imperative to exclude the presence of moderate-severe strictures prior to its use, as their presence can result in bowel obstruction from the capsule becoming lodged at the point of stenosis.

26.5.3 Endoscopy

Whereas direct observation of the perianal area and anoscopy will identify disease such as skin tags, external fistula openings and fissures, endoscopy is needed to identify the extent and severity of the disease and perform biopsies to aid in diagnosis.[51] In the clinic, flexible or rigid sigmoidoscopy can be performed as adjuncts to the physical examination to evaluate the mid-to-upper rectum and sigmoid colon. However, endoscopic evaluation of the entire colon, including the terminal ileum, with colonoscopy along with appropriate biopsies is required in patients suspected of CD. Early changes seen in the mucosa include aphthous ulcerations, erosions, and serpiginous ulcers that occur in a skip-type pattern. As the full-thickness inflammatory cycle continues, these ulcerated areas become progressive, enlarge, and coalesce, forming the cobblestone-type pattern. The presence of rectal sparing and terminal ileal disease may help differentiate CD from ulcerative colitis, although the latter findings may demonstrate similar characteristics due to medical therapy and backwash ileitis, respectively.[52] Finally, the presence of strictures or associated masses may indicate the need for surgical or therapeutic intervention.

Esophagogastroduodenoscopy (EGD) also plays a role for patients with suspected or known proximal disease and can identify ulcers, fistulas, and strictures that may be responsible for various upper GI symptoms. In addition, EGD allows for therapeutic intervention such as dilation for patients with gastric outlet obstruction.[53] Overall, upper and lower endoscopies are relatively safe procedures with complications occurring in less than 5% of patients,[54] generally consisting of bleeding, although perforation remains a very insignificant risk of any endoscopic procedure. Additionally, endoscopic evaluation provides an ability to track and quantify disease activity by use of the scoring systems such as the CD endoscopic index of severity (CDEIS) or Simple Endoscopic Score for CD (SES-CD).[55]

The Crohn's Disease Activity Index (CDAI) has long been the primary outcome measure used in clinical trials to study the impact of new medications for the treatment of CD. Regressing 18 clinical items against a 4-point global rating of disease activity created the CDAI.[17] Eight independent predictors were identified including liquid/soft stool frequency, abdominal pain severity, general well-being, extraintestinal symptoms, need for antidiarrheal drugs, and presence of an abdominal mass, hematocrit, and body weight. Regression coefficients for each of the eight predictors were ascertained to generate an overall CDAI score that ranges from 0 to 600. Benchmarks for disease activity were established as follows:

- Clinical remission CDAI less than 150.
- Mild disease CDAI of 150 to 219.
- Moderate disease CDAI of 220 to 450.
- Severe disease CDAI greater than 450.

Clinical response has been subsequently defined as a reduction from the baseline score of more than 70 to 100 points. The majority of the CDAI score stems from items recorded in a symptom-based, 1-week diary including stool frequency, pain, and overall well-being. Further studies have proven that the CDAI can be simplified to these patient-reported variables without a significant compromise in the instrument's responsiveness.[18,19]

26.6 Differential Diagnosis

The differential diagnosis in CD is wide and includes both benign and malignant processes (▶ Table 26.2). While CD has certain traits that are more suggestive of its presence such as noncontiguous multisite disease, fistulas, and creeping fat, a variety of abdominal processes may mimic CD. It is not an uncommon scenario for ileocolic CD to be ultimately diagnosed from a clinical picture that may at first resemble acute appendicitis, right-sided diverticulitis, an infectious process, or a perforated malignancy. Radiological studies may demonstrate similar patterns of bowel inflammation, laboratory examination often shows elevated CRP and/or white blood cell counts in each, and the patient demographics are routinely alike. This dilemma occurs intraoperatively; a decision must then be made regarding whether or not to proceed with resection versus closure and medical management alone based on clinical findings. If a resection is performed,

Table 26.2 Differential diagnosis of Crohn's disease

Ulcerative colitis/indeterminate colitis

Clostridium difficile infection

Acute appendicitis

Meckel's diverticulitis

Diverticulitis or diverticular-associated colitis

Other infectious colitides:
- CMV
- *Yersinia*
- *E. coli*
- *Salmonella*
- Tuberculosis

Ischemic colitis

Radiation enteritis

Behçet's disease

Malignancy

Celiac sprue

Abbreviation: CMV, cytomegalovirus.

questions arise regarding the extent of resection such as whether or not to perform an ileocecectomy versus appendectomy alone and what margins of resection are required for the situation at hand.

When confronted with suspected CD in the operating room, traditional teaching recommends performing an appendectomy if the cecum is normal, or to withhold on resection and undergo medical treatment only. However, data also support performing an ileocolic resection at the time of surgery. One series reported that almost half of patients required no further surgery as a result of their CD, compared to 92% of those undergoing appendectomy only (65% within the next 3 years).[56] Hence, early ileocolonic resection may be in the patient's long-term best interests to avoid recurrent disease and repeated trips to the operating room.

When disease is isolated to the colon, the major differentiation involves distinguishing Crohn's colitis from ulcerative colitis, though other infectious and inflammatory colitides remain in the differential. As previously noted, many of the same clinical and histopathological traits are shared in both diseases, and contribute to the initial diagnostic dilemma, as well as those patients with indeterminate colitis or those who undergo a change in diagnosis from ulcerative colitis to CD. Ultimately, the entire evaluation includes information taken from laboratory, pathologic, endoscopic, radiologic, and clinical examinations as outlined earlier that will help clarify the picture and aid in diagnosis.

26.7 Classification

Once diagnosed, patients with CD are often categorized in several different manners, the most common of which involves either the site of disease or the patient's phenotypical manifestations: fibrostenotic, fistulizing, or inflammatory.

26.7.1 Location

By location, the ileum (~60%) has the highest disease incidence. Localized inflammation in the ileocecal region occurs in approximately 45% of patients, whereas approximately 25 to 33% will have colonic involvement, 25% will have more proximal small bowel disease, and less than 10% will have upper GI or perianal disease (▶ Fig. 26.1). In general, patients with concomitant perianal disease tend to have a more severe clinical course,[57] and perianal disease in the setting of CD may precede abdominal manifestations in up to 45%.[58]

Phenotypical Manifestations

When stratifying by disease pattern or phenotype, patients may have fibrostenotic (stricturing), fistulizing (penetrating), or inflammatory (phlegmonous) characteristics. Due to the heterogeneous nature of the disease, these manifestations may occur concomitantly or independently, or may even vary along the longitudinal course of the disease. Fibrostenotic patterns may occur in any location, though these occur most commonly in the terminal ileal region, where patients present with obstructive-type symptoms such as nausea, vomiting, and decreased oral intake. Due to the recurrent chronic nature that results in progressive thickening of the bowel wall, medical management is typically unsuccessful and surgical intervention is required. Inflammatory disease may present with a wide range of symptoms such as abdominal pain, fever, an abdominal mass, and/or weight loss. Bowel movements may either be diarrhea or conversely follow an obstructive pattern due to luminal narrowing or extrinsic compression from the phlegmon. Finally, penetrating or fistulizing disease also has a variable presentation. Patients may be completely asymptomatic, as in the case of many entero-enteral fistulas, present with anorectal abscesses and/or fistulas, or more commonly complain of symptoms mirroring involvement of the secondarily involved organ–recurrent urinary tract infections or pneumaturia, vaginal discharge, diarrhea, cutaneous feculent drainage, and/or hip/back pain from

psoas involvement. While medical management continues to be a major component of each of the latter two patterns, surgery is often required for resolution of symptoms.

Montreal Classification

A summary of the revised Montreal classification is shown in ▶ Table 26.3.

26.7.2 Clinical Evaluation

Small Bowel

The distribution of disease will in large part dictate the clinical presentation. The terminal ileum, including the cecum, is the most commonly affected site, in addition to isolated more proximal small bowel disease. Patients with disease in this location will classically present with abdominal pain, fever, fatigue, nausea, and vomiting. The weight loss seen is a byproduct of both decreased oral intake and the malabsorptive process associated with CD. When the disease is in the terminal ileum and ileocecal region, patients may present with a slow onset of right lower quadrant pain following meals, an abdominal mass, and (when the psoas is involved) pain with hip extension. Obstructive symptoms may also occur in patients with either fibrostenotic or acute inflammation. Diarrhea tends to be nonbloody, though heme-positive stools may occur, and rarely gross blood is a manifestation from a small bowel source.

Colonic

Colonic involvement may occur in isolation in approximately one in four patients, though it is most often seen concomitantly in those with perianal (left-sided) or terminal ileal (cecal and

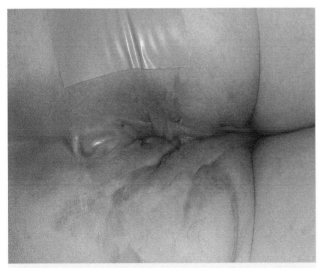

Fig. 26.1 Anal Crohn's disease.

Table 26.3 Montreal classification

Age at diagnosis (A)		
A1	16 y or younger	
A2	17–40 y	
A3	Over 40 y	
Location (L)		Upper gastrointestinal modifier (L4)
L1	L1 terminal ileum	L1 + L4
L2	L2 colon	L2 + L4
L3	L3 ileocolon	L3 + L4
L4	L4 Upper gastrointestinal	–
Behavior (B)		Perianal disease modifier (p)
B1	Nonstricturing Nonpenetrating	B1P
B2	Stricturing	B2P
B3	Penetrating	B3P

ascending colon) disease.[59] Within the colon, the distribution is somewhat variable, with approximately one-third of patients having total colonic involvement, 40% showing segmental disease, and left-sided only in up to 30%.[60] Regardless of the exact location within the large intestine, patients with colonic involvement may experience abdominal pain and, in some cases, malnutrition. Diarrhea is often of smaller volume and may be from several sources—salt/water and bile acid malabsorption, infection (CMV), or as a result of an enterocolonic fistula.[61,62] Unlike ulcerative colitis, rectal bleeding is not routine, and bowel movements are often nonbloody, except in those with moderate-to-severe Crohn's colitis. In addition, similar to disease in the small bowel, patients can experience hip pain from fistulas, cramping, and obstructive symptoms. Patients with chronic disease may also demonstrate pseudopolyps on endoscopic examination.

Anorectal

Bissell was the first to describe the anorectal component of CD, almost 2 years after the original description of the disease.[63] Despite advances in the understanding of many features of CD, perianal complaints have been recognized as one of its most challenging aspects. Isolated perianal disease is the presenting symptom in approximately 5 to 15% of CD patients; however, over the course of their lifetime, it is seen in 25 to 80%. The perianal area in CD has classically been felt to be a "window" into the abdomen, and perianal involvement is clearly more common in those with concomitant rectal or colonic disease.[64,65] In addition, active disease in the perineum is felt to act as a harbinger of an overall more virulent course.[66] The traditional anorectal complaints witnessed in non-CD patients are similar to those with the disease, including "standard" hemorrhoids, fissures, abscesses, and fistulas. However, CD patients may also manifest edematous (elephant ear) skin tags, blue discoloration of the anus, and abscesses and fistulas that are often recurrent, multiple, and located well away from the anal verge. While fissures

due to hypertonicity may be identified, more often CD fissures present as deep-seated, burrowing fissures—more like ulcers—and may be multiple, off the midline, extending in the muscle and associated with large skin tags. Finally, patients with long-standing CD may develop anal stenosis or an anal stricture (▶ Fig. 26.2) at the verge secondary to repeated bouts of chronic inflammation.

Clinical evidence of perianal CD, as manifested by many of these features, is often deemed a hallmark of disease diagnosis, although a biopsy may rarely be considered. Due to local sepsis and perianal tenderness, pain due to one or more fissures or stenosis, patients may need to undergo an examination under anesthesia to fully identify the extent of the disease. Patients presenting with perianal findings consistent with CD should undergo a full alimentary tract evaluation, as previously stated, with endoscopic and radiological evaluation. In addition, a thorough physical examination to identify any extraintestinal manifestations should be performed. A very clinically relevant, easy-to-use septic perianal CD index has been described and is recommended.[67]

Upper Gastrointestinal Disease

Upper GI CD encompasses disease from the mouth through the jejunum. The incidence of upper tract involvement varies widely, with most studies reporting overall rates of less than 5%. In patients with ileocolic disease, concomitant upper GI manifestations occur in 0.5 to 13%, yet up to 40% of patients will demonstrate early subclinical evidence of CD on radiological and endoscopic evaluation.[68] Importantly, when patients have upper GI CD, they almost uniformly have concomitant disease of lower tract and should be evaluated to determine the extent of involvement. Upper tract disease is hallmarked by both obstructive symptoms and fistulas.[69] Patients typically present with abdominal pain, cramping, nausea, vomiting, or intolerance of oral intake leading to weight loss. While fistulas may be virtually to any site, the majority involving the proximal tract are gastrocolic or ileogastric in nature. Patients may be asymptomatic or present with

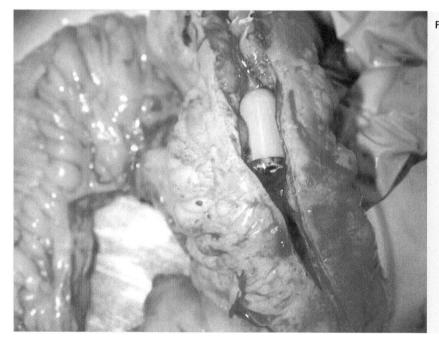

Fig. 26.2 Crohn's disease–related anal stricture.

diarrhea from high-output and colonic involvement. CD of the esophagus is exceedingly rare, involving less than 0.5% of patients. Most patients will have inflammation or ulcers, though strictures and fistulas have also been reported. As with other upper tract CD, extraesophageal disease is nearly always present.[70]

26.8 Treatment

26.8.1 Medical Management

First, despite the spectrum of disease presentations, with the exception of isolated perianal CD, the hallmark of CD remains inflammation with abdominal pain and diarrhea. As such, supportive care to include antidiarrheals and antimotility agents, along with a bland diet, is a good first-line approach to provide symptomatic control (▶ Table 26.4). It is important to exclude the concomitant presence of "super-infections" such as CMV or *Clostridium difficile* infection, as bowel-slowing medications may result in the onset of toxic megacolon (▶ Fig. 26.3) and a rapidly progressive clinical deterioration. Yet, simple over-the-counter, readily available medications such as loperamide, diphenoxylate, and bismuth, along with prescription medications such as codeine and tincture of opium, often provide tremendous relief to abdominal pain, cramping, and loose stools.

CD has also been traditionally called a "wasting disease," though increasing numbers of obese patients with CD are observed. Despite this seeming paradox, nutritional support in both groups remains paramount. Ideally, preservation of oral feeding in any form is crucial for maintenance of the absorptive and protective mechanisms provided by the GI mucosal lumen villi and microvilli. However, when enteral feeding is not possible, parenteral nutrition has become invaluable in preserving nutritional stores, aiding in positive nitrogen balance, preventing weight loss, and improving perioperative outcomes.[71] This must be weighed against the potential complications involved with intravenous routes to include infectious complications and thromboembolic events.

A tiered strategy for medical therapy is often utilized, taking into account the disease activity (flare vs. chronic), pattern (inflammatory vs. fistulizing vs. fibrotic), and location. Antibiotics and aminosalicylates are typically used in the induction and maintenance of remission, respectively, especially for patients with mild-to-moderate disease. Antibiotics are also utilized for the treatment of an acute infection for both the abdominal and perianal locations, with metronidazole and fluoroquinolones among the most commonly used antibiotics. In select cases, antibiotics can be given to patients with perianal disease including fistulas for maintenance of remission as well as decreasing pain. While the exact mechanism of action of antibiotics in CD is debated, by decreasing bacterial load and altering the bacterial milieu of the GI tract, disease activity is lessened. ▶ Table 26.5 lists the class of medications and their role in therapy.

Aminosalicylates

Aminosalicylates (5-ASA) are traditionally used as first-line maintenance agents, and are generally well tolerated by patients. Depending on the predominant location of the disease, different moieties can be formulated to allow maximal drug

Table 26.4 Medical treatment for Crohn's disease

Class of medication	Examples	Role in therapy
Steroids	Prednisone Prednisolone Methylprednisolone Budesonide[a]	Induction of remission
Immunomodulators	6-mercaptopurine Methotrexate Azathioprine Tacrolimus Cyclosporine[b]	Maintenance of remission Induction in select cases
5-ASA	Sulfasalazine Pentasa Mesalamine Olsalazine	Maintenance of remission In mild cases
Biologics	Infliximab Adalimumab Certolizumab Vedolizumab Natalizumab	Induction and maintenance of remission
Antibiotics	Metronidazole Ciprofloxacin	Induction of remission Treatment of infection

Abbreviation: ASA, aminosalicylates.
[a]Budesonide is taken enterally and has only topical effect, no systemic effect.
[b]Cyclosporine can be used as rescue therapy/induction in refractory cases, but has not been supported by evidence in the treatment of Crohn's disease.

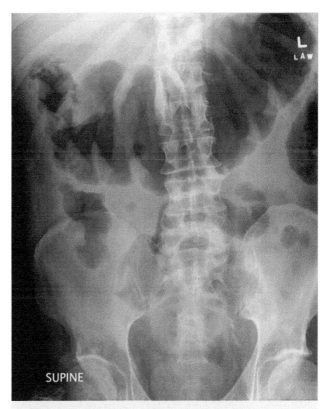

Fig. 26.3 Toxic colitis.

Table 26.5 Class of medications in treatment of Crohn's disease

Class of medication	Examples	Role in therapy
Biologics	Infliximab Adalimumab Certolizumab Natalizumab	Induction and maintenance of remission
Immunomodulators	6-mercaptopurine Methotrexate Azathioprine Tacrolimus Cyclosporine[a]	Maintenance of remission Induction in select cases
Steroids	Prednisone Prednisolone Methylprednisolone Budesonide[b]	Induction of remission
Aminosalicylates	Sulfasalazine Pentasa Mesalamine Olsalazine	Maintenance of remission In mild cases
Antibiotics	Metronidazole Ciprofloxacin	Induction of remission Treatment of infection

[a]Cyclosporine can be used as rescue therapy/induction in refractory cases, but has not been supported by evidence in the treatment of Crohn's disease.
[b]Budesonide is taken enterally and has only topical effect, no systemic effect.

concentration to be targeted at the appropriate site. 5-ASA compounds are not aspirin or nonsteroidal derivatives, though they do work to decrease proinflammatory mediators and function at the mucosal level with reduced systemic absorption. Similar to antibiotics, the mechanism of action in IBD remains unclear, though levels of nuclear factor-κB (NF-κB), TNF, and interleukin-1 have all been shown to decrease, as well as inhibiting both B- and T-cell function.[72] Additionally, they can be used in the perioperative period without increasing the risk of postoperative complications. Overall, this class of medications has been shown to prevent disease flares and minimize CD activity index for patients with mild disease, though the results have been inconsistent with questionable clinical benefit.[73] However, at most they have little downside and there are some data to suggest a decrease in disease recurrence following resection.

Steroids

Steroids remain a mainstay for both the induction and maintenance of remission; they are especially useful in the setting of disease flares, where a "burst" followed by a weaning strategy may allow some of the more well-tolerated medications to be initiated as a maintenance regimen. Purported advantages to steroids include their low cost, ability to give via the intravenous, oral, and rectal routes, and the relative speed and efficacy with which they are able to help achieve quiescent disease. However, approximately 14 to 45% of patients will ultimately have steroid recalcitrant disease, requiring either an escalation of medical therapy or surgical resection. Additionally, the wide range of potential complications of steroids ranging from adrenal suppression, insulin-resistance, ocular disease, and osteopenia to psychosis, acne and weight gain, limits durable sustained use considerably. Budesonide is a synthetic corticosteroid that is taken orally or rectally, and the steroid effect is predominantly local due to a significant first-pass metabolism in the liver. While pooled analysis demonstrated inferior effects compared to systemic steroids, it has been shown to maintain rates of remission higher than placebo and comparable to prednisolone for those with mild disease.[74]

Immunomodulators

The immunomodulator class of medications includes 6-mercaptopurine, azathioprine, methotrexate, tacrolimus, and cyclosporine. They work via different mechanisms of action, yet all serve a common purpose to alter the immune system in some capacity to blunt the patient's intrinsic response to what is considered "foreign" and to decrease inflammation. The first two (thiopurines) act via inhibition of purine synthesis, and must be monitored, as metabolites can lead to bone marrow suppression and hepatotoxicity. These drugs are useful for both induction and maintenance of remission and particularly helpful in dose reduction and weaning patients from prednisone.[75] They also have a longer onset of action, and may take months until the full effect of the medication is witnessed. Methotrexate inhibits dihydrofolate reductase, also inhibiting purine and pyrimidine synthesis, and ultimately cytokine production. Its effects are better demonstrated with intramuscular or subcutaneous injection compared to oral ingestion, where both induction and remission rates are significantly worse.[76] Side effects range from blood dyscrasias and secondary malignancies to pneumonitis and hepatic fibrosis, and serial monitoring of liver function tests is recommended.

Biological Agents

The comparatively new groups of medications are the biological agents such as infliximab, adalimumab, and certolizumab, which are monoclonal antibodies targeting TNF-α. They are also administered via subcutaneous or intravenous injection, with dosing intervals dependent on the patient response. Adalimumab is a fully human monoclonal antibody, and while still possible, provides the advantage of being less likely to develop drug antibodies than infliximab.[77] Together they are extremely useful in the induction of remission, and more and more are utilized as first-line therapy for moderate-to-severe disease (especially those with fistulizing disease), as well as in the maintenance of remission for medically refractory patients. Several large-scale multicenter randomized trials including CLASSIC I and II, CHARM, PRECiSE-1 and WELCOME have all demonstrated not only their collective efficacy, but also the ability to induce and maintain remission in patients who had previously lost response to one of the other agents.[78] However, they are not without reported significant side effects, including anaphylaxis, secondary malignancies, and opportunistic infections. Patients should be tested for latent tuberculosis (TB) prior to their administration to avoid resurgence of TB. Additionally, there is considerable debate in the literature as to their impact on perioperative complications and anastomotic leaks, with large center studies reporting contradictory results, and pooled analysis demonstrating a nonsignificant trend toward increased total complications (odds ratio [OR]: 1.72; 95% confidence interval [CI]: 0.93–3.19).[79] Despite this controversy, discretion may warrant consideration for diversion when these medications are used in the setting of higher risk anastomoses.

Anti-Integrin Antibodies

Vedolizumab is a slightly different monoclonal antibody that works via blockade of integrin α4β7 (lymphocyte Payer's patch adhesion molecule 1 or LPAM-1). Following Food and Drug Administration (FDA) approval in 2014, it has been used in both ulcerative colitis and CD patients essentially as a second- or third-line agent following medical failures. It has been demonstrated to lead to induction and maintenance of remission in 41 and 47%, respectively. Similar to early concerns with the other monoclonal antibodies, the optimal timing and impact on surgical outcomes have yet to be elucidated.

Natalizumab is another biologic agent used in CD patients. Like vedolizumab, it is almost exclusively used to induce remission as a second- or third-line agent. Unique to this agent, it has been associated with the John Cunningham (JC) virus reactivation/infection and the onset of progressive multifocal leukoencephalopathy; therefore, serologic testing for JC virus is performed prior to initiating natalizumab.

26.9 Operative Management

26.9.1 Indications for Surgery

One of the basic tenets in the management of CD is that surgery is typically reserved either for failure of medical therapy including intractable disease and steroid dependency or complications from the disease. Failure of medical management is still the most common reason for surgery in patients with CD, especially in individuals with colonic disease. Complications resulting in a potential need for operative intervention include fistula, abscess, obstruction (stricture), growth retardation, perforation, extraintestinal disease (EID), bleeding, and malignancy (▶ Table 26.6). Of note, hemorrhage in CD tends to be a more rare event, and is more commonly seen in ulcerative colitis or diverticular disease. Each of these manifestations will be outlined in the following sections. Despite improvements in medical therapy, over 70% of all CD patients will require surgery at some point in their lives, with almost half of those undergoing one operation requiring additional procedures. Therefore, having a firm understanding of the general principles and technical specifics is important to surgeons who care for these patients.

General Principles

While CD can affect the entire GI tract from mouth to anus, certain over-riding principles can help guide the planning and operative management. First, CD is a process marked by lifelong potential for recurrence; therefore, preservation of bowel when possible and consideration of future function are paramount concerns during the planning phase.[80] Next, the extent of resection required is dependent on multiple factors, including location and duration of disease, ability to exclude malignancy, and

Table 26.6 Perioperative complications of bowel resection in Crohn's patients[a]

Complication	Incidence (%)
Bleeding	1–5
Anastomotic leak	1.3–17[b]
Anastomotic stricture	6–13
Anastomotic recurrence of disease	15–39
Bowel obstruction/ileus	5–23
Abscess/intra-abdominal sepsis (excluding leak)	2.1–15
Wound infection	10–33
Thromboembolic	1.4–3.3

[a]Risk factors: malnutrition, obesity, emergent surgery, immunosuppressant use, smoking, older age, open approach, stoma surgery.
[b]Depending on location and definition (clinical vs. radiological).

prior resections that may have resulted in shortened small bowel. In addition, as the stools tend to be loose, consideration must be given to rectal compliance and sphincter function during surgical planning to avoid a "perineal colostomy," whereby in-continuity management is preserved, but the patient has no control. Furthermore, unlike ulcerative colitis, segmental resection for both small and large bowels is common with ileocolonic, colocolonic, and rectal anastomoses, all playing a role in avoiding a permanent stoma while maximizing functional bowel.[81] Patients with Crohn's pancolitis with rectal sparing may undergo a total abdominal colectomy with ileorectal anastomosis, while rectal involvement may mandate a total proctocolectomy with end ileostomy.[82] Total proctocolectomy with ileal pouch-anal anastomosis is typically discouraged, and is normally the result of an initial misdiagnosis of ulcerative colitis or indeterminate colitis.

Technical tips also come into play when planning for CD resections. For example, when performing a proctectomy, it is important to consider the potential for a delayed or nonhealed perineal wound. An intersphincteric dissection, which maximizes the amount of healthy muscle/tissue remaining, facilitates closure in attempt to avoid this complication. Some patients will require more extensive procedures such as flaps that utilize adjacent tissues including gracilis or bulbocavernosus muscles.[83] In addition, as in the small bowel, length of resection margins does not influence the risk of relapse with segmental resections, and only grossly normal bowel is all that is required.[84] Finally, diversion may be more commonly used due to both the presence of active disease and the potential negative healing effects of the CD medications.

Abdominal Fistulas

Intra-abdominal fistulas may arise from either the small or large bowel and can affect nearly every adjacent structure. Similar to any fistula, it is important to determine the site of origin of the fistula, as this section of bowel will typically require a resection to relieve symptoms. Alternatively, a section of bowel may simply be involved in the process secondarily as a "bystander," in which case the preferred treatment is to resect the fistula and primarily repair the site. It is important to ensure there is not significant active disease at the closure site; such disease may predispose to healing problems including a subsequent leak. In this case, the preferred strategy would be to perform a segmental resection.[85] Transmural bowel inflammation and communication can also occur more commonly with the skin, bladder, or vagina. Once again, the bowel is the offending organ and should be resected, and resection of the fistula with primary closure of the recipient organ defect is appropriate treatment. While the vaginal defect is often primarily closed, defects in the bladder may be treated by bladder catheter drainage until a contrast study documents healing. Similarly, skin openings are left to heal by secondary intent. In certain cases, the inflammatory process is so intense, or there is a concern for concomitant malignancy, that the entire process should be resected en bloc. When an abscess is present, it is often preferable to percutaneously drain the abscess and ensure adequate medical therapy (that often includes biologics), prior to embarking on abdominal exploration.[86] Finally, asymptomatic enteroenteric or enterocolonic fistulas are often best medically treated, especially with the relative success of anti-TNF agents.[87]

Obstruction and Stricture

Strictures in CD most commonly occur in the terminal ileum, but may arise anywhere along the GI tract. Due to the transmural inflammation, it is not uncommon to have luminal narrowing within the bowel especially following repeated flares. However, the underlying pathophysiology may be from a phlegmonous/inflammatory process or secondary to the fibrostenotic pattern of disease. In the former setting, medical management may be successful, decreasing the inflammation and resolving the intrinsic or extrinsic "compression" on the bowel wall. Conversely, patients with fibrotic strictures typically have little to no response to medical management (including anti-TNF agents) and most often require surgery.[88,89] Emerging evidence suggests early treatment of strictures with aggressive biological therapy may aid in preventing the onset of fibrosis, especially in patients younger than 40 years, prior to the onset of the irreversible cascade of fibrosis where surgery becomes inevitable.[90]

Strictures also differ somewhat based on their location. The rate of colonic strictures has been reported to be as high as 7 to 17%.[91] In general, these benign strictures are responsive to medical management as well as endoscopic dilation for moderate- to high-grade stenosis. Complicating the situation, malignancy has been shown to be present in approximately 7% of all colonic strictures,[92] and CD carries an increased risk of colorectal cancer above the general population. Furthermore, it is very difficult to differentiate malignant from benign strictures on strictly clinical basis. Therefore, all colonic strictures should undergo endoscopic evaluation and biopsy. If malignancy is detected (or the lesion appears worrisome and remains indeterminate on workup), a standard oncological resection should normally be performed. For clearly benign strictures nonresponsive to medical management, endoscopic dilation has been shown to provide symptomatic relief. Technical success occurs in approximately 70 to 90%, and provides initial symptomatic resolution in over 80% of patients.[93] Unfortunately, most patients with colonic strictures require repeated dilations. The procedure is generally safe, with hemorrhage and perforation occurring in less than 5%, which most often occurs when balloon diameters over 25 mm are used. Although concomitant direct injection of the stricture with steroids or treatment with systemic steroids immediately after dilation has demonstrated some success in case series, the true effect of injections remains uncertain.

Strictures of the small bowel have been reported in 20 to 40% of CD patients.[94] Treatment typically consists of medical management, although depending on the severity many patients will require intervention. Small bowel strictures are often amenable to dilation via double-balloon enteroscopy, especially in the 10- to 20-mm range, though perforation is a known risk.[95,96] Symptomatic relief occurs in approximately 75 to 90% following the first dilation, while approximately 30 to 40% will require repeated intervention over the next 3 years. The cumulative dilation-free rate following successful dilatation at 3 years is approximately 40 to 50%.[97] Overall complications including pain, fistula, fevers, bleeding, and perforation occur in approximately 10 to 15% of patients; major complications occur in less than 5% of patients.[98] Despite this success, many will require operative intervention when symptoms fail to resolve, repeated bouts occur, or when a stricture is associated with a nonresolving inflammatory process, malnutrition, immunosuppression, or fistula. Options then include strictureplasty (see below) or resection.

Strictureplasty preserves bowel length by avoiding resection. The Heineke–Mikulicz (▶ Fig. 26.4) method involves a longitudinal incision along the antimesenteric border of the bowel

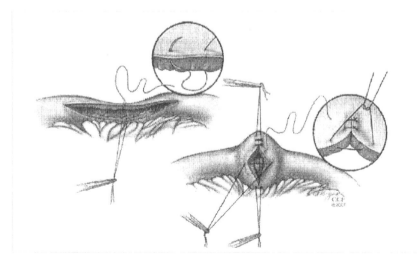

Fig. 26.4 Heineke–Mikulicz strictureplasty. (Reprinted with permission from Cleveland Clinic Center for Medical Art & Photography © 2007-2017. All rights reserved.)

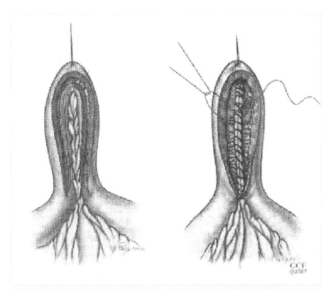

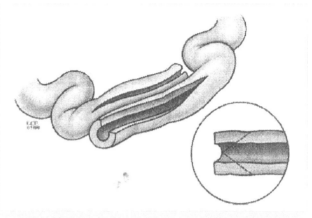

with a transverse closure, and is useful for shorter segments of bowel. Additional techniques include the Finney strictureplasty (▶ Fig. 26.5), classically used for longer strictures of 7 to 15 cm in length, where the diseased segment is opened longitudinally, the bowel is folded upon itself, and a full-thickness anastomosis is formed. In another method, an isoperistaltic Michelassi strictureplasty is created such that the narrowed diseased portion of the bowel is anastomosed to the dilated segment of an adjacent loop in a side-to-side (▶ Fig. 26.6) manner. Complications have been reported in 4 to 15% in large series, and include obstruction, bleeding, sepsis, perforation, and death.[99,100] Overall, 5-year recurrence rates for strictureplasty in jejunoileal and ileocolonic locations have been reported in between 25 and 30%, including approximately 3% site-specific recurrence. Similar to endoscopic dilation, malnutrition, presence of a phlegmon/perforation/fistula at the site, multiple strictures within a small segment, and suspicion of a malignancy are all contraindications to strictureplasty.[101]

Strictures at prior anastomotic sites may occur from recurrent disease or secondary to technical problems. They are often amenable to dilation,[102] yet they are often fibrotic in nature and nonresponsive, thus requiring resection for symptomatic strictures. To prevent postoperative stricture, side-to-side stapled anastomoses following ileocolonic resection may be associated with a lower rate of postoperative complications (OR = 0.54), leak (OR = 0.45), recurrence (OR = 0.2), and reoperation (OR = 0.18) when compared to handsewn end-to-end anastomoses.[103,104]

Hemorrhage

Although patients with CD may complain of bloody stools, hemorrhage in CD is fairly uncommon. Possible sources include deep ulcerations, toxic colitis, an underlying mass, or concomitant diverticular bleed. Significant upper GI bleeding is also rare, and is likely from a secondary source other than CD including ulcer, varices, esophageal tear, and malignancy. Similar to any other patient with a significant GI hemorrhage, patients require continued resuscitation, correction of any coagulopathy, and transfusion as indicated. Adjunctive measures such as intravascular vasopressin and infliximab have also been described,[105,106] though they should not be considered first-line agents. Endoscopy is the most useful diagnostic and therapeutic maneuver for bleeding from either an upper or lower source. When endoscopy or medical therapy is unsuccessful or bleeding recurs, segmental resection is preferred when the source is localized in the large or small bowel. In the setting of nonlocalized disease, every effort should be made to identify the source of bleeding, including upper and lower endoscopy, nuclear medicine scans, angiography, and small bowel evaluation (push endoscopy, video capsule endoscopy, or small bowel follow-through). However, in the unstable or nonlocalizable lower source, a subtotal colectomy with end ileostomy may be required.[107] In the case of upper GI bleeding, the source may be localized and controlled with endoscopy or may require a resection or ligation as in patients without CD depending on the underlying pathology.

26.10 Location, Intervention, and Results

26.10.1 Gastroduodenal Disease

As previously stated, gastroduodenal disease occurs in 0.5 to 4% of all CD patients. The most common indications likely to require advanced or surgical intervention involve stricture/obstruction, fistula, or bleeding. Isolated gastric disease is even more rare,[108] as the stomach will hardly ever be the sole source for the patient's complaints. It is important to exclude *H. pylori* infection, gastritis (NSAIDs), ulcers, and malignancy in the absence of disease elsewhere in the GI tract. Most patients will respond to medical management, especially with the anti-TNF-α therapy.[109] Gastric outlet obstruction at the level of the pylorus and first portion of the duodenum is often amenable to endoscopic balloon dilation, with avoidance of surgery in approximately half of patients.[110]

Duodenal strictures are more frequent with disease in this location, and case series have demonstrated successful amelioration of symptoms with endoscopic dilation.[111] More often, symptomatic duodenal strictures nonresponsive to medical therapy will be managed by strictureplasty, resection, or to a lesser extent, bypass (gastrojejunostomy). As previously noted, the type of strictureplasty will depend on the location, mobility of the bowel, and length of the stricture.[112] Fistulas typically arise from disease located more distally in the small bowel, and therefore require resection of the primary site with closure of the stomach or duodenum. Occasionally, the upper tract is the original site of the fistula and resection or bypass is required. With appropriate expertise, a laparoscopic approach has been associated with fewer complications and improved recovery. If bypass is performed, vagotomy is not needed; however, every effort should be made to avoid bypass if possible, as this is associated with worsening diarrhea and nutritional abnormalities.[113] For those cases where resection or closure of the duodenum is required, a jejunal serosal patch or Roux-en-Y duodenojejunostomy may help minimize wound breakdown and recurrent fistulas.[114]

26.10.2 Small Bowel Disease

Most small bowel disease is amenable to surgical resection and primary anastomosis (▶ Fig. 26.7). As previously described, strictureplasty is another option for those patients with short bowel, multiple sites of noncontiguous disease, and early recurrence—especially for noninflammatory patterns. Following resection, consideration should be given to the nutritional status of the patient, medications, and overall physiologic state, as diverting stoma may be required to minimize the incidence and consequences of an anastomotic leak. A minimally invasive approach, similar to other disease states, has been associated with improved short-term outcomes in CD patients including decreased morbidity, shorter length of stay, and reduced hospital charges for both primary and recurrent disease.[115] In addition, despite some contradictory evidence, laparoscopy and open approaches appear to have similar long-term rates of disease recurrence.[116]

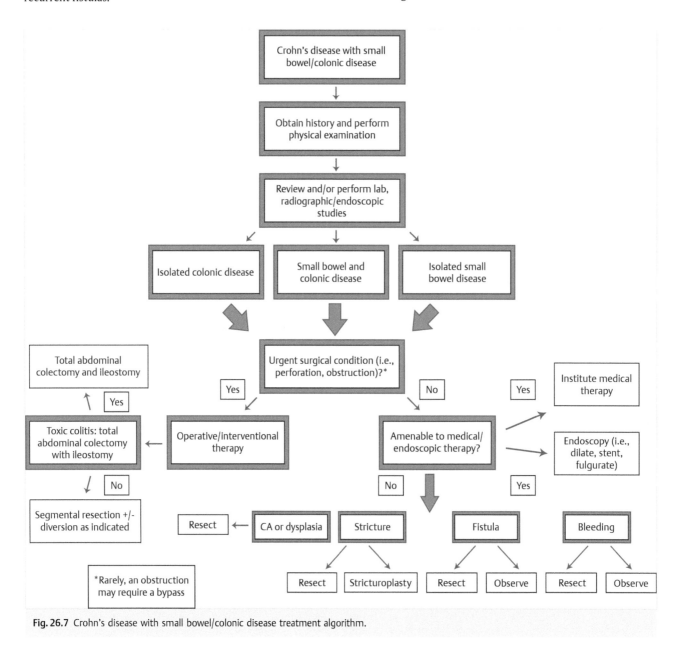

Fig. 26.7 Crohn's disease with small bowel/colonic disease treatment algorithm.

Bypass is rarely performed for small bowel disease. The rare case of a septic, obstructed patient with a large terminal ileum/ascending colon phlegmon involving the retroperitoneum that does not allow for safe mobilization or identification of the ureter and vascular anatomy may be one indication where bypass could still prove useful. These procedures have largely been abandoned as the underlying inflammatory process remains and has not been adequately addressed. Therefore, resection and strictureplasty continue to be the primary modalities to approach small bowel disease.

The surgical treatment of colonic CD is in large measure contingent upon the location of the CD. In instances of ileocolic and/or right-sided disease, an ileocolic resection with anastomosis is generally preferable. Similarly, isolated sigmoid disease, which is secondary to an enterocutaneous fistula from small bowel CD is generally managed by takedown of the fistula perhaps with a segmental sigmoid colectomy. The other scenario upon which there is general agreement is pancolonic CD, which would result in a total proctocolectomy if the rectum is involved or perhaps a subtotal colectomy and ileorectal anastomosis if the rectum is spared. The larger dilemma is when the patient has primary sigmoid CD and/or other segmental CD. In these instances, a segmental colectomy can be performed albeit with a potentially higher risk of both anastomotic leak and disease recurrence. Accordingly, it may be preferable to perform a subtotal colectomy with ileorectal anastomosis if one or more segments of the left and/or transverse colon are involved by CD. Similarly, even if the rectum is spared, severe perianal fistulizing CD may necessitate total proctocolectomy. These issues must be discussed in great detail with the patient prior to arriving upon a decision. In order to facilitate this discussion, a significant amount of preoperative imaging is necessary including both radiographic and endoscopic visualizations as well as histopathologic biopsy assessment.

The mesentery in active CD always presents a particular challenge for surgeons. Due to its thick, edematous nature with increased neovascularization, adequate hemostasis is always a point of concern. Safe division in the era of open surgery involved techniques such as overlapping clamps with both mass and individual vessel suture ligation, where appropriate. Laparoscopic approaches typically rely on advanced vessel sealing devices for hemostasis, though they may be inadequate in the CD mesentery. They can generally be safely used by subdividing the mesentery to allow smaller bites and dividing as distal (near the bowel) as possible. Surgeons must then rely on other means such as placing an ENDOLOOP (Ethicon, Cincinnati, OH) on the major vessels or by intracorporeal suturing. Crucial to whatever method is used is to avoid mesenteric hematomas, as such hematomas may result in continued bleeding as well as compromise the blood supply to the healthy remaining bowel.

The most important principle in the resection and anastomosis of small bowel in patients with small bowel CD is the ability to achieve grossly CD-free margins. There is some debate about the importance of achieving margins, which by microscopic evaluation are also uninvolved, but the body of evidence seems to favor gross rather than microscopic negative margins as the predictor of anastomotic leak and recurrence.

26.10.3 Colorectal Conditions

Toxic Colitis

Toxic colitis may occur in CD patients similar to those with ulcerative colitis (▶ Fig. 26.7).[117] Following resuscitation and intravenous steroids or immunosuppressants, emergent surgical intervention is often required for those with recalcitrant disease, perforation, or a deteriorating clinical state (▶ Fig. 26.8). The operative procedure of choice is a subtotal colectomy with end ileostomy. Debate exists as to the handling of the rectal stump, though options include a distal mucus fistula with remnant sigmoid, implantation into the subcutaneous space, or local reinforcement of the stump. Proctocolectomy should be avoided in this situation due to the prolonged operative time and increased risk of morbidity and mortality.

While acute colitis has traditionally been treated by laparotomy, an increasing body of evidence supports the benefits of laparoscopic subtotal colectomy with ileostomy. The ability to perform such a procedure is in large measure based upon the skill of the surgeon and the availability of a team to support such a procedure in what may be off hours in the operating room. Assuming the availability of a well-trained surgical team, this approach can confer significant benefits upon the patient. It is important that these patients understand that a laparotomy is possible. In addition, inability to appropriately visualize the intra-abdominal structures during laparoscopy and/or tissue which when gently handled results in potential hemorrhage and/or fecal spillage may be best managed through a larger incision. If laparoscopy can be safely performed, which it probably can in the majority of circumstances, the distal sigmoid can be stapled shut and left in situ, and the entire specimen delivered either through umbilical or superpubic incision or potentially through the stoma site. The surgeon must be cautious not to stretch the stoma site to preclude optimal stoma formation after specimen extraction. Therefore, if the colon is

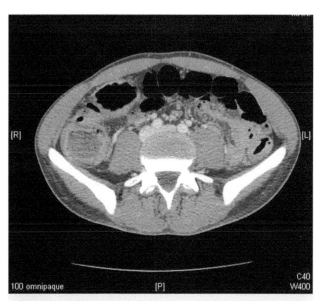

Fig. 26.8 Pneumatosis of the colon.

tremendously dilated and/or friable, the risks of stoma site dilatation and fecal contamination, respectively, should direct the surgeon to an alternate extraction incision. Regardless of the site chosen for specimen extraction, a wound protector should be used.

Ileoanal Pouch

Ileoanal pouch in the patient with CD most commonly occurs in the setting of an initial diagnosis of ulcerative colitis or indeterminate colitis. More often to the point, the pouch is performed, and the patient will subsequently manifest CD. While certain expert centers may advocate total proctocolectomy and ileal pouch construction for carefully selected patients with CD,[118] in general, this practice should be discouraged. Retrospective studies have reported 35 to 93% of patients will have CD-related complications such as pouchitis, abscesses, and pouch-anal fistulas, with another 10% requiring pouch excision or permanent diversion. Furthermore, roughly half of patients will experience urgency or continence issues. Moreover, greater than 50% of patients with CD in whom a restorative proctocolectomy was undertaken will continue to require medication to treat active CD.[91,119,120]

26.10.4 Treatment of Anorectal Conditions

A distinguishing characteristic of the surgical treatment for anorectal CD is to first consider whether or not they are symptomatic (▶ Fig. 26.9). As a follow-on principle, aggressive

intervention in the asymptomatic patient is unwarranted and potentially dangerous.

Specific Clinical Disease Processes

Anal Skin Tags and Hemorrhoids

CD patients often suffer from skin tags that appear large, edematous, and blue-colored (▶ Fig. 26.10). Similarly, they may also suffer from external hemorrhoids that may bleed, prolapse, and cause difficulty with hygiene and irritation (▶ Fig. 26.11). It is important to keep in mind that CD patients have the propensity for poor healing, especially in the face of diarrhea. Patients should be counseled as to the risk of nonhealing wounds, continence problems, and mucus drainage.[121] Therefore, at least an initial attempt at conservative treatment with warm Sitz baths and control of diarrhea is warranted. During this time, medical therapy toward CD should be also optimized, as active inflammation/proctitis will lead to increased morbidity. Should a conservative route fail, in the absence of active proctitis a standard hemorrhoidectomy may be performed. Topical metronidazole has been shown to improve post-hemorrhoidectomy pain as well as healing, with very little downside.[122] Finally, although internal hemorrhoids may occur as in any other patient, they tend to be less symptomatic and often respond to conservative measures.

Anorectal Abscess/Fistula

CD patients pose a particular challenge in the treatment of perianal fistula disease, with perianal pathology being present in

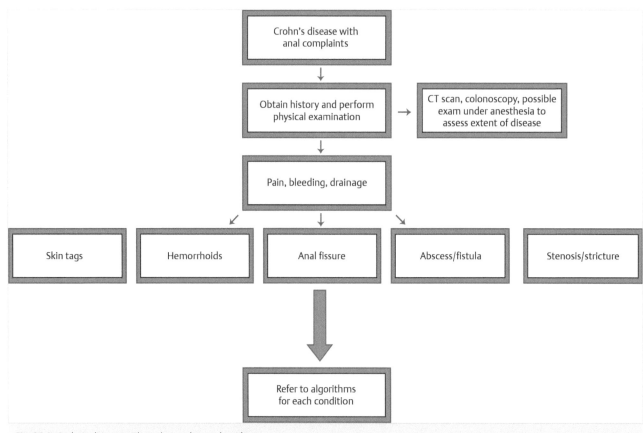

Fig. 26.9 Crohn's disease with anal complaints algorithm.

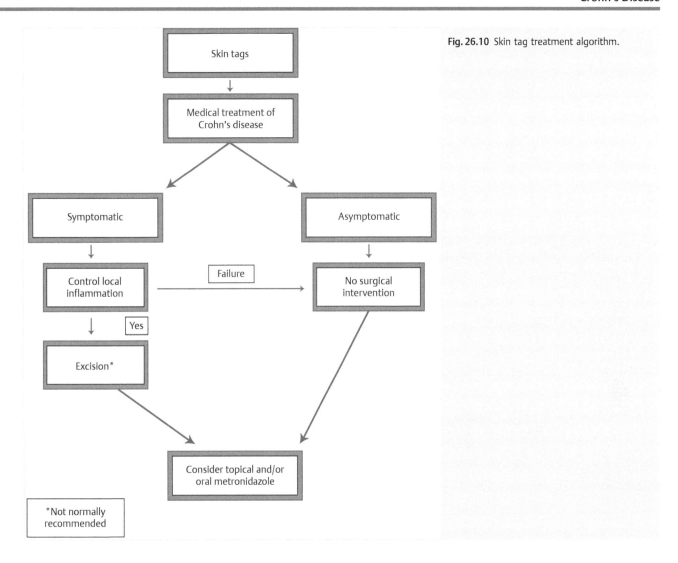

Fig. 26.10 Skin tag treatment algorithm.

up to 40 to 80% of CD patients (▶ Fig. 26.12). Unlike standard fistula disease, advances in medical treatment have been extremely helpful in addressing perianal CD. Topical 10% metronidazole (SLA Pharma; Leavesden, UK) is a simple, inexpensive, and effective means of controlling pain and discharge from anorectal CD, before, after, or as an alternative to surgery. TNF-α antibodies have been shown to decrease drainage from CD fistulas, in spite of the persistence of tracts demonstrated on ultrasound (▶ Fig. 26.13).

Surgery in anorectal CD should be very conservative, since the postoperative inflammatory response is often florid and incapacitating. Fistulas in CD characteristically "ignore" the anatomic rules of cryptoglandular tracts and are frequently termed "nonanatomic." CD fistulas are often multiple, complex, and have extensive sphincter involvement. Yet, CD patients may also have low-lying simple fistulas, where fistulotomy is safe and effective. Given the chronicity of the disease and high frequency of disease relapse, maximum preservation of sphincter function is essential. With proper patient selection, healing rates following fistulotomy are reported in greater than 50% of patients and anorectal incontinence rates as low as 10%.

Long-term loose setons (▶ Fig. 26.14), possibly combined with TNF-α therapy, result in satisfactory symptom control and

avoid sphincter division in patients with complex perianal fistulizing disease.

For more difficult CD fistulas such as a rectovaginal fistula, the principles of sphincter sparing surgery are paramount. AFPs and RVPs are most successful in longer, narrower tracts, and advancement flaps may be considered in selected patients with no active proctitis. A subset of patients has such extensive and aggressive disease that even maximum TNF-α therapy and seton placement are unsuccessful, requiring proctocolectomy and end ileostomy.

Treatment of anorectal abscesses in the setting of CD is essentially no different than those of cryptoglandular origin–incision and drainage. CD patients may have more extensive disease, and adjunct radiology testing may be useful, especially when the examination does not match the patient's symptoms. From a technical standpoint, it is important to place the incision as close to the anal verge as possible while still achieving adequate drainage, considering the possibility of fistula development.[123] Alternatively, a small pezzer mushroom-tipped catheter may be placed in the cavity, thus evacuating the abscess and allowing the cavity to close around the catheter, while allowing continued drainage.

Perianal fistulas are often deep, eroding through sphincter, and occur in the setting of extensive scarring around the

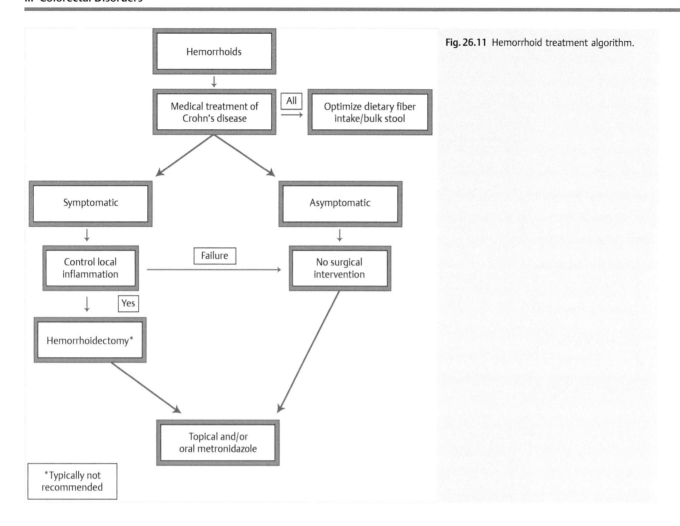

Fig. 26.11 Hemorrhoid treatment algorithm.

sphincter. Moreover, they can have high blind tracts, originate at levels well above the dentate line, and are often found in conjunction with active proctitis (▶ Fig. 26.15). Determining the anatomy of the tract is required, but attention should also be given to the presence or absence of proctitis, status of the sphincter, prior anal operations, and potential for chronic diarrhea. While aggressive fistulotomies must be avoided, distal fistulas in the absence of overt proctitis can often be treated safely with fistulotomy.[124] When the fistula is higher or more complex, endoanal advancement flaps, fistula plugs, or the ligation of the intersphincteric fistula tract (LIFT) procedure may all be performed with varying rates of success. Many patients with fistulous disease require chronic indwelling setons. Patients should be periodically reexamined both to ensure that there is adequate drainage and to look for a potential malignant growth, with case reports of squamous cell and adenocarcinoma arising in a fistulous tract. Unfortunately, fistulas and fistula procedures all vary in their outcomes, with healing rates ranging from 15 to 97% and morbidity rates from 3 to 78%, making it difficult to accurately compare results. As such, consideration should be given to a diverting stoma for recurrent or complex fistulas. Finally, a small percentage of patients may require permanent diversion or even proctectomy.[125]

Rectovaginal/Anovaginal Fistula

Rectovaginal fistulas are particularly problematic in the CD patient. Since many of these fistulas are associated with a deeply erosive process and intense inflammation, extensive tracts and hidden associated abscesses may also be present. In addition, a rectovaginal fistula may originate from small bowel, thus limiting potential diagnostic methods such as the methylene blue enema. Many patients require diversion in this setting prior to any definitive repair to aid with control of proctitis and to optimize the conditions needed for successful healing. First-line options include use of the fistula plug, endorectal advancement flap, and LIFT procedure.[126] Due to the complexity of the wounds and need for healthy tissue interposition, muscle flaps including the gracilis or bulbocavernosus are especially useful. Flaps should not be undertaken if the mucosa is actively inflamed. In general, proximal fecal diversion, preferably with loop ileostomy, should precede repeated attempts at flap closure and also any muscle interposition.

Regardless of treatment selected, a flap, plug, or tissue interposition, the failure rates of such treatments in patients with CD are universally higher than they are in patients with similar fistulas without CD.

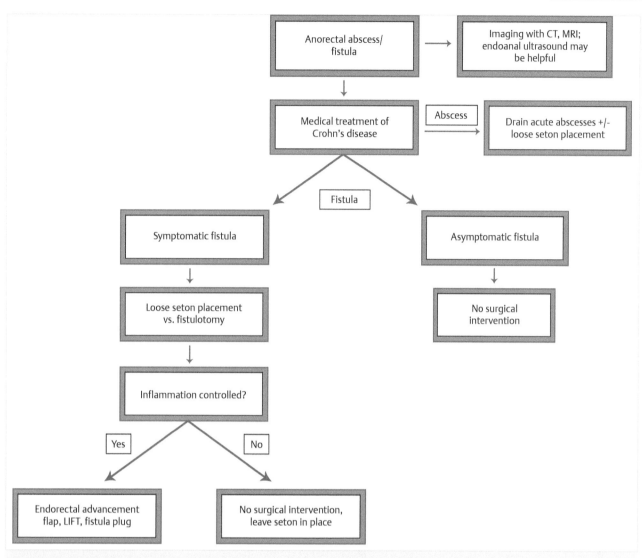

Fig. 26.12 Abscess and fistula treatment algorithm.

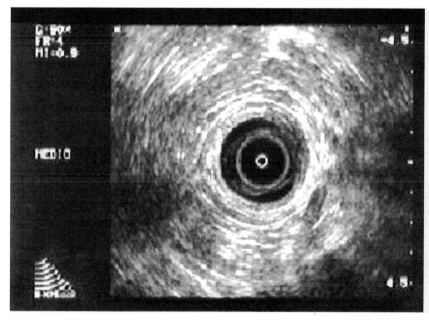

Fig. 26.13 Crohn's-related fistula shown on ultrasound.

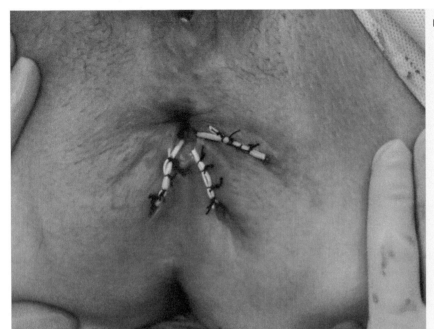

Fig. 26.14 Crohn's-related fistula with seton.

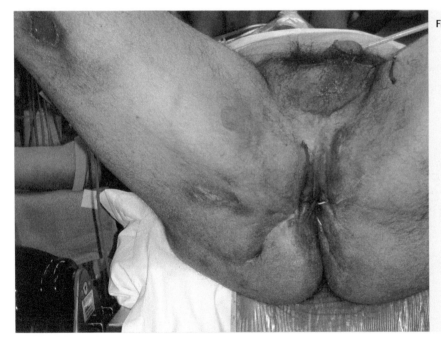

Fig. 26.15 Crohn's proctitis.

Anal Fissure

Patients with CD and anal fissures present a particular challenge (▶ Fig. 26.16). Decreasing the continence in any way may worsen an already difficult clinical situation, and limit the number of patients that may successfully undergo surgery. Despite an appearance that is hallmarked by deep, burrowing, off the midline, and sometimes multiple wounds, many anal fissures are fortunately painless and require no intervention. Excessive pain should raise the suspicion for an underlying abscess and prompt an examination under anesthesia. Initial attempts at conservative therapy with topical metronidazole, smooth muscle relaxants, and local anesthetics may be attempted to palliate symptoms and help with healing.[127] For particularly symptomatic fissures, botulinum toxin has also been used. In contrast, other authors have advocated a more aggressive surgical approach in CD patients, with one report citing 67% of patients treated surgically ultimately healed.[128] Yet given the continence risks associated with surgery, medical management is the preferred initial therapy in patients with CD-related fissures. Surgical intervention should be reserved for those patients with minimal active anorectal inflammation who fail all reasonable conservative therapy, and sphincter muscle division should be kept to a minimum.

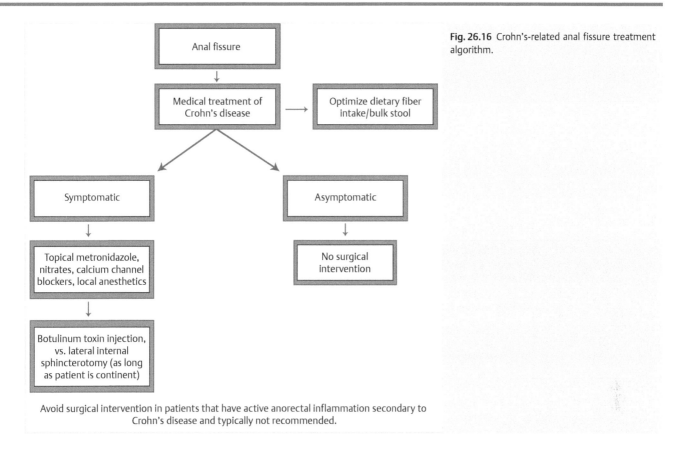

Fig. 26.16 Crohn's-related anal fissure treatment algorithm.

Anal Stenosis and Ulcer

While uncommon, anal or rectal ulcers (▶ Fig. 26.17 and ▶ Fig. 26.18), stenosis, and strictures secondary to CD can be extremely debilitating. Single institutional series have demonstrated success rates of biological agents in 18 to 60%.[129,130] Up to one-third of patients will have concomitant abscess or fistulas, and these should be appropriately drained. Due to the association of chronic inflammation with the development of malignancy, biopsy of any suspicious lesions should also be performed. For low-grade strictures, anal dilation has proven successful, though repeated sessions are the norm. Other options include steroid injection or biologics, balloon dilation, strictureplasty, flaps, and even proctectomy—depending on the severity and response to therapy.[131]

Anorectal Malignancy

Anorectal cancer may occur in any setting, including CD. Risk factors in patients with CD include the presence of chronic inflammation, long-standing open wounds, and use of immunosuppressant medication. Both squamous cell carcinoma (Marjolin's ulcer) and adenocarcinoma, and their variants, may occur.[132] Patients, especially those with long-term indwelling setons, should be periodically examined to exclude the presence of malignancy. All suspicious lesions should be biopsied and any malignancy should undergo proper staging and treatment.

26.11 Special Considerations

26.11.1 Extracolonic Manifestations

Extraintestinal Disease

Similar to ulcerative colitis, patients with CD may have manifestations from the disease process that extend outside of the GI tract (▶ Table 26.7). EID has been reported in approximately 6 to 47% of patients with IBD, and has an increased concordance among siblings and first-degree relatives—suggesting a genetic component that has been linked to the major histocompatibility complex (MHC) on chromosome 6.[133,134] EID occurs secondary to the systemic inflammatory process associated with the underlying disease and affects a wide range of organ systems (▶ Table 26.7). While the GI tract may be the primary source, the dysfunction in immune regulation incites a pathologic response that may occur in nearly every location in the body simultaneously with, preceding, or following GI manifestations.[135] Overall, rheumatologic/joint problems including peripheral or sacroiliac arthritis and arthralgias are the most common issues occurring in up to 35% of patients. Other more frequent sites of involvement include the skin, eyes, and hepatobiliary system, while the renal, pulmonary, nervous, and coagulation systems are typically involved to a lesser extent. It is important to distinguish between manifestations that parallel bowel disease activity, such as episcleritis, peripheral arthritis, and erythema nodosum, and manifestations that do not, including ankylosing spondylitis, pyoderma gangrenosum, and

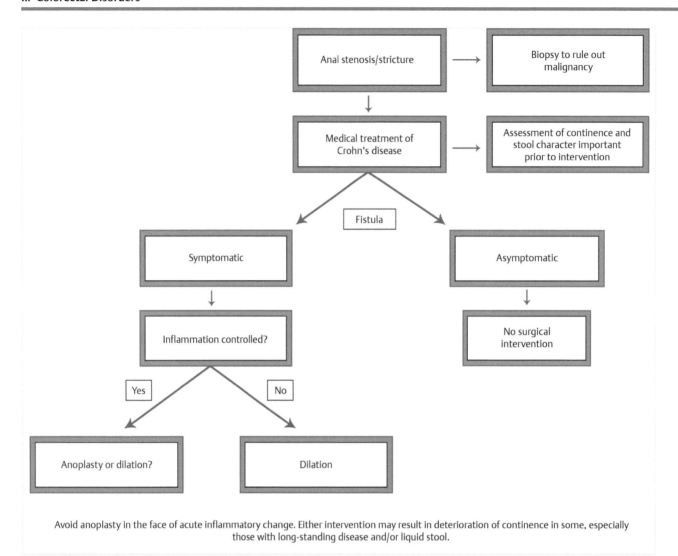

Avoid anoplasty in the face of acute inflammatory change. Either intervention may result in deterioration of continence in some, especially those with long-standing disease and/or liquid stool.

Fig. 26.17 Crohn's-related anal stenosis treatment algorithm.

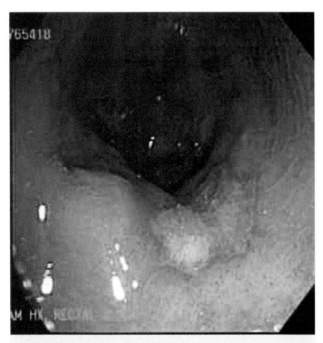

Fig. 26.18 Crohn's-related rectal ulcer.

Table 26.7 Extraintestinal manifestations of Crohn's disease

Organ system	Extraintestinal manifestations
Neurological	Demyelinating disease, neuritis
Ocular	Uveitis, iritis, episcleritis, conjunctivitis
Renal	Glomerulonephritis, amyloidosis
Skin/mucocutaneous	Erythema nodosum, pyoderma gangrenosum, aphthous ulcers
Blood	Thromboembolic disease, hemolytic anemia
Pulmonary	Bronchitis, pleuritis, tracheal stenosis
Hepatobiliary	Hepatitis, primary sclerosing cholangitis, pancreatitis, cirrhosis
Cardiac	Pericarditis, myocarditis
Musculoskeletal	Arthralgias, peripheral arthritis, ankylosing spondylitis, sacroiliitis

primary sclerosing cholangitis. Surgical intervention directed at the bowel may occasionally be required for recalcitrant EID that may appropriately go into remission following bowel resection.[136]

26.11.2 Hepatobiliary Manifestations

Malignancy

Historically, the risk of malignancy with CD was felt to be only slightly higher than the general population and significantly lower than the risk of patients with ulcerative colitis.[137] More recently, population-based data suggest that the cancer risk with long-standing CD is approximately 4- to 20-fold above that of the average population, and equivalent to patients with ulcerative colitis. Known risk factors for malignancy include pancolitis and a disease duration of greater than 8 years.[138,139,140] Endoscopic surveillance strategies to detect malignancy have had, to date, mixed results.[141] Data from a large meta-analysis found that surveillance colonoscopy has not shown to affect survival in these patients, though lesions are typically detected earlier.[142,143]

The optimal surveillance strategy for patients with CD has not been determined. As such, most recommendations favor mimicking surveillance for ulcerative colitis in patients with Crohn's colitis. In this algorithm, surveillance colonoscopy begins 8 years after disease onset for pancolitis and 15 years for patients with left-sided disease, and is repeated every 1 to 2 years. In addition, the American Society for Gastrointestinal Endoscopy, American College of Gastroenterology, and American Gastroenterological Association were unable to draw conclusions regarding the benefit of or need to perform random surveillance biopsies.[144,145,146] Treatment for malignancy in the CD patient is similar to that of the general population, with resection following standard oncological principles. As synchronous and metachronous lesions have been reported in up to 10% of patients with CD with cancer, consideration should be given to a subtotal colectomy with ileorectal anastomosis in the absence of rectal lesions.

While most evidence is from patients with ulcerative colitis, a polyp in a setting of colitis (non–adenoma dysplasia-associated lesion or mass [DALM]) has traditionally been felt to carry a significant risk of malignancy and is a strong indication for a formal resection.[138,147,148,149,150] While these non-adenoma-like DALMs should typically undergo a colectomy, more recent evidence suggests that complete endoscopic excision of an adenoma-like DALM (i.e., a sporadic adenoma occurring in a patient with colitis with or without active disease) may safely undergo a surveillance protocol.[151] Low-grade dysplasia outside the setting of a non-adenoma-like DALM and even in areas of flat mucosa warrants close follow-up, although the need for follow-up resection remains unproven.[138,150]

26.11.3 Crohn's Disease and Pregnancy

CD classically has a bimodal age distribution,[2] including reproductive-age women. While many of these women may choose not to conceive,[3,152,153,154,155,156,157,158,159,160,161,162,163,164,165] those with quiescent CD are considered to be as likely to become pregnant as the general population.[4,6,7] In fact, it has been estimated that 25% of women with known IBD will conceive.[9]

As such, obstetricians, gastroenterologists, and surgeons not infrequently find themselves caring for and advising pregnant patients who carry the burden of CD.

Unfortunately, little evidence exists to help guide clinical decision making and counseling regarding the course of CD in pregnant patients. The general consensus is that pregnant patients are as likely to flare during pregnancy as they are in a nonpregnant state[11] with rates ranging from 26 to 34%.[11,12,13] In practice, patients are often counseled that one-third of CD patients who conceive while in remission will relapse during pregnancy, and two-thirds of CD patients who conceive in the face of active disease will smolder or deteriorate.[9,16] Still, many clinicians feel that pregnancy may actually improve disease activity, presumably secondary to a state of relative immune suppression.[14] While this lack of consensus on the clinical course of CD during pregnancy is likely due to the unique experience of individual centers caring for these patients, it is also based on limited, and low-volume, level III and IV evidence.

The majority of our "understanding" of the impact of pregnancy on the course and severity of CD is predicated on several small survey-based studies conducted between 1956 and 1984.[6,11,17,18] In 1986, Miller compiled the cumulative results of these studies, including a total of 186 pregnancies.[161] Rate of disease relapse in patients with quiescent disease was 27%, which was felt to be similar to the rate of relapse in nonpregnant CD patients. Thirty-four percent of patients with active disease got better, 32% remained the same, and 33% got worse. Unfortunately, these rates were derived from patient questionnaires, which are inherently biased and subjective. The current study provides objective data regarding the severity of CD using CD-related surgical disease as a reasonable surrogate, although we cannot comment on disease status at conception or disease progression over time due to the nature of the study.

Nwokolo et al[164] published a retrospective study looking at the need for bowel resection in 88 parous CD patients with distal ileal or colonic disease. At an average follow-up of 15 years, parous patients with distal ileal disease had on average 1.17 resections, while those with colonic disease had 0.68. These data were compared to respective resection rates of 1.57 and 1.05 in previously published data in nonparous patients. Ultimately, they concluded that parity portended a better prognosis.

In contrast, a more recent population-based study by Riis[152] refuted the idea that parity decreases the rates of bowel resection in CD. His group identified 38 patients who had been diagnosed with CD prior to conception. Fifty-three percent of these patients underwent an intestinal resection within the 10-year follow-up period. Nonparous women with CD had a 43% resection rate during the same period, although this disparity was not clinically significant.[3] Ultimately, our data suggest that there is a difference in the presentation of CD between pregnant and nonpregnant women. Using a larger, population-based series, we found pregnancy portends a worse clinical picture even after controlling for age, malnutrition, smoking, and chronic steroid use, and is in contrast with other authors who have suggested that pregnancy may confer improvement in CD symptoms due to altered immune function (▶ Table 26.8).

Table 26.8 Multivariate logistic regression identifying independent predictors of overall surgical disease in women with Crohn's disease

	OR	CI	p
Pregnancy	2.9	2.3–3.7	<0.001
Malnutrition	1.5	1.4–1.6	<0.001
Age	1.01	1.01–1.02	<0.001
Smoker	1.0	0.9–1.0	0.9
Chronic steroid use	1.0	0.9–1.1	0.8

Abbreviations: CI, confidence interval; OR, odds ratio.

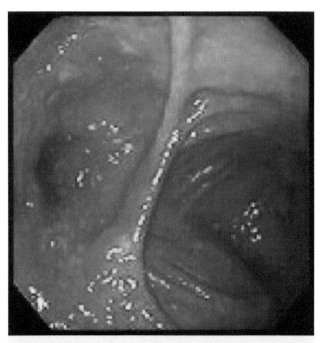

Fig. 26.19 Crohn's disease recurrence on endoscopy.

26.12 Recurrence

Unfortunately, recurrence in CD is the rule and not the exception (▶ Fig. 26.19).

26.13 Conclusion

CD remains a complex disease process with many different manifestations. Although advances in medical therapy continue to evolve and significantly alter the way patients are managed, surgeons still play a large role in both the medical and surgical therapy of the disease. Due to its recurring nature, surgeons must adhere to the principles of preventing and managing disease complications versus aiming for cure. By focusing on the maximization of functional outcomes, surgeons can optimize outcomes through a multimodality approach and minimize additional complications. All providers caring for Crohn's disease must be cognizant of the wide array of presentations and inherent difficulties in managing this disease. Medical management remains the mainstay of therapy, although the majority of patients will require surgery at some point in their life due to complications associated with the disease. Adherence to principles of surgery and a thorough understanding of the recurring nature of the disease will aid in allowing patients to have the best outcomes.

References

[1] Fielding JH. Crohn's disease in London in the latter half of the nineteenth century. Ir J Med Sci. 1984; 153(6):214–220

[2] Crohn BB, Ginzburg L, Oppenheimer GD. Regional ileitis: a pathologic and clinical entity. JAMA. 1932; 99(16):1323–1329

[3] Crohn BB, Ginzburg L, Oppenheimer GD. Landmark article Oct 15, 1932. Regional ileitis. A pathological and clinical entity. By Burril B. Crohn, Leon Ginzburg, and Gordon D. Oppenheimer. JAMA. 1984; 251(1):73–79

[4] Zani A, Cozzi DA. Giovanni Battista Morgagni and his contribution to pediatric surgery. J Pediatr Surg. 2008; 43(4):729–733

[5] Lockhart-Mummery HE, Morson BC. Crohn's disease (regional enteritis) of the large intestine and its distinction from ulcerative colitis. Gut. 1960; 1:87–105

[6] Whelan G, Farmer RG, Fazio VW, Goormastic M. Recurrence after surgery in Crohn's disease. Relationship to location of disease (clinical pattern) and surgical indication. Gastroenterology. 1985; 88(6):1826–1833

[7] Polito JM, II, Childs B, Mellits ED, Tokayer AZ, Harris ML, Bayless TM. Crohn's disease: influence of age at diagnosis on site and clinical type of disease. Gastroenterology. 1996; 111(3):580–586

[8] Russel MG, Stockbrügger RW. Epidemiology of inflammatory bowel disease: an update. Scand J Gastroenterol. 1996; 31(5):417–427

[9] Molodecky NA, Soon IS, Rabi DM, et al. Increasing incidence and prevalence of the inflammatory bowel diseases with time, based on systematic review. Gastroenterology. 2012; 142(1):46–54.e42, quiz e30

[10] Lapidus A, Bernell O, Hellers G, Persson PG, Löfberg R. Incidence of Crohn's disease in Stockholm county 1955–1989. Gut. 1997; 41(4):480–486

[11] Loftus EV, Jr, Silverstein MD, Sandborn WJ, Tremaine WJ, Harmsen WS, Zinsmeister AR. Crohn's disease in Olmsted County, Minnesota, 1940–1993: incidence, prevalence, and survival. Gastroenterology. 1998; 114(6):1161–1168

[12] Halme L, Paavola-Sakki P, Turunen U, Lappalainen M, Farkkila M, Kontula K. Family and twin studies in inflammatory bowel disease. World J Gastroenterol. 2006; 12(23):3668–3672

[13] Yang H, McElree C, Roth MP, Shanahan F, Targan SR, Rotter JI. Familial empirical risks for inflammatory bowel disease: differences between Jews and non-Jews. Gut. 1993; 34(4):517–524

[14] Halfvarson J, Bodin L, Tysk C, Lindberg E, Järnerot G. Inflammatory bowel disease in a Swedish twin cohort: a long-term follow-up of concordance and clinical characteristics. Gastroenterology. 2003; 124(7):1767–1773

[15] Sartor RB. Current theories in the etiology of Crohn's disease. Mt Sinai Newslett. 1995; 2:2–6

[16] Huttenhower C, Kostic AD, Xavier RJ. Inflammatory bowel disease as a model for translating the microbiome. Immunity. 2014; 40(6):843–854

[17] Reiff C, Kelly D. Inflammatory bowel disease, gut bacteria and probiotic therapy. Int J Med Microbiol. 2010; 300(1):25–33

[18] Macfarlane GT, Blackett KL, Nakayama T, Steed H, Macfarlane S. The gut microbiota in inflammatory bowel disease. Curr Pharm Des. 2009; 15(13):1528–1536

[19] Haag LM, Siegmund B. Exploring & exploiting our "other self": does the microbiota hold the key to the future therapy in Crohn's? Best Pract Res Clin Gastroenterol. 2014; 28(3):399–409

[20] Hugot JP, Laurent-Puig P, Gower-Rousseau C, et al. Mapping of a susceptibility locus for Crohn's disease on chromosome 16. Nature. 1996; 379(6568):821–823

[21] Cho JH. The Nod2 gene in Crohn's disease: implications for future research into the genetics and immunology of Crohn's disease. Inflamm Bowel Dis. 2001; 7(3):271–275

[22] Műzes G, Tulassay Z, Sipos F. Interplay of autophagy and innate immunity in Crohn's disease: a key immunobiologic feature. World J Gastroenterol. 2013; 19(28):4447–4454

[23] Wallace KL, Zheng LB, Kanazawa Y, Shih DQ. Immunopathology of inflammatory bowel disease. World J Gastroenterol. 2014; 20(1):6–21

[24] Gilardoni LR, Paolicchi FA, Mundo SL. Bovine paratuberculosis: a review of the advantages and disadvantages of different diagnostic tests. Rev Argent Microbiol. 2012; 44(3):201–215

[25] Wagner J, Sim WH, Lee KJ, Kirkwood CD. Current knowledge and systematic review of viruses associated with Crohn's disease. Rev Med Virol. 2013; 23 (3):145–171

[26] Sartor RB. Current concepts of the etiology and pathogenesis of ulcerative colitis and Crohn's disease. Gastroenterol Clin North Am. 1995; 24 (3):475–507

[27] Katschinski B, Fingerle D, Scherbaum B, Goebell H. Oral contraceptive use and cigarette smoking in Crohn's disease. Dig Dis Sci. 1993; 38 (9):1596–1600

[28] Cabré E, Domènech E. Impact of environmental and dietary factors on the course of inflammatory bowel disease. World J Gastroenterol. 2012; 18 (29):3814–3822

[29] Mayberry JF. Recent epidemiology of ulcerative colitis and Crohn's disease. Int J Colorectal Dis. 1989; 4(1):59–66

[30] Morpurgo E, Petras R, Kimberling J, Ziegler C, Galandiuk S. Characterization and clinical behavior of Crohn's disease initially presenting predominantly as colitis. Dis Colon Rectum. 2003; 46(7):918–924

[31] Mahadeva U, Martin JP, Patel NK, Price AB. Granulomatous ulcerative colitis: a re-appraisal of the mucosal granuloma in the distinction of Crohn's disease from ulcerative colitis. Histopathology. 2002; 41(1):50–55

[32] Yantiss RK, Odze RD. Diagnostic difficulties in inflammatory bowel disease pathology. Histopathology. 2006; 48(2):116–132

[33] Matsui T, Yao T, Sakurai T, et al. Clinical features and pattern of indeterminate colitis: Crohn's disease with ulcerative colitis-like clinical presentation. J Gastroenterol. 2003; 38(7):647–655

[34] Kim BG, Kim YS, Kim JS, Jung HC, Song IS. Diagnostic role of anti-Saccharomyces cerevisiae mannan antibodies combined with antineutrophil cytoplasmic antibodies in patients with inflammatory bowel disease. Dis Colon Rectum. 2002; 45(8):1062–1069

[35] Inoue K, Aomatsu T, Yoden A, Okuhira T, Kaji E, Tamai H. Usefulness of a novel and rapid assay system for fecal calprotectin in pediatric patients with inflammatory bowel diseases. J Gastroenterol Hepatol. 2014; 29 (7):1406–1412

[36] Nancey S, Boschetti G, Moussata D, et al. Neopterin is a novel reliable fecal marker as accurate as calprotectin for predicting endoscopic disease activity in patients with inflammatory bowel diseases. Inflamm Bowel Dis. 2013; 19 (5):1043–1052

[37] D'Haens G, Ferrante M, Vermeire S, et al. Fecal calprotectin is a surrogate marker for endoscopic lesions in inflammatory bowel disease. Inflamm Bowel Dis. 2012; 18(12):2218–2224

[38] Gisbert JP, McNicholl AG, Gomollon F. Questions and answers on the role of fecal lactoferrin as a biological marker in inflammatory bowel disease. Inflamm Bowel Dis. 2009; 15(11):1746–1754

[39] Abraham BP, Kane S. Fecal markers: calprotectin and lactoferrin. Gastroenterol Clin North Am. 2012; 41(2):483–495

[40] Joossens S, Reinisch W, Vermeire S, et al. The value of serologic markers in indeterminate colitis: a prospective follow-up study. Gastroenterology. 2002; 122(5):1242–1247

[41] Kelvin FM, Oddson TA, Rice RP, Garbutt JT, Bradenham BP. Double contrast barium enema in Crohn's disease and ulcerative colitis. AJR Am J Roentgenol. 1978; 131(2):207–213

[42] Dambha F, Tanner J, Carroll N. Diagnostic imaging in Crohn's disease: what is the new gold standard? Best Pract Res Clin Gastroenterol. 2014; 28 (3):421–436

[43] Spinelli A, Fiorino G, Bazzi P, et al. Preoperative magnetic resonance enterography in predicting findings and optimizing surgical approach in Crohn's disease. J Gastrointest Surg. 2014; 18(1):83–90, discussion 90–91

[44] Siddiki HA, Fidler JL, Fletcher JG, et al. Prospective comparison of state-of-the-art MR enterography and CT enterography in small-bowel Crohn's disease. AJR Am J Roentgenol. 2009; 193(1):113–121

[45] Gallego Ojea JC, Echarri Piudo AI, Porta Vila A. Crohn's disease: the usefulness of MR enterography in the detection of recurrence after surgery. Radiologia. 2011; 53(6):552–559

[46] Vanbeckevoort D, Bielen D, Vanslembrouck R, Van Assche G. Magnetic resonance imaging of perianal fistulas. Magn Reson Imaging Clin N Am. 2014; 22 (1):113–123

[47] Al-Hawary M, Zimmermann EM. A new look at Crohn's disease: novel imaging techniques. Curr Opin Gastroenterol. 2012; 28(4):334–340

[48] Shyn PB. 18F-FDG positron emission tomography: potential utility in the assessment of Crohn's disease. Abdom Imaging. 2012; 37(3):377–386

[49] Leighton JA, Gralnek IM, Cohen SA, et al. Capsule endoscopy is superior to small-bowel follow-through and equivalent to ileocolonoscopy in suspected Crohn's disease. Clin Gastroenterol Hepatol. 2014; 12(4):609–615

[50] Hall B, Holleran G, Costigan D, McNamara D. Capsule endoscopy: high negative predictive value in the long term despite a low diagnostic yield in patients with suspected Crohn's disease. United European Gastroenterol J. 2013; 1(6):461–466

[51] Carter D, Eliakim R. Current role of endoscopy in inflammatory bowel disease diagnosis and management. Curr Opin Gastroenterol. 2014; 30 (4):370–377

[52] Joo M, Odze RD. Rectal sparing and skip lesions in ulcerative colitis: a comparative study of endoscopic and histologic findings in patients who underwent proctocolectomy. Am J Surg Pathol. 2010; 34(5):689–696

[53] Kochhar R, Kochhar S. Endoscopic balloon dilation for benign gastric outlet obstruction in adults. World J Gastrointest Endosc. 2010; 2(1):29–35

[54] Ferreira J, Akbari M, Gashin L, et al. Prevalence and lifetime risk of endoscopy-related complications among patients with inflammatory bowel disease. Clin Gastroenterol Hepatol. 2013; 11(10):1288–1293

[55] Vucelic B. Inflammatory bowel diseases: controversies in the use of diagnostic procedures. Dig Dis. 2009; 27(3):269–277

[56] Weston LA, Roberts PL, Schoetz DJ, Jr, Coller JA, Murray JJ, Rusin LC. Ileocolic resection for acute presentation of Crohn's disease of the ileum. Dis Colon Rectum. 1996; 39(8):841–846

[57] Dias CC, Rodrigues PP, da Costa-Pereira A, Magro F. Clinical prognostic factors for disabling Crohn's disease: a systematic review and meta-analysis. World J Gastroenterol. 2013; 19(24):3866–3871

[58] Schwartz DA, Loftus EV, Jr, Tremaine WJ, et al. The natural history of fistulizing Crohn's disease in Olmsted County, Minnesota. Gastroenterology. 2002; 122(4):875–880

[59] Farmer RG, Hawk WA, Turnbull RB, Jr. Clinical patterns in Crohn's disease: a statistical study of 615 cases. Gastroenterology. 1975; 68(4 Pt 1):627–635

[60] Lapidus A, Bernell O, Hellers G, Löfberg R. Clinical course of colorectal Crohn's disease: a 35-year follow-up study of 507 patients. Gastroenterology. 1998; 114(6):1151–1160

[61] Binder HJ. Mechanisms of diarrhea in inflammatory bowel diseases. Ann N Y Acad Sci. 2009; 1165:285–293

[62] Wenzl HH. Diarrhea in chronic inflammatory bowel diseases. Gastroenterol Clin North Am. 2012; 41(3):651–675

[63] Bissell AD. Localized chronic ulcerative ileitis. Ann Surg. 1934; 99(6):957–966

[64] McKee RF, Keenan RA. Perianal Crohn's disease: is it all bad news? Dis Colon Rectum. 1996; 39(2):136–142

[65] Homan WP, Tang C, Thorgjarnarson B. Anal lesions complicating Crohn disease. Arch Surg. 1976; 111(12):1333–1335

[66] Solomon MJ. Fistulae and abscesses in symptomatic perianal Crohn's disease. Int J Colorectal Dis. 1996; 11(5):222–226

[67] Pikarsky AJ, Gervaz P, Wexner SD. Perianal Crohn disease: a new scoring system to evaluate and predict outcome of surgical intervention. Arch Surg. 2002; 137(7):774–777, discussion 778

[68] Isaacs KL. Upper gastrointestinal tract endoscopy in inflammatory bowel disease. Gastrointest Endosc Clin N Am. 2002; 12(3):451–462, vii

[69] Wagtmans MJ, van Hogezand RA, Griffioen G, Verspaget HW, Lamers CB. Crohn's disease of the upper gastrointestinal tract. Neth J Med. 1997; 50(2):S2–S7

[70] Decker GA, Loftus EV, Jr, Pasha TM, Tremaine WJ, Sandborn WJ. Crohn's disease of the esophagus: clinical features and outcomes. Inflamm Bowel Dis. 2001; 7(2):113–119

[71] Li G, Ren J, Wang G, et al. Preoperative exclusive enteral nutrition reduces the postoperative septic complications of fistulizing Crohn's disease. Eur J Clin Nutr. 2014; 68(4):441–446

[72] Caprilli R, Cesarini M, Angelucci E, Frieri G. The long journey of salicylates in ulcerative colitis: the past and the future. J Crohn's Colitis. 2009; 3(3):149–156

[73] Lim WC, Hanauer S. Aminosalicylates for induction of remission or response in Crohn's disease. Cochrane Database Syst Rev. 2010(12):CD008870

[74] Seow CH, Benchimol EI, Griffiths AM, Otley AR, Steinhart AH. Budesonide for induction of remission in Crohn's disease. Cochrane Database Syst Rev. 2008 (3):CD000296

[75] Prefontaine E, Macdonald JK, Sutherland LR. Azathioprine or 6-mercaptopurine for induction of remission in Crohn's disease. Cochrane Database Syst Rev. 2010(6):CD000545

[76] Alfadhli AA, McDonald JW, Feagan BG. Methotrexate for induction of remission in refractory Crohn's disease. Cochrane Database Syst Rev. 2005(1): CD003459

[77] Lapadula G, Marchesoni A, Armuzzi A, et al. Adalimumab in the treatment of immune-mediated diseases. Int J Immunopathol Pharmacol. 2014; 27(1) Suppl:33–48

[78] Scott FI, Osterman MT. Medical management of Crohn disease. Clin Colon Rectal Surg. 2013; 26(2):67–74

[79] Kopylov U, Ben-Horin S, Zmora O, Eliakim R, Katz LH. Anti-tumor necrosis factor and postoperative complications in Crohn's disease: systematic review and meta-analysis. Inflamm Bowel Dis. 2012; 18(12):2404–2413

[80] Wolff BG. Resection margins in Crohn's disease. Br J Surg. 2001; 88(6):771–772

[81] Bernell O, Lapidus A, Hellers G. Recurrence after colectomy in Crohn's colitis. Dis Colon Rectum. 2001; 44(5):647–654, discussion 654

[82] Tekkis PP, Purkayastha S, Lanitis S, et al. A comparison of segmental vs subtotal/total colectomy for colonic Crohn's disease: a meta-analysis. Colorectal Dis. 2006; 8(2):82–90

[83] Scammell BE, Keighley MR. Delayed perineal wound healing after proctectomy for Crohn's colitis. Br J Surg. 1986; 73(2):150–152

[84] Raab Y, Bergström R, Ejerblad S, Graf W, Påhlman L. Factors influencing recurrence in Crohn's disease. An analysis of a consecutive series of 353 patients treated with primary surgery. Dis Colon Rectum. 1996; 39(8):918–925

[85] Cellini C, Safar B, Fleshman J. Surgical management of pyogenic complications of Crohn's disease. Inflamm Bowel Dis. 2010; 16(3):512–517

[86] Sampietro GM, Casiraghi S, Foschi D. Perforating Crohn's disease: conservative and surgical treatment. Dig Dis. 2013; 31(2):218–221

[87] Poritz LS, Rowe WA, Koltun WA. Remicade does not abolish the need for surgery in fistulizing Crohn's disease. Dis Colon Rectum. 2002; 45(6):771–775

[88] Kawalec P, Mikrut A, Wiśniewska N, Pilc A. Tumor necrosis factor-α antibodies (infliximab, adalimumab and certolizumab) in Crohn's disease: systematic review and meta-analysis. Arch Med Sci. 2013; 9(5):765–779

[89] Bettenworth D, Rieder F. Medical therapy of stricturing Crohn's disease: what the gut can learn from other organs—a systematic review. Fibrogenesis Tissue Repair. 2014; 7(1):5

[90] Govani SM, Stidham RW, Higgins PD. How early to take arms against a sea of troubles? The case for aggressive early therapy in Crohn's disease to prevent fibrotic intestinal strictures. J Crohn's Colitis. 2013; 7(11):923–927

[91] Brown CJ, Maclean AR, Cohen Z, Macrae HM, O'Connor BI, McLeod RS. Crohn's disease and indeterminate colitis and the ileal pouch-anal anastomosis: outcomes and patterns of failure. Dis Colon Rectum. 2005; 48(8):1542–1549

[92] Yamazaki Y, Ribeiro MB, Sachar DB, Aufses AH, Jr, Greenstein AJ. Malignant colorectal strictures in Crohn's disease. Am J Gastroenterol. 1991; 86(7):882–885

[93] Stienecker K, Gleichmann D, Neumayer U, Glaser HJ, Tonus C. Long-term results of endoscopic balloon dilatation of lower gastrointestinal tract strictures in Crohn's disease: a prospective study. World J Gastroenterol. 2009; 15(21):2623–2627

[94] Swaminath A, Lichtiger S. Dilation of colonic strictures by intralesional injection of infliximab in patients with Crohn's colitis. Inflamm Bowel Dis. 2008; 14(2):213–216

[95] Despott EJ, Gupta A, Burling D, et al. Effective dilation of small-bowel strictures by double-balloon enteroscopy in patients with symptomatic Crohn's disease (with video). Gastrointest Endosc. 2009; 70(5):1030–1036

[96] Gill RS, Kaffes AJ. Small bowel stricture characterization and outcomes of dilatation by double-balloon enteroscopy: a single-centre experience. Therap Adv Gastroenterol. 2014; 7(3):108–114

[97] Hirai F, Beppu T, Takatsu N, et al. Long-term outcome of endoscopic balloon dilation for small bowel strictures in patients with Crohn's disease. Dig Endosc. 2014; 26(4):545–551

[98] Endo K, Takahashi S, Shiga H, Kakuta Y, Kinouchi Y, Shimosegawa T. Short and long-term outcomes of endoscopic balloon dilatation for Crohn's disease strictures. World J Gastroenterol. 2013; 19(1):86–91

[99] Yamamoto T, Fazio VW, Tekkis PP. Safety and efficacy of strictureplasty for Crohn's disease: a systematic review and meta-analysis. Dis Colon Rectum. 2007; 50(11):1968–1986

[100] Campbell L, Ambe R, Weaver J, Marcus SM, Cagir B. Comparison of conventional and nonconventional strictureplasties in Crohn's disease: a systematic review and meta-analysis. Dis Colon Rectum. 2012; 55(6):714–726

[101] Hesham W, Kann BR. Strictureplasty. Clin Colon Rectal Surg. 2013; 26(2):80–83

[102] Chen M, Shen B. Comparable short- and long-term outcomes of colonoscopic balloon dilation of Crohn's Disease and benign non-Crohn's Disease strictures. Inflamm Bowel Dis. 2014; 20(10):1739–1746

[103] He X, Chen Z, Huang J, et al. Stapled side-to-side anastomosis might be better than handsewn end-to-end anastomosis in ileocolic resection for Crohn's disease: a meta-analysis. Dig Dis Sci. 2014; 59(7):1544–1551

[104] Simillis C, Purkayastha S, Yamamoto T, Strong SA, Darzi AW, Tekkis PP. A meta-analysis comparing conventional end-to-end anastomosis vs. other anastomotic configurations after resection in Crohn's disease. Dis Colon Rectum. 2007; 50(10):1674–1687

[105] Alla VM, Ojili V, Gorthi J, Csordas A, Yellapu RK. Revisiting the past: intra-arterial vasopressin for severe gastrointestinal bleeding in Crohn's disease. J Crohn's Colitis. 2010; 4(4):479–482

[106] Ando Y, Matsushita M, Kawamata S, Shimatani M, Fujii T, Okazaki K. Infliximab for severe gastrointestinal bleeding in Crohn's disease. Inflamm Bowel Dis. 2009; 15(3):483–484

[107] Veroux M, Angriman I, Ruffolo C, et al. Severe gastrointestinal bleeding in Crohn's disease. Ann Ital Chir. 2003; 74(2):213–215, discussion 216

[108] Firth MG, Prather CM. Unusual gastric Crohn's disease treated with infliximab: a case report. Am J Gastroenterol. 2002; 97:S190

[109] Banerjee S, Peppercorn MA. Inflammatory bowel disease. Medical therapy of specific clinical presentations. Gastroenterol Clin North Am. 2002; 31(1):185–202, x

[110] Rana SS, Bhasin DK, Chandail VS, et al. Endoscopic balloon dilatation without fluoroscopy for treating gastric outlet obstruction because of benign etiologies. Surg Endosc. 2011; 25(5):1579–1584

[111] Singh VV, Draganov P, Valentine J. Efficacy and safety of endoscopic balloon dilation of symptomatic upper and lower gastrointestinal Crohn's disease strictures. J Clin Gastroenterol. 2005; 39(4):284–290

[112] Tonelli F, Alemanno G, Bellucci F, Focardi A, Sturiale A, Giudici F. Symptomatic duodenal Crohn's disease: is strictureplasty the right choice? J Crohn's Colitis. 2013; 7(10):791–796

[113] Shapiro M, Greenstein AJ, Byrn J, et al. Surgical management and outcomes of patients with duodenal Crohn's disease. J Am Coll Surg. 2008; 207(1):36–42

[114] Pettit S, Irving M. The operative management of fistulating Crohn's disease: experience with 100 consecutive cases. Surg Gynecol Obstet. 1988; 167:223–228

[115] Lesperance K, Martin MJ, Lehmann R, Brounts L, Steele SR. National trends and outcomes for the surgical therapy of ileocolonic Crohn's disease: a population-based analysis of laparoscopic vs. open approaches. J Gastrointest Surg. 2009; 13(7):1251–1259

[116] Aarons CB. Laparoscopic surgery for Crohn disease: a brief review of the literature. Clin Colon Rectal Surg. 2013; 26(2):122–127

[117] Stewart D, Chao A, Kodner I, Birnbaum E, Fleshman J, Dietz D. Subtotal colectomy for toxic and fulminant colitis in the era of immunosuppressive therapy. Colorectal Dis. 2009; 11(2):184–190

[118] Joyce MR, Fazio VW. Can ileal pouch anal anastomosis be used in Crohn's disease? Adv Surg. 2009; 43:111–137

[119] Hartley JE, Fazio VW, Remzi FH, et al. Analysis of the outcome of ileal pouch-anal anastomosis in patients with Crohn's disease. Dis Colon Rectum. 2004; 47(11):1808–1815

[120] Braveman JM, Schoetz DJ, Jr, Marcello PW, et al. The fate of the ileal pouch in patients developing Crohn's disease. Dis Colon Rectum. 2004; 47(10):1613–1619

[121] Cracco N, Zinicola R. Is haemorrhoidectomy in inflammatory bowel disease harmful? An old dogma re-examined. Colorectal Dis. 2014; 16(7):516–519

[122] Nicholson TJ, Armstrong D. Topical metronidazole (10 percent) decreases posthemorrhoidectomy pain and improves healing. Dis Colon Rectum. 2004; 47(5):711–716

[123] Lewis RT, Bleier JI. Surgical treatment of anorectal Crohn disease. Clin Colon Rectal Surg. 2013; 26(2):90–99

[124] Sneider EB, Maykel JA. Anal abscess and fistula. Gastroenterol Clin North Am. 2013; 42(4):773–784

[125] Causey MW, Nelson D, Johnson EK, et al. An NSQIP evaluation of practice patterns and outcomes following surgery for anorectal abscess and fistula in patients with and without Crohn's disease. Gastroenterol Rep (Oxf). 2013; 1(1):58–63

[126] Tozer PJ, Balmforth D, Kayani B, Rahbour G, Hart AL, Phillips RK. Surgical management of rectovaginal fistula in a tertiary referral centre: many techniques are needed. Colorectal Dis. 2013; 15(7):871–877

[127] D'Ugo S, Franceschilli L, Cadeddu F, et al. Medical and surgical treatment of haemorrhoids and anal fissure in Crohn's disease: a critical appraisal. BMC Gastroenterol. 2013; 13:47

[128] Fleshner PR, Schoetz DJ, Jr, Roberts PL, Murray JJ, Coller JA, Veidenheimer MC. Anal fissure in Crohn's disease: a plea for aggressive management. Dis Colon Rectum. 1995; 38(11):1137–1143

[129] Brochard C, Siproudhis L, Wallenhorst T, et al. Anorectal stricture in 102 patients with Crohn's disease: natural history in the era of biologics. Aliment Pharmacol Ther. 2014; 40(7):796–803

[130] Bouguen G, Trouilloud I, Siproudhis L, et al. Long-term outcome of non-fistulizing (ulcers, stricture) perianal Crohn's disease in patients treated with infliximab. Aliment Pharmacol Ther. 2009; 30(7):749–756

[131] Lawal TA, Frischer JS, Falcone RA, Chatoorgoon K, Denson LA, Levitt MA. The transanal approach with laparoscopy or laparotomy for the treatment of rectal strictures in Crohn's disease. J Laparoendosc Adv Surg Tech A. 2010; 20(9):791–795

[132] Scharl M, Frei P, Frei SM, Biedermann L, Weber A, Rogler G. Epithelial-to-mesenchymal transition in a fistula-associated anal adenocarcinoma in a patient with long-standing Crohn's disease. Eur J Gastroenterol Hepatol. 2014; 26(1):114–118

[133] Satsangi J, Grootscholten C, Holt H, Jewell DP. Clinical patterns of familial inflammatory bowel disease. Gut. 1996; 38(5):738–741

[134] Orchard TR, Thiyagaraja S, Welsh KI, Wordsworth BP, Hill Gaston JS, Jewell DP. Clinical phenotype is related to HLA genotype in the peripheral arthropathies of inflammatory bowel disease. Gastroenterology. 2000; 118(2):274–278

[135] Rothfuss KS, Stange EF, Herrlinger KR. Extraintestinal manifestations and complications in inflammatory bowel diseases. World J Gastroenterol. 2006; 12(30):4819–4831

[136] Rispo A, Musto D, Tramontano ML, Castiglione F, Bucci L, Alfinito F. Surgery-induced remission of extraintestinal manifestations in inflammatory bowel diseases. J Crohn's Colitis. 2013; 7(10):e504–e505

[137] Greenstein AJ, Sachar DB, Smith H, Janowitz HD, Aufses AH, Jr. Patterns of neoplasia in Crohn's disease and ulcerative colitis. Cancer. 1980; 46(2):403–407

[138] Jess T, Loftus EV, Jr, Velayos FS, et al. Risk of intestinal cancer in inflammatory bowel disease: a population-based study from Olmsted county, Minnesota. Gastroenterology. 2006; 130(4):1039–1046

[139] Maykel JA, Hagerman G, Mellgren AF, et al. Crohn's colitis: the incidence of dysplasia and adenocarcinoma in surgical patients. Dis Colon Rectum. 2006; 49(7):950–957

[140] Friedman S, Rubin PH, Bodian C, Goldstein E, Harpaz N, Present DH. Screening and surveillance colonoscopy in chronic Crohn's colitis. Gastroenterology. 2001; 120(4):820–826

[141] Siegel CA, Sands BE. Risk factors for colorectal cancer in Crohn's colitis: a case-control study. Inflamm Bowel Dis. 2006; 12(6):491–496

[142] Shanahan F. Review article: colitis-associated cancer—time for new strategies. Aliment Pharmacol Ther. 2003; 18 Suppl 2:6–9

[143] Collins PD, Mpofu C, Watson AJ, Rhodes JM. Strategies for detecting colon cancer and/or dysplasia in patients with inflammatory bowel disease. Cochrane Database Syst Rev. 2006(2):CD000279

[144] Hanauer SB, Meyers S. Management of Crohn's disease in adults. Am J Gastroenterol. 1997; 92(4):559–566

[145] Farraye FA, Odze RD, Eaden J, et al. AGA Institute Medical Position Panel on Diagnosis and Management of Colorectal Neoplasia in Inflammatory Bowel Disease. AGA medical position statement on the diagnosis and management of colorectal neoplasia in inflammatory bowel disease. Gastroenterology. 2010; 138(2):738–745

[146] Leighton JA, Shen B, Baron TH, et al. Standards of Practice Committee, American Society for Gastrointestinal Endoscopy. ASGE guideline: endoscopy in the diagnosis and treatment of inflammatory bowel disease. Gastrointest Endosc. 2006; 63(4):558–565

[147] Cooper DJ, Weinstein MA, Korelitz BI. Complications of Crohn's disease predisposing to dysplasia and cancer of the intestinal tract: considerations of a surveillance program. J Clin Gastroenterol. 1984; 6(3):217–224

[148] Itzkowitz SH, Harpaz N. Diagnosis and management of dysplasia in patients with inflammatory bowel diseases. Gastroenterology. 2004; 126 (6):1634–1648

[149] Greenson JK. Dysplasia in inflammatory bowel disease. Semin Diagn Pathol. 2002; 19(1):31–37

[150] Befrits R, Ljung T, Jaramillo E, Rubio C. Low-grade dysplasia in extensive, long-standing inflammatory bowel disease: a follow-up study. Dis Colon Rectum. 2002; 45(5):615–620

[151] Wanders LK, Dekker E, Pullens B, Bassett P, Travis SP, East JE. Cancer risk after resection of polypoid dysplasia in patients with longstanding ulcerative colitis: a meta-analysis. Clin Gastroenterol Hepatol. 2014; 12 (5):756–764

[152] Riis L, Vind I, Politi P, et al. European Collaborative study group on Inflammatory Bowel Disease. Does pregnancy change the disease course? A study in a European cohort of patients with inflammatory bowel disease. Am J Gastroenterol. 2006; 101(7):1539–1545

[153] Baird DD, Narendranathan M, Sandler RS. Increased risk of preterm birth for women with inflammatory bowel disease. Gastroenterology. 1990; 99 (4):987–994

[154] Khosla R, Willoughby CP, Jewell DP. Crohn's disease and pregnancy. Gut. 1984; 25(1):52–56

[155] Woolfson K, Cohen Z, McLeod RS. Crohn's disease and pregnancy. Dis Colon Rectum. 1990; 33(10):869–873

[156] Caprilli R, Gassull MA, Escher JC, et al. European Crohn's and Colitis Organisation. European evidence based consensus on the diagnosis and management of Crohn's disease: special situations. Gut. 2006; 55 Suppl 1:i36–i58

[157] Nielsen OH, Andreasson B, Bondesen S, Jacobsen O, Jarnum S. Pregnancy in Crohn's disease. Scand J Gastroenterol. 1984; 19(6):724–732

[158] Mogadam M, Korelitz BI, Ahmed SW, Dobbins WO, III, Baiocco PJ. The course of inflammatory bowel disease during pregnancy and postpartum. Am J Gastroenterol. 1981; 75(4):265–269

[159] Morales M, Berney T, Jenny A, Morel P, Extermann P. Crohn's disease as a risk factor for the outcome of pregnancy. Hepatogastroenterology. 2000; 47 (36):1595–1598

[160] Agret F, Cosnes J, Hassani Z, et al. Impact of pregnancy on the clinical activity of Crohn's disease. Aliment Pharmacol Ther. 2005; 21(5):509–513

[161] Miller JP. Inflammatory bowel disease in pregnancy: a review. J R Soc Med. 1986; 79(4):221–225

[162] Crohn BB, Korelitz BI, Yarnis H. Regional ileitis complicating pregnancy. Gastroenterology. 1956; 31(6):615–624, discussion, 625–628

[163] Homan WP, Thorbjarnarson B. Crohn disease and pregnancy. Arch Surg. 1976; 111(5):545–547

[164] Nwokolo CU, Tan WC, Andrews HA, Allan RN. Surgical resections in parous patients with distal ileal and colonic Crohn's disease. Gut. 1994; 35 (2):220–223

[165] Buyon JP. The effects of pregnancy on autoimmune diseases. J Leukoc Biol. 1998; 63(3):281–287

27 Diverticular Disease of the Colon

Janice F. Rafferty

Abstract

The term "diverticulum" indicates an abnormal pouch or sac, opening from a hollow organ such as the intestine. The advent of contrast radiology revealed a growing prevalence of this disease. These protrusions, or pseudodiverticula, are commonly associated with a muscular abnormality of the sigmoid colon. Diverticula could be associated with inflammation, perforation, adhesions, fistulas, and stenosis. When inflammation develops, the term diverticulitis is used. As anesthesia and surgical techniques became safer, physicians began to refer patients with diverticulosis for elective operation in an effort to prevent complications. Because many patients with this condition exhibit no evidence of inflammation, the encompassing term "diverticular disease" is used for the entire spectrum of the clinical consequences of colonic diverticulosis. This chapter discusses the history, anatomy, incidence, etiology, diagnosis and operative and nonoperative treatment of colonic diverticular disease.

Keywords: diverticulitis, colon, diverticulosis, treatment, emergency surgery, diagnosis, antibiotics, diet modification, uncomplicated diverticulitis, complicated diverticulitis

27.1 Introduction

The term "diverticulum" indicates an abnormal pouch or sac, opening from a hollow organ such as the intestine. It is derived from the Latin verb *divertere*, which means "to turn aside." Credit for the first description of diverticular disease has been given to Cruveilhier,[1] who in 1849 described a series of small, pear-shaped, hernia protrusions of mucosa through the muscle coat of the sigmoid colon. From a historical perspective, diverticula were initially regarded as nothing more than a curiosity of pathology, defined as mucosa protruding through the muscular wall of the bowel. The advent of contrast radiology revealed a growing prevalence of this disease. These protrusions, or pseudodiverticula, are commonly associated with a muscular abnormality of the sigmoid colon. Over time, it became evident that diverticula could be associated with inflammation, perforation, adhesions, fistulas, and stenosis. When inflammation develops, the term diverticulitis is used. Initially, diverticulosis was not treated unless complications supervened. As anesthesia and surgical techniques became safer, however, physicians began to refer patients with diverticulosis for elective operation in an effort to prevent complications. Because many patients with this condition exhibit no evidence of inflammation, the encompassing term "diverticular disease" is used for the entire spectrum of the clinical consequences of colonic diverticulosis.

27.2 History and Anatomy

In a detailed study of the anatomy and pathology of diverticular disease, Slack[2] compared the large intestine of 141 cadavers in which consecutive autopsies were performed with 36 consecutive operative specimens removed because of diverticulitis. Diverticula had broken through the circular muscle in four main positions (▶ Fig. 27.1). In approximately 40% of the cases, protrusions were also noted between the antimesenteric teniae. A sizable blood vessel was seen to course around the bowel on each side outside the muscular coat and penetrate through the mesenteric side of the antimesenteric teniae. In some cases, this vessel appeared to divide into deep and superficial branches, with the deeper one piercing the circular muscle coat and the more superficial one passing directly through the teniae. Small vessels arose from the main circumferential vessels and penetrated the circular muscle coat and the mesenteric teniae. In each case, small vessels passed along the neck of the diverticulum toward the lumen of the bowel.

27.3 Incidence

The prevalence of diverticulosis in the United States has increased dramatically since it was first described, and increases substantially with age. It is estimated that approximately 20% of patients with diverticulosis develop diverticulitis over the course of their lifetime[3] and that 30% of the population over the age of 60 years, and 60% of the population over the age of 80, may be affected.[4] Connell[5] estimated the risk of the aging population developing diverticular disease to be nearly 50%. In fact, it is impossible to estimate the precise incidence of diverticular disease in the general population. Data on the incidence and prevalence of diverticular disease of the colon represent a crude overall blend of numbers derived from radiologic, surgical, and autopsy reports on both hospitalized and ambulatory populations. In any review of statistics, autopsy studies will underestimate the incidence of diverticulosis because of the care needed to demonstrate all diverticula. Radiologic studies will overestimate the occurrence because people have colonoscopy and other imaging studies for various symptoms. What is evident is that the incidence has gradually increased in the past 100 years. For example, in 1930, Rankin and Brown[6] reported that of 24,620 barium enema examinations, 5.7% had diverticulosis, as did 5.2% of 1,925 autopsy cases at the Mayo Clinic. Heller and Hackler[7] reported that between 1909 and 1975, the autopsy incidence of diverticulosis increased from 5 to 50%. The incidence of diverticular disease is typically reported as more common in men.[8,9] Geographic location is also important, for it appears that diverticulosis is a disease of Western people. A close relationship exists between the prevalence of diverticular disease, economic development, and adoption of Western eating habits. Diverticula are common in Europe, North America, and Australia, less common in South America, and rare in Africa and Oriental countries.[10,11,12] Right-sided diverticulosis is found almost exclusively in Oriental people, and is more common than left-sided diverticula in Japan, Hawaii (among Japanese and Chinese individuals), China, Korea, Thailand, and Singapore.[6] Even so, right-sided diverticular disease of the colon seems to produce fewer clinical problems when compared with left-sided diverticular disease.

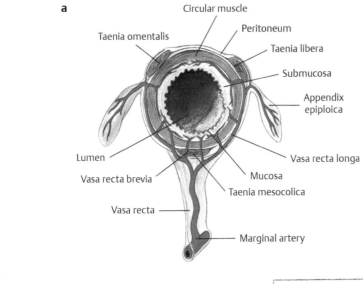

a

Circular muscle

Taenia omentalis

Peritoneum

Taenia libera

Submucosa

Appendix epiploica

Lumen

Vasa recta longa

Vasa recta brevia

Mucosa

Taenia mesocolica

Vasa recta

Marginal artery

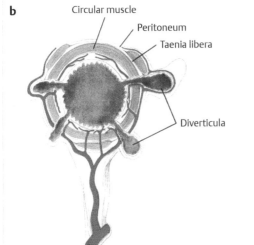

b

Circular muscle

Peritoneum

Taenia libera

Diverticula

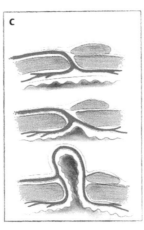

c

Fig. 27.1 (a) Cross-section of the usual anatomic layers of colonic wall with special attention to the course of vessels. **(b)** Cross-section demonstrating the location of diverticula as determined by Slack. **(c)** Relationship of the vessels to the diverticulum.

Diverticular disease currently accounts for approximately 300,000 hospitalizations per year in the United States, resulting in 1.5 million days of inpatient care.[13] Additionally, roughly 1.5 million outpatient visits each year are due to diverticular disease.[14] Over the past several years, research on natural biology of diverticulitis has been incorporated into the management recommendations for this challenging disease. Although diverticulitis may affect any location in the colon, this chapter will focus on left-sided disease.

27.4 Etiology

It is generally agreed that colonic diverticula are acquired. They are considered pulsion diverticula, which, under the influence of increased intraluminal pressure, are mucosal herniations that protrude through points of the bowel wall weakened by entry of blood vessels. Recognition of the segmentation mechanism of pressure production and its role in the localization of high intracolonic pressures has led to some understanding of the pathogenesis of diverticular disease, but the etiology of the disease to a great degree remains a mystery. Painter[15] hypothesized that it is a deficiency disease caused by inadequacy of fiber brought about by the refining of carbohydrates. In the past half century, the amount of cereal fiber consumed by individuals in the Western world has declined dramatically. Painter[15] believed that this dietary change is the most probable cause of the emergence of diverticular disease in Westernized populations in the 20th century. A colon with a wide lumen is less able to form segments efficiently, and large-bore colons are found wherever individuals eat a diet containing plenty of roughage. By contrast, consuming the over-refined, fiber-deficient diet of the industrial countries produces small hard stools that pass through a narrower colon that can segment more easily. Higher pressures are needed to transport these stiff stools, and because the fecal stream is more viscous by the time it reaches the distal colon, it causes the sigmoid to segment excessively. Thus, segmentation is postulated to be the mechanism responsible for the pathogenesis of diverticula, and a fiber-deficient diet is the likely cause of the disease. Burkitt et al[16] studied the fiber intake of African natives and compared it to that of British subjects. They found that the Africans had a higher stool weight and a shorter transit time. They attributed the low incidence of diverticular disease to this high fiber intake. Bingham[17] provided an excellent summary of the dietary fiber intake of general populations and found that Africans consume 60 to 150 g/d; Europeans, 15 to

25 g/d; Japanese, 20 g/d; Canadian vegetarians, 30 g/d; and people in the United States, 13 to 20 g/d. In a study of barium enema examinations in vegetarians and nonvegetarians, Gear et al[18] found a 12% incidence of diverticular disease in vegetarians, compared with a 33% incidence among nonvegetarians. Manousos et al[19] found that patients with diverticula consumed significantly less brown bread and vegetables but more meat than controls.

Nakaji et al[20] compared the etiology of right-sided diverticula in Japan with that of left-sided diverticula in the West. Diverticula occur predominantly in the right-sided colon (> 70%) in Japanese patients, and even among Japanese who emigrate, in contrast with the diverticula in Western patients. The increased detection rate over time is higher in urban areas than in rural areas, and it corresponds to the distribution of dietary fiber intake. Furthermore, the significant relationship of right-sided diverticula with intraluminal pressure in Japan is similar to that of left-sided diverticula in the West, and the pathological features of these diverticula are similar. The etiology of right-sided diverticula in Japan (and perhaps other Mongolian peoples) is very similar to that of left-sided diverticula in the West. The location may represent a difference in morphology of the large intestine between Mongolians (including Japanese) and Westerners, rather than environmental differences.

Other lifestyle habits also appear to have an influence on the development of symptomatic diverticular disease. In a prospective study of 47,678 American men, Aldoori et al[21] found that physical activity was inversely associated with the risk of symptoms, with a relative risk of 0.60 for individuals engaged in vigorous activity such as jogging and running. From the same cohort of men, Aldoori et al[22] found that smoking, caffeine, and alcohol intake are not associated with any substantial increase in the risk of symptomatic disease. They further examined dietary fiber calculated from food composition values from a prospective cohort of 43,881 U.S. male health professionals in the 40 to 75 years age group.[23] Their findings suggest that the insoluble component of fiber was significantly associated with a decreased risk of diverticular disease (relative ratio [RR] = 0.63), and this inverse association was particularly strong for cellulose (RR = 0.52).

Advancing age has an effect on mechanical strength of the colon wall, likely a consequence of changes in collagen structure. Wess et al[24] measured collagen from unaffected human colons and compared it to those with colonic diverticulosis obtained at necropsy. The total collagen content was constant with age. The acid solubility of the collagen, however, increased after the age of 40 years. After 60 years of age, colonic diverticulosis was associated with an increased acid solubility ratio compared with values in unaffected colons (15:3 compared with 9:2). Stumpf et al[25] showed decreased levels of mature collagen type I and increased levels of collagen type III, with a resulting lower collagen ratio I/III, in patients with diverticulitis. The expression of matrix metalloproteinase-I was significantly reduced in the diverticulitis group, while the expression of matrix metalloproteinase-13 did not differ significantly between the two groups. Their findings support the theory of structural changes in the colonic wall as one of the major pathogenic factors in the development of diverticular disease. Bode et al[26] reported the contents of types I and III collagen telopeptides and total collagen were similar in diverticulosis and healthy tissue and that type III collagen synthesis was increased in diverticulosis, but not in malignancy.

The traditional belief is that diverticula develop as a result of elevated intraluminal pressures that arise because of segmentation of the colon. Segmentation causes the colon to act not as a tube, but as a series of "little bladders," each of which has narrowed outflow (▶ Fig. 27.2).[27] High pressures develop in these segments and force the mucosa through the muscular wall of the colon. Segmentation plays a part in normal colonic physiology by shunting colon contents back and forth in the sigmoid colon, presumably to aid in the absorption of water from the fecal stream. Thus, Painter and Burkitt believe that diverticula are the outward visible sign of an inward disturbance of colonic

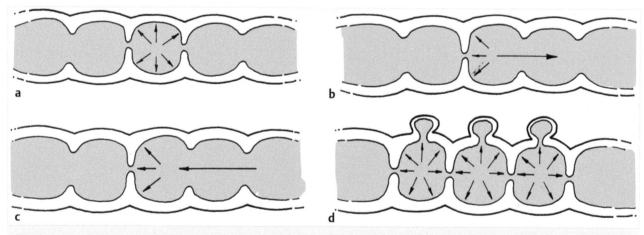

Fig. 27.2 Segmentation is concerned with the transportation and halting of feces in sigmoid colon. **(a)** Segmented colon. One segment has produced pressure by contracting. **(b)** Relaxation of contraction ring on one side of this segment allows contents to move into the next segment, which harbors lower pressure. This is a mechanism by which contents are moved. **(c)** Feces are halted. Contraction rings act as baffles that slow and finally halt contents, and a pressure change results. Segmentation is seen in sigmoid as feces are shunted back and forth. **(d)** Segmented colon acting as a series of "little bladders" whose outflow is obstructed at both ends and which extrude diverticula by generating high-localized intrasegmental pressures. Segmentation is essential to pathogenesis of diverticula. Any factor that causes segmentation to occur more frequently or more efficiently favors causation of diverticula disease.[12]

motility, due to a diet low in fiber.[27] Painter[28] summarized his extensive studies of the role of segmentation as the cause of diverticular disease and its symptoms as follows. Segmentation of the colon is the mechanism by which the colon propels its contents or halts material moving through its lumen. It involves the production of increased intraluminal pressures and has been demonstrated by recording the intracolonic pressures with open-ended tubes, while simultaneous fluoroscopy recorded the behavior of the colon. The intracolonic pressures produced by segmentation may exceed 90 mm Hg. Cineradiography also has revealed high localized intraluminal pressures that are produced by segmentation of the colon, regardless of the stimulus that evokes them.

Another theory on the etiology of diverticular change proposes that there is no muscle abnormality, but there is likely a connective tissue abnormality causing a density of diverticula in the colon. This abnormality provides inadequate support for vessels in the wall of the colon, increasing the propensity for vascular malformations and bleeding. Clinical evidence suggests that both acute and chronic pain may be caused by either inflammation or muscle spasm. This theory also proposes that perforation may be due to abnormal intraluminal pressures rather than diverticular inflammation.[29]

Nonetheless, the muscle abnormality is the most consistent and important feature in diverticular disease of the sigmoid colon.[9] When the colonic wall is sectioned, the interior aspect reveals openings that may at times be inconspicuous and detected only when fecal matter is impacted. The muscular coat is thickened, and the mucosal layer is heaped into transverse folds that project into the lumen. The luminal diameter is reduced in size. The thickened longitudinal and circular muscle layers have been considered responsible for shortening the sigmoid colon and pleating the mucosa. Narrowing of the lumen may be due to these redundant folds but in part may be secondary to pericolic fibrosis.[9]

Microscopically, pulsion diverticula are comprised of two of the four layers of the colon wall: an inner mucosal layer and an outer serosal layer. An artery, vein, and attenuated muscle may be seen close to the neck of the diverticulum (▶ Fig. 27.3). In patients with diverticular disease, both the muscularis mucosa and muscularis propria are greatly increased in thickness. There has been much conjecture about whether the muscle thickening is due to hypertrophy or hyperplasia. In their study of the thickened bowel, Whiteway and Morson[30] failed to reveal evidence of cellular hypertrophy or hyperplasia. Instead, they attributed the thickening to the presence of elastic tissue, specifically in the teniae.[31] This progressive elastosis causes longitudinal foreshortening of the colon, accentuating the semicircular corrugations of the shortened circular muscle. The source of the elastosis is uncertain, but this abnormality precedes the development of diverticulosis. It is characteristic of diverticular disease in that it is never seen in other segmental or diffuse inflammatory conditions of the colon. Why the muscle abnormality occurs predominantly in the sigmoid colon is unclear. It is postulated that the muscle of the sigmoid colon is different from that of the more proximal colon because it appears thicker and shows an increased capacity for muscular spasm.

27.5 Natural History

Despite the significant prevalence of diverticulosis of the colon in western adults—estimated to be 15 to 37%[4]—it is an asymptomatic condition in most patients. It is estimated that 10 to 25% of patients with diverticulosis will develop diverticulitis.[32] Of patients with diverticulitis of the colon, 10 to 33% eventually require operative intervention.[33] From his extensive personal studies and thorough review of the literature, Parks[4] summarized the following features of diverticular disease. The incidence increases with advancing years, with an increased risk of hemorrhage in the elderly. In young patients, the disease may pursue a more aggressive course. There seems to be an increasing incidence in women. Progression of disease relative to number and size of diverticula does not seem to occur. In the majority of patients with diverticula localized to the distal colon, the disorder will not necessarily progress relentlessly and involve additional segments; progression more often occurs within the segment of bowel initially affected. On an average, patients with extensive involvement may be younger than those with localized disease. Parks[4] also noted severe complications to occur equally in patients with distal disease and those with total colonic involvement, and after an operation to eradicate distal disease, it is unusual for inflammatory complications to develop in the proximal bowel. However, Parks described that hemorrhage occurred more readily from the proximal bowel, it was not necessarily of diverticular origin, and may be due to vascular ectasias, which are more common in the right colon.

27.6 Diagnosis

Most often, uncomplicated diverticular disease is asymptomatic and it may be discovered incidentally during an imaging study done for another reason. Some patients may experience ill-defined left-sided abdominal discomfort located most often in the left lower quadrant. Associated symptoms of anorexia, flatulence, nausea, and alteration in bowel habits may occur. Rectal bleeding is uncommon in patients with uncomplicated diverticular disease,[34] and in fact the presence of bleeding strongly suggests the presence of a concomitant lesion.[35] In patients with diverticulosis, no abnormal physical signs will be found during

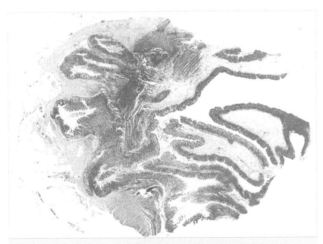

Fig. 27.3 Photomicrograph of several diverticula penetrating the colonic wall. (This image is provided courtesy of Esther Lamoureux, MD.)

physical examination. Similarly, digital rectal examination and rigid sigmoidoscopic examination are not revealing, because examination beyond the rectosigmoid junction is impossible with these modalities.

In the absence of specific symptoms and signs, the diagnosis of diverticulosis is most often established through a colonoscopy as an incidental finding; barium enema is also a good way to determine the extent and severity of the diverticulosis. Diverticula may be distributed throughout the entire colon, but it is the left colon, particularly the sigmoid, that is most often affected. A common radiologic finding is some degree of colonic spasm that in its most impressive form may produce a zigzag appearance on contrast enema. In the chronic state, the sigmoid lumen may become stenotic and the bowel wall more rigid. Colonoscopy is critical to differentiate diverticular disease from carcinoma, especially in the presence of a luminal narrowing. A review of the literature by Hunt[35] showed that carcinoma was identified by colonoscopy in 17% of 125 patients with complicated diverticular disease, with an additional diagnosis made in 32%. The cecum was only reached in 61%. In a group of 135 patients with persistent bleeding, in whom barium enema examination showed only diverticular disease, 11% had carcinoma, and an additional diagnosis was made in 37%.

The diagnosis of acute diverticulitis can often be made following a focused history and physical examination. The combination of left lower quadrant tenderness with or without other peritoneal findings, fever, and leukocytosis is suggestive of sigmoid diverticulitis. The presence of fecaluria, pneumaturia, or pyuria raises the suspicion of a fistula to the bladder. Urinalysis and plain abdominal radiographs may be helpful in excluding diagnoses in the differential, such as urinary tract infections, kidney stones, and bowel obstruction. Other diagnoses that can mimic the presentation of acute diverticulitis include irritable bowel syndrome, appendicitis, inflammatory bowel disease, ischemic bowel, neoplasia, and gynecologic disorders. Depending on the mode of presentation, other entities that may be included in the differential diagnosis are ulcerative colitis, pelvic inflammatory disease, ureteral colic, and endometriosis. With respect to age, the differential diagnosis in the elderly might include carcinoma, volvulus, and large bowel obstruction.

Clearly, the most important diagnosis to rule out is carcinoma. A number of radiologic features have been considered in establishing the differential diagnosis. For example, in a patient with diverticular disease, the affected segment of bowel is often longer than in one with carcinoma. The transition from normal to diseased bowel is more gradual in diverticular change than with carcinoma, in which it is usually abrupt. With diverticular disease, the mucosa is preserved, but it is abnormal in carcinoma. The presence of diverticula in an area of colonic narrowing favors the diagnosis of diverticular disease but in no way rules out the presence of a concomitant carcinoma. In an effort to reduce the misdiagnosis rate among patients with diverticulitis, clinical scoring systems have been proposed that rely on history, physical examination, and blood work.[36]

Computed tomography (CT) imaging has become a commonly used and widely available study to aid in the diagnosis and severity staging of patients with suspected diverticulitis, and is the most appropriate initial imaging modality in the assessment of suspected diverticulitis.[37] In the appropriate setting, multislice CT imaging with intravenous and luminal contrast has excellent sensitivity and specificity, reported as high as 98 and 99%.[38,39] With early or mild diverticulitis, CT may not be as accurate. CT findings associated with diverticulitis most commonly include diverticulosis with associated colon wall thickening, fat stranding, phlegmon, extraluminal gas, abscess, stricture, and fistula. Importantly, cross-sectional imaging can accurately diagnose other disease processes that may mimic the presentation of diverticulitis. Immunocompromised patients who may not mount a normal or significant inflammatory response may have minimal findings, however, such as extraluminal gas without other typical radiographic findings.[40] In addition, the grade of severity on CT correlates with the risk of failure of nonoperative management in the short term and with long-term complications such as recurrence, the persistence of symptoms, and the development of colonic stricture and fistula.[41,42,43]

27.7 Nonoperative Treatment

Nonoperative treatment typically includes oral or intravenous antibiotics and diet modification.[37] However, the long-held belief that diverticulitis is caused by microperforation and bacterial infection has been challenged by the concept that diverticulitis may be a primary inflammatory process.[44] A Swedish multicenter trial randomly treated 623 inpatients with CT-confirmed uncomplicated left-sided diverticulitis with intravenous fluids or intravenous fluids and antibiotics. They found that antibiotic therapy did not prevent complications, accelerate recovery, or prevent recurrences.[45] Other trials also found no significant difference between antibiotics and no antibiotics for the treatment of uncomplicated diverticulitis.[46,47] Before these reports, antibiotics were considered the unchallenged cornerstone of treatment for patients with diverticulitis.

In general, clinically stable, reliable patients with uncomplicated disease who can tolerate oral antibiotics can be treated as outpatients with a high rate of success.[48] In fact admissions for acute diverticulitis through the emergency room could probably be avoided in over 50% of patients with uncomplicated disease.[49] Patients with complicated diverticulitis (perforation with abscess), who have a high fever or white blood cell count, are elderly, or have significant health problems, as well as those who do not have adequate support at home, typically benefit from hospital admission with intravenous antibiotics and bowel rest. Antibiotics should target gram negatives and anaerobes. Multidisciplinary, nonoperative management of inpatients with acute diverticulitis is highly successful, allowing a staged surgical approach for select patients in an elective setting.

Although epidemiologic evidence suggests that a high-fiber diet prevents the formation of diverticula, there is little evidence that once diverticula are formed the use of bran and bulking agents will prevent complications associated with diverticular disease. An exception to this belief is the study by Hyland and Taylor,[50] suggesting that among those who already have diverticula, complications and recurrences of diverticulitis are reduced with a high-fiber diet. Although advocated by some, the elimination of foods with seeds is of questionable value.

Oral antibiotics and mucosal anti-inflammatory agents may have a role in prevention of symptoms associated with diverticulitis. Papi et al[51] conducted a double-blind, placebo-controlled trial to determine the efficacy of long-term intermittent administration of a poorly absorbed antibiotic in obtaining symptomatic relief in patients with uncomplicated diverticular disease. A series of 168 patients received either a fiber supplement (glucomannan, 2 g/d) plus rifaximin 400 mg twice a day for 7 days every month (84 patients) or glucomannan (2 g/d) plus placebo, two tablets twice a day for 7 days every month (84 patients). After 12 months, 70% of patients treated with rifaximin were symptom free or mildly symptomatic compared to 40% in the placebo group. Symptoms such as bloating, abdominal pain, and discomfort were primarily affected by antibiotic treatment. No advantage was accrued in preventing diverticulitis.

The role of mucosal anti-inflammatory agents in prevention of diverticulitis has also been investigated. Treatment is based on the assumption that mucosal inflammation in symptomatic uncomplicated diverticulitis may induce diverticulitis, and can be prevented by the administration of aminosalicylates such as mesalazine. Data from small studies is compelling, whereas data from randomized trials show contrasting results.[52,53,54,55] Brandimarte and Tursi[53] investigated the effectiveness of the combination of rifaximin/mesalazine, followed by mesalamine alone to evaluate tolerability and effectiveness in symptom remission, in 90 consecutive patients with symptomatic uncomplicated diverticular disease. Symptoms were scored on a quantitative scale, and included constipation, diarrhea, abdominal pain, rectal bleeding, and mucus with stool. All patients were treated with 800 mg/d rifaximin plus 2.4 g/d mesalamine for 10 days, followed by 1.6 g/d mesalamine for 8 weeks. After the eighth week of treatment, 81% of patients were completely asymptomatic with mesalamine alone, while 18.6% showed only slight symptoms. Two (2.22%) showed recurrence of diverticulitis after 4 and 6 weeks of treatment with mesalazine alone. Two patients (2.22%) were withdrawn from the study for diarrhea after starting mesalazine. Two others (2.22%) showed transitory pruritus (one) and epigastric pain (one). Their results showed that rifaximin/mesalazine followed by mesalamine alone is effective in resolving symptoms in patients with symptomatic uncomplicated diverticular disease. The roles of nonabsorbable antibiotics and topical anti-inflammatory agents in the prevention of diverticulitis are yet to be resolved.

27.7.1 Nonoperative Management of Complicated Diverticulitis

The trend toward one-stage resection for complicated diverticular disease continues to evolve. The goal of this strategy is to decrease the morbidity of a colostomy when possible, as well as a second operation to restore intestinal continuity.

Abscess formation is a common complication of acute diverticulitis and occurs in 15 to 20% of patients.[56] Patients found to have a large (> 5 cm) diverticular abscess, or an abscess located in the pelvis, are likely to benefit from image-guided percutaneous drainage.[37] This has been used extensively in the treatment of patients with an abscess accessible on cross-sectional imaging, and will allow up to 75% of patients to avoid urgent operation and undergo interval elective, one-stage colectomy.[57,58,59,60] Deciding which patients with diverticular abscesses will benefit from a percutaneous drainage procedure remains controversial, however. Those with a small (2–4 cm) abscess, or an abscess located in the mesentery, may be managed without a drainage procedure, but those who fail this strategy should be considered for drainage, or operation.

27.8 Elective Surgery for Diverticulitis

27.8.1 Elective Surgery after Recovery from Uncomplicated Diverticulitis

Determining the optimal strategy for elective colectomy in patients with diverticular disease involves a balance of the morbidity, mortality, cost, and quality of life associated with both elective and expectant management. The recommendation for elective sigmoid colon resection after recovery from uncomplicated episodes has evolved, and is now based on literature describing a relatively low rate of recurrence (up to one-third),[61] and need for emergency operation (under 6%).[62] Past recommendations included elective resection after the second episode of uncomplicated disease, but recent literature has not shown an increase in morbidity or mortality after the second, third, or fourth attacks.[63] In fact, patients who present with complicated disease most often describe it as their first episode.[64] Since the need for emergency colectomy and colostomy is rare after recovery from an uncomplicated episode, surgery for the prevention of complications is no longer recommended for the average patient. Patients with smoldering symptoms, significant impairment of lifestyle, or episodes that are increasing in frequency and severity despite no evidence of a complication should be counseled regarding elective surgery. Consideration should be given to age, comorbidities, body mass index (BMI), and tobacco use when discussing risk and outcomes with elective surgery.[65] In addition, clinical trials have shown that elective surgery following successful conservative treatment of acute diverticulitis may result in significantly better social and functional well-being.[66]

Consideration for elective surgery must also be given to those patients who are chronically immunosuppressed for organ transplant,[67] who need steroid therapy for other chronic diseases, and who have kidney failure or collagen vascular diseases as they are more likely to fail medical nonoperative management or require emergency surgery for complicated disease. Therefore, a low threshold for recommending operative intervention during the first hospitalization should be upheld for this subgroup of patients.[68]

27.8.2 Elective Surgery after Recovery from Complicated Diverticulitis

Patients who present with a pelvic abscess, or a large abscess that requires drainage, have a high recurrence rate of up to 40%, in small studies.[69] Operative management has been typically recommended after resolution of the acute episode, but nonoperative strategies have been studied, and appear to be safe in select cases,[70] but large randomized trials are lacking. Patients who present with fistula or stricture generally require resection for symptomatic relief.

Elective Resection Based on Age: Young age, defined as younger than 50 years, has been used as an indication for operation in the past; however, routine resection due to age alone is no longer recommended. It was thought to be a more virulent disease in the young, but recent studies have shown diverticulitis to be similar in frequency and severity in both younger and older patient groups, including comparable rates of the need for resection at the initial hospitalization and rates of stoma formation during subsequent attacks.[71] Young patients may have a higher risk of recurrence due to longevity compared with older patients, but the overall rate of recurrence is low, with approximately 27% developing another episode after first presentation. Furthermore, following recovery from the initial episode of acute diverticulitis, only 7.5% of young patients have been found to require subsequent emergency surgery.[61] Other retrospective data collected on young patients with CT-confirmed initial episodes of diverticulitis demonstrated a low 2.1% rate of emergency surgery at subsequent attacks, similar to risk in the older patient.[72]

Technical Considerations

Ideally, the entire thickened contracted segment involved in the inflammatory process should be resected back to non-hypertrophic colon. Over a third of patients with sigmoid diverticulitis will have pandiverticulosis, but the risk of recurrent inflammation in proximal diverticula is low. Follow-up of patients with previous resection has revealed that recurrent diverticulitis in diverticula proximal to the sigmoid is uncommon. Therefore, it is also generally agreed that every diverticulum in the proximal colon does not require resection. Due to the partial-thickness nature of a pulsion diverticulum, common sense dictates that this should not be included in the technically perfect anastomosis.

Distally, diverticular disease does not usually involve the rectum, so the rectosigmoid junction or proximal rectum should be the distal extent of resection. Patients have a higher risk of developing recurrent diverticulitis after resection if the sigmoid is used for the distal aspect of the anastomosis.[73,74]

Laparoscopic techniques for the elective resection of diverticular disease have extensively been shown to lead to a decrease in blood loss, wound infection, and incisional hernia rate, with the additional benefits offered by a minimally invasive approach: less pain, less narcotic need, and earlier return to normal activity.[75,76,77] Laparoscopic colon surgery is technically challenging; if this expertise is not available, or other technical considerations make minimally invasive surgery impossible, then traditional open techniques should be used to perform the safest possible operation with optimal outcomes for the patient.

27.8.3 Emergency Surgery for Perforated Diverticulitis

The vast majority of patients who present with diverticulitis will have focal peritonitis, and can be successfully managed nonoperatively, with or without a drain, with bowel rest and intravenous antibiotics. Approximately 25% of patients will have a far more dramatic presentation with acute illness, diffuse peritonitis, and hemodynamic changes. These patients require expeditious surgery to control the source of sepsis.

Hartmann's procedure was originally reported in 1923 as an operation to remove a rectal carcinoma.[78] It entails the resection of the perforated segment of sigmoid colon along with closure of the rectal stump and the establishment of an end sigmoid colostomy (▶ Fig. 27.4). In most circumstances, Hartmann's operation remains the procedure of choice for patients suffering from a free perforation and generalized peritonitis. Every effort should be made to optimally site the planned ostomy prior to placing the patient under general anesthesia. The advantage of this procedure is that the septic focus is removed by the primary operation, thus eliminating the continued source of contamination.

The acute inflammatory nature of the disease often permits blunt dissection to proceed without injury to adjacent structures, in particular the small bowel and left ureter. It is wise to begin dissection in normal tissues proximal and distal to the phlegmonous, perforated mass. Division of peritoneal attachments will typically permit entry into the appropriate plane (i.e., just posterior to the colon wall and anterior to the ureter and left gonadal vessels). Attachments to abdominal wall, bladder, ureter, and pelvis are systematically divided until the affected segment of perforated colon is mobilized. Difficult dissections can be facilitated by division of the colon at the proposed proximal line of resection and reflecting the colon anteriorly, which provides more working room. This proximal point of transection is ultimately brought out through the abdominal wall as an end descending colostomy. Using a proximal-to-distal dissection, the colon is lifted away from the retroperitoneal structures including the ureter, gonadal, and iliac vessels. Mesenteric vessels are sequentially ligated and

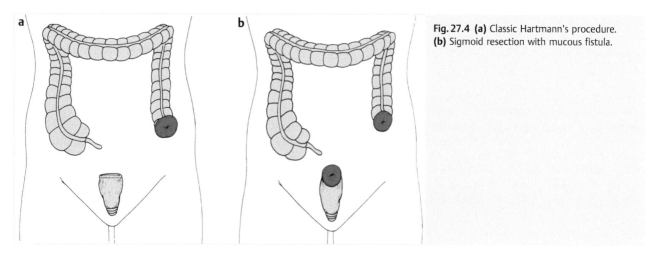

Fig. 27.4 (a) Classic Hartmann's procedure. **(b)** Sigmoid resection with mucous fistula.

divided as identified. Patience in approaching the most adherent segment from all sides eventually results in release of the fixed bowel. The distal point of transection should be at or near the sacral promontory, preserving as much rectal reservoir as possible, while ensuring the stapler is placed across soft, compliant bowel with minimal induration. If stump closure appears tenuous, a wide-bore catheter might wisely be placed via the anus to irrigate out residual stool while in the OR, and then leave it in place to decompress the rectal stump for several days. Mobilization of the retrorectal space as well as the splenic flexure should be avoided if possible, to avoid contamination, which may make restoration of intestinal continuity at a later date far more difficult.

Early "three-stage" surgery for diverticulitis involved creation of a transverse loop colostomy without resection of the perforated segment of colon, leaving behind a column of stool with continued contamination in the abdominal cavity. This option is mostly of historical interest. The preventable mortality of perforated diverticulitis is due to immediate or delayed effects of sepsis. The mortality related to cardiovascular or pulmonary disease can be difficult to modulate.

Anastomosis in this setting should be avoided due to the presence of an acutely inflamed intestine, gross fecal contamination, and free pus under emergency circumstances. Disadvantages of Hartmann's procedure include the fact that the second stage of the operation requires a major abdominal operation that can be very difficult. Timing of the second operation is critical—a prolonged waiting period, in the order of 6 to 12 months after extensive intra-abdominal contamination—typically makes the abdomen less hostile and may decrease the risk of injury to contiguous organs. The more severe the initial contamination, the longer the recommended waiting period for resolution. In rare cases, 3 months is a reasonable convalescent period, but a prolonged wait will give the patient time to heal on all fronts—recovering metabolically, nutritionally, psychologically, and from an infectious standpoint. The remaining colon must be assessed for residual diverticular disease at the time of colostomy closure. Any residual diverticular disease in the distal segment of bowel should be resected to allow safe anastomosis to the proximal rectum and decrease the risk for recurrent diverticulitis. Resecting every diverticula-bearing portion of colon proximal to the anastomosis is not essential unless the disease is so extensive that there is not a satisfactory segment of colon in which to construct an anastomosis.

The hesitance to accept a colostomy on the part of the patient can be countered with the assistance of an excellent stoma therapist and the possibility of laparoscopic closure of the colostomy. Factors associated with increased risk of death following Hartmann's procedure include persistent sepsis, fecal peritonitis, preoperative hypotension, and prolonged duration of symptom.[79] Haas and Fox reviewed the fate of the forgotten rectal pouch after Hartmann's procedure without any reconstruction.[80] They examined 45 patients at least 1 year after an operation for a variety of indications and found that 25 patients were asymptomatic. The others reported pain, mucus discharge, bleeding, or passage of bowel contents. Of the 24 patients operated on for diverticulitis, 12 had proctitis and 2 had polyps. The proctitis should be treated with reanastomosis.

Hartmann's procedure has evolved as the treatment of choice for certain patients with diffuse peritonitis. It is no longer the treatment of choice for a patient with an abscess, which should be treated primarily by percutaneous drainage; if the patient fails this intervention, then Hartmann's procedure can be considered, or if there is minimal contamination, anastomosis may be possible. There is a large body of contrasting data regarding the management of perforated diverticulitis with laparoscopic lavage in lieu of sigmoid resection. In general, in the lavage group, there is a lower rate of stoma formation and wound infection, shorter length of stay during the index admission, and similar morbidity and mortality as sigmoidectomy.[1] However, there is a statistically significantly higher rate of intra-abdominal abscess in the lavage group, leading to early termination of one large randomized trial.[2] While laparoscopic lavage may not be considered inferior to sigmoidectomy in patients with Hinchey Stage III peritonitis,[3] it does not appear to adequately control intra-abdominal sepsis. It should be used selectively after careful consideration of the patient's overall status and ability to tolerate a significant complication.[81,82,83]

References

[1] Cruveilhier J. Traité d'Anatomie Pathologique. Paris: Bailliére, 1849

[2] Slack WW. The anatomy, pathology, and some clinical features of divericulitis of the colon. Br J Surg. 1962; 50:185–190

[3] Heise CP. Epidemiology and pathogenesis of diverticular disease. J Gastrointest Surg. 2008; 12(8):1309–1311

[4] Parks TG. Natural history of diverticular disease of the colon. Clin Gastroenterol. 1975; 4(1):53–69

[5] Connell AM. Pathogenesis of diverticular disease of the colon. Adv Intern Med. 1977; 22:377–395

[6] Rankin FW, Brown PW. Diverticulitis of the colon. Surg Gynecol Obstet. 1930; 50:836–847

[7] Heller SN, Hackler LR. Changes in the crude fiber content of the American diet. Am J Clin Nutr. 1978; 31(9):1510–1514

[8] Rodkey GV, Welch CE. Changing patterns in the surgical treatment of diverticular disease. Ann Surg. 1984; 200(4):466–478

[9] Morson BC. Pathology of diverticular disease of the colon. Clin Gastroenterol. 1975; 4(1):37–52

[10] Pan GZ, Liu TH, Chen MZ, Chang HC. Diverticular disease of colon in China. A 60-year retrospective study. Chin Med J (Engl). 1984; 97(6):391–394

[11] Coode PE, Chan KW, Chan YT. Polyps and diverticula of the large intestine: a necropsy survey in Hong Kong. Gut. 1985; 26(10):1045–1048

[12] Levy N, Stermer E, Simon J. The changing epidemiology of diverticular disease in Israel. Dis Colon Rectum. 1985; 28(6):416–418

[13] Kozak LJ, DeFrances CJ, Hall MJ. National hospital survey: 2004 annual summary with detailed diagnosis and procedure data. National Center for Health Statistics. Vital Health Stat. 2006; 13:162

[14] Shaheen NJ, Hansen RA, Morgan DR, et al. The burden of gastrointestinal and liver diseases, 2006. Am J Gastroenterol. 2006; 101(9):2128–2138

[15] Painter NS. Diverticular disease of the colon. The first of the Western diseases shown to be due to a deficiency of dietary fibre. S Afr Med J. 1982; 61 (26):1016–1020

[16] Burkitt DP, Walker ARP, Painter NS. Dietary fiber and disease. JAMA. 1974; 229(8):1068–1074

[17] Bingham S. Dietary fiber intake: intake studies, problems, methods and results. In: Trowell H, Burkitt DP, Heaton K, eds. Dietary Fiber; Fiber Depleted Foods and Disease. New York, NY: Academic Press; 1985:77–104

[18] Gear JSS, Ware A, Fursdon P, et al. Symptomless diverticular disease and intake of dietary fibre. Lancet. 1979; 1(8115):511–514

[19] Manousos O, Day NE, Tzonou A, et al. Diet and other factors in the aetiology of diverticulosis: an epidemiological study in Greece. Gut. 1985; 26 (6):544–549

[20] Nakaji S, Danjo K, Munakata A, et al. Comparison of etiology of right-sided diverticula in Japan with that of left-sided diverticula in the West. Int J Colorectal Dis. 2002; 17(6):365–373

[21] Aldoori WH, Giovannucci EL, Rimm EB, et al. Prospective study of physical activity and the risk of symptomatic diverticular disease in men. Gut. 1995; 36 (2):276–282

[22] Aldoori WH, Giovannucci EL, Rimm EB, Wing AL, Trichopoulos DV, Willett WC. A prospective study of alcohol, smoking, caffeine, and the risk of symptomatic diverticular disease in men. Ann Epidemiol. 1995; 5(3):221–228

[23] Aldoori WH, Giovannucci EL, Rockett HR, Sampson L, Rimm EB, Willett WC. A prospective study of dietary fiber types and symptomatic diverticular disease in men. J Nutr. 1998; 128(4):714–719

[24] Wess L, Eastwood MA, Wess TJ, Busuttil A, Miller A. Cross linking of collagen is increased in colonic diverticulosis. Gut. 1995; 37(1):91–94

[25] Stumpf M, Cao W, Klinge U, Klosterhalfen B, Kasperk R, Schumpelick V. Increased distribution of collagen type III and reduced expression of matrix metalloproteinase 1 in patients with diverticular disease. Int J Colorectal Dis. 2001; 16(5):271–275

[26] Bode MK, Karttunen TJ, Mäkelä J, Risteli L, Risteli J. Type I and III collagens in human colon cancer and diverticulosis. Scand J Gastroenterol. 2000; 35 (7):747–752

[27] Painter NS, Burkitt DP. Diverticular disease of the colon, a 20th century problem. Clin Gastroenterol. 1975; 4(1):3–21

[28] Painter NS. The cause of diverticular disease of the colon, its symptoms and its complications. Review and hypothesis. J R Coll Surg Edinb. 1985; 30 (2):118–122

[29] Ryan P. Two kinds of diverticular disease. Ann R Coll Surg Engl. 1991; 73 (2):73–79

[30] Whiteway J, Morson BC. Pathology of the ageing–diverticular disease. Clin Gastroenterol. 1985; 14(4):829–846

[31] Whiteway J, Morson BC. Elastosis in diverticular disease of the sigmoid colon. Gut. 1985; 26(3):258–266

[32] Hackford AW, Veidenheimer MC. Diverticular disease of the colon. Current concepts and management. Surg Clin North Am. 1985; 65(2):347–363

[33] Thörn M, Graf W, Stefánsson T, Påhlman L. Clinical and functional results after elective colon resection in 75 consecutive patients with diverticular disease. Am J Surg. 2002; 183(1):7–11

[34] Kewenter J, Hellzen-Ingemarsson A, Kewenter G, Olsson U. Diverticular disease and minor rectal bleeding. Scand J Gastroenterol. 1985; 20(8):922–924

[35] Hunt RH. The role of colonoscopy in complicated diverticular disease. A review. Acta Chir Belg. 1979; 78(6):349–353

[36] Andeweg CS, Knobben L, Hendriks JC, Bleichrodt RP, van Goor H. How to diagnose acute left-sided colonic diverticulitis: proposal for a clinical scoring system. Ann Surg. 2011; 253(5):940–946

[37] Feingold D, Steele SR, Lee S, et al. Practice parameters for the treatment of sigmoid diverticulitis. Dis Colon Rectum. 2014; 57(3):284–294

[38] Laméris W, van Randen A, Bipat S, Bossuyt PM, Boermeester MA, Stoker J. Graded compression ultrasonography and computed tomography in acute colonic diverticulitis: meta-analysis of test accuracy. Eur Radiol. 2008; 18(11):2498–2511

[39] Ambrosetti P, Jenny A, Becker C, Terrier TF, Morel P. Acute left colonic diverticulitis–compared performance of computed tomography and water-soluble contrast enema: prospective evaluation of 420 patients. Dis Colon Rectum. 2000; 43(10):1363–1367

[40] Baker ME. Imaging and interventional techniques in acute left-sided diverticulitis. J Gastrointest Surg. 2008; 12(8):1314–1317

[41] Ambrosetti P. Acute diverticulitis of the left colon: value of the initial CT and timing of elective colectomy. J Gastrointest Surg. 2008; 12(8):1318–1320

[42] Ambrosetti P, Becker C, Terrier F. Colonic diverticulitis: impact of imaging on surgical management: a prospective study of 542 patients. Eur Radiol. 2002; 12(5):1145–1149

[43] Bordeianou L, Hodin R. Controversies in the surgical management of sigmoid diverticulitis. J Gastrointest Surg. 2007; 11(4):542–548

[44] de Korte N, Unlü C, Boermeester MA, Cuesta MA, Vrouenreats BC, Stockmann HB. Use of antibiotics in uncomplicated diverticulitis. Br J Surg. 2011; 98 (6):761–767

[45] Chabok A, Påhlman L, Hjern F, Haapaniemi S, Smedh K, AVOD Study Group. Randomized clinical trial of antibiotics in acute uncomplicated diverticulitis. Br J Surg. 2012; 99(4):532–539

[46] Shabanzadeh DM, Wille-Jørgensen P. Antibiotics for uncomplicated diverticulitis. Cochrane Database Syst Rev. 2012; 11:CD009092

[47] Brochmann ND, Schultz JK, Jakobsen GS, Øresland T. Management of acute uncomplicated diverticulitis without antibiotics: a single-centre cohort study. Colorectal Dis. 2016; 18(11):1101–1107

[48] Alonso S, Pera M, Parés D, et al. Outpatient treatment of patients with uncomplicated acute diverticulitis. Colorectal Dis. 2010; 12(10 Online):e278–e282

[49] Sirany AE, Gaertner WB, Madoff RD, Kwaan MR. Diverticulitis diagnosed in the emergency room: is it safe to discharge home? J Am Coll Surg. 2017; 225 (1):21–25

[50] Hyland JMP, Taylor I. Does a high fibre diet prevent the complications of diverticular disease? Br J Surg. 1980; 67(2):77–79

[51] Papi C, Ciaco A, Koch M, Capurso L. Efficacy of rifaximin in the treatment of symptomatic diverticular disease of the colon. A multicentre double-blind placebo-controlled trial. Aliment Pharmacol Ther. 1995; 9(1):33–39

[52] Barbara G, Cremon C, Barbaro MR, Bellacosa L, Stanghellini V. Treatment of diverticular disease with aminosalicylates: the evidence. J Clin Gastroenterol. 2016; 50 Suppl 1:S60–S63

[53] Brandimarte G, Tursi A. Rifaximin plus mesalazine followed by mesalazine alone is highly effective in obtaining remission of symptomatic uncomplicated diverticular disease. Med Sci Monit. 2004; 10(5):PI70–PI73

[54] Shayto RH, Abou Mrad R, Sharara AI. Use of rifaximin in gastrointestinal and liver diseases. World J Gastroenterol. 2016; 22(29):6638–6651

[55] Maconi G, Barbara G, Bosetti C, Cuomo R, Annibale B. Treatment of diverticular disease of the colon and prevention of acute diverticulitis: a systematic review. Dis Colon Rectum. 2011; 54(10):1326–1338

[56] Beckham H, Whitlow CB. The medical and nonoperative treatment of diverticulitis. Clin Colon Rectal Surg. 2009; 22(3):156–160

[57] Durmishi Y, Gervaz P, Brandt D, et al. Results from percutaneous drainage of Hinchey stage II diverticulitis guided by computed tomography scan. Surg Endosc. 2006; 20(7):1129–1133

[58] Siewert B, Tye G, Kruskal J, et al. Impact of CT-guided drainage in the treatment of diverticular abscesses: size matters. AJR Am J Roentgenol. 2006; 186 (3):680–686

[59] Brandt D, Gervaz P, Durmishi Y, Platon A, Morel P, Poletti PA. Percutaneous CT scan-guided drainage vs. antibiotherapy alone for Hinchey II diverticulitis: a case-control study. Dis Colon Rectum. 2006; 49(10):1533–1538

[60] Ambrosetti P, Chautems R, Soravia C, Peiris-Waser N, Terrier F. Long-term outcome of mesocolic and pelvic diverticular abscesses of the left colon: a prospective study of 73 cases. Dis Colon Rectum. 2005; 48(4):787–791

[61] Eglinton T, Nguyen T, Raniga S, Dixon L, Dobbs B, Frizelle FA. Patterns of recurrence in patients with acute diverticulitis. Br J Surg. 2010; 97(6):952–957

[62] Anaya DA, Flum DR. Risk of emergency colectomy and colostomy in patients with diverticular disease. Arch Surg. 2005; 140(7):681–685

[63] Salem L, Veenstra DL, Sullivan SD, Flum DR. The timing of elective colectomy in diverticulitis: a decision analysis. J Am Coll Surg. 2004; 199(6):904–912

[64] Chapman J, Davies M, Wolff B, et al. Complicated diverticulitis: is it time to rethink the rules? Ann Surg. 2005; 242(4):576–581, discussion 581–583

[65] Boostrom SY, Wolff BG, Cima RR, Merchea A, Dozois EJ, Larson DW. Uncomplicated diverticulitis, more complicated than we thought. J Gastrointest Surg. 2012; 16(9):1744–1749

[66] Forgione A, Guraya SY. Elective colonic resection after acute diverticulitis improves quality of life, intestinal symptoms and functional outcome: experts' perspectives and review of literature. Updates Surg. 2016; 68(1):53–58

[67] Lee JT, Skube S, Melton GB, et al. Elective colectomy for diverticulitis in transplant patients: is it worth the risk? J Gastrointest Surg. 2017; 21 (9):1486–1490

[68] Hwang SS, Cannom RR, Abbas MA, Etzioni D. Diverticulitis in transplant patients and patients on chronic corticosteroid therapy: a systematic review. Dis Colon Rectum. 2010; 53(12):1699–1707

[69] Kaiser AM, Jiang JK, Lake JP, et al. The management of complicated diverticulitis and the role of computed tomography. Am J Gastroenterol. 2005; 100 (4):910–917

[70] Garfinkle R, Kugler A, Pelsser V, et al. Diverticular abscess managed with long-term definitive nonoperative intent is safe. Dis Colon Rectum. 2016; 59 (7):648–655

[71] Hupfeld L, Burcharth J, Pommergaard HC, Rosenberg J. Risk factors for recurrence after acute colonic diverticulitis: a systematic review. Int J Colorectal Dis. 2017; 32(5):611–622

[72] Nelson RS, Velasco A, Mukesh BN. Management of diverticulitis in younger patients. Dis Colon Rectum. 2006; 49(9):1341–1345

[73] Benn PL, Wolff BG, Ilstrup DM. Level of anastomosis and recurrent colonic diverticulitis. Am J Surg. 1986; 151(2):269–271

[74] Thaler K, Baig MK, Berho M, et al. Determinants of recurrence after sigmoid resection for uncomplicated diverticulitis. Dis Colon Rectum. 2003; 46 (3):385–388

[75] Klarenbeek BR, Veenhof AA, Bergamaschi R, et al. Laparoscopic sigmoid resection for diverticulitis decreases major morbidity rates: a randomized control trial: short-term results of the Sigma Trial. Ann Surg. 2009; 249(1):39–44

[76] Gervaz P, Inan I, Perneger T, Schiffer E, Morel P. A prospective, randomized, single-blind comparison of laparoscopic versus open sigmoid colectomy for diverticulitis. Ann Surg. 2010; 252(1):3–8

[77] Cirocchi R, Farinella E, Trastulli S, et al. Laparoscopic versus open surgery for colonic diverticulitis. Cochrane Database Syst Rev. 2011:CD009277

[78] Hartmann H. Nouveau procedé d'ablation des cancers de la partie terminale-du colon pelvien. Congres Fr Chir. 1923; 30:2241

[79] Nagorney DM, Adson MA, Pemberton JH. Sigmoid diverticulitis with perforation and generalized peritonitis. Dis Colon Rectum. 1985; 28(2):71–75

[80] Haas PA, Fox TA, Jr. The fate of the forgotten rectal pouch after Hartmann's procedure without reconstruction. Am J Surg. 1990; 159(1):106–110, discussion 110–111

[81] Cirocchi R, DiSaverio S, WeberDG, et al. Laparoscopic lavage versus surgical resection for acute diverticulitis with generalised peritonitis: a systematic review and meta-analysis. Tech Coloproctol. 2017; 21(2):93–110

[82] Vennix S, Musters GD, Mulder IM, et al. Laparoscopic peritoneal lavage or sigmoidectomy for perforated diverticulitis with purulent peritonitis: a multicentre, parallel-group, randomised, open-label trial. Lancet. 2015; 286(10000):1269–1277

[83] Kohl A, Rosenberg J, Bock D, et al. Two-year results of the randomized clinical trial DILALA comparing laparoscopic lavage with resection as treatment for perforated diverticulitis. Br J Surg. 2018; 105(9):1128–1134

28 Volvulus of the Colon

David E. Beck and Santhat Nivatvongs

Abstract

This chapter discusses volvulus of the colon, specifically the incidence, etiology, clinical presentation, diagnosis, and treatment of sigmoid volvulus, ileosigmoid knotting, cecal volvulus, volvulus of the transverse colon, and splenic flexure volvulus.

Keywords: sigmoid volvulus, Ileosigmoid knotting, cecal volvulus, volvulus of the transverse colon, splenic flexure volvulus, etiology, clinical presentation, diagnosis, surgical treatment

28.1 Introduction

Volvulus refers to a torsion or twist of an organ on a pedicle. It can involve the stomach, spleen, gallbladder, small bowel, right colon, transverse colon, splenic flexure, or sigmoid colon.[1] Volvulus of the large bowel results from the colon's twisting on its mesentery, producing symptoms by either narrowing of the bowel lumen, strangulation of the blood vessels, or both.

Widespread differences based on geographic and epidemiologic factors are seen in the distribution of volvulus. Overall in the United States, the sigmoid colon accounts for 43 to 71% of the cases of colonic volvulus. Most of the remaining cases involve the cecum and the right colon; volvulus of the transverse colon or splenic flexure is relatively rare, accounting for only 2 to 5% and 0 to 2%, respectively.[2] In Olmstead County, Minnesota, during the period 1960 through 1980, the age-adjusted incidences of sigmoid volvulus and cecal volvulus were 1.67 and 1.20 per 100,000 persons per year, respectively.[3] In an unusual report from the high-altitude area of the Bolivian and Peruvian Andes at 13,000 feet above sea level, sigmoid volvulus accounted for 79% of all intestinal obstruction. The reason is not clear but may be related to the increased gas volume in the bowel because of high altitude.[4]

28.2 Sigmoid Volvulus

28.2.1 Incidence and Epidemiology

In the United States, sigmoid volvulus is an infrequent cause of intestinal obstruction and occurs much less often than carcinoma or diverticulitis as a cause of colonic obstruction. In an extensive review, Ballantyne[5] found that only 3.4% of 4,766 cases of intestinal obstruction and 9.6% of 1,206 cases of colonic obstruction in the United States were caused by sigmoid volvulus. The highest reported worldwide incidence appeared in a study from northern Iran by Scott,[6] who found that sigmoid volvulus was the cause of 85% of colonic obstructions. Johnson[7] reported 13 cases of sigmoid volvulus in a series of 24 bowel obstructions from Ethiopia.[7] Increased frequency of sigmoid volvulus in Pakistan, India, Brazil, and Eastern Europe also has been reported.[5] Although volvulus does occur with increased frequency in the Soviet Union,[5] the previously reported data from the 1920s,[8] in which more than 50% of cases of bowel obstruction were caused

by volvulus, may not be accurate today because of changing epidemiologic and dietary factors.

Among reported cases of sigmoid volvulus from the United States, Ballantyne[5] has isolated the following epidemiologic factors:

1. *Sex.* Sigmoid volvulus is more common in men, occurring in 63.7% of men in a collected review of 571 patients. Bruusgaard[9] had previously attributed this finding to the wider female pelvis and more relaxed abdominal musculature, which afford an early volvulus a better chance of spontaneous reduction.
2. *Age.* Analysis of data from 43 studies reveals that the average age at which sigmoid volvulus occurs in English-speaking countries is 60 to 65 years, although it tends to occur 15 to 20 years earlier in other parts of the world. Other data suggest a trend toward earlier onset in English-speaking countries as well.[10]
3. *Race.* Racial differences have been noted in many U.S. studies on sigmoid volvulus. Review of 221 patients in 10 series revealed that two-thirds (146) were black, one-third (74) were white, and 1 was Hispanic.
4. *Residence.* Review of nine U.S. studies revealed that 45.1% of 244 patients were admitted to the hospital from another institution. Of all patients, 54.9% came from private homes, 32.4% from mental institutions, and 12.7% from nursing homes.

Typically, then, the sigmoid volvulus patient in the United States is male, black, elderly, and may be institutionalized. In other parts of the world, the typical patient is also male but is younger and living at home, probably in a rural area.

28.2.2 Etiology

In order for it to twist on itself, the sigmoid colon must be long and floppy, with a narrow mesenteric root. It can be congenital or acquired, particularly after previous abdominal surgery causing scar at the root of the sigmoid mesentery.

The concept of the etiology of intestinal volvulus is based on the fact that bowel when distended becomes elongated. By direct measurement, the antimesenteric border of the bowel increased its length by 30%, whereas the mesenteric border increased by only 10%.[11] As the bowel distends, it rotates in response to the need to accommodate this disproportionate increase in the length of its antimesenteric border. Perry[11] created a model using thin latex rubber tubing gathered up on its "mesenteric" border by a stiffer adhesive rubber strip to limit the elongation of this border. A latex rubber sheet was used to produce a deep "mesentery" (▶ Fig. 28.1). Inflation of the "bowel" produced a 180-degree volvulus (▶ Fig. 28.2). The same result follows the inflation of an isolated segment of cadaver ileum in which the mesentery has been refashioned and sutured to make it deep with a narrow base (▶ Fig. 28.3). An example of this concept in vivo can be observed. In Afghanistan, for example, during the feast of Ramadan, the incidence of this type of volvulus rises sharply from bloated intestine.[12]

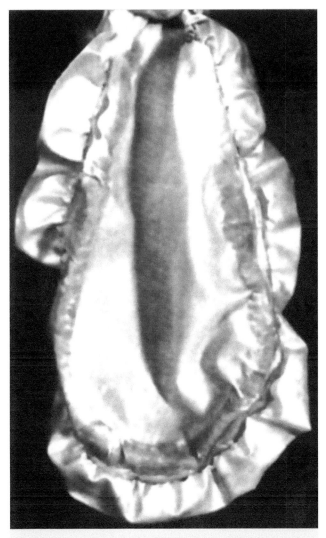

Fig. 28.1 Latex rubber model in flaccid state suspended from its base.[11] (Reproduced with permission from John Wiley and Sons.)

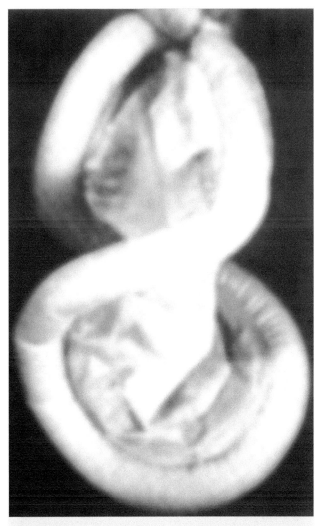

Fig. 28.2 The same model inflated with compressed air to 50 mm Hg. Note the rotation, which could be induced in either a clockwise or counterclockwise direction.[11] (Reproduced with permission from John Wiley and Sons.)

"Red gut," a disease of sheep grazing alfalfa (Lucerne), is thought to be the result of volvulus associated with bowel gas distention.[13]

It becomes clear that in order to have a volvulus, the bowel has to be distended with air to float. Colon that is full of stool cannot float and twist but by its weight may twist on itself and is not a true volvulus. In fact, the gush-out of "stool" on reducing the sigmoid volvulus is an exudate from obstruction, not the loaded stool from constipation.

A large number of precipitating or associated factors have been implicated in the genesis of sigmoid volvulus, including lead poisoning,[14] vitamin B deficiency,[14] adhesions,[15] gout,[15] Hirschsprung's disease,[16] megacolon and diabetes,[17] Parkinson's disease and other neurologic disorders,[17] Chagas' disease,[18] stroke,[19] sprue,[20] ischemic colitis,[21] peptic ulcer,[22] tuberculosis,[22] cardiovascular disease,[23] hypokalemia,[24] pregnancy,[25] and excessive enemas.[26]

28.2.3 Pathogenesis

In a patient with a sigmoid volvulus, the twist of the sigmoid may be in a clockwise or counterclockwise direction, but it is usually counterclockwise around the axis of the mesocolon with varying degrees of rotation (▶ Fig. 28.4). For significant obstruction to occur, the torsion must be at least 180 degrees. Torsion less than this is generally asymptomatic and can be considered physiologic.

The obstruction produced is a closed-loop type of mechanical obstruction that may be simple or strangulated. In the early stages of obstruction, peristalsis forces gas and fluid into the closed loop to remain trapped as the twist acts as a check valve to prevent release. Occasionally, some trapped air and gas are forced from the loop so that the diarrheal stools may occur. With simple obstruction, the bowel wall generally remains viable for a few days, largely because the sigmoid colon can tolerate more intraluminal pressure than other parts of the intestinal tract before signs of vascular compromise appear. Eventually strangulation will occur, with occlusion of the veins developing first, followed by occlusion of the arteries, mesocolic thrombosis, and infarction. Necrosis usually occurs first at the site of torsion but may include the entire loop.

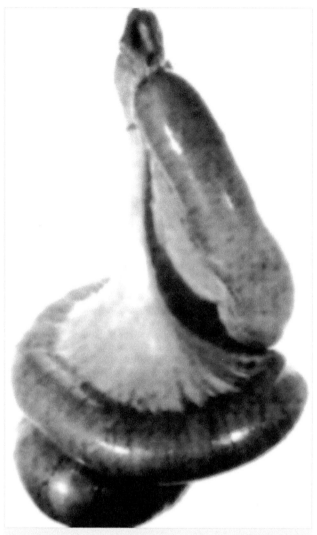

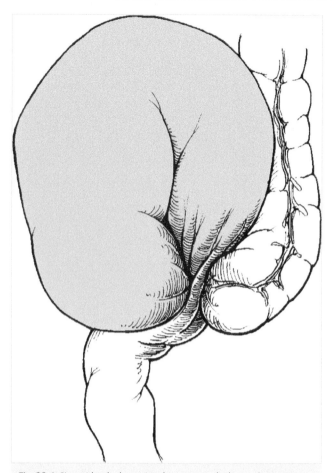

Fig. 28.4 Sigmoid volvulus twisted in counterclockwise direction. Occlusion of the veins developing first, followed by occlusion of the arteries, mesocolic thrombosis, and infarction. Necrosis usually occurs first at the site of torsion but may include the entire loop.

Fig. 28.3 The same model using cadaver ileum. Either clockwise or counterclockwise rotation could be induced on inflation.[11] (Reproduced with permission from John Wiley and Sons.)

In the acute fulminating variant of this disease, gangrene may occur much more rapidly because of a sudden, tight compression of the mesenteric vessels compounded by a rapid distention of the bowel lumen.

28.2.4 Clinical Presentation

Although a chronic, painless variant of sigmoid volvulus has been described,[27] the condition should be viewed as an acute disease. Hinshaw and Carter[28] have distinguished between two distinct clinical presentations of acute sigmoid volvulus depending on the rapidity of the twisting mesentery.

In the "acute fulminating type," the patient is generally younger, the onset of symptoms is sudden, and the course is rapid. Generally, there is little history of previous episodes, and symptoms include early vomiting, diffuse abdominal pain and tenderness, marked prostration, and the early appearance of gangrene. Distention may be minimal, and findings often are not distinctive. In its classic form, the acute fulminating variety

of sigmoid volvulus produces no distinctive diagnostic signs except for the clinical picture of an acute abdominal catastrophe; the actual diagnosis is made at celiotomy.

The second type, or "subacute progressive type," is the more common presentation. The patient is generally older, the onset more gradual, and the early course more benign. There is often a history of previous attacks and chronic constipation. Vomiting occurs late, pain is minimal, and signs of peritonitis are usually not present. Abdominal distention is generally extreme in this form, and radiographic findings are usually diagnostic.

28.2.5 Diagnosis

In the acute fulminating type, the diagnosis of acute peritonitis is evident, immediate celiotomy is mandatory, and specific diagnostic measures are generally not indicated. In the more common subacute progressive type, the diagnosis can be strongly suspected by the history and physical examination. In addition to a history of chronic constipation and possibly previous episodes, there is a recent history of gradual onset of cramping, lower abdominal pain, and progressive distention. Usually, there is obstipation and absence of flatus, although there may be occasional diarrheal stools. Vomiting is uncommon as an early symptom.

Marked abdominal distention and tympany are the most striking physical findings. Bowel sounds may be hyperactive or hypoactive but generally are not absent.

The diagnosis is usually confirmed by X-ray examination. A plain film of the abdomen classically shows a massively distended single loop of bowel on the right or left side of the abdomen with both ends in the pelvis and the bow near the diaphragm ("bent inner tube sign"; ▶ Fig. 28.5). Fluid levels may be seen in the sigmoid loop with little difference of levels in the upright position. The degree of distention of the proximal colon and small bowel on the right side of the abdomen varies. A Gastrografin enema study reveals a pathognomonic finding of the Gastrografin column, ending sharply at the level of the site of torsion ("bird's beak" or "ace of spades" deformity; ▶ Fig. 28.6). Burrell et al[29] evaluated the plain abdominal radiographs in patients with sigmoid volvulus. Three signs, the apex of the loop under the left hemidiaphragm, inferior convergence on the left, and the left flank overlap sign, are 100% specific as well as being highly sensitive. The sign that is least specific is a distended ahaustral sigmoid loop and an air:fluid ratio greater than 2:1.

In approximately 30 to 40% of the cases, plain films can be equivocal. The transverse colon or small bowel distention can superimpose on the sigmoid loops; the two limbs may overlap, deviate laterally, or be oriented in an anteroposterior plane; the sigmoid can be fluid filled; or a dilated, redundant transverse colon or a closed-loop small bowel obstruction may mimic sigmoid volvulus.[30,31] In these cases, computed tomography (CT) is the preferred confirmatory test.[32] It is noninvasive, easily obtainable, accurate, and has the advantage of identification of incidental pathology that may be missed by studies. The sigmoid afferent and efferent loops have a radial distribution around a low-attenuating adipose area (the twisted mesocolon) with a soft-tissue center (the point of torsion). Engorged and stretched vessels converge toward the center. This feature is described as the "whirl sign" (▶ Fig. 28.7). CT scan can also identify signs of strangulation.[33] In the study by Swenson,[34] the positive diagnostic yield of CT was 89%.

28.2.6 Treatment

Management of Nonstrangulated Sigmoid Volvulus

The goals of therapy in nonstrangulated sigmoid volvulus are directed at relief of acute torsion and prevention of recurrences. Ideally, the volvulus should be derotated and the colon

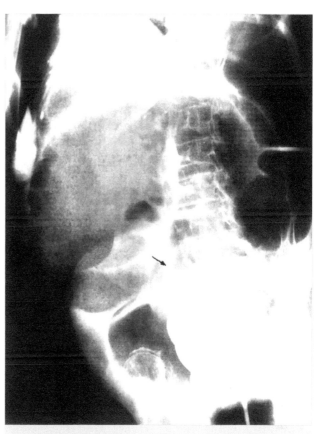

Fig. 28.6 "Bird's beak" deformity at the site of volvulus (*arrow*).

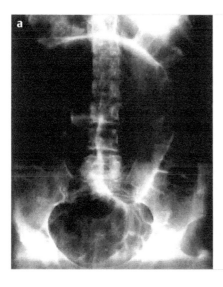
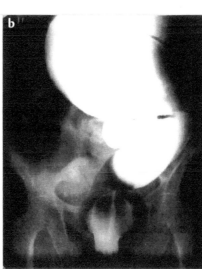

Fig. 28.5 Plain film **(a)** and contrast study **(b)** showing massively dilated sigmoid loop.

decompressed. A few days later, after a full colonic preparation, sigmoid resection is performed. However, there are other lesser procedures to prevent recurrences such as tube sigmoid colostomy,[35] mesosigmoidoplasty,[36] and sigmoid colopexy.[37]

Rigid Sigmoidoscopic Decompression

In 1947, Bruusgaard[9] described his experience with nonoperative reduction by sigmoidoscopy and passage of a rectal tube into the obstructed loop. The procedure was performed on 136 cases and was successful 123 times for a 90% success rate; 4 deaths occurred, with a mortality rate of 2.9%. In the 1950s and 1960s, greater experience was gained with the nonoperative method. Several larger series with equally impressive results were reported. Drapanas and Stewart[38] reported successful

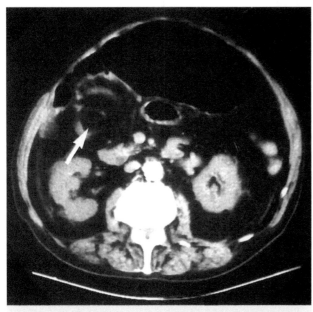

Fig. 28.7 A typical "whirl sign" of cecal volvulus (*arrow*). (This image is provided courtesy of Richard Devine, MD.)

decompression with rectal intubation in 82 of 98 cases (84% success) with a 1.2% mortality rate; Wuepper et al[19] were successful with this method in 44 of 54 cases, and had a mortality rate of 5.5%; and Shepherd[39] was successful in 78 of 89 cases, with a 3.4% mortality rate. In addition, in 1973 Arnold and Nance[23] had a 77% success rate in 114 cases.

Comparative figures for survival with operative detorsion have consistently yielded higher mortality rates than nonoperative reduction. Hinshaw and Carter[28] reported a 22% mortality rate for operative detorsion in 18 patients. Shepherd[39] reported a 16% mortality rate for 49 patients, and Sutcliffe[40] reported 2 deaths in 19 patients (11% mortality rate). Gama et al[18] and Sharpton and Cheek[41] have reported mortality rates as low as 5 and 8%, respectively, and Gulati et al[42] have reported a 35% mortality rate for 34 patients.

Nonoperative decompression thus has become the preferred initial treatment for nonstrangulated sigmoid volvulus. This approach, however, should not be used in three situations: (1) when there are clinical signs of nonviable bowel, (2) if a trial of sigmoidoscopy has failed to achieve immediate reduction, and (3) when volvulus repeatedly recurs. In these situations, it is safest to proceed with immediate celiotomy.

The technique of sigmoidoscopic decompression is as follows. Preparation of the patient for surgery is begun so that if the nonoperative technique fails, operative intervention will not be delayed. Preferably the patient is placed in the prone jackknife position because this position facilitates the decompression by allowing the colon to fall away. The lateral decubitus position is acceptable if the patient cannot tolerate the jackknife position. The rigid sigmoidoscope is carefully inserted until the site of torsion is seen, and the mucosa is inspected carefully for signs of ischemia or necrosis. If the mucosa appears intact, a soft, well-lubricated 40- to 60-cm rectal tube is passed gently beyond the site of torsion until there is an immediate return of gas and stool from the obstructed loop. The rectal tube can be passed through the sigmoidoscope or along the side of the sigmoidoscope. The tube is then secured to the perianal skin and is left in place for at least 48 hours (▶ Fig. 28.8). Reports showed a wide range of success rates in sigmoidoscopic decompression

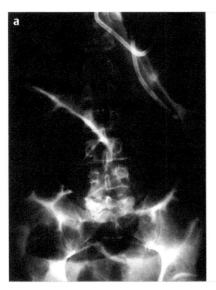
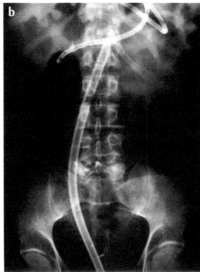

Fig. 28.8 (a) Abdominal film of patient with sigmoid volvulus. **(b)** Abdominal film of same patient after sigmoidoscopic decompression with a rectal tube in place.

between 38 and 100%.[2,37,43,44,45,46] When decompression is unsuccessful, strangulation of the sigmoid volvulus must be suspected, or the volvulus is beyond reach of the sigmoidoscope. Flexible sigmoidoscopy and colonoscopy are now widely used and have largely replaced the rigid sigmoidoscope.

Colonoscopic and Flexible Sigmoidoscopic Decompression

Despite the fact that many failures of sigmoidoscopic decompression of a sigmoid volvulus are related to gangrenous changes at the site of torsion, a significant number of failures occur because the rigid 25-cm sigmoidoscope does not reach the site of obstruction.

In 1976, Ghazi et al[47] presented the first case of colonoscopic decompression of sigmoid volvulus with the site of obstruction measured at 105 cm from the insertion of the colonoscope. Subsequent favorable reports with both the full-length colonoscope[48,49,50] and the flexible sigmoidoscope[51] have appeared. A review of 25 cases of sigmoid volvulus revealed that 24 of the cases were safely decompressed colonoscopically, with the only failure occurring when the colonoscope was deliberately withdrawn when cyanotic mucosa was identified 80 cm from the anus.[49] Renzulli et al[52] reported a success rate of only 58% in a small series of 12 patients. In a review of 189 patients with sigmoid volvulus from Veterans Affairs hospitals, using endoscopy (rigid sigmoidoscopy, flexible sigmoidoscopy, or endoscopy), the success rate was 81%.[53] Colonoscopic and flexible sigmoidoscopic decompression differs from rigid sigmoidoscopic decompression in that the colonoscope itself is passed through the site of torsion, often with gentle air insufflation as the scope is passed beyond the obstruction. Some authors have attached an external suction device to the biopsy portion of the colonoscope to facilitate removal of liquid, stool, and debris from the unprepared colon.[54] Others have attached to the colonoscope a jejunostomy-type tube that is left as a decompressing stent that can be passed as far proximally as the cecum.[55] A rectal tube can be passed after the volvulus has been reduced by passing the tube alongside with the flexible scope in place or after it has been withdrawn.

The precautions taken for rigid sigmoidoscopic decompression also apply to colonoscopic and flexible sigmoidoscopic decompression. If reduction does not occur promptly, the procedure should be terminated in favor of surgery. The procedure should also be abandoned in the presence of bloody drainage or cyanotic mucosa.

Flexible endoscopy is a sensitive means of diagnosing both acute sigmoid volvulus and intermittent sigmoid volvulus. Twisting spirals of mucosa are seen if the volvulus is still present. Even if the volvulus has spontaneously reduced, the mucosa at the site of volvulus demonstrates discrete and localized signs of inflammation. In addition, the vascular markings are obscured and the mucosal folds are thickened. There may also be some granularity or friability. These findings are limited only to short segments of approximately 4 to 5 cm at both the rectosigmoid and the descending sigmoid junctions.[3]

Surgical Management

Although the mortality rate of sigmoidoscopic deflation without further treatment is relatively low, at 5 to 8%, most deaths are the result of coexisting disease rather than a direct result of the procedure itself or complications related to the procedure.[56] The recurrence from sigmoidoscopic deflation alone is high, 40 to 70%.[2,39,44] With this high recurrence, it is obvious that further management is desirable. The mortality of surgery for sigmoid volvulus depends on whether the colon is gangrenous, and on the severity of intercurrent disease. Elective colon resection for sigmoid volvulus is most efficient. When properly performed, recurrence should not occur, although this complication has been reported.[39,46]

Most authors have emphasized the need for elective resection in all patients who had an episode of sigmoid volvulus, although some have reserved elective resection for selected lower-risk patients. Shepherd[39] reported on 74 elective resections performed 5 to 8 days after conservative treatment, with a mortality rate of 2.8%. Even in patients who have been classified as higher risk, the elective mortality rate should be lower than the risk of death from complications of recurrent volvulus.

In a recent study by Yassaie et al,[57] 31 patients with sigmoid volvulus who underwent successful endoscopic detorsion and no further interventions before discharge were evaluated. Recurrent sigmoid volvulus was diagnosed in 19 (61%) of these patients at a median of 31 days. Of these 19 patients, 7 underwent colectomy and 12 had repeat endoscopic detorsion alone, of whom 5 (48%) were diagnosed with a third episode of volvulus at a median interval of 5 months and 3 (25%) required emergent sigmoid colectomy. In a study by Swenson et al,[34] 10 (48%) of 21 patients with sigmoid volvulus treated nonoperatively returned with recurrent volvulus at a median of 106 days (range 8–374 days) after discharge. Tan et al[58] observed recurrent sigmoid volvulus in 28 (61%) of 46 patients who were discharged after endoscopic reduction alone.

Sigmoid Colon Resection

For a nonstrangulated colon, sigmoid colon resection can be performed as an elective procedure a few days later, after a bowel preparation. If an urgent exploratory celiotomy is necessary, the left colon and rectum can be irrigated with povidone–iodine via a rectal tube. The mortality rate for sigmoid colon resection with primary anastomosis has been reported to be between 0 and 12.5%.[39,43,59,60,61] For gangrenous bowel, sigmoid resection with a colostomy and Hartmann's procedure is the safest, although some authors perform an anastomosis. The operative mortality is between 0 and 38%.[39,43,59,60,61,62] Even without gangrenous colon, emergency sigmoid resection with primary anastomosis has a high anastomotic leak rate.[63]

Much of the mortality associated with elective sigmoid resection after volvulus can be reduced by taking advantage of the unique anatomic features of the sigmoid in these patients. Because the sigmoid is long and freely movable, the mesosigmoid is also long, and the points of peritoneal fixation are close together, the redundant loop usually can be delivered out of the abdominal cavity through a limited incision (▶ Fig. 28.9). The peritoneum is entered through a short transverse incision made in the left lower quadrant, dividing through the left rectus muscle. The redundant loop is delivered, the mesocolon is divided to free a proximal and a distal end, and the anastomosis is made on the surface of the abdomen. The bowel is then

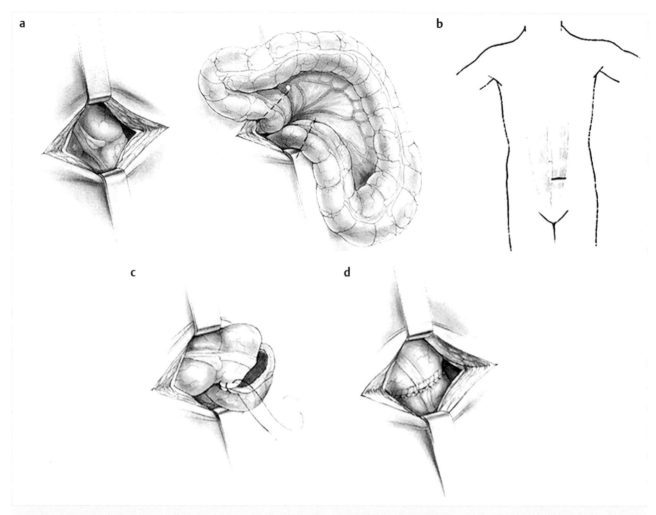

Fig. 28.9 Elective sigmoid resection after nonoperative decompression for volvulus. **(a)** Limited left lower quadrant incision. **(b)** Delivery of redundant sigmoid. **(c)** Anastomosis at level of abdominal wall after resection of redundant sigmoid. **(d)** Anastomotic segment dropped back into abdominal cavity.

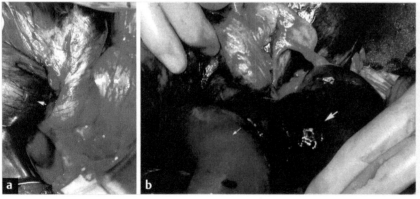

Fig. 28.10 Simultaneous sigmoid and cecal volvulus. **(a)** Sigmoid volvulus with gangrene (*arrow*). **(b)** Cecal volvulus with gangrene (*large arrow*). Note the inflamed terminal ileum (*small arrow*).

dropped back into the peritoneal cavity and the incision is closed. In elderly debilitated patients, this procedure can often be performed with local anesthesia.

At operation, it is important to examine the entire abdomen to make certain that there is no volvulus at any other part. Simultaneous sigmoid and cecal volvulus is rare but has been reported.[64] An example of this condition can be seen in ▶ Fig. 28.10.

In the series reported by Grossmann et al,[53] 178 of 228 (78%) patients underwent a colostomy, with 44% considered to be urgent. Evidence of ischemia was present in 86 of 178 cases (48%), and frank necrosis of the colon was observed in 59 of 178 cases

(33%). Sigmoid resection was performed in 173 of 178 patients (97%): 107 of 173 patients (62%) had resection with colostomy; 66 of 173 patients (38%) had primary anastomosis; colostomy without sigmoid resection was performed in 2 of 178 patients (1%); and 3 of 178 patients (2%) underwent sigmoidopexy. There were no operative deaths. Twenty-five of 178 patients (14%) died within 30 days of surgery.

Laparoscopy

There are limited data on emergent laparoscopic sigmoid volvulus surgery. A recent comparison of open and laparoscopic cases found a twofold increase in anastomotic leak in the laparoscopic group and similar overall postoperative morbidity.[64] Of note, the extensive bowel length and distention in volvulus cases make laparoscopic procedures challenging. As described previously, the operation can usually be performed through a small incision and with modern postoperative pain management, many of the potential advantages of laparoscopy are difficult to demonstrate.

Nonresective Procedures

Even elective sigmoid colon resection has significant morbidity and mortality. In very ill patients, a resection should be avoided, unless the bowel is gangrenous. Surgeons should know other effective but less radical procedures to prevent a recurrence.

Sigmoid Decompression and Colopexy

This is a unique procedure claimed to produce no recurrence and no death in 20 patients with nongangrenous sigmoid volvulus. The only complication was one wound infection.[35] The author first deflated the sigmoid volvulus with an 18-gauge needle. With the collapsed sigmoid colon, his success in sigmoidoscopic insertion of a rectal tube was 100%, and there was no incidence of stool leakage from the needle. Four to 5 days later, the patient was explored and a sigmoid colopexy performed.

The sigmoid colon was placed against the lateral and anterior abdominal wall at the left iliac fossa to determine the site of colopexy. Strips of Gore-Tex band were cut from a bifurcated vascular graft with the size and length suitable to encircling the colon and sutured to the abdominal wall without obstructing the bowel lumen. Usually six to eight strips were sutured at one end to the abdominal wall with interrupted 2–0 Prolene sutures. An arterial forceps was pushed through the mesocolon. The bands were then pulled through, wrapped around half the colonic circumference, and sutured with interrupted 2–0 Prolene to the abdominal wall (▶ Fig. 28.11). Prolene or Vicryl mesh would be a more practical option.

The authors believe that decompression of the volvulus should be attempted with a rigid or a flexible sigmoidoscope first. If this is not successful, a percutaneous needle deflation should then be performed, followed by placement of a rectal tube.

Mesosigmoidoplasty

The concept of this technique is to reduce the length of the mesosigmoid and broaden its attachment. It can be used in an elective or emergency situation but without gangrene. The sigmoid colon must be decompressed. The peritoneum over the mesosigmoid is incised vertically in the midline starting from the base up to 2.5 cm from the mesenteric border of the sigmoid colon (▶ Fig. 28.12). The flaps of peritoneum on each side are

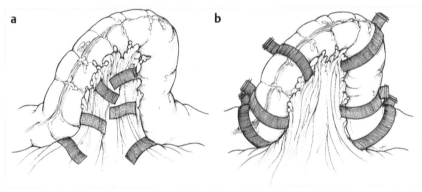

Fig. 28.11 **(a)** Strips of Gore-Tex band are sutured to the intra-abdominal wall and the loose ends are delivered through the sigmoid mesentery. **(b)** Gore-Tex bands sutured around the sigmoid colon.

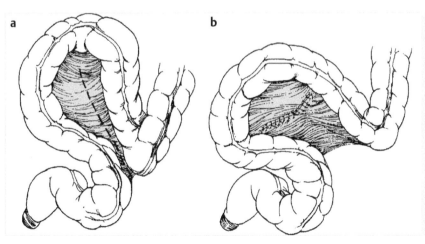

Fig. 28.12 Mesosigmoidoplasty. **(a)** Sigmoid colon showing long mesosigmoid colon and narrow attachment at the base. Note longitudinal line of incision of peritoneum. **(b)** The longitudinal incision of peritoneum is closed transversely. Note the reduction in height of sigmoid loop and broadened base.

raised laterally. The flaps are then approximated transversely with continuous suture using synthetic absorbable sutures. The procedure is repeated over the other side of the mesosigmoid.

Subrahmanyam[36] performed this technique in 126 patients (48 elective, 78 emergency). There was one death from aspiration pneumonia and two recurrences after 2 and 6 months. The mean follow-up was 8.2 years. This technique may not be feasible in obese patients with fatty mesocolon.[65]

Bach et al[66] modified this technique by cutting the sigmoid mesentery in its full thickness longitudinally. The key to this modified technique is to preserve the first branch of the sigmoid vessel at the base of the mesentery, and the last vascular arcade near the colonic wall. Following the principles of mesosigmoidoplasty, the longitudinal slot of the mesosigmoid was sutured horizontally, using absorbable sutures on each aspect of the mesosigmoid (medial and lateral), taking only the peritoneal layer. Twelve patients were successfully operated on. A short-term follow-up in eight patients from 4 to 8 months later showed no problems with recurrence, abdominal discomfort, or change in bowel habits.

Balloon Catheter Sigmoidostomy

The aim of this technique is to fix the redundant sigmoid colon to the anterior abdominal wall. A balloon catheter is placed through the abdominal wall and inserted into the colon. The balloon is inflated with water, and traction on the catheter attaches the colon to the abdominal wall. The balloon catheter is removed 2 weeks later. Tanga[35] reported favorable results in 10 patients with a one-stage procedure consisting of detorsion and bladder catheter sigmoidostomy analogous to detorsion and cecostomy performed to treat cecal volvulus.

T-Fasteners Sigmoidopexy

This innovated technique was devised by Brown et al[67] to endoscopically tag the stomach wall to the anterior abdominal wall for the percutaneous gastrostomy to prevent leaking around the tube. Gallagher et al[68,69] applied this technique to fix the sigmoid colon to the anterior abdominal wall with the aid of colonoscopy, for sigmoid volvulus. The procedure is used exclusively for patients with sigmoid volvulus who are not candidates for general anesthetic.

The instruments consist of a T-fastener with cotton pledget, a washer to hold the pledget to the skin, a needle with slot to house the T-fastener, and a stylet for ejecting the fastener (Ross Laboratories, Columbus, OH).

The technique requires a successful detorsion and decompression of the viable sigmoid colon using a colonoscope. With the colonoscope as a guide, the T-fastener is deployed via the needle. The T-fastener then pulls the sigmoid colon up against the abdominal wall and is tightened on the skin over the cotton pledget (▶ Fig. 28.13). Three to four T-fasteners are placed 4 to 5 cm apart, in a triangular disposition.[69,70] These fasteners are cut at the skin level after 28 days.[70] They will eventually pass through with stool. By this time, the sigmoid colon should adhere to the anterior abdominal wall. The procedure is performed under mild sedation.

Pinedo et al[70] successfully performed this technique in two patients with a follow-up of 7 to 18 months. Gallagher et al[69] reported six patients: one patient died of peritonitis, one patient developed a small bowel obstruction that resolved with

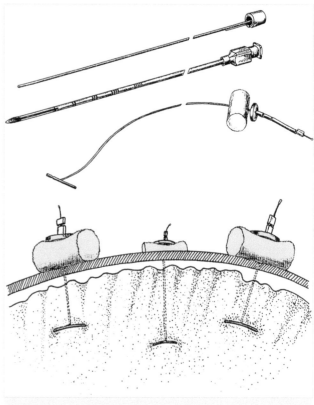

Fig. 28.13 T-fasteners.[65]

conservative management, one patient had a recurrent volvulus of more proximal sigmoid colon at 8 months—successfully treated with a repeated procedure.

Nonresectional operative procedures are inferior to sigmoid colectomy for the prevention of recurrent volvulus; however, they may be the preferred option in patients who are in extremely poor condition.

28.3 Ileosigmoid Knotting

Ileosigmoid knotting is a unique entity in which a loop of ileum and the sigmoid colon wrap around each other. It was once called "double volvulus," but this term has been abandoned. It is rare in the Western world but is not uncommon in Africa, Asia, and the Middle East.[66] Ileosigmoid knotting accounted for 8.8% of 773 cases of sigmoid volvulus and 1.7% of 4,005 cases of all mechanical obstruction in the series from Turkey reported by Alver et al.[71] Other series dealing with this condition had a higher incidence, between 18 and 27% of all cases of volvulus.

Ironically, review of the world literature in 1932 showed that out of 161 cases, all but 7 came from Russia or Scandinavia.[39] At that time, no cases had been reported from America or Africa. The first case reports from the southern hemisphere appear to be from Sri Lanka in 1940 and India in 1953. From Africa, the first account was in 1952 from Uganda.[39]

28.3.1 Mechanism

Experience suggests that the knot is not initiated by the colon but by a hyperactive ileum that winds itself around the pedicle of a passive sigmoid loop. Bulk may be an important factor in stimulating small bowel activity. In the volvulus-belt region, it is customary to eat most of the day's food in one large evening meal. Several pounds of food are washed down with large quantities of liquid. The most common intestinal knotting occurs in the early hours of the morning.[39] Alver et al[71] summarize the different patterns of knotting (▶ Fig. 28.14).

28.3.2 Clinical Features

There are many differences between the clinical features of knotting and those of volvulus. Sigmoid volvulus is seen five times as often as intestinal knotting in males, whereas in females intestinal knotting is seen nearly twice as often as sigmoid volvulus in the series from Uganda.[39] The age of patients with ileosigmoid knotting is also younger than patients with volvulus, 42 versus 53 years. The absence of previous attacks is also striking, in contrast with sigmoid volvulus in which over 30% of the patients give a history of recurrent attacks of volvulus. Pain is the main complaint in every case. The onset is acute and occurs most commonly in the early hours of the morning, awakening the patient from sleep. Initial central colic gives way to constant agonizing generalized pain. Almost 75% of patients from Uganda arrive at the hospital on the day of onset compared with 25% of patients with volvulus of the sigmoid colon who arrive at the hospital in the first 24 hours.[39]

Vomiting usually occurs at the onset of pain. In sigmoid volvulus, vomiting is a late feature and is often absent. Another striking feature of ileosigmoid knotting is that distention is not a common complaint by the patient, in contrast to sigmoid volvulus in which distention is obvious. The patient usually arrives at the hospital in shock, with pale, cold, clammy skin. In the majority of cases, gangrene is present and a generalized peritonitis is found. It is usually abundantly obvious that a grave abdominal catastrophe has occurred. In regions where this condition is not uncommon, the diagnosis can be made with confidence from the clinical picture.

28.3.3 Surgical Treatment

Ileosigmoid knotting requires an emergency operation, because it cannot be reduced via an endoscope. The mortality of this condition is exceedingly high, 67%.[71] With no other operation is death on the operating table seen so often. The abdominal cavity usually contains several liters of heavily bloodstained fluid. The bowel wall and the lumen are also full of blood, and there is little doubt that most deaths are due to hemorrhagic shock.[39]

If the bowels are viable, the knot can be safely untied. After the bowel is decompressed, both the small bowel and the colon are resected with or without anastomosis, depending on the patient's condition and the condition of the bowel. The operating mortality for nongangrenous bowel is 28% in the series by Alver et al.[71]

Untying the knot in gangrenous bowel is difficult and time-consuming and carries the hazard of rupturing the gangrenous loop even after deflation. It also risks bacterial toxins and breakdown products escaping into the general circulation, causing irreversible septic shock.[39] The gangrenous bowel should be

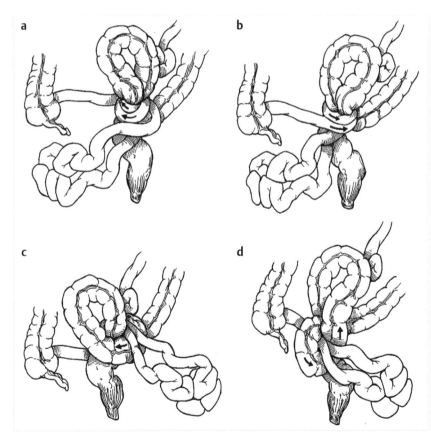

Fig. 28.14 Schematic diagrams showing the types of ileosigmoid knotting. The ileum (active component) wraps itself around the sigmoid colon (passive component) in a clockwise **(a)** and counterclockwise **(b)** direction. The sigmoid colon (active component) wraps itself around a loop of ileum (passive component) in a clockwise **(c)** and counterclockwise **(d)** direction.

removed en bloc with its mesentery. Anastomosis of the bowel should be avoided. The operative mortality in this situation is 40 to 50%.[39,71,72] Alver et al[73] reported 12 cases of internal herniation concurrent with ileosigmoid knotting or sigmoid volvulus. Only cases of internal herniation through a congenital defect, mostly the mesentery, were included. The age of the patients ranged from 25 to 72 years. Of note was the finding of gangrene of the small bowel or sigmoid colon in all of the patients at the time of the operation that required an en bloc resection. Postoperative morbidity and mortality were 33.3% in both.

28.3.4 Sigmoid Volvulus in Pregnancy

Sigmoid volvulus in pregnancy is a rare occurrence; there were only 73 cases reported in a review by Alshawi.[74] It is a potentially serious condition and should be recognized as a surgical emergency. Prompt management is necessary to minimize maternal and fetal morbidity and mortality.[74] Alshawi[74] proposed that in the first trimester, a nonoperative procedure using colonoscopic detorsion and rectal tube decompression be recommended until the second trimester when sigmoid resection is performed for recurrent cases. In the third trimester, the treatment is nonoperative until fetal maturity and delivery when sigmoid resection can be performed.

28.4 Cecal Volvulus

28.4.1 Incidence and Epidemiology

Cecal volvulus occurs less commonly than sigmoid volvulus and accounts for approximately 1% of all cases of intestinal obstruction.[75] Most reported cases have involved patients younger than those having sigmoid volvulus, with ages ranging from 30 to 70 years,[76,77,78] although some authors have noted the occurrence of cecal volvulus in older patients as well.[79,80] Most patients having recurrent or intermittent forms of cecal volvulus are younger, with 92% younger than 36 years in one study.[81] A clear predominance of women over men has been reported by most authors.[79]

28.4.2 Etiology and Pathogenesis

Unlike the acquired anatomic features of sigmoid volvulus, a distinct congenital anatomic variant is present in cecal volvulus patients, involving incomplete peritoneal fixation of the right colon and resulting in an abnormal ascending colon. Cadaver studies have reported that this variant is present in 10 to 22% or more of the population.[82,83]

Given the anatomic prerequisite of a mobile cecum, a number of associated or precipitating factors have been implicated in the development of cecal volvulus. Among the frequently cited factors are congenital bands,[82] adhesions from previous surgery,[50,84] and trauma and manipulation from a recent abdominal operation.[85] Coarse high-fiber diets have been implicated in the development of cecal volvulus in eastern Europe,[85] although they have not been described as a factor elsewhere. Increased peristalsis caused by diarrhea or cathartics has been suggested as a predisposing factor,[86] as has overeating.[87] Distention related to obstruction has been implicated,[88] as has pregnancy or space-occupying pelvic lesions.[89] Rare congenital factors include nonrotation of the midgut[90] and torsion around a vitelline duct remnant.[91] Clinically, the most important precipitating factor may be the presence of distal colonic obstruction. This obstruction reportedly can occur in as many as one-third[88] to one-half[92] of the cases of cecal volvulus.

A cecal volvulus tends to twist in a clockwise fashion, in contrast to the counterclockwise twist of a sigmoid volvulus. The resulting obstruction, however, is similarly of the closed loop and complete type. A cecal bascule is an anterior and superior folding of the mobile cecum over the fixed distal ascending colon (▶ Fig. 28.15). Although tension gangrene may develop, there is no major vessel obstruction. Some authors exclude this condition from being a cecal volvulus because it is not a true volvulus.[79]

28.4.3 Clinical Presentation

The clinical presentation of cecal volvulus may be divided into three major types: acute fulminating, acute obstructive, and intermittent or recurrent.[77,81] In the acute fulminating type, vascular obstruction occurs early, and the clinical picture is that of an acute surgical abdomen, with the need for immediate surgical intervention apparent. The acute obstructive type is more indolent and progressive, with findings related to the development of a closed-loop cecal obstruction and distal small bowel obstruction. In this variant, the patient generally presents with vague cramping, abdominal pain, nausea with or without vomiting, and slowly increasing abdominal distention. Abdominal X-ray films and a Gastrografin enema study often are needed to confirm the diagnosis.

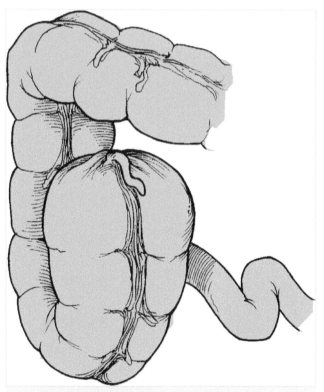

Fig. 28.15 Cecal bascule type of cecal volvulus.

In the intermittent form, the symptoms may vary from mild indigestion to severe cramping pains, but the symptoms last for only short periods and subside spontaneously, making the diagnosis difficult.

28.4.4 Diagnosis

The diagnosis of cecal volvulus should be suspected from the history and usually can be confirmed by X-ray studies. Abdominal plain films may be confusing, because the lack of lateral fixation allows visualization of the mobile cecum anywhere in the abdomen. Closed loop filled with fluid may obscure the image on the radiograph. Regardless of location, however, the most important single finding is the presence of a large dilated cecum. The loop often may be ovoid and midabdominal, or it may occupy the left upper quadrant, with its convex surface facing the left lower quadrant (due to its clockwise rotation). Distended loops of small bowel are usually present (▶ Fig. 28.16a). As in sigmoid volvulus, contrast studies are pathognomonic, with a characteristic "ace of spades" or "bird's beak" deformity seen at the site of torsion (▶ Fig. 28.16b). CT of the abdomen reveals a typical "whirl sign" in the right abdomen with marked distention of the colon (▶ Fig. 28.7).

CT of the abdomen gives the presence and location of the volvulus and gives the added benefit of allowing early identification of ischemia and perforation. Three-dimensional (3D) reconstruction may further improve diagnostic capabilities by allowing visualization of the entire small bowel in a single image.[93]

28.4.5 Treatment

Nonoperative Reduction

Radiographic attempts at reduction of right-sided colonic volvulus are generally unsuccessful and potentially hazardous.[94] Although success in colonoscopic decompression of cecal volvuli has been sporadically reported,[49,75] the chance of success is slim. It only introduces more air into the colon and delays the operation. More appealing is the percutaneous decompression of the cecal volvulus.[95] CT-guided percutaneous decompression of the acute massive dilatation of the cecum has been reported,

using a no. 22 Chiba needle[96] or a trocar with insertion of a 12-Fr suprapubic cystostomy catheter.[97] This approach should only be used as a last resort.

28.4.6 Operative Treatment

Most patients with cecal volvulus require urgent or emergency operation. Seventeen of 20 patients with cecal volvulus in the series reported by Geer et al[98] required emergency operative intervention.

Little argument exists over the need for resectional therapy for gangrenous cecal volvulus or that the operation should consist of a right hemicolectomy. In most circumstances, an anastomosis should be avoided. The ileum is brought out as an ileostomy and the colon closed or brought out as mucous fistula. The mortality of ileocolectomy for gangrenous cecal volvulus is 22 to 40%.[99,100] (B) Contrast study of same patient showing the site of torsion.

Several options are available for the viable bowel. Ileocolectomy will cure the problem and eliminate a recurrence. However, the mortality rate is significant, 0 to 22%.[84,99,101] The high mortality rate in some series has discouraged some surgeons from performing a resection. However, the decision should be individualized. If the bowel is markedly edematous or does not have good color, an anastomosis should not be performed. The proximal end should be brought out as an ileostomy and the distal end closed. In the majority of cases, an ileocolectomy with a primary anastomosis can be performed.

Cecostomy is appealing in its simplicity and fixation to the abdominal wall to prevent a recurrence. It has become the procedure of choice for some surgeons,[95,98] but the high infection rate, the significant recurrence of 13% in one series, and the nuisance of postoperative care have made it not as popular as it should be. Cecopexy has its advocates. The relatively high recurrent rate of 13 to 28.5%[79,99,102,103] has prompted some surgeons to perform a simultaneous cecopexy and tube cecostomy.[81] Simple cecopexy involves suture of the peritoneum to the taenia of the right colon, using interrupted 3–0 or 4–0 nonabsorbable sutures. The peritoneal flap, if used, is made at the level of the ileocecal valve and is extended to cover the ascending colon up to but not including the hepatic flexure. After the flap has

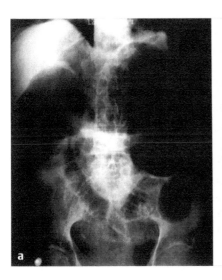
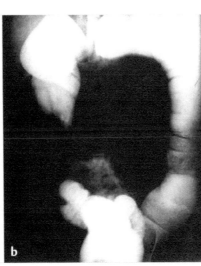

Fig. 28.16 Cecal volvulus. **(a)** Abdominal film of patient with cecal volvulus showing dilated, abnormally positioned cecum with dilated distal small bowel loops. **(b)** Contrast study of same patient showing the site of torsion.

been tailored to cover half the circumference of the right colonic segment, it is sutured in place with interrupted nonabsorbable sutures (▸ Fig. 28.17).

Detorsion of the cecal volvulus without any kind of colonic fixation is unreliable and should not be used alone. Cecal volvulus in pregnancy is rare.[104,105] Unlike sigmoid volvulus in which a nonsurgical correction with endoscopic detorsion is reasonably successful, most if not all cecal volvuli require surgical intervention. For a second and third trimester, a celiotomy can be performed under general anesthesia, and proceed with an ileocolonic resection, or nonresection procedure as appropriate. Detorsion of the cecal volvulus in the first trimester will have to be done under spinal anesthesia. Unless it is gangrenous, a nonresective procedure such as a tube cecostomy or a colopexy seems to be a good option for the situation.

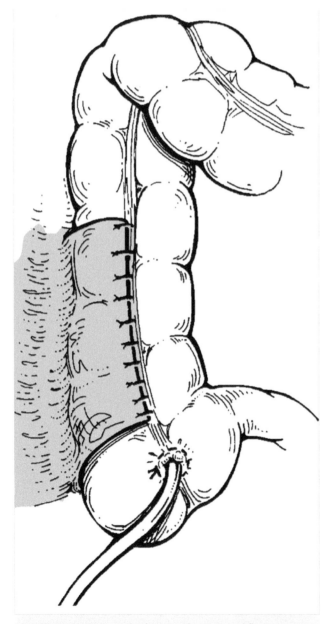

Fig. 28.17 Cecostomy and colopexy with a peritoneal flap.

28.5 Volvulus of Transverse Colon

28.5.1 Incidence and Epidemiology

Volvulus of the transverse colon is rare. Only 69 cases were reported in the literature before 1983.[106] A review of 306 cases of colonic volvulus from the 1960s revealed that only 4% of the cases involved the transverse colon.[107] Age and sex distribution tend to parallel that for cecal volvulus rather than sigmoid volvulus, because patients with transverse colonic volvulus tend to be younger and more often are females.[108,109]

28.5.2 Etiology and Pathogenesis

A short transverse mesocolon and wide points of fixation of the hepatic and splenic flexures normally prevent the transverse colon from twisting. For transverse colonic volvulus to occur, certain congenital, physiologic, or mechanical factors must alter these relationships. Congenital factors include a freely movable right colon, a long mesotransverse colon, close proximity of fixation,[108,109] or other visceral abnormalities, including the Chilaiditi syndrome[110,111] (hepatodiaphragmatic interposition of the colon). Physiologic factors include chronic constipation from a variety of causes, high-fiber diet,[109] and megacolon from Hirschsprung's disease[112] or scleroderma.[113] Mechanical factors generally include some form of distal colonic obstruction, either from adhesion, neoplasm, stricture, or sigmoid volvulus.[1,109,110,114]

28.5.3 Clinical Presentation and Diagnosis

Eisenstat et al[1] have described an acute fulminating and a subacute progressive variant of transverse colonic volvulus similar to types previously described for cecal volvulus and sigmoid volvulus. Patients with the acute type present with sudden severe pain, minimal distention, and rapid deterioration. The course of patients with the subacute type mimics the development of a distal small bowel obstruction, with gradual onset of pain, vomiting, and distention.

Diagnosis is made on clinical grounds and is confirmed by radiographic evaluation of middle colonic obstruction, particularly the presence of distention of the proximal colon, with an empty distal bowel and two air–fluid levels seen in the upright and lateral decubitus positions.[115] The two air–fluid levels represent proximal and distal transverse colonic limbs analogous to those seen with a sigmoid volvulus but distinct from the single air–fluid level seen with a cecal volvulus. Contrast studies will demonstrate the characteristic bird's beak deformity at the site of torsion (▸ Fig. 28.18).

28.5.4 Treatment

Colonoscopic decompression and detorsion of transverse colonic volvulus have been reported[116,117] and may be the preferred initial procedure for the high-risk patient who has no evidence of nonviable bowel. The tendency for the volvulus to recur is documented by Anderson et al,[118] who found recurrent transverse colonic volvulus in three of four patients treated by operative detorsion, with or without simple colopexy. Many

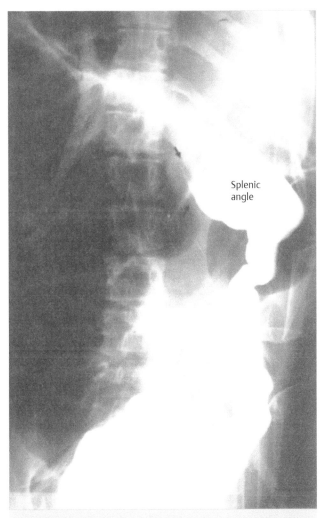

Fig. 28.18 Bird's beak deformity of transverse colonic volvulus. (This image is provided courtesy of Alain Ouimet, MD.)

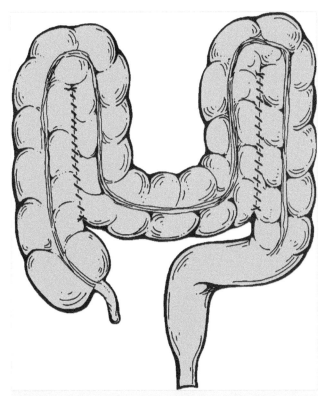

Fig. 28.19 Parallel colopexy. Redundant transverse colonic loop is sutured to the adjacent ascending and descending ends of the colon.

authors recommend resection as definitive treatment, either as a segmental colectomy or as an extended right hemicolectomy.[1,108,109,116,117]

A number of colopexy procedures have been attempted previously, including suturing of the greater omentum or mesocolon to the anterior abdominal wall, right cecopexy with or without a peritoneal flap, and cecostomy.[106] Mortensen and Hoffman[119] have described a parallel colopexy in which the redundant U-loop of transverse colon is sutured to the adjacent ascending and descending limbs of the colon with a continuous absorbable seromuscular suture (▶ Fig. 28.19). This procedure may prove to be a useful alternative to resection in select cases. However, until more experience is available with this procedure or the other colopexy methods, segmental resection or extended right hemicolectomy should be considered the preferred treatment for nonstrangulated transverse colonic volvulus.

Cases involving gangrene or perforation should be managed by resection with colostomy and closure of the distal end or mucous fistula, or by extended right hemicolectomy and ileocolonic anastomosis. Mortality can be significant, as reported by Kerry and Ransom,[107] who noted a 33% mortality rate among

their cases of transverse colonic volvulus. Early diagnosis and aggressive therapy should dramatically lessen this figure.

28.6 Splenic Flexure Volvulus

28.6.1 Incidence and Epidemiology

Fewer than 25 cases of splenic flexure volvulus have been reported, including one case of "traveling volvulus," involving the sigmoid and splenic flexure.[120] The average patient age among 22 reported cases was 50.5 years, and women outnumbered men by two to one.[121,122]

28.6.2 Etiology, Pathogenesis, and Clinical Presentation

Splenic flexure volvulus normally is prevented by the limited mobility of this point of the colon because of the phrenicocolic, gastrocolic, and splenocolic ligaments, along with the retroperitoneal position of the descending colon. For splenic flexure volvulus to occur, the normal anatomic arrangements must be altered, either by congenital deficiency or by surgery, making the splenic flexure more mobile. Sixteen of 22 reported patients in a review by Naraynsingh and Raju[123] had had previous abdominal surgery. Congenital bands or adhesions also have been implicated in the etiology.[122,123] Associated factors have included constipation and neuropsychiatric disorders.[124] The clinical presentation of splenic flexure volvulus is similar to that seen with transverse colonic or cecal volvulus (▶ Fig. 28.20).

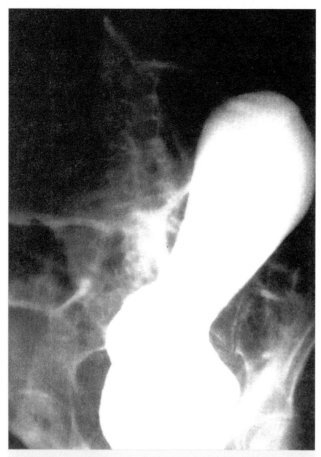

Fig. 28.20 Barium enema demonstrating obstruction of splenic flexure volvulus. (This image is provided courtesy of John Keyserlingk, MD.)

Radiographic diagnosis of a splenic flexure volvulus is suggested when the following are seen: (1) a markedly dilated, air-filled colon with an abrupt termination at the anatomic splenic flexure; (2) two widely separated air–fluid levels, one in the transverse colon and the other in the cecum; (3) an empty descending and sigmoid colon; and (4) a characteristic bird's beak deformity at the anatomic splenic flexure indicated by contrast enema examination.[125]

28.6.3 Treatment

Treatment is surgical and has consisted of either resection or detorsion with lysis of adhesions and/or fixation of the splenic flexure. One recurrence has been reported after simple colopexy.[121] The only death occurred in an untreated patient. The low mortality rate may relate to the fact that strangulation of the splenic flexure occurs infrequently.[120] Although experience with simple colopexy for sigmoid volvulus and transverse colonic volvulus suggests that recurrence may be a problem, the limited experience to date suggests that either resection or detorsion and fixation are acceptable alternative procedures.[120,122,123]

References

[1] Eisenstat TE, Raneri AJ, Mason GR. Volvulus of the transverse colon. Am J Surg. 1977; 134(3):396–399

[2] Brothers TE, Strodel WE, Eckhauser FE. Endoscopy in colonic volvulus. Ann Surg. 1987; 206(1):1–4

[3] Ballantyne GH. Volvulus of the large intestine. [Expert Commentary]. Perspect Colon Rectal Surg. 1990; 3:56–60

[4] Asbun HJ, Castellanos H, Balderrama B, et al. Sigmoid volvulus in the high altitude of the Andes. Review of 230 cases. Dis Colon Rectum. 1992; 35 (4):350–353

[5] Ballantyne GH. Review of sigmoid volvulus. Clinical patterns and pathogenesis. Dis Colon Rectum. 1982; 25(8):823–830

[6] Scott GW. Volvulus of the sigmoid flexure. Dis Colon Rectum. 1965; 8:30–34

[7] Johnson LP. Recent experience with sigmoid volvulus in Ethiopia; its incidence and management by primary resection. Ethiop Med J. 1965; 4:197–204

[8] Perlmann J. Klinische Beitra¨ge zur Pathologie und chirurgischen Behandlung des Darmverschlusses. Arch Klin Chir. 1925; 137:245–264

[9] Bruusgaard C. Volvulus of the sigmoid colon and its treatment. Surgery. 1947; 22(3):466–478

[10] Northeast ADR, Dennison AR, Lee EG. Sigmoid volvulus: new thoughts on the epidemiology. Dis Colon Rectum. 1984; 27(4):260–261

[11] Perry EG. Intestinal volvulus: a new concept. Aust N Z J Surg. 1983; 53 (5):483–486

[12] Duke JH, Jr, Yar MS. Primary small bowel volvulus: cause and management. Arch Surg. 1977; 112(6):685–688

[13] Gumbrell RC, Jagusch KT. Letter: "Red gut" syndrome in lambs grazing lucerne. N Z Vet J. 1973; 21(8):178–179

[14] Berger KE, Lundberg EA. Intestinal volvulus precipitated by lead poisoning; report of five cases. J Am Med Assoc. 1951; 147(1):13–16

[15] String ST, DeCosse JJ. Sigmoid volvulus. An examination of the mortality. Am J Surg. 1971; 121(3):293–297

[16] Shepherd JJ. The epidemiology and clinical presentation of sigmoid volvulus. Br J Surg. 1969; 56(5):353–359

[17] Berenyi MR, Schwarz GS. Megasigmoid syndrome in diabetes and neurologic disease. Review of 13 cases. Am J Gastroenterol. 1967; 47(4):311–320

[18] Gama AH, Haddad J, Simonsen O, et al. Volvulus of the sigmoid colon in Brazil: a report of 230 cases. Dis Colon Rectum. 1976; 19(4):314–320

[19] Wuepper KD, Otteman MG, Stahlgren LH. An appraisal of the operative and nonoperative treatment of sigmoid volvulus. Surg Gynecol Obstet. 1966; 122 (1):84–88

[20] Glazer I, Adlersberg D. Volvulus of the colon; a complication of sprue. Gastroenterology. 1953; 24(2):159–172

[21] Meyers MA, Ghahremani GG, Govoni AF. Ischemic colitis associated with sigmoid volvulus: new observations. AJR Am J Roentgenol. 1977; 128(4):591–595

[22] Friedlaender E. The surgical treatment of acute volvulus of the megasigmoid by primary resection. J Int Coll Surg. 1961; 35:296–301

[23] Arnold GJ, Nance FC. Volvulus of the sigmoid colon. Ann Surg. 1973; 177 (5):527–537

[24] Forward AD. Hypokalemia associated with sigmoid volvulus. Surg Gynecol Obstet. 1966; 123(1):35–42

[25] Lord SA, Boswell WC, Hungerpiller JC. Sigmoid volvulus in pregnancy. Am Surg. 1996; 62(5):380–382

[26] Schagen van Leeuwen JH. Sigmoid volvulus in a West African population. Dis Colon Rectum. 1985; 28(10):712–716

[27] Verheyden CN, Newcomer AD, Beart RW, Jr. Painless chronic sigmoid volvulus. JAMA. 1978; 240(5):464–465

[28] Hinshaw DB, Carter R. Surgical management of acute volvulus of the sigmoid colon; a study of 55 cases. Ann Surg. 1957; 146(1):52–60

[29] Burrell HC, Baker DM, Wardrop P, Evans AJ. Significant plain film findings in sigmoid volvulus. Clin Radiol. 1994; 49(5):317–319

[30] Ott DJ, Chen MY. Specific acute colonic disorders. Radiol Clin North Am. 1994; 32(5):871–884

[31] Young WS, Engelbrecht HE, Stoker A. Plain film analysis in sigmoid volvulus. Clin Radiol. 1978; 29(5):553–560

[32] Vogel JD, Feingold DL, Stewart DB, et al. Clinical practice guidelines for colon volvulus and acute colonic pseudo-obstruction. Dis Colon Rectum. 2016; 59 (7):589–600

[33] Catalano O. Computed tomographic appearance of sigmoid volvulus. Abdom Imaging. 1996; 21(4):314–317

[34] Swenson BR, Kwaan MR, Burkart NE, et al. Colonic volvulus: presentation and management in metropolitan Minnesota, United States. Dis Colon Rectum. 2012; 55(4):444–449

[35] Tanga MR. Sigmoid volvulus: a new concept in treatment. Am J Surg. 1974; 128(1):119–121

[36] Subrahmanyam M. Mesosigmoplasty as a definitive operation for sigmoid volvulus. Br J Surg. 1992; 79(7):683–684

[37] Salim AS. Management of acute volvulus of the sigmoid colon: a new approach by percutaneous deflation and colopexy. World J Surg. 1991; 15 (1):68–72, discussion 73

[38] Drapanas T, Stewart JD. Acute sigmoid volvulus. Concepts in surgical treatment. Am J Surg. 1961; 101:70–77

[39] Shepherd JJ. Treatment of volvulus of sigmoid colon: a review of 425 cases. BMJ. 1968; 1(5587):280–283

[40] Sutcliffe MML. Volvulus of the sigmoid colon. Br J Surg. 1968; 55 (12):903–910

[41] Sharpton B, Cheek RC. Volvulus of the sigmoid colon. Am Surg. 1976; 42 (6):436–440

[42] Gulati SM, Grover NK, Tagore NK, Taneja OP. Volvulus of the sigmoid colon in Delhi, India. Dis Colon Rectum. 1974; 17(2):219–225

[43] Ballantyne GH, Brandner MD, Beart RW, Jr, Ilstrup DM. Volvulus of the colon. Incidence and mortality. Ann Surg. 1985; 202(1):83–92

[44] Mangiante EC, Croce MA, Fabian TC, Moore OF, III, Britt LG. Sigmoid volvulus. A four-decade experience. Am Surg. 1989; 55(1):41–44

[45] Keller A, Aeberhard P. Emergency resection and primary anastomosis for sigmoid volvulus in an African population. Int J Colorectal Dis. 1990; 5(4):209–212

[46] Jacobs DM, Bubrick MP. Volvulus of the large intestines. Perspect Colon Rectal Surg. 1990; 3:34–55

[47] Ghazi A, Shinya H, Wolfe WI. Treatment of volvulus of the colon by colonoscopy. Ann Surg. 1976; 183(3):263–265

[48] Biery DL, Hoffman SMJ. Colonoscopic reduction of sigmoid volvulus. J Am Osteopath Assoc. 1978; 77(7):543–545

[49] Orchard JL, Mehta R, Khan AH. The use of colonoscopy in the treatment of colonic volvulus: three cases and review of the literature. Am J Gastroenterol. 1984; 79(11):864–867

[50] Wertkin MG, Aufses AH, Jr. Management of volvulus of the colon. Dis Colon Rectum. 1978; 21(1):40–45

[51] Previti FW, Holt RW. Detorsion of sigmoid volvulus by flexible fiberoptic sigmoidoscopy. J Med Soc N J. 1981; 78(4):288–290

[52] Renzulli P, Maurer CA, Netzer P, Büchler MW. Preoperative colonoscopic derotation is beneficial in acute colonic volvulus. Dig Surg. 2002; 19(3):223–229

[53] Grossmann EM, Longo WE, Stratton MD, Virgo KS, Johnson FE. Sigmoid volvulus in Department of Veterans Affairs Medical Centers. Dis Colon Rectum. 2000; 43(3):414–418

[54] Wissler DW, Morrissey JF. Use of an external suction-irrigation device in endoscopy. Gastrointest Endosc. 1980; 26(1):11–12

[55] Bernton E, Myers R, Reyna T. Pseudoobstruction of the colon: case report including a new endoscopic treatment. Gastrointest Endosc. 1982; 28(2):90–92

[56] Gibney EJ. Volvulus of the sigmoid colon. Surg Gynecol Obstet. 1991; 173 (3):243–255

[57] Yassaie O, Thompson-Fawcett M, Rossaak J. Management of sigmoid volvulus: is early surgery justifiable? ANZ J Surg. 2013; 83(1–2):74–78

[58] Tan KK, Chong CS, Sim R. Management of acute sigmoid volvulus: an institution's experience over 9 years. World J Surg. 2010; 34(8):1943–1948

[59] Bagarani M, Conde AS, Longo R, Italiano A, Terenzi A, Venuto G. Sigmoid volvulus in west Africa: a prospective study on surgical treatments. Dis Colon Rectum. 1993; 36(2):186–190

[60] Naaeder SB, Archampong EQ. One-stage resection of acute sigmoid volvulus. Br J Surg. 1995; 82(12):1635–1636

[61] Degiannis E, Levy RD, Sliwa K, Hale MJ, Saadia R. Volvulus of the sigmoid colon at Baragwanath Hospital. S Afr J Surg. 1996; 34(1):25–28

[62] Isbister WH. Large bowel volvulus. Int J Colorectal Dis. 1996; 11(2):96–98

[63] Raveenthiran V. Restorative resection of unprepared left-colon in gangrenous vs. viable sigmoid volvulus. Int J Colorectal Dis. 2004; 19(3):258–263

[64] Moore JH, Cintron JR, Duarte B, Espinosa G, Abcarian H. Synchronous cecal and sigmoid volvulus. Report of a case. Dis Colon Rectum. 1992; 35(8):803–805

[65] Basato S, Lin Sun Fui S, Pautrat K, Tresallet C, Pocard M. Comparison of two surgical techniques for resection of uncomplicated sigmoid volvulus: laparoscopy or open surgical approach? J Visc Surg. 2014; 151(6):431–434

[66] Bach O, Rudloff U, Post S. Modification of mesosigmoidoplasty for nongangrenous sigmoid volvulus. World J Surg. 2003; 27(12):1329–1332

[67] Brown AS, Mueller PR, Ferrucci JT, Jr. Controlled percutaneous gastrostomy: nylon T-fastener for fixation of the anterior gastric wall. Radiology. 1986; 158(2):543–545

[68] Gallagher HJ, Aitken D, Chapman A, Ambrose NS. Endoscopic T-bar sigmoidopexy. A novel and effective treatment of sigmoid volvulus. Colorectal Dis. 2000; 2 Suppl:68

[69] Gallagher HJ, Aitken D, Chapman AH, Ambrose NS. Additional experience of endoscopic T-bar sigmoidopexy [letter to editor]. Dis Colon Rectum. 2002; 45(11):1565–1566, author reply 1566

[70] Pinedo G, Kirberg A. Percutaneous endoscopic sigmoidopexy in sigmoid volvulus with T-fasteners: report of two cases. Dis Colon Rectum. 2001; 44 (12):1867–1869, discussion 1869–1870

[71] Alver O, Oren D, Tireli M, Kayabaşi B, Akdemir D. Ileosigmoid knotting in Turkey. Review of 68 cases. Dis Colon Rectum. 1993; 36(12):1139–1147

[72] Mallick IH, Winslet MC. Ileosigmoid knotting. Colorectal Dis. 2004; 6 (4):220–225

[73] Alver O, Oren D, Apaydin B, Yiğitbaşi R, Ersan Y. Internal herniation concurrent with ileosigmoid knotting or sigmoid volvulus: presentation of 12 patients. Surgery. 2005; 137(3):372–377

[74] Alshawi JS. Recurrent sigmoid volvulus in pregnancy: report of a case and review of the literature. Dis Colon Rectum. 2005; 48(9):1811–1813

[75] Anderson MJ, Sr, Okike N, Spencer RJ. The colonoscope in cecal volvulus: report of three cases. Dis Colon Rectum. 1978; 21(1):71–74

[76] Hendrick JW. Treatment of volvulus of the cecum and right colon. Arch Surg. 1964; 88:364–373

[77] Hinshaw DB, Carter R, Joergenson EJ. Volvulus of the cecum or right colon; a study of fourteen cases. Am J Surg. 1959; 98(2):175–183

[78] Jeck HS. Volvulus of the cecum; with a review of the recent literature and report of a case occurring as a postoperative complication. Am J Surg. 1958; 96(3):411–414

[79] Anderson JR, Welch GH. Acute volvulus of the right colon: an analysis of 69 patients. World J Surg. 1986; 10(2):336–342

[80] Wolf RY, Wilson H. Emergency operation for volvulus of the cecum. Review of 22 cases. Am Surg. 1966; 32(2):96–102

[81] Barss JA, Coury JJ, Koch DA, Sites EC, Hazledine HJ. Intermittent volvulus of the right colon. Am J Surg. 1959; 97(3):316–320

[82] Wolfer JA, Beaton LE, Anson BJ. Volvulus of the cecum: anatomic factors in its etiology. Report of a case. Surg Gynecol Obstet. 1942; 74:882–893

[83] Donhauser JL, Atwell S. Volvulus of the cecum with a review of 100 cases in the literature and a report of six new cases. Arch Surg. 1949; 58(2):129–148

[84] Burke JB, Ballantyne GH. Cecal volvulus. Low mortality at a city hospital. Dis Colon Rectum. 1984; 27(11):737–740

[85] Jordan GL, Jr, Beahrs OH. Volvulus of the cecum as a postoperative complication; report of six cases. Ann Surg. 1953; 137(2):245–249

[86] Grover NK, Gulati SM, Tagore NK, Taneja OP. Volvulus of the cecum and ascending colon. Am J Surg. 1973; 125(6):672–675

[87] Rahbar A, Easley GW, Mendoza CB, Jr. Volvulus of the cecum. Am Surg. 1973; 39(6):325–330

[88] Krippaehne WW, Vetto RM, Jenkins CC. Volvulus of the ascending colon. A report of twenty-two cases. Am J Surg. 1967; 114(2):323–332

[89] Sorg J, Whitaker WG, Jr, Richmond L. Volvulus of the right colon in the postpartum and postoperative patient. J Med Assoc Ga. 1977; 66(7):519–523

[90] Berger RB, Hillemeier AC, Stahl RS, Markowitz RI. Volvulus of the ascending colon: an unusual complication of non-rotation of the midgut. Pediatr Radiol. 1982; 12(6):298–300

[91] Bedard CK, Ramirez A, Holsinger D. Ascending colon volvulus due to a vitelline duct remnant in an elderly patient. Am J Gastroenterol. 1979; 71 (6):617–620

[92] Ritvo M, Farrell GE, Jr, Shauffer IA. The association of volvulus of the cecum and ascending colon with other obstructive colonic lesions. Am J Roentgenol Radium Ther Nucl Med. 1957; 78(4):587–598

[93] Moore CJ, Corl FM, Fishman EK. CT of cecal volvulus: unraveling the image. AJR Am J Roentgenol. 2001; 177(1):95–98

[94] Nay HR, West JP. Treatment of volvulus of the sigmoid colon and cecum. Arch Surg. 1967; 94(1):11–13

[95] Patel D, Ansari E, Berman MD. Percutaneous decompression of cecal volvulus. AJR Am J Roentgenol. 1987; 148(4):747–748

[96] Crass JR, Simmons RL, Frick MP, Maile CW. Percutaneous decompression of the colon using CT guidance in Ogilvie syndrome. AJR Am J Roentgenol. 1985; 144(3):475–476

[97] Casola G, Withers C, vanSonnenberg E, Herba MJ, Saba RM, Brown RA. Percutaneous cecostomy for decompression of the massively distended cecum. Radiology. 1986; 158(3):793–794

[98] Geer DA, Arnaud G, Beitler A, et al. Colonic volvulus. The Army Medical Center experience 1983–1987. Am Surg. 1991; 57(5):295–300

[99] Todd GJ, Forde KA. Volvulus of the cecum: choice of operation. Am J Surg. 1979; 138(5):632–634

[100] Rabinovici R, Simansky DA, Kaplan O, Mavor E, Manny J. Cecal volvulus. Dis Colon Rectum. 1990; 33(9):765–769

[101] Madiba TE, Thomson SR. The management of cecal volvulus. Dis Colon Rectum. 2002; 45(2):264–267

[102] Benacci JC, Wolff BG. Cecostomy. Therapeutic indications and results. Dis Colon Rectum. 1995; 38(5):530–534

[103] Tejler G, Jiborn H. Volvulus of the cecum. Report of 26 cases and review of the literature. Dis Colon Rectum. 1988; 31(6):445–449

[104] John H, Gyr T, Giudici G, Martinoli S, Marx A. Cecal volvulus in pregnancy. Case report and review of literature. Arch Gynecol Obstet. 1996; 258(3):161–164

[105] Montes H, Wolf J. Cecal volvulus in pregnancy. Am J Gastroenterol. 1999; 94(9):2554–2556

[106] Gumbs MA, Kashan F, Shumofsky E, Yerubandi SR. Volvulus of the transverse colon. Reports of cases and review of the literature. Dis Colon Rectum. 1983; 26(12):825–828

[107] Kerry R, Ransom HK. Volvulus of the colon: etiology, diagnosis and treatment. Arch Surg. 1969; 29:78–85

[108] Fishman EK, Goldman SM, Patt PG, Berlanstein B, Bohlman ME. Transverse colon volvulus: diagnosis and treatment. South Med J. 1983; 76(2):185–189

[109] Zinkin LD, Katz LD, Rosin JD. Volvulus of the transverse colon: report of case and review of the literature. Dis Colon Rectum. 1979; 22(7):492–496

[110] Boley SJ. Volvulus of the transverse colon. Am J Surg. 1958; 96(1):122–125

[111] Orangio GR, Fazio VW, Winkelman E, McGonagle BA. The Chilaiditi syndrome and associated volvulus of the transverse colon. An indication for surgical therapy. Dis Colon Rectum. 1986; 29(10):653–656

[112] Plorde JJ, Raker EJ. Transverse colon volvulus and associated Chilaiditi's syndrome: case report and literature review. Am J Gastroenterol. 1996; 91(12):2613–2616

[113] Martin JD, Jr, Ward CS. Megacolon associated with volvulus of transverse colon. Am J Surg. 1944; 64:412–416

[114] Budd DC, Nirdlinger EL, Sturtz DL, Fouty WJ, Jr. Transverse colon volvulus associated with scleroderma. Am J Surg. 1977; 133(3):370–372

[115] Newton NA, Reines HD. Transverse colon volvulus: case reports and review. AJR Am J Roentgenol. 1977; 128(1):69–72

[116] Chang TH. Acute volvulus of the transverse colon: report of an unusual case. W V Med J. 1985; 81(5):95–98

[117] Joergensen K, Kronborg O. The colonoscope in volvulus of the transverse colon. Dis Colon Rectum. 1980; 23(5):357–358

[118] Anderson JR, Lee D, Taylor TV, Ross AH. Volvulus of the transverse colon. Br J Surg. 1981; 68(3):179–181

[119] Mortensen NJM, Hoffman G. Volvulus of the transverse colon. Postgrad Med J. 1979; 55(639):54–57

[120] Anderson MF, Pickney L. The traveling volvulus. Dis Colon Rectum. 1979; 22(4):276–278

[121] Goldberg M, Lernau OZ, Mogle P, Dermer R, Nissan S. Volvulus of the splenic flexure of the colon. Am J Gastroenterol. 1984; 79(9):693–694

[122] Welch GH, Anderson JR. Volvulus of the splenic flexure of the colon. Dis Colon Rectum. 1985; 28(8):592–593

[123] Naraynsingh V, Raju GC. Splenic flexure volvulus. Postgrad Med J. 1985; 61(721):1007–1008

[124] Ballantyne GH. Volvulus of the splenic flexure: report of a case and review of the literature. Dis Colon Rectum. 1981; 24(8):630–632

[125] Mindelzun RE, Stone JM. Volvulus of the splenic flexure: radiographic features. Radiology. 1991; 181(1):221–223

29 Large Bowel Obstruction

Sharmini Su Sivarajah and David G. Jayne

Abstract

Acute large bowel obstruction is a common surgical emergency associated with high morbidity and mortality. Symptoms include abdominal distension and constipation. Survival is maximized by appreciation of the etiology and pathophysiology of large bowel obstruction along with the risks of various treatment options.

Keywords: large bowel obstruction, etiology, pathophysiology, left colonic obstruction, right colonic obstruction, sigmoid colon obstruction, management, pseudo-obstruction, volvulus, diverticular disease

29.1 Introduction

Acute large bowel obstruction is a common surgical emergency associated with high morbidity and mortality rates unless treatment is expedient. Large bowel obstruction can be defined as an impediment to the passage of intraluminal contents in the colon and/or rectum resulting in abdominal distension and constipation. Patients are often elderly and unwell. The chances of survival will be maximized if one appreciates the etiology and pathophysiology of large bowel obstruction along with the risks of various treatment options.

The most common cause of large bowel obstruction in adults (78%) is adenocarcinoma of the colon and rectum.[1] It is followed by benign conditions, including diverticulitis, colonic volvulus, metastatic cancer, and inflammatory bowel disease.[1] Of note, the etiology of large bowel obstruction varies worldwide, as does the patient population affected. In Africa and India, the primary cause of large bowel obstruction is volvulus (60%) affecting patients who are young and fit.[2]

29.2 Mechanical Large Bowel Obstruction

29.2.1 Etiology and Pathophysiology

Large bowel obstruction can be divided into mechanical and nonmechanical causes (pseudo-obstruction). In this section, we will focus on mechanical causes and the pathophysiology; pseudo-obstruction will be discussed later.

Mechanical large bowel obstruction causes changes in intestinal motility, the intraluminal colonic milieu, and colonic blood flow. Proximal to the site of obstruction, the bowel becomes dilated and fluid is sequestered due to disturbed reabsorption. Up to 10 L of fluid can be sequestered into the bowel over a 24-hour period and major fluid loss can occur. This is made worse by limited oral intake and vomiting. There is decreased intravascular volume and electrolyte disturbance, which causes hypovolemic shock.

Initially, peristaltic activity may be increased in an attempt to overcome the obstruction, with the patient experiencing colicky abdominal pain. With time, the intestinal smooth muscle becomes enervated and peristalsis stops. The bowel empties distal to the obstruction (the patient can present with diarrhea initially), before becoming collapsed. In cases where adynamic obstruction occurs, abdominal discomfort is secondary to the distension due to the reduced or absent peristaltic activity.

Systemic inflammatory response syndrome (SIRS) supervenes as the intraluminal pressure increases, causing microvascular changes with loss of mucosal integrity and translocation of bacteria into the bloodstream.

With worsening distension of the bowel wall, venous return becomes disrupted and leads to progressive congestion, loss of fluid into bowel lumen, and third space (due to the leakage of serosal fluid into the abdomen causing ascites). Intestinal ischemic occurs with worsening venous engorgement that jeopardizes the arterial inflow into the capillary bed. Eventually, the bowel wall becomes necrotic and perforation occurs.

In "closed-loop" obstruction, two limbs of the bowel are involved and obstructed. This can occur when a loop of bowel is trapped by a band adhesion or an internal hernia. In this situation, increase in distension and intraluminal pressure will be swift with sudden vascular occlusion.

The most common cause of mechanical large bowel obstruction is primary colonic carcinoma. Buechter et al[1] reported 127 patients presenting with large bowel obstruction with 90% being due to colonic carcinoma. ▶ Table 29.1 lists the causes of mechanical large bowel obstruction including rare causes such as diverticular disease, hernia, inflammatory bowel disease, foreign body, colonic intussusception, and deep penetrating endometriosis.

Table 29.1 Etiology of mechanical large bowel obstruction

Causes of mechanical large bowel obstruction
Primary colonic carcinoma (60–80%)
Volvulus (11–15%)
Diverticulitis (4–10%)
Hernia
Inflammatory bowel disease
Intraluminal foreign body
Extrinsic compression from masses (benign or malignant) and abscesses
Colonic intussusception
Diaphragmatic disease of the colon
Deep penetrating endometriosis
Iatrogenic causes
Postoperative adhesions
Radiation stricture
Anastomotic stricture

Carcinoma

Large bowel obstruction due to carcinoma is not common. In a series of 908 cases, Serpell et al[3] reported that 16% of patients presented with complete obstruction and 31% had partial obstruction. Of 4,583 patients in the Large Bowel Cancer Project in the United Kingdom, obstruction was noted in 16%.[4] In this series, the splenic flexure was the site of obstruction in 49% of cases, followed by the left colon (23%), the right colon (23%), and the rectum and rectosigmoid colon (6%). In the series by Buechter et al,[1] the sigmoid colon was the most common site of obstruction, accounting for 38%, followed by the descending colon, splenic flexure, transverse colon, rectum, cecum, ascending colon, and hepatic flexure. The sigmoid colon was also noted by Kyllönen[5] as the predominant site of obstruction. Due to the fact that the lumen of the sigmoid and descending colon is smaller and the stool more solid in this region, obstruction in the left colon manifests earlier than that caused by obstruction in the right colon.

Volvulus

Approximately 10 to 15% of large bowel obstruction is due to acute colonic volvulus.[6] Volvulus is an axial rotation of a segment of bowel about its mesentery. It is improbable for the volvulus to settle without intervention if the twist is greater than 360 degrees. Narrowing at the site of torsion produces signs and symptoms of obstruction. The torsion of the mesentery causes vascular compromise at the site of volvulus, which leads to ischemia, necrosis, and perforation.

Sigmoid volvulus is three to four times more prevalent than cecal volvulus (60–75 vs. 25–33%, respectively). It is rare to acquire a volvulus at the transverse colon or splenic flexure (< 1%).[7,8] A very mobile redundant colon on a mesentery and a fixed point about which the colon can twist are usually the main precipitating factors leading to a colonic volvulus. Sigmoid volvulus commonly occurs in the elderly, who tend to have poor mobility and a history of constipation, as well as a chronically dilated and elongated sigmoid colon. Volvulus is associated with certain comorbidities such as Parkinson's disease, Alzheimer's disease, and multiple sclerosis. Electrolyte disturbance, particularly hypokalemia, should be excluded. Studies have also shown that a high dietary fiber intake is associated with sigmoid volvulus and this might explain why volvulus is the most common cause of bowel obstruction in Africa and India.[9] Factors that provoke a dilatation of the right colon, such as pregnancy and colonoscopy, can increase the risk of cecal volvulus (Chapter 28).[10]

Diverticular Disease

Some degree of colonic obstruction occurs in approximately two-thirds of the patients with acute diverticulitis. This partial obstruction is usually caused by inflammation with spasm and edema together with an element of adynamic ileus. Complete obstruction occurs in approximately 10% of cases and is the second most frequent cause of acute colonic obstruction. Complete obstruction usually implies abscess formation with encroachment of the lumen or repeated episodes of diverticulitis with fibrosis and stenosis.

Large bowel obstruction caused by diverticulitis can occur at any location, but the most common location is the sigmoid colon (▸ Fig. 29.1). In Asian countries, however, it is not uncommon for obstruction to occur in the right colon.[11] In patients presenting with a first attack of diverticulitis, it is recommended that they undergo visualization of the colon, usually by colonoscopy, to exclude a coexisting carcinoma that may then present as obstruction (Chapter 25).[12]

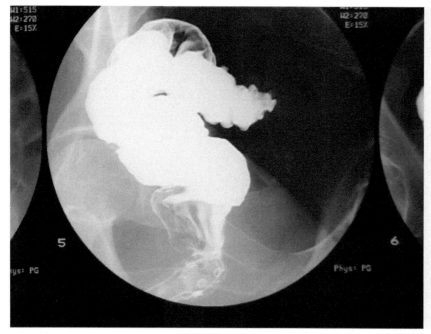

Fig. 29.1 Single contrast rectal enema demonstrating a tapering stricture in the sigmoid colon due to diverticular disease.

Hernias

Hernias tend to be associated with small bowel obstruction and less commonly are a cause of large bowel obstruction. However, large bowel obstruction can occur secondary to inguinal, femoral, umbilical, Spigelian, incisional, lumbar, and diaphragmatic hernias.[8] The most common internal hernia to produce large bowel obstruction involves the foramen of Winslow hernia, a condition in which small bowel, and in one-third of cases the right colon, herniate through the normal communication between the greater and lesser peritoneal cavities, between the free edge of the lesser omentum and the hepatoduodenal ligament.[13]

Crohn's Disease

Colonic involvement with Crohn's disease occurs in about 20 to 50% of patients.[14,15] Colonic obstruction in patients with Crohn's disease is usually due to strictures formed after repeated attacks of transmural inflammation of the colon causing fibrosis and scarring. Symptoms of progressive bowel obstruction become apparent as the bowel becomes strictured and the lumen narrows. Patients with Crohn's disease have a two to three times higher risk of developing colon carcinoma compared with age-matched standard population.[16] It is therefore important to exclude malignancy in such patients.

Intraluminal Contents

The rectum (70%) and sigmoid colon (20%) are the most common sites of colonic obstruction due to intraluminal contents such as bezoars (▶ Fig. 29.2).[7,8] The most likely causes include gallstones, enteroliths, intentionally inserted foreign body, medications, and illegal drugs. Fecal impaction is seen the most frequently in the elderly, the chronically debilitated patients, and among patients taking constipating medications, such as opiates.[6,17]

External Compression

External compression of the bowel, usually from adjacent masses, can cause large bowel obstruction. The possible underlying causes are extensive and include endometriosis, lymphadenopathy, pancreatitis, intra-abdominal abscess, peritoneal carcinomatosis, and direct invasion from gynecologic or prostatic malignancies.[6]

Intussusception

Intussusception is the invagination (telescope or accordion) of a proximal segment of the bowel (intussusceptum) into an adjacent distal segment (intussuscipiens).[18] As the intussusceptum enters the intussuscipiens, the mesentery is carried with it and becomes trapped between the overlapping layers of the bowel. This causes vascular compression with eventual ischemic necrosis unless timely intervention is undertaken. The classic CT appearance of intussusception (▶ Fig. 29.3) includes the following:

1. Target appearance (intraluminal soft tissue mass and eccentric fat density).
2. Reniform pattern (bilobed density with peripheral high-density attenuation and low attenuation centrally).
3. Sausage pattern (alternating areas of low and high attenuation related to the bowel wall, mesenteric fat and fluid, intraluminal fluid, contrast material or air).[19]

Adult intussusception is rare. In 30 years at Massachusetts General Hospital in Boston, there were 58 cases of surgically proven adult intussusception.[20] Adult intussusception accounts for 1 to 5% of all intestinal obstruction and 5% of all intussusceptions; the other 95% of intussusceptions occur in children.[20,21] In adults, approximately 90% of the cases are secondary to a definable lesion, while in children the opposite is true.[20,21] In adults, primary colon carcinoma is the most common cause,[22] followed by a number of benign pathologies, including lipomas and adenomatous polyps.[23] Various other lesions have been described as a cause for colonic intussusception, including gastrointestinal stromal tumors and a variety of appendiceal lesions, such as an inverted appendiceal stump, endometriosis involving the appendix and mucocele of the appendix [24,25]. Other reported

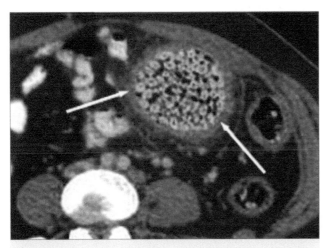

Fig. 29.2 Intraluminal colonic obstruction caused by a bezoar (*white arrows*).

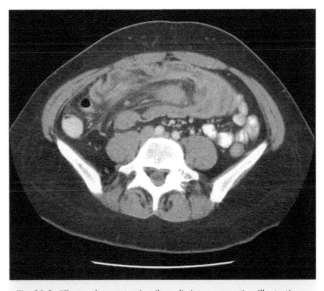

Fig. 29.3 CT scan demonstrating ileocolic intussusception illustrating a "sausage pattern" as the terminal ileum invaginates into the colon.

causes of colonic intussusception include eosinophilic colitis, pseudomembranous colitis, and epiploic appendagitis.[22,26,27,28]

Adult intussusception can occur at any age, with a mean of 47 to 54 years.[20,21] Of the 58 cases reported by Azar and Berger,[20] 44 were small bowel and 14 colonic; 48% of the small bowel lesions were malignant, compared with 43% of the colonic lesions. Intussusception may present as acute or chronic.

Diaphragmatic Disease of the Colon

Debenham was the first to describe nonsteroidal anti-inflammatory drug (NSAID) induced enteropathy.[29] Lang et al reported evidence of ulceration and stricture formation in the small bowel in long-term users of NSAIDs[30] and it was subsequently referred to as "diaphragm disease." The condition is thought to occur due to NSAID-induced inhibition of prostaglandins in the bowel mucosa.[31] Newer preparations of NSAIDs, such as the "slow release" or "modified release" agents, have some protective effect against the upper gastrointestinal side effects of NSAIDs. As a result, there is an increasing incidence of colonic enteropathy, although this is still rare.

Diaphragmatic disease of the colon is more prevalent in women and is commonly seen in patients in their seventh decade of life. Patients usually present chronically rather than acutely. Symptoms tend to relate to loss of blood and protein from these ulcers. Stricturing can occasionally cause large bowel obstruction.

Histological analysis of the diaphragms typically shows areas of ulceration and granulation, supporting the reactive theory of "healing by fibrosis."[32,33,34] Several studies have shown that colonic enteropathic ulceration can progress to diaphragm disease on serial follow-up.[35] The presence of a circumferential "rim ulcer" seen at the edge of the diaphragms suggests that the luminal contents containing active NSAID products come into contact with the diaphragmatic orifice.[36] To differentiate diaphragms from a prominent plica fold, it is essential to identify the histological hallmark of submucosal fibrosis with intact muscularis propria. Collagen fibers are often predominant and concentrate toward the apex of the strictures.

The main treatment for this condition is to discontinue the usage of NSAIDs with resolution of inflammation as soon as the medication is withdrawn.[37,38,39] Other described therapies are aimed at reducing inflammation, such as steroids[40,41] and 5-aminosalicylic acid.[36] However, the fibrotic process that led to the formation of diaphragms is permanent and cannot always be reversed. In this event, mechanical dilation of the diaphragms is necessary using endoscopy techniques[42] and failing this surgical resection may be necessary.

Deep Penetrating Endometriosis

Intestinal involvement occurs in approximately 12 to 37% of women with endometriosis. Most cases are asymptomatic or subclinical.[43,44] The most common site of involvement is at the rectosigmoid colon (70%). The rest occur in the small bowel (7%), cecum (3.6%), and appendix (3%).[43,45]

Extraintestinal involvement can also involve other organs, such as the bladder, kidneys, and peritoneum.[43] Endometriosis is commonly seen in women of reproductive age, with a median

of 34 to 40 years, although it can occur in postmenopausal women.[45] There are three main theories to explain the etiology of endometriosis. The first theory advocates that retrograde menstruation causes endometrial tissue to implant into the peritoneum. The second theory claims that endometriosis is a result of metaplastic peritoneal tissue. Finally, it has been proposed that endometrial tissues can be transplanted hematogenously or lymphatically, which may explain some cases of distant involvement.[45]

Symptoms indicating intestinal involvement can be vague and may include abdominal pain, nausea, vomiting, tenesmus, and change in bowel habit.[43,44,45,46,47] Symptoms typically fluctuate with the menstrual cycle, being worse at times of menstruation. Endometrial tissue in the bowel tends to involve either the serosa or subserosa. It is rare for endometrial tissue to involve the mucosa and if it does the patient will present with rectal bleeding.

Only 0.1 to 0.7% of cases of endometriosis present with bowel obstruction.[44,45,46] It has been hypothesized that the endometrial tissue implanted on the bowel is sensitive to ovarian hormones. The cyclical nature of hormonal changes causes repeated attacks of inflammation, fibrosis, and resultant hypertrophy of the bowel smooth muscle.[45] These changes lead to narrowing of the bowel lumen causing obstruction.

Differentiating large bowel endometriosis from other pathologies can be difficult because the symptoms are often nonspecific. Most patients are misdiagnosed as irritable bowel syndrome, inflammatory bowel disease, ischemic colitis, or even malignancy. Imaging and endoscopic evaluation have a limited role in diagnosing colonic endometriosis. Colonoscopy may reveal a site of narrowing; however, the mucosal biopsy is often normal as the stricture is due to the pressure effect from the muscular and serosal involvement (▶ Fig. 29.4). Barium enema or CT will only reveal external compression. The definitive diagnosis can often only be made at the time of surgery and confirmed on histopathology.[48]

Treatment for endometriosis is generally conservative using medication such as NSAIDS, oral contraceptive pills, and gonadotropin-releasing hormone (GnRH) agonists. However, surgical intervention is warranted if a patient presents with symptoms of bowel obstruction.

Adhesions

Adhesions are a very rare cause of large bowel obstruction. Studies have reported adhesive bands causing large bowel obstruction in the right, transverse, and sigmoid colon.[8,49,50]

Sarcoidosis

Hilzenrat et al[51] reported a case of colonic obstruction secondary to sarcoidosis. Two areas of narrowing were observed in the rectum and at the splenic flexure, through which a colonoscopy could not pass, but biopsies demonstrated sarcoidosis. Despite the abdominal and proximal bowel distension, treatment with oral prednisolone resulted in symptomatic improvement in 3 days. Follow-up colonoscopy 1 month later was essentially normal and the patient avoided operation.

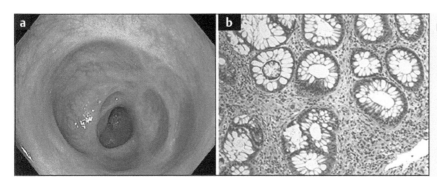

Fig. 29.4 **(a)** Colonoscopy. **(b)** Pathology.

29.2.2 Clinical Manifestations

A patient with large bowel obstruction usually presents with abdominal pain, distension, and constipation. Vomiting in a patient with large bowel obstruction is a late manifestation unless there is an associated small bowel obstruction. Abdominal tenderness associated with peritoneal irritation is caused by distension of the colon and the small bowel and perhaps by edema of the mesentery. Marked abdominal pain, peritoneal irritation out of proportion, and a white blood count greater than 20,000/mL suggest ischemia or gangrene of the bowel.

Colonic distension produces pain, usually colicky, in the lower abdomen. The pain may be associated with reflexive nausea. Somatic pain occurs when an inflammatory process such as sigmoid diverticulitis reaches the peritoneum and is sensed by afferent fibers there.[52]

The clinical picture of large bowel obstruction is often dictated by whether the ileocecal valve is competent, with 75% of patients having a competent ileocecal valve. In this scenario, closed-loop large bowel obstruction will occur as the obstruction cannot decompress into the small bowel.[7] Cecal distension increases the bowel wall tension and, without intervention, will progress to ischemia and necrosis. The size of the cecum at risk of perforation ranges from 9 to 12 cm.[8]

An important cause of colonic dilatation and perforation, which should not be confused with an underlying obstructing etiology, is toxic megacolon. Toxic megacolon is usually a consequence of failed treatment of inflammatory bowel disease (ulcerative colitis) or an acute infective etiology, with the associated inflammation leading to weakening of the bowel wall. If perforation occurs, mortality ranges from 19 to 41%.[53] Toxic megacolon may be diagnosed according to a well-defined set of clinical parameters, including pyrexia, tachycardia, raised white cell count, and anemia.[54]

29.2.3 Diagnosis and Clinical Evaluation

Surgical assessment should include any recent change of bowel function or habit, weight loss over the preceding few months, signs of lethargy, patient or family history of colorectal cancer or other malignancies, and finally the results of any recent diagnostic tests. At initial presentation, the patient may show signs of dehydration, which may include a dry, furred tongue, sunken dull eyes, a characteristic fetor or decreased tissue turgor. All these signs advocate loss of extracellular fluid. At a later stage, the patient could develop hypovolemic

shock with signs of tachycardia, hypotension, and cold peripheries. On physical examination, the surgeon should actively seek for signs of peritonitis, scars indicating previous abdominal surgery, and evidence of any hernias. A digital rectal examination should always be performed. The rectum is often empty when there is large bowel obstruction. It is possible to feel a palpable tumor within the cul-de-sac on rectal examination.[55]

Blood and urine test should be taken to look for signs of anemia, electrolyte disturbances, coagulation abnormalities, dehydration, ischemia, and perforation. Arterial or venous blood gas will show a raised lactate or a negative base excess. These findings will suggest dehydration and/or ischemia. Before any intervention, a large-bore intravenous line should be obtained with fluid and electrolyte replacement started. Any clinically significant anemia should be corrected with blood transfusion. A chest radiograph and electrocardiogram should be obtained if surgical intervention is being considered.[55]

A plain film of the abdomen is the simplest test for diagnosing obstruction of the large bowel, although it does not provide reliable information about the site of the obstruction (▶ Fig. 29.5).[56] Initially, the large bowel is distended. If there is a cutoff between the distended colon and the collapsed colon, the diagnosis of large bowel obstruction can be entertained, although the specific cause cannot be established. In the presence of an incompetent ileocecal valve, air will fill the small bowel and a picture of small bowel obstruction may supervene.

Distension of the right and transverse colon associated with minimal gas in the left colon suggests acute pseudo-obstruction. Water-soluble or contrast enema distinguishes between a mechanical cause and pseudo-obstruction, and in the former, may identify the site of obstruction and the underlying pathology (▶ Fig. 29.6). Previously, a single contrast enema was recommended as the preferred means of diagnosing large bowel obstruction.[57] The sensitivity of a contrast enema in the diagnosis of large bowel obstruction is 80%, with specificity of 100%.[57,58,59] More recently, the CT scan has become the preferred imaging modality (▶ Fig. 29.7). Multidetector CT is a well-tolerated, quick examination that allows the images to be obtained in one breath hold without the need of rectal contrast agent or air insufflation. CT can reveal the cause of large bowel obstruction and whether it is intraluminal, mural, or extramural.[60] CT has been reported to have a sensitivity and specificity of 96 and 93%, respectively.[59,61]

Flexible sigmoidoscopy allows a direct visualization of the distal colon and the obstructing lesion and can exclude other

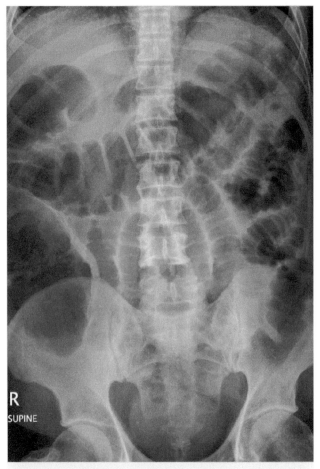

Fig. 29.5 Abdominal X-ray demonstrating dilated large and small bowel due to colonic obstruction with an incompetent ileocecal valve.

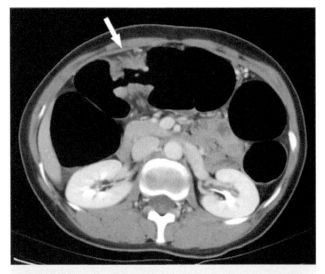

Fig. 29.7 CT scan showing a stricturing lesion in the transverse colon (*white arrow*).

causes of obstruction. One of its disadvantages is that it is not readily available at all hours for emergencies, but it has the advantages that it allows direct inspection of the obstructing

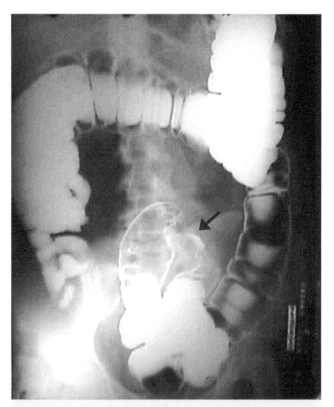

Fig. 29.6 Barium enema demonstrating an "apple-core" lesion (*arrow*) in the sigmoid colon due to a cancer.

lesion and biopsy. In some cases, endoscopic decompression may be achievable, for example, by insertion of an endoluminal stent through an obstructing cancer or untwisting of a colonic volvulus.

29.2.4 Management

There are some fundamental principles that must be followed in managing patients with large bowel obstruction regardless of the underlying cause. The principle of "drip and suck" is the foundation of conservative management. Fluid and electrolyte losses should be replaced and urine output closely monitored. The patient should also be given adequate analgesia (usually intravenous opiates) as well as anti-emetics.

Aims of Surgery

One of the major aims of surgery is to avoid fatal outcomes due to cardiovascular collapse or perforation secondary to bowel distension. It is also essential to consider the oncological principles if the obstruction is due to a malignancy. For patients who are high risk or suffer from disseminated disease, it may be prudent to offer a temporary solution to relieve the obstruction that will allow an extended period of optimization and neoadjuvant therapy with subsequent elective surgery at a later date.

Preoperative Preparation

It is important that patients receive adequate fluid resuscitation and electrolyte replacement. Blood results of urea and electrolytes (U&Es) and arterial blood gas (ABGs) should guide the rate of fluid replacement. Patients should have a urinary catheter so that hourly measurement of urine output (> 0.5 mL/kg) can be assessed. In addition, critical care should be consulted early, especially in patients with preexisting cardiac or renal disease, as they may benefit from more invasive monitoring. Patients should be kept "nil by mouth," but can be allowed sips of clear fluids for comfort. Placement of a nasogastric tube is advisable to relieve nausea and/or vomiting and minimize the risk of aspiration, especially when there is evidence of small bowel distension. The nasogastric tube may be either left on free drainage or aspirated regularly. The total measurement of the gastric losses can aid fluid replacement therapy.[62]

Operative Management

There is good evidence that elective surgery has superior outcomes to emergency surgery and hence, elective surgery should be chosen wherever possible. The preoperative mortality for emergency surgery and elective surgery for colorectal cancer is 50 and 5%, respectively, and the morbidity is double in a patient undergoing emergency surgery as compared to elective surgery.[63,64,65] Predictive factors for postoperative mortality in large bowel obstruction include age of 70 years or above, America Society of Anesthesiologists (ASA) score III–IV, presence of proximal colon damage, and preoperative renal failure.[66] During the past 20 years, endoluminal therapies have been pursued as they have several advantages, including temporary relief of obstruction and as a bridge to elective surgery.

Obstruction of the Right or Transverse Colon

Obstruction involving the cecum to the splenic flexure can be treated by (extended) right hemicolectomy with immediate ileocolic anastomosis. As long as complete oncologic resection can be achieved, this should be the standard treatment for obstructing colon cancers, with the benefit of immediate restoration of intestinal continuity.[58] Anastomotic leak rates of 2.8 to 4.6% have been published when primary ileocolic anastomosis is undertaken in the emergency setting.[58] However, if the patient presents with hemodynamic instability and/or fecal peritonitis at the time of surgery, a right hemicolectomy with an end ileostomy should be advocated instead as the initial management to avoid the risk of anastomotic leak in an unfit patient.

Left Colon Obstruction

The surgical treatment of distal colonic obstruction has evolved in the past 60 years from a three-stage procedure (proximal colostomy, second-stage resection, and third-stage stoma closure) to management as a one-stage procedure. Previous studies have shown that staged resection does not improve survival and is instead associated with high morbidity and mortality rates.[57,58, 67,68,69] Recent technological advances, which include the development of endoluminal stents, have led to many changes in the management strategies for left colonic obstruction.[57,58,64,68,69,70] This has led to diversity in the management of distal malignant colonic obstruction, which includes the following procedures.

Single or Staged Procedure

Traditionally, the three-stage procedure (proximal stoma, tumor resection, and stoma reversal) was proposed as a safe method to decrease mortality in acute obstruction. However, a Cochrane review in 2004[71] and a randomized trial studied by Kronborg[72] did not confirm any true advantage from a stoma compared with those receiving a primary resection.

Kronborg[72] reported on 121 patients who either had a three-stage or a two-stage procedure, of whom most had cancer as the cause of obstruction. Mortality was similar in the two groups (13 and 12%). However, only 6% of patients who had the three-stage procedure ended up with a permanent stoma compared to 28% of patients who had Hartmann's procedure as their initial operation. None of the patients underwent a single-stage operation. Other studies have shown comparable mortality with low anastomotic leak rates after primary resection,[73,74, 75,76] but with a high proportion of patients ending up with a permanent stoma after staged procedures.[77,78] It should be noted that staged procedures cause further morbidity and mortality during the second/third procedures. In addition, the overall hospital stay is longer compared to patients receiving a primary anastomosis.

Although the data on single versus multistage procedures might suggest an advantage for the single-stage approach, the published studies all suffer from potential biases. Surgeons will tend to perform a primary resection and anastomosis in younger and healthier patients and, unsurprisingly, the outcomes for staged procedures will appear worse. The Cochrane review from 2004 comparing primary with staged resection for large bowel obstruction could not find any studies worthy of inclusion. Results were inconclusive and there was no evidence to recommend either primary or staged resection. It was concluded that it is unlikely that a large enough trial could be performed to address the question.[75]

In emergency surgery where there is obstruction or perforation due to a left colonic lesion, Hartmann's procedure is the most frequent approach.[57,66,72,79] Hartmann's procedure is a less complex procedure to perform in the emergency setting because it avoids the morbidity associated with an anastomosis and requires less colorectal surgical expertise. It is also recommended in patients who are of high risk.[70,75]

Currently, staged management (proximal stoma and resection later) tends to be reserved for mid or low rectal cancers causing obstruction, so that neoadjuvant treatment can be administered if tumor downstaging is required, followed by elective resection. Formation of a defunctioning proximal stoma is also used if the tumor is unresectable or if the patient is unfit for a major resection in the absence of colonic perforation. In cases of uncomplicated malignant left-sided large bowel obstruction, primary resection with anastomosis is the preferred option because it carries a low mortality and morbidity rate and is safe under favorable circumstances.[57] However, if there is fecal peritonitis, shock, severe sepsis, ASA IV patient, or widespread peritoneal malignancy, Hartmann's procedure is preferred as it removes the additional risks associated with a primary anastomosis.

On-Table Lavage and Mechanical Decompression

Intraoperative colonic lavage requires externalization of the colon proximal to the stenosis and often necessitates the mobilization of both flexures. The obstructing lesion is resected and the proximal colon exteriorized with its end sealed in a plastic sheath that opens into a bucket. A bladder catheter is secured with a purse-string suture into the appendiceal stump, or through a small enterotomy in patients with previous appendectomy. A clamp is placed across the terminal ileum to prevent retrograde flow of fluid into the small bowel. Warm saline of 6 to 8 L is irrigated through the bladder catheter until the fluid runs clear,[58] which takes about 20 to 60 minutes. Once irrigation is complete, the anastomosis is made according to surgeon's preference, and may be protected by a proximal stoma. Colonic lavage does prolong operative time, as well as increase the risk of fecal contamination into the peritoneal cavity.

Manual colonic decompression requires the same steps as above. Instead of using lavage, the colon is emptied by expressing the stool contents manually. This is repeated until the colon is evacuated of all content, whether solid, liquid, or gas.[58]

In the past, there was a belief that bowel preparation was essential for a safe anastomosis and this underpinned the rationale for the three-staged procedure.[80,81] The introduction of intraoperative colonic irrigation was the first step toward recreating the ideal situation for an anastomosis. This technique was first reported by Muir in 1968,[82] but is also attributed to Dudley et al.[83] Currently, there is a change of approach with the realization that bowel preparation may do more harm than good[84] and consequently the need for lavage in the emergency situation is questionable. Two studies have compared manual decompression with on-table lavage. A prospective randomized trial reported no significant differences in outcomes between the two groups.[85] In the other study, the only significant difference was of increased operating time with on-table lavage,[86] with lavage taking 25 minutes longer than manual decompression.

Trompetas et al[70] conducted a systematic review in 2004 and showed no evidence that mechanical bowel preparation is associated with a decrease in anastomotic leak rate after colorectal surgery. Ortiz et al[87] reported that resection and primary anastomosis at the same operation can be safely performed without intraoperative irrigation. Overall, it seems that on-table lavage and manual decompression are equally effective in patients with left-sided colonic obstruction and the use of these techniques is at the discretion of the surgeon, but is not essential.[57]

There are currently no reports to suggest that primary anastomosis should routinely be covered by a defunctioning loop stoma. There is also no guidance as to the circumstances that would merit a diversion.

Subtotal or Segmental Colectomy

When there is a choice, subtotal colectomy and segmental resection are equally effective and safe.[57] The Subtotal Colectomy versus On-table Irrigation and Anastomosis (SCOTIA) randomized trial[88] reported 91 patients comparing subtotal colectomy and segmental resection. There was no significant difference between the two procedures in terms of mortality and anastomotic leakage. Length of hospital stay was similar. The only significant difference was in bowel function. In the subtotal colectomy group, there were more frequent bowel motions and greater usage of antidiarrheal agents compared to the segmental resection group. Even though bowel function improved over time, it remained significantly different between the two groups at 4 months postoperatively.

Subtotal colectomy has the advantage of excising a nonprepared, distended colon that can harbor patches of transmural ischemia or synchronous tumors not detected during surgery. Nevertheless, segmental colectomy provides better functional and quality-of-life outcomes compared with subtotal colectomy, with acceptable morbidity and mortality of 7 and 2%, respectively.[70,88,89] However, if there is evidence of cecal perforation/ischemia or there are synchronous neoplasms in the colon, a subtotal colectomy is the procedure of choice.

Endoluminal Stenting as a Bridge to Surgery

Recent controversies surround the role of primary surgical resection and colonic stenting. Colonic stenting can be used as a "bridge to surgery" in a patient with left-sided obstruction, converting an emergency open operation and end colostomy into an elective, possibly laparoscopic, operation with a primary anastomosis ± a defunctioning stoma (▶ Fig. 29.8).[62] The rate of technical success in stent placement is high (between 83 and 100%) if undertaken by an experienced operator.[90,91,92] Unfortunately, stenting carries risk of complications, including bleeding (5%) and perforation (4%).[93] Stent migration can also occur, which will result in a loss of efficacy in about 5 to 10% of cases.[92,93] Mortality after stenting ranges from 0 to 1% and is largely secondary to perforation. Overall, colonic stenting allows elective resection in about 85% of cases.[92,93,94,95]

Pirlet et al[96] designed a study to test the hypothesis that colonic stenting before resection would decrease the rate of stoma formation as well as reduce morbidity and mortality when compared with emergency surgical resection. Relief of obstruction after colonic stenting was only achieved in 40% of patients and the morbidity rate was considerably high (50%). The stoma rate in the stent and surgery groups was 43 and 57%, respectively. In this study, there was a high proportion of patients who did not achieve adequate resolution of

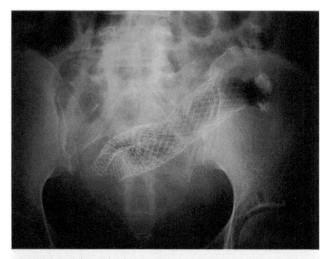

Fig. 29.8 Endoluminal colonic stent across an obstructing sigmoid cancer.

obstruction after colonic stenting, which led the investigators to terminate the study early.

In another study of colonic stenting for obstruction, van Hooft et al[97] used the global health status as the primary outcome measure. No differences in morbidity, mortality, and general health status were observed between the groups. Stoma formation rate was significantly higher in the emergency surgery group. However, the anastomotic leak rate was five times higher in the stent group compared with the emergency surgery group. Due to the considerably high morbidity observed in the stent group, the study was terminated.

Ho et al[98] undertook a trial and demonstrated a 40% reduction in morbidity following stenting as compared to emergency surgery. The success rate of colonic stenting was marginally higher than 50%, and the stoma rate was lower compared to the emergency surgery group. Overall morbidity rates were lower in the stented group, with the main differences seen in the frequency of urinary tract and abdominal wall infections. There was no significant difference in major complications requiring surgical revision between the two groups: 10% in the stent group and 11% in the emergency surgery group.

Iversen et al reported no significant difference in overall survival and no adverse oncologic consequences in patients who received colonic stenting as a bridge to surgery compared to those undergoing emergency surgery,[99] although others have described a higher rate of lymphatic invasion in bridge-to-surgery patients.[100]

Tan et al[101] conducted a meta-analysis and concluded that there were no significant differences between colonic stenting and emergency surgery, although the rate of stoma formation was significantly lower in the stent group. The postoperative mortality and complications, including anastomotic leak, were similar in both groups.

A systematic review and meta-analysis has been published including only multicenter randomized controlled trials (RCTs).[102] The clinical success rate for resolution of the obstruction was 52.5% in the stent group as compared to 99% in the emergency surgery group. Thirty-day postoperative morbidity was 48.4% in the stent group as compared to 51.0% in the emergency surgery group. Thirty-day mortality was similar between the two groups: 8.2% in the stent group and 9.0% in the emergency surgery group. Primary anastomosis was only achievable in 64.9% of patients in the stent group, compared with 55.0% in the emergency surgery group. The anastomotic leak rates were 9.0% in the stent group and 3.7% in the emergency group.

Recently, preliminary results from the largest multicenter, randomized controlled ColoRectal Stenting Trial (CReST) study have shown that stenting achieves relief of obstruction in 82% of patients with a significant reduction of stoma formation: 69% in the emergency surgery versus 45% with colonic stenting. A total of 246 patients from 39 units were randomized between 2009 and 2014 with 98% complying with allocated treatment. Ninety-two percent were treated with curative intent. The 30-day postoperative mortality was 5.3 and 4.4% in the stenting and emergency surgery groups, respectively.[103]

In a study from Belgium comprising 97 patients with tumor stenting as a bridge to surgery and subsequent surgical resection, patients were followed for 10 years.[104] Technical success in stent placement, performed by two experienced interventional gastroenterologists, was 95%. Stent migration occurred in

9%, and perforation in 14%. Survival rates at 1, 3, 5, and 10 years for stented patients were 96%, 66%, 55%, and 41%, respectively, all of which were numerically superior and statistically not different than overall colorectal cancer survival rates based on the Belgian Cancer Registry. The authors concluded that in patients with bowel obstruction from colorectal cancers that appear resectable for cure, colorectal stenting as a bridge to surgery might impair oncologic outcomes, particularly because of the risk for stent-induced complications such as perforation.

Open or Laparoscopic Resection

Laparoscopic surgery is technically difficult and often avoided in patients with bowel obstruction. Nevertheless, with increased experience and the development of new instruments, laparoscopic surgery can be performed in a proportion of patients with colonic obstruction.[105]

Palliative Patients

Endoluminal Stenting

Endoluminal stenting can be used for permanent palliation in patients with stenosis secondary to an unresectable colorectal cancer. The technical success rates for insertion of metallic stents range from 80 to 100% and symptomatic improvement occurs in more than 75% of patients.[106,107] Although most patients will achieve relief of symptoms, restenosis is common, usually by tumor ingrowth. If restenosis occurs, it can often be managed by inserting another stent or endoscopic dilatation. The tumor ingrowth might also be treated with laser ablation.[106,107,108]

Xinopoulos et al[109] reported a study of 30 patients with inoperable malignant obstruction who were randomized to either colonic stenting or defunctioning proximal stoma. There was no difference of costs between the two procedures. Stent insertion was successful in 93% of patients and resulted in a shorter length of hospital stay as well as better quality of life.

There are a few studies comparing survival in palliative patients who either had stents placed or palliative resectional surgery.[110] In patients with unresectable metastatic disease, various studies have shown shorter length of hospital stays, lower rates of stoma formation, and an earlier start of chemotherapy in the stent group.[111,112] However, Lee et al[111] and others[113] have shown better prognosis in patients who undergo resection of the primary tumor compared to those who are stented. The mean survival rate ranged from 15.9 to 23.7 months in the resection group, which was higher than the mean survival rate of 4.4 to 7.6 months in the stent group.

The design of studies investigating patients with unresectable metastatic disease is less than ideal because there is a lack of homogeneity in patient inclusion and treatments. Nevertheless, colonic stenting is a feasible option for many patients with reasonable outcomes in terms of efficacy and relief of symptoms.

Local Therapies

In a palliative setting, laser photocoagulation of colorectal malignancies has been suggested as an alternative to surgery. It can treat bleeding and relieve obstructive symptoms in stenosing lesions. It has also been used as an adjunct in patients who have colonic stenting and develop tumor ingrowth. Gevers et al[114] conducted a large retrospective study of 219 patients collected over a 9-year period and reported relief of symptoms in 198 (90.4%) patients. Repeated treatments were needed for obstructing and circumferential tumors. Five patients died from laser ablation.

Cryosurgery may also be useful as a palliative treatment in rectal cancer.[115] Local symptoms such as rectal bleeding and mucous discharge can be controlled in 62% of patients. Sixteen percent obtain moderate palliation and the remaining 22% have no improvement. It appears to be mainly useful in low rectal tumors, especially after the acute obstruction has been relieved.

Surgery

In patients with severe comorbidity that prevents surgical resection and patients with extensive malignant disease, an ileocolic or colocolic bypass can provide symptomatic relief. An alternative is a defunctioning loop ileostomy or loop colostomy. The decision to offer operative intervention should be tempered by the high risk of morbidity and mortality, although the use of laparoscopic techniques for stoma formation may help reduce these risks.

Special Situations

Colonic Volvulus

Plain X-rays will reveal a distended loop of colon that resembles a coffee bean or bent inner tire tube projecting toward the upper abdomen, sometimes above the transverse colon, described as the "northern exposure sign" (▶ Fig. 29.9).[116,117] Both contrast enema and CT imaging will be helpful in diagnosing a colonic volvulus (▶ Fig. 29.10). At the point of colonic torsion, a water-soluble contrast enema will demonstrate a smooth, tapered point of obstruction known as a "bird's beak."[116,117]

Sigmoid volvulus can usually be treated by untwisting of the volvulus using a flatus tube or endoscopically with a flexible sigmoidoscope or colonoscope. After successful detorsion of the sigmoid colon, a flatus tube should be left in place for 1 to 3 days to maintain the reduction and to allow continuing colonic decompression.[118] If this fails, a laparotomy may be necessary because of the risk of colonic ischemia and perforation (▶ Fig. 29.11). In cases of cecal volvulus, untwisting the torsion by colonoscopy is unpredictable and carries a high risk of complication. Hence, endoscopic reduction of cecal volvulus is generally not recommended.[119] Once the diagnosis has been made, an exploratory laparotomy should be considered (Chapter 28).

Sigmoid volvulus has a 90% recurrence rate when treated by decompression techniques and all patients should be considered for definitive surgery if they are physically fit because of the risk of perforation, which might be as high as 25 and 35%.[120] Sigmoid colectomy with primary anastomosis is the procedure of choice and prevents recurrent episodes of volvulus[118] in the presence of viable colon. Bowel preparation or on-table lavage is not necessary. Other procedures include Hartmann's procedure, a double-barreled stoma as the Paul-Mikulicz procedure, or a subtotal colectomy and ileosigmoid anastomosis. The type of procedure should be individualized and will depend on the overall condition of the patient and the viability of the remaining colon. Nonresectional procedures including detorsion alone, sigmoidoplasty and mesosigmoidoplasty are inferior to sigmoid colectomy for the prevention of recurrent volvulus. Nevertheless, for cecal volvulus, surgical options such as detorsion, cecopexy, cecostomy, and segmental resection of the colon may be a suitable alternative to resection.[119]

If the patient is unfit for resectional surgery or general anesthesia, fixation of the involved sigmoid colon by percutaneous endoscopic sigmoidopexy has been advocated as a less invasive option. However, before this is performed, the sigmoid loop must

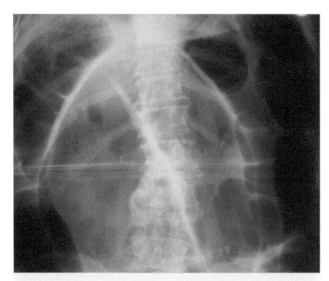

Fig. 29.9 Abdominal X-ray demonstrating a sigmoid volvulus with the distended sigmoid loop projecting toward the upper abdomen.

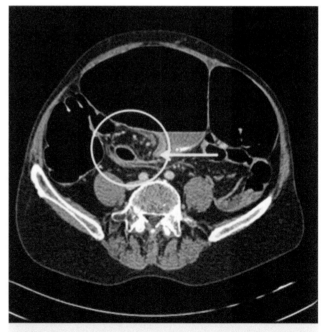

Fig. 29.10 CT scan showing a sigmoid volvulus with the classical "whirl sign" (*yellow circle and arrow*).

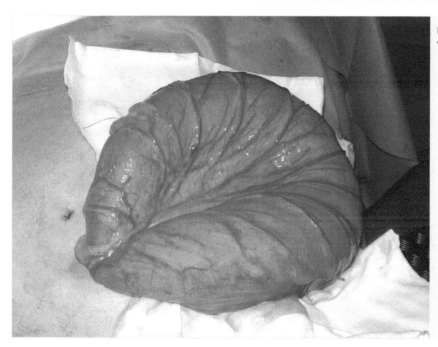

Fig. 29.11 Operative photograph of sigmoid volvulus.

be decompressed and untwisted. The redundant bowel is then triangulated and fixed using two or three percutaneous endoscopic gastrostomy (PEG) tubes or abdominal wall fixation devices.[121]

29.3 Nonmechanical Obstruction (Intestinal Pseudo-obstruction)

Nonmechanical obstruction or intestinal pseudo-obstruction is defined as a clinical syndrome characterized by the disturbance of intestinal propulsion, which may mirror an intestinal obstruction with no apparent mechanical cause. It presents in acute, subacute, or chronic forms. Both large and small bowels can be involved. The precise underlying pathophysiological mechanisms are unclear. By definition, it includes a wide range of conditions, ranging from simple constipation to more severe and complicated forms such as chronic intestinal pseudo-obstruction (CIPO).[122]

29.3.1 Acute Intestinal Pseudo-obstruction (Ogilvie's Syndrome)

In 1944, Ogilvie[123] first described acute pseudo-obstruction of the colon, a condition in which the colon becomes massively dilated in the absence of a mechanical obstruction. It is commonly seen in critically ill medical or surgical patients. This condition has received many terminologies such as ileus,[124] colonic ileus,[125] and acute colonic pseudo-obstruction. Unfortunately, these terms have been used interchangeably and have led to confusion. Ileus refers to motor inactivity, whereas intestinal pseudo-obstruction suggests uncoordinated contractions with inhibited propulsion. The mechanism of intestinal pseudo-obstruction is not clear; many believe that it is related to sacral parasympathetic nerve dysfunction.[126,127,128] There is an assumption that the normal parasympathetic outflows from sacral segments 2, 3, and 4 are disturbed,

which will cause functional obstruction. In fact, an acute pseudo-obstruction of the colon is a form of ileus that usually starts in the distal transverse colon. The impaired distal part of the colon is collapsed and contains minimal air, while the proximal colon is functionally normal. This is different from generalized ileus in which the small bowel, the colon, and the rectum are distended and dilated with air. The pathophysiology of acute pseudo-obstruction is currently thought to involve the following:

1. A noxious stimulus affects the splanchnic afferents and inhibits the reflex motor response.
2. Both the sympathetic and parasympathetic motor inputs are stimulated excessively, causing lack of contraction and relaxation of the bowel.
3. Nitric oxide release from inhibitory neurons decreases relaxation of the bowel.
4. The situation is exacerbated by either endogenous or exogenous opioids, which cause excess stimulation of peripheral μ-opioid receptors.[122]

Ogilvie proposed that disruption of the sympathetic supply to the bowel with unopposed parasympathetic innervation resulted in "enterospasm" and dilation of the colon.[123] Almost 20 years later, Catchpole suggested that an increase in sympathetic input to the bowel was the main mechanism for ileus after surgical insult.[124] He tested his hypothesis by using guanethidine, a sympathetic blocking agent, followed by neostigmine, an inhibitor of acetyl cholinesterase enzyme. His experiments concluded that the main cause of ileus was the domination of the sympathetic nervous influence on the bowel. Subsequently, other studies have provided similar evidence to support this finding.[129]

There are many conditions that can cause acute pseudo-obstruction of the colon (▶ Table 29.2). It is commonly seen in male patients who are older than 60 years. Most of them are suffering from a severe illness needing hospitalization. About 3 to 15% of patients will suffer the risk of spontaneous cecal perforation in acute colonic pseudo-obstruction, with a mortality of 50%.[130] Local stimuli activate the inhibitory reflex through

Table 29.2 Etiology of acute pseudo-obstruction of the large bowel

Causes of acute colonic pseudo-obstruction

1. Surgical
   a) Intra-abdominal sepsis
   b) Abdominal and pelvic surgery
   c) Organ transplantation
   d) Thoracic and cardiovascular surgery
   e) Trauma and fractures
   f) Burns
   g) Craniotomy
   h) Caesarean section and hysterectomy; complications of pregnancy and normal pregnancy
2. Medical
   a) All malignancies
   b) Cardiopulmonary causes such as pneumonia, myocardial infarction (MI), heart failure, and congestive obstructive pulmonary disease (COPD)
   c) Metabolic disturbance
   d) Parkinson's disease, multiple sclerosis, and dementia
   e) Organ failure
   f) Alcoholism
   g) Medication such as narcotics, anticholinergics, anti-Parkinsonian, laxative abuse

Table 29.3 Causes of secondary chronic intestinal pseudo-obstruction

Autoimmune disease	Scleroderma, dermatomyositis, lupus, mixed connective tissue disorder, and rheumatoid arthritis
Endocrine disorders	Diabetes, hypothyroidism, hypoparathyroidism, pheochromocytoma
Neurological disorders	Stroke, encephalitis, calcification of basal ganglia, paraneoplastic syndrome secondary to central nervous system neoplasm, bronchial carcinoid and leiomyosarcomas, Parkinson's disease, multiple system atrophy, Hirschsprung's disease, and von Recklinghausen's disease
Muscular disorder	Myotonic dystrophy, systemic sclerosis, desmin myopathy, Duchenne's muscular dystrophy or myotonic dystrophy
Infection	Chagas' disease, Epstein–Barr virus, or cytomegalovirus
Drugs	Clonidine, phenothiazines, antidepressants, anti-Parkinsonians, antineoplastics, bronchodilators, anthraquinones
Other	Ehlers–Danlos, jejunal diverticulosis, amyloidosis, celiac disease, mitochondrial neuro-gastrointestinal encephalopathy (MNGIE), and radiation enteritis

the splanchnic nerves that will cause ileus. The splanchnic nerves provide both afferent and efferent pathways.[131] Handling the bowel at operation will cause an increase in inflammatory mediators, such as intercellular adhesion molecule-1 (ICAM-1), monocyte chemoattractant protein 1 (MCP-1), inducible nitric oxide synthase (iNOS), and cyclooxygenase-2 (COX-2) messenger ribonucleic acid (mRNA). There will also be massive monocyte infiltration into the bowel wall.[132] The severity of postoperative ileus correlates with the degree of intestinal inflammatory response.[133,134] Several studies[134,135] have shown that the increased and frequent use of opioids for the treatment of postoperative pain can increase the inflammatory response to surgery and, thus, worsen the "normal" postoperative ileus, which might then induce acute intestinal pseudo-obstruction.

29.3.2 Chronic Intestinal Pseudo-obstruction

CIPO is a rare disorder that is due to possibly three mechanisms: (1) an underlying neuropathic disorder (involving the enteric or extrinsic nervous system), (2) a myopathic disorder (involving the smooth muscle), or (3) a disturbance to the interstitial cells of Cajal (ICC). Not surprisingly, there are parallels in the mechanisms of CIPO and gastroparesis. CIPO also affects the young and pediatric population and accounts for about 20% of all adult chronic intestinal failure.[136]

Many CIPO cases are idiopathic.[137] They usually present sporadically; however, there are familial forms that are inherited as an autosomal dominant, autosomal recessive, or X-linked recessive.[138] The remainder are secondary to various diseases documented in ▶ Table 29.3. Most adult cases of CIPO are sporadic and secondary, while most childhood cases are primary and sporadic.

More than one factor of the neuromuscular apparatus of the bowel can be affected in certain diseases. For example, in scleroderma there will be an intrinsic neuropathic phase before the

involvement of smooth muscle causing myopathy. Similarly, in mitochondrial cytopathy and amyloidosis, neuropathy initially occurs, followed by myopathy. In diabetes, both the extrinsic nerves and the ICC are affected.

Prognosis is exceptionally poor in children with the mortality rate in the first year of life for congenital CIPO reaching 10 to 25%.[139] In adults, the mortality rate is about 20 to 30% after 10 years of disease duration.[140] Many patients will eventually need long-term home parenteral nutrition (HPN) as malnourishment occurs in 80% of children[139] and in one-third of adults.

Any part of the gastrointestinal tract can be affected, but the symptoms are worse if the small bowel is affected by CIPO.[141] Patients with CIPO have a similar presentation to those with acute intestinal pseudo-obstruction. One cross-sectional study of 20 patients with CIPO has shown that the median age at onset of symptoms is 17 years, with a wide range from 2 weeks to 59 years.[142] This emphasizes that the CIPO population is diverse, which is in contrast to patients who suffer from acute intestinal pseudo-obstruction in which most patients are infirm.

A study carried out by St. Mark's Hospital[142] has shown that abdominal pain occurs in 80% of patients, vomiting in 75%, constipation in 40%, and diarrhea in 20%. Between each episode, the patient may be completely asymptomatic, though such episodes are rare. Typically, patients suffer a protracted clinical course, which includes chronic nausea, vomiting, weight loss, diffuse abdominal pain with distension and constipation. Diarrhea or steatorrhea can be associated with bacterial overgrowth. Upper gastrointestinal symptoms, such as dysphagia, are occasionally reported. All these symptoms imply delayed transit in the proximal and distal intestine.[136,143] In time, symptoms and signs of malnutrition and malabsorption will become apparent as the disease becomes more advanced. This is made worse by the fact that oral intake is likely to worsen digestive symptoms. Hence, patients tend to avoid eating altogether.

When encountering patients who might have CIPO, diagnosis is essentially one of exclusion after patients have undergone extensive investigations, trials of prokinetic agents, and even surgical interventions. If CIPO is suspected, various basic laboratory tests are required to exclude secondary causes, including full blood count, serum electrolytes, glucose, calcium, magnesium, phosphorus, serum albumin, thyroid function tests, coagulation, and inflammatory markers (i.e., erythrocyte sedimentation rate and C-reactive protein). In addition, there are specialized tests that may help in diagnosing the specific cause of CIPO, such as fasting cortisol, antinuclear antibody, anti–double-stranded DNA and SCL-70 panel for scleroderma or systemic sclerosis. For the diagnosis of paraneoplastic syndrome, serum anti-Hu can be calculated.[144]

Small bowel manometry can also help in diagnosing CIPO because the pressure profiles are different in mechanical obstruction compared to functional obstruction. It is also helpful in differentiating dysmotility of myogenic origin from neurogenic origin. However, this investigation is not readily available and the findings have low specificity. Thus, it should only be considered as a diagnostic adjunct especially in patients who have no diagnosis with frequent presentations.[141] Patients with colonic involvement usually present with delayed colonic transit. Anorectal physiology tests may show loss of sensation, absence of a rectoanal inhibitory reflex, and a decrease in resting tone and squeeze pressure.

Full-thickness intestinal biopsy has lost popularity as it often does not aid diagnosis and is an invasive procedure. In primary myopathic disorders, biopsies will show smooth muscle atrophy, whereas in primary neuropathic disorders there will be evidence of neuropathic degeneration. In addition, biopsies can show evidence of amyloid, lymphoma, or even fibrosis, which is seen predominantly in primary systemic sclerosis.[145] Lately, there have been advancements in histopathology and molecular testing, as well as a wider role for laparoscopic surgery, which are improving the accuracy of diagnosing CIPO. It has been recommended that patients who suffer from severe derangements of gut dysmotility of unknown origin, and who are unresponsive to medical therapy, should be offered invasive investigations.[138,142]

29.3.3 Management

Acute Pseudo-obstruction

Acute pseudo-obstruction of the colon is a self-limited condition if the underlying cause is eliminated. However, waiting for the condition to spontaneously resolve is not recommended because the colonic dilatation can persist. Air in the distended colon is swallowed air; therefore, the first step in the management is placement of a nasogastric tube. All exacerbating medications, especially opiates, should be discontinued and fluid and electrolyte disorders corrected. The main goal of treatment is to prevent cecal perforation. It is generally accepted that the critical size of the cecum is 12 cm.[128]

Treatment with colonoscopy decompression is effective in 85 to 88% of cases with a low morbidity rate[127,128,146] but should be undertaken by an experienced endoscopist. Colonoscopy in acute pseudo-obstruction has a reported perforation rate of 1 to 3%.[147] It is performed without bowel preparation and with minimal air insufflation. The goal of colonoscopy is to intubate the right colon and place a decompression tube while removing as much gas as possible on withdrawal. Repeating the procedure may be necessary because of recurrence.[128,146] Tsirline et al[148] reported retrospective data on 100 patients over a 10-year period and concluded that colonoscopic decompression is superior to neostigmine, both after one intervention (75.0 vs. 35.5%; $p = 0.0002$) and two interventions (84.6 vs. 55.6%; $p = 0.0031$). Currently, with more experience in endoscopic techniques, it is suggested that colonoscopic decompression is comparable to neostigmine infusion or subcutaneous neostigmine as first-line therapy after failed conservative measures.

Prokinetic drugs such as erythromycin,[149] metoclopramide,[150] and cisapride have all shown variable and unpredictable efficacy. Cisapride was found to cause cardiac arrhythmias and was withdrawn from use in 2000.[151] Recently, there is growing interest in μ-opioid-receptor antagonists such as methylnaltrexone[152] and alvimopan,[153] given the association between acute pseudo-obstruction and opiate use. A case study has reported that methylnaltrexone is effective in relieving acute pseudo-obstruction in a patient who was on opioid therapy.[152] A double-blinded study of 133 patients has also demonstrated efficacy of methylnaltrexone in the treatment of opioid-induced constipation.[154] The peripherally acting alvimopan has been shown to be effective in postoperative ileus,[153] but there are no studies to demonstrate whether it has any influence on acute pseudo-obstruction. Hence, further studies are needed to clarify the issues of safety and efficacy of drugs explicitly for acute pseudo-obstruction.[155,156,157,158]

Neostigmine has been used with impressive results and has been advocated as first-line treatment. Neostigmine is a parasympathomimetic drug used in a dose of 2.0 to 2.5 mg given intravenously over 3 minutes.[130,159] The response is usually within minutes. Severe abdominal cramps may be followed by the passage of a large amount of gas. The procedure should be performed with close monitoring due to cardiac arrhythmias and hypotension. Atropine should be readily available in the event of severe bradycardia. Neostigmine should not be given to patients who have been on beta-blockers and those who are acidotic or have had a recent myocardial infarction. Patients who suffer from renal insufficiency and bronchospasm are also contraindicated. Prolonged, recurrent acute pseudo-obstruction in the colon may signify intra-abdominal complications such as abscess or peritonitis, in which case further investigations are indicated.

Ponec et al[155] conducted a small, prospective, randomized trial to evaluate the success rate of neostigmine in patients with acute pseudo-obstruction of the colon. The study involved 21 patients, all with abdominal distension and radiographic evidence of colonic dilatation, with a cecal diameter of at least 10 cm, and no response to at least 24 hours of conservative treatment. Patients were randomly assigned to receive 2.0 mg of neostigmine intravenously ($n = 11$) or intravenous saline ($n = 10$). Ten of the 11 patients who received neostigmine had prompt colonic decompression as compared with none of the 10 patients who received placebo ($p < 0.001$). The median time to response was 4 minutes (range: 3–30 min). Side effects to neostigmine include abdominal pain, excess salivation, and vomiting. Symptomatic bradycardia developed in two patients, requiring treatment with atropine.

Before treating a patient with neostigmine, it is important to rule out a mechanical obstruction. If there is any doubt, Gastrografin enema or CT scan should be performed. Gastrografin may result in therapeutic success.[156] If neostigmine and/or colonoscopic decompression fail, a prospective, randomized, placebo-controlled trial involving 25 patients has shown that oral polyethylene glycol (PEG) solution can prevent relapse; no patients receiving PEG had recurrence of symptoms compared to 33% in the placebo group.[157] Recently, another drug, pyridostigmine (a long-acting acetyl cholinesterase inhibitor) has been shown to relieve symptoms in seven patients who suffer from recurrent pseudo-obstruction.[158]

If the cecum is 12 cm or larger and nonoperative treatments are not successful, a tube cecostomy may be considered. The traditional use of a bladder catheter is not effective because of its very small lumen. Using an endotracheal tube is a better technique.[156] A transverse colostomy is seldom necessary. A colectomy is indicated only when there is impending colonic ischemia or perforation. In this situation, operative options are dependent upon the length and section of colon involved. A laparoscopic tube cecostomy can also be performed.[159]

Chronic Pseudo-obstruction

When a patient presents with chronic pseudo-obstruction, conservative management is similar to that employed in acute pseudo-obstruction. Once chronic pseudo-obstruction is diagnosed (often after many years), treatment consists of nutritional, pharmacological, and surgical interventions. The main aims include maximizing nutrition, restoring gut motility, and decreasing complications due to bacterial stasis. In secondary CIPO, the underlying cause should be identified and treated.

A formal nutrition evaluation with an experienced dietician is needed for patients with CIPO. Overall, oral intake should be maximized as tolerated. Any nutrition deficiencies should be corrected and patients advised to take small and frequent meals (5–6 per day). Foods high in fat and fiber should be avoided, whereas liquid calories and protein should be increased. Nutrition supplements can be used as an adjunct especially in patients who are malnourished. The ability to maintain oral intake is an independent predictor of survival in patients with CIPO.[140]

Enteral feeding should be considered only if oral intake is inadequate to sustain nutrition requirements. Scolapio et al[160] have conducted a retrospective study that demonstrated that patients with CIPO can successfully maintain their nutrition requirement with tube feeds using a standard nonelemental formula. Permanent enteral access can be secured by either nasogastric or nasojejunal feeding without significant discomfort. If there is delayed gastric emptying, then the stomach can be bypassed with permanent enteral access into the small intestine. Large bolus feeding is usually less well tolerated than continuous feeding or cyclical feeding (12 hours of continuous feeding during the night). HPN is given as a last resort unless enteral intake is inadequate, because HPN is associated with complications, including cellulitis, sepsis, thrombus formation,

nonalcoholic fatty liver disease, and pancreatitis.[140] Nevertheless, most patients with CIPO will eventually require HPN given the progressive nature of the disease. Even when receiving HPN, patients should be encouraged to maximize and continue with oral intake as tolerated.[140]

Nasogastric suction, rectal tubes, or endoscopy are sometimes used to decompress distended intestinal segments and can be useful in controlling symptoms in some patients. Occasionally, a venting enterostomy is placed for decompression of a distended intestinal segment. These are typically secured in the stomach, although there are some cases where feeding J-tubes are used.[161] A surgically placed gastrostomy tube can decrease hospital admissions, from 1.2 to 0.2 admissions per patient-year.[162] However, there are no studies or guidance to advise on when these interventions should be undertaken.

All patients with CIPO have some form of deranged gastrointestinal tract motility regardless of whether the underlying cause is myopathic or neuropathic in nature. There are many prokinetic drugs that have been used to normalize gut motility. Unfortunately, few studies are available to prove adequate efficacy of these drugs in patients with CIPO. Patients with CIPO tend to have bouts of nausea and vomiting during an episode of pseudo-obstruction and these symptoms can occur on a near daily basis, but no single drug has been found to consistently control symptoms.

Bacterial overgrowth and diarrhea can result from intestinal stasis, and if not treated adequately can lead to malabsorption, weight loss, and multiple vitamin deficiencies. To treat symptoms of diarrhea and bacterial overgrowth, rotating antibiotics may provide a way forward to improve nutrition in many patients with CIPO. Currently, there are no controlled trials to determine which antibiotics work best; however, patients can be prescribed a different antibiotic every month for the duration of about 1 week over a 5- to 6-month cycle.[163]

Abdominal pain is the most common symptom in patients with CIPO.[136,142] Most patients will eventually turn to opiates for pain relief. Unfortunately, there are not many medications that can provide adequate relief in CIPO. In placebo-controlled trials, prucalopride[164] and somatostatin[165] have both demonstrated substantial benefit in reducing pain. Tricyclic antidepressants and serotonin–norepinephrine reuptake inhibitors have been used, but may cause side effects from constipation and drowsiness. Hence, it is advisable to start on a low dose and titrate up as necessary. Another drug that is commonly prescribed is tramadol, a μ-opioid receptor agonist, which is known to be less constipating than opiates. If opiates are prescribed, clinicians should be aware of their constipating side effects and the development of drug tolerance if taken long term. A study involving children with idiopathic CIPO evaluated the efficacy of transdermal buprenorphine, a partial agonist at the μ-opioid receptor and an antagonist at the κ- and δ-opioid receptors. Relief was sustained in 75% of children and none required a higher dose.[166]

Small bowel transplantation is recognized as a possible option in patients with severe CIPO suffering with life-threatening HPN complications.[167] About 9% of total small bowel transplants are patients with CIPO, both adults and children. In current United Network for Organ Sharing data, the 1- and 5-year survival rates for children who receive small bowel transplant for functional disorders are 75 and 57%, respectively.[168]

References

[1] Buechter KJ, Boustany C, Caillouette R, Cohn I, Jr. Surgical management of the acutely obstructed colon. A review of 127 cases. Am J Surg. 1988; 156(3, Pt 1):163–168

[2] Sule AZ, Ajibade A. Adult large bowel obstruction: a review of clinical experience. Ann Afr Med. 2011; 10(1):45–50

[3] Serpell JW, McDermott FT, Katrivessis H, Hughes ESR. Obstructing carcinomas of the colon. Br J Surg. 1989; 76(9):965–969

[4] Phillips RKS, Hittinger R, Fry JS, Fielding LP. Malignant large bowel obstruction. Br J Surg. 1985; 72(4):296–302

[5] Kyllönen LE. Obstruction and perforation complicating colorectal carcinoma. An epidemiologic and clinical study with special reference to incidence and survival. Acta Chir Scand. 1987; 153(10):607–614

[6] Taourel P, Kessler N, Lesnik A, Pujol J, Morcos L, Bruel JM. Helical CT of large bowel obstruction. Abdom Imaging. 2003; 28(2):267–275

[7] Welsh J. Bowel Obstruction: Differential Diagnosis and Clinical Management. Philadelphia, PA: Saunders; 1989

[8] Gore R, Levine M. Textbook of Gastrointestinal Radiology. 3rd ed. Philadelphia, PA: Saunders and Elsevier; 2008

[9] Cirocchi R, Farinella E, La Mura F, et al. The sigmoid volvulus: surgical timing and mortality for different clinical types. World J Emerg Surg. 2010; 5:1

[10] Peterson CM, Anderson JS, Hara AK, Carenza JW, Menias CO. Volvulus of the gastrointestinal tract: appearances at multimodality imaging. Radiographics. 2009; 29(5):1281–1293

[11] Law WL, Lo CY, Chu KW. Emergency surgery for colonic diverticulitis: differences between right-sided and left-sided lesions. Int J Colorectal Dis. 2001; 16(5):280–284

[12] Sai VF, Velayos F, Neuhaus J, Westphalen AC. Colonoscopy after CT diagnosis of diverticulitis to exclude colon cancer: a systematic literature review. Radiology. 2012; 263(2):383–390

[13] Martin LC, Merkle EM, Thompson WM. Review of internal hernias: radiographic and clinical findings. AJR Am J Roentgenol. 2006; 186(3):703–717

[14] Berg DF, Bahadursingh AM, Kaminski DL, Longo WE. Acute surgical emergencies in inflammatory bowel disease. Am J Surg. 2002; 184(1):45–51

[15] Swaminath A, Lichtiger S. Dilation of colonic strictures by intralesional injection of infliximab in patients with Crohn's colitis. Inflamm Bowel Dis. 2008; 14(2):213–216

[16] Laukoetter MG, Mennigen R, Hannig CM, et al. Intestinal cancer risk in Crohn's disease: a meta-analysis. J Gastrointest Surg. 2011; 15(4):576–583

[17] Stewart RB, Moore MT, Marks RG, Hale WE. Correlates of constipation in an ambulatory elderly population. Am J Gastroenterol. 1992; 87(7):859–864

[18] Bar-Ziv J, Solomon A. Computed tomography in adult intussusception. Gastrointest Radiol. 1991; 16(3):264–266

[19] Horton KM, Fishman EK. MDCT and 3D imaging in transient enteroenteric intussusception: clinical observations and review of the literature. AJR Am J Roentgenol. 2008; 191(3):736–742

[20] Azar T, Berger DL. Adult intussusception. Ann Surg. 1997; 226(2):134–138

[21] Begos DG, Sandor A, Modlin IM. The diagnosis and management of adult intussusception. Am J Surg. 1997; 173(2):88–94

[22] Gayer G, Zissin R, Apter S, Papa M, Hertz M. Pictorial review: adult intussusception–a CT diagnosis. Br J Radiol. 2002; 75(890):185–190

[23] Kim YH, Blake MA, Harisinghani MG, et al. Adult intestinal intussusception: CT appearances and identification of a causative lead point. Radiographics. 2006; 26(3):733–744

[24] Duncan JE, DeNobile JW, Sweeney WB. Colonoscopic diagnosis of appendiceal intussusception: case report and review of the literature. JSLS. 2005; 9(4):488–490

[25] Laalim SA, Toughai I, Benjelloun B, Majdoub KH, Mazaz K. Appendiceal intussusception to the cecum caused by mucocele of the appendix: laparoscopic approach. Int J Surg Case Rep. 2012; 3(9):445–447

[26] Yamada H, Morita T, Fujita M, Miyasaka Y, Senmaru N, Oshikiri T. Adult intussusception due to enteric neoplasms. Dig Dis Sci. 2007; 52(3):764–766

[27] Box JC, Tucker J, Watne AL, Lucas G. Eosinophilic colitis presenting as a left-sided colocolonic intussusception with secondary large bowel obstruction: an uncommon entity with a rare presentation. Am Surg. 1997; 63(8):741–743

[28] Ikuhara M, Tsang TK, Tosiou A, White EM, Buto SK, Meyer KC. Intussusception in an adult with pseudomembranous colitis. J Clin Gastroenterol. 1995; 21(4):336–338

[29] Debenham GP. Ulcer of the cecum during oxyphenbutazone (Tandearil) therapy. Can Med Assoc J. 1966; 94(22):1182–1184

[30] Lang J, Price AB, Levi AJ, Burke M, Gumpel JM, Bjarnason I. Diaphragm disease: pathology of disease of the small intestine induced by non-steroidal anti-inflammatory drugs. J Clin Pathol. 1988; 41(5):516–526

[31] Bjarnason I, Hayllar J, MacPherson AJ, Russell AS. Side effects of nonsteroidal anti-inflammatory drugs on the small and large intestine in humans. Gastroenterology. 1993; 104(6):1832–1847

[32] Gargot D, Chaussade S, d'Alteroche L, et al. Nonsteroidal anti-inflammatory drug-induced colonic strictures: two cases and literature review. Am J Gastroenterol. 1995; 90(11):2035–2038

[33] Ribeiro A, Wolfsen HC, Wolfe JT, III, Loeb DS. Colonic strictures induced by nonsteroidal anti-inflammatory drugs. South Med J. 1998; 91(6):568–572

[34] Israel LH, Koea JB, Stewart ID, Wright CL, Frankish PD. Nonsteroidal anti-inflammatory drug-induced strictures of the colon: report of a case and review of the literature. Dis Colon Rectum. 2001; 44(9):1362–1364

[35] Monahan DW, Starnes EC, Parker AL. Colonic strictures in a patient on long-term non-steroidal anti-inflammatory drugs. Gastrointest Endosc. 1992; 38(3):385–388

[36] Halter F, Weber B, Huber T, Eigenmann F, Frey MP, Ruchti C. Diaphragm disease of the ascending colon. Association with sustained-release diclofenac. J Clin Gastroenterol. 1993; 16(1):74–80

[37] Whitcomb DC, Martin SP, Trellis DR, Evans BA, Becich MJ. 'Diaphragmlike' stricture and ulcer of the colon during diclofenac treatment. Arch Intern Med. 1992; 152(11):2341–2343

[38] Byrne MF, McGuinness J, Smyth CM, et al. Nonsteroidal anti-inflammatory drug-induced diaphragms and ulceration in the colon. Eur J Gastroenterol Hepatol. 2002; 14(11):1265–1269

[39] Hakeem A, Subramonia S, Badrinath K, Menon A. NSAIDs-induced diaphragm-like colonic strictures: a case report. BMJ Case Rep. 2009; 2009: bcr02.2009.1595

[40] Weinstock LB, Hammoud Z, Brandwin L. Nonsteroidal anti-inflammatory drug-induced colonic stricture and ulceration treated with balloon dilation and prednisone. Gastrointest Endosc. 1999; 50(4):564–566

[41] Penner RM, Williams CN. Resolution of multiple severe nonsteroidal anti-inflammatory drug-induced colonic strictures with prednisone therapy: a case report and review of the literature. Can J Gastroenterol. 2003; 17(8):497–500

[42] Smith JA, Pineau BC. Endoscopic therapy of NSAID-induced colonic diaphragm disease: two cases and a review of published reports. Gastrointest Endosc. 2000; 52(1):120–125

[43] Jarmin R, Idris MA, Shaharuddin S, Nadeson S, Rashid LM, Mustaffa WM. Intestinal obstruction due to rectal endometriosis: a surgical enigma. Asian J Surg. 2006; 29(3):149–152

[44] de Jong MJ, Mijatovic V, van Waesberghe JH, Cuesta MA, Hompes PG. Surgical outcome and long-term follow-up after segmental colorectal resection in women with a complete obstruction of the rectosigmoid due to endometriosis. Dig Surg. 2009; 26(1):50–55

[45] Nasim H, Sikafi D, Nasr A. Sigmoid endometriosis and a diagnostic dilemma - A case report and literature review. Int J Surg Case Rep. 2011; 2(7):181–184

[46] Katsikogiannis N, Tsaroucha A, Dimakis K, Sivridis E, Simopoulos C. Rectal endometriosis causing colonic obstruction and concurrent endometriosis of the appendix: a case report. J Med Case Reports. 2011; 5:320

[47] Pramateftakis MG, Psomas S, Kanellos D, et al. Large bowel obstruction due to endometriosis. Tech Coloproctol. 2010; 14 Suppl 1:S87–S89

[48] Bidarmaghz B, Shekhar A, Hendahewa R. Sigmoid endometriosis in a postmenopausal woman leading to acute large bowel obstruction: a case report. Int J Surg Case Rep. 2016; 28:65–67

[49] Brodey PA, Schuldt DR, Magnuson A, Esterkyn S. Complete colonic obstruction secondary to adhesions. AJR Am J Roentgenol. 1979; 133(5):917–918

[50] Holt RW, Wagner RC. Adhesional obstruction of the colon. Dis Colon Rectum. 1984; 27(5):314–315

[51] Hilzenrat N, Spanier A, Lamoureux E, Bloom C, Sherker A. Colonic obstruction secondary to sarcoidosis: nonsurgical diagnosis and management. Gastroenterology. 1995; 108(5):1556–1559

[52] Harris N, McNeely W, Shepord J, Ebeling S. Case record of the Massachusetts General Hospital. Weekly clinicopathological exercises. Case 26-2002. An 87-year-old woman with abdominal pain, vomiting, bloody diarrhea, and an abdominal mass. N Engl J Med. 2002; 347(8):601–606

[53] Gan SI, Beck PL. A new look at toxic megacolon: an update and review of incidence, etiology, pathogenesis, and management. Am J Gastroenterol. 2003; 98(11):2363–2371

[54] Jalan KN, Sircus W, Card WI, et al. An experience of ulcerative colitis. I. Toxic dilation in 55 cases. Gastroenterology. 1969; 57(1):68–82

[55] Sharma S, Milsom J. The evolution of surgery for the treatment of malignant large bowel obstruction. Tech Gastrointest Endosc. 2014; 16:112–118

[56] Stewart J, Finan PJ, Courtney DF, Brennan TG. Does a water soluble contrast enema assist in the management of acute large bowel obstruction: a prospective study of 117 cases. Br J Surg. 1984; 71(10):799–801

[57] Finan PJ, Campbell S, Verma R, et al. The management of malignant large bowel obstruction: ACPGBI position statement. Colorectal Dis. 2007; 9 Suppl 4:1–17

[58] Gainant A. Emergency management of acute colonic cancer obstruction. J Visc Surg. 2012; 149(1):e3–e10

[59] Frager D, Rovno HD, Baer JW, Bashist B, Friedman M. Prospective evaluation of colonic obstruction with computed tomography. Abdom Imaging. 1998; 23(2):141–146

[60] Jaffe T, Thompson WM. Large-bowel obstruction in the adult: classic radiographic and CT findings, etiology, and mimics. Radiology. 2015; 275(3):651–663

[61] Godfrey EM, Addley HC, Shaw AS. The use of computed tomography in the detection and characterisation of large bowel obstruction. N Z Med J. 2009; 122(1305):57–73

[62] Soressa U, Mamo A, Hiko D, Fentahun N. Prevalence, causes and management outcome of intestinal obstruction in Adama Hospital, Ethiopia. BMC Surg. 2016; 16(1):38

[63] Tekkis PP, Kinsman R, Thompson MR, Stamatakis JD, Association of Coloproctology of Great Britain, Ireland. The Association of Coloproctology of Great Britain and Ireland study of large bowel obstruction caused by colorectal cancer. Ann Surg. 2004; 240(1):76–81

[64] Alves A, Panis Y, Mathieu P, Mantion G, Kwiatkowski F, Slim K, Association Française de Chirurgie. Postoperative mortality and morbidity in French patients undergoing colorectal surgery: results of a prospective multicenter study. Arch Surg. 2005; 140(3):278–283, discussion 284

[65] Paulson EC, Mahmoud NN, Wirtalla C, Armstrong K. Acuity and survival in colon cancer surgery. Dis Colon Rectum. 2010; 53(4):385–392

[66] Biondo S, Parés D, Frago R, et al. Large bowel obstruction: predictive factors for postoperative mortality. Dis Colon Rectum. 2004; 47(11):1889–1897

[67] Frago R, Biondo S, Millan M, et al. Differences between proximal and distal obstructing colonic cancer after curative surgery. Colorectal Dis. 2011; 13(6):e116–e122

[68] Ansaloni L, Andersson RE, Bazzoli F, et al. Guidelines in the management of obstructing cancer of the left colon: consensus conference of the world society of emergency surgery (WSES) and peritoneum and surgery (PnS) society. World J Emerg Surg. 2010; 5:29

[69] Breitenstein S, Rickenbacher A, Berdajs D, Puhan M, Clavien PA, Demartines N. Systematic evaluation of surgical strategies for acute malignant left-sided colonic obstruction. Br J Surg. 2007; 94(12):1451–1460

[70] Trompetas V. Emergency management of malignant acute left-sided colonic obstruction. Ann R Coll Surg Engl. 2008; 90(3):181–186

[71] De Salvo GL, Gava C, Pucciarelli S, Lise M. Curative surgery for obstruction from primary left colorectal carcinoma: primary or staged resection? Cochrane Database Syst Rev. 2002(1):CD002101

[72] Kronborg O. Acute obstruction from tumour in the left colon without spread. A randomized trial of emergency colostomy versus resection. Int J Colorectal Dis. 1995; 10(1):1–5

[73] Sjödahl R, Franzén T, Nyström PO. Primary versus staged resection for acute obstructing colorectal carcinoma. Br J Surg. 1992; 79(7):685–688

[74] Kressner U, Antonsson J, Ejerblad S, Gerdin B, Påhlman L. Intraoperative colonic lavage and primary anastomosis–an alternative to Hartmann procedure in emergency surgery of the left colon. Eur J Surg. 1994; 160(5):287–292

[75] Zorcolo L, Covotta L, Carlomagno N, Bartolo DC. Safety of primary anastomosis in emergency colo-rectal surgery. Colorectal Dis. 2003; 5(3):262–269

[76] Meyer F, Marusch F, Koch A, et al. German Study Group "Colorectal Carcinoma (Primary Tumor)". Emergency operation in carcinomas of the left colon: value of Hartmann's procedure. Tech Coloproctol. 2004; 8 Suppl 1: s226–s229

[77] Isbister WH, Prasad J. Hartmann's operation: a personal experience. Aust N Z J Surg. 1995; 65(2):98–100

[78] Kristiansen VB, Lausen IM, Frederiksen HJ, Kjaergaard J. [Hartmann's procedure in the treatment of acute obstructive left-sided colonic cancer]. Ugeskr Laeger. 1993; 155(47):3816–3818

[79] Biondo S, Kreisler E, Millan M, et al. Impact of surgical specialization on emergency colorectal surgery outcomes. Arch Surg. 2010; 145(1):79–86

[80] Schrock TR, Deveney CW, Dunphy JE. Factor contributing to leakage of colonic anastomoses. Ann Surg. 1973; 177(5):513–518

[81] Smith SR, Connolly JC, Gilmore OJ. The effect of faecal loading on colonic anastomotic healing. Br J Surg. 1983; 70(1):49–50

[82] Muir EG. Safety in colinic resection. Proc R Soc Med. 1968; 61(4):401–408

[83] Dudley HA, Racliffe AG, McGeehan D. Intraoperative irrigation of the colon to permit primary anastomosis. Br J Surg. 1980; 67(2):80–81

[84] Wille-Jørgensen P, Guenaga KF, Matos D, Castro AA. Pre-operative mechanical bowel cleansing or not? an updated meta-analysis. Colorectal Dis. 2005; 7(4):304–310

[85] Lim JF, Tang CL, Seow-Choen F, Heah SM. Prospective, randomized trial comparing intraoperative colonic irrigation with manual decompression only for obstructed left-sided colorectal cancer. Dis Colon Rectum. 2005; 48(2):205–209

[86] Nyam DC, Seow-Choen F, Leong AF, Ho YH. Colonic decompression without on-table irrigation for obstructing left-sided colorectal tumours. Br J Surg. 1996; 83(6):786–787

[87] Ortiz H, Biondo S, Ciga MA, Kreisler E, Oteiza F, Fraccalvieri D. Comparative study to determine the need for intraoperative colonic irrigation for primary anastomosis in left-sided colonic emergencies. Colorectal Dis. 2009; 11(6):648–652

[88] Single-stage treatment for malignant left-sided colonic obstruction: a prospective randomized clinical trial comparing subtotal colectomy with segmental resection following intraoperative irrigation. The SCOTIA Study Group. Subtotal Colectomy versus On-table Irrigation and Anastomosis. Br J Surg. 1995; 82(12):1622–1627

[89] Hennekinne-Mucci S, Tuech JJ, Bréhant O, et al. Emergency subtotal/total colectomy in the management of obstructed left colon carcinoma. Int J Colorectal Dis. 2006; 21(6):538–541

[90] Cheung HY, Chung CC, Tsang WW, Wong JC, Yau KK, Li MK. Endolaparoscopic approach vs conventional open surgery in the treatment of obstructing left-sided colon cancer: a randomized controlled trial. Arch Surg. 2009; 144(12):1127–1132

[91] Lee JH, Ross WA, Davila R, et al. Self-expandable metal stents (SEMS) can serve as a bridge to surgery or as a definitive therapy in patients with an advanced stage of cancer: clinical experience of a tertiary cancer center. Dig Dis Sci. 2010; 55(12):3530–3536

[92] Branger F, Thibaudeau E, Mucci-Hennekinne S, et al. Management of acute malignant large-bowel obstruction with self-expanding metal stent. Int J Colorectal Dis. 2010; 25(12):1481–1485

[93] Sebastian S, Johnston S, Geoghegan T, Torreggiani W, Buckley M. Pooled analysis of the efficacy and safety of self-expanding metal stenting in malignant colorectal obstruction. Am J Gastroenterol. 2004; 99(10):2051–2057

[94] West M, Kiff R. Stenting of the colon in patients with malignant large bowel obstruction: a local experience. J Gastrointest Cancer. 2011; 42(3):155–159

[95] Kim SY, Kwon SH, Oh JH. Radiologic placement of uncovered stents for the treatment of malignant colorectal obstruction. J Vasc Interv Radiol. 2010; 21(8):1244–1249

[96] Pirlet IA, Slim K, Kwiatkowski F, Michot F, Millat BL. Emergency preoperative stenting versus surgery for acute left-sided malignant colonic obstruction: a multicenter randomized controlled trial. Surg Endosc. 2011; 25(6):1814–1821

[97] van Hooft JE, Bemelman WA, Oldenburg B, et al. collaborative Dutch Stent-In study group. Colonic stenting versus emergency surgery for acute left-sided malignant colonic obstruction: a multicentre randomised trial. Lancet Oncol. 2011; 12(4):344–352

[98] Ho KS, Quah HM, Lim JF, Tang CL, Eu KW. Endoscopic stenting and elective surgery versus emergency surgery for left-sided malignant colonic obstruction: a prospective randomized trial. Int J Colorectal Dis. 2012; 27(3):355–362

[99] Iversen LH, Kratmann M, Bøje M, Laurberg S. Self-expanding metallic stents as bridge to surgery in obstructing colorectal cancer. Br J Surg. 2011; 98(2):275–281

[100] Kim HJ, Choi GS, Park JS, Park SY, Jun SH. Higher rate of perineural invasion in stent-laparoscopic approach in comparison to emergent open resection for obstructing left-sided colon cancer. Int J Colorectal Dis. 2013; 28(3):407–414

[101] Tan CJ, Dasari BV, Gardiner K. Systematic review and meta-analysis of randomized clinical trials of self-expanding metallic stents as a bridge to surgery versus emergency surgery for malignant left-sided large bowel obstruction. Br J Surg. 2012; 99(4):469–476

[102] Cirocchi R, Farinella E, Trastulli S, et al. Safety and efficacy of endoscopic colonic stenting as a bridge to surgery in the management of intestinal obstruction due to left colon and rectal cancer: a systematic review and meta-analysis. Surg Oncol. 2013; 22(1):14–21

[103] Hill JKC, Morton D, Magill L, et al. CREST: Randomised phase III study of stenting as a bridge to surgery in obstructing colorectal cancer—Results of the UK ColoRectal Endoscopic Stenting Trial (CREST). Proceedings of the American Society of Clinical Oncology Annual Meeting; June 3–7, 2016. Chicago, IL; 2018

[104] Verstockt B, Van Driessche A, De Man M, et al. Ten-year survival after endoscopic stenting as a bridge to surgery in obstructing colon cancer. Gastrointest Endosc. 2018; 87(3):705–713

[105] Gash K, Chambers W, Ghosh A, Dixon AR. The role of laparoscopic surgery for the management of acute large bowel obstruction. Colorectal Dis. 2011; 13(3):263–266

[106] Camúñez F, Echenagusia A, Simó G, Turégano F, Vázquez J, Barreiro-Meiro I. Malignant colorectal obstruction treated by means of self-expanding metallic stents: effectiveness before surgery and in palliation. Radiology. 2000; 216(2):492–497

[107] Law WL, Chu KW, Ho JW, Tung HM, Law SY, Chu KM. Self-expanding metallic stent in the treatment of colonic obstruction caused by advanced malignancies. Dis Colon Rectum. 2000; 43(11):1522–1527

[108] Pothuri B, Guirguis A, Gerdes H, Barakat RR, Chi DS. The use of colorectal stents for palliation of large-bowel obstruction due to recurrent gynecologic cancer. Gynecol Oncol. 2004; 95(3):513–517

[109] Xinopoulos D, Dimitroulopoulos D, Theodosopoulos T, et al. Stenting or stoma creation for patients with inoperable malignant colonic obstructions? Results of a study and cost-effectiveness analysis. Surg Endosc. 2004; 18 (3):421–426

[110] Faragher IG, Chaitowitz IM, Stupart DA. Long-term results of palliative stenting or surgery for incurable obstructing colon cancer. Colorectal Dis. 2008; 10(7):668–672

[111] Lee WS, Baek JH, Kang JM, Choi S, Kwon KA. The outcome after stent placement or surgery as the initial treatment for obstructive primary tumor in patients with stage IV colon cancer. Am J Surg. 2012; 203(6):715–719

[112] Watt AM, Faragher IG, Griffin TT, Rieger NA, Maddern GJ. Self-expanding metallic stents for relieving malignant colorectal obstruction: a systematic review. Ann Surg. 2007; 246(1):24–30

[113] Frago R, Kreisler E, Biondo S, Salazar R, Dominguez J, Escalante E. Outcomes in the management of obstructive unresectable stage IV colorectal cancer. Eur J Surg Oncol. 2010; 36(12):1187–1194

[114] Gevers AM, Macken E, Hiele M, Rutgeerts P. Endoscopic laser therapy for palliation of patients with distal colorectal carcinoma: analysis of factors influencing long-term outcome. Gastrointest Endosc. 2000; 51(5):580–585

[115] Meijer S, Rahusen FD, van der Plas LG. Palliative cryosurgery for rectal carcinoma. Int J Colorectal Dis. 1999; 14(3):177–180

[116] Raveenthiran V, Madiba TE, Atamanalp SS, De U. Volvulus of the sigmoid colon. Colorectal Dis. 2010; 12 7 Online:e1–e17

[117] Agrez M, Cameron D. Radiology of sigmoid volvulus. Dis Colon Rectum. 1981; 24(7):510–514

[118] Bruzzi M, Lefèvre JH, Desaint B, et al. Management of acute sigmoid volvulus: short- and long-term results. Colorectal Dis. 2015; 17(10):922–928

[119] Vogel JD, Feingold DL, Stewart DB, et al. Clinical practice guidelines for colon volvulus and acute colonic pseudo-obstruction. Dis Colon Rectum. 2016; 59 (7):589–600

[120] Atamanalp SS. Sigmoid volvulus: diagnosis in 938 patients over 45.5 years. Tech Coloproctol. 2013; 17(4):419–424

[121] Melling J, Makin C. Sigmoid volvulus, acquired megacolon and pseudo-obstruction. Surgery. 2011; 29:387–390

[122] Delgado-Aros S, Camilleri M. Pseudo-obstruction in the critically ill. Best Pract Res Clin Gastroenterol. 2003; 17(3):427–444

[123] Ogilvie H. Large-intestine colic due to sympathetic deprivation; a new clinical syndrome. BMJ. 1948; 2(4579):671–673

[124] Catchpole BN. Ileus: use of sympathetic blocking agents in its treatment. Surgery. 1969; 66(5):811–820

[125] Gierson ED, Storm FK, Shaw W, Coyne SK. Caecal rupture due to colonic ileus. Br J Surg. 1975; 62(5):383–386

[126] Trevisani GT, Hyman NH, Church JM. Neostigmine: safe and effective treatment for acute colonic pseudo-obstruction. Dis Colon Rectum. 2000; 43 (5):599–603

[127] Vanek VW, Al-Salti M. Acute pseudo-obstruction of the colon (Ogilvie's syndrome). An analysis of 400 cases. Dis Colon Rectum. 1986; 29(3):203–210

[128] Nivatvongs S, Vermeulen FD, Fang DT. Colonoscopic decompression of acute pseudo-obstruction of the colon. Ann Surg. 1982; 196(5):598–600

[129] Smith J, Kelly KA, Weinshilboum RM. Pathophysiology of postoperative ileus. Arch Surg. 1977; 112(2):203–209

[130] Rex DK. Colonoscopy and acute colonic pseudo-obstruction. Gastrointest Endosc Clin N Am. 1997; 7(3):499–508

[131] Sengupta J, Gebhart G. Gastrointestinal afferent fibres and sensation. In: Johnson LR, ed. Physiology of the Gastrointestinal Tract. New York, NY: Raven Press; 1994:483–520

[132] Türler A, Moore BA, Pezzone MA, Overhaus M, Kalff JC, Bauer AJ. Colonic postoperative inflammatory ileus in the rat. Ann Surg. 2002; 236(1):56–66

[133] Kalff JC, Schraut WH, Simmons RL, Bauer AJ. Surgical manipulation of the gut elicits an intestinal muscularis inflammatory response resulting in postsurgical ileus. Ann Surg. 1998; 228(5):652–663

[134] Brix-Christensen V, Tønnesen E, Sanchez RG, Bilfinger TV, Stefano GB. Endogenous morphine levels increase following cardiac surgery as part of the antiinflammatory response? Int J Cardiol. 1997; 62(3):191–197

[135] Yoshida S, Ohta J, Yamasaki K, et al. Effect of surgical stress on endogenous morphine and cytokine levels in the plasma after laparoscopic or open cholecystectomy. Surg Endosc. 2000; 14(2):137–140

[136] Stanghellini V, Cogliandro RF, De Giorgio R, et al. Natural history of chronic idiopathic intestinal pseudo-obstruction in adults: a single center study. Clin Gastroenterol Hepatol. 2005; 3(5):449–458

[137] Maldonado JE, Gregg JA, Green PA, Brown AL, Jr. Chronic idiopathic intestinal pseudo-obstruction. Am J Med. 1970; 49(2):203–212

[138] De Giorgio R, Sarnelli G, Corinaldesi R, Stanghellini V. Advances in our understanding of the pathology of chronic intestinal pseudo-obstruction. Gut. 2004; 53(11):1549–1552

[139] Mousa H, Hyman PE, Cocjin J, Flores AF, Di Lorenzo C. Long-term outcome of congenital intestinal pseudoobstruction. Dig Dis Sci. 2002; 47 (10):2298–2305

[140] Amiot A, Joly F, Alves A, Panis Y, Bouhnik Y, Messing B. Long-term outcome of chronic intestinal pseudo-obstruction adult patients requiring home parenteral nutrition. Am J Gastroenterol. 2009; 104(5):1262–1270

[141] De Giorgio R, Cogliandro RF, Barbara G, Corinaldesi R, Stanghellini V. Chronic intestinal pseudo-obstruction: clinical features, diagnosis, and therapy. Gastroenterol Clin North Am. 2011; 40(4):787–807

[142] Mann SD, Debinski HS, Kamm MA. Clinical characteristics of chronic idiopathic intestinal pseudo-obstruction in adults. Gut. 1997; 41(5):675–681

[143] Antonucci A, Fronzoni L, Cogliandro L, et al. Chronic intestinal pseudo-obstruction. World J Gastroenterol. 2008; 14(19):2953–2961

[144] Gabbard SL, Lacy BE. Chronic intestinal pseudo-obstruction. Nutr Clin Pract. 2013; 28(3):307–316

[145] Di Nardo G, Blandizzi C, Volta U, et al. Review article: molecular, pathological and therapeutic features of human enteric neuropathies. Aliment Pharmacol Ther. 2008; 28(1):25–42

[146] Geller A, Petersen BT, Gostout CJ. Endoscopic decompression for acute colonic pseudo-obstruction. Gastrointest Endosc. 1996; 44(2):144–150

[147] Harrison ME, Anderson MA, Appalaneni V, et al. ASGE Standards of Practice Committee. The role of endoscopy in the management of patients with known and suspected colonic obstruction and pseudo-obstruction. Gastrointest Endosc. 2010; 71(4):669–679

[148] Tsirline VB, Zemlyak AY, Avery MJ, et al. Colonoscopy is superior to neostigmine in the treatment of Ogilvie's syndrome. Am J Surg. 2012; 204(6):849–855, discussion 855

[149] Bonacini M, Smith OJ, Pritchard T. Erythromycin as therapy for acute colonic pseudo-obstruction (Ogilvie's syndrome). J Clin Gastroenterol. 1991; 13 (4):475–476

[150] Lipton AB, Knauer CM. Pseudo-obstruction of the bowel. Therapeutic trial of metoclopramide. Am J Dig Dis. 1977; 22(3):263–265

[151] Jain A, Vargas HD. Advances and challenges in the management of acute colonic pseudo-obstruction (Ogilvie syndrome). Clin Colon Rectal Surg. 2012; 25(1):37–45

[152] Weinstock LB, Chang AC. Methylnaltrexone for treatment of acute colonic pseudo-obstruction. J Clin Gastroenterol. 2011; 45(10):883–884

[153] Holzer P. Opioid antagonists for prevention and treatment of opioid-induced gastrointestinal effects. Curr Opin Anaesthesiol. 2010; 23(5):616–622

[154] Grant D, Abu-Elmagd K, Reyes J, et al. Intestine Transplant Registry. 2003 report of the intestine transplant registry: a new era has dawned. Ann Surg. 2005; 241(4):607–613

[155] Ponec RJ, Saunders MD, Kimmey MB. Neostigmine for the treatment of acute colonic pseudo-obstruction. N Engl J Med. 1999; 341(3):137–141

[156] Schermer CR, Hanosh JJ, Davis M, Pitcher DE. Ogilvie's syndrome in the surgical patient: a new therapeutic modality. J Gastrointest Surg. 1999; 3(2):173–177

[157] Sgouros SN, Vlachogiannakos J, Vassiliadis K, et al. Effect of polyethylene glycol electrolyte balanced solution on patients with acute colonic pseudo obstruction after resolution of colonic dilation: a prospective, randomised, placebo controlled trial. Gut. 2006; 55(5):638–642

[158] O'Dea CJ, Brookes JH, Wattchow DA. The efficacy of treatment of patients with severe constipation or recurrent pseudo-obstruction with pyridostigmine. Colorectal Dis. 2010; 12(6):540–548

[159] Duh QY, Way LW. Diagnostic laparoscopy and laparoscopic cecostomy for colonic pseudo-obstruction. Dis Colon Rectum. 1993; 36(1):65–70

[160] Scolapio JS, Ukleja A, Bouras EP, Romano M. Nutritional management of chronic intestinal pseudo-obstruction. J Clin Gastroenterol. 1999; 28 (4):306–312

[161] Faure C, Goulet O, Ategbo S, et al. French-Speaking Group of Pediatric Gastroenterology. Chronic intestinal pseudoobstruction syndrome: clinical analysis, outcome, and prognosis in 105 children. Dig Dis Sci. 1999; 44 (5):953–959

[162] Pitt HA, Mann LL, Berquist WE, Ament ME, Fonkalsrud EW, DenBesten L. Chronic intestinal pseudo-obstruction. Management with total parenteral nutrition and a venting enterostomy. Arch Surg. 1985; 120(5):614–618

[163] Smith DS, Williams CS, Ferris CD. Diagnosis and treatment of chronic gastroparesis and chronic intestinal pseudo-obstruction. Gastroenterol Clin North Am. 2003; 32(2):619–658

[164] Emmanuel AV, Kamm MA, Roy AJ, Kerstens R, Vandeplassche L. Randomised clinical trial: the efficacy of prucalopride in patients with chronic intestinal pseudo-obstruction—a double-blind, placebo-controlled, cross-over, multiple n = 1 study. Aliment Pharmacol Ther. 2012; 35(1):48–55

[165] Perlemuter G, Cacoub P, Chaussade S, Wechsler B, Couturier D, Piette JC. Octreotide treatment of chronic intestinal pseudoobstruction secondary to connective tissue diseases. Arthritis Rheum. 1999; 42(7):1545–1549

[166] Prapaitrakool S, Hollmann MW, Wartenberg HC, Preckel B, Brugger S. Use of buprenorphine in children with chronic pseudoobstruction syndrome: case series and review of literature. Clin J Pain. 2012; 28(8):722–725

[167] Bond GJ, Reyes JD. Intestinal transplantation for total/near-total aganglionosis and intestinal pseudo-obstruction. Semin Pediatr Surg. 2004; 13(4):286–292

[168] Lao OB, Healey PJ, Perkins JD, Horslen S, Reyes JD, Goldin AB. Outcomes in children after intestinal transplant. Pediatrics. 2010; 125(3):e550–e558

30 Mesenteric Vascular Diseases

David E. Beck and Philip H. Gordon

Abstract

Mesenteric vascular disease can result in injury to the small or large bowel. Mesenteric disease is present in 18% of patients older than 65 years and in 70% of those undergoing aortofemoral bypass. The disease varies in anatomic and symptom complexes. The estimated frequencies of causes of acute mesenteric ischemia are arterial occlusion (50%), nonocclusive mesenteric ischemia (20 to 30%), venous occlusion (5 to 15%), as well as extravascular sources such as incarcerated hernia, volvulus, intussusception, and adhesive bands. It is important to recognize the common anatomic and physiologic principles involved in each syndrome.

Keywords: mesenteric vascular disease, intestinal ischemia, superior mesenteric artery embolism, superior mesenteric artery thrombosis, nonocclusive mesenteric ischemia and infarction, mesenteric venous thrombosis, aortoiliac injury, cardiopulmonary bypass, obstructing carcinoma, ischemic proctitis

30.1 Introduction

Mesenteric vascular disease encompasses a family of diseases of which the end result is injury to the small or large bowel resulting from diminished blood flow or inadequate oxygen and nutrient delivery. Mesenteric disease is present in 18% of patients older than 65 years and in 70% of those undergoing aortofemoral bypass.[1] The diseases vary from anatomically definable and clinically reproducible symptom complexes, such as those seen in superior mesenteric artery (SMA) embolism, to more erratic and unpredictable patterns, such as those of ischemic colitis. The estimated frequencies of causes of acute mesenteric ischemia are arterial occlusion 50%, nonocclusive mesenteric ischemia 20 to 30%, and venous occlusion 5 to 15%, as well as extravascular sources such as incarcerated hernia, volvulus, intussusception, and adhesive bands.[2] Although it is important to view these diseases clinically as individual entities often requiring different clinical approaches, it is equally important to recognize the common anatomic and physiologic principles involved in each syndrome.

30.2 Vascular Anatomy

The intestinal tract has a generous overlapping blood supply, with blood flow averaging 1,500 to 1,800 mL/min. Wide variations in blood flow are possible in response to meals or exercise. The three main vessels supplying circulation to the bowel include the celiac axis, the SMA, and the inferior mesenteric artery (IMA). Because of the important collateral blood flow emanating from the hypogastric arteries at the level of the sigmoid colon, the hypogastrics also should be considered to be part of this system.

The celiac artery consists of three main trunks, which are the splenic, common hepatic, and left gastric arteries. The main collateral communication between the celiac and the SMA system is via the pancreaticoduodenal loop and to a lesser extent from the dorsal pancreatic artery. The pancreaticoduodenal artery originates as anterior and posterior superior pancreaticoduodenal branches that arise from the gastroduodenal artery, which is itself a branch of the common hepatic artery. This loop communicates around the duodenal sweep between the pancreatic border of the duodenum and the pancreas and unites with inferior pancreaticoduodenal vessels coming from the SMA. The pancreaticoduodenal loop can dilate considerably in the presence of ischemic disease. Another collateral vessel, the dorsal pancreatic artery, is a branch that traverses the pancreas, coming from either the splenic artery or the common hepatic artery to join and collateralize with the SMA system below via the middle colic artery.

The SMA gives off the inferior pancreaticoduodenal artery as its first branch, and it then supplies virtually the entire blood supply to the jejunum and ileum via individual mesenteric arteries. At the level of the distal ileum, a large ileocolic artery nourishes the terminal ileum and cecum. The ascending colon and transverse colon receive blood from branches that arise from the SMA more proximally. The right colic artery arises from the midportion of the SMA to supply the ascending colon. The middle colic artery is frequently spared from SMA embolism because it originates from the most proximal portion of the SMA before dividing into right and left branches.

The left branch of the middle colic artery traverses the mesocolon along the left side of the transverse colon, the splenic flexure, and the descending colon to ultimately collateralize with the IMA at the level of the midportion of the descending colon. The IMA communication between the left colic artery and the SMA circulation has been variously called the marginal artery, the arc of Riolan, the central anastomotic artery, and the meandering mesenteric artery. Two or more anastomotic arteries may be present.[3] Discussion of the anatomy and varying nomenclature is elaborated in Chapter 1. The IMA also gives off sigmoidal branches and superior rectal branches; the latter branches communicate with the hypogastric system by means of middle and inferior rectal vessels (see Chapter 1).

In general, acute occlusion of any of the three main mesenteric vessels, either celiac, SMA, or IMA, is capable of causing varying degrees of acute infarction, whereas gradual occlusion of any one, two, or even three of these vessels can occur without injury, depending largely on the extent of the collateral circulation.

The arcade system and overlapping circulation within the small bowel end at the level of the villus, where the arterioles effectively become end vessels. A single arteriole, designated the main arteriole, enters through the core of the villus. This vessel arborizes into a tuft arrangement of capillaries at the tip of the villus and subsequently drains into venules that converge at the villus base to form the collecting venule.[4] There is evidence for a countercurrent exchange mechanism similar to that seen in the renal nephron; in the villus, the mechanism involves the central arteriole and the venules lying in close proximity at the base of the villus.[5] During low-flow states, oxygen is shunted by diffusion from arteriole to venule, and this renders the villus tip vulnerable to ischemic injury.[6] The high metabolic rate of the villus and the oxygen shunting make the villus the first part of the intestine to feel the impact of ischemic injury (▶ Fig. 30.1).

30.3 Pathophysiology of Intestinal Ischemia

The gut receives 20% of resting and 35% of postprandial cardiac output. Of this, 70% supplies the mucosa.[1] Kaleya and Boley[7] summarized the microcirculation and collateral flow within the intestinal wall. An extensive network of vessels within the bowel wall arises from the vasa recta and vasa brevia on the mesenteric border of the bowel. These vessels give rise, sequentially, to the external muscular vascular plexus, then penetrate the muscular coat and form a rich submucosal plexus. The submucosal plexus is more extensive in the small bowel than in the colon and may make the small intestine more resistant to ischemia than the colon. A central arteriole originates from the submucosal plexus, loses its muscular coat, and arborizes into an extremely rich subepithelial capillary network within each individual villus. The flow through this redundant system is controlled by a network of resistance and capillary vessels, which, in turn, are affected by many functional, humoral, local, and neural influences. There are two primary mechanisms for the control of splanchnic vascular resistance. The first is neural. The sympathetic nervous system is important for the maintenance of resting splanchnic arteriolar tone and the primary mechanism of sympathetic control is neural. The second is humoral, consisting of a variety of circulating hormones, including catecholamines, vasoactive peptides, and inflammatory mediators such as histamine and the arachidonic acid metabolites. The important vasoconstrictor peptides include angiotensin II and vasopressin. Local factors play a role in intestinal blood flow. Prostaglandins, leukotrienes, and some thromboxane analogs produce splanchnic vasoconstriction. Local factors that accompany ischemia have potent vasodilatory effects on intestinal vessels. Hyperkalemia, hyperosmolarity, decreased local oxygen tension, adenosine, and high concentrations of carbon dioxide, causing local acidosis, dilate resistance vessels and produce local hyperemia. Exogenously administered vasodilators (e.g., papaverine) prevent and reverse the persistent vasoconstriction that follows a drop in SMA blood flow.

Inadequate intestinal perfusion is a consequence of either focal vascular occlusions or a low-flow state. Within 15 minutes of absolute ischemia, structural damage to the villi of the small bowel can be demonstrated; within 3 hours, mucosal sloughing occurs. At 6 hours, transmural necrosis is complete.[1] The nature and rapidity of these processes are affected by two other factors: collateral circulation and disorders of splanchnic autoregulation. Despite the variety of conditions that predispose to ischemia, the histopathology and sequence of events remain consistent and predictable. Intestinal ischemia induces a spectrum of injury, from subtle changes in capillary permeability to transmural necrosis, and the final outcome depends on local as well as systemic factors.[7] There basically are two separate factors responsible for the subsequent damage: tissue hypoxia and reperfusion injury. Hypoxia occurs during the period of ischemia and reperfusion injury when some flow is reestablished. The early phase of acute intestinal ischemia involves mechanisms that ultimately cause volume loss and acidosis. Reversal of the ischemic injury is possible early in the process. Later in the course, bacterial invasion with endotoxic release, septicemia, and shock becomes more prominent and indicates full-thickness irreversible injury.

Following an episode of intestinal ischemia, the first event involves loss of circulatory blood volume with intense outpouring of fluid and protein through the injured villus. The most tenable explanation for this early extravasation of fluid is that the ischemic villus tip loses its absorptive function, while the crypt cells are relatively spared of injury and can continue their secretory functions.[8] Loss of circulating blood volume and distention caused by intraluminal exudation contribute to a further decrease in perfusion. As submucosal layers are rendered ischemic, bowel edema develops, and this is followed by transudation of fluid into the peritoneal cavity, complicating the already serious hypovolemia. The intense volume loss alone can lead to profound hypovolemia, with the metabolic sequelae of hypoxia at the tissue level and lactic acidosis.

The changes that occur when intestine is deprived of an adequate blood supply are both metabolic and morphologic.[7]

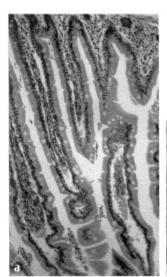
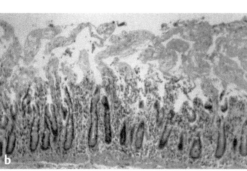

Fig. 30.1 (a) Microscopic section of normal small bowel villus pattern. **(b)** Section of small bowel having sustained ischemic injury, showing sloughing and loss of villus tips with preservation of cellular elements of villus at the base.

Ultrastructural changes occur within 10 minutes and, by 30 minutes, extensive changes, including accumulation of fluid between cells and the basement membranes, are present. The tips of the villi then begin to slough, and a membrane of necrotic epithelium, fibrin, inflammatory cells, and bacteria accumulates. Later, edema appears, followed by bleeding into the submucosa. Cellular death progresses from the lumen outward until transmural necrosis of the bowel wall occurs.

Vasoactive substances released in response to intestinal ischemia act to further diminish perfusion. Release of myocardial depressant factor probably contributes to worsening the already diminished cardiac output. Other mediators such as cytokines, platelet-activating factor, and tumor necrosis factor are also released.[1] Histamine release during ischemic reperfusion appears to play an important role in the progression of the shock state. Diamine oxidase, an enzyme that acts to inactivate histamine, has been shown to have a protective effect in intestinal ischemia.[9] Also implicated in circulatory collapse following intestinal infarction is the vasoactive intestinal polypeptide (VIP), which acts as a potent vasodilator and contributes to the intense outpouring of intraluminal fluids.[10,11]

Bacterial invasion does not occur until 24 hours or more into the course of the ischemic episode. In studies with an isolated colonic ischemia model, Bennion et al[12,13] showed that by 72 hours the total number of anaerobic bacteria had increased, while aerobic bacteria counts had decreased. All anaerobe species were found to be increased, especially *Bacteroides*, as well as a variety of clostridial species, including *Clostridium difficile*. In the same animal model, cultures of portal venous blood and liver became infected with a mixed anaerobic flora by 24 hours. Systemic bacteremia followed portal venous bacteremia at 48 hours when aortic and peritoneal cultures grew mixed anaerobes. This suggests that ischemia-induced mucosal injury first causes portal vein bacteremia, followed by systemic bacteremia once the hepatic reticuloendothelial system becomes overwhelmed. These findings precede perforation, which causes more widespread bacterial dissemination within the peritoneal cavity from gross spillage of bowel contents.

Recent attention has been directed at the role of oxygen-free radicals in the pathogenesis of reperfusion injury. Partial reduction of molecular oxygen results in the production of oxygen-free radicals. These superoxide radicals mark the beginning of a metabolic cascade that results in the formation of highly toxic hydroxyl-free radicals. The enzymes, superoxide dismutase and catalase, provide a defense against superoxide radicals by converting the radicals to peroxide and water. Cytotoxic effects of oxygen-derived free radicals result from peroxidation of the lipid components of cellular membranes and the degradation of the hyaluronic acid and collagen components of basement membranes and extracellular matrices.[14,15] The resulting increased vascular permeability and mucosal membrane injury lead to enhanced transcapillary fluid transudation and interstitial edema. Studies by Granger et al[16] have provided evidence that free radical scavenger enzymes substantially block the increased vascular permeability induced by ischemia, while antihistamines, indomethacin, and methylprednisolone do not.

Parks et al[17] subsequently have shown that experimentally generated oxygen-free radicals cause increased vascular permeability in nonischemic bowel comparable to that seen with ischemia. The source of superoxide production in intestinal ischemia appears to be the enzyme xanthine oxidase. Xanthine oxidase is abundant in small bowel mucosa, where it is most heavily concentrated in the villus tip. Substrates for the reaction include hypoxanthine, which is a catabolic product of adenosine triphosphate, and molecular oxygen available with reperfusion. The tissue damage occurs during reperfusion and not during the period of ischemia.[1]

Andrei et al[18] documented a fatal case of small bowel ischemia following laparoscopic cholecystectomy. Their literature review revealed at least six cases of small bowel ischemia following laparoscopic cholecystectomy. It is postulated this was due to the physiological adverse effects of pneumoperitoneum associated intra-abdominal hypertension, compromising the mesenteric circulation.

30.4 Diagnostic Studies

Improved results in the treatment of most types of mesenteric vascular disease must come from earlier diagnosis. Diagnostic laboratory studies for mesenteric ischemia are based on measurements of physiologic derangements. Specific radiographic studies and other diagnostic procedures will be covered in the discussion of each disease process.

The white blood cell count generally is a reliable indicator of ischemic injury and often can be used to monitor the progress or the worsening of the disease. However, some studies have shown that as many as 25% of patients will have significant ischemic injury without elevation of the white blood cell count,[7] emphasizing the need to consider other subjective and objective findings. Hematocrit may be a helpful guide to the status of ischemic disease because it can reflect the intense hypovolemia seen with significant small bowel injuries. Hematocrit levels as high as 60% can be seen in some patients, and this hemoconcentration may further contribute to the ischemic process by causing sludging and microvascular thrombosis.

Arterial blood gases show a metabolic acidosis pattern associated with intestinal infarction. The acidosis may precede the development of shock and may be of diagnostic significance.[19] Some studies have shown a disproportionately high elevation of serum phosphate levels in the presence of intestinal ischemia, suggesting that serum phosphate may serve as a marker for the disease. Serum phosphate elevation, while not specific for bowel ischemia, is useful because it is so readily determined, and the phosphate elevation may precede irreversible ischemic injury.[20]

A number of enzyme levels have been studied, but many are nonspecific and others are not readily available. Amylase, lactic dehydrogenase, and serum glutamate oxaloacetate transaminase levels often are elevated, but these elevations are nonspecific and generally are not reliable. Animal studies have shown that serum intestinal alkaline phosphatase (SIAP) levels are elevated in the presence of mesenteric ischemic disease but not in the presence of inflammatory disease or perforation.[21] This could make SIAP levels a useful and specific marker in the future, although the test is not available for clinical use at this time. Creatine phosphokinase (CPK) isoenzyme levels also have been shown to be elevated in the presence of ischemic bowel disease,[22,23] and assays for these enzymes are readily available. Animal studies have shown that fractionating the CPK into BB and MB bands can be especially helpful in the first 24 hours.[23] The CPK-BB isoenzyme tends to be elevated in the first 12 hours, whereas the CPK-MB band becomes elevated in the second 12 hours, making these potentially useful diagnostic markers for early intestinal ischemia.

The level of diamine oxidase, a histamine catabolizing enzyme, has been shown to be elevated early in the face of intestinal ischemia, probably in response to the intensive release of histamine by the ischemic process.[24] If this enzyme assay becomes available in the future, it may be helpful in differentiating ischemic injury from other inflammatory processes. The level of VIP also has been shown to be elevated, particularly early in ischemic disease,[10] but an assay for VIP is not yet available in most medical centers.

Acosta et al[25] assessed the value of the fibrinolytic marker D-dimer testing to diagnose SMA occlusion by means of likelihood ratios. Nine of 101 patients included had acute SMA occlusion. The median D-dimer concentration was 1.6 mg/L, which was higher than that in 25 patients with inflammatory disease or in 14 patients with intestinal obstruction. The combination of a D-dimer level greater than 1.5 mg/L, atrial fibrillation, and female sex resulted in a likelihood ratio for acute SMA occlusion of 17.5, whereas no patient with a D-dimer concentration of 0.3 mg/L or less had acute SMA occlusion.

Scholz[26] described the following radiologic findings that may be expected in acute bowel ischemia with any modality that images the intestine: gasless abdomen, rapid transit, slow transit, ileus, bowel obstruction, unchanging loop of small bowel, blood blister formation, thumbprinting, thick folds, "stack of coins," thickening of bowel wall, persisting enhancement of thick bowel wall on computed tomography (CT), and prompt reversal of these findings if ischemia is reversed. The following findings indicate that bowel infarction is present or was present and that fibrotic healing has occurred: focal ulcer, shaggy mucosa, "collar button" ulcers, mesenteric or portal vein gas, intramural fistula, intraluminal mucosal cast, intraperitoneal air, stricture, and pseudodiverticulum. Wiesner et al[27] published an extensive review of CT findings in acute bowel ischemia. These may consist of various morphologic changes, including homogeneous or heterogeneous hypoattenuating or hyperattenuating wall thickening, dilatation, abnormal or absent wall enhancement, mesenteric stranding, vascular engorgement, ascites, pneumatosis, and portal venous gas. Acute bowel ischemia may affect the small and/or large bowel and may be diffuse or localized, segmental or focal, and superficial or transmural; therefore, it can mimic various intestinal diseases. Acute bowel ischemia may involve more typical regions such as the left-sided colon; under such circumstances or if there are more specific CT findings such as pneumatosis or portal venous gas, the correct diagnosis will usually be suspected by the radiologist in an appropriate clinical setting. The CT appearance of acute bowel ischemia will depend on its cause, severity, localization, extent, and distribution, as well as the presence and degree of submucosal or intramural hemorrhage, superimposed bowel wall infection, and/or bowel wall perforation. Therefore, the CT findings in acute bowel ischemia may be as heterogeneous and nonspecific in these patients as their clinical and laboratory findings are. Klein et al[28] reviewed the value of all diagnostic imaging of 54 patients with mesenteric infarction. The authors found CT (82%) and angiography (87.5%) to be highly sensitive but favored CT because it can also be used to rule out other causes of the acute abdomen. Chou et al[29] evaluated the CT features of small bowel ischemia and necrosis and correlated the findings with clinical outcome or patient prognosis in 68 surgically or angiographically proved cases of small bowel ischemia. The CT features of intestinal ischemia were divided into three groups: (1) thinned bowel wall with poor enhancement, intramural gas, or portal venous gas; (2) thickened small bowel wall without superior mesenteric vein thrombosis; and (3) thickened small bowel wall with superior mesenteric vein thrombosis or intussusception. The evaluated factors include small bowel wall or mucosal enhancement pattern, small bowel dilatation, mesenteric edema, and CT evidence of narrowing or occlusion of the SMA or vein. Oral contrast material was not administered. Intramural gas and small bowel dilatation were associated with a higher bowel necrosis rate (8 of 8 and 17 of 21, respectively) in group 1. Poor mucosal enhancement of the thickened bowel wall indicated a higher bowel necrosis rate in groups 2 (6 of 7) and 3 (12 of 12) than did normal mucosal enhancement. Only intramural gas was accompanied by a higher mortality (six of eight).[29]

Sreenarasimhaiah[2] summarized the value of imaging studies. CT imaging has evolved over several years into a very useful modality for diagnosis of mesenteric ischemia and is the test of choice in the diagnosis of acute mesenteric ischemia. Findings include focal or segmental bowel wall thickening, submucosal edema or hemorrhage, pneumatosis, and portal venous gas. Contrast-enhanced CT detects acute mesenteric ischemia with sensitivity rates exceeding 90%. CT has been able to detect nonvascular visceral abnormalities. CT angiography is also available. Magnetic resonance imaging (MRI) with angiography is another noninvasive modality that rivals conventional angiography. In mesenteric venous disease, excellent visualization of the vascular anatomy is possible in addition to assessment of portal venous patency, flow direction, splanchnic thrombosis, and changes suggestive of portal hypertension. Three-dimensional gadolinium-enhanced reconstruction of vascular anatomy with a single breath hold and ultrafast scanning with digital subtraction angiography are also available. MRI with angiography has high sensitivity and specificity similar to those of CT angiography with the advantage of safer gadolinium agents and lack of ionizing radiation. Although MRI with angiography is an excellent tool for the evaluation of chronic mesenteric ischemia, it should not be the first technique used in the diagnosis of acute mesenteric ischemia, because of its potentially insufficient resolution to adequately identify nonocclusive low-flow states or distal emboli. Burkart et al[30] studied MR measurements of mesenteric venous flow and found the imaging technique promising as a noninvasive screening test for chronic mesenteric ischemia. Duplex scanning may be of value in identifying major vessel occlusion.[7] Laparoscopy may also be useful in the diagnosis but is limited by its inability to assess mucosal necrosis.

30.5 Clinical Syndromes

30.5.1 Superior Mesenteric Artery Embolism

SMA embolism is the most dramatic of the mesenteric vascular diseases and accounts for 33 to 50% of acute mesenteric ischemia.[1,7,31] Most commonly, this originates as a consequence of atrial fibrillation or acute myocardial infarction. It affords the potential for complete reversal and resolution if diagnosis and treatment are carried out promptly.[32]

The disease is characterized by a sudden onset of severe abdominal pain that generally is out of proportion to the physical examination. Associated findings include forceful gastric emptying with vomiting in approximately one-half of the patients and diarrhea in one-third. The white blood cell count usually is elevated, and frequently a history of cardiac disease and/or previous embolic phenomena is present. Plain radiography may show dilated thickened bowel loops, a ground-glass appearance due to ascites, thumbprinting, and toxic dilatation or gas in the bowel wall, portal vein, or peritoneum. All these features indicate infarction, but one-fourth of patients with infarction have a normal plain abdominal radiograph.[1] Duplex ultrasonography of the mesenteric vessels is highly sensitive and specific; however, it is often technically limited by accompanying abdominal distention and overlying bowel gas. The historical gold standard for the diagnosis of mesenteric ischemia was selective catheterization and mesenteric angiography, but CT angiography with its better image quality, availability, and relative ease of image acquisition has challenged angiography. Conventional CT may also show ascites, intestinal wall thickening, mucosal thumbprints, pneumatosis, and portal vein gas but may be normal in 30% of patients with proven mesenteric ischemia.[1] Diagnosis is confirmed by arteriogram. Characteristically, a sharp cutoff or meniscus sign is present at the site of the embolus several centimeters from the takeoff of the SMA. The most proximal branches supplying the proximal jejunum and the right transverse colon usually are not affected. This differentiates SMA embolism from SMA thrombosis, where the occlusion occurs at the origin of the vessel (▶ Fig. 30.2).

Some favorable early results also have been seen with thrombolytic therapy.[33,34,35,36] However, most patients with SMA embolism will need surgery, particularly when progression of the ischemic injury is suspected. The characteristic finding at surgery is a normal proximal jejunum with pulses present, reflecting the more distal placement of the embolus beyond the origin of the SMA. The ischemic changes are seen from the level of the midportion of the jejunum to the transverse colon, and no pulses are found in any of the vessels to this large section of the small and large bowels. This differs from SMA thrombosis, which is accompanied by ischemic changes involving the entire jejunum, the ileum, and the right colon.

Treatment of SMA embolism includes embolectomy or arterial reconstruction. Resection should be limited to those cases in which intestinal segments are frankly infarcted (▶ Fig. 30.3).[1,31] Early embolectomy alone usually is sufficient to restore perfusion (▶ Fig. 30.4). Care must be taken to evacuate all distally propagated thrombi, and narrowing must be avoided when closing the arteriotomy site. The need for small bowel resection often may be avoided by reevaluating the viability of the bowel 15 to 30 minutes after restoration of blood flow.

Traditional methods of determining bowel viability following reperfusion are inaccurate. Reliance on the return of normal

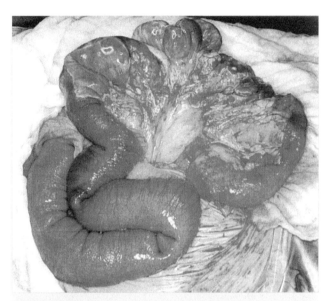

Fig. 30.3 Well-delineated necrotic small bowel.

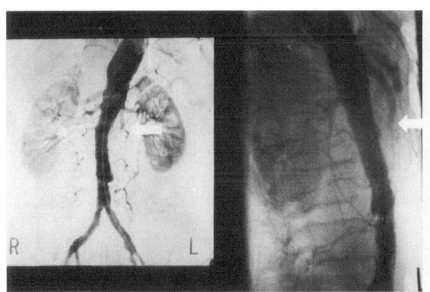

Fig. 30.2 Arteriogram showing superior mesenteric artery embolism with arrow pointing to site of occlusion forming a meniscus sign.

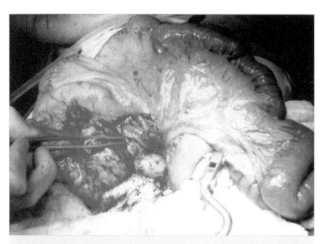

Fig. 30.4 Operative photography of superior mesenteric artery embolectomy site following restoration of blood flow. Ischemic sites are prominent at center of field indicating areas of small bowel that needed resection.

color, the presence of mesenteric pulsations, and peristalsis promotes unnecessary bowel resection in up to 50% of cases.[37] It is much more accurate to determine viability by fluorescein dye injection or by Doppler ultrasonography. Both techniques are relatively simple and allow for more precise delineation of nonperfused and nonviable bowel.[31,37,38] The use of surface oximetry to assess the adequacy of intestinal tissue oxygenation is especially promising. Sheridan et al[39] have used a modified Clark oxygen electrode to measure tissue oxygen tension (PtO_2) and have established a reference range for intraoperative PtO_2 for the entire gastrointestinal (GI) tract. The papaverine infusion may be continued for 12 to 24 hours, and repeat angiograms may be obtained to ascertain that the vasoconstriction has been abolished.[31] Heparin is controversial because GI hemorrhage is a significant risk. Thrombolytic therapy with streptokinase, urokinase, or recombinant tissue plasminogen activators in cases of acute and subacute SMA embolism or thrombosis has been described.[1]

The use of second-look laparotomy may maximize intestinal salvage for those cases in which viability is uncertain. The decision to perform a second-look procedure should be made at the time of the original operation. Re-exploration has been advocated 12 to 48 hours later, regardless of apparent clinical improvement or stabilization of the patient's overall condition. To avoid a formal second-look operation following massive resection for bowel infarction Slutzki et al[40] used laparoscopic inspection to assess the integrity of the anastomosis and viability of the remaining bowel. At the primary operation, two 10-/12-mm laparoscopic trocars were inserted in the lower quadrants, and 48 to 72 hours later the abdominal contents were inspected laparoscopically in five consecutive patients. The authors found the technique safe and reliable in all patients. Because of concern about decreasing mesenteric blood flow, care was taken to limit the pressure to 15 mm Hg during the procedure.[40]

Anadol et al[41] compared open and laparoscopic "second-look" procedures in patients with mesenteric ischemia. In the open group (41 patients), the abdomen was closed and a second-look laparotomy was performed in 23 patients. In the laparoscopic group (36 patients), a 10-mm trocar was inserted before closing the abdomen and second-look intervention was performed by a laparoscope in 23 patients. Sixteen of the re-laparotomies in the open group (70%) revealed nothing and were unnecessary. Two patients (8%) in the laparoscopic group needed re-resection, while 20 patients (87%) were rescued from unnecessary laparotomies.

Some authors are comfortable enough with Doppler assessment of bowel viability that they no longer recommend second-look procedures.[42] In a review of the literature, Bergan[43] demonstrated that second-look operations are useful only for select patients. Of 49 patients who had survived SMA embolectomy, a second-look operation was not performed in 42 of these survivors. Among those seven patients in whom the second-look procedure was performed, resection was necessary in only two, suggesting that the yield from this operation is modest when it is not performed on an individualized basis. The use of a second-look operation is clearly indicated whenever bowel of questionable viability has been left behind.[31] Sales et al[44] reported on a series of 29 patients who underwent small bowel resection primarily for mesenteric artery occlusive disease. All patients were given an ostomy, and the authors believe that this policy decreased the mortality rate (34%) in their series. All the surviving patients had intestinal continuity restored.

Bingol et al[45] reported 24 patients who underwent SMA embolectomy. The patients were divided into three groups according to the onset of symptoms and operation time. Group I ($n = 12$) patients were operated on in the first 6 hours after onset of symptoms; group II ($n = 9$) patients were operated on between 6 and 12 hours after onset of symptoms; and group III ($n = 3$) patients underwent embolectomy after 12 hours. Low-dose (5–10 mg) local tissue-type plasminogen activator (t-PA) administration directly into the SMA was an additional procedure with the embolectomy in all patients. The macroscopic view of the intestine was normal in 15 patients (12 patients in group I and 3 patients in group II) 30 minutes after the administration of local t-PA. Segmental resection was necessary in four patients in group II. Extended resection was necessary in two patients in group II and three patients in group III and all the patients died during the early postoperative period. They suggest that exploratory laparotomy should be done in patients with sudden abdominal pain, nausea, vomiting, mild leucocytosis, and metabolic acidosis who have previous valvular heart disease or atrial fibrillation. Ultimately, selective low-dose t-PA (5–10 mg) administration reduces the length of intestinal portion to be resected.

Savassi-Rocha and Veloso[46] reported a case of SMA embolism in which arterial flow was reestablished by selective intra-arterial infusion of streptokinase. They found 18 similar cases in the literature. This procedure could be an alternative to embolectomy in selected patients, that is, patients with an early diagnosis, no evidence of intestinal necrosis, and with partial occlusion and/or occlusion of secondary branches of the SMA. Frequent arteriographies and intensive care are necessary in this approach. The patient should be continuously monitored because of the possibility of treatment failure and the need for embolectomy.

30.5.2 Superior Mesenteric Artery Thrombosis

SMA thrombosis is distinguishable from embolism because of the more insidious onset of symptoms and the prominence of hypovolemic signs initially and cardiovascular collapse later. It accounts for 5 to 50% of acute mesenteric ischemia.[1,7,31] The usual presentation involves the gradual onset of abdominal pain associated with progressive distention and clinical signs of dehydration. Frequently there is anorexia, nausea and vomiting, and diarrhea with occult or gross blood. Leukocytosis is usually present. Often there is a history compatible with chronic intestinal insufficiency.[1,1] Although a diagnosis can be made by arteriogram, most patients are so acutely ill at the time of presentation that surgery is inevitable, and often the definitive diagnosis is made at the time of operation. Arteriography usually shows a cutoff of SMA blood flow at its origin. When advanced disease is present, plain abdominal X-ray films may show air in the portal vein and the liver (▶ Fig. 30.5).

As with SMA embolism, initial operative management for arterial thrombosis must include revascularization of any extensive segment of ischemic bowel. Thromboendarterectomy for acute mesenteric arterial thrombosis has been associated with a high failure rate. Aortomesenteric bypass may be beneficial even if viability is not completely restored and resection becomes necessary.[31] The graft may salvage marginally viable proximal jejunum, which ultimately may allow the patient to be maintained on oral alimentation. In addition, the graft may lessen the risk of anastomotic leak, since healing may be impaired if an anastomosis is performed in a potentially compromised but still viable small bowel. It has been argued that emergency bypass is doomed to failure because the gut has already infarcted, early graft thrombosis is almost universal, and the patient is likely to succumb from the systemic effects of reperfusion.[1] For these reasons, extensive resection is probably preferable to time-consuming attempts at revascularization. Johnston et al[48] reported on nine patients who underwent a bypass graft because of acute mesenteric thrombosis with an operative mortality of 22%. Survival at 1 year was 65% and survival at 5 years was 52%.

30.5.3 Nonocclusive Mesenteric Ischemia and Infarction

Nonocclusive mesenteric infarction has been diagnosed with increasing frequency in intensive care unit settings among patients critically ill from other unrelated diseases. It accounts for 20 to 30% of cases of mesenteric ischemia.[1,7,31] The signs and symptoms of nonocclusive mesenteric ischemia or infarction are similar to those of thrombotic infarction, except that nonocclusive disease tends to occur in a specific group of vulnerable patients. The disease should be suspected in any patient with cardiovascular disease and abdominal pain. Although the diagnosis is difficult to make, it is important to differentiate from other causes of ischemia because therapy is primarily nonoperative. Arteriography in these patients generally does not reveal an occlusion but shows reduced blood flow secondary to severe mesenteric vasospasm. Newer studies show that the renin–angiotensin axis, not catecholamines, may be the primary mediator of the splanchnic vasoconstriction seen in response to the severe physiologic stress associated with this condition.[49,50]

Predisposing factors to nonocclusive ischemia include (1) patients with congestive heart failure who are taking digitalis and diuretics, (2) patients with valvular heart disease and low output syndromes, (3) patients with digitalis intoxication and cardiac arrhythmia, (4) patients in shock or with prolonged hypovolemia, and (5) patients experiencing postoperative hypotension. The common denominator for all these predisposing factors is the low-flow state.

Initial treatment should focus on the underlying problem contributing to the presentation. The correction of hypovolemia, treatment of arrhythmias, and relief of congestive heart failure are crucial beginnings. Antibiotics may be helpful since the ischemia may result in a loss of the mucosal barrier to bacteria. A number of vasodilator drugs have been tried, but the one most frequently used is papaverine (30–60 mg/h), usually given by angiographic catheter infusion until clinical and radiologic resolution, for up to 5 days.[51,52] Epidural block and intraoperative splanchnic block also have been used to relieve the reflex component of the vasospasm. In many patients, nonthrombotic ischemia cannot be differentiated from infarction, and laparotomy is necessary for this distinction to be made. At laparotomy, all necrotic bowels should be resected; splanchnic block or epidural block may be added at that time. The prognosis for nonocclusive mesenteric ischemia tends to be poor largely because of the severity of the underlying illness that precipitates the ischemic event.

Ward et al[53] adopted an aggressive approach to the management of these patients. In a review of 34 patients with

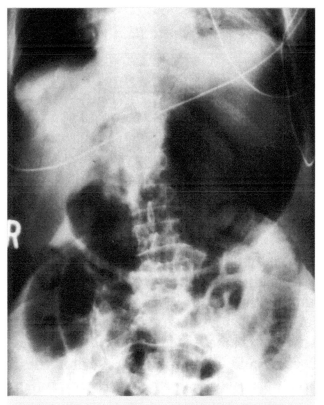

Fig. 30.5 Abdominal X-ray film of patient with massive small bowel infarction showing a dilated stomach and gas in the portal vein.

nonocclusive mesenteric ischemia, 7 patients underwent visceral arteriography, 2 of whom required operation and both died. Of the 29 patients who were explored, 21 had segmental injury and 8 had massive injury. Of the 21 with segmental injury, 12 (57%) had a primary anastomosis, 5 of whom died (42%). Nine of 21 patients (43%) underwent delayed anastomosis, and 2 of them died (22%). None with massive injury underwent primary anastomosis. A second-look operation was performed on 22 of 29 patients (76%). Eleven of the 22 (50%) underwent further bowel resection. Overall, 55% survived.

Schuler and Hudlin[54] described the presentation and management of five cases of nonocclusive ischemic cecal necrosis. Four of the patients presented with right-sided abdominal pain, tenderness, and leucocytosis. The preoperative diagnosis was incorrect in all patients. Two patients were thought to have appendicitis, two were thought to have carcinoma, and one was thought to have a perforated viscus. Each patient underwent a right hemicolectomy and four survived. Each of the patients had ischemic necrosis without evidence of emboli or vasculitis or hypotension. Ischemic necrosis of the cecum is an infrequent variant of ischemic colitis that should be considered in the differential diagnosis of the elderly patient presenting with right lower quadrant pain.

Neri et al[55] reviewed the diagnostic and treatment methods that emerged from their experience in 371 patients with a diagnosis of aortic dissection. Mesenteric ischemia was present in 19% of patients. In 9% of patients, bowel ischemia was not associated with a false lumen anatomy or an extension of the dissection process. The mortality rate in patients with nonocclusive mesenteric ischemia was 86%; sepsis and multiple organ failure were the cause of death in all nonsurvivors. Surgical treatment was beneficial only in the early phases of the disease. In patients who underwent operation, the significant risk factors were severe coagulation disorders, postoperative cerebral ischemia, maximal oxygen extraction rate of more than 0.40, aortic calcinosis, chronic obstructive pulmonary disease, thrombosis of the false lumen, inotropic support, and chronic renal insufficiency.

30.5.4 Mesenteric Venous Thrombosis

Mesenteric venous thrombosis accounts for 5 to 30% of all cases of gut ischemia.[7,31] Bradbury et al[1] classified the causes of mesenteric venous thrombosis (▶ Table 30.1). To this list, Flaherty et al[56] added a previously unrecognized cause of ischemia characterized by a vasculitis of mesenteric veins and their intramural tributaries. The authors proposed the term "mesenteric inflammatory veno-occlusive disease" to describe the entity.

Mesenteric venous thrombosis is characterized by the insidious onset of abdominal discomfort. The subacute nature of the symptoms may persist for 1 to 4 weeks. Progression of the disease is accompanied by more severe symptoms of crampy or diffuse abdominal pain, distention, or vomiting. The chief symptom of colicky pain is usually universal, nonlocalizing, and out of proportion to the meager findings of the physical examination. Mesenteric venous occlusion can often be differentiated from the previously described arterial occlusive syndromes by one of several commonly associated diseases that are present in most of the patients (▶ Table 30.1). Between 15 and 44% of patients with primary venous thrombosis will have suffered

Table 30.1 Classification of the causes of mesenteric venous thrombosis[1]

Primary (30%)	Secondary (60%)
Splenectomy	Portal hypertension; prehepatic, hepatic, and posthepatic
Polycythemia rubra vera	
Sickle-cell disease	Injection sclerotherapy of esophageal varices
Antithrombin III deficiency	
Protein C deficiency	Portosystemic shunt insertion
Protein S deficiency	Intra-abdominal sepsis; appendicitis, diverticulitis, pelvic abscess, visceral perforation, cholangitis
Dysfibrinogenemia	
Platelet disorders	
Myeloproliferative disease	Acute and chronic pancreatitis
Heparin cofactor II deficiency	Intra-abdominal neoplasia
Pregnancy	Gastroenteritis; bacterial, viral, and parasite
Puerperium	
Contraceptive pill use	Inflammatory bowel disease
Carcinomatosis	Abdominal trauma
	Malignancy
Idiopathic (10%)	

previous thromboembolic disease.[1] The physical examination is so nonspecific that it belies the seriousness of the situation. Physical findings vary with the stage of disease and may manifest as abdominal tenderness, distention, decreased bowel sounds, guarding, rebound tenderness, a temperature greater than 38 °C, and clinical signs of shock in 25% of patients.

In general, diagnostic laboratory studies are disappointing, the exception being diagnostic peritoneal lavage, which uniformly returns serosanguineous fluid.[57,58] A leukocytosis of 10,000 to 30,000/mm^3 with a leftward shift is often present. Evaluation for a hypercoagulable state should be made if the diagnosis is suspected. Radiographs, whether plain or with contrast, rarely assist in the diagnostic process. CT has established the diagnosis in 90% of cases by demonstrating thrombus directly.[1] Small bowel follow-through findings may include marked thickening of the bowel wall and valvulae conniventes because of congestion and edema, separation of loops caused by mesenteric thickening, a long transition zone between involved and uninvolved bowel with progressive narrowing of the lumen by thickened wall, and thumbprints. Angiographic findings may include the demonstration of a thrombus in the superior mesenteric vein with partial or complete occlusion, failure to visualize the superior mesenteric or portal vein, slow or absent filling of mesenteric veins, arterial spasm, failure of arterial arcades to empty, and a prolonged blush in the involved segment.[7] Diagnosis frequently is made at the time of operation.

Treatment of mesenteric venous thrombosis includes fluid resuscitation, antibiotics, and prompt heparinization.[1] The development of an acute abdomen requires operative intervention. Operative findings include the presence of congested, cyanotic, bluish-black, edematous bowel with arterial pulsations present in the mesentery. Thrombosed veins may be clearly visible, and sectioning across the mesentery shows thrombus extruding from the mesenteric veins and brisk arterial bleeding. Occasionally, a venous thrombectomy is helpful. If a long segment of bowel is involved and there is complete thrombosis of the superior mesenteric vein with possible extension to the portal vein, venous thrombectomy is indicated. A second-look operation should be performed, at which time a better assessment of the extent of nonviable bowel is made. Heparin therapy is instituted.[7] For short segments of bowel involvement, thrombectomy would not appear to be indicated. A wide resection of involved bowel is recommended with a primary end-to-end anastomosis. If there is doubt regarding the wisdom of restoring intestinal continuity, the bowel can be brought to the surface as a stoma or reexamined at a "second look." Anticoagulant therapy with heparin is indicated and should be initiated during or immediately after operation,[1,59,60] and anticoagulation therapy should be continued for several months postoperatively unless specifically contraindicated by other associated diseases. Following resection, about half of the patients experience recurrence if anticoagulants are not administered, and of those with recurrence, approximately 50% are found to have an associated deep venous thrombosis or pulmonary embolus.[61] In the study cited, treatment with anticoagulants dramatically decreased mortality; without operation and without anticoagulant therapy, the natural history of mesenteric venous thrombosis resulted in a 95% mortality rate; with operation but without anticoagulant therapy, the mortality rate was 65%; and with operation, followed by immediate anticoagulant therapy, the mortality rate was 35%.[61]

Rhee et al[62] evaluated the outcome of 72 patients with mesenteric venous thrombosis—53 acute and 19 chronic. A laparotomy was performed in 34 patients, 31 undergoing bowel resection and 1 an unsuccessful mesenteric venous thrombectomy. Mesenteric venous thrombosis recurred in 36%. The 30-day mortality rate was 27%. The long-term survival of patients with acute mesenteric venous thrombosis was worse than for chronic disease (36 vs. 83% at 3 years).

Divino et al[63] analyzed nine patients treated surgically for mesenteric venous thrombosis. The most common presenting symptom was abdominal pain with bloody diarrhea in three patients; preoperative diagnosis of mesenteric vein thrombosis was suspected in two. Radiologic tests included plain X-rays, CT, and ultrasound. The time to operation ranged from 3 hours to 7 days after admission. All patients underwent resection of infarcted bowel with primary anastomosis and immediate postoperative anticoagulation. No patient underwent a second-look operation. The postoperative morbidity and mortality rates were 55 and 11%, respectively.

An algorithm outlining a possible approach to the management of mesenteric ischemia was published by Bradbury et al (▶ Fig. 30.6).[1]

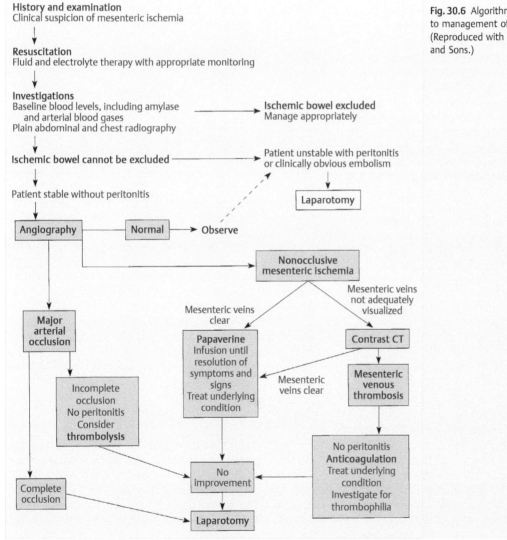

Fig. 30.6 Algorithm outlining possible approach to management of mesenteric ischemia.[1] (Reproduced with permission from John Wiley and Sons.)

30.5.5 Chronic Mesenteric Vascular Disease

A detailed account of chronic mesenteric vascular disease or "intestinal angina" is beyond the scope of this text, and the reader is referred to textbooks of vascular surgery. However, any discussion of acute mesenteric vascular disease would be incomplete without a brief overview of the salient points of chronic mesenteric vascular disease.

Mesenteric angina is poorly understood partly due to problems involved in diagnosing and defining the disease as a clinical syndrome. The disease is difficult to induce experimentally because the rich mesenteric collateral circulation has made it difficult to develop a satisfactory animal model. Diagnosis is further complicated by the lack of correlation between arteriographic findings and clinical symptoms. Finally, clinical studies on this disease are remarkably limited, particularly when compared with the wealth of material available on vascular disease involving other organs or organ systems.

Croft et al[64] reviewed autopsy material on 203 patients and tried to correlate arteriographic findings with clinical symptoms and autopsy findings. Critical stenosis on two of three vessels was seen in only four of their patients, and correlation with symptoms was not found. Other researchers have reported that complaints of intestinal angina precede acute intestinal infarction in a sizable percentage of cases. Kwaan and Connolly[47] noted that they found conspicuous warning signs present for several months in all 25 patients operated on for acute intestinal infarction.

The classic triad of symptoms is postprandial pain, fear of eating, and involuntary weight loss. The most consistent symptom complex involves the presence of postprandial pain in association with weight loss and malabsorption. The postprandial pain often is associated with "food fear," causing the patient to refuse to eat because of the fear of subsequent pain. The pain, which is directly related to eating, is experienced soon after a meal and lasts for several hours. Because patients with chronic mesenteric vascular disease frequently are cachectic in appearance, they sometimes are evaluated for the presence of widespread malignancy rather than vascular disease. Color flow duplex scanning is increasingly used as the first-line investigation of patients suspected of having mesenteric ischemia. When an arteriogram is performed, high-grade stenosis or complete occlusion of three mesenteric vessels suggests that significant ischemic disease may be present. No relationship has been found between the loss of intestinal absorptive function and the degree of reduced flow seen on angiography.[65] Because of the prevalence of asymptomatic arterial stenosis, the diagnosis is difficult and the indications for surgery are unclear. In general, surgery should be considered when a patient has a clinical presentation that is compatible with intestinal ischemia, arteriographic evidence of critical stenosis in two of three vessels, and no plausible explanation for the abdominal pain.

A patient with intestinal angina and weight loss, in whom other causes have been excluded, and in whom angiography shows occlusive disease of at least two of three major visceral arteries, should be considered for revascularization. Few patients meet these criteria. Surgical options for reconstruction include bypass grafting, endarterectomy, and reimplantation. Bypass grafting has been the preferred procedure,[48,66] with most authors recommending prosthetic grafts over autogenous vein grafts. Prosthetic grafts have less tendency for kinking when used between the aorta and the mobile SMA. They also are more readily available than vein grafts. Total revascularization of all affected vessels is preferred to single-vessel revascularization, since this may decrease the incidence of late recurrence.[48,67,68] Because of the presence of significant atherosclerotic disease in the adjacent aorta, reimplantation is seldom performed.

Illuminati et al[69] reported on 11 patients who underwent revascularization of 11 digestive arteries for symptomatic chronic mesenteric occlusive disease. Eleven superior mesenteric arteries and 1 celiac axis were revascularized. The revascularization techniques included retrograde bypass grafting in seven cases, antegrade bypass grafting in two, percutaneous arterial angioplasty in one, and arterial reimplantation in one case. There was no operative mortality. Cumulative survival rate was 88.9% at 36 months. Primary patency rate was 90% at 36 months. The symptom-free rate was 90% at 36 months. They found that direct reimplantation and antegrade and retrograde bypass grafting all allowed good midterm results: the choice of the optimal method depends on the anatomic and general patient's status. Angioplasty alone yields poor results and should be limited to patients at poor risk for operation.

Leke et al[70] reported their experience with a tailored surgical approach of 16 patients operated on for chronic mesenteric ischemia. The patients ranged in age from 32 to 80 years and 75% of patients were females. The most common preoperative complaints were postprandial abdominal pain and weight loss. Revascularization was tailored to the arterial anatomy and included bypass to the SMA alone (eight), bypass to the celiac artery and SMA (six), SMA reimplantation onto the aorta (one), SMA/IMA reimplantation (one), and transaortic endarterectomy of the celiac artery/SMA (one). There was one perioperative death (mortality 5.6%). Follow-up duplex scans at a mean of 34 months showed no graft thromboses.

Some early success has been reported following angioplasty for chronic mesenteric vascular disease.[71,72,73] Success rates of 70 to 100% have been reported with recurrence rates of 10 to 50% within 4 to 28 months.[1] If the patient's symptoms later recur following angioplasty, the history of having undergone successful angioplasty suggests that the patient may expect a favorable result from surgical reconstruction.

Kasirajan et al[74] evaluated the efficacy of percutaneous angioplasty and stenting in comparison with traditional open surgical revascularization for the treatment of chronic mesenteric ischemia. Although the results of percutaneous angioplasty and stenting and open surgery were similar with respect to morbidity, death, and recurrent stenosis, percutaneous angioplasty and stenting was associated with a significantly higher incidence of recurrent symptoms and thus their suggestion that open surgery should be preferentially offered to patients deemed fit for open revascularization.

Results of Therapy

The prognosis for mesenteric infarction is extraordinarily grave, and this disease is associated with mortality rates that are among the highest of any disease in the surgical literature. ▶ Table 30.2 summarizes the poor prognosis of patients with mesenteric infarction; the range in mortality is from 24 to 90%. The seemingly hopeless prognosis reflects the late presentation and diagnosis for most patients.[75,76,77,78]

Table 30.2 Mesenteric infarction mortality rates

Author(s)	Type of ischemia	No. of patients	Mortality rate (%)
Guttormson and Bubrick[75]	IC	20	65
Levy et al[76]	All	45	
Brewster et al[77,a]	All	24	24
Parish et al[78]	IC	16	25
Inderbitzi et al[79]	All	100	62
	SMA e	60	68
	SMA t	15	50
	NOMI	6	90
	MVT	19	67
Longo et al[80]	NOMI, IC	31	30
Sales et al[44]	All	29	29
Rhee et al[62]	MVT	31	34
Kaleya and Boley[7]	All	65	27
	SMA e	23	45
	SMA t	6	39
	NOMI	26	33
	MVT	6	46
Ward et al[53]	NOMI	29	33
Longo et al[81]	IC	19	31
Klempnauer et al[82]	All	90	89
	SMA e	21	66
	SMA t	27	76
	NOMI	12	81
	MVT	30	83
Divino et al[63]	MVT	9	27
Neri et al[55]	NOMI	73	11
Edwards et al[83]	SMA e + t, IC	76	86
Scharff et al[84]	IC	129	29
Kasirajan et al[85]	SMA e	20	60
	SMA t	55	56
	NOMI	6	38
	MVT	6	33
	Volvulus	3	33
	Hernia	8	13
Schoots et al[86,b]	SMA e	705	79
	SMA t	980	83
	MVT	394	45
	NOMI	556	78

Abbreviations: IC, ischemic colitis; MVT, mesenteric venous thrombosis; NOMI, nonocclusive mesenteric insufficiency; SMA e, superior mesenteric artery embolus; SMA t, superior mesenteric artery thrombosis.
[a]All patients following aortic reconstruction.
[b]Review of literature.

Inderbitzi et al[79] reported that the outcome of mesenteric ische-mia varies with the pathology responsible; the mortality rate is reported as 50% in patients with embolic arterial occlusion, 95% in those with thrombotic arterial occlusion, 67% in those with nonocclusive mesenteric ischemia, and 30% in those with mesen-teric thrombosis. Despite this, salvage is possible in some pa-tients, particularly those who are younger and potentially more vigorous and for whom survival with either minimal residual small bowel or home hyperalimentation may be feasible.[80,81]

Klempnauer et al[82] treated 90 patients with acute mesenteric ischemia by vascular reconstruction, bowel resection, or both. The overall mortality rate was 66%. The 2- and 5-year survival rates were 70 and 90%, respectively, and mortality was related to cardiovascular comorbidity and malignant disease. Twenty percent of patients suffered from the short bowel syndrome.

Levy et al[76] conducted a retrospective analysis of 92 patients with acute mesenteric ischemia. In the early part of their re-view when 17 patients were treated with resection only, the mortality rate was 82%. Improved results were documented when, in addition to resection, revascularization, second-look operations, and delayed anastomosis were used (overall mor-tality, 24%). Gentile et al[66] performed 29 bypasses to only the SMA in 26 patients, with 3 perioperative deaths (10%). Graft pa-tency and survival rates at 4 years were 89 and 82%, respec-tively. Symptomatic improvement was reported in all patients available for follow-up.

Edwards et al[83] examined trends in management and associ-ated outcomes in 76 patients treated for acute mesenteric is-chemia. At presentation, 64% demonstrated peritonitis and 30% exhibited hypotension. The interval from symptoms onset to treatment exceeded 24 hours in 63% of cases. Etiology was mes-enteric thrombosis in 58% of patients and embolism in 42% of patients. Thirty-five patients (46%) had prior conditions placing them at high risk for the development of acute mesenteric is-chemia including chronic mesenteric ischemia ($n = 26$) and in-adequately anticoagulated chronic atrial fibrillation ($n = 9$). Surgical management consisted of exploration alone in 16 pa-tients, bowel resection alone in 18 patients, and revasculariza-tion in 43 patients, including 28 who required concomitant bowel resection. Overall, intestinal necrosis was present in 81% of cases. Perioperative mortality was 62% and long-term paren-teral nutrition was required in 31% of survivors. Peritonitis (odds ratio = 9.4) and bowel necrosis (odds ratio = 10.4) at pre-sentation were independent predictors of death or survival de-pendent upon TPN (total parenteral nutrition).[84]

Kasirajan et al[85] undertook a study to identify predictors of in-hospital death and length of stay in 107 patients diagnosed with acute bowel gangrene. Among the baseline factors that had a significant univariable association with mortality (51%) were age, symptom duration, preoperative and postoperative pH and lactic acid, history of hypertension, and renal failure. Symptom duration and history of hypertension were independ-ent risk factors for mortality. Longer length of stay was invaria-bly associated with symptom duration, systemic acidosis, vascular etiology, amount of resected bowel, and need for sec-ond-look procedures. The presence of multiple risk factors pre-dictive of a high mortality rate may aid more realistic decision making for physicians, patients, and family members.

There are large differences in prognosis after acute mesenter-ic ischemia depending on etiology. Schoots et al[86] analyzed the published data on survival following acute mesenteric ischemia over the past four decades in relation to disease etiology and mode of treatment. They conducted a systematic review of the available literature from 1966 to 2002 and performed quantita-tive analysis of data derived from 45 observational studies con-taining 3,692 patients with acute mesenteric ischemia. They showed that the prognosis after acute mesenteric venous thrombosis is better than that following acute arterial mesen-teric ischemia, the prognosis after mesenteric arterial embolism is better than that after arterial thrombosis or nonocclusive is-chemia, the mortality rate following surgical treatment of arte-rial embolism and venous thrombosis (54.1 and 32.1%, respectively) is less than that after surgery for arterial thrombo-sis and nonocclusive ischemia (77.4 and 72.7%, respectively), and the overall survival after acute mesenteric ischemia has im-proved over the past four decades but overall is still only 28.4%. Surgical treatment of arterial embolism has improved outcome, whereas the mortality rate following surgery for arterial throm-bosis and nonocclusive ischemia remains poor.

Johnston et al[48] reviewed the results of 21 patients who underwent arterial bypass grafts for the treatment of chronic ischemia. There were no intraoperative deaths. Survival at 1 year was 100%, 86% at 3 years, and 79% at 5 years. During fol-low-up, graft thrombosis occurred in three patients. Of the pa-tients who underwent only a single SMA or celiac bypass, two of five died of bowel infarction; only 1 of 16 patients who underwent both celiac and SMA bypass had to undergo a re-peat procedure because of graft occlusion. The authors' review of the literature, which encompassed eight other reports, re-vealed operative mortality rates ranging from 0 to 12%. In a series of 58 patients, McAfee et al[68] reported a 5-year survival rate of 73% for three-vessel repairs, 57% for two-vessel repairs, and 0% for one-vessel repair.

30.5.6 Ischemic Colitis

Colonic ischemia is the most common form of ischemic injury to the gut. It is usually focal, nonocclusive, and commonly involves a "watershed" area, typically the splenic flexure. A precipitating cause is found in fewer than 20% of patients. The syndrome of is-chemic colitis has been defined only relatively recently. In 1963, Boley et al[87] described a reversible component to colonic ische-mia, and 3 years later Marston et al[88] reported on the three stages of ischemic colitis and described the natural history of the disease. The incidence of ischemic colitis in general populations ranged from 4.5 to 44 cases per 100,000 person-years.[89] The risk was increased twofold to fourfold by either prevalent irritable bowel syndrome (IBS) or chronic obstructive pulmonary disease. Most cases occur between the sixth and ninth decades of life, with men slightly more prone to this disease than women.[90] However, other investigators found no significant sex predilec-tion, while still others found the risk increased in females and in persons aged 65 years and older.[7,89]

Etiology

Ischemic colitis is usually not associated with major vascular occlusion. The colon has a generous overlapping blood sup-ply, with contributions from the SMA, IMA, and hypogastric arteries. Two regions that are believed to be anatomically vulnerable to ischemic disease are "Griffith's point," at the splenic flexure corresponding to the junction of the SMA (left branch of middle colic) and the IMA (ascending branch of left colon), and "Sudeck's critical point," corresponding to the junction of the IMA (last sigmoid branch) and hypogastric systems. A watershed phenomenon has been described to explain the vulnerability of these points, since perfusion between the overlapping circulations may be inadequate during periods of hemodynamic insult. Because of the vulnerability of the colon at the sigmoid and splenic flexure, these areas have historically been considered to be the most frequent sites of clinical ischemic colitis. The sigmoid site is probably not a clinically significant factor.

Occlusive events and low-flow states both have been associated with ischemic injury to the colon. The severity of ischemic colitis is influenced by several factors, including the duration of the decrease in blood flow, the caliber of occluded vessel, the rapidity of onset of ischemia, the metabolic requirements of the affected bowel, the presence of associated conditions such as colonic distention, the adequacy of collateral circulation, and the concentration and virulence of colonic bacteria.[91] Colonic bacteria become a factor in the severity of the disease once the mucosal barrier has been compromised. For this reason, colonic ischemia may be less severe when it occurs postoperatively in patients who have undergone preoperative mechanical and antibiotic bowel cleansing.

Finally, distention of the involved colon segment is of importance because distention of the colonic lumen will compromise the transmural blood flow to that segment.[92]

A number of predisposing factors that are associated with the development of ischemic colitis have been defined (Box 30.1).[93] In the largest series of patients with ischemic colitis studied for coagulation defects in the United States, the prevalence of clotting disorders was 28%, higher than that in the general population (8.4%).[94] Koutroubakis et al[95] investigated the role of acquired and hereditary thrombotic risk factors in patients with a definite diagnosis of colon ischemia. The prevalence of antiphospholipid antibodies was significantly higher in patients with colon ischemia compared with inflammatory and healthy controls (19.4 vs. 0% and 1.9%). Among genetic factors, only factor V Leiden was significantly associated with colon ischemia (22.2 vs. 0% and 3.8%). A combination of thrombophilic disorders was found in 25% of the cases. A comprehensive thrombophilic screening in colon ischemia revealed a congenital or acquired thrombophilic state in 72% of patients. This may represent evidence supporting the possible role of acquired and hereditary thrombotic risk factors in the pathogenesis of ischemic colitis.[95] Low plasma protein Z levels may play a role in the disease development in some cases with ischemic colitis. Protein Z deficiency was found in patients' cases with ischemic colitis (18.2%) compared to diverticulitis (7.7%) and controls (3.0%).[96]

Colonic ischemia: etiologic factors[93]

- Idiopathic (spontaneous)
- Major vascular occlusion
  - Trauma
  - Thrombosis, embolization of mesenteric arteries
  - Arterial embolus
  - Cholesterol embolus
  - Aortography
  - Colectomy with inferior mesenteric artery ligation
  - Midgut ischemia
  - Post-abdominal aortic reconstruction
  - Mesenteric venous thrombosis
    - Hypercoagulable states
    - Portal hypertension
    - Pancreatitis
- Small vessel disease
  - Diabetes mellitus
  - Rheumatoid arthritis
  - Amyloidosis
  - Radiation injury
  - Systemic vasculitis disorders
    - Systemic lupus erythematosus
    - Polyarteritis nodosa
    - Allergic granulomatosis
    - Scleroderma
    - Behçet's syndrome
    - Takayasu's arteritis
    - Thromboangiitis obliterans
    - Buerger's disease
- Shock
  - Cardiac failure
  - Hypovolemia
  - Sepsis
  - Neurogenic insult
  - Anaphylaxis
- Medications
  - Digitalis preparations
  - Diuretics
  - Catecholamines
  - Estrogens
  - Danazol
  - Gold
  - Nonsteroidal anti-inflammatory drugs
  - Neuroleptics
- Colonic obstruction
  - Colon carcinoma
  - Adhesions
  - Stricture
  - Diverticular disease
  - Rectal prolapse
  - Fecal impaction
  - Volvulus
  - Strangulated hernia
  - Pseudo-obstruction
- Hematologic disorders
  - Sickle-cell disease
  - Protein C deficiency
  - Protein S deficiency
  - Antithrombin III deficiency
- Cocaine abuse
- Long-distance running

A host of drugs have reportedly been responsible for the development of ischemic colitis. Acute ischemic colitis has also been caused by an allergy to amoxicillin.[97] The damage to the gut seemed to occur as a result of the hypotension suffered during an anaphylactic episode. A case of ischemic colitis possibly linked to the use of a weight loss drug phentermine has been reported.[98] Ischemic colitis has reportedly been associated with paclitaxel and carboplatin chemotherapy.[99,100]

The Food and Drug Administration (FDA) MedWatch system received 20 spontaneous reports of ischemic colitis associated with the use of tegaserod (Zelnorm), an agent used for the short-term treatment of constipation-predominant IBS in women.[101] The manufacturer of the drug states that in over 11,600 patients using tegaserod with a total of 3,456 patient-years of exposure, no case of ischemic colitis was reported. They further note that patients with IBS are approximately three to four times as likely to receive a diagnosis of ischemic colitis as are patients without IBS. They also report that during postmarketing surveillance, 21 cases of ischemic colitis were reported worldwide. On the basis of worldwide use of tegaserod, a postmarketing incidence of seven cases of ischemic colitis for 100,000 patient-years can be calculated. This approximates the incidence of ischemic colitis in the general population (7–47 cases per 100,000 patient-years) and significantly lower than that in the population of patients with IBS (43–179 cases per 100,000 patient-years). Tegaserod therapy should be reserved for specific patients (women with IBS and constipation) who have more moderate to severe symptoms.[102] The duration of treatment should not exceed 12 weeks and therapy should be stopped after 4 weeks if there has been no response. Patients should be warned that they may experience potentially serious diarrhea or rarely intestinal ischemia. They should be advised to seek prompt medical attention if serious diarrhea, lightheadedness, or postural symptoms develop during treatment. The drug should be immediately stopped if rectal bleeding or new or worsening abdominal pain develops.

Frossard et al[103] reported two cases of ischemic colitis in young women attributed to a high level of circulating estrogens due to pregnancy in the first case and the second due to oral contraceptive medication. Ischemic colitis has been reported with alosetron, a potent and selective serotonin antagonist that is used to treat diarrhea-predominant IBS.[104] Meloxicam used to treat osteoarthritis has reportedly been a cause of ischemic colitis.[105]

Cocaine use can result in visceral infarction, intestinal ischemia, and GI tract perforation. Linder et al[106] reported cocaine-associated colonic ischemia in three patients, and including theirs, 28 cases have been reported in the literature. Cocaine is a potentially life-threatening cause of ischemic colitis.

Dowd et al[107] reported four cases linking ischemic colitis and orally administered nasal decongestants containing pseudoephedrine. On colonoscopy, all four patients had colitis primarily affecting the splenic flexure in the anatomical watershed area. Colonoscopic biopsies were consistent with ischemic injury. All cases responded to abstinence from pseudoephedrine and medical supportive therapy. None had a relapse since discontinuing the pseudoephedrine (8–12 months). The vasoconstrictive action of pseudoephedrine may predispose susceptible patients to develop ischemic colitis in the watershed area of the splenic flexure. Knudsen et al[108] reported on the development of eight serious cases of ischemic colitis in patients with migraine treated with sumatriptan.

To the already long list of conditions that predispose to intestinal ischemia, operative procedures such as cardiac bypass and gynecologic operations as well as colonoscopy and barium enema should be added.[2] Mesenteric colitis following colonoscopy has been reported.[109] Transient ischemic colitis following an airplane flight as the only predisposing factor has been reported.[110] Ischemic colitis has been reported in patients with strict dieting.[111] Ischemic colitis has been associated with herbal product ingestion.[112]

Dee et al[113] found that 3.1% of patients developed ischemia of the small or large bowel or both within 20 days after renal transplantation and 54.5% died as a result. The most prominent segment involved was the terminal ileum and ascending colon. Right colon involvement is associated with severe forms of ischemic colitis and occurs frequently in patients with chronic renal failure requiring hemodialysis.[114]

A case of ischemic colitis associated with pheochromocytoma has been reported.[115] Mesenteric inflammatory veno-occlusive disease is a rare cause of mesenteric ischemia that is diagnosed by histologic examination of the operative specimen. Complete resolution of the process following resection confirms a relatively benign course of this disease.[116]

Ischemic colitis is a rare but serious consequence of long-distance running.[117] Physiologic shunting due to splanchnic vasoconstriction, intravascular volume depletion due to chronic dehydration, and possibly some element of hypercoagulability due to secondary polycythemia may have been causative factors. Ischemic colitis associated with the use of electrical muscle stimulation device exercise equipment has been reported.[118] Ischemic colitis has been reported after flexible endoscopy in patients with connective tissue disorders,[119,120] and the hemolytic uremic syndrome.[121]

Walker et al[122] sought predictors of colon ischemia in a group of 700 persons at least 20 years old with presumed colon ischemia and 6,440 controls. Patients with colon ischemia were nearly three times as likely to have IBS as controls. A history of nonspecific colitis, lower GI hemorrhage, systemic rheumatologic disorders, ischemic heart disease in the preceding 6 months, and abdominal surgery in the past month were also much more common in colon ischemia cases than controls. Use of a drug to treat diarrhea was strongly associated with risk. The most prevalent risk factor for colon ischemia was the use of drugs with the side effect of constipation, found in one-third of cases and one in nine controls. Cases had seen physicians, particularly gastroenterologists, much more commonly in the preceding 6 months than had controls. They concluded that clinically evident colon ischemia arose preferentially in persons with prior abdominal symptoms, many of whom carried a diagnosis of IBS. Drugs that reduce bowel motility may constitute a widespread and potentially avoidable risk factor. The frequency of a preceding doctor visit, without a specific diagnosis, suggested that colon ischemia might have a prolonged subacute presentation.

Classification

The three degrees of severity of ischemic colitis as classified by Marston et al[88] include transient ischemia, ischemic stricture as

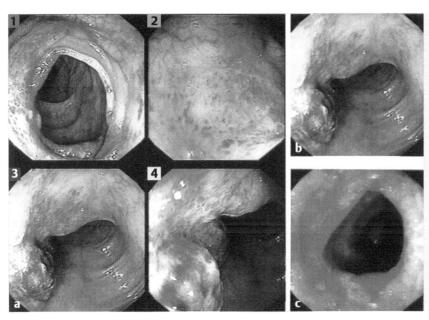

Fig. 30.7 (a) Acute, mild stage characterized by hyperemia, edema, and petechiae. 1: mass, mid-transverse colon; 2: mass, mid-transverse colon; 3: mass, mid-ascending colon; 4: mass, mid-ascending colon. **(b)** Acute stage with edema and submucosal hemorrhage. **(c)** Subacute stage consisting of edema, exudation, and ulceration. (These images are provided courtesy of David Morowitz, MD.)

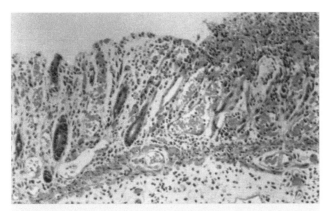

Fig. 30.8 Microscopic section of transient ischemic colitis showing sloughing and infiltration of the mucosa.

a late sequela of a partial-thickness injury, and the gangrenous form. Gangrenous injury is seen in 15 to 20% of cases. Of the 80 to 85% of nongangrenous cases, most are transient and reversible. Chronic damage in the form of persistent segmental colitis occurs in 20 to 25% and strictures in 10 to 15% of cases.[93]

The transient form is characterized by its reversibility and is associated with mucosal edema, congestion, superficial ulcerations, and petechiae (▶ Fig. 30.7). Histologically, the changes are confined predominantly to the mucosa and submucosa and consist of an intense inflammatory reaction with superficial sloughing of the mucosa, submucosal hemorrhage, and edema (▶ Fig. 30.8). Multiple superficial ulcerations may develop. Gradually, the blood is resorbed, and the edema resolves with complete structural and functional recovery in 1 to 2 weeks. Characteristic radiographic findings are either thumbprinting caused by submucosal hemorrhage or pseudotumors that reflect distortion of the bowel lumen by the same process (▶ Fig. 30.9). Reoperative processes can return these changes to normal if perfusion is restored at this stage. On occasion, patchy areas of acute ischemic colitis may be found on screening colonoscopy on many asymptomatic patients (▶ Fig. 30.10a–c). The

ischemic stricture represents a partial-thickness injury that involves the mucosa and muscular layers and results in fibrosis and narrowing of the lumen over a period of weeks to months. Endoscopically, the stricture is characterized by fixed narrowing of the lumen and a mucosa that is replaced by granulation tissue (▶ Fig. 30.11). Histologically, marked fibrosis is seen within the muscularis, the mucosa is replaced by granulation tissue, and hemosiderin-laden macrophages are prevalent (▶ Fig. 30.12). On barium enema, the stricture appears as an area of irreversible narrowing of the lumen. Dilatation proximal to the stricture suggests that the stricture may be significant, while the presence of a simple asymptomatic stricture may not be of clinical importance (▶ Fig. 30.13).

Gangrenous ischemic colitis is characterized by full-thickness necrosis and infarction. Gross examination reveals the segment to be dilated with patchy or confluent gray-green or black discoloration (▶ Fig. 30.14). Histologic sections reveal intense inflammation with transmural necrosis (▶ Fig. 30.15). Contrast studies should be avoided in the presence of suspected gangrenous changes. Patients with gangrenous change will go on to perforation, sepsis, and death unless surgical intervention is undertaken promptly.

Despite similarities in the initial presentation of most episodes of colonic ischemia, the outcome of any single event cannot be predicted at its onset unless the initial physical findings indicate an intra-abdominal catastrophe. The clinical spectrum of colonic ischemia along with the relative frequencies of each type as reported by Brandt and Boley[123] is shown in ▶ Fig. 30.16.

Patterns of Involvement

The reported anatomic site of involvement of ischemic colitis has varied considerably from series to series. Historically, ischemic colitis has been described as usually involving, or at least being most severe, near the splenic flexure where the arterial supply is a watershed area between the territories of the SMA and IMA. Numerous reports support this pattern of involvement.[124,125,126] In a review of 1,024 patients in the literature, Reeders et al[90] found the incidence to be as follows: right colon,

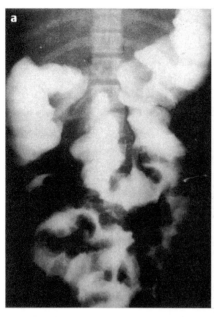
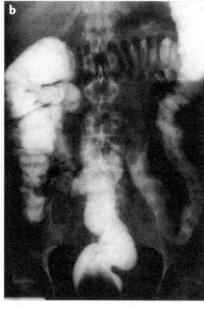

Fig. 30.9 **(a)** X-ray film of patient with ischemic colitis with thumbprinting seen in sigmoid colon. **(b)** X-ray film of patient with ischemic colitis segment showing pseudotumor formation in descending colon and sigmoid.

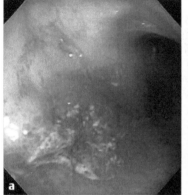
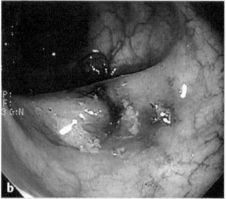
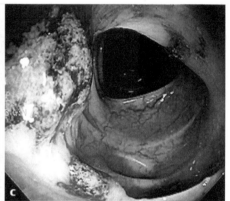

Fig. 30.10 **(a)** Mild ischemic colopathy. **(b)** Isolated ischemic patch. **(c)** More dramatic patchy acute ischemic colitis.

8%; transverse colon, 15%; splenic flexure, 23%; descending colon, 27%; and sigmoid colon, 23%. Rectal ischemia has been described in 4% of the cases in the above review, and only rarely does it progress to gangrene.[127] A different pattern was found by Guttormson and Bubrick,[75] who noted that ischemic disease can occur on the right side with equal or greater frequency, despite the richer blood supply to this segment of colon. Longo et al[80] also reported in their series that the anatomic distribution of disease was different than that usually reported with ischemic colitis: right colon, 46%; splenic flexure, 4%; descending colon, 7%; rectosigmoid, 40%; and pancolitis, 8%. Others have also found a predilection for the right side of the colon.[128]

Clinical Manifestations

The presentation of this disease is variable. It frequently occurs in the elderly and debilitated patient, often in association with severe comorbid disease. The medical diseases found most frequently by Longo et al[80] were cardiovascular, 55%; diabetes mellitus, 23%; pulmonary, 21%; renal failure, 6%; and hematologic, 6%. The precipitating factors may not be evident. The outcome rests on numerous factors, including severity, extent, and rapidity of the ischemic insult in addition to the therapy given.[93]

The symptoms of ischemic colitis include the sudden onset of crampy abdominal pain, usually on the left side if the disease involves the left side of the colon. There may be bloody diarrhea and often fever and abdominal distention. Blood loss is usually minimal. An urge to defecate may accompany the pain. Anorexia, nausea, and vomiting secondary to associated ileus may be present. Newman and Cooper[129] compared the incidence and clinical characteristics of lower GI bleeding due to ischemic colitis with those of lower GI bleeding of other causes. Of 124 patients with lower GI bleeding, 24 cases were due to ischemic colitis, 62 to diverticulosis, 11 to inflammatory bowel disease, and 27 to other causes. The average age of patients in each group was 65.5, 76.5, 40.5, and 77.5 years, respectively. Patients with ischemic colitis were statistically younger than those with diverticular bleeding and others. The three patients with ischemic colitis underwent blood transfusion, while 23 with diverticulosis, 15 others, and none with IBD received blood. Three patients with ischemic colitis and one patient from the other group died. More women[75] than

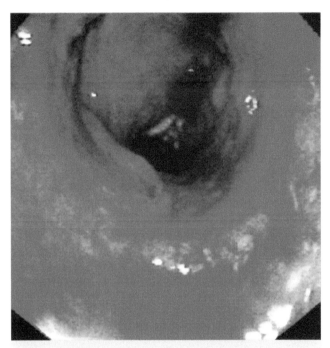

Fig. 30.11 Chronic stage with mucosal granularity, decreased haustration, and stricture.

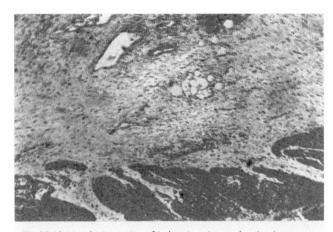

Fig. 30.12 Histologic section of ischemic stricture showing intense fibrosis.

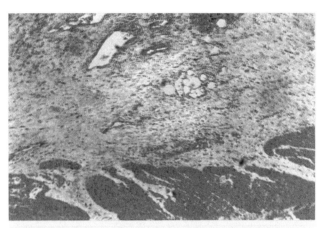

Fig. 30.13 X-ray film showing ischemic stricture of junction of descending and sigmoid colon.

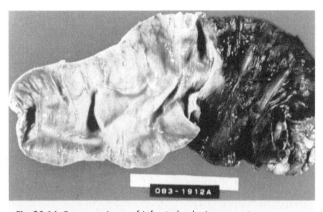

Fig. 30.14 Gross specimen of infarcted colonic segment.

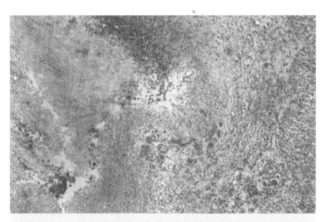

Fig. 30.15 Histologic section of infarcted segment of colon showing intense full-thickness inflammatory changes and necrosis.

men[49] had lower GI bleeding—in total and within each group. Of women with lower GI bleeding, many more with ischemic colitis (44.4%) than with diverticulosis (3.0%), IBD (0%), or others (5.6%) were taking estrogen. In their series, ischemic colitis was the second most common cause of lower GI bleeding.

Ardigo et al[130] reported two cases of spontaneous anal passage of a large bowel "cast" caused by acute ischemic injury. Their literature review revealed six cases of passage of a large bowel cast. In the eight total patients, infarcted muscularis propria was found in seven patients, five patients had a diversion procedure, and seven survived.

Abdominal examination may reveal mild distention and varying degrees of tenderness that usually correspond to the site of the ischemic colon. Rectal examination reveals stools positive for occult blood. Patients with the gangrenous variety may exhibit the picture of an abdominal catastrophe with signs of sepsis and shock. For patients hospitalized with another critical illness, a nonresolving ileus might raise the suspicion of an ischemic colitis.

Ullery et al[131] reviewed charts of 100 patients with an ICD-9 code for mesenteric or intestinal ischemia. Compared to patients with mesenteric ischemia, those with colonic ischemia were older (61 vs. 77 years), were more likely to present with GI bleeding (11 vs. 90%), and were less likely to report abdominal pain as

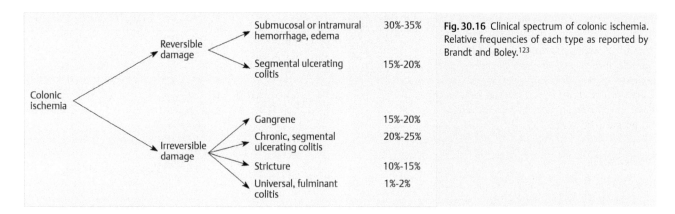

Fig. 30.16 Clinical spectrum of colonic ischemia. Relative frequencies of each type as reported by Brandt and Boley.[123]

their primary complaint (89 vs. 10%), or to receive a correct emergency department diagnosis (75 vs. 9%). Preventza et al[132] investigated the demographics, etiology, clinical features, and prognosis of ischemic colitis in 39 young adults (<50 years of age). The mean age at diagnosis was 38 years; the female-to-male ratio was 1:8. Fifty-two percent of women were using oral contraceptives at the time of diagnosis. Other potential associations identified were vascular thromboembolism (4 of 39), vasoactive drugs (4 of 39), hypovolemia (4 of 39), and vasculitis (2 of 39); 19 patients (49%) had no identifiable predisposing factors.

Dominant presenting symptoms were abdominal pain (77%), bloody diarrhea (54%), and hematochezia (51%). Most patients were diagnosed at colonoscopy, and most disease was left sided. Twenty-nine patients were successfully managed with intravenous fluids, broad-spectrum antibiotics, and bowel rest; 10 patients required operation. There was one disease-related death in the operative group.

Diagnosis

Unfortunately, there are no specific diagnostic tests. Patients usually exhibit leukocytosis. Abdominal series may reveal thickened bowel, suggest thumbprinting, or exhibit a distended colon. In a rare circumstance, toxic megacolon may supervene.[133] A plain radiograph that demonstrates free air secondary to perforation, air within the bowel wall, or portal venous gas signifies colonic infarction and mandates emergency laparotomy. CT demonstrates only nonspecific findings, such as a thickened bowel wall.[134] Ultrasonography has been reported to aid in the diagnosis but is not widely used.[135]

There are no reliable serum markers of intestinal viability. Lange and Jackel[136] reported that a raised serum lactate concentration is the best marker for mesenteric ischemia. In a study of 85 patients with acute abdominal symptoms, the authors found that a raised plasma lactate concentration was always a sign of a life-threatening condition and usually indicated the need for an emergency operation. As a marker of mesenteric ischemia, its sensitivity was 100% and its specificity was 42%.

In the past, diagnosis was made by barium enema or exploratory laparotomy, but in recent years colonoscopy has been used with increased accuracy.[75,137] Hemorrhagic nodules seen at colonoscopy represent bleeding into the submucosa. Sequential colonoscopies may confirm the diagnosis of colonic ischemia and help ascertain the outcome of the ischemic injury. The initial examination should be performed early because thumbprinting

dissipates within days as the submucosal hemorrhages are either absorbed or evacuated into the colon lumen when the overlying mucosa ulcerates and sloughs. If ischemic colitis is not demonstrated, colonoscopy can help identify other forms of inflammatory bowel disease or rule out a malignancy. Areas of gray and green or black mucosa and submucosa are seen in patients with transmural infarction. Biopsy may be helpful in differentiating the disease from inflammatory processes, such as granulomatous colitis or atypical ulcerative colitis. Histologic evidence of mucosal infarction or ghost cells is pathognomonic of ischemia but is rare.[93] Biopsies usually display nonspecific inflammatory changes. Other changes include vascular congestion, damage in the superficial half of the mucosa, loss of mucin and surface epithelial cells, and degeneration of normal crypt architecture. In the stricture phase, fibrosis dominates the biopsy picture.

The diagnosis of ischemic colitis depends on the recognition of clinical features.[2] In patients in whom colonic ischemia is suspected but no signs of peritonitis are present, a sigmoidoscopy should be performed to identify mucosal changes. CT imaging is usually nonspecific and may only show thickening of the bowel wall. Mesenteric angiography usually has no role in the diagnosis of colon ischemia, because the mesenteric vessels and arcades are usually patent.

An excellent discussion of the differential diagnosis was presented by Gandhi et al.[93] According to them, acute mesenteric arterial insufficiency is characterized by significant abdominal pain. Patients also often have a history of previous distal emboli, dysrhythmias, or atherosclerotic heart disease. The diagnosis is established by arteriography. Mesenteric venous occlusion is characterized by the insidious onset of abdominal discomfort. Progression of disease is accompanied by more severe symptoms of crampy or diffuse abdominal pain, distention, or vomiting. Approximately 20% of cases are idiopathic, but the remainder is associated with liver disease, inflammatory bowel disease, hematologic disease, or hypercoagulable states, particularly malignancy. Ultrasonographic or CT scanning may reveal a lack of patency of the mesenteric veins, and venous filling will not be seen on arteriography. In the younger population, the possibility of inflammatory bowel disease should be entertained. Patients with acute diverticulitis usually present with abdominal pain that is localized to the left lower quadrant; it may be related to a recent bowel movement. Up to 25% of patients will have had a previous attack. Physical examination reveals localized peritonitis in the left lower quadrant. Contrast enemas and a CT scan may reveal the diagnosis. Infectious colitis may also be mistaken for the ischemic variety. Watery diarrhea, fever, leukocytosis, and recent antibiotic usage characterize pseudomembranous colitis. Proctosigmoidoscopic examination may illustrate diffuse edema, multiple ulcerations, and the presence of pseudomembranes. Evidence of trophozoites in fresh stool specimens documents amebic colitis. Other etiologies of acute abdominal pain, such as bowel obstruction, peptic ulcer disease, volvulus, and pancreatitis, must also be excluded.

Treatment

Treatment of ischemic colitis can be conservative when the diagnosis is made early. Occasionally, mild cases can be managed on an outpatient basis with liquid diet, close observation, and possibly antibiotics. More serious cases require hospitalization, and more aggressive treatment includes bowel rest, nasogastric suction, and intravenous fluid replacement. Parenteral hyperalimentation may be helpful when a protracted course is suspected or the disease has been associated with underlying nutritional deficiencies. Antibiotics that are effective against both aerobic and anaerobic bacteria should be started. Cardiac function and oxygen delivery are optimized, and medications that may contribute to colonic ischemia are withdrawn if possible. Agents such as papaverine and dextran have been used to improve flow, but their value has not been proved. Patients who fail to improve on a conservative regimen should be treated surgically.

Patients with chronic segmental colitis should be treated symptomatically. Local steroid enemas may be of some benefit.[93] The successful treatment of a patient with chronic segmental ischemic colitis suffering from persistent fever and diarrhea with 1,500-mg mesalamine/day has been reported.[138] Colonoscopy revealed multiple ulcers including a broad longitudinal one and erosions on friable and edematous mucosa of the sigmoid colon and rectum. A follow-up colonoscopy revealed a healing mucosa. Recurrent episodes of sepsis in otherwise asymptomatic patients with unhealed areas of segmental colitis may be an indication for resection.

Specific indications for operation include peritonitis, perforation, recurrent fever or sepsis, clinical deterioration in patients refractory to medical management with continuation of symptoms beyond 2 to 3 weeks, and gangrene visualized endoscopically. Other indications include fulminant colitis, massive hemorrhage, chronic protein losing colopathy, and symptomatic ischemic stricture.[2] At operation, a wide resection of nonviable bowel should be performed. Intraoperative assessment of colonic viability may prove difficult. A palpable pulse in the SMA will rule out a correctable cause of midgut ischemia. With a normal-appearing serosa, determination of viability may be achieved with colonoscopy, evaluation of the antimesenteric serosal surface by hand-held continuous wave Doppler, tonometric measurement of intramural pH, pulse oximetry of transcolonic oxygen saturation, or intravenous fluorescein.[93] It is still wise to open the resected specimen to inspect for mucosal injury. This is especially critical if an anastomosis is being considered. The surgeon should not be fooled by the dark appearance of mucosa secondary to melanosis coli, in which case the blood supply is normal and extended resection because of "black" mucosa is not necessary.

Primary anastomosis is usually unsafe in this setting, because postoperative progression of the ischemia can compromise the anastomotic site. The proximal limb of bowel is brought out as a colostomy and the distal limb as a mucous fistula or oversewn as a Hartmann procedure. Concern about ongoing ischemia may mandate a planned second look 24 to 48 hours later.

Operation generally is not indicated for patients who have radiographic evidence of strictures but no associated clinical symptoms. Strictures associated with obstruction or protracted bleeding should be resected.

Occasionally, resection is indicated because malignancy at the stricture site cannot be ruled out. The chronic subtype of ischemic colitis may lead to the sequelae of persistent segmental colitis or colonic strictures, occasionally requiring operation.[93]

Results

The prognosis on the outcome for ischemic colitis varies considerably.

Abel and Russell[139] reported the management of 18 patients with ischemic colitis, 9 of whom were treated conservatively with a mortality rate of 45% and 9 of whom required an operation with a mortality rate of 55%. Reeders et al[90] reported the results of treatment of 199 patients with ischemic colitis. Thirty-five patients underwent immediate operation for peritonitis, and all died. The remaining 164 patients were initially managed nonoperatively. Ninety-eight patients continued conservative treatment throughout their hospitalization, 57% of whom died. Among the remaining 66 patients initially treated nonoperatively who ultimately required an operation for progression of the disease, 51% died.

Longo et al[80] identified 47 patients with nonocclusive ischemia of the large intestine. Overall, 15 of 16 patients were successfully treated nonoperatively with bowel rest and antibiotics, 1 of whom died. Among the 31 patients requiring resection, intestinal continuity was reestablished in 14. Second-look laparotomies in eight patients revealed further ischemia in two (20%). The mortality rate in the operative group was 29%. No patient developed recurrent ischemia in a mean follow-up of 5.3 years. The authors found that while the course may be self-limited, elderly and diabetic patients as well as those developing ischemia following aortic surgery or hypotension continued to have a poor prognosis.

Parish et al[78] reported on 38 patients identified with ischemic colitis. Among patients with spontaneous disease, the mortality rate was 24% compared with 54% in postoperative patients. Of the 16 patients requiring operative intervention, the mortality rate was 62%. In patients who required reoperation, the operative mortality rate was 88%. The mortality rate for nonoperative treatment was 14%. Guttormson and Bubrick[75] reviewed 39 patients with ischemic colitis and found an overall mortality rate of 53% (42% nonoperative treatment and 65% operative treatment). The authors' data showed a close association between ischemic colitis and a number of serious systemic diseases, including renal failure, arteriosclerotic heart disease, vascular disease, and hematologic, vasculitic, and connective tissue disorders.

Longo et al[140] studied the outcome of 43 patients with ischemic colitis. Diagnosis was established by colonoscopy in 72%, whereas in the remainder diagnosis was made in the operating room. Ischemic colitis developed in the hospital in 40% of patients during admission for an unrelated illness. Segmental colitis was present in 72% of patients and 35% of these patients were successfully managed nonoperatively. In the patients with segmental colitis who required operation, the 30-day mortality rate was 22%. Among 17 patients with segmental ischemia treated by resection and stoma, 75% underwent eventual stoma closure.

Guivarc'h et al[141] reported their experience in 88 cases of ischemic colitis including 76 cases of gangrene with 17 perforations, 6 cases with stenosis, and 6 cases that regressed. The left colon was involved in 59 cases with extension to the transverse colon in 20, the right colon in 10, and global involvement in 18. Abdominal pain, diarrhea, and abdominal distention occurred in 81, 62, and 78% of the cases, respectively. Colonoscopy was performed in 61 cases, a barium enema in 27. A colectomy was required in 77 patients: 50 left colectomies with 16 extensions to the transverse colon, 17 total colectomies, and 10 right colectomies. Morbidity was 53% in cases with perforated gangrene and 28% without perforation. There was no morbidity in stenosis and regressive forms. Intestinal continuity was conserved or re-established in 51 of the 62 survivors.

Scharff et al[84] studied the outcome of 129 patients with colon ischemia. The mean age was 66 years; 47% were male. Risk factors included chronic renal failure (33%), receiving vasoactive drugs (57%), and atherosclerosis (56%). Of 43% with melena, 88% of patients survived. Of 33% with an acute abdomen, 51% died. Initially, 54% were treated nonoperatively, of which 24% required operation. Of 76 patients who were treated operatively, 41% died. Eleven patients at operation had ischemia without colon infarction or perforation; 45% died. The overall mortality was 29%. Mortality rates remained high, despite treatment.

Medina et al[142] reviewed the clinical characteristics of patients and analyzed predictive factors of poor outcome in 53 cases of ischemic colitis. Hypertension (51%) was the main risk factor associated with ischemic colitis. Peritonitis was present only in the severe group. Colonoscopy and histologic studies were the most used diagnostic procedures. Peripheral vasculopathy and right colonic involvement were risk factors for severe outcome. Five patients died during admission and among these the right colon was affected in four.

30.5.7 Colonic "Cast" Slough

The spontaneous passage per rectum of a full-thickness colon "cast" is a rare consequence of acute colonic ischemia. Foley et al[143] reported a patient who had undergone Hartmann's procedure for a perforated diverticular abscess, which was reversed 6 months later. On the first postoperative night after reversal, the patient had a brief hypotensive episode, and 3 weeks later passed a 21-cm full-thickness infarcted piece of colon. The patient did not develop peritonitis and for 11 months experienced only mild symptoms. Under colonoscopic surveillance, the granulation tissue conduit connecting the remaining viable bowel became increasingly stenosed proximally and difficult to dilate. After three rapidly consecutive episodes of large bowel obstruction, the patient required a laparotomy to resect the stricture and restore bowel continuity. From a literature review, this was the eighth case of its kind and the first in which such prolonged conservative management has been possible.

30.5.8 Idiopathic Mesenteric Phlebosclerosis

A new clinicopathologic disease was described by Iwashita et al[144] and they proposed the term "idiopathic mesenteric phlebosclerosis." In fact, the entity was originally described by Koyama et al[145] and later reviewed by Yoshinaga et al,[146] who found 18 cases. Iwashita et al identified seven patients with calcifications in the small mesenteric veins and their intramural branches. Clinical findings included abdominal pain and diarrhea of a gradual onset and chronic course. A positive fecal occult blood test and mild anemia were often found. Patients had linear calcifications and stenosis in the right colon, which were discovered by plain abdominal radiography and barium enema, respectively. Endoscopic findings included edematous, dark-colored mucosa and ulcerations. Four patients underwent a subtotal colectomy because of persistent abdominal pain or ileus. The histopathologic findings were macroscopically characterized by a dark purple- or dark brown-colored colonic surface, the swelling and disappearance of plicae semilunares coli, and marked thickening of the colonic wall, while they were microscopically characterized by marked fibrous thickening of the venous walls with calcifications, marked submucosal fibrosis, deposition of collagen in the mucosa, and foamy macrophages within the vessel walls.

30.5.9 Ischemic Colitis and Aortoiliac Surgery

Ischemic colitis is an infrequent but highly lethal complication following aortic surgery. It is unique because in part it may be a direct consequence of an anatomic change in blood flow resulting from ligation of the IMA (see Chapter 1). Ernst et al[147] and Hagihara et al[148] have evaluated patients endoscopically following abdominal aortic aneurysm resection and have found that the incidence of clinical ischemic disease was 1 to 2% and that the incidence of endoscopic disease was 6.8%. Endoscopic evidence of ischemic colitis was found in 60% of patients following emergency repair of abdominal aortic aneurysm, reflecting in part the hypovolemia, shock, and also the absence of mechanical or antibiotic bowel preparation prior to emergency operation. In a review of 2,137 patients undergoing aortic reconstructive operations, Brewster et al[77] found a 1.1% incidence of intestinal ischemia. Björck et al[149] studied the incidence and clinical presentation of intestinal ischemia after 2,930 aortoiliac/femoral operations. The estimated incidence of bowel ischemia was 2.8%. Among patients operated on for a ruptured aneurysm in shock, the estimated incidence of bowel ischemia was 7.3%. Of the 63 patients with intestinal ischemia, only 15 patients presented with early passage of bloody stools. In 60 patients (95%), the lesion affected the left colon within the reach of the sigmoidoscope. Champagne et al[150] reviewed 88 patients who underwent emergent aortic reconstruction because of ruptured abdominal aortic aneurysms. Operative mortality was 42%. Colonoscopy was performed in 62 of 72 patients who survived more than 24 hours. Bowel ischemia was documented in 36% of patients. Of these, 62% had grade I or II ischemia at both initial and repeat endoscopy. Exploratory laparotomy with bowel resection was undertaken in 35% because of grade III ischemia. Two procedures were performed because of worsening ischemia discovered at repeat colonoscopy. In patients with colonoscopic findings of bowel ischemia, the mortality rate was 50%. In those with grade III necrosis who underwent resection, the mortality rate was 55%. Elevated lactate levels, immature white blood cells, and increased fluid sequestration were all variables associated with the occurrence of colon ischemia. When the cardinal symptoms are not present, the surgeon may be alerted to the diagnosis by general signs of deterioration, such as oliguria, circulatory instability, septicemia, and coagulopathy.

In a review by Longo et al[81] of 4,957 patients who underwent operation of the abdominal aorta for abdominal aortic aneurysm, 58 (1.2%) had subsequent ischemic colitis. The mean time to diagnosis of ischemic colitis was 5.5 days after aortic surgery (range, 1–21 days). Of 17 patients initially treated nonoperatively, only 1 required a sigmoid resection. One of these patients required a resection for stricture 14 months later. Bowel resection with fecal diversion was required in 32 of 49 patients (65%)—13 for ischemia without infarction and 19 with infarction. The overall mortality rate was 54%, but that rate was 89% if bowel resection for bowel infarction was required (19 patients). Only 2 of 12 (16%) of those who required fecal diversion and survived underwent eventual stoma closure. Among seven patients who received second-look laparotomy for ischemic colitis, additional bowel resection was required in six. No patient had aortic graft infection diagnosed during the index hospitalization. The overall mean hospitalization duration after the diagnosis of ischemic colitis was 38 days (range, 1–164 days). The high overall mortality rate is almost identical to that of previous reports.[151] In view of high mortality rates, routine postoperative colonoscopy could be justified on high-risk patients (those with multiple risk factors and/or ruptured aneurysms) to enable timely reoperative intervention in patients suspected of full-thickness necrosis. Caution is advised in patients with ischemic colitis undergoing colonoscopy in that distention of the bowel with air may diminish colonic blood flow and further exacerbate the ischemia.[152]

Brandt et al[153] suggested that flexible sigmoidoscopy reliably predicts full-thickness colonic ischemia following repair of ruptured aortic aneurysms. They believe patients with nonconfluent ischemia limited to the mucosa can be safely followed by serial endoscopic examinations. However, in contrast, Houe et al[154] reviewed seven prospective nonrandomized reports on routine colonoscopy after abdominal aortic surgery. Endoscopy may disclose ischemic colitis but cannot separate transmural from clinically less important mucosal ischemia. Endoscopy had no impact on mortality in any of the prospective series.

For patients developing clinical ischemic colitis following aortic surgery, the mortality rate has been reported to be high after elective aneurysm resection and significantly higher after emergency operation, even as high as 60 to 100%.[155] Brewster et al[77] reported an overall mortality rate of 25% that rose to 50% if reoperation for bowel resection was required. Maupin et al[156] reviewed 103 patients who underwent operation for a ruptured abdominal aortic aneurysm. Of the 71 survivors, ischemic colitis developed in 27%. For those who required bowel resection, the mortality rate was 58%, and hence the authors recommended flexible fiberoptic sigmoidoscopy in the early postoperative period to detect ischemic colitis prior to the onset of clinical sepsis. Bast et al[157] conducted a prospective study of the incidence and risk factors for ischemic disease of the colon and rectum following operation for abdominal aortic aneurysm. In their series of 100 patients, routine postoperative colonoscopy revealed ischemic colonic disease, defined as ulceration or necrosis in 4.5% of patients undergoing elective operation and 17.6% of patients undergoing operation for ruptured aneurysms. Ligation of a patent IMA was not in this study related to the development of ischemic disease, nor was a prolonged (>1 hour) cross-damping of the aorta. Zelenock et al[155] conducted a prospective study of 100 patients undergoing aortic reconstructive surgery in which patients underwent colonoscopy within 24 to 48 hours. Only three patients developed endoscopic evidence of ischemia, and no patient required bowel resection. The authors attributed their good results to utilization of adjunctive procedures to enhance colonic perfusion in 12 patients (IMA reimplantation, bypass to internal iliac artery, and anastomosis of aortofemoral bypass limb to adjacent common iliac artery).

Piotrowski et al[158] conducted a retrospective review of 101 patients who were treated for abdominal aortic aneurysm, 71 (70%) of whom survived for longer than 24 hours postoperatively. Colonic ischemia, primarily left sided, was a perioperative complication in 24 patients (35%) and required colectomy in 11 patients (44%). Colectomy carried a 44% mortality rate compared to 20% in patients without this complication. Colonic ischemia occurred more frequently in patients with preoperative shock and a greater intraoperative blood loss, but showed no correlation with patient age, comorbid medical conditions, laboratory values, time to operation, or treatment of the IMA. Most patients with postoperative bowel ischemia, including 8 of the 11 patients whom required colectomy, were found to have chronic IMA occlusion. Revascularization of patent IMAs had little effect on outcome. Of the 17 patent IMAs, 9 were reimplanted, and 5 patients (55%) developed bowel ischemia, 2 of who required colectomy. Eight were ligated and three (39%) developed bowel ischemia, one of whom required colectomy. The authors concluded that preoperative shock was the most important factor predicting the development of colonic ischemia following ruptured abdominal aortic aneurysm.

Lane and Bentley[159] described two cases of rectal stricture formation following aortic aneurysm repair. A combination of hypotension, compromised internal iliac circulation, and poor collateral supply following IMA ligation can result in acute ischemic proctitis—an infrequently described clinical entity. Ulceration and necrosis are the sequelae of prolonged ischemia and fibrous stricture formation may result. One patient responded to dilatation and posterior midrectal myotomy; the other failed to respond to conservative measures and eventually had an end colostomy fashioned following intractable symptoms.

Järvinen et al[160] defined the incidence and attendant mortality of intestinal infarction of 1,752 patients who underwent abdominal aortic reconstruction as recorded in the Finnish National Vascular Registry. Among the 1,752 operations, 27 patients had intestinal ischemia for an incidence of bowel infarction of 1.2%. Among patients operated on for a ruptured aneurysm it was 3.1%, whereas it was 1% for patients with nonruptured aneurysm, and 0.6% of those operated on for aortoiliac occlusive disease developed intestinal infarction. In 14 patients (67%), the lesion affected the left colon. The overall 30-day mortality rate was 13% but reached 67% among those with intestinal infarction.

The frequency of ischemic colitis following aortoiliac surgery varies from 7% after repair of ruptured aortic aneurysm to 0.6% after bypass for aortoiliac occlusive disease.[161] In order to analyze the predisposing factors and outcome of ischemic colitis, Van Damme et al[161] reviewed their clinical experience of 28 cases (16 ruptured aortic aneurysms, 7 elective aortic aneurysms, and 5 aortoiliac occlusive disease) of clinically evident colonic ischemia. Transmural necrosis was observed in 21 patients, 15 of which underwent Hartmann's procedure with a mortality of 66%. All nonoperated grade III patients died. Overall, 16 of the 28 patients died at hospital (57% mortality rate). Associated colon revascularization could not avoid the evolution of colon necrosis in four patients. Reimplantation of a patent IMA or internal iliac artery was performed in only 4.8% of all aortic reconstructions and did not influence the development of ischemic colitis. The authors conclude that a more liberal use of postoperative sigmoidoscopy could allow detecting colonic ischemia at an earlier stage and reduce ensuing mortality.

Colonic necrosis can complicate endovascular abdominal aortic aneurysm repair even when both internal iliac arteries are preserved.[162] Advantageously, the clinical signs of severe colonic ischemia in endograft patients are not obscured by aftereffects of a laparotomy.

Although the most likely etiology of colonic ischemia following aortic surgery appears to be a sudden loss of blood flow from a patent IMA, a number of other factors have been described. These factors include failure to resume hypogastric flow, absence of or injury to the collateral circulation, operative trauma to the colon, cholesterol emboli, or an aortoiliac steal syndrome in which blood flow is shunted from the colon to the extremities through the newly revascularized iliac or femoral vessels.[163,164] Klok et al[165] noted that all patients undergoing aortic reconstructive operations develop a significant drop in sigmoidal intramucosal pH. Return to a normal baseline within 6 to 12 hours after declamping probably predicts a postoperative course without ischemic colitis. Björck and Hedberg[166] also found that sigmoid intramucosal pH could be used to monitor patients undergoing aortic operations. In a study of 34 patients, 8 patients developed major complications, 4 of whom had ischemic colitis and 5 of whom died. Sigmoid acidosis (pH < 7.1) served as an early warning. If acidosis was reversed within 24 hours, no major complications developed; if prolonged, it was predictive of major morbidity.

Risk factors to the development of ischemia include prolonged cross-clamp time, rupture of the aortic aneurysm, hypotension, hypoxemia, arrhythmia, retroperitoneal hematoma with compression of the viscera and its blood supply, inadequacy of colonic collaterals, intraoperative injury or interruption of the marginal artery of Drummond or meandering mesenteric arcade, operative trauma to the colon, bowel distention, lack of preoperative bowel preparation,[93] and ligation of a patent IMA. Ligation of the IMA was the most important feature in one series (74%).[77] Decisions on whether or not to reimplant the IMA should be based on Doppler ultrasonography, fluorescein dye injections, or IMA stump pressure.[37,167]

Prevention of ischemic colitis can result from IMA reimplantation. Criteria for reimplantation of a patent IMA recommended by Brewster et al[77] include severe SMA disease, an enlarged IMA or meandering mesenteric artery, exclusion of hypogastric circulation, loss of Doppler signal in sigmoid mesentery, poor IMA back-bleeding (stump pressure < 40 mmHg), and a history of prior colon resection. Mechanical and antibiotic bowel preparation should also be considered in the preoperative preparation for elective aortic reconstruction. Intraoperative methods used to diminish the likelihood of colonic ischemia include preservation of the meandering mesenteric artery, avoidance of distal embolization of atherosclerotic debris, gentle handling of the colon, and intraoperative anticoagulation.[93]

IMA reimplantation does not ensure colon viability in aortic surgery. Mitchell and Valentine[168] identified 10 patients with aortic surgery, 5 of whom underwent successful IMA reimplantation for inadequate Doppler signals on the antimesenteric border of the sigmoid colon. The other five patients did not undergo IMA reimplantation because they were deemed to have adequate blood perfusion. Transmural colon necrosis occurred in 6 of the 10 study patients, 4 of whom had IMA reimplantation. Three of the four patients with colon ischemia presenting less than 24 hours after aortic revascularization survived, but both patients with late colon ischemia died of multisystem organ failure. Although transmural necrosis is a highly morbid complication after aortic surgery, timely colectomy may lead to survival in some patients.

Signs and symptoms may be difficult to detect in a patient who has just undergone a major reconstructive aortic operation. Bloody diarrhea during the first day or two after an aortic operation should alert the clinician of the diagnosis of ischemic colitis. Metabolic acidosis, leukocytosis, oliguria, tachycardia, and hypotension may develop with aggressive disease. Treatment follows the recommendation above with nonoperative treatment for mild forms of the disease and resection for severe irreversible transmural disease. In the latter case, primary anastomosis is contraindicated because of the potential for leakage and contamination of the aortic prosthesis.

Controversy exists as to the cause of ischemic colitis complicating endovascular aneurysm repair. Occlusion of the hypogastric arteries during endovascular repair of aortoiliac aneurysm results in a significant incidence of buttock claudication, and has been suggested as a causative factor in the development of postprocedural colonic ischemia, in addition to factors such as systemic hypotension, embolization of atheromatous debris, and interruption of IMA inflow. To analyze the relationship between perioperative hypogastric artery occlusion and postoperative ischemic colitis, Geraghty et al[169] reviewed their experience with bifurcated endovascular grafts in 233 patients. Unilateral perioperative hypogastric artery occlusion during the course of endovascular aortoiliac aneurysm repair occurred in 18.9%, and 0.4% underwent bilateral hypogastric artery occlusion. In 1.7%, signs and symptoms of ischemic colitis developed 2±1.4 days postoperatively. In all patients, the diagnosis was confirmed at sigmoidoscopy, and initial treatment included bowel rest, hydration, and intravenous antibiotic agents. Three patients with bilateral patent hypogastric arteries required colonic resection 14.7±9.7 days after the initial diagnosis and two of these three patients died in the postoperative period. Pathologic findings confirmed the presence of atheroemboli in the colonic vasculature in all three patients who underwent colonic resection. The fourth patient had undergone multiple manipulations of the left hypogastric artery in an unsuccessful attempt to preserve patency of this vessel during aortoiliac aneurysm repair. This patient recovered completely with nonoperative management. Perioperative unilateral hypogastric artery occlusion was not associated with a significantly higher incidence of postoperative ischemic colitis. Their extensive experience suggests that embolization of atheromatous debris to the hypogastric artery tissue beds during endovascular manipulations, rather than proximal hypogastric artery occlusion, is the primary cause of clinically significant ischemic colitis after endovascular aneurysm repair.

Ischemic Colitis Following Cardiopulmonary Bypass

Colonic ischemia following cardiopulmonary bypass is a rare development (0.06–0.2%), but when it occurs, it carries a high mortality rate (76%).[93] The clinical picture is subtle. Contributing factors of systemic hypovolemia, hypotension, and hypothermia result in reduction of blood flow through the intestinal microcirculation. Other insults may include long bypass times, use of inotropes that may induce splanchnic vasoconstriction, and the intra-aortic pump. The combination of these factors may result in sepsis and multiple organ failure. Timely operative intervention may be lifesaving.

Ischemic Colitis Proximal to Obstructing Carcinoma

An acute colitic process believed to be ischemic in nature may develop proximal to an obstructing carcinoma of the colon. Symptoms are usually attributed to the carcinoma. The major importance for recognition of this entity is that an anastomosis constructed in an unrecognized ischemic colon is in jeopardy of failure. When that condition is suspected, a biopsy may aid in the diagnosis. Other obstructing processes such as diverticulitis, volvulus, fecal impaction, or strictures from previous ischemic insults, operations, or radiation therapy may cause diminished colonic blood flow by the effects of sustained increased intraluminal pressure.[93]

30.5.10 Total Colonic Ischemia

A fulminating form of colonic ischemia involving all or most of the colon and rectum has been identified.[124,170] These patients manifest a sudden onset of universal colitis with bloody diarrhea, fever, abdominal pain, and tenderness, often with signs of peritonitis. Contributing factors include large and small vessel arterial disease, decreased perfusion pressure, inadequacy of collateral circulation, and plasma viscosity.[124] These patients are systemically ill, and management necessitates total abdominal colectomy and ileostomy. Ischemic pancolitis is rare with only a limited number of documented cases.[140,141,170] All 12 cases reported by Longo et al[140] required operation and 75% died. Both patients reported by Al-Saleh et al[170] survived. In a surgical series of 88 cases of ischemic colitis reported by Guivarc'h et al,[141] 17 of the 18 patients with global involvement required total colectomy. Although indications for operation do not differ from those with segmental ischemia, Al-Saleh et al[170] recommend vigilant examination of the entire colon at laparotomy as well as pre- or intraoperative colonoscopy in order to recognize the diffuse nature of the disease and institute appropriate management.

30.5.11 Ischemic Proctitis

Ischemic proctitis is a rare condition that affects elderly patients with arteriosclerosis. It is most commonly seen following aortic operations in which hypotension develops secondary to blood loss. It has been reported to occur as a result of hypovolemic shock sustained through trauma.[171] Ischemic proctitis has also been reported in association with adventitial fibromuscular dysplasia.[172] Ischemic necrosis has complicated systemic lupus erythematosus.[173] Up to 1992, 37 cases had been reported.[174] In a review of 328 patients with ischemic colitis, Bharucha et al[175] identified 10 patients with isolated proctosigmoiditis defined as involvement extending to no more than 30 cm above the dentate line. In the six patients with acute rectal ischemia (symptoms < 4 weeks), clearly identifiable precipitating factors such as a major illness or hemodynamic disturbance were identified in four patients but in only one of four patients with chronic ischemic proctosigmoiditis (symptoms 24 weeks). Bloody diarrhea is the most common symptom. The diagnosis of ischemia is made by the mucosal appearance of the sigmoid and is differentiated from infectious proctitis by stool culture. Plain radiographic signs of ischemic proctitis are unlikely to be recognized until necrosis is established and extramural air is visible adjacent to the rectal wall.[176] CT may reveal rectal wall thickening and/or perirectal stranding.[175] Angiography may demonstrate atheromatous disease of the aortoiliac vessels. Biopsy and histopathologic changes may help differentiate this entity from idiopathic inflammatory bowel disease, especially if the hallmark feature of superficial epithelial necrosis is present. Mild ischemic proctitis may be treated with antibiotics and intravenous fluids, but full-thickness ischemia requires a Hartmann resection with low division of the rectum. Cataldo and Zarka[177] reported the use of topical instillation of 4% formalin in the treatment of refractory hemorrhagic ischemic proctitis. Complete proctectomy or abdominoperineal resection should not be necessary. Kishikawa et al[178] reported a case of chronic ischemic proctitis that occurred spontaneously, and the following information was extracted from their review of the literature on this subject. Symptoms include diarrhea, fecal incontinence, abdominal pain, rectal pain, and bloody diarrhea. The endoscopic findings of chronic ischemic proctitis include atrophic mucosa with scattered white scars reflecting repeated episodes of ischemia and healing. Chronic ischemic proctitis should be suspected whenever ulcer formation or erosion is observed endoscopically in the context of atrophic mucosa and multiple whitish scars in the rectosigmoid colon with mucosal crypt atrophy or fibrosis evident in biopsy specimens. On CT, ischemic proctitis should be considered when mural thickening confined to the rectum and sigmoid colon is associated with perirectal fat stranding especially in elderly patients with known cardiovascular risk factors. Patients with ischemic proctitis fall into two groups: those with atherosclerotic disease who have been hospitalized for some other disorder (myocardial infarction, pneumonia, and heart failure)[1] and those with mesenteric venous occlusion.[2] Cocaine is the only agent that induces focal rectal ischemia and this effect of the drug demonstrates the importance of vasoconstriction in the pathogenesis of ischemic proctitis. Ischemic proctitis has been associated with mesenteric venous occlusion. Treatment of ischemic proctitis, acute or chronic, depends on the level of ischemia. Superficial mucosa ischemia should be treated conservatively with close monitoring for signs of sepsis or perforation. Operation is required for necrosis of the bowel wall. Nelson et al[174] performed resection in four of six cases of acute ischemic proctitis.

References

[1] Bradbury AW, Brittenden J, McBride K, Ruckley CV. Mesenteric ischaemia: a multidisciplinary approach. Br J Surg. 1995; 82(11):1446–1459

[2] Sreenarasimhaiah J. Diagnosis and management of intestinal ischaemic disorders. BMJ. 2003; 326(7403):1372–1376

[3] Moskowitz M, Zimmerman H, Felson B. The meandering mesenteric artery of the colon. Am J Roentgenol Radium Ther Nucl Med. 1964; 92:1088–1099

[4] Jacobson LF, Noer RJ. The vascular pattern of the intestinal villi in various laboratory animals and man. Anat Rec. 1952; 114(1):85–101

[5] Hallbäck DA, Hultén L, Jodal M, Lindhagen J, Lundgren O. Evidence for the existence of a countercurrent exchanger in the small intestine in man. Gastroenterology. 1978; 74(4):683–690

[6] Lundgren O. The circulation of the small bowel mucosa. Gut. 1974; 15(12):1005–1013

[7] Kaleya RN, Boley SJ. Acute mesenteric ischemia. Crit Care Clin. 1995; 11(2):479–512

[8] Robinson JWL, Winistörfer B, Mirkovitch V. Source of net water and electrolyte loss following intestinal ischaemia. Res Exp Med (Berl). 1980; 176(3):263–275

[9] Kusche J, Lorenz W, Stahlknecht CD, et al. Intestinal diamine oxidase and histamine release in rabbit mesenteric ischemia. Gastroenterology. 1981; 80(5, pt 1):980–987

[10] Bateson PG, Buchanan KD, Stewart DM, Parks TG. The release of vasoactive intestinal peptide during altered mid-gut blood flow. Br J Surg. 1980; 67(2):131–134

[11] Modlin IM, Bloom SR, Mitchell S. Plasma vasoactive intestinal polypeptide (VIP) levels and intestinal ischaemia. Experientia. 1978; 34(4):535–536

[12] Bennion RS, Wilson SE, Serota AI, Williams RA. The role of gastrointestinal microflora in the pathogenesis of complications of mesenteric ischemia. Rev Infect Dis. 1984; 6 Suppl 1:S132–S138

[13] Bennion RS, Wilson SE, Williams RA. Early portal anaerobic bacteremia in mesenteric ischemia. Arch Surg. 1984; 119(2):151–155

[14] Brawn K, Fridovich I. Superoxide radical and superoxide dismutases: threat and defense. Acta Physiol Scand Suppl. 1980; 492:9–18

[15] Parks DA, Bulkley GB, Granger DN. Role of oxygen-derived free radicals in digestive tract diseases. Surgery. 1983; 94(3):415–422

[16] Granger DN, Rutili G, McCord JM. Superoxide radicals in feline intestinal ischemia. Gastroenterology. 1981; 81(1):22–29

[17] Parks DA, Granger DN, Bulkley GB. Superoxide radicals and mucosal lesions in the ischemic small intestine. Fed Proc. 1982; 44:1742

[18] Andrei VE, Schein M, Wise L. Small bowel ischemia following laparoscopic cholecystectomy. Dig Surg. 1999; 16(6):522–524

[19] Brooks DH, Carey LC. Base deficit in superior mesenteric artery occlusion, an aid to early diagnosis. Ann Surg. 1973; 177(3):352–356

[20] Jamieson WG, Marchuk S, Rowsom J, Durand D. The early diagnosis of massive acute intestinal ischaemia. Br J Surg. 1982; 69 Suppl:S52–S53

[21] Barnett SM, Davidson ED, Bradley EL, III. Intestinal alkaline phosphatase and base deficit in mesenteric occlusion. J Surg Res. 1976; 20(3):243–246

[22] Lamar W, Woodard L, Statland BE. Clinical implications of creatine kinase-BB isoenzyme. N Engl J Med. 1978; 299(15):834–835

[23] Graeber GM, Cafferty PJ, Reardon MJ, Curley CP, Ackerman NB, Harmon JW. Changes in serum total creatine phosphokinase (CPK) and its isoenzymes caused by experimental ligation of the superior mesenteric artery. Ann Surg. 1981; 193(4):499–505

[24] Wollin A, Navert H, Bounous G. Effect of intestinal ischemia on diamine oxidase activity in rat intestinal tissue and blood. Gastroenterology. 1981; 80(2):349–355

[25] Acosta S, Nilsson TK, Björck M. D-dimer testing in patients with suspected acute thromboembolic occlusion of the superior mesenteric artery. Br J Surg. 2004; 91(8):991–994

[26] Scholz FJ. Ischemic bowel disease. Radiol Clin North Am. 1993; 31(6):1197–1218

[27] Wiesner W, Khurana B, Ji H, Ros PR. CT of acute bowel ischemia. Radiology. 2003; 226(3):635–650

[28] Klein HM, Lensing R, Klosterhalfen B, Töns C, Günther RW. Diagnostic imaging of mesenteric infarction. Radiology. 1995; 197(1):79–82

[29] Chou CK, Mak CW, Tzeng WS, Chang JM. CT of small bowel ischemia. Abdom Imaging. 2004; 29(1):18–22

[30] Burkart DJ, Johnson CD, Reading CC, Ehman RL. MR measurements of mesenteric venous flow: prospective evaluation in healthy volunteers and patients with suspected chronic mesenteric ischemia. Radiology. 1995; 194(3):801–806

[31] Stoney RJ, Cunningham CG. Acute mesenteric ischemia. Surgery. 1993; 114(3):489–490

[32] Acosta S, Ogren M, Sternby NH, Bergqvist D, Björck M. Incidence of acute thrombo-embolic occlusion of the superior mesenteric artery–a population-based study. Eur J Vasc Endovasc Surg. 2004; 27(2):145–150

[33] Boley SJ, Feinstein FR, Sammartano R, Brandt LJ, Sprayregen S. New concepts in the management of emboli of the superior mesenteric artery. Surg Gynecol Obstet. 1981; 153(4):561–569

[34] Vujic I, Stanley J, Gobien RP. Treatment of acute embolus of the superior mesenteric artery by topical infusion of streptokinase. Cardiovasc Intervent Radiol. 1984; 7(2):94–96

[35] Pillari G, Doscher W, Fierstein J, Ross W, Loh G, Berkowitz BJ. Low-dose streptokinase in the treatment of celiac and superior mesenteric artery occlusion. Arch Surg. 1983; 118(11):1340–1342

[36] Jamieson AC, Thomas RJS, Cade JF. Lysis of a superior mesenteric artery embolus following local infusion of streptokinase and heparin. Aust N Z J Surg. 1979; 49(3):355–356

[37] Bulkley GB, Zuidema GD, Hamilton SR, et al. Intraoperative determination of small bowel viability following ischemic injury. Ann Surg. 1981; 193:628–637

[38] O'Donell JA, Hobson RW. Operative confirmation in evaluation of intestinal ischemia. Surgery. 1980; 87:109–112

[39] Sheridan WG, Lowndes RH, Young HL. Intraoperative tissue oximetry in the human gastrointestinal tract. Am J Surg. 1990; 159(3):314–319

[40] Slutzki S, Halpern Z, Negri M, Kais H, Halevy A. The laparoscopic second look for ischemic bowel disease. Surg Endosc. 1996; 10(7):729–731

[41] Anadol AZ, Ersoy E, Taneri F, Tekin EH. Laparoscopic "second-look" in the management of mesenteric ischemia. Surg Laparosc Endosc Percutan Tech. 2004; 14(4):191–193

[42] Cooperman M. Intestinal Ischemia. New York, NY: Futura Publishing; 1983:147

[43] Bergan JJ. Acute intestinal infarction. In: Rutherford R, ed. Vascular Surgery. 2nd ed. Philadelphia, PA: WS Saunders; 1984:955

[44] Sales JP, Frileux P, Cugnenc PH, Parc R. Mesenteric infarction: improved survival rate after temporary enterostomy. Br J Surg. 1993; 80(8):1029

[45] Bingol H, Zeybek N, Cingöz F, Yilmaz AT, Tatar H, Sen D. Surgical therapy for acute superior mesenteric artery embolism. Am J Surg. 2004; 188(1):68–70

[46] Savassi-Rocha PR, Veloso LF. Treatment of superior mesenteric artery embolism with a fibrinolytic agent: case report and literature review. Hepatogastroenterology. 2002; 49(47):1307–1310

[47] Kwaan JH, Connolly JE. Prevention of intestinal infarction resulting from mesenteric arterial occlusive disease. Surg Gynecol Obstet. 1983; 157(4):321–324

[48] Johnston KW, Lindsay TF, Walker PM, Kalman PG. Mesenteric arterial bypass grafts: early and late results and suggested surgical approach for chronic and acute mesenteric ischemia. Surgery. 1995; 118(1):1–7

[49] Bailey RW, Bulkley GB, Hamilton SR, Morris JB, Haglund UH. Protection of the small intestine from nonocclusive mesenteric ischemic injury due to cardiogenic shock. Am J Surg. 1987; 153(1):108–116

[50] Bailey RW, Bulkley GB, Hamilton SR, Morris JB, Smith GW. Pathogenesis of nonocclusive ischemic colitis. Ann Surg. 1986; 203(6):590–599

[51] Clark RA, Gallant TE. Acute mesenteric ischemia: angiographic spectrum. AJR Am J Roentgenol. 1984; 142(3):555–562

[52] Kaleya RN, Sammartano RJ, Boley SJ. Aggressive approach to acute mesenteric ischemia. Surg Clin North Am. 1992; 72(1):157–182

[53] Ward D, Vernava AM, Kaminski DL, et al. Improved outcome by identification of high-risk nonocclusive mesenteric ischemia, aggressive reexploration, and delayed anastomosis. Am J Surg. 1995; 170(6):577–580, discussion 580–581

[54] Schuler JG, Hudlin MM. Cecal necrosis: infrequent variant of ischemic colitis. Report of five cases. Dis Colon Rectum. 2000; 43(5):708–712

[55] Neri E, Sassi C, Massetti M, et al. Nonocclusive intestinal ischemia in patients with acute aortic dissection. J Vasc Surg. 2002; 36(4):738–745

[56] Flaherty MJ, Lie JT, Haggitt RC. Mesenteric inflammatory veno-occlusive disease. A seldom recognized cause of intestinal ischemia. Am J Surg Pathol. 1994; 18(8):779–784

[57] Grendell JH, Ockner RK. Mesenteric venous thrombosis. Gastroenterology. 1982; 82(2):358–372

[58] Benjamin E, Oropello JM, Iberti TJ. Acute mesenteric ischemia: pathophysiology, diagnosis, and treatment. Dis Mon. 1993; 39(3):131–210

[59] Khodadadi J, Rozencwajg J, Nacasch N, Schmidt B, Feuchtwanger MM. Mesenteric vein thrombosis. The importance of a second-look operation. Arch Surg. 1980; 115(3):315–317

[60] Sack J, Aldrete JS. Primary mesenteric venous thrombosis. Surg Gynecol Obstet. 1982; 154(2):205–208

[61] Kitchens CS. Evolution of our understanding of the pathophysiology of primary mesenteric venous thrombosis. Am J Surg. 1992; 163(3):346–348

[62] Rhee RY, Gloviczki P, Mendonca CT, et al. Mesenteric venous thrombosis: still a lethal disease in the 1990s. J Vasc Surg. 1994; 20(5):688–697

[63] Divino CM, Park IS, Angel LP, Ellozy S, Spiegel R, Kim U. A retrospective study of diagnosis and management of mesenteric vein thrombosis. Am J Surg. 2001; 181(1):20–23

[64] Croft RJ, Menon GP, Marston A. Does "intestinal angina" exist? A critical study of obstructed visceral arteries. Br J Surg. 1981; 68(5):316–318

[65] Marston A, Clarke JM, Garcia Garcia J, Miller AL. Intestinal function and intestinal blood supply: a 20 year surgical study. Gut. 1985; 26(7):656–666

[66] Gentile AT, Moneta GL, Taylor LM, Jr, Park TC, McConnell DB, Porter JM. Isolated bypass to the superior mesenteric artery for intestinal ischemia. Arch Surg. 1994; 129(9):926–931, discussion 931–932

[67] Hollier LH, Bernatz PE, Pairolero PC, Payne WS, Osmundson PJ. Surgical management of chronic intestinal ischemia: a reappraisal. Surgery. 1981; 90 (6):940–946

[68] McAfee MK, Cherry KJ, Jr, Naessens JM, et al. Influence of complete revascularization on chronic mesenteric ischemia. Am J Surg. 1992; 164(3):220–224

[69] Illuminati G, Caliò FG, D'Urso A, Papaspiropoulos V, Mancini P, Ceccanei G. The surgical treatment of chronic intestinal ischemia: results of a recent series. Acta Chir Belg. 2004; 104(2):175–183

[70] Leke MA, Hood DB, Rowe VL, Katz SG, Kohl RD, Weaver FA. Technical consideration in the management of chronic mesenteric ischemia. Am Surg. 2002; 68(12):1088–1092

[71] Furrer J, Gruntzig A, Kugelmeier J, et al. Treatment of abdominal angina with percutaneous dilation of an arteria mesenterica superior stenosis. Cardiovasc Intervent Radiol. 1980; 3:43–44

[72] Golden DA, Ring EJ, McLean GK, Freiman DB. Percutaneous transluminal angioplasty in the treatment of abdominal angina. AJR Am J Roentgenol. 1982; 139(2):247–249

[73] Birch SJ, Colapinto RF. Transluminal dilation in the management of mesenteric angina. Journal de l'Association Canadienne des Radtologistes. 1982; 33:46–47

[74] Kasirajan K, O'Hara PJ, Gray BH, et al. Chronic mesenteric ischemia: open surgery versus percutaneous angioplasty and stenting. J Vasc Surg. 2001; 33(1):63–71

[75] Guttormson NL, Bubrick MP. Mortality from ischemic colitis. Dis Colon Rectum. 1989; 32(6):469–472

[76] Levy PJ, Krausz MM, Manny J. Acute mesenteric ischemia: improved results: a retrospective analysis of ninety-two patients. Surgery. 1990; 107(4):372–380

[77] Brewster DC, Franklin DP, Cambria RP, et al. Intestinal ischemia complicating abdominal aortic surgery. Surgery. 1991; 109(4):447–454

[78] Parish KL, Chapman WC, Williams LF, Jr. Ischemic colitis. An ever-changing spectrum? Am Surg. 1991; 57(2):118–121

[79] Inderbitzi R, Wagner HE, Seiler C, Stirnemann P, Gertsch P. Acute mesenteric ischaemia. Eur J Surg. 1992; 158(2):123–126

[80] Longo WE, Ballantyne GH, Gusberg RJ. Ischemic colitis: patterns and prognosis. Dis Colon Rectum. 1992; 35(8):726–730

[81] Longo WE, Lee TC, Barnett MG, et al. Ischemic colitis complicating abdominal aortic aneurysm surgery in the U.S. veteran. J Surg Res. 1996; 60(2):351–354

[82] Klempnauer J, Grothues F, Bektas H, Pichlmayr R. Long-term results after surgery for acute mesenteric ischemia. Surgery. 1997; 121(3):239–243

[83] Edwards MS, Cherr GS, Craven TE, et al. Acute occlusive mesenteric ischemia: surgical management and outcomes. Ann Vasc Surg. 2003; 17(1):72–79

[84] Scharff JR, Longo WE, Vartanian SM, Jacobs DL, Bahadursingh AN, Kaminski DL. Ischemic colitis: spectrum of disease and outcome. Surgery. 2003; 134 (4):624–629, discussion 629–630

[85] Kasirajan K, Mascha EJ, Heffernan D, Sifuentes J, III. Determinants of in-hospital mortality and length of stay for acute intestinal gangrene. Am J Surg. 2004; 187(4):482–485

[86] Schoots IG, Koffeman GI, Legemate DA, Levi M, van Gulik TM. Systematic review of survival after acute mesenteric ischaemia according to disease aetiology. Br J Surg. 2004; 91(1):17–27

[87] Boley SJ, Schwartz S, Lash J, Sternhill V. Reversible vascular occlusion of the colon. Surg Gynecol Obstet. 1963; 116:53–60

[88] Marston A, Pheils MT, Thomas ML, Morson BC. Ischaemic colitis. Gut. 1966; 7(1):1–15

[89] Higgins PD, Davis KJ, Laine L. Systematic review: the epidemiology of ischaemic colitis. Aliment Pharmacol Ther. 2004; 19(7):729–738

[90] Reeders JWAJ, Tytgat GNJ, Rosenbusch G, et al. Ischemic Colitis. Dordrecht, The Netherlands: Martinus Nijhoff; 1984:30, 157

[91] Kaleya RN, Boley SJ. Colonic ischemia. Perspect Colon Rectal Surg. 1990; 3:62–81

[92] Saegesser F, Sandblom P. Ischemic lesions of the distended colon: a complication of obstructive colorectal cancer. Am J Surg. 1975; 129(3):309–315

[93] Gandhi SK, Hanson MM, Vernava AM, Kaminski DL, Longo WE. Ischemic colitis. Dis Colon Rectum. 1996; 39(1):88–100

[94] Midian-Singh R, Polen A, Durishin C, Crock RD, Whittier FC, Fahmy N. Ischemic colitis revisited: a prospective study identifying hypercoagulability as a risk factor. South Med J. 2004; 97(2):120–123

[95] Koutroubakis IE, Sfiridaki A, Theodoropoulou A, Kouroumalis EA. Role of acquired and hereditary thrombotic risk factors in colon ischemia of ambulatory patients. Gastroenterology. 2001; 121(3):561–565

[96] Koutroubakis IE, Theodoropoulou A, Sfiridaki A, Kouroumalis EA. Low plasma protein Z levels in patients with ischemic colitis. Dig Dis Sci. 2003; 48 (9):1673–1676

[97] Pérez-Carral C, Carreira J, Vidal C. Acute ischaemic colitis due to hypotension and amoxicillin allergy. Postgrad Med J. 2004; 80(943):298–299

[98] Comay D, Ramsay J, Irvine EJ. Ischemic colitis after weight-loss medication. Can J Gastroenterol. 2003; 17(12):719–721

[99] Tashiro M, Yoshikawa I, Kume K, Otsuki M. Ischemic colitis associated with paclitaxel and carboplatin chemotherapy. Am J Gastroenterol. 2003; 98 (1):231–232

[100] Daniele B, Rossi GB, Losito S, Gridelli C, de Bellis M. Ischemic colitis associated with paclitaxel. J Clin Gastroenterol. 2001; 33(2):159–160

[101] Brinker AD, Mackey AC, Prizont R. Tegaserod and ischemic colitis. N Engl J Med. 2004; 351(13):1361–1364, discussion 1361–1364

[102] Wooltorton E. Tegaserod (Zelnorm) for irritable bowel syndrome: reports of serious diarrhea and intestinal ischemia. CMAJ. 2004; 170(13):1908

[103] Frossard JL, Spahr L, Queneau PE, Armenian B, Bründler MA, Hadengue A. Ischemic colitis during pregnancy and contraceptive medication. Digestion. 2001; 64(2):125–127

[104] Friedel D, Thomas R, Fisher RS. Ischemic colitis during treatment with alosetron. Gastroenterology. 2001; 120(2):557–560

[105] Garcia B, Ramaholimihaso F, Diebold MD, Cadiot G, Thiéfin G. Ischaemic colitis in a patient taking meloxicam. Lancet. 2001; 357(9257):690

[106] Linder JD, Mönkemüller KE, Raijman I, Johnson L, Lazenby AJ, Wilcox CM. Cocaine-associated ischemic colitis. South Med J. 2000; 93(9):909–913

[107] Dowd J, Bailey D, Moussa K, Nair S, Doyle R, Culpepper-Morgan JA. Ischemic colitis associated with pseudoephedrine: four cases. Am J Gastroenterol. 1999; 94(9):2430–2434

[108] Knudsen JF, Friedman B, Chen M, Goldwasser JE. Ischemic colitis and sumatriptan use. Arch Intern Med. 1998; 158(17):1946–1948

[109] Rice E, DiBaise JK, Quigley EM. Superior mesenteric artery thrombosis after colonoscopy. Gastrointest Endosc. 1999; 50(5):706–707

[110] Butcher JH, Davis AJM, Page A, Green B, Shepherd HA. Transient ischaemic colitis following an aeroplane flight: two case reports and review of the literature. Gut. 2002; 51(5):746–747

[111] Shibata M, Nakamuta H, Abe S, et al. Ischemic colitis caused by strict dieting in an 18-year-old female: report of a case. Dis Colon Rectum. 2002; 45(3):425–428

[112] Ryan CK, Reamy B, Rochester JA. Ischemic colitis associated with herbal product use in a young woman. J Am Board Fam Pract. 2002; 15(4):309–312

[113] Dee SL, Butt K, Ramaswamy G. Intestinal ischemia. Arch Pathol Lab Med. 2002; 126(10):1201–1204

[114] Flobert C, Cellier C, Berger A, et al. Right colonic involvement is associated with severe forms of ischemic colitis and occurs frequently in patients with chronic renal failure requiring hemodialysis. Am J Gastroenterol. 2000; 95 (1):195–198

[115] Sohn CI, Kim JJ, Lim YH, et al. A case of ischemic colitis associated with pheochromocytoma. Am J Gastroenterol. 1998; 93(1):124–126

[116] Bao P, Welch DC, Washington MK, Herline AJ. Resection of mesenteric inflammatory veno-occlusive disease causing ischemic colitis. J Gastrointest Surg. 2005; 9(6):812–817

[117] Lucas W, Schroy PC, III. Reversible ischemic colitis in a high endurance athlete. Am J Gastroenterol. 1998; 93(11):2231–2234

[118] Tsujimoto T, Takano M, Ishikawa M, et al. Onset of ischemic colitis following use of electrical muscle stimulation (EMS) exercise equipment. Intern Med. 2004; 43(8):693–695

[119] Church JM. Ischemic colitis complicating flexible endoscopy in a patient with connective tissue disease. Gastrointest Endosc. 1995; 41(2):181–182

[120] Versaci A, Macrì A, Scuderi G, et al. Ischemic colitis following colonoscopy in a systemic lupus erythematosus patient: report of a case. Dis Colon Rectum. 2005; 48(4):866–869

[121] Schwarz DA, Stark M, Wright J. Segmental colonic gangrene: a previously unreported complication of adult hemolytic uremic syndrome. Surgery. 1994; 116(1):107–110

[122] Walker AM, Bohn RL, Cali C, Cook SF, Ajene AN, Sands BE. Risk factors for colon ischemia. Am J Gastroenterol. 2004; 99(7):1333–1337

[123] Brandt LJ, Boley SJ. Colonic ischemia. Surg Clin North Am. 1992; 72(1):203–229

[124] Welch GH, Shearer MG, Imrie CW, Anderson JR, Gilmour DG. Total colonic ischemia. Dis Colon Rectum. 1986; 29(6):410–412

[125] West BR, Ray JE, Gathright JB. Comparison of transient ischemic colitis with that requiring surgical treatment. Surg Gynecol Obstet. 1980; 151(3):366–368

[126] Sakai L, Keltner R, Kaminski D. Spontaneous and shock-associated ischemic colitis. Am J Surg. 1980; 140(6):755–760

[127] Boley SJ, Corman M, Moosa AR, et al. Symposium. Management of colonic ischemia. Contemp Surg. 1989; 34:73–104

[128] Landreneau RJ, Fry WJ. The right colon as a target organ of non-occlusive mesenteric ischemia. Arch Surg. 1990; 125:591–594

[129] Newman JR, Cooper MA. Lower gastrointestinal bleeding and ischemic colitis. Can J Gastroenterol. 2002; 16(9):597–600

[130] Ardigo GJ, Longstreth GF, Weston LA, Walker FD. Passage of a large bowel cast caused by acute ischemia: report of two cases. Dis Colon Rectum. 1998; 41(6):793–796

[131] Ullery BS, Boyko AT, Banet GA, Lewis LM. Colonic ischemia: an under-recognized cause of lower gastrointestinal bleeding. J Emerg Med. 2004; 27(1):1–5

[132] Preventza OA, Lazarides K, Sawyer MD. Ischemic colitis in young adults: a single-institution experience. J Gastrointest Surg. 2001; 5(4):388–392

[133] Markoglou C, Avgerinos A, Mitrakou M, et al. Toxic megacolon secondary to acute ischemic colitis. Hepatogastroenterology. 1993; 40(2):188–190

[134] Philpotts LE, Heiken JP, Westcott MA, Gore RM. Colitis: use of CT findings in differential diagnosis. Radiology. 1994; 190(2):445–449

[135] Ranschaert E, Verhille R, Marchal G, Rigauts H, Ponette E. Sonographic diagnosis of ischemic colitis. J Belge Radiol. 1994; 77(4):166–168

[136] Lange H, Jäckel R. Usefulness of plasma lactate concentration in the diagnosis of acute abdominal disease. Eur J Surg. 1994; 160(6–7):381–384

[137] Tada M, Misaki F, Kawai K. Analysis of the clinical features of ischemic colitis. Gastroenterol Jpn. 1983; 18(3):204–209

[138] Sano S, Nishimori I, Miyao M, et al. Successful use of mesalamine in the treatment of chronic segmental lesion in a case of ischemic colitis. J Gastroenterol Hepatol. 2003; 18(7):882–883

[139] Abel ME, Russell TR. Ischemic colitis. Comparison of surgical and nonoperative management. Dis Colon Rectum. 1983; 26(2):113–115

[140] Longo WE, Ward D, Vernava AM, III, Kaminski DL. Outcome of patients with total colonic ischemia. Dis Colon Rectum. 1997; 40(12):1448–1454

[141] Guivarc'h M, Roullet-Audy JC, Mosnier H, Boché O. [Ischemic colitis. A surgical series of 88 cases]. J Chir (Paris). 1997; 134(3):103–108

[142] Medina C, Vilaseca J, Videla S, Fabra R, Armengol-Miro JR, Malagelada JR. Outcome of patients with ischemic colitis: review of fifty-three cases. Dis Colon Rectum. 2004; 47(2):180–184

[143] Foley CL, Taylor CJ, Aslam M, Reddy KP, Birch HA, Owen ER. Failure of conservative management after the passage of a distal colonic "cast": report of a case. Dis Colon Rectum. 2005; 48(5):1090–1093

[144] Iwashita A, Yao T, Schlemper RJ, et al. Mesenteric phlebosclerosis: a new disease entity causing ischemic colitis. Dis Colon Rectum. 2003; 46(2):209–220

[145] Koyama N, Koyama H, Hanajima T, et al. Chronic ischemic colitis causing stenosis. Report of a case. Stomach Intestine (Tokyo). 1991; 26:455–460

[146] Yoshinaga S, Harada N, Araki Y, et al. Chronic ischemic colonic lesion caused by phlebosclerosis: a case report. Gastrointest Endosc. 2001; 53(1):107–111

[147] Ernst CB, Hagihara PF, Daughtery ME, Sachatello CR, Griffen WO, Jr. Ischemic colitis incidence following abdominal aortic reconstruction: a prospective study. Surgery. 1976; 80(4):417–421

[148] Hagihara PF, Ernst CB, Griffen WO, Jr. Incidence of ischemic colitis following abdominal aortic reconstruction. Surg Gynecol Obstet. 1979; 149(4):571–573

[149] Björck M, Bergqvist D, Troëng T. Incidence and clinical presentation of bowel ischaemia after aortoiliac surgery–2930 operations from a population-based registry in Sweden. Eur J Vasc Endovasc Surg. 1996; 12(2):139–144

[150] Champagne BJ, Darling RC, III, Daneshmand M, et al. Outcome of aggressive surveillance colonoscopy in ruptured abdominal aortic aneurysm. J Vasc Surg. 2004; 39(4):792–796

[151] Schroeder T, Christoffersen JK, Andersen J, et al. Ischemic colitis complicating reconstruction of the abdominal aorta. Surg Gynecol Obstet. 1985; 160(4):299–303

[152] Kozarek RA, Earnest DL, Silverstein ME, Smith RG. Air-pressure-induced colon injury during diagnostic colonoscopy. Gastroenterology. 1980; 78(1):7–14

[153] Brandt CP, Piotrowski JJ, Alexander JJ. Flexible sigmoidoscopy. A reliable determinant of colonic ischemia following ruptured abdominal aortic aneurysm. Surg Endosc. 1997; 11(2):113–115

[154] Houe T, Thorböll JE, Sigild U, Liisberg-Larsen O, Schroeder TV. Can colonoscopy diagnose transmural ischaemic colitis after abdominal aortic surgery? An evidence-based approach. Eur J Vasc Endovasc Surg. 2000; 19(3):304–307

[155] Zelenock GB, Strodel WE, Knol JA, et al. A prospective study of clinically and endoscopically documented colonic ischemia in 100 patients undergoing aortic reconstructive surgery with aggressive colonic and direct pelvic revascularization, compared with historic controls. Surgery. 1989; 106(4):771–779, discussion 779–780

[156] Maupin G-E, Rimar SD, Villalba M. Ischemic colitis following abdominal aortic reconstruction for ruptured aneurysm. A 10-year experience. Am Surg. 1989; 55(6):378–380

[157] Bast TJ, van der Biezen JJ, Scherpenisse J, Eikelboom BC. Ischaemic disease of the colon and rectum after surgery for abdominal aortic aneurysm: a prospective study of the incidence and risk factors. Eur J Vasc Surg. 1990; 4(3):253–257

[158] Piotrowski JJ, Ripepi AJ, Yuhas JP, Alexander JJ, Brandt CP. Colonic ischemia: the Achilles heel of ruptured aortic aneurysm repair. Am Surg. 1996; 62(7):557–560, discussion 560–561

[159] Lane TM, Bentley PG. Rectal strictures following abdominal aortic aneurysm surgery. Ann R Coll Surg Engl. 2000; 82(6):421–423

[160] Järvinen O, Laurikka J, Salenius JP, Lepäntalo M. Mesenteric infarction after aortoiliac surgery on the basis of 1752 operations from the National Vascular Registry. World J Surg. 1999; 23(3):243–247

[161] Van Damme H, Creemers E, Limet R. Ischaemic colitis following aortoiliac surgery. Acta Chir Belg. 2000; 100(1):21–27

[162] Hinchliffe RJ, Armon MP, Tse CC, Wenham PW, Hopkinson BR. Colonic infarction following endovascular AAA repair: a multifactorial complication. J Endovasc Ther. 2002; 9(4):554–558

[163] Connolly JE, Stemmer EA. Intestinal gangrene as the result of mesenteric arterial steal. Am J Surg. 1973; 126(2):197–204

[164] Cordoba A, Gordillo O. Mesenteric arterial steal syndrome secondary to bilateral lumbar sympathectomy. Int Surg. 1979; 64(4):67–69

[165] Klok T, Moll FL, Leusink JA, Theunissen DJ, Gerrits CM, Keijer C. The relationship between sigmoidal intramucosal pH and intestinal arterial occlusion during aortic reconstructive surgery. Eur J Vasc Endovasc Surg. 1996; 11(3):304–307

[166] Björck M, Hedberg B. Early detection of major complications after abdominal aortic surgery: predictive value of sigmoid colon and gastric intramucosal pH monitoring. Br J Surg. 1994; 81(1):25–30

[167] Ernst CB, Hagihara PF, Daugherty ME, Griffen WO, Jr. Inferior mesenteric artery stump pressure: a reliable index for safe IMA ligation during abdominal aortic aneurysmectomy. Ann Surg. 1978; 187(6):641–646

[168] Mitchell KM, Valentine RJ. Inferior mesenteric artery reimplantation does not guarantee colon viability in aortic surgery. J Am Coll Surg. 2002; 194(2):151–155

[169] Geraghty PJ, Sanchez LA, Rubin BG, et al. Overt ischemic colitis after endovascular repair of aortoiliac aneurysms. J Vasc Surg. 2004; 40(3):413–418

[170] Al-Saleh N, Wehrli BM, Driman DK, Taylor BM. Ischemic pancolitis: recognizing a rare form of acute ischemic colitis. Can J Surg. 2004; 47(5):382–383

[171] Ahmed I, Kerwat R, Morgan AR, Beynon J. Rectal ischaemia following hypovolaemic shock. Br J Surg. 1996; 83(4):508

[172] Quirke P, Campbell I, Talbot IC. Ischaemic proctitis and adventitial fibromuscular dysplasia of the superior rectal artery. Br J Surg. 1984; 71(1):33–38

[173] Lazaris ACh, Papanikolaou IS, Theodoropoulos GE, Petraki K, Davaris PS. Ischaemic necrosis of the rectum and sigmoid colon complicating systemic lupus erythematosus. Acta Gastroenterol Belg. 2003; 66(2):191–194

[174] Nelson RL, Briley S, Schuler JJ, Abcarian H. Acute ischemic proctitis. Report of six cases. Dis Colon Rectum. 1992; 35(4):375–380

[175] Bharucha AE, Tremaine WJ, Johnson CD, Batts KP. Ischemic proctosigmoiditis. Am J Gastroenterol. 1996; 91(11):2305–2309

[176] Mackay C, Murphy P, Rosenberg IL, Tait NP. Case report: rectal infarction after abdominal aortic surgery. Br J Radiol. 1994; 67(797):497–498

[177] Cataldo PA, Zarka MA. Formalin instillation for ischemic proctitis with unrelenting hemorrhage: report of a case. Dis Colon Rectum. 2000; 43(2):261–263

[178] Kishikawa H, Nishida J, Hirano E, et al. Chronic ischemic proctitis: case report and review. Gastrointest Endosc. 2004; 60(2):304–308

31 Radiation Injuries to the Small and Large Intestines

David E. Beck and Santhat Nivatvongs

Abstract

Radiation therapy is an important treatment option in patients with carcinoma of the cervix, uterus, ovaries, prostate, testicles, bladder, and rectum. Much has been written about the pathology and clinical symptomatology of radiation injury to individual organ systems. Some of the most serious injuries occur in the gastrointestinal tract, with damage to the small bowel, colon, and rectum. Despite improved technology and a better understanding of the effects of radiation on normal tissues, radiation injury is still a formidable problem. Many patients who are cured of carcinoma still suffer considerable morbidity and occasional mortality from the radiation itself.

Keywords: radiation, small intestine, large intestine, pathology, predisposing factors, incidence, clinical manifestations, medical management, surgical management, radiation proctitis

31.1 Introduction

Radiation therapy is an important treatment option in patients with carcinoma of the cervix, uterus, ovaries, prostate, testicles, bladder, and rectum.[1,2,3,4] The injurious effects of X-rays on normal intestine were noted only 2 years after Roentgen's discovery of X-rays, when Walsh[5] described the case of a coworker who developed bowel dysfunction while exposed to X-rays. The coworker's symptoms cleared when he was kept from further exposure. Much has been written about the pathology and clinical symptomatology of radiation injury to individual organ systems. Some of the most serious injuries occur in the gastrointestinal tract, with damage to the small bowel, colon, and rectum. Despite improved technology and a better understanding of the effects of radiation on normal tissues, radiation injury is still a formidable problem. Many patients who are cured of carcinoma still suffer considerable morbidity and occasional mortality from the radiation itself.

31.2 Incidence and Clinical Manifestations

The true incidence of radiation injury is difficult to assess accurately. Most large series estimate the incidence of chronic radiation injury to be between 5 and 11%, with approximately 20% of these requiring an operation.[6] Krook et al[7] reported a 6.7% incidence of bowel complications in patients who received postoperative chemoradiation for rectal adenocarcinoma.

Although the acute effects of radiation begin within hours of the commencement of radiation therapy, most patients will not experience the symptoms of acute radiation injury until 3,000 to 4,000 cGy have been delivered. Acute colitis and proctitis are manifested by abdominal pain, diarrhea, tenesmus, and rectal bleeding. There is little value in pursuing an aggressive diagnostic evaluation in this clinical setting. Approximately 50 to 70% of all patients undergoing therapeutic pelvic irradiation will develop these symptoms. A decrease in the daily dosage of the radiation is usually successful, and it is distinctly uncommon to have to discontinue the therapy.[6]

Late complications can lead to a multitude of clinical problems. Patients may present with bowel obstruction, stricture, fistula formation, perforation, hemorrhage, and malabsorption. They may also experience fecal incontinence, either because of direct radiation damage to the anal sphincter or as a consequence of late radiation effects on pelvic nerves.[8] One must keep in mind that patients who survive 5 or more years after their first malignancy may be at risk for the development of subsequent malignancies within the radiation fields.[6]

Eighty-five percent of all patients who develop radiation injury present between 6 and 24 months after completion of radiation therapy.[9,10,11] The remaining 15% of patients may develop complications years or even decades after treatment.[12] In general, patients with rectal ulceration or proctitis present somewhat earlier in their course than with strictures and fistulas.[13,14]

Damage to the small intestine is more serious and constitutes 30 to 50% of the radiation injuries severe enough to require operation.[15,16] Urinary tract complications, including ureteral obstruction secondary to fibrosis, cystitis, and fibrotic changes in the bladder (with bladder dysfunction and fistula formation), occur in up to 28% of patients having late gastrointestinal complications.[17,18]

Late complications can appear clinically as anorexia, malnourishment, colicky abdominal pain, bowel dysfunction (including diarrhea, obstipation, fecal urgency, and frequency of defecation with or without incontinence), rectal pain, rectal bleeding, dysuria, hematuria, chronic urinary tract infections, sepsis, and shock. Since many of these symptom complexes may also be seen in patients with recurrent malignancy, it is often difficult to distinguish late radiation injury from recurrent carcinoma.

A systemic review of 21 randomized controlled trials in 2015 evaluated the quality of toxicity information.[19] There was a lack of reporting standards, and studies that used patient-reported outcomes identified higher rates of toxicity symptoms than clinician-reported studies.

31.3 Mechanisms of Radiation Injury

Ionizing radiation injures cells by the transfer of energy to critical biologic macromolecules, including DNA, proteins, and membrane lipids. Some damage occurs directly from absorption of energy by the target molecules. Indirect damage is caused by diffusible oxygen-free radicals, highly reactive intermediates generated from the absorption of radiant energy by low-molecular-weight compounds. Water is, by far, the most abundant component of the cell, and the radiologic products of water are responsible largely for indirect, free radical damage. When target macromolecules are irradiated directly or react with high-energy free radical intermediates, the targets themselves become ionized or transformed into free radicals.

Although radiation can exert its damaging effects by these two different mechanisms, the end result is the same.[20]

Damage to lipid membranes results, in part, from lipid peroxidation. Functionally, these changes are expressed as altered membrane fluidity and increased permeability, which can trigger the release of potent physiologic mediators that enhance the damage.[20]

31.4 Pathology

The gastrointestinal tract is second only to the kidneys in radiosensitivity, and gastrointestinal tract injury is the major limiting factor affecting tolerance to radiation of the abdomen and pelvis.[21,22] Although the small intestine is more radiosensitive than the large intestine, it is injured less frequently because of its mobility within the abdominal cavity. The sites of most severe injury after pelvic irradiation are in the lower sigmoid colon and upper rectum, probably because of their proximity to the field of radiation. Overt injury to the small intestine is less common but, when it occurs, is usually situated 6 to 10 cm from the ileocecal valve. These areas show the most severe derangement of vascular architecture and maximum reduction in microvascular volume.[23]

At the cellular level, the injurious effect of radiation is still not fully understood. Ionizing radiation generates free radicals from intracellular water; they, in turn, can interact with DNA to block transcription and replication. Cells with a high proliferation rate such as those in the intestinal mucosa are more susceptible to such disruptions.[24,25] More latent effects can occur in the vascular connective tissue, giving rise to complications later.[24]

Grossly, early radiation injuries result in an edematous, thickened, and hyperemic mucosa. Areas of superficial ulceration or necrosis may also be present (▶ Fig. 31.1).[26] In the small bowel, the villi become blunted, and in both the small and large bowels, the crypts become shortened, and cryptal microabscesses can form. Microscopically, the microvilli of the surface epithelium are shortened, prominent large nuclei are present, and the mitochondria and endoplasmic reticulum are dilated.[15] The submucosa may show some cytologic atypia with bizarre, enlarged fibroblasts that could be mistaken for malignant cells

(▶ Fig. 31.2). A loss of the normal fibrillar pattern of collagen and the deposition of large amounts of hyalin may also be present in the submucosa.[27] A hyalin-type substance thickens artery walls as well.[22,28] Spasm and thrombosis may occur in the arterioles (▶ Fig. 31.3), and vascular ectasias may develop.[22,28] Infiltration by leukocytes can be seen throughout the full thickness of the bowel wall.

Late injuries are characterized by a severe degree of fibrosis. Grossly, the bowel appears pale and opaque, and is usually shortened. The mesentery becomes thickened and may also be shortened.[15] Gross radiation changes may be indistinguishable from those of Crohn's disease, but the fat does not generally extend over the surface of the bowel as it does in Crohn's disease (▶ Fig. 31.4).[29] Loops of small intestine may be fused with fibrous adhesions and normal tissue planes obliterated, giving rise to a "frozen pelvis" comparable to that seen with recurrent malignancy.[15,29] Strictures, generally long and tapered, may appear; ulcers may develop and can be deep and progress to a fistula or perforation.[29,30]

Histologically, the villi show thickening and flattening, with areas of atrophy and degeneration. There is a marked submucosal fibrosis with hyalinization.[14] Telangiectasias may be prominent in the submucosa but may also occur throughout

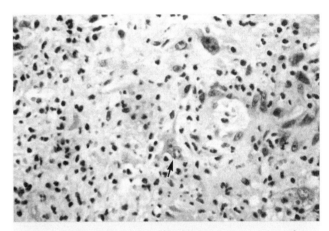

Fig. 31.2 Enlarged bizarre-shaped fibroblast (*arrow*) seen in tissue from an acute radiation injury.

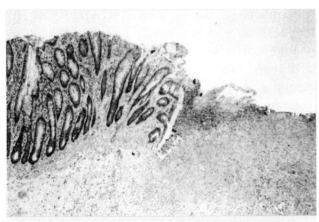

Fig. 31.1 Superficial ulceration showing loss of mucosa and inflammatory reaction in an acute radiation injury.

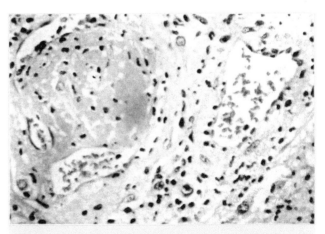

Fig. 31.3 Thrombosis and recanalization changes in arteriole in irradiated tissue.

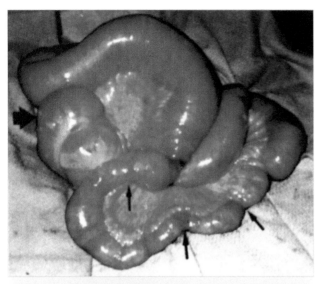

Fig. 31.4 Specimen from ileocolic resection for chronic radiation enteritis. *Small arrows* point to areas of stricture without fat wrapping in the ileum. *Large arrow* points to cecum. Note dilatation of the proximal nonstrictured small bowel.

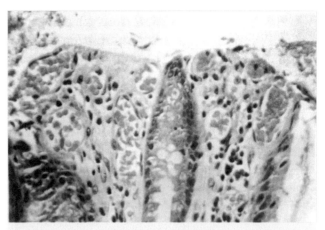

Fig. 31.5 Mucosal telangiectasias seen in a chronic radiation injury.

the bowel wall (▶ Fig. 31.5). The arterioles show hyaline thickening of the media with intimal proliferation.[27] Areas of venous and lymphatic sclerosis are noted, and venous and lymphatic ectasias can appear in the submucosa.[14] The smooth muscle of both the small and large intestines may become hypertrophic, and the ganglion cells in the rectum may also undergo hypertrophy and degenerate; the latter change can affect function.[8,16] The serosa and perirectal connective tissue usually show fibrosis with arterial hyalinization and intimal fibrosis.[29]

A microradiography study using barium sulfate infusion by Carr et al[23] showed that in radiation-injured bowel that requires resection, alterations in microvascular architecture are present in all sections, but these appearances vary with the type of lesion. At the site of fully developed strictures, a reduction in vascularity affects all the layers of the intestinal wall. Histologically, these areas show pronounced fibrosis in the submucosa and muscularis propria together with severe vascular changes that consist of occlusive fibrin thrombi in capillaries and sometimes-occlusive intimal fibrosis in the small intramural arterial vessels. In sections taken from sites adjacent to perforations, avascularity zones are apparent. The mucosal vascular pattern is abnormal, and the severity of change parallels the reduction in vascularity in the remainder of the section. Capillary microthrombi are present in these mucosal vessels with or without accompanying mucosal necrosis.

31.5 Pathogenesis

Malabsorption with intractable diarrhea is one of the most serious consequences of radiation injury to the intestine. Several factors may be involved in the genesis of this problem, including increased bowel motility.[31] The change in motility may stem from increased prostaglandin release, which can stimulate the smooth muscle of the small bowel.[31,32] Loss of the brush border and its digestive enzymes may occur, causing a decrease in carbohydrate

absorption and osmotic diarrhea.[28] Bacterial overgrowth in the intestine can also cause malabsorption and subsequent diarrhea.[33] Injury to the terminal ileum can cause a decrease in the absorption of bile salts, which has a dual effect. An increased bile salt load to the colon causes intraluminal sodium retention with an increase in intraluminal water retention. In addition, the bile salt pool decreases in size, with a decrease in the absorption of fats and the development of steatorrhea.[33]

Although injury to the small intestine is chiefly responsible for malabsorption and diarrhea, injury to the rectum is responsible for the development of incontinence and the frequency and urgency of defecation. Stenosis of the rectosigmoid area sometimes is severe enough to cause these symptoms.[27] Anal manometric study in patients with radiation proctitis showed a decrease in rectal volume and compliance. The physiologic length of the internal sphincter decreased, while the squeeze pressure and external sphincter muscle function were normal. Rectosphincteric reflex was abnormal in several patients.[8,16] Correlating these findings with histologic studies showed hypertrophy of smooth muscle and abnormalities in the myenteric plexus, including hypertrophy of the nerve fibers and a decrease in the number of ganglion cells within the plexus of Auerbach.[34] A similarity between these findings and those of Hirschsprung's disease was apparent.

Another complication of intestinal radiation is the development of a primary carcinoma in the radiated tissue. This was first noted by Slaughter and Southwick[35] in 1957. In 1965, Black and Ackerman[36] developed criteria for the diagnosis of radiation-induced carcinoma. These criteria include a 10-year latency period from the time of radiation therapy and severe radiation changes in the adjacent tissues. Sandler and Sandler[37] demonstrated that patients who have had radiation therapy have a relative risk for developing a primary carcinoma in the radiated field 2.0 to 3.6 times that of the normal population. Patients who have undergone radiation in the pelvic region have careful surveillance beginning 10 years after completion of radiation therapy. Most of these neoplasms are likely to arise in the rectum and, therefore, should be within reach of a rigid or flexible sigmoidoscope.

Although one would expect high-dose radiation to be essential for the induction of colorectal carcinoma, in fact, the opposite may be true. Palmer and Spratt[38] found that patients who received low-dose radiation for benign gynecologic conditions had a greater chance (3.32%) of developing rectal carcinoma than those who received high-dose radiation (1.42%) to treat carcinoma of the cervix. Radiation-induced colorectal carcinomas were more often of mucinous histologic type (25–60% of cases) than carcinomas in nonradiated patients (10% of cases).[6] The fact that these carcinomas are of a different histologic type and that all colon carcinomas induced by radiation in rats are mucinous adenocarcinomas[39] lends further support to the concept that these carcinomas are radiation induced.

Another pathologic process that can be confused with adenocarcinoma is colitis cystica profunda, which has been noted to occur in irradiated tissue. It is a rare condition characterized by the presence of epithelial mucous cysts that are generally deep to the mucosa.[40,41] Although the glandular elements in the submucosa and muscularis propria may appear as adenocarcinoma, cytologic evidence of malignancy must be present before the lesions may be called adenocarcinoma.

31.6 Predisposing Factors

The cumulative total dosage of radiation delivered to the tissues is an important determinant of any subsequent radiation damage. Strockbine et al[42] in a review of 831 patients noted no intestinal injuries when the total radiation dose was less than 3,000 rads but found an injury rate of 36% among patients receiving 7,000 rads. Assessment of the minimal and maximal tolerance doses for the gastrointestinal tract has shown that the small bowel is the most radiosensitive area.

Although total dosage is an important etiologic factor in the development of radiation injuries, patients receiving low-dose radiation can still suffer radiation damage to normal tissues.[11,27] This damage can occur because cell injury is also dependent on the rate at which the radiation is delivered. Malignant cells do not self-repair as well as normal cells between doses of radiation; so malignant cells do not repopulate between doses as well as normal cells. Consequently, the normal cell population is better able to tolerate radiation that is given more frequently, especially when smaller doses are used.[24,43] Doses of less than 200 rads per day comprise the regimen usually given for external beam radiation. Dosage rates are especially important when intracavitary radiation is used. Lee et al[44] have shown that dosage rates greater than 60 rads per hour are associated with a higher incidence of bladder and rectal injuries.

It has long been known that some patients tolerate radiotherapy better than others. One important predisposing factor is existing vascular damage from hypertension, diabetes mellitus, collagen vascular disease, and atherosclerosis.[1,10,19,28,45,46,47,48,49] Second is a previous abdominal or pelvic operation that led to adhesions that immobilize the small bowel such that the same segment receives radiation with each treatment.[20,50] A thin habitus has also been associated with a greater frequency of chronic radiation damage.[48]

A strong correlation has also been made between radiation injury and various chemotherapeutic agents. Doxorubicin (Adriamycin), actimycin, bleomycin, and 5-fluorouracil (5-FU) enhance cell injury in the gastrointestinal tract; this necessitates reduction in radiation dosage when these agents are being used.[51,52] Olsalazine is contraindicated during pelvis radiation

therapy because it increases the risk of proctitis.[53] Animal studies have shown that intraluminal contents, including pancreatic secretions, can predispose the patient to radiation injuries.[54]

31.7 Small Intestine Injuries

31.7.1 Diagnosis

Injuries to the small bowel are not readily identified as it is the most difficult part of the gastrointestinal tract to study radiographically and it cannot be reached readily endoscopically. Small bowel studies are notoriously inexact; extensive narrowing may be present with normal radiologic findings. Positive findings, when present, are generally those of ischemia with "'thumbprinting,'" nodular filling defects, and separation of loops secondary to edema and/or fibrosis (▶ Fig. 31.6).[55] Strictures and fistulas also can be seen, but fistulograms are often necessary to localize enterocutaneous fistulas. The recent progress in CT enterography will lead to its replacing other radiologic tests for evaluating the small intestine.[56,57] Radiation-induced lesions may be especially difficult to distinguish from neoplastic invasion on X-ray studies. Most lesions secondary to radiation appear in the terminal ileum, whereas 58% of those caused by malignancy occur in the duodenum or jejunum.[58] Angiography can help distinguish the two entities. Characteristic findings of radiation injury include arterial stenosis, decreased vascularity, luminal irregularities, and stenosis in the veins, with a decrease in the capillary phase in the bowel wall. In contrast, arteries supplying a malignancy tend to be dilated and are associated

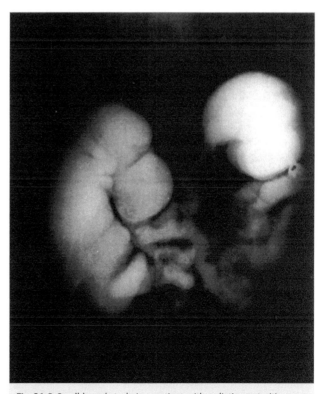

Fig. 31.6 Small bowel study in a patient with radiation enteritis showing "thumbprinting," submucosal edema, and fluid between small bowel loops.

with a large number of tiny "tumor" vessels within the carcinoma during the capillary phase.[59] The recent progress of technology using integrated PET-CT imaging is valuable for the differentiation of posttreatment changes from recurrent carcinoma.[60]

The clinical manifestation of radiation damage to the small bowel can be divided into two groups according to the time of appearance. Acute enteral complications of radiation therapy occur either during or immediately following a course of radiation therapy. Nausea, vomiting, cramps, and intermittent diarrhea are all symptoms of acute radiation enteritis. Such symptoms are probably caused by a breakdown in the intestinal mucosa that is no longer able to absorb the usual fluids and nutrients. The mucosa is also unable to prevent the efflux of fluids from the underlying supporting stroma. These changes in the intestinal epithelium result in disorders of motility and transport of fluid and solutes.[24,61]

Long-term complications of radiation therapy are usually manifestations of progressive vasculitis and interstitial fibrosis initiated by radiation therapy, often delivered many years before clinical signs develop. Partial or complete intestinal obstruction due to strictures or decreased motility, intestinal perforation, gastrointestinal bleeding, and malabsorption and enteric fistulas are all long-term enteral complications of patients treated with abdominal or pelvic radiation therapy.[24,61]

31.7.2 Medical Management

No effective medical treatment is available. Conservative therapy can control many of the symptoms of radiation enteropathy. Antispasmodics, anticholinergics, opiates, a low-residue diet, and a diet low in fats and lactose can improve symptoms of abdominal pain and diarrhea.[62,63] Lactose deficiency from villus blunting with emergent lactose intolerance is seen in 20% of subsequent patients.[64,65] Malabsorption studies should be done on patients who do not respond to the aforementioned measures. If a study reveals that a patient has abnormal bile salt absorption, the specific bile salt–binding resin, cholestyramine, can often decrease the diarrhea significantly.[63,66,67] Cholestyramine is usually well tolerated, although it binds oral medications and should not be given concomitantly with other drugs.[66] Oral antibiotics can help patients who have suspected bacterial overgrowth of the small bowel from intestinal stasis. 5-ASA and steroids are effective.[68,69]

In some patients, elemental diets have been shown to decrease stool output while maintaining nutrition.[70] For other patients either short-term or long-term total parenteral nutrition (TPN) may be needed. Some patients, in whom both medical and surgical therapies have failed, have done well with home TPN.[71,72] TPN is often the initial treatment of choice for an enterocutaneous fistula, especially in the malnourished patient, although spontaneous closure is uncommon.[73] TPN is invaluable for preparing the malnourished patient for operation.

31.7.3 Surgical Management

Selection of appropriate procedures should consider general as well as local aspects. Literature data indicate that over 40% of patients with radiation enteritis will not survive 2 years following operation, and over 60% of the deceased succumb to their primary malignancy.[74] Operation is clearly indicated for obstruction, perforation, fistula that is unresponsive to TPN, abscess, and intractable bleeding or diarrhea. Although the number of patients requiring operation is small, the morbidity rate has been reported to be as high as 65%[73] and the mortality rate as high as 45%.[75] Decisions concerning timing of operation and type of operation can be critical.

Often it is impossible to distinguish radiation injury from recurrent malignancy, thus influencing surgical decision-making. Walsh and Schofield[76] reported on 53 patients with small bowel obstruction who underwent exploratory laparotomy and found that 17 of the 53 patients had recurrent malignancy, whereas the others had obstruction from other causes. Most of the patients with malignancy received good palliation from the operation, and the authors concluded that operation should not be denied solely because of concern about recurrent carcinoma.

The most controversial issue relating to the surgical management of patients with small bowel radiation injury is whether to bypass or resect the abnormal bowel. The argument against resection with primary anastomosis is that dividing the mesenteric vessels will further jeopardize an already compromised bowel and that dissection around adhesions increases the risk of subsequent fistula formation.[73] On the other hand, bypassing an irradiated segment leaves behind a diseased portion of bowel with the potential for fistula formation and the development of a blind-loop syndrome.[77,78]

Surgical decision-making was influenced by a retrospective multicenter study with literature meta-analysis published in 1976,[72] which rather indiscriminately compared the surgical outcome of resection versus bypass, that is, without consideration of the intestinal segment involved. The conclusion that bypass was superior to resection in terms of surgical complication and operative mortality had substantial impact for more than a decade.[74]

Overall, an individualized approach selectively using bypass and resection is probably the safest course. For those cases in which most of the small bowel is involved and dense adhesions have formed in the pelvis, dissection should be avoided and a bypass procedure performed instead. On the other hand, resection is preferable if disease is confined to a short segment of small intestine or if wide resection and ileocolic anastomosis to the colon can be done. In the latter cases, frozen-section biopsy of the grossly normal colon segment can be helpful to rule out fibrosis, obliteration of vessels, or other evidence of significant radiation injury.[28,62,79]

Strictureplasty is not recommended as a primary procedure for radiation strictures. However, in patients with limited intestinal reserve where strictures are located within long segments of diseased bowel which, if resected or bypassed, would have significant nutritional or metabolic consequences, strictureplasty may be an effective and safe tool to conserve intestinal length.[80]

Despite high initial mortality and morbidity rates, life expectancy in patients with chronic radiation enteritis without recurrence of their primary neoplastic disease is good. Resection seems to provide a lower reoperative rate and a better 5-year survival and better quality of life than bypass procedure.[81,82]

Regardless of the procedure, special mention must be made of enterolysis. A high incidence of fistula formation and perforation has been reported after enterolysis because of either ischemia or small enterotomies made during the procedure.[1,10] Enterolysis should be undertaken with great caution and generally only if the surgeon is willing to resect the involved bowel if necessary.

The management of small bowel fistulas can be particularly difficult. The fistula may be due to recurrent malignancy as well as radiation injury. It is useful to divide the management of patients with enteric fistulas into three phases: (1) stabilization, (2) definition of the fistula, and (3) definitive therapy.[83] Stabilization of the patient includes fluid and electrolyte resuscitation, control of fistula output, and nutritional repletion of the chronically debilitated patient. To define the extent of the fistula, contrast studies, including large and small bowel X-ray films and fistulograms, are employed. Every effort is made to ascertain the full extent of the often-complex small bowel fistulas encountered. Despite prolonged TPN, no radiation-induced small bowel fistula has ever closed with conservative management alone. However, TPN with gut rest may be a valuable initial treatment. Poor results have been obtained with attempts at resection of the fistula or partial bypass; the best results have followed total exclusion of the involved segment of bowel.[73,83,84] Smith et al[83] reported a 92% success rate of total exclusion, bringing out one end of the excluded segment as a mucous fistula (▶ Fig. 31.7). This compares favorably with a 67% success rate with resection and a 69% success rate with partial bypass.

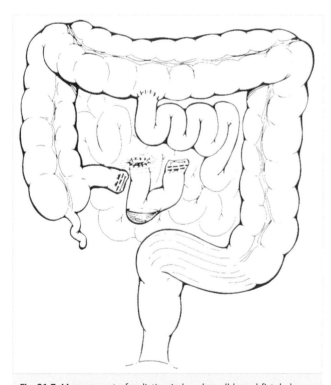

Fig. 31.7 Management of radiation-induced small bowel fistula by total exclusion of the involved segment, bringing out one end as a mucous fistula.

31.8 Colon and Rectal Injuries

31.8.1 Diagnosis

Injuries of the colon and rectum are more easily diagnosed than small bowel injuries. A digital examination alone can define areas of anorectal stenosis, and a bimanual examination can detect a frozen pelvis. Sometimes these examinations are painful, in which case they should be performed with the patient under general or regional anesthesia.

Proctoscopy or colonoscopy is essential to diagnosis, but each must be performed with caution because fixation of the bowel may make it vulnerable to perforation. The rectal mucosa can undergo a wide range of changes, with varying degrees of edema, increased friability, petechial hemorrhages, and diffuse oozing.[27,32,85] Ulcerations may be present, usually on the anterior wall. The ulcers tend to have a sloughing gray base with flat edges.[18] Biopsy may be required to rule out malignancy, but care must be taken in performing these biopsies, or a rectal fistula can result.

Proctitis associated with radiation therapy has been divided into three stages by Dean and Taylor.[86] Stage I consists of vascular congestion and friability of the rectal mucosa. The areas of severe injury are usually located on the anterior wall at the level of the cervix. Often there is a circumscribed area of thickening with a mucoid exudate present (▶ Fig. 31.8). This stage is clinically accompanied by rectal bleeding, diarrhea, tenesmus, sphincter irritability, and mucoid discharge. Stage II is an ulcerative stage resulting from thrombosis of the small mucosal vessels. The mucosa is thickened and generally is covered with an exudate, but ischemia is more marked in this stage. Rectal pain is more severe and is associated with more bleeding and diarrhea. Stage III is characterized by progression of the ischemia with endarteritis, necrosis, and, sometimes, fistula formation. Rectal strictures are found in this stage (▶ Fig. 31.9). Clinically, erosions can lead to massive hemorrhage, and the strictures

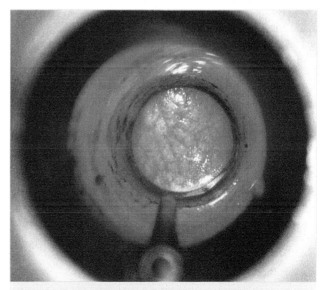

Fig. 31.8 Proctoscopic view of stage I radiation-induced proctitis with vascular congestion, edema, and friability.

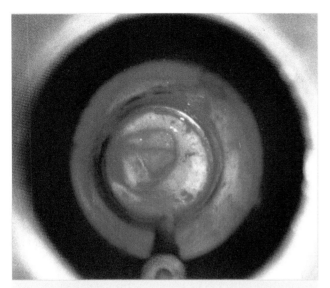

Fig. 31.9 Proctoscopic view of stage III radiation-induced proctitis with severe fibrosis and stricture.

can cause diarrhea with urgency, incomplete evacuation, and fecal or purulent drainage. Dean and Taylor[86] considered stages I and II amenable to medical therapy, whereas stage III generally requires surgical intervention.

DeCosse et al[10] have divided patients with radiation-induced rectal injury into two groups. Group I consists of those with proctitis, rectal ulceration, or stenosis. In these patients, symptoms of bleeding, tenesmus, and rectal pain do not correlate with the degree of injury. When present, rectal stenosis is generally located proximal to the ulcers, usually 8 to 12 cm from the anal verge. The process is often reversible in these patients. Group II injuries consist of rectovaginal fistulas. These injuries are irreversible and require surgical intervention.

Radiation injuries to the colon proximal to the rectosigmoid can be diagnosed by flexible colonoscopy and barium enema. Colonoscopy reveals a pale arid opaque mucosa at the injury site, suggesting fibrosis and submucosal edema. The surrounding tissue may appear more normal, but prominent submucosal telangiectasias may be present. The mucosa may be erythematous, granular, and friable when more active and acute distress is present.[73,87] Barium enema studies reveal shortening and narrowing of the rectosigmoid region with loss of the normal curvature.[9,15] The presacral space may increase secondary to thickening of the rectal wall and the perirectal tissues. These changes are best seen on lateral and oblique projections.[11,55] The examination may reveal rigidity and lack of distensibility of the rectum. Atrophy of the mucosa may give a pipe stem appearance.[9] When active disease is present, the mucosa may show a granular irregularity similar to that seen in other inflammatory bowel diseases with pseudopolypoid protrusions.[9] Multiple areas of stricture may be present, and they can be difficult to distinguish from recurrent carcinoma (▶ Fig. 31.10).[34]

31.8.2 Medical Management

Antispasmodic agents, anticholinergics, and opiates can be helpful in treating patients with large bowel injuries. Use of a low-residue diet and stool softeners is beneficial because of the

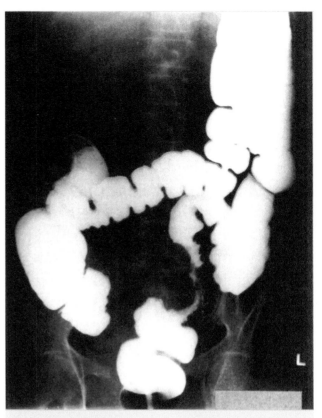

Fig. 31.10 Barium enema examination in a patient with radiation proctocolitis showing long rectosigmoid stricture.

friability of the rectal mucosa and its vulnerability to damage from the fecal stream.

Sucralfate enema, given twice daily, has been shown to be of benefit.[88] Aminosalicylic acid (ASA) derivatives, given rectally or orally, have not been shown to be of benefit.[89]

Vitamin A stimulates various aspects of wound repair and wound healing. Levitsky et al[90] reported a case of a patient with HIV infection who developed a symptomatic anal ulcer after receiving radiotherapy for anal squamous cell carcinoma. Vitamin A 8000 IU was given orally twice daily. Within 7 weeks, the patient's anorectal symptoms and anal ulcer were completely resolved.

A prospective, randomized, double-blind, placebo-controlled trial of retinol palmitate (vitamin A) for chronic radiation proctopathy with symptoms of diarrhea, rectal pain, rectal urgency, rectal bleeding, and fecal incontinence was reported.[91] Nineteen patients were randomized: 10 to retinyl palmitate 10,000 IU by mouth daily for 90 days, 9 to placebo. The results showed that the retinol palmitate group had significantly reduced symptoms. This series is small but may serve as the basis for a larger, multicenter trial for the future.[91]

One of the mechanisms of radiation injury to the gastrointestinal tract is the indirect damage of the cell caused by diffusible oxygen-free radicals.[20] Antioxidants, which have a scavenging property for reactive oxygen metabolites,[92] have been found to prevent tissue damage in radiation injury and ischemia–reperfusion injury.[93]

Kennedy et al[93] conducted a prospective study using vitamins E and C in patients suffering from radiation injury of the rectum. Twenty patients (10 prostate carcinomas, 10 gynecological malignancies) who had received previous radiation treatment were referred for treatment with symptoms of rectal pain, bleeding, or diarrhea with and without urgency. Symptoms had been present for at least 6 months. The radiation exposure ranged from 1 to 36 years (average, 4 years). All of these patients had received some form of therapy for their symptoms and had failed to respond. In this study, the treatment was initiated with vitamin E 400 IU, taken orally three times a day, and vitamin C 500 mg taken orally three times a day. Other medications were discontinued.

The results showed that at 4 to 6 weeks of follow-up, there was a significant improvement in the bleeding, diarrhea, and urgency. However, there was no significant improvement of rectal pain. All 10 patients who underwent a second follow-up interview reported sustained improvement in their symptoms 1 year later. The favorable results of vitamin E and vitamin C need to be confirmed by a double-blind placebo-controlled trial.[93]

A Cochrane review in 2016 looked at 16 studies and 993 patients to assess the effectiveness and safety of nonsurgical interventions for bleeding, pain, fecal urgency, and incontinence after pelvic radiotherapy for cancer.[94] Nine studies assessed treatments for rectal bleeding and found that argon plasma coagulation made a significant difference followed by oral sucralfate and topical formalin. Studies that assessed treatments for pelvic symptoms favored hyperbaric oxygen.[95]

31.8.3 Surgical Management

Most colorectal radiation injuries do not require surgery, and operation on the previously irradiated colon has been associated with substantially high morbidity and mortality rates. However, if obstruction, perforation, fistula, persistent bleeding, intractable pain, or severe fecal incontinence develops, operative intervention is required.

For patients having proctocolitis with severe bleeding or intractable pain despite conservative treatment, a diverting colostomy should be performed. It will allow edema and infection to subside and will usually give immediate symptomatic relief. Preliminary experience with endoscopic laser coagulation of abnormal rectal vessels and bleeding suggests that it can be useful in controlling bleeding when used either alone or with colostomy. Jao et al[96] reviewed their experience with 62 patients treated surgically for radiation injury to the colon and rectum; 27 of the patients had colostomy alone as the initial treatment. Of the 24 patients who survived for follow-up, 5 had no further operation, 15 had the colostomy closed after a mean interval of 9.6 months, and 9 required resection.

In patients requiring colostomy for radiation proctitis, the stoma itself has been associated with high incidence of complications, including peristomal fistula, stomal retraction, and necrosis. Mobilization of healthy proximal bowel and exteriorization of a significant length should minimize the occurrence of these problems.[73,75] An ileostomy is easier to manage, and its construction does not interfere with the blood supply to the colon if a coloanal procedure is performed in the future.

Takedown of the colostomy or an ileostomy should not be attempted for at least 6 months and it should be performed only after the rectal area has healed. Radiographic and endoscopic studies should be performed on the distal segment to rule out the interim development of stricture or fistula. Careful consideration must be always given to the possible progression of the disease (with recurrence of its symptoms) after colostomy takedown.

Although a permanent colostomy may be preferable for some patients with refractory disease, it will not control symptoms satisfactorily in some patients and will not be well accepted by others. Such patients should be considered for resection and anastomosis. Clinical studies have shown that colorectal anastomosis can be performed safely in the presence of moderate, acute, or chronic radiation change; anastomosis is clearly more hazardous when performed for clinically demonstrable radiation colitis or proctitis. Conventional anterior resection with low anastomosis in cases of radiation injury has been associated with complication rates as high as 71%.[96] Although setting absolute guidelines for safe anastomosis after radiation therapy is not possible because of differences in radiation techniques and differences in individual responses, the following general guidelines are reasonable: (1) an anastomosis can be usually performed safely if the colon and rectum have received less than 4,000 to 4,500 rads; (2) constructing a protective loop ileostomy is advised if anastomosis will be performed after radiation in the range of 4,000 to 5,500 rads; and (3) anastomosis is generally unsafe after administration of 5,500 to 6,000 rads or more even if a protective loop ileostomy is added.

In 1978, Parks et al[97] reported on five patients having an ultra-low anterior resection and coloanal sleeve anastomosis. Four of the patients had rectovaginal fistulas and one had intractable pain from a radiation ulcer. All five patients had satisfactory result. The operation is performed with the patient in the lithotomy position, although the mucosal dissection can be accomplished initially with the patient in the prone jackknife position. In the abdominal phase, the colon is mobilized to include the splenic flexure, and the rectum is dissected close to the bowel. Dissection is continued beyond the necrotic rectal tissue, stricture, ulcer, or fistula. The rectum is divided at this level. The colon is divided proximally at a nonirradiated site, and the rectosigmoid is removed. From the perineal approach, the submucosa of the distal rectum is infiltrated with an epinephrine solution, and the mucosa is dissected circumferentially with a scissors up to the point of proximal dissection. The proximal colon is then pulled through the denuded region with stay sutures, and a coloanal anastomosis is performed at the dentate line, with the use of interrupted 3–0 braided synthetic absorbable sutures. A temporary loop ileostomy is performed, to protect the anastomosis (▶ Fig. 31.11).

Since the description by Parks et al,[97] other authors have reported similarly good results with this technique.[98,99,100,101,102] Cooke and De Moor[100] reported good continence in the follow-up of 21 of 28 patients at one year. They did note that liquid stool with variable degrees of incontinence persisted in 79% of the patients who had an anastomosis at the dentate line for low-lying fistulas. This was not a problem for patients having anastomosis at a higher level. Cooke and de Moor[100] were also concerned about ischemia when the blood supply to the distal colon was based on the left colic artery. They had better results with the blood supply based on the left branch of the middle colic artery. Several authors have noted that the anorectum can form a narrow rigid tunnel just below the pelvic peritoneum in patients having a frozen pelvis.[100,102] This tunnel can be enlarged by sharp dissection of the fibrous tissue anteriorly in the midline. Nowacki et al[102] also noted that

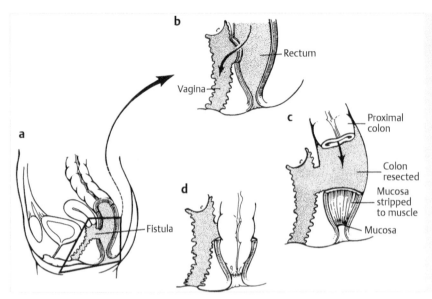

Fig. 31.11 (a–d) The trend for the coloanal anastomosis currently is to use a coloanal J reservoir. It may minimize urgency and frequency symptoms.

sometimes mucosectomy cannot be performed by the dissection method described by Parks et al; in these situations, curettes may be used to remove the mucosa.

Radiation-induced rectovaginal fistulas generally require operation for closure. Local repair of the fistulas inevitably fails. Boronow[103] described five points to follow when treating rectovaginal fistulas: (1) recurrent carcinoma should be ruled out; (2) the fecal stream must be diverted; (3) acute radiation injuries should be allowed to subside; (4) a new blood supply must be brought into the fistula repair area; and (5) the fistula itself should be closed. Based on these principles, various techniques for bringing new blood supply to the area have been tried. These sources of blood supply include gracilis muscle, adductor muscle, rectus muscle, omentum, and labial fat pads. Most repairs are performed through an episiotomy-type incision, with transverse repair of the colonic fistula. The new tissue with its blood supply is brought in and positioned in the rectovaginal septal region at the site of the fistula, and the vaginal mucosa is closed. Although these methods have had some success, the Parks coloanal sleeve anastomosis is especially well suited for this problem and should be considered the procedure of choice.

For low rectal strictures unresponsive to medical management, a diverting colostomy may be acceptable as definitive therapy for many patients. For patients wanting to maintain continuity, resection with the Parks sleeve anastomosis is usually the best choice. The Bricker-type fold-over anastomosis[104] and the Duhamel procedure[105] have now been outdated.

31.8.4 Radiation Proctitis

Injury to the rectum is unavoidable when the patients receive pelvic irradiation. Acute radiation proctitis occurs during, or soon after, completing the course of radiotherapy. It is characterized histologically by epithelial meganucleosis, lack of mitotic activity, and patchy fibroblastic proliferation in the lamina propria with normal blood vessels.

Chronic radiation proctitis is characterized histologically by narrowing of the arterioles from subintimal fibrosis, telangiectasia of capillaries and postcapillary venules, endothelial degeneration, and platelet thrombi formation associated with severe fibrosis of the lamina propria and crypt distortion. These changes correspond to the progressive ischemia and resulting symptoms are managed by patients with chronic radiation proctitis.[106]

Clinical Manifestations

The incidence of both acute and chronic radiation proctitis correlates with the dose of the radiation. Smit et al[107] reported an incidence of 20% when the total dose to the anterior rectal wall was 7,500 cGy or below compared with 60% when the dose was above 7,500 cGy.

Patients may present with symptoms of radiation proctitis from as early as the first week of therapy to as late as 30 years posttreatment. Patients who present during or soon after therapy may complain of diarrhea (with or without blood), nausea, abdominal cramping, tenesmus, sphincter irritability, mucoid discharge, and, less commonly, constipation. Hematuria and dysuria may be present because of concurrent radiation injury of urinary tract. In general, these patients do well in the short term, with conservative medical therapy, typically resolving over 2 to 6 months. Approximately 20% of the patients with acute radiation proctitis require temporary cessation of radiation treatments. Fortunately, the majority of these symptoms resolve within 1 to 2 weeks and the treatments can resume. Once the acute radiation proctitis has resolved, many patients remain asymptomatic and suffer no further manifestation of radiation injury.[106]

Approximately 1 to 20% of patients who receive radiation therapy develop chronic radiation proctitis. The clinical presentation is determined by the location and severity of the radiation injury. These include rectal bleeding, most commonly from mucosal telangiectasias; intense fibrosis causing frozen pelvis; major tissue destruction resulting in vaginal, enteric, or cutaneous fistulas; or severe stricture formation presenting as partial to complete obstruction of the rectum. Patient complaints vary widely from severe pain to no pain and from constipation to diarrhea with or without incontinence. A rectum that appears severely affected by radiation damage on endoscopic examination but does not bother the patient does not warrant treatment.[106]

Surgical Management

The safest operation for treatment of severe and intractable radiation proctitis is fecal diversion via a stoma. Fecal diversion, in most cases, allows the rectal mucosal edema and secondary infection to subside: Bleeding usually ceases and pain is typically relieved. Surgical therapy is indicated for obstruction, stricture, perforation of rectal vaginal fistula, fecal incontinence, intractable pain, and persistent bleeding. If the patient is young, with good fecal continence, the Parks coloanal anastomosis, preferably a colonic J pouch, should be considered. Patients with severe disease should have a proctectomy.

Low rectal complications from radiation for carcinoma of the prostate present a difficult problem. Larson et al[108] conducted a retrospective study on 5,719 patients who underwent radiation therapy at the Mayo Clinic for carcinoma of the prostate, between 1990 and 2003. Fourteen patients developed rectal complications: 10 patients (71%) had documented rectourethral fistulas; 4 patients (29%) had either transfusion-dependent, persistent rectal bleeding or fecal incontinence. The treatment included fecal diversion alone (20%), urinary and fecal diversion alone (50%), and primary repair with or without a tissue flap and fecal diversion (29%) in the 14 affected patients. Symptomatic improvement and resolution of these three complications occurred in 12 (85%) of the patients. However, only two (15%) were able to retain their intestinal continuity to achieve this outcome.

Treatment for Hemorrhagic Radiation Proctitis

Minor bleeding from radiation proctitis can be improved by treating the constipation or diarrhea. A 5-ASA enema has not been found to be helpful. Sucralfate, 2 g suspended in 20 mL tap water delivered as an enema twice a day, has been reported to promote healing.[109]

Persistent and severe bleeding due to radiation proctitis is uncommon and can be a challenge. Currently, there are nonoperative techniques that should be tried first before considering a colostomy or a proctectomy.

Argon plasma coagulation is highly effective in controlling hemorrhagic radiation proctitis.[110,111,112,113] Villavicencio et al[110] performed this on an outpatient via a flexible endoscope. The Argon gas flow rate used ranged from 1.2 to 2 L/min, the electrical power setting ranged from 45 to 50 W, and the probe size ranged from 2.7 to 3.2 mm diameter. An effort was made to treat individual telangiectasias, and whenever possible to avoid "painting" the rectal mucosa to minimize ulceration. The pulse duration was usually less than 1 second unless telangiectasias were virtually confluent, in which case longer pulse durations are used. All lesions were treated in a single session whenever possible. Telangiectasias in the skin of the anal canal are not treated, but the area coagulated is extended to the dentate line when necessary. The authors have treated 12 patients, all of whom were anemic, and 4 had received blood transfusions. The mean number of treatment sessions was 1.7, and 10 patients were successfully treated in a single session. Rectal bleeding resolved within 1 month of the last treatment in 19 patients, usually on the day of the last procedure. Short-term side effects occurred in three (14%) patients (rectal pain, tenesmus, and/or

abdominal distention); long-term complications (rectal pain, tenesmus, and diarrhea) developed in four patients (19%).

Topical application of diluted formalin has been found to stop active bleeding from radiation proctitis. Saclarides et al[114] reported success in stopping bleeding in 75% of the patients with a single treatment. The rest of the patients improved but continued to have bleeding. The 4% formalin solution is prepared by mixing 200 mL of 10% buffered formalin with 300 mL water. The patient was prepared with cleansing enemas before the procedure. The procedure was performed in the operating room under local, caudal, or general anesthesia. Approximately 400 to 500 mL was instilled in 30 to 50 mL aliquots via a rigid sigmoidoscope. Each aliquot is kept in contact with rectal mucosa for 30 seconds. Saline should be used liberally to irrigate the rectum between formalin aliquots and to wash the perineum in the event that the formalin has escaped externally. The authors used this technique only in severe cases. In the milder case, they used a formalin-soaked cotton-tip applicator. This is a technique favored by Seow-Choen et al.[115] They performed this procedure under caudal anesthesia in lithotomy position. Gauze sponges soaked in 4% formalin were held in direct contact with bleeding sites through a rigid sigmoidoscope until the bleeding site ceased to bleed, which usually took 2 to 3 minutes. The process was repeated at other sites until all the bleeding had stopped. Seven of the eight patients had cessation of bleeding in one session and had not rebled through 1 to 6 months of follow-up. The eighth patient required a second session for mild recurrent bleeding 2 weeks later. Other authors also found this method of treatment to be effective.[116,117,118,119]

Histologic study of the rectal mucosa after formalin application was undertaken by Chautems et al.[118] Endoscopic biopsies were performed at three different occasions: for four patients, immediately before 4% formaldehyde application; for four patients, immediately after the application; and for three patients, 1 month later and at 1 year. The results showed that unspecified radiation-induced reactions were found on the baseline biopsies. The rectal mucosa was erythematous and friable. It contained edematous granulation tissue with a mild acute inflammation, small neovessels, bizarre atypical radiation fibroblast, and mild fibrosis. On the biopsies performed after the application of 4% formaldehyde, multiple fresh thromboses appeared in the areas of neovascularization. This occurred only in the superficial mucosa. On the biopsies of the rectum performed 1 month or 12 months later, there were signs of chronic changes related to the radiotherapy, and there were no signs of acute inflammation or thrombosed vessels. This was characterized by mild fibrosis of the lamina propria, hyalinized vessel wall, and muscular degeneration of the muscularis mucosa.

31.9 Increased Risk of Rectal Carcinoma after Prostate Radiation

Radiation therapy for prostate carcinoma has been associated with an increased rate of pelvic malignancies, particularly bladder carcinoma. The association between radiation therapy and colorectal carcinoma yields conflicting results.[120] In a study by Brenner et al,[121] a 105% increase in the incidence of rectal carcinoma was found in prostate carcinoma patients following radiation (vs. surgery) after more than 10 years of follow-up; in addition, a 24% (nonsignificant) increase in the incidence of colon carcinoma was found after radiation. In the other study by Neugut et al,[122] no increased incidence of rectal carcinoma was found in prostate carcinoma patients after radiation (vs. no radiation), even in those with long-term follow-up. Both of these studies have limitations that may explain the discrepant result. Most importantly, the mean years of follow-up are limited in both studies. The study of Brenner et al[121] included patients diagnosed from 1973 through 1993, but the mean survival time after prostate carcinoma diagnosis was only 4 years. The mean follow-up time was not presented in the study of Neugut et al[122]; however, it included patients diagnosed from 1973 through 1990 and was published 4 years earlier than the study of Brenner et al; so follow-up would be even shorter. Given that biologically, the latency period between radiation exposure and radiation-induced malignancy is at least 5 years, neither study had sufficient follow-up time to determine the true effect of radiation. Similarly, both studies included cases of rectal carcinoma discovered at 2 months[121] and 6 months[122] after prostate diagnosis; yet, such early rectal carcinomas could not have resulted from radiation exposure, rather they may have been missed. Neither study excluded patients with prior history of colorectal carcinoma.[120]

Baxter et al[120] conducted a retrospective cohort study using Surveillance, Epidemiology, and End Results (SEER) registry data from 1973 to 1994. The study focused on men with prostate carcinoma, but with no previous history of colorectal carcinoma, treated with either surgery or radiation who survived at least 5 years. The authors evaluated the effect of radiation on the development of carcinoma for three sites: definitely irradiated sites (rectum), potentially irradiated sites (rectosigmoid, sigmoid, and cecum), and nonirradiated sites (the rest of the colon). Using a proportional hazards model, they evaluated the effect of radiation on the development of colorectal carcinoma over time.

The result showed that a total of 30,552 men received radiation, and 55,263 underwent surgery only. Colorectal carcinomas developed in 1,437 patients: 267 in irradiated sites, 686 in potentially irradiated sites, and 484 in nonirradiated sites. Radiation was independently associated with the development of carcinoma over time in irradiated sites but not in the remainder of the colon. The adjusted hazard ratio for the development of rectal carcinoma was 1.7 for the radiated group, compared with surgery-only group. The authors concluded that there was a significant increase in the development of rectal carcinoma after radiation for prostate cancer. Radiation had no effect on the development of carcinoma in the remainder of the colon, indicating that the effect is specific to directly irradiated tissue.

This study represents a significant improvement over prior analysis of the secondary consequences of radiation for prostate carcinoma. First, this study is based on a large number of men with prostate carcinoma, all of whom had their prostate disease confirmed microscopically, underwent treatment for their disease, and had long-term follow-up; the mean follow-up time was 9 years in the radiation group and 9.5 years in the surgery-only group. The authors included only men who survived at least 5 years; thus, biologically, all radiated patients were at risk for radiation-induced rectal carcinoma. They excluded men with previous colorectal carcinoma as well as men

who developed a colorectal carcinoma in the first 5 years after prostate carcinoma treatment. Allowing for this lag time serves two purposes: (1) it excludes men diagnosed with colorectal carcinoma only because of more intense evaluation associated with complications of their prostate carcinoma treatment and (2) it is consistent with the hypothesis that radiation-induced carcinogenesis takes at least 5 years to manifest. The authors found no increase in the incidence of colon carcinoma in potentially irradiated sites and nonirradiated sites; by using other parts of the colon as control measures, they reduced the likelihood that any observed radiation effect in the rectum was merely because of confounding and demonstrated that carcinogenic effect of radiation is specific to irradiated sites.[120]

31.10 Prevention

31.10.1 Radiation Technique

Because of the high morbidity and mortality associated with late radiation complications, prevention of these injuries has received increasing attention. Fractionating radiation doses and other refinements in radiotherapy techniques have helped decrease radiation complications. However, by identifying those patients most at risk, further precautions can be taken. Green et al[123,124] successfully developed a program for minimizing small bowel injury in high-risk patients. They initially identified high-risk patients by performing small bowel contrast studies. When small intestine adhesions were identified in the pelvis, Green[123] modified the total dose, altered the size of the radiated field, and used various positioning techniques such as the prone position and bladder distention to minimize small bowel exposure.

Use of the hyperfractionation technique has been suggested for other patients with increased risk factors. This involves giving the patient less than the usual 180 to 200 rads per day and spreading the dose across several daily treatments.[1] The use of barium-soaked vaginal packing around the radium source has also been recommended as a way to displace the bladder anteriorly and the rectum posteriorly away from the radium source.[86] Emptying the rectum before insertion of intracavitary radiation has also been recommended as a way to protect it from radiation.[73]

A number of other methods for minimizing injury have been tried or are being considered. Hypoxia renders tissue less susceptible to radial injury, but it has not been useful as it also makes the carcinoma less radiosensitive.[15] Elemental diets, TPN, and protease have been suggested as beneficial by decreasing pancreatic secretions or altering function.[1]

31.10.2 Radioprotective Agents

There have been reports that have addressed pharmacologic manipulations of the luminal environment of the animal intestine. An alkaline lumen provides some reduction in radiation mucosal damage. Alterations in osmolarity have little influence. The absence of either bile salts or proteolytic enzymes at the time of radiation delivery leads to significantly diminished damage. Studies on use of 5-ASA-type drugs to prevent radiation proctitis are largely unsuccessful.[53,125,126]

Balsalazide is a new-generation 5-ASA drug that yields a high concentration of active drug in the distal colon. Jahraus et al[127] conducted a randomized, double-blind, placebo-controlled trial. Twenty-seven patients with carcinoma of the prostate received 2,250 mg capsules of balsalazide twice daily for 5 days before radiotherapy and continued for 2 weeks after completion of radiation treatment. The results showed that with the exception of nausea or vomiting seen in three patients on balsalazide and two patients on placebo, all toxicities were appreciably lower in patients taking balsalazide. Proctitis was prevented most significantly with a mean proctitis index of 35 in balsalazide-treated patients and 74 in placebo patients. These results were encouraging but have not been confirmed in a cooperative group trial to assess its efficiency in a multi-institutional setting.

Glutamine and an elemental diet have been shown to protect the intestine from radiation damage.[128,129] Oral luminal adrenocortical steroid, methylprednisolone, provides some damage reduction.[20]

From all these observations, it is possible that the small bowel lumen can be physiologically or pharmacologically perturbed at the time of radiation exposure to reduce mucosal damage. The small bowel, however, does not lend itself to such manipulations by oral route in the clinical situation. Absorption, secretion, peristalsis, and, perhaps, enzymatic activity combine to frustrate efforts to bathe the entire small bowel mucosa with a chosen concentration of any substance.

31.10.3 Surgical Techniques

Three surgical techniques that are practical and useful to exclude the small intestine from the pelvis and thus avoid or minimize radiation injury are the omental envelope,[130,131,132] the absorbable mesh sling,[133] and pelvic space tissue expander.[134,135]

Omental Envelope

This technique can be accomplished only if the greater omentum has substantial size that can cover the upper to midabdominal cavity. The greater omentum is freed from any adhesion except at its pedicle to the greater curvature of the stomach. The cecum and terminal ileum are mobilized out of the pelvis. The entire small intestine is then covered with the entire greater omentum. The right free edge of the omentum is sutured to the anteromedial aspect of the ascending colon, beginning at the hepatic flexure and ending at the cecum (▶ Fig. 31.12). This is accomplished with a continuous 3–0 braided or monofilament synthetic absorbable suture, taking full-thickness bites of the edge of the omentum to the seromuscular bites on the wall of the colon.

Similarly, the left free edge of the omentum is sutured to the descending colon, beginning near the splenic flexure and ending at the level of descending sigmoid junction. The inferior free edge of the omentum begins at the previous suture at the cecum and continues transversely at the level of the pelvic brim, suturing the inferior free edge of the omentum to the posterior parietal peritoneum and ending in the midline on the sacral promontory where it meets the suture from the left side (▶ Fig. 31.12).

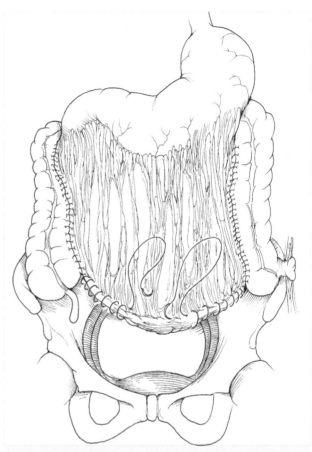

Fig. 31.12 Omental envelope. The apron of the greater omentum is sutured to the left and right colon and transversely, the pelvic brim and promontory of the sacrum.

If further descent of the omentum is required, it can be achieved by mobilizing the splenic and hepatic flexures of the colon and also by detaching the omentum from the greater curvature of the stomach. A final inspection is made to ascertain that no gaps exist in the suture lines so that herniation of the small intestine may be avoided.[131] The series by Choi and Lee[132] compared 32 patients with omental envelope to 25 patients without. The former group demonstrated that an omental envelope can protect the small bowel from radiation injury in both early and late follow-up. There has been no significant complication as the result of the omental hammock.

Pelvic Mesh Sling

A sheet of 7 × 9 in. polyglycolic acid (Vicryl) mesh is sewn into the sacral promontory periosteum using 2–0 monofilament synthetic absorbable sutures (▶ Fig. 31.13a). The cecum and terminal ileum are mobilized to assure a more cephalad position. The suture on the right side incorporates the edge of the mesh to the sacral promontory and transversely to the posterior parietal peritoneum and continues cephalad to the right gutter on to the psoas and quadratus lumborum fascia (▶ Fig. 31.13b). The suture then progresses to the posterior sheath of the anterior abdominal wall to meet the similar suture on the left side. The incision above the umbilicus is closed to allow suturing the

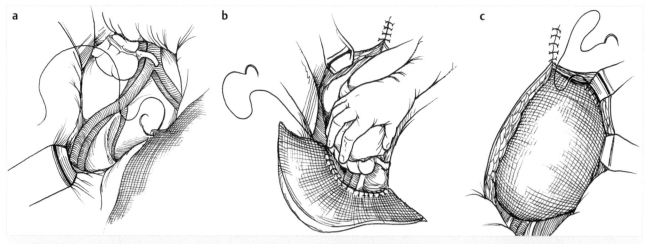

Fig. 31.13 Pelvic mesh sling. **(a)** The mesh is sewn into the sacral promontory periosteum and carried laterally on each side. **(b)** With the terminal ileum and cecum retracted, the suture is continued cephalad to the right gutter, then progresses to the posterior sheath of the anterior abdominal wall to meet a similar suture on the left side. **(c)** At completion, the bowel contents are in the "sling" with finishing sutures tied in the midline under a roof created by closure of the midline incision, which is usually above the umbilicus.

mesh across the anterior abdominal wall. At completion, bowel contents are in the "sling" (▶ Fig. 31.13c).

Devereux et al[136] used this technique in 60 patients who received an average 5,500 cGy in fractionated doses for rectal carcinoma and gynecologic malignancies. None has developed radiation enteritis with a mean follow-up of 28 months. Similar good results have also been obtained by Rodier et al.[137] In 60 patients with gynecologic malignancies who received irradiation between 4,250 and 5,800 cGy in fractions of 180 to 200 cGy per day, 5 days a week, 7% developed radiation enteritis, with a mean follow-up of 17.8 months (range, 1–57 months).

Tissue Expander in Pelvis

The logic for using tissue expander is to fill the pelvis cavity and exclude the small bowel from the radiation field. In the past, a saline-filled prosthesis for breast augmentation was used. There are now available custom-designed pelvic tissue expanders with sewing straps.[133] Sezeur et al[135] used a silicone rubber molded balloon that can be filled with saline solution up to 600 mL, and has a spherical shape. A sheet of absorbable mesh is placed between the small bowel and the balloon. It is then fixed to the posterior and lateral pelvic walls to prevent small bowel herniation. The balloon is then filled with saline solution to the appropriate size, displacing the small bowel and ovary from the radiation field. They used this technique in 22 patients; one patient required its removal because of small bowel injury during the procedure. The rest of the patients showed no signs or symptoms of radiation enteritis, with a mean follow-up of 24.5 months (range, 10–73). One disadvantage of using the tissue expander is that it must be removed at completion of the radiotherapy.

References

[1] Morgenstern L, Hart M, Lugo D, Friedman NB. Changing aspects of radiation enteropathy. Arch Surg. 1985; 120(11):1225–1228

[2] Andre N, Schmiegel W. Chemoradiotherapy for colorectal cancer. Gut. 2005; 54(8):1194–1202

[3] Wheeler JM, Dodds E, Warren BF, et al. Preoperative chemoradiotherapy and total mesorectal excision surgery for locally advanced rectal cancer: correlation with rectal cancer regression grade. Dis Colon Rectum. 2004; 47 (12):2025–2031

[4] Moore HG, Gittleman AE, Minsky BD, et al. Rate of pathologic complete response with increased interval between preoperative combined modality therapy and rectal cancer resection. Dis Colon Rectum. 2004; 47(3):279–286

[5] Walsh D. Deep tissue traumatism from roentgen ray exposure. BMJ. 1897; 2 (1909):272–273

[6] Otchy DP, Nelson H. Radiation injuries of the colon and rectum. Surg Clin North Am. 1993; 73(5):1017–1035

[7] Krook JE, Moertel CG, Gunderson LL, et al. Effective surgical adjuvant therapy for high-risk rectal carcinoma. N Engl J Med. 1991; 324(11):709–715

[8] Kollmorgen CF, Meagher AP, Wolff BG, Pemberton JH, Martenson JA, Illstrup DM. The long-term effect of adjuvant postoperative chemoradiotherapy for rectal carcinoma on bowel function. Ann Surg. 1994; 220(5):676–682

[9] Gilinsky NH, Burns DG, Barbezat GO, Levin W, Myers HS, Marks IN. The natural history of radiation-induced proctosigmoiditis: an analysis of 88 patients. Q J Med. 1983; 52(205):40–53

[10] DeCosse JJ, Rhodes RS, Wentz WB, Reagan JW, Dworken HJ, Holden WD. The natural history and management of radiation induced injury of the gastrointestinal tract. Ann Surg. 1969; 170(3):369–384

[11] Palmer JA, Bush RS. Radiation injuries to the bowel associated with the treatment of carcinoma of the cervix. Surgery. 1976; 80(4):458–464

[12] Harling H, Balslev I. Long-term prognosis of patients with severe radiation enteritis. Am J Surg. 1988; 155(3):517–519

[13] Schofield PF, Holden D, Carr ND. Bowel disease after radiotherapy. J R Soc Med. 1983; 76(6):463–466

[14] Wellwood JM, Jackson BT. The intestinal complications of radiotherapy. Br J Surg. 1973; 60(10):814–818

[15] Kinsella TJ, Bloomer WD. Tolerance of the intestine to radiation therapy. Surg Gynecol Obstet. 1980; 151(2):273–284

[16] Varma JS, Smith AN, Busuttil A. Correlation of clinical and manometric abnormalities of rectal function following chronic radiation injury. Br J Surg. 1985; 72(11):875–878

[17] Cochrane JP, Yarnold JR, Slack WW. The surgical treatment of radiation injuries after radiotherapy for uterine carcinoma. Br J Surg. 1981; 68(1):25–28

[18] Kagan AR, Nussbaum H, Gilbert H, et al. A new staging system for irradiation injuries following treatment for cancer of the cervix uteri. Gynecol Oncol. 1979; 7(2):166–175

[19] Gilbert A, Ziegler L, Martland M, et al. Systemic review of radiation therapy toxicity reporting in randomized controlled trials of rectal cancer: a comparison of patient-reported outcomes and clinician toxicity reporting. Int J Radiat Oncol Biol Phys. 2015; 92(3):555–567

[20] Delaney JP, Bonsack ME, Felemovicius I. Luminal route for intestinal radioprotection. Am J Surg. 1993; 166(5):492–501

[21] Roswit B, Malsky SJ, Reid CB. Severe radiation injuries of the stomach, small intestine, colon and rectum. Am J Roentgenol Radium Ther Nucl Med. 1972; 114(3):460–475

[22] Girvin GW, Schnug GE, Cavanagh CR, McGonigle DJ. Complications of abdominal irradiation. Am Surg. 1971; 37(8):498–502

[23] Carr ND, Pullen BR, Hasleton PS, Schofield PF. Microvascular studies in human radiation bowel disease. Gut. 1984; 25(5):448–454

[24] Smith DH, DeCosse JJ. Radiation damage to the small intestine. World J Surg. 1986; 10(2):189–194

[25] Yeoh EK, Horowitz M. Radiation enteritis. Surg Gynecol Obstet. 1987; 165 (4):373–379

[26] Schmitz RL, Chao JH, Bartolome JS, Jr. Intestinal injuries incidental to irradiation of carcinoma of the cervix of the uterus. Surg Gynecol Obstet. 1974; 138 (1):29–32

[27] Villasanta U. Complications of radiotherapy for carcinoma of the uterine cervix. Am J Obstet Gynecol. 1972; 114(6):717–726

[28] Localio SA, Pachter HL, Gouge TH. The radiation-injured bowel. Surg Annu. 1979; 11:181–205

[29] Berthrong M. Pathologic changes secondary to radiation. World J Surg. 1986; 10(2):155–170

[30] Joelsson I, Räf L. Late injuries of the small intestine following radiotherapy for uterine carcinoma. Acta Chir Scand. 1973; 139(2):194–200

[31] Yeoh EK, Lui D, Lee NY. The mechanism of diarrhoea resulting from pelvic and abdominal radiotherapy; a prospective study using selenium-75 labelled conjugated bile acid and cobalt-58 labelled cyanocobalamin. Br J Radiol. 1984; 57(684):1131–1136

[32] Cunningham IGE. The management of radiation proctitis. Aust N Z J Surg. 1980; 50(2):172–178

[33] Ludgate SM, Merrick MV. The pathogenesis of post-irradiation chronic diarrhoea: measurement of SeHCAT and B12 absorption for differential diagnosis determines treatment. Clin Radiol. 1985; 36(3):275–278

[34] Varma JS, Smith AN. Anorectal function following colo-anal sleeve anastomosis for chronic radiation injury to the rectum. Br J Surg. 1986; 73 (4):285–289

[35] Slaughter DP, Southwick HW. Mucosal carcinomas as a result of irradiation. AMA Arch Surg. 1957; 74(3):420–429

[36] Black WC, III, Ackerman LV. Carcinoma of the large intestine as a late complication of pelvic radiotherapy. Clin Radiol. 1965; 16:278–281

[37] Sandler RS, Sandler DP. Radiation-induced cancers of the colon and rectum: assessing the risk. Gastroenterology. 1983; 84(1):51–57

[38] Palmer JP, Spratt DW. Pelvic carcinoma following irradiation for benign gynecological diseases. Am J Obstet Gynecol. 1956; 72(3):497–505

[39] Denman DL, Kirchner FR, Osborne JW. Induction of colonic adenocarcinoma in the rat by X-irradiation. Cancer Res. 1978; 38(7):1899–1905

[40] Gardiner GW, McAuliffe N, Murray D. Colitis cystica profunda occurring in a radiation-induced colonic stricture. Hum Pathol. 1984; 15(3):295–298

[41] Valiulis AP, Gardiner GW, Mahoney LJ. Adenocarcinoma and colitis cystica profunda in a radiation-induced colonic stricture. Dis Colon Rectum. 1985; 28(2):128–131

[42] Strockbine MF, Hancock JE, Fletcher GH. Complications in 831 patients with squamous cell carcinoma of the intact uterine cervix treated with 3,000 rads or more whole pelvis irradiation. Am J Roentgenol Radium Ther Nucl Med. 1970; 108(2):293–304

[43] Bourne RG, Kearsley JH, Grove WD, Roberts SJ. The relationship between early and late gastrointestinal complications of radiation therapy for carcinoma of the cervix. Int J Radiat Oncol Biol Phys. 1983; 9(10):1445–1450

[44] Lee KH, Kagan AR, Nussbaum H, Wollin M, Winkley JH, Norman A. Analysis of dose, dose-rate and treatment time in the production of injuries by radium treatment for cancer of the uterine cervix. Br J Radiol. 1976; 49 (581):430–444

[45] Yoonessi M, Romney S, Dayem H. Gastrointestinal tract complications following radiotherapy of uterine cervical cancer: past and present. J Surg Oncol. 1981; 18(2):135–142

[46] Potish RA. Prediction of radiation-related small-bowel damage. Radiology. 1980; 135(1):219–221

[47] Potish RA, Jones TK, Jr, Levitt SH. Factors predisposing to radiation-related small-bowel damage. Radiology. 1979; 132(2):479–482

[48] Potish RA. Importance of predisposing factors in the development of enteric damage. Am J Clin Oncol. 1982; 5(2):189–194

[49] van Nagell JR, Jr, Maruyama Y, Parker JC, Jr, Dalton WL. Small bowel injury following radiation therapy for cervical cancer. Am J Obstet Gynecol. 1974; 118(2):163–167

[50] Loludice T, Baxter D, Balint J. Effects of abdominal surgery on the development of radiation enteropathy. Gastroenterology. 1977; 73(5):1093–1097

[51] Danjoux CE, Catton GE. Delayed complications in colo-rectal carcinoma treated by combination radiotherapy and 5-fluorouracil–Eastern Cooperative Oncology Group (E.C.O.G.) pilot study. Int J Radiat Oncol Biol Phys. 1979; 5(3):311–315

[52] Phillips TL, Fu KK. Quantification of combined radiation therapy and chemotherapy effects on critical normal tissues. Cancer. 1976; 37(2) Suppl:1186–1200

[53] Martenson JA, Jr, Hyland G, Moertel CG, et al. Olsalazine is contraindicated during pelvic radiation therapy: results of a double-blind, randomized clinical trial. Int J Radiat Oncol Biol Phys. 1996; 35(2):299–303

[54] Mulholland MW, Levitt SH, Song CW, Potish RA, Delaney JP. The role of luminal contents in radiation enteritis. Cancer. 1984; 54(11):2396–2402

[55] Rogers LF, Goldstein HM. Roentgen manifestations of radiation injury to the gastrointestinal tract. Gastrointest Radiol. 1977; 2(3):281–291

[56] Hara AK, Leighton JA, Heigh RI, et al. Crohn disease of the small bowel: preliminary comparison among CT enterography, capsule endoscopy, small-bowel follow-through, and ileoscopy. Radiology. 2006; 238(1):128–134

[57] Boudiaf M, Jaff A, Soyer P, Bouhnik Y, Hamzi L, Rymer R. Small-bowel diseases: prospective evaluation of multi-detector row helical CT enteroclysis in 107 consecutive patients. Radiology. 2004; 233(2):338–344

[58] Yuhasz M, Laufer I, Sutton G, Herlinger H, Caroline DF. Radiography of the small bowel in patients with gynecologic malignancies. AJR Am J Roentgenol. 1985; 144(2):303–307

[59] Dencker H, Holmdahl KH, Lunderquist A, Olivecrona H, Tylén U. Mesenteric angiography in patients with radiation injury of the bowel after pelvis irradiation. Am J Roentgenol Radium Ther Nucl Med. 1972; 114(3):476–481

[60] Delbeke D. Integrated PET-CT imaging: implications for evaluation of patients with colorectal carcinoma. Semin Colon Rect Surg. 2005; 16(2):69–81

[61] Scully RE, Mark FJ, McNeely WR, McNeely BW. Case records of the Massachusetts General hospital, case 9–1994. N Engl J Med. 1994; 330:627–630

[62] Morgenstern L, Thompson R, Friedman NB. The modern enigma of radiation enteropathy: sequelae and solutions. Am J Surg. 1977; 134(1):166–172

[63] McLaren JR. Sequelae of abdominal radiation and their medical management. Compr Ther. 1977; 3(2):25–33

[64] Yeoh E, Horowitz M, Russo A, et al. Effect of pelvic irradiation on gastrointestinal function: a prospective longitudinal study. Am J Med. 1993; 95(4):397–406

[65] Danielsson A, Nyhlin H, Persson H, Stendahl U, Stenling R, Suhr O. Chronic diarrhoea after radiotherapy for gynaecological cancer: occurrence and aetiology. Gut. 1991; 32(10):1180–1187

[66] Heusinkveld RS, Manning MR, Aristizabal SA. Control of radiation-induced diarrhea with cholestyramine. Int J Radiat Oncol Biol Phys. 1978; 4(7–8):687–690

[67] Condon JR, Wolverson RL, South M, Brinkley D. Radiation diarrhea and cholestyramine. Postgrad Med J. 1978; 54:838

[68] Baum CA, Biddle WL, Miner PB, Jr. Failure of 5-aminosalicylic acid enemas to improve radiation proctitis. Dig Dis Sci. 1989; 34(5):758–760

[69] Triantafillidis JK, Dadioti P, Nicolakis D, Mericas E. High doses of 5-aminosalicylic acid enemas in chronic radiation proctitis: comparison with betamethasone enemas. Am J Gastroenterol. 1990; 85(11):1537–1538

[70] Beer WH, Fan A, Halsted CH. Clinical and nutritional implications of radiation enteritis. Am J Clin Nutr. 1985; 41(1):85–91

[71] Miller DG, Ivey M, Young J. Home parenteral nutrition in treatment of severe radiation enteritis. Ann Intern Med. 1979; 91(6):858–860

[72] Scolapio JS, Ukleja A, Burnes JU, Kelly DG. Outcome of patients with radiation enteritis treated with home parenteral nutrition. Am J Gastroenterol. 2002; 97(3):662–666

[73] Russell JC, Welch JP. Operative management of radiation injuries of the intestinal tract. Am J Surg. 1979; 137(4):433–442

[74] Meissner K. Late radiogenic small bowel damage: guidelines for the general surgeon. Dig Surg. 1999; 16(3):169–174

[75] Galland RB, Spencer J. Surgical aspects of radiation injury to the intestine. Br J Surg. 1979; 66(2):135–138

[76] Walsh HPJ, Schofield PF. Is laparotomy for small bowel obstruction justified in patients with previously treated malignancy? Br J Surg. 1984; 71 (12):933–935

[77] Smith ST, Seski JC, Copeland LJ, Gershenson DM, Edwards CL, Herson J. Surgical management of irradiation-induced small bowel damage. Obstet Gynecol. 1985; 65(4):563–567

[78] Swan RW, Fowler WC, Jr, Boronow RC. Surgical management of radiation injury to the small intestine. Surg Gynecol Obstet. 1976; 142(3):325–327

[79] Dirksen PK, Matolo NM, Trelford JD. Complications following operation in the previously irradiated abdominopelvic cavity. Am Surg. 1977; 43(4):234–241

[80] Dietz DW, Remzi FH, Fazio VW. Strictureplasty for obstructing small-bowel lesions in diffuse radiation enteritis–successful outcome in five patients. Dis Colon Rectum. 2001; 44(12):1772–1777

[81] Onodera H, Nagayama S, Mori A, Fujimoto A, Tachibana T, Yonenaga Y. Reappraisal of surgical treatment for radiation enteritis. World J Surg. 2005; 29 (4):459–463

[82] Regimbeau JM, Panis Y, Gouzi JL, Fagniez PL, French University Association for Surgical Research. Operative and long term results after surgery for chronic radiation enteritis. Am J Surg. 2001; 182(3):237–242

[83] Smith DH, Pierce VK, Lewis JL, Jr. Enteric fistulas encountered on a gynecologic oncology service from 1969 through 1980. Surg Gynecol Obstet. 1984; 158(1):71–75

[84] Piver MS, Lele S. Enterovaginal and enterocutaneous fistulae in women with gynecologic malignancies. Obstet Gynecol. 1976; 48(5):560–563

[85] Jackson BT. Bowel damage from radiation. Proc R Soc Med. 1976; 69(9):683–686

[86] Dean RE, Taylor ES. Surgical treatment of complications resulting from irradiation therapy of cervical cancer. Am J Obstet Gynecol. 1960; 79:34–42

[87] Reichelderfer M, Morrissey JF. Colonoscopy in radiation colitis. Gastrointest Endosc. 1980; 26(2):41–43

[88] Kochhar R, Sriram PV, Sharma SC, Goel RC, Patel F. Natural history of late radiation proctosigmoiditis treated with topical sucralfate suspension. Dig Dis Sci. 1999; 44(5):973–978

[89] Baum CA, Biddle WL, Miner PB, Jr. Failure of 5-aminosalicylic acid enemas to improve chronic radiation proctitis. Dig Dis Sci. 1989; 34(5):758–760

[90] Levitsky J, Hong JJ, Jani AB, Ehrenpreis ED. Oral vitamin a therapy for a patient with a severely symptomatic postradiation anal ulceration: report of a case. Dis Colon Rectum. 2003; 46(5):679–682

[91] Ehrenpreis ED, Jani A, Levitsky J, Ahn J, Hong J. A prospective, randomized, double-blind, placebo-controlled trial of retinol palmitate (vitamin A) for symptomatic chronic radiation proctopathy. Dis Colon Rectum. 2005; 48(1):1–8

[92] Niki E. Lipid antioxidants: how they may act in biological systems. Br J Cancer Suppl. 1987; 8:153–157

[93] Kennedy M, Bruninga K, Mutlu EA, Losurdo J, Choudhary S, Keshavarzian A. Successful and sustained treatment of chronic radiation proctitis with antioxidant vitamins E and C. Am J Gastroenterol. 2001; 96(4):1080–1084

[94] van de Wetering FT, Verleye L, Andreyev HJ, et al. Non-surgical interventions for late rectal problems (proctopathy) of radiotherapy in people who have received radiotherapy to the pelvis. Cochrane Database Syst Rev. 2016; 4:CD003455

[95] Borek C. Radiation and chemically induced transformation: free radicals, antioxidants and cancer. Br J Cancer Suppl. 1987; 8:74–86

[96] Jao SW, Beart RW, Jr, Gunderson LL. Surgical treatment of radiation injuries of the colon and rectum. Am J Surg. 1986; 151(2):272–277

[97] Parks AG, Allen CLO, Frank JD, McPartlin JF. A method of treating post-irradiation rectovaginal fistulas. Br J Surg. 1978; 65(6):417–421

[98] Allen-Mersh TG, Wilson EJ, Hope-Stone HF, Mann CV. The management of late radiation-induced rectal injury after treatment of carcinoma of the uterus. Surg Gynecol Obstet. 1987; 164(6):521–524

[99] Browning GGP, Varma JS, Smith AN, Small WP, Duncan W. Late results of mucosal proctectomy and colo-anal sleeve anastomosis for chronic irradiation rectal injury. Br J Surg. 1987; 74(1):31–34

[100] Cooke SAR, de Moor NG. The surgical treatment of the radiation-damaged rectum. Br J Surg. 1981; 68(7):488–492

[101] Gazet JC. Parks' coloanal pull-through anastomosis for severe, complicated radiation proctitis. Dis Colon Rectum. 1985; 28(2):110–114

[102] Nowacki MP, Szawlowski AW, Borkowski A. Parks' coloanal sleeve anastomosis for treatment of postirradiation rectovaginal fistula. Dis Colon Rectum. 1986; 29(12):817–820

[103] Boronow RC. Management of radiation-induced vaginal fistulas. Am J Obstet Gynecol. 1971; 110(1):1–8

[104] Bricker EM, Johnston WD, Patwardhan RV. Repair of postirradiation damage to colorectum: a progress report. Ann Surg. 1981; 193(5):555–564

[105] Starr DS, Lawrie GM, Morris GC, Jr. Treatment of postradiation stricture of the rectum by the modified Duhamel procedure. Am J Surg. 1979; 137(6):795–797

[106] Lisehora GB, Rothenberger DA. Radiation proctitis. Semin Colorect Surg. 1993; 4:240–248

[107] Smit WG, Helle PA, van Putten WL, Wijnmaalen AJ, Seldenrath JJ, van der Werf-Messing BH. Late radiation damage in prostate cancer patients treated by high dose external radiotherapy in relation to rectal dose. Int J Radiat Oncol Biol Phys. 1990; 18(1):23–29

[108] Larson DW, Chrouser K, Young-Fadok T, Nelson H. Rectal complications after modern radiation for prostate cancer: a colorectal surgical challenge. J Gastrointest Surg. 2005; 9(4):461–466

[109] Kochhar R, Sharma SC, Gupta BB, Mehta SK. Rectal sucralfate in radiation proctitis. Lancet. 1988; 2(8607):400

[110] Villavicencio RT, Rex DK, Rahmani E. Efficacy and complications of argon plasma coagulation for hematochezia related to radiation proctopathy. Gastrointest Endosc. 2002; 55(1):70–74

[111] Venkatesh KS, Ramanujam P. Endoscopic therapy for radiation proctitis-induced hemorrhage in patients with prostatic carcinoma using argon plasma coagulator application. Surg Endosc. 2002; 16(4):707–710

[112] Tjandra JJ, Sengupta S. Argon plasma coagulation is an effective treatment for refractory hemorrhagic radiation proctitis. Dis Colon Rectum. 2001; 44 (12):1759–1765, discussion 1771

[113] Taïeb S, Rolachon A, Cenni JC, et al. Effective use of argon plasma coagulation in the treatment of severe radiation proctitis. Dis Colon Rectum. 2001; 44 (12):1766–1771

[114] Saclarides TJ, King DG, Franklin JL, Doolas A. Formalin instillation for refractory radiation-induced hemorrhagic proctitis. Report of 16 patients. Dis Colon Rectum. 1996; 39(2):196–199

[115] Seow-Choen F, Goh HS, Eu KW, Ho YH, Tay SK. A simple and effective treatment for hemorrhagic radiation proctitis using formalin. Dis Colon Rectum. 1993; 36(2):135–138

[116] de Parades V, Etienney I, Bauer P, et al. Formalin application in the treatment of chronic radiation-induced hemorrhagic proctitis–an effective but not risk-free procedure: a prospective study of 33 patients. Dis Colon Rectum. 2005; 48(8):1535–1541

[117] Parikh S, Hughes C, Salvati EP, et al. Treatment of hemorrhagic radiation proctitis with 4 percent formalin. Dis Colon Rectum. 2003; 46(5):596–600

[118] Chautems RC, Delgadillo X, Rubbia-Brandt L, Deleaval JP, Marti MCL, Roche B. Formaldehyde application for haemorrhagic radiation-induced proctitis: a clinical and histological study. Colorectal Dis. 2003; 5(1):24–28

[119] Counter SF, Froese DP, Hart MJ. Prospective evaluation of formalin therapy for radiation proctitis. Am J Surg. 1999; 177(5):396–398

[120] Baxter NN, Tepper JE, Durham SB, Rothenberger DA, Virnig BA. Increased risk of rectal cancer after prostate radiation: a population-based study. Gastroenterology. 2005; 128(4):819–824

[121] Brenner DJ, Curtis RE, Hall EJ, Ron E. Second malignancies in prostate carcinoma patients after radiotherapy compared with surgery. Cancer. 2000; 88 (2):398–406

[122] Neugut AI, Ahsan H, Robinson E, Ennis RD. Bladder carcinoma and other second malignancies after radiotherapy for prostate carcinoma. Cancer. 1997; 79(8):1600–1604

[123] Green N. The avoidance of small intestine injury in gynecologic cancer. Int J Radiat Oncol Biol Phys. 1983; 9(9):1385–1390

[124] Green N, Melbye RW, Iba G, Kussin L. Radiation therapy for carcinoma of the prostate: the experience with small intestine injury. Int J Radiat Oncol Biol Phys. 1978; 4(11–12):1049–1053

[125] Resbeut M, Marteau P, Cowen D, et al. A randomized double blind placebo controlled multicenter study of mesalazine for the prevention of acute radiation enteritis. Radiother Oncol. 1997; 44(1):59–63

[126] Baughan CA, Canney PA, Buchanan RB, Pickering RM. A randomized trial to assess the efficacy of 5-aminosalicylic acid for the prevention of radiation enteritis. Clin Oncol (R Coll Radiol). 1993; 5(1):19–24

[127] Jahraus CD, Bettenhausen D, Malik U, Sellitti M, St Clair WH. Prevention of acute radiation-induced proctosigmoiditis by balsalazide: a randomized, double-blind, placebo controlled trial in prostate cancer patients. Int J Radiat Oncol Biol Phys. 2005; 63(5):1483–1487

[128] Jensen JC, Schaefer R, Nwokedi E, et al. Prevention of chronic radiation enteropathy by dietary glutamine. Ann Surg Oncol. 1994; 1(2):157–163

[129] McArdle AH, Reid EC, Laplante MP, Freeman CR. Prophylaxis against radiation injury. The use of elemental diet prior to and during radiotherapy for invasive bladder cancer and in early postoperative feeding following radical cystectomy and ileal conduit. Arch Surg. 1986; 121 (8):879–885

[130] Lechner P, Cesnik H. Abdominopelvic omentopexy: preparatory procedure for radiotherapy in rectal cancer. Dis Colon Rectum. 1992; 35 (12):1157–1160

[131] DeLuca FR, Ragins H. Construction of an omental envelope as a method of excluding the small intestine from the field of postoperative irradiation to the pelvis. Surg Gynecol Obstet. 1985; 160(4):365–366

[132] Choi HJ, Lee HS. Effect of omental pedicle hammock in protection against radiation-induced enteropathy in patients with rectal cancer. Dis Colon Rectum. 1995; 38(3):276–280

[133] Waddell BE, Lee RJ, Rodriguez-Bigas MA, Weber TK, Petrelli NJ. Absorbable mesh sling prevents radiation-induced bowel injury during "sandwich" chemoradiation for rectal cancer. Arch Surg. 2000; 135 (10):1212–1217

[134] Waddell BE, Rodriguez-Bigas MA, Lee RJ, Weber TK, Petrelli NJ. Prevention of chronic radiation enteritis. J Am Coll Surg. 1999; 189(6):611–624

[135] Sezeur A, Martella L, Abbou C, et al. Small intestine protection from radiation by means of a removable adapted prosthesis. Am J Surg. 1999; 178 (1):22–25, discussion 25–26

[136] Devereux DF, Chandler JJ, Eisenstat T, Zinkin L. Efficacy of an absorbable mesh in keeping the small bowel out of the human pelvis following surgery. Dis Colon Rectum. 1988; 31(1):17–21

[137] Rodier JF, Janser JC, Rodier D, et al. Prevention of radiation enteritis by an absorbable polyglycolic acid mesh sling. A 60-case multicentric study. Cancer. 1991; 68(12):2545–2549

32 Intestinal Stomas

David E. Beck

Abstract

Abdominal stomas serve a critical function in the management of benign and malignant diseases. Currently, 130,000 patients undergo ostomy surgery in the United States annually. Many patients have major complications from the operation and problems with the stoma. The judicious assessment of the need for the stoma, careful surgical technique, and skilled wound ostomy continence or enterostomal nursing are essential for a satisfactory outcome.

Keywords: intestinal stoma, ileostomy, colostomy, loop ileostomy, bowel obstruction, stoma ischemia, stenosis, recession, parastomal hernia, fistula

32.1 Introduction

Although the advent of restorative proctocolectomy and stapled low anterior anastomosis has lessened the need for permanent ileostomy and permanent end colostomy, the abdominal stoma still serves a critical function in the management of benign and malignant diseases. Currently, approximately 130,000 patients undergo ostomy surgery in the United States, annually.[1] Many of these patients will have major complications from the operation, and all of them will experience at least some problems, as a result of the stoma. These problems are biopsychosocial in nature and may include surgical complications; peristomal skin complications; and problems with odor, noise, anxiety, depression, sexual dysfunction, and social isolation.[2,3,4] The judicious assessment of the need for the stoma, careful surgical technique, and skilled wound ostomy continence (WOC) or enterostomal nursing are essential for a satisfactory outcome.

32.2 Ileostomy

32.2.1 History

It was Baum who performed the first ever ileostomy in 1879 on a patient with an obstructing carcinoma of the ascending colon. The patient survived the ileostomy procedure but died from complications of a second operation that involved resecting the primary carcinoma and creating an ileocolic anastomosis. Kraussold, Billroth, Bergman, and Maydl were among the other 19th century surgeons who subsequently performed the ileostomy surgery. Maydl's patient is generally considered to be the first to survive and fully recover from an ileostomy performed in combination with resection for colon carcinoma.[5]

In 1913, Brown[6] reported on 10 patients in whom he constructed an ileostomy. He made the stoma as an end ileostomy, closing off the distal end and bringing 2 in. of the proximal end out through the lower part of the incision. He inserted a catheter into the lumen and allowed it to separate as the surrounding tissue sloughed, and the bowel became granulated, contracted, and eventually formed a mucocutaneous junction with the abdominal wall skin. Brown achieved a favorable result in all of his patients.

The results of ileostomy surgery as reported by subsequent authors were uniformly disappointing. A variety of techniques were introduced, including the method of placing the terminal ileum through a separate right lower quadrant incision as an end ileostomy and various loop ileostomy techniques. The most significant achievement during this period, however, occurred in the late 1920s, when Dr. Alfred Strauss of Chicago performed an ileostomy and later a colectomy for ulcerative colitis on a young chemist named Koenig. Koenig subsequently designed an ileostomy appliance bag, commercially known as the Koenig-Rutzen bag. This appliance was used widely until the introduction of karaya in the 1950s.

In the following years, ileostomy-related fluid and electrolyte problems were identified and the need for earlier operation in patients with severe ulcerative colitis was recognized. The problem of high ileostomy output remained an obstacle to full rehabilitation for many patients until the 1950s, when Warren and McKittrick[7] related the problem of ileostomy dysfunction to partial obstruction of the stoma at the level of the abdominal wall. A few years later, Crile and Turnbull[8] showed that excessive ileostomy fluid loss in the early postoperative period resulted from serositis of the exposed ileal serosal surface. The authors subsequently showed that covering the exposed serosa with an everted layer of mucosa could prevent or minimize ileostomy dysfunction. The simplified full-thickness eversion technique described by Brooke[9] has since gained universal acceptance. Later technical developments include Goligher's description of the extraperitoneal ileostomy in 1958[10] and the description by Kock et al[11] of the continent ileostomy in the early 1970s.

Two events that were critical to the success of ileostomy surgery and the rehabilitation of the ileostomy patient were the formation of the first ileostomy club at Mount Sinai Hospital in New York in 1951 and the initiation of an educational program for enterostomal therapists (later to be known as enterostomal therapy [ET] nurses and subsequently as wound ostomy continence nurses [WOCN]) by Rupert Turnbull at the Cleveland Clinic in 1961. Today the United Ostomy Associations of America comprises over 300 affiliated support groups.[1] The specialty of WOCN has matured and expanded as well with the opportunity of these specially trained nurses to become board certified. For more than 30 years, over 7,600 dedicated nurses have been certified (*http://www.wocncb.org/*; accessed December 6, 2016).

32.2.2 Stomal Physiology

Physiologically left-sided colostomy output is very similar to that of normal bowel movements. There are essentially no significant physiologic abnormalities associated with left-sided colostomy; for that reason the physiology segment of this chapter will be dedicated to ileostomy output.

Ileostomy output clearly changes as the patient recovers from the operation and appears to have three distinct phases of adaptation. In the first 3 days, the output is bilious and liquid in nature and increases daily with the maximum output occurring on the third or fourth day. During the second phase, which occurs from the fourth to the sixth day following operation, the output stabilizes, thickens, and even decreases slightly. Phase III, adaptation, occurs from the first week to the eighth week following operation and is associated with a steady decrease in volume and thickening of the stoma output.[12,13] After complete adaptation, the output from an end ileostomy created without significant ileal resection stabilizes between 200 and 700 mL/day.

Tang et al[12] studied the ileostomy output of 60 patients who underwent restorative proctectomy with defunctioning ileostomy. By the fourth postoperative day, 65% of patients had a functioning ileostomy. Ileostomy output peaked at the fourth day with a median of 700 mL (range, 10–3,250 mL) per 24-hour period. Output decreased after the fifth day, and by the 10th postoperative day, a median of 300 mL (range, 100–750 mL) per 24-hour period was reached despite normal intake. The authors noted that the critical period for acute dehydration was the third to eighth day and recommended aggressive fluid and electrolyte replacement. They therefore suggested that patients should not be discharged before 9 or 10 days after ileostomy construction. Modern surgical practice in the United States has many of these patients leaving the hospital at 2 to 6 days, stressing the importance of patient education and home health care. Small bowel adaptation following ileostomy creation results in increased reabsorption of water and electrolytes. In a normal individual, between 1,500 and 2,000 mL/day, the terminal ileum exits into the colon. With ileostomy adaptation, 70 to 80% of this output is reabsorbed.

Historically, ileostomies were created without eversion and matured spontaneously in the first 1 to 2 weeks following operation. This was commonly associated with ileostomy dysfunction. In the 1950s, Warren and McKittrick related ileostomy dysfunction to partial obstruction due to stomal edema.[7] This stomal edema was further clarified by Crile and Turnbull[8] when they showed that ileostomy effluent damaged the ileal serosa leading to serositis and subsequent edema and ileostomy obstruction. The primarily "matured" ileostomy described by Brooke has essentially eliminated ileostomy dysfunction.[9]

Most patients are able to tolerate an unrestricted diet following postoperative recovery. Dietary changes have little effect on ileostomy output with the exception that fasting can decrease ileostomy output to between 50 and 100 mL/day. Studies have shown that an elemental diet will decrease volume and concentration of digestive enzymes as well as bile acids.[14] Diets high in fat, perhaps due to fat malabsorption and alterations in bile salt circulation, have been shown to increase stoma output to 20% above baseline.[14,15] In addition, increases in oral fiber intake greater than 16 g/day have also been shown to increase output, stool frequency, and flatus.[16]

Nutrition

Individuals with ileostomies associated with less than 100 cm of resected terminal ileum are able to maintain essentially normal nutrition. Although rare, fat malabsorption, from impaired bile salt absorption or reduced bile salt pool, may cause osmotic diarrhea. Bile salt output may increase either by absorptive inhibition or perhaps by direct secretory stimulation on intestinal mucosa.[14,17] Lactase deficiency and/or enterokinase deficiency may be more evident in individuals with an ileostomy. In the absence of significant terminal ileal resection, nutritional consequences of ileostomy are minimal and patients are able to maintain a normal weight and body composition. Resection of greater than 100 cm of terminal ileum or bacterial overgrowth may result in B12 malabsorption, and vitamin B supplementation may be necessary to prevent megaloblastic anemia.

Metabolic Changes

Normal individuals lose between 2 and 10 mEq of sodium in their stool on a daily basis, while the ileostomates lose approximately 60 mEq/day. In the review by Soybel,[13] the daily steady state of fecal losses following ileostomy compared to normal stool were water, 100 to 150 mL versus 650 mL; sodium, 1 to 5 mmol versus 81 mmol; potassium, 5 to 15 mmol versus 6 mmol; and chloride, 1 to 2 mmol versus 34 mmol. Symptomatic salt depletion, however, is rare due to renal compensation. Individuals with ileostomies have been shown to have chronically elevated mineralocorticoid levels that increase water and sodium reabsorption, compensating for the increased losses in the stool. Renal compensation combined with a normal diet makes chronic dehydration and salt depletion a rare circumstance in individuals with well-adapted ileostomies. Additionally, calcium and magnesium levels are unaffected unless extensive terminal ileum has been resected.

Although the sodium concentration of ileostomy fluid rises and falls in relation to total body sodium levels, the usual sodium concentration is about 115 mEq/L. Others have reported the intestinal loss of sodium in patients with a conventional ileostomy to be 62 mmol/24 hours. (For univalent molecules [e.g., Na+, K+] 1 mEq/L = 1 mmol/L; for divalent molecules [e.g., Ca++, Mg++] 2 mEq/L = 1 mmol/L.) With dehydration, the sodium concentration falls and the potassium level rises; changes in the sodium/potassium ratio reflect the participation of the terminal ileum in sodium conservation during times of salt depletion. Normally, the sodium/potassium ratio is about 12 and rarely rises above 15.[9] The pH is generally on the acidic side, just slightly below 7.

The bacteriologic composition of the ileostomy fluid is different from that of normal small or large intestine. Gorbach et al[18] showed that the total number of bacteria in ileostomy effluent is approximately 80 times greater than that in the normal ileum. The ileostomy effluent contains a 100-fold increase in the number of aerobes, a 2,500-fold increase in coliform bacteria, and increases in total anaerobes compared to the normal ileum.

The single most important factor influencing ileostomy output is the amount of uninjured intestine proximally.[13] Increased body mass is associated with increased output. Water intake plays virtually no role. Elemental diets are associated with decreased volume, while high fat content is associated with higher losses. Increases in fiber content increase ileostomy output by as much as 20 to 25% when dietary bran supplementation exceeds 16 g/day. Losses of nutrients such as carbohydrates and protein are also increased with diets high in fiber or fat. Overproduction of gastric acid contributes to the volume of ileostomy output. Ileostomy output decreases when patients receive antisecretory agents such as omeprazole, but such benefits are reaped only with patients with large ileostomy output (22.61 L/day) or those who have had significant amounts of small bowel resected.

Intestinal transit does slow in individuals with end ileostomy. Using radioisotopes, Soper et al demonstrated that gastric emptying was normal. However, oral stomal transit time was significantly increased compared to normal controls (348 vs. 243 minutes).[19] Similar findings were observed in a study of transit times in individuals undergoing proctocolectomy and ileostomy.[20] Similarly, Bruewer et al demonstrated, by lactose breath test, that oral pouch transit time was prolonged in individuals undergoing proctocolectomy and ileal pouch–anal anastomosis.[21] Adaptation occurs over a period greater than 1 year and the mechanism remains unknown. Theories include epithelial hypertrophy with an increased absorptive surface.[22] In addition, an inverse relationship between nutrition and electrolyte absorption and intestinal transit time has been identified.[23]

Bacterial flora in the ileostomy approaches that of the colon. Gorbach et al found an 80-fold increase in total number of organisms in the terminal ileum.[18] Specifically coliforms were 2,500 times more common than normal ileal fluid. However, ileostomy bacterial content was still considerably less than that of normal stool. *Bacteroides fragilis*, a normal inhabitant of colonic stool, was rarely found in ileostomy output.

Individuals with inflammatory bowel disease, particularly associated with ileal resection and/or ileostomy, are at an increased risk for urinary stone formation. The incidence in these individuals ranges from 3 to 13%, whereas it is 4% in the normal population.[24] Uric acid stones are rare in the normal population, but comprise 60% of stones in individuals with an ileostomy.[25] Low urinary volume and pH combined with increased concentrations of calcium and oxalate are thought to be responsible for this phenomenon.[26] In addition, decreased urinary volume and decreased urinary pH facilitate stone precipitation.[26] Prophylaxis and treatment consist of increasing daily fluid intake to increase urinary volume and urinary pH.

The association between ileostomies and gallstone formation has not been well established. Individuals with well-adapted ileostomies are found to have bile acid secretions similar to those with an intact colon.[27,28] However, significant terminal ileal resection or extensive terminal ileal disease does affect the enterohepatic circulation. Bile absorption and/or depletion may occur, resulting in increased saturation of bile that leads to bile salt precipitation and subsequent stone formation. Despite this, Ritchie found no increase in incidence in cholecystectomy rates in ileostomy patients compared with that in the normal population.[29] However, Kurchin et al recommended prophylactic cholecystectomy in female individuals undergoing proctocolectomy or small intestinal resection for inflammatory bowel disease because of a threefold increase in asymptomatic gallstones.[30]

Ileostomy Dysfunction

Significant diarrhea may occur in individuals with ileostomies for many reasons. It develops more rapidly and has greater physiologic consequences than when it occurs in individuals with a normal colon. Diarrhea may result from significant ileal resection, partial small obstruction, bacteria overgrowth, recurrent or persistent regional enteritis, or infections. In most cases, treatment is similar to those given to individuals with an intact colon. Specific attention must be paid to fluid and electrolyte repletion, however, because these individuals are at significant risk for dehydration and metabolic abnormalities.

Kusuhara et al[31] found that the administration of a somatostatin analog, SMS 201–995 (100 mg thrice a day for 5 days), reduced the daily output of proximal ileostomies from 997 to 736 g along with a decrease in daily sodium and chloride excretion. The authors suggested a possible role for this agent in the management of a proximal ileostomy.

Bacterial overgrowth may develop when stasis occurs in the small bowel and can lead to deconjugation of bile salts and subsequent osmotic diarrhea as well as B12 malabsorption. Unconjugated bile salts impair sugar, water, sodium, and potassium reabsorption in the small intestine.[32] In addition, anaerobic bacteria bind to the B12-intrinsic factor complex inhibiting reabsorption. Treatment is directed at eliminating the cause of stagnation in the small intestine and, if appropriate, antibiotics are used to decrease bacterial load.

32.2.3 Types of Ileostomies

End Ileostomy

An end ileostomy is indicated after a total proctocolectomy for inflammatory bowel disease or familial polyposis, and in some cases after more limited resection for other colonic diseases. The procedure is rarely performed today without concomitant resection. It is potentially reversible when it has been performed with a partial or total colectomy (when the hazards of primary anastomosis between the ileum and colon or rectum were considered to be unacceptably high), such as in cases of ischemic infarction, peritonitis, or severe nutritional deficiency.

When the ileostomy is performed for benign inflammatory conditions, it is desirable to preserve as much ileum as possible; consequently, the ileum should be divided within 1 to 2 cm of the ileocecal valve. If the resection is performed for benign conditions, it is possible to preserve the ileocolic artery, although collateral flow from the next proximal mesenteric vessel is sufficient to nourish the entire distal ileum.

Once the blood supply and mesentery have been taken, the ileum is divided between either staples or intestinal clamps. The small mesenteric vessels and fat are trimmed proximally for a distance of 5 to 6 cm. A 1-cm strip of mesentery is left attached to the terminal bowel in order to prevent ischemia. A 2.5- to 3-cm circumferential incision is made in the skin around the previously marked site in the right lower quadrant (▶ Fig. 32.1a). Care should be exercised not to remove excess subcutaneous fat because its presence is beneficial in the support of the ileostomy appliance.[33] The fascia is exposed, and a vertical incision is made through the fascia (▶ Fig. 32.1b). The rectus muscle is spread apart with a hemostat or scissors, and the incision is carefully extended through the posterior rectus sheath and peritoneum, with electrocautery or scissors (▶ Fig. 32.1c). The opening is extended to produce a defect of 3 to 4 cm that corresponds to the width of the tips of the index and middle fingers of a surgeon with average-size hands.

The ileum is drawn through the circular incision in the right lower quadrant so that the ileal mesentery is oriented cephalad, toward the diaphragm (▶ Fig. 32.1d). Exteriorization of 5 to 6 cm of ileum should be accomplished (▶ Fig. 32.1e). The mesenteric defect may be closed by suturing the cut edge of the mesentery to the anterior abdominal wall 2 cm lateral to the midline incision from the ileostomy site to the ligamentum

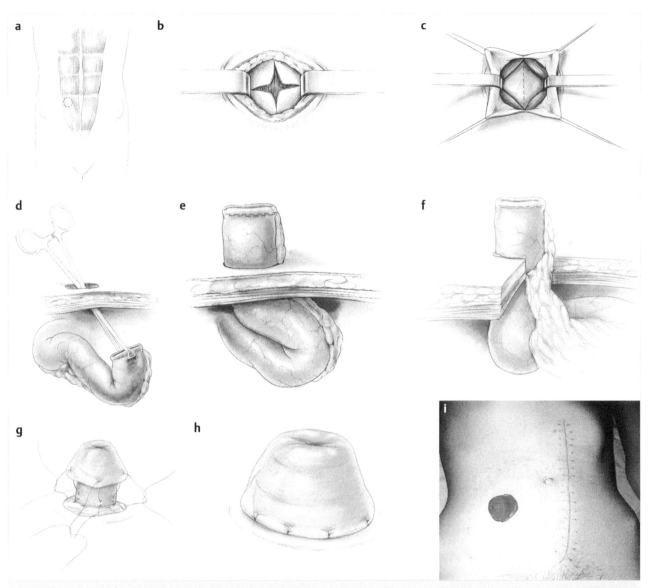

Fig. 32.1 Technique of Brooke end ileostomy construction (intraperitoneal method). **(a)** Skin and subcutaneous fat are resected over rectus muscle in preselected right lower quadrant site. **(b)** Cruciate incision is made in fascia. **(c)** Rectus muscle is retracted and peritoneal cavity is entered. **(d,e)** Ileum is delivered through ileostomy site. **(f)** Ileal mesentery is fixed to peritoneum from the ileostomy to the ligamentum teres. **(g,h)** Brooke maturation is done. **(i)** Well-constructed ileostomy showing satisfactory protrusion above skin level.

teres (▶ Fig. 32.1f). The primary Brooke-type maturation of the ileostomy can either be performed at this point or after the abdominal wall has been closed. The advantage of waiting until the abdomen is closed is that it prevents the spilling of ileostomy contents into the abdominal cavity and onto the wound. The advantage of maturing the stoma immediately is that it allows the surgeon to make adjustments, as needed, if inspection of the ileostomy suggests that its viability is tenuous. The mucosal surface should always be pink and should bleed freely at its edges. The primary maturation is performed by placing interrupted three-point buttressing sutures of absorbable suture between the tip of the ileum, the seromuscular layer of the ileum at the level of the fascia, and the deep dermis (▶ Fig. 32.1g). Interrupted sutures connecting the full-thickness bowel wall directly to the dermis of the skin are then added to secure the ileostomy (▶ Fig. 32.1h). The ileostomy should protrude at least

2 cm beyond the abdominal wall (▶ Fig. 32.1i). An appliance bag is fitted immediately in the operating room.

The Brooke ileostomy is now the most widely used technique for the construction of an end ileostomy. In most patients, it is relatively simple to perform and problems with retraction, serositis, or obstruction are uncommon. In some patients, however, the terminal ileal segment may be so edematous that full-thickness eversion using the Brooke technique is not possible. In these instances, the Turnbull technique may be useful.[8] This involves resecting the distal serosa and muscularis and everting the mucosa over the proximal ileum.

The Guy rope suture technique is an alternative method of creating eversion in a thickened terminal ileum without the need for seromuscular resection. With this technique, three permanent 3–0 absorbable sutures are placed between the distal edge of the ileum and the full thickness of the skin. In

759

addition, three temporary internal Guy traction sutures are placed 1.5 to 2 cm apart inside the ileal lumen. Upward traction on the Guy sutures with simultaneous outward traction on the permanent external sutures helps evert the thickened segment without damage or tearing of the mucosa.[34] Carlsen and Bergan[35] reviewed the complications of 358 end ileostomies: 224 were primary constructions, 96 were reconstructed by laparotomy, and 38 were local reconstruction. Only two ileostomies were primarily located on the left side. The mean length was 5 cm. The authors performed 11.6% of reoperations after primary ileostomy and 7.3 and 7.9% of reoperations after reconstruction by laparotomy and local approach, respectively. There were 12.9 and 8.7% reoperations after emergency and elective primary operations, respectively. Closing the lateral gutter or fixation of ileum to the rectus fascia did not significantly influence the number of reoperations. Postoperative discoloration of the ileostomy was not predictive of ileostomy dysfunction. Stenosis of the ileostomy, peristomal fistulas, and peristomal dermatitis were seen in 23 (10.3%), 21 (9.4%), and 18 (8%) of the patients after primary ileostomies, respectively. Patients with Crohn's disease had significantly more of these problems than patients with ulcerative colitis. Only a few patients had retraction of the ileostomy (2.7%), stomal prolapse (1.8%), or parastomal herniation (1.8%). Women had significantly more parastomal herniation than men; otherwise, there were no differences between the sexes.

Loop Ileostomy

The loop ileostomy is used to protect an ileoanal or high-risk colonic anastomosis. Although a loop transverse colostomy had traditionally been used to protect a low-lying colorectal anastomosis, Williams et al[36] recommended the loop ileostomy whenever a stoma is needed to divert stool from the distal colorectum. The authors compared the loop ileostomy to the loop colostomy and found that the ileostomy had significantly less odor, required significantly fewer appliance changes, and had fewer overall problems than the colostomy. Others have advocated loop ileostomy as a superior method for diverting the bowel to cover a colonic or rectal anastomosis and found septic complications following ileostomy closure less frequent than those following colostomy closure. However, postoperative bowel obstruction and other serious complications such as severe dehydration requiring antidiarrheal medication and hospitalization, skin breakdown, and even cholelithiasis may occur, rarely.[37]

Winslet et al[38] assessed the defunctioning efficiency of the loop ileostomy using a radioisotope and dye technique. The median defunctioning capacity in patients without episodes of fecal discharge per rectum (n = 18) was 99% and was not affected by body position or the formation of a dependent stoma. In four patients who passed fecal material per rectum but who had no stomal retraction, the median defunctioning efficiency was 99%, and continued fecal discharge was considered to be due to mucopurulent secretion from active distal disease. In four patients who passed fecal material per rectum and also had a retracted stoma, the defunctioning efficiency was significantly reduced (median, 85%), owing to the overspill into the distal limb. Chen and Stuart[39] reviewed the choice of a defunctioning stoma in restorative resection for colorectal carcinoma. The authors found the morbidity of stoma construction and closure comparable, but favored loop ileostomy because it is generally easier to manage.

Loop ileostomies are most commonly created at the time of laparotomy and bowel resection; therefore, exposure is generally through a midline incision. A segment of ileum several centimeters proximal to the ileocecal valve (which reaches the predetermined stoma site without tension; ▶ Fig. 32.2a) is chosen and encircled with a Penrose drain or umbilical tape or grasped with a Babcock clamp. The distal limb is tagged with a suture or scored to ensure correct orientation. A disc of skin is excised and a defect in the abdominal wall is created similar to or slightly larger than that of an end ileostomy. The loop is then

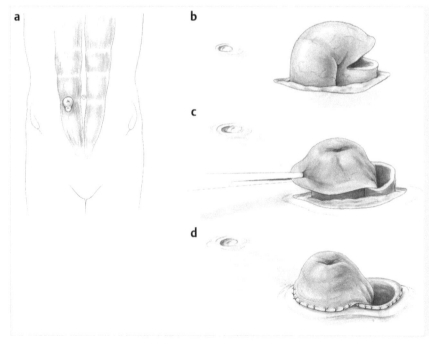

Fig. 32.2 Loop ileostomy maturation. (a) Site of completed loop over rectus muscle. (b) Incision is made in distal limb just above skin level. (c) Proximal limb is everted. (d) Both limbs are sutured to skin.

passed through the abdominal wall with care to avoid twisting. The suture marking the distal limb should be clearly visible. The loop is matured by making an incision across the distal aspect of ileum from one mesenteric border to the other at skin level (▶ Fig. 32.2b). This allows the functional limb to be the larger of the two stomas. The functional, or proximal, limb will assume a cephalad position, and the defunctionalized loop will assume a caudad position. The distal loop is sutured to the dermis of the skin with 3–0 absorbable suture. The cephalad, proximal end is then everted to assume the appearance of an end ileostomy by placing three-point anchoring sutures through the ileostomy tip, the ileum at the fascia level, and the dermal layer of the skin (▶ Fig. 32.2c). Interrupted sutures securing the remainder of the afferent opening to the skin level are placed to complete the stoma maturation (▶ Fig. 32.2d). In most circumstances, a stomal support rod is not necessary.

Some authors[36,40,41] prefer to rotate the loop 180 degrees so that the afferent loop is in the caudad position and the defunctionalized efferent limb is cephalad to allow for maximal fecal diversion when the patient is upright. However, this increases the risk of bowel obstruction and does not improve diversion rates.[42]

Prasad et al[43] described a rodless end-loop ileostomy procedure in which the ileum is divided between surgical staples after only a short segment of mesentery has been taken and the stapled proximal end is brought out and matured as a Brooke ileostomy. The antimesenteric corner of the distal stapled end is brought out inferiorly, and a small distal ileostomy opening is created and matured primarily at the skin level (▶ Fig. 32.3). Sitzmann[44] described a similar technique in which the staple line of the distal limb is left closed and the limb is tacked to the afferent limb at the level of the fascia.

Loop-end ileostomies may be created in any situation where a loop ileostomy is indicated. They may be particularly helpful in individuals with thick abdominal walls or short ileal mesenteries. In addition, if there is a significant likelihood that the "temporary" ileostomy may become permanent, an end-loop stoma may make long-term management easier for the ostomate. The end-loop ileostomy is constructed by dividing the ileum with staples and by elevating the ileum at a point where the bowel is redundant enough to permit elevation above the abdominal wall. This ileostomy is matured in the same way as a conventional incontinuity loop ileostomy (▶ Fig. 32.4).[35]

32.2.4 Loop Ileostomy Takedown

Before closing a diverting ileostomy, it is important to ensure that there is no distal stricture as may be seen in patients with a diverting ileostomy constructed at the time of an ileal-pouch anal reservoir. Takedown of a loop ileostomy generally can be performed through a peristomal incision and usually does not necessitate a formal laparotomy. In some patients, particularly in those who are obese or have unusually dense adhesions, it may be necessary to open the previous abdominal incision and mobilize additional small bowel in order to safely perform the procedure.

An incision is made at the mucocutaneous junction and extended down to the fascia and the peritoneum by sharp dissection, with meticulous care taken to avoid bowel injury. Once the proximal and distal limbs of the loop have been freed down to the peritoneal level, the remaining peritoneal attachments to the abdominal wall can be divided by blunt or sharp dissection. The ileal segment has been adequately mobilized when it can be elevated from the incision and the wound edges are clear to the peritoneum (▶ Fig. 32.5a,b). The surgeon then has three options of closure: anterior ileal wall closure, stomal resection with end-to-end anastomosis, and functional end-to-end stapled anastomosis.

The choice of anterior wall closure as opposed to resection and anastomosis is one that can be made at the time of surgery. It is often feasible to simply trim the stomal margin and then transversely close the bowel in either one or two layers or with staples (▶ Fig. 32.5c,d). If induration or distortion of the lumen

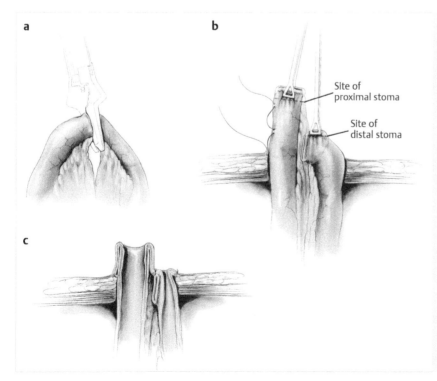

Fig. 32.3 Modified loop ileostomy (end loop). **(a)** Ileostomy loop is divided between staples. **(b)** Proximal end is elevated above skin level and everted. **(c)** Both ends are sutured to skin.

Site of proximal stoma

Site of distal stoma

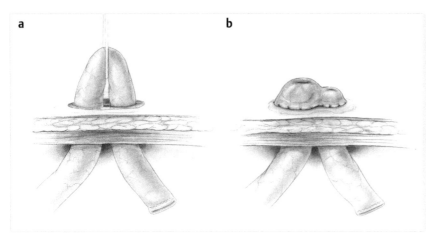

Fig. 32.4 An end-loop ileostomy. **(a)** Loop of ileum is elevated proximal to stapled end. **(b)** Completed maturation of loop.

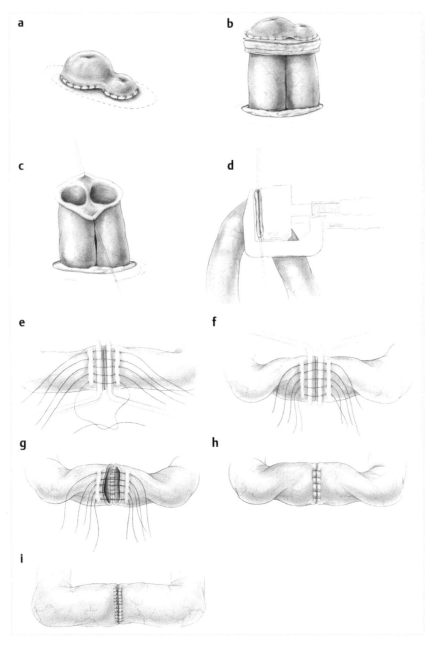

Fig. 32.5 Loop ileostomy takedown. **(a)** Elliptical incision is made around ileostomy. **(b)** Ileum is mobilized circumferentially and elevated. **(c,d)** Stoma with skin edge is resected, and anterior wall is closed. **(e–i)** Ileostomy is resected, and proximal and distal ends reunited with end-to-end handsewn anastomosis.

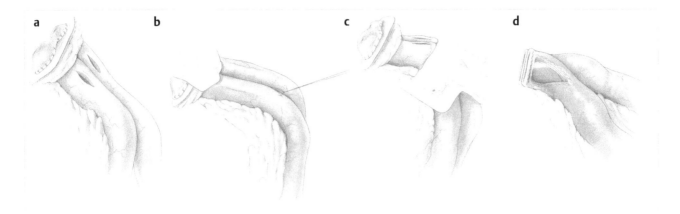

Fig. 32.6 Stapled ileostomy takedown. **(a)** Ileostomy is mobilized, and stab incisions are made on antimesenteric surface. **(b)** Stapler is positioned through stab wounds and fired. **(c)** Ileostomy is resected with linear stapler to include stab wounds in resection. **(d)** Functional end-to-end anastomosis.

is present, however, it is safe to resect the edges of both limbs and perform a primary end-to-end anastomosis using healthy ileal tissue proximally and distally (▶ Fig. 32.5e–i).

Kestenberg and Becker[45] proposed the technique of stapled functional end-to-end anastomosis because of the dissatisfaction they experienced with long operating times, anastomotic edema, stricture, and partial obstruction following end-to-end anastomosis. A simplified method involves mobilizing both proximal and distal limbs of the ileostomy and inserting a linear cutting stapler in both limbs of the ileostomy and firing the linear stapler. The residual opening can be closed in two layers with sutures or with a stapler (▶ Fig. 32.6).

van de Pavoordt et al[46] reviewed their experience with closure of loop ileostomies. Ninety-three percent of the stoma closures were done through simple transverse incisions. The overall complication rate was 17%. Of the early postoperative complications (13%), the major complication was small bowel obstruction, commonly in patients in whom the stoma was protecting a pelvic ileal reservoir. Abdominal septic complications occurred in 1% of patients. The wound infection rate after healing by both secondary intention and primary skin closure was 3%. Only one incisional hernia was observed in the late postoperative period; in three patients, a posterior rectus sheath defect at the stoma site was found incidentally at laparotomy, without clinical evidence of an incisional hernia.

An additional adjunct to ileostomy closure is the application of sodium hyaluronate/carboxymethyl cellulose (SH/CMC) sheets (Seprafilm Genzyme, Cambridge, MA) during creation of the ileostomy. Bertoni et al[47] retrospectively reviewed a series of ileostomy closures and compared 146 patients in which SH/CMC was used to 147 patients without SH/CMC. The SH/CMC patients had a shorter closure time. Other studies showed that use of SH/CMC resulted in lower perioperative complications and facilitation of early stomal closure.[48,49]

32.3 Colostomy

32.3.1 History

In 1776, Pillore, a French surgeon, created a cutaneous cecostomy for a wine merchant suffering from obstructing rectal carcinoma. Although the patient died 2 weeks later from a small bowel perforation induced by forced catharsis, the cecostomy was the first recorded instance of a successful colonic stoma being performed.[50] At autopsy, the cecostomy was healthy. A number of sporadic reports of colostomies followed, and these generally involved construction of a loop colostomy for obstruction in adults or imperforate anus in infants. In 1793, Duret, a naval surgeon from Brent, performed the first successful left iliac colostomy for a case of imperforate anus in a 3-day-old child. The patient lived up to the age of 45 years. In 1839, Ammusat, a Parisian surgeon, reported 29 cases of colostomy, with all of them sited in the lumbar area. Twenty-one of these cases involved infants with an imperforate anus; of these, four survived.

In 1884, Maydl introduced the technique of loop colostomy supported by a rod, when he suggested using a goose quill to support the loop against the abdominal wall. In 1881, Schitininger described the creation of an end sigmoid colostomy and an oversewn distal stump. This operation was the forerunner of the Hartmann procedure described in 1923, which consisted of sigmoid resection with end colostomy and an oversewn rectal stump.[50] The operation of colostomy for obstruction came into widespread use in the 20th century.

Miles[51] has been credited for the 1908 description of the operation of end sigmoid colostomy and abdominoperineal resection. In fact, C.H. Mayo had previously described the technique in 1904. This operation, with the loop colostomy that preceded it, ushered in a new surgical era. The end sigmoid colostomy and loop diverting colostomy as described by Miles, Maydl, and others have now been performed by thousands of surgeons on hundreds of thousands of patients in this century with relatively few technical modifications. In the last two decades, the need for end sigmoid colostomy has diminished as surgical stapling techniques have made low anterior anastomosis more feasible.[52]

32.3.2 Fecal Diversion

Although the standard method of diverting the fecal stream away from the left colon has traditionally been the transverse loop colostomy, the indications for fecal diversion as well as the choice of a loop colostomy as the best means to achieve this have become controversial. The most common indications for diversion in the past have been obstruction or inflammation of the left colon, trauma to the colon, anterior resection of the rectum, and perineal sepsis. The increasing popularity of Hartmann's procedure with end colostomy for diverticulitis or obstructing carcinoma, the more aggressive use of primary resection and anastomosis in some of these cases, and the increasing reliance on primary closure for many colon injuries have no doubt decreased the popularity of loop colostomy in the emergency setting.

Fielding et al[53] prospectively studied more than 2,000 patients having elective colorectal anastomoses and found that 15.8% received a synchronous covering stoma to protect the anastomosis. No differences in mortality were observed between patients who had a covering stoma and those who did not, although significant differences in surgical practice were identified in different surgeons. The authors concluded that the covering diverting stoma was not necessary for surgeons who were able to keep their patients' leak rates at an acceptably low level.

Although many patients with colon and rectal injuries, particularly those with multiple abdominal injuries, need some type of fecal diversion, surgeons have increasingly recognized that the isolated and uncomplicated colonic injury treated promptly can be managed successfully with primary closure.[54]

The methods of diversion not involving resection include the "medical colostomy," ileostomy, cecostomy, and diverting colostomy. The concept of a "medical colostomy" using a chemically defined diet was recommended by Gordon for such anorectal procedures as sphincteroplasty, postanal repair, skin grafting following excision of a neoplasm or hidradenitis suppurativa, and repair of rectovaginal fistula.[55] It puts the gastrointestinal tract at rest so that the repaired area does not have to be challenged with bowel movements. Today it is not necessary for most anal sphincter and rectovaginal fistula repairs, but may be beneficial in the treatment of extrasphincteric fistulas. Robertson[56] achieved similar benefits with an elemental diet in 16 patients with inflammatory bowel disease, anorectal sphincter surgery, or wounds that had to be protected from fecal soiling. None of the patients on the elemental diet had bowel movements within 3 days of operation, and most had bowel movements only at 5- to 6-day intervals. Nutritional support, either by total parenteral nutrition or the elemental diet, is a useful alternative in select patients who need a brief period of gastrointestinal tract rest but do not otherwise need total prolonged fecal diversion.

The value of the loop ileostomy was discussed earlier and should be considered as an alternative to loop colostomy, in most patients. Both the loop ileostomy and loop colostomy, however, can pose management problems for the patient, and neither is an ideal stoma for long-term use. The comparative study by Williams et al[36] showed that both loop ileostomy and loop transverse colostomy successfully defunctionalized the distal bowel. The ileostomy had fewer peristomal problems and fewer management problems than the colostomy, although dehydration from diarrhea or high ileostomy output could be a potential problem with the ileostomy, particularly in elderly patients.

Corman[57] stated that "cecostomy could be removed from our surgical armamentarium with very little consequence to health care delivery." Others[58,59] have been more supportive of the cecostomy as a method of decompressing select patients without subjecting them to the morbidity of a loop colostomy. Attention has focused on less invasive ways of performing cecostomy, including the computed tomography (CT)-guided percutaneous method[60] and the percutaneous endoscopic method for nonobstructing colonic dilatation.[61]

Winkler and Volpe[62] reviewed loop transverse colostomy among 29 patients in a community hospital and found that 5 patients died, 8 had complications, and only 18 patients underwent colostomy closure. The authors concluded that the first stage in the management of these patients should be resection of the diseased segment and that the colostomy should be end bearing and placed as close to the disease process as possible. Hopkins[63] supported the concept that temporary loop colostomy may not be "temporary" in many patients by reporting that colostomy closure was not performed in 19 of 45 patients (42%) having transverse colostomy for malignancy. Abrams et al[64] similarly found that colostomy closure was not performed in 156 of 248 patients (63%) having transverse and left colostomies. The difficulties in managing a loop transverse colostomy compared to an end sigmoid colostomy are so substantial that the surgeon must always consider that the loop colostomy may ultimately subject the patients to a less-than-ideal colostomy for life. Although much of the controversy on indications and methods for fecal diversion involves personal preferences on the part of individual authors, some general principle should be applicable for most patients. The principle of resecting primary disease and performing an end-bearing stoma in preference to a loop colostomy or other proximal diverting method is a sound principle that should be adhered to whenever possible. For other patients needing fecal diversion, the loop colostomy or loop ileostomy can be performed. In deciding whether to perform a fecal diversion for patients undergoing anterior resection or for patients with trauma, the surgeon must weigh the risks and consequences of anastomotic or colonic closure leakage against the morbidity and mortality of later colostomy takedown. These risks vary among patients and also among surgeons. The medical colostomy is a useful means of avoiding a surgical stoma in patients who need only short-term diversion to protect perineal wounds or perineal incisions. Tube cecostomy is of limited value and should be used only for decompression and not for fecal diversion.

Cecostomy

Since the turn of the century, tube cecostomy has been advocated mainly as a decompression procedure for acute colonic obstruction and as a safety valve for colonic resection. It has also been suggested for perforation or impending perforation of the cecum, for cecal volvulus, adynamic ileus of the colon, and toxic dilatation in inflammatory bowel disease. The procedure is best performed as a tube cecostomy rather than a primary stoma. When a primary stoma is needed, it is better to perform a loop ileostomy or a loop transverse colostomy, as both are more diverting and are easier for the patients to manage.

The virtues of tube cecostomy, as cited by its proponents, are that it is easy to perform, can be carried out under local anesthesia, the cecum is the portion of colon most likely to perforate, it does not interfere with subsequent resection of the left side of the colon, and it may eventually close spontaneously. In cases of extreme obesity of the abdominal wall and when gross distention of the bowel has "used up" the leaves of the transverse mesocolon, transverse colostomy may be impossible. Under these circumstances, cecostomy may be the only method of relieving obstruction.

The use of cecostomy has frequently been criticized and has lost favor with many surgeons. Detractors point out that it provides less effective decompression than does a transverse colostomy and that it does not allow complete diversion.

Tube cecostomy can be performed as a primary operation through a right lower quadrant (McBurney) or a right lateral transverse incision. Once the peritoneum is opened, the distended cecum is easily delivered through this incision. The serosal surface should be secured to the peritoneal surface with interrupted absorbable sutures. Two pursestring sutures of nonabsorbable material such as 3–0 silk are then placed around the apex of the cecum, and a no. 30-Fr bladder catheter or no. 36 to 40 Pezzer catheter is inserted inside the pursestring sutures. The two pursestring sutures are tied, and the tube is secured in place. It is best to deliver the catheter through a stab wound either cephalad or caudad to this incision so that the incision can be closed primarily. The tube can be removed after 7 to 10 days, and the cecocutaneous fistula should be closed spontaneously.

Rosenberg and Gordon[65] conducted a retrospective review of 59 tube cecostomies to evaluate operative indications, outcome, and associated morbidity. Tube cecostomy was performed as a complementary procedure in 81.4% of cases; in the other 18.6%, it represented either the only operative intervention or the initial stage of a two-stage procedure. Complications included local infection in 32% of cases, pericatheter leak in 25%, skin excoriation in 24%, and pain in 12%. Catheters remained in place for an average of 14 days, but function was adequate in only 40% of cases. Cecal drainage persisted from 24 hours to 90 days after the tube was removed.

Two additional procedures were required to close persistent cecal fistulas. In addition, other reported complications included wound dehiscence, recurrence of a fistula after closure of the cecostomy, subcutaneous emphysema, prolapse of the omentum, stitch granuloma, evisceration, retraction, and hernia formation at the cecostomy site. Aseptic decompression of a distended cecum can be difficult and peritonitis and poor tube function after cecostomy have been responsible for a substantial number of deaths. Tube cecostomy fails to decompress the bowel adequately in as many as 50% of cases. The authors concluded that the high morbidity associated with this procedure militates against its use. Benacci and Wolff[59] were more encouraging about cecostomy. In a retrospective chart review of 67 patients who had catheter tube cecostomy placement, clinical indications for tube cecostomy were colonic pseudoobstruction (39%), distal colonic obstruction (16%), cecal perforation (15%), cecal volvulus (13%), preanastomotic decompression (12%), and miscellaneous (5%). Operation was emergent in 64% of patients and elective in 36% of patients. Tube cecostomy was the primary procedure in 70% of patients and complementary in 36% of patients. Minor complications were seen in 45%, including pericatheter leak (15%), superficial wound infection (12%), tube occlusion (7%), skin excoriation (4%), premature tube dislodgement (4%), colocutaneous fistula (3%), and ventral hernia (12%). No patients required reoperation for tube-related morbidity.

The authors concluded that catheter tube cecostomy is of therapeutic value in select clinical situations.

A protective diversionary cecostomy or transverse colostomy is now rarely warranted for left-sided colon procedures as this can be safely performed without diversion. A review of contemporary literature suggests that reasonable current indications for tube cecostomy include volvulus, pseudoobstruction (if an attempt at colonoscopic decompression has failed), cecal perforation associated with an obstructed left-sided lesion, and to relieve obstruction in morbidly obese patients when transverse colostomy is technically impossible.

Loop Transverse Colostomy

In the past, the loop transverse colostomy was a commonly used method to achieve temporary or short-term fecal diversion, whether necessitated by obstruction, inflammation, trauma, low colorectal anastomoses, or perineal wounds. Fontes et al[66] studied the ability of the emergency loop colostomy to achieve total fecal diversion in 62 patients. The authors found that fecal diversion was virtually complete in all patients for the first 3 months but that the diversion became incomplete in about 15% of the patients in subsequent months, probably because of recession and retraction of the stoma. Schofield et al[67] found that they could achieve total fecal diversion from a right transverse colostomy by rotating the stoma counterclockwise for 90 degrees so that proximal limb was in the most dependent position caudad to the distal limb. Morris and Rayburn[68] studied 23 patients with loop colostomies by giving them barium by mouth. In no patient was barium found in the distal limb, indicating full diversion. At least 17 other individual techniques have been recorded in the literature to ensure complete fecal diversion from a loop colostomy.[66] Most of these manipulations appear to be unnecessary, as a traditional loop colostomy should be able to achieve complete fecal diversion for at least a few months postoperatively. Complete diversions should rarely, if ever, be necessary for a longer period of time.

Loop Colostomy Construction

Although a seemingly endless number of techniques have been described for construction of a loop colostomy, three generic methods are used most often. The first involves construction of the loop colostomy over a fascial bridge without the use of a supporting rod or prosthetic bridge material. The second method involves the use of a rod or bridge, and the third method involves creating an end loop or divided type of colostomy. The dissatisfaction with the postoperative management problems caused by loops and bridges has no doubt led to the proliferation of techniques.

In addition to the three types of loop colostomies, a fourth type of diverting temporary colostomy has been described by Turnbull et al[69] as part of an operation for the treatment of toxic megacolon complicating ulcerative colitis. That procedure consisted of a skin-level (trephine) colostomy along with a loop ileostomy as the preliminary operative treatment of critically ill patients with toxic megacolon. This procedure is infrequently performed today, and a skin-level temporary colostomy with its attendant management problems is rarely indicated. However, a trefine stoma may be useful in selected cases of carcinomatous where it may be the only option for fecal diversion.

Loop Colostomy over Fascial Bridge

A transverse incision is made in the right upper quadrant at the previously marked stoma site. The incision is extended across the rectus fascia anteriorly and the rectus muscle fibers are separated. If the patient does not have a concomitant lower transverse incision, rectus can be divided between clamps and ligated to allow for a larger opening. If, however, a simultaneous lower transverse incision through the rectus muscle below the umbilicus has been made, then it is best not to devascularize rectus muscle in the right upper quadrant because of the risk of leaving an ischemic muscle segment between the two transverse incisions. The peritoneum is incised either sharply or with a fine hemostat, and the peritoneal cavity is entered.

The right transverse colon should be grasped with a Babcock forceps and elevated out of the incision, with care taken to identify the taeniae and confirm that the segment is colon. The incision may have to be enlarged if there is too much tension on the bowel as it leaves the abdominal wall. On occasion, it may be necessary to extend the incision and take down the hepatic flexure of the right colon to allow the right transverse colon enough mobility to be delivered through the incision, but this maneuver is usually not necessary.

Once the transverse colon has been elevated from the abdomen, the gastrocolic omentum adherent to the superior surface of the colon is cleaned away, and a short segment of mesocolon (< 5 cm) is taken between clamps and ligated with sutures. The fascial bridge is defined by grasping the fascia and peritoneum together with either an Allis or Kocher clamp. Two or three sutures of heavy nonabsorbable material such as braided nylon or slowly absorbable material are placed through both the fascia and peritoneum of the superior lip of the incision, then through the window created between the colon and the mesocolon, and then through the fascia and peritoneum of the inferior lip on the opposite side. After all sutures have been placed, they are tied on the same side as the incision. The fascia should be felt carefully to make sure it is not constricting the lumen or blood supply of either loop. If the fascial or peritoneal openings are tight, they should be incised either medially or laterally but not along the fascial bridge. If the abdominal wall incision appears too large on either side, it can be partially closed with an interrupted nonabsorbable or slowly absorbable suture.

An incision is made across the apex of the colon. A primary maturation is performed with a 3–0 absorbable material such as Vicryl or chromic catgut. The residual lateral or medial extension of the incision can be closed with a running subcuticular absorbable suture (▶ Fig. 32.7).

Loop Transverse Colostomy over Rod

This procedure is identical to that described for the fascial bridge technique, except that the colostomy is supported through the mesocolic defect by a plastic rod, bridge, or other type of supporting material (▶ Fig. 32.8). Regardless of type, the supporting structure is removed approximately 3 to 10 days after surgery, at which time the colostomy is adherent enough to the incision that it should not recede. Schofield et al[67] described the operation of dependent proximal loop colostomy. This stoma avoids the complications of prolapse and paracolostomy hernia and is easy to

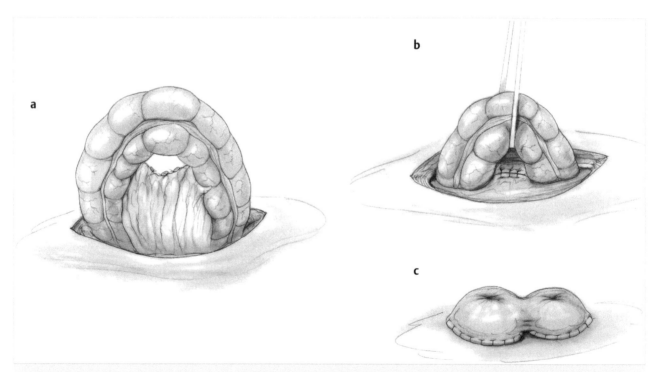

Fig. 32.7 Loop colostomy constructed over fascial bridge. **(a)** Window in mesocolon is formed and colon is elevated. **(b)** Fascial bridge is created through mesocolic window with interrupted sutures. **(c)** Colon is opened and sutured to skin.

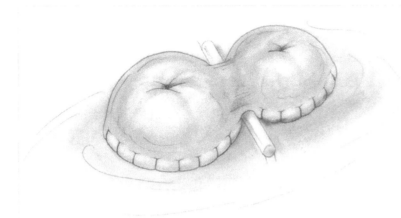

Fig. 32.8 Loop colostomy constructed over glass rod.

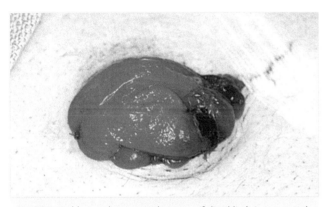

Fig. 32.9 End-loop colostomy with corner of distal limb incorporated into stoma. Overall appearance is like an end colostomy.

close. It defunctions the distal colon as evidenced by the study of 10 patients given a radioactive tracer, chromium 51, by mouth and none spilled over into the distal loop.

Divided-Loop Colostomy

The divided-loop colostomy is analogous to the divided-loop ileostomy described by Prasad et al.[70] In this technique, the transverse colon is divided between surgical staples. The proximal end is brought out as an end stoma through the incision, and the tip of the distal limb is brought out alongside the proximal stoma. The corner is opened and matured as a small distal stoma (▶ Fig. 32.9). The end-loop colostomy eliminates the risk of distal segment prolapse and creates a stoma easier to care for postoperatively.

Unti et al[71] conducted a retrospective review of their 7-year experience in 229 patients with end-loop colostomies,[72] ileocolostomies,[70] and ileostomies.[23] A total of 30 stoma-related complications were observed in 27 stomas, for an overall complication rate of 13.1%. The most common complications were skin excoriation secondary to leakage (3.5%), retraction (3.5%), partial necrosis (2.6%), and peristomal sepsis (1.8%). Mucocutaneous separation, prolapse, and stenosis were each seen in less than 1% of patients. No cases of stomal herniation, obstruction, or hemorrhage were encountered. Twelve deaths occurred, but none was attributed to stoma-related complications.

Hidden Colostomy

Sometimes a patient is found to have an unresectable carcinoma of the colon or rectum in association with extensive metastases or carcinomatosis. If the primary lesion is not causing complete or partial obstruction, the surgeon must decide between doing nothing and risking that the patient will need a second operation later for obstruction or creating a colostomy at the first operation, knowing that the patient may never need it. The hidden colostomy can be a useful technique in this setting.

The colostomy is performed as a loop over a fascial bridge proximal to the carcinoma, which is usually in the rectum. The colon is not elevated above the skin level but is instead buried in the subcutaneous fat where it can easily be identified later. Then if obstruction occurs, the colostomy can be opened at the bedside with the patient under local anesthesia. The resulting stoma is not anatomically ideal, but the patient is usually terminal or near terminal when it is performed, and overall it serves the patient well.

Loop Colostomy Closure

The decision to perform a temporary loop colostomy must always involve some consideration of the morbidity, the mortality, and the cost of colostomy closure. Parks and Hastings[73] reported that complications related to colostomy takedown decreased if colostomy closure was put off for 90 days or more. Williams et al[74] analyzed the morbidity, mortality, and cost of colostomy closure in patients having a colostomy constructed for either trauma or nontraumatic diseases and found no significant differences in complication rates, although the authors noted that the colostomy was less likely to be closed if it was performed for nontraumatic disease. Thal and Yeary[75] reported no deaths and a relatively low complication rate of only 10.2% among 137 patients having a colostomy closed following diverting colostomy for trauma. They emphasized the importance of meticulous surgical technique and attention to detail during the procedure.

Altomare et al[37] reviewed the closure of 87 protective colostomies and identified hypoalbuminemia and interval to closure as risk factors. Operative mortality was 4.6%, major complications developed in 13% (fecal fistula, sepsis, intestinal obstruction, and myocardial insufficiency), and minor complications were recorded in 29% of patients. Colostomy closures within 30 days had a mortality rate of 12.5%, a major complication rate of 25%, and a minor complication rate of 50%. For closures performed between 31 and 90 days, rates were 5.2, 10.5, and 36.8%, respectively. For closure after 90 days, rates were 0, 9.3, and 9.3%, respectively. Their review of the literature, which included 26 reports, revealed a range of death rates from 0 to 4.6%, fecal fistula from 2 to 43%, and total complications from 5 to 61%. The authors emphasized that these data underscore the very significant morbidity and mortality associated with colostomy closure, and therefore the same skill and meticulous approach are required for this operation as for any major procedure performed on the colon.

Velmahos et al[76] reported conflicting recommendations from randomized trials of trauma patients in which they compared early (within 15 days of initial operation) and late (> 90 days after the initial operation) closure. The authors found no significant difference in morbidity between the two groups, with an overall complication rate of 26.3%. Technically, the early closure of colostomies was far easier than late closure, required significantly less operating time, and resulted in less intraoperative blood loss. The closure of end colostomies was more time consuming, both early and late, and caused more bleeding. Total hospitalization was marginally shorter overall for early closure, but late closure of end colostomies resulted in prolonged hospitalization. The authors recommend early closure of colostomies and the use of loop colostomies whenever possible as both are safe and beneficial for patients with colonic injury after trauma. Contraindications to early closure include a nonhealing distal bowel, persistent would sepsis, and persistent postoperative instability.

The loop colostomy can be closed by any of the following three methods: mobilization of the colostomy with closure of the anterior wall of the colon, mobilization with functional end-to-end surgical staple closure, and resection of the colostomy with primary end-to-end anastomosis. The three techniques are analogous to those used for loop ileostomy takedown. If the colon is satisfactorily mobilized proximally and distally; if the colon edges are satisfactorily debrided so that sutures or staples are placed only through healthy, noninflamed tissue; if the blood supply to both ends of the colon is satisfactory; and if there is no tension on the suture line, then all three methods should give comparably good results.

32.3.3 End Sigmoid Colostomy

End sigmoid colostomy may be temporary or permanent. It is performed as a permanent procedure following abdominoperineal resection of the rectum for malignant disease, and it is also indicated as a definitive stoma for incontinent patients who are not suitable candidates for other procedures. End sigmoid colostomy may be performed as a temporary stoma following resection of the rectosigmoid for benign or malignant disease, and it may serve as a means of achieving temporary diversion for other conditions such as radiation proctitis. The end colostomy allows the patient to take advantage of the absorptive capacity of the proximal colon, making it the easiest type of intestinal stoma for the patient to manage.

A key technical consideration in end sigmoid colostomy construction involves deciding whether to fashion the colostomy as an extraperitoneal or intraperitoneal structure. Goligher[10] first described the extraperitoneal approach after observing that patients with both ileostomy and colostomy seemed especially predisposed to postoperative intestinal obstruction. The extraperitoneal colostomy was designed to prevent obstruction from occurring so frequently. Subsequently, Whittaker and Goligher[77] reviewed their experience with 251 patients and found that patients having an extraperitoneal iliac colostomy did not have a lower incidence of mechanical obstruction, but they did have a significantly lower incidence of pericolostomy herniation, prolapse, and recession compared to patients having an intraperitoneal colostomy.

The extraperitoneal colostomy is a good option for patients needing a permanent iliac colostomy. Extraperitoneal colostomy is also good for patients with ascites. The leaking of fluid is minimized or eliminated. For those patients needing only a temporary stoma, the intraperitoneal method is preferable, because takedown of the colostomy and subsequent reanastomosis are less difficult when the proximal colon has been left in an intraperitoneal position.

Technique of Extraperitoneal Colostomy Construction

The technique of extraperitoneal end sigmoid colostomy construction is the same whether it is performed as part of an abdominoperineal resection or as a permanent end colostomy for benign disease. Either a lower midline or transverse incision is suitable once it has been determined that the preselected stoma site will not be too close to either incision. A minimum of 3 cm and preferably 5 to 8 cm should separate the edge of the stoma from the abdominal incision.

Once the abdomen is opened, the sigmoid colon is mobilized by incising the lateral peritoneal reflection along the white line of Toldt, carefully identifying the left ureter as it crosses the left common iliac artery. The intraperitoneal rectosigmoid is then resected and the rectal stump, if retained, closed with staples. Otherwise, a complete proctectomy is performed as described in Chapter 22 for resection of rectal carcinoma. The colostomy site is then created by excising a disk of skin and separating subcutaneous fat down to the level of the fascia. It is important that a layer of fat be retained between the abdominal incision and the colostomy site so that the two wounds are not in direct communication at the subcutaneous level. Goligher[10] originally recommended that the extraperitoneal colostomy be placed a little more laterally so that the rectus muscle is not included. Subsequent experience has shown that the extraperitoneal tunnel can be readily extended into the rectus sheath; this allows the stoma to be positioned medially through the rectus muscle. Although either method is acceptable, the more medial placement of the stoma is preferable because the rectus muscle adds extra support to the stoma. Sjödahl et al[78] reported a dramatic reduction in parastomal hernia development when a permanent stoma was brought out through the rectus muscle. In a review of 130 patients, the prevalence of parastomal hernia was 2.8% when the stoma was constructed through the rectus muscle versus 21.6% when brought out lateral to the rectus muscle. In contrast, Ortiz et al[79] found no correlation between the presence of parastomal hernia and the position of the stoma in the abdominal wall.

The left lateral peritoneal leaf is then grasped with a forceps, and an extraperitoneal tunnel is created by a combination of sharp and blunt dissection to connect with the colostomy wound in the abdominal wall. The tunnel is gently developed by finger dissection and the colon delivered through the tunnel so that 3 to 5 cm of colon comfortably protrudes above the skin level. The colon is then secured to the fascia with interrupted or running sutures of 3–0 polyglycolic acid. The pelvic peritoneum should be secured over the colon, and, if the procedure is performed as part of an abdominoperineal resection, the process of pelvic reperitonealization is completed at this time.

Primary maturation of the colostomy is performed using interrupted 3–0 absorbable sutures with the matured colostomy fashioned to protrude 1 to 2 cm above the abdominal wall. Maturation is accomplished by placing four anchoring stitches through the full thickness of the colon, then the colonic wall below the skin level, then the dermis. Interrupted simple sutures are placed between each of the four quadrants to complete the maturation (▶ Fig. 32.10).

The intraperitoneal colostomy differs only in that the colon is delivered through the rectus muscle, and the defect in the left lateral peritoneal gutter may be closed with interrupted slowly absorbable sutures. However, most surgeons currently leave this space open.

Several techniques of end colostomy maturation using stapling devices have been described using either the linear skin stapler[80] or the circular stapling device.[81] Neither of these methods allows the surgeon the opportunity to optimize stomal contour and stomal protrusion for the individual abdominal wall. In addition, the use of staplers adds significant cost to the procedure.

Porter et al[82] reported on 126 patients who underwent 130 end colostomies, 44 for benign, and 86 for malignant disease, and were followed up for an average of 35 months. The left or sigmoid colon was used in 99 and the transverse colon in 31 patients. Stomas were made electively in 98 patients and urgently in 32 patients. Seventy-six stomas were brought out through the incision and 54 from separate sites. There were 69 complications in 55 patients (44%), including 11 strictures, 9 wound infections, 14 hernias, 9 small bowel obstructions, 4 prolapses,

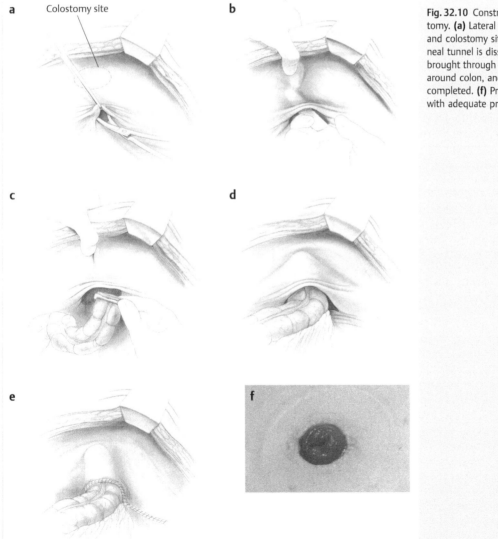

a Colostomy site
b
c
d
e
f

Fig. 32.10 Construction of extraperitoneal colostomy. **(a)** Lateral peritoneal reflection is incised, and colostomy site is prepared. **(b)** Extraperitoneal tunnel is dissected bluntly. **(c,d)** Colon is brought through tunnel. **(e)** Peritoneum is closed around colon, and pelvic floor reconstruction is completed. **(f)** Properly constructed colostomy with adequate protrusion above skin level.

2 abscesses, 1 peristomal fistula, 17 skin erosions, and 2 poor stoma locations. Fifteen complications required reoperation. Five of these procedures included stoma revision. Total numbers of complications were not related to the stoma site, the disease process, the urgency of the procedure, or the segment of colon used. Wound infections, however, were increased in urgently made stomas. The incidence of hernia was equivalent in stomas brought out through the incision or at a separate site. Forty-one patients (30%) had 43 colostomies closed at an average of 3.5 months after creation. Thirteen patients had 14 complications (five wound infections, six hernias, two small bowel obstructions, and one rectovaginal fistula). One patient died. Four patients required reoperation. There were no anastomotic leaks. Complications were equivalent in Hartmann's closures and transverse colostomy closures. Complications were similar in stomas created for carcinoma and those created for diverticular disease.

32.3.4 Continent Colostomies

Numerous devices have been introduced for use with an end sigmoid colostomy to help the patient achieve greater control of both gas and stool output from the stoma. Interest in magnetic devices was stimulated by the work of Feustel and Hennig,[83] who described a magnetic ring system in the early 1970s. The system consists of a magnetic ring that is implanted subcutaneously, and the colonic stoma is brought through the ring. An external magnetic cap fitted over the stoma mechanically prevents the expulsion of stool. A disposable charcoal filter disk on the undersurface of the cap permits gas to escape.

Khubchandani et al,[84] using careful patient selection methods, reported favorable results among 14 patients. Husemann and Hager[85] reported the results of 240 patients who underwent implantation of the Erlangen magnetic device. Forty-five rings were explored because of infection, pressure necrosis, parastomal hernia, invagination, prolapse, and stenosis. Although continence was obtained in 68% of patients, only 43% of surviving patients still use the system. Reasons given for not using the cap were pain and weight. Although the magnetic ring device has been successful in some patients, it has two main disadvantages. It requires a magnetic material to be permanently implanted in the abdominal wall and placement must be nearly perfect to allow for satisfactory function. For these reasons, the device has failed to gain widespread popularity.

In Prager's preliminary experience[86] with a two-part silicone device, three of five patients were able to achieve continence by inserting a specially designed inflatable plug into the stoma. The Conseal colostomy system (Coloplast, Inc., Tampa, FL) is composed of an open-cell polyurethane foam with a water-repellent cover. The cover contains a charcoal filter that enables intestinal gas to pass without odor while preventing the passage of fecal material. The Conseal plug expands to form a bell-shaped plug when it is inserted into the stoma (▶ Fig. 32.11). Clague and Heald[87] evaluated the Conseal system in a multicenter trial of 100 patients and found that it was successful in approximately one-third of the patients. Patients who irrigated their colostomy tended to retain the plug longer than those who used the natural method. Codina Cazador et al[88] conducted another multicenter trial in which

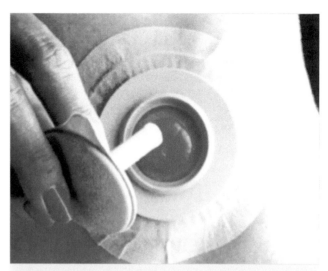

Fig. 32.11 Conseal system. Skin barrier is positioned around stoma, and plug is about to be inserted into stoma and snapped on to flange of skin barrier.

43 patients were evaluated. No complications arose, and complete fecal continence was obtained in 71%. This continence device did not achieve its original promise.

A number of methods have been used to achieve continence without using external devices, the most promising being the intestinal smooth muscle graft. Schmidt[89] reported an 80% success rate with this procedure among 500 patients. The procedure consists of a free transplant of a 10- to 15-cm segment of colonic smooth muscle that is sutured to become ruffled into a muscle mass of about half that length. The graft is wrapped around the bowel and sutured to produce continence.

32.3.5 End Colostomy Takedown

End colostomy takedown with intraperitoneal anastomosis involves mobilizing proximal and distal colonic segments and creating an end-to-end anastomosis using either staples or sutures. The previous abdominal incision, either vertical or transverse, needs to be reopened, and often, extensive adhesions need to be taken down. The colostomy is mobilized by making an incision at the mucocutaneous junction and then dissecting down to the fascia and peritoneum until the colon is free. The mucous fistula or distal rectosigmoid is also mobilized, and the anastomosis can usually be performed without difficulty.

Before the advent of circular staplers, end sigmoid colostomy takedown with extraperitoneal anastomosis to a low-lying rectal stump was often an exceptionally difficult and hazardous procedure. This procedure has been greatly simplified by the introduction of the newer circular stapling devices. After the proximal sigmoid has been mobilized and prepared for anastomosis, the distal stump needs to be dissected only enough to define the apex and free the colon from adhesions that will inhibit smooth placement of the stapling device. The stapler is inserted per anum, and the device is opened so that the trocar can penetrate the apex of the rectal stump and bring the barrel of the device through that hole. A pursestring suture is placed on the proximal sigmoid and tied around the anvil shaft. This shaft is reengaged into the central shaft of the cartridge, and the anvil is approximated to the cartridge. The stapler is fired and then removed. The procedure should carry minimal morbidity as long as the apex of the rectal stump has been carefully defined and a clean circular anastomosis has been obtained. This particular operation lends itself well to a laparoscopic approach. In the event that considerable residual sigmoid colon remains, the circular stapler may not reach the apex of the sigmoid stump. Also there may be kinking of rectum in the hollow of the sacrum. In either event, an additional portion of rectosigmoid will require resection.

The purported ease and safety of closure of loop colostomy are cited as reasons for avoiding end colostomy, with or without resection. Data comparing the complications of loop colostomy closure and end colostomy takedown and anastomosis are sparse. Mileski et al[90] analyzed data from 93 consecutive colostomy closures, 62 of which were loop and 31 were end colostomies. The two groups were comparable with respect to age, underlying disease, and risk factors, such as coronary artery disease, diabetes, hypertension, steroid dependence, hypoalbuminemia, and smoking. Closure of end colostomies took longer and was associated with more blood loss than closure of loop colostomies. However, the mortality rates for closure of loop (4.8%) and end (3.2%) colostomies were not significantly different. The complication rates were identical (16%). Although none of the other risk factors was associated with increased rates of mortality or morbidity, the detrimental effects of steroid dependence and preoperative hypoalbuminemia were striking. Four deaths and 60% of the complications occurred in patients with steroid dependence or hypoalbuminemia, or both. The rates of wound infection after primary or secondary closure of the stoma site were not significantly different. The authors concluded that loop colostomy closure is not associated with fewer complications than closure of end colostomy, even though the latter takes longer to perform and is more difficult. Primary closure of the stomal site is safe and reduces the length of hospital stay.

Mosdell and Doberneck[91] reviewed the charts of 59 patients undergoing Hartmann's procedure and 43 patients undergoing ostomy closure after divided colostomy, loop colostomy, or divided ileostomy-colostomy. Ostomy closure after Hartmann's procedure was accomplished in 46 patients. These 46 patients (group I) were compared with the 43 patients having ostomy closure following divided colostomy, loop colostomy, or divided ileostomy-colostomy (group II). No deaths occurred in either group. The morbidity rate was 30% in group I and 19% in group II. Major complications involved wound, lung, small bowel, and colonic anastomoses. Anastomotic stricture rate was 9% in group I and 5% in group II. Small bowel and anastomotic complications in both groups occurred only when ostomy closure was performed after a delay of less than 6 months after ostomy construction. Stricture occurred only after end-to-end colocolostomy and coloproctostomy and did not occur after ileostomy or ileoproctostomy. All strictures were successfully treated by reoperation. Anastomotic leak and pelvic abscess did not occur in either group. The authors concluded that ostomy closure after Hartmann's procedure may be more difficult and time consuming than ostomy closure after loop colostomy, divided colostomy, or divided ileostomy-colostomy, but that ostomy closure after Hartmann's procedure does not result in a higher morbidity rate. The authors advise an interval of 6 months between ostomy construction and ostomy closure and submit that

all patients whose general condition permits reoperation may safely undergo ostomy closure. Pearce et al[92] reviewed the outcome of 145 patients undergoing Hartmann's resection. The mortality rate of the primary procedure was 8%. Eighty patients also underwent reanastomosis. The interval between the primary and secondary procedures was found to be the most important risk factor. Six of 12 patients had clinical evidence of a leak when this interval was less than 3 months, compared with 7 of 28 patients for 3 to 6 months, and none of 40 when the second operation was delayed for greater than 6 months. All deaths (three patients) and clinical septicemia (four patients) occurred in the two "early" groups. All colovaginal fistulas (three patients) and strictures (three patients) were associated with stapled anastomoses. No association was found between the complication rate following reanastomosis and the initial pathology or experience of the surgeon undertaking the secondary operation.

Keck et al[93] reviewed the case records of 111 patients undergoing Hartmann's procedure mostly for advanced carcinoma and complicated diverticular disease. Of 96 patients who survived, 50 (52%) underwent reversal. Of those with diverticular disease, 40 of 48 (83%) underwent reversal. Mortality for Hartmann's reversal was 2%, anastomotic leak rate was 4%, and overall complication rate was 26%. Early reversal was performed in 13 patients and late reversal in 37 patients. There was no difference in these groups in mortality, morbidity, or anastomotic leakage. However, bed stay was longer in the early group and graded operative difficulty greater. In particular, cases in which adhesion density was most severe and in which accidental enterotomy occurred were more common in the early group.

Livingston et al[94] questioned whether the risks after colostomy closure were exaggerated. The authors reviewed 121 patients who underwent colostomy closure for trauma. There was no mortality and a 4.9% incidence of major morbidity. Although there was no apparent relationship between the interval between colostomy creation and closure, three of the six major complications occurred in patients whose colostomies were closed soon after complicated initial injuries. The authors recommended that if the primary operation is complicated by intra-abdominal sepsis or major wound problems, 6 months should ensue before attempting closure. Long-term follow-up of these patients (mean, 39 months) disclosed a low incidence of late complications secondary to colostomy closure. Although the trend toward the increased use of primary repair of colon injuries in selected patients is supported, the authors' study indicates that the risk of colostomy closure has been exaggerated and should not be a factor in the decision to create a colostomy after colon trauma.

Khoury et al[95] retrospectively reviewed the records of 46 patients who underwent colostomy closure. Patients ranged in age from 24 to 87 years, and 54% were women. Stomas had been created during emergency operations in 87%. Most operations (54%) were performed for complications of acute diverticulitis. Of the 46 procedures, 40 (87%) were end colostomies and 6 were loop colostomies. Stomas were closed at a range of 11 to 1,357 days after creation (mean, 207 days; median, 116 days). Inpatient complications occurred in 15% of patients, including congestive heart failure (2%), cerebrovascular accident (4%), pneumonia (2%), enterocutaneous fistula (2%), and pulmonary embolus with death (2%). The most common long-term complication was midline wound hernia, which occurred in 10% of surviving patients. Overall complications occurred in 24%. The authors concluded that colostomy closure is a major operation.

32.4 Complications

Colostomy complications are similar to those associated with ileostomies. The most frequently encountered problems include ischemia, recession, prolapse, and parastomal hernia. Allen-Mersh and Thomson[96] reviewed 156 operations on 23 patients over a 3-year period for correction of late colostomy complications and found that problems included stenosis in 65 patients, paracolostomy hernia in 42, and prolapse in 16.

Leenen and Kuypers[97] studied 266 patients with 345 stomas on the small and large bowel to determine possible etiologic factors for stomal complications. The overall complication rate for creating a stoma was 36%. No differences in overall complication rate were encountered when comparing acute and elective management; however, high-output stomas and necrosis were encountered more often in the acutely managed group. Preoperative contamination was followed more often by stomal retraction. Septic events, however, occurred less frequently than in the noncontaminated procedures. Moderate obesity had no significant influence on the outcome of the procedure. Adipose patients had a statistically significant greater number of necroses. The outcome of stoma surgery was greatly influenced by bowel quality. Crohn's disease and bowel ischemia were encountered in 50% of patients with stoma complications. In ischemic disease, significantly more necrosis was found. Retraction of the stoma occurred more often in patients with Crohn's disease. Patients with chronic ulcerative colitis did not have a higher complication rate.

Although complications of ileostomy are common, they can be minimized by careful surgical techniques and good ET nursing. Carlstedt et al[98] reviewed the ileostomy complications in 203 patients operated on with proctocolectomy and ileostomy for ulcerative colitis and Crohn's disease. The crude rate of ileostomy complications necessitating reconstruction was 34% and was significantly higher in patients with Crohn's disease compared with patients with ulcerative colitis. The cumulative rate of surgical revision after 8 years was 75% in the former group and 44% in the latter. Ileostomy stenosis and sliding recession were the two most common indications for reconstruction. Eighty-three percent of the revisions were performed as local procedures, making a formal laparotomy unnecessary. Causative factors such as surgical technique, length of concomitant ileal resection, and postoperative weight gain were analyzed for possible influence on the rate of reconstruction, but no significant association was identified.

Khoo et al[99] prospectively assessed the morbidity of creating and closing loop ileostomies in a consecutive series of 203 patients having an ileoanal pouch procedure. There was one death as a result of liver failure. One patient developed a persistent pouch-vaginal fistula that resulted in pouch excision. The remaining 201 patients had their ileostomy closed at a mean time of 10 weeks after the primary procedure. Only 7% needed reoperation to correct ileostomy-related problems. After ileostomy closure, complications were noted in only 2% of patients.

Stothert et al[100] reviewed the outcome of 49 high-risk patients having 51 stomas created as an emergency measure and found a morbidity of more than 50%. Feinberg et al[101] found complications referable either to a temporary loop ileostomy or its closure in 69 of 117 patients undergoing loop ileostomy in association with the pelvic reservoir procedure and ileoanal anastomosis. Grobler et al,[102] in a randomized trial of loop ileostomy in restorative proctocolectomy, found that 52% of patients developed ileostomy-related complications. On the other hand, Wexner et al[103] found that loop ileostomy was a safe option for fecal diversion in a study of 83 patients who required temporary fecal diversion after either ileoanal or low colorectal anastomosis (72 patients), for perianal Crohn's disease (5 patients), or for other reasons (6 patients). All loop ileostomies were supported with a rod, and fecal diversion was maintained for a mean of 10 weeks. Sixty-seven patients had reestablishment of intestinal continuity. Stoma closure was effected through a parastomal incision in 64 patients; in 3, a laparotomy was required. The closure was stapled side to side in 49 patients, while a hand-sewn anastomosis was performed in the other 18 patients. All skin wounds were left open. Nine patients (10.8%) developed 10 complications. Four patients developed dehydration and electrolyte abnormalities secondary to high stoma output, two had anastomotic leaks that spontaneously healed following conservative management, one patient developed a superficial wound infection that spontaneously drained and one patient developed a partial small bowel obstruction that resolved without operation after a 4-day hospitalization. One stoma retracted after supporting rod removal and prompted premature closure. There were no instances of stomal ischemia, hemorrhage, prolapse, or mortality in this series.

Leong et al[104] conducted an actuarial analysis of complications of 150 permanent end ileostomies constructed over a 10-year period. By 20 years, the incidence of stomal complications approached 76% in patients operated on for ulcerative colitis and 59% in those with Crohn's disease. Revisional surgery rates were higher in patients with ulcerative colitis than in those with Crohn's disease (28 vs. 16%). Complications encountered were skin problems (cumulative probability, 34%), intestinal obstruction (23%), retraction (17%), parastomal herniation (16%), fistula or suppuration (12%), prolapse (11%), stenosis (5%), and necrosis (1%). Closure of the lateral space did not reduce the probability of developing intestinal obstruction (18% at 20 years in those with closure vs. 3% in those without). Fixation of the mesentery did not reduce the probability of developing prolapse of the ileostomy (11% in those with fixation vs. none in those without). The incidence of parastomal herniation was not reduced by siting through the rectus abdominis (21% in those sited through the body of the rectus abdominis vs. 7% in those sited through the oblique muscles). Some of the surgical dogmas relating to ileostomy construction are not supported by the results of this study.

In a review by Senapati et al,[105] of 310 patients who underwent restorative proctocolectomy, 296 had a covering ileostomy and 14 did not. The stoma had been closed in 88.9% at a median interval from formation of 12 weeks. Ileostomy-related complications before closure occurred in 5.7%. Laparotomy for obstruction due to the ileostomy was required in 2.4%. Retraction requiring revision occurred in 1.0%, an abscess behind the stoma in 0.3%, and miscellaneous appliance problems in 2.4%. Following closure, 22.4% developed an ileostomy-related complication. There were 30 cases of small bowel obstruction, treated conservatively in 19 (7.2%) and by laparotomy in 11 (4.2%). Peritonitis requiring laparotomy occurred in 1.1%, and 0.8% developed an enterocutaneous fistula. There were 5.3% wound infections and 6.1% other miscellaneous problems. Significant complications associated with a temporary ileostomy were less frequent in this series than in some other reports. Obstruction was the most common complication and fistula was rare.

In a review of the complications of temporary loop ileostomy by Kaidar-Person et al,[106] factors suggested to predispose to stoma complications were high body mass index, inflammatory bowel disease, use of steroids and immunosuppressive therapy, diabetes, old age, emergency operation, operative technique, and surgeon experience. Preoperative evaluation and proper marking of the stoma site before an operation were associated with fewer adverse outcomes. In the review of 14 publications, the reported morbidity ranged from 3 to 100% (with many in the 35–45% range). Major complications included stenosis, small bowel obstruction, retraction, necrosis, prolapse, stricture, fistula, and parastomal hernia. Small bowel obstruction ranged from 0 to 17% (mostly in the 3–8% range), high output 1 to 72% (mostly in the 3–5% range), appliance leakage 7 to 68% (mostly in the 17–38% range), skin irritation 2% to 41% (mostly in the 4–7% range), and reoperation rate 1% to 9%. Minor complications included dermatitis, electrolyte imbalance, and dehydration from high stoma output. The latter may often necessitate early closure of the stoma. Although not a complication, nonclosure of a temporary ileostomy ranged from 0 to 19%.

32.4.1 Bowel Obstruction

Small intestinal obstruction is a relatively common occurrence among ileostomy patients. It is usually caused by extrinsic compression from adhesions or an internal hernia, intraluminal compression from impacted boluses of food, or recurrent Crohn's disease.

Although food bolus obstruction is usually self-limited, it is clinically indistinguishable from complete extrinsic small intestinal obstruction. Food bolus obstructions tend to be complete and present as an impaction at a point of angulation or stricture at the fascial level. Since the impaction may occur after the ingestion of exotic or high-fiber foods, such as coconut, the patient often relates the onset of pain to a time just after eating these foods. The patient frequently has a history of similar episodes.

The onset of pain and obstructive symptoms tends to be sudden, and cessation of ileostomy output usually follows. With a partial high-grade obstruction, the patient describes passing a large volume of watery effluent from the stoma and may confuse this event with gastroenteritis. Whether the obstruction is complete or partial, significant dehydration can result from associated nausea and vomiting, as well as from the secretion of fluid into the dilated small bowel proximal to the obstruction. Toxicity is generally not present, and perforation and peritonitis are uncommon.

Management of food bolus obstruction should include fluid and electrolyte restoration, nasogastric suction, and close observation. Gentle irrigation of the ileostomy with a soft, well-lubricated rubber catheter, using 4 oz of either saline or liquid glycerine often dislodges the impaction and relieves the obstruction. Alternatively, lavage of the ileostomy with up to 500 mL of saline may be tried using an enema bag, a cone-tip irrigator, and an irrigation sleeve. Operation is rarely needed.

Mechanical extrinsic obstruction is less common but potentially more serious than intraluminal obstruction. Patients who have had operations for inflammatory bowel disease have a greater predilection for obstruction than those who have undergone abdominal operations and bowel resection for other disease. Hughes et al[107] found a 9.1% incidence of small bowel obstruction requiring operation among 463 patients having resectional therapy for inflammatory bowel disease compared to a 2.3% incidence of operation among 2,474 patients having resection for colon and rectal neoplasms. Two-thirds of the obstructions in this series were related to adhesions, and the other third was related to the stoma. Fasth and Hultén[41] noted a lower incidence of obstruction, approximately 3%, for patients with loop ileostomies.

Intestinal obstruction has been reported as an especially frequent complication following restorative proctocolectomy for inflammatory bowel disease. The obstructive events are related either to the temporary ileostomy or to the adhesions. Obstructive phenomena have been reported in up to 43.5% of patients having such restorative procedures.[108] Francois et al[109] reviewed the Mayo Clinic experience with small bowel obstruction complicating ileal pouch–anal anastomosis and found that 17% of their patients developed small bowel obstruction; 7.5% of these patients required operation. In this series, obstruction was more likely to occur in patients who had a temporary Brooke ileostomy (12.5%) than those who had a loop ileostomy (4.6%). Although the loop ileostomy with an open mesenteric defect laterally appears especially vulnerable to obstruction, it is clear that patients having either a Brooke end ileostomy or loop ileostomy are at risk.

Anderson et al[110] described a simple technique to minimize the risk of volvulus following establishment of a loop ileostomy. A broad antimesenteric attachment of the seromuscular layer of ileum to the parietes at the stoma site is achieved with absorbable sutures, creating a broader fulcrum. After adopting this technique, no complications were noted in 30 patients followed up for a minimum of 4 years.

The patient with mechanical small bowel obstruction is often indistinguishable from the patient with food bolus obstruction. The initial management is the same, consisting of fluid and electrolyte resuscitation, nasogastric suction, and a brief trial of irrigation or lavage of the stoma. If pain persists despite nasogastric tube decompression and lavage of the stoma, then early operation is the safest course. If, however, the patient is comfortable with the nasogastric tube in place and if the abdomen is soft and free of signs of peritonitis, then the patient may be observed for a period of 24 to 48 hours. Immediate operation must be considered if the patient develops increasing pain, increased distention, leukocytosis, or fever. For all patients with an uncertain obstruction and unsatisfactory course, early operation is often the safest approach. Although Francois et al[109] emphasized that necrosis from small bowel obstruction complicating the loop or Brooke ileostomy was rare in their series, the

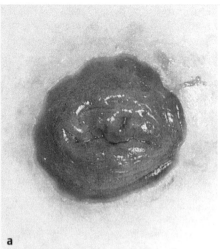
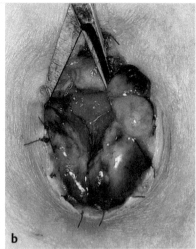

Fig. 32.12 (a) Ischemic colostomy. **(b)** Only distal-most portion of transverse colostomy is necrotic.

consequences of additional small bowel loss from infarction in a patient who already has an ileostomy are significant and the need for resection must be avoided.

32.4.2 Stoma Ischemia

Stoma ischemia is present when a healthy stoma turns dark purple or black, usually within the first 24 hours after operation. Ischemia may be limited to the part of the stoma above the skin level, or it may extend deep to the fascial level, the peritoneal level, or the proximal intra-abdominal ileum. When a stoma becomes dark, the first priority is to assess the proximal extent of the ischemia. If the ischemia extends below the fascia and peritoneum, immediate revision is indicated to prevent perforation and peritonitis. Viability of the proximal mucosa can be assessed by inserting a test tube and illuminating it with a penlight or inserting an endoscope into the bowel lumen. If the ischemia is limited to the level of the fascia or above, it is best to monitor this condition nonoperatively and revise the stoma at a later time if stenosis or other complications develop. A two-piece pouching system instead of a single appliance may be especially helpful in this case because it allows easy access to the stoma without removing the adhesive covering the peristomal skin. Another handy test in evaluating stoma ischemia is a pinprick test in which arterial bleeding may be seen from the muscle, even in the presence of mucosal necrosis. With ischemia limited to the mucosa, spontaneous resolution can usually be expected.

Ischemia following construction of a colostomy, especially an end sigmoid colostomy, is seen more frequently than ischemia following ileostomy construction. This occurs in part because the left colon is less mobile than the ileum and in part because the colon is often brought through a thickened abdominal wall under some tension. When an end sigmoid colostomy is performed for carcinoma, the left colic artery has usually been taken, often as part of a high ligation of the inferior mesenteric artery. In this case, the blood supply through the marginal artery may be inadequate to nourish the stomal end.

A healthy stoma should be pink at all times. If the stoma is dusky or black in the first 24 hours, the extent of the ischemia must be evaluated (▶ Fig. 32.12a). The technique of using a penlight inside a test tube described to evaluate ileostomy

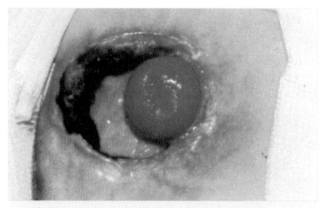

Fig. 32.13 Ileostomy with gaping mucocutaneous separation.

viability also works well for the colostomy. If uncertainty remains, 5 mL fluorescein dye can be injected intravenously for 10 minutes.[111] A long-wave ultraviolet lamp is used to inspect the stoma after a test tube is inserted. If strong fluorescence of the mucosa is noted, viability is assured. A negative result is indeterminate. It might best be remembered that a dark or even black stoma postoperatively, especially a moist one, may not be a necrotic stoma or infarcted bowel, but perhaps melanosis coli.[112] This should be considered as it requires no treatment and its recognition will obviate a needless operation. If in the early postoperative period, the cyanosis, ischemia, or necrosis is above the fascial level, it is best to do nothing but manage the wound locally and let a mucocutaneous junction form by secondary intention (▶ Fig. 32.12b). Stricture or recession is often the late consequence of ischemia, but such problems can be revised electively later. If necrosis extends below the level of the fascia and peritoneum, however, immediate laparotomy and colostomy revision should be undertaken to avoid perforation and peritonitis.

32.4.3 Mucocutaneous Separation

Mucocutaneous separation of the stoma from the skin may occur as a result of tension (i.e., creation of a skin opening too large for the exteriorized bowel) or superficial infection (▶ Fig. 32.13). Good ET nursing is especially important when this problem occurs, and stenosis at the skin level is always possible as a late consequence. The subcutaneous tissue between the stoma and skin should be kept clean by packing the area with a paste material (e.g., Stomahesive) or absorptive powder until a new junction forms secondarily.

32.4.4 Stoma Stenosis

Stoma stenosis occurs as a consequence of ischemia or infection, although occasionally it can result from the opening in the skin or fascia being made too small at the time of stoma construction (▶ Fig. 32.14). The stenosis can be managed initially with simple and gentle dilatation of the stoma in conjunction with a low-fiber diet. If the patient has recurrent obstructive episodes or pain, however, the stoma should be revised. Skin-level stenosis can be managed by detaching the skin from the mucosa, and by excising a small amount of skin to increase the

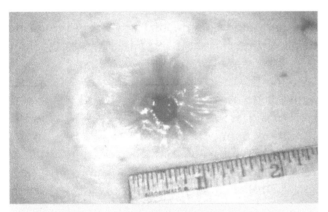

Fig. 32.14 Ileostomy stenosis with marked skin scarring.

trephine size. This incision can be extended down to the fascia, if necessary, where the fascial opening can be enlarged. The fascia and skin are re-sutured primarily and a new Brooke-type stoma fashioned. Malt et al[113] described a technique for relieving stricture at the fascial level by performing a fasciotomy similar to those performed for compartment syndromes of the calf or forearm. With this technique, incisions are made above and below the ileostomy and away from the peristomal skin. A scissors is then slid through the grain of the anterior rectus sheath to the ileum and the stricture is relieved (▶ Fig. 32.15).

32.4.5 Recession (Retraction)

Recession, or retraction, of an ileostomy or colostomy can occur in as many as 10 to 15% of patients.[114] The recession can be intermittent or fixed. Intermittent recession, or telescoping, results from having too large a gap through the abdominal wall or from having inadequate fixation and adhesion formation between the stoma and the abdominal wall. With intermittent recession, the stoma length and protrusion are generally satisfactory when patients assume the upright position, but the stoma becomes flush with the skin or may recede below the skin level when patients lie supine and the abdominal muscles are relaxed. This often leads to soiling and leakage, since it is difficult to maintain a satisfactory appliance seal whenever the stoma does not protrude above the skin level. Fixed ostomy recession usually implies that the stoma was designed too short at the time of construction or that it became too short when the width of the abdominal wall increased after a period of postoperative weight gain (▶ Fig. 32.16). Some patients with either fixed or intermittent ileostomy recession can be managed with skilled ET nursing. A convex faceplate placed firmly against the skin sometimes allows patients to maintain a satisfactory seal and

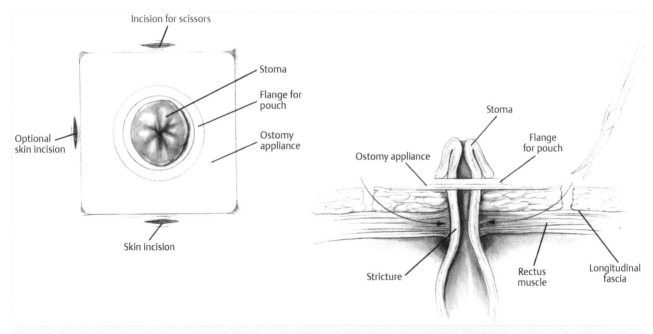

Fig. 32.15 Repair of fascial stenosis. Incisions are made outside of ostomy appliance, and fascia is split with scissors to relieve stenosis.[113]

not need operative revision. If the patient continues to have leakage and soiling, then the ileostomy should be revised.

The simplest type of revision is performed locally by making a circumferential incision around the stoma at the mucocutaneous junction and extending the incision down to the level of fascia and peritoneum to free up the entire distal bowel that is then refixed to the peritoneum and fascia, and a new Brooke maturation is performed (▶ Fig. 32.17).

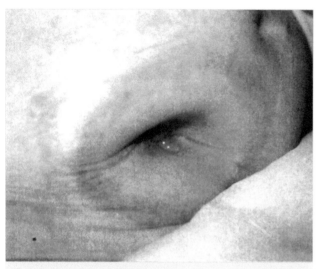

Fig. 32.16 Fixed recession of ileostomy.

32.4.6 Ostomy Prolapse

Introduction

Stomal prolapse may develop in any type of abdominal stoma. Rates are variable, but substantially lower than those of parastomal hernias. In a review of the United Ostomy Association Registry, Fleshman and Lewis found the rates as follows: ileostomy 3%, colostomy 2%, and urostomy less than 1%.[115] Similarly, a Cook County Hospital registry including 1,616 stomas found the overall incidence to be 2%. Age and lack of preoperative stoma site markings were predictive risk factors.[116] However, registries tend to include predominantly individuals with permanent stomas, thus underestimating the risk of complications associated with temporary stomas.

The stoma at highest risk for prolapse has been the transverse loop colostomy and the distal defunctionalized limb is usually responsible. Reasons for this are unclear, but a large stoma aperture (particularly when stomas are created in an emergency setting) and a poorly fixed, redundant, distal transverse colon have been implicated. Incidence varies, but rates of prolapse as high as 47% have been found in association with loop colostomies.[117]

Some authors divide prolapse into two types, fixed and sliding. Fixed prolapse is defined as permanent eversion of a greater than desired segment of bowel. This occurs because too much bowel has been everted at the time of stoma construction. It is uncommon and rarely requires treatment. The remainder of this segment will focus on sliding prolapse. Sliding prolapse occurs when long segments of ileum or colon protrude

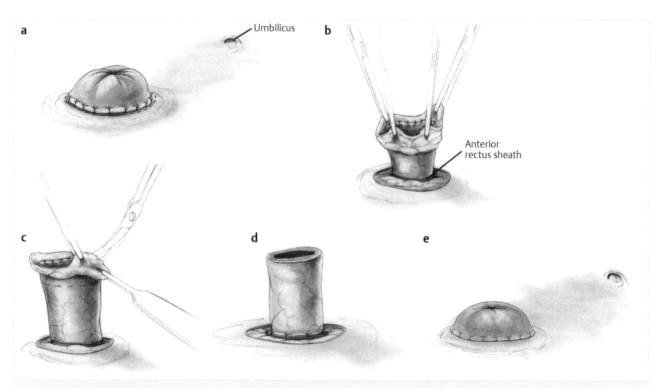

Fig. 32.17 Ileostomy revision. **(a)** Circumferential incision around stoma. **(b,c)** Stoma is mobilized to fascia and peritoneum, and tip is resected. **(d)** Ileum is fixed to fascia. **(e)** New Brooke maturation is done.

through the stoma orifice intermittently, usually in response to Valsalva or increased abdominal pressure. Segments greater than 40 to 50 cm have been observed (▶ Fig. 32.18 and ▶ Fig. 32.19).

Particularly when prolapse develops in colostomies, a parastomal hernia may also be present. It is essential that any concomitant hernia be identified prior to treatment, as the presence of a parastomal hernia will dictate the type of repair required. Allen-Mersh and Thomson identified a 50% incidence of hernia associated with colostomy prolapse, most commonly associated with end colostomies.[96]

Symptoms

Stomal prolapse always presents as a stomal mass, but other symptoms include dislodgement of the appliance, bowel obstruction, and pain due to venous engorgement of the constricted, prolapsed segment. Diagnosis is ascertained by history and physical examination. The frequency and consequences of

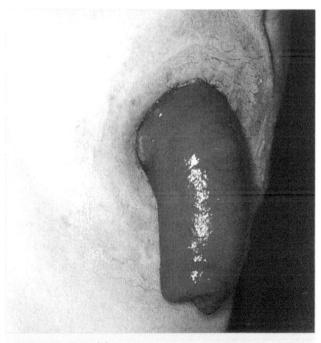

Fig. 32.18 Prolapsed ileostomy.

symptoms are important because minimally symptomatic, infrequent prolapse does not require repair.

When examining the abdomen, the prolapse should be reduced and a finger placed in the stomal orifice. Diligent inspection and palpation of the peristomal skin will determine the presence or absence of a hernia. If a hernia is present, its presence and symptoms should dictate the type of repair performed. The prolapse will, by necessity, be repaired during the process.

Treatment

Less than 10% of prolapse will be complicated by incarceration and/or strangulation. In these situations, treatment is urgent. In viable, incarcerated stomas, table sugar may be sprinkled (large amounts) on the stoma to draw out water and decrease edema. This may allow for reduction of the prolapse with subsequent elective operation. If this is unsuccessful or if viability is in question, then it will be necessary to proceed with operation. If the bowel is nonviable, then an extra-abdominal resection and cutaneous recreation of the stoma is the preferred option. Otherwise any of the options mentioned in the ensuing sections may be applied.

When prolapse or any stoma complication develops, the surgeon should first determine if the stoma can be reversed and intestinal continuity can be reestablished. If this can be done safely, it should be the first surgical option even if earlier than previously planned. If this is not an option, then repair should be undertaken.

Regardless of the planned preoperative approach, all of the following should be accomplished prior to operation. A comprehensive history and physical must be performed not only to determine the patient's ability to tolerate an operation but also to determine preoperative stoma-related problems so that these can be addressed (i.e., odor, leakage, poorly fitting appliance, and poor stoma visualization). In addition, any disability or dysfunction that will limit stoma care, such as arthritis or poor vision, should be elicited. All patients should also be attended to by a trained stoma therapist and/or the surgeon preoperatively, in the event resiting of a stoma becomes necessary. Finally, at the time of operation, all patients need to be prepped and draped for laparotomy and transabdominal repair even if preoperative plan dictates a parastomal approach. Repair takes one of three forms: resection, revision, or resiting. Resection is most commonly employed for end stomas. Resection simply involves

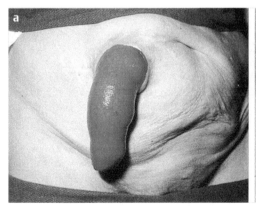
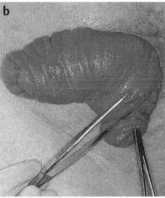

Fig. 32.19 (a) Dramatic end-colostomy prolapse. (b) End transverse colostomy with prolapse of ascending colon and cecum. Forceps indicate the ileocecal valve and hemostat in appendical orifice.

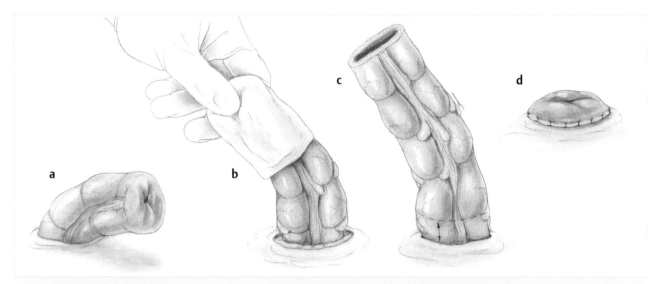

Fig. 32.20 Repair of prolapsed end colostomy. **(a,b)** Mucocutaneous junction of colostomy is incised and colon elevated. **(c)** Redundant colon is resected. **(d)** New colostomy is matured.

mucocutaneous disconnection (care should be taken to prevent creating an oversized skin defect), eversion of the prolapsed segment, resection of any exteriorized bowel, and recreation of the stoma.

Simple prolapse can easily be repaired through a paracolostomy incision. The colon is mobilized in the same fashion as for local colostomy revision, with dissection down to the peritoneal cavity to free the colon circumferentially. The colon, with all its redundancy, is then delivered through the abdominal wall. The redundant sigmoid is resected, leaving a 5-cm protrusion above the abdominal wall. The sigmoid is fixed to the fascia with 3–0 nonabsorbable sutures, and a primary maturation is performed with 3–0 chromic catgut suture (▶ Fig. 32.20).

Revision is most appropriate for prolapse of the distal limb of a transverse loop colostomy. In this case, through peristomal skin incision, the distal limb is dissected free and separated from the proximal limb. The open end is then closed and returned to the abdominal cavity. The fascial and skin defects are then tailored to an appropriate size and an end colostomy created. Care should be taken to ensure proper orientation of the proximal and distal limbs as dropping the proximal, functional end of a transverse colostomy into the peritoneal cavity will have predictable, devastating consequences.

Prolapse is more common with a transverse colostomy than with an end colostomy, but transverse colostomy prolapse can be managed conservatively since the stoma is usually temporary (▶ Fig. 32.21). When operation is indicated, several procedures have been proposed. Zinkin and Rosin[118] described a modification of an old procedure called "button colopexy" for patients who are not candidates for extensive revision. This procedure can be performed on an outpatient basis. It is performed by pressing the proximal and distal loop of bowel against the anterior abdominal wall by a finger inserted in the lumen, and then securing each loop against the abdominal wall with large nonabsorbable sutures tied over a button. Another option for the transverse colostomy prolapse in high-risk patients

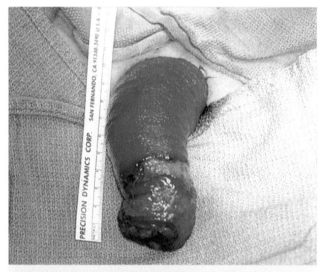

Fig. 32.21 Prolapsed, partially ulcerated distal limb of transverse colostomy.

is dividing the loop colostomy into two limbs. The prolapsing proximal or distal colon limb is dissected free, the redundant tip is resected, and a new end colostomy is fashioned with a long Hartmann's pouch or a small mucous fistula.

Finally, resiting is best reserved for prolapsed stomas with other associated problems. As previously mentioned, this is an option for prolapse in association with hernia. However, resiting may be beneficial in other situations. If the stoma was originally poorly sited and this has led to significant problems, then resiting may be appropriate. In addition, a transverse loop colostomy may be associated with other significant problems such as odor, leakage, or the need for an overly large unsightly appliance. Here, right colectomy and ileostomy may be the procedure of choice if reestablishment of continuity is not appropriate.

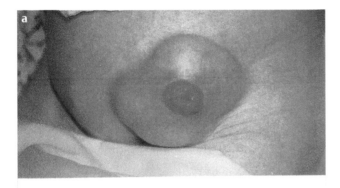

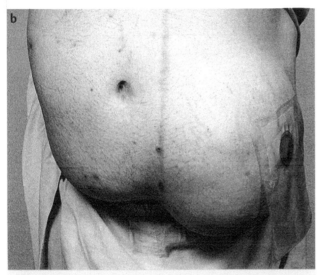

Fig. 32.22 **(a)** Large parastomal hernia around end sigmoid colostomy. **(b)** Huge paracolostomy hernia with laterally displaced ostomy opening.

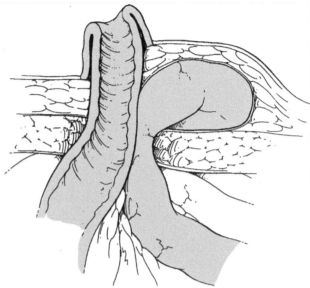

Fig. 32.23 True parastomal hernia.[128]

32.4.7 Parastomal Hernia

Parastomal hernias may develop around both ileostomies and colostomies (▶ Fig. 32.22). The risk of parastomal hernia is increased with high intra-abdominal pressure, chronic cough, obesity, malnutrition, and use of immunosuppressive drugs and steroids. The probability of the occurrence of the risk of this complication may be reduced by locating the stoma through the rectus muscle. The incidence varies, but paraileostomy hernias are less frequent (0–28%) compared with colostomies (0–58%).[119] Advanced age of colostomates versus ileostomates, solid nature of feces, and larger size of colostomies versus ileostomies have all been implicated as causative factors.[119]

The most frequent complication of colostomy is parastomal hernia (▶ Fig. 32.22). Parastomal hernia may be caused by poor operative technique, infection, incorrect location, too large a hole (early hernia), or by high intra-abdominal pressure due to obesity, constipation, prostatism, or chronic cough (late hernia).[120]

Carne et al[121] reviewed the technical factors related to the construction of the stoma that may influence the incidence and success of the different methods of repair. They found parastomal hernia affects 1.8 to 28.3% of end ileostomies and 0 to 6.2% of loop ileostomies. Following colostomy formation, the rates

are 4.0 to 48.1% and 0 to 30.8%, respectively. Site of stoma formation (through or lateral to rectus abdominus), trephine size, fascial fixation, and closure of lateral space are not proven to affect the incidence of hernia. The role of extraperitoneal stoma construction is uncertain. Mesh repair gives a lower rate of recurrence (0–33%) than direct tissue repair (46–100%), or stoma relocation (0–76.2%).

Hernias commonly present as a mass in the peristomal skin or are discovered incidentally on physical examination. Additional symptoms include difficulty maintaining an appliance seal, pain, small bowel obstruction, stoma outlet obstruction, skin excoriation, and difficulty with stoma irrigation.

A careful physical examination with a finger in the stoma is often all that is necessary to diagnose and characterize a parastomal hernia. Hernias have been divided into four types.[119] Type I is a "true" parastomal hernia, where small bowel protrudes within a peritoneal sac through a fascial defect (▶ Fig. 32.23). In Type II, peritoneal contents protrude between the two layers of everted bowel in association with a prolapsed stoma (▶ Fig. 32.24). Type III describes subcutaneous protrusion of the stoma between the fascia and the peristomal skin with no real fascial defect (▶ Fig. 32.25). Type IV is a "pseudohernia" or a diffuse bulge due to weakness in the abdominal wall musculature and requires no treatment (▶ Fig. 32.26).

As previously mentioned, a careful physical examination can distinguish between the four hernia types. Occasionally an abdominal CT scan may be helpful if classification is difficult. It is essential to classify these hernias preoperatively as treatment will vary significantly. Prior to recommending operation, it is important to note that stomal hernia repair may be associated with significant complications and success rates are variable. Consequently, not all parastomal hernias require repair. Asymptomatic patients may need no treatment. Minimally symptomatic patients can be treated with appliance modification with or without a support belt with the aid of a stoma therapist (▶ Fig. 32.27).[79,120,121,122,123,124,125,126,127,128]

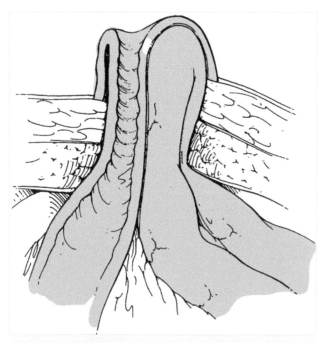

Fig. 32.24 Intrastomal hernia (may be associated with prolapse).

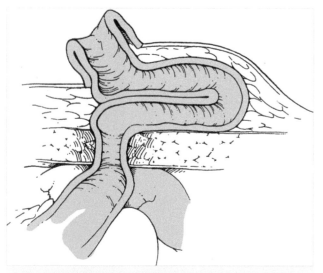

Fig. 32.25 Subcutaneous prolapse (pseudohernia) with intact fascial ring.[128]

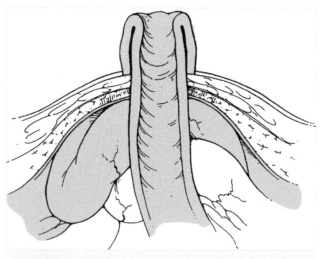

Fig. 32.26 Pseudohernia due to weakness of abdominal wall without fascial defect.[128]

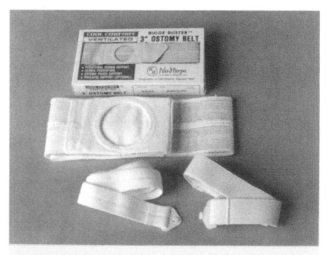

Fig. 32.27 Ostomy belts. Upper belt is designed to support parastomal hernia. Lower belts are attached to pouching systems.

If conservative measures fail, or if bowel obstruction or significant skin excoriation develops, operation is indicated. In several series, long-term follow-up of stomas revealed between 15 and 32% of ostomates with hernias requiring operative repair.[129,130]

Three surgical approaches are available for the treatment of paraileostomy or paracolostomy hernias: local repair, transperitoneal repair, or stoma resiting (▶ Fig. 32.28). Mesh can be used with any of the three techniques. Regardless of the selected approach, all patients should be prepared for laparotomy and stoma resiting. Each patient should have one or two alternate stoma sites identified and marked by a stoma therapist or surgeon prior to operation. In cases where stoma

placement is difficult or the abdominal wall has multiple scars and/or skin creases, patients may need to wear an appliance at the prospective, new stoma sites for a day prior to operation to assess satisfaction.

Local approaches may vary, but all follow similar principles. An incision is made in the peristomal skin outside the footprint of the appliance; the hernia sac is separated from the surrounding, subcutaneous tissue, and reduced. Finally, the defect is repaired. Currently, mesh is used in nearly all the repairs, as recurrence is almost inevitable without prosthetic material.

Although some parastomal hernias can be repaired by excision of the sac and local resuture of the fascia, recurrences are especially common if this method is used for larger hernias or hernias associated with weakened fascia. Repair of these hernias requires either the use of mesh or moving the stoma. Allen-Mersh and Thomson[96] found that relocating the stoma above and medial to the previous stoma tended to be less successful than resiting either to the right side of the abdomen or the umbilicus. Relocating is technically easier to do through the

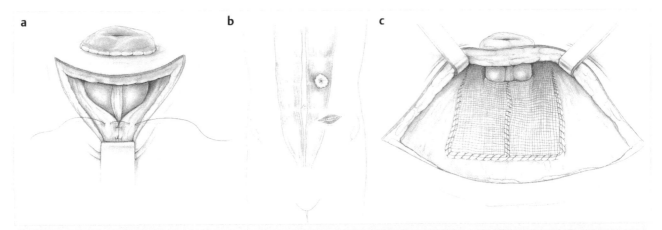

Fig. 32.28 Parastomal colostomy hernia. Types of repair: **(a)** Direct resuture of fascia after resecting hernia sac. **(b)** Repair of hernia after relocating stoma. **(c)** Repair with synthetic mesh.

umbilicus, but stomal management is much easier from the patient's perspective if the stoma is on the right side. For some larger hernias, synthetic or biologic mesh can be used to close the hernia defect and the colon can be placed through (keyhole) or underneath the mesh with the bowel exiting the medial or the lateral border of the mesh (Sugarbaker's technique; ▸ Fig. 32.28a–c).[131,132]

The technique described by Sugarbaker reduces the hernia, lateralizes the intra-abdominal bowel, and uses a large piece of intra-abdominal mesh to repair the hernia (▸ Fig. 32.29).[132] The technique has been used with an open and laparoscopic approach.

Stephenson and Phillips[133] described an approach to the repair of a parastomal hernia that avoids laparotomy and maintains the existing stoma site. Under local anesthesia, the stoma is mobilized around the mucocutaneous junction. The stoma is then brought out through a fresh adjacent area of abdominal wall and the defect repaired with a tension-free mesh. A drain is brought out at a distance not to interfere with appliance application. The stoma is then resited at its original position and anchored in place. Eight patients so treated had no recurrences at a mean follow-up of 15 months.

The transabdominal approach consists of the same steps performed through a midline laparotomy. The mesh may be placed intraperitoneally or in a supraperitoneal position below the posterior rectus fascia. Geisler et al[134] reported 11 patients undergoing parastomal hernia with an overall recurrence for mesh repair at a parastomal site of 63%. Wound infection occurred in sites of parastomal repair in 13% of parastomal hernia sites. Wound infection rates were statistically independent of type of hernia, variety of mesh, or operative approach.

Steele et al[135] reviewed the rate of complications and outcomes with polypropylene mesh in parastomal hernia repairs in 58 patients. After closure of the fascia, the stoma was pulled through the center of the mesh, which was placed either above or below the fascia. There were 31 end colostomies, 24 end ileostomies, and 3 loop transverse colostomies. Mean follow-up was 51 months. Overall complications related to the polypropylene mesh were 36% (recurrence: 26%, surgical bowel obstruction: 9%, prolapse: 3%, wound infection: 3%, fistula: 3%, and mesh erosion: 2%). None of the patients had extirpation of their mesh. Complications were significantly associated with younger

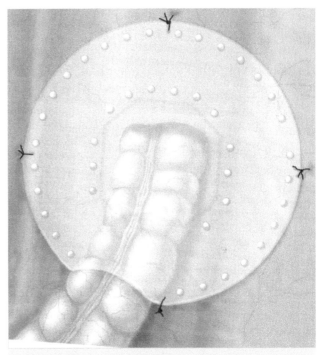

Fig. 32.29 Peristomal hernia repair with mesh. Sugarbaker technique.

age (60 vs. 67 years). Carcinoma patients with stomas had fewer complications. Inflammatory bowel disease, stomal type, mesh location, urgent procedures, steroid use, and surgical approaches were not significantly associated with an increased complication rate. Of the 15 patients with recurrence, 7 underwent successful repair for an overall success rate of 86%.

A number of small laparoscopic series with short-term follow-up and systemic reviews have been published. A meta-analysis of 15 studies and 469 patients found an overall recurrence rate of 17.4%. The recurrence rate for a modified laparoscopic Sugarbaker's approach was 10.2%, whereas the recurrence rate was 27.9% for a keyhole approach.[136] Surgical site infection occurred in 3.8% and mesh infection was observed in 1.7%. A laparoscopic technique is not feasible in all patients and in one study 15% of 55 patients had to be converted to an open procedure.[137]

A systematic review in 2011[138] 1 of four retrospective studies included 57 patients in which biologic mesh was used to repair parastomal hernias. The studies used a variety of techniques for mesh placement with open and laparoscopic techniques. The recurrence rate was 15.7% and the wound-related complication rate was 26.2%. No mortality or graft infections were reported. The authors concluded that the results were similar to those published with synthetic mesh.

Jänes et al[139] determined the effect of stomal complications using a mesh at the primary operation. They randomized 27 patients to have a conventional stoma and 27 to have the mesh. No infection, fistula formation, or pain occurred (observation time, 2–28 months). At the 12-month follow-up, parastomal hernia was present in 8 of the 18 patients without a mesh and in none of the 16 patients in whom the mesh was used.

Finally, stoma resiting is a straightforward approach and involves stoma takedown, necessary lysis of adhesions, and recreation of the stoma at a premarked, new location. The hernia and old stoma defect are closed appropriately, and may include mesh if a satisfactory repair cannot be otherwise obtained. Success rates are variable, but local repair alone fails in up to 64% of patients,[96] while success following prosthetic repair, either local or transabdominal, is associated with a greater than 80% success rate.[140,141] Stomal resiting is associated with a 30% recurrence rate.[130] The risk of recurrence after parastomal hernia repair is considerable and is higher for fascial repair (76%) than for stoma relocation (33%).[142] However, complications are more common after stoma relocation (88%) than fascial repair (50%). This high rate reflects incisional hernia, which develops in 52% of patients. Botet et al[120] reported their experience with a technique of stoma translocation without laparotomy. The original stoma was closed and dissected free from the abdominal wall. A disk of skin was excised 6 cm from the original site and a fascial opening created. The colon was drawn through the new site, the original colostomy opening sutured, and the colostomy matured. In 11 patients so treated, there were no recurrences with a follow-up ranging from 2 to 36 months.

The incidence of parastomal hernias and the challenges of repair have spurred interest in the placement of prophylactic mesh at the initial creation of ostomies. Two recent systematic reviews and meta-analysis have reviewed the published data.[140,141] Cross et al reviewed 10 randomized trials that included 649 patients.[143] The use of mesh reduced the rate of parastomal hernia repair by 65% (p = 0.02) without any difference in infection, stomal stenosis, or necrosis. Mesh type or position and study quality did not have an independent effect on this relationship. Chapman et al reviewed seven randomized controlled trials (432 patients).[144] Mesh reduced the incidence of clinically detected parastomal hernia (10.8 vs. 32.4%, p = 0.001) and the rate of radiologically detected parastomal hernia (34.6 vs. 55.3%, p = 0.01). There was no increase in the incidence of stomal-related complications with the use of prophylactic mesh.

32.4.8 Fistula

Although superficial fistulas can occur around a stoma because of stitch abscess, trauma, or other minor problems, a peristomal fistula is usually a serious problem. Fistulas can be especially troublesome when they occur after an ileostomy for Crohn's disease, as they almost invariably indicate recurrent disease. Many superficial fistulas heal spontaneously, but major fistulas below the skin level usually require formal stomal reconstruction, and the stoma often needs to be moved.[114]

Greatorex[145] described a simple method of closing a fistula by debriding the fistula tract with a pipe cleaner soaked in 6% aqueous phenol solution. The procedure is based on the principle that many simple fistula tracts will close after careful debridement and the addition of a sclerosing agent. Fibrin glue can be used as an alternative to phenol.

32.4.9 Stomal Varices

Varices are abnormal portosystemic vascular connections and develop in response to increase in portal pressure. Sclerosing cholangitis, alcoholic cirrhosis, and extensive metastatic disease to the liver are the most common causes in ostomates. Other risk factors for the development of parastomal varices include splenomegaly, esophageal varices, advanced histologic stage at liver biopsy, low serum albumin, thrombocytopenia, and an increased prothrombin time.[146] In individuals with ileostomies or colostomies, the surgical proximity of the portal (intestine) and systemic (skin) vessels leads to the possibility of varices in individuals with liver disease. This should be kept in mind when choosing surgical options for the treatment of ulcerative colitis accompanied by sclerosing cholangitis. An ileal-pouch anal anastomosis, avoiding a permanent ileostomy, eliminates the risk of stomal varices in these individuals. The actual incidence of peristomal varices is unknown, but may be as high as 27% in patients with known hepatic dysfunction.[147]

The management of bleeding from ileostomy varices poses a dilemma as recurrent bleeding is almost the rule following local treatment (43–100%),[148] and yet definitive control by portal decompression carries significant morbidity and mortality for most patients.[149] Grundfest-Broniatowski and Fazio[150] have emphasized the hazards of portacaval shunting for bleeding stomal varices, particularly since shunting does not appear to improve overall survival in these patients. The authors recommend a conservative approach consisting of appliance refitting if the bleeding is related to trauma, local pressure, epinephrine compresses, and transfusions, if needed. Ligation of the varices with or without stoma revision generally stops hemorrhage in those patients who continue to bleed. Mucocutaneous disconnection interrupts the high-pressure portosystemic collaterals; only rarely is it necessary to resort to shunting. Stomal sclerotherapy with 3% sodium tetradecyl sulfate, ethanol, and saline in a 1:1:1 mixture,[151] or 0.5 to 1% polidocanol (Ethoxysclerol), or almond oil containing 5% phenol[152] has been used with some success. Roberts et al[148] recommended shunts after failure of local therapy. If decompressive shunt therapy is to be done, it is best to create a splenorenal shunt away from the right upper quadrant, as many of these patients ultimately become candidates for liver transplantation. For the occasional patient who continues to bleed despite conservative measures and is not a suitable candidate for portacaval shunting, percutaneous transhepatic embolization of varices has been reported to be successful and may be considered as an option.[153]

Roberts et al[148] reviewed their experience with 12 patients who had bleeding stomal varices. Stomal variceal bleeding

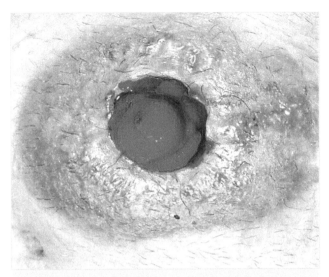

Fig. 32.30 Ileostomy with typical circumferential caput medusae. (Courtesy: Patricia Roberts, MD.)

occurred between 1 and 11 years (median, 5.5 years) after creation of the stoma. At the time of diagnosis, a typical caput medusae is seen around the stoma (▶ Fig. 32.30). Control of bleeding initially consisted of direct pressure; recurrent bleeding occurred in one patient who died before definitive therapy could be performed. The remaining 11 patients underwent a total of 18 additional procedures to control bleeding stomal varices, including 9 local procedures (suture ligation of the stoma in 4, mucocutaneous disconnection in 3, cauterization of the stoma in 1, and transposition of the stoma in 1), 8 portosystemic shunts, and 1 liver transplantation. Seven patients died of hepatic failure a median of 4 years (range, 1–9 years) after treatment. Recurrent bleeding occurred in three patients after local treatment and in one patient after a portosystemic shunt. Although local procedures may be effective for the initial control of bleeding, recurrent bleeding often occurs. Mortality is high because of the severity of the underlying liver disease.

More recently, the use of transjugular, intrahepatic, portosystemic shunting (TIPS) has increased substantially. It has been successfully applied to the treatment of variceal bleeding from many sites in individuals with portal hypertension, including stomal variceal hemorrhage.[154,155] TIPS allows for the treatment of the primary cause of variceal bleeding (portal hypertension) without the need for laparotomy. It has the additional advantage of not altering perihepatic anatomy in patients who are candidates for future liver transplantation.

In summary, the selection of treatment for individuals with bleeding stomal varices, whether from an ileostomy, urostomy, or colostomy, should be based on the patients' underlying disease process and general medical condition. Simple, local measures are often a good first step to control hemorrhage, but bleeding will ultimately recur. It may be all that is necessary in individuals with end-stage liver disease who are not transplant candidates. Eliminating the underlying cause, however, is essential for long-term prevention of bleeding. Portosystemic shunting, either by TIPS in individuals who are transplant candidates, or by formal, surgical shunts in patients who are not, will ultimately be necessary.

32.4.10 Ulceration

Ulceration is either due to local trauma, infection, recurrent Crohn's disease, or pyoderma gangrenosum. Ulceration around the stoma implies recurrent Crohn's disease or pyoderma, whereas ulceration on the stoma itself may be the result of other causes. Ulcers should be treated symptomatically with good enterostomal care. Resection is not indicated unless ulcerations extend deep into the ileostomy or peristomal abdominal wall ulceration becomes unmanageable.

Pyoderma gangrenosum is an uncommon, ulcerative cutaneous condition of uncertain etiology. It is an uncommon cause of recalcitrant peristomal ulceration and is associated with active inflammatory bowel disease and immunosuppression. Best results have been achieved with closure of the stoma, relocation, and/or resection of active disease.[156,157] If stoma closure is not possible, topical and systemic treatments with steroids and immunosuppressants have been effective. Additional information on this uncommon condition is presented later.

32.4.11 Diversion Colitis

Diversion colitis is an iatrogenic, nutritional complication following the creation of a diverting colostomy. It can occur regardless of whether the colostomy is performed as a loop colostomy or end colostomy with a defunctionalized Hartmann's pouch or mucous fistula. The colitis is a unique type of inflammatory process that can appear within weeks of fecal diversion and resolves rapidly once continuity has been reestablished. The histologic findings tend to be nonspecific and undistinguishable from ulcerative colitis. Diversion colitis develops due to the fact that the colon and rectum require luminal stool to meet the nutritional needs of the colonocytes. N-butyrate, a short-chain fatty acid, is the primary fuel source for colonic mucosal cells and is available only through luminal absorption from stool.

Korelitz et al[158] proposed that short-chain fatty acids produced by anaerobic bacteria serve as a trophic factor for the distal colon and rectal mucosa. Harig et al[159] administered short-chain fatty acids to the diverted segment of four patients with diversion colitis, and in each case the inflammation resolved. The best treatment for diversion colitis is to reestablish colonic continuity. If this is not possible, then short-chain fatty acid enemas may be of benefit. However, in most cases no treatment is necessary. Diversion colitis is often found incidentally on preoperative endoscopy of the defunctionalized limb. Patients occasionally suffer minor inconvenience of mild tenesmus and small mucousy, bloody stools. Reassurance is usually all that is required.

The most important fact regarding diversion colitis or proctitis is to realize that it exists and that patients have not developed ulcerative proctitis precluding stoma takedown. The opposite is in fact true; stoma takedown and reestablishment of intestinal continuity will resupply the colon with N-butyrate and the diversion colitis will resolve.

32.5 Outcomes of Stomal Construction and Closure

The overall morbidity of closure of a temporary ileostomy ranges from 2 to 33%.[106] In particular, small bowel obstruction occurs in 0 to 13% (mostly in the 6–10% range), wound infection in 0 to 18% (mostly in the 3–7% range), and relaparotomy in 0 to 13% (mostly in the 4–7% range). The incidence of incisional hernia at the previous stoma site varies from less than 1 to 12%.

Pokorny et al[160] analyzed 533 patients with stoma closure. The overall stoma closure–related mortality was 3%; the overall stomal closure–related surgical complication rate was 20%. Wound infections (9%) and anastomotic leakage (5%) were the most common surgical complications. Age was the only significant risk factor for survival. Use of a soft silicone drain for intraperitoneal drainage (odds ratio: 1.62) was the only risk factor for complications. In patients with carcinoma as the primary disease (odds ratio < 1.61), they observed significantly fewer complications. Stomal closure is so often considered a minor procedure but as clearly and appropriately pointed out in this article, it is associated with significant morbidity and mortality. This should not be unexpected because these patients are undergoing bowel operations and therefore should be accorded the same considerations and respect as any other patient undergoing bowel operation. Moug et al[161] reported on 100 consecutive patients undergoing elective closure of a loop ileostomy. The overall postoperative complication rate was 32% and mortality rate was 3%. Minor complications included wound infection, nausea and vomiting, and cardiac arrhythmia. Major complications were obstruction, ischemic bowel, sepsis, and anastomotic leak. The likelihood of postoperative complications increases significantly with increasing deprivation category scores. The overall complication rate in patients with low,[1,2] intermediate,[3,4,5] and high[6,7] scores were 0, 26, and 46%, respectively. Thus, high levels of socioeconomic deprivation significantly increased risk of postoperative complications after elective closure of loop ileostomies.

Bosshardt[162] reviewed his facility's experience with 383 fecal ostomies to determine the effect of advanced age on surgical outcome measures in a tertiary-managed care medical center. There were 103 patients aged 70 years or older and 280 patients were younger than 70 years. There were 220 elective procedures and 163 emergency procedures. The diagnosis leading to creation of the ostomy was more often malignancy in older patients (75%) compared with younger patients (45%). Both age groups underwent a similar proportion of emergency procedures (older vs. younger patients, 44 vs. 42%), but more older patients were left with permanent stomas (59 vs. 41%). Older patients also had more preoperative comorbidities, higher American Society of Anesthesiologists score, longer hospital stays, and more postoperative complications. Thirty-day mortality was 6.8% in the older group versus 0.4% in the younger group. Fewer older patients were eligible for ostomy reversal (41 vs. 59%) and a smaller proportion of eligible older patients actually underwent the reversal procedure (78 vs. 95%). The complication rate associated with ostomy reversal was not significantly different in the two age groups. They concluded that patients aged 70 years and older undergo proportionally more permanent fecal ostomy procedures than younger patients. Furthermore, older patients tolerate ostomy reversal with minimal morbidity and should not be denied consideration based on age alone if they are eligible candidates.

Park et al[116] analyzed 1,616 patients with enteric stomas and found 34% of patients with complications. Among the total complications, 28% occurred early (< 1 month postoperation) and 6% occurred late (> 1 month). The most common early complications were skin irritations (12%), pain associated with poor stoma location (7%), and partial necrosis (5%). The most common late complications were skin irritation (6%), prolapse (2%), and stenosis (2%). The enteric stoma with the most complications was the loop ileostomy (75%). The enteric stoma with the least complications was the end transverse colostomy (6%). The general surgery service had the most complications (47%), followed by gynecology (44%), surgical oncology (37%), colorectal (32%), pediatric surgery (29%), and trauma (25%). Age, operating service, enteric stoma type and configuration, and preoperative enterostomal therapist marking were found to be variables that influenced stoma complications. They concluded that preoperative enterostomal site marking, especially in older patients, and avoiding the ileostomy, particularly in the loop configuration, can help minimize complications.

With respect to stoma-related complications and type of stoma, Edwards et al[163] presented a contrary view. For patients requiring defunctioning following anterior resection and total mesorectal excision, they conducted a randomized study to receive either loop ileostomy or loop transverse colostomy. Follow-up after stoma closure was a median of 36 months. There were 70 patients randomized (loop transverse colostomy: 36 and loop ileostomy: 34), of whom 63 underwent stoma closure (loop transverse colostomy: 31 and loop ileostomy: 32). There were no significant differences in the difficulty of formation or closure or in the postoperative recovery between the groups. However, there were 10 complications related directly to the stoma in the loop transverse colostomy group: fecal fistula,[1] prolapse,[2] parastomal hernia,[2] incisional hernia during follow-up.[5] None of these complications occurred in the loop ileostomy group. They concluded that the choice of diversion is loop ileostomy as a method of defunctioning a low anastomosis.

Kairaluoma et al[164] examined the outcome of 349 intestinal stomas constructed in 342 patients. In 141 of these patients, the stoma could be considered as temporary. The 30-day mortality rate was 7%. The overall complication rate was 50%. Pure stoma-related complications were observed in 12% of the patients. The final closure rate of temporary stomas was 67%. The closure rate was significantly higher if the temporary stomas were of the double-barrel type. There was no significant difference in the closure rate between patients with benign and malignant diseases, but the rate decreased significantly in age groups over 70 years. They concluded that 40% of stomas constructed are considered as temporary but only two-thirds of temporary stomas are closed subsequently.

Duchesne et al[165] analyzed 164 ostomy patients to document the frequency and types of ostomy complications and the risk factors associated with them. Complications occurred in 25% of patients; 39% occurred within 1 month of the procedure. Complications included prolapse in 22%, necrosis in 22%, stenosis in 17%, irritation in 17%, infection in 15%, bleeding in 5%, and retraction in 5%. Gender, carcinoma, trauma, diverticulitis, emergency operation, ileostomy, and ostomy location/type were not associated with a stoma complication.

Significant predictors of ostomy malfunction included inflammatory bowel disease (odds ratio < 4.49) and obesity (odds ratio < 2.66). The care of an ET nurse was found to prevent complications (odds ratio = 0.15).

32.6 Enterostomal Care and Rehabilitation

The history of enterostomal therapy has been documented by Cataldo.[166] He noted that the earliest stomas were not the artistry of pioneering surgeons but were created by acts of nature (i.e., the end results of strangulated hernia or penetrating trauma). Patients were left to their own devices to determine how to care for this new intrusion in their life. This, of course, is no longer true, and stoma care is an integral part of the overall management of these patients.

Whether the stoma is permanent or temporary, patients with abdominal stomas have multiple adjustment demands. Physical alterations resulting from construction of the stoma require immediate and long-term attention and will have an impact on the patient's biopsychosocial status for the duration of the stoma.

Rehabilitation of the person with an abdominal stoma begins preoperatively with a multidisciplinary health care team.[167,168] The medical physician, surgeon, WOC (ET) nurse specialist, and, most important, the patient and family offer unique contributions to the positive outcome of a well-rehabilitated person. In addition, individualized patient needs may necessitate a referral to a social worker, dietitian, home care nurse, counselor, or a well-rehabilitated ostomy patient visitor. Of particular importance within the team is the collaboration between the surgeon and the ET nurse specialist.

Research addressing the unique rehabilitation issues of this patient group both preoperatively and postoperatively highlights the need for family support and pertinent information based on their learning needs.[169] The following is a discussion of ostomy patient needs and interventions in the preoperative, postoperative, and long-term phases of rehabilitation.

32.6.1 Preoperative Considerations

Expected outcomes in the preoperative period include (1) well-informed patient and family, (2) properly selected and marked stoma site, and (3) manageable level of anxiety. Outcomes may not always be achievable during this phase because of acute illness. However, the plan of preoperative care is generally developed with these outcomes in mind.[161,163,164]

Assessment and Planning

Preoperative assessment and planning are essential for successful rehabilitation of the ostomy patient. Ideally, education begins in the clinic setting prior to hospital admission when the patient is better able to absorb information provided by the enterostomal nurse. When this is not possible, education provided at the bedside the day prior to or on the day of operation must take into account the heightened level of stress experienced by the patient and significant others. Family members are encouraged to attend preoperative teaching sessions as they not only provide much needed emotional support but also validate and reinforce information the patient may not have assimilated. The participation of family members in all phases of patient teaching also allows the ET nurse to address the needs and concerns of significant others which may not always reflect those of the ostomy patient. In addition, a study performed by Persson et al[170,171,172] showed that spouses of patients undergoing ostomy surgery for rectal carcinoma felt that when they were excluded from information sessions, they felt isolated and experienced greater fear. This situation can become a vicious cycle where the patient and significant others cease to communicate in an effort to protect each other from further stress and worry. In emergency situations, it may not be possible for the Wound Ostomy Continence (WOC or ET) nurse to mark the stoma site or provide education and counseling. The surgeon must, therefore, select an appropriate stoma site.

Patient assessment in the preoperative period includes emotional and physical factors that will affect the individual's ability to manage routine ostomy care as well as the ability to adjust and return to a previous lifestyle. Any physical limitations such as manual dexterity or diminished eyesight must be noted to prepare for future teaching sessions. When communicating with a patient who has difficulty hearing, care must be taken to share delicate information while maintaining confidentiality in a busy hospital ward or clinic setting. The patient's previous contact with an individual who had an ostomy should be discussed to dispel any fear or misconception resulting from the experience.

Preoperative assessment of the patient's learning style and education assists the WOC nurse in preparing to teach in all three domains required to master the care of an ostomy: cognitive, affective, and psychomotor.[173] Some patients will prefer to read as much information as possible or view videos, while others will depend solely on demonstrations provided by the WOC nurse. Patients who are illiterate may be reluctant to divulge this fact; therefore, the WOC nurse must be sensitive to behavior, which indicates any learning disability. A patient's profession or hobby can contribute to the ability to master some of the technical components of ostomy care. An example of this would be that of a seamstress who would have little difficulty measuring and cutting a stoma opening in a pouch. In order to accurately gauge learning needs, both verbal and nonverbal cues must be observed while interacting with a patient. In some instances, patients may indicate a need to limit information, particularly when they are feeling overwhelmed. Of utmost importance is the need to individualize teaching. A patient's religious background may present as an issue if the presence of a stoma restricts certain aspects of religious practice. The patient's emotional status, coping mechanisms, social support, financial concerns, and relationship issues should also be included in the preoperative assessment.

Knowledge of common concerns for the ostomy patient in the short and long term provides guidance for the physician and WOC nurse. Numerous studies have been published on psychosocial issues of ostomy patients. Jeter[174] stressed the importance of preoperative teaching and counseling to fully recover and enjoy a satisfactory quality of life for patients undergoing operations for colorectal carcinoma resulting in a stoma. Common misconceptions about ostomies should be dispelled. An effort should be made to allay patients' fears associated with colorectal carcinoma and ostomy operations.

Fears cited by Jeter[174] include those of the primary disease, long-term prognosis after operation, fear of operation, postoperative pain, inability to manage the appliance, rejection by family, inability to retain employment, and sexuality, as well as concern for social adjustment. Jeter listed certain concepts and facts that are considered essential for patients and family members to learn before hospital discharge. The list includes how to change appliances, where to buy ostomy supplies, signs and symptoms of early postoperative complications, person(s) to whom complications or ostomy problems should be reported, and sources of financial aid if necessary. Additional types of information that can be considered "nice to know" but not essential include United Ostomy Association of America or local ostomy support group meeting dates, foods that cause gas and odor, travel information, details about operation, ostomy accessory items, and potential long-term complications.

A study examined the concerns of patients before and after discharge from the hospital and found eight common areas. They include, in order of importance, fear of stool leakage, odor, ability to participate in sports, necessity for further treatment, wearing a pouch, changing the pouch, change in body appearance, and participating in sexual love play and intercourse.[175] Information related to these topics is included throughout this chapter.

Interventions

Much research has been performed in the area of adaptation to life with a stoma. Piwonka and Merino[169] found that regardless of time since operation, factors that remained the most influential on psychological adaptation were ostomy self-care, body image, and perceived social support. The importance of teaching technical skills must therefore be balanced with the need to explore psychosocial concerns. Information provided in the preoperative period is essential to patient understanding, decreased anxiety, and informed consent. Topics included are anatomy and physiology, terminology, disease process, planned operation changes in function, complications, and expected results. Not surprisingly, it is equally important to discuss what is to be removed as well as what is not to be removed during the operation. A discussion of ostomy function, diet, pouches, and general ostomy management is also provided.[167,176]

Emotional concerns are addressed when the clinician seeks the patient's view of the coming operation and how it will affect the person's lifestyle and quality of life. Discussion of work, play, sexuality, and other patient-introduced concerns is also important. Diagrams, written pamphlets, and videotapes are useful and may be obtained from manufacturers at no charge. Educational materials are available from organizations such as the American Cancer Society, American College of Surgeons, and United Ostomy Association of America. However, nothing replaces personal contact with the surgeon and WOC nurse. The therapeutic relationship is intensely important at this most vulnerable time. Experienced clinicians know that a few well chosen, honest words of hope can arrest a great deal of anxiety, particularly during the preoperative period.

Stoma site selection and construction have a direct bearing on the quality of life for the person with a stoma. Leakage, odor, difficulty with pouch changes, increased equipment costs, and stoma revisions occur as a result of poor stoma location.[177,178] Patients who experience recurrent leakage from poorly sealed pouches may become reclusive and limit their social contact for fear of an embarrassing incident.[179] Therefore, the primary technical intervention during this period is stoma site marking. Turnbull and Weakley[180] first emphasized the importance of stoma site selection and marking during the preoperative period. Recommendations of the past are the standards of today as experts agree that stoma sites are to be marked preoperatively, usually by the ET nurse specialist, and often in conjunction with the surgeon.[177,181]

Primary requirements for the ideal stoma site include placement within the rectus muscle with approximately 6 to 7 cm of flat skin around the site. This will provide an anatomically stable area. The rectus muscle is palpated while the patient is supine, lifting his or her head off the pillow. The intraperitoneal stoma should pass through the rectus muscle to minimize future prolapse or parastomal hernia. Extraperitoneal stomas may be placed just lateral to the rectus muscle to facilitate making the extraperitoneal tunnel, although medial placement through the rectus muscle is preferable. The abdomen is assessed while the patient is supine, sitting, standing, and bending forward (▶ Fig. 32.31). If the patient wears a brace or is in a wheelchair, the abdomen is assessed with these devices in use. When possible, trousers or skirts should be worn to establish the location of the beltline as this not only affects

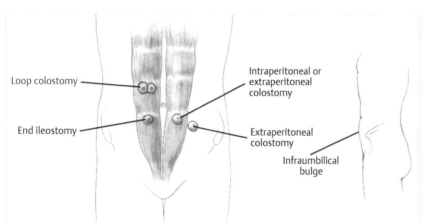

Fig. 32.31 Diagram of usual stoma sites for ileostomies and colostomies.

Loop colostomy

End ileostomy

Intraperitoneal or extraperitoneal colostomy

Extraperitoneal colostomy

Infraumbilical bulge

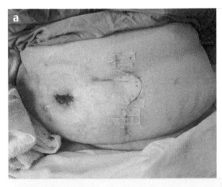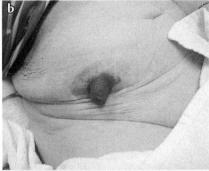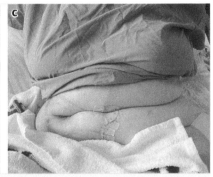

Fig. 32.32 **(a)** Poorly sited stoma in obese patient (supine). **(b)** Stoma difficult to visualize even with patient in semi Fowler's position (45 degree). **(c)** Stoma cannot be visualized when patient is seated upright (90 degree).

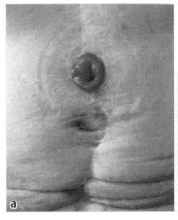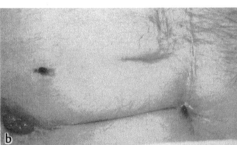

Fig. 32.33 Improperly placed stoma. **(a)** Improper placement of stoma above umbilicus and through midline incision will make it difficult to fit secure pouching system. **(b)** Unsuitable stoma because of placement that is too low, too lateral, and across transverse incision. Skin markings for suitable stoma sites on either right or left side are shown.

flange placement of the appliance but also the manner in which the pouch will be accommodated by clothing.

Abdominal topography is also evaluated. The area of the peristomal plane should ideally be free of incisions, sutures, drains, rods, bony prominences, umbilicus scars, and waistline and skin folds as they form defects in the abdominal contours that may result in pouch leakage (▶ Fig. 32.32 and ▶ Fig. 32.33). The natural elevation of the infraumbilical area enables the patient to visualize the stoma well, which is critical to self-care.[182] Therefore, the site is usually marked at the apex of the infraumbilical bulge. Exceptions to this evaluation occur in the obese patient, younger child, or patient with a barrel-shaped abdomen. It is generally important to mark these stomas in the upper quadrants so that the patient is able to see, and therefore care for, the stoma independently.[177]

Other challenges in stoma site selection include patients with multiple surgical scars. An adolescent patient with Crohn's disease and multiple previous abdominal operations may have few good locations available (▶ Fig. 32.34). When two stomas are planned, they should be located far enough apart so that each stoma may be pouched separately, if necessary. This holds true when one of the stomas is a mucous fistula as mucous discharge and odor may necessitate pouching (▶ Fig. 32.35). For the patient undergoing pelvic exenteration, the colostomy should be placed lower than the urinary diversion to allow for clearance if an ostomy belt is used.

Site selection can be marked with a variety of methods, but the most common and simplest would be to use indelible ink or silver nitrate. A waterproof clear film dressing can be used

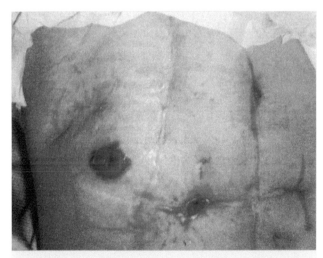

Fig. 32.34 Stoma placement must be individualized in patients with Crohn's disease and multiple previous scars and active fistula.

to protect the site if marking takes place well in advance of the operation.

32.6.2 Postoperative Aspects of Care

Expected outcomes for the patient and family in the postoperative period include (1) mastery of basic ostomy care knowledge and skills, (2) ability to express concerns and adaptive approaches toward resolution, and (3) knowledge of resources needed for effective ostomy management in the home care and community settings.[177],[183].

Immediate Postoperative Care

Technical management of the patient postoperatively starts in the operating room with a properly fitted and applied pouching system. The pouch contains effluent, protects the peristomal skin and incision, and avoids soiling of monitoring leads and clothing in the area. Most pouching systems will maintain a seal for at least 3 to 4 days when used appropriately. Pouches applied early postoperatively are clear for later observation of mucosal vascularity. They are also drainable, which avoids frequent adhesive removal once the stoma begins to pass gas and stool. Pre-sized systems are not recommended in the operating room as postoperative mucosal edema may occur that could result in stomal laceration and

bleeding. Similarly, convex pouching systems are generally not used as the application of pressure to a newly sutured mucocutaneous suture line may result in separation.[183] Rather, a sizable system is selected that will be cut to the size of the patient's stoma. Using this approach provides further benefits as inventory in the operating room is decreased and a standardized procedure reduces application errors.

Once the pouch has been selected, the stoma is measured. The correct size of the stoma is determined by using a measuring guide, and by selecting the size opening on the guide that will allow the pouch to cover peristomal skin up to the mucocutaneous juncture (▶ Fig. 32.36). The skin surrounding the stoma is cleansed with tap water or with an appropriate commercial solution, then allowed to completely dry prior to pouch application. For pouch application procedure, see "Changing a Pouching System" (p. 799) section.

Rods and bridges used in stomal construction are obstacles to effective pouch adherence and delay routine patient teaching.

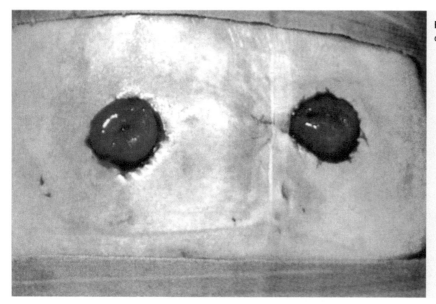

Fig. 32.35 Dual stomas in patients having colostomy and mucous fistula.

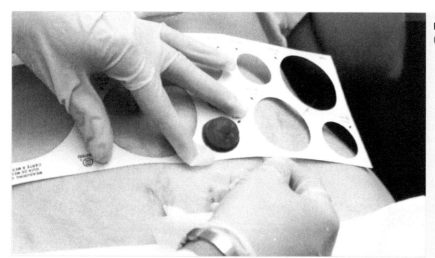

Fig. 32.36 Technique of measuring stoma (stoma-measuring guide).

They may also put tension on the stoma during pouching. When the rod is placed in a cephalad-to-caudad position or on the plane with the umbilicus, the patient may experience discomfort and limited mobility. If a rod is used, there are two options for pouch application. The device may be placed into the pouch or the pouch may be applied over the device. The potential for leakage is less when the rod or bridge is placed into the pouch. During application of the pouch, the rod is guided into the aperture of the pouch first. Then the pouch is secured around the stoma, and the rod is adjusted to its original position. A label or notation is made directly on the front of the pouch as an indication to future caregivers that a supporting device is inside the pouch. The date for rod removal and the name of the person doing it must be established as part of the patient ostomy care plan to avoid unnecessary delay in teaching and promote patient comfort.

Information and Emotional Support

Currently, the average hospital postoperative stay for patients undergoing abdominoperineal resection and sigmoid colostomy, total proctocolectomy and ileostomy, or restorative ileoanal reservoir is from 3 to 6 days. During this period, the patient experiences multiple educational and adjustment issues that will be ongoing in the posthospital period. However, basic skills to master in self-care are pouch emptying, pouch changing, skin care, and care of the incision. One technique used to begin teaching postoperatively is a "tour" of the abdomen. The ET nurse and patient embark on this "tour" by examining the stoma and peristomal skin. A discussion of normal values is initially undertaken. The color of the stoma and quality of the skin are discussed and, later, documented. The integrity of the mucocutaneous juncture and abdominal incision is assessed and documented. As the patient recovers, specific areas are included in postoperative teaching and support. A few are discussed here. However, ▶ Table 32.1 provides a comprehensive listing of topics to be included. Prioritizing patient needs is important, as hospital stays have become brief. Essential information, such as pouch emptying and changing, is completed prior to discharge.

Emotional care of the patient that promotes adaptation is important to be included in the care plan. One dimension of the ET nurse's role is supportive counseling. The patient is encouraged to explore the ostomy experience in discussion sessions with the ET nurse. The patient is allowed to identify concerns and to begin to resolve them. Focus is also on the concerns and fears of the family. By exploring these feelings and meanings for the patient, problems become more manageable, and the patient moves toward adaptation.[168]

Unique Aspects of Care

Ileostomies may be temporary or permanent. Temporary ileostomies have been more frequently performed as a component of the restorative ileoanal reservoir. Issues unique to the patient with ileostomy include maintenance of peristomal skin integrity, fluid and electrolyte balance, prevention of small bowel obstruction, and psychosocial issues inherent to younger populations (i.e., childbearing, raising children, and professional and work situations). The expected function of a conventional ileostomy is 800 to 1000 mL per 24 hours or pouch emptying six to eight times in 24 hours. A drainable pouch is used and changed once every 4 to 7 days (▶ Table 32.2).

Transverse colostomies are generally intended to be temporary or palliative. They function similarly to ileostomies but with less fluid output. Stools may be malodorous. The pouch may be emptied four to six times in 24 hours. The change interval is also 4 to 7 days.

Many of the operative procedures resulting in a transverse colostomy are performed on an emergency basis and present pouching challenges as these stomas are often exteriorized at the waistline or proximal to the ribcage. Changes in abdominal contour or contact with a rigid ribcage can cause stressors to the pouching system which will limit adhesion and cause subsequent leakage and skin irritation. The surgeon should consider these factors and construct a stoma in a lower quadrant whenever possible.

Table 32.1 Postoperative components of the rehabilitation care plan for ostomates

Technical skills	Information	Emotion
Pouch emptying	Normal anatomy	Individualized care
Pouch changing	Function and appearance of the stomas	Family inclusion
Peristomal skin cleansing	Diet	Time to discuss concerns
Stoma measurement	Odor and gas control	Role modeling support (i.e., caregivers and ostomy group members)
Ongoing stoma and peristomal skin assessment	Fluid and electrolyte needs	Discussion of sexuality and return to previous lifestyle
	Recognition of departures from normal	
	Community resources (e.g., ostomy groups and supplies)	

Table 32.2 Stoma management: quick reference guide

Type of stoma	Output characteristics	Management approach
Ileostomy	Liquid to paste	Drainable pouch with skin barrier
	Active enzymes	Change pouching system every 4 to 7 d Deodorizers: oral or pouch (powder, liquid, and tablet)
Transverse colostomy	Liquid to semiformed	Drainable pouch with skin barrier
	Low active enzymes	Change pouching system every 4 to 7 d Deodorizers: oral or pouch (powder and liquid) No routine colostomy irrigations
Descending or sigmoid colostomy	Semiformed Minimal active enzymes	Natural method of control Drainable pouch with skin barrier Change pouching system every 4 to 7 d Deodorizer: oral or pouch (liquid) Colostomy irrigation method Irrigate every 1 to 2 d Closed or drainable pouch Skin barrier optional Stoma plug optional Diet to promote constipation

Descending and sigmoid colostomies are usually permanent and most frequently performed in older individuals. Concomitant health problems, such as arthritis, diabetes, or impaired vision, may provide additional challenges during rehabilitation. Descending and sigmoid colostomies begin to function 3 to 7 days postoperatively. Therefore, teaching in the hospital is shortened as the patient will have little experience with pouch emptying. Stools are not corrosive to the peristomal skin, yet protection is recommended to keep the skin clean and dry. Stool may be malodorous and a deodorizer required. As normal bowel function returns, there may be one to three stools a day. The question of whether to irrigate or use the natural method of colostomy control is usually discussed briefly preoperatively as management options. However, current practice defers this decision to the outpatient clinic. Once the patient recovers from the operation and is able to provide self-care, discussion regarding colostomy irrigation is undertaken.

Peristomal Skin Care

Gold standard in peristomal skin care is that less is more. The goal is to prevent irritation and loss of skin integrity, thus avoiding pain, infection, and further pouching complications. The use of tap water, soft material, and gentle skin cleansing is recommended. The addition of soap is optional, but if used should be mild and free of perfumes, oil, and dye. Patients may need to be reminded that peristomal skin care is not a sterile procedure and therefore showering is an acceptable method of cleaning the skin. Careful hair removal of skin beneath the appliance is recommended to prevent folliculitis and will improve patient comfort with pouch removal. Coarse body hair can be clipped. The parastomal skin can be shaved with a safety razor using soap or with the use of a barrier powder on clean dry skin. Mechanical trauma is best avoided with careful removal of all the adhesive components of the appliance. Patients must be taught to gently pull the appliance away with one hand while the other hand anchors the adjacent skin. Reducing contact with chemicals will decrease the possibility of a local reaction and subsequent sensitization.

Diet, Gas, and Noise

Diet is a key to many postoperative concerns. Odor, gas, noise, diarrhea, bowel obstruction, and social activities may all be affected by fluid and food choices. Postoperatively, increased levels of gas and noise are expected as the surgical ileus resolves. However, complaints of excessive gas in the posthospital phase require assessment. They are frequently the result of eating habits and food choices (Box 32.1). Dietary restrictions are recommended in the literature, but few studies have been performed to substantiate these restrictions. Due to postoperative edema of the intestinal tract, patients with ileostomies are often advised to limit fiber intake for 6 to 8 weeks following operation.[184]

Box 32.1 Foods affecting bowel function

- Foods that increase odor
  - Asparagus
  - Broccoli
  - Brussels sprouts
  - Cabbage
  - Cauliflower
  - Dried peas, beans, and lentils
  - Eggs
  - Fish
  - Garlic, onions
  - Some spices
  - Turnip
  - Some strong cheeses (e.g., Roquefort)
  - Some medications
  - Some vitamin preparations
- Foods that increase gas
  - Beans
  - Beer/carbonated soda
  - Alcohol
  - Broccoli
  - brussels sprouts
  - Cabbage
  - Cauliflower
  - Corn
  - Cucumbers
  - Pickles, sauerkraut
  - Mushrooms
  - Dried peas, lentils
  - Radishes
  - Spinach
  - Dairy products
  - Onions
  - Turnips
  - Eggs
  - Melons
  - Peppers
  - Onions, chives
  - Chewing gum
- Foods that may help control gas
  - Fresh parsley
  - Yogurt
  - Buttermilk
- Foods that thicken stool (decrease output)
  - Applesauce
  - Bananas
  - Cheese
  - Boiled milk

- Marshmallows
- Pasta
- Creamy peanut butter
- Pretzels
- Rice
- Bread
- Tapioca
- Toast
- Yogurt
- Bagels
- Soda crackers
- Potatoes
- Barley
- Oatmeal or oat bran
- Foods that loosen stool (increase output)
  - Green beans
  - Beer, alcohol
  - Broccoli
  - Fresh fruits
  - Grape juice
  - Raw vegetables
  - Prunes/juice
  - Spicy foods
  - Fried foods
  - Chocolate
  - Spinach
  - Leafy green vegetables
  - Aspartame/Nutrasweet®
  - Licorice
  - Coffee
  - High-sugar foods
  - Caffeinated beverages
- High-fiber foods that may cause blockages
  - Dried fruit
  - Grapefruits, apples
  - Nuts
  - Corn
  - Raisins
  - Celery
  - Popcorn
  - Coconut
  - Seeds
  - Coleslaw
  - Asian vegetables
  - Meats with casings
  - Oranges
  - Mushrooms

All ostomy patients are instructed to chew food very well, eat at regular intervals, and drink eight 8-oz glasses (2 L) of fluid per day and to gradually return to a regular diet. The fact that most ostomates can return to a regular diet is supported by a survey of members of the United Ostomy Association which was performed to identify the dietary restrictions of patients with ileostomies (13%), colostomies (83%), and urostomies (4%). The findings indicated that 88% of respondents had resumed a regular diet following their ostomy surgery.[184]

Small Bowel Obstruction

Small bowel obstruction is a complication of abdominal operations. In stoma patients, food boluses and adhesions are a frequent cause. Patients are instructed to recognize early the signs of obstruction (i.e., pain, decreased stomal output, stoma swelling, nausea, and vomiting). If obstruction occurs, a liquid diet is recommended with relaxation techniques (i.e., a warm bath). The pouch should be removed, if necessary, and the aperture cut larger to avoid laceration. The patient's physician should be contacted when the patient experiences prolonged obstruction, vomiting, or when pain is severe. An ileostomy lavage may be necessary (see "Ileostomy Lavage Procedure" (p.800) section). Most commonly, the obstruction resolves with conservative management. Interestingly, the patient is usually able to identify the offending food. Patients are instructed to chew foods thoroughly and increase fluid intake when eating or eliminate offending foods from the diet.[185]

Fluid and Electrolytes

Fluid and electrolyte balance is particularly important to patients with ileostomy or high-output transverse colostomy. Education includes information about dehydration as well as fluid and electrolyte balance. As previously stated, patients are encouraged to drink eight 8-oz glasses of fluids in a 24-hour period. If sodium depletion is in question, soups, bouillon, and Gatorade may be taken. Sources of potassium include orange juice, bananas, strong tea, and Gatorade.

Odor

Most pouching systems are odor proof. Therefore, the only time a patient should experience odor is when the pouch is emptied. If this is offensive, pouch deodorizers, oral odor control tablets, or room deodorizers may be used. A liquid or powder deodorizer may be squirted into the bottom of the pouch following each emptying procedure. Oral deodorizers may also be effective, but should be manufactured specifically for the intended use. Room sprays are not always handy or effective, but are frequently used. If odor is detected under other circumstances, it is usually observed to be caused by leakage or an emptying spout that has not been properly cleaned. When a pouch leaks, it should be changed rather than taped for future attention. Pouch spouts may be kept clean by cuffing the spout back during emptying. Otherwise, spouts are cleaned with tissue and water after each emptying. Some patients attempt to manage odor by rinsing the pouch. However, rinsing with water is awkward and may result in decreased wear time.

Activities

Following abdominal operations, lifting restrictions serve to allow for healing and aid in avoiding abdominal hernia. Generally, heavy lifting (> 15 lb) should be avoided during the first 4 to 6 weeks postoperatively. It is useful to give examples of lifting activities to be avoided (i.e., wet laundry, shoveling snow, lifting the garage door, carrying groceries). Following this period, however, patients may gradually return to previous physical activities involving lifting or heavy pushing and pulling. Sports, workouts, and other strenuous activities are generally permitted at that point.

There are no restrictions on sexuality following operation except that sexual intercourse is to be avoided until the patient has recovered. Abdominal tenderness, incision discomfort, and perineal pain may curtail sexual intercourse for a few weeks or more following discharge from the hospital.

Discharge Instructions

Most patients experience a degree of anxiety caring for their stomas without nursing assistance for the first time. Referral to a home care agency for short-term support is suggested to ease the transition from the hospital setting to the community. A referral to social services is initiated when planning for an interim or long-term care facility or to respond to questions regarding insurance coverage. Follow-up appointments with the physicians and WOC nurse are also made. The WOC nurse usually sees the patient in the clinic within 2 weeks of discharge. Depending on the institution, ostomy supplies may be provided or patients purchase supplies in amounts required for a short period, as adjustments will most likely be made at clinic appointments. The ostomy patient should be sent home with written instructions, a recent stoma pattern, a list of local suppliers, product codes, and reading material pertinent to their operative procedure. Exercise and social contacts are important for physical and psychological recovery. Patients are encouraged to walk, see friends, and get out of the house as tolerated.

32.6.3 Posthospitalization Management

Expected outcomes in the long term include (1) prevention of complications, (2) resumption of previous or desired lifestyle, and (3) psychological adaptation to life with a stoma.

Generally, patients who avoid major complications with the stoma, peristomal skin, or pouching system are able to view the stoma as manageable sooner and move to resume previous lifestyles and psychological adaptation more easily. Therefore, prevention and planning pre- and postoperatively are the keys to the outcomes seen during the posthospitalization phase. Lack of a properly constructed and sited stoma or effective enterostomal care results in complications, delayed patient adaptation, and additional expense (i.e., equipment, outpatient visits, or revision of the stoma).[177,183]

Technical and Educational Aspects

The recovering patient may be independent in care or require assistance with the stoma from a spouse or friend. In a long-term care facility, the nursing staff may be the caregivers. Whatever the circumstances, there is an ongoing need for refitting the pouching system as the stoma shrinks, abdominal contours change, and questions regarding peristomal skin care or treatment occur. This is also a particularly important time to educate the patient, as this is the time when the patient and the family express their questions and concerns.

Basic information should be reviewed. However, the goals of complication prevention and independence are primary in this period. Initially, patients in the hospital were taught to empty and change the pouching system. As the patient recovers and learning is increased, the standard for success is raised. When a problem occurs, patients are soon able to recognize and participate in technical problem solving. If pouch leakage occurs, the patient should assess the back of the appliance to determine where erosion took place. This can help establish what changes need to be made to the system to improve the seal. Leakage can take place if the pouch is not fitted properly or does not conform to the shape of the parastomal skin. The patient should also know that weight gain affects the peristomal plane and the abdominal contours, which also requires a refitting.[183] Peristomal skin condition should be routinely checked by the patient at each pouch change. If a small area of erythema or denudation develops, the patient can independently intervene with an absorptive hydrocolloid powder. Under humid conditions, if an itchy, erythematous rash with satellite lesions develops, the patient should consider a candidiasis etiology and initiate use of an antifungal agent.[186]

Colostomy Irrigation

Advanced knowledge for the patient with a descending or sigmoid colostomy includes discussion of management options: the natural method or colostomy irrigation. As the patient begins to resume his or her previous lifestyle, schedules, activities, sports, or other preferences may dictate how the stoma is managed. In the past, most patients were taught to irrigate as the acceptable means of management. However, today the pros and cons of irrigation are discussed, and the patient makes the final decision.

The natural method of colostomy control allows the colostomy to function normally with a pouching system in use. There is a wide variety of pouches available to patients with colostomies such as one- or two-piece systems as well as a drainable or closed pouch (with or without charcoal filter). The pouch may need to be emptied one to three times in a 24-hour period. The appliance is changed every 5 to 7 days. Special instructions on diet are provided to avoid constipation. Many patients decide to continue with this method because it is simple and less time consuming. Although much has been written about the option of colostomy irrigation to "control" the bowel function, a technique that will permit many patients to be free of evacuations at unwanted times, we have observed that given the choice, most patients opt for the natural evacuation format. The availability of a variety of appliances permits patients to successfully manage their colostomy.

Alternatively, colostomy irrigation may be selected. The purpose of routine irrigation of a colostomy is to regulate the bowel and avoid stool discharges between irrigations. The procedure is intended as a convenience for patients. Those who have a high level of success are independent patients with previously predictable bowel function, good prognosis, absence of severe physical or mental limitations, good dietary habits, and absence of medications or current treatment that may result in loose stools. Contraindications for routine irrigation include diarrhea regardless of etiology, radiation enteritis, parastomal hernia, or the need for fluid restrictions due to renal failure. Precautions should be taken when there is a history of diverticulitis, angina, myocardial infarct, or spastic bowel.[187] Patients considering routine irrigation are educated regarding the procedure, time requirements, and expected results. (see "Colostomy Irrigation Procedure" (p. 799) section).

Since there is a possibility of stool leakage between irrigations, patients are instructed to use a pouching system. Discussion with the ostomate who chooses to irrigate include the need to consider long-term issues such as expected changes with aging that could interfere with the ability to irrigate independently. Individuals who select irrigation as a form of colostomy management must ensure that the medical nursing staff is advised of the need for continued irrigations in the event of hospitalization, or admission to a long-term care facility.[188]

Jao et al[189] retrospectively reviewed colostomy irrigation as a management option in 223 patients who had undergone abdominoperineal resection at the Mayo Clinic. Of that group, 134 (60%) of the patients irrigated and had good continence with only minor leakage of stool between irrigations. Of those who irrigated, 48 (22%) had regular stool leakage between irrigations and 41 (18%) patients discontinued irrigation for a number of reasons. Dini et al[190] assessed 509 patients having a colostomy for rectal carcinoma as potential candidates for irrigation. Fifty-two patients were considered unsuitable and 40 refused to learn the technique. The remaining 417 patients (82%) adopted the irrigation method. Of these, 97% achieved full continence for periods of 24 to 48 hours. There was no case of colonic perforation; 31.6% had been irrigating from 1 to 5 years and 10.3% for more than 5 years. There was a reduction of more than 50% per 24-hour period in the number of appliances used by patients. The authors concluded that irrigation is a simple, safe, and cost-effective means of managing a colostomy and that with careful selection of patients, irrigation should be recommended as a routine part of rehabilitation. Sanada et al[191] studied 214 ostomates to assess daily activities and psychosocial differences between patients who adopted natural evacuation and those who irrigated their colostomy. The authors found that colostomy irrigation imposes less distress on the patient, causes fewer skin problems, and is less of a financial burden. In daily activities, irrigation causes fewer difficulties compared to natural evacuation in the areas of bathing and sleeping. Furthermore, the authors found that the frequency of going outdoors remained the same as in preoperative days and that the patients were able to adjust to daily activities postoperatively. From a psychosocial standpoint, irrigation patients had a higher degree of self-esteem and had fewer anxieties and fewer worries than those using natural evacuation. The instruction of evacuation control, management of gas odor, and a great deal of psychosocial support must be given to natural evacuation patients (▶ Fig. 32.37).[191]

Surveillance

Over the long term, research has supported the need for outpatient follow-up. Follick et al[192] reported that of 131 ostomy patients belonging to an ostomy support group, 84% reported problems in at least one aspect of ostomy management. Fifty-three percent experienced peristomal skin irritation, 38% identified leakage, 37% reported pouching problems, 37% experienced odor, and 34% complained of noise. In a survey from the Cleveland Clinic, ileostomy patients were surveyed to identify problems encountered. Forty-nine percent identified peristomal skin irritation, 42% stated noise and odor, and 29% had difficulty managing the pouching system.[193] Based on this level of technical morbidity, outpatient services are required to intervene with proper treatment and attempt to prevent complications through routine preventive education and follow-up.

WOC or ET nurse specialists generally have routine surveillance programs. The intervals for follow-up may be within 2 weeks of discharge from the hospital, 1 month later, 6 weeks following that

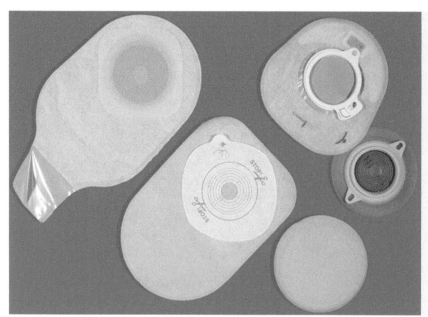

Fig. 32.37 Colostomy pouching options for patients using irrigation methods.

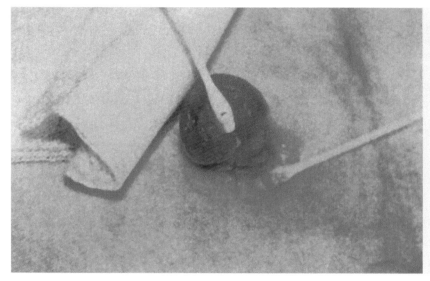

Fig. 32.38 Stoma laceration caused by pouching system.

appointment, 3 months, 6 months, and annually. The condition of the stoma and peristomal skin is assessed as well as self-care techniques, activity levels, and intimacy concerns.

Follow-up education and reinforcement regarding dehydration and electrolyte replacement are also provided. This is particularly important in warm weather or during strenuous physical activities.

Ostomy equipment is expensive. In the United States, Medicare currently reimburses 80% of medically necessary equipment. However, "medically necessary" does not include all equipment available. Examples of currently reimbursable items under Medicare are cleansers, preparations, pouch covers, and additional closure clamps. Further, there is a guideline for the appropriate utilization of equipment. Organizations such as the United Ostomy Associations of America and the Wound, Ostomy Continence Nurses Society have lobbied to change some of the funding obstacles presented by Medicare.[187] The maximum number of supplies allocated has been increased in some instances. For example, utilization of the number of drainable pouches which was initially limited to 10 per month has been increased to 20. If there is a need for a greater number of supplies than is allowed by Medicare, the patient's physician can provide a letter indicating the medical necessity for these additional items.[194] In Canada, funding for ostomy supplies is a provincial mandate. There are variations between provinces ranging from programs allocating 75% coverage to no provincial coverage whatsoever.[195] The details required to determine whether private insurance will offer coverage are most frequently found under the prosthetic device or durable medical equipment portion of the policy.[196]

32.6.4 Local Stoma and Peristomal Skin Problems

Stoma Laceration

Stoma laceration can be caused by a pouching system that fits too closely, slides against the stoma, or from an improperly fitted belt (▶ Fig. 32.38). Patients with visual impairment can cause stoma trauma with improper application of the appliance. The most common site for laceration is inferolaterally. Correcting the stoma size opening and possibly discontinuing the use of a belt should alleviate further problems. When visual acuity is an issue, home health aide may be required to assist the patient with appliance change and prevent further trauma. Use of a hydrocolloid powder on lacerations will assist with healing.

Contact Dermatitis

Contact dermatitis occurs in stoma patients as a response of the skin to contact with external agents. The etiology may be either an irritant or an allergic reaction.[197] Irritant contact dermatitis —the most common type—is caused by mechanical injury to the skin from pouch removal, contact of the skin with stomal effluent, or irritation from solvents, cements, or other products acting alone or in combination (▶ Fig. 32.39). Treatment of irritant contact dermatitis should include removal of the irritant chemicals, pouch refitting, and often patient education. Peristomal skin medications are usually not necessary, as the problem should resolve when the underlying cause has been removed. If the skin is erythematous and moist, applying the Stanley procedure will help absorb moisture and provide an intact surface for adhesion of the appliance. This involves the application of three layers of a skin-barrier powder and/or alcohol-free skin prep onto any denuded peristomal skin. Each layer is allowed to completely dry between applications.

Allergic contact dermatitis is an allergic reaction to a specific stomal product (▶ Fig. 32.40). Because allergic contact dermatitis is relatively rare, it is important to search for an irritant cause first. If the condition is considered to be allergic, then patch testing should be performed to identify the causative agent and to confirm that the reaction is allergic. It is important not to attribute what might be a simple irritant contact dermatitis to an allergic reaction, as this restricts the patient's ability to use the adhesive material that has been implicated in the allergic reaction, even though the material may otherwise have been useful for the patient.

Yeast Infection

Monilial yeast infections are frequent and commonly occur in the peristomal skin surrounding all types of stomas (▶ Fig. 32.41). Although Candida infections tend to occur in the debilitated host, most peristomal monilial infections are due to local conditions such as pouch system leakage with proliferation of yeast under the pouch adhesive. Monilial yeast infection is characterized by bright red primary and satellite papular lesions. Usually the patient complains of itching and burning around the irritated skin. The condition is managed by applying nystatin powder (e.g., Mycostatin) at the time of routine pouch changing until the infection has resolved.

Pseudoepithelial Hyperplasia

Pseudoepithelial hyperplasia (PEH) presents as a wart-like thickening of epithelium that has been repeatedly exposed to highly liquid or corrosive effluent (▶ Fig. 32.42). The affected area can be painful and bleed easily depending on the severity of PEH. The definitive treatment is to choose a pouching system that will protect the parastomal skin from contact with the offending effluent. Silver nitrate sticks or electrocautery can be used to control bleeding.[191] More frequent appliance changes may be required initially to protect the affected area and provide comfort.[191] In a suspicious situation, biopsy may be appropriate to rule out carcinoma.

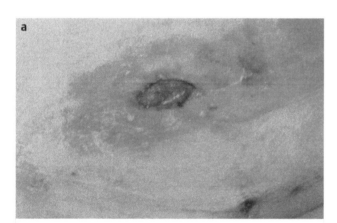

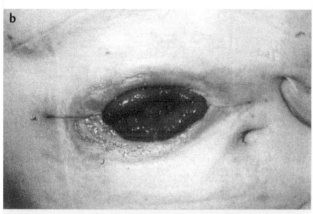

Fig. 32.39 Contact dermatitis. **(a)** Mechanical contact dermatitis caused by improper removal of pouching system. **(b)** Chemical contact dermatitis caused by irritation from fecal effluent.

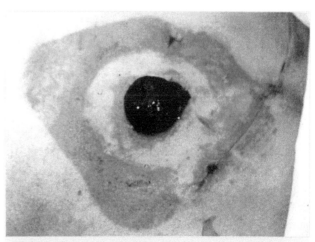

Fig. 32.40 Allergic contact dermatitis caused by reaction to pouch adhesive.

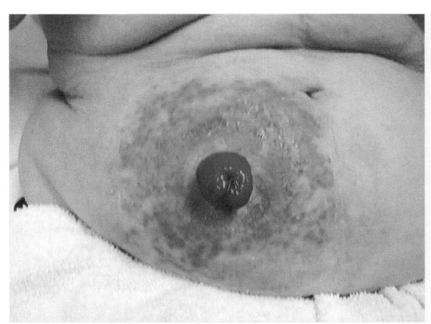

Fig. 32.41 Candidiasis around ileostomy.

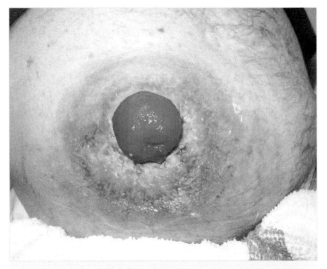

Fig. 32.42 Hyperplasia caused by chronic exposure of skin to effluent.

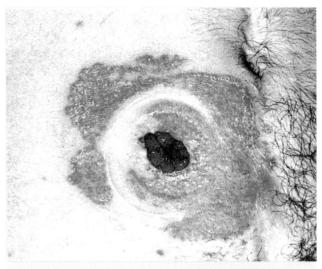

Fig. 32.43 Psoriasis surrounding umbilicus and peristomal skin.

Pyoderma Gangrenosum

Pyoderma gangrenosum may be associated with Crohn's disease, chronic ulcerative colitis, or a malignancy (▶ Fig. 32.43). It was first described by Brunsting in 1930 and occurs in approximately 2% of patients whose Crohn's disease or ulcerative colitis results in the creation of a stoma.[195,196,197,198,199] It presents clinically as an irregular ulcerated gangrenous area with ragged purple edges. Initially the skin may appear ecchymotic, and the patient complains of pain. Later the lesions undergo tunneling, resulting in increasingly large necrotic ulcers surrounded by a violaceous area. A number of treatments have been utilized. These include corticosteroids (topical, systemic, and intralesional), antibiotics, and or biologicals (e.g., tumor necrosis factor antagonists). Topical management includes providing an adequate appliance seal and controlling

wound pain and infection while applying principles of moist wound healing. In some cases, the use of sodium cromoglycate spray in combination with betamethasone dipropionate ointment has been effective and does not interfere with the pouch seal. In accordance with wound care principles, proper cleaning and an antimicrobial absorbent silver dressing (e.g., Aquacel Ag or Acticoat) can decrease the bacterial burden and promote healing.[200] Further exudate control can be achieved by covering the primary dressing with a hydrocolloid such as Duoderm (Convatec) or Comfeel (Comfeel) prior to the application of the pouch. Intralesional injection of steroids (e.g., triamcinolone acetonide solution, 10 mg/mL administered at 2-week intervals on two or three occasions) may prove ideal because it is administered intermittently when the ostomy appliance is changed and it does not interfere with the adhesion of the divide. A systematic review of nine interventional studies found that tumor necrosis factor antagonists achieved a complete response in 21 to 25% of patients and 92 to 100% of patients in 13 noninterventional studies.[201] Topical tacrolimus has also been effective.[202]

Kiran et al[203] reported on the outcome of peristomal pyoderma gangrenosum. Diagnosis was predominantly clinically based on a classic presentation of painful, undermined, peristomal ulceration. The underlying diagnosis was Crohn's disease in 11 patients, ulcerative colitis in 3 patients, indeterminate colitis in 1 patient, and posterior urethral valves in 1 patient. At the time of development of peristomal pyoderma gangrenosum, the underlying disease was active in 69% of patients. Stoma care, ulcer debridement with unroofing of undermined edges, and intralesional corticosteroid injection were associated with 40% complete response rate and a further 40% partial response rate. Of five patients who received infliximab, four responded to therapy. Complete response after all forms of therapy, including stoma relocation in seven patients, was 87%. They concluded that local wound management and WOC are extremely important for patients with peristomal pyoderma gangrenosum. Relocation of this stoma is reserved for persistent ulceration failing other therapies because peristomal pyoderma gangrenosum may occur at the new stoma site.

Psoriasis

Psoriasis may present on the peristomal skin as sharply demarcated, erythematous, weeping, papular lesions, or plaques with scales (▶ Fig. 32.44). Treatment includes the use of a solid-form skin barrier such as a Hollister psoriasis dressing. Occasionally adjunctive treatment with corticosteroids may be indicated.

Recurrent Peristomal Carcinoma

Recurrence of carcinoma in the peristomal field or on the stoma itself poses a serious management problem because pouch leakage odor and discomfort may be difficult to control (▶ Fig. 32.45a). Frequent pouch refittings are often needed. Ideally, a recurrent malignancy should be managed by resection and relocation of the stoma, but this is not always feasible because recurrent stomal carcinoma is often a sign of widespread end-stage malignant metastatic disease.[138]

Adenocarcinoma arising at the ileostomy stoma–cutaneous junction is exceedingly rare. The coexistence of ileal carcinoma and chronic ulcerative colitis is distinctly uncommon, and the development of ileal carcinoma in a patient following resection for chronic ulcerative colitis is exceptionally rare. Review of the literature until 1993 repealed only 12 such cases.[204] Primary adenocarcinoma of a Brooke ileostomy has been reported in four cases of patients undergoing total proctocolectomy and ileostomy for familial adenomatous polyposis.[204] A more recent review of the subject reported another case and noted there were 35 other such cases.[205] The most common presenting signs and symptoms include bleeding, ulceration, and the presence of a friable mass at the ileostomy (▶ Fig. 32.45b). In addition, pain, intermittent ileostomy obstruction, stenosis, and retraction have been observed. These manifestations may occur decades following the initial operation for chronic ulcerative colitis.[206]

Review of the literature until 2003 reveals one article that addresses the occurrence of metachronous adenocarcinoma

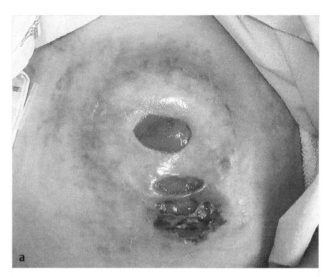

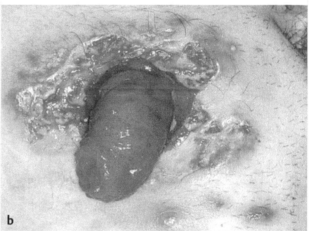

Fig. 32.44 (a) Pyoderma gangrenosum around sigmoid colostomy in patient with Crohn's disease. **(b)** Pyoderma gangrenosum around ileostomy in patient with Crohn's disease.

occurring at a colostomy site. The authors found only seven other cases reported to the surgical association in Japan between 1983 and 1997.[207] One cannot rely on biopsy of suspicious lesions, since in half the reported cases biopsies revealed only inflammation. Subsequent resections performed for ileostomy revision in these patients revealed adenocarcinoma in the resected specimens. It is therefore recommended that the presence of atypia within a biopsy specimen necessitates further biopsy. Treatment consists of wide excision of the abdominal wall circumferential to the ileostomy, adjacent ileal resection, and creation of a new ileostomy. Of the 16 patients with adenocarcinoma in an ileostomy found in the literature by Carey et al,[208] only two patients were found to have lymph node metastases. Two patients developed local recurrence, and four patients died—one of an unresectable local recurrence and three others of widespread metastases.

32.6.5 Quality of Life

Over time, people change, as do their needs. When faced with the diagnosis of carcinoma or debilitating chronic disease and

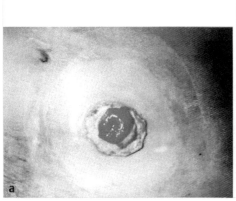
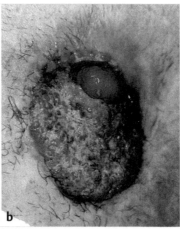

Fig. 32.45 **(a)** Recurrent adenocarcinoma around sigmoid colostomy. **(b)** Exophytic polypoid friable mass adjacent to and partially surrounding the ileostomy.[195]

the hope of cure, a stoma may seem a small price to pay. However, in the longer term, some patients do well and some find life more difficult. Quality is measured by considering physical health, functional status, and the psychological well-being of an individual. Psychological adaptation is reflected in a return to previous activities and social relationships, which is generally quite possible. In patients who have been ill for extended periods prior to operation, the level of social activities and sports participation increases following recovery. However, there are reports of significant morbidity in ostomy patient adaptation. Therefore, psychological adaptation cannot be left to happenstance. Recognizing the pitfalls and supportive interventions assists adaptation in the long term.

Sexuality is a frequently reported concern. In men, the concern about impotence and infertility requires attention. Damage to nerves during operation for carcinoma of the rectum may impair erection and ejaculation. However, in benign disease, the incidence of sexual dysfunction following proctectomy is significantly less. Based on the disease and risk of sexual dysfunction, patients may wish to "bank" sperm or avoid proctectomy with Hartmann's pouch. In women, dyspareunia may result because of the decreased lubrication or decrease in vaginal size that may occur following proctectomy for malignancy. However, preoperative libido and an interested partner are probably the two most important factors in reestablishing sexual intimacy following operation. Individuals, both heterosexual and homosexual, who have undergone a proctectomy and who had once engaged in anal intercourse must be informed that the stoma cannot be used as a substitute for the anus.[209]

An alteration in body image has a huge impact on the ostomate's ability to progress through the rehabilitation process. Helman[210] referred to body image as an individual's perception of a combination of concepts or "maps" that help us understand the structure and function of our bodies. When a patient undergoes surgery resulting in the creation of a stoma, the map of his body is changed. Furthermore, the creation of stoma can make a private issue public in the event of leakage, and an internal function external with the constant need for an external collecting device. Ostomy patients are subject to the stigma attached to any deviation from norm that dictates youth and physical beauty. They experience the dichotomy of looking normal on the outside while not feeling normal because of the hidden changes of their body.[210] This shift in body image can have an impact on interpersonal relationships due to fear and embarrassment.

Carlsson[211] studied a group of 21 patients with ileostomies between the ages of 36 and 65 years and found that their most intense concerns were intimacy, access to quality medical care, energy level, loss of sexual drive, producing odor, being a burden to others, ability to perform sexually, attractiveness, and feelings about their body.

Psychosocial support continues over the long term. Providing the opportunity for patients and family to express concerns and for problem solving is essential. Frequently, concerns about technical issues that may impair social contacts can be resolved. Ostomy support group members may demonstrate a positive attitude to encourage the patient. Occasionally it is appropriate to refer a patient for therapeutic counseling. Whatever the circumstances, quality referrals and ongoing monitoring can assist the patient in psychological adaptation.

Karadağ et al[212] examined the problems faced by patients with irrigating colostomies ($n = 16$), nonirrigating colostomies ($n = 15$), and ileostomies ($n = 15$). The digestive disease quality of life questionnaire 15 (DDQ-15) was used to analyze quality of life before and 3 months after stoma therapy. A second questionnaire consisting of 11 questions with yes/no answers was also used before and 3 months after stoma therapy to define more specifically the stoma-related problems of each patient as well as the frequency of each issue in a patient group at a given time. Cumulatively the mean quality-of-life score was significantly higher after stoma therapy than before. Before stoma therapy, the irrigating colostomy patients had the highest quality-of-life score and the ileostomy group the lowest. Quality-of-life scores 3 months after stoma therapy were significantly higher in all patients than before. Again, the irrigating colostomy patients had a significantly higher score than the nonirrigating colostomy and ileostomy patients. Cumulatively all of the items improved significantly after stoma therapy, such as getting dressed, bathing, and participating in sports. These findings confirm that colostomy or ileostomy has a profoundly negative impact on quality of life, but specialized counseling of these patients by a dedicated team improves quality of life significantly.

More recently, Karadağ et al[213] documented their results with colostomy irrigation on the quality of life. When successful, irrigation offers a regular, predictable elimination pattern and only a small covering is needed for security between irrigations. The DDQ-15 and shortform-36 were used to analyze quality of life before and 12 months after stoma therapy in a series of 25 irrigating patients with permanent end colostomies. During the same time period, 10 similar patients with left-sided colostomies who also received counseling but did not consent to colostomy irrigation were also analyzed for comparison. Colostomy irrigation was found to be effective for achieving fecal continence in selected patients with end colostomies with no complications or significant side effects. The DDQ-15 score improved significantly in both groups after stoma therapy. The post–stoma therapy DDQ-15 score of the irrigating group was also significantly higher than that of the nonirrigating group. Although none of the post–stoma therapy item scales of short-form-36 differs significantly between the two groups, stoma therapy with colostomy irrigation resulted in significant improvements in role limitation due to physical problems, social functioning, role limitation due to emotional problems, general mental health, vitality, and bodily pain. On the contrary, the nonirrigation patient group showed significant improvements only in social functioning and general mental health.

32.6.6 Special Procedures

Changing a Pouching System

The pouch is changed once every 4 to 7 days or whenever it is leaking. It is best to change the pouch when there is the least amount of output from the stoma. This is usually early in the morning or before meals. The best place to perform a pouch change is in the bathroom, where there is good visibility and counter space. Patients in wheelchairs should perform the procedure in the chair. (When the patient is in a health care facility and a nurse is providing care, the best position for the patient is supine. Universal precautions are then used.)

Setup equipment:
1. Pouching system.
2. Stoma measuring guide.
3. Closure clip.
4. Soft tissues.
5. Scissors, if needed.
6. Pouch pattern (optional).
7. Paste (optional).
8. Powder (optional).
9. Preps (optional).
10. Plastic disposal bag.

Assemble equipment:
1. Close the spout on the pouching system by securing the closure clip.
2. If the opening on the pouching system requires cutting, use the pouch pattern to trace the size onto the pouch skin barrier. Cut out the opening.
3. Remove the paper covering the adhesive.
4. If a skin barrier paste is to be used, apply a small ring of paste around the opening on the pouch.

Remove the soiled pouch:
1. Moisten the adhesive and gently begin removing the pouch. Support the skin while pulling the adhesive away.
2. Discard the soiled pouch in the plastic bag. Save the closure clip and any other reusable parts.

Apply the clean pouching system:
1. Use a dry tissue to remove any mucus, stool, or paste from the stoma and skin.
2. Cleanse the peristomal skin by rinsing with water and a soft tissue. Avoid scrubbing and the use of greasy soaps.
3. Keep soft tissues handy to contain stool if the stoma begins to function.
4. Ensure the peristomal skin is completely dry.
5. Apply powder on any reddened or irritated skin—remove excess with a tissue.
6. Apply the pouch. Smooth the edges to avoid wrinkles in the adhesive.
7. Apply gentle pressure over the system with your hand to be sure that the seal is in contact with the skin.
8. During changing of the appliance, oftentimes the ileostomy functions, thus soiling the field. One trick that can be used to control ileostomy effluent is the insertion of a tampon while the skin is being cleaned and the faceplate is being reapplied. Then just prior to application of the appliance, the tampon is removed, thereby allowing a clean field of work. The use of a water-soluble lubricant will aid in the insertion of the tampon.

Colostomy Irrigation Procedure

Routine colostomy irrigation is performed to regulate bowel function. It is performed at approximately the same time each day and requires approximately 1 hour. A patient teaching sheet for colostomy irrigation follows:
1. Prepare equipment by setting up an irrigation set with a cone tip.
2. Fill the water bag with approximately 1,000 mL tepid tap water. Hang the bag on a hook in the bathroom so that it is visible.
3. Sit on a chair in front of the toilet.
4. Remove the colostomy pouch.
5. Put on the irrigation sleeve, centering the stoma in the middle of the ring.
6. Place the end of the sleeve in the toilet. Sleeves may be attached by belts or adhesive or attached to a flange.
7. Remove air in the tubing by running water through and into the sleeve.
8. Lubricate the cone tip with a water-soluble lubricant.
9. Insert the cone tip gently into the stoma.
10. Hold the tip firmly in the stoma so that no water is running back during the procedure.
11. Run the water into the colon slowly. It usually requires 5 minutes. If cramping is a problem, stop the water flow until comfortable. If you begin to feel light-headed, stop the water, sit quietly, or have a glass of water. Light-headedness is usually a sign of water running in too quickly or using cold water.

12. Once the water is into the colon, remove the cone tip and clip the top of the sleeve closed.
13. It is important to sit on the toilet for approximately 15 minutes while the initial return passes into the sleeve and then into the toilet. The toilet may be flushed during the procedure.
14. When there is no further discharge of stool from the colon, rinse out the sleeve and clip the bottom closed. It is now permissible to leave the bathroom with the sleeve in place.
15. Usually, the sleeve is worn for approximately 45 minutes to collect stool that may be discharged. At the end of this period, a clean pouching system can be applied. The sleeve is rinsed and cleaned with a mild soap.

Ileostomy Lavage Procedure

An ileostomy lavage may be performed in an attempt to dislodge a food bolus obstruction. It is most frequently performed in the emergency room.
1. Setup equipment: 500 mL of saline, disposable irrigation sleeve, 60-mL syringe, cone tip or catheter, basin, and water-soluble lubricant.
2. Remove the ileostomy pouching system.
3. Rinse and dry the peristomal skin.
4. Attach the disposable irrigation sleeve.
5. Lubricate the cone tip or catheter.
6. Fill the syringe with saline and attach to the catheter.
7. Insert the cone tip or catheter into the stoma and slowly instill the fluid.
8. Repeat instillations of saline and allow the fluid to drain.

This is not a retention enema. The patient may become very uncomfortable if fluid is retained. Allow the saline to discharge between installations.

32.6.7 Stoma Management Products

Adhesives

Adhesives are used to attach the pouching system to peristomal skin and include paper tape used to support the pouching system. Most pouches have adhesive backings. Adhesive is also a component of a solid-form skin barrier. Yet adhesive may be required when solid skin barriers are not in use or when additional tack is needed. Faceplates require application of adhesive. Adhesives are available in disk, tape, spray, and cement forms.

Deodorizers

Internal and external forms of deodorant are available. Internal forms are over-the-counter preparations (e.g., bismuth subgallate and chlorophyllin) taken orally multiple times a day. External deodorizers are available in liquid, powder, tablet, and spray forms. Liquid, powder, and tablet forms are indicated for use within the pouch. Sprays are used as room deodorizers.

Irrigation Equipment

Colostomy irrigation or bowel preparation equipment is packaged in a set, and replacement parts are available.

Pouching Systems

Also known as appliances, pouching systems are external collection devices that contain effluent. They may be disposable or reusable, adhesive or nonadhesive, drainable or closed at the bottom, or clear or opaque. Closed pouches are indicated for patients who have a colostomy, irrigate, or have a mucous fistula. Most closed and drainable pouches are offered with or without a charcoal filter to release gas without odor. There are also "clipless" drainable pouches whose spouts are secured without the use of a rigid plastic clip. Pouching systems can be one piece or two pieces (▶ Fig. 32.46). The majority of ostomy patients prefer a two-piece system.

Skin Barriers

Skin barriers protect the peristomal skin from effluent and adhesives. Skin barriers are available as pastes, powders, sealants, and rings and wafers.

Pastes

Paste skin barriers are used to caulk or fill in uneven surfaces in the peristomal field, usually at the base of the stoma. Examples include Stomahesive Paste and Hollister Premium Barrier Paste.

Powders

Commonly made of pectin or karaya, powder barriers are absorptive substances used to treat peristomal skin. They are composed of materials similar to skin-barrier wafers.

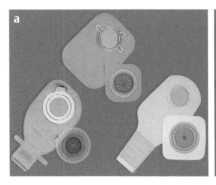
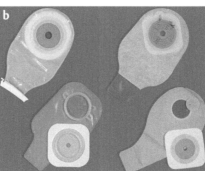

Fig. 32.46 Pouching systems. **(a)** Clipless drainable and closed pouch. **(b)** Drainable systems one and two pieces.

Sealants

These products consist of a copolymer liquid film used on the peristomal skin or any skin surface that is to be taped. Sealants reduce mechanical injury, protect the skin from moisture, and fix powders and medications on the skin. Skin-barrier sealants are available in 2 × 2-in. wipes, dabber bottles, and sprays. Most contain alcohol and therefore they should not be used on reddened or irritated skin.

Rings and Wafers

Also referred to as solid-form skin barriers, these products are available in disks, wafers, and strips for protection of peristomal skin from effluent and perspiration. They are available as single pieces or attached to the adhesive backing of a pouch. They may be composed of pectin and gelatin or karaya. Solid skin barriers come with a plastic flange for attaching the pouch (▶ Fig. 32.47 and ▶ Fig. 32.48).

Accessories

Belts

Two types of belts are available: ostomy and abdominal support belts. Ostomy belts attach to or around the pouching system, creating pressure at the stoma base. Abdominal support belts are 3 to 9 in. wide and have an opening that surrounds the pouching system in the peristomal field (see ▶ Fig. 32.27).

Closure Clips

Plastic, rubber, and metal clips are used to close the bottom of a spout on the drainable pouch.

Colostomy Plugs

Occlusive colostomy plugs are inserted into the stoma and snapped onto an intact skin barrier flange. They are indicated only after careful assessment of the patient and require close follow-up.

Pouch Covers

These are fabric garments designed to fit around the base of the pouching system and cover the plastic of the pouch so that the patient's skin is not in contact with plastic.

Skin Care Products

Adhesive solvents, skin cleansers, moisturizers, and antifungal preparations are available. Indiscriminate use is to be avoided. They are not considered essential in routine patient management.

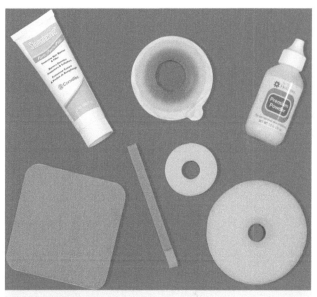

Fig. 32.47 Wafer skin barriers.

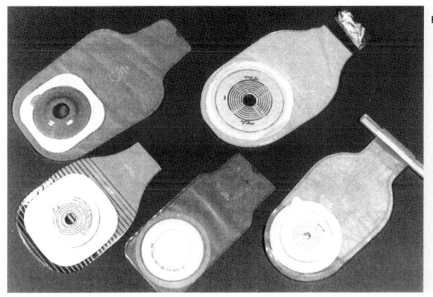

Fig. 32.48 Pouch skin barrier combinations.

References

[1] http://www.ostomy.org/About_the_UOAA.htm. Accessed December 6, 2016

[2] Klopp AL. Body image and self-concept among individuals with stomas. J Enterostomal Ther. 1990; 17(3):98–105

[3] Rolstad BS, Wilson G, Rothenberger DA. Sexual concerns in the patient with an ileostomy. Dis Colon Rectum. 1983; 26(3):170–171

[4] Keltikangas-Järvinen L, Loven E, Möller C. Psychic factors determining the long-term adaptation of colostomy and ileostomy patients. Psychother Psychosom. 1984; 41(3):153–159

[5] Franks K. Colectomy or resection of the large intestine for malignant disease. Med Chir Trans. 1889; 72:211–232

[6] Brown JY. The value of complete physiological rest of the large bowel in the treatment of certain ulcerative and obstructive lesions of this organ. Surg Gynecol Obstet. 1913; 16:610–613

[7] Warren R, McKittrick LS. Ileostomy for ulcerative colitis; technique, complications, and management. Surg Gynecol Obstet. 1951; 93(5):555–567

[8] Crile G, Jr, Turnbull RB, Jr. The mechanism and prevention of ileostomy dysfunction. Ann Surg. 1954; 140(4):459–466

[9] Brooke BN. The management of an ileostomy, including its complications. Lancet. 1952; 2(6725):102–104

[10] Goligher JC. Extraperitoneal colostomy or ileostomy. Br J Surg. 1958; 46 (196):97–103

[11] Kock NG, Brevinge H, Philipson BM, Ojerskog B. Continent ileostomy. The present technique and long term results. Ann Chir Gynaecol. 1986; 75 (2):63–70

[12] Tang CL, Yunos A, Leong APK, Seow-Choen F, Goh HS. Ileostomy output in the early postoperative period. Br J Surg. 1995; 82(5):607–608

[13] Soybel DI. Adaptation to ileal diversion. Surgery. 2001; 129(2):123–127

[14] Ladas SD, Isaacs PE, Murphy GM, Sladen GE. Fasting and postprandial ileal function in adapted ileostomates and normal subjects. Gut. 1986; 27 (8):906–912

[15] Hallgren T, Oresland T, Andersson H, Hultén L. Ileostomy output and bile acid excretion after intraduodenal administration of oleic acid. Scand J Gastroenterol. 1994; 29(11):1017–1023

[16] Steinhart AH, Jenkins DJA, Mitchell S, Cuff D, Prokipchuk EJ. Effect of dietary fiber on total carbohydrate losses in ileostomy effluent. Am J Gastroenterol. 1992; 87(1):48–54

[17] MacGregor IL, Wiley ZD, Sleisenger MH. The role of bile acids in determining ileal flow rates in normal subjects and following ileostomy. Digestion. 1978; 18(3–4):192–200

[18] Gorbach SL, Nahas L, Weinstein L, Levitan R, Patterson JF. Studies of intestinal microflora. IV. The microflora of ileostomy effluent: a unique microbial ecology. Gastroenterology. 1967; 53(6):874–880

[19] Soper NJ, Orkin BA, Kelly KA, Phillips SF, Brown ML. Gastrointestinal transit after proctocolectomy with ileal pouch-anal anastomosis or ileostomy. J Surg Res. 1989; 46(4):300–305

[20] Pemberton JH, van Heerden JA, Beart RW, Jr, Kelly KA, Phillips SF, Taylor BM. A continent ileostomy device. Ann Surg. 1983; 197(5):618–626

[21] Bruewer M, Stern J, Herrmann S, Senninger N, Herfarth C. Changes in intestinal transit time after proctocolectomy assessed by the lactulose breath test. World J Surg. 2000; 24(1):119–124

[22] Mibu R, Itoh H, Nakayama F. Effect of total colectomy and mucosal proctectomy on intestinal absorptive capacity in dogs. Dis Colon Rectum. 1987; 30 (1):47–51

[23] Wright HK, Cleveland JC, Tilson MD, Herskovic T. Morphology and absorptive capacity of the ileum after ileostomy in man. Am J Surg. 1969; 117 (2):242–245

[24] Scott R, Freeland R, Mowat W, et al. The prevalence of calcified upper urinary tract stone disease in a random population–Cumbernauld Health Survey. Br J Urol. 1977; 49(7):589–595

[25] Smith LH. Application of physical, chemical and metabolic factors to the management of urolithiasis. In: Fleisch H, Robertson WG, Smith LH, Vahlenslеck W, eds. Urolithiasis Research. New York, NY: Premium Press; 1976:199–211

[26] Christie PM, Knight GS, Hill GL. Comparison of relative risks of urinary stone formation after surgery for ulcerative colitis: conventional ileostomy vs. J-pouch. A comparative study. Dis Colon Rectum. 1996; 39(1):50–54

[27] Miettinen TA, Peltokallio P. Bile salt, fat, water, and vitamin B 12 excretion after ileostomy. Scand J Gastroenterol. 1971; 6(6):543–552

[28] Huibregtse K, Hoek F, Sanders GT, Tytgat GN. Bile acid metabolism in ileostomy patients. Eur J Clin Invest. 1977; 7(2):137–140

[29] Ritchie JK. Ileostomy and excisional surgery for chronic inflammatory disease of the colon: a survey of one hospital region. Gut. 1971; 12(7):528–540

[30] Kurchin A, Ray JE, Bluth EI, et al. Cholelithiasis in ileostomy patients. Dis Colon Rectum. 1984; 27(9):585–588

[31] Kusuhara K, Kusunoki M, Okamoto T, Sakanoue Y, Utsunomiya J. Reduction of the effluent volume in high-output ileostomy patients by a somatostatin analogue, SMS 201–995. Int J Colorectal Dis. 1992; 7(4):202–205

[32] Gracey M, Burke V, Oshin A. Reversible inhibition of intestinal active sugar transport by deconjugated bile salt in vitro. Biochim Biophys Acta. 1971; 225(2):308–314

[33] Keating J, Kelly EW, Hunt I. Save the skin and improve the scar: a simple technique to minimize the scar from a temporary stoma. Dis Colon Rectum. 2003; 46(10):1428–1429

[34] Kittur DS, Talamini M, Smith GW. Eversion of difficult ileostomies by guy rope suture technique. Am J Surg. 1989; 157(6):593–594

[35] Carlsen E, Bergan A. Technical aspects and complications of end-ileostomies. World J Surg. 1995; 19(4):632–636

[36] Williams NS, Nasmyth DG, Jones D, Smith AH. De-functioning stomas: a prospective controlled trial comparing loop ileostomy with loop transverse colostomy. Br J Surg. 1986; 73(7):566–570

[37] Altomare DF, Pannarale OC, Lupo L, Palasciano N, Memeo V, Rubino M. Protective colostomy closure: the hazards of a "minor" operation. Int J Colorectal Dis. 1990; 5(2):73–78

[38] Winslet MC, Drolc Z, Allan A, Keighley MR. Assessment of the defunctioning efficiency of the loop ileostomy. Dis Colon Rectum. 1991; 34(8):699–703

[39] Chen F, Stuart M. The morbidity of defunctioning stomata. Aust N Z J Surg. 1996; 66(4):218–221

[40] Alexander-Williams J. Loop ileostomy and colostomy for faecal diversion. Ann R Coll Surg Engl. 1974; 54(3):141–148

[41] Fasth S, Hultén L. Loop ileostomy: a superior diverting stoma in colorectal surgery. World J Surg. 1984; 8(3):401–407

[42] Marcello PW, Roberts PL, Schoetz DJ, Jr, Coller JA, Murray JJ, Veidenheimer MC. Obstruction after ileal pouch-anal anastomosis: a preventable complication? Dis Colon Rectum. 1993; 36(12):1105–1111

[43] Prasad ML, Pearl RK, Orsay CP, Abcarian H. Rodless ileostomy. A modified loop ileostomy. Dis Colon Rectum. 1984; 27(4):270–271

[44] Sitzmann JV. A new alternative to diverting double barreled ileostomy. Surg Gynecol Obstet. 1987; 165(5):461–464

[45] Kestenberg A, Becker JM. A new technique of loop ileostomy closure after endorectal ileoanal anastomosis. Surgery. 1985; 98(1):109–111

[46] van de Pavoordt HDWM, Fazio VW, Jagelman DG, Lavery IC, Weakley FL. The outcome of loop ileostomy closure in 293 cases. Int J Colorectal Dis. 1987; 2 (4):214–217

[47] Bertoni DM, Hammond KL, Beck DE, et al. Use of sodium hyaluronate/carboxymethylcellulose bioresorbable membrane in loop ileostomy construction facilitates stoma closure. Ochsner J. 2017; 17:146–149

[48] Tang CL, Seow-Choen F, Fook-Chong S, Eu KW. Bioresorbable adhesion barrier facilitates early closure of the defunctioning ileostomy after rectal excision: a prospective, randomized trial. Dis Colon Rectum. 2003; 46(9):1200–1207

[49] Memon S, Heriot AG, Atkin CE, Lynch AC. Facilitated early ileostomy closure after rectal cancer surgery: a case-matched study. Tech Coloproctol. 2012; 16(4):285–290

[50] Abrams JS. Abdominal stomas. Indications, operative techniques and patient care. In: Wright J, ed. Spontaneous Fistula to Continent Ileostomy. Littleton, MA: PSG; 1984:19–24

[51] Miles WE. A method of performing abdominoperineal excision for carcinoma of the rectum and of the terminal portion of the pelvic colon. Lancet. 1908; 2:1812–1813

[52] Heald RJ. Towards fewer colostomies–the impact of circular stapling devices on the surgery of rectal cancer in a district hospital. Br J Surg. 1980; 67 (3):198–200

[53] Fielding LP, Stewart-Brown S, Hittinger R, Blesovsky L. Covering stoma for elective anterior resection of the rectum: an outmoded operation? Am J Surg. 1984; 147(4):524–530

[54] Stone HH, Fabian TC. Management of perforating colon trauma: randomization between primary closure and exteriorization. Ann Surg. 1979; 190 (4):430–436

[55] Gordon PH. The chemically defined diet and anorectal procedures. Can J Surg. 1976; 19(6):511–513

[56] Robertson HD. Use of an elemental diet as a nutritionally complete "medical colostomy". South Med J. 1983; 76(8):1005–1007

[57] Corman ML. Colon and Rectal Surgery. 2nd ed. Philadelphia, PA: JB Lippincott; 1989

[58] Goldstein SD, Salvati EP, Rubin RJ, Eisenstat TE. Tube cecostomy with cecal extraperitonealization in the management of obstructing left sided carcinoma of the large intestine. Surg Gynecol Obstet. 1986; 162(4):379–380

[59] Benacci JC, Wolff BG. Cecostomy. Therapeutic indications and results. Dis Colon Rectum. 1995; 38(5):530–534

[60] Haaga JR, Bick RJ, Zollinger RM, Jr. CT-guided percutaneous catheter cecostomy. Gastrointest Radiol. 1987; 12(2):166–168

[61] Ponsky JL, Aszodi A, Perse D. Percutaneous endoscopic cecostomy: a new approach to nonobstructive colonic dilation. Gastrointest Endosc. 1986; 32 (2):108–111

[62] Winkler MJ, Volpe PA. Loop transverse colostomy. The case against. Dis Colon Rectum. 1982; 25(4):321–326

[63] Hopkins JE. Transverse colostomy in the management of cancer of the colon. Dis Colon Rectum. 1971; 14(3):232–236

[64] Abrams BL, Alsikafi FH, Waterman NG. Colostomy: a new look at morbidity and mortality. Am Surg. 1979; 45(7):462–464

[65] Rosenberg L, Gordon PH. Tube cecostomy revisited. Can J Surg. 1986; 29 (1):38–40

[66] Fontes B, Fontes W, Utiyama EM, Birolini D. The efficacy of loop colostomy for complete fecal diversion. Dis Colon Rectum. 1988; 31(4):298–302

[67] Schofield PF, Cade D, Lambert M. Dependent proximal loop colostomy: does it defunction the distal colon? Br J Surg. 1980; 67(3):201–202

[68] Morris DM, Rayburn D. Loop colostomies are totally diverting in adults. Am J Surg. 1991; 161(6):668–671

[69] Turnbull RB, Jr, Weakley FL, Hawk WA, Schofield P. Choice of operation for the toxic megacolon phase of nonspecific ulcerative colitis. Surg Clin North Am. 1970; 50(5):1151–1169

[70] Prasad ML, Pearl RK, Abcarian H. End-loop colostomy. Surg Gynecol Obstet. 1984; 158(4):380–382

[71] Unti JA, Abcarian H, Pearl RK, et al. Rodless end-loop stomas. Seven-year experience. Dis Colon Rectum. 1991; 34(11):999–1004

[72] Slater NJ, Hansson BME, Buyne OR, Hendriks T, Bleichrodt RP. Repair of parastomal hernias with biologic grafts: a systematic review. J Gastrointest Surg. 2011; 15(7):1252–1258

[73] Parks SE, Hastings PR. Complications of colostomy closure. Am J Surg. 1985; 149(5):672–675

[74] Williams RA, Csepanyi E, Hiatt J, Wilson SE. Analysis of the morbidity, mortality, and cost of colostomy closure in traumatic compared with nontraumatic colorectal diseases. Dis Colon Rectum. 1987; 30(3):164–167

[75] Thal ER, Yeary EC. Morbidity of colostomy closure following colon trauma. J Trauma. 1980; 20(4):287–291

[76] Velmahos GC, Degiannis E, Wells M, Souter I, Saadia R. Early closure of colostomies in trauma patients–a prospective randomized trial. Surgery. 1995; 118(5):815–820

[77] Whittaker M, Goligher JC. A comparison of the results of extraperitoneal and intraperitoneal techniques for construction of terminal iliac colostomies. Dis Colon Rectum. 1976; 19(4):342–344

[78] Sjödahl R, Anderberg B, Bolin T. Parastomal hernia in relation to site of the abdominal stoma. Br J Surg. 1988; 75(4):339–341

[79] Ortiz H, Sara MJ, Armendariz P, de Miguel M, Marti J, Chocarro C. Does the frequency of paracolostomy hernias depend on the position of the colostomy in the abdominal wall? Int J Colorectal Dis. 1994; 9(2):65–67

[80] Antrum RM, Price JJ. Use of skin staples for fashioning colostomies. Br J Surg. 1988; 75(8):736

[81] Burke TW, Weiser EB, Hoskins WJ, Heller PB, Nash JD, Park RC. End colostomy using the end-to-end anastomosis instrument. Obstet Gynecol. 1987; 69(2):156–159

[82] Porter JA, Salvati EP, Rubin RJ, Eisenstat TE. Complications of colostomies. Dis Colon Rectum. 1989; 32(4):299–303

[83] Feustel H, Hennig G. Kontinente Kolostomie durch Magnetverschluss. Dtsch Med Wochenschr. 1975; 100(19):1063–1064

[84] Khubchandani IT, Trimpi HD, Sheets JA. The magnetic stoma device: a continent colostomy. Dis Colon Rectum. 1981; 24:344–350

[85] Husemann B, Hager T. Experience with the Erlangen magnetic ring colostomy-closure system. Int Surg. 1984; 69(4):297–300

[86] Prager E. The continent colostomy. Dis Colon Rectum. 1984; 27:235–237

[87] Clague MB, Heald RJ. Achievement of stomal continence in one-third of colostomies by use of a new disposable plug. Surg Gynecol Obstet. 1990; 170:390–394

[88] Codina Cazador A, Piñol M, Marti Rague J, Montane J, Nogueras FM, Suñol J. Multicentre study of a continent colostomy plug. Br J Surg. 1993; 80 (7):930–932

[89] Schmidt E. The continent colostomy. World J Surg. 1982; 6(6):805–809

[90] Mileski WJ, Rege RV, Joehl RJ, Nahrwold DL. Rates of morbidity and mortality after closure of loop and end colostomy. Surg Gynecol Obstet. 1990; 171 (1):17–21

[91] Mosdell DM, Doberneck RC. Morbidity and mortality of ostomy closure. Am J Surg. 1991; 162(6):633–636, discussion 636–637

[92] Pearce NW, Scott SD, Karran SJ. Timing and method of reversal of Hartmann's procedure. Br J Surg. 1992; 79(8):839–841

[93] Keck JO, Collopy BT, Ryan PJ, Fink R, Mackay JR, Woods RJ. Reversal of Hartmann's procedure: effect of timing and technique on ease and safety. Dis Colon Rectum. 1994; 37(3):243–248

[94] Livingston DH, Miller FB, Richardson JD. Are the risks after colostomy closure exaggerated? Am J Surg. 1989; 158(1):17–20

[95] Khoury DA, Beck DE, Opelka FG, Hicks TC, Timmcke AE, Gathright JB, Jr. Colostomy closure. Ochsner Clinic experience. Dis Colon Rectum. 1996; 39 (6):605–609

[96] Allen-Mersh TG, Thomson JPS. Surgical treatment of colostomy complications. Br J Surg. 1988; 75(5):416–418

[97] Leenen LP, Kuypers JH. Some factors influencing the outcome of stoma surgery. Dis Colon Rectum. 1989; 32(6):500–504

[98] Carlstedt A, Fasth S, Hultén L, Nordgren S, Palselius I. Long-term ileostomy complications in patients with ulcerative colitis and Crohn's disease. Int J Colorectal Dis. 1987; 2(1):22–25

[99] Khoo REH, Cohen MM, Chapman GM, Jenken DA, Langevin JM. Loop ileostomy for temporary fecal diversion. Am J Surg. 1994; 167(5):519–522

[100] Stothert JC, Jr, Brubacher L, Simonowitz DA. Complications of emergency stoma formation. Arch Surg. 1982; 117(3):307–309

[101] Feinberg SM, McLeod RS, Cohen Z. Complications of loop ileostomy. Am J Surg. 1987; 153(1):102–107

[102] Grobler SP, Hosie KB, Keighley MRB. Randomized trial of loop ileostomy in restorative proctocolectomy. Br J Surg. 1992; 79(9):903–906

[103] Wexner SD, Taranow DA, Johansen OB, et al. Loop ileostomy is a safe option for fecal diversion. Dis Colon Rectum. 1993; 36(4):349–354

[104] Leong APK, Londono-Schimmer EE, Phillips RKS. Life-table analysis of stomal complications following ileostomy. Br J Surg. 1994; 81(5):727–729

[105] Senapati A, Nicholls RJ, Ritchie JK, Tibbs CJ, Hawley PR. Temporary loop ileostomy for restorative proctocolectomy. Br J Surg. 1993; 80(5):628–630

[106] Kaidar-Person O, Person B, Wexner SD. Complications of construction and closure of temporary loop ileostomy. J Am Coll Surg. 2005; 201(5):759–773

[107] Hughes ESR, McDermott FT, Masterton JP. Intestinal obstruction following operation for inflammatory disease of the bowel. Dis Colon Rectum. 1979; 22(7):469–471

[108] Bubrick MP, Jacobs DM, Levy M. Experience with the endorectal pull-through and S pouch for ulcerative colitis and familial polyposis in adults. Surgery. 1985; 98(4):689–699

[109] Francois Y, Dozois RR, Kelly KA, et al. Small intestinal obstruction complicating ileal pouch-anal anastomosis. Ann Surg. 1989; 209(1):46–50

[110] Anderson DN, Driver CP, Park KGM, Davidson AI, Keenan RA. Loop ileostomy fixation: a simple technique to minimise the risk of stomal volvulus. Int J Colorectal Dis. 1994; 9(3):138–140

[111] Snyder CL, Kaufman DB. A simple technique for assessing the viability of stomas of the intestines. Surg Gynecol Obstet. 1991; 172(5):399–400

[112] Fleischer I, Bryant D. Melanosis coli or mucosa ischemia? A case report. Ostomy Wound Manage. 1995; 41(4):44, 46–47

[113] Malt RA, Bartlett MK, Wheelock FC. Subcutaneous fasciotomy for relief of stricture of the ileostomy. Surg Gynecol Obstet. 1984; 159(2):175–176

[114] Todd IP. Mechanical complications of ileostomy. Clin Gastroenterol. 1982; 11 (2):268–273

[115] Fleshman JW, Lewis MG. Complications and quality of life after stoma surgery: a review of 16,470 patients in the UOA Data Registry. Semin Colon Rectal Surg. 1991; 2:66–72

[116] Park JJ, Del Pino A, Orsay CP, et al. Stoma complications: the Cook County Hospital experience. Dis Colon Rectum. 1999; 42(12):1575–1580

[117] Cheung MT. Complications of an abdominal stoma: an analysis of 322 stomas. Aust N Z J Surg. 1995; 65(11):808–811

[118] Zinkin LD, Rosin JD. Button colopexy for colostomy prolapse. Surg Gynecol Obstet. 1981; 152(1):89–90

[119] Rubin MS. Parastomal hernias. In: Cataldo PA, MacKeigan JM, eds. Intestinal Stomas: Principles, Techniques, and Management. 2nd ed. New York, NY: Marcel Dekker; 2004:277–305

[120] Botet X, Boldó E, Llauradó JM. Colonic parastomal hernia repair by translocation without formal laparotomy. Br J Surg. 1996; 83(7):981

[121] Carne PW, Robertson GM, Frizelle FA. Parastomal hernia. Br J Surg. 2003; 90 (7):784–793

[122] Birnbaum W, Ferrier P. Complications of abdominal colostomy. Am J Surg. 1952; 83(1):64–67

[123] Grier WRN, Grier WR, Postel AH, Syarse A, Localio SA. An evaluation of colonic stoma management without irrigations. Surg Gynecol Obstet. 1964; 118:1234–1242

[124] Marks CG, Ritchie JK. The complications of synchronous combined excision for adenocarcinoma of the rectum at St Mark's Hospital. Br J Surg. 1975; 62 (11):901–905

[125] von Smitten K, Husa A, Kyllönen L. Long-term results of sigmoidostomy in patients with anorectal malignancy. Acta Chir Scand. 1986; 152:211–213

[126] Williams JG, Etherington R, Hayward MWJ, Hughes LE. Paraileostomy hernia: a clinical and radiological study. Br J Surg. 1990; 77(12):1355–1357

[127] Londono-Schimmer EE, Leong APK, Phillips RKS. Life table analysis of stomal complications following colostomy. Dis Colon Rectum. 1994; 37(9):916–920

[128] Lavery IC, Erwin-Toth P. Stomal therapy. In: Cataldo P, Mackeigan JM, eds. Intestinal Stomas: Principles, Therapy, and Management. 2nd ed. New York, NY: Marcell Dekker; 2004:65-90

[129] Balslev AI. Parakolostomihernier. Ugeskr Laeger. 1973; 135:2799–2804

[130] Cheung MT, Chia NH, Chiu WY. Surgical treatment of parastomal hernia complicating sigmoid colostomies. Dis Colon Rectum. 2001; 44(2):266–270

[131] Bayer I, Kyzer S, Chaimoff C. A new approach to primary strengthening of colostomy with Marlex mesh to prevent paracolostomy hernia. Surg Gynecol Obstet. 1986; 163(6):579–580

[132] Sugarbaker PH. Prosthetic mesh repair of large hernias at the site of colonic stomas. Surg Gynecol Obstet. 1980; 150(4):576–578

[133] Stephenson BM, Phillips RKS. Parastomal hernia: local resiting and mesh repair. Br J Surg. 1995; 82(10):1395–1396

[134] Geisler DJ, Reilly JC, Vaughan SG, Glennon EJ, Kondylis PD. Safety and outcome of use of nonabsorbable mesh for repair of fascial defects in the presence of open bowel. Dis Colon Rectum. 2003; 46(8):1118–1123

[135] Steele SR, Lee P, Martin MJ, Mullenix ES. Is parastomal hernia repair with polypropylene mesh safe? Am J Surg. 2003; 185(5):436–440

[136] DeAsis FJ, Lapin B, Gitelis ME, Ujiki MB. Current state of laparoscopic parastomal hernia repair: A meta-analysis. World J Gastroenterol. 2015; 21 (28):8670–8677

[137] Hansson BM, de Hingh IH, Bleichrodt RP. Laparoscopic parastomal hernia repair is feasible and safe: early results of a prospective clinical study including 55 consecutive patients. Surg Endosc. 2007; 21(6):989–993

[138] Slater NJ, Hansson BME, Buyne OR, Hendriks T, Bleichrodt RP. Repair of parastomal hernias with biologic grafts: A systemic review. J Gastrointest Surg. 2011; 15:1252–1258

[139] Jänes A, Cengiz Y, Israelsson LA. Randomized clinical trial of the use of a prosthetic mesh to prevent parastomal hernia. Br J Surg. 2004; 91(3):280–282

[140] Stelzner S, Hellmich G, Ludwig K. New method for paracolostomy hernia repair? Dis Colon Rectum. 1999; 42(6):823

[141] Amin SN, Armitage NC, Abercrombie JF, Scholefield JH. Lateral repair of parastomal hernia. Ann R Coll Surg Engl. 2001; 83(3):206–208

[142] Rubin MS, Schoetz DJ, Jr, Matthews JB. Parastomal hernia. Is stoma relocation superior to fascial repair? Arch Surg. 1994; 129(4):413–418, discussion 418–419

[143] Cross AJ, Buchwald PL, Frizelle FA, Eglinton TW. Meta-analysis of prophylactic mesh to prevent parastomal hernia. Br J Surg. 2017; 104(3):179–186

[144] Chapman SJ, Wood B, Drake TM, Young N, Jayne DG. Systemic review and meta-analysis of prophylactic mesh during primary stomal formation to prevent parastomal hernia. Dis Colon Rectum. 2017; 60(1):107–115

[145] Greatorex RA. Simple method of closing a para-ileostomy fistula. Br J Surg. 1988; 75(6):543

[146] Wiesner RH, LaRusso NF, Dozois RR, Beaver SJ. Peristomal varices after proctocolectomy in patients with primary sclerosing cholangitis. Gastroenterology. 1986; 90(2):316–322

[147] Strong SA. Colonic anorectal and peristomal varices. Semin Colorectal Surg. 1994; 5:50–58

[148] Roberts PL, Martin FM, Schoetz DJ, Jr, Murray JJ, Coller JA, Veidenheimer MC. Bleeding stomal varices. The role of local treatment. Dis Colon Rectum. 1990; 33(7):547–549

[149] Peck JJ, Boyden AM. Exigent ileostomy hemorrhage. A complication of proctocolectomy in patients with chronic ulcerative colitis and primary sclerosing cholangitis. Am J Surg. 1985; 150(1):153–158

[150] Grundfest-Broniatowski S, Fazio V. Conservative treatment of bleeding stomal varices. Arch Surg. 1983; 118(8):981–985

[151] Morgan TR, Feldshon SD, Tripp MR. Recurrent stomal variceal bleeding. Successful treatment using injection sclerotherapy. Dis Colon Rectum. 1986; 29 (4):269–270

[152] Hesterberg R, Stahlknecht CD, Röher HD. Sclerotherapy for massive enterostomy bleeding resulting from portal hypertension. Dis Colon Rectum. 1986; 29(4):275–277

[153] Samaraweera RN, Feldman L, Widrich WC, et al. Stomal varices: percutaneous transhepatic embolization. Radiology. 1989; 170(3, Pt 1):779–782

[154] Fitzgerald JB, Chalmers N, Abbott G, et al. The use of TIPS to control bleeding caput medusae. Br J Radiol. 1998; 71(845):558–560

[155] Shibata D, Brophy DP, Gordon FD, Anastopoulos HT, Sentovich SM, Bleday R. Transjugular intrahepatic portosystemic shunt for treatment of bleeding ectopic varices with portal hypertension. Dis Colon Rectum. 1999; 42 (12):1581–1585

[156] Barbosa NS, Tolkachjov SN, El-Azhary RA, et al. Clinical features, causes, treatments, and outcomes of peristomal pyoderma gangrenosum (PPG) in 44 patients: The Mayo Clinic experience, 1996 through 2013. J Am Acad Dermatol. 2016; 75(5):931–939

[157] Poritz LS, Lebo MA, Bobb AD, Ardell CM, Koltun WA. Management of peristomal pyoderma gangrenosum. J Am Coll Surg. 2008; 206(2):311–315

[158] Korelitz BI, Cheskin LJ, Sohn N, Sommers SC. The fate of the rectal segment after diversion of the fecal stream in Crohn's disease: its implications for surgical management. J Clin Gastroenterol. 1985; 7(1):37–43

[159] Harig JM, Soergel KH, Komorowski RA, Wood CM. Treatment of diversion colitis with short-chain-fatty acid irrigation. N Engl J Med. 1989; 320(1):23–28

[160] Pokorny H, Herkner H, Jakesz R, Herbst F. Mortality and complications after stoma closure. Arch Surg. 2005; 140(10):956–960, discussion 960

[161] Moug SJ, Robertson E, Angerson WJ, Horgan PG. Socioeconomic deprivation has an adverse effect on outcome after ileostomy closure. Br J Surg. 2005; 92 (3):376–377

[162] Bosshardt TL. Outcomes of ostomy procedures in patients aged 70 years and older. Arch Surg. 2003; 138(10):1077–1082

[163] Edwards DP, Leppington-Clarke A, Sexton R, Heald RJ, Moran BJ. Stoma-related complications are more frequent after transverse colostomy than loop ileostomy: a prospective randomized clinical trial. Br J Surg. 2001; 88 (3):360–363

[164] Kairaluoma M, Rissanen H, Kultti V, Mecklin JP, Kellokumpu I. Outcome of temporary stomas. A prospective study of temporary intestinal stomas constructed between 1989 and 1996. Dig Surg. 2002; 19(1):45–51

[165] Duchesne JC, Wang YZ, Weintraub SL, Boyle M, Hunt JP. Stoma complications: a multivariate analysis. Am Surg. 2002; 68(11):961–966, discussion 966

[166] Cataldo PA. History of enterostomal therapy. Perspect Colon Rectal Surg. 1996; 9:117–123

[167] Walsh BA, Grunert BK, Telford GL, Otterson MF. Multidisciplinary management of altered body image in the patient with an ostomy. J Wound Ostomy Continence Nurs. 1995; 22(5):227–236

[168] Rolstad BS. Facilitating psychosocial adaptation. J Enterostomal Ther. 1987; 14(1):28–34

[169] Piwonka MA, Merino JM. A multidimensional modeling of predictors influencing the adjustment to a colostomy. J Wound Ostomy Continence Nurs. 1999; 26(6):298–305

[170] Standards of Care. Patient with Ileostomy. Costa Mesa, CA: Wound Ostomy and Continence Nurses Society (WOCN); 1990

[171] Standards of Care. Patient with Colostomy. Costa Mesa, CA: Wound Ostomy and Continence Nurses Society (WOCN); 1989

[172] Persson E, Severinsson E, Hellström AL. Spouses' perceptions of and reactions to living with a partner who has undergone surgery for rectal cancer resulting in a stoma. Cancer Nurs. 2004; 27(1):85–90

[173] O'Shea HS. Teaching the adult ostomy patient. J Wound Ostomy Continence Nurs. 2001; 28(1):47–54

[174] Jeter KF. Perioperative teaching and counseling. Cancer. 1992; 70(5) Suppl:1346–1349

[175] Pieper B, Mikols C. Predischarge and postdischarge concerns of persons with an ostomy. J Wound Ostomy Continence Nurs. 1996; 23(2):105–109

[176] Klopp AL. Gastrointestinal and digestive care plans: fecal ostomy. In: Gulanick M, Klopp A, Galanes S, et al, eds. Nursing Care Plans: Nursing Diagnosis and Intervention. 3rd ed. St. Louis, MO: Mosby; 1994:308–310

[177] Corman ML. Preoperative considerations. In: MacKeigan JM, Cataldo PA, eds. Intestinal Stomas: Principles, Techniques, and Management. St Louis, MO: Quality Medical Publishing; 1993:52–59

[178] Lavery IC, Erwin-Toth P. Stoma therapy. In: MacKeigan JM, Cataldo PA, eds. Intestinal Stomas: Principles Techniques and Management. St Louis, MO: Quality Medical Publishing; 1993:60–84

[179] Banks N, Razor B. Preoperative stoma site assessment and marking: trained RNs can improve ostomy outcome. AJN. 2003; 103:64A–64B

[180] Turnbull R, Weakley F. Atlas of Intestinal Stomas. St. Louis, MO: CV Mosby, 1967:7–9

[181] Weakley FL. A historical perspective of stomal construction. J Wound Ostomy Continence Nurs. 1994; 21(2):59–75

[182] Boarini J. Gastrointestinal cancer: colon, rectum, and anus. In: Groenwald SL, Frogge MH, Goodman M, et al., eds. Cancer Nursing: Principles and Practice. 2nd ed. Boston: Jones and Bartlett; 1990:792–807

[183] Rolstad BS, Boarini J. Principles and techniques in the use of convexity. Ostomy Wound Manage. 1996; 42(1):24–26, 28–32, quiz 33–34

[184] Floruta CV. Dietary choices of people with ostomies. J Wound Ostomy Continence Nurs. 2001; 28(1):28–31

[185] Rolstad BS, Hoyman K. Continent diversions and reservoirs. In: Hampton B, Bryant R, eds. Ostomies and Continent Diversions: Nursing Management. St. Louis, MO: Mosby-Year Book; 1992:129–162

[186] Erwin-Toth P, Doughty DB. Principles and procedures of stomal management. In: Hampton B, Bryant R, eds. Ostomies and Continent Diversions: Nursing Management. St. Louis, MO: Mosby-Year Book; 1992:103

[187] Association Francaise d'Enterostoma-Therapeutes. Guide des Bonnes Pratiques en Stomatherapie Chez L'adulte-Enterostomies. Citron Marine, France; 2003:135

[188] Turnbull G. Managing oversight of colostomy irrigation in long term care facilities. OWM. 2002; 49:13–14

[189] Jao S-W, Beart RW, Jr, Wendorf LJ, Ilstrup DM. Irrigation management of sigmoid colostomy. Arch Surg. 1985; 120(8):916–917

[190] Dini D, Venturini M, Forno G, Bertelli G, Grandi G. Irrigation for colostomized cancer patients: a rational approach. Int J Colorectal Dis. 1991; 6(1):9–11

[191] Sanada H, Kawashima K, Tsuda M, Yamaguchi A. Natural evacuation versus irrigation. Ostomy Wound Manage. 1992; 38(4):24, 26–30, 32 passim

[192] Follick MJ, Smith TW, Turk DC. Psychosocial adjustment following ostomy. Health Psychol. 1984; 3(6):505–517

[193] McLeod RS, Lavery IC, Leatherman JR, et al. Patient evaluation of the conventional ileostomy. Dis Colon Rectum. 1985; 28(3):152–154

[194] Turnbull GB. The evolution, current status, and regulation of ostomy products in the United States. J Wound Ostomy Continence Nurs. 2001; 28(1):18–24

[195] Milne CT, Corbett LQ, Dubuc DL. Wound, Ostomy, and Incontinence Nursing Secrets. Philadelphia, PA: Hanley Belfus Inc.; 2003:305

[196] Thompson G. Financial resources for persons with an ostomy. CAET J. 1999; 18:7–16

[197] Tucker SB, Smith DB. Dermatologic conditions complicating ostomy care. In: Smith DB, Johnson DE, eds. Ostomy Care and the Cancer Patient. Orlando, FL: Grune & Stratton; 1986:139–153

[198] Canadian Ostomy Assessment Guide. Peristomal Skin Guide. Ville St-Laurent: Canvatec 2000:4

[199] Brady E. Severe peristomal pyoderma gangrenosum: a case study. J Wound Ostomy Continence Nurs. 1999; 26(6):306–311

[200] Sibbald RG, Orsted H, Schultz GS, Coutts P, Keast D, International Wound Bed Preparation Advisory Board, Canadian Chronic Wound Advisory Board. Preparing the wound bed 2003: focus on infection and inflammation. Ostomy Wound Manage. 2003; 49(11):24–51

[201] Peyrin-Biroulet L, Van Assche G, Gómez-Ulloa D, et al. Systematic review of tumor necrosis factor antagonists in extraintestinal manifestations in inflammatory bowel disease. Clin Gastroenterol Hepatol. 2017; 15 (1):25–36.e27

[202] Barrie A, Regueiro M. Biologic therapy in the management of extraintestinal manifestations of inflammatory bowel disease. Inflamm Bowel Dis. 2007; 13 (11):1424–1429

[203] Kiran RP, O'Brien-Ermlich B, Achkar JP, Fazio VW, Delaney CP. Managment of peristomal pyoderma gangrenosum. Dis Colon Rectum. 2003; 48(7):1397–1403

[204] Vasilevsky CA, Gordon PH. Adenocarcinoma arising at the ileocutaneous junction occurring after proctocolectomy for ulcerative colitis. Br J Surg. 1986; 73(5):378

[205] Starke J, Rodriguez-Bigas M, Marshall W, Sohrabi A, Petrelli NJ. Primary adenocarcinoma arising in an ileostomy. Surgery. 1993; 114(1):125–128

[206] Iizuka T, Sawada T, Hayakawa K, Hashimoto M, Udagawa H, Watanabe G. Successful local excision of ileostomy adenocarcinoma after colectomy for familial adenomatous polyposis: report of a case. Surg Today. 2002; 32 (7):638–641

[207] Shibuya T, Uchiyama K, Kokuma M, et al. Metachronous adenocarcinoma occurring at a colostomy site after abdominoperineal resection for rectal carcinoma. J Gastroenterol. 2002; 37(5):387–390

[208] Carey PD, Suvarna SK, Baloch KG, Guillou PJ, Monson JR. Primary adenocarcinoma in an ileostomy: a late complication of surgery for ulcerative colitis. Surgery. 1993; 113(6):712–715

[209] Zmijewski HC. Sexual counseling by the ET nurse: if not you, then who? J Wound Ostomy Continence Nurs. 2002; 29(4):184–185

[210] Helman CG. The body image in health and disease: exploring patients' maps of body and self. Patient Educ Couns. 1995; 26(1–3):169–175

[211] Carlsson E. Body Composition and Quality of Life in Patients with IBD, Ileostomy and Short Bowel Syndrome. Tryckt av Intellect Docusys; 2003:36

[212] Karadağ A, Menteş BB, Uner A, Irkörücü O, Ayaz S, Ozkan S. Impact of stomatherapy on quality of life in patients with permanent colostomies or ileostomies. Int J Colorectal Dis. 2003; 18(3):234–238

[213] Karadağ A, Menteş BB, Ayaz S. Colostomy irrigation: results of 25 cases with particular reference to quality of life. J Clin Nurs. 2005; 14(4):479–485

33 Constipation

Rajeev Peravali and David G. Jayne

Abstract

Constipation is an age-old, global problem for which a variety of treatments have been tried. Patients, often young women, may be in distress for days and even weeks before having a bowel movement. The use of a great variety of different laxatives and/or suppositories, with or without the regular use of enemas, has become normal practice for many of these troubled patients. This chapter addresses constipation and its etiology, investigation, diagnosis, and treatment.

Keywords: constipation, etiology, diagnosis, surgical treatment, medical treatment, biofeedback, diet, laxatives, colonic inertia, defecography

33.1 Introduction

Constipation is an age-old and worldwide problem for which a variety of treatments have been tried. In ancient times, the Chinese technique for treating constipation consisted of massaging the abdomen with wooden rollers. Today patients, often young women, may be in distress for days and even weeks before having a bowel movement. The use of a great variety of different laxatives and/or suppositories, with or without the regular use of enemas, has become normal practice for many of these troubled patients.

The perception of what constitutes a normal bowel habit varies widely among populations. The prevalence of constipation in the United Kingdom, defined by Rome II criteria, has been estimated at 8.2%.[1] In another UK survey, 39% of men and 52% of women reported straining at stool on more than one in four occasions.[2] The prevalence of chronic constipation in the United States varies from 2 to 28%.[3,4,5,6,7,8]

33.2 Definition

Constipation is a symptom. The meaning differs between patients and also between different cultures and regions. In a Swedish population study, it was found that a need to take laxatives was the most common manifestation of constipation (57% of respondents). In the same study, women (41%) were twice as likely as men (21%) to regard infrequent bowel motions as representing constipation, whereas equal proportions of men and women regarded hard stools (43%), straining during bowel movements (24%), and pain when passing a motion (23%) as being symptomatic.[9,10,11,12,13,14,15,16] Due to this ambiguity, an international panel of experts developed the Rome definition. The most current Rome III definition is shown in ▶ Table 33.1.

Table 33.1 Rome III criteria for functional constipation

General criteria

- Constipation for at least 3 mo during a period of 6 mo
- Specific criteria apply to at least one out of every four defecations.
- Insufficient criteria for inflammatory bowel syndrome
- No stools, or rarely loose stools

Specific criteria (two or more present)

- Straining
- Lumpy or hard stools
- Feeling of incomplete evacuation
- Sensation of anorectal blockade or obstruction
- Manual or digital maneuvers applied to facilitate defecation
- Fewer than three defecations per week

Probert et al[2] compared a validated estimate of the whole gut transit time with self-perceived constipation and the "Rome" definition and found little agreement between the definitions. Of 101 women classified as constipated by one or both of the subjective definitions, 64 had normal transit times. Based on these and other data, the authors questioned the validity of the "Rome" definition and any other definition based on individual's perceptions, except for infrequency of defecation. Many individuals perceive themselves as constipated, only because they have straining and incomplete evacuation. These symptoms also occur in irritable bowel syndrome. Therefore, it seems reasonable to use stool frequency as a clinical guide. Drossman et al[11] surveyed 789 students and hospital employees and found that 4.2% passed two or fewer stools per week. At present, some use the term constipation exclusively for the description of slow colonic transit, resulting in a stool frequency of fewer than two times per week and reserve the term disturbed or obstructed defecation for all the symptoms associated with impaired evacuation. Devroede[17] believes that a patient should be considered constipated under any of the following circumstances: (1) if the stool weight is less than 35 g/day; (2) if fewer than three stools for women and five for men are passed per week while following a high residue diet (30 g of dietary fiber); or (3) if more than 3 days pass without a bowel movement. Agachan et al[18] developed a constipation scoring system based on the following aspects: stool frequency, evacuation difficulties, abdominal pain, time spent in the lavatory per attempt, assistance required for evacuation, number of unsuccessful attempts per 24 hours, and duration of constipation. This system can be quite useful for both clinical and research purposes.

33.3 Etiology

The causes of constipation are numerous and diverse. Various classifications have been described.[19,20,21] The classification presented in Box 33.1, although not exhaustive, is fairly comprehensive.

Box 33.1 Classification of Causes of Constipation

- Mechanical obstruction:
  - Colorectal tumor
  - Diverticulosis
  - Strictures
  - External compression from tumor/other
  - Large rectocele
  - Megacolon
  - Postsurgical abnormalities
  - Anal fissure
- Neurological disorders/neuropath:
  - Autonomic neuropathy
  - Cerebrovascular disease
  - Cognitive impairment/dementia
  - Depression
  - Multiple sclerosis
  - Parkinson disease
  - Spinal cord pathology
- Endocrine/metabolic conditions:
  - Chronic kidney disease
  - Dehydration
  - Diabetes mellitus
  - Heavy metal poisoning
  - Hypercalcemia
  - Hypermagnesemia
  - Hyperparathyroidism
  - Hypokalemia
  - Hypomagnesemia
  - Hypothyroidism
  - Multiple endocrine neoplasia II
  - Porphyria
  - Uremia
- Gastrointestinal disorders and local painful conditions:
  - Irritable bowel syndrome
  - Abscess
  - Anal fissure
  - Fistula
  - Hemorrhoids
  - Levator ani syndrome
  - Megacolon
  - Proctalgia fugax
  - Rectal prolapse
  - Rectocele
  - Volvulus
- Myopathy:
  - Amyloidosis
  - Dermatomyositis
  - Scleroderma
  - Systemic sclerosis
- Dietary:
  - Dieting
  - Fluid depletion
  - Low fiber
  - Anorexia, dementia, depression
- Prescription drugs
  - Antidepressants
  - Antiepileptics
  - Antihistamines
  - Antiparkinson drugs
  - Antipsychotics
  - Antispasmodics
  - Calcium-channel blockers
  - Diuretics
  - Monoamine oxidase inhibitors
  - Opiates
  - Sympathomimetics
  - Tricyclic antidepressants

33.3.1 Diet and Habits

Of outstanding importance are the epidemiologic studies of Burkitt, Painter, Walker, and others,[21,22,23] which have shown that the fiber content of our foodstuffs is the prime factor that determines the fecal weight or bulk and the rate of transit through the colon. Inadequate dietary fiber, common in the Western diet, produces sparse, inspissated stools, whereas populations with a high fiber diet may have a normal bowel habit of two or three large, soft motions per day.[24] Because peristaltic movements are stimulated by distention of the intestine, they tend to be sluggish when the food bulk is insufficient to cause a normal amount of distention. Excessive ingestion of foods that harden stools, such as processed cheese, and inadequate fluid intake may be contributing factors. Lack of exercise also decreases colonic activity.

Repeatedly ignoring the call to stool results in insensitivity of the reflex initiated by a fecal mass in the rectum. This in turn results in adaptation of the sensory mechanism so that arrival of further propulsive waves fails to produce an adequate call to stool. Ultimately, all natural periodic urges disappear.

There is often a perception by patients that a daily bowel movement is necessary for good health. This belief may lead to the chronic abuse of harsh laxatives. After the bowel has been completely emptied by a purgative, it generally takes 2 days for fecal material to accumulate in sufficient quantity to stimulate the desire for a bowel action. Although this may seem self-evident, the absence of a bowel movement often increases the distress of a patient whose attention is focused on his or her bowel function. Further purgation (because of the failure to have a bowel movement the very next day) will unnecessarily abuse the intestine and ultimately lead to a complete loss of natural bowel habits (cathartic colon).

Environmental circumstances such as unfavorable working conditions, travel, and admission to hospital may cause the patient to ignore the call to stool. Some are obviously only temporary problems.

33.3.2 Structural or Functional Disorders

Constipation may be only one of several symptoms with which a patient with disorders of bowel structure will present. Constipation in association with other symptoms will lead the examining physician to the appropriate diagnosis, often with the aid of certain investigative modalities. Clearly, obstructive lesions explain constipation, but patients with these lesions may have alternating constipation and diarrhea. Similarly, individuals with painful anal lesions suppress the call to stool because of the fear of the pain of defecation. This suppression aggravates the problem because the stool becomes harder and more difficult to pass (a detailed discussion of each cause in this section is provided under the specific heading either later in this chapter or in relevant chapters).

Through the use of radiopaque markers, a slow transit rate —particularly along the transverse, descending, and sigmoid colon—can be demonstrated. Its exact cause is unclear. Patients with idiopathic megabowel have a dilated rectum or distal colon, but ganglion cells are present. Transit studies can also show abnormalities. Patients with irritable bowel syndrome have the dominant complaint of abdominal pain, with constipation only an associated finding in those with constipation-predominant disease. Constipation is not an uncommon symptom associated with diverticular disease and may result from the tendency of the colon to form closed high-pressure segments. Aganglionosis, whether it occurs congenitally in patients with Hirschsprung's disease or is acquired because of the neurotoxin of *Trypanosoma cruzi*, will cause constipation.

33.3.3 Neurologic Abnormalities

Defects of innervation such as those that follow pelvic surgery and occur with diseases of the spinal cord and brain are factors contributing to constipation. Severe constipation occurs in all patients who sustain a spinal cord injury. Menardo et al[25] and Levi et al[26] demonstrated that patients with injuries between C4 and T12 have a marked prolongation of transit at the level of the left colon and rectum, with minor degrees of transit delay at the level of the right colon. Several surveys have revealed that constipation in patients with spinal cord injury has a significant impact on their quality of life.[27,28]

33.3.4 Psychiatric Disorders

Psychiatric disturbances are often associated with constipation. However, the medications used in the treatment of psychiatric illnesses very frequently contribute to or cause constipation in their own right. Some patients may become obsessed with their bowel function or lack thereof and resort to excessive laxative abuse. In addition, certain psychiatric patients will deny bowel actions while, in fact, their bowels are moving. Such patients can be detected with the use of radiopaque markers.

33.3.5 Iatrogenic Causes

A host of medications can contribute to constipation (frequent offenders are listed in Box 33.1). Bedpans are uncomfortable and should be replaced by bedside commodes whenever feasible.

33.3.6 Endocrine and Metabolic Causes

Patients with various endocrine abnormalities with their characteristic clinical patterns may experience constipation. Also included in this group are those patients who are pregnant.

33.4 Investigation

33.4.1 Patient Evaluation

Clinical history and examination is the starting point of evaluation, and in many cases can differentiate slow transit constipation from obstructed defecation, although these subtypes coexist. Attention should be paid to any causative factors and "alarm" symptoms must be excluded.

> **Red Flags**
>
> - Heme-positive stool
> - Iron-deficiency anemia
> - Patients older than 50 years with no previous colon cancer screening
> - Recent onset of constipation
> - Rectal bleeding
> - Weight loss

33.4.2 History

Stool Frequency

When a patient has two or fewer bowel actions a week, the diagnosis of constipation is considered. The question is whether the reported stool frequency is reliable enough to diagnose constipation. Ashraf et al[28] investigated 45 patients complaining of infrequent defecation with fewer than two bowel actions weekly and found a striking discrepancy between the reported stool frequencies on the one hand and objective measures on the other hand. More than half of the patients who professed constipation were found to have underestimated stool frequency by three or more bowel actions weekly. In this group, a past history of psychiatric problems was common, and bowel symptoms correlated poorly with colonic transit time.

Stool Consistency

This is an indicator of colonic transit and can be classified with the use of a reference chart, such as the Bristol Stool Chart that categorizes stool consistency into seven subtypes (▶ Fig. 33.1).

Symptom Onset

Onset of symptoms is important because onset in childhood may point to a congenital cause such as Hirschsprung's disease, whereas a more recent onset might point to one of the specific disorders of bowel structure. A recent onset in an adult, especially with blood loss and mucus, is more commonly associated with significant colorectal pathology.

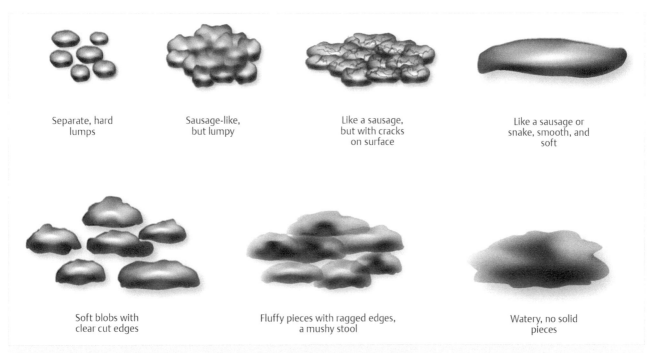

Separate, hard lumps

Sausage-like, but lumpy

Like a sausage, but with cracks on surface

Like a sausage or snake, smooth, and soft

Soft blobs with clear cut edges

Fluffy pieces with ragged edges, a mushy stool

Watery, no solid pieces

Fig. 33.1 Bristol Stool Scale.[29] (Adapted with permission from Taylor and Francis; © 1997.)

Other Specific Questions

Specific questions about dietary and bowel habits, laxative ingestion, other associated symptoms, and prior abdominal or pelvic surgery may lead to the correct diagnosis. Characteristic symptoms such as prolonged and repeated straining at stool, rectal fullness, sense of incomplete evacuation, and necessity for manual assistance may suggest a defecation disorder.

33.4.3 Physical Examination

In most patients with constipation, abdominal findings will be unremarkable. A stool-filled colon may be palpated. Rarely, a mass suggestive of a carcinoma or hepatomegaly suggestive of metastases may be found.

The anal region should be inspected carefully for findings such as fissures, hemorrhoids, fistulas, and abscesses. Digital examination might reveal a mass suggestive of a rectal neoplasm or a fecaloma. In female patients with a rectocele, the pocket-like defect of the anterior rectal wall can be demonstrated just above the anal sphincter. Almy[30] pointed out that the absence of stool in the rectum suggests that the difficulty lies above the rectum and makes a disorder of defecation unlikely. This observation is not valid if the patient is using laxatives, enemas, or suppositories.

Anal sensitivity and reflexes should be checked. Deficient sensation may represent a neurogenic disorder and cutaneosphincteric reflexes may be absent. In patients with Hirschsprung's disease, profuse fecal discharge occurs characteristically after rectal examination.

33.4.4 Stool Examination

Gross examination of the stool might reveal a large, hard mass or possibly the pellet-like stools characteristically seen in patients with diverticular disease or irritable bowel syndrome. Stool also should be examined for occult blood, and any positive findings should be investigated further. It has been suggested that determination of stool weight and examination of stool form are mandatory in the evaluation of constipation, because both aspects are closely correlated with colonic transit time, but this is rarely practical within the normal clinic setting.[28,31]

33.4.5 Biochemical Examination

Routine biochemical examination, including values for electrolytes, calcium, phosphate, urea, creatinine, thyroid stimulating hormone, and free thyroxine, is necessary to exclude those endocrine and metabolic disorders that can cause constipation.

Special biochemical investigations such as of gastrointestinal neuropeptides are of interest, but they are not readily available. Interest has grown in the effect of these neuropeptides on gastrointestinal motility. Using sensitive and specific radioimmunoassays, the concentration of gastrointestinal neuropeptides can be determined quantitatively.[32] The effect of these neuropeptides on the motor activity of the upper gastrointestinal tract (stomach, duodenum, and small intestine) has been established,[32] but the exact role of some of these peptides in the regulation of colonic motor activity has not been determined (▶ Table 33.2).

It has been suggested that gastrin and motilin have a stimulating effect on the peristaltic activity of the colon.[32] Patients with constipation have a smaller rise in circulating blood levels of gastrin and motilin after a meal,[33] whereas reduced motilin levels have been reported in pregnancy, when there is a tendency toward constipation.[34] However, it is still unknown whether or not these phenomena are primary or secondary. The pharmacokinetics, catabolism, and release of these hormones are very complex. For example, the release of vasoactive intestinal peptide (VIP) from intramural neurons, especially those neurons in the lamina propria and circular muscle of the gut, is induced by stimulation of preganglionic parasympathetic fibers.[32] This finding demonstrates the complex interaction between hormonal and neurogenic factors. Further investigation is necessary to determine the exact role of gastrointestinal hormones, especially in patients with slow-transit constipation.

Table 33.2 Effect of gastrointestinal neuropeptides on colonic motility

In vivo effect	Gastrointestinal neuropeptides
Stimulation	Gastrin
	Motilin
	Cholecystokinin
	Oxytocin
	Corticotropin releasing factor
	Neuropeptide Y
	Serotonin
Inhibitors	Glucagon
	Somatostatin
	Secretin
	Calcitonin gene-related peptide
	Enkephalins
	Peptide YY
Unknown	Galanin
	Gastrin-releasing polypeptide (VIP)
	Neurotensin
	Substance P
	Bombesin
None	Gastric inhibitory polypeptide
	Pancreatic polypeptide

33.4.6 Proctosigmoidoscopy

Endoscopic examination is mandatory to rule out the presence of a neoplasm. Nevertheless, in the vast majority of patients complaining of constipation, proctosigmoidoscopic examination will not reveal any abnormality. Frequently, patients with long-standing laxative abuse, mainly involving laxative ingredients of the anthracene family, will demonstrate melanosis coli—a discoloration of the mucosa that may range from light brown to black. In other patients, a solitary rectal ulcer, sometimes associated with anterior mucosal prolapse, will be found.

33.4.7 Luminal Imaging

Although plain films of the abdomen occasionally show the extent of fecal accumulation, the main diagnostic tool to demonstrate structural abnormalities in the colon is colonoscopy, which has the advantage over other modalities in obtaining mucosa imaging and biopsy for histological analysis. Contrast studies, such as barium enema, are largely obsolete and have been surpassed by CT colonography as the preferred radiological imaging technique, although it is generally reserved for patients who are unfit or unable to tolerate colonoscopic examination.

33.4.8 Defecating Proctogram

Defecography or evacuation proctography is an established radiologic technique to image the dynamic changes in rectal anatomy during expulsion of barium paste (▶ Fig. 33.2). This

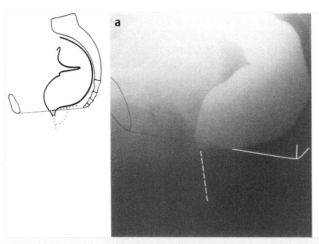
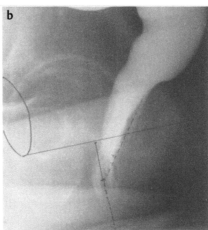
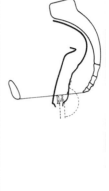

Fig. 33.2 Defecography in a normal patient. **(a)** At rest, X-ray film and diagram showing a normal anorectal angle of 92 degrees. **(b)** During straining, X-ray film and diagram showing anorectal angle widens to 137 degrees.

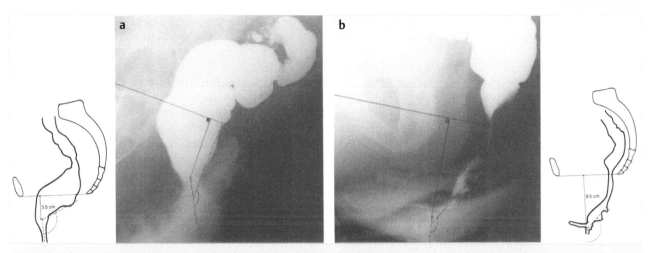

Fig. 33.3 Defecography in an incontinent patient. **(a)** At rest, loss of anorectal angle and widening of anal canal, pool of barium escaping beyond anal sphincter, and pathologic descent of perineum (anus well below pubococcygeal line) are noted. **(b)** During straining.

method offers the possibility of visualizing abnormalities such as anterior rectal wall prolapse, rectal intussusception, rectocele, and enterocele.[35,36] It also allows measurement of the anorectal angle, which is determined by the tone of the puborectalis and levator ani muscles. The angle becomes more obtuse during attempted evacuation due to relaxation of the pelvic floor. Failure to increase the anorectal angle on straining, sometimes associated with accentuation of the puborectalis impression, is considered a radiologic sign of anismus. In patients with fecal incontinence, the anorectal angle may be widened even at rest (▶ Fig. 33.3). It has been argued, however, that visual assessment of the anorectal angle is rather subjective and, therefore, unreliable. Several authors found wide interobserver and intraobserver variations in the measurement of this angle and concluded that its quantification has only limited clinical value.[37,38] Defecography also enables the determination of the position of the pelvic floor by calculating the distance between the anorectal junction and the pubococcygeal line. Demonstrating a drop in the anorectal junction of several centimeters or more below the pubococcygeal line signifies the pathologic descent of the pelvic floor. Evacuation proctography also provides a valid estimate of the rate and degree of rectal emptying.[39] These parameters can also be assessed utilizing scintigraphic methods.[40] The investigation of rectal emptying is considered a major step in the evaluation of constipation, because many patients with infrequent bowel movements also present varying degrees of defecatory impairment. It has been argued, however, that the estimation of time and degree of rectal emptying is rather inaccurate.[41] Furthermore, it is questionable whether a delayed and incomplete evacuation on proctography really represents impaired rectal emptying. Karlbom et al[42] analyzed the relations between proctography findings, rectal emptying, and colonic transit time in 80 constipated patients. The correlation between a sense of obstruction and rectal evacuation as evaluated by defecography was found to be very poor. Patients who claimed emptying difficulties actually had the most efficient evacuation. It has also been suggested that incomplete and prolonged evacuation on proctography may be caused by inability to raise intra-abdominal pressure, thereby simply reflecting inadequate straining.[43] Despite these and other objections, evacuation

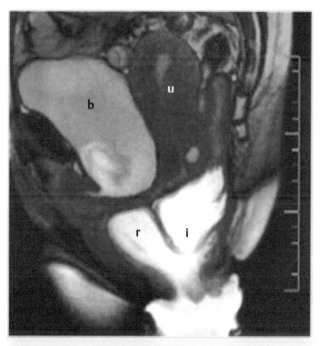

Fig. 33.4 Defecating MRI demonstrating bladder (b), uterus (u), rectocele (r), and intussusception (i).

proctography is still considered as one of the most useful tools in the investigation of patients with constipation and disturbed defecation.

33.4.9 Magnetic Resonance Proctography

More recently, MR proctography has gained popularity as an effective method for evaluating dynamic pelvic floor function (▶ Fig. 33.4). The main advantage over barium proctography is that it does not involve radiation exposure. It makes visualization of the bony landmarks easier and therefore the measurement of anorectal and pelvic floor movements during straining more accurate. Importantly, it allows visualization of the whole pelvis, including the bladder and uterus. It can provide useful information on extrarectal lesions that might cause constipation. It is becoming the investigation of choice in patients with multicompartmental pelvic floor dysfunction.

33.4.10 Colonic Transit Time

A major step in the evaluation of constipation is the measurement of colonic transit time. The technique can establish an abnormality but also can demonstrate a normal transit time in a patient with a bowel neurosis or in the occasional patient who denies having bowel actions. With the original method described by Hinton et al,[44] 20 radiopaque markers of similar specific gravity to feces were ingested on one occasion on the first day before breakfast. Stools were collected and studied with radiography for 7 days or longer until all the pellets had been observed on a radiograph. A variation of this method has been described by Cummings and Wiggins.[45] Markers of different shapes were ingested on three consecutive days. Subsequently, all markers present in a single stool collected on the fourth day were counted. This technique reduces the effect of day-to-day variation in transit time by providing 3-day transit studies from one radiograph. Although these marker-appearance methods do not provide accurate data on transit through the different colonic regions, they can be used as a simple test to assess whole-gut transit time. With the Hinton technique, Evans et al[46] found that 95% of normal male and female individuals pass less than 20% of markers within 12 hours and more than 80% of markers within 120 hours. This finding was similar to the original observation of Hinton et al[44] in male individuals. It has been argued that it is more convenient to measure the disappearance of a marker from the colon rather than its appearance in the stool. Therefore, Martelli et al[47] described a technique whereby the patient ingests a single dose of 20 markers. The progression of the markers is followed by daily films of the abdomen until complete expulsion is noted or for a maximum of 7 days after ingestion of the markers. Normally all the markers have passed within 7 days. The arrival and disappearance of markers in three regions of the colon (right, left, and rectosigmoid) are assessed. For this purpose, the spinal processes and two lines from the fifth lumbar vertebra to the pelvic inlet serve as landmarks (▶ Fig. 33.5). Transit time is considered prolonged when more than 20% of the markers are still present within the colon, 5 days after ingestion. A drawback of interpretation of such studies is that evaluation of transit of contents in any segment is dependent on the amount of markers received from the proximal bowel. To reduce the radiation exposure, Metcalf et al[48] developed a somewhat different technique by giving differently shaped markers on three successive days and taking an abdominal radiograph on the fourth day after ingestion and if necessary on days 7 and 10. Chaussade et al[49] modified this technique by giving identical markers on three consecutive days. The quantification of regional colonic transit with these methods has been validated in healthy individuals. It is questionable, however, whether infrequent radiographs allow correct assessment of the site of delay in constipated patients with irregular mass movements, because the results will be very different if a radiograph is

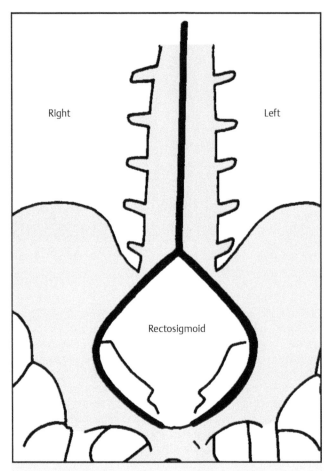

Fig. 33.5 Landmarks for markers used to determine transit time.

taken just before or just after such an event. It has been suggested that the use of radioisotopes provides more accurate information about regional colonic transit, because multiple images can be obtained with a low radiation dose. An additional advantage of scintigraphy is the clear delineation of the different colonic regions, even in patients with a significant overlap of bowel segments. The use of a radiolabeled meal also yields information about gastric emptying and small bowel transit.[50] The radioisotope can also be administered in a coated capsule, which is designed to dissolve at the pH found in the distal part of the small bowel,[51] or as a liquid through a tube placed to instill it in the cecum or the ascending colon.[52]

Another technique to measure intestinal transit was developed by Ewe et al.[53] They followed a metal particle on its way through the gastrointestinal tract by means of a portable detector. Basile et al[54] used a magnetized steel sphere and localized this particle with biomagnetic instruments. With this technique they were able to demonstrate that the total colonic transit time in healthy volunteers was 44 ± 5 hours (mean ±SD). Similar figures have been reported by others. The normal values for whole-gut transit time, total colonic transit time, and segmental colonic transit time are listed in ▶ Table 33.3, ▶ Table 33.4, and ▶ Table 33.5.

Table 33.3 Normal values for whole-gut transit time, expressed in hours

Authors	No. of subjects	Method	Mean ± SD	Upper limit
Cummings and Wiggins[45]	12	Radiopaque markers	54 ± 9	72
Metcalf et al[48]	21	Radiopaque markers	53 ± 8	70
Evans et al[46]	43	Radiopaque markers	120 ± NS	168
Basile et al[54]	12	Magnetic markers	56 ± 5	NS
van der Sijp et al[50]	12	Radioisotopes	NS	103

Abbreviations: SD, standard deviation; NS, not stated.

Table 33.4 Normal values for total colonic transit time, expressed in hours

Authors	No. of subjects	Method	Sex	Mean ± SD	Upper limit
Arhan et al[55]	38	Radiopaque markers		39 ± 5	93
Metcalf et al[48]	73	Radiopaque markers	Male	31 ± 18	66
			Female	39 ± 18	75
Chaussade et al[49]	22	Radiopaque markers		34 ± 16	67
Meir et al[57]	128	Radiopaque markers	Male	30 ± 2	44
			Female	41 ± 3	77
Basile et al[54]	12	Magnetic markers		44 ± 5	NS
Escalante et al[58]	18	Radiopaque markers		28 ± NS	NS
Danquechin Dorval et al[59]	82	Radiopaque markers	Male	25 ± NS	77
			Female	47 ± NS	91
Bouchoucha et al[60]	11	Radiopaque markers		36 ± 3	NS

Table 33.5 Normal values of segmental colonic transit time, expressed in hours

Authors	No. of subjects	Sex	Right colon	Left colon	Rectosigmoid
Arhan et al[55]	38		14	14	11
Metcalf et al[48]	73	Male	9	9	13
		Female	13	14	12
Chaussade et al[56]	22		7	9	18
Basile et al[54]	12		27	15	12
Escalante et al[58]	18		7	10	11
Danquechin Dorval et al[59]	82		8	13	12
		Male	7	8	8
		Female	10	21	17
Bouchoucha et al[60]	11		7	16	14

A relatively simple method for assessing colonic transit is using the Sitzmarks (Konsyl Pharmaceuticals, Texas) method. A single Sitzmarks capsule containing 24 radiopaque markers is taken on day 0 by mouth with water and a plain abdominal X-ray is taken on day 5 (▶ Fig. 33.6). The patient is instructed to refrain from laxatives, enemas, or suppositories for 5 days. Patients who expel at least 80% of the markers have grossly normal transit. For patients who have more than 20% of markers remaining a further capsule is given along with a bulking agent and a further X-ray is performed at day 10 to determine the location and extent of the markers. If the markers are scattered throughout the colon, slow transit is suggested. If most of the markers are gathered in the rectosigmoid, a functional outlet obstruction may be present.

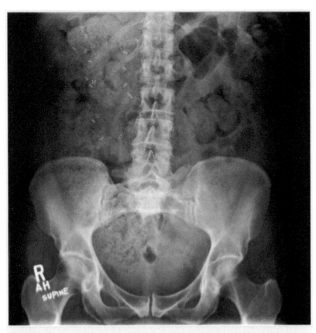

Fig. 33.6 Colonic transit study demonstrating numerous retained markers in the right colon on day 5 in keeping with slow transit constipation.

33.4.11 Anorectal Manometry

A number of authors advocate the use of anorectal manometry during the initial evaluation of constipation and disturbed defecation to develop individualized and more effective modes of treatment.[61,62]

In patients with Hirschsprung's disease, rectal distention does not induce internal sphincter relaxation. This is referred to as the rectoanal inhibitory reflex (RAIR). Absence of RAIR response to rectal distension is a reliable test in the diagnosis of Hirschsprung's disease.[63,64] Although manometry is clearly useful in discriminating Hirschsprung's disease from other forms of constipation, its role in the evaluation and management of non-Hirschsprung's constipation remains unclear. There are few data correlating manometric findings with clinical symptoms and outcome of treatment. Studying encopretic children, Loening-Baucke et al[63] demonstrated that the response to different treatment modalities could be predicted by manometric findings. Borowitz et al[65] studied 44 children with chronic constipation and encopresis. Spasm of the external anal sphincter during attempted defecation was correlated with the patient's age at onset and duration of symptoms, but manometric findings were not predictive of the ability to defecate. They also questioned the conceptual understanding of childhood constipation, based on the assumption that a diminished sense of rectal distention and paradoxical contraction of the external anal sphincter are the principal causes of constipation and obstructed defecation. In adults, similar conflicting findings have been observed. Pluta et al[66] studied 24 female patients with severe and disabling slow-transit constipation who underwent a subtotal colectomy followed by ileorectal anastomosis. No correlation was noted between the results of the operation and the manometric parameters, except in one case. Patients requiring

abnormally high pressures inside a distending rectal balloon for sensory perception and internal anal sphincter relaxation did worse than the others. Another striking predictive factor, noted by these authors, was a history of psychiatric illness.

Many demonstrable pressure abnormalities can be detected by anorectal manometry in patients with idiopathic constipation. The reflex may be normal, the amplitude of relaxation may be less than that in normal controls, or the reflex may be totally absent. The resting pressure of the anal canal may be greater than expected and occasionally is accompanied by a rectoanal inhibitory reflex with an amplitude greater than normal.[67]

In several studies, elevated anal resting pressures have been found in patients with idiopathic constipation, but in other studies no pressure abnormalities could be detected. Although some authors suggested a normal amplitude of the internal sphincter reflex, these findings are not supported by the results of two other studies that showed the amplitude of relaxation is less in patients with idiopathic constipation than in normal controls. In patients with severe chronic constipation without megarectum, the threshold for the internal sphincter reflex apparently was normal, whereas in patients with a megarectum the threshold was elevated.

Despite the conflicting published data, manometry should continue as part of the evaluation of the severely constipated patient. Only by the continued study of these patients will there be a resolution of the discrepancies that have been reported to date.

During the last decade, attention has been focused on rectal wall properties. Grotz et al investigated rectal wall contractility in controls and in patients with chronic severe constipation. They found that in patients with constipation, the increase in rectal tone following a meal and after the administration of a cholinergic agonist was significantly blunted. According to these authors, the reduced rectal tone contributes to the inability of these patients to expel stool.[68] Other workers from the Netherlands used an electronic barostat assembly to examine rectal tone in response to an evoked urge to defecate. Under radiological control, an infinitely compliant polyethylene bag was inserted over a guide wire into the proximal part of the rectum. Additionally, a latex balloon was introduced into the distal part of the rectum. This latex balloon was inflated until an urge to defecate was experienced. Simultaneously, rectal wall tone was assessed by measuring the variations in bag volume. These variations were expressed as percentage changes from the baseline volume. Comparing female controls and women with obstructed defecation, a significant difference was found regarding mean distending volume required to elicit an urge to defecate (median values: 125 vs. 320 mL of air). Twenty-four patients (24%) did not feel an urge to defecate at all. In all controls, the evocation of an urge to defecate induced a pronounced increase in rectal tone, proximal to the distending balloon. In symptomatic patients, this increase in rectal tone was significantly lower. Thirty-one patients (31%) showed no increase in rectal tone at all.[69] It has been shown that rectal tone increases after a meal. This phenomenon is absent or blunted in women with obstructed defecation.[70] These data indicate that the sensorimotor function of the rectum is impaired in patients with obstructed defecation. Afferent parasympathetic nerves are thought to mediate rectal filling sensations. These nerves run from the rectum through branches, which are situated on each side of the rectum around the cervix uteri and both lateral vaginal surfaces. This extensive network of nerve fibers can be damaged during hysterectomy and also during rectopexy with division of the lateral ligaments. It is well known that in some women, obstructed defecation starts following pelvic surgery. Varma and Smith studied rectal function in 14 women with intractable constipation following hysterectomy. These patients had significantly decreased rectal sensory perception.[71] It has been shown that constipation occurs more frequently the more radical a hysterectomy is performed.[72] Based on an experimental study in dogs, Shafik et al addressed the important role of the parasympathetic nervous system in the defecation mechanism.[73] These and other data do suggest that a deficit of the afferent parasympathetic nerves contributes to the impaired sensorimotor function of the rectum in women with obstructed defecation.

33.4.12 Electromyography

Electromyography (EMG) can be used as a functional test for the investigation of muscle activity and is a reliable method for the evaluation of electrical activity in the external anal sphincter and puborectalis muscles (Chapter 2).[74]

Through electrophysiologic techniques it has been shown that damage can occur to the nerve supply of the external sphincter and the puborectalis muscle in patients with chronic constipation; this damage is probably due to perineal descent during defecation straining.[75] Paradoxical contraction of the pelvic floor during attempted evacuation is considered as the principal cause of functional obstructed defecation, that is, obstructed defecation not associated with a structural abnormality. The terms most frequently used to describe this condition are anismus, spastic pelvic floor syndrome, and nonrelaxing puborectalis syndrome. Despite many limitations, EMG is probably the most specific test providing the best assessment of pelvic floor activity during straining (▶ Fig. 2.29).

33.4.13 Balloon Expulsion Test

The balloon expulsion test is another method commonly used to reach the diagnosis of anismus. This simple test was introduced by Preston and Lennard-Jones in 1985.[76] It has been reported that almost all controls are able to expel a water-filled rectal balloon, whereas many constipated patients fail to do so. Although this observation underscores the difference between controls and patients, it does not signify that the inability to expel a balloon represents anismus. Normal rectal evacuation requires adequate intrarectal pressure, which can be raised by increasing intrapelvic pressure, achieved by voluntary contraction of the diaphragm and abdominal wall muscles. Propulsive contractile activity of the rectal wall is another contributing factor. It has been reported that constipated patients with both prolonged evacuation and pelvic floor descent on proctography are not able to void a small nondeformable rectal balloon because they fail to raise intrarectal pressure.[77] This finding suggests that failure to raise intrapelvic pressure is a major cause of inadequate evacuation.

The aforementioned diagnostic tests are generally recommended, because it is difficult to differentiate subgroups of constipation based on symptoms alone. Despite this recommendation,

the clinical utility of these tests is still not known. Recently, Rao et al conducted a systematic review of studies assessing the clinical value of these tests in patients with constipation. Their search revealed no methodologically sound studies, and identified several pitfalls. First, no single test appears to provide a pathophysiological basis for constipation. Often, several tests are required to identify the underlying mechanism. Second, the inclusion criteria for patients with constipation were either not defined or when available there were significant interstudy differences. Third, a reference or gold standard test is still missing. Despite these pitfalls, the authors concluded that, "there is good evidence to support the use of these tests in order to define subtypes of constipation and aid treatment."[77]

33.4.14 Special Examinations

Routine Histologic Examination

In patients with solitary rectal ulcer syndrome, performing a biopsy is mandatory to confirm the diagnosis and exclude an underlying carcinoma. Histologic examination will reveal fibromuscular obliteration of the lamina propria, hypertrophy of the muscularis mucosa, and displacement of glands into the submucosa (▶ Fig. 33.7).[78,79]

When Hirschsprung's disease is suspected, a biopsy is indicated because, classically, aganglionosis is diagnostic of Hirschsprung's disease (▶ Fig. 33.8). There is no consensus as to whether the best biopsy technique is the superficial punch biopsy, deep full-thickness biopsy, or mucosal suction biopsy. Usually biopsy specimens are taken 2 to 3 cm above the dentate line, as recommended by Aldridge and Campbell,[80,81] who demonstrated a normal hypoganglionic zone in the region of the internal sphincter. This hypoganglionic zone extends proximally from the dentate line an average of 4 mm in the myenteric plexus, 7 mm in the deep submucous plexus, and 10 mm in the superficial submucous plexus. In two studies, it was suggested that the optimal level at which the biopsy should be taken is 1.0 to 1.5 cm above the dentate line.[81,82] The authors chose this lower range because taking rectal biopsy specimens at a higher level may result in a missed diagnosis of ultrashort-segment aganglionosis.[83] It is not certain how the measurements in these reports from pediatric patients might apply to the adult.

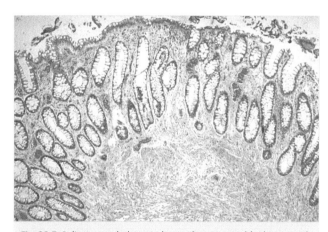

Fig. 33.7 Solitary rectal ulcer syndrome demonstrated by biopsy with thickened lamina propria.

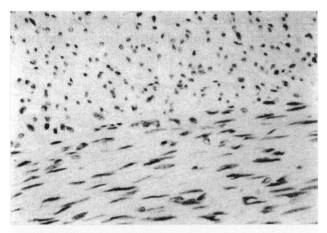

Fig. 33.8 Hirschsprung's disease.

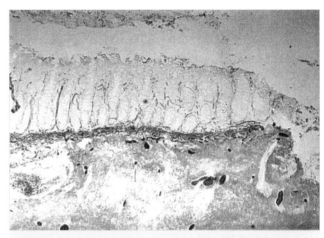

Fig. 33.9 Acetylcholinesterase staining used to demonstrate parasympathetic nerves. Note axon bundles with dark staining in center of microphotograph, with staining of small filaments in periphery.

Several difficulties arise in the histopathologic interpretation of biopsy specimens. First, the distal segment of bowel does not contain neurons for up to 25 mm from the distal edge of the internal sphincter, and the normal value for adults is unknown. Second, the severity of the clinical course correlates poorly with the length of the aganglionic segment. A third problem with the histopathologic interpretation lies in the potential existence of "skip" lesions. A fourth problem concerns the qualitative appearance of the nervous plexus. Fifth, although hypoganglionosis causes constipation, the range in the normal number of ganglion cells is not known.[84] Finally, the diagnostic accuracy with routine hematoxylin and eosin staining on superficial biopsies is low, as was demonstrated in a study showing an accuracy of only 61%.[82]

Ultrastructural studies of colonic biopsies from patients with a history of long-term laxative abuse, primarily involving anthraquinone derivatives or bisacodyl, indicated that submucosal nerve fibers might be severely damaged. These alterations may correlate morphologically to the clinically evident disturbance of gut motility.[85]

Acetylcholinesterase Staining

Increased acetylcholinesterase activity has been demonstrated in patients with Hirschsprung's disease.[86,87,88,89] With acetylcholinesterase staining, an increased number of enlarged, brown-stained nerve fibers can be found in either the submucosa or the lamina propria (▶ Fig. 33.9). According to Ikawa et al,[82] this technique has many advantages over routine hematoxylin and eosin staining. The authors demonstrated 99% accuracy in the differentiation of patients with Hirschsprung's disease from patients with idiopathic constipation. Park et al[90] demonstrated a 97% diagnostic accuracy compared with a 74% accuracy of hematoxylin and eosin staining. Routine hematoxylin and eosin staining of superficial biopsy specimens failed to reveal ganglion cells in 39% of their patients without Hirschsprung's disease, all of whom required repeat superficial biopsy studies or even deep full-thickness biopsies while under general anesthesia. Using acetylcholinesterase staining, this problem can be eliminated. Even if the submucosa is not included in the superficial biopsy, the diagnosis still can be made by studying the lamina propria. The

histochemical demonstration of acetylcholinesterase activity in suction rectal biopsy specimens is considered an accurate technique and has been recommended in screening for Hirschsprung's disease.[91]

Monoclonal Antineurofilament Antibodies

It has been proposed that a distinct visceral neuropathy may be present in patients with idiopathic slow-transit constipation and in patients with idiopathic megacolon. However, with the use of conventional light microscopy (hematoxylin and eosin staining), no abnormalities have been found. Examining resected colon specimens with silver staining (Smith's method), Preston et al[92] demonstrated complete loss of the argyrophil plexus with a marked increase in Schwann cells, indicating that extrinsic damage to the plexus had occurred. Based on these findings, the authors theorized that the myenteric plexus abnormality is not the primary cause but may be the result of long-standing laxative use. Using conventional light microscopy, Krishnamurthy et al[93] found no apparent abnormalities of the myenteric plexus in 12 patients who underwent subtotal colectomy for constipation. In contrast, silver stains of the myenteric plexus showed quantitatively reduced numbers of argyrophilic neurons in 10 patients, morphologically abnormal argyrophilic neurons in 11, decreased numbers of axons in 11, and increased numbers of variable-size nuclei within ganglia in all 12. Thus, severe idiopathic constipation is associated with a pathologically identifiable abnormality of the myenteric plexus.[93]

Koch et al[80] found decreased colonic VIP in patients with idiopathic chronic constipation. This finding could not be confirmed by Tzavella et al,[94] who found normal levels of VIP and decreased levels of the excitatory neurotransmitter substance P in rectal biopsies from patients with slow-transit constipation.

An immunostaining technique using monoclonal antibodies raised against neurofilament (NF2F11; Sanbio) has been described for the investigation of bowel innervation anomalies.[95] In the normally functioning bowel, some axons of the submucous plexus and the myenteric plexus do stain with these monoclonal antibodies (▶ Fig. 33.10a). In contrast to this subtotal (partial)

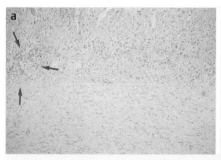 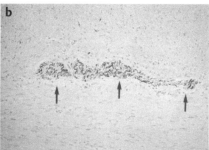 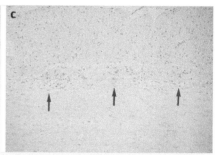

Fig. 33.10 Monoclonal antineurofilament antibody. **(a)** Normal subtotal staining of axonal fibers in myenteric plexus (*arrows*). **(b)** Hirschsprung's disease, deep stain (increased) in myenteric plexus (*arrows*). **(c)** Idiopathic slow-transit constipation: absence of staining in myenteric plexus (*arrows*).

staining in normal bowel, heavy total axon-bundle staining has been found in the aganglionic segment of patients with Hirschsprung's disease (▶ Fig. 33.10b).

Schouten et al[96] were able to demonstrate that in 29 out of 39 patients with slow-transit constipation, the apparently normal axon bundles in the myenteric plexus stained markedly less than normal or failed to stain at all with the monoclonal antibody. In 17 patients, this reduced or absent neurofilament expression was found along the entire length of the colon, whereas in 12 patients only a portion of the colon was affected. The same picture was found in the proximal ganglionic segment in 18 of 22 patients with persistent constipation after colectomy for aganglionosis (▶ Fig. 33.10c).[97]

Because intrinsic innervation is lacking in patients with Hirschsprung's disease, the stained axon bundles in the aganglionic segment can only be of extrinsic origin. Therefore, the lack of axonal staining in patients with constipation indicates a disturbed extrinsic innervation. It is unlikely that this is a secondary phenomenon caused by laxatives because the same condition was found in neonates with severe constipation who were never treated with laxatives. Two studies have revealed increased serotonin levels in the colonic mucosa and normal serotonin levels in the colonic muscularis propria of patients with slow-transit constipation.[98,99] The question is why colonic motility is reduced and transit is prolonged despite local high and normal serotonin levels. It has been suggested that abnormal expression of the serotonin receptors in the colonic wall contributes to colonic inertia. Recently, Zhao et al were able to demonstrate a reduced expression of serotonin receptors in the left colon of patients with this type of constipation.[100] Wedel et al compared the colonic enteric nervous system of patients with slow-transit constipation with the enteric nervous system of controls. They performed a morphometric analysis of the submucous plexus and the myenteric plexus. This analysis was based on Protein Gene Product 9.5 immunohistochemistry. In patients with slow-transit constipation, the total ganglionic area and neuronal number per intestinal length as well as the mean neuron count per ganglion were significantly decreased within the myenteric plexus and the external part of the submucous plexus. The ratio of glia cells to neurons was increased in myenteric ganglia but not in submucous ganglia. The observed quantitative alterations of the colonic enteric nervous system resemble the histologic features by oligoneuronal hypoganglionosis.[101] Two recent studies provide further evidence for these findings. Bassotti et al examined the

surgical specimens from 26 patients with slow-transit constipation. They used conventional and immunohistochemical methods. Comparing patients and controls they found a significant decrease in enteric neurons, glial cells, and interstitial cells of Cajal in the constipated patients.[102] Similar findings have been reported by Lee et al.[103] Although all these data provide evidence for the neuropathologic deficit in patients with slow-transit constipation, it is still not known whether these alterations of the colonic enteric nervous system are secondary to long-standing constipation or represent a primary defect.

33.4.15 Psychological Evaluation

The exact role of psychological factors as related to bowel function has not been defined clearly, but suggestions of such influence have been made. Tucker et al[104] suggested that stool weight and bowel frequency correlated with personality as much as with variations in fiber intake. Heavier stools tended to be produced by individuals who were more socially outgoing, more energetic and optimistic, and less anxious and who described themselves in more favorable terms than others. A common cause of withholding stool during childhood has been attributed to conflict between parent and child over bowel function.

It is well known that constipation and disturbed defecation occur primarily in women. It is still not clear why these conditions are characterized with such preponderance. One explanation might be the relationship between hysterectomy and changes in bowel habits. Another explanation for the female preponderance might be the fact that women are prone to develop a symptomatic rectocele. It is unlikely, however, that the adverse side effects of hysterectomy and the defecation difficulties due to rectoceles account for all the cases of constipation and disturbed defecation. It is well known that many patients use somatization as a defensive strategy for dealing with psychological distress. This unconscious defense mechanism can be uncovered by several psychological tests such as the Minnesota Multiphasic Personality Inventory (MMPI). In 1989, Devroede et al[105] used the MMPI to compare women with idiopathic (functional) constipation and women with arthritis. The authors reported that many constipated women demonstrated a "conversion V" profile pattern, which indicates the presence of a somatization defense structure. This finding has been confirmed by others.[106] In 1990, Drossman et al[107] demonstrated that a history of sexual and physical abuse is a frequent experience in women seen in a referral-based gastrointestinal practice and is particularly common in those with functional gastrointestinal disorders. Of 209 consecutive female patients, 89 (44%) reported a history of abuse, but only 17% had informed their physicians. This extremely high prevalence of a past history of sexual abuse is similar to that found by Leroi et al,[108] who reported that 40% of patients suffering from functional disorders of the lower gastrointestinal tract gave a history of having been victims of sexual abuse in contrast to only 10% of patients with organic disease. The prevalence was similar in private practice and university hospital settings. The most frequent symptom of abused patients was constipation. The prevalence of abuse was four times greater in patients with lower rather than upper functional motor disorders. The risk of having a history of sexual abuse was nine times greater among patients with manometric evidence of anismus. The clinical implications of these findings are noteworthy. Because the vast majority of abused patients do not report their hidden history, this type of information must be actively sought.

Dykes et al[109] performed a psychological enquiry among patients with chronic constipation. These patients were assessed for evidence of previous and current affective disorders. A previous episode of psychiatric illness was noted in 64% of the patients, whereas a current affective disorder was observed in 61% of the subjects. Based on these findings, the authors suggest that patients who present to surgical departments with chronic intractable constipation should routinely have a psychological assessment. It is well known that the vast majority of patients with constipation, especially those with a slow colonic transit, are women.[110] It has been suggested that aspects of female identity provide clues to the underlying nature of this condition. Mason et al conducted a study to examine possible emotional difficulties related to female identity in women with idiopathic constipation and compared the findings with an age-matched group of healthy women and with an age-matched group of women with Crohn's disease. Women with idiopathic constipation were found to have increased psychological and social morbidity, characterized by anxiety, depression, and social dysfunction. They also had increased somatization, less satisfaction in their sexual life, and an altered perception about female self.[111] It has been shown that this type of morbidity is associated with altered rectal mucosa blood flow, indicating autonomic dysfunction.[112] Chan et al observed defective use of coping strategies in patients with functional constipation. These differing coping mechanisms were reflected in an absent or blunted rectal sensory perception.[113] It has been shown that biofeedback alone is not successful in the treatment of abused patients with anismus.[114] The clinical outcome could be improved by adding psychotherapy to biofeedback conditioning.

Patients with mental illness are liable to the development of megacolon, and constipation may be a presenting symptom of a depressive illness. Patients with anorexia often develop intractable constipation, presumably caused in part by inadequate food intake. A patient may deny the passage of stool, although a transit study may demonstrate clearly that defecation actually has occurred. The denial of passage of stool emphasizes the need to obtain objective evidence of a prolonged transit time before any operative treatment is contemplated.

33.5 Why Treat Constipation?

33.5.1 Dispelling Myths

Patients must be reassured first that there is a wide variation of normality with regard to the frequency of bowel movements. The folklore and mythology associated with the need for daily evacuation must be dispelled. Advertising encourages self-purgation by making people feel guilty about constipation and by portraying daily bowel movements as the secret to a healthy and happy life. Erroneous concepts such as the belief that toxic substances may be absorbed into the body without a daily bowel movement must be cast aside.

33.5.2 Associated Symptoms and Daily Activity

Martelli et al[47] noted that constipation is not without associated symptoms and complications. The authors noted the disappearance of a multitude of symptoms after successful surgical treatment of constipation. Symptoms described included hard stools, stools difficult to evacuate, abdominal distention and bloating, and anorexia. Signs included fecalomas, abdominal masses, and abdominal tenderness. To this list, Thompson[115] added foul breath, furred tongue, flatulence, headache, and irritability. Regardless of the cause of constipation, absence of the numerous associated symptoms should allow the patient to function better in his usual daily activity.

33.5.3 Potential Disease

Although the immediate adverse effect of low-fiber diets may be constipation, the long-term adverse effects may include diverticular disease and malignancy, as noted in studies that link the low-fiber content of the usual Western diet with an increased risk of colon carcinoma and diverticulosis.[22] Three studies suggest the link between carcinoma and constipation.[116,117,118] More women with carcinoma of the colon had antecedent constipation than a comparable group of controls without constipation. More men with carcinoma of the rectum had a history of constipation. In a study by Wynder and Shigematsu,[118] having three stools per week for a long period of time was considered a risk factor. However, in a penetrating review, Cranston et al[119] examined the evidence linking dietary fiber to gastrointestinal disease. They noted that fiber increases stool weight, decreases whole-gut transit time, and lowers colonic intraluminal pressure. Although fiber may be of benefit in the treatment of constipation, irritable bowel syndrome, and diverticular disease, its role in the prevention or treatment of other gastrointestinal disease has not been established.

The most recent effort to evaluate the association between dietary fiber intake and risk of colorectal carcinoma was reported by Park et al.[120] From 13 prospective cohort studies included in the Pooling Project of Prospective Studies of Diet and Carcinoma, 725,628 men and women were followed up for up to 6 to 20 years across studies. In this large pooled analysis, dietary fiber intake was inversely associated with risk of colorectal carcinoma in age-adjusted analyses. However, after accounting for other dietary risk factors, high dietary fiber intake was not associated with reduced risk of colorectal carcinoma.

No available data substantiate the claim that volvulus of the large bowel is frequently preceded by long-standing constipation. In many cases, hard stools with straining are the initiating factors in the development of fissures and hemorrhoids.

33.5.4 Economic Considerations

Constipation creates an economic problem of staggering proportions. In 2005, purchases of laxatives in ethical and proprietary markets (drugstores and hospitals), excluding other points of sale, totaled an astounding sum of $79,504,000 in Canada and $650,624,300 in the United States (D. Rhodes, personal communication, 2006; IMS Canada Drug Store and Hospital purchases, 2005; IMS America, Drug Store audit and provider perspective). Because these values do not include the consumption of all laxatives, the true figures are undoubtedly much higher. A common misconception is that nonprescription medication is totally safe and without adverse effects. However, if a bowel movement is induced by a laxative, it may be several days before enough stool is present for another bowel movement. Therefore, when an individual attempts to maintain a daily bowel movement with the prolonged use of laxatives, a vicious cycle may develop in which either more of the same laxative or a more potent one must be used. A "cathartic colon" then may develop. Such long-standing use of laxatives creates a varying degree of financial burden on a given patient.

33.6 Diagnosis and Treatment

Careful history and selective investigations will enable the appropriate subclassification of idiopathic chronic constipation. In general, three subgroups are recognized:

1. Constipation-predominant irritable bowel syndrome (IBS-C). This is constipation without prolongation of transit or disordered evacuatory pelvic floor mechanisms. Often IBS-C is associated with abdominal pain and bloating.
2. Slow transit constipation. Characterized by prolongation of colonic transit or colonic inertia.
3. Obstructed defecation. Constipation characterized by normal transit time but an inability to initiate defecation due to a disordered pelvic floor function.

Subdivision, as above, is important to direct therapy, but it needs to be recognized that significant overlap between the subgroups exists. It is known that some patients with slow transit constipation have obstructed defecation and vice versa and all may have an element of abdominal pain and bloating.

Almy[30] described the goals in the treatment of a patient with chronic constipation as follows: restoration of normal frequency and consistency of stools, freedom from the discomforts ordinarily associated with constipation, maintenance of reasonably regular elimination without artificial aids, and relief of any generalized illness of which constipation may be a symptom. Although these goals are the ideal, they should be achieved if at all possible.

Traditionally, the mainstay of treatment has included laxatives, suppositories, and enemas. It is now being recognized that surgery has an increasing role to play in the management of these patients. Therefore, medical treatment is discussed first, followed by consideration of the role of surgery as appropriate for the latter two subgroups described previously.

33.6.1 Medical Treatment

General Recommendations

Specific metabolic and endocrinologic problems such as hypothyroidism must be treated on their own merits. A favorite recommendation is for the patient to sit on the toilet at regular intervals and for prolonged periods, regardless of whether there is an urge to defecate or not. However, the value of such a ritual is open to debate. Antispasmodics may relieve cramping in individuals with irritable bowel syndrome.

Dietary and Lifestyle Changes

Because the most common causes of constipation are faulty diet and habits, management often requires no more than careful examination and reassurance, together with simple guidance. Patients should be advised not to ignore the call to stool because neglect only disrupts the normal adaptive relaxation mechanism of the rectum, yielding fecal stasis. Regular exercise should be encouraged; some patients claim an easier and more satisfactory bowel action with nothing more than a regular walk in the morning or evening. Environmental factors such as working conditions are often difficult to change. Other factors, such as meal patterns (e.g., omission of breakfast), shift work, and dependence on fast foods, may contribute to abnormal bowel function. If the patient's history reveals excessive ingestion of foods that cause hardened stools, such as processed cheese, such foods might be eliminated or at least reduced in quantity. An adequate daily intake of fluids is encouraged up to 2 to 3 L if need be. Finally, cultural habits and norms may influence an individual's perception of what is abnormal as opposed to normal function.

Fiber-containing foodstuffs have hydrophilic properties that soften the stool. The increased volume of feces favors the stimulation of a natural peristaltic reflex. Cereals, especially bran, are good agents in this regard. The most inexpensive cereal with the highest concentration of crude fiber is unprocessed bran, or Miller's bran.[121] This easily obtainable material is effective in lowering intraluminal pressure and decreasing transit time in patients with constipation and diverticular disease. Coarser bran is more beneficial because of its greater water-holding capacity.[122] Of the various fiber components, pectin has the greatest water-holding capacity but produces the smallest change in fecal weight, whereas bran has the lowest water-holding capacity and the largest fecal weight changes.[123] An inverse relationship between water holding and fecal bulking suggests that dietary fiber does not exert its effect on fecal weight simply by retaining water in the gut. There are four ways in which dietary fiber might cause stool bulking.[124] First, the amount of fiber determines the number of bacteria, which are estimated to form 30 to 50% of feces, and there is a direct relationship between stool weight and pentose-containing polysaccharides. Second, water may be absorbed by undigested hydrophilic components of fiber, but the importance of this is questionable. Third, short-chain fatty acids produced by fermentation of dietary fiber accelerate transit and leave less time for the colonic mucosa to reabsorb water. Fourth, stool weight may increase merely because of the increase in undigested residue. In any event, the diet should contain generous portions of vegetables and fruits. Foods with fat (not excessive) are of value. Patients who are unable to achieve adequate intake of fiber-containing foods should supplement their diets with hydrophilic preparations such as psyllium seed extracts, which act in a similar fashion.

In their diet trial, Devroede et al recommended that patients ingest an average of 14.4 g of crude fiber per day.[105] Today the concept of ingesting dietary fiber is generally accepted. Dietary fiber is the residue derived from plant foods that is resistant to human digestive enzymes.[125] The main components of dietary fiber include the structural materials of the plant cell wall (i.e., cellulose, hemicellulose, pectin substances, and lignin) and nonstructural polysaccharides (i.e., gums, mucilages, algal polysaccharides, and modified celluloses). Furthermore, fiber can be considered insoluble or water soluble. The physical and chemical properties of each component of fiber are important in determining the physiologic response to it. For example, the water-insoluble fibers, which include lignin, cellulose, and hemicelluloses, accelerate intestinal transit, augment fecal weight, slow down starch hydrolysis, and delay glucose absorption. Water-soluble fibers, which include pectin and gums, delay intestinal transit, gastric emptying, and glucose absorption and decrease serum cholesterol concentration.

Foods rich in dietary fiber contain a mixture of these fiber components, which are present in the form of a matrix. Food sources of fiber are complex, and the amount of fiber detected varies depending on the plant species and the method used to analyze the fiber content. Crude fiber analysis does not accurately reflect the total amount of dietary fiber in food materials and, in general, underestimates the total amount of fiber in a range from unity to a ratio of 7:1, depending on the specific components of a given food.[126]

"How much dietary fiber should the average person consume daily?" is a difficult question to answer. It has been estimated that the average dietary fiber consumed is approximately 19 g/day. For a beneficial effect on stool weight, consumption of 30 to 60 g/day has been suggested, but this estimate would vary from individual to individual. Soluble fiber, which can be readily degraded by bacteria, increases fecal bulk. However, insoluble fiber, which is resistant to bacterial degradation, is responsible for the major contribution to fecal bulk. During a diet trial, patients are instructed to record each bowel movement. They also are instructed to stop taking drugs, if not essential, particularly laxatives, and not to resort to enemas. A diet containing 30 g of dietary fiber from a wide variety of sources is continued for 1 month. Dietary recommendations emphasize the ingestion of sources of insoluble fiber.[127] Sources of fiber and sample diets are shown in ▶ Table 33.6. Patients who fail to respond to a change in diet (e.g., three or more stools per week) may require further studies such as colonic transit time evaluation and manometry. Patients who do respond are encouraged to adopt a high-fiber diet with a generous fluid intake as a daily habit, to prevent constipation.

Table 33.6 Fiber content of various foods

1 cup (250 mL) cornflakes = 7 g fiber (total) vs. 1 cup (250 mL) raisin bran = 6.7 g fiber (total)
1 slice white bread = 6 g fiber (total) vs. 1 slice whole wheat bread = 2.0 g fiber (total)
1 cup (250 mL) shredded lettuce = 0.9 g fiber (total) vs. 1 cup coleslaw = 1.9 g fiber (total)
1 chocolate chip cookie = 0.4 g fiber (total) vs. 1 date square = 2.1 g fiber (total)

	Dietary fiber (g)	
	Total	Insoluble
High-fiber breakfast cereals and breads		
Fiber, 1.5 cup (125 mL—refer to label)	14.0	
All Bran, 0.5 cup (125 mL)	11.8	10.2
Grape Nuts, 0.5 cup (125 mL)	6.0	4.8
Harvest Crunch (raisin-almond), 0.5 cup (125 mL)	3.1	2.1
Muffets[2]	4.9	4.2
Fruit and Fiber (date raisin nut), 0.5 cup (125 mL)	4.2	
Shredded wheat (spoon size), 0.5 cup (125 mL)	3.2	2.6
Shredded wheat (1 biscuit)	3.0	2.5
Multigrain bagel (large—refer to label)	7.0	
Whole wheat bread (1 slice)	2.0	
Bran muffin (commercial mix)	1.5	
High-fiber fruit		
Pear, 1 fresh (170 g)	5.1	3.4
Prunes (cooked), 0.5 cup (125 mL)	4.8	
Orange, 1 (150 g)	4.4	
Mango, 1 fresh	4.1	2.2
Raspberries (raw), 0.5 cup (125 mL)	3.2	1.0
Raisins, 0.5 cup (125 mL)	3.1	2.0
Apple, 1 with skin (138 g)	2.6	
Fig, 1 dried	2.3	
Blueberries (raw), 0.5 cup (125 mL)	2.0	1.5
Banana, 1 medium	2.0	1.1
Strawberries (raw), 0.5 cup (125 mL)	1.7	1.0
Peaches canned slices, 0.5 cup (125 mL)	1.7	0.6
Applesauce, 0.5 cup (125 mL)	1.5	1.0
High-fiber snacks		
Peanuts, 0.5 cup (125 mL)	5.6	2.8
Nuts, mixed, no peanuts, 0.5 cup (125 mL)	4.2	

Table 33.6 continued

1 cup (250 mL) cornflakes = 7 g fiber (total) vs. 1 cup (250 mL) raisin bran = 6.7 g fiber (total)
1 slice white bread = 6 g fiber (total) vs. 1 slice whole wheat bread = 2.0 g fiber (total)
1 cup (250 mL) shredded lettuce = 0.9 g fiber (total) vs. 1 cup coleslaw = 1.9 g fiber (total)
1 chocolate chip cookie = 0.4 g fiber (total) vs. 1 date square = 2.1 g fiber (total)

	Dietary fiber (g)	
	Total	Insoluble
Popcorn, 1 cup	1.4	
High-fiber vegetables		
Beans, red kidney, 0.5 cup (125 mL)	6.1	3.3
Peas, green, fresh (cooked), 0.5 cup (125 mL)	5.6	4.2
Corn, fresh, 1 cob (120 g)	4.5	
Lentils (cooked), 0.5 cup (125 mL)	4.4	4.2
Chick peas (cooked), 0.5 cup (125 mL)	4.0	3.0
Lima beans (cooked), 0.5 cup (125 mL)	4.0	
Cabbage, red (shredded raw), 1 cup (250 mL)	3.8	
Potato baked with skin	3.4	1.1
Corn, fresh, niblets (cooked), 0.5 cup (125 mL)	3.2	
Sweet potato (mashed cooked), 0.5 cup (125 mL)	3.1	1.9
Brussels sprouts, fresh (cooked), 0.5 cup (125 mL)	3.0	1.6
Carrots, fresh (cooked), 0.5 cup (125 mL)	2.2	1.0
Turnip (cooked), 0.5 cup (125 mL)	2.4	
Broccoli, fresh (cooked), 0.5 cup (125 mL)	2.4	1.5
Squash, winter (cooked), 0.5 cup (125 mL)	1.9	1.3
Tomato, 1 medium	1.5	1.0
Celery (chopped raw), 0.5 cup (125 mL)	1.0	0.6
Lettuce (chopped), 1 cup (250 mL)	0.9	0.5

Laxatives

Laxatives are compounds that facilitate the passage and elimination of feces from the colon and rectum. In addition to the treatment of constipation, valid indications for the use of laxatives include preparation for gastrointestinal investigations and surgery.

With the almost countless number of laxatives available on the market today, classification of such drugs becomes extremely important but correspondingly difficult. More than 700 proprietary laxative preparations are available in almost every dosage form. The most meaningful method is based on the mechanism of action of the drug. The classification shown in ▶ Table 33.7 is a modification of the ones presented by Brunton[128] and Curry.[129] The use of all cathartics is contraindicated in a patient with abdominal cramps, colic, nausea, vomiting, or any undiagnosed abdominal pain. Because the drugs in each group act similarly, they are described in groups.

Stimulants

Drugs in this group chemically stimulate the intestinal wall to increased peristaltic activity and hence cause gripping, intestinal cramps, increased mucous secretion, and excessively rapid evacuation in some patients. The mechanism of action is by irritation of the intestinal mucosa or by selective action on the enteric nervous system or intestinal smooth muscle. Increased water and electrolyte excretion is attributed to more rapid transit of feces through the intestine. The initiation of the irritant activity may occur in either the small intestine or the large bowel. Although it might be expected that the colon always must be the site of laxative irritant activity, this is not the case. Any agent that increases the propulsive activity of the small intestine necessarily accelerates large bowel peristalsis. These agents are useful in the treatment of acute constipation as well as constipation caused by prolonged bed rest or hospitalization and preparation for radiologic examinations. Abuse, however, may lead to cathartic colon, that is, a poorly functioning large intestine; hence prolonged use should be discouraged. It may be that it was induced by laxatives that are no longer in use.[130] Anthranoid-containing laxatives—aloe, cascara, frangula, and rheum—may play a role in colorectal carcinoma. Clinical epidemiologic studies have evaluated the carcinoma risk in patients who have abused anthranoid laxatives over a long period. Pseudomelanosis coli is a reliable parameter of chronic laxative abuse (more than 9–12 months) and is specific for anthranoid drugs. In a retrospective study of 3,049 patients who underwent diagnostic colorectal endoscopy, the incidence of pseudomelanosis coli was 3.13% in patients without pathologic changes.[131] In those with colorectal adenomas, the incidence increased to 8.64%, and in those with colorectal carcinoma, it was 3.29%. In a prospective study of 1,095 patients, the incidence of pseudomelanosis coli was 6.9% for patients with no abnormality seen on endoscopy, 9.8% for patients with adenomas, and 18.6% for patients with colorectal carcinomas. From these data, a relative risk of 3.04 can be calculated for colorectal carcinoma, as a result of anthranoid laxative abuse.

Mechanical Cleansers

Laxatives in this group increase propulsive activity by either increasing the bulk of the stool or changing the consistency of the stool. Traditional teaching dictates that hypertonic salts attract and retain a large volume of isotonic fluid in the gastrointestinal tract, thus stimulating peristalsis in the small intestine, reducing transit time, and causing the passage of a watery stool. Saline cathartics stimulate the release of cholecystokinin, stimulating small bowel motility, and inhibiting absorption of fluid and electrolytes from the jejunum and ileum.[132] These laxatives should be given with adequate amounts of water for two reasons: (1) the holdover in the stomach is shortened and (2) the patient suffers less dehydration. With oral administration, laxation occurs in 3 to 6 hours.

The laxative effect of bulk-forming agents is due to the absorption and retention of large amounts of water. Mechanical distention caused by this increased residue of unabsorbed material promotes peristalsis and facilitates the passage of stool. The laxative effect usually occurs within 24 hours of ingestion but may take up to 3 days. Side effects are relatively rare. Minor adverse effects include frequent flatulence and borborygmi.

Table 33.7 Modified classification of laxatives based on Brunton[128] and Curry[129]

Stimulants	Mechanical cleansers	Miscellaneous
Anthracene (emodin, anthraquinone)	Saline laxative	Lactulose
• Cascara sagrada	• Magnesium sulfate (Epsom salt, Milk of Magnesia, magnesium citrate, magnesium cardonate, sodium sulfate [Glauber's salt], sodium phosphate, potassium sodium tartrate [Rochelle salt])	**Obsolete cathartics** Calomel, aloe, podophyllum, jalap, colocynth, elaterin, ipomea, gambage, croton oil, sulfur
• Senna (Senokot)	Bulk forming agents	
• Danthron	• Psyllium seed preparations (plantago), Metamucil, Konsyl, LA formula, Hydrocil, Mucilose, Sibliny	
• Rhubarb	• Synthetic mucilloids (methylcellulose, sodium carboxymethyl cellulose)	
Castor oil	• Agar	
Diphenylmethane cathartics	• Tragacanth	
• Bisacodyl (Dulcolax)	Mineral oil	
• Phenolphthalein	Surface-active agents	
• Oxyphensatin acetate	• Dioctyl sodium sulfosuccinate (Colace, Doxinate, Bulax, DOSS)	
	• Poloxalkol	
	• Dioctyl calcium sulfosuccinate (Surfak)	

Esophageal, gastric, small intestinal, and colonic obstructions and fecal impactions have been reported with their use. Therefore, this group of agents should be taken with generous amounts of fluids to avoid such problems.

Liquid petrolatum retards the absorption of water from the stool and thus softens fecal material. The onset of action is approximately 6 to 8 hours. This substance can be administered orally or as an enema. The usual dose is 15 to 45 mL. Mineral oil should not be taken at bedtime because of the dangers of aspiration and is best taken between meals to obviate any tendency for interference with absorption of fat-soluble vitamins. A patient with dysphagia should not take it because of the threat of lipoid pneumonia. Pruritus ani and anal leakage are minor annoying side effects.

With its sodium or calcium salt, dioctyl sulfosuccinate lowers surface tension at the oil–water interface of the stool, thereby softening the stool by permitting a greater penetration of feces by water and fat. It has been suggested that dioctyl sulfosuccinate stimulates fluid and electrolyte secretion as well.[133] The calcium salt has been reported as more effective than the sodium salt.[134] The usual daily dose is 100 to 200 mg. They act within 24 to 48 hours.

Lactulose is a synthetic disaccharide not digested by small intestinal or pancreatic enzymes. In the colon, it is metabolized by microflora with resultant acidification of the stool and release of gas. It is effective in treating constipation and changes the nature of the colonic flora. The resultant anions may cause osmotic catharsis; for this reason, the agent might be classified with the saline laxatives. However, it is too costly for routine administration, and with long-term use, superinfection is a risk.

Several potential adverse effects may result from overconsumption of laxatives. In fact, the ill effects of laxative abuse may be greater than those of constipation. Such effects include

(1) dehydration and electrolyte disturbance; (2) hypokalemia; (3) hypermagnesemia; (4) nausea, vomiting, and abdominal distress; (5) malabsorption; (6) paraffinomas; (7) lipoid pneumonia; (8) intestinal obstruction; (9) specific toxic effect; (10) anal stenosis; (11) dependence; and (12) colonic structural injury. Colonic nerve plexus damage attributed to the long-term use of sennosides has been questioned, and experimental evidence does not support this hypothesis.[130] The morphologic changes noted may very well be on an entirely different basis.

Other Pharmacologic Agents

The use of agents that enhance the normal propulsive action of the bowel is more appealing than the use of agents whose mechanism of action is by irritation. A number of agents that fall into this category are summarized in ▶ Table 33.8. Johanson et al[135] evaluated the efficacy, safety, and tolerability of tegaserod (Zelnorm, Novartis), a serotonin subtype 4 receptor, partial agonist in patients with chronic constipation in a randomized double blind, placebo-controlled study. Responder rates for complete spontaneous bowel movements (CSBMs) during weeks 1 to 4 were significantly greater in the tegaserod 2 mg twice daily (41.4%) and 6 mg twice daily groups (43.2%) versus placebo (25.1%). This effect was maintained over 12 weeks. No rebound effect was observed after treatment withdrawal. Tegaserod was well tolerated; headache and nasopharyngitis, the most frequent adverse events, were more common in the placebo group than in either tegaserod group. Kamm et al[136] also investigated the efficacy, safety, and tolerability of tegaserod in the treatment of chronic constipation. They randomized 1,264 patients to tegaserod or placebo. Responder rates for the primary efficacy variable were 35.6% for tegaserod 2 mg twice daily, 40.2% for 6 mg twice daily, and 26.7% for placebo. Tegaserod

Table 33.8 Agents affecting neurotransmission

General class	Mechanisms of action	Subclass	Example
Cholinomimetics	Stimulate cholinergic receptors, predominantly muscarinics	Cholinergic agents	Bethanechol
		Cholinesterase inhibitors	Neostigmine
Prokinetic agents	Facilitate release of acetylcholine and antagonize dopamine receptors		Metoclopramide
	Facilitate only neurotransmitter		Cisapride
Opioid antagonists	Selectively inhibit peripheral opioid receptors		Naloxone

Source: Modified from Ogorek and Reynolds.[140]

6 mg twice daily reduced straining, abdominal bloating/distension, and abdominal pain/discomfort during the 12-week treatment period compared with placebo. Significant improvements were also seen in stool form and in global assessment of bowel habits and constipation. The most common adverse events, headache and abdominal pain, were more frequent with placebo than with tegaserod. In 2007, the FDA withdrew approval due to significantly increased risk of serious cardiovascular events compared with placebo (0.1 vs. 0.01%). A highly selective 5HT4 receptor agonist—prucalopride (Resolor)—has a much safer cardiovascular side effect profile and in 2010 was recommended by the National Institute for Health and Care Excellence (NICE) for the treatment of constipation in women. Three randomized control trials have looked at the efficacy of prucalopride in chronic constipation.[137,138,139] The major inclusion criterion was the presence of chronic constipation, defined as two or fewer spontaneous complete bowel movements (SCBMs) per week for at least 6 months prior to screening plus any one of the following: hard/very hard stools, a sensation of incomplete evacuation, or straining, during defecation in relation to at least 25% of bowel movements. After a 2-week baseline period, eligible patients were randomized to either placebo or 2 or 4 mg of prucalopride for 12 weeks. The primary endpoint, in each study, was the proportion of patients passing at least three SCBMs per week during the 12 weeks of the trial, based on an intention-to-treat analysis. All three trials (which assessed 620, 641, and 713 patients, respectively) demonstrated a significant increase in the proportion of patients achieving at least three SCBMs per week compared with placebo. Response rates ranged from 19.5 to 31% with 2 mg prucalopride, 24 to 28% with 4 mg prucalopride, and 9.6 to 12% with placebo. Clinically relevant and statistically significant improvements were also demonstrated in a number of secondary endpoints, including satisfaction with bowel function, perception of constipation severity, and patient-assessed symptom scores. Even though men and women were enrolled in these studies, over 85% of evaluated patients were female. While this led to the approval of the drug being restricted to women, it needs to be stressed that this should not be taken to imply prucalopride is not effective in men but, rather, that it has not been adequately tested in this gender.

In 2014, NICE also approved the use of lubiprostone for chronic constipation. Lubiprostone is a bicyclic fatty acid derived from prostaglandin E1 that acts by specifically activating ClC-2 chloride channels on the apical aspect of gastrointestinal epithelial cells, producing a chloride-rich fluid secretion. These secretions soften the stool, increase motility, and promote spontaneous bowel movements. Several studies have established the role of lubiprostone in chronic constipation. A double-blind, placebo-controlled, dose-finding study of lubiprostone randomized 129 patients who met Rome II criteria for chronic constipation to lubiprostone at doses of 12, 24, or 36 μg twice daily or placebo for 3 weeks and recorded the frequency of spontaneous bowel movements, use of rescue medications, symptoms, and adverse events. The primary endpoint was the average daily number of bowel movements. Lubiprostone improved spontaneous bowel movement frequency in a dose-dependent manner and the overall number of bowel movements for all three doses of lubiprostone was greater than placebo at week 2. There was no statistically significant difference between the groups in serious and minor adverse events.[141] Based on the results of this study, it was determined that the lubiprostone dose of 24 μg twice daily had the best risk–benefit profile and it was chosen for subsequent phase III studies.

Additional randomized controlled trials with similar study designs have shown a significantly higher percentage of patients treated with lubiprostone had a spontaneous bowel movement within 24 hours compared with placebo (56.7 vs. 36.9%, 62.9 vs. 31.9%). There were also significant improvements in straining effort, stool consistency, and global satisfaction with bowel function compared with placebo.

Linaclotide is another drug that has had recent approval in the United States and United Kingdom. Linaclotide is a 14-amino acid synthetic peptide that is structurally related to the endogenous guanylin peptide family. It binds to and activates the guanylate cyclase C receptor on the luminal surface of the intestinal epithelium. Activation of guanylate cyclase C results in the generation of cyclic guanosine monophosphate (cGMP), the levels of which increase both extracellularly and intracellularly. Within the intestinal epithelial cells, the increase in cGMP triggers a signal-transduction cascade that activates the cystic fibrosis transmembrane conductance regulator.[142,143] This activation causes secretion of chloride and bicarbonate into the intestinal lumen, increasing luminal fluid secretion and accelerating intestinal transit.[144] In animal models, linaclotide has been shown to increase gastrointestinal transit and to reduce visceral pain.[145,146] Two randomized control trials looked at the efficacy of linaclotide in chronic constipation.[147] Patients received either placebo or linaclotide, 145 or 290 μg, once daily for

12 weeks. The primary efficacy end point was three or more CSBMs per week and an increase of one or more CSBMs from baseline during at least 9 of the 12 weeks. In the two trials, the primary end point was reached by 21.2 and 16.0% of the patients who received 145 μg of linaclotide and by 19.4 and 21.3% of the patients who received 290 μg of linaclotide, as compared with 3.3 and 6.0% of those who received placebo ($p < 0.01$ for all comparisons of linaclotide with placebo). Improvements in all secondary end points were significantly greater in both linaclotide groups than in the placebo groups. Its effects on abdominal pain make it a particularly attractive option in IBS-C.

Suppositories

Suppositories are useful for evacuating the lower bowel, and their use instead of an enema has been advocated. Although they are probably not as effective as enemas, they are more acceptable to both patient and nurse. The insertion of an inert cylinder such as a glycerin suppository often initiates a defecation response, usually within 30 minutes, which apparently is a reflex act. Other suppositories contain bisacodyl, dioctyl sodium sulfosuccinate, senna, or carbon dioxide.

Enemas

Clinical indications for enemas include preparation for endoscopic examination, surgery, or childbirth, removal of fecal impaction and barium, and certain cases of acute constipation. Warm tap water or warm saline enemas are preferred. Soapsuds and hydrogen peroxide enemas are quite irritating to the colonic mucosa and should be avoided. Hypertonic phosphate salts also are irritating to the colonic mucosa and tend to stimulate the rectum to produce a large amount of mucus, which may interfere with evaluation of the state of the mucosa. Enemas work within approximately five minutes and act by causing distention and by osmotic activity. Hypertonic enemas may give rise to sodium retention. However, the practical advantage of the packaged enemas makes their use ideal in a busy office practice. Enemas should be administered with the patient lying on his or her left side or prone and with the enema bag two feet above the level of the rectum. Material should be introduced slowly with as many temporary interruptions as necessary to prevent cramps. Repositioning the patient on his or her right side might help ensure adequate distribution of the enema fluid. Certain dangers are involved with enemas, including electrolyte depletion, water intoxication, colonic perforation, and even psychological dependence.

33.6.2 Surgical Treatment

The indications for operation in patients with constipation of recent origin are relatively clear, and they are related to the underlying cause of the constipation such as carcinoma or diverticular disease. On the other hand, the indications for operation in patients with chronic constipation are poorly defined and controversial at best. During the last two decades, there has been an increasing recognition of serious psychological and psychiatric disorders, particularly in female patients with functional disorders of the lower digestive tract. According to some authors, it is naive to believe that operation could cure these conditions. Despite an increasing skepticism regarding the potential role of surgery, some surgeons still believe that there is a sound indication for operative treatment in selected cases. The high cost of treating constipation and the uncontrolled use of laxatives seems to support the contention that no patient should need to resort to a lifelong consumption of laxatives and administration of enemas if another solution is available. Martelli et al[47] classified patients with constipation of unknown origin in terms of the segment of bowel with the disordered function. The authors described three groups: (1) outlet obstruction—impaired rectal evacuation; (2) hindgut dysfunction—the right colon empties very well, but markers accumulate in the left colon, sigmoid colon, and rectum; and (3) colonic inertia—the entire large bowel fails to propel contents. Prior to operation, delineation of patients with colonic inertia from those with obstructed defecation is advocated. At first sight, distinction between the first two types of constipation seems logical because it has an obvious impact on the treatment. However, many patients present with symptoms suggestive of both abnormalities. Although it has been suggested that good results can be achieved by adequate selection of patients, it is still not known how to treat patients with both colonic inertia and obstructed defecation.

Slow-Transit Constipation (Colonic Inertia)

At the beginning of the 20th century, Sir William Arbuthnot Lane[148] was probably the first to perform colectomy with ileorectal anastomosis in patients with colonic inertia. Initially, colectomy was performed only in patients with idiopathic megacolon because many surgeons were reluctant to remove a normal size colon. It has been shown that colectomy also might be beneficial in patients with severe constipation without megacolon. The effort to compare results is probably not entirely justified because series are not comparable. In particular, some series are of patients with megacolon, others are of patients without megacolon, and most are of both. In addition, the extent of resection varies from series to series and within a given series. Despite the fact that the reported results are apparently good, the exact role of colectomy has yet to be defined.[149,150,151,152,153,154,155]

Slow-Transit Constipation with Megacolon and/or Megarectum

Some patients with severe, intractable constipation have a markedly dilated rectum and/or colon. This condition, also called idiopathic megarectum and/or megacolon, affects males and females in equal proportion. Most patients have the onset of symptoms in childhood or early adult life. Various segments of the large bowel may become dilated, but the process usually begins in the rectum. The etiology of this condition is still unknown. It has been suggested that rectal dilation may result from a behavioral defecatory problem in childhood. Although the muscle layers of the dilated segment and their intrinsic and extrinsic innervation appear grossly normal, subtle neural and muscular abnormalities have been reported.[156,157] Koch et al[158] reported that VIP levels are decreased in the external muscle layer from idiopathic megacolon. Similar findings have been reported by Gattuso et al.[159] Koch et al[160] were able to demonstrate that diminished VIP levels are associated with a depletion of the tissue antioxidant, glutathione. This depletion probably permits the free radical-induced alteration of VIP-containing neurons. In another study, the same authors observed a diminished release of nitric oxide in circular smooth muscle from patients with idiopathic megacolon.[161] Meier-Ruge examined surgical specimens obtained from patients with idiopathic megacolon. In all specimens, she observed a lack of connective tissue in the muscularis propria. Normally, this connective tissue, consisting of collagen Type III, enables contraction and relaxation of the circular and longitudinal muscle layers. According to Meier-Ruge, the absence of this tissue affects normal peristalsis, resulting in stasis of fecal material and dilatation of the large bowel, despite a normal enteric nervous system.[162] Recently, Lee et al reported a decreased density of interstitial cells of Cajal in resected sigmoid specimens of patients with acquired megacolon.[103] Based on a retrospective study among 63 operated patients with megarectum and/or megacolon, Gattuso and Kamm concluded that patients with megarectum differ clinically, diagnostically, and in their outcome from those with megacolon. Patients with megarectum are younger and develop symptoms in childhood. Half of the patients with megacolon become symptomatic as adults. All patients with megarectum present with fecal impaction associated with soiling and fecal incontinence. Manual disimpaction is frequently reported by these patients.[163] The diagnosis of idiopathic megabowel can only be made after exclusion of recognized neurologic, toxic, and degenerative pathology such as Hirschsprung's disease, myotonic dystrophy, Chagas' disease, and systemic sclerosis. Digital examination almost invariably shows that the rectum is full of feces.[163] Radiographic findings are also characteristic, because almost all patients have rectal dilation down to the pelvic floor, with no distal narrow segment. Patients with idiopathic megarectum have normal small bowel transit and abnormal colonic transit, with delay occurring predominantly in the dilated segment.[164] The initial management of patients with idiopathic megarectum and/or megacolon should be medical. The aim of treatment is to prevent fecal impaction, either by inducing a semiliquid stool using osmotic laxatives or by regular use of enemas or suppositories. The use of senna laxatives may prove helpful to these patients. In some patients, however, manual disimpaction is inevitable. This is not without risk, because it has been shown that manual disimpaction, performed under general anesthesia, may damage the anal sphincters. This damage further affects continence and compromises the outcome of operative treatment.[165] If laxatives and enemas are poorly tolerated or ineffective, operative treatment should be considered.

Colectomy with cecorectal or ileorectal anastomosis is the most commonly performed operation in patients with idiopathic megarectum and/or megacolon.[166] Stabile et al[167] reported a series of 40 patients in whom the rectum was moderately dilated, measuring 7 to 10 cm in diameter on a lateral radiograph. Twenty-two patients had a cecorectal anastomosis, 11 had an ileorectal anastomosis, and 7 had a sigmoid resection. When considering all patients, 80% developed a normal stool frequency, and most patients no longer needed to use laxatives. These results are similar to those previously reported by Lane and Todd.[168] In patients with a grossly dilated rectum, a colectomy with ileorectal anastomosis seems less appropriate. In these patients, the Duhamel procedure is the most commonly performed operation. The outcome of this operation appears to be less favorable than previously reported. In a series of 20 patients, Stabile et al[169] documented persistent constipation in seven patients and, of these, five required further operation. Based on the assumption that the physiological abnormalities are confined to the dilated part of the bowel, it seems reasonable to perform a coloanal anastomosis after complete resection of the distal dilated segment down to the level of the pelvic floor. Stabile et al[170] reported that five of seven patients experienced a return to normal bowel frequency after coloanal anastomosis. Stewart et al[171] observed a favorable outcome in 8 of 10 patients who underwent coloanal anastomosis. The overall results, as reported in the literature, are listed in ▶ Table 33.9. In their review of the literature, Pfeifer et al[172] found 84 patients with megabowel in whom the success rate for subtotal colectomy and ileorectal anastomosis was 88%. O Súilleabháin et al[173] reported on several operative procedures used to treat idiopathic megabowel in 28 patients. All patients had conservative treatment for 6 months. Those failing to improve underwent full-thickness biopsy of the anorectal junction, anorectal physiology studies, colonic transit studies, and evacuation proctography. Surgery involved excision of the abnormal large bowel and formation of an anastomosis (coloanal or ileoanal) using "normal" bowel, identified either by a defunctioning stoma or colonic motility studies. Eight patients responded to conservative management. Two of the 17 patients who underwent full-thickness biopsy were cured by the procedure. Anorectal physiology and colonic transit and evacuation studies did not aid selection

Table 33.9 Results of colonic resection for slow-transit constipation with megacolon

Authors	Treatment	No. of cases	Success rate (%)[a]
Lane and Todd[168]	Subtotal colectomy	9	88
	Hemicolectomy	2	50
	Sigmoid resection	3	33
Hughes et al[149]	Subtotal colectomy	7	100
Belliveau et al[150]	Subtotal colectomy	29	76
Hughes et al[151]	Segmental resection	5	100
Klatt[152]	Subtotal colectomy	3	100
Barnes et al[164]	Subtotal colectomy	16	69
	Segmental colectomy	4	50
Vasilevsky et al[156]	Subtotal colectomy	14	93
Stabile et al[169]	Subtotal and segmental resection	40	80
Stabile et al[169]	Duhamel procedure	20	35
Stabile et al[170]	Coloanal anastomosis	7	71
Keighley[174]	Ileoanal anastomosis	6	83
	Coloanal anastomosis	10	70
Stewart et al[171]	Coloanal anastomosis	10	80

[a]Regular defecation without the use of laxatives.

of the operative procedure performed in 15 patients: proctectomy and coloanal anastomosis (six), restorative proctocolectomy (three), panproctocolectomy (one), and defunctioning stoma (five). At a median follow-up of 3.6 years, 13 of 15 evaluable patients had a satisfactory outcome. They concluded, approximately 40% of patients with megabowel referred for surgery responded to conservative treatment. The remaining patients may be treated successfully by operation.

Based on a recent systematic review, Gladman et al concluded that the outcome data of surgery for idiopathic megarectum and/or megacolon should be interpreted with caution due to limitations of the reviewed studies.[175] None of these studies were comparative. Most series involved only a small number of patients without long-term follow-up.[173] Although recommendations based on clear evidence cannot be given, Gladman et al advocated subtotal colectomy with ileorectal anastomosis as the optimum procedure in patients with a non-dilated rectum. For patients presenting with a dilatation of their colon and rectum, restorative proctocolectomy seems to be the most suitable procedure. For patients with dilatation confined to the rectum, Gladman et al advocated a vertical reduction rectoplasty. This novel procedure involves transsection of the rectum in a vertical direction along its antimesenteric border and excision of the anterior portion, thereby reducing rectal capacity. In a small series, significant improvements in bowel frequency were obtained in eight out of ten patients.[175]

An alternative to these major resections involves the formation of a stoma either as a primary procedure or after a previous operation has failed. One should realize that only the creation of a stoma proximal to the dilated segment would relieve the constipation.

Slow-Transit Constipation without Megacolon

Slow-transit constipation without megacolon is a condition that is almost entirely confined to women.[176] Other terms used to describe this syndrome are colonic inertia or Arbuthnot Lane's disease. In tertiary referral centers, about 20 to 40% of the patients with constipation will be found to have slow-transit constipation. In the majority of patients, symptoms arise de novo in childhood. A proportion of patients present later in life. Some of these patients have no obvious trigger for their complaints, whereas others report symptoms following events such as hysterectomy and childbirth.[177] Patients with this syndrome have infrequent defecation with two or fewer bowel actions each week. Although these patients have a normal size colon, their colonic transit time is markedly prolonged. In most patients, the constipation is associated with a general sense of malaise, bloating, abdominal pain, nausea, and vomiting, which interferes with the ability to work and enjoy social activities. Many of these women have associated gynecologic problems such as irregular menstrual periods, ovarian cysts, and galactorrhea.[176] In addition, a delay in gastric emptying and small bowel transit has been found, indicating that inertia of the large bowel might be the colonic manifestation of a pan-gastrointestinal motility disorder.[177,178,179] Hemingway et al[180] used cholecystokinin-augmented hepatic 2,6-dimethyliminodiacetic acid (HIDA) scans to measure gall bladder ejection fraction in patients with constipation. The authors found a significant difference between patients with idiopathic slow-transit constipation and those with other causes of constipation, indicating that colonic inertia is associated with biliary dyskinesia. Penning et al[181] evaluated gall bladder motility in 16 patients with slow-transit constipation and in 20 healthy controls. They observed that patients with slow-transit constipation have smaller fasting gall bladder volumes, impaired gall bladder responses to vagal cholinergic stimulation, but normal gall bladder responses to hormonal stimulation with cholecystokinin. These findings indicate that gall bladder motility is disturbed in patients with slow-transit constipation, probably due to impaired neural responsiveness. Mollen et al[182] reported abnormalities of antroduodenal motility, characterized by absence or prolonged duration of the migrating motor complex, an increased number of clustered contractions, and a decreased motility during late phase 2 of the migrating motor complex. Similar findings have been reported by others.[183] In contrast with these observations, Penning et al[184] reported that patients with slow-transit constipation have generally well-preserved antroduodenal motility with only minor alterations. It is still unclear whether these anomalies of the proximal digestive tract are primary or not. These abnormalities may very well be primary, because it has been shown that delayed gastric emptying persists in the majority of the patients after subtotal colectomy with ileorectal anastomosis.[185] Alternatively they may be secondary to the colonic inertia itself, because it has been shown that inflation of a balloon in the rectum inhibits the motor activity of the entire gastrointestinal tract.[186] The observation that women with slow-transit constipation may also have functional urologic problems has prompted the investigation of sacral spinal cord function. In 15 women with colonic inertia, Varma and Smith[71] observed blunted rectal defecatory sensation and increased rectal compliance. In addition, the latency of the pudendoanal reflex was significantly prolonged. Based on these findings, a central neurogenic deficit was postulated. Kerrigan et al[187] assessed the integrity of evoked spinal reflexes relaying in the conus medullaris (S2–S4). One or more of these reflexes were absent in 75% of the authors' patients. The results of this study indicate that the integration of sensory information within the sacral cord may be impaired in slow-transit constipation. Extramural damage to the pelvic parasympathetic nerves has also been considered a major contributing factor. Colonic branches, arising from the inferior hypogastric plexus, enter the wall of the large bowel at the rectosigmoid junction and extend in the intramuscular plane both caudad and cephalad. In humans, it has been demonstrated that these intramural nerves extend cephalad up to 80% of the large intestine.[188] Canine studies sectioning pelvic nerves have demonstrated abolition of high amplitude propagating contractions (HAPCs), a decrease in proximal colonic motility, and abnormal bowel movements, characterized by the passage of smaller harder stools with associated straining.[189] In patients with slow-transit constipation, the number, amplitude, and duration of HAPCs are reduced.[190,191] In many patients with slow-transit constipation, rectal sensory perception is reduced. In some patients, this rectal hyposensitivity may be partly explained by abnormal rectal compliance. In other patients, however, rectal wall properties are normal. This latter finding is suggestive of impairment of afferent nerves.[192] A significant group of patients with slow-transit constipation have symptoms that started after pelvic surgery, especially hysterectomy, or after childbirth. It has been assumed that extramural damage to the parasympathetic nerves occurs during hysterectomy and childbirth.[193] Women with slow-transit constipation show impaired sweating after acetylcholine application. It has been suggested that this abnormality is the manifestation of a systemic autonomic dysfunction.[194]

On the other hand, alterations in the enteric nervous system have also been cited as a possible explanation for the disturbed motility in colonic inertia. Silver-staining methods and modern techniques with monoclonal antibodies raised against neurofilament have revealed distinctive abnormalities in the enteric nervous system.

According to Wedel et al, the underlying defect is morphologically characterized by oligoneuronal hypoganglionosis of the myenteric plexus and the external submucous plexus, associated with an increased number of thickened submucous nerve fibers.[101] Bassotti et al also observed abnormalities of the enteric nervous system. These abnormalities were not confined to the neurons of the myenteric and submucous plexus. They also found a decreased number of interstitial cells of Cajal as well as a decreased number of enteric glial cells.[102] A decreased density of interstitial cells of Cajal has also been reported by others.[103,195] Toman et al could not confirm these reports. They used quantitative immunohistochemistry and did not find a decreased number of interstitial cells of Cajal in patients as compared to controls.[196] The neuroendocrine system of the digestive tract has also been subject of several studies. Most of these studies have concentrated on the colonic neuroendocrine system and their results are rather contradictory. Both peptide YY cell density and serotonin cell density in the large bowel have been reported to increase or decrease in patients with slow-transit constipation.[197] Another study has shown that the large bowel of patients with slow-transit constipation is more densely innervated by nitric oxide nerves.[198] Although some of the reported data are conflicting, most studies indicate that there is a subgroup of patients in whom constipation is associated with a dysfunctioning enteric nervous system. Slater et al,[199] in an effort to better understand the pathophysiology of idiopathic slow-transit constipation, studied abnormalities in the contractile properties of colonic smooth muscle. The authors found a hypersensitivity to cholinergic stimulation and suggested the existence of a smooth muscle myopathy in this condition. Rao et al[200] performed ambulatory 24-hour colonic manometry in 21 patients with slow-transit constipation and 20 healthy controls. Constipated patients showed fewer pressure waves than controls during daytime. Motility induced by waking or meal was decreased in patients. HAPCs were detected in 43% of the patients compared to 100% of the controls and with a much lower incidence. Similar findings have been reported by others.[201] To date, these techniques have been applied only to resected colon specimens. These methods are, therefore, not suitable to determine preoperatively whether the neuropathologic abnormalities affect only a portion of the colon or its entire length. It has been shown that levels of substance P are decreased in both rectal mucosa and submucosa of patients with slow-transit constipation.[202] It seems likely that this finding will become more diagnostically relevant, because biopsies can easily be obtained in contrast to transmural sampling. It remains unclear whether the alterations in the enteric nervous system are congenital or acquired due to a possible neurotoxic effect of certain laxatives. These and other controversies indicate that the precise pathogenesis of slow-transit constipation is still an enigma.

Dietary measures and medical treatment including laxatives and enemas usually fail to relieve the distressing symptoms of this syndrome. Battaglia et al[203] assessed the medium- and long-term effects of biofeedback and muscle training in patients with slow-transit constipation in 10 patients who were unresponsive to conventional treatments. At 1 year follow-up, beneficial effect was seen in only 20% of these patients and there was no improvement in colonic transit time.

For these reasons, operative intervention is frequently considered. The most common technique is subtotal colectomy with ileorectal anastomosis. According to enthusiastic reports, this procedure seems to be highly effective with success rates of greater than 90%, as shown in ▶ Table 33.10. In their review of the literature, Pfeifer et al[172] found 444 patients without megabowel, and the success rate for subtotal colectomy and ileorectal anastomosis was 83%. Because the selection of patients with constipation for colectomy may prove difficult, Sunderland et al[204] evaluated the role of video proctography. The authors suggested that when true idiopathic slow-transit constipation is identified on the basis of delayed markers and the ability to expel liquid on proctography, an excellent result could be anticipated from colectomy and ileorectal anastomosis. Mollen et al[205] assessed the results of preoperative functional evaluation of patients with severe slow-transit constipation in relation to functional outcome in 21 patients who underwent colectomy and ileorectal anastomosis. Mean colorectal transit time was 156 hours (normal < 45 hours). Small bowel transit time was normal in 10 patients and delayed in five patients. Morbidity was 33%. Small bowel obstruction occurred in six patients; relaparotomy was done in four patients. Follow-up varied from 14 to 153 (mean 62) months. After 3 months, defecation frequency was increased from one bowel movement per 5.9 days to 2.8 times per day. Seventeen patients continued to experience abdominal pain, and 13 still used laxatives and enemas. Satisfaction rate was 76%. After 1 year, defecation frequency was back at the preoperative level in five patients. An ileostomy was created in two more patients because of incontinence and persistent diarrhea but 52% still felt improved. They concluded the patients should be informed that despite an increase in defecation frequency, abdominal symptoms might persist.

Despite the fact that the reported results of subtotal colectomy are apparently good, some authors have questioned the exact role of this procedure in patients with colonic inertia. In 1988, Kamm et al[212] reviewed the results obtained in 44 female patients. Subtotal colectomy produced improvement in 22 patients (50%) as defined by more frequent stools. However, 17 patients experienced diarrhea, three-fourths of the patients had persistent abdominal pain, six patients had some degree of incontinence, five patients had persistent constipation, eight patients required an operation for obstruction caused by adhesions, and six patients required an ileostomy—three for persistent constipation and three for intractable diarrhea. Ten patients needed psychiatric treatment. The authors also found that impaired balloon expulsion and signs of anismus did not correlate with the clinical outcome.

Similar findings have been documented by Ghosh et al. They also reported a high complication rate during long-term follow-up.

Table 33.10 Results of subtotal colectomy with ileorectal anastomosis for colonic inertia (without megacolon)

Authors	No. of cases	Mean follow-up (y)	Success rate (%)
Hughes et al[149]	10	NS	80
Klatt[152]	6	2.1	100
Krishnamurthy et al[93]	12	NS	100
Todd[206]	16	NS	88
Preston and Lennard-Jones[207]	16	3.5	81
Roe et al[208]	7	0.7	71
Beck et al[155]	14	1.2	100
Leon et al[209]	13	2.6	77
Walsh et al[210]	19	3.2	65
Akervall et al[211]	12	3.4	66
Kamm et al[212]	33	2.0	50
Vasilevsky et al[156]	24	4.0	71
Zenilman et al[213]	12	2.0	100
Yoshioka and Keighley[214]	32	3.0	58
Coremans[215]	10	3.8	60
Kuijpers[216]	12	NS	50
Pemberton et al[217]	38	NS	100
Takahashi et al[218]	37	3.0	97
Redmond et al[219]	34	7.5	90
Piccirillo et al[220]	54	2.2	94
Pluta et al[66]	24	5.5	92
de Graaf et al[221]	24	4.0	33
Nyam et al[222]	74	5.5	90
Fan and Wang[223]	24	1	88
Mollen et al[205]	21	5	76
Nylund et al[224]	40	11	73
Pikarsky et al[225]	30	9	100
Webster and Dayton[226]	55	1	89
Glia et al[227]	17	5	86

Note: Regular defecation without the use of laxatives. NS, not significant.

For example, 71% of their patients experienced at least one episode of small intestinal obstruction and 42% of these episodes resulted in laparotomy. The incidence of this complication is significantly higher among patients with slow-transit constipation as compared to patients who underwent colectomy for another reason.[228] Recently, FitzHarris et al reviewed the charts and operative reports of all their patients who underwent subtotal colectomy for slow-transit constipation during one decade. Seventy-five patients returned their questionnaire. Although 81% of these patients were at least somewhat pleased with the final outcome, 41% cited persistent abdominal pain, 21% fecal incontinence, and 46% diarrhea. These problems adversely affected their quality of life.[229]

These data suggest that subtotal colectomy in patients with colonic inertia produces new problems of its own. Persistent constipation and abdominal discomfort after this procedure might be derived from small bowel involvement, which is masked by the predominant symptom of constipation, becoming apparent only after the colon has been resected.[230] Glia et al found a trend toward better long-term results after subtotal colectomy with ileorectal anastomosis in constipated patients with normal antroduodenal motility as compared to those with abnormal manometric findings.[227] In a study, de Graaf et al[221] evaluated the clinical outcome of subtotal colectomy in a consecutive series of 24 patients with colonic inertia. Seventeen patients regained normal stool frequency. However, persistent abdominal discomfort and disabling diarrhea with incontinence were noted in 63 and 25%, respectively. Similar results have been reported by others. It has been suggested that these rather disappointing results are due to poor selection of patients. In a prospective study, Wexner et al[231] evaluated 163 patients with chronic constipation. All patients underwent colonic transit time studies, anorectal manometry, evacuation proctography, and EMG of the pelvic floor. Colonic inertia was defined as a diffuse marker delay on transit study without evidence of paradoxic puborectalis contraction on proctography. Only 16 patients fulfilled these criteria and underwent a subtotal colectomy. At a mean follow-up of 15 months, patient satisfaction was good or excellent in 94% of the cases. Pluta et al[66] noted that patients with a psychiatric history or physiologic evidence of a defect in afferent innervation of the rectum had poorer results. Akervall et al[211] found that patients with normal rectal sensory function had a satisfactory functional result after subtotal colectomy, whereas patients with blunted sensation did not improve. The authors suggested that determination of the distention pressures required to elicit rectal sensation is an important step in selecting patients suitable for subtotal colectomy and ileorectal anastomosis. Similar findings have been reported by others.[232]

Many experts consider anismus an absolute contraindication to colectomy and expect it to fail. However, objective evidence for this conclusion can only be provided by a prospective study aimed at evaluating the effect of colectomy both in patients with and without evidence of anismus. Duthie and Bartolo[233] performed a subtotal colectomy in 32 patients with slow-transit constipation. One-half of their patients demonstrated proctographic evidence of anismus. No specific attempt had been made to improve pelvic floor function prior to operation. The clinical outcome was reassessed after five years. Overall, 67% of the patients thought that their life had been significantly improved. Comparing patients with and without radiologic signs of anismus, no differences were noted with regard to the final results. Similar findings have been reported by others.[234] Based on these observations, it might be concluded that anismus in the setting of slow-transit constipation may in essence be ignored when considering operative intervention.

Most surgeons perform subtotal colectomy, mainly based on the recommendations of Preston et al,[153] who concluded that subtotal colectomy was successful in 11 of 16 patients. However, eight of these 16 patients continued having abdominal pain, 10 had bloating, and 6 experienced episodes of fecal incontinence. These symptoms were not included in the evaluation of the clinical outcome. Five further patients underwent partial colectomy. In two of these patients, a partial left-sided colectomy was performed and in three patients a sigmoid resection was performed. None of these five patients were selected on the basis of segmental colonic transit time studies.

In contrast to the detailed discussion regarding the clinical outcome after subtotal colectomy, the authors stated that only patients who had partial colectomy did not improve. Despite a hesitation to perform a segmental resection, most surgeons point to the significance of segmental colonic transit time studies. However, it probably does not make sense to quantify regional transit if subtotal colectomy is the only preferable option for patients with slow-transit constipation. de Graaf et al[221] conducted a prospective study to investigate the value of segmental colonic transit times in the decision-making process prior to operative intervention. Based on the results of the transit time studies, 18 patients underwent partial left-sided colectomy and 24 underwent subtotal colectomy. Comparing both groups, no significant differences were found with regard to recurrent constipation and persistent abdominal pain. Kamm et al[234] and Lundin et al[235] noted the same favorable experience with left hemicolectomy in selected patients. It would seem germane to consider regional transit in the decision-making process. If markers pass through the right colon but are only held up in the descending and sigmoid colon, a left hemicolectomy would be deemed appropriate because it would accomplish the task of removing the poorly functioning portion of the colon while obviating the potential complications of subtotal colectomy.

It has been demonstrated that proximal gastrointestinal function is normal in the majority of patients with onset of their symptoms after pelvic surgery or childbirth.[236] Based on this finding, it has been argued that these patients are more suitable for surgical treatment.

Because the functional results of total colectomy and ileorectal anastomosis in the treatment of chronic constipation caused by colonic inertia are often considered unsatisfactory due to the frequency of postoperative diarrhea and the high rate of postoperative small bowel obstruction, Sarli et al[237] assessed the functional results of eight females who underwent subtotal colectomy with antiperistaltic cecorectal anastomosis. Before antiperistaltic cecorectal anastomosis, all ten patients were laxative dependent, with a mean bowel frequency of 10 days; eight of them had distention, seven bloating, and three abdominal pain. One month after antiperistaltic cecorectal anastomosis, bowel frequency was a mean of 2.2 per day with a semiliquid stool consistency. After 1 year, bowel frequency was a mean of 1.3 per day with a solid stool consistency; laxatives continued to be used by two patients with paradoxical puborectalis contraction. All 10 patients reported a good or improved quality of life.

After subtotal colectomy with ileorectal anastomosis, approximately 10% of the patients require a stoma because of intractable diarrhea or persistent constipation associated with abdominal discomfort. The creation of a stoma can also be considered as a primary procedure. Little information is available regarding the results of stoma formation in patients with slow-transit constipation. van der Sijp et al[238] studied 39 patients who were treated at some stage with either a colostomy or an ileostomy. The authors noted that many symptoms persisted after the creation of a stoma. However, those with the best results were patients who had a primary stoma as the first treatment for their colonic inertia.

Restorative Proctocolectomy

In the desperate situation in which a patient has severe idiopathic constipation for which all medical treatment has failed and total colectomy and ileorectal anastomosis have not resolved the problem, Nicholls and Kamm[239] described the use of the proctocolectomy with a restorative ileoanal reservoir. The authors suggest that in the very small group of patients who do not show improvement after colectomy and ileorectal anastomosis and who are not prepared to accept an ileostomy, consideration should be given to a pouch procedure that the authors have performed with satisfactory results. Hosie et al[240] performed a restorative proctocolectomy in 13 patients. Eight of those patients had recurrent constipation after colectomy and five had constipation and overflow incontinence associated with megarectum and megacolon. Despite a high complication rate, 85% of the patients experienced improved symptoms and quality of life. In their review of the literature, Pfeifer et al[172] found 10 patients who underwent a pouch procedure with an 82% success rate. Thakur et al[241] reviewed the hospital records of five patients with persistent symptomatic idiopathic colonic inertia. Each of the patients had undergone extensive medical management, and eventually four underwent one or more colonic resections to relieve the recurrent abdominal distention and pain. Three of the patients eventually received a distal ileostomy, which functioned well. Anorectal manometric studies were within normal range for each of the five patients. Restorative proctocolectomy (J-pouch) was performed for each. With a mean follow-up of 42 months after restorative proctocolectomy, each of the five patients was relieved of constipation and small bowel distension. The average number of bowel movements per 24 hours at 6 months was 4.8. All patients were able to discriminate flatus from stool, could hold back for up to 1.5 hours after the initial urge to defecate, and had total daytime continence. Each returned to work or school within 3 months and each reported greater satisfaction of bowel function than with the ileostomy.

Kalbassi et al assessed the outcome of proctocolectomy among 15 patients. Two patients required pouch excision because of intractable pelvic pain. The authors noted improvement in lifestyle scores in the categories of physical function, social function, and pain.[242] It is not clear whether this procedure is an appropriate option, because the reported results are rather conflicting.

Sacral Neuromodulation and Posterior Tibial Nerve Stimulation (PTNS)

Sacral neuromodulation has been used successfully in the treatment of patients with urologic disorders and of those with fecal incontinence. Some of these patients noted increased stool frequency and improved rectal evacuation. Based on this observation, Malouf et al implanted a temporary percutaneous electrode in the third sacral foramen of eight women with slow-transit constipation. The electrode was attached to an external stimulator for 3 weeks. A bowel symptom diary card, anorectal physiology studies, and a radiopaque marker transit study were completed before and during the test stimulation. Only two patients clinically responded, both reporting a marked improvement in stool frequency and symptoms. These two patients had an immediate return to prestimulation symptoms after removal of the stimulating leads. Colonic transit did not return to normal in any patient, including the two responders. The test stimulation resulted in a significant improvement of rectal sensory perception, which was the only parameter to change.[243] Kenefick et al[244] described four women with a permanent implant for intractable slow-transit constipation. A good clinical response was obtained in three of them at a median follow-up of 4.5 months. The number of evacuations per week increased from a mean of 1.1 to 5.8. The Cleveland Clinic constipation score improved from 21.5 to 9.2. Kenefick et al[245] also carried out a double-blind crossover study in two women, who were implanted with a permanent stimulator 12 months previously. The study consisted of 2-week interval with subsensory stimulation either "on" or "off." The patients and the investigator were blinded. The number of evacuations per week changed from one to five and from two to five, respectively, when the stimulator was turned on. Abdominal pain and bloating improved with increased frequency of defecation. This finding suggests that there was no placebo effect. Although randomized control trials are lacking, a review of the literature by Sharma et al[246] looked at 10 studies that discussed the results of SNS with constipation. A total of 225 temporary neuromodulations and 125 permanent implants were performed. Bowel diaries showed improvement in assessment criteria in more than 50% of patients on temporary neuromodulation and the results were maintained in approximately 90% of patients who underwent permanent implantation over medium- to long-term follow-up. Improvements in transit studies and anorectal physiology after neuromodulation were noted in some studies. Knowles et al reported the CONFIDeNT randomized trial in which 115 patients underwent controlled PTNS and 112 received sham treatment. PTNS did not show any significant clinical benefit over sham electrical stimulation. Moreover, a subsequent post hoc analysis revealed that concomitant obstructive defecation symptoms negatively affected the clinical outcome of PTNS. Thus, PTNS cannot be recommended for the treatment of constipation in the UK or the EU and it is not FDA approved for this indication in the USA.[247,248,249]

Antegrade Continent Enema Procedure

The antegrade continent enema procedure involves the formation of a continent conduit suitable for intermittent catheterization, allowing antegrade irrigation of the colon. The procedure was first described by Malone in 1990 for the treatment of neuropathic constipation in pediatric practice. There are some data regarding the short-term outcome of this procedure in the treatment of constipation in adults. Hill et al[250] described early results in six patients, all of whom were successfully relieved of constipation. Krogh and Laurberg[251] reported a successful outcome in four of six patients after a follow-up of up to 39 months. Rongen et al[252] reported a successful outcome in eight

of twelve patients after a median follow-up of 532 days. Recently, Lees et al[253] described the long-term results of this procedure, obtained in 32 patients. They observed a high rate of conduit reversal or major revision. Satisfactory function was ultimately achieved in 47% of the patients. This long-term result indicates that this procedure is less beneficial for patients with slow-transit constipation than previously thought.

Anorectal Outlet Obstruction

Anismus

In 1964, Wasserman[254] described four patients with obstructed defecation due to a "type of stenosis of the anorectum caused by a spasm of a component of the external anal sphincter muscle" and named it "puborectalis syndrome." Since then, a wide variety of appellations have been devised to describe this condition. The most frequently used terms are anismus, spastic pelvic floor syndrome, and nonrelaxing puborectalis syndrome. Most experts believe that symptoms such as prolonged and repeated straining at stool, the necessity of manual assistance, the sensation of incomplete evacuation, and the need for suppositories and enemas are suggestive of this condition. It has to be emphasized, however, that an almost identical pattern of symptoms might be observed in women with a large rectocele. Therefore, the history of the patient is inconclusive in establishing nonrelaxation of the pelvic floor during attempted evacuation. Although paradoxic contraction of the puborectalis muscle has been reported to be easily assessed by physical examination during straining, most investigators do not rely on palpation and advocate the use of specific tests to document anismus. EMG, evacuation proctography, and balloon expulsion test are the most commonly used methods. Much controversy, however, exists relative to the optimal diagnostic test. No single method has been proven to be pathognomonic for anismus or superior to the others. Despite several limitations, EMG is considered the most specific test, providing the best assessment of puborectalis activity during straining. In most studies, EMG is performed with the patient in the left lateral position. However, straining in this position after the painful insertion of a needle and without a natural desire to defecate is rather unphysiologic. Duthie and Bartolo[255] found evidence of anismus on EMG recordings in 11 patients with constipation during attempted defecation on a commode in the laboratory. However, during home recordings, the pelvic floor relaxed during straining in all but three patients. These findings support the view that the inability to relax the pelvic floor might represent the inability to comply with the request in the unfamiliar and unphysiologic circumstances of the laboratory.

If anismus represents the principal cause of obstructed defecation, then increased EMG activity of the puborectalis muscle should be observed exclusively in patients with evacuation difficulties. Moreover, recruitment of EMG activity should be associated with a more acute anorectal angle on evacuation proctography and subsequent failure to expel a rectal balloon. Between 1985 and 1993, ten studies were published regarding EMG evidence of anismus in controls. In only three studies did none of the controls show evidence of paradoxic contraction of the pelvic floor. In the other seven studies, the incidence of anismus varied between 12 and 61%.[256] Pezim et al,[257] for example, reported that nearly 50% of their controls exhibited either a paradoxic increase in EMG activity or no suppression during straining. Jones et al[258] found EMG evidence of anismus in 76% of patients with constipation, 50% of patients with solitary rectal ulcer syndrome, and 48% of subjects with anorectal pain. All patients with anorectal pain had a normal defecation pattern. In 74 patients with functional constipation, Kuijpers[216] found evidence of anismus on EMG and evacuation proctography in 74 and 74% of patients, respectively. Such an excellent agreement between EMG and the other diagnostic tests could not be demonstrated by others.[259,260] In a prospective evaluation of a consecutive series of 112 patients with constipation associated with obstructed defecation, Jorge et al[261] observed evidence of anismus based on EMG and evacuation proctography in 38 and 36% of patients, respectively. Based on these data, one might suppose that the correlation between the two tests is almost optimal. However, 33% of the patients with evidence of anismus on evacuation proctography showed a normal EMG, whereas 30% of the patients with an EMG diagnosis had a normal evacuation proctography. These observations support the view that the signs of anismus are not specific for constipation and/or obstructed defecation and that EMG results are poorly correlated with evacuation proctography and balloon expulsion test. A study conducted by Schouten et al[262] also revealed that EMG has a very poor agreement with the other diagnostic modalities.

The efficacy of biofeedback has been used as an argument to support the clinical significance of anismus (▶ Table 33.11). Loening-Baucke[263] investigated the results of biofeedback in 38 children presenting with chronic constipation and encopresis. All these children showed contraction of the pelvic floor during straining. Twenty-eight children learned to relax their pelvic floor. Despite this beneficial effect of biofeedback, 14 of these children did not recover from constipation. The author also reported that the non-recovered patients who learned to relax their pelvic floor had significantly decreased rectal and anal responsiveness to rectal distention when compared with the recovered patients. Keck et al[264] reported the results of biofeedback in 12 constipated patients. Although all subjects could be taught to relax their sphincter in response to bearing down, only one patient reported resolution of symptoms. Turnbull and Ritvo[265] reported a successful outcome after biofeedback in 8 of 10 female patients with constipation. However, five of these patients showed persisting and continuing anismus on objective testing. These findings are not in accordance with the assumption that anismus is the principal cause of obstructed defecation and that biofeedback is successful solely because it corrects the "paradoxic" contraction of the pelvic floor.

Lubowski et al[266] developed a new scintigraphic method to assess both colonic and rectal function during normal defecation. The authors found that colonic emptying is an integral part of normal defecation and that defecation is not a process of rectal emptying alone. They suggested that "obstructed defecation may occur in some patients as a result of a disorder of colonic function rather than a disorder of the rectum or the pelvic floor muscles." It seems obvious that the popular concept that obstructed defecation is mainly due to pelvic floor muscle incoordination has little scientific basis. In an earlier EMG study of the pubococcygeus muscles in patients with obstructed defecation, Lubowski et al[267] concluded that the puborectalis muscle did not cause obstructed defecation and that the concept of "paradoxic" contraction of this muscle is questionable.

In recent years, attention has been focused on the rectal wall properties in women with obstructed defecation. As discussed earlier in this chapter, there is growing evidence that rectal sensory perceptions and rectal motility are impaired in these patients, probably due to extramural damage to the efferent and afferent nerves. It seems likely that this damage to the rectal innervation results in "rectal akinesia," as described by Faucheron and Dubreuil.[268]

Biofeedback Training

During the last two decades, biofeedback therapy has gained popularity as the foremost treatment for obstructed defecation. Bleijenberg and Kuijpers[269] achieved good results in 7 of 10 women with spastic pelvic floor syndrome. It has been argued, however, that the length of the hospital admission (2 weeks) and the rather extensive psychotherapy may have been more beneficial than the biofeedback itself. In the same period, Weber et al[276] reported a successful outcome in 12 of 25 constipated patients (48%) after biofeedback on an outpatient basis. Since then, spectacular results have been reported with success rates of up to 100% (▶ Table 33.12). There are some data indicating that biofeedback is more effective in patients with obstructed defecation than in patients with colonic inertia. At 1-year control, Battaglia et al found that 50% of their patients with obstructed defecation still maintained a beneficial effect from biofeedback, whereas only 20% of those with slow-transit constipation did so.[203] Chiarioni et al reported similar findings. Six months after biofeedback, the outcome was successful in 71% of the patients with obstructed defecation. Only 8% of the patients with slow-transit constipation were satisfied with the effect of biofeedback.[271] Palsson et al reviewed the literature in order to assess the efficacy of biofeedback for functional anorectal disorders. They qualified 38 studies on obstructed defecation and/or functional constipation for review. The overall average probability of successful treatment was 62.4%.[272] In contrast to the high percentage of controlled studies found in the pediatric literature, only four adult studies randomly assigned patients to different treatment protocols. Koutsomanis et al[273] randomly assigned 60 patients with obstructed defecation either to EMG biofeedback with balloon defecation training or to balloon defecation training alone and found no significant differences. In a randomized study of 20 patients with obstructed defecation, Bleijenberg and Kuijpers[270] found EMG biofeedback to be superior to balloon defecation training. Heymen at al compared four different biofeedback protocols and found no differences among

Table 33.11 Effect of biofeedback training on paradoxic puborectalis contraction and symptoms of obstructed defecation

Author(s)	No. of cases	Evidence of anismus (%)		Successful outcome
		Before	After	
Loening-Baucke[263]	38	100	24	37
Dahl et al[260]	14	100	0	93
Turnbull and Ritvo[265]	10	100	70	80
Papachrysostomou and Smith[282]	22	100	0	86
Keck et al[264]	12	100	0	8
Glia et al[275]	20	100	10	75

Table 33.12 Outcome of biofeedback training in patients with obstructed defecation

Authors	No. of cases	Follow-up (mo)	Success rate (%)
Bleijenberg and Kuijpers[269]	10	>6	70
Weber et al[276]	25	6	48
Dahl et al[260]	14	6	93
Kawimbe et al[277]	15	6	100
Loening-Baucke[263]	38	1	37
Lestàr et al[278]	16	15	69
Turnbull and Ritvo[265]	10	3	71
West et al[279]	18	12	100
Wexner et al[280]	18	9	89
Fleshman et al[281]	9	6	89
Keck et al[264]	12	8	8
Papachrysostomou and Smith[282]	22	NS	86
Koutsomanis et al 1995[273]	60	3	40
Ho et al[283]	62	15	90
Park et al[284]	57	24	55
Glia et al[275]	20	6	75
Rao et al[285]	25	NS	76
Karlbom et al[286]	28	14	43
McKee et al[287]	28	NS	21
Lau et al[288]	108	NS	55
Dailianas et al[289]	11	6	64
Rhee et al[290]	45	NS	69
Battaglia et al[203]	14	12	50
Chiarioni et al[271]	34	6	71

Abbreviation: NS, not stated.

Table 33.13 Results of division of the puborectalis muscle for anismus

Authors	No. of cases	Procedure	Success rate (%)
Keighley and Shoulder[154]	7	PPD	14
Barnes et al[291]	9	PPD	24
Kawano et al[292]	7	PPR	43
Kamm et al[293]	18	CLD	24
Yu and Cui[294]	18	PPR	85

Abbreviations: CLD, complete lateral division; PPD, posterior partial division; PPR, posterior partial resection.

admit to any clinical improvement. Ho et al[283] studied 62 patients with obstructed defecation. In 40 patients, signs of anismus were observed, whereas 20 subjects had no evidence of anismus. The outcome of biofeedback was similar in both groups. Dahl et al[260] reported that paradoxic anal contraction disappeared in all their patients after biofeedback. All but one patient improved considerably and learned to defecate spontaneously (▶ Table 33.13). In other studies, symptom relief has been noted without evidence of correction of anismus.[263,264,265] Rao et al[285] reported that biofeedback improves objective parameters such as balloon expulsion time and rectal sensory perception. It has been demonstrated that coexistent abnormalities such as rectocele and rectal intussusception do not adversely affect the outcome of biofeedback in patients with obstructed defecation.[288] Leroi et al[114] reported that biofeedback alone was not successful in the majority of sexually abused women with anismus. The authors noted that the outcome was markedly better if biofeedback was combined with psychotherapy. This finding suggests that the resolution of symptoms may be attributed to other factors, such as the psychological effects of encouragement and positive verbal feedback.

It has been noted that many patients use the biofeedback sessions to talk about psychosocial distress. So, it might be possible that the behavioral and psychological aspects of therapy are just as important for a successful outcome.

Botulinum Toxin

In 1988, Hallan et al[295] reported seven patients with anismus, diagnosed by EMG and evacuation proctography. The symptoms of anismus resolved in six patients after the injection of botulinum toxin into the left and right sides of both the puborectalis muscle and the external sphincter. The most important side effect was fecal incontinence, occurring in two patients. Joo et al[296] reported their experience with four patients who failed to respond to biofeedback. All four patients improved between 1 and 3 months after botulinum injections. This improvement was sustained for a longer period of time in only two subjects. Maria et al[297] treated three patients with animus by injecting 30 units of Type A botulinum toxin in both limbs of the puborectalis muscle. These three patients experienced symptomatic relief. In one patient, the treatment had to be repeated twice because of recurrent symptoms.[297] Ron et al[298] treated 25 patients with obstructed defecation by local injection of 10 units of botulinum toxin to each side of the puborectalis muscle. Only 37% of the patients were satisfied with the overall results. Straining, which was the main complaint,

the treatment strategies.[274] Glia et al[275] found EMG biofeedback to be superior to pressure biofeedback with balloon training. Of these four studies, the study of Koutsomanis et al is the only one with a sufficient sample size to provide meaningful conclusions.

There is much controversy regarding the objective effects of biofeedback on anorectal function. Kawimbe et al[277] observed a significant reduction in the anismus index after biofeedback training, which was intended as a relearning process in which the inappropriate contraction of the pelvic floor was gradually suppressed. There was an associated reduction in the time spent straining stool and in the difficulty of defecation as well as an increased stool frequency. Papachrysostomou and Smith[282] demonstrated that various parameters related to the obstructive defecation syndrome showed significant change at the end of the biofeedback training period. However, these changes were also observed in those patients (14%) who did not decreased in only 29% of the cases. Defecation frequency did not increase after the injection. Based on these disappointing results, the authors concluded that "injection of botulinum toxin into the puborectalis muscle has limited therapeutic effect on patients suffering from anismus."

In contrast, the Oxford group from the United Kingdom suggests an excellent response to botulinum toxin if other concordant diagnoses are excluded. Fifty-six patients with proctographic anismus were treated with Botox. Twenty-two (39%) responded initially and 21/22 (95%) underwent repeat treatment. At a median follow-up of 19.2 (range, 7.0–30.4) months, 20/21 (95%) had a sustained response and required no further treatment. Isolated obstructed defecation symptoms (OR = 7.8, p = 0.008), but not proctographic or physiological factors, predicted response on logistic regression analysis. In 33 (97%) of 34 nonresponders, significant abnormalities were demonstrated at EUA: 31 (94%) had a grade 3 to 5 rectal prolapse, one had internal anal sphincter myopathy, and one had a fissure. Exclusion of these alternative diagnoses revised the initial response rate to 96%.[299] This study suggests that in patients with proctographical anismus, Botox is good treatment modality possibly in parallel to biofeedback therapy.

Division of the Puborectalis Muscle (▶ Table 33.13)

In the 1960s, Wasserman[254] and Wallace and Madden[300] advocated partial resection of the puborectalis muscle at the posterior midline in patients with anismus. Although their early results were promising, two other studies revealed very disappointing results after partial division of the puborectalis muscle.[153,291] Dissatisfied with the poor outcome after partial division at the posterior midline, Kamm et al[293] reported on 15 patients with severe constipation and 3 patients with megarectum who underwent an almost complete uni- or bilateral division of the puborectalis muscle. Only four patients had symptomatic improvement. It was remarkable that this information did not correlate with the ability to expel a balloon. In contrast to the current opinion that division of the puborectalis muscle is not appropriate, Yu and Cui[294] from China believe that there is still a sound indication for this procedure. The authors reported on 18 patients with anismus associated with puborectalis hypertrophy in which a partial resection at the posterior

midline was performed. According to Yu and Cui,[294] this procedure was successful in 83% of the patients studied. Despite these reports, the treatment of anismus with surgery is of historical interest only and its use has been largely abandoned due to the success of more conservative treatments.

Sacral Neuromodulation

Ganio et al[301] reported their experience with sacral neuromodulation in 16 patients with chronic outlet constipation. Following successful test stimulation, all these patients were implanted with a permanent stimulator. Prior to the procedure, the overall Wexner score was 14.6 (range, 8–20). This score dropped to 2.7 (range, 3–16) at 12 months of follow-up.[301] Unfortunately, these promising results have not been confirmed by others.

Rectal Intussusception

Intussusception of the rectum, or internal procidentia, is considered to be a preliminary stage in the development of complete rectal prolapse. Although complete rectal prolapse is readily apparent, the diagnosis of intussusception may be difficult to demonstrate by physical examination, endoscopy, or barium contrast examination. Evacuation proctography is the most useful diagnostic procedure for identifying intussusception. The radiologic features are characteristic. The rectum begins to intussuscept a few centimeters above the pelvic floor. A typical funnel-like configuration is seen in ▶ Fig. 33.11.

In the past, rectal intussusception was considered one of the principal causes of obstructed defecation. In 1984, Hoffman et al[302] suggested that a modified Ripstein procedure was adequate to relieve symptoms of obstructed defecation. However, the authors' follow-up was short and concerned only a small group of patients. Johansson et al[303] reported a series of 23 patients who presented for operation because of obstructed defecation. Thirty-five percent of those patients had worsening of their symptoms after rectopexy. Similar results have been described by others.[304] There is growing evidence that a posterior rectopexy induces rectal evacuation disturbances, especially when the lateral ligaments of the rectum

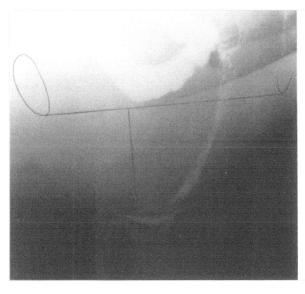

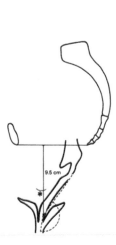

Fig. 33.11 Defecography in a patient with rectal intussusception.

are divided.[305,306] Moreover, it has been shown that rectal intussusception is a common finding on evacuation proctography in normal volunteers.[307] The benefit of surgical correction of rectal intussusception was therefore questioned. More recently, however, there has been a renewed interest with the advent of new operations to treat intussusception. In 2003, Longo described the stapled transanal rectal resection (STARR) procedure based on the observation that stapled hemorrhoidopexy often improved defecation in patients with rectocele and intussusception.[308] Using two firings of a transanal circular stapler, Longo described a full-thickness, circumferential resection of the intussusception and any accompanying rectocele. Evolution of the technique led to the development of a dedicated curved stapling device and the description of the TranStar procedure, whereby the distal rectal ampulla could be resected transanally using sequential, circumferential stapler firings. The use of STARR and TranStar for obstructed defecation has been the source of much controversy. Several small studies have reported a significant benefit[309,310] and a large, prospective European registry has shown significant improvement in constipation scores and quality of life following STARR and TranStar.[311] However, there have also been reports of complications, including intractable pain, defecatory urgency, and worsening of incontinence.[312] The procedure should therefore be used selectively, and only after thorough pelvic floor investigation. It should probably be avoided in patients with known anal sphincter dysfunction who appear to be more at risk of postoperative urgency and incontinence. Others have adopted an alternative approach to the surgical correction of intussusception, with the use of laparoscopic ventral mesh rectopexy. Initially described by D'Hoore et al as a treatment for full-thickness rectal prolapse, the operation has been used in patients with obstructed defecation due to intussusception with reasonable results.[313] In this procedure, partial laparoscopic mobilization of the rectum and dissection of the rectovaginal septum enables placement of a strip of mesh, which is secured to the anterior rectum and posterior vaginal vault. Attachment of the proximal end of the mesh to the sacral promontory re-suspends the rectum, correcting the intussusception and any associated rectocele and enterocele. Several reports testify to the benefits of the procedure in treating obstructed defecation. However, concerns have been expressed about serious mesh-related complications, including mesh migration and rectal erosion.[314] Whether the use of biological meshes reduces the risk of these complications is not yet established.

Rectocele

A rectocele is a herniation of the anterior rectal wall into the posterior wall of the vagina. The significance of rectoceles in the pathogenesis of obstructed defecation remains debatable. Some experts believe that rectoceles are merely a secondary manifestation of chronic straining on a rectovaginal septum weakened both by obstetric trauma and progressive pelvic floor deficiency, as part of the aging process. Others believe that rectoceles are indeed an important cause of obstructed defecation. Although rectoceles are common, they usually do not become symptomatic until the fourth or fifth decade of life. During straining, the apex of the rectocele moves inferiorly and anteriorly. Stool is trapped in this sacculation, and straining aggravates the problem by pushing the stool further from the anal

opening. Most patients with a symptomatic rectocele have a normal daily urge to defecate, but they "can't get it out." To aid defecation, some patients use manual pressure on the side or front of the anal outlet or they insert a finger against the posterior vaginal wall. A rectocele may be associated with other symptoms such as tenesmus, incomplete evacuation, pain, bleeding, protrusion, and soiling. The diagnosis is made by obtaining an adequate history and by bimanual or rectovaginal palpation. A hooked finger pressed on the anterior rectal wall can detect the pocket-like defect located just above the anal sphincter. The presence of a rectocele, along with any contrast trapping, can be readily appreciated on a defecating proctogram (▶ Fig. 33.12).

A wide variety of anatomic and functional changes on defecography have been observed in patients with a so-called symptomatic rectocele.[315] However, whether a rectocele is responsible for evacuatory symptoms or is a secondary phenomenon can be difficult to determine. It is generally accepted that rectoceles less than 2 cm in size are not clinically significant.[316] Only rectoceles more than 3 cm in depth are considered abnormal. It has been shown that larger rectoceles are more likely to retain contrast than smaller ones.[317] However, the size of the rectocele and the extent of barium trapping have not been shown to correlate with the degree of symptoms or with the outcome of rectocele repair.[318,319] Johansson et al[319] have suggested that anismus is a causative factor in the formation of a rectocele. The authors stated that rectocele repair in patients with concomitant anismus cannot be successful, because the underlying cause for obstructed defecation persists. In contrast, van Dam et al[320] conducted a prospective study to evaluate the prevalence of anismus in patients with a symptomatic rectocele and to investigate the impact of anismus on the outcome of rectocele repair. They concluded that results of rectocele repair in

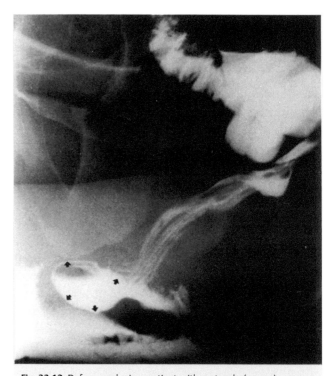

Fig. 33.12 Defecography in a patient with rectocele (*arrows*).

patients with anismus were similar to those obtained in patients without evidence of anismus. This finding was irrespective of the method of diagnosing anismus.

Several authors have tried to assess specific features encountered in women with a symptomatic rectocele. Siproudhis et al[321] found that patients with a rectocele differed significantly from those without a rectocele in having frequent vaginal digitation, more frequent symptoms of urinary incontinence, and a history of hysterectomy. Delayed rectal emptying, incomplete rectal emptying, and manometric signs of anismus were more frequently encountered in the rectocele group. Murthy et al[322] adopted a selective approach, based on several criteria, including the sensation of a vaginal mass or bulge that required digital support, barium trapping in the rectocele, and the presence of a very large rectocele associated with anterior rectal wall prolapse. These authors claimed that the selection of patients based on these criteria results in a very good clinical outcome. Karlbom et al[323] observed that the need for vaginal or perineal digitation preoperatively was related to a good result, whereas a previous hysterectomy, a large rectal area on defecography, and the preoperative use of enemas and laxatives related to a poor outcome. In contrast, Mellgren et al[324] found that preoperative vaginal digitation was not mandatory for a good postoperative result. The authors also demonstrated that delayed colonic transit was related to a less favorable outcome. This finding has been confirmed by others.[325] Stojkovic et al compared women with a successful rectocele repair to those with persistent symptoms.[325] There was no difference in age between the two groups. There was also no difference in size of rectocele, degree of emptying, the presence of another defecographic abnormality, and the need to self-digitate between the two groups.[326]

Some authors are reluctant to repair a completely emptying rectocele, whereas others report that some patients still derive benefit from operative treatment. These reflections illustrate that many questions regarding the specific features of rectoceles and the selection criteria for repair are still unanswered. Rectoceles can be repaired by several approaches: transvaginal, transanal (or a combination of both), transperineal, and abdominal. The use of a mesh to reinforce rectocele repair has fallen into disrepute due to the high incidence of mesh-related complications, resulting in several high-profile, class action lawsuits.

Transvaginal Repair

For more than one century, the history of rectocele repair was written by gynecologists. They performed a posterior colporrhaphy combined with levator plication and some form of perineorrhaphy. Nonrandomized studies suggest that this approach is associated with a 25% incidence of dyspareunia and that one-third of the patients suffer from persistent evacuation difficulties.[327] Arnold et al[327] performed a retrospective review of 64 rectocele repairs. Both the transvaginal and the transanal approaches were used in 26 and 35 patients, respectively. They found no difference in complications between the techniques. Forty-seven patients could be contacted for follow-up. Although improvement was reported by 80% of the patients, persistent obstructed defecation was noted by 54% of the women. New-onset dyspareunia was noted by 22% of the patients. There was

no difference in results and complications between the two approaches.[327] Nieminen et al[328] compared the transvaginal approach to the transanal approach. Thirty female patients with a symptomatic rectocele were enrolled in a randomized controlled trial. The need to digitally assist rectal emptying decreased in the transvaginal group from 73 to 7% and in the transanal group from 66 to 27%. The respective recurrence rates were 7 and 40%. In contrast with other studies, none of the patients reported new-onset dyspareunia.[328] In attempt to reduce recurrence rates, mesh was introduced for transvaginal rectocele repair. De Tayrac et al[329] used a polypropylene mesh. Mesh infection and rectovaginal fistulas were not encountered with the procedure being successful in 92% of the patients. Altman et al[330] designed a study to evaluate transvaginal rectocele repair using porcine collagen mesh (Pelvicol, CR Bard, Murray Hill, NJ). The outcome was assessed in 29 women. At 12-month follow-up, defecography revealed a persistent or recurrent rectocele in 15 patients. At 6-month follow-up, many patients experienced a significant decrease in rectal evacuation difficulties. This beneficial effect was less pronounced at 12-month follow-up. New-onset dyspareunia was not observed. Based on these findings, the authors concluded that, although transvaginal rectocele repair with a collagen mesh improves anatomic support, there is a substantial risk for recurrence. It is obvious that further evaluation is warranted before the use of biomaterial mesh can be adopted into clinical practice.[330]

Transanal Repair

Marks[331] was one of the first to note persistent evacuation difficulties following traditional transvaginal rectocele repair. He also noted that many women with a symptomatic rectocele had a "thinning" of the anterior rectal wall, including the muscle layers, and an enlarged rectal ampulla. Based on these observations, he advocated repair of the rectal side of the rectocele. Although there are several variations and modifications, the principal goal of the procedure is to remove or plicate redundant rectal mucosa and to plicate the anterior rectal wall.

Advantages attributed to the transanal approach are that it is a procedure of lesser magnitude than the gynecologic approach, it affords the opportunity to correct associated anorectal pathology, and there is a more direct access to the suprasphincteric area. The disadvantage of this approach is the inability to correct a cystocele simultaneously.

For transanal repair, the patient is placed in the prone jackknife position. The submucosal plane of the anterior wall is infiltrated with an epinephrine-containing solution such as 0.5% lidocaine (Xylocaine) in 1:200,000 epinephrine. A midline incision is made at a point starting just above the dentate line and is carried upward in the rectum approximately 7 to 8 cm, depending on the size of the rectocele (▶ Fig. 33.13a). Alternatively, a rectangular flap of mucosa and submucosa is elevated. Mucosal flaps are developed on each side. A further option is a simple transverse mucosal incision 1 cm above the dentate line.[332] Meticulous hemostasis is obtained with cautery. The musculofascial defect in the anterior wall is plicated in a transverse manner with interrupted absorbable sutures such as 2–0 Vicryl (▶ Fig. 33.13b, c). If weakness of the anterior wall persists, another row of similar sutures can be placed (▶ Fig. 33.13d). This row may be supplemented with three or four vertical sutures of the same

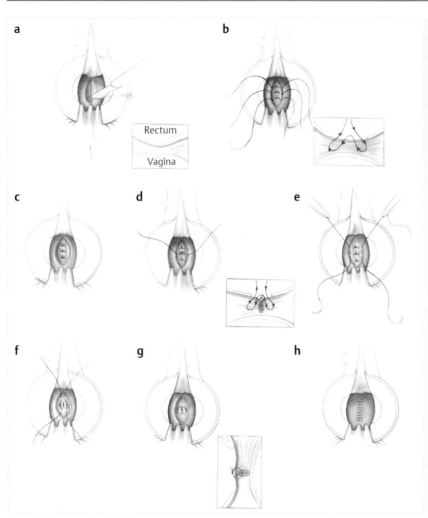

Rectum

Vagina

Fig. 33.13 Rectocele repair. **(a)** Mucosal incision over rectocele. **(b,c)** Transverse plication of defect. **(d)** Second row of sutures for persistent anterior defect. **(e)** Supplemental repair by vertical sutures. **(f,g)** Sullivan's technique for repair of rectocele. **(h)** Mucosal reapproximation.

material[333,334] (▶ Fig. 33.13e). The technique adopted by Sullivan et al[335] consists of longitudinal plication of the circular muscle of the anterior rectal wall with five or more slowly absorbed sutures such as 2–0 Dexon or Vicryl (▶ Fig. 33.13f, g). For large rectoceles, the authors recommend the initial use of three or four transverse sutures to pull the levator ani muscles medially. The transverse apposition is then reinforced by a longitudinal plication (▶ Fig. 33.13f, g). The authors subsequently abandoned the use of transverse sutures in favor of longitudinal plication based on a prospective study of 100 patients, in which sepsis and separation of the wound was noted when the combined technique was used. Sarles et al[332] used interrupted polyglycolic acid sutures (2–0), with "bites" of rectal muscle wall taken every 5 mm. Their rationale was that the anatomic lesion was due to weakness of the circular muscle, the horizontal fibers of which are spread apart and attenuated by progressive distention of the anterior rectal wall. Thus, vertical plication sutures are more likely to reconstitute the rectovaginal septum. The excess mucosa is excised, and the mucosal flaps are closed with a continuous absorbable suture (▶ Fig. 33.13h).

Block[337] described a modification, characterized by simple plication of the redundant mucosa without excision. This technique is less popular because some patients complain of persistent tenesmus, and urge to defecate if the excess mucosa is not

removed. In addition, necrosis of the plicated rectal mucosa may result in postoperative infection.[338] Transanal repair can also be performed using a linear stapler.[339] A major concern after transanal repair is the impairment of fecal continence. Arnold et al reported that 38% of their patients developed incontinence.[327] This serious side effect may occur because of an occult sphincter defect that becomes symptomatic or may develop as a result of the anal dilatation and stretching during the procedure. It has been shown that transanal rectocele repair results in a decline of anal resting pressure as well as anal squeeze pressure.[340] van Dam et al[341] evaluated the impact of a combined transvaginal/transanal rectocele repair on fecal continence in a consecutive series of 89 women. They observed deterioration of continence in 7% of the patients. Another concern after transanal repair is the development of dyspareunia. Sehapayak et al[334] observed this complication in 20% of their patients. van Dam et al[341] found new-onset dyspareunia following a combined transvaginal/transanal repair in 17 out of 41 sexually active patients (41%). Similar figures have been reported by others.[342] Most series, except those reported by Arnold et al,[327] have revealed promising short-term results after transanal rectocele repair. Recent studies, however, do suggest that the medium- and long-term outcome is less favorable (▶ Table 33.14).

Table 33.14 Results of rectocele repair

Authors	No. of cases	Procedure	Follow-up (y)	Success rate (%)[a]
Sullivan et al[335]	151	TAR	1.5	80
Capps[333]	51	TAR	ns	94
Khubchandani et al[336]	59	TAR	1.5	80
Sehapayak[334]	355	TAR	ns	85
Sarles et al[332]	16	TAR	1.6	94
Arnold et al[327]	35	TAR	ns	46
	29	TVR	ns	46
Janssen and van Dijke[343]	76	TAR	1.0	87
Mellgren et al[324]	25	TVR	1.0	88
Karlbom et al[323]	244	TAR	0.9	79
Van Dam et al[341]	75	TAR + TVR	4.0	71
Murthy et al[322]	31	TAR	2.5	92
Khubchandani et al[336]	123	TAR	NS	82
Tjandra et al[344]	59	TAR	1.5	78
Ayav et al[339]	21	TAR[b]	5	71
Heriot et al[345]	45	TAR	2	55
Thornton et al[342]	40	TAR	3.5	63
Abbas et al[346]	107	TAR	4	72
Hirst et al[347]	42	TAR	2	48
Roman and Michot[348]	71	TAR	6	50

Abbreviations: ns, not significant; TAR, transanal repair; TVR, transvaginal repair; NS, not stated.
[a]Excellent (asymptomatic) or good (considerable improvement).
[b]Using a linear stapler.

STARR Procedure

Although the STARR procedure is not advocated solely for the treatment of rectocele, it is used for obstructed defecation when there is internal rectal prolapse, which is often accompanied by a rectocele. The STARR gained popularity, particularly in Europe, when it was first introduced. The technique was first developed using two firings of the PPH-01 circular stapler to achieve a circumferential resection of the internal prolapse, along with any accompanying rectocele. The CONTOUR TRANSSTAR stapler was subsequently developed to enable a complete circumferential resection with successive firings of a curved stapler.[349,350] Many studies attest to the efficacy of STARR and TRANSTAR in improving obstructed defecation and quality of life as measured by patient-reported scores.[351,352,353] But, there have also been concerns expressed about serious complications, including rectovaginal fistula and rectal perforation.[354] Moreover, fecal urgency, possibly related to resection of the rectal ampulla resulting in reduced rectal compliance and increased sensitivity, can occur frequently in the early postoperative period, although it tends to decline on longer-term follow-up.[40] Fecal incontinence following STARR procedure has been reported,[354,355] but this is mainly seen in patients

with preexisting anal sphincter weakness and for this reason STARR should be used with great caution in such patients. If necessary, STARR can be combined with other gynecological procedures, such as vaginal hysterectomy for uterine prolapse, without any additional morbidity. Similar to all proctological interventions, patient selection for STARR is of great importance in achieving a satisfactory outcome.

Transperineal Repair

Rectoceles can also be repaired by a transperineal approach. This type of repair is usually performed through a transverse perineal incision. The rectovaginal plane is dissected and the rectocele is plicated with a running suture. After this plication, a levatorplasty may be performed. Transperineal repair seems to be as effective as the transanal and the transvaginal repair in relieving the symptoms of obstructed defecation.[356] Hirst et al[347] reported a successful outcome in 64% of their patients. In another study, the short-term outcome was good in 91% of the cases. However, 5 years after the procedure, the success rate had dropped to 70%. The same study revealed new-onset dyspareunia in 17% of the cases.[348] Similar figures have been reported by others.[357] The transperineal route avoids anal instrumentation and allows the surgeon to perform a sphincter repair in patients who have associated fecal incontinence.[320] Ayabaca et al reported that fecal continence improved in 74% of their patients after a transperineal rectocele repair with concomitant sphincteroplasty.[358] In 1996, Watson et al were the first to describe a transperineal mesh repair, which was successful in eight out of nine women.[359] More recently, similar results have been reported by others. One year after mesh repair, Mercer-Jones et al noted a successful outcome in 77% of their patients. They encountered two superficial infections and one deep wound infection, all responding to antibiotic therapy. In their series, no mesh had to be removed.[360] Lechaux et al reported a successful outcome in 80% of the cases.[361] An abdominal approach is most often employed by gynecologists when repair of an accompanying enterocele or vault prolapse is indicated. Usually, the dissection is performed in the rectovaginal space to expose the posterior vaginal wall.

Abdominal Repair

Correction of a rectocele by an abdominal approach is most often employed by gynecologists, when repair of an accompanying enterocele or vault prolapse is indicated. Usually the dissection is performed in the rectovaginal space to expose the posterior vaginal wall down to the perineal body. The fascial defect resulting in the rectocele is repaired by reattaching the posterior vagina bilaterally to the superior fascia of the levator ani, from the perineal body to the uterosacral ligament. In a retrospective matched cohort study, Thornton et al compared transanal repair to abdominal correction. They found a statistically greater alleviation of obstructed defecation after transanal repair (68 vs. 28%, respectively). New onset dyspareunia was encountered by 36% of the patients following transanal repair and by 22% of the patients after abdominal correction.[342] In another study, Vermeulen et al evaluated the results of anterolateral rectopexies for rectocele repair. Twenty patients were included. Defecography, performed postoperatively, revealed that all rectoceles were restored or at least diminished to normal size. Despite this observation, only 40% of the patients experienced resolution of symptoms. New-onset dyspareunia was encountered by 50%.[362]

Although the role of rectocele as a cause of difficult defecation has been long misunderstood or unrecognized, it should not be dismissed. By the same token, the presence of a rectocele in a patient with constipation does not necessarily indicate that the anatomic abnormality is causative. The simple detection of a rectocele is not in its own right an indication for operation. Sarles et al[332] listed three points of importance in correctly defining the role of rectocele in constipation: (1) the necessity for digital vaginal maneuver for evacuation, (2) defecography not only demonstrating the rectocele but also presenting evidence of retention of stool, and (3) defecography permitting the recognition of associated lesions, especially internal rectal procidentia.

Short-Segment Hirschsprung's Disease

When classic Hirschsprung's disease is treated by restorative anterior resection of the rectum (Rehbein's procedure), a short aganglionic segment remains, and symptoms of constipation persist. These residual symptoms can be treated by anorectal dilatation. Based on these findings, Bentley recommended using anorectal myectomy for the treatment of short-segment Hirschsprung's disease, which is one of the causes of anorectal outlet obstruction.[363] He assumed that the therapeutic effect of the anorectal myectomy could be compared to that of gastroesophageal myotomy (Heller's procedure) in patients with esophageal achalasia. Because his preliminary results were promising, other authors started to treat patients with short-segment Hirschsprung's disease as well as patients with non-Hirschsprung's constipation by anorectal myectomy. Anorectal myectomy can be expected to be effective only if patients with high anal basal tone in association with normal transit and impaired rectal emptying are selected. Anorectal myectomy alone or in combination with anterior resection was curative in a small number of patients reported by Fishbein et al.[364]

Idiopathic Megarectum

The entity of idiopathic megarectum was described in the section on slow-transit constipation. The question of which patients might be candidates for operative therapy is difficult to answer. Indications for operation are based on colonic function, taking into account an abnormally low frequency of defecation, delayed transit time of radiopaque markers, and/or abnormalities detected with anorectal manometry. These abnormalities include an absent or aberrant rectoanal inhibitory reflex, spontaneous variations of pressure in the rectum and anal canal, a hypertonic anal canal, and pressure exceeding predistention values before returning to the resting level (overshoot).

Anorectal Myectomy

Anorectal myectomy appears to have a limited role in the treatment of megarectum. The technique consists of submucosal resection of a 1-cm-wide strip of internal sphincteric muscle up to at least 6 cm above the dentate line (▶ Fig. 33.14).

In the series by Martelli et al,[67] anorectal myectomy was performed in 62 patients; 62% of the 50 patients who had fewer than three stools per week had more than three stools per week 1 year after myectomy. The six patients operated on because of the abnormal transit of radiopaque markers and the six operated on because of abnormal manometric findings were asymptomatic. Of the 26% of patients who were incontinent preoperatively, two-thirds became continent postoperatively. However, 16% of the patients who were continent preoperatively became incontinent postoperatively. Poisson and Devroede[365] stated that the results of anorectal myectomy were disappointing. In their experience, this condition responds well to a Boley pull-through procedure. Yoshioka and Keighley[366] reported the results of anorectal myectomy in 29 patients with chronic constipation. The improvement in 62% of patients correlated with a decrease in the maximal resting anal pressure associated with outlet obstruction. The results of other reports are summarized in ▶ Table 33.15. Martelli et al[67] recommended performing a Soave procedure in patients who have undergone

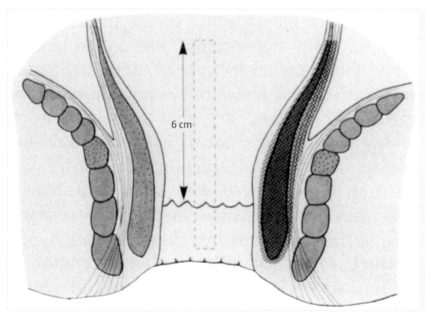

Fig. 33.14 Anorectal myectomy.

6 cm

Table 33.15 Clinical results of anorectal myectomy

Author(s)	Short-segment Hirschsprung's disease		Non-Hirschsprung's constipation	
	No. of patients	Success rate (%)	No. of patients	Success rate (%)
Thomas et al[368]	11	45		
Lynn and van Heerden[369]	28	93		
Clayden and Lawson[370]	10	100	11	82
Shermeta and Nilprabhassorn[371]	9	78		
Martelli et al[47]			62	77
McCready and Beart[372]	13	62		
Freeman[373]			61	86
Hamdy and Scobie[374]	6	66		
Mishalany and Wooley[375]			25	76
Pinto et al[376]	12	17	39	17

an anorectal myectomy with no success and in whom markers have demonstrated delayed transit time in the descending and sigmoid colon. Kimura et al[367] performed posterior myectomy of the remaining aganglionic rectal muscular cuff in patients with persistent rectal achalasia after the Soave endorectal pull-through procedure. Following this procedure, five patients had remarkable relief of constipation, distention, and enterocolitis.

Theory based on rather extensive experience with lateral internal sphincterotomy in the treatment of fissure-in-ano suggests that a lateral internal sphincterotomy results in fewer problems than a posterior sphincterotomy. In addition, a sphincterotomy probably also would suffice rather than performing a myectomy.

Adult Hirschsprung's Disease

A certain number of patients with Hirschsprung's disease do not present themselves for medical care until adulthood. Recognition of this childhood disease in an adult is difficult. The patients are usually men in their 20s with a lifelong history of constipation necessitating frequent use of laxatives and enemas. Plain films of the abdomen show distention of the distal colon. A barium enema study reveals a narrowed rectum with proximal colonic distention. The diagnosis depends on the patient's history, barium enema results, anorectal manometry, and rectal biopsy, which reveals the absence of ganglion cells, hypertrophy and hyperplasia of nerve fibers, and an increase of acetylcholinesterase-positive nerve fibers in the lamina propria and muscularis mucosa. Reported complications of adult Hirschsprung's disease are severe fecal impaction leading to obstruction, hemorrhage, volvulus of the colon secondary to an elongated colonic mesentery, ischemia secondary to compromise of the vasculature by colonic distention, perforation, superficial inflammation, ulceration of the mucosa by fecalomas, compromise of venous return, and decreased diaphragmatic excursion leading to pulmonary atelectasis.[377] Several procedures have been used to treat adult Hirschsprung's disease.

Although conclusions are difficult to reach regarding the appropriate operative therapy, the operation of choice is the Duhamel procedure.[378,379,380,381] In a comprehensive review of the literature, Wheatley et al[382] found that for the Duhamel operation, the complication rate was 10% for major complications and 2% for minor complications, and the results were good in 91%, fair in 7%, and poor in 2%. A more recent report by Kim et al[381] on 11 patients undergoing a Duhamel procedure revealed three major postoperative complications—two fistula-in-ano and one ileus, each resolving without operation. The long-term results were excellent except in one patient who developed impotence. Luukkonen et al[383] reported eight patients with adult Hirschsprung's disease, seven of whom underwent a Duhamel procedure and one who underwent an anterior resection later converted to a Soave procedure. None of the patients experienced constipation, but five had occasional soiling. These results can be compared to Swenson's operation, in which major complications occurred in 33%, minor complications in 7%, and impotence in 7%, with results good in 80% and poor in 20%. Endorectal pull-through operations result in major complications in 25% and minor complications in 13%, with results good in 85%, fair in 6%, and poor in 9%. The Duhamel operation obviates any extensive pelvic dissection and avoids the damage to the sensory fibers of the rectum that may be encountered during the Swenson procedure. It also avoids the mucosal dissection of the rectum required by the Soave procedure. Wu et al[384] reported on three patients who underwent resection of the diseased bowel, rectal mucosectomy, and coloanal anastomosis with good results.

Introduction of stapling devices has facilitated performance of the Duhamel procedure. An improved technique involving use of the curved EEA, GIA, and TA 55 staplers has simplified the operation.[385] The operation is performed with the patient in the modified lithotomy position. The colon is mobilized, freeing a portion of the aganglionic segment of bowel and any markedly dilated bowel that appears decompensated proximal to the aganglionic segment. The presacral space is entered and a tunnel is created down to the levator ani muscle. Extensive dissection in the pelvis should be avoided, with only enough room made for delivery of the proximal bowel into this space. Mobilization of the proximal colon should be carried out only if there is inadequate length to reach the lower rectum. A 2–0 Prolene pursestring suture is inserted at the proximal line of resection. Attention is then directed to the perineum, where a suitable retractor (Parks or Pratt) is inserted into the anal canal. A curved circular stapler with the trocar in place is inserted through the anus. The trocar can be extruded through the posterior rectal wall just above the levator ani muscle (▶ Fig. 33.15a). The trocar is removed (depending on the instrument used), the anvil is re-engaged in the central shaft, and the anastomosis is created (▶ Fig. 33.15b). Inspection reveals that proximal tissue removed is the familiar "ring," but that distal tissue comes out in the form of a disk, because no suture was applied (▶ Fig. 33.15c). With the 90- or 100-mm anastomotic stapler, a single application through the anus should suffice to create the side-to-side anastomosis (▶ Fig. 33.15d, e) between the rectum and the proximal ganglionic bowel. A second application, if necessary, is made by making an opening in the proximal colon and the adjacent rectum. It is probably better not to divide the rectum before this point because it is a convenient "handle" during this step of the procedure. The rectal stump is then transected with a linear stapling instrument. If an

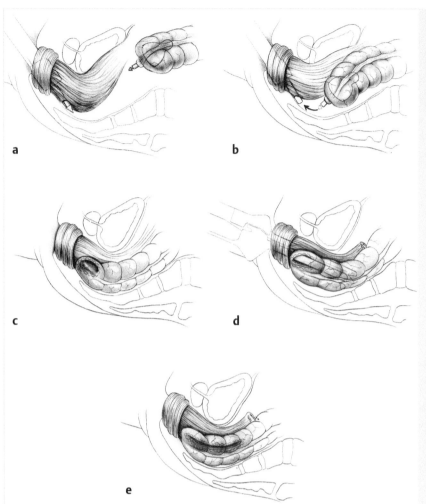

Fig. 33.15 Duhamel procedure. **(a)** Insertion of CEEA stapler through anus and extrusion of trocar through posterior rectal wall. **(b)** Engagement of anvil into central shaft. **(c)** Completed end-to-side anastomosis. **(d)** Division of common wall with GIA 90 or 100 instrument. **(e)** Completed procedure.

abdominal application of the anastomotic stapler was necessary, the residual opening is closed with sutures or another application of the linear stapling instrument. At the end of the procedure, the pelvis is filled with saline, and sigmoidoscopy is performed. The bowel is insufflated with air to ensure that no leak is present. No "covering" colostomy is necessary.

Megacolon Secondary to Chagas' Disease

Chagas' disease is an endemic clinical entity caused by *Trypanosoma cruzi*, a parasite that is transmitted to humans by the hematophagic Triatominae insects. It affects several million people in Latin America, mostly in Brazil, Argentina, Chile, Paraguay, and Bolivia. Megacolon, the most common complication of intestinal trypanosomiasis, results in severe constipation, for which operation is indicated. The two main complications are fecaloma and volvulus of the sigmoid colon. A variety of procedures have been proposed for the correction of this disabling condition, including sigmoidectomy, rectosigmoidectomy, left colectomy, and subtotal colectomy. On long-term follow-up, however, these operations have proved to be inadequate in a significant number of cases, apparently due to preservation of the dyskinetic rectum that continues to act as a functional obstacle to the progression of the fecal bolus. Pull-through operations, which include the removal of

all or almost all of the dyskinetic rectum, or the exclusion of the rectum, as in the Duhamel-Haddad operation, have been demonstrated to be superior.[386] Functional results are satisfactory. Anal continence is normal in the vast majority of cases, and sexual disturbances are rare.

Neuronal Intestinal Dysplasia

Neuronal intestinal dysplasia is a specific congenital innervation defect of the intestinal wall belonging to the group of dysganglionosis.[387] Type A is characterized by aplasia or hypoplasia of the sympathetic innervation leading to constipation and spasticity of the intestinal wall. This form is observed only in children and not in adults. Type B is characterized by dysplasia of the submucous plexus because of impaired development. The clinical manifestation is a weak propulsive motility and consequently constipation. This form is observed in adults as well as in children. Classic histologic features show hyperplasia and giant ganglia with 7 to 10 nerve cells that show a variable enzyme activity. Enzyme histochemical examination reveals a dense network of parasympathetic nerve fibers with increased acetylcholinesterase activity. Conservative treatment is usually unavailing and operative intervention is needed—most often subtotal colectomy.

33.7 Special Considerations

33.7.1 Prevention

In certain clinical circumstances, straining at stool presents an added hazard to the patient. Patients who have had a myocardial infarction and patients with cerebral and cardiovascular disease and thromboembolic disease are at special risk. These patients should be given bulk-forming agents, either those found in natural foodstuffs or in a psyllium seed preparation.

33.7.2 Fecal Impaction

Fecal impaction is a serious crisis that may constitute an intestinal obstruction. Ninety-eight percent of fecal impaction occurs in the rectum. The most common complications associated with fecal impaction include fecal incontinence, urinary tract infections, intestinal obstruction, and ischemic necrosis and stercoral ulcerations that may lead to bleeding or perforation.[388] Fecal impaction in an undistressed individual can be evacuated with high doses of stimulant laxatives, such as senna. More often, administration of enemas is required, and tap water or sodium phosphate enemas are effective. The use of mineral oil and dioctyl sodium sulfosuccinate has been advocated, although the effectiveness of these agents is probably due to the fluid volume. In an acutely distressed individual, digital evacuation can be achieved with the use of moderate sedation, although general anesthetic is often required. For more proximal impactions, water-soluble contrast material in 20 to 50% solutions will stimulate hyperperistalsis and draw water into the bowel and lubricate the fecal mass.[389] Whole-gut irrigation with 2 L of isosmotic solution of polyethylene glycol has been used in nonemergency cases without complete obstruction.

Recurrent fecal impaction should be prevented by reviewing the background factors that have led to the impaction and eliminating or avoiding them in the future. Dietary management and prescription of suppositories and senna preparations may be necessary. Stool softeners are useful, especially in the unusual case in which fecalomas pack the large bowel all the way to the cecum. Endoscopic or radiologic examination of the colon is indicated to rule out the presence of a neoplasm. An endocrine or metabolic screen may also be appropriate.

33.7.3 Psychiatric States

As noted previously, various psychiatric states are associated with constipation. The clinician also should remember that various antidepressant drugs are constipating. Constipation resulting from the latter cause is amenable to stimulant laxatives. An organic cause of constipation must not be overlooked in psychiatric patients.

33.7.4 Spinal Cord Injuries

Severe constipation often follows spinal cord injury. Several mechanisms may be involved in the pathogenesis, including the lack of conscious urge to defecate; forced body immobilization; associated motor paralysis of the abdominal and perineal muscles; and possible motor alterations at the level of the colon, rectum, and anus. Although a minor degree of transit delay may be present in the right colon in virtually all patients, there is either no or abnormally slow transit in the left colon and rectum.[18] Constipation in patients with paraplegia and transection of the spine between C4 and T12 vertebral levels is due to alteration in bowel segments innervated by the parasympathetic sacral outflow.

Longo et al,[389] in a review of the functional alterations of the denervated hindgut, summarized their findings as follows. The foregut and midgut are innervated by parasympathetic fibers in the vagus and sympathetic fibers from the lower six thoracic vertebrae. In contrast, the hindgut is innervated by parasympathetic fibers arising from the sacral plexus and by sympathetic fibers from the lumbar spinal column. Consequently, in most spinal cord injuries, the foregut and midgut remain normally innervated, whereas the hindgut loses input from cerebral and spinal cord sources. In high-cord lesions, this results in decreased colonic motility. In low-cord injuries, there is loss of inhibitory influences that normally regulate left colonic and rectosigmoid sphincter activity downward. In both high- and low-cord injuries, reflex activity of the anorectum is left unregulated by cerebral input. Once stimulated by distention, the rectum spontaneously evacuates its contents. Thus, fecal impaction and incontinence in these patients principally result from loss of inhibitory influences on rectosigmoid sphincter activity and rectal reflex activity.

Constipation is a major problem in the management of patients with spinal cord transection. To avoid overflow, fecal incontinence, and the necessity for frequent disimpaction, these patients may benefit from a bowel training regimen in which the defecation reflex is initiated at fixed time intervals.

Approximately the third or fourth night after the injury, a laxative is given and followed, if necessary, by a suppository the next morning. Administration of the laxative and/or the suppository is continued until a regular bowel habit is achieved. Digital removal and one or two enemas may be required in the first or second week. The goal is bowel evacuation every other day. Diet should contain plentiful amounts of fiber-containing foods. A chemical stimulant such as senna or bisacodyl should be administered on alternate nights. Stimulation to initiate defecation might include body movement, eating, drinking, massage of the abdomen, anal digital stimulation, or insertion of a suppository.

In patients who do not respond to simple measures, the next step is usually to try and stimulate the lower bowel and achieve effective rectal evacuation with the use of transanal irrigation systems and retrograde enemas.[383] Retrograde techniques are usually preferred, but some patients may benefit from antegrade enema administration via a Malone appendicostomy or Chait cecostomy button, which are increasingly being performed using minimally invasive surgery. A recent study investigating the cost-effectiveness of transanal irrigation for neurogenic bowel dysfunction has shown that irrigation is predicted to reduce fecal incontinence episodes by 36%, urinary tract infections by 29%, the likelihood of needing a stoma by 35%, and produce a significant improvement in quality of life. The lifetime cost-saving was calculated to be cost-effective.[390,391]

There will be some patients who fail to respond to the aforementioned measures, or for some other reason prefer to undergo fecal diversion with a stoma. The formation of an intestinal stoma is effective in the treatment of colonic dysmotility associated with spinal cord injuries. Safadi et al[392] reviewed the records of 45 spinal cord injury patients with intestinal stomas. A left-sided colostomy was performed in 21 patients, right-sided colostomy in 20, and ileostomy in 7. Three of the patients in the right colostomy group ultimately underwent total abdominal colectomy and ileostomy. The indications for stoma formation and colonic transit times were different in the three groups. Bloating, constipation, chronic abdominal pain, and difficulty in evacuation with prolonged colonic transit time were the main indications in 95% of patients in the right colostomy group, 43% of patients in the left colostomy group, and 29% in the ileostomy group. Management of complicated decubitus ulcers, perineal, and pelvic wounds was the primary indication in 43% of patients in the left colostomy group, 5% in the right colostomy group, and none in the ileostomy group. Preoperative total and right colonic transit times were longer in the right colostomy group compared with the left colostomy group: 128 versus 83 hours and 54 versus 29 hours, respectively. At a mean follow-up of 5.5 years after stoma formation, most patients were satisfied with their stoma (right colostomy, 88%; left colostomy, 100%; ileostomy, 83%) and the majority would have preferred to have the stoma earlier (right colostomy, 63%; left colostomy, 77%; ileostomy, 63%). The quality-of-life index significantly improved in all groups (right colostomy, 49–79; left colostomy, 50–86; and ileostomy, 60–82), as well as the health status index (right colostomy, 58–83; left colostomy, 63–92; and ileostomy, 61–88). The average daily time for bowel care was significantly shortened in all groups (right colostomy, 102–11 minutes; left colostomy, 123–18 minutes; and ileostomy, 73–13 minutes). They concluded, regardless of the type of stoma, most patients had functional improvement postoperatively. The successful outcome noted in all groups suggests that preoperative symptoms and colonic transit time studies may have been helpful in the optimal choice of stoma site selection.

33.7.5 Geriatric Population

Read et al[393] conducted a survey of 453 people living in Sheffield, United Kingdom, and found that the prevalence of constipation was 12% but increased to 41% of patients in acute geriatric wards and to more than 80% of patients in long-term geriatric wards. The authors attributed the abnormally increased incidence in hospitalized patients to immobility, chronic illness, neurologic or psychiatric disease, colonic disease, and drug ingestion rather than solely a consequence of aging. In his doctoral thesis on constipation in the elderly, Kinnunen[394] recorded the complaint of constipation and the use of laxatives separately. He found incidences of 79 and 76%, respectively, in a geriatric hospital, 59 and 60% in an "old people's home," 29 and 31% in a day hospital, 38 and 20% in elderly people living at home, and 12 and 5% in middle-aged people living at home. An increased risk of constipation was found in persons with poor mobility and advancing age and in those living in institutions.

Delay in transit time, incomplete emptying, diminished awareness, and neglect of the call to stool are the four most commonly occurring causes of constipation in the elderly.[395] Because this group comprises elderly, physically inactive individuals, often immobile in bed, a loss of muscle tone makes it difficult to empty the bowel completely without straining at stool. A possible cause or explanation of the association of constipation and old age may be autonomic nerve fiber degeneration, especially in diabetics[396]

or those who suffer strokes.[393] Jones and Godding[20] pointed out that there are several complications of constipation more likely to occur in the elderly. They include cardiovascular changes, gastrointestinal effects (including pain that simulates angina pectoris), and fecal impaction. As a consequence of fecal impaction, fecal incontinence may occur; if its cause is unrecognized, it may result in unnecessary institutionalization of a patient. Kinnunen[394] conducted a retrospective screening of one-year duration on 245 hospitalized geriatric patients and identified 65 periods of diarrhea that continued for at least 3 days, 32% of which recurred. Fecal impaction was associated with diarrhea in 55% of the patients, and laxative-induced diarrhea was found in 20%. Other consequences of impaction included intestinal obstruction, restlessness, confusional states, rectal hemorrhage resulting from stercoral ulceration, and urinary retention.

In a review of colonic disease in the elderly, Brocklehurst[397] stressed three important complications of constipation:
1. Fecal impaction and intestinal obstruction.
2. Idiopathic megacolon and sigmoid volvulus.
3. Fecal incontinence.

Therapeutic measures have emphasized reassurance with bowel retraining, encouragement of physical activity, intake of adequate fluids and dietary alterations, and avoidance of constipation and treatment of known underlying diseases, especially hypothyroidism. Such recommendations infer a readily curable problem, but when the patient is elderly, such hope is unrealistic.[398] Elderly patients usually require laxatives; the agents of choice are stimulant laxatives, such as senna or bisacodyl. Saline purgatives may disturb water and electrolyte balance, and the hazards of liquid paraffin are well recognized. Bulk-forming agents must be accompanied by adequate amounts of fluids but are contraindicated when fecal accumulations are already present. The use of stool softeners may be inappropriate if the stool is already soft; instead, the neuromuscular responses in the colon need stimulation. Successful therapy is an individual trial-and-error proposition. Encouragement comes from a study at one geriatric center, where supplementation of the total dietary fiber proved effective in preventing constipation in 60% of the residents, with the institution's pharmacy reporting a saving of $44,000 in expenditures for laxatives.[399] Similar results were experienced by Hope and Down,[400] who found that in elderly institutionalized patients, a daily fiber intake of 25 g per person and controlled fluid intake improved bowel function and almost eliminated aperient use with no adverse effects on body weight or nutritional or mineral status. Kinnunen[394] found magnesium hydroxide to be more efficient than bulk-forming laxatives in treating long-term constipation in elderly patients.

For the nursing home patient who is debilitated and unable to heed the call to stool promptly, an acceptable routine for management includes the regular use of suppositories or enemas. Tap water enemas administered every 3 to 5 days will keep the colon empty and the patient comfortable.

33.7.6 Obstetric Patients

Multiple etiologic factors are implicated in the occurrence of constipation during pregnancy. Decreased physical activity, changes in hormonal concentration (possibly contributing to atony of the gut muscle), decreased bulk in the diet, and the use of drugs such as iron all may contribute. During pregnancy, the aim should be prevention of constipation, and this is best accomplished with dietary fiber. Anderson and Whichelow[401] have shown that therapeutic supplementation bringing dietary fiber intake to 27 g/day is effective in treating constipation in pregnancy. Increased fluid intake is widely recommended. Laxatives are best avoided, but, if necessary, the choice is between bisacodyl and senna. Senna is safe for both mother and baby with no known adverse effects on nutrition or lactation.[401] Soft stools passed without straining may help prevent the problems of hemorrhoids and anal fissures so frequently associated with pregnancy. In the puerperium, a simple, safe, and inexpensive method of preventing constipation is the use of senna.[402]

33.7.7 Terminally Ill Patients

Lamerton[403] reported that patients who are dying, especially from carcinomatosis, present an often neglected problem. Their constipation, frequently aggravated by the universal administration of an opiate analgesic, leads to the distressing symptoms of abdominal distention and excessive gas, with added pain and even vomiting. These patients will benefit from a suppository (glycerin or bisacodyl) or from an enema. Greater attention should be paid to making their dying days more comfortable and peaceful. They should receive a laxative prophylactically with the opiate analgesic.

Patients with carcinoma often suffer from constipation, a symptom that can be considered in one of three categories[403]: (1) the direct result of the malignancy itself, with intraluminal or extraluminal encroachment on the bowel or interference with its innervation; (2) the result of the effects of therapy (e.g., chemotherapy); or (3) the result of factors indirectly related to the carcinoma. An example of the last category is the general debility accompanying advanced disease, marked by diminished oral intake, immobility, and depression, which predisposes to constipation. An intestinal visceral neuropathy may be a paraneoplastic effect of some carcinomas.[404] The results of organ failure such as uremia can have a compounding effect. Therapy with opiates or drugs with anticholinergic effects (e.g., antidepressants and neuroleptics) further complicates the problem.

References

[1] Higgins PD, Johanson JF. Epidemiology of constipation in North America: a systematic review. Am J Gastroenterol. 2004; 99(4):750–759

[2] Probert CS, Emmett PM, Heaton KW. Some determinants of whole-gut transit time: a population-based study. QJM. 1995; 88(5):311–315

[3] Heaton KW. T. L. Cleave and the fibre story. J R Nav Med Serv. 1980; 66 (1):5–10

[4] Pare P, Ferrazzi S, Thompson WG, Irvine EJ, Rance L. An epidemiological survey of constipation in canada: definitions, rates, demographics, and predictors of health care seeking. Am J Gastroenterol. 2001; 96(11):3130–3137

[5] Stewart WF, Liberman G, Sandler RS, et al. A large U.S. national epidemiological study of constipation gastroenterology. Gastroenterology. 1998; 114 Suppl 1:A44

[6] Everhart JE, Go VL, Johannes RS, Fitzsimmons SC, Roth HP, White LR. A longitudinal survey of self-reported bowel habits in the United States. Dig Dis Sci. 1989; 34(8):1153–1162

[7] Talley NJ, Fleming KC, Evans JM, et al. Constipation in an elderly community: a study of prevalence and potential risk factors. Am J Gastroenterol. 1996; 91(1):19–25

[8] Sonnenberg A, Koch TR. Physician visits in the United States for constipation: 1958 to 1986. Dig Dis Sci. 1989; 34(4):606–611

[9] Suares NC, Ford AC. Prevalence of, and risk factors for, chronic idiopathic constipation in the community: systematic review and meta-analysis. Am J Gastroenterol. 2011; 106(9):1582–1591, quiz 1581, 1592

[10] Wald A, Scarpignato C, Mueller-Lissner S, et al. A multinational survey of prevalence and patterns of laxative use among adults with self-defined constipation. Aliment Pharmacol Ther. 2008; 28(7):917–930

[11] Drossman DA, Li Z, Andruzzi E, et al. U.S. householder survey of functional gastrointestinal disorders. Prevalence, sociodemography, and health impact. Dig Dis Sci. 1993; 38(9):1569–1580

[12] Harari D, Gurwitz JH, Avorn J, Bohn R, Minaker KL. Bowel habit in relation to age and gender. Findings from the National Health Interview Survey and clinical implications. Arch Intern Med. 1996; 156(3):315–320

[13] Pekmezaris R, Aversa L, Wolf-Klein G, Cedarbaum J, Reid-Durant M. The cost of chronic constipation. J Am Med Dir Assoc. 2002; 3(4):224–228

[14] Chang L, Toner BB, Fukudo S, et al. Gender, age, society, culture, and the patient's perspective in the functional gastrointestinal disorders. Gastroenterology. 2006; 130(5):1435–1446

[15] Sonnenberg A, Koch TR. Epidemiology of constipation in the United States. Dis Colon Rectum. 1989; 32(1):1–8

[16] Drossman DA, Thompson WG, Talley NJ, Funch-Jensen P, Janssens J, Whitehead WE. Identification of sub-groups of functional gastrointestinal disorders. Gastroenterol Int. 1990; 3:159–172

[17] Devroede G. Constipation: mechanisms and management. In: Sleisenger MH, Fordtran JS, eds. Gastrointestinal Disease, 3rd ed. Philadelphia, PA: WB Saunders; 1983

[18] Agachan F, Chen T, Pfeifer J, Reissman P, Wexner SD. A constipation scoring system to simplify evaluation and management of constipated patients. Dis Colon Rectum. 1996; 39(6):681–685

[19] Hinton JM, Lennard-Jones JE. Constipation: definition and classification. Postgrad Med J. 1968; 44(515):720–723

[20] Jones FA, Godding EW. Management of Constipation. London: Blackwell Scientific Publications; 1972

[21] Burkitt DP. Epidemiology of cancer of the colon and rectum. Cancer. 1971; 28(1):3–13

[22] Painter NS, Burkitt DP. Diverticular disease of the colon: a deficiency disease of Western civilization. BMJ. 1971; 2(5759):450–454

[23] Schneeman BO. Soluble vs. insoluble fiber—different physiological responses. Food Technol. 1987; 41:81–82

[24] Walker ARP, Walker BF, Richardson BD. Bowel transit times in Bantu populations. BMJ. 1970; 3(5713):48–49

[25] Menardo G, Bausano G, Corazziari E, et al. Large-bowel transit in paraplegic patients. Dis Colon Rectum. 1987; 30(12):924–928

[26] Levi R, Hultling C, Nash MS, Seiger A. The Stockholm spinal cord injury study: 1. Medical problems in a regional SCI population. Paraplegia. 1995; 33:308–315

[27] Glickman S, Kamm MA. Bowel dysfunction in spinal-cord-injury patients. Lancet. 1996; 347(9016):1651–1653

[28] Ashraf W, Park F, Lof J, Quigley EMM. An examination of the reliability of reported stool frequency in the diagnosis of idiopathic constipation. Am J Gastroenterol. 1996; 91(1):26–32

[29] Lewis SJ, Heaton KW. Stool form scale as a useful guide to intestinal transit time. Scand J Gastroenterol. 1997; 32(9):920–924

[30] Almy TP. Constipation. In: Sleisenger MH, Fordtran JS, eds. Gastrointestinal Disease. Philadelphia, PA: WB Saunders; 1973

[31] Heaton KW, O'Donnell LJ. An office guide to whole-gut transit time. Patients' recollection of their stool form. J Clin Gastroenterol. 1994; 19(1):28–30

[32] Thompson JC, Marx M. Gastrointestinal hormones. Curr Probl Surg. 1984; 21 (6):1–80

[33] Preston DM, Adrian TE, Christofides ND, Lennard-Jones JE, Bloom SR. Positive correlation between symptoms and circulating motilin, pancreatic polypeptide and gastrin concentrations in functional bowel disorders. Gut. 1985; 26 (10):1059–1064

[34] Christofides ND, Ghatei MA, Bloom SR, Borberg C, Gillmer MDG. Decreased plasma motilin concentrations in pregnancy. Br Med J (Clin Res Ed). 1982; 285(6353):1453–1454

[35] Agachan F, Pfeifer J, Wexner SD. Defecography and proctography. Results of 744 patients. Dis Colon Rectum. 1996; 39(8):899–905

[36] Mellgren A, Bremmer S, Johansson C, et al. Defecography. Results of investigations in 2,816 patients. Dis Colon Rectum. 1994; 37(11):1133–1141

[37] Ferrante SL, Perry RE, Schreiman JS, Cheng SC, Frick MP. The reproducibility of measuring the anorectal angle in defecography. Dis Colon Rectum. 1991; 34(1):51–55

[38] Penninckx F, Debruyne C, Lestar B, Kerremans R. Intraobserver variation in the radiological measurement of the anorectal angle. Gastrointest Radiol. 1991; 16(1):73–76

[39] Halligan S, McGee S, Bartram CI. Quantification of evacuation proctography. Dis Colon Rectum. 1994; 37(11):1151–1154

[40] Barkel DC, Pemberton JH, Pezim ME, Phillips SF, Kelly KA, Brown ML. Scintigraphic assessment of the anorectal angle in health and after ileal pouch-anal anastomosis. Ann Surg. 1988; 208(1):42–49

[41] Freimanis MG, Wald A, Caruana B, Bauman DH. Evacuation proctography in normal volunteers. Invest Radiol. 1991; 26(6):581–585

[42] Karlbom U, Påhlman L, Nilsson S, Graf W. Relationships between defecographic findings, rectal emptying, and colonic transit time in constipated patients. Gut. 1995; 36(6):907–912

[43] Halligan S, Thomas J, Bartram C. Intrarectal pressures and balloon expulsion related to evacuation proctography. Gut. 1995; 37(1):100–104

[44] Hinton JM, Lennard-Jones JE, Young AC. A new method for studying gut transit times using radioopaque markers. Gut. 1969; 10(10):842–847

[45] Cummings JH, Wiggins HS. Transit through the gut measured by analysis of a single stool. Gut. 1976; 17(3):219–223

[46] Evans RC, Kamm MA, Hinton JM, Lennard-Jones JE. The normal range and a simple diagram for recording whole gut transit time. Int J Colorectal Dis. 1992; 7(1):15–17

[47] Martelli H, Devroede G, Arhan P, Duguay C, Dornic C, Faverdin C. Some parameters of large bowel motility in normal man. Gastroenterology. 1978; 75(4):612–618

[48] Metcalf AM, Phillips SF, Zinsmeister AR, MacCarty RL, Beart RW, Wolff BG. Simplified assessment of segmental colonic transit. Gastroenterology. 1987; 92(1):40–47

[49] Chaussade S, Guerre J, Couturier D. Measurement of colonic transit. Gastroenterology. 1987; 92(6):2053

[50] van der Sijp JRM, Kamm MA, Nightingale JMD, et al. Radioisotope determination of regional colonic transit in severe constipation: comparison with radio opaque markers. Gut. 1993; 34(3):402–408

[51] Stivland T, Camilleri M, Vassallo M, et al. Scintigraphic measurement of regional gut transit in idiopathic constipation. Gastroenterology. 1991; 101(1):107–115

[52] Krevsky B, Maurer AH, Fisher RS. Patterns of colonic transit in chronic idiopathic constipation. Am J Gastroenterol. 1989; 84(2):127–132

[53] Ewe K, Press AG, Dederer W. Gastrointestinal transit of undigestible solids measured by metal detector EAS II. Eur J Clin Invest. 1989; 19(3):291–297

[54] Basile M, Neri M, Carriero A, et al. Measurement of segmental transit through the gut in man. A novel approach by the biomagnetic method. Dig Dis Sci. 1992; 37(10):1537–1543

[55] Arhan P, Devroede G, Jehannin B, et al. Segmental colonic transit time. Dis Colon Rectum. 1981; 24(8):625–629

[56] Chaussade S, Khyari A, Roche H, et al. Determination of total and segmental colonic transit time. Results in 91 patients with a new simplified method. Dig Dis Sci. 1989; 34(8):1168–1172

[57] Meir R, Beglinger C, Dederding JP, et al. [Age- and sex-specific standard values of colonic transit time in healthy subjects]. Schweiz Med Wochenschr. 1992; 122(24):940–943

[58] Escalante R, Sorgi M, Salas Z. [Total and segmental colonic transit time. Clinical and prospective study using radiopaque markers in normal subjects]. G.E.N. 1993; 47(2):88–92

[59] Danquechin Dorval E, Barbieux JP, Picon L, Alison D, Codjovi P, Rouleau P. [Simplified measurement of colonic transit time by one radiography of the abdomen and a single type of marker. Normal values in 82 volunteers related to the sexes]. Gastroenterol Clin Biol. 1994; 18(2):141–144

[60] Bouchoucha M, Devroede G, Renard P, Arhan P, Barbier JP, Cugnenc PH. Compartmental analysis of colonic transit reveals abnormalities in constipated patients with normal transit. Clin Sci (Lond). 1995; 89(2):129–135

[61] Loening-Baucke V. Factors determining outcome in children with chronic constipation and faecal soiling. Gut. 1989; 30(7):999–1006

[62] Benninga MA, Büller HA, Taminiau JA. Biofeedback training in chronic constipation. Arch Dis Child. 1993; 68(1):126–129

[63] Loening-Baucke V, Pringle KC, Ekwo EE. Anorectal manometry for the exclusion of Hirschsprung's disease in neonates. J Pediatr Gastroenterol Nutr. 1985; 4(4):596–603

[64] Low PS, Quak SH, Prabhakaran K, Joseph VT, Chiang GS, Aiyathurai EJ. Accuracy of anorectal manometry in the diagnosis of Hirschsprung's disease. J Pediatr Gastroenterol Nutr. 1989; 9(3):342–346

[65] Borowitz SM, Sutphen J, Ling W, Cox DJ. Lack of correlation of anorectal manometry with symptoms of chronic childhood constipation and encopresis. Dis Colon Rectum. 1996; 39(4):400–405

[66] Pluta H, Bowes KL, Jewell LD. Long-term results of total abdominal colectomy for chronic idiopathic constipation. Value of preoperative assessment. Dis Colon Rectum. 1996; 39(2):160–166

[67] Martelli H, Devroede G, Arhan P, Duguay C. Mechanisms of idiopathic constipation: outlet obstruction. Gastroenterology. 1978; 75(4):623–631

[68] Grotz RL, Pemberton JH, Levin KE, Bell AM, Hanson RB. Rectal wall contractility in healthy subjects and in patients with chronic severe constipation. Ann Surg. 1993; 218(6):761–768

[69] Schouten WR, Gosselink MJ, Boerma MO, Ginai AZ. Rectal tone in response to an evoked urge to defecate. Dis Colon Rectum. 1998; 41:473–479

[70] Gosselink MJ, Schouten WR. The gastrorectal reflex in women with obstructed defecation. Int J Colorectal Dis. 2001; 16(2):112–118

[71] Varma JS, Smith AN. Neurophysiological dysfunction in young women with intractable constipation. Gut. 1988; 29(7):963–968

[72] Gurnari M, Mazziotti F, Corazziari E, et al. Chronic constipation after gynaecological surgery: a retrospective study. Br J Gastroenterol. 1988; 20:183–186

[73] Shafik A, El-Sibai O, Ahmed I. Parasympathetic extrinsic reflex: role in defecation mechanism. World J Surg. 2002; 26(6):737–740, discussion 741

[74] Swash M, Snooks SJ. Electromyography in pelvic floor disorders. In: Henry MM, Swash M, eds. Coloproctology and the Pelvic Floor. London: Butterworth; 1985

[75] Snooks SJ, Barnes PRH, Swash M, Henry MM. Damage to the innervation of the pelvic floor musculature in chronic constipation. Gastroenterology. 1985; 89(5):977–981

[76] Preston DM, Lennard-Jones JE. Anismus in chronic constipation. Dig Dis Sci. 1985; 30(5):413–418

[77] Rao SSC, Ozturk R, Laine L. Clinical utility of diagnostic tests for constipation in adults: a systematic review. Am J Gastroenterol. 2005; 100(7):1605–1615

[78] Madigan MR, Morson BC. Solitary ulcer of the rectum. Gut. 1969; 10(11):871–881

[79] Martin CJ, Parks TG, Biggart JD. Solitary rectal ulcer syndrome in Northern Ireland. 1971–1980. Br J Surg. 1981; 68(10):744–747

[80] Koch TR, Carney JA, Go L, Go VL. Idiopathic chronic constipation is associated with decreased colonic vasoactive intestinal peptide. Gastroenterology. 1988; 94(2):300–310

[81] Aldridge RT, Campbell PE. Ganglion cell distribution in the normal rectum and anal canal. A basis for the diagnosis of Hirschsprung's disease by anorectal biopsy. J Pediatr Surg. 1968; 3(4):475–490

[82] Ikawa H, Kim SH, Hendren WH, Donahoe PK. Acetylcholinesterase and manometry in the diagnosis of the constipated child. Arch Surg. 1986; 121(4):435–438

[83] Venugopal S, Mancer K, Shandling B. The validity of rectal biopsy in relation to morphology and distribution of ganglion cells. J Pediatr Surg. 1981; 16(4):433–437

[84] Weinberg AG. The anorectal myenteric plexus: its relation to hypoganglionosis of the colon. Am J Clin Pathol. 1970; 54(4):637–642

[85] Riemann JF, Schmidt H, Zimmermann W. The fine structure of colonic submucosal nerves in patients with chronic laxative abuse. Scand J Gastroenterol. 1980; 15(6):761–768

[86] Causse E, Vaysse P, Fabre J, Valdiguie P, Thouvenot JP. The diagnostic value of acetylcholinesterase/butyrylcholinesterase ratio in Hirschsprung's disease. Am J Clin Pathol. 1987; 88(4):477–480

[87] Goto S, Ikeda K, Nagasaki A, Tomokiyo A, Kusaba M. Hirschsprung's disease in an adult. Special reference to histochemical determination of the acetylcholinesterase activity. Dis Colon Rectum. 1984; 27(5):319–320

[88] Meier-Ruge W, Lutterbeck PM, Herzog B, Morger R, Moser R, Schärli A. Acetylcholinesterase activity in suction biopsies of the rectum in the diagnosis of Hirschsprung's disease. J Pediatr Surg. 1972; 7(1):11–17

[89] Robey SS, Kuhajda FP, Yardley JH. Immunoperoxidase stains of ganglion cells and abnormal mucosal nerve proliferations in Hirschsprung's disease. Hum Pathol. 1988; 19(4):432–437

[90] Park WH, Choi SO, Kwon KY, Chang ES. Acetylcholinesterase histochemistry of rectal suction biopsies in the diagnosis of Hirschsprung's disease. J Korean Med Sci. 1992; 7(4):353–359

[91] Barr LC, Booth J, Filipe MI, Lawson JON. Clinical evaluation of the histochemical diagnosis of Hirschsprung's disease. Gut. 1985; 26(4):393–399

[92] Preston DM, Butler MG, Smith B, Lennard-Jones JE. Neuropathology of slow transit constipation. Gut. 1983; 24:A997

[93] Krishnamurthy S, Schuffler MD, Rohrmann CA, Pope CE, II. Severe idiopathic constipation is associated with a distinctive abnormality of the colonic myenteric plexus. Gastroenterology. 1985; 88(1, Pt 1):26–34

[94] Tzavella K, Riepl RL, Klauser AG, Voderholzer WA, Schindlbeck NE, Müller-Lissner SA. Decreased substance P levels in rectal biopsies from patients with slow transit constipation. Eur J Gastroenterol Hepatol. 1996; 8 (12):1207–1211

[95] Kluck P, van Muyen GNP, van der Kamp AWM, et al. Diagnosis of Hirschsprung's disease with monoclonal antineurofllament antibodies on tissue sections. Lancet. 1984; 24:652–653

[96] Schouten WR, ten Kate FJ, de Graaf EJ, Gilberts EC, Simons JL, Klück P. Visceral neuropathy in slow transit constipation: an immunohistochemical investigation with monoclonal antibodies against neurofilament. Dis Colon Rectum. 1993; 36(12):1112–1117

[97] Klück P, Tibboel D, Leendertse-Verloop K, van der Kamp AW, ten Kate FJ, Molenaar JC. Disturbed defecation after colectomy for aganglionosis investigated with monoclonal antineurofilament antibody. J Pediatr Surg. 1986; 21 (10):845–847

[98] Lincoln J, Crowe R, Kamm MA, Burnstock G, Lennard-Jones JE. Serotonin and 5-hydroxyindoleacetic acid are increased in the sigmoid colon in severe idiopathic constipation. Gastroenterology. 1990; 98(5, Pt 1):1219–1225

[99] Zhao R, Baig MK, Wexner SD, et al. Enterochromaffin and serotonin cells are abnormal for patients with colonic inertia. Dis Colon Rectum. 2000; 43 (6):858–863

[100] Zhao RH, Baig MK, Thaler KJ, et al. Reduced expression of serotonin receptor (s) in the left colon of patients with colonic inertia. Dis Colon Rectum. 2003; 46(1):81–86

[101] Wedel T, Roblick UJ, Ott V, et al. Oligoneuronal hypoganglionosis in patients with idiopathic slow-transit constipation. Dis Colon Rectum. 2002; 45 (1):54–62

[102] Bassotti G, Villanacci V, Maure CA, Fisogni S, Di Fabio F, et al. The role of glial cells and apoptosis of enteric neurons in the neuropathology of intractable slow transit constipation. Gut. 2006; 55(1):41–46

[103] Lee JI, Park H, Kamm MA, Talbot IC. Decreased density of interstitial cells of Cajal and neuronal cells in patients with slow-transit constipation and acquired megacolon. J Gastroenterol Hepatol. 2005; 20(8):1292–1298

[104] Tucker DM, Sandstead HH, Logan GM, Jr, et al. Dietary fiber and personality factors as determinants of stool output. Gastroenterology. 1981; 81 (5):879–883

[105] Devroede G, Girard G, Bouchoucha M, et al. Idiopathic constipation by colonic dysfunction. Relationship with personality and anxiety. Dig Dis Sci. 1989; 34(9):1428–1433

[106] Heymen S, Wexner SD, Gulledge AD. MMPI assessment of patients with functional bowel disorders. Dis Colon Rectum. 1993; 36(6):593–596

[107] Drossman DA, Leserman J, Nachman G, et al. Sexual and physical abuse in women with functional or organic disorders of the lower gastrointestinal tract. Ann Intern Med. 1990; 113:828–833

[108] Leroi AM, Bernier C, Watier A, et al. Prevalence of sexual abuse among patients with functional disorders of the lower gastrointestinal tract. Int J Colorectal Dis. 1995; 10(4):200–206

[109] Dykes S, Smilgin-Humphreys S, Bass C. Chronic idiopathic constipation: a psychological enquiry. Eur J Gastroenterol Hepatol. 2001; 13(1):39–44

[110] Knowles CH, Scott SM, Rayner C, et al. Idiopathic slow-transit constipation: an almost exclusively female disorder. Dis Colon Rectum. 2003; 46 (12):1716–1717

[111] Mason HJ, Serrano-Ikkos E, Kamm MA. Psychological morbidity in women with idiopathic constipation. Am J Gastroenterol. 2000; 95(10):2852–2857

[112] Emmanuel AV, Mason HJ, Kamm MA. Relationship between psychological state and level of activity of extrinsic gut innervation in patients with a functional gut disorder. Gut. 2001; 49(2):209–213

[113] Chan AO, Cheng C, Hui WM, et al. Differing coping mechanisms, stress level and anorectal physiology in patients with functional constipation. World J Gastroenterol. 2005; 11(34):5362–5366

[114] Leroi AM, Duval V, Roussignol C, Berkelmans I, Peninque P, Denis P. Biofeedback for anismus in 15 sexually abused women. Int J Colorectal Dis. 1996; 11 (4):187–190

[115] Thompson WG. Constipation and catharsis. Can Med Assoc J. 1976; 114 (10):927–931

[116] Bjelke E. Epidemiologic studies of cancer of the stomach, colon, and rectum; with special emphasis on the role of diet. Scand J Gastroenterol Suppl. 1974; 31 Suppl:1–235

[117] Higginson J. Etiological factors in gastrointestinal cancer in man. J Natl Cancer Inst. 1966; 37(4):527–545

[118] Wynder EL, Shigematsu T. Environmental factors of cancer of the colon and rectum. Cancer. 1967; 20(9):1520–1561

[119] Cranston D, McWhinnie D, Collin J. Dietary fibre and gastrointestinal disease. Br J Surg. 1988; 75(6):508–512

[120] Park Y, Hunter DJ, Spiegelman D, et al. Dietary fiber intake and risk of colorectal cancer. JAMA. 2005; 294:2849–2857

[121] Laxatives and dietary fiber. Med Lett. 1973; 15:98

[122] Kirwan WO, Smith AN, McConnell AA, Mitchell WD, Eastwood MA. Action of different bran preparations on colonic function. BMJ. 1974; 4 (5938):187–189

[123] Stephen AM, Cummings JH. Water-holding by dietary fibre in vitro and its relationship to faecal output in man. Gut. 1979; 20(8):722–729

[124] Ornstein MH, Baird IM. Dietary fibre and the colon. Mol Aspects Med. 1987; 9(1):41–67

[125] Trowell H. The development of the concept of dietary fiber in human nutrition. Am J Clin Nutr. 1978; 31(10) Suppl:S3–S11

[126] McNutt K. Prospective-fiber. J Nutr Ed 1976;8:150

[127] Dubuc MB, Lahaie LC. Nutritive value of foods. Ottawa: National Library; 1987:16–158

[128] Brunton LL. Laxatives. In: Gilman AG, Goodman LS, Bal TN, Murd F, eds. Goodman and Gilman's the Pharmacological Basis of Therapeutics, 7th ed. New York, NY: Macmillan; 1985:994–1003

[129] Curry CE. Handbook of Non-Prescription Drugs, 8th ed. Washington, DC: American Pharmaceutical Association; 1986:75–97

[130] Müller-Lissner SA. Adverse effects of laxatives: fact and fiction. Pharmacology. 1993; 47 Suppl 1:138–145

[131] Siegers CP, von Hertzberg-Lottin E, Otte M, Schneider B. Anthranoid laxative abuse–a risk for colorectal cancer? Gut. 1993; 34(8):1099–1101

[132] Harvey RF, Read AE. Mode of action of the saline purgatives. Am Heart J. 1975; 89(6):810–812

[133] Donowitz M, Binder HJ. Effect of dioctyl sodium sulfosuccinate on colonic fluid and electrolyte movement. Gastroenterology. 1975; 69(4):941–950

[134] Fain AM, Susat R, Herring M, Dorton K. Treatment of constipation in geriatric and chronically ill patients: a comparison. South Med J. 1978; 71 (6):677–680

[135] Johanson JF, Wald A, Tougas G, et al. Effect of tegaserod in chronic constipation: a randomized, double-blind, controlled trial. Clin Gastroenterol Hepatol. 2004; 2(9):796–805

[136] Kamm MA, Müller-Lissner S, Talley NJ, et al. Tegaserod for the treatment of chronic constipation: a randomized, double-blind, placebo-controlled multinational study. Am J Gastroenterol. 2005; 100(2):362–372

[137] Tack J, van Outryve M, Beyens G, Kerstens R, Vandeplassche L. Prucalopride (Resolor) in the treatment of severe chronic constipation in patients dissatisfied with laxatives. Gut. 2009; 58(3):357–365

[138] Quigley EM, Vandeplassche L, Kerstens R, Ausma J. Clinical trial: the efficacy, impact on quality of life, and safety and tolerability of prucalopride in severe chronic constipation–a 12-week, randomized, double-blind, placebo-controlled study. Aliment Pharmacol Ther. 2009; 29(3):315–328

[139] Johanson JF, Morton D, Geenen J, Ueno R. Multicenter, 4-week, double-blind, randomized, placebo-controlled trial of lubiprostone, a locally-acting type-2 chloride channel activator, in patients with chronic constipation. Am J Gastroenterol. 2008; 103(1):170–177

[140] Ogorek CP, Reynolds JC. Chronic constipation. Diagnosis and treatment. Endosc Rev. 1987; 4(6):47

[141] Lembo AJ, Johanson JF, Parkman HP, Rao SS, Miner PB, Jr, Ueno R. Long-term safety and effectiveness of lubiprostone, a chloride channel (ClC-2) activator, in patients with chronic idiopathic constipation. Dig Dis Sci. 2011; 56 (9):2639–2645

[142] Seidler U, Blumenstein I, Kretz A, et al. A functional CFTR protein is required for mouse intestinal cAMP-, cGMP- and Ca(2 +)-dependent HCO3- secretion. J Physiol. 1997; 505(Pt 2):411–423

[143] Tien XY, Brasitus TA, Kaetzel MA, Dedman JR, Nelson DJ. Activation of the cystic fibrosis transmembrane conductance regulator by cGMP in the human colonic cancer cell line, Caco-2. J Biol Chem. 1994; 269(1):51–54

[144] Andresen V, Camilleri M, Busciglio IA, et al. Effect of 5 days linaclotide on transit and bowel function in females with constipation-predominant irritable bowel syndrome. Gastroenterology. 2007; 133(3):761–768

[145] Eutamene H, Bradesi S, Larauche M, et al. Guanylate cyclase C-mediated antinociceptive effects of linaclotide in rodent models of visceral pain. Neurogastroenterol Motil. 2010; 22(3):312–e84

[146] Bryant AP, Busby RW, Bartolini WP, et al. Linaclotide is a potent and selective guanylate cyclase C agonist that elicits pharmacological effects locally in the gastrointestinal tract. Life Sci. 2010; 86(19–20):760–765

[147] Lembo AJ, Schneier HA, Shiff SJ, et al. Two randomized trials of linaclotide for chronic constipation. N Engl J Med. 2011; 365(6):527–536

[148] Lane WA. Chronic intestinal stasis. BMJ. 1912; 2:1125–1130

[149] Hughes ESR, McDermott FT, Johnson WR, Polglase AL. Surgery for constipation. Aust N Z J Surg. 1981; 51(2):144–148

[150] Belliveau P, Goldberg SM, Rothenberger DA, Nivatvongs S. Idiopathic acquired megacolon: the value of subtotal colectomy. Dis Colon Rectum. 1982; 25(2):118–121

[151] Hughes ESR, McDermott FT, Johnson WR, Polglase A. Surgery for constipation. In: Heberer G, Denecke H, eds. Colorectal Surgery. Berlin: Springer-Verlag; 1982:11–17

[152] Klatt GR. Role of subtotal colectomy in the treatment of incapacitating constipation. Am J Surg. 1983; 145(5):623–625

[153] Preston DM, Hawley PR, Lennard-Jones JE, Todd IP. Results of colectomy for severe idiopathic constipation in women (Arbuthnot Lane's disease). Br J Surg. 1984; 71(7):547–552

[154] Keighley MRB, Shouler P. Outlet syndrome: is there a surgical option? J R Soc Med. 1984; 77(7):559–563

[155] Beck DE, Jagelman DG, Fazio VW. The surgery of idiopathic constipation. Gastroenterol Clin North Am. 1987; 16(1):143–156

[156] Vasilevsky CA, Nemer FD, Balcos EG, Christenson CE, Goldberg SM. Is subtotal colectomy a viable option in the management of chronic constipation? Dis Colon Rectum. 1988; 31(9):679–681

[157] Gattuso JM, Kamm MA, Abassi M, Talbot IC. First description of the pathology of idiopathic megarectum and megacolon. Gut. 1993; 34:S49

[158] Koch TR, Schulte-Bockholt A, Telford GL, Otterson MF, Murad TM, Stryker SJ. Acquired megacolon is associated with alteration of vasoactive intestinal peptide levels and acetylcholinesterase activity. Regul Pept. 1993; 48(3):309–319

[159] Gattuso JM, Hoyle CHV, Milner P, Kamm MA, Burnstock G. Enteric innervation in idiopathic megarectum and megacolon. Int J Colorectal Dis. 1996; 11 (6):264–271

[160] Koch TR, Schulte-Bockholt A, Otterson MF, et al. Decreased vasoactive intestinal peptide levels and glutathione depletion in acquired megacolon. Dig Dis Sci. 1996; 41(7):1409–1416

[161] Koch TR, Otterson MF, Telford GL. Nitric oxide production is diminished in colonic circular muscle from acquired megacolon. Dis Colon Rectum. 2000; 43(6):821–828

[162] Meier-Ruge WA. [Idiopathic megacolon. New findings on histopathology and musculo-mechanical causes]. Chirurg. 2000; 71(8):927–931

[163] Gattuso JM, Kamm MA. Clinical features of idiopathic megarectum and idiopathic megacolon. Gut. 1997; 41(1):93–99

[164] Barnes PR, Lennard-Jones JE, Hawley PR, Todd IP. Hirschsprung's disease and idiopathic megacolon in adults and adolescents. Gut. 1986; 27(5):534–541

[165] Gattuso JM, Kamm MA, Morris G, Britton KE, Britton KE. Gastrointestinal transit in patients with idiopathic megarectum. Dis Colon Rectum. 1996; 39 (9):1044–1050

[166] Gattuso JM, Kamm MA, Halligan SM, Bartram CI, Bartram CI. The anal sphincter in idiopathic megarectum: effects of manual disimpaction under general anesthetic. Dis Colon Rectum. 1996; 39(4):435–439

[167] Stabile G, Kamm MA, Hawley PR, Lennard-Jones JE. Colectomy for idiopathic megarectum and megacolon. Gut. 1991; 32(12):1538–1540

[168] Lane RH, Todd IP. Idiopathic megacolon: a review of 42 cases. Br J Surg. 1977; 64(5):307–310

[169] Stabile G, Kamm MA, Hawley PR, Lennard-Jones JE. Results of the Duhamel operation in the treatment of idiopathic megarectum and megacolon. Br J Surg. 1991; 78(6):661–663

[170] Stabile G, Kamm MA, Phillips RKS, Hawley PR, Lennard-Jones JE. Partial colectomy and coloanal anastomosis for idiopathic megarectum and megacolon. Dis Colon Rectum. 1992; 35(2):158–162

[171] Stewart J, Kumar D, Keighley MRB. Results of anal or low rectal anastomosis and pouch construction for megarectum and megacolon. Br J Surg. 1994; 81 (7):1051–1053

[172] Pfeifer J, Agachan F, Wexner SD. Surgery for constipation: a review. Dis Colon Rectum. 1996; 39(4):444–460

[173] O Súilleabháin CB, Anderson JH, McKee RF, Finlay IG. Strategy for the surgical management of patients with idiopathic megarectum and megacolon. Br J Surg. 2001; 88(10):1392–1396

[174] Keighley MR. Megacolon and megarectum. In: Keighley MR, Williams NS, eds. Surgery of the Anus, Rectum and Colon, Vol 1. London: WB Saunders; 1993:658–673

[175] Gladman MA, Scott SM, Lunniss PJ, Williams NS. Systematic review of surgical options for idiopathic megarectum and megacolon. Ann Surg. 2005; 241 (4):562–574

[176] Gladman MA, Williams NS, Scott SM, Ogunbiyi OA, Lunniss PJ. Medium-term results of vertical reduction rectoplasty and sigmoid colectomy for idiopathic megarectum. Br J Surg. 2005; 92(5):624–630

[177] Surrenti E, Rath DM, Pemberton JH, Camilleri M. Audit of constipation in a tertiary referral gastroenterology practice. Am J Gastroenterol. 1995; 90 (9):1471–1475

[178] Watier A, Devroede G, Duranceau A, et al. Constipation with colonic inertia. A manifestation of systemic disease? Dig Dis Sci. 1983; 28(11):1025–1033

[179] Panagamuwa B, Kumar D, Ortiz J, Keighley MR. Motor abnormalities in the terminal ileum of patients with chronic idiopathic constipation. Br J Surg. 1994; 81(11):1685–1688

[180] Hemingway D, Neilly JB, Finlay IG. Biliary dyskinesia in idiopathic slow-transit constipation. Dis Colon Rectum. 1996; 39(11):1303–1307

[181] Penning C, Gielkens HA, Delemarre JB, Lamers CB, Masclee AA. Gall bladder emptying in severe idiopathic constipation. Gut. 1999; 45(2):264–268

[182] Mollen RM, Hopman WP, Kuijpers HH, Jansen JB. Abnormalities of upper gut motility in patients with slow-transit constipation. Eur J Gastroenterol Hepatol. 1999; 11(7):701–708

[183] Glia A, Lindberg G. Antroduodenal manometry findings in patients with slow-transit constipation. Scand J Gastroenterol. 1998; 33(1):55–62

[184] Penning C, Gielkens HA, Hemelaar M, et al. Prolonged ambulatory recording of antroduodenal motility in slow-transit constipation. Br J Surg. 2000; 87 (2):211–217

[185] Mollen RM, Hopman WP, Oyen WJ, Kuijpers HH, Edelbroek MA, Jansen JB. Effect of subtotal colectomy on gastric emptying of a solid meal in slow-transit constipation. Dis Colon Rectum. 2001; 44(8):1189–1195

[186] Warren SJ, Lord MG, Rogers J, Williams NS. Neural medication of the human rectocolon inhibitory reflex. Gut. 1994; 35:S31

[187] Kerrigan DD, Lucas MG, Sun WM, Donnelly TC, Read NW. Idiopathic constipation associated with impaired urethrovesical and sacral reflex function. Br J Surg. 1989; 76(7):748–751

[188] Knowles CH, Martin JE. Slow transit constipation: a model of human gut dysmotility. Review of possible aetiologies. Neurogastroenterol Motil. 2000; 12(2):181–196

[189] Ishikawa M, Mibu R, Iwamoto T, Konomi H, Oohata Y, Tanaka M. Change in colonic motility after extrinsic autonomic denervation in dogs. Dig Dis Sci. 1997; 42(9):1950–1956

[190] Waldron DJ, Kumar D, Hallan RI, Wingate DL, Williams NS. Evidence for motor neuropathy and reduced filling of the rectum in chronic intractable constipation. Gut. 1990; 31(11):1284–1288

[191] Bassotti G, de Roberto G, Castellani D, Sediari L, Morelli A. Normal aspects of colorectal motility and abnormalities in slow transit constipation. World J Gastroenterol. 2005; 11(18):2691–2696

[192] Gladman MA, Dvorkin LS, Lunniss PJ, Williams NS, Scott SM. Rectal hyposensitivity: a disorder of the rectal wall or the afferent pathway? An assessment using the barostat. Am J Gastroenterol. 2005; 100(1):106–114

[193] Knowles CH, Scott SM, Lunniss PJ. Slow transit constipation: a disorder of pelvic autonomic nerves? Dig Dis Sci. 2001; 46(2):389–401

[194] Altomare D, Pilot MA, Scott M, et al. Detection of subclinical autonomic neuropathy in constipated patients using a sweat test. Gut. 1992; 33 (11):1539–1543

[195] Lyford GL, He CL, Soffer E, et al. Pan-colonic decrease in interstitial cells of Cajal in patients with slow transit constipation. Gut. 2002; 51(4):496–501

[196] Toman J, Turina M, Ray M, Petras RE, Stromberg AJ, Galandiuk S. Slow transit colon constipation is not related to the number of interstitial cells of Cajal. Int J Colorectal Dis. 2006; 21(6):527–532

[197] El-Salhy M. Chronic idiopathic slow transit constipation: pathophysiology and management. Colorectal Dis. 2003; 5(4):288–296

[198] Tomita R, Fujisaki S, Ikeda T, Fukuzawa M. Role of nitric oxide in the colon of patients with slow-transit constipation. Dis Colon Rectum. 2002; 45 (5):593–600

[199] Slater BJ, Varma JS, Gillespie JI. Abnormalities in the contractile properties of colonic smooth muscle in idiopathic slow transit constipation. Br J Surg. 1997; 84(2):181–184

[200] Rao SSC, Sadeghi P, Beaty J, Kavlock R. Ambulatory 24-hour colonic manometry in slow-transit constipation. Am J Gastroenterol. 2004; 99(12):2405–2416

[201] Hagger R, Kumar D, Benson M, Grundy A. Colonic motor activity in slow-transit idiopathic constipation as identified by 24-h pancolonic ambulatory manometry. Neurogastroenterol Motil. 2003; 15(5):515–522

[202] Goldin E, Karmeli F, Selinger Z, Rachmilewitz D. Colonic substance P levels are increased in ulcerative colitis and decreased in chronic severe constipation. Dig Dis Sci. 1989; 34(5):754–757

[203] Battaglia E, Serra AM, Buonafede G, et al. Long-term study on the effects of visual biofeedback and muscle training as a therapeutic modality in pelvic floor dyssynergia and slow-transit constipation. Dis Colon Rectum. 2004; 47 (1):90–95

[204] Sunderland GT, Poon FW, Lauder J, Finlay IG. Videoproctography in selecting patients with constipation for colectomy. Dis Colon Rectum. 1992; 35 (3):235–237

[205] Mollen RM, Kuijpers HC, Claassen AT. Colectomy for slow-transit constipation: preoperative functional evaluation is important but not a guarantee for a successful outcome. Dis Colon Rectum. 2001; 44(4):577–580

[206] Todd IP. Constipation: results of surgical treatment. Br J Surg. 1985; 72 Suppl:S12–S13

[207] Preston DM, Lennard-Jones JE. Severe chronic constipation of young women: 'idiopathic slow transit constipation'. Gut. 1986; 27(1):41–48

[208] Roe AM, Bartolo DC, Mortensen NJ. Diagnosis and surgical management of intractable constipation. Br J Surg. 1986; 73(10):854–861

[209] Leon SH, Krishnamurthy S, Schuffler MD. Subtotal colectomy for severe idiopathic constipation. A follow-up study of 13 patients. Dig Dis Sci. 1987; 32 (11):1249–1254

[210] Walsh PV, Peebles-Brown DA, Watkinson G. Colectomy for slow transit constipation. Ann R Coll Surg Engl. 1987; 69(2):71–75

[211] Akervall S, Fasth S, Nordgren S, Oresland T, Hultén L. The functional results after colectomy and ileorectal anastomosis for severe constipation (Arbuthnot Lane's disease) as related to rectal sensory function. Int J Colorectal Dis. 1988; 3(2):96–101

[212] Kamm MA, Hawley PR, Lennard-Jones JE. Outcome of colectomy for severe idiopathic constipation. Gut. 1988; 29(7):969–973

[213] Zenilman ME, Dunnegan DL, Super NJ, Becker JM. Successful surgical treatment of idiopathic colonic dysmotility. Arch Surg. 1989; 124:947–951

[214] Yoshioka K, Keighley MR. Clinical results of colectomy for severe constipation. Br J Surg. 1989; 76(6):600–604

[215] Coremans GE. Surgical aspects of severe chronic non-Hirschsprung constipation. Hepatogastroenterology. 1990; 37(6):588–595

[216] Kuijpers HC. Application of the colorectal laboratory in diagnosis and treatment of functional constipation. Dis Colon Rectum. 1990; 33(1):35–39

[217] Pemberton JH, Rath DM, Ilstrup DM. Evaluation and surgical treatment of severe chronic constipation. Ann Surg. 1991; 214(4):403–411, discussion 411–413

[218] Takahashi T, Fitzgerald SD, Pemberton JH. Evaluation and treatment of constipation. Rev Gastroenterol Mex. 1994; 59(2):133–138

[219] Redmond JM, Smith GW, Barofsky I, Ratych RE, Goldsborough DC, Schuster MM. Physiological tests to predict long-term outcome of total abdominal colectomy for intractable constipation. Am J Gastroenterol. 1995; 90 (5):748–753

[220] Piccirillo MF, Reissman P, Wexner SD, Wexner SD. Colectomy as treatment for constipation in selected patients. Br J Surg. 1995; 82(7):898–901

[221] de Graaf EJR, Gilberts ECAM, Schouten WR. Role of segmental colonic transit time studies to select patients with slow transit constipation for partial left-sided or subtotal colectomy. Br J Surg. 1996; 83(5):648–651

[222] Nyam DC, Pemberton JH, Ilstrup DM, Rath DM. Long-term results of surgery for chronic constipation. Dis Colon Rectum. 1997; 40(3):273–279

[223] Fan CW, Wang JY. Subtotal colectomy for colonic inertia. Int Surg. 2000; 85 (4):309–312

[224] Nylund G, Oresland T, Fasth S, Nordgren S. Long-term outcome after colectomy in severe idiopathic constipation. Colorectal Dis. 2001; 3(4):253–258

[225] Pikarsky AJ, Singh JJ, Weiss EG, Nogueras JJ, Wexner SD. Long-term follow-up of patients undergoing colectomy for colonic inertia. Dis Colon Rectum. 2001; 44(2):179–183

[226] Webster C, Dayton M. Results after colectomy for colonic inertia: a sixteen-year experience. Am J Surg. 2001; 182(6):639–644

[227] Glia A, Akerlund JE, Lindberg G. Outcome of colectomy for slow transit constipation in relation to the presence of small bowel motility. Dis Colon Rectum. 2004; 47:96–102

[228] Ghosh S, Papachrysostomou M, Batool M, Eastwood MA. Long-term results of subtotal colectomy and evidence of noncolonic involvement in patients with idiopathic slow-transit constipation. Scand J Gastroenterol. 1996; 31 (11):1083–1091

[229] FitzHarris GP, Garcia-Aguilar J, Parker SC, et al. Quality of life after subtotal colectomy for slow-transit constipation: both quality and quantity count. Dis Colon Rectum. 2003; 46(4):433–440

[230] Schuffler MD, Krishnamurthy S. Constipation and colectomy. Dig Dis Sci. 1988; 33(9):1197–1198

[231] Wexner SD, Daniel N, Jagelman DG. Colectomy for constipation: physiologic investigation is the key to success. Dis Colon Rectum. 1991; 34(10):851–856

[232] Aldulaymi BH, Rasmussen OO, Christiansen J. Long-term results of subtotal colectomy for severe slow-transit constipation in patients with normal rectal function. Colorectal Dis. 2001; 3(6):392–395

[233] Duthie GS, Bartolo DCC. Slow transit constipation and anismus. In: Wexner SD, Bartolo DCC, eds. Constipation: Etiology, Evaluation and Management. Oxford: Butterworth-Heinemann; 1995

[234] Kamm MA, van der Sijp JR, Hawley PR, Phillips RK, Lennard-Jones JE. Left hemicolectomy with rectal excision for severe idiopathic constipation. Int J Colorectal Dis. 1991; 6(1):49–51

[235] Lundin E, Karlbom U, Påhlman L, Graf W. Outcome of segmental colonic resection for slow-transit constipation. Br J Surg. 2002; 89(10):1270–1274

[236] MacDonald A, Baxter JN, Bessent RG, Gray HW, Finlay IG. Gastric emptying in patients with constipation following childbirth and due to idiopathic slow transit. Br J Surg. 1997; 84(8):1141–1143

[237] Sarli L, Costi R, Sarli D, Roncoroni L. Pilot study of subtotal colectomy with antiperistaltic cecoproctostomy for the treatment of chronic slow-transit constipation. Dis Colon Rectum. 2001; 44(10):1514–1520

[238] van der Sijp JRM, Kamm MA, Evans RC, Lennard-Jones JE. The results of stoma formation in severe idiopathic constipation. Eur J Gastroenterol Hepatol. 1992; 4:137–140

[239] Nicholls RJ, Kamm MA. Proctocolectomy with restorative ileoanal reservoir for severe idiopathic constipation. Report of two cases. Dis Colon Rectum. 1988; 31(12):968–969

[240] Hosie KB, Kmiot WA, Keighley MR. Constipation: another indication for restorative proctocolectomy. Br J Surg. 1990; 77(7):801–802

[241] Thakur A, Fonkalsrud EW, Buchmiller T, French S. Surgical treatment of severe colonic inertia with restorative proctocolectomy. Am Surg. 2001; 67 (1):36–40

[242] Kalbassi MR, Winter DC, Deasy JM. Quality-of-life assessment of patients after ileal pouch-anal anastomosis for slow-transit constipation with rectal inertia. Dis Colon Rectum. 2003; 46(11):1508–1512

[243] Malouf AJ, Wiesel PH, Nicholls T, Nicholls RJ, Kamm MA. Short-term effects of sacral nerve stimulation for idiopathic slow transit constipation. World J Surg. 2002; 26(2):166–170

[244] Kenefick NJ, Nicholls RJ, Cohen RG, Kamm MA. Permanent sacral nerve stimulation for treatment of idiopathic constipation. Br J Surg. 2002; 89 (7):882–888

[245] Kenefick NJ, Vaizey CJ, Cohen CRG, Nicholls RJ, Kamm MA. Double-blind placebo-controlled crossover study of sacral nerve stimulation for idiopathic constipation. Br J Surg. 2002; 89(12):1570–1571

[246] Sharma A, Bussen D, Herold A, Jayne D. Review of sacral neuromodulation for management of constipation. Surg Innov. 2013; 20(6):614–624

[247] Wexner SD. Percutaneous tibial nerve stimulation in faecal incontinence. Lancet. 2015; 386(10004):1605–1606

[248] Horrocks EJ, Chadi SA, Stevens NJ, Wexner SD, Knowles CH. Factors Associated With Efficacy of Percutaneous Tibial Nerve Stimulation for Fecal Incontinence, Based on Post-Hoc Analysis of Data From a Randomized Trial. Clin Gastroenterol Hepatol. 2017; 15(12):1915–1921

[249] Knowles CH, Horrocks EJ, Bremner SA, Stevens N, Norton C, O'Connell PR, Eldridge S, CONFIDeNT study group. Percutaneous tibial nerve stimulation versus sham electrical stimulation for the treatment of faecal incontinence in adults (CONFIDeNT): a double-blind, multicentre, pragmatic, parallel-group, randomised controlled trial. Lancet. 2015; 386 (10004):1640–1648

[250] Hill J, Stott S, MacLennan I. Antegrade enemas for the treatment of severe idiopathic constipation. Br J Surg. 1994; 81(10):1490–1491

[251] Krogh K, Laurberg S. Malone antegrade continence enema for faecal incontinence and constipation in adults. Br J Surg. 1998; 85(7):974–977

[252] Rongen MJ, van der Hoop AG, Baeten CG. Cecal access for antegrade colon enemas in medically refractory slow-transit constipation: a prospective study. Dis Colon Rectum. 2001; 44(11):1644–1649

[253] Lees NP, Hodson P, Hill J, Pearson RC, MacLennan I. Long-term results of the antegrade continent enema procedure for constipation in adults. Colorectal Dis. 2004; 6(5):362–368

[254] Wasserman IF. Puborectalis syndrome: rectal stenosis due to anorectal spasm. Dis Colon Rectum. 1964; 7:87–98

[255] Duthie GS, Bartolo DCC. Anismus: the cause of constipation? Results of investigation and treatment. World J Surg. 1992; 16(5):831–835

[256] Schouten WR. Diagnosis and treatment of constipation and disturbed defecation. Perspect Colon Rectal Surg. 1996; 9:71–85

[257] Pezim ME, Pemberton JH, Levin KE, Litchy WJ, Phillips SF. Parameters of ano-rectal and colonic motility in health and in severe constipation. Dis Colon Rectum. 1993; 36(5):484–491

[258] Jones PN, Lubowski DZ, Swash M, Henry MM. Is paradoxical contraction of puborectalis muscle of functional importance? Dis Colon Rectum. 1987; 30 (9):667–670

[259] Miller R, Duthie GS, Bartolo DCC, Roe AM, Locke-Edmunds J, Mortensen NJ. Anismus in patients with normal and slow transit constipation. Br J Surg. 1991; 78(6):690–692

[260] Dahl J, Lindquist BL, Tysk C, Leissner P, Philipson L, Järnerot G. Behavioral medicine treatment in chronic constipation with paradoxical anal sphincter contraction. Dis Colon Rectum. 1991; 34(9):769–776

[261] Jorge JMN, Wexner SD, Ger GC, Salanga VD, Nogueras JJ, Jagelman DG. Cine-defecography and electromyography in the diagnosis of nonrelaxing puborectalis syndrome. Dis Colon Rectum. 1993; 36(7):668–676

[262] Schouten WR, Briel JW, Auwerda JJA, et al. Anismus: fact or fiction? Dis Colon Rectum. 1997; 40(9):1033–1041

[263] Loening-Baucke V. Persistence of chronic constipation in children after biofeedback treatment. Dig Dis Sci. 1991; 36(2):153–160

[264] Keck JO, Staniunas RJ, Coller JA, et al. Biofeedback training is useful in fecal incontinence but disappointing in constipation. Dis Colon Rectum. 1994; 37 (12):1271–1276

[265] Turnbull GK, Ritvo PG. Anal sphincter biofeedback relaxation treatment for women with intractable constipation symptoms. Dis Colon Rectum. 1992; 35(6):530–536

[266] Lubowski DZ, Meagher AP, Smart RC, Butler SP. Scintigraphic assessment of colonic function during defaecation. Int J Colorectal Dis. 1995; 10(2):91–93

[267] Lubowski DZ, King DW, Finlay IG. Electromyography of the pubococcygeus muscles in patients with obstructed defaecation. Int J Colorectal Dis. 1992; 7 (4):184–187

[268] Faucheron JL, Dubreuil A. Rectal akinesia as a new cause of impaired defecation. Dis Colon Rectum. 2000; 43(11):1545–1549

[269] Bleijenberg G, Kuijpers HC. Treatment of the spastic pelvic floor syndrome with biofeedback. Dis Colon Rectum. 1987; 30(2):108–111

[270] Bleijenberg G, Kuijpers HC. Biofeedback treatment of constipation: a comparison of two methods. Am J Gastroenterol. 1994; 89(7):1021–1026

[271] Chiarioni G, Salandini L, Whitehead WE. Biofeedback benefits only patients with outlet dysfunction, not patients with isolated slow transit constipation. Gastroenterology. 2005; 129(1):86–97

[272] Palsson OS, Heymen S, Whitehead WE. Biofeedback treatment for functional anorectal disorders: a comprehensive efficacy review. Appl Psychophysiol Biofeedback. 2004; 29(3):153–174

[273] Koutsomanis D, Lennard-Jones JE, Roy AJ, Kamm MA. Controlled randomised trial of visual biofeedback versus muscle training without a visual display for intractable constipation. Gut. 1995; 37(1):95–99

[274] Heymen S, Wexner SD, Vickers D, Nogueras JJ, Weiss EG, Pikarsky AJ. Prospective, randomized trial comparing four biofeedback techniques for patients with constipation. Dis Colon Rectum. 1999; 42(11):1388–1393

[275] Glia A, Gylin M, Gullberg K, Lindberg G. Biofeedback retraining in patients with functional constipation and paradoxical puborectalis contraction: comparison of anal manometry and sphincter electromyography for feedback. Dis Colon Rectum. 1997; 40(8):889–895

[276] Weber J, Ducrotte P, Touchais JY, Roussignol C, Denis P. Biofeedback training for constipation in adults and children. Dis Colon Rectum. 1987; 30 (11):844–846

[277] Kawimbe BM, Papachrysostomou M, Binnie NR, Clare N, Smith AN. Outlet obstruction constipation (anismus) managed by biofeedback. Gut. 1991; 32 (10):1175–1179

[278] Lestàr B, Penninckx F, Kerremans R. Biofeedback defaecation training for anismus. Int J Colorectal Dis. 1991; 6(4):202–207

[279] West L, Abell TL, Cutts T. Long-term results of pelvic floor muscle rehabilitationin the treatment of constipation. Gastroenterology. 1992; 102:A533

[280] Wexner SD, Cheape JD, Jorge JMN, Heymen S, Jagelman DG. Prospective assessment of biofeedback for the treatment of paradoxical puborectalis contraction. Dis Colon Rectum. 1992; 35(2):145–150

[281] Fleshman JW, Dreznik Z, Meyer K, Fry RD, Carney R, Kodner IJ. Outpatient protocol for biofeedback therapy of pelvic floor outlet obstruction. Dis Colon Rectum. 1992; 35(1):1–7

[282] Papachrysostomou M, Smith AN. Effects of biofeedback on obstructive defecation–reconditioning of the defecation reflex? Gut. 1994; 35(2):252–256

[283] Ho YH, Tan M, Goh HS. Clinical and physiologic effects of biofeedback in outlet obstruction constipation. Dis Colon Rectum. 1996; 39(5):520–524

[284] Park UC, Choi SK, Piccirillo MF, Verzaro R, Wexner SD. Patterns of anismus and the relation to biofeedback therapy. Dis Colon Rectum. 1996; 39 (7):768–773

[285] Rao SSC, Welcher KD, Pelsang RE. Effects of biofeedback therapy on anorectal function in obstructive defecation. Dig Dis Sci. 1997; 42(11):2197–2205

[286] Karlbom U, Hållden M, Eeg-Olofsson KE, Påhlman L, Graf W. Results of biofeedback in constipated patients: a prospective study. Dis Colon Rectum. 1997; 40(10):1149–1155

[287] McKee RF, McEnroe L, Anderson JH, Finlay IG. Identification of patients likely to benefit from biofeedback for outlet obstruction constipation. Br J Surg. 1999; 86(3):355–359

[288] Lau CW, Heymen S, Alabaz O, Iroatulam AJ, Wexner SD. Prognostic significance of rectocele, intussusception, and abnormal perineal descent in biofeedback treatment for constipated patients with paradoxical puborectalis contraction. Dis Colon Rectum. 2000; 43(4):478–482

[289] Dailianas A, Skandalis N, Rimikis MN, Koutsomanis D, Kardasi M, Archimandritis A. Pelvic floor study in patients with obstructive defecation: influence of biofeedback. J Clin Gastroenterol. 2000; 30(2):176–180

[290] Rhee PL, Choi MS, Kim YH, et al. An increased rectal maximum tolerable volume and long anal canal are associated with poor short-term response to biofeedback therapy for patients with anismus with decreased bowel frequency and normal colonic transit time. Dis Colon Rectum. 2000; 43 (10):1405–1411

[291] Barnes PRH, Hawley PR, Preston DM, Lennard-Jones JE. Experience of posterior division of the puborectalis muscle in the management of chronic constipation. Br J Surg. 1985; 72(6):475–477

[292] Kawano M, Fujioshi T, Takagi K. Puborectalis syndrome. J Jpn Soc Coloproctol. 1987; 40:612

[293] Kamm MA, Hawley PR, Lennard-Jones JE. Lateral division of the puborectalis muscle in the management of severe constipation. Br J Surg. 1988; 75 (7):661–663

[294] Yu DH, Cui FD. Surgical treatment of puborectalis syndrome. J Pract Surg. 1990; 10:1599–1600

[295] Hallan RI, Williams NS, Melling J, Waldron DJ, Womack NR, Morrison JFB. Treatment of anismus in intractable constipation with botulinum A toxin. Lancet. 1988; 2(8613):714–717

[296] Joo JS, Agachan F, Wolff B, Nogueras JJ, Wexner SD. Initial North American experience with botulinum toxin type A for treatment of anismus. Dis Colon Rectum. 1996; 39(10):1107–1111

[297] Maria G, Brisinda G, Bentivoglio AR, Cassetta E, Albanese A. Botulinum toxin in the treatment of outlet obstruction constipation caused by puborectalis syndrome. Dis Colon Rectum. 2000; 43(3):376–380

[298] Ron Y, Avni Y, Lukovetski A, et al. Botulinum toxin type-A in therapy of patients with anismus. Dis Colon Rectum. 2001; 44(12):1821–1826

[299] Hompes R, Harmston C, Wijffels N, Jones OM, Cunningham C, Lindsey I. Excellent response rate of anismus to botulinum toxin if rectal prolapse misdiagnosed as anismus ('pseudoanismus') is excluded. Colorectal Dis. 2012; 14(2):224–230

[300] Wallace WC, Madden WM. Experience with partial resection of the puborectalis muscle. Dis Colon Rectum. 1969; 12(3):196–200

[301] Ganio E, Masin A, Ratto C, et al. Sacral nerve modulation for chronic outlet constipation. Available at: http://www.colorep.it. Accessed January 15, 2018

[302] Hoffman MJ, Kodner IJ, Fry RD. Internal intussusception of the rectum. Diagnosis and surgical management. Dis Colon Rectum. 1984; 27(7):435–441

[303] Johansson C, Ihre T, Ahlbäck SO. Disturbances in the defecation mechanism with special reference to intussusception of the rectum (internal procidentia). Dis Colon Rectum. 1985; 28(12):920–924

[304] Fleshman JW, Kodner IJ, Fry RD. Internal intussusception of the rectum: a changing perspective. Neth J Surg. 1989; 41(6):145–148

[305] Speakman CT, Madden MV, Nicholls RJ, Kamm MA. Lateral ligament division during rectopexy causes constipation but prevents recurrence: results of a prospective randomized study. Br J Surg. 1991; 78(12):1431–1433

[306] Brodén G, Dolk A, Holmström B. Evacuation difficulties and other characteristics of rectal function associated with procidentia and the Ripstein operation. Dis Colon Rectum. 1988; 31(4):283–286

[307] Shorvon PJ, McHugh S, Diamant NE, Somers S, Stevenson GW. Defecography in normal volunteers: results and implications. Gut. 1989; 30 (12):1737–1749

[308] Longo A. Obstructed defecation because of rectal pathologies. Novel surgical treatment: stapled transanal rectal resection (STARR). Proceedings of the 14th Annual International Colorectal Disease Symposium, Ft Lauderdale, Florida, February 13–15, 2003

[309] Boccasanta P, Venturi M, Stuto A, et al. Stapled transanal rectal resection for outlet obstruction: a prospective, multicenter trial. Dis Colon Rectum. 2004; 47(8):1285–1296, discussion 1296–1297

[310] Mathur P, Ng K-H, Seow-Choen F. Stapled mucosectomy for rectocele repair: a preliminary report. Dis Colon Rectum. 2004; 47(11):1978–1980, discussion 1980–1981

[311] Jayne DG, Schwandner O, Stuto A. Stapled transanal rectal resection for obstructed defecation syndrome: one-year results of the European STARR Registry. Dis Colon Rectum. 2009; 52(7):1205–1212, discussion 1212–1214

[312] Dodi G, Pietroletti R, Milito G, Binda G, Pescatori M. Bleeding, incontinence, pain and constipation after STARR transanal double stapling rectotomy for obstructed defecation. Tech Coloproctol. 2003; 7(3):148–153

[313] D'Hoore A, Cadoni R, Penninckx F. Long-term outcome of laparoscopic ventral rectopexy for total rectal prolapse. Br J Surg. 2004; 91(11):1500–1505

[314] Evans C, Stevenson AR, Sileri P, et al. A multicenter collaboration to assess the safety of laparoscopic ventral rectopexy. Dis Colon Rectum. 2015; 58 (8):799–807

[315] van Dam JH, Ginai AZ, Gosselink MJ, et al. Role of defecography in predicting clinical outcome of rectocele repair. Dis Colon Rectum. 1997; 40(2):201–207

[316] Halligan S, Bartram CI. Is barium trapping in rectoceles significant? Dis Colon Rectum. 1995; 38(7):764–768

[317] Kelvin FM, Maglinte DD, Hornback JA. Pelvic floor prolapse: assessment with evacuation proctography. Radiology. 1992; 184:547–551

[318] Siproudhis L, Ropert A, Lucas J, et al. Defecatory disorders, anorectal and pelvic floor dysfunction: a polygamy? Radiologic and manometric studies in 41 patients. Int J Colorectal Dis. 1992; 7(2):102–107

[319] Johansson C, Nilsson BY, Holmström B, Dolk A, Mellgren A. Association between rectocele and paradoxical sphincter response. Dis Colon Rectum. 1992; 35(5):503–509

[320] van Dam JH, Schouten WR, Ginai AZ, Huisman WM, Hop WCJ. The impact of anismus on the clinical outcome of rectocele repair. Int J Colorectal Dis. 1996; 11(5):238–242

[321] Siproudhis L, Dautrème S, Ropert A, et al. Dyschezia and rectocele–a marriage of convenience? Physiologic evaluation of the rectocele in a group of 52 women complaining of difficulty in evacuation. Dis Colon Rectum. 1993; 36(11):1030–1036

[322] Murthy VK, Orkin BA, Smith LE, Glassman LM. Excellent outcome using selective criteria for rectocele repair. Dis Colon Rectum. 1996; 39(4):374–378

[323] Karlbom U, Graf W, Nilsson S, Påhlman L. Does surgical repair of a rectocele improve rectal emptying? Dis Colon Rectum. 1996; 39(11):1296–1302

[324] Mellgren A, Anzén B, Nilsson BY, et al. Results of rectocele repair. A prospective study. Dis Colon Rectum. 1995; 38(1):7–13

[325] Stojkovic SG, Balfour L, Burke D, Finan PJ, Sagar PM. Does the need to self-digitate or the presence of a large or nonemptying rectocoele on proctography influence the outcome of transanal rectocoele repair? Colorectal Dis. 2003; 5(2):169–172

[326] Zbar AP, Lienemann A, Fritsch H, Beer-Gabel M, Pescatori M. Rectocele: pathogenesis and surgical management. Int J Colorectal Dis. 2003; 18 (5):369–384

[327] Arnold MW, Stewart WRC, Aguilar PS. Rectocele repair. Four years' experience. Dis Colon Rectum. 1990; 33(8):684–687

[328] Nieminen K, Hiltunen KM, Laitinen J, Oksala J, Heinonen PK. Transanal or vaginal approach to rectocele repair: a prospective, randomized pilot study. Dis Colon Rectum. 2004; 47(10):1636–1642

[329] De Tayrac R, Picone O, Chauveaud-Lambling A, Fernandez H. A 2-year anatomical and functional assessment of transvaginal rectocele repair using a polypropylene mesh. Int Urogynecol J Pelvic Floor Dysfunct. 2006; 17(2):100–105

[330] Altman D, Zetterström J, López A, et al. Functional and anatomic outcome after transvaginal rectocele repair using collagen mesh: a prospective study. Dis Colon Rectum. 2005; 48(6):1233–1241, discussion 1241–1242, author reply 1242

[331] Marks MM. The rectal side of the rectocele. Dis Colon Rectum. 1967; 10 (5):387–388

[332] Sarles JC, Arnaud A, Selezneff I, Olivier S. Endo-rectal repair of rectocele. Int J Colorectal Dis. 1989; 4(3):167–171

[333] Capps WF, Jr. Rectoplasty and perineoplasty for the symptomatic rectocele: a report of fifty cases. Dis Colon Rectum. 1975; 18(3):237–243

[334] Sehapayak S. Transrectal repair of rectocele: an extended armamentarium of colorectal surgeons. A report of 355 cases. Dis Colon Rectum. 1985; 28 (6):422–433

[335] Sullivan ES, Leaverton GH, Hardwick CE. Transrectal perineal repair: an adjunct to improved function after anorectal surgery. Dis Colon Rectum. 1968; 11(2):106–114

[336] Khubchandani IT, Sheets JA, Stasik JJ, Hakki AR. Endorectal repair of rectocele. Dis Colon Rectum. 1983; 26(12):792–796

[337] Block IR. Transrectal repair of rectocele using obliterative suture. Dis Colon Rectum. 1986; 29(11):707–711

[338] Cundiff GW, Fenner D. Evaluation and treatment of women with rectocele: focus on associated defecatory and sexual dysfunction. Obstet Gynecol. 2004; 104(6):1403–1421

[339] Ayav A, Bresler L, Brunaud L, Boissel P. Long-term results of transanal repair of rectocele using linear stapler. Dis Colon Rectum. 2004; 47(6):889–894

[340] Ho YH, Ang M, Nyam D, Tan M, Seow-Choen F. Transanal approach to rectocele repair may compromise anal sphincter pressures. Dis Colon Rectum. 1998; 41(3):354–358

[341] van Dam JH, Huisman WM, Hop WCJ, Schouten WR. Fecal continence after rectocele repair: a prospective study. Int J Colorectal Dis. 2000; 15(1):54–57

[342] Thornton MJ, Lam A, King DW. Laparoscopic or transanal repair of rectocele? A retrospective matched cohort study. Dis Colon Rectum. 2005; 48(4):792–798

[343] Janssen LW, van Dijke CF. Selection criteria for anterior rectal wall repair in symptomatic rectocele and anterior rectal wall prolapse. Dis Colon Rectum. 1994; 37(11):1100–1107

[344] Tjandra JJ, Ooi BS, Tang CL, Dwyer P, Carey M. Transanal repair of rectocele corrects obstructed defecation if it is not associated with anismus. Dis Colon Rectum. 1999; 42(12):1544–1550

[345] Heriot AG, Skull A, Kumar D. Functional and physiological outcome following transanal repair of rectocele. Br J Surg. 2004; 91(10):1340–1344

[346] Abbas SM, Bissett IP, Neill ME, Macmillan AK, Milne D, Parry BR. Long-term results of the anterior Délorme's operation in the management of symptomatic rectocele. Dis Colon Rectum. 2005; 48(2):317–322

[347] Hirst GR, Hughes RJ, Morgan AR, Carr ND, Patel B, Beynon J. The role of rectocele repair in targeted patients with obstructed defaecation. Colorectal Dis. 2005; 7(2):159–163

[348] Roman H, Michot F. Long-term outcomes of transanal rectocele repair. Dis Colon Rectum. 2005; 48(3):510–517

[349] Ribaric G, D'Hoore A, Schiffhorst G, Hempel E, TRANSTAR Registry Study Group. STARR with CONTOUR® TRANSTAR™ device for obstructed defecation syndrome: one-year real-world outcomes of the European TRANSTAR registry. Int J Colorectal Dis. 2014; 29(5):611–622

[350] Isbert C, Reibetanz J, Jayne DG, Kim M, Germer CT, Boenicke L. Comparative study of Contour Transtar and STARR procedure for the treatment of obstructed defecation syndrome (ODS)–feasibility, morbidity and early functional results. Colorectal Dis. 2010; 12(9):901–908

[351] Zhang B, Ding JH, Yin SH, Zhang M, Zhao K. Stapled transanal rectal resection for obstructed defecation syndrome associated with rectocele and rectal intussusception. World J Gastroenterol. 2010; 16(20):2542–2548

[352] Lenisa L, Schwandner O, Stuto A, et al. STARR with Contour Transtar: prospective multicentre European study. Colorectal Dis. 2009; 11(8):821–827

[353] Arroyo A, González-Argenté FX, García-Domingo M, et al. Prospective multicentre clinical trial of stapled transanal rectal resection for obstructive defaecation syndrome. Br J Surg. 2008; 95(12):1521–1527

[354] Pescatori M, Gagliardi G. Postoperative complications after procedure for prolapsed hemorrhoids (PPH) and stapled transanal rectal resection (STARR) procedures. Tech Coloproctol. 2008; 12(1):7–19

[355] Goede AC, Glancy D, Carter H, Mills A, Mabey K, Dixon AR. Medium-term results of stapled transanal rectal resection (STARR) for obstructed defecation and symptomatic rectal-anal intussusception. Colorectal Dis. 2011; 13(9):1052–1057

[356] Samaranayake CB, Luo C, Plank AW, Merrie AE, Plank LD, Bissett IP. Systematic review on ventral rectopexy for rectal prolapse and intussusception. Colorectal Dis. 2010; 12(6):504–512

[357] Lamah M, Ho J, Leicester RJ. Results of anterior levatorplasty for rectocele. Colorectal Dis. 2001; 3(6):412–416

[358] Ayabaca SM, Zbar AP, Pescatori M. Anal continence after rectocele repair. Dis Colon Rectum. 2002; 45(1):63–69

[359] Watson SJ, Loder PB, Halligan S, Bartram CI, Kamm MA, Phillips RK. Transperineal repair of symptomatic rectocele with Marlex mesh: a clinical, physiological and radiologic assessment of treatment. J Am Coll Surg. 1996; 183(3):257–261

[360] Mercer-Jones MA, Sprowson A, Varma JS. Outcome after transperineal mesh repair of rectocele: a case series. Dis Colon Rectum. 2004; 47(6):864–868

[361] Lechaux JP, Lechaux D, Bataille P, Bars I. [Transperineal repair of rectocele with prosthetic mesh. A prospective study]. Ann Chir. 2004; 129(4):211–217

[362] Vermeulen J, Lange JF, Sikkenk AC, van der Harst E. Anterolateral rectopexy for correction of rectoceles leads to good anatomical but poor functional results. Tech Coloproctol. 2005; 9(1):35–41, discussion 41

[363] Bentley JFR. Posterior excisional anorectal myotomy in management of chronic fecal accumulation. Arch Dis Child. 1966; 41:144

[364] Fishbein RH, Handelsman JC, Schuster MM. Surgical treatment of Hirschsprung's disease in adults. Surg Gynecol Obstet. 1986; 163(5):458–464

[365] Poisson J, Devroede G. Severe chronic constipation as a surgical problem. Surg Clin North Am. 1983; 63(1):193–217

[366] Yoshioka K, Keighley MRB. Anorectal myectomy for outlet obstruction. Br J Surg. 1987; 74(5):373–376

[367] Kimura K, Inomata Y, Soper RT. Posterior sagittal rectal myectomy for persistent rectal achalasia after the Soave procedure for Hirschsprung's disease. J Pediatr Surg. 1993; 28(9):1200–1201

[368] Thomas CG, Jr, Bream CA, DeConnick P. Posterior sphincterotomy and rectal myotomy in the management of Hirschsprung's disease. Ann Surg. 1970; 171(5):796–810

[369] Lynn HB, van Heerden JA. Rectal myectomy in Hirschsprung disease: a decade of experience. Arch Surg. 1975; 110(8):991–994

[370] Clayden GS, Lawson JON. Investigation and management of long-standing chronic constipation in childhood. Arch Dis Child. 1976; 51(12):918–923

[371] Shermeta DW, Nilprabhassorn P. Posterior myectomy for primary and secondary short segment aganglionosis. Am J Surg. 1977; 133(1):39–41

[372] McCready RA, Beart RW, Jr. Adult Hirschsprung's disease: results of surgical treatment at Mayo Clinic. Dis Colon Rectum. 1980; 23(6):401–407

[373] Freeman NV. Intractable constipation in children treated by forceful anal stretch or anorectal myectomy: preliminary communication. J R Soc Med. 1984; 77 Suppl 3:6–8

[374] Hamdy MH, Scobie WG. Anorectal myectomy in adult Hirschsprung's disease: a report of six cases. Br J Surg. 1984; 71(8):611–613

[375] Mishalany HG, Woolley MG. Chronic constipation. Manometric patterns and surgical considerations. Arch Surg. 1984; 119(11):1257–1259

[376] Pinho M, Yoshioka K, Keighley MR. Long-term results of anorectal myectomy for chronic constipation. Dis Colon Rectum. 1990; 33(9):795–797

[377] McGarity WC, Cody JE. Complications of Hirschsprung's disease in the adult. Am J Gastroenterol. 1974; 61(5):390–393

[378] Elliot MS, Todd IP. Adult Hirschsprung's disease: results of the Duhamel procedure. Br J Surg. 1985; 72(11):884–885

[379] Hung WT, Chiang TP, Tsai YW, et al. Adult Hirschsprung's disease. J Pediatr Surg. 1989; 24(4):363–366

[380] Steichen FM, Talbert JL, Ravitch MM. Primary side-to-side colorectal anastomosis in the Duhamel operation for Hirschsprung's disease. Surgery. 1968; 64(2):475–483

[381] Kim CY, Park JG, Park KW, Park KJ, Cho MH, Kim WK. Adult Hirschsprung's disease. Results of the Duhamel's procedure. Int J Colorectal Dis. 1995; 10 (3):156–160

[382] Wheatley MJ, Wesley JR, Coran AG, Polley TZ, Jr. Hirschsprung's disease in adolescents and adults. Dis Colon Rectum. 1990; 33(7):622–629

[383] Luukkonen P, Heikkinen M, Huikuri K, Järvinen H. Adult Hirschsprung's disease. Clinical features and functional outcome after surgery. Dis Colon Rectum. 1990; 33(1):65–69

[384] Wu JS, Schoetz DJ, Jr, Coller JA, Veidenheimer MC. Treatment of Hirschsprung's disease in the adult. Report of five cases. Dis Colon Rectum. 1995; 38(6):655–659

[385] Gordon PH. An improved technique for the Duhamel operation using the EEA stapler. Dis Colon Rectum. 1983; 26(10):690–692

[386] Cutait DE, Cutait R. Surgery of chagasic megacolon. World J Surg. 1991; 15 (2):188–197

[387] Stoss F, Meier-Ruge W. Experience with neuronal intestinal dysplasia (NID) in adults. Eur J Pediatr Surg. 1994; 4(5):298–302

[388] Wrenn K. Fecal impaction. N Engl J Med. 1989; 321(10):658–662

[389] Longo WE, Ballantyne GH, Modlin IM. The colon, anorectum, and spinal cord patient. A review of the functional alterations of the denervated hindgut. Dis Colon Rectum. 1989; 32(3):261–267

[390] Gor RA, Katorski JR, Elliott SP. Medical and surgical management of neurogenic bowel. Curr Opin Urol. 2016; 26(4):369–375

[391] Emmanuel A, Kumar G, Christensen P, et al. Long-term cost-effectiveness of transanal irrigation in patients with neurogenic bowel dysfunction. PLoS One. 2016; 11(8):e0159394

[392] Safadi BY, Rosito O, Nino-Murcia M, Wolfe VA, Perkash I. Which stoma works better for colonic dysmotility in the spinal cord injured patient? Am J Surg. 2003; 186(5):437–442

[393] Read NW, Celik AF, Katsinelos P. Constipation and incontinence in the elderly. J Clin Gastroenterol. 1995; 20(1):61–70

[394] Kinnunen O. Constipation in the elderly, with special reference to treatment with magnesium hydroxide and a bulk laxative. Acta Universitatis Ouluensis. Series D. Medica. Oulu University Library © 1990: 1-72

[395] Hinton JM. Studies with drugs and hormones on the human colon. Proc R Soc Med. 1967; 60:215

[396] Katz LA, Spiro HM. Gastrointestinal manifestations of diabetes. N Engl J Med. 1966; 275(24):1350–1361

[397] Brocklehurst JC. Colonic disease in the elderly. Clin Gastroenterol. 1985; 14 (4):725–747

[398] Palmer ED. "Presbycolon" problems in the nursing home. JAMA. 1976; 235 (11):1150–1151

[399] Hull C, Greco RS, Brooks DL. Alleviation of constipation in the elderly by dietary fiber supplementation. J Am Geriatr Soc. 1980; 28(9):410–414

[400] Hope AK, Down EC. Dietary fibre and fluid in the control of constipation in a nursing home population. Med J Aust. 1986; 144(6):306–307

[401] Anderson AS, Whichelow MJ. Constipation during pregnancy: dietary fibre intake and the effect of fibre supplementation. Hum Nutr Appl Nutr. 1985; 39(3):202–207

[402] Jones FA, Godding EW. Management of Constipation. London: Blackwell Scientific Publications; 1972

[403] Lamerton R. Resurrected by an enema. Nurs Times. 1976; 72(42):1653

[404] Portenoy RK. Constipation in the cancer patient: causes and management. Med Clin North Am. 1987; 71(2):303–311

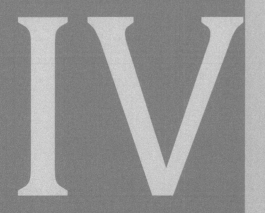

Part IV

Other Considerations

IV

34 Traumatic Injuries of the Colon, Rectum, and Anus

David E. Beck

Abstract

Trauma is the leading cause of death for young people and the third overall for all age groups in the United States. In penetrating abdominal trauma, the colon and rectum are often injured. Blunt trauma as well as diagnostic and therapeutic endoscopic procedures may cause perforation. Management of battle injuries has been the driving force of surgical progress throughout history with a reducing mortality rate from colonic injuries.

Keywords: traumatic injury, penetrating trauma, blunt trauma, operative injury, obstetric injury, foreign body ingestion, sexual assault, child abuse, ultrasound, laparoscopy

Significant portions of this chapter were adopted from the third edition chapter written by Dr. Lee E. Smith.

34.1 Introduction

Trauma ranks as the number 1 cause of death for people in the age group of 1 to 46 years and the third overall for all age groups in the United States.[1] It accounts for more lost years of useful life than any other cause. With penetrating abdominal trauma, the colon and rectum are often injured because of the large area they occupy. Diagnostic and therapeutic endoscopic procedures may cause perforation from within the lumen, and external penetrating or blunt injury may cause perforation from without.

The desire to improve the results for traumatic injuries received in battle has been the driving force of surgical progress throughout history. The mortality rate from colonic injuries has decreased with each war from the Civil War to the Vietnam War (▶ Table 34.1).

34.2 Etiology

34.2.1 Penetrating Trauma

External penetrating trauma may result from a bullet, shotgun pellets, a knife, a piercing instrument, or impalement.[2,3,4,5,6] A bullet wound is the most frequent wound type, outnumbering knife wounds by a ratio of 10:1.[7] Inexpensive low-velocity weapons known as "Saturday night specials" have been the usual weapons used in criminal assault in the past. In recent years, high-velocity weapons (with bullets traveling at more than 2,000 ft/s) have become increasingly available and are now common throughout society. Velocity is the dominant factor in determining the amount of tissue damage within the body.[8,9] The other factor that determines wound ballistics (motion of the bullet within the tissues) is the mass of the bullet. Velocity (*V*) and mass (*M*) can be expressed in the formula for kinetic energy (KE):

$$KE = \frac{1}{2}M \times V^2$$

The prime factor in kinetic energy is velocity, since it is expressed as the square. As the bullet travels through tissue, it creates a temporary high-pressure cavity around itself, resulting in secondary tissue damage away from the direct path of the bullet. The bullet may tumble (yaw) in its trajectory, also expanding the injury diameter (▶ Fig. 34.1).

Shotguns are smooth-bore weapons that discharge a number of small projectiles. The velocity of the pellets diminishes rapidly so that deep penetration in most instances does not occur if the weapon is fired more than 7 yards away from the person, but if a shotgun wound is inflicted at close range, extensive tissue loss occurs. Close-range shotgun wounds require extensive local debridement.

Large, bowel impalement injuries are caused by falling onto or running into an object that penetrates the abdomen or rectum. The rectal injury usually occurs after the individual falls with the legs astride the penetrating object such as a picket fence or a stake.

Table 34.1 Mortality from colonic trauma in war[2,3,4,5,6]

War	Mortality rate (%)
U.S. Civil War	90
Spanish-American War	90
World War I	58
World War II	37
Korean War	15
Vietnam War	9

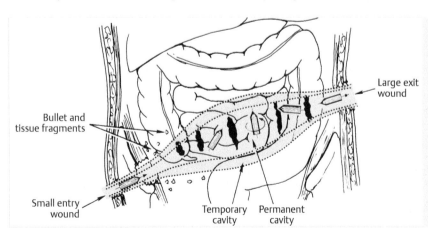

Fig. 34.1 Bullet traversing the abdomen. Note tumbling and yawing of the bullet. Area of destruction also results from a combination of cavitation and trajectory of secondary particles.

34.2.2 Blunt Trauma

Blunt trauma accounts for approximately 4% of colorectal injuries. Most injuries in this category result from motor vehicle accidents, with the steering wheel being the primary source of injury. Seat belts do save lives, but colonic or rectal injury can occur secondary to the use of seat belts, which cause pelvic fracture with a rectal tear or a compression of the colon between the anterior abdominal wall and the vertebral column, resulting in a "blow out" injury.[10] Direct force across the abdomen occurs when the belt either rides up from below the iliac crest or the person has slid down on the seat beneath the belt, creating free abdominal exposure. Shearing from rapid deceleration may cause an injury in which the fixed mesenteric peritoneum suspends the free-floating colon. In addition, hematoma and vascular injury may cause delayed perforation; thus, perforation after blunt trauma must be considered to avoid delay in treatment.[11,12] Automobiles striking pedestrians, motorcycle accidents, falls, being crushed under a heavy object, and athletic injuries result in similar damage. Also, blunt trauma to the perineum can disrupt the rectosigmoid and anal canal from the levator muscular sling.[11,12]

34.2.3 Iatrogenic Injury

Few organ systems are as accessible for diagnosis and treatment as is the large bowel. This accessibility places it at risk for unintended injury. Diagnostic and therapeutic procedures performed for colon and rectal disease can result in injury if they are performed improperly or if the tissues investigated are weakened by disease.

Injury from Operative Procedures

Intraoperative injury to the colon and rectum can occur during any procedure in the pelvis or abdomen because the colorectum extends into every quadrant. By proximity, gynecologic procedures can lead to colorectal injury. Perforation may occur during routine dilatation and curettage of the uterus, and the adjacent colorectum is vulnerable to puncture. More complicated procedures that are performed frequently, such as total abdominal hysterectomy and vaginal hysterectomy, also may result in colorectal injury or fistulization. During laparoscopic sterilization, electrocoagulation may be used, possibly leading to bowel injury; deaths associated with this procedure have been reported.[13] Intrauterine devices have been known to erode into the peritoneal cavity and subsequently into the colon, creating a localized septic inflammatory process.[14]

Anorectal injuries can result from simple anorectal surgery, including operations for hemorrhoids, fistulas, and fissure. Resulting complications may include anal stenosis, ectropion, or incontinence. Already there are several reports of leaks and sepsis following the new stapling procedures for hemorrhoids.[15,16,17,18] The surgical correction of these complications is specifically addressed in Chapters 6, 7, and 33.

Urologic surgery can cause colorectal trauma. Percutaneous nephrostomy is ordinarily a safe and reliable procedure for decompressing the urinary collecting system; however, LeRoy et al[19] reported on two perforations of the colon that occurred during nephrostomy. Perineal prostatectomy, suprapubic prostatectomy,

or transurethral resection of the prostate can be associated with injury of the adjacent rectum.[20,21]

During surgery in which electrocautery is used, explosions have occurred in the presence of combustible colonic gases, resulting in large perforations and deaths.[22,23] Both the hydrogen from a mannitol bowel preparation or unabsorbed carbohydrates and the methane sometimes naturally present within the colon are combustible.

Colorectal injury can occur with neurosurgical and orthopaedic operations. Inserting ventriculoperitoneal shunts in infants with hydrocephalus is a standard treatment to reduce intracerebral pressure, but on rare occasions the bowel has been perforated during placement of the peritoneal limb.[7,24,25] During internal fixation of a hip fracture, there have been instances of nails being too deep, causing injury to the rectum.[26]

Colorectal stents have been employed in obstruction secondary to carcinoma for either palliation or as a bridge to surgery. Khot et al[27] reviewed the literature and found 29 case series covering 598 stent insertion attempts. Perforation occurred in 22 (4%) cases.

Endoscopically Induced Trauma

Injury associated with endoscopic procedures is uncommon.[28] Proctosigmoidoscopic perforation usually occurs near the peritoneal reflection, and in most instances the tear is in diseased bowel, with a mortality rate greater than 25%. Perforation is also associated with biopsy or snare polypectomy and if it is below the 10-cm level from the anal verge infrequently causes serious complications. In other studies, the mortality rate was only 8% if operation for the perforation was performed within 6 hours, but if the delay between perforation and operation was greater than 12 hours, death ensued in 20% of cases.[29] The major complications of colonoscopy are hemorrhage and perforation,[30,31,32] which were discussed in Chapter 4.

Injury from Rectal Thermometer

Obtaining rectal temperature is a routine procedure. Rectal thermometers are well-known causes of perforation during the first few days of a newborn's life. In 1965, Fonkalsrud and Clatworthy[33] reported on 10 accidental perforations of the intestine in infants. The authors pointed out that the distance between the anus and the peritoneal cul-de-sac over the rectosigmoid in newborns is less than 3 cm and that half the perforations occur at this low level. Horwitz and Bennett[34] reported on an outbreak of peritonitis in a neonatal nursery that was caused by a nurse perforating the rectum with a thermometer while taking rectal temperatures (▶ Fig. 34.2).

Perforation by Therapeutic Enema

Even procedures such as giving a simple enema are subject to human error. Usually, perforation results from insertion of the enema tip by an unskilled or careless attendant or during self-insertion. A spectrum of anorectal injuries can occur during insertion of an enema tip.[35,36] Perforation from enemas can be classified into five types: (1) anal perforation, (2) submucosal perforation, (3) extraperitoneal perforation, (4) intraperitoneal perforation, and (5) perforation into adjacent organs. The majority of rectal perforations

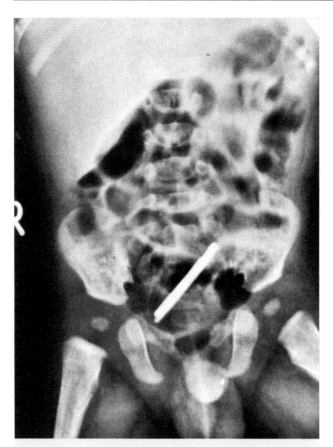

Fig. 34.2 Broken rectal thermometer in the rectosigmoid.

from enema tips are on the anterior wall. Extraperitoneal perforation can cause abscess, fistula, or severe hemorrhage. Gayer et al[37] reported 14 rectal perforations secondary to cleansing enemas. Abdominal pain and fever were the common symptoms. All had computed tomography (CT) with the findings of extraluminal air in the perianal and perirectal fat. No leak was seen on any CT. The CT was of help, because the physician did not suspect the etiology. Ten were subjected to surgery, but 5 died. The four who were treated conservatively all died.

Installation of the wrong liquid, such as scalding water, can cause severe burns; the wrong solution, such as formaldehyde instead of paraldehyde, can cause sloughing and rectal bleeding.

Injury from Barium Enema

A variety of complications have been associated with barium enema studies.[38] Two of the most serious of these complications are mechanical perforation of the bowel, either intraperitoneally or extraperitoneally by direct penetration of the enema tip, and overinflation of the rectal balloon, causing pneumatic rupture of the rectum.[39] Other complications include the formation of barium granulomas within the rectal wall, necrotizing proctitis, and barium embolism.

Kiser et al[40] reported that one perforation of the colon occurred in 1,250 barium enemas administered at the Ellis Fischell State Cancer Center in Columbia, Missouri. Most perforations are ruptures through ulcers, neoplasms, diverticula, hernias, inflammatory bowel disease, or other areas of disease. Rosenklint et al[41] reported on six extraperitoneal perforations that occurred from

barium extravasation during 20,000 barium enema examinations. Four of the six patients died, and the other two have permanent colostomies. None of the patients had disease in the colon or rectum. Obtaining tissue for a simple rectal biopsy weakens the bowel enough that a barium enema may complete a perforation. A 7-day wait allows sealing and helps protect against perforation. Biopsy specimens obtained through the rigid sigmoidoscope easily can be 5 mm in size; those taken through the colonoscope can be only 2 to 3 mm.[42] Thus, deeper biopsies afford greater risk to proceed to full-thickness perforation.

When small amounts of barium are injected submucosally, a simple barium granuloma results, which may be asymptomatic or cause pain. Sterile barium causes little inflammatory reaction when injected into the subcutaneous and retroperitoneal tissues, the wall of the rectum, or the peritoneal cavity. Several years later, it may present as isolated rectal nodules in a patient who has been asymptomatic.[43,44] Larger amounts of barium injected in the same manner can result in severe inflammatory reaction, abscess formation, or even necrotizing proctitis. Ultimately, retroperitoneal barium causes dense retroperitoneal fibrosis. Perforation above the peritoneal reflection results in intraperitoneal contamination by both barium and residual stool from the bowel. Even when perforation reaches into the free peritoneal cavity, the injury may not be suspected immediately because of the lack of symptoms suggesting that a free perforation has occurred. However, symptoms of peritoneal irritation occurring minutes or hours after the enema should be considered as possibly resulting from the barium enema study. During repeat abdominal radiograph, most of these cases show the presence of free air and/or evidence of barium outside the lumen of the bowel. Perforation also may be retroperitoneal.

Unlike the sometimes benign course of endoscopic biopsy perforation, the combination of barium and feces is a dreaded complication.[44,45,46,47] When barium is combined with significant bacterial contamination from the bowel, a massive, and often overwhelming, inflammatory response occurs. Sisel et al[48] experimented on rabbits, producing colonic rupture after a barium enema or an enema performed with a water-soluble contrast material. Without treatment, both types were uniformly fatal. Surgical repair of the rupture with concomitant peritoneal lavage resulted in only a 10% survival rate in animals with feces and barium contamination. Fifty percent of the animals with Gastrografin and feces contamination survived if surgery was performed promptly. Zheutlin et al[49] reported on a collected series of 53 patients in whom barium mixed with feces spilled into the peritoneal cavity. The mortality rate in this group was 51%. Nelson et al[50] reported a 100% mortality rate with this type of perforation. Based on these data, water-soluble contrast material is the preferred type for use in patients with suspected perforations, or suspected leaks in recent anastomoses.

Barium embolism is rare, but when it happens, a fatal outcome is likely. The pathophysiology begins with intravasation of barium into the veins of the rectum, resulting in pulmonary embolism and sudden death.[51] Not performing a barium enema on patients with acute inflammatory bowel disease or on patients who have had recent endoscopic procedures with biopsy or polypectomy will decrease the incidence of this rare occurrence.

A barium enema sometimes is used therapeutically to reduce intussusceptions in infants. Unfortunately, the hydrostatic force introduced into the colon perforated 6 of 1,000 colons in one series.[52]

Obstetric Trauma

Cephalopelvic disproportion and the stretching of local anatomy that takes place during childbirth result in trauma to some degree in almost every vaginal delivery.[53,54] A deep laceration may occur in the perineum after parturition that involves not only the vagina, but also the perineal body, the rectum, and the anal canal, including the anal sphincter mechanism. An episiotomy during delivery will decrease the tendency for third-degree lacerations involving the anal sphincter. If the episiotomy is performed in the posterior midline of the vagina, harm to the sphincteric mechanism is more likely than if it is directed laterally. The size of the infant, the flexibility of the pelvic tissues, the parity of the patient, the weight of the patient, the skill of the obstetrician, and the decision whether or not to use instrumentation are factors that influence incidence of anorectal trauma during childbirth.[54]

Precise repair of a third-degree tear is a necessary skill for those who practice obstetrics; a colorectal surgeon seldom is needed to repair such an injury on an emergency basis. Most repairs will heal uneventfully; however, if incontinence is a postdelivery problem, a secondary repair by sphincteroplasty is indicated. See Chapter 14 for details of repair.

Rectovaginal fistulas may also result from difficult parturition, and laceration. Pressure necrosis of the rectovaginal wall, forceps delivery, and midline episiotomies are often associated factors. See Chapter 15 for repair details.

Irradiation-Induced Proctitis

Irradiation of neoplasms of the pelvis may cause both immediate and delayed complications. Irradiation proctitis is an anticipated sequela after radiation of common neoplasms that originate from the uterus, ovary, bladder, prostate, anus, or rectum. Quan[55] reviewed 65 patients who underwent irradiation therapy for pelvic malignancy, 52 of whom had carcinoma of the cervix. Often, radiation damages both the bladder and the intestine simultaneously. The acute findings are edema, inflammation, erythema, and friability of the rectal mucosa, which may progress to ulceration or necrosis.[56] As the rectum heals, granulation tissue, fibrosis, and telangiectasia may result. Full rectal wall necrosis may develop, and in women a rectovaginal fistula may occur if necrosis is severe anteriorly. The radiation injury site may form a stricture as part of the healing phase. Microscopic examination of these tissues reveals underlying irradiation-induced endarteritis leading to tissue hypoxia, resulting in the above sequence of macroscopic events. Likewise, lymphatic channels are destroyed.

The onset of symptoms after radiotherapy varies from immediately to years after treatment, with rectal bleeding as the most common symptom. The anterior rectal wall usually demonstrates the most severe radiation-induced changes. The extent of damage depends on the size of the area treated, the total dose delivered, overall treatment time, and fractionation of the dosage. Individual techniques affect the outcome as well.

Mild proctitis usually requires no treatment. Sherman et al[57] reported good results from using corticosteroid enemas in the management of patients with acute and chronic irradiation proctitis. Henriksson et al[58] performed a double-blind, placebo-controlled trial using oral sucralfate, an aluminum hydroxide complex of sulfonated sucrose, for 2 weeks after onset of radiation and continued for 6 weeks. Bowel movements were significantly improved with treatment and fewer patients required antidiarrheal medications. Colonic obstruction caused by irradiation colitis or proctitis is rare, but if such complications do occur, colostomy is indicated.[59] When bleeding becomes incessant oozing from the injured surface, the laser, the argon plasma coagulator, or topical formalin have been effectively used over the entire surface to stop the hemorrhage.[60,61,62]

van Nagell et al[63] reported on rectal injury in a series of patients with uterine carcinoma requiring irradiation. An increasing incidence of proctitis was noted in patients who had preexisting hypertensive vascular disease or diabetes mellitus. No rectal injuries occurred when the total dose to the rectum was less than 4,000 rad. The authors also stressed that severe proctitis often preceded bladder or other bowel complications. Fractionation of the remaining irradiation dosage over longer periods of time prevented much of the later irradiation changes. A 2-week rest period in the middle of the treatment course using topical steroids and cleansing enemas lessened acute injury symptoms.

34.2.4 Ingested Foreign Bodies

Perforation of the gastrointestinal tract from ingestion of foreign bodies is rare. Natural foods, such as pits, thorns, seeds, or soft bones, undergo significant digestion by the time they reach the colon. However, hard particulate matter, such as chicken and other animal bones, toothpicks, portions of glass, shells, or other sharp objects, may pass through the intestinal tract into the colon and cause injury to the rectum and anus. Infants, children, and mentally deranged adults are at higher risk because of objects they may put in their mouths and subsequently swallow. Of course, anyone could inadvertently swallow an object that enters the mouth; parts of dentures sometimes break off and are swallowed. To prevent such injuries, potentially dangerous objects should be kept out of the reach of infants, children, and mentally incompetent adults.

The complications secondary to ingested foreign bodies include perforation, hemorrhage, abscess formation, bowel obstruction, and death.[64,65] Less than 1% of foreign bodies that become entrapped cause perforation. Observation and expeditious gastrointestinal endoscopy are the two best forms of therapy. The physician must decide if it is preferable to watch the foreign body pass spontaneously or to perform endoscopic removal within 1 or 2 hours of ingestion. Surgical intervention is required for the 1% of patients who experience perforation or obstruction because of these objects. Seventy-five percent of gastrointestinal perforations occur at the ileocecal valve and the appendix. Sequential abdominal roentgenograms show that most objects exit the gastrointestinal tract within 1 week. Failure of the foreign body to exit is another indication for surgery. Close observation for the development of the rare complication is a safe approach. Early endoscopic removal of selected easily reached objects may be an acceptable approach.

Illegal drug traffic has led drug dealers to develop multiple ways to import their product secretly. A health hazard is created if a packet of a pure narcotic is placed into a body orifice (▶ Fig. 34.3). If swallowed, large packets of the drug may obstruct the gastrointestinal tract. During the attempt to remove

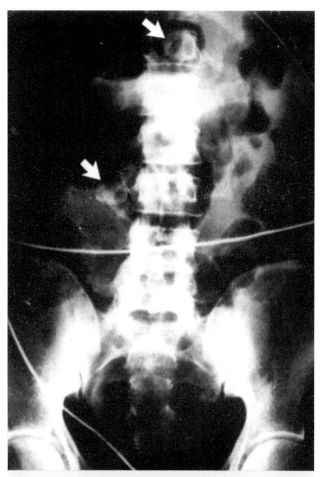

Fig. 34.3 Ingested packets of narcotic (*arrows*). These are associated with local bowel obstruction, often at the ileocecal value. Rupture of a packet results in a drug overdose.

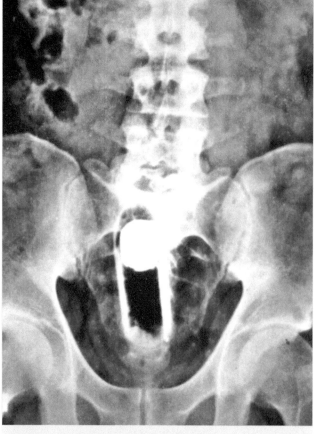

Fig. 34.4 Vibrator lodged in the rectosigmoid. Objects such as this are pushed into the anus and cannot be retrieved.

them endoscopically or surgically, special care should be exercised to avoid rupturing the packets because if they open in the gut, the patient may suffer overdose.

34.2.5 Foreign Bodies and Sexual Trauma

An amazing variety of objects have been inserted into the rectum and have become entrapped above the anal sphincter musculature. Practically any object that can be contemplated as fitting into the rectum has been used for sexual stimulation. Some of the more "fashionable" rectal foreign bodies include vibrators, plastic phalluses, cucumbers, baby powder cans, balls, bottles of all shapes and sizes, glasses, flashlight batteries, flashlights, test tubes, screwdrivers, ballpoint pens, paperweights, and thermometers (▶ Fig. 34.4). The entrapment of the object causes the patient not only social embarrassment, but also significant physical pain.

Serious injuries to the rectum, rectosigmoid, and other intraperitoneal structures can occur. Death resulting from placement of foreign bodies in the rectum has been reported by numerous authors.[66,67,68,69,70] Eftaiha et al[69] found it useful to classify the level of entrapment of the foreign body. Most objects lying in

the rectum at the low or middle level (up to 10 cm) can be removed transanally, but celiotomy may be needed to remove objects that become lodged in the upper rectum or lower sigmoid.

Sohn et al,[70] Beall and DeBakey,[71] and Barone et al[67] have reported independently on rectosigmoid perforation caused by insertion of foreign bodies. Such injury may be incurred by the patient in an attempt at autoeroticism or may be delivered by a sexual partner or during a criminal assault. Splitting of the rectosigmoid results in peritoneal contamination and peritonitis. Presenting with an acute abdomen, the patient may hide the history of sexual or assaultive action. Plain radiographs should be part of the emergency evaluation when such injuries are reported or suspected. Anteroposterior and lateral abdominal and pelvic views should be used to determine the type, number, and location of the foreign bodies; however, radiolucent objects may not be visualized.

34.2.6 Sexual Assault

Sexual assault is a common violent crime. Over 300,000 adults over the age of 12 years report being assaulted each year.[72] The assault may be criminal and intended to harm, or it may be the result of a vigorous sexual act that was intended to be enjoyed by both partners. Whatever the motive, sexual assault can cause significant injury to the extraperitoneal or intraperitoneal rectum or rectosigmoid.

Sohn et al[70] reported on an act termed "fist fornication" or "fisting" in 11 patients over a 4-year interval. Fist fornicators force a closed clenched fist through the intact anus into the rectum for sexual gratification. The rectum or sigmoid colon was the site of injury. Six patients had mucosal lacerations in the rectum that bled, but no sphincteric laceration was noted. Only simple suturing of the mucosal laceration was necessary for these patients. Four patients developed an acute abdomen requiring celiotomy, resection, and a Hartmann pouch. One patient had complete anal sphincteric incontinence from severe sphincteric laceration.

34.2.7 Child Abuse

Anorectal trauma in children is rare, but when found, it is usually due to abuse.[73] Sexually abused boys experience anorectal trauma in 7 to 16% of cases of this type of abuse, and they are abused at a younger age than girls. Anal sexual acts account for injury in 54.5% of abused boys. Only 3.7% of abused girls suffer anal injury.[74]

Black et al[74] reported on 617 rape victims. Twenty-four percent were younger than 16 years, and 33% had anal trauma. The medical community must be alert to recognize these criminal acts and report them to prevent more physical and emotional morbidity to the child and his or her siblings.[75] The examiner should keep accurate records as legal evidence, and a one-on-one interview should take place.

Signs of trauma around the anus or elsewhere on the body should be noted. Anal trauma may be the only visible trauma site because no resistance is offered if the assailant is known to the victim. Sperm and acid phosphatase should be sought in any material retrieved.[76] Venereal disease testing should be performed if the circumstances make the physician suspicious.

Sedation may be necessary to perform an anal or rectal examination if there is pain or great distress. Obtaining abdominal films to look for free air is warranted if the abdomen is tender.

34.2.8 Unusual Perforations

Hard impacted stool sometimes perforates the rectum, or the rectosigmoid colon by ischemic necrosis, a condition termed "stercoral perforation." The blood supply to a site in the colorectum is impaired by pressure of the hard bolus of stool pressed against an unyielding organ.[77,78]

Rarely, spontaneous perforation will occur in the rectosigmoid or cecum from either distention or spasm. The possibility of perforation is well recognized in preexisting disease such as inflammatory bowel disease, diverticulitis, or carcinoma, but sometimes spontaneous perforation occurs in the absence of pathologic disease.[79]

Cain et al[80] reported on five bizarre cases of trauma resulting from children sitting on a swimming pool drain. Suction caused perforation of the rectosigmoid, followed by small bowel evisceration and loss of much small bowel.

Electrocution may immediately or subsequently perforate the bowel but most often the colon. If celiotomy is performed as part of therapy, careful exploration for burned bowel is mandatory.[81] During sexual antics, people have directed compressed

air toward and into the anus so that a hole is blown in the proximal colon.[82] Thermal injury of the gastrointestinal tract is rare, but there has been a report of instillation of hot water into a stoma, causing a mucosal burn that subsequently formed a stenosis.[83] Improper insertion of a stomal irrigation tube or forceful insertion of a catheter to empty a continent reservoir pouch (Kock's pouch) may cause perforation, which may be unrecognized initially since little or no pain may occur. The design of cone tips for ostomy irrigation prevents deep insertion and bowel injury.

34.3 Management

Progress continues in the management of the traumatized patient. The Advanced Trauma Life Support (ATLS) courses promote a systematic approach, which is divided into four phases: primary survey, resuscitation, secondary survey, and definitive care (▶ Table 34.2).[84] These principles can be applied to both the military combat situation and civilian trauma.

The primary survey comprises rapid clinical diagnosis of life-threatening conditions such as an occluded airway, inadequate respirations, cardiac failure, arrhythmias, and hemorrhage. The resuscitation phase involves using procedures immediately to save lives. Chest tube placement, pericardiocentesis, intubation of the airway, control of obvious severe hemorrhage, and placement of lines must be performed without delay before time-consuming laboratory examinations are begun.

During the secondary survey, the colorectal injuries are identified, leading to the final phase, definitive care. These two phases are dealt with in depth in the following sections. Without the secondary survey, more subtle perineal and rectal wounds may be overlooked, and delay in diagnosis and late treatment lead to increased morbidity and mortality.[85]

34.3.1 Diagnosis of Trauma (Secondary Survey Phase)

History

An alert and cooperative patient may be questioned about the circumstances of the trauma. However, the patient with a head injury or multiple trauma may be unable to communicate. At times, the trauma is obvious, but a history from someone at the scene (if available) may prove helpful. The observer—a paramedic, ambulance driver, litter bearer, helicopter pilot, corpsman,

Table 34.2 Phases of management in trauma

Phase	Action	Pertinence of colorectal injury
1	Primary survey: diagnosis of life-threatening conditions	
2	Resuscitation	
3	Secondary survey: diagnosis of trauma	Diagnosis of colorectal injury
4	Definitive care	Surgery to repair colorectal injury

or a relative—may be able to relate important details of the trauma, specifically the type of trauma, the wounding agent, and the interval of time that has elapsed. For example, knowing whether the injury was caused by an ice pick or a bayonet, a low-velocity 22-caliber pistol or a high-velocity M16 rifle, a fall from 5 or 50 feet, or a fall from a golf cart or a motorcycle traveling at high speed, or whether it occurred 20 minutes or 20 hours previously would aid in making the decisions about appropriate diagnostic tests and the extent of treatment.

Patients with isolated anorectal trauma may complain of perineal, anorectal, or abdominal pain. Usually pain begins precisely at the time of injury. Less often, the pain may be delayed in a patient with small extraperitoneal perforations of the rectum or after a foreign body cannot be removed from the rectum. Dull lower abdominal pain may be the only manifestation of an upper rectal or rectosigmoid tear with perforation. Rectal bleeding denotes rectal trauma, and its presence warrants a thorough examination.[67,69,86] Wounds of the colon and rectum may be lethal if not recognized promptly. The patient who is hemodynamically stable may deteriorate 1 or 2 days later if sepsis results from an overlooked rectal or colonic injury, which may be recognized only when such a patient becomes septic and hypotensive. Crepitus and soft-tissue manifestations may denote gas gangrene. When sepsis is not recognized until it is in its late stages, patient survival is less likely.

Physical Examination

During resuscitation, a nasogastric tube and transurethral catheter are inserted as part of the "place a tube in every orifice" dictum. Blood in the nasogastric aspirate directs the examiner to look for intra-abdominal injury. Blood in the urine calls attention to the retroperitoneum and the pelvis. The bladder may be penetrated via the rectum in patients with impalement or other penetrating injuries, so examination of the urine is imperative.[87] In the patient with multiple trauma, anorectal and other pelvic organ injuries may be overlooked because of preoccupation of the resuscitation team with cranial and thoracic injury or massive hemorrhage. Thus, looking at the back and perineum should be part of the routine assessment. Furthermore, a wound below the nipple line on the chest or just below the scapular tips represents abdominal entry in 15% of stab wounds and 50% of gunshot wounds.[88] Abdominal injury is considered with any thoracoabdominal penetration. This area extends from the nipples to the inguinal ligaments and from the scapular tips to the buttocks.

Multiple trauma from high-speed vehicle injuries or major blunt injuries on the battleground is a prime example of a situation in which less obvious wounds may be overlooked. A conscious patient can indicate whether or not abdominal pain is present. Thorough examination includes inspection of the abdominal wall and palpation for crepitus and hematoma formation. In a patient with penetrating trauma, both the entry and exit wounds should be sought. The surmised track of the penetration provides clues as to organs that may be injured and directs the exploration at laparotomy.

Anal examination can be performed with the patient in the supine or lateral position. It should be noted whether the anus is in its normal position, for blunt trauma sometimes detaches it from muscular sling.[89] Even with no observable evidence of

perineal trauma, a digital examination should be performed in the usual fashion. In a series by Mangiante et al,[90] blood was evident on rectal examination in 80% of patients with rectal gunshot wounds. A loose sphincteric tone might suggest a central nervous system injury. Specifically, in patients with blunt trauma the levator attachments should be palpated to verify that they are intact. Hematoma may create bogginess around the prostate, or the prostate may be dislocated by severe blunt trauma. In female patients, a vaginal examination should be performed to be certain that the injury does not involve the genital tract. If rectal injury is suspected because bright red blood is present, anoscopy and sigmoidoscopy should be performed to attempt visualization of the lower part of the rectum and anal canal. Positioning of the multiply traumatized patient is difficult, but before operation it is necessary to know whether and where the rectum is injured. Irrigation and suction may allow clearance of stool and blood to at least the peritoneal reflection level (15 cm). The injured site can be specifically identified in 91% of rectal injuries.[84] The insufflation of large volumes of air should be avoided when the rectum is filled with blood, because stool and contaminated blood can be forced into the peritoneal cavity or extraperitoneal soft tissues if a perforation is present.

Pelvic and rectal trauma also should direct the examiner to evaluate for neurologic integrity. The sciatic nerve is at risk, and appropriate neurologic assessment should be performed. Impotence may be a neurologic sequela of pelvic trauma that is not noted until later.[4]

Radiologic Study

Flat and upright abdominal films and lateral films of the pelvis usually are helpful. They aid in defining the location and trajectory of a bullet. Visualization of free intraperitoneal air, extraperitoneal or extrarectal soft-tissue densities, or extraluminal gas shadows may point to colonic or rectal injury. Diastasis of the symphysis pubis or pelvic fracture often is associated with injury to the rectum or other pelvic organs.[85]

If the patient's condition permits and the clinical suspicion so indicates, diagnostic contrast studies can be performed; however, they are not performed if the patient has an acute abdomen and operative intervention is planned. Use of water-soluble substances such as diatrizoate sodium (e.g., Gastrografin or Hypaque) is preferred over the use of barium. The radiologist, aware of the possibilities of colorectal injury, should instill the contrast material carefully during the fluoroscopic examination and should stop immediately at the first sign of bowel perforation.

Computed Tomography and Sonography

CT scans are currently readily available and rapid. They have become the diagnostic procedure of choice in stable patients. They are highly sensitive in the nonoperative diagnosis of solid organ injury. Very small volumes of free air are detectable, suggesting a hollow viscous injury. Fluid collections in the absence of solid organ injury may mean hollow organ injury. Given time, a triple contrast CT, using oral, intravenous, and rectal contrast may be performed. This gives some evaluation of retroperitoneal portions of the colon. Accuracy of CT in the detection of blunt bowel and mesenteric injuries has been reported as 80% for sensitivity and 78% for specificity.[91]

These special studies are also of particular value in the evaluation of patients who are delayed in presentation.[92] Septic sites in both the pelvis and abdomen, such as pelvic or ischioanal abscesses, may be identified by either CT or ultrasonography. Furthermore, percutaneous drainage of fluid collections can be guided by CT or ultrasound.

Ultrasound in the form of focused assessment with sonography for trauma (FAST) has been adopted by the ATLS protocol.[93] A positive FAST examination (hemoperitoneum) is useful and reliable in the hemodynamically unstable blunt trauma patient. However, if the FAST examination is negative or equivocal, it should be followed by a diagnostic peritoneal lavage (DPL). A FAST examination is hampered by subcutaneous or intra-abdominal air, obesity, and pelvic fractures. It is also operator dependent.

Peritoneal Lavage

DPL can be used to evaluate both blunt and penetrating abdominal trauma in patients who are hemodynamically unstable or who require urgent surgical intervention for associated extra-abdominal injuries. DPL can rapidly confirm or exclude the presence of intraperitoneal hemorrhage. Thus, the patient with a closed head injury, the unstable patient who has been in a motor vehicle accident, or the patient with a pelvic fracture and potential retroperitoneal hemorrhage can be appropriately triaged to emergency laparotomy.

Laparoscopy

Minimally invasive techniques should be more specific as compared to peritoneal lavage. Presuming a trajectory directs where to look for wounds, laparoscopy often gives a definitive diagnosis. Injury to the flank is problematic and may give a tangential trajectory, not entering the peritoneal cavity. Diagnostic laparoscopy may spare the victim a laparotomy. The same dilemma is created by a back wound. Thus, laparoscopy may permit a look at the retroperitoneum as well as the intraperitoneum.

Laparoscopy is a valuable diagnostic technique when assessing stab wounds. Because two-thirds of stab wounds do not result in intra-abdominal injury, a stepwise approach is taken. A means of determining entry into the abdomen is exploration of the wound tract under local anesthesia. If penetration of the fascia is recognized, further examination by laparoscopy is useful. If the peritoneum is entered, laparotomy is then needed.

34.3.2 Surgical Treatment (Definitive Care Phase)

A spectrum of treatments exists for traumatic wounds that involve the colon, rectum, and anus. The most important factors in determining treatment for penetrating injuries are the following:

- The general physical condition of the patient.
- The mechanism by which the injury was incurred.
- The interval between the injury and operative intervention.
- The presence of shock or hemodynamic instability.

- The presence of peritoneal contamination.
- Any injury or avulsion of the mesentery of the colon or rectum.
- The presence of multiple organ injury.

The difference in the mortality rates of war and civilian trauma series is based on the velocity of the missiles, the extent of contamination after injury to the colon, the interval between the injury and definitive care, and the early use of antibiotics. In a series of war injuries, Dent and Jena[94] reported that two factors resulted in increased mortality: high-velocity bullets and colonic injury. The mortality rate with high-velocity wounds of the colon was 52%, yet the mortality rate from all other penetrating wounds was only 6%.

An isolated colonic injury occurs in approximately 25% of penetrating wounds. Both the morbidity and mortality rates of colonic injuries are directly related to the number of other organs traumatized. Two-thirds of the deaths in patients who have colorectal trauma are due to injury to other organs in the body. The other organs most frequently injured are the small intestine, liver, stomach, lung, and bladder.[95]

Intraperitoneal Rectal and Colonic Injury

Penetrating trauma usually demands exploration.[96] Gunshot wounds of the anterior abdomen enter the peritoneal cavity 85% of the time and after entry strike an important structure 95% of the time. On the other hand, stab wounds enter the peritoneal cavity only 66% of the time, and of this number serious injury occurs in less than 50%.[97] Thus, only a quarter of the time may a celiotomy be required for a stab wound of the abdomen. Yet once the peritoneal cavity has been soiled, an acute abdomen will ensue. Exploratory laparotomy for repair of the injury to the intraperitoneal rectum or colon is necessary.

Preoperative broad-spectrum antibiotics for both anaerobic and aerobic flora should be given early after the injury.[98,99,100,101,102,103] Broad-spectrum single-drug agents that are effective include cefotetan, cefoxitin, and ampicillin/sulbactam.

The conduct of the operation is the same whether the patient is in a war zone or in a civilian institution. The patient should be positioned in stirrups especially if there is a question about rectal or other pelvic injury. The ability to perform endoscopy on the operating table with the abdomen open should always be available. The operation is performed through a midline incision that may be extended to the xiphoid or the symphysis pubis to gain better access to the injured organs. First stopping hemorrhage to aid in resuscitation is accomplished and hemodynamic stability is established. Then contamination from an open intestine must be controlled. Noncrushing bowel clamps isolate the open wound. Holes are closed quickly with running sutures or staples to stop contamination. Thereafter, complete exploration identifies all injuries before repair of any one is undertaken. The "rule of two" applies when following a bullet track. Both an entry wound and an exit wound should be found in each organ. If an odd number of holes are found, either a tangential wound occurred or the bullet is still located in the organ. The surgeon must be convinced that no hole has been missed. Hematoma around the colon and retroperitoneal air require exposure of the retroperitoneal colon. The missile may be left in place unless the colon is traversed. A feces-contaminated bullet may act as a nidus for subsequent infections.[104] The wound and the abdominal cavity should be irrigated liberally to remove spillage from the colon. The entry and exit wounds should be debrided.

Mature judgment and a disciplined approach allow the patient to be placed in the proper treatment group. Better categorization of colonic injury has been attempted by Flint et al,[105] who recommend a three-level grading system. Grade 1 is an isolated colonic injury with minimal contamination, no shock, and minimal delay. Grade 2 includes through-and-through perforations and lacerations with moderate contamination. Grade 3 comprises severe tissue loss, devascularization, and heavy contamination.

Another method to quantitate severity of injury, a scale called the Penetrating Abdominal Trauma Index (PATI), has been created by Moore et al.[106] The organ injury is estimated on a scale from 1 to 5: 1, minimal; 2, minor; 3, moderate; 4, major; and 5, maximal. In addition to this general PATI scale, a colon injury scale (CIS) was devised: grade 1, serosal injury; grade 2, single wall injury; grade 3, less than 25% wall involvement; grade 4, greater than 25% wall involvement; and grade 5, whole colonic wall involvement and blood supply injury. The authors plan their surgical management based on the score of injury. Grades 1 to 3 may be eligible for primary repair. New statistical models to accurately predict mortality from trauma have been devised. The newest is a physiologic trauma score, which is easily calculable at bedside, used along with other commonly used indices.[107]

In the civilian population, penetrating trauma of the colorectum occurs frequently from a low-velocity weapon, the interval from injury to treatment is short, and only the colon or rectum is perforated by a small single bullet. Such an injury is often ideal for primary closure (▶ Fig. 34.5).[83,108] The wound can be debrided and blood supply assured. Primary repair can be running or interrupted sutures, single or double layer, but the standard requirements are that the closure is watertight, there is no tension on the anastomosis, and the blood supply is intact.

Although the literature supports primary repair in most colon injuries, unfavorable cases must be recognized and primary repair avoided. Relative contraindications to the use of primary closure without colostomy are the following: (1) delay in operation associated with spreading peritonitis, (2) high-velocity bullet wounds, (3) explosive or shotgun injuries with shattering wounds of the colon and rectum, (4) tissue destruction with extensive intramural hematomas or mesenteric vascular damage, and (5) multiple organ injury.[109] Stone and Fabian[110] defined the criteria for obligatory colostomy formation. The patients who did not meet the criteria for exclusion were randomized to primary closure alone (▶ Fig. 34.5) or primary closure plus colostomy or ileostomy (▶ Fig. 34.6). In the final analysis, the complication and mortality rates were comparable. ▶ Table 34.3 presents a composite list of criteria for ostomy formation.[109,110,111]

Some differences between war injuries and civilian injuries must be emphasized. In battle, special conditions are to be expected. Multiple casualties may be admitted almost simultaneously; delays in operation occur because of triage priorities; follow-up is seldom performed by the same physician; transportation from the war zone as soon as the patient is stabilized is imperative; and stops while in transit, especially if an ocean must be crossed, are almost a certainty. After World War II, some authors advocated primary closure of colonic wounds without fecal diversion, but the mortality rates with this method exceeded 20%.[71,112,113,114,115] Thus, results dictated that primary closure of colorectal injuries alone is not safe. In general, wounds must be resected with ostomy creation, exteriorized, or, if that is not possible, protected by diversion (▶ Fig. 34.6 and ▶ Fig. 34.7). The evidence to support this policy is based on reports from war zones in the past.[6,116,117,118,119] The dictum of colostomy applied to war wounds has carried over to civilian wounds, even though there has been a safe record for primary repair in properly selected colon injuries.

Controversy still exists as to whether colon injuries require a colostomy or whether primary repair is preferable. Many retrospective and some prospective studies have shown a trend toward favoring primary repair. These studies have been faulted by inherent biases in the trial designs. Six prospective randomized trials have been conducted to answer this question. These are listed in ▶ Table 34.4.

Stone and Fabian,[126] in the first of the prospective randomized trials, decided on six conditions that were necessary to be included: (1) shock never less than 80 mmHg, (2) blood loss less than 1,000 cm³, (3) no more than two intra-abdominal organs injured, (4) no significant fecal soilage, (5) less than 8 hour delay to operation, and (6) an extent of injury to the colon or abdominal wall that did not require a resection of the structure. Forty-eight percent of patients were thus excluded.

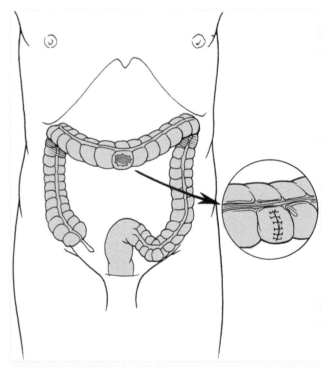

Fig. 34.5 Primary repair.

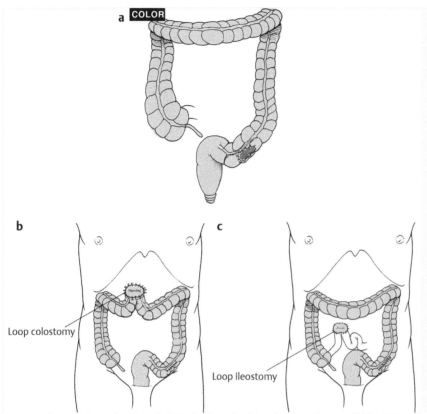

Fig. 34.6 Primary repair with proximal diversions. **(a)** Sigmoid colon wound. **(b)** Primary repair with loop colostomy. **(c)** Primary repair with loop ileostomy.

Table 34.3 Criteria for use of an ostomy

Injuring agent factors

High-velocity bullet wounds

Shotgun wounds

Explosive blast wounds

Crush injury

Patient factors

Presence of tumor

Radiated tissue

Medical condition

Advanced age

Injury factors

Inflamed tissue

Advanced infection

Distal obstruction

Local foreign body

Impaired blood supply

Mesenteric vascular damage

Shock with blood pressure < 80/60 mm Hg

Hemorrhage > 1,000 mL

More than two organs injured (especially kidney, pancreas, spleen, and liver)

Interval to operation > 12 h

Extensive injury requiring resection

Major abdominal wall loss

Thoracoabdominal penetration

No selective criteria were part of the experimental design by Chappuis et al.[127] Their incidence of complications was not increased by primary repair. Unfortunately, the study size (56 patients) was small. The prospective randomized study by Falcone et al[128] had exclusion criteria of no delay greater than 8 hours and patients not deemed admissible by the surgeons. Again the number of patients enrolled in the study, only 22 patients, was a very small sample. In a trial reported in 1995 by Sasaki et al,[129] 71 patients were randomized, with 60% receiving primary repair. The authors' analysis of multiple factors showed only one factor, the PATI score, which correlated with complications. A PATI score of greater than 25 meant morbidity. Those patients with PATI scores greater than 25 had a 33% complication rate after primary repair and 93% after diversion. There were only 7 stab wounds and 2 shotgun injuries as opposed to 62 gunshot wounds. Thus, the mechanism of injury was not delineated with regard to stab and shotgun wounds.

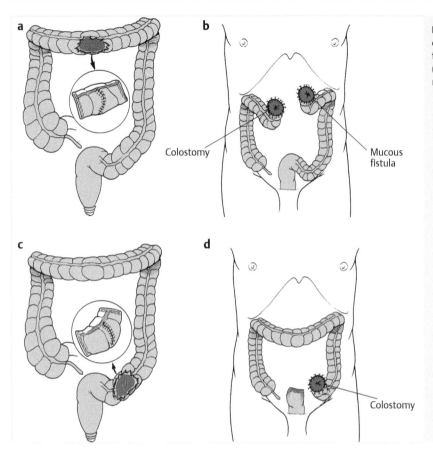

Fig. 34.7 (a) Transverse colon wound with excision, **(b)** followed by colostomy and mucous fistula. **(c)** Sigmoid colon wound with excision, **(d)** followed by sigmoid colostomy and Hartmann's closure.

Colostomy

Mucous fistula

Colostomy

Table 34.4 Prospective randomized trials of primary repair versus colostomy

Authors	Year	No. of patients	Primary repair no (%)	Diverting ostomy no (%)	Morbidity primary repair (%)	Morbidity ostomy (%)	Mortality primary repair (%)	Mortality ostomy (%)
Stone and Fabian[110]	1979	139	67 (48)	72 (52)	43 (64)	71 (99)	1 (2)	1 (1)
Chappuis et al[127]	1991	56	28 (50)	28 (50)	10 (20)	18 (64)	0	0
Falcone et al[128]	1992	22	11 (50)	11 (50)	8 (73)	10 (91)	1 (9)	0
Sasaki et al[129]	1995	71	43 (60)	28 (40)	9 (21)	24 (86)	0	0
Gonzalez et al[130]	2000	181	92 (51)	89 (49)	21 (23)	21 (24)	5 (5)	3 (3)
Kamwendo et al[131]	2003	240	120 (50)	120 (50)	31(26)	22 (18)	0	2 (1.7)

The authors' study group was young, so advanced age must be investigated. Because the authors' patients were all operated on within 90 minutes, the problem of delay in surgery was not a factor in this study. Of special note in this study is that the extent of colon injury did not predict outcome.

Gonzalez et al[130] published a trial in 2000 with 181 patients. Their randomization was independent of severity of colon injury, presence of hypotension, blood loss, extent of fecal contamination, and the time from injury to operation. An area of controversy in this study is the removal of five patients initially entered, but who died in less than 24 hours of other causes. The PATI score for the diversion group was 22.7 and that for the primary group was 23.7. Septic complications were 18 (21%) in the diversion group and 16 (18%) in the primary repair group. Their conclusion was that all penetrating colon injuries should be managed by primary repair.

Kamwendo et al[131] studied 240 patients in South Africa with half randomized to primary repair. The results were stratified by length of time from injury to surgery (greater or less than 12 hours). Significant differences were not found between groups for rates of sepsis, wound complications, or mortality.

Singer and Nelson[132] performed systematic review of six randomized trials found in ► Table 34.4. The total patients were 709 with 361 randomized to the primary closure group and 348 randomized to the fecal diversion group. The outcomes evaluated were mortality, total complications, infectious complications, intra-abdominal infections, wound complications, penetrating abdominal trauma index, and length of stay. The mortality in both the primary anastomosis group and the diverted group was the same. However, all other complication groups showed primary anastomosis to be superior, including the septic complications of intra-abdominal wound infection,

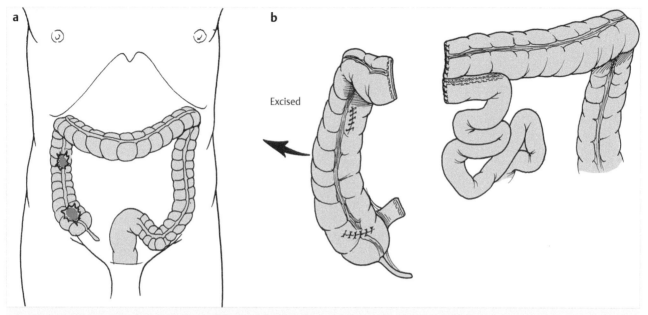

Fig. 34.8 **(a)** Two wounds in the right colon. **(b)** Resection of right colon with functional end-to-end anastomosis.

dehiscence, generalized sepsis, and peristomal abscess. Thus, they conclude that primary anastomosis is arguably the choice in all penetrating abdominal trauma. More recently, Fealk et al[125] came to the same conclusion. They believe that the emerging dictum for traumatic colon injuries is primary repair. Questions remain as to whether primary repair is the safest option for all colon injuries. The PATI score, CIS grade, and multiple other factors should be included in the decision-making algorithm with an emphasis on primary repair.

Primary resection has the most value when there is a large hole or an area in which several holes in the colon are adjacent and lend themselves to excision in a short segment (▶ Fig. 34.8). The open ends are anastomosed only if the patient otherwise meets the criteria for a primary repair. Drains are not used because they do not prevent infections and, if placed near an anastomosis, promote leaks. Stewart et al[133] reported a 14% leak rate after primary resection and anastomosis in 60 patients with destructive colon wounds. The key factors in their review were the presence of underlying medical illness or massive blood transfusion. The leak rate in patients who had one or more of these factors was 42%. The results of ileocolostomy were just as bad as those of colocolostomy. The authors' criteria for primary repair or primary anastomosis are not based on the site of injury in the colon but rather on the criteria set forth in ▶ Table 34.3.

The exteriorized repair is out of favor with most trauma surgeons and is mentioned for historic interest.[134,135] Iatrogenic injuries, such as those associated with colonoscopy, often can be closed primarily.[136,137] However, the criteria in ▶ Table 34.3 apply to the management decisions.

War Injured

In civilian literature, there is a low rate of suture line leaks of primary repair or resection and primary anastomosis (2–7%).[138,139] However, 16 to 30% of patients from the Iraq and Afghanistan wars initially managed with primary repair or anastomosis experienced leaks, which required fecal diversion.[140,141] Independent

risk factors for anastomotic failures included hypotension, hemodynamic instability, advanced age, high abdominal trauma index, more than 4 units RBC in the first 24 hours, abdominal compartment syndrome, prolonged ICU stay, and a higher number of suture lines.[142]

Technical Variations

Colonic anastomosis can be accomplished by a hand-sewn or a stapled anastomosis. The two methods are equivalent in elective colon resections. In trauma patients, the evidence is less compelling, but a 2001 prospective multicenter trial found no difference in complication rates from stapled (26.6%) and hand-sewn anastomosis (20.3%).[143]

Antibiotic therapy should adequately cover aerobes and anaerobes. A single broad-spectrum antibiotic should cover non-destructive colon injuries; however, combinations such as ampicillin/sulbactam are favored for destructive colon injuries. Strong class 1 evidence has shown that the duration of antibiotics should be 24 hours or less.[138]

The fascia of the incision should be closed with a monofilament suture. The skin and subcutaneous tissue are left open if fecal contamination is present, and secondary closure may be effected in 5 to 6 days if the patient is doing well. Modern management of wounds including negative pressure dressings has significantly reduced morbidity and improved outcomes.[138]

The primary complication of colonic surgery for trauma is sepsis. Leak of any repair or anastomosis, intra-abdominal abscess, fistula formation, and wound infection must be managed by proper drainage. Diversion of the fecal stream is warranted in patients with anastomotic leaks.

Damage Control

In an attempt to reduce overall morbidity and mortality, the techniques of damage control surgery have been routinely incorporated into the care of the multiply injured patients.[138] Using this technique, surgeons delay definitive reconstruction in the unstable, hypothermic, and coagulopathic patient, with the main primary surgical focus being on stopping hemorrhage and controlling enteric contamination.[144] The overarching goal of damage control surgery is to avoid or rapidly correct the lethal triad of hypothermia, coagulopathy, and acidosis. After accomplishing the initial objectives, the patient can be warmed, fully resuscitated, and stabilized in the ICU prior to proceeding with a definitive surgical procedure over the next 12 to 48 hours. This application of damage control surgery has expanded to the patient with colon and rectal pathology in both the elective setting and following trauma.[145] Following stabilization, operative re-evaluation can then take into account all the other factors that typically weigh into this decision of management strategy, as well as the condition of the bowel following what may have been a massive volume resuscitation. Most patients can undergo anastomosis within 12 to 48 hours after the initial damage control procedure. However, patients unsuitable for anastomosis should likely undergo fecal control with a diverting stoma.[146]

Extraperitoneal Rectal Injury

If the injury to the rectum is partial thickness or a hematoma is found without mucosal injury, no treatment is required. With a small full-thickness perforation in a relatively clean bowel, such as in one prepared for polypectomy, the defect can be closed primarily and the patient placed on antibiotics. Even with penetrating injuries with minimal contamination, Levine et al[147] primarily repaired five rectal injuries by transanal approach. Two were the result of gunshot, two from prostate biopsy, and one from a foreign object. These five were carefully selected from a total of 30 such injuries. In cases of significant soft-tissue injury or pelvic fracture, thorough debridement of devitalized tissue and foreign bodies, adequate retrorectal drainage, closure of the rectal wound (if possible), irrigation of the distal colon and rectum, and construction of a proximal diverting colostomy have evolved as the therapeutic principles of choice (▶ Fig. 34.9).[148] Copious irrigation with saline or antibiotic solutions into the contaminated tissues should be performed.[120,121,149] To gain access to the anus, the patient must be positioned in stirrups.

Studies from wartime experience have shown that the treatment just described is associated with the lowest mortality and morbidity rates. Armstrong et al[2] showed from the Vietnam War experience that of 32 patients with missile injuries to the extraperitoneal rectum, 4 died, indicating a mortality rate of 12.5%. An associated intraperitoneal injury occurred in 18 of

these patients. If colostomy alone was performed, the incidence of pelvic abscess was 36%, but when colostomy, closure of the primary wound, and transperineal drainage were added to the regimen, the incidence of pelvic abscess was 0%. Armstrong et al[2] used the washout technique to clear stool from the distal segment of the injured rectum, thus preventing persistent contamination of the perirectal tissues. Washout is aided by dilatation of the anus to allow egress of the feces and solution introduced via the distal limb of the ostomy. For low rectal wounds, the closure of the injured site may be accomplished by per anal suturing technique. The authors recommended using a pericoccygeal drain but did not advocate the performance of coccygectomy, since excision of the coccyx opens new tissue planes and creates the possibility of osteomyelitis. Allen[112] reported on 65 cases of high-velocity extrarectal injuries from combat in Vietnam. He stressed the importance of adequate debridement, posterior-dependent drainage, and evacuation of all retained fecal material from the distal segment. Foreign bodies such as bone, clothing, missiles, and stool must be removed from the pelvis.

Several other authors writing from both civilian and military experience reported a death rate of greater than 20% in patients with extraperitoneal rectal injuries and showed the importance of performing distal washout to decrease the incidence of further sepsis.[112,122,123,124] Other authors fear that washout will push feces out the perforation hole into adjacent tissues. However, if the hole is closed well, the washout should be of benefit. A diverting descending colostomy also is recommended. When a loop colostomy was created, complications occurred in 47% of the patients, with a 5.5% mortality rate, compared with patients with a completely diverting colostomy in whom complications from sepsis occurred in 29%, with a 0% mortality rate. Although creation of a mucous fistula is preferred, constructing a Hartmann pouch is also acceptable. Other organs frequently injured in rectal trauma include the bladder, urethra, vagina, small bowel, and colon.[92,109,110] Death rates reflect the association with injuries to other organs and with sepsis, that is, with wound infection, urinary tract infection, respiratory distress syndrome, pancreatitis, osteomyelitis, fistulas, strictures, dehiscence, and pelvic abscess.[111,112] If damage to the sacrum opens the dura and the central nervous system is exposed to contamination, ligation of the dura may become necessary.[45] The late complications include fecal incontinence, impotence, urinary incontinence, perianal pain, and perineal deformity.

Extensive damage to the rectum and perineum such as with crush compression requires debridement of necrotic tissue and foreign bodies. The sphincter may be sewn together with

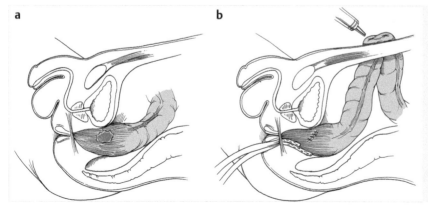

Fig. 34.9 (a) Wound in the extraperitoneal rectum. **(b)** Colostomy, washout, closed wound, and drains.

absorbable sutures. Uncontrollable bleeding may require that packs be left in place. Return to the operating room is necessary to complete debridement and remove packs applied earlier for bleeding. Sometimes abdominoperineal resection may be the best first procedure to perform if the sphincter is not repairable and sepsis and bleeding are out of control.

Attention to a few details prevents local sepsis. Suture materials, when necessary, should be absorbable rather than permanent, since permanent ones may induce chronic sinus tract formation. At the end of the repairs, our policy is to irrigate the peritoneal cavity with up to 10 L of saline solution. The fascia and peritoneum of the incision are closed in one layer, but the skin and subcutaneous tissue are left open if there is intra-abdominal contamination. Entry and exit wounds should be debrided, the peritoneum and fascia should be closed in the base of these wounds, and the skin and subcutaneous tissues should be left open. The incision nearest to the colostomy must be closed for a short length to allow the ostomy appliance to fit better.

Schrock and Christensen[6] and Gustavson[150] have pointed out the septic complications and the mortality rate in patients with extraperitoneal rectal injuries. In a series from Vietnam by Lavenson and Cohen,[123] the complication rate caused by sepsis was 60%. Schrock and Christensen[6] noted that half of their patients with rectal injuries were hospitalized for more than 50 days and 4 patients were hospitalized for more than 100 days. Use of systemic antibiotics is absolutely necessary, and those effective against both anaerobic and aerobic floras should be used.[67,100,101]

Massive rectal bleeding that is not responsive to transfusion can be localized by arteriography via the inferior mesenteric artery and iliac vessels. Once the bleeding point has been localized, embolization of autologous clots or Gelfoam may be used to reduce or stop the bleeding. If therapeutic arteriography fails to work, suture ligation or temporary packing of the rectum with gauze usually suffices to control diffuse bleeding. Splitting the symphysis pubis to gain direct visualization of the pelvis allows direct hemostasis. Ligation of the internal iliac arteries has had mixed results in affecting uncontrollable hemorrhage.[4] Rarely, massive rectal bleeding secondary to trauma is unresponsive to supportive or arteriographic measures; abdominoperineal resection as an emergency procedure then may be required to stop the bleeding.[113] Extensive wounds secondary to a shattered rectum with marked contamination are another indication for performing abdominoperineal resection.[123] The management of rectal impalement is similar to that for other perforations. Initially leaving the impaling object in place is the key to treatment of such injuries.[151] The intra-abdominal organs can be examined and explored, and the impaling object can be removed under direct visualization, reducing contamination and damage to the colon and adjacent organs. The specific repair depends on the contamination and the amount of injury to the rectum, colon, and other organs.

Management of Barium Enema Perforation

If the extraperitoneal rectum has been perforated during the performance of a barium enema examination, a regimen of intravenous fluids, broad-spectrum antibiotics, and observation should be started. Fortunately, in this situation the bowel has been cleared of stool in preparation for the study. If peritoneal findings or signs of sepsis appear, a diverting colostomy with distal irrigation and drainage should be performed.[66] Removal of the barium is necessary. However, the barium sometimes is tightly adherent to the wall of loops of bowel. To remove this contamination, excising the bowel and diversion may be necessary. Prevention of this complication depends on several factors:

- Keeping the "head of pressure" of the barium less than 1 m.
- Not overinflating the balloon.
- Keeping the balloon tip minimally inserted.
- Deferring the barium enema in patients who have recently undergone a biopsy or polypectomy of the colon or rectum.

Management of Blunt Trauma

In deciding whether a patient had an intraperitoneal or an extraperitoneal rectal injury from blunt abdominal trauma, Perry et al[152] and Gumbert et al[153] used DPL to detect colorectal injuries intraperitoneally. If such lavage is properly performed, the incidence of false-positive and false-negative lavages is approximately 4%. In recent years, ultrasonography has become a primary diagnostic tool in the assessment of blunt abdominal trauma.[154] However, this study is operator dependent. Some investigators have used CT to diagnose perforation[155]; however, ultrasonography is often available to the surgeon and thus is faster to obtain and inexpensive. The ability to better assess the patient has led to decreasing the number of laparotomies.

Injuries to the colon and rectum constitute only approximately 10% of all blunt injuries to the abdomen, and only 3% are full-thickness perforations.[11] Carrillo et al[12] believe that primary repair without ostomy can be performed if criteria similar to those for penetrating trauma are observed (i.e., no gross fecal contamination, few associated extra-abdominal injuries, a stable vital condition, and no delay in operation).[11]

The literature generally supports the view that intraperitoneal soilage or a large wound is more safely managed with a diverting colostomy, which is believed to be superior to a loop colostomy in preventing sepsis and further complications. When a blunt force is great enough to fracture the pelvic bones and cause major perineal wounds, the resultant trauma should be treated as a major extraperitoneal rectal injury, with the use of colostomy.[96] Mesenteric injury and contamination mandate resection of open colonic wounds with colostomy formation. If a nonexpanding intraperitoneal hematoma is found during laparotomy, it should not be opened. The rectum should be evaluated for injury by sigmoidoscopy. Major bleeding from the pelvis or presacral plexus often accompanies penetrating injuries into the pelvis. Control of bleeding can be accomplished by packing, angiographic embolization, balloon tamponade and thumbtack occlusion. Sometimes, a balloon catheter can be introduced to the site of bleeding, the balloon can be inflated, and if in good position, it can be sewn in place. If stable after 5 days, the balloon can be deflated. It is left in place in case rebleeding ensues. The mortality rate in patients with a blunt colon injury, as in patients with penetrating trauma, is proportional to the number and severity of injuries to other organs.[156]

Strate and Grieco[156] reported on 109 patients with colonic or rectal injuries. Of the four colon-related deaths, two patients died from anastomotic leaks after resection and primary anastomosis. The other two deaths resulted from a delay in readmission and misdiagnosis. Patients with blunt trauma may present with a delayed colocutaneous fistula and posttraumatic stenosis.[157]

Anal Sphincter Injury

The anal sphincter can be injured by a blunt or penetrating force. If there is an isolated sphincteric injury, performing primary repair without colostomy is acceptable, but if the perineal injury is extensive, an associated colostomy becomes necessary. Polyglycolic acid or polyglactin sutures should be used instead of permanent sutures to prevent chronic suture sinuses. Other surgeons prefer to use a delayed repair, especially if the patient has other life-threatening injuries and the abdomen is already open, because sphincteric injuries alone are rarely life-threatening.[158,159] If the patient's condition is critical, a delayed repair is preferable. A diverting colostomy can be constructed quickly and protects the anorectal area.

After healing, a posttraumatic assessment by anorectal physiologic testing (manometry and electromyography), anal endosonography, and sometimes examination under general anesthesia are complementary in determining the structural and functional integrity of the anal sphincters. In the study by Engel et al,[160] overlapping repair for traumatic external sphincter damage led to a good clinical outcome in 69% of patients; however, perfect continence was achieved in only 33%.

Sphincteric injury from a blast in war is particularly troubling. In 1970, Lung et al[4] studied wounds of the rectum sustained by 24 patients during the Vietnam War and stressed using a primary repair of the anal sphincteric musculature. However, the authors noted that hospitalizations were complicated and prolonged, with a mean time of 207 days and an average of 3.2 operations per patient. For details of sphincteric repair, refer to Chapter 15.

Removal of Foreign Bodies

After the diagnosis of a foreign body in the rectum has been made, the task of removing the object must be undertaken.[161] Although certain tried methods are discussed in this section, new ideas may be formulated for ways to remove foreign bodies and minimize the trauma.

Appropriate relaxation and sedation of the patient are necessary for removal of the object. If these measures fail, anesthesia to relax the patient and to relax the anal sphincter muscles totally is required. The anesthetic can be administered in the physician's office, the outpatient area of the emergency room, or the operating room. Use of local anesthetic serves a twofold purpose: analgesia and sphincteric relaxation. After local anesthesia has been achieved, the examiner can insert instruments more easily to examine the patient and to remove the object. Often intravenous sedation can be administered adjunctively. Use of a tranquilizer for sedation is helpful, and narcotics may be necessary if the patient complains of pain. Since the patient is awake, he or she can voluntary perform a Valsalva maneuver, assisting the extraction. Objects that lodge in the low or middle rectum usually can be removed via the anus with the patient under local anesthesia.

A major effort should be made to remove the object through the anus with the anal sphincter kept intact. However, performing an internal anal sphincterotomy or opening the external sphincter muscles to allow extraction of large foreign bodies may be necessary. Thereafter, the muscles must be repaired. Having the patient in the lithotomy position is beneficial because performance of the Valsalva maneuver and abdominal manipulation may prove useful. Regardless of the method used for extraction, complete lubrication of the anal area is a great aid.

A variety of unique ways to remove foreign bodies through the anus have been suggested. Peet[162] recommended using obstetric forceps to remove impacted foreign bodies from the rectum. Vadlamudi et al[163] recommended using a bladder catheter inserted above the object, then inflating the balloon and using it to pull the object down for retrieval. This method breaks the suction formed by the foreign body against the rectosigmoid wall. Hughes et al[164] recommended the use of special well-padded pliers for removal of hollow objects, and Sachdev[165] has used plaster of Paris inserted into hollow objects, with a string or a clamp inserted into the plaster for use as a handle after it hardens. Occasionally, the proctoscope (and less often the colonoscope) may be used to retrieve foreign bodies. The Sengstaken–Blakemore tube passed through the proctoscope and wedged into a glass provides a handle for removal. After removal of the object via the anus, proctosigmoidoscopy should be performed to check for perforations and bleeding. The patient should be admitted for inpatient observation if there has been difficulty with extraction, because delayed symptoms of perforation may not be evident for several hours.

If a physician fails to remove the object with the patient under local anesthesia, the next step is to attempt removal after administering a caudal or regional anesthetic, which should be performed in the operating room. The approach is the same as that used with a patient under local anesthesia.

Celiotomy is used only as a last resort, after the failure of all anal manipulations, and is performed with the patient under general anesthesia. Objects that lodge in the upper rectum or the lower rectosigmoid may require abdominal celiotomy. The patient is prepared for celiotomy in the usual fashion, which includes the use of antibiotics. The patient's legs are placed in stirrups because the procedure requires both an abdominal and transanal approach. Often no mobilization of the rectum or the sigmoid is necessary. The foreign body can be "milked down" into the middle or lower rectum through the intact rectosigmoid so that the surgeon can remove the object by hand or with instruments. If this procedure fails, a colotomy on the anterior wall of the rectum or the rectosigmoid may be needed for manual extraction of the object. In patients with rectosigmoid perforation caused by a foreign body, the injury is managed as with other intraperitoneal injuries of the colon and rectum. Primary closure alone is rarely recommended because delay is involved and a large contusion with contamination of the peritoneal cavity is usually associated. Most often the laceration or split is repaired, but possibly excised. The wound is usually deep in the pelvis and cannot be exteriorized; therefore, constructing a proximal diverting colostomy and mucous fistula is recommended. The distal washout technique discussed earlier may be used. Sphincteric avulsion caused by a large object or a fist forced through the anus may be repaired primarily.[38]

Lake et al reviewed 93 cases of transanally introduced, retained foreign bodies.[166] They identified 87 patients. Bedside extraction was successful in 74%. Ultimately, 23 patients were taken to the operating room for removal of their foreign body. In total, 17 examinations under anesthesia and 8 laparotomies were performed (2 patients initially underwent examination under anesthesia before laparotomy). In the eight patients who underwent exploratory laparotomy, only one had successful delivery of the foreign object into the rectum for transanal extraction. The remainder required repair of perforated bowel or retrieval of the foreign body via a colotomy. In that review, a majority of cases had objects retained within the rectum; the rest were located in the sigmoid colon. Fifty-five percent of patients (6/11) presenting with a foreign body in the sigmoid colon required operative intervention versus 24% of patients (17/70) with objects in their rectum ($p = 0.04$). This is the largest single institution series of retained colorectal foreign bodies.

References

[1] National Trauma Institute. Trauma Statistics & Facts. Available at: http://nationaltraumainstitute.org/home/trauma_statistics.html. Accessed April 5, 2017

[2] Armstrong RG, Schmitt HJ, Jr, Patterson LT. Combat wounds of the extraperitoneal rectum. Surgery. 1973; 74(4):570–574

[3] Ganchrow MI, Lavenson GS, Jr, McNamara JJ. Surgical management of traumatic injuries of the colon and rectum. Arch Surg. 1970; 100(4):515–520

[4] Lung JA, Turk RP, Miller RE, Eiseman B. Wounds of the rectum. Ann Surg. 1970; 172(6):985–990

[5] Morton JH. Perineal and rectal damage following nonpenetrating abdominal trauma. J Trauma. 1972; 12(4):347–352

[6] Schrock TR, Christensen N. Management of perforating injuries of the colon. Surg Gynecol Obstet. 1972; 135(1):65–68

[7] Abu-Dalu K, Pode D, Hadani M, Sahar A. Colonic complications of ventriculoperitoneal shunts. Neurosurgery. 1983; 13(2):167–169

[8] Amato JL, Billy LJ, Lawson NS, Rich NM. High velocity missile injury. An experimental study of the retentive forces of tissue. Am J Surg. 1974; 127(4):454–459

[9] Sykes LN, Champion HR, Fouty W. Wound ballistics. Contemp Surg. 1986; 29:23

[10] Appleby JP, Nagy AG. Abdominal injuries associated with the use of seatbelts. Am J Surg. 1989; 157(5):457–458

[11] Ross SE, Cobean RA, Hoyt DB, et al. Blunt colonic injury: a multicenter review. J Trauma. 1992; 33(3):379–384

[12] Carrillo EH, Somberg LB, Ceballos CE, et al. Blunt traumatic injuries to the colon and rectum. J Am Coll Surg. 1996; 183(6):548–552

[13] Peterson HB, Ory HW, Greenspan JR, Tyler CW, Jr. Deaths associated with laparoscopic sterilization by unipolar electrocoagulation devices, 1978 and 1979. Am J Obstet Gynecol. 1981; 139(2):141–143

[14] Cohen PL, Sutcliffe TJ. Bowel perforation by an intra-uterine contraceptive device. S Afr Med J. 1982; 62(26):973

[15] Molloy RG, Kingsmore D. Life threatening pelvic sepsis after stapled haemorrhoidectomy. Lancet. 2000; 355(9206):810

[16] Roos P. Haemorrhoid surgery revised [letter]. Lancet. 2000; 355(9215):1648

[17] Ripetti V, Caricato M, Arullani A. Rectal perforation, retropneumoperitoneum, and pneumomediastinum after stapling procedure for prolapsed hemorrhoids: report of a case and subsequent considerations. Dis Colon Rectum. 2002; 45(2):268–270

[18] Wong LY, Jiang JK, Chang SC, Lin JK. Rectal perforation: a life-threatening complication of stapled hemorrhoidectomy: report of a case. Dis Colon Rectum. 2003; 46(1):116–117

[19] LeRoy AJ, Williams HJ, Jr, Bender CE, Segura JW, Patterson DE, Benson RC. Colon perforation following percutaneous nephrostomy and renal calculus removal. Radiology. 1985; 155(1):83–85

[20] Borland RN, Walsh PC. The management of rectal injury during radical retropubic prostatectomy. J Urol. 1992; 147(3, Pt 2):905–907

[21] Lassen PM, Kearse WS, Jr. Rectal injuries during radical perineal prostatectomy. Urology. 1995; 45(2):266–269

[22] Bonnet YY, Haberer JP, Schutz R, et al. Intestinal gas explosion during operation. Ann Fr Anesth Reanim. 1983; 2:431

[23] Zanoni CE, Bergamini C, Bertoncini M, Bertoncini L, Garbini A. Whole-gut lavage for surgery. A case of intraoperative colonic explosion after administration of mannitol. Dis Colon Rectum. 1982; 25(6):580–581

[24] Fischer G, Goebel H, Latta E. Penetration of the colon by a ventriculo-peritoneal drain resulting in an intra-cerebral abscess. Zentralbl Neurochir. 1983; 44(2):155–160

[25] Sathyanarayana S, Wylen EL, Baskaya MK, Nanda A. Spontaneous bowel perforation after ventriculoperitoneal shunt surgery: case report and a review of 45 cases. Surg Neurol. 2000; 54(5):388–396

[26] Seitz WHJ, Jr, Berardis JM, Giannaris T, Schreiber G. Perforation of the rectum by a Smith-Petersen nail. J Trauma. 1982; 22(4):339–340

[27] Khot UP, Lang AW, Murali K, Parker MC. Systematic review of the efficacy and safety of colorectal stents. Br J Surg. 2002; 89(9):1096–1102

[28] Befeler D. Proctoscopic perforation of the large bowel. Dis Colon Rectum. 1967; 10(5):376–378

[29] Andresen AFR. Perforations from proctoscopy. Gastroenterology. 1947; 9 (1):32–43

[30] Jacobsohn WZ, Levy A. Colonoscopic perforation: its emergency treatment. Endoscopy. 1976; 8(1):15–17

[31] Smith LE, Nivatvongs S. Complications in colonoscopy. Dis Colon Rectum. 1975; 18(3):214–220

[32] Smith LE. Fiberoptic colonoscopy: complications of colonoscopy and polypectomy. Dis Colon Rectum. 1976; 19(5):407–412

[33] Fonkalsrud EW, Clatworthy HW, Jr. Accidental perforation of the colon and rectum in newborn infants. N Engl J Med. 1965; 272:1097–1100

[34] Horwitz MA, Bennett JV. Nursery outbreak of peritonitis with pneumoperitoneum probably caused by thermometer-induced rectal perforation. Am J Epidemiol. 1976; 104(6):632–644

[35] Hool GJ, Bokey EL, Pheils MT. Enema-nozzle injury of the rectum. Med J Aust. 1980; 1(8):364–381

[36] Weiss Y, Grünberger P, Aronowitz S. Asymptomatic rectal perforation with retroperitoneal emphysema. Dis Colon Rectum. 1981; 24(7):545–547

[37] Gayer G, Zissin R, Apter S, Oscadchy A, Hertz M. Perforations of the rectosigmoid colon induced by cleansing enema: CT findings in 14 patients. Abdom Imaging. 2002; 27(4):453–457

[38] Critchlow JF, Houlihan MJ, Landolt CC, Weinstein ME. Primary sphincter repair in anorectal trauma. Dis Colon Rectum. 1985; 28(12):945–947

[39] Nelson JA, Daniels AU, Dodds WJ. Rectal balloons: complications, causes, and recommendations. Invest Radiol. 1979; 14(1):48–59

[40] Kiser JL, Spratt JS, Jr, Johnson CA. Colon perforations occurring during sigmoidoscopic examinations and barium enemas. Mo Med. 1968; 65 (12):969–974

[41] Rosenklint A, Buemann B, Hansen P, Baden H. Extraperitoneal perforation of the rectum during barium enema. Scand J Gastroenterol. 1975; 10(1):87–90

[42] Harned RK, Consigny PM, Cooper NB, Williams SM, Woltjen AJ. Barium enema examination following biopsy of the rectum or colon. Radiology. 1982; 145(1):11–16

[43] Kay S, Choy SH. Results of intraperitoneal injection of barium sulfate contrast medium; an experimental study. AMA Arch Pathol. 1955; 59 (3):388–392

[44] Sanders AW, Kobernick SD. Fate of barium sulfate in the retroperitoneum. Am J Surg. 1957; 93(5):907–910

[45] Beerman PJ, Gelfand DW, Ott DJ. Pneumomediastinum after double-contrast barium enema examination: a sign of colonic perforation. AJR Am J Roentgenol. 1981; 136(1):197–198

[46] Levy MD, Hanna EA. Extraperitoneal perirectal extravasation of barium during a barium enema examination: natural course and treatment. Am Surg. 1980; 46(7):382–385

[47] Peterson N, Rohrmann CA, Jr, Lennard ES. Diagnosis and treatment of retroperitoneal perforation complicating the double-contrast barium-enema examination. Radiology. 1982; 144(2):249–252

[48] Sisel RJ, Donovan AJ, Yellin AE. Experimental fecal peritonitis. Influence of barium sulfate or water-soluble radiographic contrast material on survival. Arch Surg. 1972; 104(6):765–768

[49] Zheutlin N, Lasser EC, Rigler LG. Clinical studies on effect of barium in the peritoneal cavity following rupture of the colon. Surgery. 1952; 32 (6):967–979

[50] Nelson RL, Abcarian H, Prasad ML. Iatrogenic perforation of the colon and rectum. Dis Colon Rectum. 1982; 25(4):305–308

[51] Rosenberg LS, Fine A. Fatal venous intravasation of barium during a barium enema. Radiology. 1959; 73:771–773

[52] Ein SH, Mercer S, Humphry A, Macdonald P. Colon perforation during attempted barium enema reduction of intussusception. J Pediatr Surg. 1981; 16(3):313–315

[53] Sultan AH, Kamm MA, Bartram CI, Hudson CN. Anal sphincter trauma during instrumental delivery. Int J Gynaecol Obstet. 1993; 43(3):263–270

[54] Richter HE, Brumfield CG, Cliver SP, Burgio KL, Neely CL, Varner RE. Risk factors associated with anal sphincter tear: a comparison of primiparous patients, vaginal births after cesarean deliveries, and patients with previous vaginal delivery. Am J Obstet Gynecol. 2002; 187(5):1194–1198

[55] Quan SH. Factitial proctitis due to irradiation for cancer of the cervix uteri. Surg Gynecol Obstet. 1968; 126(1):70–74

[56] Sedgwick DM, Howard GC, Ferguson A. Pathogenesis of acute radiation injury to the rectum. A prospective study in patients. Int J Colorectal Dis. 1994; 9(1):23–30

[57] Sherman LF, Prem KA, Mensheha NM. Factitial proctitis: a restudy at the University of Minnesota. Dis Colon Rectum. 1971; 14(4):281–285

[58] Henriksson R, Franzén L, Littbrand B. Effects of sucralfate on acute and late bowel discomfort following radiotherapy of pelvic cancer. J Clin Oncol. 1992; 10(6):969–975

[59] Otchy DP, Nelson H. Radiation injuries of the colon and rectum. Surg Clin North Am. 1993; 73(5):1017–1035

[60] Ahlquist DA, Gostout CJ, Viggiano TR, Pemberton JH. Laser therapy for severe radiation-induced rectal bleeding. Mayo Clin Proc. 1986; 61(12):927–931

[61] Alexander TJ, Dwyer TM. Endoscopic Nd:YAG laser treatment of severe radiation injury of the gastrointestinal tract. Gastrointest Endosc. 1985; 31:152

[62] Buchi KN, Dixon JA. Argon laser treatment of hemorrhagic radiation proctitis. Gastrointest Endosc. 1987; 33(1):27–30

[63] van Nagell JR, Jr, Parker JC, Jr, Maruyama Y, Utley J, Luckett P. Bladder or rectal injury following radiation therapy for cervical cancer. Am J Obstet Gynecol. 1974; 119(6):727–732

[64] Fry RD. Anorectal trauma and foreign bodies. Surg Clin North Am. 1994; 74(6):1491–1505

[65] Schwartz GF, Polsky HS. Ingested foreign bodies of the gastrointestinal tract. Am Surg. 1976; 42(4):236–238

[66] Abcarian H, Lowe R. Colon and rectal trauma. Surg Clin North Am. 1978; 58(3):519–537

[67] Barone JE, Sohn N, Nealon TF, Jr. Perforations and foreign bodies of the rectum: report of 28 cases. Ann Surg. 1976; 184(5):601–604

[68] Benjamin HB, Klamecki B, Haft JS. Removal of exotic foreign objects from the abdominal orifices. Am J Proctol. 1969; 20(6):413–417

[69] Eftaiha M, Hambrick E, Abcarian H. Principles of management of colorectal foreign bodies. Arch Surg. 1977; 112(6):691–695

[70] Sohn N, Weinstein MA, Gonchar J. Social injuries of the rectum. Am J Surg. 1977; 134(5):611–612

[71] Beall AC, DeBakey ME. Injuries and foreign bodies of the colon and rectum. In: Turell R, ed. Diseases of the colon and anorectum. 2nd ed. Philadelphia, PA: WB Saunders; 1969

[72] RAINN. Sexual Violence Has Fallen by More Than Half since 1993. Available at: https://www.rainn.org/statistics/scope-problem. Accessed April 8, 2017

[73] McCann J, Voris J. Perianal injuries resulting from sexual abuse: a longitudinal study. Pediatrics. 1993; 91(2):390–397

[74] Black CT, Pokorny WJ, McGill CW, Harberg FJ. Ano-rectal trauma in children. J Pediatr Surg. 1982; 17(5):501–504

[75] Schiff AF. Attending the child "rape" victim. South Med J. 1979; 72(8):906–910

[76] Dziegelewski M, Simich JP, Rittenhouse-Olson K. Use of a Y chromosome probe as an aid in the forensic proof of sexual assault. J Forensic Sci. 2002; 47(3):601–604

[77] Bauer JJ, Weiss M, Dreiling DA. Stercoraceous perforation of the colon. Surg Clin North Am. 1972; 52(4):1047–1053

[78] Wang SY, Sutherland JC. Colonic perforation secondary to fecal impaction: report of a case. Dis Colon Rectum. 1977; 20(4):355–356

[79] Lyon DC, Sheiner HJ. Idiopathic rectosigmoid perforation. Surg Gynecol Obstet. 1969; 128(5):991–1000

[80] Cain WS, Howell CG, Ziegler MM, Finley AJ, Asch MJ, Grant JP. Rectosigmoid perforation and intestinal evisceration from transanal suction. J Pediatr Surg. 1983; 18(1):10–13

[81] Williams DB, Karl RC. Intestinal injury associated with low-voltage electrocution. J Trauma. 1981; 21(3):246–250

[82] Raina S, Machiedo GW. Multiple perforations of colon after compressed air injury. Arch Surg. 1980; 115(5):660–661

[83] Jackson FR, Ott DJ, Gelfand DW. Thermal injury of the colon due to colostomy irrigation. Gastrointest Radiol. 1981; 6(3):231–233

[84] Committee on Trauma, American College of Surgeons. Advanced Trauma Life Support. Chicago, IL: The College; 1981

[85] Berman AT, Tom L. Traumatic separation of the pubic symphysis with associated fatal rectal tear: a case report and analysis of mechanism of injury. J Trauma. 1974; 14(12):1060–1067

[86] Wolfe WG, Silver D. Rectal perforation with profuse bleeding following an enema. Case report and review of the literature. Arch Surg. 1966; 92(5):715–717

[87] Johnson PA. Rectal impalement with perforation of the bladder. BMJ. 1971; 2(5764):748–749

[88] Moore JB, Moore EE, Thompson JS. Abdominal injuries associated with penetrating trauma in the lower chest. Am J Surg. 1980; 140(6):724–730

[89] Kusminsky RE, Shbeeb I, Makos G, Boland JP. Blunt pelviperineal injuries. An expanded role for the diverting colostomy. Dis Colon Rectum. 1982; 25(8):787–790

[90] Mangiante EC, Graham AD, Fabian TC. Rectal gunshot wounds. Management of civilian injuries. Am Surg. 1986; 52(1):37–40

[91] Elton C, Riaz AA, Young N, Schamschula R, Papadopoulos B, Malka V. Accuracy of computed tomography in the detection of blunt bowel and mesenteric injuries. Br J Surg. 2005; 92(8):1024–1028

[92] Nguyen BD, Beckman I. Silent rectal perforation after endoscopic polypectomy: CT features. Gastrointest Radiol. 1992; 17(3):271–273

[93] Medscape. Diagnostic Peritoneal Lavage. Available at: http://emedicine.medscape.com/article/82888-overview. Accessed April 9, 2017

[94] Dent RI, Jena GP. Missile injuries of the abdomen in Zimbabwe-Rhodesia. Br J Surg. 1980; 67(5):305–310

[95] Grablowsky OM, Gage JO, Ray JE, Hanley PH. Traumatic colonic and rectal injuries. Dis Colon Rectum. 1973; 16(4):296–299

[96] Moore EE, Moore JB, Van Duzer-Moore S, Thompson JS. Mandatory laparotomy for gunshot wounds penetrating the abdomen. Am J Surg. 1980; 140(6):847–851

[97] Thompson JS, Moore EE, Van Duzer-Moore S, Moore JB, Galloway AC. The evolution of abdominal stab wound management. J Trauma. 1980; 20(6):478–484

[98] Wittmann DH, Schein M, Condon RE. Management of secondary peritonitis. Ann Surg. 1996; 224(1):10–18

[99] Thadepalli H, Gorbach SL, Broido PW, Norsen J, Nyhus L. Abdominal trauma, anaerobes, and antibiotics. Surg Gynecol Obstet. 1973; 137(2):270–276

[100] Fullen WD, Hunt J, Altemeier WA. Prophylactic antibiotics in penetrating wounds of the abdomen. J Trauma. 1972; 12(4):282–289

[101] Altemeier WA. Bacteriology of traumatic wounds. JAMA. 1944; 124:413

[102] Mandal AK, Thadepalli H, Matory E, Lou MA, O'Donnell VA, Jr. Evaluation of antibiotic therapy and surgical techniques in cases of homicidal wounds of the colon. Am Surg. 1984; 50(5):254–257

[103] Polk HC, Jr, Miles AA. The decisive period in the primary infection of muscle by Escherichia coli. Br J Exp Pathol. 1973; 54(1):99–109

[104] Poret HA, III, Fabian TC, Croce MA, Bynoe RP, Kudsk KA. Analysis of septic morbidity following gunshot wounds to the colon: the missile is an adjuvant for abscess. J Trauma. 1991; 31(8):1088–1094, discussion 1094–1095

[105] Flint LM, Vitale GC, Richardson JD, Polk HC, Jr. The injured colon: relationships of management to complications. Ann Surg. 1981; 193(5):619–623

[106] Moore EE, Dunn EL, Moore JB, Thompson JS. Penetrating abdominal trauma index. J Trauma. 1981; 21(6):439–445

[107] Kuhls DA, Malone DL, McCarter RJ, Napolitano LM. Predictors of mortality in adult trauma patients: the physiologic trauma score is equivalent to the Trauma and Injury Severity Score. J Am Coll Surg. 2002; 194(6):695–704

[108] Shannon FL, Moore EE. Primary repair of the colon: when is it a safe alternative? Surgery. 1985; 98(4):851–860

[109] Thompson JS, Moore EE, Moore JB. Comparison of penetrating injuries of the right and left colon. Ann Surg. 1981; 193(4):414–418

[110] Stone HH, Fabian TC. Management of perforating colon trauma: randomization between primary closure and exteriorization. Ann Surg. 1979; 190(4):430–436

[111] Adkins RB, Jr, Zirkle PK, Waterhouse G. Penetrating colon trauma. J Trauma. 1984; 24(6):491–499

[112] Allen BD. Penetrating wounds of the rectum. Tex Med. 1973; 69(9):77–81

[113] Getzen LC, Pollak EW, Wolfman EF, Jr. Abdominoperineal resection in the treatment of devascularizing rectal injuries. Surgery. 1977; 82(3):310–313

[114] Imes PR. War surgery of the abdomen. Surg Gynecol Obstet. 1945; 81:608–616

[115] Woodhall JP, Ochsner A. The management of perforating injuries of the colon and rectum in civilian practice. Surgery. 1951; 29(2):305–320

[116] Whelan TJ, ed. Emergency War Surgery. Washington, DC: U.S. Government Printing Office; 1975

[117] Josen AS, Ferrer JM, Jr, Forde KA, Zikria BA. Primary closure of civilian colorectal wounds. Ann Surg. 1972; 176(6):782–786

[118] LoCicero J, III, Tajima T, Drapanas T. A half-century of experience in the management of colon injuries: changing concepts. J Trauma. 1975; 15(7):575–579

[119] Trunkey D, Hays RJ, Shires GT. Management of rectal trauma. J Trauma. 1973; 13(5):411–415

[120] Tuggle D, Huber PJ, Jr. Management of rectal trauma. Am J Surg. 1984; 148(6):806–808

[121] Weil PH. Injuries of the retroperitoneal portions of the colon and rectum. Dis Colon Rectum. 1983; 26(1):19–21

[122] Lavenson GS, Cohen A. Management of rectal injuries. Am J Surg. 1971; 122(2):226–230

[123] Vannix RS, Carter R, Hinshaw DB, Joergenson EJ. Surgical management of colon trauma in civilian practice. Am J Surg. 1963; 106:364–371

[124] Wanebo HJ, Hunt TK, Mathewson C, Jr. Rectal injuries. J Trauma. 1969; 9 (8):712–722

[125] Fealk M, Osipov R, Foster K, Caruso D, Kassir A. The conundrum of traumatic colon injury. Am J Surg. 2004; 188(6):663–670

[126] Stone HH, Fabian TC. Colon trauma: further support for primary repair. Am J Surg. 1979; 190:430–433

[127] Chappuis CW, Frey DJ, Dietzen CD, Panetta TP, Buechter KJ, Cohn I, Jr. Management of penetrating colon injuries. A prospective randomized trial. Ann Surg. 1991; 213(5):492–497, discussion 497–498

[128] Falcone RE, Wanamaker SR, Santanello SA, Carey LC. Colorectal trauma: primary repair or anastomosis with intracolonic bypass vs. ostomy. Dis Colon Rectum. 1992; 35(10):957–963

[129] Sasaki LS, Allaben RD, Golwala R, Mittal VK. Primary repair of colon injuries: a prospective randomized study. J Trauma. 1995; 39(5):895–901

[130] Gonzalez RP, Falimirski ME, Holevar MR. Further evaluation of colostomy in penetrating colon injury. Am Surg. 2000; 66(4):342–346, discussion 346–347

[131] Kamwendo NY, Modiba MC, Matlala NS, Becker PJ. Randomized clinical trial to determine if delay from time of penetrating colonic injury precludes primary repair. Br J Surg. 2002; 89(8):993–998

[132] Nelson R, Singer M. Primary repair for penetrating colon injuries. Cochrane Database Syst Rev. 2003; 3(3):CD002247

[133] Stewart RM, Fabian TC, Croce MA, Pritchard FE, Minard G, Kudsk KA. Is resection with primary anastomosis following destructive colon wounds always safe? Am J Surg. 1994; 168(4):316–319

[134] Nallathambi MN, Ivatury RR, Shah PM, Gaudino J, Stahl WM. Aggressive definitive management of penetrating colon injuries: 136 cases with 3.7 per cent mortality. J Trauma. 1984; 24(6):500–505

[135] Nallathambi MN, Ivatury RR, Rohman M, Stahl WM. Penetrating colon injuries: exteriorized repair vs. loop colostomy. J Trauma. 1987; 27(8):876–882

[136] Vincent M, Smith LE. Management of perforation due to colonoscopy. Dis Colon Rectum. 1983; 26(1):61–63

[137] Gedebou TM, Wong RA, Rappaport WD, Jaffe P, Kahsai D, Hunter GC. Clinical presentation and management of iatrogenic colon perforations. Am J Surg. 1996; 172(5):454–457, discussion 457–458

[138] Causey MW, Rivadeneira DE, Steele SR. Historical and current trends in colon trauma. Clin Colon Rectal Surg. 2012; 25(4):189–199

[139] Greer LT, Gillern SM, Vertrees AE. Evolving colon injury management: a review. Am Surg. 2013; 79(2):119–127

[140] Demetriades D, Murray JA, Chan L, et al. Committee on Multicenter Clinical Trials. American Association for the Surgery of Trauma. Penetrating colon injuries requiring resection: diversion or primary anastomosis? An AAST prospective multicenter study. J Trauma. 2001; 50(5):765–775

[141] Duncan JE, Corwin CH, Sweeney WB, et al. Management of colorectal injuries during operation Iraqi freedom: patterns of stoma usage. J Trauma. 2008; 64 (4):1043–1047

[142] Ott MM, Norris PR, Diaz JJ, et al. Colon anastomosis after damage control laparotomy: recommendations from 174 trauma colectomies. J Trauma. 2011; 70(3):595–602

[143] Demetriades D, Murray JA, Chan LS, et al. Handsewn versus stapled anastomosis in penetrating colon injuries requiring resection: a multicenter study. J Trauma. 2002; 52(1):117–121

[144] Cotton BA, Reddy N, Hatch QM, et al. Damage control resuscitation is associated with a reduction in resuscitation volumes and improvement in survival in 390 damage control laparotomy patients. Ann Surg. 2011; 254 (4):598–605

[145] McPartland KJ, Hyman NH. Damage control: what is its role in colorectal surgery? Dis Colon Rectum. 2003; 46(7):981–986

[146] Ott MM, Norris PR, Diaz JJ, et al. Colon anastomosis after damage control laparotomy: recommendations from 174 trauma colectomies. J Trauma. 2011; 70(3):595–602

[147] Levine JH, Longo WE, Pruitt C, Mazuski JE, Shapiro MJ, Durham RM. Management of selected rectal injuries by primary repair. Am J Surg. 1996; 172 (5):575–578, discussion 578–579

[148] Levy RD, Strauss P, Aladgem D, Degiannis E, Boffard KD, Saadia R. Extraperitoneal rectal gunshot injuries. J Trauma. 1995; 38(2):273–277

[149] Grasberger RC, Hirsch EF. Rectal trauma. A retrospective analysis and guidelines for therapy. Am J Surg. 1983; 145(6):795–799

[150] Gustavson RG. Rectal injuries. Am Surg. 1973; 39(8):456–458

[151] Kaufer N, Shein S, Levowitz BS. Implacement injury of the rectum: an unusual case. Dis Colon Rectum. 1967; 10(5):395–396

[152] Perry JF, Jr, DeMeules JE, Root HD. Diagnostic peritoneal lavage in blunt abdominal trauma. Surg Gynecol Obstet. 1970; 131(4):742–744

[153] Gumbert JL, Froderman SE, Mercho JP. Diagnostic peritoneal lavage in blunt abdominal trauma. Ann Surg. 1967; 165(1):70–72

[154] McKenney M, Lentz K, Nunez D, et al. Can ultrasound replace diagnostic peritoneal lavage in the assessment of blunt trauma? J Trauma. 1994; 37 (3):439–441

[155] Sherck J, Shatney C, Sensaki K, Selivanov V. The accuracy of computed tomography in the diagnosis of blunt small-bowel perforation. Am J Surg. 1994; 168(6):670–675

[156] Strate RG, Grieco JG. Blunt injury to the colon and rectum. J Trauma. 1983; 23(5):384–388

[157] McKenzie AD, Bell GA. Nonpenetrating injuries of the colon and rectum. Surg Clin North Am. 1972; 52(3):735–746

[158] Goligher JC. Injuries of the rectum and colon. In: Goligher JC, ed. Surgery of the Anus, Rectum and Colon. 3rd ed. Springfield, IL: Charles C Thomas, 1975

[159] Large PG, Mukheiber WJ. Injury to rectum and anal canal by enema syringes. Lancet. 1956; 271(6943):596–599

[160] Engel AF, Kamm MA, Hawley PR. Civilian and war injuries of the perineum and anal sphincters. Br J Surg. 1994; 81(7):1069–1073

[161] Shillingstad RB, Marks JM, Ponsky JL. Endoscopic management of gastrointestinal foreign bodies. Contemp Surg. 1997; 50:87–92

[162] Peet TND. Removal of impacted rectal foreign body with obstetric forceps. BMJ. 1976; 1(6008):500–501

[163] Vadlamudi KK, Van Bockstaele PG, McManus JE. Bladder catheter in removal of a foreign body from rectum. JAMA. 1972; 221(12):1412

[164] Hughes JP, Marice HP, Gathright JB, Jr. Method of removing a hollow object from the rectum. Dis Colon Rectum. 1976; 19(1):44–45

[165] Sachdev YV. An unusual foreign body in the rectum. Dis Colon Rectum. 1967; 10(3):220–221

[166] Lake JP, Essani R, Petrone P, Kaiser AM, Asensio J, Beart RW, Jr. Management of retained colorectal foreign bodies: predictors of operative intervention. Dis Colon Rectum. 2004; 47(10):1694–1698

35 Colorectal Complications of Colonic Disease and Complication Management

David E. Beck

Abstract

A number of uncommon but very serious and life-threatening conditions can occur in the large and small intestines. Many of these require emergency operations. The management of free intraperitoneal perforation, neutropenic colitis, gastrointestinal bleeding and operative complications are reviewed in this chapter.

Keywords: colon disease, free perforation, neutropenic enterocolitis, massive gastrointestinal bleeding, complication

35.1 Free Perforation

Free perforation of the large bowel from colonic diseases is uncommon, but it is a very serious and life-threatening condition that usually requires an emergency operation. Untreated, the patient will die from generalized peritonitis or sepsis. This chapter discusses patients with free intraperitoneal perforation causing generalized purulent or fecal peritonitis. Patients with a confined or extraperitoneal perforation are not considered.

35.1.1 Etiologies

Diverticular Disease

Most diverticula are situated in the sigmoid colon. Perforation of mesenteric diverticula is confined to the extraperitoneum or between the leaves of the sigmoid colon mesentery, causing an abscess or a phlegmon. Intraperitoneal perforation causing purulent or fecal peritonitis is uncommon. Krukowski and Matheson[1] found that this type of problem was seen, on an average, less than once per year at the Lahey Clinic in Boston, twice per year at the Mayo Clinic, and seven times per year at Birmingham, United Kingdom. In a prospective study of acute diverticulitis treated throughout Australia and New Zealand, 248 patients were accepted for the survey.[2] Of them, 214 had peritonitis: serous in 82 (38%), purulent in 104 (49%), and fecal in 28 (13%).

Carcinoma

Perforation from carcinoma of the colon and rectum is also uncommon. It occurs in 3.3 to 9.5%[3,4] of the cases. There are two types of perforation that may develop: perforation of the carcinoma itself and, less often, perforation of the colon proximal to the carcinoma, especially the cecum, which may occur from overdistention by air.

In the series of 1,551 patients by Mandava et al,[4] 51 (3.3%) presented with perforation, 61% had localized perforation with abscess, and 39% had free perforation. The site of perforation was most often at the carcinoma site (82%). In the remaining patients (18%), perforation occurred proximal to the obstructed primary lesion.

Ulcerative Colitis

Free perforation resulting from ulcerative colitis without toxic megacolon is unusual and usually occurs in the course of a severe attack of colitis, often during the initial attack itself.[5] Among the 1,928 patients with ulcerative colitis in one study, perforation of the colon was noted in only 5 (0.3%), mostly in the sigmoid colon.[5]

Crohn's Colitis

Free perforation resulting from small bowel Crohn's disease is rare. In one series, it occurred in 1 to 2% of the cases.[6] Free perforation in a patient with Crohn's colitis is even more unusual. A 10-year review at the Royal Infirmary of Edinburgh identified 198 patients diagnosed as having Crohn's disease of the colon.[7] Six patients (3%) developed free perforation. Out of 679 patients with large bowel Crohn's disease in the series from Oslo, Norway, 7 (1%) had free perforations.[5] The locations of intra-abdominal fistulas in patients operated on for complications of Crohn's disease are listed in ▸ Table 35.1.

Toxic Megacolon

Toxic megacolon is a serious condition in which the inflamed colon becomes dilated, causing abdominal distention and serious illness. Although it is typically associated with ulcerative colitis, Crohn's disease, other bacterial colitides, including *Clostridium difficile* colitis, are emerging as important causes of

Table 35.1 Location of 290 intra-abdominal fistulas in 22 patients operated on for complications of Crohn's disease[103]

Location	No. of fistulas (%)
Internal	
Enteroduodenal	14 (5)
Enteroenteric	51 (18)
Enterocolonic	83 (29)
Enterosigmoid	49 (17)
Enterovesical	36 (12)
Colosigmoid	5 (2)
Enterosalpingeal	2 (2)[a]
Total internal	240 (83)
External	
Enterocutaneous	46 (16)
Enterovaginal	4 (2)[a]
Total external	50 (17)
Total fistulas	290

[a]The percentage is based on the number of fistulas in women.

toxic megacolon. Delayed operative intervention may lead to perforation. In a series of 70 patients with toxic megacolon reported by Heppell et al,[8] 15 (21%) had sealed or free perforation.

35.1.2 Clinical Manifestations

Free perforation of the colon and rectum into the peritoneal cavity has a sudden onset, with classic signs and symptoms of acute abdominal pain, distention, peritoneal irritation, fever, and chills. In spite of its severity, the typical presenting signs and symptoms of perforation may be absent and nonspecific. In elderly debilitated patients or patients receiving steroids, the traditional signs and symptoms of an inflammatory process or peritonitis are often muted, and the perforation may go unrecognized until the condition has progressed to unexplained sepsis and multiple organ failure. A sudden or gradual deterioration in a patient should alert physicians and surgeons to the clinical diagnosis of an "acute abdomen."

35.1.3 Diagnosis and Clinical Evaluation

Upright and flat plate films of the abdomen and lateral decubitus X-ray films demonstrate a pneumoperitoneum, the pathognomonic sign of a perforated viscus, in only 20 to 50% of the cases.[3,7] Bleeding, presumably from the site of perforation, may be present but usually is minimum or moderate in amount. Proctoscopy, flexible sigmoidoscopy, and colonoscopy are contraindicated because of the risk of enlarging the size of the perforation and further contamination of the peritoneal cavity. Computed tomography (CT) scan of the abdomen is often unnecessary, but is frequently the first test obtained. A water-soluble enema such as Hypaque or Gastrografin is helpful in locating the site of perforation and is particularly useful in establishing the diagnosis in patients with peritonitis confined to the left lower quadrant.[9]

35.1.4 Management

Free perforation of the colon and rectum into the peritoneal cavity is a true emergency condition. The operative mortality rate is high, ranging from 6 to 29% for diverticular disease,[1] 14 to 71% for carcinoma,[3,4,10] and 27% for toxic megacolon.[8] Once free perforation is diagnosed or suspected, exploratory surgery should be performed as soon as possible. The aim of the operation is to remove the perforated colon or rectum to stop further contamination and to wash the entire abdominal cavity, including performing debridement of fibrin and necrotic tissues. A primary anastomosis is rarely possible. The significant prognostic factors are age older than 65 years, organ failure, and septic state.[11]

35.2 Neutropenic Enterocolitis

Although rare in adults, neutropenic enterocolitis is a potentially fatal condition that deserves to be included as a separate entity. Neutropenic enterocolitis is now a commonly recognized complication of potent combinations of chemotherapy. Surgeons will be increasingly called upon to evaluate neutropenic patients with abdominal pain. Although most cases are associated with chemotherapy, the disease has been described with immunosuppression therapy in transplant recipients, benign cyclic neutropenia, and aplastic anemia.[12,13]

Neutropenia is defined as less than 1,000 neutrophils/mm^3 and severe neutropenia as less than 100 neutrophils/mm^3.[14] The condition was first described by Cooke in 1933[15] and the term neutropenic enterocolitis was first used by Moir and Bale in 1976.[16] This entity has also been called typhlitis (*typhlon* in Greek is cecum), necrotizing enterocolitis, agranulocyte colitis, and neutropenic enteropathy.[13] The process has a predilection for the terminal ileum and cecum, but any segment of the bowel can be involved.[13]

The exact pathogenesis of neutropenic enterocolitis is unknown. The neutropenia may allow bacterial invasion of the bowel wall leading to necrosis of various layers of the bowel.[12,13] The common signs and symptoms are abdominal pain, fever, diarrhea, abdominal distention, blood in stool, nausea, and vomiting.[17] Although these symptoms are nonspecific, their presence in patients with neutropenia should alert physicians and surgeons to suspect neutropenic enterocolitis.

The accurate diagnosis is often difficult since other acute abdominal diseases can also occur, such as pancreatitis, appendicitis, and hepatic abscess.[13] Besides, the lack of significant intraperitoneal inflammatory response due to neutropenia makes it difficult to diagnose the extent of the acute abdomen. The severity of the enterocolitis ranges from mucosal ulceration to transmural necrosis and perforation. CT scan showed abnormality of the ileocecal area in only 46% of the patients in the series by Wade et al.[13] However, CT scan is the most accurate method of diagnosis. In a typical case, the CT scan shows a dilated cecum with thickened wall and spiculation of pericolonic fat.[17] The finding of pneumatosis intestinalis supports the diagnosis but is not specific.[18]

The management of neutropenic enterocolitis is most challenging. Needless surgery must be avoided in these very sick patients. On the other hand, delayed operation only increases the risk of mortality. Not all neutropenic patients with abdominal pain require operation. Medical treatment includes nasogastric suction to rest the bowel, broad-spectrum antibiotics, fluid, electrolytes, intravenous nutrition, and consideration of granulocyte transfusion.[12,19,20] In the meta-analysis of randomized controlled trials,[21] ciprofloxacin combined with a beta-lactam antimicrobial agent is superior to the more commonly used aminoglycoside/beta-lactam in the management of hospitalized febrile neutropenic patients. In addition, this combination is less nephrotoxic and is less expensive.

There are evidences suggesting that the disease may resolve when the number of white blood cells rises.[13] If the condition does not improve within a few days, operation is indicated.[20] Patients with signs of localized or generalized peritonitis should be operated on. The bowel should be resected without anastomosis. All dead bowels, regardless of how extensive, have to be resected. A questionable viable small bowel may require a second-look operation within 24 hours.[22]

Wade et al[13] reported 50 patients with neutropenic enterocolitis. The overall mortality rate was 60%. The mortality rate of 37 patients treated medically was 70% and of 17 patients treated surgically, 41%. Abdominal distention was a significant risk to the outcome; 60% of the patients who died had abdominal distention compared with 20% of the patients who did not have abdominal distention and survived. Localization of pain or tenderness and diarrhea had no predictive value to the outcome. Overwhelming sepsis was the major cause of death.

35.3 Massive Gastrointestinal Bleeding

35.3.1 General Considerations

Massive colonic bleeding is defined as bleeding that has become life threatening, usually requiring approximately 5 units of transfused blood. The site of the bleeding is difficult to pinpoint, because bleeding from the gastroduodenum and small bowel can present as bright red rectal bleeding. During the past 20 years, the diagnosis of massive colonic bleeding has changed remarkably. The use of arteriography and nuclear medicine tracers not only identifies the source and site of bleeding in many cases, but may prove therapeutic as well. The recent introduction of emergency colonoscopy has changed the method of diagnosis and treatment further.

Angiectasia

Prompted by the reports of small cecal vascular abnormalities by other authors,[23,24] Boley et al[25] set out to study the blood vessels of the right colon in 1977. They found that in patients with a clinical and angiographic diagnosis of bleeding from colonic vascular lesions, the most consistent and apparently the earliest abnormality noted in all lesions was the presence of dilated, often huge, submucosal veins. The colonic mucosa overlying the lesion was very thin, often separated from the dilated vessels by a single layer of endothelium. Boley et al[25] believed that the lesions were acquired vascular ectasias, resulting from degenerative changes that accompany aging. This theory accounts both for the higher incidence in older persons and for the multiplicity of lesions.

According to the authors' concept, the direct cause of the ectasias is chronic, partial, and intermittent low-grade obstruction of the submucosal veins, especially where these veins pierce the circular and longitudinal muscular layers of the colon. This obstruction occurs repeatedly over many years during muscular contraction and distention of the cecum and the right colon. Because of the lower pressure within the veins, they can become occluded while higher arterial pressure maintains arterial inflow. Ultimately, repeated episodes of transiently elevated pressure within a submucosal vein result in dilatation and tortuosity of these vessels and later of the venules and capillaries of the mucosal units draining into it. Finally, as the responsible rings dilate, competency of the precapillary sphincters is lost, producing a small arteriovenous communication (▶ Fig. 35.1). The latter is for the "early" filling veins. Examination of colon resected from those patients older than 60 years without a history of gastrointestinal (GI) bleeding or obstruction found submucosal vascular ectasia in 53% and mucosal ectasia in 27% of specimen. These findings support the concept that these are degenerative lesions of aging in an older population.

Although aortic stenosis and GI bleeding have been noted and blamed as the cause of angiectasia, Boley et al[25] believed that the low perfusion pressure from aortic stenosis might cause ischemic necrosis of the single layer of endothelium that often separates ectatic vessels from the colonic lumen. Angiectasia tends to cause slow repeated bleeding from the large bowel. Patients present with anemia or weakness. This is in sharp contrast to diverticular bleeding that is abrupt, more impressive, and less chronic.[26] With increased awareness of angiectasia, more and more lesions have been recognized. Colonoscopy is a safe and effective test for making the diagnosis.[26,27]

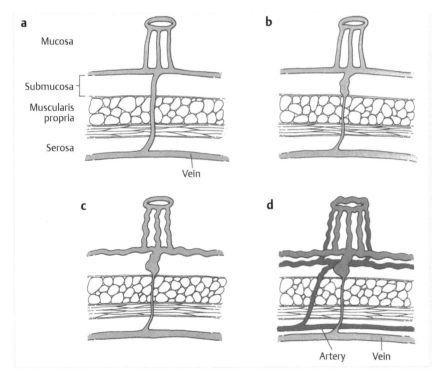

Fig. 35.1 Diagrammatic illustration of proposed concept of development of angiectasia. **(a)** Normal state of vein perforating muscular layer of the colonic wall. **(b)** Vein is obstructed partially as a result of muscular contraction or increased intraluminal pressure. **(c)** After repeated episodes over many years, the submucosal and mucosal venules become dilated and tortuous. **(d)** Ultimately, the capillary ring becomes dilated, the precapillary sphincter becomes incompetent, and a small arteriovenous communication is present through the ectasia.

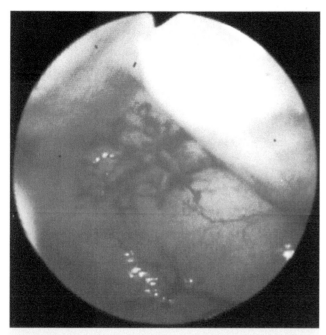

Fig. 35.2 Angiectasia of the cecum as seen through the colonoscope.

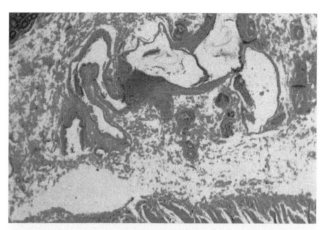

Fig. 35.3 Histology of angiectasia shows tortuous and dilated capillaries in the lamina propria.

Angiectasia can be recognized easily via colonoscopy as a distinct red mucosal patch consisting of capillaries (▶ Fig. 35.2). The size may vary from 2 mm to 1.5 cm. The histology of angiectasia shows tortuous and dilated capillaries in the lamina propria (▶ Fig. 35.3). Angiectasia discovered incidentally does not need to be treated. When angiectasias with active bleeding are found during colonoscopy in patients with massive lower gastrointestinal bleeding (LGIB), colon resection should be considered. Electrocoagulation can be performed, but the current bleeding is in the range of 40 to 50% with a significant risk of perforation.[26] More than 70% of angiectasia was found in the right colon on colonoscopy, 22% in the descending and sigmoid colon, and 6% in the transverse colon in the series of 437 lesions studied by Jensen and Machicado.[28]

Diverticular Disease

Approximately 50% of the people older than 60 years have radiologic evidence of diverticula. Up to 20% bleed during their lifetime, and 5% have massive bleeding, which recurs in 25%, if the colon is not resected.[29] Although most diverticula are in the sigmoid colon, 50 to 95% of bleeding diverticula are to the right of the splenic flexure.[30,31] Before the 1960s, it was thought that inflammation of the diverticula caused bleeding. Noer et al[32] were the first to note that most bleeding comes from noninflamed diverticula.

McGuire[31] studied 79 patients with severe bleeding diverticulosis and found that bleeding stopped spontaneously in 76%. Emergency operation was required in 24%. In patients who required no more than 3 units of blood transfusion on any day, 98.5% stopped spontaneously. In patients who required four or more transfusions on any day, 60% required emergency operation. In those patients who did not require operation, the recurrence rate was 38%, and in 79% of these patients, again, bleeding stopped spontaneously. Bokhari et al[33] reported that of 115 elderly patients with a mean age of 79 years admitted to the hospital with bleeding diverticulosis and who required

blood transfusion, 18% required colon resection. The postoperative mortality rate was 9%.

In the study of acute bleeding diverticulosis by Meyer et al,[34] who used arteriographic and microangiographic techniques, the serial histologic sections revealed that the bleeding was the result of rupture of the vasa recta, which passed around the dome of the diverticulum. The vasa recta at the site of rupture had eccentric intimal thickening associated with thinning of the media and duplication of the internal elastic lamina. These arterial changes probably represent a nonspecific response to repeated arterial injury. The increased frequency of bleeding from the right-sided colonic diverticula remains a puzzling fact. Although the anatomic relationships of the vasa recta to diverticula are similar throughout the colon, one feature distinguishes right-sided from left-sided diverticula. Those on the right have wider necks and domes. Their vasa recta are, therefore, exposed over a greater length to any injurious factors arising from the colon. The nature of the injurious factors has not been determined yet. In addition, the true cause of the bleeding may be an unrecognized vascular ectasia.[35]

Carcinoma

Colonic bleeding is common with carcinoma of the colon and rectum, and ranges from a small amount of intermittent bright red rectal blood to chronic occult or gross bleeding causing anemia. The incidence of massive bleeding from a patient with colorectal carcinoma varies from series to series. In the series reported by Rossini et al,[36] 311 patients with massive colonic bleeding underwent emergency colonoscopy; carcinoma caused the bleeding in 21%. Jensen and Machicado,[28] using urgent colonoscopy, found that severe bleeding was caused by colorectal carcinomas and polyps in 11% of the patients. Leitman et al,[35] using emergency arteriography, found carcinoma as the cause of massive bleeding in 10% of 55 patients.

Polyps

Although polyps of the colon and rectum are common, their causing massive bleeding is uncommon, with the incidence ranging from 2 to 10%.[28,35,36]

Ischemic Colitis

Ischemic colitis may be acute, transient, or agressive.[37] The patient usually presents with bleeding per rectum, diarrhea, and abdominal pain; acute abdomen usually designates gangrene or perforation. In a series of 54 patients with massive lower GI hemorrhage who were undergoing emergency arteriography, Leitman et al[35] found 3 patients with intestinal ischemia. Using urgent colonoscopy in 74 patients with severe hematochezia, Jensen and Machicado[28] found no case of ischemic colitis. On the other hand, Rossini et al[36] reported that 21 out of 311 patients with massive, active lower GI hemorrhage had ischemic colitis.

Inflammatory Bowel Disease

Ulcerative colitis is characterized by bloody diarrhea in more than 95% of the cases, but severe or massive hemorrhage is quite rare, occurring less commonly than other complications such as toxic megacolon, colonic perforation, or neoplastic degeneration.[38] Nevertheless, massive hemorrhage occasionally represents the principal indication for emergency operation. The frequency of severe hemorrhage reported in the literature ranges from 0 to 4.5%. However, this relatively rare complication accounts for approximately 10% of all urgent colectomies for ulcerative colitis.[35] In the series by Rossini et al,[36] 45 of 311 patients (14%) with massive LGIB diagnosed by emergency colonoscopy had ulcerative colitis.

The incidence of massive bleeding in patients with Crohn's disease has been reported as 1 to 13%.[39] Active bleeding caused by Crohn's colitis is uncommon. In the series reported by Robert et al,[40] 21 of 1,526 patients (1.3%) with Crohn's disease developed severe GI hemorrhage. The frequency of bleeding was significantly higher among patients with colonic involvement (17 of 929, 1.9%) than among those with small bowel disease alone (4 of 597, 0.7%). Primary bleeding episodes subsided without operation in 10 of 21 patients, but 3 of the 10 patients (30%) rebled massively. By contrast, primary excisional surgery was followed by recurrent hemorrhage in only 1 of the 11 cases (9%). Although the differences in mortality and in recurrent bleeding rates were not statistically significant, they favor surgical removal of the diseased bowel at the time of the first episode of massive hemorrhage.[40] A review of literature by Cirocco et al[41] showed that operation was necessary to prevent life-threatening hemorrhage in 30 of 33 patients (91%).

35.3.2 Clinical Manifestations

Massive LGIB is generally defined as bleeding per rectum that requires 3 to 6 units of transfused blood within 24 hours[34] or bleeding that results in a hemoglobin level of below 10 g/dL.[35] A large amount of blood acts as a cathartic and will be evacuated accordingly. The color of the stool ranges from bright red to dark red, depending on the speed of bleeding. Symptoms of these patients reflect the underlying disease. Bleeding caused by diverticular disease, ulcerative colitis, polyps, or carcinomas is usually asymptomatic except for some abdominal cramps from the cathartic effect of the blood. Bleeding caused by ischemic colitis is usually associated with severe abdominal cramps. Other signs of severe blood loss such as tachycardia, pallor, and weakness are apparent.

35.3.3 Diagnosis and Management

Massive bleeding per rectum is a life-threatening condition. The most important parts of management are the initial resuscitation with blood and volume replacement and the monitoring of vital systems. These steps must be performed immediately. Any blood dyscrasia should be ruled out and treated accordingly. The next critical item is making an accurate and early diagnosis. The diagnosis of massive colonic bleeding is usually difficult because the diagnostic techniques are not completely efficient or reliable. Knowing the exact site of bleeding is more important than knowing what causes the bleeding.

In approximately 85% of all patients who have acute GI bleeding, the bleeding stops spontaneously. This fact should be known by all involved in the care of these patients.[42] Shock from massive GI bleeding is usually from gastroduodenal rather than small intestinal or colonic sources.

Nasogastric Suction

The most common cause of massive GI bleeding remains peptic ulcer disease. All patients with GI hemorrhage should have a nasogastric tube placed in the stomach to rule out an upper GI source. If blood returns, a gastroduodenal source is confirmed. The nasogastric return must contain bile to rule out a bleeding duodenal ulcer. A bloody nasogastric aspirate has the highest specificity for high-risk lesions. A clear nasogastric aspirate reduces the possibility significantly.[43] If any doubt remains, gastroduodenoscopy should be performed.

Proctoscopy

The rectum and anal canal can be examined quickly with a proctoscope to rule out a local source of the bleeding and to confirm the presence of blood proximal to the rectum. Most of the blood can be washed out, and an adequate examination can be usually done without much difficulty. Any active bleeding from a specific source in the anorectum can be treated with electrocautery or suture ligation.

Computed Tomography Angiography

Widespread availability and recent advances in CT have led to the development and validation of CT angiography (CTA) techniques. Sixty-four-row CTA allows thinner collimation, faster scanning times, greater anatomic coverage, and better multiplanar reformatted images, greatly expanding its diagnostic role for the evaluation of intestinal bleeding.[44] With its widespread availability, CTA has largely supplanted ^{99m}Tc-labeled red blood cell (RBC) scanning as the initial means of evaluating most patients presenting with acute LGIB who do not have a contraindication such as renal insufficiency or allergy to contrast dye. Besides the detection of active bleeding, CTA has the added advantages of being able to localize the site of bleeding and identify any coexisting pathology. A positive CTA should prompt further therapeutic efforts, such as angiographic embolization, or if the patient is showing signs of massive hemorrhage, targeted surgical resection of the culprit segment of intestine. The rate of bleeding able to be detected by CTA has been reported to be as low as 0.3 mL/min.[45] The sensitivity of CTA for localization of a LGIB source is 91 to

92% when active bleeding is present, though it drops to as low as 45 to 47% when bleeding is intermittent.[46] In a prospective trial, Ren et al found that CTA had an accuracy of 90.5% in the detection of active GI bleeding, and treatment planning was correctly established on the basis of CTA findings with an accuracy of 98.4%. Another prospective study comparing the diagnostic performance of CTA with angiography, colonoscopy, and surgical findings reported a sensitivity of 100%, specificity of 96%, positive predictive value (PPV) of 95%, negative predictive value (NPV) of 100%, and accuracy of 93%.[47] A prospective trial published by Obana et al[48] found that the detection rate of colonic diverticular bleeding by CTA alone was only 15.4%, but jumped to 46.2% when combined with colonoscopy. Nagata et al[49] evaluated rates of detection of an LGIB source comparing early colonoscopy following urgent CTA with early colonoscopy alone and found that the detection rate was higher with colonoscopy following CTA than with colonoscopy alone for vascular lesions (35.7 vs. 20.6%; p = 0.01), leading to more endoscopic therapies (34.9 vs. 13.4%; $p < 0.01$). A major advantage of CTA in the evaluation of the patient with LGIB is its ready availability and ease with which the study can be performed and rapidly interpreted, leading to earlier and more targeted therapeutic intervention. It is a noninvasive study that does not require mechanical bowel preparation and carries very little risk. The main disadvantage is the small risk of contrast nephropathy, which may limit its use in patients with renal insufficiency.

Technetium-99 m Scintigraphy

The detection of colonic bleeding with nuclear medicine tracers depends on the intravenous infusion of technetium, which will stay within the blood pool for a reasonable period of time so that the source of the bleeding, which often is intermittent, can be detected. This procedure was first performed using sulfur colloid. However, because sulfur colloid collects in the liver and spleen, bleeding that occurs in the upper or middle abdomen such as in the stomach, duodenum, and transverse colon was often obscured. For this reason, RBCs labeled with technetium-99 m (^{99m}Tc) are now used. A small sample of the patient's own RBCs is withdrawn, labeled with ^{99m}Tc sodium pertechnetate, and reinjected. Scintigraphic images are then obtained in the hope of identifying the source of bleeding. Even if the patient is not bleeding at the moment of injection, bleeding over the next 12 or more hours can be detected by repeat scanning. With ^{99m}Tc-labeled RBCs, bleeding at a rate of 0.1 mL/min can be detected (▶ Fig. 35.4).[36] Nuclear medicine tracers are efficient for detecting bleeding that has slowed down and bleeding that is intermittent, but it requires several hours to follow the patient. RBC-tagged scanning is 30 to 90% accurate in localizing the bleeding point.[50,51] One of the major problems is that the tagged RBC study depends heavily on the technique and the radiologist. The poor results may be the result of an incorrect scanning interval because of the intermittent nature of bleeding or because the blood moves distally by peristalsis.

In the series by Nicholson et al,[52] the test sensitivity was as high as 97%, and the specificity was 85%. The predictive values were 94 and 92% when the scans were positive and negative, respectively. These impressive results are also shared by other authors.[53,54] Suzman et al[54] emphasize using a delayed periodic scintigraphic imaging technique. In this technique, the images

are acquired at 5-minute intervals for the first hour and at 15-minute intervals for up to 4 hours and stored in a dynamic mode. If needed, the patient is imaged every 90 minutes thereafter for up to 24 hours. Scan results demonstrating extravasation to tagged erythrocytes into the bowel lumen are read as positive. Fifty patients who required surgical intervention to control hemorrhage had a bleeding site confirmed by both clinical and pathologic examinations. Forty-eight of these patients (96%) had a bleeding site determined preoperatively. Of 37 patients with bleeding sites localized preoperatively by scintigraphy, 36 (97.3%) had correct localization based on surgical pathology. Only one patient required a subtotal colectomy solely because of nonlocalized bleeding. There was no recurrent postoperative bleeding, and there was no mortality in either operated or nonoperated patients.

Selective Mesenteric Arteriography

Selective mesenteric arteriography is an invasive method that can detect LGIB provided that the bleeding is active and brisk (0.5–1 mL/min) at the time of the test. Intermittent bleeding or minimal rates of bleeding may be missed by this method. In a patient with active bleeding, the contrast medium can be seen extravasated into the bowel lumen (▶ Fig. 35.5). Arteriography, when positive, can localize the site of the bleeding. The angiographic pattern of the vasculature may also suggest a malignancy, a diverticulum, a vascular malformation, or angiectasia. In a patient with massive and continuing bleeding, mesenteric arteriography should be used as the primary test, provided that the facilities for the technique are available and can be mobilized quickly. Another important advantage of mesenteric arteriography is its potential therapeutic applications. It is

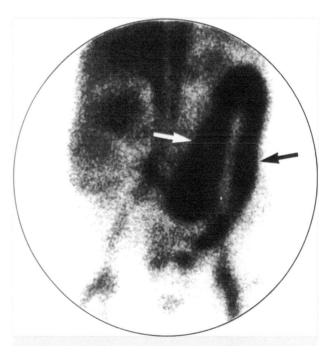

Fig. 35.4 A technetium-99m-labeled red blood cell–tagged scan shows hyperactivity of the blood in the left transverse colon, splenic flexure, and descending colon (*arrows*). (These images are provided courtesy of Michael McKusick, MD.)

important to adequately resuscitate the patient with adequate intravenous fluid and blood transfusion to maintain good blood pressure. Once the bleeding site is detected, the transcatheter treatment using a vasopressin drip or emboli can be accomplished.[35] If successful, it may convert an emergency exploratory celiotomy into an elective one, or it may avert an operation altogether (▶ Fig. 35.6). The action of vasopressin is twofold. It produces both arteriolar contraction and bowel wall contraction, which help stop the bleeding.[55,56]

However, the use of selective vasoconstrictive agent infusion is associated with high recurrence rates and complication of ischemia of the GI tract. Recently, improved microcatheters that allow selective cannulation of secondary vessels and embolization

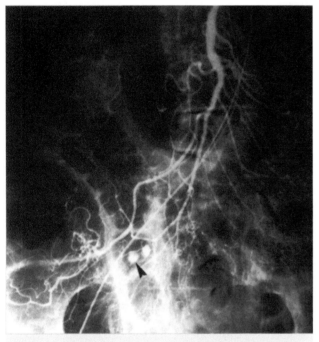

Fig. 35.5 Mesenteric arteriography shows extravasation of contrast material into bowel lumen from diverticular bleeding in transverse colon (*arrow*). (This image is provided courtesy of Michael McKusick, MD.)

agents such as polyvinyl alcohol (PVA) and metal coils have been used with much greater success.

The incidence of ischemia has markedly decreased due to the use of larger PVA or metal coils and increased experience. Most series since 1997 reported ischemia that required resection of less than 5%.[55]

Khanna et al[55] conducted a meta-analysis of 25 identified publications reporting the use of embolization and an unpublished series of 12 consecutive patients with LGIB from their own institution. Six published series and the authors' series met selection criteria for the analysis. The results showed that embolization for diverticular bleeding was successful in 85% of patients (no recurrence after 30 days). In contrast, rebleeding after embolization for angioectasia and other nondiverticular bleeding occurred in 45%.

Angiographic evidence of angiectasia included clusters of small arteries frequently located along the entire mesenteric border of the cecum and ascending colon, a vascular tuft (representing the degeneration of mucosal venules), and an early filling vein (▶ Fig. 35.7). Because the natural history of ectasias is one of recurrent bleeding, Boley et al[57] recommended that all patients who have bleeding and have an ectasia demonstrated by angiography should undergo colonic resection. It is difficult to determine the frequency of bleeding in patients with diverticular disease and angiectasia, because both occur in the elderly and often the bleeding stops during angiography or colonoscopy.

One advantage of angiography as opposed to scintigraphy or colonoscopy for this particular patient population is that no special preparation is necessary such as labeling of erythrocytes and bowel cleansing. Even hemodynamically unstable patients can be studied while resuscitation efforts are under way, including the administration of intravenous fluids and/or blood products. It is critical that no oral contrast agents be administered before angiography because it may obscure subtle bleeding.[58]

Urgent Colonoscopy

The use of a colonic lavage (GoLytely or CoLyte) as a gut cleanser has opened a new approach to colonic bleeding. In the hands of a growing number of physicians, urgent colonoscopy has become the first choice of investigative modality in the diagnosis

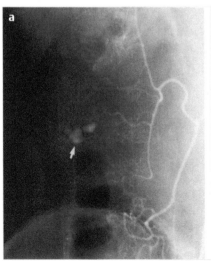
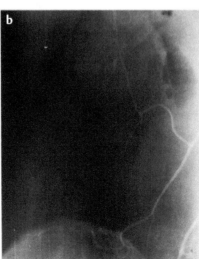

Fig. 35.6 (a) Mesenteric arteriography shows bleeding in the ascending colon from colonoscopic polypectomy (*arrow*). **(b)** Bleeding stopped by vasospasm after vasopressin (Pitressin) drip.

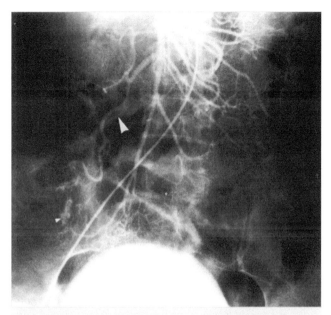

Fig. 35.7 Mesenteric arteriography shows vascular tuft in the right colon from angiectasia (*small arrowhead*) and early filling vein (*large arrowhead*). (This image is provided courtesy of Michael McKusick, MD.)

Table 35.2 Clinical diagnosis at emergency colonoscopy for massive colonic bleeding[57]

Condition	No. of cases
Diverticular disease	56
Solitary diverticulum of the right colon	4
Ulcerative colitis	45
Ulcerative colitis plus carcinoma or polyp	2
Radiation colitis	15
Ischemic colitis	21
Ulcerated carcinoma	66
Polyp	34
Angioma	2
Solitary ulcer	5
Angiectasia	16
Anastomotic recurrence of carcinoma	22
Recurrence of Crohn's disease (ileotransversostomy)	4
Endometriosis	3
Postpolypectomy hemorrhage (4–5 d after operation)	14
Lymphoma	1
Ureterosigmoidostomy plus ulcerated carcinoma	1
Total	311

and therapy of massive colonic bleeding. As soon as the patient has been resuscitated and upper GI bleeding has been ruled out, GoLytely or CoLyte is rapidly instituted via the nasogastric tube or orally. The entire colon can be cleansed within 2 hours. Alternatively, oral Phospho-soda can be administered to accomplish the same goal. Colonoscopy can be performed immediately. In a series reported by Jensen and Machicado,[59] in 80 consecutive patients with severe, ongoing rectal bleeding (mean, 6 units of transfused blood) from an unknown source, urgent colonoscopy was performed after oral purge. In all cases, the cecum was reached. Seventy-four percent of the patients had bled from the colon (angiomas, 30%; diverticulosis, 17%; polyps or carcinomas, 11%; focal ulcers, 9%; others, 7%), 11% had upper GI lesions, and 9% had presumed small bowel lesions. In only 6% was the cause of bleeding not identified. No complications resulted from colonoscopic hemostatic procedures, although four patients had clinically significant fluid overload and early heart failure during the cleansing procedure. Rossini et al[36] performed 409 emergency colonoscopies for massive colonic bleeding. The sites and causes of bleeding were found in 311 cases (76%). There was a wide range of causes of the bleeding (▶ Table 35.2). In 85% of the cases, the bleeding was in the left colon, 4% in the transverse colon, and 11% in the right colon. Only two patients had complications: one developed increasing hemorrhage from ulcerative colitis and one developed diverticulitis. There was no perforation.

One of the greatest advantages of successful colonoscopy is its providing an access to therapy. Colonoscopic hemostatic techniques can be divided into two categories: nonthermal and thermal modalities. The nonthermal techniques involve injection of vasoconstricting agents such as a dilute epinephrine solution and vasodestructive agents alone or in combination with such agents as absolute alcohol, morrhuate sodium, and sodium tetradecyl sulfate. A wide variety of thermal modalities,

including electrocoagulation, laser photocoagulation, and heater probe coagulation, are available.

Urgent colonoscopy for massive colonic bleeding has emerged as a practical and efficient method to diagnose and control some causes of colonic bleeding. The GI bleeding team established at the Mayo Clinic on October 1, 1988, provides a very useful team approach to the treatment of GI bleeding. The bleeding-team contact begins within an hour of the patient's clinical presentation. The triage team determines whether the patient should be admitted to the intensive care unit or whether the team should proceed with evaluation, deciding on the timing of colonoscopy. Emergency colonoscopy is performed after a rapid (1- to 2-hour) lavage with GoLytely or CoLyte.[60] Several lessons can be learned from this study. A total of 417 patients were evaluated. Fifty-six percent of the patients were seen from 8 a.m. to 5:00 p.m., 34% from 5:00 p.m. to 12 a.m., and 10% from 12 a.m. to 8 a.m. Of the 417 patients, 56% developed bleeding during hospitalization. Upper GI bleeding accounted for 82%. The five most common etiologies included gastric ulcers (83 patients), duodenal ulcers (67 patients), gastric erosions (41 patients), esophageal varices (35 patients), and diverticulosis (29 patients). Nonsteroidal anti-inflammatory drugs (NSAIDs) were implicated in 53% of gastroduodenal ulcers.

Twenty-nine patients with bleeding diverticulosis involved the oldest patient group, with an average age of 77 years. Diverticula were limited to the left colon in 52% (15 patients). Eventual cessation of bleeding was commonplace and occurred in 27 patients (93%). Four patients (14%) experienced rebleeding during the hospitalization. Only one patient required operation for rebleeding.

From the Mayo Clinic study, it is unclear whether urgent colonoscopy for acute colonic bleeding will alter outcome, especially if majority of the bleeding is from diverticulosis. The very high rates of spontaneous cessation, the low relative transfusion requirements, and absent mortality argue for initial observation as an appropriate and cost-effective approach. Colonoscopy might more appropriately be performed on an elective basis.

With the better technique of RBC-tagged scan, using dynamic scanning technique, the very high accuracy of both the detection of GI bleeding and the localization of the site of bleeding has made it the choice as the primary test.[54,61] Another advantage of RBC-tagged scanning is that when the scan is negative, those patients (7.3%) rarely require operative intervention.[51] At the present time, it appears that the trend has shifted from urgent or emergent colonoscopy to an emergency RBC-tagged scan or selective mesenteric arteriography as the primary test for acute LGIB.[54,55]

Exploratory Celiotomy

Determining when to operate on patients with massive and continuous colonic bleeding requires astute clinical judgment. Generally, an exploratory celiotomy is considered seriously when a patient requires 5 units of blood transfused within 24 hours or less, if the patient's condition deteriorates. Ironically, greater aggressiveness in deciding to operate earlier is appropriate in treating older and unfit patients. Patients who have recurrent active bleeding that has stopped spontaneously or after nonoperative treatment also should undergo an operation.

Known Bleeding Site

A segmental resection is indicated when the site of bleeding is known, whether the knowledge comes from scintigraphic, arteriographic, or colonoscopic information. The rate of recurrent bleeding after definitive resection has ranged from 0 to 11% (average, 4%), and the reported operative mortality rate has ranged from 0 to 22% (average, 10%).[36,62,63,64,65,66]

Unknown Bleeding Site

It is not uncommon that despite all the efforts and the availability of modern technology, the site of the bleeding is still not ascertained and the bleeding continues. Under these circumstances, exploratory celiotomy should be performed. The entire GI tract must be examined carefully for abnormalities. Small bowel lesions such as leiomyoma, lymphoma, and those of Crohn's disease are occasional sources. If they are not present, an intraoperative endoscopy should follow. A sterilized colonoscope is introduced via an enterotomy in the proximal jejunum. An alternative is to pass a clean but nonsterilized colonoscope through the mouth into the stomach and duodenum. The surgeon then guides the scope throughout the entire small bowel into the cecum. The entire small bowel mucosa is examined. At the same time, the surgeon can examine the bowel by transillumination.[67,68] Angiectasia can be recognized by its abnormal vasculature. If these are found, they can be ligated with interrupted sutures. Other abnormalities can also be effectively visualized.[69] If colonoscopy has not been accomplished preoperatively, an intraoperative colonoscopy also should be performed.

When intraoperative endoscopy or thorough examination of the entire GI tract is negative and evidence points to colonic bleeding at an unknown site, a subtotal colectomy is performed. Some investigators have argued that blind segmental resection of the right colon may be a better surgical option than blind total colectomy, especially if there are suggestions of right-sided bleeding such as blood primarily in the right colon. This argument is strengthened by a negative preoperative examination of the left colon. Blind right hemicolectomy has had the lowest mortality (less than 5%), and the lowest frequency of rebleeding among segmental resections, and it does not incur the risk of incontinence or diarrhea, especially in elderly patients.[66] However, the risk of rebleeding is still significant, and the author feels more confident with a total abdominal colectomy. Farner et al[70] conducted a retrospective study comparing 50 limited colon resections to 27 total/subtotal colon resections for acute LGIB (receiving two or more units of packed RBCs). They found that recurrent bleeding after the operation was more common in the limited colon resection group (18 vs. 4%; $p < 0.05$).

Torrential LGIB from an unknown site should be explored as soon as possible. If there is no obvious source of bleeding in the small intestine, a total abdominal colectomy should be performed. The recurrent bleeding has ranged from 0 to 6%, and the mortality rate from 0 to 50% (average, 22%).[34,53,62,66,71,72,73,74] Because most of the high morbidity and mortality are from anastomotic leaks,[73,74,75] an anastomosis should not be performed in this circumstance. Another risk factor is the delay of surgery. The operation should be performed before 10 units of blood are needed.[74] A schematic approach to massive colonic bleeding is shown in ▶ Fig. 35.8.

35.4 Operative Complications

Colorectal surgery, by its nature, is prone to complications. The distal GI tract is a potential source of infection and improper operative technique can lead to ischemia, which may result in a leak or a stricture. Operations change the anatomy and the physiology of the large bowel and each procedure is associated with common and unique potential complications. Knowledge of etiology, methods of management, and means of prevention are critical to minimize the impact of complications.

35.4.1 Anorectal Operations

Early complications include bleeding, pain, urinary retention, and infection.

Bleeding

Early postoperative bleeding, which is usually the result of a technical error, is not common. The most common source is from the external hemorrhoidal area and is easily detected and controlled by placement of a suture. The suturing can be performed at bedside or in a treatment room with local anesthetic used. In other cases, the patient should be returned to the operating room, where the anorectum is examined with the patient under local, regional, or general anesthesia. Acute bleeding from the anal canal usually is from insecure suture ligation of the hemorrhoidal pedicles.

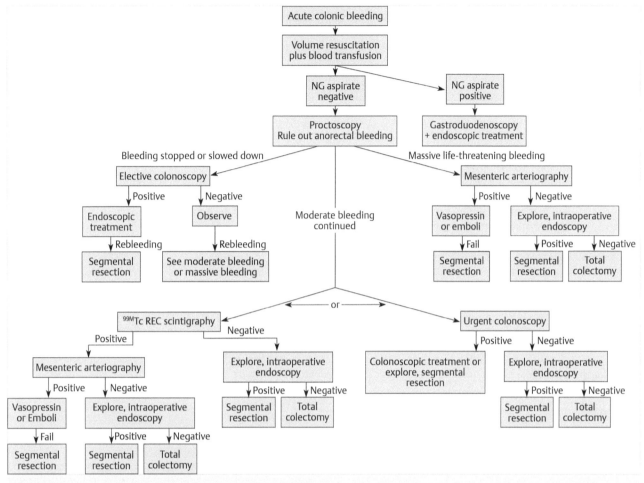

Fig. 35.8 Schematic approach to treatment of massive colonic bleeding.

Severe Anal Pain

For most patients, the pain following anorectal operations is moderate and requires analgesics during the first 1 to 2 postoperative days. Intolerable pain despite adequate analgesics is uncommon. However, because such pain may be a sign of a perianal hematoma, inspection of the anal wound is required. Even a light dressing around the anus may aggravate the pain, and so it should be removed a few hours after the operation. Anorectal packing has no place in modern anorectal surgery. Warm heat directed toward the perineum will help relieve the pain during the first 24 hours after operation. The next day, warm sitz baths can be used as treatment. Most pain following hemorrhoidectomy comes from anal sphincter spasm. Another source of pain is the closure of the anoderm and anal verge with tension. It is better to leave the wound open than to close it with tension.

Anal dilatation does not reduce postoperative hemorrhoidal pain and risks incontinence.[76] The use of multimodality techniques with long-acting analgesics (i.e., liposomal bupivacaine) and acetaminophen and nonsteroidal drugs as described in Chapters 5 and 6 has diminished this problem.

Urinary Retention

To minimize urinary retention, a preoperative assessment with good history taking will identify patient with voiding problems such as prostatic hypertrophy and urethral stricture. These should be corrected prior to embarking on an elective rectal procedure. Urinary retention after hemorrhoidectomy is common, but it is unusual following fistulotomy and lateral internal sphincterotomy. Following hemorrhoidectomy, urinary retention has been reported to be as low as 3.5 to 10% if the patient is given a limited amount of intravenous fluid during the operation.[77,78] A retrospective review of 1,026 patients who underwent anal operative care over a 5-year period at the Mayo Clinic revealed a urinary retention rate of 34% for hemorrhoidectomy, 4% for internal sphincterotomy, 5% for incision and drainage of perianal abscesses, and 2% for fistulotomy.[79] Anorectal surgery may dull the sacral parasympathetic nerve fibers controlling contraction of the detrusor muscle of the bladder. Pain from surgery may stimulate the sympathetic nerve to the urethral sphincter, causing spasms.[80]

The rationale of fluid restriction is to avoid distention of the bladder for as long as possible because many patients are unable to void for several hours after anorectal operations. Friend and Medwell[81] have shown that for hemorrhoidectomy in an outpatient setting, urinary retention is uncommon (1%) and that it is not related to the amount of fluid given during the procedure. The type of anesthesia does not seem to affect urinary retention. The reason for the low incidence of urinary retention in the outpatient setting is unclear, but could involve the psychological effect of the home or hotel environment. The authors believe that if the incisions are not beyond the anorectal ring, urinary retention is uncommon. The rare urinary retention is observed in a transsphincteric fistulotomy in which pain is significant, whereas the frequent urinary retention is observed in a transanal excision of low rectum in which there is almost no pain.

Avoiding catheterization, unless the bladder is markedly distended, is the goal. However, excessive bladder distention may cause damage. A single episode of overdistention of the bladder produces chronic changes of irreversible damage to the detrusor muscle.[82] Avoidance of acute bladder overdistention by the judicious use of sterile intermittent catheterization in the postoperative period would appear to involve a low risk of inducing bacteremia and may prevent bladder decompensation.[83] Using bethanechol chloride (Urecholine) to stimulate the detrusor muscle does not help prevent or correct urinary retention after hemorrhoidectomy.[84,85] Similarly, using prazosin, an alpha-adrenergic blocker, to release the bladder neck spasm is also not effective.[86]

For practicality, all patients should void just before undergoing operation. The intravenous fluid during surgery as well as the first few hours after the operation should be limited to 300 mL. Patients should not be pushed or rushed to void, which may cause anxiety. Anal dressing should be removed and a pad used instead.

Infection

It is common for a patient to have a transient low-grade fever after anorectal operations, particularly hemorrhoidectomy, during the first 1 to 2 days as a response to the anal wound. Despite an unprepared bowel and the fecal load, abscess formation following anorectal operations is rare. In a series of 500 closed hemorrhoidectomies reported on by Buls and Goldberg,[78] there were no abscesses recorded. In a study by Bonardi et al,[87] 36 patients had serial blood drawn every 6 hours for 24 hours after hemorrhoidectomy; 39% of the patients developed a fever above 99 °F (37.2 °C) in the first 6 hours, 67% between 99 °F (37.2 °C) and 101 °F (38.3 °C), and one patient had a temperature higher than 101 °F (38.3 °C). Three patients (8%) had positive blood cultures in the immediate postoperative samples but none in the subsequent samples. The significance of fever and bacteremia after hemorrhoidectomy is probably trivial because none of the patients developed further septic complications.

In patients with high fever, other signs of sepsis such as chills, leukocytosis, malaise, and jaundice may be signs of serious complications. Parikh et al[88] reported that two cases of liver abscesses occurred within 1 week after an uncomplicated hemorrhoidectomy. In both cases, the diagnosis was confirmed by CT scan of the abdomen and both were successfully treated with CT-guided percutaneous drainage and antibiotics. The bacteria found were *Streptococcus viridans*, *Peptostreptococcus*, and *Klebsiella pneumoniae*. Pyogenic liver abscess after hemorrhoidectomy is extremely rare. Only four cases have been reported. It is important to be aware of the possibility, because the mortality rate of undrained liver abscesses is between 94 and 100%. Even with treatment, the mortality rate reached 20%.

Delayed complications are defined as those that occur more than 1 week after the operation. These include bleeding, fecal impaction, wound abscess, incontinence, stricture, skin tags, ectropion, mucosal prolapse, and the unhealed wound. Most patients would have been discharged from the hospital by the time they present.

Bleeding

Delayed massive bleeding occurs in 0.8 to 4% of patients after hemorrhoidectomy, usually between 4 and 14 days.[78,89,90] The rate of occurrence is much lower for other anorectal procedures. It has been speculated that the bleeding is caused by the breakdown of the granulating wound during defecation or by infection disrupting the blood vessels and the pedicle of the wound in the anal canal. The patient should be admitted to the hospital and given appropriate intravenous fluids. Patients may be hypotensive, and some may require blood transfusions.[90] Of note is that one-third of patients with post-hemorrhoidectomy bleeding were being anticoagulated with medication such as acetylsalicylic acid (ASA), NSAIDs, or warfarin (Coumadin) in the series reported by Rosen et al.[90]

Most bleeding stops after bed rest. If bleeding continues, some surgeons have used a 30-mL balloon bladder catheter to create a tamponade of the anal canal.[91] However, this method is crude and may cause severe anorectal pain. Rosen et al[90] successfully treated delayed post-hemorrhoidectomy bleeding with packing in 20 of 20 patients. They used a rolled, slightly moistened absorbable gelatin sponge (Gelfoam) packing in the anal canal. However, late complications requiring reoperation developed in 15%.

Another option is taking the patient to the operating room, where the anal canal can be explored with the patient under local, regional, or general anesthesia. Hemostasis is controlled with 3–0 Vicryl or Dexon sutures. Frequently, after all blood clots have been removed, the bleeding point cannot be identified except for a friable anal wound. In these situations, a deep stick-tie should be placed at the pedicle of the anal wound; if oozing blood is noted, the suture line should be redone. Besides providing an immediate control of bleeding, cleaning the anorectum stops the patients from passing old blood, which often makes it difficult to tell whether the bleeding has stopped.

High-risk patients for postoperative bleeding include those on chronic hemodialysis or anticoagulants. Sheikh et al[92] performed these anorectal procedures in 18 patients with chronic renal failure, who were undergoing hemodialysis. Two patients developed postoperative hemorrhage. Only one of them required surgical hemostasis in the operating room on the third postoperative day. None of the patients had delayed wound healing. The authors recommend certain measures to minimize the problems. The final preoperative dialysis should be performed within 24 hours. The bleeding diathesis in patients with chronic renal failure is due to a platelet defect that is corrected by dialysis. They recommend a template bleeding time assessment in addition to standard prothrombin time and partial thromboplastin time testing. Profound anemia (average, 6.1 g/dL in this series) is generally well tolerated by these patients. Preoperative transfusions to raise the hemoglobin level are usually unnecessary and even inadvisable, because transfusion subjects the patient to risk of potassium administration, congestive heart failure, and hepatitis. Intraoperative fluid administration should be severely restricted, and solutions containing potassium avoided. Arteriovenous fistula thrombosis is a frequent and troublesome complication requiring careful positioning of the involved area during surgery. Infusion or measuring blood pressure in that arm should be avoided. It is desirable to delay hemodialysis in the immediate postoperative period because heparin is required for the extracorporeal circuit.[92]

Fecal Impaction

Many patients develop constipation after anorectal procedures, particularly hemorrhoidectomy, partly because of the fear of pain and the lack of the urge to defecate. Patients who require a large amount of analgesics, particularly morphine, are also prone to constipation. Codeine is contraindicated in anorectal surgery because it severely disturbs the motility of the GI tract. Prevention of constipation is the best treatment. Eating plenty of fruits and vegetables along with other high roughage foods is ideal advice. Psyllium seed preparations may not prove beneficial for all patients, especially if such preparations have not been prescribed preoperatively. Laxatives should be given early usually on the first postoperative day, and the dosage should be increased gradually to the maximum until the patient has a good bowel movement. Polyethylene glycol (17 g orally once or twice a day in fluid) assists in keeping the stool soft.

Fecal impaction may be difficult to diagnose in the postoperative period. Usual symptoms are increasing pain or pressure in the perineum and sometimes diarrhea from overflow of stool around the impaction. Pain out of proportion is a good indication of fecal impaction. Digital rectal examination will reveal a fecal bolus in the anorectum. If the pain is severe, the surgeon may use a small cotton swab lubricated with KY jelly instead of the finger. If the patient has fecal impaction, and laxatives and enemas have failed to work, it may be necessary to evacuate the impaction in the operating room with the patient under anesthesia. Tap water or other kinds of enemas often do not work in that situation because water cannot be passed into the rectum.

Fecal impaction is a serious complication following anorectal operations. Fortunately, it is uncommon. Impaction occurs in only 0.4% of patients, usually after hemorrhoidectomy.[78] The low incidence should be credited to careful attention to bowel movements after anorectal operations, a common practice among colorectal surgeons.

Anal Wound Abscess

Despite continuing fecal contamination after operation, abscess in the anal wound is rare. In a report on 500 patients who underwent closed hemorrhoidectomy, Buls and Goldberg[78] recorded no abscesses. Walker et al[93] reported a perianal abscess in 2% of 306 patients, following internal sphincterotomy for anal fissure and anal stenosis.

Fecal Incontinence

Most patients experience some degree of incontinence, particularly of gas and liquid stool, after anorectal procedures for anal fissure, fistula-in-ano, and hemorrhoids. Anal sensation is partially impaired, leading to some degree of incontinence in up to 50% of patients after hemorrhoidectomy, but it usually resolves within 6 weeks.[94] Persistent incontinence after operation for a transsphincteric or extrasphincteric fistulotomy may be improved by a sphincteroplasty (see Chapter 14).

Anal Stricture

Stricture or narrowing of the anal canal after hemorrhoidectomy is the direct result of excising too much anoderm and mucosa. Even in circumferential prolapsed hemorrhoids, a standard three-quadrant hemorrhoidectomy is all that is necessary. The redundant mucosa can be trimmed, but there is no need to denude the anal canal.

Mild anal stricture can be treated by the surgeon with a Hegar dilator, or a rectal dilator can be inserted by the patient at home. Severe stricture will require a lateral internal sphincterotomy or a lateral sphincterotomy with an island flap anoplasty.

Anal Skin Tags

Some excess skin around the anus does not cause any problem. After hemorrhoidectomy, the anal verge frequently becomes swollen and engorged with edema. On occasion, a thrombosed external hemorrhoid develops. With time, this swollen skin will partially resolve, and the patient is left with a residual skin tag. The skin tag may lead to irritation, discomfort, and difficulty in personal hygiene. Unless symptomatic, skin tags can be left alone; otherwise, a simple excision can be performed in the office with the patient under local anesthesia.

Ectropion

Ectropion is a deformity of the anal canal characterized by protrusion of rectal mucosa through the anus at rest (▶ Fig. 35.9). It is a complication resulting from an improperly performed Whitehead hemorrhoidectomy, in which the mucosa is pulled down to the anoderm for suturing instead of mobilizing the anoderm upward for suturing to the rectal

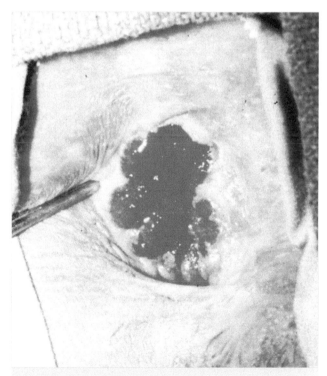

Fig. 35.9 Ectropion following a hemorrhoidectomy.

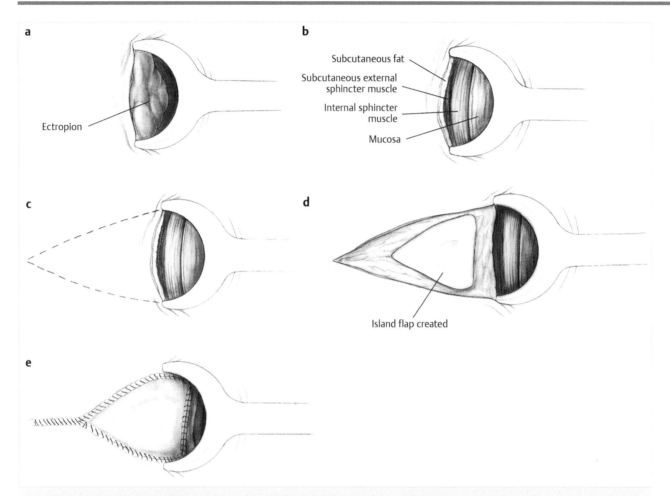

Fig. 35.10 Island flap anoplasty. **(a)** Ectropion is exposed with the Hill–Ferguson retractor. **(b)** Ectropion in left half is excised up into midanal canal. Care is taken not to injure external and internal sphincter muscles. **(c)** Pear-shaped island skin flap is outlined. **(d)** Island flap is created. **(e)** Flap is slid to cover entire defect with running 3–0 Vicryl or Dexon sutures. Better yet, using interrupted subcuticular stitches with inverted knots, 3–0 PDS or Maxon, makes the wound heal neater. For circumferential ectropion, the other half is performed in the same manner.

mucosa.[95] The mucosa secretes mucus, which causes irritation and a "wet" anus. Excision with resuture of the mobilized skin into the upper anal canal may solve the problem. In most severe cases, an island flap anoplasty is the procedure of choice (▶ Fig. 35.10).

Mucosal Prolapse

This is a late complication of hemorrhoidectomy resulting from inadequate excision of the redundant rectal mucosa or from the rectal mucosa being pulled down too far during suturing. In mild cases, rubber band ligation is effective. In severe cases, excision or anoplasty is necessary.

Unhealed Wound

Healing following a closed hemorrhoidectomy occurs rapidly. If the wound is closed without tension, it should heal completely within 2 weeks. If the wound is partially separated, it will take longer to heal. For open hemorrhoidectomy, the wound should heal within 4 to 6 weeks. Occasionally, the wounds following both open and closed hemorrhoidectomy do not heal, leaving an unhealed ulcer. The same is true for fistulotomy wounds, which in most cases are open ones. Most of the unhealed wounds are found in the posterior midline of the anal canal. Initially anal hygiene and curettage of granulation tissue should be tried. If this fails after several months of adequate local care, excision with a sliding skin flap to cover the wound should be performed. Because an unhealed wound that progresses may be an indication of Crohn's disease, a complete GI investigation may be necessary.

35.4.2 Colorectal Operations

Thromboembolism

Thromboembolism is a general complication that may follow any operation and as such will not be discussed here. However, because thromboembolism that occurs in inflammatory bowel disease (IBD) is unique, it is essential for surgeons to have some knowledge of this phenomenon and to recognize the problem.

The incidence of thromboembolism associated with IBD is 1 to 7% in various series.[96] In autopsy studies, it has been reported as 7 to 39%.[96] In a series from the Mayo Clinic, an incidence of 1.3% among 7,199 patients with IBD was reported.[97] Thromboembolism proved to be a grave complication in IBD patients because 25% of them died. In one autopsy series, pulmonary embolism and venous thrombosis ranked third in frequency (9%) as a cause of death in patients with ulcerative colitis, behind peritonitis (38%), and malignant neoplasm (12%).[98]

Thromboses can be venous or arterial. These have been reported to be found in the brain, retinal arteries, mesenteric veins,[99] portal veins,[100] skin, and peripheral deep veins. Of 92 thromboembolic episodes in the Mayo Clinic series, 66% were peripheral or deep venous thromboses, pulmonary emboli, or both.[97] Risk of thromboembolic complications seems to increase with increased disease activities, and thrombosis may recur with another episode. Of 113 patients with thromboembolic complications and other vasculitis, 72 (64%) had active disease at the time and 7 (6%) had a history of recurrent thromboembolic episodes with exacerbated IBD.

The mechanism of thrombosis in IBD is not clear. Most authors point to a hypercoagulable state associated with exacerbations of IBD, including thrombocytosis; elevations in factors V and VIII, and fibrinogen; and a decrease in antithrombin. In contrast, patients with inactive chronic IBD showed no evidence of coagulopathy that might predispose to clotting.[96] A study by Hudson et al[101] showed that the most consistent abnormality is an increase in plasma VII:C concentrations, particularly in patients with Crohn's disease. Increased concentrations of plasma might lead to complications such as microvascular damage and inflammation in the intestinal wall by augmenting focal fibrin deposition on the luminal surface of inflamed vessels. There is no evidence that the plasma concentration is an acute phase reactant.

No controlled trials of anticoagulation have been performed in patients with thrombosis associated with IBD. No data exist on the acute effects of colectomy on the course of thrombosis, and there are no comparisons of lasting medical treatment versus immediate colectomy for thrombosis. In an autopsy series reported by Graef et al,[98] medically treated patients had a significantly higher incidence of venous thrombosis (45%) than those who underwent operation (29%). In the series reported by Talbot et al,[97] 15 stable patients underwent resection of diseased bowel after an episode of deep venous thrombosis or pulmonary embolism. None died postoperatively, and of the 13 patients who were followed up, 12 remained free of recurrent thrombosis 2 to 9 years later. Operation in the acute setting, however, actually may increase the risk of thrombosis and is no guarantee that further trouble will not develop.

The use of subcutaneous heparin for prophylaxis in hospitalized patients with acute IBD should be evaluated, with the judgment made against the risk of severe colonic bleeding. Using heparin may help prevent thrombosis in the postoperative period. For patients with severe deep venous thrombosis of the lower extremities and the pelvis, a caval filter should be considered before colonic resection is performed.

Splenic Injury

Operative injury to the spleen accounts for 20 to 40% of all splenectomies performed in hospitals, in the United States. Neither the incidence of this mishap nor its complications have lessened appreciably in the last three decades.[102]

Splenic injury can occur during both colorectal operations (0.8%) and operations in which mobilization of the spleen is performed (3%).[103] The injury is invariably an avulsion of the splenic capsule caused by tearing the normal splenic attachments (i.e., gastrosplenic, splenocolic, phrenicosplenic, and phrenicocolic ligaments), or it may be caused by traction on the greater omentum. In one series, half of the splenic injuries were due to traction on an omental band leading to the spleen.[103] Injury can occur even before mobilization of the splenic flexure. A common site of capsular tear is a small area (~1 cm) on the anterior or medial aspect of the lower pole of the spleen. Often, there is a definite peritoneal band running medially from the lower pole of the spleen to the greater omentum and adjacent to the greater curvature of the stomach. The band does not become prominent until the stomach is drawn across to the right. Very little traction is needed to pull the band from the spleen and cause bleeding. This band, for which there seems to be no detailed description in most textbooks, usually will be noted if the surgeon looks for it. Lord and Gourevitch[104] have given it the name "lieno-omental band of peritoneum" (▸ Table 35.1).

Another area where a splenic tear commonly occurs is the hilum. The greater omentum, as it passes to the left, becomes continuous with the gastrosplenic ligament. In most individuals, the greater omentum divides, giving rise to an anterior sheet of omentum that hangs down as an apron of variable length from the greater curvature, partially marking the gastrosplenic ligament.[104] This anterior or presplenic omental fold can be torn if the stomach or the greater omentum is pulled to the right.

To avoid capsular tear, these omental folds should be incised before any traction is placed on the greater omentum and stomach and before mobilization of the splenic flexure is begun. For safe exploration of the left upper quadrant and mobilization of the splenic flexure, it is important to have adequate exposure and assistant help. Placing the patient in stirrups, with the operator standing between the patient's legs, will facilitate the procedure, especially in obese patients.

Every attempt should be made to save the spleen. Most capsular tears can be managed by compressing the bleeding points with microfibrillar collagen pledgets (e.g., Avitine). It may be necessary to completely mobilize the spleen in order to adequately compress it. A splenectomy is reserved as a last resort only. Most extensive iatrogenic splenic injuries can be controlled by a partial splenectomy. Morgenstern and Shapiro[105] have recommended the following very useful techniques: control of splenic vasculature and control of parenchymatous bleeding.

Control of Splenic Vasculature

The entire spleen should be mobilized medially toward the anterior abdominal wall. The splenic artery is identified as it courses above the pancreas. This artery should be isolated and encircled with a vessel loop for occlusion if necessary. No attempt is made to isolate the fragile splenic veins. The use of vascular clamps for temporary control of the splenic pedicle is not advised because they produce trauma and may result in venous injury. The splenic arterial branches are carefully dissected at or near the splenic hilum. The most constant branch is the superior polar artery, which arises one to several centimeters from the hilum as the first branch of the splenic artery before it enters the spleen. For injury of the superior pole, the superior polar vessel is doubly tied with 2–0 silk. Tying the segmental artery results in almost immediate branching of the dearterialized segment. Arteries to the lower pole of the spleen may be identified and ligated if branching takes place outside the spleen. For a lower pole injury, if segmental arteries cannot be identified, it may be necessary to tie the main splenic artery distal to the superior pole. Once the segmental branch or branches have been ligated, a scalpel incision is made into the splenic parenchyma at the line of demarcation.

Control of Parenchymatous Bleeding

If excessive bleeding occurs as the initial incision is made, partial control may be achieved by temporarily occluding the splenic artery with the thumb on the vessel loop. The dissection is performed with the back of the scalpel handle, a suction tip, or a peanut sponge. As the vessels are encountered, they are clipped and divided. Large segmental veins should be spared. Following the transection of the splenic parenchyma, a number of bleeding sites will remain. Arterial bleeders are grasped with forceps and clipped. If this is not successful, a figure-of-eight suture should be used. Open linear venous channels are controlled with running sutures. The residual sinusoidal bleeding can be controlled by the use of topical microfibrillar collagen pledgets. Electrocautery is unsatisfactory for maintaining splenic parenchymal hemostasis. However, occasionally it may be useful for minor capsular bleeding points. Heat-induced coagulum poses the threat of delayed bleeding when it sloughs. If such control cannot be achieved, through and through parenchymal sutures are necessary, with 2–0 chromic catgut used on a straight or curved GI needle.

Prevention and Treatment of Postsplenectomy Infection

Fulminant, potentially life-threatening infection is a major long-term risk after splenectomy. Splenic macrophages have an important filtering and phagocytic role in removing bacteria and parasitized RBCs from the circulation. Although the liver can perform this function in the absence of a spleen, higher levels of specific antibody and an intact complement system are probably required. The ability of a splenic patient to mount an adequate protective antibody response may relate more to the indication for or age at splenectomy and to the presence of underlying immune suppression than to the absence of the spleen.

Most instances of serious infection are due to encapsulated bacteria such as *Streptococcus pneumoniae* (*pneumococcus*), *Haemophilus influenzae* type B, and *Neisseria meningitidis* (*meningococcus*). Pneumococcal infection is most common and carries a mortality rate of up to 60%. Infection with *H. influenzae* type B is much less common but nonetheless significant, particularly in children. *Meningococcus* may also be associated with serious infection. Other infections include *Escherichia coli*, malaria, babesiosis (a rare tick-borne infection), and *Capnocytophaga canimorsus* (DF-2 bacillus), which is associated with dog bites.[106]

Immunization

The current available polyvalent pneumococcal vaccine contains purified capsular polysaccharide from the 23 most prevalent serotypes. The vaccine is greater than 90% effective in healthy adults younger than 55 years. The patient should be immunized as soon as possible after recovery from the operation and before discharge from hospital. Immunization, however, should be delayed at least 6 months after immune-suppressive chemotherapy, during which time prophylactic antibiotics should be given. Re-immunization of asplenic patients is currently recommended every 5 to 10 years.[106] Additional immunizations should be administered for influenza and meningitis.

Current recommendations for immunizations, antibiotic prophylaxis, and treatment of acute infections should be reviewed when an asplenic patient is encountered.

Presacral Hemorrhage

During mobilization of the rectum, presacral bleeding can occur if the presacral fascia is stripped and the presacral vein is torn. Although the bleeding is brisk, it usually can be controlled with packing, a stick-tie, or electrocautery, balloon tamponade, breast implant tamponade, and muscle fragment welding.[107, 108,109,110,111] Bleeding from the spongy bone of the sacrum is usually mild and only a nuisance. On rare occasions, it can be massive and life threatening.

A study by Wang et al[112] revealed that in 15% of Chinese patients the basivertebral vein connects the presacral vein and the internal vertebral vein and is usually located at the level of S3–S5 (▶ Fig. 35.11). Bleeding from this vein is not only massive, but also cannot be controlled by packing, electrocautery, stick-tie, or occlusion with bone wax because of the high pressure. The only effective method of temporarily stopping this type of bleeding is occluding the bleeding point with the index finger. For the permanent arrest of this type of hemorrhage, a thumbtack can be used.[113]

To be successful, the pin has to be driven into the hole in the sacrum to plug it. A thumbtack made of material compatible with the body, such as titanium, is preferred (▶ Fig. 35.12 and ▶ Fig. 35.13).[37,40] Unfortunately, a laparoscopic delivered presacral tack is not currently commercially available. Other successful methods are also available. Xu and Lin[110] originally used a piece of rectus muscle fragment, holding it against the bleeding point of the perineal vein with a long forceps. The muscle was then indirectly electrocoagulated using high current until it melted and sealed the bleeding point. Harrison et al[114] successfully used this technique in eight patients with basivertebral bleeding. Remzi et al[115] harvested a 4 × 2 × 1 cm piece of rectus abdominis and sutured the presacral fascia onto the bleeding point to tamponade it. They reported success in two patients.

The diagnosis of bleeding from the basivertebral vein is not difficult. The blood rapidly fills the pelvis. The location is almost always between S3 and S5. The bleeding point can be felt with the index finger as a crater or an opening about 5 mm in size. This potentially fatal complication can be avoided by preserving the presacral fascia during mobilization of the rectum. Sharp dissection of the posterior rectum with scissors or electrocautery is recommended rather than blunt dissection by hand.

Anastomotic Bleeding

Early postoperative bleeding from a colorectal or an ileocolic anastomosis is uncommon regardless of technique provided there is no bleeding diathesis. All techniques of anastomosis

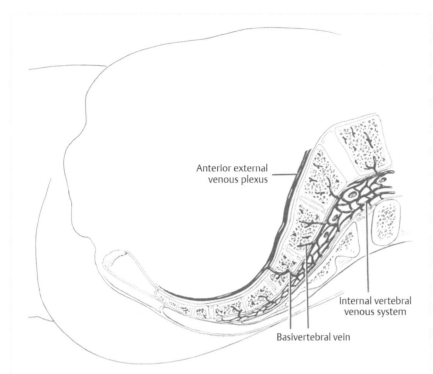

Fig. 35.11 Venous system of sacrum.[113] (Reproduced with permission from Wolters Kluwer.)

Anterior external
venous plexus

Internal vertebral
venous system

Basivertebral vein

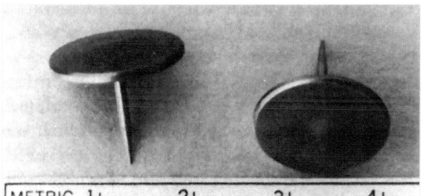

Fig. 35.12 Homemade titanium thumbtacks, not commercially available. Hemorrhage occlude pin, commercially available from Surgin Surgical Instrument, Inc. (Tustin, CA) comes with set of two pins.[113] (Reproduced with permission from Wolters Kluwer.)

involve some degree of hemostasis. The oozing of blood at the cut ends of the bowel should not be disturbed unless there is an active arterial pumper, in which case the pumper is individually ligated or cauterized. Suture line bleeding following the application of the anastomotic stapler can be controlled easily with suture ligatures or reinforcement of the anastomosis with an absorbable suture.

The diagnosis of anastomotic bleeding in the early postoperative period is difficult and usually is determined by deduction. Always, upper GI bleeding must be excluded. Proctoscopy or flexible sigmoidoscopy should be performed to rule out the presence of any lesion in the anorectum. Even if the anastomosis is in the lower left colon, it can be examined. Colonoscopy should not be performed for a high anastomosis in the early postoperative period because of the danger of disruption of the anastomosis. Selective arteriography is one option, with the possibility of stopping the bleeding with vasopressin. However, vasopressin may involve the risk of ischemia and eventual anastomotic leak.

Initially, the management of anastomotic hemorrhage is conservative. The patient must be closely monitored and resuscitated. Bleeding diathesis must be corrected. Bleeding from a low anastomosis in the anorectum can be controlled by a perianal approach with fulguration or suture of the bleeding point. Most high colonic anastomoses require an exploratory celiotomy. Reinforcement sutures are applied, but a resection and reanastomosis may be necessary.

Injury to Ureter

Because of the proximity of the ureters to the colon, intraoperative injury to the ureters can occur particularly when there are

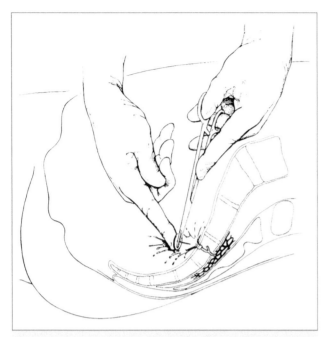

Fig. 35.13 Technique of occluding basivertebral vein of sacrum with thumbtack.[113] (Reproduced with permission from Wolters Kluwer.)

severe adhesions in that region from multiple previous operations, a malignancy, an inflammatory process, or previous radiation. However, intraoperative ureteral injuries are not common during colorectal operations. It is important to note that only 20 to 30% of iatrogenic ureteral injuries are recognized or detected at the time of operation.[116] This is crucial because immediate repair of the injury results in good healing. When recognition of the problem is delayed, the outcome becomes unpredictable and the incidence of nephrectomy increases sevenfold. It is helpful to remember that "the venial sin is injury to the ureter, but the mortal sin is failure of recognition."[117]

Mechanisms of Injury

For practical purposes, the ureter can be considered as two segments of approximately equal length: the abdominal ureter and the pelvic ureter. The abdominal ureter originates from the renal pelvis and courses downward on the anterior surface of the psoas muscle. As the ureter enters the pelvis, it crosses the iliac artery at the junction of the internal and external iliac arteries. The ureter then tracks posteriorly and inferiorly along the curvature of the pelvis down to the levator ani muscle, where it crosses under the superior vesical artery before entering the posterior aspect of the bladder. In the female, the pelvic ureter lies in the uterosacral ligament as it courses behind the ovary and then continues inferiorly in the portion of the broad ligament.

Most intraoperative ureteral injuries result from gynecologic procedures and occur at the pelvic brim, but they also may result from colorectal operations. In a series reported by Higgins,[117] 61 of 87 iatrogenic ureteral injuries resulted from gynecologic procedures, 12 from colorectal procedures (11 abdominoperineal resections and 1 sigmoid colostomy), 8 from vascular procedures, 5 from urologic procedures, and 1 from an

orthopaedic procedure. In colonic operations, the left ureter is more commonly injured than the right.[118] Types of injuries include ligation, crush injury, transection (partial or complete), and ischemic injury.[119]

There are four specific situations that involve the risk of injury to the ureter during colorectal procedures: (1) ligation of the inferior mesenteric artery, (2) procedures performed near the cul-de-sac, where the ureter crosses the vas deferens of the sacral promontory, (3) division of the lateral stalks of the rectum, and (4) reperitonealization when the ureter may be included in ligatures.[117]

Recognition of Intraoperative Injury

Visual inspection is the most reliable means of assessing ureteral integrity. If there is doubt, methylene blue can be injected intravenously. Extravasation of blue-tinged urine or dye will confirm diagnosis. For delayed diagnosis, retrograde pyelography is the most sensitive radiographic tool for identifying ureteral extravasation or obstruction from ligation.[119] Ureteral catheters do not reduce the incidence of injury, but significantly improve the intraoperative identification of an injury.

Ureteral Repair

Repair of ureteral injuries requires good judgment, experience, and skill. It should be performed by a surgeon who is thoroughly familiar with this type of repair. In general, injuries detected intraoperatively or within the first few days postoperatively in a stable patient should be repaired immediately. When patient is unstable or the detection is delayed for several days or weeks, the patient should undergo immediate proximal urinary diversion followed by delayed repair. In most cases, proximal urinary diversion can be achieved by placement of a percutaneous nephrostomy catheter.[119]

When the ureter has been inadvertently ligated intraoperatively, often all that is necessary is removal of the suture. If the ureter has been crushed by a clamp, the likelihood of injury is higher. The adventitia must be inspected carefully for discoloration because ischemic injury may take several days to manifest itself fully. If the adventitia is nonviable, a repair should be performed.

The general principles of ureteral repair include debridement of nonviable tissues, tension anastomosis, and mucosa-to-mucosa reapproximation. Partial transection often can be managed by primary closure with interrupted 4–0 or 5–0 absorbable sutures. Usually complete transection and ischemic injuries can be repaired by resection of the injured segment followed by ureteroureterostomy. All ureteral repairs (primary closures or ureteroureterostomies) should be drained. All complete transections and most partial transections should be stented, such as with a double-J stent. Complete transection of the pelvic ureter or extensive ischemic injury will often be best handled by ureteral reimplantation.[119] Various methods of repairs for ureteral injuries have been described by Hamawy et al.[120]

When a difficult operation is anticipated, as may occur with a large malignant mass, an inflammatory mass in the pelvis, or in those who have undergone severe radiation, the risk of ureteral injury can be minimized by preoperative placement of ureteral catheters. This measure will make identification of the ureters easier, although there is no guarantee that injury can be eliminated completely. The complications of preoperative ureteral placement are trivial.[121] In the series reported by Bothwell et al,[121] ureteral catheterization was attempted in 92 patients who underwent a left colectomy. It was successful bilaterally in 87% and unilaterally in 98%. A transmural ureteral injury occurred in 0.43%. Surgical injury to the ureter occurred in one patient (1.1%) despite ureteral placement.

Bladder Dysfunction

Problems with bladder function are encountered in 20 to 30% of patients undergoing colon and rectal procedures.[122] Several causes of urinary retention include anesthesia and sedation, stimulation of the anovesical reflex by operation, local pain, and anal packing.

Micturition is a reflex process. Parasympathetic nerves innervate the detrusor muscle. Sympathetic nerves innervate the bladder neck, trigone, and urethral area.[122] Injury to the autonomic nerves in the pelvis causes bladder dysfunction. Moreover, loss of the posterior support of the bladder after low anterior resection or abdominoperineal resection may add to the problem.[123,124] Kinn and Ohman[123] studied 26 patients who underwent resection for rectal carcinoma. All patients had undergone urodynamic studies preoperatively and 6 months postoperatively; interviews concerning bladder and sexual function also were obtained. Seven of 26 patients had impaired urinary voiding in the early postoperative course. At follow-up after 6 months, however, there was no significant decrease of detrusor contractility that would indicate persistent parasympathetic denervation. No patients had total detrusor paralysis. The low incidence of bladder dysfunction in the late postoperative phase probably indicates a time-related nerve regeneration, which is also supported by histologic studies.

In all patients with pelvic dissection, the bladder catheter is left in place for 24 to 48 hours. Usually, the bladder dysfunction improves gradually. In some patients, the dysfunction persists when they are ready to be discharged. In this situation, instructions should be given for intermittent self-catheterization. Permanent bladder dysfunction is rare after a colorectal procedure. In symptomatic cases in men, the indication for prostatic surgery should be liberal because even minor obstruction added to slight neurogenic detrusor muscle dysfunction could cause severe voiding difficulties.[123]

Sexual Dysfunction

As in bladder dysfunction, injuries to pelvic parasympathetic and sympathetic nerves give rise to impotence. The degree and pattern of impotence depends on the nerve involved and can be partial or complete. Potency is defined as the ability to achieve an erection sufficient for vaginal penetration and orgasm. Usually for most patients, sexual dysfunction following operation resolves gradually during the first year. Thus, the minimum follow-up interval for determining whether a patient is potent is 1 year.[125]

Penile erection is mediated by a coordinated vascular and neurologic event that results in increased inflow of blood to the corpora cavernosa, dilatation of venous sinusoids within the pelvis, and decreased outflow from the corpora cavernosa.[125] In addition to the important role of the parasympathetic nerves in initiating the vascular events required to achieve full erection, the somatic nervous system (pudendal nerve) also plays an important role in penile rigidity. Stimulation of the dorsal nerve of the penis will trigger the bulbocavernosus reflex. Contraction of the ischiocavernosus muscle compresses the proximal corpora cavernosa and further increases the intracavernous pressure to a level well above the systolic pressure, resulting in the penile rigidity commonly occurring during the heights of masturbation or sexual intercourse.[125,126] The pudendal nerves, which are well protected by the endopelvic fascia, are not usually damaged during a colorectal procedure. The neurologic input for erection is primarily from the parasympathetic nerves (nervi erigentes). Emission and ejaculation are mediated predominantly by sympathetic nerves that travel from the thoracolumbar region of the spinal cord along the sympathetic ganglia and down the hypogastric nerves to the pelvic plexus.[52]

Injury to the hypogastric nerves in the retroperitoneal space just above the promontory of the sacrum may result in ejaculatory dysfunction. Excessive traction on the rectum with anterior displacement of the rectum secondary to mobilization posterior to the rectum may result in neurapraxia or avulsion of sacral roots two, three, and four (nervi erigentes). Depending on the severity of injury, this could result in temporary or permanent bladder and/or erectile dysfunction. Such injuries may be prevented by recognizing these possibilities and avoiding excessive traction.[125]

Direct injuries to the pelvic plexus may occur during division of the rectal ligaments. The location of the pelvic plexus may be identified intraoperatively by its relationship to the tip of the seminal vesicles. Experience with radical prostatectomy has shown that it is possible to preserve erectile function (and therefore, possible bladder function) despite wide unilateral resection of these nerves. Injuries to the cavernous nerves during perineal dissection of the rectum may result in erectile dysfunction as well. After division of the rectourethralis muscle in the midline anterior to the rectum, the neurovascular bundles may be seen in association with the lateral prostatic fascia coursing from the urethra along the posterolateral surface of the prostate. These neurovascular bundles are anterolateral to the rectum. Excessive use of cauterization or blind blunt dissection in this region may result in injury to these nerves.[125]

It is important to remember that during any pelvic operation, ligation of the anterior division or distal branch of the internal iliac artery may result in vasculogenic impotence, especially if bilateral ligation of the internal pudendal vessels occurs.[125]

The incidence of sexual dysfunction following operation of the rectum depends on many factors. These include the age of the patient, the nature of the disease, and the extent of the procedure. A review of the literature by Walsh and Schlegel[125] showed that erectile dysfunction occurred in 46% of 641 men undergoing abdominoperineal resection for carcinoma and in 15% of those who underwent low anterior resection. Ejaculatory dysfunction occurred in 35 and 44% in the two groups, respectively. Havenga et al[127] of Memorial Sloan Kettering Cancer Center in New York reported the results of radical total mesorectal excision with an abdominoperineal resection and low anterior resection, with autonomic nerve preservation for carcinoma of the rectum. The authors retrospectively studied postoperative sexual and urinary function in 136 patients (82 men and 54 women). Patients who had preoperative dysfunction were excluded. The ability to engage in intercourse was maintained by 86% of the patients younger than 60 years of age and by 67% of patients 60 years of age or older. Eighty-seven percent of male patients maintained their ability to achieve orgasm. An abdominoperineal resection had a higher incidence of erectile dysfunction than an anterior resection. Of the female patients, 85% were able to experience arousal with vaginal lubrication, and 91% could achieve orgasm. Serious urinary dysfunction such as a neurogenic bladder was not encountered. Excellent results were also obtained by Masui et al[128] when the autonomic nerve–preserving technique was used.

Sexual dysfunction following proctectomy for benign diseases such as ulcerative colitis has a much lower incidence. The incidence of impotence in men who had undergone an ileoanal pouch procedure was 1.6 to 2.0% and retrograde ejaculation was 2.0 to 2.3%.[129] The incidence of dyspareunia in women was 7.0 to 8.3%.[129,130,131] These lower incidences reflect the less extensive dissection and the younger age group of patients, usually in their early 30 s. Lindsey et al[132] found no difference in damage to pelvic sexual nerves between close rectal dissection (dissection within mesorectum, close to rectal wall) and anatomical mesorectal plane, in rectal excision for IBD. In their series of 156 patients, total impotence occurred in 3.8%; they were all in the 50- to 70-year-old age group, and there were no ejaculatory difficulties. Minor diminution of erectile function occurred in 13.5%, where sexual activity was still possible. The median follow-up was 74.5 months. Age was the most important risk factor for postoperative impotence.

Peroneal Nerve Injury

The so-called synchronous or modified lithotomy position is now standard for an abdominoperineal resection, total proctocolectomy, low anterior resection with stapled anastomosis, low anterior resection with coloanal anastomosis, and ileoanal pouch procedures. The patient is placed on his or her back with both legs on stirrups. Lloyd Davies stirrups were previously used for positioning the patient. The problem with this equipment is its lack of support of the feet, which makes it necessary to put the patient's calves on the resting pads. If the positioning is not carefully adjusted or if the procedure lasts longer than 6.5 hours,[133] the risk of excessive compression to the calf muscle or peroneal nerve is increased. This varies according to how the patient is positioned and how heavy the patient is. Lloyd Davies stirrups have now been replaced by Allen stirrups or Yellofins stirrups in the United States.

The common peroneal nerve leaves the posterior aspect of the knee and extends laterally around the head of the fibula, where it is extremely superficial and prone to injury. The surgeon must be thoroughly familiar with the patient's history, physical and laboratory findings, and even occupation. Before operation, the patient with a peripheral nerve lesion may have had any of the several conditions (e.g., diabetes, arteriosclerosis, herniated disk, aneurysm, neuritis, or neuroma) that could be responsible for the nerve dysfunction now manifested. Diseased nerves will not withstand even short periods of compression, ischemia, or slight degrees of trauma that would be withstood readily by normal nerves.[134] The common sign of peroneal nerve injury is foot drop, often associated with an area of sensory loss in the lateral surface of the leg and dorsum of the foot.

A rapid test can be performed to rule out a peroneal nerve injury. If dorsiflexion of the big toe is present, the peroneal nerve is intact.[134] In the series reported by Herrera-Ornelas et al,[135] of 10 injuries in 8 patients, 7 resolved without deficit on conservative management alone.

Compartment Syndrome

Another important complication is prolonged compression of the calf muscle that results in development of a compartment syndrome. Acute compartment syndrome is a condition in which raised pressure within closed and unyielding facial space reduces capillary perfusion below a level that is necessary for tissue viability leading to muscle and nerve ischemia within a few hours.

Pressure has been seen to arise in the compartments of the leg after some ileoanal pouch procedures lasting 6 to 9 hours.[136] The compartment pressure is increased when there is head-down tilt into the Trendelenburg position. Pressures have been shown to rapidly return to normal on taking the legs down from the stirrups and placing the legs into the supine position. This maneuver has been recommended during operations lasting for more than 5 hours.[136] Trendelenburg with a 15-degree head-down tilt results in an immediate fall in leg perfusion. Perfusion returns to normal on positioning the legs flat. Acidosis, intraoperative hypotension, and vasoconstricting agents may increase intracompartmental ischemia.

The height of elevation of the legs above the level of the heart is crucial. For every centimeter the calves are raised above the right atrium, arteriolar pressure is reduced by 0.78 mm Hg. A 15-degree head-down tilt has been shown to cause an additional significant decline in blood flow to the limb. If the extreme knee-chest position is used, it can lead to direct compression of blood supply to the lower limb. The calf compartmental pressure can rise from a normal value of 20 up to 240 mm Hg in the lithotomy position. Compartmental pressure may increase even further when adequate tissue perfusion is restored by returning the patient to the supine position, because a reperfusion injury develops. This postoperative hyperemia reaches its peak 2 hours after completing operation.

Cited risk factors for the compartment syndrome include lithotomy position, compromise of blood supply to the periphery, compression of pelvic blood vessels, hypotension, hypovolemia, vasoconstriction, hypothermia, obesity, and ischemic time greater than 6 hours.[137]

The diagnosis of an impending compartment syndrome may be considered with any of the "6 Ps":
- Progressive pain out of proportion to the clinical situation.
- Paresthesia in peripheral nerve distribution.
- Paresis and pain on passive stretch of muscles.
- Pink skin.
- Presence of pulse until the compartment pressure exceeds arterial inflow pressure.
- Compartment pressure of greater than 30 mm Hg in any osteofascial compartment.

The presence of myoglobin in the urine suggests an impending compartment syndrome. Serum creatine kinase may be elevated. A definitive diagnosis is made by directly measuring the compartment pressure. The critical compartment pressure value is controversial. A pressure of less than 45 mm Hg can be tolerated and a fasciotomy spared, while others recommend a fasciotomy at 30 mm Hg. A pressure of 50 to 55 mm Hg for 4 to 8 hours will certainly cause irreversible muscle damage.[137]

A compartment syndrome may be difficult to differentiate from a nerve injury or an arterial occlusion. Primary nerve injury is expected to produce a deficit in neuromuscular function, but it should not be progressive after the initial injury. Furthermore, signs and symptoms of ischemia and increased tissue pressure should be absent in primary nerve injury.

Acute arterial occlusion may mimic a compartment syndrome by producing signs of compartment ischemia and loss of neuromuscular function. Peripheral pulses are frequently normal in a compartment syndrome because intracompartmental pressure is usually insufficient to affect arterial flow. The presence of Doppler signal distal to the compartment provides no information about the adequacy of compartment perfusion but may indicate an arterial occlusion. When in doubt about the diagnosis of a compartment syndrome, it may be necessary to perform tissue pressure measurements of the calf and direct nerve stimulation.[138]

Once the diagnosis of a compartment syndrome has been established, operative decompression is indicated. It is preferable to open all compartments—anterior, lateral, superficial, and deep posterior—through a single lateral incision without removing the fibula.[139] Any devitalized tissue should be debrided. The wound should be left open. The patient should be taken to the operating room 3 to 5 days later for reexamination and possible closure if this can be performed without tension.

These measures include the careful positioning of the lower extremities to avoid excessive angulation of the hips, the use of stirrups that support the leg at the ankle rather than at the calf, and maintaining the Trendelenburg position for only that portion of the operation during which pelvic dissection is actually occurring to avoid intraoperative hypotension.

The Allen or Yellofins Universal stirrups are designed so that compression of the legs does not occur because the legs rest on the feet (▶ Fig. 35.14) and have gel pads (viscoelastic polymer) as protector. The knees should be slightly flexed and in a neutral position, without internal or external rotation of the hip.

The legs must be comfortably rested on the feet and there should be no pressure of the calves resting on the stirrups. Because the stirrups that support the leg are short, compression of the peroneal nerve is eliminated. When the legs are properly placed, the risk of leg injury in the lithotomy position should be very low.

Femoral Neuropathy

Femoral nerve injury is uncommon, but it may be underestimated because the majority of cases are not severe and are self-limited. The injury is caused by the commonly used Balfour and Bookwalter self-retaining abdominal retractors. In the first period of a prospective study conducted by Goldman et al,[129] during two 5-year periods, there were 282 cases of postoperative femoral neuropathy following 3,736 abdominal hysterectomies. The neuropathy was attributed to the use of the self-retaining retractor. In the second 5-year period, no self-retaining retractors were used. The authors reported a 0.7% incidence of femoral neuropathy. Recently, Brasch et al[140] reported three cases of femoral neuropathy following colon resections.

Anatomically, the femoral nerve is the largest branch of the lumbar plexus. Branches of the lumbar plexus innervate the psoas major muscle before formation of the femoral nerve. The nerve passes obliquely downward through the psoas major muscle to emerge laterally between the psoas major and iliacus, deep to the iliacus fascia. The femoral nerve enters the thigh lateral to the femoral artery and sheath, where it divides into terminal motor and sensory branches. The signs and symptoms of femoral neuropathy consist of paresis, quadriceps femoris atrophy, hypoesthesia of the anteromedial thigh, and absent or decreased patellar tendon reflex. In a series of 17 patients with femoral neuropathy reported by Kvist-Poulsen and Borel,[141] 94% of patients exhibited sensory deficits and 41% had a decreased or absent patellar reflex or an inability to perform straight leg raising. The prognosis is good. In a series of 282 patients, 265 spontaneously recovered, whereas 17 exhibited mild symptoms for as long as 116 days.[129] A review of 40 patients with postoperative femoral neuropathy in the literature by Celebrezze et al[142] revealed that 24 patients fully recovered spontaneously; 2 patients

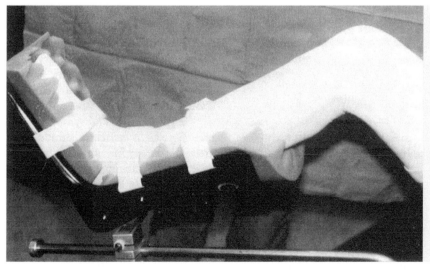

Fig. 35.14 Allen stirrups, showing leg resting on foot without compression of calf.

had permanent deficits; 8 patients had permanent sensory deficit; 5 patients had partial motor deficit; and 1 patient was lost to follow-up.

Retractor injury results from direct compression of the psoas major muscle or impingement of femoral nerve and psoas major against the lateral pelvic wall. Patients who are thin, of short stature, or have poorly developed rectus muscles are prone to this injury. Retractor injury is preventable, given a thorough understanding of femoral nerve anatomy and repeated evaluation of the placement blades during the operative procedure. Retractor pressure should be minimized and the shortest blade used to permit adequate exposure.[140]

Anastomotic Leak

A bowel anastomosis should heal per primam: the capacity of anastomotic healing is dependent on the patient's general and local conditions, such as malnutrition, particularly hypoalbuminemia, diabetes, irradiation, shock, severe blood loss, and immune deficiency. Technical factors at the time of anastomosis are of equal importance, and these vary depending on how the anastomosis is performed. Important technical factors that must be considered during bowel anastomosis include blood supply, tension, condition of bowel lumen, condition of bowel ends, and technique of anastomosis.

The mesentery at or near the transected bowel must be properly dissected, with the surgeon making certain that there is at least an arcade of vessels supplying the area. The fatty tissue should be cleared no more than 5 to 6 mm from the edge. Adequate blood supply is one of the most important factors for proper anastomotic healing. Too much tension at the anastomosis not only causes dehiscence of the anastomosis but also compromises its blood supply. Both bowel ends must be in healthy condition. Bowel that is inflamed and thickened from diverticulitis or radiation enteritis and IBD must be adequately resected until each end has become soft and thin. A generalized edema and thickened bowel from chronic obstruction or malnutrition is a sign of a potential problem.

When performed properly, the bowel anastomosis should heal well. There is no longer an issue of whether the anastomosis is performed with one layer or two layers, with interrupted or continuous sutures, and with a stapling device. These methods are all acceptable. Most anastomotic leaks are from resection of rectosigmoid colon with low anastomosis. The incidence varies from 3 to 15% and the mortality is 2 to 7%.[143,144,145] This wide variation reflects the site of anastomosis, definition of leak, the diligence in its detection, and whether the procedure is performed as an elective or emergency situation. The highest risk of anastomotic leak is at the level below 7 cm.[143,144,145] In a prospective study by Law et al,[146] 196 patients with carcinoma of rectum at 3 to 12 cm from the anal verge were treated by low anterior resection with total mesorectum excision. The only significant factors affecting anastomotic leak were male gender and a diverting stoma. Although surgical technique is important, there are other adverse factors as well, such as chronic obstructive pulmonary disease, peritonitis, bowel obstruction, malnutrition, the use of corticosteroids, and perioperative blood transfusions, smoking, and excessive alcohol abuse.[147]

An anastomotic leak usually becomes apparent between 5 and 7 days postoperatively. Early dehiscence (within 48 hours)

is usually serious because adhesions have not developed. Fecal spillage gives rise to generalized peritonitis. The early signs of an anastomotic leak are those of sepsis, including fever, leukocytosis, localized or generalized tenderness, generalized ileus with abdominal distention, and tachycardia or even shock. The evaluation for an anastomotic leak depends on the patient's condition. In generalized peritonitis, indication of an urgent or emergent exploratory celiotomy, along with other signs of sepsis, is obvious. Any investigation to confirm the diagnosis is unnecessary and only delays treatment. Antibiotic coverage for both aerobes and anaerobes should be started immediately.

For an anastomotic leak that develops after 48 hours, pus or fecal material may be apparent if drain is still in place. Plain abdominal films are useful in stapled anastomoses. If anastomotic dehiscence has occurred, the line or the ring of staples is broken. If the anastomotic leak is not apparent but is suspected, a gentle Gastrografin enema is the most accurate method of identifying the leak. Proctoscopy or flexible sigmoidoscopy may or may not be useful in identifying the dehiscence. A CT scan cannot be used to determine the location of an anastomotic leak, unless intraluminal contrast is administered, but the presence of accumulated fluid may suggest that a leak has occurred.

For practical purposes, the discussion will be limited to leaks that cause generalized peritonitis in the anterior or low anterior resection. The goal of management is to limit morbidity and mortality and to effectively treat the leak and the resulting sepsis.[148,149] The level of treatment depends on the intraoperative findings.

A leak that is caused by necrosis or ischemia at the anastomosis requires its disconnection and a Hartmann procedure. A dehiscence of more than one-third of the circumference should also be disconnected, and a Hartmann procedure performed. Smaller leaks (< 1 cm) can be locally repaired with sutures if the edges of the bowel are healthy, and covered with a piece of omentum if it is available. The area is drained, and a loop ileostomy is performed. If the surrounding area of the anastomosis is cemented from dense inflammation, a suction drain should be placed nearby and a loop ileostomy performed.

The fibrins coated on the peritoneum and on the bowel wall should be scraped off with wet sponges as much as possible. The debris in the abscess cavity is curetted and a suction drain placed. The abdominal cavity is irrigated with copious amounts of normal saline solution.

Anastomotic Stricture

Several factors that contribute to the formation of anastomotic strictures include ischemia, radiation, anastomotic leakage, and recurrent disease (e.g., carcinoma or Crohn's disease). The complication rate has been especially prevalent following low anterior resection of the rectum. From a survey of the members of the American Society of Colon and Rectal Surgeons, Smith[150] found a stenosis incidence of 9% of 3,594 patients who underwent an anastomosis with the end-to-end anastomosis (EEA) stapler. Graffner et al[151] reported that the risk of stricture formation is increased by the establishment of a proximal diverting colostomy. In a series of 73 patients, Gordon and Vasilevsky[152] reported a 20% incidence of stenosis using the circular stapler. Stenosis was defined as failure of the 19-mm sigmoidoscope to pass freely through the anastomosis. Review of the literature reveals that the incidence of rectal anastomotic narrowing varies from 0 to

30%.[153] Few authors have given their definition of stenosis. Kyzer and Gordon[153] considered as stenotic any anastomosis that does not accept the 19-mm sigmoidoscope. Leff et al[154] and Fazio[155] have defined a stricture as a narrowing that does not allow passage of the 15-mm sigmoidoscope. It was postulated that the narrowing was based on ischemia caused by excessive clearing of the mesentery adjacent to the anastomosis.[153] By limiting the clearing of the bowel edges, Kyzer and Gordon[153] noted that the incidence of narrowing was reduced to 12.5%, and in the last 72 cases, this incidence was further reduced to 4.2%.

Fortunately, most anastomotic strictures are asymptomatic and dilate spontaneously during the first postoperative year. When strictures are symptomatic, several procedures have been tried, namely, Hegar dilators, operative intervention, and, more recently, balloon dilatation. Some strictures are thin or membranous and can easily be corrected by a single digital dilatation or sigmoidoscopy, following which bulk-forming agents help maintain patency. Kyzer and Gordon[153] reported a series of 215 anastomoses created, following which 27 patients developed stenosis, but only 8 were permanent and only 3 were symptomatic. Each of those patients was treated with balloon dilatation. Johansson[156] performed endoscopic balloon dilatation of postoperative or radiation-induced rectal strictures on 49 occasions on 18 patients. Of the 114 evaluable patients, 12 were relieved of symptoms. The method is simple and can be accomplished with a number of commercially available balloons. It can be performed as an outpatient procedure. The complication rate is acceptable, and one perforation was reported in the Johansson series. In the colon, anastomotic strictures are uncommon. In a series of 223 anastomoses reported by Kyzer and Gordon,[157] no strictures were noted. The authors' review of the literature revealed reports of stenosis ranging from 0 to 1.1%.

Fecal Incontinence

The technical ability to construct anastomoses at lower and lower levels in the pelvis has resulted in the potential imposition of yet another complication, namely, fecal incontinence. It has been suggested that as many as 5% of patients may have total incontinence and 25% may have changed bowel habits, such as soiling or an increase in stool frequency that may affect their daily lifestyle.[158] Another review suggested 10 to 50% of patients who have undergone sphincter-saving operations complain of "incomplete function"[159]; incontinence rates as high as 60 to 80% following low anterior resection have also been suggested. Restoration of normal anorectal function parameters over a period of 1 year following operation is believed to occur, but approximately 47% continue to suffer incontinence.[160]

Many factors may contribute to postoperative dysfunction. Stapling devices may harm the sphincter muscles, and rectal mobilization may damage innervation of the sphincter. The high frequency of bowel movements after operation is related to loss of reservoir capacity. Decreased compliance of the neorectum is a consistent finding in all studies.[161]

Otto et al[158] studied 17 patients with rectal neoplasms and found that immediately after operation, 14 of 17 patients showed a certain degree of incontinence but recovered during follow-up with only 2 patients reporting minor soiling. Anorectal manometric evaluation revealed that resting and squeeze pressures were moderately reduced after operation and increased during the following 6 months without regaining preoperative levels. This suggests damage to sphincter muscle fibers or innervation. The rectoanal inhibitory reflex was present in 94.4% of patients before operation and in about 25% after operation, but was not associated with incontinence. Rectal sensation was significantly reduced as a result of what was believed to be a loss in reservoir capacity, and its recovery was well correlated with a decrease in the frequency of bowel movements.

In a clinic-physiologic study, Ikeuchi et al[159] found that stapled coloanal anastomoses resulted in a poorer outcome than anterior resection or low anterior resection in terms of soiling and urgency at 12 months. The authors noted that incomplete evacuation was frequently observed in the stapled coloanal anastomoses and low anterior resection groups. Anal manometric parameters recovered in the anterior resection group but not in the other two groups. The authors concluded that the clinical outcome was related to the anastomotic level. This is not universally agreed upon.[160]

Ikeuchi et al[159] related the length of the rectal remnant to the pelvic nervous system. Following anterior resection, the external and internal sphincters, the superior inferior rectal branch, and approximately 10 cm of the rectum remained; following low anterior resection, the external and internal sphincters, the inferior rectal nerve branch, and 4 cm of the rectum remained; and following stapled coloanal anastomoses, the external and internal sphincters, part of the inferior rectal branches, and 2 cm of the rectum remained. Clinically, the daily frequencies of bowel movement and incomplete evacuation were disturbed in the patients who underwent the low anterior resection or stapled coloanal anastomosis procedures. With anterior resection, the remnant rectum and superior rectal branch were longer than with low anterior resection and stapled coloanal anastomosis. The soiling frequency also increased as a result of dissection of the inferior rectal branch. The ability to differentiate between flatus and feces recovered with time. In the early postoperative period, significant differences were observed according to the anastomotic level. No physiologic parameter was shown to be closely related to the change in the frequency of urgency in these patients. However, preservation of the inferior rectal branch may have been involved in the recovery from urgency in the low anterior group by 12 months. Both the maximum resting pressure and maximum squeeze pressure showed identical patterns of recovery, indicating that anal sphincter was preserved in all three procedures. Threshold volume was reportedly correlated with difficult evacuation in patients with a coloanal anastomosis. Threshold volume in the stapled coloanal anastomotic group was significantly lower than in either of the other groups. The only parameter that was significantly higher in the stapled coloanal anastomotic group than in the other groups was the soiling frequency. The authors' study demonstrated that the preserved anal sphincter alone was not sufficient to control either bowel movement frequency or urgency. The reservoir function of the neorectum, which is composed of the colorectal muscle layer and nervous components, plays a role in the maintenance of fecal function.

In another physiologic study, Rao et al[160] concluded that major incontinence is secondary to neurotensin of the inferior mesenteric ganglia and the hypogastric plexus, whereas minor incontinence represents a localized neurotensin/neurapraxia of the inferior mesenteric plexus. Surely other factors play a role in postoperative incontinence, and only time and further studies will clarify the pathogenesis of the problem.

Ileus

Postoperative ileus is a form of temporary bowel motor dysfunction that regularly follows operative procedures in the abdomen. It also occurs after operations remote from the abdomen such as lower extremity arthroplasty[161] and particularly surgery of the brain.[162] The definitions of ileus and methods of assessment are not well defined. Management was discussed in Chapter 5.

Early Mechanical Small Bowel Obstruction

Mechanical small bowel obstruction can occur after any exploratory celiotomy, particularly procedures performed below the transverse mesocolon. Early postoperative small bowel obstruction from operations on organs above the mesocolon, such as biliary tract procedures, is uncommon.[163] In the series reported by Stewart et al,[163] the incidence of early postoperative small bowel obstruction (within 30 days after operation) that required reoperation after a right colectomy was 1.5% and for a left colectomy and resection of rectum it was 3%. A series from Menzies and Ellis[164] showed that the incidence of small bowel obstruction in all cases of exploratory celiotomy was 3.2%. However, operations accounting for the majority of early postoperative adhesive obstructions are large bowel, rectal, and appendiceal procedures as well as gynecologic surgery. In the series by Menzies and Ellis,[164] 39% of small bowel obstructions occurred within 1 year of the abdominal surgery, 21% within 1 month, and 21% more than 10 years after operation.

Diagnosis

The diagnosis of early postoperative small bowel obstruction is difficult and is usually impossible to differentiate from postoperative ileus. For this reason, Pickleman and Lee[165] defined an early postoperative small bowel obstruction as one occurring between 7 and 30 days after the operation. A typical patient with early postoperative small bowel obstruction cannot tolerate removal of the nasogastric tube after 7 days following the operation or would have already started a liquid or soft diet and has developed abdominal distention associated with nausea and vomiting. Ninety percent of postoperative small bowel obstructions occurred during the first 2 weeks after the operation.[165]

Because the clinical signs of small bowel obstruction (abdominal distention, colicky pain, nausea, and vomiting) are nonspecific, the plain film radiographic demonstration of dilated loops of small intestine with air–fluid levels, and minimal or no colonic gas has been considered essential. Unfortunately, plain film examination is diagnostic in only 46 to 80% of cases. The lower percentage probably reflects radiographic findings at the patients' initial presentation, and the high percentage includes patients who underwent follow-up plain film studies.[166]

Management

The management of an early postoperative small bowel obstruction is nasogastric suction and administration of fluid and electrolytes. Nasogastric suction can be continued as long as there is no increased distention of the abdomen, abdominal cramps are not worse, and the body temperature and white blood count are not elevated. With careful monitoring, the obstruction can be treated with nasogastric decompression safely for 10 to 14 days.[165] A total parenteral nutrition should be considered after 1 week of unresolved small bowel obstruction.

In a series of 101 patients with early postoperative small bowel obstruction reported by Pickleman and Lee,[165] obstruction was successfully resolved in 78 patients by nasogastric decompression: 70% resolved within 1 week, 26% within 2 weeks, and 4% within 3 weeks. Five percent of patients died during treatment, but none of the deaths resulted from strangulation or gangrene of the bowel. Among 23 patients with obstruction who underwent exploratory celiotomy, 14 patients (61%) had obstructive bands, 7 patients (31%) had a phlegmon, 1 patient (4%) had an abscess, and 1 patient (4%) had intussusception. Three patients (13%) died after the operation, but none of the deaths was from strangulation or ischemia.

When to Operate?

There are three situations in early postoperative small bowel obstruction that require surgical intervention: unresolved obstruction after a prolonged nasogastric tube, a high-grade or complete small bowel obstruction, and ischemic or strangulated small bowel. All these conditions require an expert judgment based on clinical evaluation and interpretation of essential workup. As shown by Pickleman and Lee,[165] 2 weeks' time should be a cut-off point to consider an exploratory celiotomy, but sooner if the condition deteriorates.

A high-grade or total small bowel obstruction seldom responds to prolonged conservative treatment and has a danger of becoming ischemia or perforation. A plain and upright abdomen and erect chest X-ray as an initial evaluation with subsequent serial films give useful and important information. A gasless colon and a stepladder pattern to air–fluid levels on the dilated small intestine signifies complete small bowel obstruction; the "ground glass" appearance and the gasless small bowel and large bowel are the picture of a closed-loop obstruction. Nauta[167] used clinical examination, leukocyte count, and the plain film radiography to determine when to operate and when to treat conservatively. In a retrospective review of 413 patients with small bowel obstruction (not an early postoperative small bowel obstruction), 72 patients underwent immediate operation because of the diagnosis of a complete small bowel obstruction, 47 patients required an operation after a period of observation ranging from 3 to 15 days, and 294 patients resolved without an operation. Of the 72 patients who underwent immediate operation, 22 bowel resections were required: 6 for obstructive carcinoma, 12 for ischemic bowel, and 4 for extensive adhesions. Two postoperative deaths occurred within 30 days, both in the bowel resection group; one of these was from an aspiration pneumonia established preoperatively and the other was from acute renal failure established preoperatively. In the 294 patients who were successfully treated conservatively, the readmission and reoperation rates were comparable with those reported in a series in which earlier operation was undertaken (56 patients were readmitted with 7 requiring operation in a 6-year period). The author concluded that plain abdominal films of the abdomen can accurately differentiate between complete and partial small bowel obstruction and that partial small bowel obstruction can be safely treated conservatively with close observation. Although this series does not fit the topic of early postoperative small bowel obstruction, it gives a good lesson on how to simply use abdominal films to diagnose a complete small bowel obstruction that requires an immediate operation.

Ischemic bowel is an urgent indication for surgery. The diagnosis, however, is difficult. A prospective study was conducted by Sarr et al[168] to evaluate numerous parameters that might be useful in predicting strangulation versus a simple small bowel obstruction before exploratory celiotomy. No parameter has proved to be more sensitive than 52%, either when used alone or in combination. Parameters studied included continuous abdominal pain (as opposed to colicky pain), bloody bowel movements, duration of symptoms, location of abdominal pain, time interval since last bowel movement, surgical history, fever (> 100 °F), white blood count greater than 10,000, and tachycardia. Some laboratory studies, such as those used to determine the presence of metabolic acidosis and elevation of serum creatine phosphokinase, have a predictive value of 75%. Hyperamylasemia and hyperphosphatemia were of no diagnostic value. Even the preoperative diagnosis of senior experienced surgeons proved disappointing: sensitivity for recognition of strangulation was only 48 ± 22%.

Review of literature by Sajja et al[169] showed that in multiple series of early postoperative small bowel obstruction that required an operation, the incidence of intestinal strangulation ranges from 0 to 12% and the mortality ranges from 2 to 18%. The incidence of strangulation is relatively low in early postoperative small bowel obstruction compared to small bowel obstruction from incarcerated hernias because more of these are from adhesions.[169]

CT has played an important role in the diagnosis of complicated small bowel obstruction. Mallo et al[170] conducted a systematic and comprehensive review of the scientific literature using MEDLINE and Cochrane databases for a period from 1966 to 2004. A report on CT diagnosis of ischemia in small bowel obstruction included 743 patients. The sensitivity was 83% (range, 63–100%) and the specificity was 92% (range, 61–100%). The PPV was 79% (range, 69–100%) and the NPV was 93% (range, 33–100%). For complete or high-grade obstruction including 408 patients, the sensitivity was 92% (range, 81–100%) and the specificity was 94% (range, 68–100%). The PPV was 92% (range, 84–100%) and the NPV was 93% (range, 76–100%). The CT abdomen has largely replaced the small bowel follow-through or enteroclysis study. The emerging CT enterography[168,171] may improve the accuracy of the conventional CT abdomen for the diagnosis of complicated small bowel obstruction.

Preventing Adhesions

Because of the frequency of postoperative adhesions and the substantial suffering and morbidity endured by patients in addition to the enormous cost in terms of medical care and lost income, the prevention of adhesion formation has been the subject of countless studies. None has offered much hope until the publication by Becker et al[172] who studied the use of a sodium hyaluronate and carboxymethylcellulose, bioresorbable

membrane (Seprafilm, Genzyme Corp., Cambridge, MA). The authors randomly assigned 183 patients with ulcerative colitis or familial adenomatous polyposis (FAP), who were scheduled for colectomy and ileal pouch-anal anastomosis diverting loop ileostomy to receive or not to receive the membrane placed under the midline incision. At the ileostomy closure 8 to 12 weeks later, laparoscopy was used to evaluate the incidence, extent, and severity of adhesion formation. Data analyzed from 175 assessable patients revealed that only 6% of control patients had no adhesions, whereas 51% of patients receiving the membrane were free of adhesions. Dense adhesions were observed in 58% of control patients but in only 15% of those receiving the membrane. This study represents the first controlled prospective evaluation of postoperative abdominal adhesion formation and prevention after general abdominal surgery using standardized direct peritoneal visualization. The membrane was safe with no reported adverse effects.

The results that it is safe and has fewer adhesions have been confirmed by the prospective, randomized, multicenter, controlled studies conducted by Beck et al[173] and Cohen et al.[174] However, wrapping the anastomosis with Seprafilm should be avoided as it has a higher risk of anastomosis leak rate.[173] In the most recent report on the subject, Fazio et al[175] published their prospective, randomized, multicenter, multinational, single-blind, controlled study on 1,701 patients who underwent intestinal resection to determine whether Seprafilm usage would translate into a reduction in adhesive small bowel obstruction. Before closure of the abdomen, patients were randomized to receive Seprafilm or no treatment. Seprafilm was applied to adhesiogenic tissues throughout the abdomen. The mean follow-up time for the occurrence of adhesive small bowel obstruction was 3.5 years. There was no difference between the treatment and control groups in overall rate of bowel obstruction. However, the incidence of adhesive small bowel obstruction requiring reoperation was significantly lower for Seprafilm patients compared with no treatment patients (1.8 vs. 3.4%).

Abdominal Wound Infection

Prevention of abdominal wound infections after colorectal surgery is related to antibiotic and mechanical preparation as described in Chapter 5. Surgical operations call upon the phagocytes involved in host defense responses to respond to traumatized tissue and contaminating bacteria; if either element is present in excess, host defense may be strained. If both are present in excess, defense mechanism may be overwhelmed, resulting in a wound abscess. Antibiotics help in defense against bacteria but can do nothing to minimize the effects of excessive trauma to the wound tissues. The amount of tissue damage correlates negatively with the number of bacteria required to induce infection. Following closure of the wound, its environment is sealed off from the body as a result of local intravascular coagulation and the mechanisms of early inflammation. Any blood remaining within the wound may harbor and nourish bacteria. Pathogens within the wound are protected from host defense and antimicrobial agents by the inflammatory diffusion barrier, explaining why postoperative administration of antibiotics is ineffective in preventing wound infection. Administered preoperatively at the right time, antibiotics diffuse into the peripheral compartment, or in this case, the wound fluid during the operation. The antibiotics must be present in a wound early enough to reduce the ability of contaminating bacteria to cause postoperative infection. If the antibiotic is given too early, it may diffuse into and then be eliminated from the tissues before the incision is made and may not be available in the wound during the vulnerable period. Prophylactic antibiotics are effective only when given immediately preoperatively but not when given after the termination of the operation.[176]

Operative wounds have been classified into four different types.[177] In a clean wound (type I), the bowel content is not exposed (e.g., an exploratory celiotomy or a simple lysis of adhesions). With a clean contaminated wound (type II), the bowel is open, but there is no gross spilling of the GI content (e.g., colon resection and anastomosis). In a contaminated wound (type III), there is a gross spilling of GI content during the procedure. With a dirty wound (type IV), there is existing infection (e.g., perforated diverticulitis).

The incidence of wound infection in a clean wound is very low (1–3%) and usually results from exogenous contamination with gram-positive organisms such as *Staphylococcus*.[178] In type II, III, and IV wounds, the risk of wound infection is between 3 and 16%.[177,179] The common pathogens found in the colon and rectum are *E. coli*, *Klebsiella*, *Enterobacter*, *Bacteroides fragilis*, *Peptostreptococcus*, and *Clostridia*.[176]

The reliable management of dirty wounds is to delay the wound closure or to leave it open altogether, which may take a few months to heal. However, if the healing wound is clean, a secondary skin closure can be done. An alternative is to use vacuum-assisted wound closure. This technique has been successfully used in trauma patients who require leaving the abdomen open.[180] Nosocomial infection is still a major cause of surgical wound infection.[181] However, this fact is frequently overlooked. Every effort must be made to minimize this type of infection, and adherence to a few basic principles will help.

From the working group that developed guidelines for prevention of surgical infection at the Centers for Disease Control and Prevention, Polk et al[181] outlined the preparation of patients for operation as follows: (1) For elective operation, all bacterial infections that are identified should be treated and controlled before the operation, excluding ones for which the operation is performed. (2) The preoperative hospital stay should be as short as possible. Many tests and therapies can be performed on an outpatient basis. (3) For elective operation, a grossly malnourished patient should receive preoperative oral or parenteral hyperalimentation. (4) For elective operation, the patient should bathe or be bathed the night before the operation with an antiseptic soap. Unless hair near the operative site is thick enough to interfere with the surgical procedure, it should not be removed. If hair removal is necessary, it should be performed as close to the time of operation as possible, preferably immediately before. The entire operative field and the adjacent area should be scrubbed with a detergent solution and then covered with an antiseptic solution. Tincture of chlorhexidine iodophors and tincture of iodine are recommended. Plain soap, alcohol, or hexachlorophene is not recommended as a single agent for operative site preparation unless the patient's skin is sensitive to the recommended antiseptic products. Other control measures that must be observed are the preparation of the surgical team and the checking of ventilation and air quality

in the operating room, which should be established and standardized in all hospitals.

Factors that have proven or probable influence on the frequency of wound infections are the use of antibiotic prophylaxis, the duration of surgery, the defense mechanisms of the host, the use of ultraclean air in the operating room, the presence of hypovolemia, diabetes mellitus, or adiposity in the patient, the patient's nutritional status, the use of blood transfusion, and pain control. The importance of each factor, however, is difficult to detemine.[182]

The maintenance of a normal temperature in the patient during surgery has been reported to decrease the infection rate by two-thirds[183] and the use of supplemental oxygen decreased the rate by half using 30% oxygen during and 2 hours after surgery.[184]

The decisive period for the development of surgical wound infection is during surgery, and for the first few hours thereafter.[182]

Abdominal Wound Dehiscence

Abdominal wound dehiscence formerly was a fairly common complication of intra-abdominal operations and was associated with a high morbidity and mortality. At present, it is an uncommon problem, partly because of better suture materials, improved techniques, and better antibiotics to control wound infection. In most series, the incidence of abdominal dehiscence varies from 0 to 4%.[185,186,187,188] However, the incidence of incisional hernia is much higher and is directly related to the duration of follow-up. The incidence ranged from 3% in the series reported by Schoetz et al[185] to 21% in the series reported by Wissing et al.[189] This wide range of complications probably reflects the different techniques of closure and the varying suture size and material used. The most common cause of abdominal wound dehiscence is related to improper closure technique.[186] Three major causes of wound dehiscence are tissue tear, suture break, and knot slippage. Other factors include the following: male older than 60 years, severe obstructive pulmonary disease, malnutrition, emergency abdominal procedures, complicated neoplasia and IBD, and acute abdominal distention.[187,188] Patients with jaundice also were found to have healing of abdominal incision as well as visceral wounds, seriously impaired.[190] In some patients, dehiscence occurred as a result of deep abdominal wound infection, with necrosis of the fascia.

Unless there is evisceration, the dehiscence may not be apparent. Initially the patient develops ileus, which causes abdominal distention. Nausea and vomiting may mimic small bowel obstruction. Later, serosanguineous fluid leaks through the abdominal wound. Examination of the abdominal wound reveals separation of the fascia. Skin sutures should not be removed because this maneuver will only convert a fascial dehiscence to a complete evisceration. There is no urgency to repair a fascial dehiscence, especially in a relatively sick patient. One can accept an incisional hernia that can be repaired at a later date. In the face of a complete evisceration, it is best to take the patient to the operating room for exploration under general anesthesia. Clinical observation showed that in 88 patients, the sutures in a disrupted wound were intact; having pulled through the fascia,[191] the wound should be properly resutured. Although tension sutures probably do not prevent the dehiscence from recurring, they should be considered in some conditions such as severe obstructive pulmonary disease. Many studies have been conducted in a randomized prospective manner and are helpful when applied to the techniques of abdominal wound closure.

It is now generally accepted that closure of the peritoneal layer is unnecessary.[192] Ellis and Heddle[190] used a mass closure technique that included all layers of the abdominal wall apart from the skin and incorporates wide bites of tissue on either side of the line of incision, placed close together under no tension. Only one burst abdomen (0.4%) was noted. This rate compared favorably with 2.5% incidence of burst abdomen in two-layer closure. Mass closure, however, is not perfect; 3% of these patients developed an incisional hernia within 6 months of follow-up.

In a prospective randomized trial on retention sutures, the flush-tied sutures (tight) were associated with a higher incidence of wound dehiscence than were loosely tied sutures (over three fingers).[193] Experimental studies in male rats showed that tight closure of sutures on fascia caused overlap of tissue, whereas loosely closed sutures afforded proper alignment of the wound edges and had greater proliferative activity in the cleft of the wounds. The tensile strength and energy-to-failure studies showed loosely approximated wounds to be far stronger. However, no statistically significant difference was found in hydroxyproline assays of the two groups.[194] In practice, it is important to approximate the abdominal fascia, not to strangulate it.

A randomized prospective multicentric study was organized to compare results between techniques using continuous sutures and interrupted sutures in closing abdominal midline incisions.[195] The suture material employed was polyglycolic acid. This study included 3,135 patients who were randomized between the two methods of closure and stratified according to the type of wound (i.e., clean, clean contaminated, and contaminated). The overall dehiscence rate was 1.6% in the continuous suture group versus 2% in the interrupted suture group. In six trials comparing continuous versus interrupted technique (irrespective of suture type), there was no statistical difference in the rate of wound infection or wound dehiscence.[196] Meta-analyses of various randomized trials showed that continuous slowly absorbable sutures (such as PDS) gave the best results in terms of less pain, fewer sinuses, with a follow-up of 1 year.[197]

Most surgeons favor running sutures for closing abdominal wounds, as they are cheaper and faster. The use of running sutures consumes only half the time needed for interrupted sutures. Continuous sutures, however, are more prone to be pulled too tight either by the surgeon or the assistant. Earlier studies recommended tissue bites 1.5 cm from the fascial edges.[186] However, the STITCH trial was a double-blinded multicenter randomized controlled trial designed to compare a standardized large bite technique with a standardized small bite technique at surgical and gynecological departments in 10 hospitals in the Netherlands. Patients aged 18 years or older who were scheduled to undergo elective abdominal surgery with midline laparotomy were randomly assigned to receive small tissue bites of 5 mm every 5 mm or large bites of 1 cm every 1 cm. Between October 20, 2009, and March 12, 2012, 560 patients were randomly assigned to the large bites group ($n = 284$) or the small bites group ($n = 276$). The small bite group patients had a higher ratio of suture length to wound length and a longer closure time (14 vs. 10 minutes; $p < 0.0001$). At 1-year follow-up, 57 (21%) of 277 patients in the large bite group and 35 (13%) of 268 patients in the small bite group had incisional hernia ($p = 0.022$). Rates of adverse events did not differ

significantly between groups. This study demonstrated that the small bite suture technique is more effective than the traditional large bite technique for prevention of incisional hernia in midline incisions and is not associated with a higher rate of adverse events.[198]

An extensive review of the literature by Poole,[199] which included 111 references, concluded that chromic catgut should be abandoned for abdominal wound closure because of its unreliable strength by early suture dissolution or breakage. Braided organic nonabsorbable materials, such as silk and cotton, have fallen into disfavor because of the intense inflammatory response they elicit and because of the propensity for bacteria to grow in the interstices of the suture, resulting in an increased incidence of wound infection and delayed check in the formation of suture sinuses.[185] Most studies indicate that synthetic absorbable sutures have demonstrated strength equal to that of permanent sutures.[196] Monofilament sutures are preferred for their lack of reactivity, prolonged tensile strength, and resistance to infection. There is a higher incidence of incisional hernia formation when braided absorbable suture material is used.[200]

Laboratory evaluation of a monofilament PDS has shown that its strength prior to implantation exceeds that of nonabsorbable monofilament sutures. Furthermore, its strength is maintained in vivo much longer than that of braided synthetic absorbable sutures. Size 00 PDS suture retained 70% of its breaking strength following in vivo residence of 28 days and still retained 13% of its original strength at 56 days. In contrast, braided synthetic absorbable sutures retained only 1 to 5% of strength at 28 days. Cellular responses are found only in the vicinity of the implant site and are predominately mononuclear in character.[201] A no. 1 monofilament synthetic absorbable suture is available and is suitable for a secured abdominal wound closure. A prospective study conducted by Israelsson and Jonsson[202] comparing continuous sutures in midline abdominal incisions using PDS-2 vs. no. 1 nylon showed that PDS suture was as good as nylon.

Retention Sutures

Retention sutures are heavy, nonabsorbable sutures that are placed with wide tissue bites through all layers of the abdominal wall including the skin and are tied over a buttress device for skin protection to reduce tension on the wound edges. They are often used to repair postoperative fascial dehiscence. They have also been recommended to reduce the rate of wound dehiscence after major abdominal operations, particularly in those patients who are at increased risk.[203]

Rink et al[203] conducted a controlled randomized study in 95 patients with infective or malignant intra-abdominal diseases that required major abdominal operations and showed that retention sutures cause inconvenience and pain. However, whether retention sutures are beneficial in preventing evisceration in a subgroup of patients with high risk of wound complications, such as patients who have been on long-term steroids, is not known.

Unhealed Perineal Wound

After a controlled trial designed to compare the results of healing following packing the perineal wound open and after closure with drainage of the pelvis following an abdominoperineal resection or a total proctocolectomy, Irvin and Goligher[204] concluded that primary closure was the procedure of choice. At the present time, most surgeons completely close the perineal wound in abdominoperineal resection for carcinoma of the rectum and in total proctocolectomy for ulcerative colitis and Crohn's disease. A closed suction drain is placed in the presacral space and preferably brought out through a separate stab wound in the lower abdomen. Campos et al[205] found that closure of the pelvic peritoneum and perineal wound with a drain results in a higher rate of perineal wound infection and in a longer hospital stay than closure of the perineum without closure of the pelvic peritoneum. Other complications, including bowel obstruction, are not significantly different.

Bullard et al[206] reviewed 160 patients who underwent abdominoperineal resection with primary closure of perineal wound, for carcinoma of rectum. Seventy-three percent of patients received preoperative radiation. Major wound complication rate was 35%. Delayed healing was the most common complication (24%), followed by infection (10%). Radiation therapy increased the risk of major wound complication (41 vs. 19%), and risk of infection (14 vs. 0%). Christian et al[207] reviewed their experience in patients who underwent abdominoperineal resection. In the subgroup of 120 patients with carcinoma of rectum, the predictors for major wound complications were increased BMI and diabetes. Chemoradiation did not appear to increase the complications.

In patients with preoperative sepsis of the perineum, such as those with multiple perineal fistulas or perianal abscesses, the perineal subcutaneous tissue and the skin should be packed open. When there is significant fecal spillage of the pelvis and perineum during the procedure, or in patients who continue to ooze blood in the pelvis or perineum at the end of the procedure, the surgeon must judge whether the wound should be packed open or closed with suction drainage. Delalande et al[208] showed that although the incidence of wound infection was higher after primary closure, the long-term benefit was better, particularly if the patient required postoperative adjuvant therapy because the delayed wound healing in the group whose wounds were packed was long. The authors argued that it is worthwhile to take a chance and reopen the wound if it becomes infected.

Primary healing of the closed perineal wound is achieved in 45 to 95% of patients.[209,210,211,212] Patients with IBD have a greater tendency toward perineal wound breakdown than patients with carcinoma of the rectum unless a high dose of preoperative radiation has been given. Most postoperative perineal wounds that are infected should be opened, and those wounds that were left open initially should eventually heal, although this may take a few months. From 4 to 20% of perineal wounds remain open 1 year after the operation.[213]

Patients with unhealed perineal wounds require evaluation of the GI tract to rule out recurrence or flare-up of Crohn's disease; such patients with carcinoma should be evaluated for a recurrent carcinoma of the pelvis or the perineum. The wound should be curetted and examined for any foreign bodies such as stitches. The wound should be carefully packed and the hair in that region shaved. If these basic measures fail, a further procedure should be considered. If small and shallow wounds are present, it may be wise to have the patient live with them.

Recent advances in reconstructive surgery have allowed various muscle flap procedures to be performed with reliable success. Baird et al[214] used the inferior gluteal myocutaneous flap with eventual healing in 15 out of 16 patients who have had recalcitrant perineal wounds. Anthony and Mathes[213] used the gracilis, gluteus maximus (inferior and superior half), gluteal thigh, and rectus abdominis muscle flaps with long-term (3.5-year follow-up) success of 92%. Others also found them useful as a primary closure or treatment on nonhealing perineal wounds.[215,216] The flap of choice depends on three factors: muscle flaps available, the size of the wound, and amount of skin required for closure.[213]

A persistent perineal size is a common problem after an abdominoperineal resection. It is usually small and deep, with the track running into the presacral space. In this situation, the sinus track can be unrooted by excising the coccyx and caudal part of the sacrum. A vacuum-assisted closure (VAC) is then employed. The VAC removes exudate serum and clears bacteria, and thus accelerates wound healing and eventually closes the wound in 95% of cases.[217]

For large sacral and perineal defects following an abdominoperineal resection with or without radiation, the trend is to use the rectus abdominis myocutaneous flap. This type of flap has been used extensively in the head and neck, chest wall, breast, extremity, and groin. It provides a wide arc of rotation based on the deep inferior epigastric vessels. It provides a large bulk of tissue to fill the pelvis and perineum and results in minimal donor site morbidity.[218,219]

Postoperative Perineal Hernia

Perineal hernia, a protrusion of intra-abdominal viscera through a defect in the pelvic floor, is a rare complication following abdominoperineal resection or pelvic exenteration. In an excellent review, So et al[220] discussed the subject of postoperative perineal hernia and elaborated on their experience with this problem. The following account draws heavily from their review. The exact incidence is unknown, but symptomatic herniation is estimated to occur in less than 1% of patients with abdominoperineal resection and in approximately 3% after pelvic exenteration. Barium X-ray studies reveal perineal hernias in 7%, but most are asymptomatic and do not require repair. So et al[220] summarized the factors that have been postulated to predispose a patient to perineal hernia formation. These include coccygectomy, previous hysterectomy, pelvic irradiation, excessive length of small bowel mesentery, the larger size of the female pelvis, failure to close the peritoneal defect, and excision of the levators. Symptoms associated with a perineal hernia include a dragging feeling, a sensation of bulging, and discomfort in the perineum. More serious problems such as skin breakdown, urinary symptoms, and bowel obstruction may occur.

Management of the condition is difficult. Symptoms may be controlled with a T bandage or a firm pair of underpants. Repair of this hernia poses a challenging surgical problem. The surgical principles are the same as those for other hernias (i.e., mobilize the sac, reduce its contents, excise the sac, and repair the defect). A perineal approach is attractive because it is simple and the abdominal cavity is not entered. Nevertheless, exposure is limited, so it may be difficult to exclude recurrent carcinoma, to mobilize adherent small bowel, or to repair injured viscera.

With an abdominal approach, mesh can be sutured to the bony pelvis under direct vision. It is best reserved for patient with recurrent hernia or for those in whom laparotomy is necessary for other reasons. A combined abdominoperineal approach may provide the best exposure, although it is probably unnecessary except in unusual circumstances.

Operative techniques via the perineum may include simple layered closure, insertion of a synthetic mesh, creation of a gluteus maximus flap, and retroflexion of uterus. Via the abdominal approach, a layered closure may be performed, a mesh inserted, or the bladder or uterus retroflexed. It is not likely that the levators can be approximated because following excision for malignancy, the defect is likely too large. The bladder or uterus may be sutured to the posterior pelvic wall, thus obliterating the defect. A prosthetic mesh may be sutured to the musculofascial tissue around the pelvic outlet via a perineal or transabdominal approach. Flaps of fascia lata, gracilis, rectus abdominis, or gluteus maximus can be used to close the pelvic defect.

Beck et al[221] recommended that the mesh be sutured from the vagina or the prostatic capsule to the presacral fascia and periosteum at or below the level of S3 (▶ Fig. 35.15). Care should be taken to avoid large vessels. The attachment should be below the level of the ureters. An obturator may be placed into the vagina to aid in the operative identification of the vaginal cuff, and ureteral stents may be inserted preoperatively to identify the ureters. Suction drainage can be used to obliterate dead space below the mesh. Beck et al[221] used Marlex mesh to repair perineal hernias in eight patients—two perineal and six abdominal. Both perineal hernias and one abdominal hernia recurred (37.5%) and were re-repaired through the abdominal approach. The authors believe that the best method of repair involves the placement of a mesh across the pelvic inlet through an abdominal approach. Brotschi et al[222] used a gracilis muscle graft tunneled subcutaneously from the thigh and attached to the sacrum.

So et al[220] reported on 21 patients with perineal hernia. The authors' estimated incidence of symptomatic perineal recurrence following abdominoperineal resection was 0.62%. The original perineal wound was left partially open in 69% and completely open in 10% of patients. The peritoneal defect was closed in 53%, and the levators closed in 21% of patients. A perineal repair was accomplished in 13 patients, an abdominal approach was used in 3 patients, and a combined approach was used in 3 patients. Methods of repair included simple closure of pelvic defect in 10 patients, mesh insertion in 5, gluteus flap in 1, retroflexion of the uterus in 1, and retroflexion of the bladder in 1. The recurrence rate was 16% after a median 12-month follow-up. All patients had undergone a perineal repair.

Sarr et al[223] used a combined abdominal and perineal approach allowing mobilization and reduction of herniated viscera. The mesh was sutured transabdominally to the sacrum posteriorly and to the lateral pelvic wall, to the pelvic rami anteriorly from above and from below.

It appears that the perineal approach (with or without mesh) is successful in the majority of cases and that the abdominal approach is best reserved for recurrent hernias or when access to the abdomen or pelvic contents is required. One of the editors (SDW) prefers placement of synthetic dual sided mesh followed by bilateral gluteal flaps in the perineal approach with the patient in the prone jackknife position. The gluteal flaps add bulk between the mesh and the skin, which may reduce mesh erosion and enhance patient comfort while seated. However, the patient is maintained in bed rest on an air mattress for 3 days following this procedure, after which sitting is discouraged for at least 2 additional weeks.

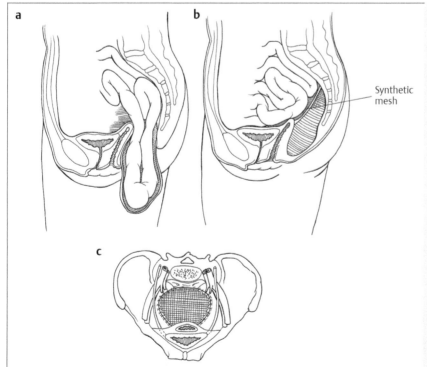

Fig. 35.15 Synthetic mesh repair of perineal hernia. **(a)** Sagittal view of pelvis demonstrating perineal hernia with incarcerated small bowel. **(b)** Sagittal view of pelvis with synthetic mesh in place. **(c)** View of the pelvis from above with synthetic mesh in place.

Synthetic mesh

References

[1] Krukowski ZH, Matheson NA. Emergency surgery for diverticular disease complicated by generalized and faecal peritonitis: a review. Br J Surg. 1984; 71(12):921–927

[2] Killingback M. Management of perforative diverticulitis. Surg Clin North Am. 1983; 63(1):97–115

[3] Badía JM, Sitges-Serra A, Pla J, Ragué JM, Roqueta F, Sitges-Creus A. Perforation of colonic neoplasms. A review of 36 cases. Int J Colorectal Dis. 1987; 2 (4):187–189

[4] Mandava N, Kumar S, Pizzi WF, Aprile IJ. Perforated colorectal carcinomas. Am J Surg. 1996; 172(3):236–238

[5] Softley A, Clamp SE, Bouchier IAD, Myren J, Watkinson G, de Dombal FT. Perforation of the intestine in inflammatory bowel disease. An OMGE survey. Scand J Gastroenterol Suppl. 1988; 144 Suppl 144:24–26

[6] Abascal J, Diaz-Rojas F, Jorge J, et al. Free perforation of the small bowel in Crohn's disease. World J Surg. 1982; 6(2):216–220

[7] Bundred NJ, Dixon JM, Lumsden AB, Gilmour HM, Davies GC. Free perforation in Crohn's colitis. A ten-year review. Dis Colon Rectum. 1985; 28 (1):35–37

[8] Heppell J, Farkouh E, Dubé S, Péloquin A, Morgan S, Bernard D. Toxic megacolon. An analysis of 70 cases. Dis Colon Rectum. 1986; 29(12):789–792

[9] Wexner SD, Dailey TH. The initial management of left lower quadrant peritonitis. Dis Colon Rectum. 1986; 29(10):635–638

[10] Kriwanek S, Armbruster C, Dittrich K, Beckerhinn P. Perforated colorectal cancer. Dis Colon Rectum. 1996; 39(12):1409–1414

[11] Kriwanek S, Armbruster C, Beckerhinn P, Dittrich K. Prognostic factors for survival in colonic perforation. Int J Colorectal Dis. 1994; 9(3):158–162

[12] Mulholland MW, Delaney JP. Neutropenic colitis and aplastic anemia: a new association. Ann Surg. 1983; 197(1):84–90

[13] Wade DS, Douglass H, Jr, Nava HR, Piedmonte M. Abdominal pain in neutropenic patients. Arch Surg. 1990; 125(9):1119–1127

[14] Bodey GP, Buckley M, Sathe YS, Freireich EJ. Quantitative relationships between circulating leukocytes and infection in patients with acute leukemia. Ann Intern Med. 1966; 64(2):328–340

[15] Cooke JV. Acute leukemia in children. JAMA. 1993; 101:432–435

[16] Moir DH, Bale PM. Necropsy findings in childhood leukaemia, emphasizing neutropenic enterocolitis and cerebral calcification. Pathology. 1976; 8 (3):247–258

[17] Keidan RD, Fanning J, Gatenby RA, Weese JL. Recurrent typhlitis. A disease resulting from aggressive chemotherapy. Dis Colon Rectum. 1989; 32 (3):206–209

[18] Kernagis LY, Levine MS, Jacobs JE. Pneumatosis intestinals: correlation of CT findings with viability of the bowel. Am J Roent. 2003; 180:733–736

[19] Crawford J, Armitage J, Balducci L, et al. National comprehensive cancer network. Myeloid growth factors. J Natl Compr Canc Netw. 2013; 11 (10):1266–1290

[20] Rodrigues FG, Dasilva G, Wexner SD. Neutropenic enterocolitis. World J Gastroenterol. 2017; 23(1):42–47

[21] Bliziotis IA, Michalopoulos A, Kasiakou SK, et al. Ciprofloxacin vs an aminoglycoside in combination with a beta-lactam for the treatment of febrile neutropenia: a meta-analysis of randomized controlled trials. Mayo Clin Proc. 2005; 80(9):1146–1156

[22] Cunningham SC, Fakhry K, Bass BL, Napolitano LM. Neutropenic enterocolitis in adults: case series and review of the literature. Dig Dis Sci. 2005; 50:215–220

[23] Margulis AR, Heinbecker P, Bernard HR. Operative mesenteric arteriography in the search for the site of bleeding in unexplained gastrointestinal hemorrhage: a preliminary report. Surgery. 1960; 48:534–539

[24] Baum S, Nusbaum M, Blakemore WS, Finkelstein AK. The preoperative radiographic demonstration of intra-abdominal bleeding from undetermined sites by percutaneous selective celiac and superior mesenteric arteriography. Surgery. 1965; 58(5):797–805

[25] Boley SJ, Sammartano R, Adams A, DiBiase A, Kleinhaus S, Sprayregen S. On the nature and etiology of vascular ectasias of the colon. Degenerative lesions of aging. Gastroenterology. 1977; 72(4)(,)(Pt 1):650–660

[26] Church JM. Angiodysplasia. Semin Colon Rectal Surg. 1994; 5:43–49

[27] Roberts PL, Schoetz DJ, Jr, Coller JA. Vascular ectasia. Diagnosis and treatment by colonoscopy. Am Surg. 1988; 54(1):56–59

[28] Jensen DM, Machicado GA. Endoscopic diagnosis and treatment of bleeding colonic angiomas and radiation telangiectasia. Perspect Colon Rect Surg. 1989; 2:99–113

[29] McGuire HH, Jr, Haynes BW, Jr. Massive hemorrhage for diverticulosis of the colon: guidelines for therapy based on bleeding patterns observed in fifty cases. Ann Surg. 1972; 175(6):847–855

[30] Casarella WJ, Galloway SJ, Taxin RN, Follett DA, Pollock EJ, Seaman WB. "Lower" gastrointestinal tract hemorrhage: new concepts based on arteriography. Am J Roentgenol Radium Ther Nucl Med. 1974; 121(2):357–368

[31] McGuire HH, Jr. Bleeding colonic diverticula. A reappraisal of natural history and management. Ann Surg. 1994; 220(5):653–656

[32] Noer RJ, Hamilton JE, Williams DJ, Broughton DS. Rectal hemorrhage: moderate and severe. Ann Surg. 1962; 155:794–805

[33] Bokhari M, Vernava AM, Ure T, Longo WE. Diverticular hemorrhage in the elderly: is it well tolerated? Dis Colon Rectum. 1996; 39(2):191–195

[34] Meyers MA, Alonso DR, Gray GF, Baer JW. Pathogenesis of bleeding colonic diverticulosis. Gastroenterology. 1976; 71(4):577–583

[35] Leitman IM, Paull DE, Shires GT, III. Evaluation and management of massive lower gastrointestinal hemorrhage. Ann Surg. 1989; 209(2):175–180

[36] Rossini FP, Ferrari A, Spandre M, et al. Emergency colonoscopy. World J Surg. 1989; 13(2):190–192

[37] Chou YH, Hsu SC, Wang CY, Chen CL, How SW. Ischemic colitis as a cause of massive lower gastrointestinal bleeding and peritonitis. Report of five cases. Dis Colon Rectum. 1989; 32(12):1065–1070

[38] Robert JH, Sachar DB, Aufses AH, Jr, Greenstein AJ. Management of severe hemorrhage in ulcerative colitis. Am J Surg. 1990; 159(6):550–555

[39] Renison DM, Forouhar FA, Levine JB, Breiter JR. Filiform polyposis of the colon presenting as massive hemorrhage: an uncommon complication of Crohn's disease. Am J Gastroenterol. 1983; 78(7):413–416

[40] Robert JR, Sachar DB, Greenstein AJ. Severe gastrointestinal hemorrhage in Crohn's disease. Ann Surg. 1991; 213(3):207–211

[41] Cirocco WC, Reilly JC, Rusin LC. Life-threatening hemorrhage and exsanguination from Crohn's disease. Report of four cases. Dis Colon Rectum. 1995; 38(1):85–95

[42] Gostout CJ. Acute gastrointestinal bleeding: a common problem revisited. Mayo Clin Proc. 1988; 63(6):596–604

[43] Aljebreen AM, Fallone CA, Barkun AN. Nasogastric aspirate predicts high-risk endoscopic lesions in patients with acute upper-GI bleeding. Gastrointest Endosc. 2004; 59(2):172–178

[44] Ren JZ, Zhang MF, Rong AM, et al. Lower gastrointestinal bleeding: role of 64-row computed tomographic angiography in diagnosis and therapeutic planning. World J Gastroenterol. 2015; 21(13):4030–4037

[45] Kuhle WG, Sheiman RG. Detection of active colonic hemorrhage with use of helical CT: findings in a swine model. Radiology. 2003; 228(3):743–752

[46] Raphaeli T, Menon R. Current treatment of lower gastrointestinal hemorrhage. Clin Colon Rectal Surg. 2012; 25(4):219–227

[47] Martí M, Artigas JM, Garzón G, Alvarez-Sala R, Soto JA. Acute lower intestinal bleeding: feasibility and diagnostic performance of CT angiography. Radiology. 2012; 262(1):109–116

[48] Obana T, Fujita N, Sugita R, et al. Prospective evaluation of contrast-enhanced computed tomography for the detection of colonic diverticular bleeding. Dig Dis Sci. 2013; 58(7):1985–1990

[49] Nagata N, Niikura R, Aoki T, et al. Role of urgent contrast-enhanced multidetector computed tomography for acute lower gastrointestinal bleeding in patients undergoing early colonoscopy. J Gastroenterol. 2015; 50(12):1162–1172

[50] Forde KA, Webb WA. Acute lower gastrointestinal bleeding. Perspect Colon Rectal Surg. 1988; 1(1):105–112

[51] Bentley DE, Richardson JD. The role of tagged red blood cell imaging in the localization of gastrointestinal bleeding. Arch Surg. 1991; 126(7):821–824

[52] Nicholson ML, Neoptolemos JP, Sharp JF, Watkin EM, Fossard DP. Localization of lower gastrointestinal bleeding using in vivo technetium-99m-labelled red blood cell scintigraphy. Br J Surg. 1989; 76(4):358–361

[53] Ryan P, Styles CB, Chmiel R. Identification of the site of severe colon bleeding by technetium-labeled red-cell scan. Dis Colon Rectum. 1992; 35(3):219–222

[54] Suzman MS, Talmor M, Jennis R, Binkert B, Barie PS. Accurate localization and surgical management of active lower gastrointestinal hemorrhage with technetium-labeled erythrocyte scintigraphy. Ann Surg. 1996; 224(1):29–36

[55] Khanna A, Ognibene SJ, Koniaris LG. Embolization as first-line therapy for diverticulosis-related massive lower gastrointestinal bleeding: evidence from a meta-analysis. J Gastrointest Surg. 2005; 9(3):343–352

[56] Athanasoulis CA. Angiography in the management of patients with gastrointestinal bleeding. Adv Surg. 1983; 16:1–23

[57] Boley SJ, DiBiase A, Brandt LJ, Sammartano RJ. Lower intestinal bleeding in the elderly. Am J Surg. 1979; 137(1):57–64

[58] Zuckerman DA, Bocchini TP. The role of angiography in the diagnosis and treatment of vascular disorders of the lower gastrointestinal tract. Semin Colon Rectal Surg. 1994; 5:15–26

[59] Jensen DM, Machicado GA. Diagnosis and treatment of severe hematochezia. The role of urgent colonoscopy after purge. Gastroenterology. 1988; 95 (6):1569–1574

[60] Gostout CJ, Wang KK, Ahlquist DA, et al. Acute gastrointestinal bleeding. Experience of a specialized management team. J Clin Gastroenterol. 1992; 14 (3):260–267

[61] Margolin DA, Opelka FG. The role of radionuclide scintigraphy in the management of lower gastrointestinal bleeding. Semin Colon Rectal Surg. 1997; 8:156–160

[62] Colacchio TA, Forde KA, Patsos TJ, Nunez D. Impact of modern diagnostic methods on the management of active rectal bleeding. Ten year experience. Am J Surg. 1982; 143(5):607–610

[63] Britt LG, Warren L, Moore OF, III. Selective management of lower gastrointestinal bleeding. Am Surg. 1983; 49(3):121–125

[64] Browder W, Cerise EJ, Litwin MS. Impact of emergency angiography in massive lower gastrointestinal bleeding. Ann Surg. 1986; 204(5):530–536

[65] Parkes BM, Obeid FN, Sorensen VJ, Horst HM, Fath JJ. The management of massive lower gastrointestinal bleeding. Am Surg. 1993; 59(10):676–678

[66] Klas JV, Madoff RD. Surgical options in lower gastrointestinal bleeding. Semin Colon Rectal Surg. 1997; 8:172–177

[67] Bowden TA, Jr, Hooks VH, III, Mansberger AR, Jr. Intraoperative gastrointestinal endoscopy. Ann Surg. 1980; 191(6):680–687

[68] Lau WY, Wong SY, Yuen WK, Wong KK. Intraoperative enteroscopy for bleeding angiodysplasias of small intestine. Surg Gynecol Obstet. 1989; 168 (4):341–344

[69] Szold A, Katz LB, Lewis BS. Surgical approach to occult gastrointestinal bleeding. Am J Surg. 1992; 163(1):90–92, discussion 92–93

[70] Farner R, Lichliter W, Kuhn J, Fisher T. Total colectomy versus limited colonic resection for acute lower gastrointestinal bleeding. Am J Surg. 1999; 178 (6):587–591

[71] Gianfrancisco JA, Abcarian H. Pitfalls in the treatment of massive lower gastrointestinal bleeding with "blind" subtotal colectomy. Dis Colon Rectum. 1982; 25(5):441–445

[72] Farrands PA, Taylor I. Management of acute lower gastrointestinal haemorrhage in a surgical unit over a 4-year period. J R Soc Med. 1987; 80(2):79–82

[73] Setya V, Singer JA, Minken SL. Subtotal colectomy as a last resort for unrelenting, unlocalized, lower gastrointestinal hemorrhage: experience with 12 cases. Am Surg. 1992; 58(5):295–299

[74] Bender JS, Wiencek RG, Bouwman DL. Morbidity and mortality following total abdominal colectomy for massive lower gastrointestinal bleeding. Am Surg. 1991; 57(8):536–540, discussion 540–541

[75] Terry BG, Beart RW, Jr. Emergency abdominal colectomy with primary anastomosis. Dis Colon Rectum. 1981; 24(1):1–4

[76] Mortensen PE, Olsen J, Pedersen IK, Christiansen J. A randomized study on hemorrhoidectomy combined with anal dilatation. Dis Colon Rectum. 1987; 30(10):755–757

[77] Bailey HR, Ferguson JA. Prevention of urinary retention by fluid restriction following anorectal operations. Dis Colon Rectum. 1976; 19:250–252

[78] Buls JG, Goldberg SM. Modern management of hemorrhoids. Surg Clin North Am. 1978; 58(3):469–478

[79] Zaheer S, Reilly WT, Pemberton JH, Ilstrup D. Urinary retention after operations for benign anorectal diseases. Dis Colon Rectum. 1998; 41(6):696–704

[80] Petros JG, Mallen JK, Howe K, Rimm EB, Robillard RJ. Patient-controlled analgesia and postoperative urinary retention after open appendectomy. Surg Gynecol Obstet. 1993; 177(2):172–175

[81] Friend WG, Medwell SJ. Outpatient anorectal surgery. Perspect Colon Rectal Surg. 1989; 2(1):167–173

[82] Hinman F. Editorial: postoperative overdistention of the bladder. Surg Gynecol Obstet. 1976; 142(6):901–902

[83] Blute ML. Urinary retention in men after total hip arthroplasty. In: Coventry MB, ed. Year Book of Orthopedics. Chicago, IL: Year Book Medical Publishers; 1987:121–122

[84] Bowers FJ, Hartmann R, Khanduja KS, Hardy TG, Jr, Aguilar PS, Stewart WR. Urecholine prophylaxis for urinary retention in anorectal surgery. Dis Colon Rectum. 1987; 30(1):41–42

[85] Finkbeiner AE. Is bethanechol chloride clinically effective in promoting bladder emptying? A literature review. J Urol. 1985; 134(3):443–449

[86] Cataldo PA, Senagore AJ. Does alpha sympathetic blockade prevent urinary retention following anorectal surgery? Dis Colon Rectum. 1991; 34 (12):1113–1116

[87] Bonardi RA, Rosin JD, Stonesifer GL, Jr, Bauer FW. Bacteremias associated with routine hemorrhoidectomies. Dis Colon Rectum. 1976; 19:233–236

[88] Parikh SR, Molinelli B, Dailey TH. Liver abscess after hemorrhoidectomy. Report of two cases. Dis Colon Rectum. 1994; 37(2):185–189

[89] Ganchrow MI, Mazier WP, Friend WG, Ferguson JA. Hemorrhoidectomy revisited: a computer analysis of 2,038 cases. Dis Colon Rectum. 1971; 14 (2):128–133

[90] Rosen L, Sipe P, Stasik JJ, Riether RD, Trimpi HD. Outcome of delayed hemorrhage following surgical hemorrhoidectomy. Dis Colon Rectum. 1993; 36 (8):743–746

[91] Basso L, Pescatori M. Outcome of delayed hemorrhage following surgical hemorrhoidectomy. Dis Colon Rectum. 1994; 37(3):288–289

[92] Sheikh F, Khubchandani IT, Rosen L, Sheets JA, Stasik JJ. Is anorectal surgery on chronic dialysis patients risky? Dis Colon Rectum. 1992; 35(1):56–58

[93] Walker WA, Rothenberger DA, Goldberg SM. Morbidity of internal sphincterotomy for anal fissure and stenosis. Dis Colon Rectum. 1985; 28 (11):832–835

[94] Roe AM, Bartolo DCC, Vellacott KD, Locke-Edmunds J, Mortensen NJ. Submucosal versus ligation excision haemorrhoidectomy: a comparison of anal sensation, anal sphincter manometry and postoperative pain and function. Br J Surg. 1987; 74(10):948–951

[95] Wolff BG, Culp CE. The Whitehead hemorrhoidectomy. An unjustly maligned procedure. Dis Colon Rectum. 1988; 31(8):587–590

[96] Koenigs KP, McPhedran P, Spiro HM. Thrombosis in inflammatory bowel disease. J Clin Gastroenterol. 1987; 9(6):627–631

[97] Talbot RW, Heppell J, Dozois RR, Beart RW, Jr. Vascular complications of inflammatory bowel disease. Mayo Clin Proc. 1986; 61(2):140–145

[98] Graef V, Baggenstoss AH, Sauer WG, Spittell JA, Jr. Venous thrombosis occurring in nonspecific ulcerative colitis. A necropsy study. Arch Intern Med. 1966; 117:377–382

[99] Fichera A, Cicchiello LA, Mendelson DS, Greenstein AJ, Heimann TM. Superior mesenteric vein thrombosis after colectomy for inflammatory bowel disease: a not uncommon cause of postoperative acute abdominal pain. Dis Colon Rectum. 2003; 46(5):643–648

[100] Remzi FH, Fazio VW, Oncel M, et al. Portal vein thrombi after restorative proctocolectomy. Surgery. 2002; 132(4):655–661, discussion 661–662

[101] Hudson M, Chitolie A, Hutton RA, Smith MSH, Pounder RE, Wakefield AJ. Thrombotic vascular risk factors in inflammatory bowel disease. Gut. 1996; 38(5):733–737

[102] Morgenstern L. The avoidable complications of splenectomy. Surg Gynecol Obstet. 1977; 145(4):525–528

[103] Langevin JM, Rothenberger DA, Goldberg SM. Accidental splenic injury during surgical treatment of the colon and rectum. Surg Gynecol Obstet. 1984; 159(2):139–144

[104] Lord MD, Gourevitch A. The peritoneal anatomy of the spleen, with special reference to the operation of partial gastrectomy. Br J Surg. 1965; 52:202–204

[105] Morgenstern L, Shapiro SJ. Techniques of splenic conservation. Arch Surg. 1979; 114(4):449–454

[106] Working Party of the British Committee for Standards in Haematology Clinical Haematology Task Force. Guidelines for the prevention and treatment of infection in patients with an absent or dysfunctional spleen. BMJ. 1996; 312 (7028):430–434

[107] Zama N, Fazio VW, Jagelman DG, Lavery IC, Weakley FL, Church JM. Efficacy of pelvic packing in maintaining hemostasis after rectal excision for cancer. Dis Colon Rectum. 1988; 31(12):923–928

[108] Metzger PP. Modified packing technique for control of presacral pelvic bleeding. Dis Colon Rectum. 1988; 31(12):981–982

[109] McCourtney JS, Hussain N, Mackenzie I. Balloon tamponade for control of massive presacral haemorrhage. Br J Surg. 1996; 83(2):222

[110] Xu J, Lin J. Control of presacral hemorrhage with electrocautery through a muscle fragment pressed on the bleeding vein. J Am Coll Surg. 1994; 179 (3):351–352

[111] Braley SC, Schneider PD, Bold RJ, Goodnight JE, Jr, Khatri VP. Controlled tamponade of severe presacral venous hemorrhage: use of a breast implant sizer. Dis Colon Rectum. 2002; 45(1):140–142

[112] Wang QY, Shi WJ, Zhao YR, Zhou WQ, He ZR. New concepts in severe presacral hemorrhage during proctectomy. Arch Surg. 1985; 120(9):1013–1020

[113] Nivatvongs S, Fang DT. The use of thumbtacks to stop massive presacral hemorrhage. Dis Colon Rectum. 1986; 29(9):589–590

[114] Harrison JL, Hooks VH, Pearl RK, et al. Muscle fragment welding for control of massive presacral bleeding during rectal mobilization: a review of eight cases. Dis Colon Rectum. 2003; 46(8):1115–1117

[115] Remzi FH, Oncel M, Fazio VW. Muscle tamponade to control presacral venous bleeding: report of two cases. Dis Colon Rectum. 2002; 45 (8):1109–1111

[116] Zinman LM, Libertino JA, Roth RA. Management of operative ureteral injury. Urology. 1978; 12(3):290–303

[117] Higgins CC. Ureteral injuries during surgery. A review of 87 cases. JAMA. 1967; 199(2):82–88

[118] Melick WF. Complications of colonic and rectal surgery: the causes and management of postoperative urologic complications. Dis Colon Rectum. 1973; 16(1):7–11

[119] Presti JC, Carroll PR. Intraoperative management of the injured ureter. Perspect Colon Rectal Surg. 1988; 1(2):98–106

[120] Hamawy K, Smith JJ, III, Libertino JA. Injuries of the distal ureter. Semin Colon Rectal Surg. 2000; 11:163–179

[121] Bothwell WN, Bleicher RJ, Dent TL. Prophylactic ureteral catheterization in colon surgery. A five-year review. Dis Colon Rectum. 1994; 37(4):330–334

[122] Roach MB, Donaldson DS. Urologic complications of colorectal surgery. In: Hicks TC, Beck DE, Opelka PG, Timmke AE, eds. Complications of Colon and Rectal Surgery. Baltimore, MD: Williams & Wilkins; 1996:99–117

[123] Kinn AC, Ohman U. Bladder and sexual function after surgery for rectal cancer. Dis Colon Rectum. 1986; 29(1):43–48

[124] Cass AS, Bubrick MP. Ureteral injuries in colonic surgery. Urology. 1981; 18 (4):359–364

[125] Walsh PC, Schlegel PN. Radical pelvic surgery with preservation of sexual function. Ann Surg. 1988; 208(4):391–400

[126] Aboseif SR, Matzel KE, Lue TF. Sexual dysfunction after rectal surgery. Perspect Colon Rectal Surg. 1990; 3(1):157–172

[127] Havenga K, Enker WE, McDermott K, Cohen AM, Minsky BD, Guillem J. Male and female sexual and urinary function after total mesorectal excision with autonomic nerve preservation for carcinoma of the rectum. J Am Coll Surg. 1996; 182(6):495–502

[128] Masui H, Ike H, Yamaguchi S, Oki S, Shimada H. Male sexual function after autonomic nerve-preserving operation for rectal cancer. Dis Colon Rectum. 1996; 39(10):1140–1145

[129] Goldman JA, Feldberg D, Dicker D, Samuel N, Dekel A. Femoral neuropathy subsequent to abdominal hysterectomy. A comparative study. Eur J Obstet Gynecol Reprod Biol. 1985; 20(6):385–392

[130] Platell CF, Thompson PJ, Makin GB. Sexual health in women following pelvic surgery for rectal cancer. Br J Surg. 2004; 91(4):465–468

[131] Young-Fadok TM, Wolff BG. Long-term functional outcome with ileal pouch-anal anastomosis. Semin Colorectal Surg. 1996; 7:114–120

[132] Lindsey I, George BD, Kettlewell MGW, Mortensen NJMEC. Impotence after mesorectal and close rectal dissection for inflammatory bowel disease. Dis Colon Rectum. 2001; 44(6):831–835

[133] Lydon JC, Spielman FJ. Bilateral compartment syndrome following prolonged surgery in the lithotomy position. Anesthesiology. 1984; 60(3):236–238

[134] Nicholson MJ, McAlpine FS. Neural injuries associated with surgical positions and operations. In: Martin JT, ed. Positioning in Anesthesia and Surgery. Philadelphia, PA: WB Saunders; 1978:193–224

[135] Herrera-Ornelas L, Tolls RM, Petrelli NJ, Piver S, Mittelman A. Common peroneal nerve palsy associated with pelvic surgery for cancer. An analysis of 11 cases. Dis Colon Rectum. 1986; 29(6):392–397

[136] Schofield PF, Grace RH. Acute compartment syndrome of the legs after colorectal surgery. Colorectal Dis. 2004; 6(4):285–287

[137] Mumtaz FH, Chew H, Gelister JS. Lower limb compartment syndrome associated with the lithotomy position: concepts and perspectives for the urologist. BJU Int. 2002; 90(8):792–799

[138] Masten FA III. Compartmental Syndromes. New York, NY: Grune & Stratton; 1980:1–162

[139] Matsen FA, III, Winquist RA, Krugmire RB, Jr. Diagnosis and management of compartmental syndromes. J Bone Joint Surg Am. 1980; 62(2):286–291

[140] Brasch RC, Bufo AJ, Kreienberg PF, Johnson GP. Femoral neuropathy secondary to the use of a self-retaining retractor. Report of three cases and review of the literature. Dis Colon Rectum. 1995; 38(10):1115–1118

[141] Kvist-Poulsen H, Borel J. Iatrogenic femoral neuropathy subsequent to abdominal hysterectomy: incidence and prevention. Obstet Gynecol. 1982; 60 (4):516–520

[142] Celebrezze JP, Jr, Pidala MJ, Porter JA, Slezak FA. Femoral neuropathy: an infrequently reported postoperative complication. Report of four cases. Dis Colon Rectum. 2000; 43(3):419–422

[143] Pollard CW, Nivatvongs S, Rojanasakul A, Ilstrup DM. Carcinoma of the rectum. Profiles of intraoperative and early postoperative complications. Dis Colon Rectum. 1994; 37(9):866–874

[144] Eriksen MT, Wibe A, Norstern J, Haffner J, Wiig JN, Norwegian Rectal Cancer Group. Anastomotic leakage following routine mesorectal excision for rectal cancer in a national cohort of patients. Colorectal Dis. 2005; 7:51–57

[145] Matthiessen P, Hallböök O, Andersson M, Rutegård J, Sjödahl R. Risk factors for anastomotic leakage after anterior resection of the rectum. Colorectal Dis. 2004; 6(6):462–469

[146] Law WI, Chu KW, Ho JW, Chan CW. Risk factors for anastomotic leakage after low anterior resection with total mesorectal excision. Am J Surg. 2000; 179(2):92–96

[147] Sørensen LT, Jørgensen T, Kirkeby LT, Skovdal J, Vennits B, Wille-Jørgensen P. Smoking and alcohol abuse are major risk factors for anastomotic leakage in colorectal surgery. Br J Surg. 1999; 86(7):927–931

[148] Soeters PB, de Zoete JPJGM, Dejong CHC, Williams NS, Baeten CGMI. Colorectal surgery and anastomotic leakage. Dig Surg. 2002; 19(2):150–155

[149] Parc Y, Frileux P, Schmitt G, Dehni N, Ollivier JM, Parc R. Management of postoperative peritonitis after anterior resection: experience from a referral intensive care unit. Dis Colon Rectum. 2000; 43(5):579–587, discussion 587–589

[150] Smith LE. Anastomosis with EEA stapler after anterior colonic resection. Dis Colon Rectum. 1981; 24(4):236–242

[151] Graffner H, Fredlund P, Olsson SA, Oscarson J, Petersson BG. Protective colostomy in low anterior resection of the rectum using the EEA stapling instrument. A randomized study. Dis Colon Rectum. 1983; 26(2):87–90

[152] Gordon PH, Vasilevsky CA. Experience with stapling in rectal surgery. Surg Clin North Am. 1984; 64(3):555–566

[153] Kyzer S, Gordon PH. Experience with the use of the circular stapler in rectal surgery. Dis Colon Rectum. 1992; 35(7):696–706

[154] Leff EI, Hoexter B, Labow SB, Eisenstat TE, Rubin RJ, Salvati EP. The EEA stapler in low colorectal anastomoses: initial experience. Dis Colon Rectum. 1982; 25(7):704–707

[155] Fazio VW. Advances in the surgery of rectal carcinoma utilizing the circular stapler. In: Spratt JS, ed. Neoplasms of the Colon, Rectum, and Anus. Philadelphia, PA: WB Saunders; 1984:268–288

[156] Johansson C. Endoscopic dilation of rectal strictures: a prospective study of 18 cases. Dis Colon Rectum. 1996; 39(4):423–428

[157] Kyzer S, Gordon PH. The stapled functional end-to-end anastomosis following colonic resection. Int J Colorectal Dis. 1992; 7(3):125–131

[158] Otto IC, Ito K, Ye C, et al. Causes of rectal incontinence after sphincter-preserving operations for rectal cancer. Dis Colon Rectum. 1996; 39(12):1423–1427

[159] Ikeuchi H, Kusunoki M, Shoji Y, Yamamur T, Utsunomiya J. Clinico-physiological results after sphincter-saving resection for rectal carcinoma. Int J Colorectal Dis. 1996; 11(4):172–176

[160] Rao GN, Drew PJ, Lee PWR, Monson JR, Duthie GS. Anterior resection syndrome is secondary to sympathetic denervation. Int J Colorectal Dis. 1996; 11(5):250–258

[161] Bederman SS, Betsy M, Winiarsky R, Seldes RM, Sharrock NE, Sculco TP. Postoperative ileus in the lower extremity arthroplasty patient. J Arthroplasty. 2001; 16(8):1066–1070

[162] Condon RE, Frantzides CT, Cowles VE, Mahoney JL, Schulte WJ, Sarna SK. Resolution of postoperative ileus in humans. Ann Surg. 1986; 203 (5):574–581

[163] Stewart RM, Page CP, Brender J, Schwesinger W, Eisenhut D. The incidence and risk of early postoperative small bowel obstruction. A cohort study. Am J Surg. 1987; 154(6):643–647

[164] Menzies D, Ellis H. Intestinal obstruction from adhesions: how big is the problem? Ann R Coll Surg Engl. 1990; 72(1):60–63

[165] Pickleman J, Lee RM. The management of patients with suspected early postoperative small bowel obstruction. Ann Surg. 1989; 210(2):216–219

[166] Frager DH, Baer JW. Role of CT in evaluating patients with small-bowel obstruction. Semin Ultrasound CT MR. 1995; 16(2):127–140

[167] Nauta RJ. Advanced abdominal imaging is not required to exclude strangulation if complete small bowel obstructions undergo prompt laparotomy. J Am Coll Surg. 2005; 200(6):904–911

[168] Sarr MG, Bulkley GB, Zuidema GD. Preoperative recognition of intestinal strangulation obstruction. Prospective evaluation of diagnostic capability. Am J Surg. 1983; 145(1):176–182

[169] Sajja SBS, Schein M. Early postoperative small bowel obstruction. Br J Surg. 2004; 91(6):683–691

[170] Mallo RD, Salem L, Lalani T, Flum DR. Computed tomography diagnosis of ischemia and complete obstruction in small bowel obstruction: a systematic review. J Gastrointest Surg. 2005; 9(5):690–694

[171] Boudiaf M, Jaff A, Soyer P, Bouhnik Y, Hamzi L, Rymer R. Small-bowel diseases: prospective evaluation of multi-detector row helical CT enteroclysis in 107 consecutive patients. Radiology. 2004; 233(2):338–344

[172] Becker JM, Dayton MT, Fazio VW, et al. Prevention of postoperative abdominal adhesions by a sodium hyaluronate-based bioresorbable membrane: a prospective, randomized, double-blind multicenter study. J Am Coll Surg. 1996; 183(4):297–306

[173] Beck DE, Cohen Z, Fleshman JW, Kaufman HS, van Goor H, Wolff BG, Adhesion Study Group Steering Committee. A prospective, randomized, multicenter, controlled study of the safety of Seprafilm adhesion barrier in abdominopelvic surgery of the intestine. Dis Colon Rectum. 2003; 46 (10):1310–1319

[174] Cohen Z, Senagore AJ, Dayton MT, et al. Prevention of postoperative abdominal adhesions by a novel, glycerol/sodium hyaluronate/carboxymethylcellulose-based bioresorbable membrane: a prospective, randomized, evaluator-blinded multicenter study. Dis Colon Rectum. 2005; 48(6):1130–1139

[175] Fazio VW, Cohen Z, Fleshman JW, et al. Reduction in adhesive small-bowel obstruction by Seprafilm adhesion barrier after intestinal resection. Dis Colon Rectum. 2006; 49(1):1–11

[176] Ulnalp K, Condon RE. Antibiotics prophylaxis for scheduled operative procedures. Surg Clin North Am. 1992; 6:613–625

[177] Farnell MB, Worthington-Self S, Mucha P, Jr, Ilstrup DM, McIlrath DC. Closure of abdominal incisions with subcutaneous catheters. A prospective randomized trial. Arch Surg. 1986; 121(6):641–648

[178] Nichols RL, Holmes JWC. Prophylactic and therapeutic antibiotics in colon and rectal surgery. Perspect Colon Recta. 1990; 3(1):183–195

[179] Olson M, O'Connor M, Schwartz ML. Surgical wound infections. A 5-year prospective study of 20,193 wounds at the Minneapolis VA Medical Center. Ann Surg. 1984; 199(3):253–259

[180] Miller PR, Meredith JW, Johnson JC, Chang MC. Prospective evaluation of vacuum-assisted fascial closure after open abdomen: planned ventral hernia rate is substantially reduced. Ann Surg. 2004; 239(5):608–614, discussion 614–616

[181] Polk HC, Jr, Simpson CJ, Simmons BP, Alexander JW. Guidelines for prevention of surgical wound infection. Arch Surg. 1983; 118(10):1213–1217

[182] Gottrup F. Prevention of surgical-wound infections. N Engl J Med. 2000; 342 (3):202–204

[183] Kurz A, Sessler DI, Lenhardt R, Study of Wound Infection and Temperature Group. Perioperative normothermia to reduce the incidence of surgical-wound infection and shorten hospitalization. N Engl J Med. 1996; 334 (19):1209–1215

[184] Greif R, Akça O, Horn EP, Kurz A, Sessler DI, Outcomes Research Group. Supplemental perioperative oxygen to reduce the incidence of surgical-wound infection. N Engl J Med. 2000; 342(3):161–167

[185] Schoetz DJ, Jr, Coller JA, Veidenheimer MC. Closure of abdominal wounds with polydioxanone. A prospective study. Arch Surg. 1988; 123(1):72–74

[186] Richards PC, Balch CM, Aldrete JS. Abdominal wound closure. A randomized prospective study of 571 patients comparing continuous vs. interrupted suture techniques. Ann Surg. 1983; 197(2):238–243

[187] Penninckx FM, Poelmans SV, Kerremans RP, Beckers JP. Abdominal wound dehiscence in gastroenterological surgery. Ann Surg. 1979; 189(3):345–352

[188] Greenburg AG, Saik RP, Peskin GW. Wound dehiscence. Pathophysiology and prevention. Arch Surg. 1979; 114(2):143–146

[189] Wissing J, van Vroonhoven TJ, Schattenkerk ME, Veen HF, Ponsen RJ, Jeekel J. Fascia closure after midline laparotomy: results of a randomized trial. Br J Surg. 1987; 74(8):738–741

[190] Ellis H, Heddle R. Closure of the abdominal wound. J R Soc Med. 1979; 72 (1):17–18

[191] Alexander HC, Prudden JF. The causes of abdominal wound disruption. Surg Gynecol Obstet. 1966; 122(6):1223–1229

[192] Hugh TB, Nankivell C, Meagher AP, Li B. Is closure of the peritoneal layer necessary in the repair of midline surgical abdominal wounds? World J Surg. 1990; 14(2):231–233, discussion 233–234

[193] Rosenberg IL, Brennan TG, Giles GR. How tight should tension sutures be tied? A controlled clinical trial. Br J Surg. 1975; 62(12):950–951

[194] Stone IK, von Fraunhofer JA, Masterson BJ. The biomechanical effects of tight suture closure upon fascia. Surg Gynecol Obstet. 1986; 163(5):448–452

[195] Fagniez PL, Hay JM, Lacàine F, Thomsen C. Abdominal midline incision closure. A multicentric randomized prospective trial of 3,135 patients, comparing continuous vs interrupted polyglycolic acid sutures. Arch Surg. 1985; 120(12):1351–1353

[196] Hodgson NC, Malthaner RA, Ostbye T. The search for an ideal method of abdominal fascial closure: a meta-analysis. Ann Surg. 2000; 231(3):436–442

[197] van 't Riet M, Steyerberg EW, Nellensteyn J, Bonjer HJ, Jeekel J. Meta-analysis of techniques for closure of midline abdominal incisions. Br J Surg. 2002; 89 (11):1350–1356

[198] Deerenberg EB, Harlaar JJ, Steyerberg EW, et al. Small bites versus large bites for closure of abdominal midline incisions (STITCH): a double-blind, multicentre, randomised controlled trial. Lancet. 2015; 386(10000):1254–1260

[199] Poole GV, Jr. Mechanical factors in abdominal wound closure: the prevention of fascial dehiscence. Surgery. 1985; 97(6):631–640

[200] Rucinski J, Margolis M, Panagopoulos G, Wise L. Closure of the abdominal midline fascia: meta-analysis delineates the optimal technique. Am Surg. 2001; 67(5):421–426

[201] Ray JA, Doddi N, Regula D, Williams JA, Melveger A. Polydioxanone (PDS), a novel monofilament synthetic absorbable suture. Surg Gynecol Obstet. 1981; 153(4):497–507

[202] Israelsson LA, Jonsson T. Closure of midline laparotomy incisions with polydioxanone and nylon: the importance of suture technique. Br J Surg. 1994; 81(11):1606–1608

[203] Rink AD, Goldschmidt D, Dietrich J, Nagelschmidt M, Vestweber KH. Negative side-effects of retention sutures for abdominal wound closure. A prospective randomised study. Eur J Surg. 2000; 166(12):932–937

[204] Irvin TT, Goligher JC. A controlled clinical trial of three different methods of perineal wound management following excision of the rectum. Br J Surg. 1975; 62(4):287–291

[205] Robles Campos R, Garcia Ayllon J, Parrila Paricio P, et al. Management of the perineal wound following abdominoperineal resection: prospective study of three methods. Br J Surg. 1992; 79(1):29–31

[206] Bullard KM, Trudel JL, Baxter NN, Rothenberger DA. Primary perineal wound closure after preoperative radiotherapy and abdominoperineal resection has a high incidence of wound failure. Dis Colon Rectum. 2005; 48(3):438–443

[207] Christian CK, Kwaan MR, Betensky RA, Breen EM, Zinner MJ, Bleday R. Risk factors for perineal wound complications following abdominoperineal resection. Dis Colon Rectum. 2005; 48(1):43–48

[208] Delalande JP, Hay JM, Fingerhut A, Kohlmann GC, Paquet JC. French Association for Surgical Research. Perineal wound management after abdominoperineal rectal excision for carcinoma with unsatisfactory hemostasis or gross septic contamination; Primary closure vs. packing. A multicenter, control trial. Dis Colon Rectum. 1994; 37:890–896

[209] Baudot P, Keighley MRB, Alexander-Williams J. Perineal wound healing after proctectomy for carcinoma and inflammatory disease. Br J Surg. 1980; 67 (4):275–276

[210] Elliot MS, Todd IP. Primary suture of the perineal wound using constant suction and irrigation, following rectal excision for inflammatory bowel disease. Ann R Coll Surg Engl. 1985; 67(1):6–7

[211] Oakley JR, Fazio VW, Jagelman DG, Lavery IC, Weakley FL, Easley K. Management of the perineal wound after rectal excision for ulcerative colitis. Dis Colon Rectum. 1985; 28(12):885–888

[212] Tompkins RG, Warshaw AL. Improved management of the perineal wound after proctectomy. Ann Surg. 1985; 202(6):760–765

[213] Anthony JP, Mathes SJ. The recalcitrant perineal wound after rectal extirpation. Applications of muscle flap closure. Arch Surg. 1990; 125(10):1371–1376, discussion 1376–1377

[214] Baird WL, Hester TR, Nahai F, Bostwick J, III. Management of perineal wounds following abdominoperineal resection with inferior gluteal flaps. Arch Surg. 1990; 125(11):1486–1489

[215] Galandiuk S, Jorden J, Mahid S, McCafferty MH, Tobin G. The use of tissue flaps as an adjunct to pelvic surgery. Am J Surg. 2005; 190(2):186–190

[216] Menon A, Clark MA, Shatari T, Keh C, Keighley MRB. Pedicled flaps in the treatment of nonhealing perineal wounds. Colorectal Dis. 2005; 7(5):441–444

[217] Pemberton JH. How to treat the persistent perineal sinus after rectal excision. Colorectal Dis. 2003; 5(5):486–489

[218] Loessin SJ, Meland NB, Devine RM, Wolff BG, Nelson H, Zincke H. Management of sacral and perineal defects following abdominoperineal resection and radiation with transpelvic muscle flaps. Dis Colon Rectum. 1995; 38 (9):940–945

[219] Temple L, Lindsay RL, Temple WJ, Magi E, Ketcham AS. Rectus myocutaneous flaps for primary repair of composite defects of the pelvis. Perspect Colon Rectal Surg. 1993; 6:171–174

[220] So JB, Palmer MT, Shellito PC. Postoperative perineal hernia. Dis Colon Rectum. 1997; 40(8):954–957

[221] Beck DE, Fazio VW, Jagelman DG, Lavery IC, McGonagle BA. Postoperative perineal hernia. Dis Colon Rectum. 1987; 30(1):21–24

[222] Brotschi E, Noe JM, Silen W. Perineal hernias after proctectomy. A new approach to repair. Am J Surg. 1985; 149(2):301–305

[223] Sarr MG, Stewart JR, Cameron JC. Combined abdominoperineal approach to repair of postoperative perineal hernia. Dis Colon Rectum. 1982; 25 (6):597–599

36 Unexpected Intraoperative Findings and Complex Preoperative Decisions

David E. Beck

Abstract

Despite advances in preoperative evaluation, unexpected disease states or anatomic variations will be identified intraoperatively, which requires the surgeon to make important decisions rapidly. Challenging complex preoperative decisions as well as unusual or unexpected intraoperative findings are discussed with suggestions for managing them. Several of these were selected for their controversial nature. While not particularly uncommon, they continue to present a dilemma for the surgeon.

Keywords: intraoperative findings, unexpected, complex preoperative decision, colorectal carcinoma, unexpected rectal mass, appendix, Meckel's diverticulum, rectal injury

36.1 Introduction

The ever-expanding technology available to the practicing physician has greatly improved the identification of intra-abdominal pathology in advance of a laparotomy. This often leads to complex preoperative decisions. Nevertheless, from time to time surprises do arise with additional disease states or anatomic variations and the surgeon must make important decisions rapidly. This chapter highlights some complex preoperative decisions as well as unusual or unexpected findings and offers suggestions for managing them. We recognize that the management of many of these problems is controversial; in fact, that is precisely why these subjects have been selected. Although we are well aware that the list of surprises could extend almost without limit, we have chosen to focus on subjects that are not particularly uncommon yet present a dilemma to the surgeon. Suggested therapy may represent only a consensus of the authors.

The gynecologist or urologist often discovers large bowel pathology under one of the following circumstances: (1) during the operative treatment of established gynecologic pathology, (2) when acute or chronic pelvic sepsis is demonstrated as due to complications of large bowel disease, (3) when the true nature of an abdominal pelvic neoplasm is determined at laparotomy. Since bowel preparation may not have been performed in such situations, definitive treatment may result in higher postoperative morbidity than would result under ideal conditions. The dilemma involved is that the surgeon is faced with one of several challenging situations: (1) unprepared bowel, which may have an increased sepsis in colorectal operations; (2) established sepsis with the obvious concern of creating an anastomosis; or (3) possible catastrophic outcome if sepsis should ensue following an associated operation (e.g., as for an abdominal aortic aneurysm [AAA]). Some of the following case examples will be all too familiar to many readers.

36.1.1 Colorectal Carcinoma

During operations for colorectal cancer, intraoperative findings may be challenging.

36.1.2 Case 1: Carcinoma of Rectum and Unexpected Synchronous Colon Carcinoma

At laparotomy, a 72-year-old patient being operated on for carcinoma of the rectosigmoid is found to have a previously unsuspected mass in the hepatic flexure deemed to represent a synchronous carcinoma. There is no evidence of metastatic disease. What is the most appropriate operation?

With a patient having synchronous carcinomas, a number of options are open. The surgeon could proceed with the planned low anterior resection and assess the right colonic mass postoperatively through a barium enema or colonoscopic evaluation. Alternatively, the surgeon could allow recovery period of several weeks before a right hemicolectomy is performed. Both options are inappropriate.

The two preferred options are (1) to proceed immediately with a total abdominal colectomy and ileorectal anastomosis or (2) to perform two resections, the planned low anterior resection and a right hemicolectomy. There is no question that the first option is appealing because it rids the patient of both carcinomas through only one anastomosis. Furthermore, it might be best for a patient who already harbors two malignancies of the colon to be liberated from an organ with demonstrated propensity to neoplasia. The short rectal stump would make follow-up of the remaining bowel simple for both the patient and the surgeon. The risk of one anastomosis may be less than the risk of two anastomoses. For patients with carcinomas that are both located more proximally in the bowel (i.e., anywhere from the cecum to the proximal to middle sigmoid colon), this option would seem to be the treatment of choice. If synchronous carcinomas are located in an area of similar lymph node drainage, the respective hemicolectomy is indicated. For patients with malignancies involving different drainage areas in the lymphatic system of the colon, subtotal colectomy or total proctocolectomy and ileostomy (if the distal rectum is involved) can be performed.

There are several proponents of subtotal colectomy.[1,2,3] However, an overriding consideration, especially in the older patient, is the postoperative functional results.[4] Exactly how much distal bowel is necessary for an adequate reservoir is uncertain and will vary from patient to patient. Experience with patients with familial adenomatous polyposis suggests that an anastomosis performed at the level of the sacral promontory has resulted in an acceptable frequency of defecation. It must be noted that for the most part this experience has been accumulated in young individuals.

The patient in question is older, and the proposed anastomosis would need to be performed at a considerably lower level. Under these circumstances, it would be anticipated that functional results would not be good, and therefore we would lean toward a double resection (i.e., the planned low anterior resection and a concomitant right hemicolectomy at the same operation). With the use of repeated colonoscopy, little trouble would be encountered in following the residual colon for metachronous neoplasia.

36.1.3 Case 2: Carcinoma of Right Colon and Unexpected Hepatic Metastasis

Most large hepatic masses will be identified on the preoperative CT scan. However, small lesions may be missed. Two unexpected 1-cm masses are found at the edge of the right lobe of the liver during laparotomy for resection of a right colonic carcinoma. Preoperative CT scan was normal. What is the recommended management?

The philosophy of the management of patients with metastatic disease to the liver has changed dramatically in the past 20 years. The goal of therapy in any operation for malignancy is the removal of all detectable disease. In this situation, the operation would encompass both a right hemicolectomy and an excision of the two small masses.

If the lesions had been larger (an uncommon finding with preoperative scanning), a procedure of greater magnitude (e.g., a right hepatic lobectomy) may have been required. Prior to hepatic resection, it would be necessary to determine the extent of other metastatic disease, if present. It also would be appropriate to discuss with the patient the potential risks of a partial hepatic resection of this magnitude. In addition, current practice in many centers is to consider four courses of adjuvant chemotherapy prior to liver resection.

Even in the presence of metastatic disease in the liver, the primary colonic carcinoma should be removed because of the risk of later complications such as bleeding and obstruction. Liver lesions not resected should be biopsied to confirm the presence of metastatic disease. The evaluation and treatment of colorectal metastasis is discussed in Chapters 21 and 22.[5,6,7]

36.1.4 Case 3: Carcinoma of Rectum with Incidental Cholelithiasis

A 79-year-old man is undergoing anterior resection with a low pelvic anastomosis for adenocarcinoma of the rectum located 9 cm from the dentate line. The liver is normal, but the gallbladder contains multiple stones. There is no clear-cut history of symptomatic gallbladder disease. Should the gallbladder be removed?

The decision of whether to proceed with cholecystectomy must take into account the added morbidity and mortality of this procedure, the risks of symptomatic gallbladder disease developing in the immediate or late postoperative period.

Most studies have emphasized that although complication rates range from 20 to 41% when cholecystectomy is added to another intra-abdominal procedure, complications specifically related to the cholecystectomy occur in less than 3% of these cases, and the mortality rate is not increased.[8,9,10,11,12,13,14,15,16,17,18,19,20,21,22,23,24,25,26] All of this assumes, however, that the cholecystectomy is performed during a procedure that has gone well, that the patient is stable, and that the incision does not need to be significantly extended. The assumption is that the scope and magnitude of the operation are not significantly increased or that the operation was inordinately prolonged. Shennib et al,[27] in a study of 25 patients who underwent simultaneous cholecystectomy

and colectomy, concluded that the addition of cholecystectomy was safe when performed during the course of an elective colonic resection if the patient was stable. The authors do not recommend performing cholecystectomy during the course of emergency colectomy in an ill patient with an unprepared bowel.

It is possible that patients with cholelithiasis discovered incidentally at the time of another abdominal operation may be at greater risk for developing symptomatic gallbladder disease than similar individuals not undergoing operation. In one study, the risk of cholecystitis or symptomatic gallbladder disease developing within 6 months of operation was found to be as high as 70% among 23 patients with cholelithiasis who did not have incidental cholecystectomy during an abdominal operation.[24] Acute cholecystitis developing in the immediate postoperative period in similar patients also has been noted.[24] Whether this relationship is fortuitous in the above studies or whether it is related to postoperative mechanical or metabolic factors is unclear.

Overall, it does appear reasonable and appropriate to proceed with cholecystectomy in the patient described here if favorable conditions exist. This would mean that the anterior resection and anastomosis proceeded without complication, that the patient's condition remained stable throughout the procedure, and that the gallbladder can be reached easily through the original incision. Usually, cholecystectomy is technically feasible from either vertical or transverse incisions as long as the initial incision is generous and the patient is not obese. If the incision needs to be significantly extended to achieve adequate exposure for cholecystectomy, the overall scope of the operation is being expanded and the possibility of having a significant increase in postoperative complications becomes a factor. In these circumstances, it is best to leave the gallbladder intact.

If the cholelithiasis was not known preoperatively, from a medicolegal point of view it appears safe to proceed with a previously unplanned cholecystectomy when unsuspected cholelithiasis is identified, since a surgeon is ordinarily protected by the legal doctrine of "extension of informed consent."[28] The low morbidity and negligible mortality when cholecystectomy is performed, along with the alternative risks of postoperative symptomatic gallbladder disease when cholecystectomy is not performed, reinforce the validity of an intraoperative decision to proceed with cholecystectomy. Nevertheless, since this does constitute removal of an organ without the patient's prior consent, it is especially important that the cholecystectomy be performed only under favorable conditions without increasing the magnitude of the operation. Legally, the safest course is to discuss the possibility of cholecystectomy or removal of other tissues with the patient at the time that consent for colectomy is obtained.

36.1.5 Case 4: Carcinoma of Rectum with Invasion of Urinary Bladder

An otherwise healthy 56-year-old man is scheduled to undergo a low anterior resection of the rectum. Preoperative imaging demonstrates that the carcinoma invades the base of the bladder and the prostate.[29,30,31,32,33,34,35,36,37] There is no evidence of distal spread. Should a pelvic exenteration be performed?

The recommendations made here are what we believe to be in the best interest of the patient. However, following them may result in procedures being performed without the patient's fully informed consent. This discussion is not intended to cover that legal aspect of the problem.

Pelvic exenteration for colorectal carcinoma involves en bloc removal of the colon and/or anorectum, the bladder and distal ureters with creation of an ileal conduit, a pelvic lymph node dissection, and removal of internal reproductive organs as indicated. It is a formidable procedure with high morbidity and mortality rates. A review of the literature by Eckhauser et al[38] showed a mortality rate of 12%. In a large series of pelvic exenterations for colorectal, gynecologic, and urologic diseases reported by Jakowatz et al,[29] there was a major complication rate of 49%, including gastrointestinal fistulas or obstruction, urinary tract fistulas, infection or obstruction, wound dehiscence, and/or hemorrhages. The complications rate was highest (67%) when patients received preoperative radiation and lowest (26%) when radiation was not given. However, the operative mortality rate was only 2.9%. Other reports support the justification of pelvic exenteration or en bloc excision of a T4 lesion, if the procedure can be performed with an intention of cure.[30,31,32,33]

There are two major justifications for aggressive surgical treatment of patients with locally advanced primary and recurrent rectal carcinoma in the absence of gross distant metastases. First, many of these patients will die with catastrophic symptomatic consequences of uncontrolled pelvic carcinoma, primarily pain and tenesmus. Symptoms are only temporarily abated with radiation therapy alone. Second, autopsy studies suggest that 25 to 50% of such patients have carcinoma limited to the pelvis at the time of death. Hence, aggressive efforts at local control may not only avoid painful recurrence in such patients but also disease-free and overall survival may be improved.[34]

Colorectal carcinoma with direct invasion into the bladder but without distant metastases is uncommon, accounting for only 5% of cases.[35] This type of lesion cannot be cured by nonoperative management such as chemotherapy or radiation therapy. Preoperative radiation for a clinically resectable lesion will not change the extent of the resection,[36] and it may only increase the complication rate.[29] When patients are properly selected, the 5-year survival rate can be expected to be 45 to 50%.[35,37] Ideally, the lesion should be limited locally without lymph node metastases. En bloc resection of the rectum and the adjacent involved organs was performed in 65 patients in a series reported by Orkin et al.[37] Of those patients, 26% underwent a cystectomy. There were no perioperative deaths. Postoperative complications developed in 20% of patients, and the overall 5-year survival rate was 52%. Talamonti et al[39] reviewed the records of 70 patients who underwent resection of a carcinoma of the colon and rectum with en bloc total cystectomy (36 patients) or partial cystectomy (34 patients) because of malignancy directly extending into the urinary bladder. Sixty-four patients with negative resection margins had a median survival of 34 months and a 5-year actuarial survival rate of 51.8%. In contrast, the median survival period for six patients who had positive margins was 11 months, with no survivors at 5 years.

The only hope for cure in colorectal carcinoma with invasion into the bladder is to perform pelvic exenteration. This is an extensive operation with potentially high morbidity, mortality,

and prolonged postoperative recovery. In properly selected patients, the operation is worthwhile in terms of long-term survival and symptomatic relief. Patients with distant metastases should not be considered for pelvic exenteration.

At the time of exploration, the surgeon must accurately establish the extent of pelvic disease and the surgeon's ability to remove it. Actual histologic invasion of adjacent structures can be very difficult to differentiate from inflammatory reaction without pathologic confirmation. Complete excision of the neoplasm with a portion or all of any apparently involved organs appears to result in the best possibility of complete excision and thus cure. A team approach consisting of a colorectal surgeon, a gynecologic surgeon, and a urologic surgeon helps achieve optimal results.[37]

The bulkiness of the lesion should not deter surgeons. Size and local extension do not correlate with long-term survival. The most important predictors of survival are lymph node status and involvement of the resection margins. In fact, the overall survival in patients with T4 carcinomas who underwent radical resection is not significantly different from that in those with T3 carcinomas, even in N1 stages.[32]

Armed with this information, what should the surgeon do for the patient? Ideally, a discussion is held with the patient preoperatively, but since the intraoperative findings were a surprise, this cannot be done. The options are to proceed with an exenteration or close the abdomen and discuss the recommendation with the patient. It is technically easier to proceed at the original operation because repeat operations are more difficult. Most often, a portion of the mobilization has already been accomplished, and it is quite possible that the best technical operation can be accomplished at this time. However, because of the magnitude of the procedure, the potential high complication rate, and the lifestyle alteration for the patient, we would favor aborting the procedure and discussing the advantages of a pelvic exenteration with the patient.

36.1.6 Case 5: Concomitant Carcinoma of Rectum and Abdominal Aortic Aneurysm

A 75-year-old man is scheduled to undergo low anterior resection of the rectum for a carcinoma. Preoperative scanning reveals a 6-cm AAA. What is the appropriate management?

The occurrence of synchronous colorectal carcinoma and AAA is uncommon. At the Mayo Clinic from 1975 to 1986, approximately 3,500 patients with AAA underwent repair, but only 17 patients were found to have a simultaneous colorectal carcinoma.[40] Most lesions were discovered before the operation and thus the management could be planned. More recently, Baxter et al[41] reviewed 435 Mayo Clinic patients with a history of colorectal carcinoma and AAA, of which 83 patients had concomitant AAA and colorectal carcinoma. In 64 patients, the colorectal carcinoma was treated first, and 44 of these patients had an AAA < 5 cm in diameter (average = 3.8 cm). No AAA ruptured in the postoperative period. Median delay in colorectal carcinoma surgery from diagnosis was 4 days. There were 20 patients with AAA of 5 cm or greater (average = 5.4 cm) who were treated for colorectal carcinoma first. In two of these patients (with AAA sized 5 and 6.4 cm), the AAA ruptured in the early postoperative period. Median delay in colorectal carcinoma resection was 8 days. There were 12 patients who had both an AAA and colorectal carcinoma treated at the same time. The average size of the AAA was 6.4 cm. Median delay from colorectal carcinoma diagnosis to resection was 15 days. No documented cases of graft infection occurred in this group; median follow-up was 3.2 years. There were seven patients who underwent AAA repair before resection of their colorectal carcinoma; in two patients, colorectal carcinoma was found at the time of resection. The average size of the AAA was 6 cm and median delay to treatment of colorectal carcinoma was 122 days, a statistically significantly longer delay than in the other two groups. They concluded that in patients with colorectal carcinoma and AAA of 5 cm or more, treatment of colorectal carcinoma first might result in life-threatening rupture, whereas treatment of the AAA first might significantly delay treatment of the colorectal carcinoma. Concomitant treatment seems to be a safe alternative. If anatomically suitable, the AAA may be considered for endovascular repair, followed by a staged colon resection. The presence of an AAA less than 5 cm does not affect colorectal carcinoma treatment. Herald et al[42] also described the use of endovascular placement of a graft for the treatment of AAA in association with rectal carcinoma. Minimally invasive endovascular repair is currently the procedure of choice.[43,44]

In general, it has been recommended to treat the lesion that causes symptoms first, with an option to manage the second lesion at the same time or at a later date.[45] Frequently, however, the patients are generally free of symptoms, and one lesion is discovered incidentally at the elective resection of the other. What should be done? If neither symptoms nor aneurysm size establishes priority, the relative indolent course of colon carcinoma favors aneurysm repair with colectomy in 2 to 4 weeks.[40]

Historically, the advantages of concomitant resections of colorectal carcinoma and AAA are avoidance of a second operation and elimination of the possibility of a ruptured AAA postoperatively if left untreated. The major risk of this approach is a possible aortic graft infection, which can be life threatening. The risk of ruptured AAA after laparotomy is real.[40,46] Some attribute this to the increased activity of the proteolytic enzymes collagenase and elastase,[45,46,47,48] although this is only speculation. In a series by Nora et al,[40] eight patients had colorectal resection without resection of the AAA. Three patients died from complications of the aneurysm, including two ruptured aneurysms and one thrombotic aneurysm. The remaining five patients also died, four from disseminated carcinoma, with death occurring 6, 12, 18, and 48 months later; the other patient died from sepsis 36 hours postoperatively. It appears that for long-term survival both lesions must be resected aggressively.[40] The size of the aneurysm plays an important role in the decision-making process. It is generally agreed that an AAA > 7 cm poses a risk of rupture in the near future and tends to rupture soon after colonic resection.[49] Therefore, such an aneurysm should be resected first, unless the colorectal carcinoma is obstructing. Velanovich and Andersen[45] recommended that when both lesions are asymptomatic and the aneurysm is 4 to 5 cm in diameter, it should be resected first, if the colorectal carcinoma has a less than 5% chance of obstruction or perforation, as is found in noncircumferential lesions. When the aneurysm is greater than 5 cm, it should be resected first if the carcinoma has a less than 22% chance of obstructing or perforating, as with circumferential

lesions. Simultaneous resection should be considered for patients with aneurysms greater than 5 cm and carcinomas with a greater than 75 to 80% chance of obstruction or perforation, provided the dual procedures can be performed with a less than 10% operative mortality and less than 50% complication rate. If it is deemed that there is an impending obstruction by the carcinoma, both the aneurysm and the carcinoma should be resected simultaneously.[50] The AAA should be resected first and the retroperitoneum closed, with interposition of omentum between the graft and the peritoneum before resection of the colon and rectum to minimize the risk of graft infection. An elective simultaneous resection of AAA and a right colectomy can be safely performed. The risk of anastomotic leak is higher for a left colectomy. For a low anterior resection, unless the procedure is easy, a complementary loop ileostomy should be considered, or a colostomy and Hartmann's pouch procedure should be performed.

A 5-cm-diameter AAA has a 4.1% annual risk of rupture if left untreated, and this risk increases exponentially with increasing aneurysm diameter so that a 7-cm AAA has a 19% yearly risk of rupture.[51] In situations where the carcinoma shows no symptoms of obstruction and the aneurysm is also asymptomatic and less than 6 cm in diameter, it has traditionally been taught that the aneurysm should be resected first because of the risk of postlaparotomy rupture of the aneurysm, which has been reported to be as high as 33.8%.[45]

The surgeon must be certain that the two ends of bowel have good blood supply. After sacrificing the inferior mesenteric artery, there is usually enough blood supply from the marginal artery of Drummond as well as branches from the iliac arteries. It has been shown that colonic ischemia is usually the result of perioperative low cardiac output and the use of alpha-adrenergic vasopressive agents.[52,53] In this situation, an anastomosis should not be performed.

In the patient with a small AAA, the carcinoma should be resected first and the AAA should be resected at a later date.

The ability to perform minimally invasive endovascular aortic repair has largely eliminated the above discussion.[43,44] Larger or systematic aneurysms are percutaneously repaired and a colectomy can follow in short period.

36.2 Unexpected Colorectal Mass

36.2.1 Case 6: Sigmoid Mass that Proves to Be Endometrioma Instead of Carcinoma

A 42-year-old woman presented with a 6-month history of abdominal cramps. Barium enema study revealed narrowing in the sigmoid colon, and colonoscopy was unsuccessful because the scope could not be negotiated through the narrow portion. A laparotomy was performed for the presumed diagnosis of carcinoma of the sigmoid, but extrinsic pressure from a partially encompassing blue–brown mass was seen. Further inspection revealed purple specks on the pelvic structures. A presumptive diagnosis of endometriosis was made. What would be the appropriate management?

Endometriotic implants on pelvic structures are a common finding during pelvic laparotomy for gynecologic disease. Once the intestinal involvement has become symptomatic, the only successful treatment that prevents subsequent recurrence of symptoms is resection of the affected segment combined with total abdominal hysterectomy and bilateral salpingo-oophorectomy.[8,9,10] If the diagnosis of endometriosis had been suspected preoperatively and the patient was informed of the possibility, resection is the treatment of choice. However, under the current circumstances, we would suggest limitation of treatment to sigmoid resection. We would be reluctant to perform a total abdominal hysterectomy and bilateral salpingo-oophorectomy without the patient's knowledge. Simple retreat with hope of relief of symptoms by hormonal administration is inappropriate because once intestinal symptoms have developed, scarring has advanced to the point where endocrine treatment will be ineffective.[11,12] Similar operative treatments would be endorsed for the patient who still desires a family. If the implant is well circumscribed, local excision of the colonic endometrioma may be effective.[9,13] Gonadotropin-releasing hormone antagonists such as leuprolide (Lupron) and nafarelin (Synarel) have demonstrated efficacy in the treatment of small endometrial implants but do not have a major impact on large deposits.[10]

36.2.2 Case 7: Exploration for Appendicitis that Proves to Be Carcinoma of Cecum

The patient is a 51-year-old man presenting with right lower quadrant pain and scheduled to undergo laparoscopy and an appendectomy for acute appendicitis. The patient is found to have a mass interpreted as a walled-off perforated carcinoma of the cecum. How should the patient's management be handled?

The discovery of unexpected disease at laparoscopy or laparotomy often taxes the judgment and ingenuity of the surgeon. This is especially true for emergency operations, which are often performed at night. However, the almost universal preoperative emergency room CT scan often suggests unusual pathology. It is estimated that 10 to 15% of right colonic carcinomas will first appear as acute abdomen. It was not uncommon for a patient to undergo exploration for a preoperative diagnosis of appendicitis only for the surgeon to find a carcinoma of the cecum causing obstruction and resulting appendicitis, a perforated carcinoma of the cecum or ascending colon with a normal appendix, an acute appendicitis with a more distal obstructing carcinoma of the hepatic flexure or the sigmoid colon, or an adenocarcinoma of the appendix itself. The surgeon is faced with the unprepared bowel and the prospect of contamination from perforation of the bowel if a resection is performed immediately. One choice would be to close the abdomen and return after the patient has undergone adequate bowel preparation, which offers a theoretic advantage for operation. However, there is the risk of progression of the inflammatory process with potential aggravation during bowel preparation. A free perforation may even result. Therefore, whenever the surgeon is faced with the situation that carcinoma is suspected, a right hemicolectomy should be performed.

Next, the surgeon must decide whether laparoscopy or a McBurney incision is adequate for the revised operation. Some surgeons would convert to a formal midline incision to gain greater exposure. However, extension of the extraction site (McBurney's incision) across the rectus muscle to the midline creates more than ample exposure for performing a right hemicolectomy. In an elderly patient with a less certain diagnosis, a lower midline incision might be considered. After that procedure has been performed, the surgeon is faced with the question of whether to perform a primary anastomosis or to bring out the two ends of bowel. Considerable evidence suggests that it is safe to proceed with a primary anastomosis following emergency right hemicolectomy.[14] Appropriate operative treatment should not be postponed because of lack of bowel preparation. Even the presence of walled-off pus rarely contraindicates resection and anastomosis. In the face of generalized peritonitis following excision of the diseased segment of bowel, consideration should be given to performing an end-loop stoma. Of course, appropriate antibiotic coverage is indicated.

Usually, the major problem under these circumstances is making the diagnosis. The ileocecal region is notorious for inflammatory masses that are difficult to distinguish from carcinoma. When appendicitis is present, it is understandable that the surrounding induration may be attributed to the associated inflammatory process without suspicion of an underlying malignancy. The degree of difficulty in making a diagnosis at the time of appendectomy is underscored by the fact that less than one-half of the cases reported in the literature were diagnosed at initial laparotomy. The average delay in diagnosis is 4 to 6 months.[15,16,17] Postoperative clues to the true nature of the underlying disease include cecal fistulas, recurrent abscesses, and discharging sinus following appendectomy. These circumstances dictate further investigation of the colon.

36.2.3 Case 8: Pelvic Laparotomy for Gynecologic Mass that Proves to Be Carcinoma of Sigmoid

A 43-year-old woman is undergoing laparotomy for a pelvic mass presumed to be of ovarian origin. The gynecologist finds the ovaries to be normal, and the mass proves to be a hard 7-cm lesion in the middle sigmoid colon that is compatible with either carcinoma or diverticular disease. You are called to the operating room and asked to consider removing the lesion. The bowel has not been prepared and hard stool can be palpated throughout the colon. What is your decision?

The options in this case include (1) performing a resection and a colostomy, (2) performing a resection and an anastomosis, (3) doing nothing and having the patient return for an elective resection at a later date, after the bowel has been prepared and the patient has been evaluated fully, or (4) performing a resection, on-table lavage, and anastomosis. If the lesion were in the right colon, a right hemicolectomy with anastomosis would seem appropriate since this procedure can be accomplished without preparation and with minimum morbidity.[14,18]

Emergency or unplanned resection of the left colon is much more controversial, particularly in the presence of fecal loading. If the patient has an impending obstruction, resection must be performed immediately. In this circumstance, waiting for time to perform a mechanical bowel preparation and elective resection may not be feasible, and the bowel preparation actually may provoke complete obstruction. Whether obstruction is imminent or not, once a decision has been made to proceed with resection, a second choice must be made between performing an anastomosis or creating a colostomy. Although primary anastomosis in select patients has been advocated by some authors,[19] others have emphasized the prevalence of septic complications and anastomotic leaks when anastomosis is performed in unprepared bowel.[20,21] If a colostomy is to be performed, creating an end colostomy and Hartmann's pouch is preferable. The alternative of creating a proximal colostomy with distal anastomosis leaves a column of stool and bacteria between the colostomy and the anastomosis, and does not completely protect against septic anastomotic complications. In addition to resection and anastomosis or resection and colostomy, a third option is resection with anastomosis and intraoperative fecal washout.[22] One variation is to perform a subtotal excision of the colon to a point in the distal sigmoid colon and to achieve washout of the rectosigmoid per annum to permit a safe anastomosis of the ileum to the distal sigmoid.

Since favorable results have been reported with each of these options, any one of them can be considered acceptable. A growing number of surgeons will favor resection, on-table lavage, and primary anastomosis. Some surgeons prefer resection and anastomosis and this course of action is supported by publications stating that bowel preparation is not mandatory. If concern of integrity of anastomosis arises, a diverting ileostomy might be in order. This topic has been described in detail in Chapter 4 on bowel preparation.

36.2.4 Case 9: Exploration for Acute Appendicitis that Proves to Be Sigmoid Phlegmon

A 40-year-old man is undergoing exploration for appendicitis through McBurney's incision. The appendix, cecum, and terminal ileum are found to be perfectly normal. A small amount of serous fluid is found in the peritoneal cavity, but the sigmoid colon is noted to be acutely inflamed. What should the management be?

There is controversy regarding the most effective method of managing the perforated diverticular segment. When there is a major unsealed perforation with fecal contamination, immediate resection for the involved segment is appropriate. But in the vast majority of cases with generalized peritonitis from perforated diverticular disease, there is no evidence of fecal contamination, and the perforation is already sealed or cannot be found at laparotomy. Possibly only a phlegmon is present. In this circumstance, it is unclear whether immediate definitive resection is required. Many surgeons favor this policy because the patient is already committed to undergoing laparotomy. On the other hand, some would argue that if the diagnosis had been known preoperatively and if the patient was responding to medical treatment, an urgent operation would not have been offered to the patient and therefore no resection should be performed. It is perhaps important to know whether the patient had experienced previous symptoms of diverticular disease because this would tip the scale in favor of resection. In the minds of some surgeons, a patient younger than the age of 40 years and even younger than the age of 50 years should undergo resection. Stefansson et al[23] found that in patients with a phlegmonous diverticulitis or abscess, the postoperative complications were threefold greater (13 vs. 4%) in those who did not undergo resection. If

resection is considered, then a decision must be made as to which of the several options would be the most appropriate—Hartmann's procedure, a primary resection with anastomosis with or without on-table lavage, or a primary resection and anastomosis with proximal diversion. If the patient were previously symptomatic, resection with on-table lavage would probably best serve the patient. Even if the patient had not had symptoms attributable to diverticular disease, the complication rate for phlegmonous diverticulitis reported by Stefansson et al[23] would persuade us to choose the resection option.

36.3 Appendix

36.3.1 Case 10: Propriety of Incidental Appendectomy

The patient is a 72-year-old man who is undergoing sigmoid resection for an annular carcinoma. Should an incidental appendectomy be performed?

When not inflamed, the appendix is easy to remove. Therefore, it is one of the most common organs removed incidentally after completion of the primary abdominal operation mission. The rationale for removing a normal appendix is to avoid the development of appendicitis in the future. The diagnosis of acute appendicitis has remained a problem for the past 100 years, with a false-positive rate of 20 to 25% and a delay in diagnosis leading to perforation in as many as 25 to 30% of patients.[54] Approximately 7% of the population will have acute appendicitis sometime during their lifetime.[55] The morbidity rate of appendicitis is significant. In nonperforated appendicitis, the infection rate is 8%.[56] For perforated appendicitis, the septic rate is 32%, with a wound infection rate of 25% and an intra-abdominal abscess rate of 7%.[57] Incidental appendectomy thus eliminates future problems that may occur.

Whether an incidental appendectomy should be performed has been a subject of debate for many years. There are both pros and cons,[58,59] largely based on philosophical reasons rather than facts, which are impossible to obtain. Several prospective-controlled studies have shown that incidental appendectomy does not increase morbidity and mortality rates compared with the primary abdominal operation alone.[60,61,62] It must be emphasized that in these studies when incidental appendectomy was performed, the appendix was readily exposed and removed without much time and effort. One should also note that some series show a higher rate of infection when the incidental appendectomy is performed in patients older than 50 years.[63,64]

Approximately 250,000 cases of appendicitis occurred annually in the United States between 1979 and 1984. The highest incidence of appendectomy for appendicitis is found in persons who range in age from 10 to 19 years (23.3 per 100,000 population per year). Men have a higher rate of appendicitis than women in all age groups. Appendicitis rates are 1.5 times higher in whites than in nonwhites. The highest rate (15.4 per 10,000 population per year) is in the West North Central region of the United States and is 11.3% higher in the summer than in the winter months.[65]

The highest rate of incidental appendectomy is found in women from 35 to 44 years of age (43.8 per 10,000 population per year) or 12.1 times higher than the rate in men of the same age. Presumably, this rate is influenced by the same rate of gynecologic procedures in this specific population. Between 1970 and 1984, the incidence of appendicitis decreased by 14.6%; the reasons for this decline are unknown. A life-table model suggests that the lifetime risk of appendicitis is 8.6% for men and 6.7% for women; the lifetime risk of appendectomy is 12% for men and 23.1% for women. Overall, an estimated 36 incidental procedures are performed to prevent one case of appendicitis.[65]

The preventive value of each incidental appendectomy performed in different age groups can be estimated using the life-table analysis. For example, 1,000 incidental appendectomies can be expected to prevent 52 cases of appendicitis when performed in women from 15 to 19 years of age, 24 cases when performed in women from 35 to 39 years of age, and 8 cases when performed in women from 60 to 64 years of age.[65]

Although the highest rate of appendicitis is observed in persons from 10 to 19 years of age, most incidental appendectomies are performed in persons older than 35 years of age, which is well past the age of greatest risk for appendicitis, and in women, who are at lower risk than men. To prevent a single lifetime case of acute appendicitis in persons 35 years of age, 59 incidental appendectomies are required. For those 59 years of age, 166 procedures are required. Although the overall rate of incidental appendectomy declined sharply between 1979 and 1984, little change is noted among the elderly, for whom the procedure has the lowest preventive value.[65]

In the less recent literature, several papers showed that patients with previous appendectomy had a higher incidence of carcinoma of the colon than a comparable control group.[66,67,68] It was believed that lymphoid tissues of the appendix produced immunity against development of malignant disease of the colon and other sites in the body. This issue was put to rest by the prospective study by Moertel et al,[69] who found no evidence to suggest that appendectomy posed a higher risk for development of large bowel carcinoma.

A study by Rutgeerts et al[70] of Belgium revealed that appendectomy is a protective factor against ulcerative colitis. The authors found that in a group of 174 patients with ulcerative colitis, only 1 patient had undergone appendectomy, compared with 25% of the case–control group. The authors postulated that normal adult appendiceal lymphocyte reactivity is predominated by helper T cells. The appendix is mainly a helper organ. Resection of the appendix could tip the balance in favor of preventing or suppressing an inappropriate response.[70,71]

It is reasonable to remove a normal appendix up to the age of 35 to 40 years, provided it can be performed without difficulty and without the necessity to extend the abdominal incision. However, with a patient of any age, if the appendix contains a mass, an appendicolith, or a calculus, an appendectomy should be performed since carcinoid, adenocarcinoma, lymphoma, mucinous cystadenomas, parasites, metastatic carcinoma, and many other abnormalities may be found.[72,73] Appendicoliths and calculi of the appendix often are associated with complicated appendicitis, being present in 18% of patients with perforated appendicitis and in 42% of patients with appendiceal abscesses.[74] Some authors have reported on patients with appendiceal calculi who developed abdominal pain mimicking appendicitis but who did not require an operation, only to return some time later with acute appendicitis.[74,75] Since appendiceal fecaliths and calculi play a role in the pathogenesis of acute appendicitis and are associated with complicated appendicitis, particularly perforation and abscess, an incidental appendectomy should be considered seriously.

36.3.2 Case 11: Exploration for Appendicitis with Unexpected Pseudomyxoma Peritonei

A 39-year-old man is undergoing an emergency laparotomy for suspected appendicitis. A cecal mass is identified. During mobilization of the mass, it ruptures, and pools of mucin are discovered. How should this patient be managed?

The true source of this mucin is unknown. It may be mucin accumulated within the dilated lumen of an obstructed appendix, a mucocele, or produced by proliferative epithelial cells, a cystadenoma, or mucinous cystadenocarcinoma. Since this is an unexpected finding, these sources may be indistinguishable. Appendicitis is the presenting clinical diagnosis in 25%.[76,77,78,79, 80,81,82,83,84,85,86,87,88,89,90] Gelatinous deposits or mucinous ascites is termed pseudomyxoma peritonei. If the mucin is secondary to rupture of a simple mucocele, the removal of the appendix is curative. On the other hand, mucin on the basis of cystadenocarcinoma often persists or recurs. The primary treatment of these mucin-producing lesions is resection, and the prognosis is based on the completeness of removal.[91,92] On occasion, a thin-walled, distended appendix is recognized; removal of the obstructed appendix is curative. However, sometimes the appendix is surrounded by neoplastic deposits. Then a right colectomy, applying the principles of en bloc resection, is the treatment of choice.

If a diffuse process is discovered on further exploration, and all disease cannot be removed, the patient may be closed and sent to a surgeon who is familiar with debulking and chemotherapy for these neoplasms. Generally, all gross gelatinous implants should be removed. The omentum is part of the diffuse process and should be removed.[93,94] Some authors suggest using an irrigation of 5% dextrose solution, a mucolytic agent.[95] If the patient is female, the ovaries should be removed in cases of pseudomyxoma peritonei because they may be a hidden source of the process or harbor metastases.[96]

Adjuvant therapy is unproven because of the small number of these cases. Because adjuvant treatments may include intraperitoneal chemotherapy, appropriate catheters for introduction and removal of the agents should be placed in the peritoneal cavity and brought out through separate stab wounds. Other adjuvant therapy includes radiogold colloid or systemic chemotherapy, but rarely radiation therapy. Recurrence leads to repeated debulking, cytoreductive operations, and chemotherapy, either systemic or intraperitoneal.[94,95,97,98]

36.4 Meckel's Diverticulum

36.4.1 Case 12: Propriety of Incidental Meckel's Diverticulectomy

A 52-year-old woman is undergoing resection for recurrent bouts of diverticulitis. At laparotomy, Meckel's diverticulum is noted in the ileum 2 feet from the ileocecal junction. Should the diverticulum be resected?

Meckel's diverticulum is the persistence of a portion of the embryonic omphalomesenteric duct. The incidence of this disease is 0.3 to 4% at autopsy and 0.14 to 4.5% at laparotomy. Most Meckel's diverticula are located in the terminal ileum within 90 cm of the ileocecal junction, although there have been reports of their occurrence in the appendix and the jejunum.[76]

Complications from Meckel's diverticula occur most often in children. The most common complication is small bowel obstruction, followed by bleeding. In the adult, inflammation is the most common problem, followed by small bowel obstruction and bleeding. Inflammation of Meckel's diverticulum most often is caused by ectopic tissues, namely, gastric and pancreatic cells, which occur in 23% of cases.[77] The gastric cells are much more common and may lead to bleeding, ulceration, and perforation. Most obstruction is caused by a fibrous band from Meckel's diverticulum, intussusception, and volvulus.[76,78]

Recognizing a 2% incidence of Meckel's diverticula in the general population, the surgeon can use life-table analysis to calculate the risk of the development of future complications from Meckel's diverticulum. At age 10 years, the risk is 3%. This gradually drops to 0% at 75 years. At age 50 years, the risk is 1% (▶ Fig. 36.1).[79] In a collective series, the average risk of morbidity from incidental Meckel's diverticulectomy was 4% (range, 2–30%) and the mortality rate was 0.2% (range, 0–0.8%).[80] It appears that incidental Meckel's diverticulectomy for a normal Meckel's diverticulum in patients older than 50 years of age is not indicated. However, if there is evidence of ectopic tissue, which usually can be palpated as thickened tissue, or if there is a fibrous band or a very long Meckel diverticulum that may cause bowel obstruction or volvulus, excision should be considered strongly.[81]

Park et al[82] reviewed the Mayo Clinic experience with patients who had Meckel's diverticulum to determine which diverticula should be removed when discovered incidentally during abdominal surgery. They found 1,476 patients to have Meckel's diverticulum during operation from 1950 to 2002. Among the 1,476 patients, 16% of Meckel's diverticula were symptomatic. The most common clinical presentation in adults was bleeding and in children it was obstruction. Among patients with a symptomatic Meckel diverticulum, the male-to-female ratio was approximately 3:1. Clinical or histologic features most commonly associated with symptomatic Meckel's diverticula were patients aged younger

than 50 years (odds ratio = 3.5), male sex (odds ratio = 1.8), diverticulum length greater than 2 cm (odds ratio = 2.2), and the presence of histologically abnormal tissue (odds ratio = 13.9). After analyzing their data, they neither support nor reject the recommendation that all Meckel's diverticula found incidentally should be removed, although the procedure today has little risk. If a selective approach is taken, they recommend removing all incidental Meckel's diverticula that have any of the four features most commonly associated with symptomatic Meckel's diverticula.

36.5 Unexpected Findings

36.5.1 Case 13: Rectal Prolapse and Unexpected Ovarian Mass

During an abdominal procedure to repair a rectal prolapse in a 67-year-old woman, a mass is found in the right ovary. With the patient under general anesthesia, the bowel is prepared and the patient's condition is stable. There is no obvious evidence of other intra-abdominal disease. How should the surgeon proceed?

An initial impression may be supported by deciding whether the mass is neoplastic, inflammatory, functional, or congenital. It is likely that an inflammatory mass would be associated with fever, pain, and an elevated white blood cell count. A congenital or functional mass might be cystic and regular in shape. Patients younger than 40 years would be more likely to have a benign mass. Benign masses may be removed locally, with care taken to preserve the ovary in young patients. This elderly patient would be more likely to have an ovarian carcinoma or metastatic carcinoma. An elderly patient would have atrophic, tiny ovaries, and a hard, enlarged ovary points to a neoplasm. The large variety of ovarian neoplasms have been classified, and the reader is referred to the World Health Organization classification and the International Federation of Gynecologists and Obstetrics classification.[83,84]

All adnexal masses must be considered to be neoplasms until proven otherwise because approximately 30 to 40% of them are malignant. The greatest frequency of ovarian carcinoma is in the sixth and seventh decades, as in the case of this patient.

Careful exploration of the abdomen should be performed to locate unrecognized primary malignancies or metastases. Any suspicious site should be excised or biopsied. Consultation with a surgeon experienced with gynecologic oncology is ideal but not always possible.

If the mass appears to be benign, unilateral salpingo-oophorectomy is appropriate therapy. The principal operation for ovarian carcinoma is total hysterectomy with bilateral salpingo-oophorectomy.[85] The procedure may be quite complicated if the carcinoma is adherent to other organs or to the retroperitoneum. The formal operation may be performed for aggressive removal of the mass(es) (debulking) and omentectomy.

To obtain the most information from the operation, staging procedures should be performed.[85,86] Since ovarian metastases float freely in the abdomen, biopsies of the diaphragm, omentum, and retroperitoneal nodes are recommended. Washings of the peritoneal cavity may provide cytologic evidence.

The remaining question is: What is to be done for the prolapse? If the mass was deemed benign, the surgeon should proceed with the operation planned for the prolapse. If the mass

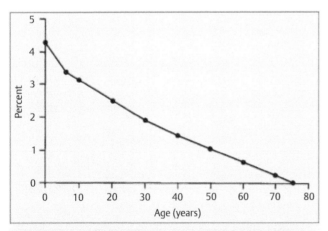

Fig. 36.1 Risk of developing a complication from a Meckel's diverticulum from age 0 to 75 years.[77]

proved malignant and it was clear that the patient's condition was incurable, consideration can still be given to repair of the prolapse, since the symptoms of rectal procidentia may make the patient's quality of life miserable, and some patients will live for several years. If the patient showed marked symptoms from prolapse, a proctopexy without bowel resection might be performed. If the surgeon believes that a curative total abdominal hysterectomy and a bilateral salpingo-oophorectomy have been performed, it is reasonable to proceed with repair of the prolapse, but a procedure might be selected for a repair that does not involve the use of a foreign body. If the malignant disease is widely disseminated, consideration can be given to terminating the operation and not treating the prolapse.

36.6 Rectal Injury

36.6.1 Case 14: Vaginal Hysterectomy and Intraoperative Perforation of Rectum

While a 55-year-old woman is undergoing a vaginal hysterectomy, the gynecologist notices an inadvertent perforation of the rectum. You are asked to step in and help solve the problem. Inspection confirms the findings of fecal material in the vagina, but the source is not evident. What course of action would you take?

First, the patient should be administered intravenous antibiotics that are appropriate for a colorectal operation. Second, sigmoidoscopy should be performed. The specific site of perforation may be localized; if found, its size can be appreciated. If the patient is immunocompromised or has diseased bowel at the site of the injury, the surgeon diverts the fecal stream. However, the other questions ordinarily associated with trauma, including time from injury to operation and the velocity of the injury agent, are as favorable as can be expected.

Contamination is the major factor influencing modification of the operative approach. Ideally, the gynecologist will have performed a preoperative bowel preparation. In general, gynecologists who expect a difficult dissection will plan ahead for inadvertent enterotomy by bowel preparation.

A low-lying, distal rectal, and distal vaginal perforation may be repaired in layers via the anus and/or the vagina.[87,88,89] The contamination will predicate the need for colostomy. If an upper rectal wound has occurred, laparotomy is necessary to repair it and a colostomy often is warranted. The vaginal and rectal repairs may be separated by omentum or a peritoneal flap.

If trauma to the bowel at any point in the free peritoneal cavity occurs, primary closure is the treatment of choice. On the other hand, if perforation is found below the peritoneal reflection in conjunction with gross contamination of the freshly opened planes for the pelvic surgery and the dissection to find and repair the hole, morbidity from infection is likely. This is the ideal model for subsequent cellulitis, abscess, and suture leak. Since a leak will quickly convert the situation to a rectovaginal fistula, diversion of the fecal stream is the safest approach.[89]

In addition, the contaminated planes should be drained. Our choice is a soft, closed sum p-type drain that can be brought out through separate stab wounds on the abdominal wall.

An important issue for patients with major contamination is distal rectal washout. If a local repair is selected, an effort should be made to evacuate the rectal ampulla in order to remove retained stool. If a primary repair was instituted at laparotomy, the colon proximal to the injury can be emptied by an on-table preparation if there is a fecal load.[87] A tube for infusion can be placed into the terminal ileum and advanced into the cecum; thus, liters of saline can be flooded through the bowel. The saline may be allowed to egress from the colorectum by insertion of an anal retractor so that the sphincter mechanism is gently opened. If the situation merits the construction of a colostomy, the distal bowel can be irrigated to empty it of any stool.

36.7 Conclusion

It is hoped that discussions of these challenging case examples will serve as a useful backdrop enabling surgeons faced with similar difficult operative decisions to reach practical and appropriate conclusions.

References

[1] Enker WE, Dragacevic S. Multiple carcinomas of the large bowel: a natural experiment in etiology and pathogenesis. Ann Surg. 1978; 187(1):8–11

[2] Fogler R, Weiner E. Multiple foci of colorectal carcinoma; argument for subtotal colectomy. N Y State J Med. 1980; 80(1):47–51

[3] Welch JP. Multiple colorectal tumors. An appraisal of natural history and therapeutic options. Am J Surg. 1981; 142(2):274–280

[4] Ottinger LW. Frequency of bowel movements after colectomy with ileorectal anastomosis. Arch Surg. 1978; 113(9):1048–1049

[5] Adson MA, van Heerden JA, Adson MH, Wagner JS, Ilstrup DM. Resection of hepatic metastases from colorectal cancer. Arch Surg. 1984; 119(6):647–651

[6] Foster JH, Berman MM. Solid Liver Tumours. Major Problems in Clinical Surgery. Philadelphia, PA: WB Saunders, 1977

[7] Taylor B, Langer B, Falk RE, Ambus U. Role of resection in the management of metastases to the liver. Can J Surg. 1983; 26(3):215–217

[8] Dmowski WP. Current concepts in the management of endometriosis. Obstet Gynecol Annu. 1981; 10:279–311

[9] Croom RD, III, Donovan ML, Schwesinger WH. Intestinal endometriosis. Am J Surg. 1984; 148(5):660–667

[10] Bailey HR. Colorectal endometriosis. Perspect Colon Rectal Surg. 1992; 5:251–259

[11] Meyers WC, Kelvin FM, Jones RS. Diagnosis and surgical treatment of colonic endometriosis. Arch Surg. 1979; 114(2):169–175

[12] Perry EP, Peel ALG. The treatment of obstructing intestinal endometriosis. J R Soc Med. 1988; 81(3):172–173

[13] Forsgren H, Lindhagen J, Melander S, Wågermark J. Colorectal endometriosis. Acta Chir Scand. 1983; 149(4):431–435

[14] Peck JJ. Management of carcinoma discovered unexpectedly at operation for acute appendicitis. Am J Surg. 1988; 155(5):683–685

[15] Hill J, Leaper DJ. Acute appendicitis and carcinoma of the colon. J R Soc Med. 1986; 79(11):678–680

[16] Sumpio BE, Ballantyne GH, Zdon MJ, Modlin IM. Perforated appendicitis and obstructing colonic carcinoma in the elderly. Dis Colon Rectum. 1986; 29 (10):668–670

[17] Arnbjörnsson E. Acute appendicitis as a sign of a colorectal carcinoma. J Surg Oncol. 1982; 20(1):17–20

[18] Kovalicik PJ, Simstein NL, Cross GH. Ileocecal masses discovered unexpectedly at surgery for appendicitis. Am Surg. 1978; 44(5):279–281

[19] Goodall RG, Park M. Primary resection and anastomosis of lesions obstructing the left colon. Can J Surg. 1988; 31(3):167–168

[20] Irvin GL, III, Horsley JS, III, Caruana JA, Jr. The morbidity and mortality of emergent operations for colorectal disease. Ann Surg. 1984; 199(5):598–603

[21] Terry BG, Beart RW, Jr. Emergency abdominal colectomy with primary anastomosis. Dis Colon Rectum. 1981; 24(1):1–4

[22] Thow GB. Emergency left colon resection with primary anastomosis. Dis Colon Rectum. 1980; 23(1):17–24

[23] Stefansson T, Pahlman L, Ekbom A, Yuen J. Surgery in Acute Diverticulitis, a Retrospective Population Based Study. 130 Patients Operated in the University Hospital in Uppsala, Sweden, 1969–1989. Uppsala: Acta Universitatis Upsaliensis Uppsala; 1994

[24] Thompson JS, Philben VJ, Hodgson PE. Operative management of incidental cholelithiasis. Am J Surg. 1984; 148(6):821–824

[25] Kovalcik PJ, Burrell MJ, Old WL, Jr. Cholecystectomy concomitant with other intra-abdominal operations. Assessment of risk. Arch Surg. 1983; 118 (9):1059–1062

[26] Juhasz ES, Wolff BG, Meagher AP, Kluiber RM, Weaver AL, van Heerden JA. Incidental cholecystectomy during colorectal surgery. Ann Surg. 1994; 219 (5):467–472, discussion 472–474

[27] Shennib H, Fried GM, Hampson LG. Does simultaneous cholecystectomy increase the risk of colonic surgery? Am J Surg. 1986; 151(2):266–268

[28] Rosoff AJ. Informed consent: A guide for health care providers. Rockville, MD: Aspen Systems Corp; 1981

[29] Jakowatz JG, Porudominsky D, Riihimaki DU, et al. Complications of pelvic exenteration. Arch Surg. 1985; 120(11):1261–1265

[30] Rodriguwz-Bigas MA, Petrelli NJ. Pelvic exenteration and its modifications. Am J Surg. 1996; 171(2):293–298

[31] Izbicki JR, Hosch SB, Knoefel WT, Passlick B, Bloechle C, Broelsch CE. Extended resections are beneficial for patients with locally advanced colorectal cancer. Dis Colon Rectum. 1995; 38(12):1251–1256

[32] Poeze M, Houbiers JGA, van de Velde CJH, Wobbes T, von Meyenfeldt MF. Radical resection of locally advanced colorectal cancer. Br J Surg. 1995; 82 (10):1386–1390

[33] Plukker JT, Aalders JG, Mensink HJA, Oldhoff J. Total pelvic exenteration: a justified procedure. Br J Surg. 1993; 80(12):1615–1617

[34] Cohen AM, Minsky BD. Aggressive surgical management of locally advanced primary and recurrent rectal cancer. Current status and future directions. Dis Colon Rectum. 1990; 33(5):432–438

[35] Boey J, Wong J, Ong GB. Pelvic exenteration for locally advanced colorectal carcinoma. Ann Surg. 1982; 195(4):513–518

[36] Lopez MJ, Kraybill WG, Downey RS, Johnston WD, Bricker EM. Exenterative surgery for locally advanced rectosigmoid cancers. Is it worthwhile? Surgery. 1987; 102(4):644–651

[37] Orkin BA, Dozois RR, Beart RW, Jr, Patterson DE, Gunderson LL, Ilstrup DM. Extended resection for locally advanced primary adenocarcinoma of the rectum. Dis Colon Rectum. 1989; 32(4):286–292

[38] Eckhauser FE, Lindenauer SM, Morley GW. Pelvic exenteration for advanced rectal carcinoma. Am J Surg. 1979; 138(3):412–414

[39] Talamonti MS, Shumate CR, Carlson GW, Curley SA. Locally advanced carcinoma of the colon and rectum involving the urinary bladder. Surg Gynecol Obstet. 1993; 177(5):481–487

[40] Nora JD, Pairolero PC, Nivatvongs S, Cherry KJ, Hallett JW, Gloviczki P. Concomitant abdominal aortic aneurysm and colorectal carcinoma: priority of resection. J Vasc Surg. 1989; 9(5):630–635, discussion 635–636

[41] Baxter NN, Noel AA, Cherry K, Wolff BG. Management of patients with colorectal cancer and concomitant abdominal aortic aneurysm. Dis Colon Rectum. 2002; 45(2):165–170

[42] Herald JA, Young CJ, White GH, Solomon MJ. Endosurgical treatment of synchronous rectal cancer and abdominal aortic aneurysm, without laparotomy. Surgery. 1998; 124(5):932–933

[43] Mohandas S, Malik HT, Syed I. Concomitant abdominal aortic aneurysm and gastrointestinal malignancy: evolution of treatment paradigm in the endovascular era - review article. Int J Surg. 2013; 11(2):112–115

[44] Lin PH, Barshes NR, Albo D, et al. Concomitant colorectal cancer and abdominal aortic aneurysm: evolution of treatment paradigm in the endovascular era. J Am Coll Surg. 2008; 206(5):1065–1073, discussion 1074–1075

[45] Velanovich V, Andersen CA. Concomitant abdominal aortic aneurysm and colorectal cancer: a decision analysis approach to a therapeutic dilemma. Ann Vasc Surg. 1991; 5(5):449–455

[46] Swanson RJ, Littooy FN, Hunt TK, Stoney RJ. Laparotomy as a precipitating factor in the rupture of intra-abdominal aneurysms. Arch Surg. 1980; 115 (3):299–304

[47] Busuttil RW, Abou-Zamzam AM, Machleder HI. Collagenase activity of the human aorta. A comparison of patients with and without abdominal aortic aneurysms. Arch Surg. 1980; 115(11):1373–1378

[48] Cohen JR, Mandell C, Margolis I, Chang J, Wise L. Altered aortic protease and antiprotease activity in patients with ruptured abdominal aortic aneurysms. Surg Gynecol Obstet. 1987; 164(4):355–358

[49] Lobbato VJ, Rothenberg RE, LaRaja RD, Georgiou J. Coexistence of abdominal aortic aneurysm and carcinoma of the colon: a dilemma. J Vasc Surg. 1985; 2 (5):724–726

[50] Morris HL, da Silva AF. Co-existing abdominal aortic aneurysm and intraabdominal carcinoma. Br J Surg. 1998; 85:1185–1190

[51] Taylor LM, Jr, Porter JM. Basic data related to clinical decision-making in abdominal aortic aneurysms. Ann Vasc Surg. 1987; 1(4):502–504

[52] Meissner MH, Johansen KH. Colon infarction after ruptured abdominal aortic aneurysm. Arch Surg. 1992; 127(8):979–985

[53] Barnett MG, Longo WE. Intestinal ischemia after aortic surgery. Semin Colon Rectal Surg. 1993; 4:229–234

[54] Nivatvongs S. Diseases of the appendix. Curr Opin Gastroenterol. 1989; 5:76–79

[55] Fisher KS, Ross DS. Guidelines for therapeutic decision in incidental appendectomy. Surg Gynecol Obstet. 1990; 171(1):95–98

[56] Coleman RJ, Blackwood JM, Swan KG. Role of antibiotic prophylaxis in surgery for nonperforated appendicitis. Am Surg. 1987; 53(10):584–586

[57] Pieper R, Forsell P, Kager L. Perforating appendicitis. A nine-year survey of treatment and results. Acta Chir Scand Suppl. 1986; 530:51–57

[58] Nockerts SR, Detmer DE, Fryback DG. Incidental appendectomy in the elderly? No. Surgery. 1980; 88(2):301–306

[59] Tranmer BI, Graham AM, Sterns EE. Incidental appendectomy?: Yes. Can J Surg. 1981; 24(2):191–192

[60] Parsons AK, Sauer MV, Parsons MT, Tunca J, Spellacy WN. Appendectomy at cesarean section: a prospective study. Obstet Gynecol. 1986; 68(4):479–482

[61] Strom PR, Turkleson ML, Stone HH. Safety of incidental appendectomy. Am J Surg. 1983; 145(6):819–822

[62] Ikard RW. Prospective analysis of the effect of incidental appendectomy on infection rate after cholecystectomy. South Med J. 1987; 80(3):292–295

[63] Warren JL, Penberthy LT, Addiss DG, McBean AM. Appendectomy incidental to cholecystectomy among elderly Medicare beneficiaries. Surg Gynecol Obstet. 1993; 177(3):288–294

[64] Andrew MH, Roty AR, Jr. Incidental appendectomy with cholecystectomy: is the increased risk justified? Am Surg. 1987; 53(10):553–557

[65] Addiss DG, Shaffer N, Fowler BS, Tauxe RV. The epidemiology of appendicitis and appendectomy in the United States. Am J Epidemiol. 1990; 132(5):910–925

[66] Gross L. Incidence of appendectomies and tonsillectomies in cancer patients. Cancer. 1966; 19(6):849–852

[67] McVay JR, Jr. The appendix in relation to neoplastic disease. Cancer. 1964; 17:929–937

[68] Bierman HR. Human appendix and neoplasia. Cancer. 1968; 21(1):109–118

[69] Moertel CG, Nobrega FT, Elveback LR, Wentz JR. A prospective study of appendectomy and predisposition to cancer. Surg Gynecol Obstet. 1974; 138 (4):549–553

[70] Rutgeerts P, D'Haens G, Hiele M, Geboes K, Vantrappen G. Appendectomy protects against ulcerative colitis. Gastroenterology. 1994; 106(5):1251–1253

[71] Logan R. Appendectomy and ulcerative colitis: what connection? Gastroenterology. 1994; 106(5):1382–1384

[72] Chan W, Fu KH. Value of routine histopathological examination of appendices in Hong Kong. J Clin Pathol. 1987; 40(4):429–433

[73] Westermann C, Mann WJ, Chumas J, Rochelson B, Stone ML. Routine appendectomy in extensive gynecologic operations. Surg Gynecol Obstet. 1986; 162 (4):307–312

[74] Nitecki S, Karmeli R, Sarr MG. Appendiceal calculi and fecaliths as indications for appendectomy. Surg Gynecol Obstet. 1990; 171(3):185–188

[75] Brady BM, Carroll DS. The significance of the calcified appendiceal enterolith. Radiology. 1957; 68(5):648–653

[76] DeBartolo HM, Jr, van Heerden JA. Meckel's diverticulum. Ann Surg. 1976; 183(1):30–33

[77] Lüdtke FE, Mende V, Köhler H, Lepsien G. Incidence and frequency or complications and management of Meckel's diverticulum. Surg Gynecol Obstet. 1989; 169(6):537–542

[78] Bemelman WA, Hugenholtz E, Heij HA, Wiersma PH, Obertop H. Meckel's diverticulum in Amsterdam: experience in 136 patients. World J Surg. 1995; 19 (5):734–736, discussion 737

[79] Soltero MJ, Bill AH. The natural history of Meckel's Diverticulum and its relation to incidental removal. A study of 202 cases of diseased Meckel's Diverticulum found in King County, Washington, over a fifteen year period. Am J Surg. 1976; 132(2):168–173

[80] Peoples JB, Lichtenberger EJ, Dunn MM. Incidental Meckel's diverticulectomy in adults. Surgery. 1995; 118(4):649–652

[81] Longo WE, Vernava AM, III. Clinical implications of jejunoileal diverticular disease. Dis Colon Rectum. 1992; 35(4):381–388

[82] Park JJ, Wolff BG, Tollefson MK, Walsh EE, Larson DR. Meckel diverticulum: the Mayo Clinic experience with 1476 patients (1950–2002). Ann Surg. 2005; 241(3):529–533

[83] Jones HW III. Ovarian cysts and tumors. In: Jones HW III, Wentz AC, Burnett LS, eds. Novak's textbook of gynecology. 11th ed. Baltimore, MD: Williams & Wilkins, 1988:783

[84] Pernoll ML, Benson RC, eds. Current obstetric and gynecologic diagnosis and treatment. Los Altos, CA: Appleton & Lange, 1987:670–714

[85] Lewis JL Jr. Unexpected adenocarcinoma of ovary and uterus. In: Nichols DH, Anderson GW, eds. Clinical Problems, Injuries, and complications of Gynecologic Surgery. Baltimore, MD: Williams & Wilkins, 1988:265–267

[86] Ozols RF, Rubin SC, Gillian T. Epithelial ovarian cancer. In: Hoskins WJ, Perez CA, Young RD, eds. Principles and practices of Gynecologic Oncology, 2nd ed. Philadelphia, PA: Lippincott-Raven, 1997:939–941

[87] Nelson RL, Abcarian H, Prasad ML. Iatrogenic perforation of the colon and rectum. Dis Colon Rectum. 1982; 25(4):305–308

[88] Grasberger RC, Hirsch EF. Rectal trauma. A retrospective analysis and guidelines for therapy. Am J Surg. 1983; 145(6):795–799

[89] Haas PA, Fox TA, Jr. Civilian injuries of the rectum and anus. Dis Colon Rectum. 1979; 22(1):17–23

[90] Yeh HC, Shafir MK, Slater G, Meyer RJ, Cohen BA, Geller SA. Ultrasonography and computed tomography in pseudomyxoma peritonei. Radiology. 1984; 153(2):507–510

[91] Novell R, Lewis A. Role of surgery in the treatment of pseudomyxoma peritonei. J R Coll Surg Edinb. 1990; 35(1):21–24

[92] Smith JW, Kemeny N, Caldwell C, Banner P, Sigurdson E, Huvos A. Pseudomyxoma peritonei of appendiceal origin. The Memorial Sloan-Kettering Cancer Center experience. Cancer. 1992; 70(2):396–401

[93] Gough DB, Donohue JH, Schutt AJ, et al. Pseudomyxoma peritonei. Long-term patient survival with an aggressive regional approach. Ann Surg. 1994; 219(2):112–119

[94] Sugarbaker PH, Landy D, Jaffe G, Pascal R. Histologic changes induced by intraperitoneal chemotherapy with 5-fluorouracil and mitomycin C in patients with peritoneal carcinomatosis from cystadenocarcinoma of the colon or appendix. Cancer. 1990; 65(7):1495–1501

[95] Mann WJ, Jr, Wagner J, Chumas J, Chalas E. The management of pseudomyxoma peritonei. Cancer. 1990; 66(7):1636–1640

[96] Young RH, Gilks CB, Scully RE. Mucinous tumors of the appendix associated with mucinous tumors of the ovary and pseudomyxoma peritonei. A clinicopathological analysis of 22 cases supporting an origin in the appendix. Am J Surg Pathol. 1991; 15(5):415–429

[97] Sindelar WF, DeLaney TF, Tochner Z, et al. Technique of photodynamic therapy for disseminated intraperitoneal malignant neoplasms. Phase I study. Arch Surg. 1991; 126(3):318–324

[98] Nasr MF, Kemp GM, Given FT, Jr. Pseudomyxoma peritonei: treatment with intraperitoneal 5-fluorouracil. Eur J Gynaecol Oncol. 1993; 14(3):213–217

37 Miscellaneous Conditions of the Colon and Rectum

Steven D. Wexner and Joshua I.S. Bleier

Abstract

This chapter will address miscellaneous conditions of the colon and rectum including coccygodynia, endometriosis, proctalgia fugax, levator syndrome, melanosis coli, colitis cystica profunda, descending perineal syndrome, pneumatosis coli, hidradenitis, diversion colitis, and segmental or diverticula-associated colitis.

Keywords: coccygodynia, endometriosis, proctalgia fugax, levator syndrome, melanosis coli, colitis cystica profunda, descending perineal syndrome, pneumatosis coli, hidradenitis, diversion colitis

37.1 Coccygodynia

Coccygodynia (coccydynia, coccalgia) denotes pain in the coccyx, which may be functional or organic in origin. Patients complain of aching, cramping, or sharp pain that is localized in the region of the coccyx or sometimes radiates to the buttocks or down the backs of the thighs. At times, the attacks of pain can become sharp, shooting, or breathtaking. Patients with symptoms of coccygodynia usually seek the opinions of numerous orthopaedic surgeons, gynecologists, neurologists, and colon and rectal surgeons to try to seek help.

A recent review by Lirette provides an excellent summary of the overview and management of coccydynia.[1] While the term was first coined by Simpson in 1859, the accounts of coccygeal pain date back as early as the 16th century. Treatment is often difficult because of the multifactorial nature of its etiology. Both physical and psychological factors can contribute. The condition is five times more common in women than in men, and teens and adults are more likely to present with coccygeal pain as compared to children. Significant weight loss, leading to lack of cushioning, may also be an etiologic factor. Some authors attribute female predominance to the more posterior location of the sacrum and coccyx and the characteristics of the ischial tuberosities that leave a woman's coccyx more exposed and susceptible to trauma both in common situations (sitting position) and during childbirth. The coccyx is larger in women than in men and is therefore more susceptible to injuries. A high incidence of the disorder has also been reported in debilitated elderly patients.[2]

37.1.1 Anatomic Review

The coccyx is composed of one to four bony segments joined to the distal portion of the sacrum by means of the sacrococcygeal joint, the latter joint constituting a synarthrosis or fibrous joint. Sacrococcygeal ligaments bind the sacrococcygeal joint and this fibrous tissue encloses the sacral cornua that form the last intervertebral foramen, through which the fifth sacral roots exit. The first and second coccygeal segments are potentially mobile, a fact that predisposes them to possible pathologic hypermobility. Posterior luxation is a common feature with obesity or a

history of trauma. The S5 roots exit above the first coccygeal vertebra to contribute to the coccygeal plexus, which is formed from the anterior division of L5 and a small filament from L4 that joins with the coccygeal nerve. These nerves lie anterior to the sacrum and coccyx but posterior to the pelvic organs, an area rich in somatic and autonomic nerve endings. These autonomic structures consist of the so-called ganglion impar (ganglion of Walther) and the superior and inferior hypogastric plexus. Pain around the coccyx is felt with stimulation of S4, S5, and coccygeal roots. In some patients, the coccalgia is related to the S3 distribution, because the stimulation of this root is felt in the perianal region, rectum, and genitalia.

37.1.2 Etiology and Pathogenesis of Coccygodynia

The classification of coccygodynia is based on the chronology of the disorder. The most common sources of acute pain are the coccygeal disks or joints in 70% of the cases with four different causes: coccygeal spicules, anterior luxation, coccygeal hypermobility, and subluxation or luxation. Acute local trauma related to a fall in the sitting position or childbirth is a common etiology. This presentation usually responds well to conservative management with anti-inflammatory drugs and rest, and the duration of pain is limited. The condition is considered chronic when it has persisted for more than 2 months and the underlying cause is often uncertain. Treatment response is variable.

Coccygodynia has been classified according to the characteristics of pain. Conditions associated with somatic pain have included idiopathic hypermobility of the coccyx, luxation of the coccyx, myofascial syndromes, depression and somatization, septic conditions, arthritis, osteitis, and sacral hemangioma. Those conditions associated with neuropathic pain include idiopathic lumbar disk herniation, intradural schwannoma, neurinoma, arachnoid cysts, and glomus neoplasms. Mixed presentations may be associated with chordoma, bone metastases, and neoplastic visceral processes.

37.1.3 Diagnosis

Diagnosis is based on the clinical manifestations. Patients should be questioned about the characteristics of pain, because the information obtained might help determine the underlying pathogenic mechanism. All patients should be asked for a history of precipitating trauma and the time at which it occurred, presence of sudden and acute pain when passing from sitting to standing, and type of seat that makes the pain worse. Comprehensive personality/behavioral assessment may be recommended to show possible abnormal personality traits or psychological impairment as indicative of anxiety or depression.

In cases of coccygodynia involving somatic pain, the coccyx is found to be painful and tender to palpation. The pain is intensified on sitting on a hard surface and the diagnosis of coccygodynia should be questioned when the pain fails to disappear on lying down. Somatic pain at coccygeal level is related to body posture and is accentuated with coccygeal movements during rectal digital examination.

Neuropathic pain manifests as poorly localized coccygeal pain accompanied by a burning or lancing sensation and is occasionally associated with loss of sensitivity or paresthesias. In such cases, the pain increases in response to palpation, but no pain is recorded on mobilizing the coccyx. The pain tends to exhibit a segmental distribution when originating from the sacral root or peripheral nerve. In cases of spinal involvement, the pain characteristically intensifies with coughing, sneezing, or defecation. In cases of spinal (lumbar) involvement, the pain can also be triggered by lumbar movements.

Radiographic studies usually include a lateral X-ray view of the coccyx. X-rays can identify fractures, luxations, osteoarthritis, and osteolytic lesions caused by neoplasms. In dynamic radiographic imaging, hypermobility of the coccyx is defined as more than 25 degrees of flexion on the lateral view. Luxation is defined as more than 25% movement (backward displacement) of the coccyx from the standing to the sitting view. Measurement of the intercoccygeal angle, the angle formed between the first coccygeal segment and the last coccygeal segment, can provide an objective measurement of forward inclination of the coccyx. Magnetic resonance imaging (MRI) might be used for better visualization of the shape of the coccyx, especially the tip, for visualization of a dorsal bursitis and also to discard cysts, neoplasms, or neural lesions. Isotope bone scans of the sacrococcygeal area might be useful. Less common causes of coccydynia include infectious etiologies such as pilonidal disease, masses, and pelvic floor spasm; imaging is highly useful in this regard. Kim and Suk[3] compared the clinical and radiological differences between 19 patients with traumatic coccygodynia and 13 patients with idiopathic coccygodynia. A visual analog scale (VAS) based on the pain score assessed the outcome of treatment. There were no statistically significant differences between the traumatic and idiopathic coccygodynia groups in terms of age, sex ratio, and the number of coccyx segments. There were significant differences between the traumatic and idiopathic coccygodynia groups in terms of the pain score (pain on sitting: 82 vs. 47), pain on defecation (39 vs. 87), the intercoccygeal angle (47.9 vs. 72.2 degrees), and the satisfactory outcome of conservative treatment (47.4 vs. 92.3%).

37.1.4 Functional Coccygodynia

No organic pathology has been described for functional coccygodynia, a condition more frequently seen in highly nervous people. Spasm of the coccygeus and piriformis muscles has been mentioned as an accompaniment. The condition has been tagged as "TV watcher's disease," with the implication that sitting for long periods of time on sofas or soft chairs may be a causative factor. Sitting on hard chairs, frequent changes of position, supportive measures for reassurance, and, occasionally, tranquilizers are recommended measures. Performing surgery (coccygectomy) is never indicated because the pain often decreases without treatment or is increased by any treatment.

Maroy[4] described a novel and imaginative systematic study of the association of coccygodynia with depression. For 6 months, he followed 313 patients who had signs of depression or spontaneous or evoked pain in the coccygeal area. A highly significant correlation was found between the following evoked parameters: pain and depressive status in noncoccygodynic patients, coccygodynia and evoked pain, and coccygeal and paracoccygeal muscular spasm. Seventy-nine percent of patients with spontaneous pain and 66% without pain had coccygeal pain evoked by rectal digital examination, and 71% of patients with spontaneous pain and 56% without spontaneous pain had paracoccygeal pain evoked by rectal digital examination. Among severely depressed patients, 76% had evoked pain and 80% coccygeal pain (either spontaneous or evoked). By comparison, in 120 consecutive patients who had colonic radiographic examination and no depressive signs, only two had coccygeal pain during rectal touch. In 57%, all signs disappeared within 6 months when the patients were treated with various antidepressants. Two percent were failures, 14% were lost to followup, and 27% did not return after the first consultation. In a few patients, signs recurred after treatment was stopped but disappeared when treatment was administered again. Ninety-six percent of the 59% of patients followed to the end of the study completely recovered. Accordingly, Maroy has proposed rectal pain evoked by digital examination as an "objective" diagnostic sign for masked depression.

37.1.5 Organic Coccygodynia

Organic coccygodynia may arise either from rigidity of the sacrococcygeal joint or from traumatic arthritis. Fracture and dislocation of the coccyx with displacement are usually a result of direct violence but may occur during difficult childbirth. Coccygodynia has also been attributed to so-called pericoccygeal glomus tumors.[5] However, an autopsy study of 20 coccyges from fetuses, infants, and adults revealed intracoccygeal glomera in 6 of 9 pediatric specimens and all 11 adult specimens. All were microscopic structures, and none appeared to cause bony destruction or erosion. Their role in the pathogenesis of coccygodynia is therefore questionable.

The symptoms of local pain during sitting and during defecation are attributed to spasm of the surrounding muscles. Pain is exquisite, and tenderness is sharply localized over the coccyx. In a patient with a recent injury, swelling and ecchymosis may be found over the lower sacral region. The diagnosis is made if abnormal mobility at the coccygeal articulation and accompanying sensitivity and tenderness are present.[6] Other symptoms include pelvic floor muscle spasms, referred pain from lumbar pathology, arachnoiditis of the lower sacral nerve roots, local posttraumatic lesions, and somatization.[2] Marx[7] suggested that if the injection of a mixture of local anesthetic (4 mL 1% lidocaine and 4 mL 0.5% bupivacaine) with a depository steroid (100-mg prednisone) into the pericoccygeal soft tissue resulted in relief of pain within a few minutes, the diagnosis of coccygodynia is confirmed. Coccygeal pain resulting from acute trauma responds well to conservative management with nonsteroidal anti-inflammatory drugs (NSAIDs) and sitting aids (donut pillow).

Treatment generally consists of reduction by digital manipulation through the rectum, but that may fail because of the muscle forces continually in play.[6] Bed rest for approximately 1 week is usually sufficient to alleviate majority of the symptoms. Tight cross-strapping of the buttocks lessens pain in some patients, but exacerbates it in others. The patient should sit on an inflated rubber ring. Sitting on one buttock at an angle may be sufficient to eliminate the discomfort of sitting squarely on both ischial tuberosities. Some patients prefer a hard surface that allows the ischia to bear most of the body weight.[6] Sitz baths help relieve muscle spasm, and stool softeners should be provided so that constipation does not aggravate symptoms.

Other therapeutic possibilities include blockade of the ganglion of Walther (or ganglion impar), electrical spinal cord stimulation, and selective nerve root stimulation.[2] Coccygectomy should be considered for those patients who have severe disability following a coccygeal fracture. To determine whether surgery probably will be beneficial, Steindler advised infiltrating the region of the coccyx with a local anesthetic; if temporary relief is obtained, then, according to them, coccygectomy probably will relieve the pain.[6] Wray et al[8] conducted a 5-year prospective trial involving 120 patients to investigate the etiology and treatment of coccydynia. The cause lies in some localized musculoskeletal abnormality in the coccygeal region. The condition is genuine and distressing and they found no evidence of neurosis in their patients. Physiotherapy was of little help in treatment, but 60% of the patients responded to local injections of corticosteroid and local anesthesia. Manipulation and injection was even more successful and cured about 85%. Coccygectomy was required in almost 20% and had a success rate of over 90%.

Operation is generally contraindicated for acute sacrococcygeal injuries even when the coccyx is severely anteriorly angulated. Operation is also contraindicated when the low back is painful because occasionally coccygodynia or rectal pain is an early symptom of pathologic change in the lumbosacral disc.[9]

Operative removal of the coccyx is accomplished through a paramedian incision that extends from the sacrococcygeal junction distally.[6] The sacrococcygeal joint is disarticulated and dissection is continued distally along each side of the bone. The sharp distal margin of the sacrum should be beveled so that no prominence remains. The pelvic diaphragm is repaired by reanchoring the structures stripped from the coccyx, and the gluteus maximus muscle is reattached to the posterior sacral aponeurosis.

Grosso and van Dam[10] reported on nine patients who underwent total coccygectomy. There was one postoperative wound infection. With an average follow-up of 56 months, three patients reported complete relief of pain, five reported marked improvement, and one reported slight improvement.

Doursounian et al[11] operated on 61 patients with instability-related coccygodynia. There were 49 women and 12 men, with a mean age of 45.3 years. Twenty-seven patients had hypermobility of the coccyx and 33 had subluxation. In all cases, the unstable portion was removed through a limited incision directly over the coccyx. Follow-up was between 12 months and more than 30 months. The outcome was rated excellent or good in 53 patients, fair in 1, and poor in 7. There were nine patients with infection requiring reoperation. Hodges et al[12] assessed the outcomes after conservative and surgical therapy in 32 patients presenting with symptoms of coccydynia. Patients completed visual analog pain scales and the Oswestry functional capacity index. Of the 32 patients, 13% were treated with NSAIDs alone, 53% were treated with NSAIDs, followed by local injections, and 34% underwent coccygectomy after failure of NSAIDs or local injection. Patients undergoing operation had significantly greater pretreatment VAS scores (8.3 vs. 5.4). Surgical patients also had greater Oswestry Low Back Disability (OSW) scores, but not significantly (36.6 vs. 24.2). Marked improvement was reported by 82% of the surgical patients. Wound infections developed in 27% of the surgical patients and 9% developed wound dehiscence. All infections resolved following irrigation and debridement and a short course of oral antibiotics. Ramsey et al[13] reviewed the clinical results of the treatment of coccygodynia. Twenty-four patients were treated with local injections and 15 patients treated with coccygectomy. Local injections were successful in 78% and coccygectomy was successful in 87% of the patients. Perkins et al[14] reviewed 13 patients of a mean age of 45 years who underwent coccygectomy. Pain was assessed by the numerical rating scale and function by OSW at a mean of 43 months. There were two complications and the numerical rating scale improved from 7.3 to 3.6 and the OSW improved from 55 to 36.

A newer approach to the treatment of coccydynia involves radiofrequency ablation. A cohort of 12 patients, inclusive of 10 males and 2 females, at Johns Hopkins in Walter Reed National Military Medical Center were treated with pulsed or conventional radiofrequency treatment. This therapy was aimed at ablation of the sacrococcygeal nerves in patients who have failed more conservative measures. In this study, the average benefit was a 55% pain relief based on VAS scores. Patients who underwent prognostic neural blockade were more likely to experience a positive outcome.[15]

De Andrés and Chaves[2] offered the algorithm presented in ▶ Fig. 37.1 for the diagnosis and therapeutic approach to coccygodynia.

37.2 Endometriosis

Endometriosis is characterized by the presence of ectopic endometrial glands and stroma outside of the uterine cavity. This relatively common disorder may affect up to 15% of all women of reproductive age, and may be responsible for one-third of women experiencing infertility. Its manifestations can range from asymptomatic to intractable and disabling pain. The degree of symptoms does not always correspond to the extent of disease seen at surgery. Diagnosis is clinically suspected and usually confirmed at the time of laparoscopy or laparotomy.

The exact etiology of endometriosis is unknown, though it is postulated to arise from either coelomic metaplasia, in which peritoneal epithelium undergoes metaplastic change into endometrial tissue[17] or implantation of viable endometrial cells through retrograde menstruation from the fallopian tubes. Endometriosis is most commonly found in the pelvis, affecting the ovaries in 60 to 75% of cases. The next most common sites in decreasing order of frequency are the uterosacral ligaments, cul-de-sac, uterus, and rectosigmoid colon in 3 to 10% of cases. Less commonly, endometriosis may affect the appendix, ureter, bladder, surgical scars, and, rarely, via hematogenous dissemination, the lungs, resulting in catamenial pneumothorax. ▶ Table 37.1 shows the sites and incidence of endometriosis. An estimate of the incidence of endometriosis is approximately 4 to 17% of women in the reproductive age group. Although the incidence of colorectal involvement in women with endometriosis has been reported as high as 50%, involvement severe enough to necessitate bowel resection is less than 10%.[18]

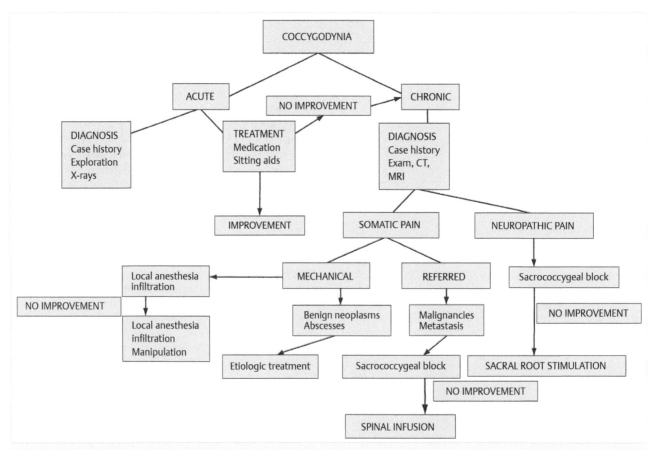

Fig. 37.1 Algorithm for diagnosis and therapeutic approach to coccydynia.

Table 37.1 Sites and incidence of endometriosis

Site	Incidence (%)
Ovaries	60–75
Uterosacral ligament	30–65
Cul-de-sac (pouch of Douglas)	20–30
Uterus	4–20
Rectosigmoid colon	3–10
Appendix	2
Ureter	1–2
Cecum and terminal ileum	1
Bladder	<1
Abdominal scars	<1

Source: Adapted from Snyder 2016.[16]

37.2.1 Colorectal Involvement

Pathology

The lesions of endometriosis are typically multiple and vary in size from minute hard nodules to extensive areas of cystic hemorrhagic necrosis and fibrosis. They are generally serosal, sometimes intramural, and only rarely mucosal. At operation, intestinal endometriosis appears either as a puckered scarred area, often on the antimesenteric surface of the bowel, or as a nodular constricting lesion extending into the wall or encircling it.[18] Further inspection may reveal rusty brown or purplish specks. Frequently, implants are seen on other pelvic structures. Palpation discloses thickening of the colonic wall. The focus of endometriosis may enlarge to present as a mass, hence the designation as an endometrioma. The mucosal surface is usually intact, but on occasion ulceration may be evident.

Microscopically, multiple foci of endometrial glands and stroma are present in the muscularis propria and in the subtending mesentery in which there is reactive fibrosis and scarring. Smooth muscle hyperplasia is produced by the endometrioma.[19] The overlying mucosa is usually normal. However, the mucosa overlying endometrial deposits may be abnormal with crypt irregularity with branching and sometimes shortening of the tubules, crypt abscesses and an increase in lamina propria mononuclear cells, or mucosal atrophy.[20] Endometriosis of the large bowel can masquerade as inflammatory bowel disease or ischemic changes, but the possibility should be borne in mind, particularly with very focal histologic changes.[21]

Clinical Features

Endometriosis is characteristically a disease of the reproductive years of life and occurs most frequently in women 30 to 40 years of age. Prystowsky et al,[22] in a review of 1,573 consecutive patients with endometriosis diagnosed at laparoscopy or celiotomy, found that only 85 patients (5.4%) had gastrointestinal involvement and only 11 patients (0.7%) required bowel resection as a result of recurrent usually obstructive gastrointestinal symptoms and/or suspicion of malignancy. In a review of 1,616 operations for endometriosis, Bailey[18] reported only 16 bowel resections (1%). Endometriosis may mimic malignancy in that it is characterized by local disease and distant "spread." Gastrointestinal involvement commonly affects those segments of bowel in proximity to the genital organs, with the rectosigmoid region more frequently involved than the ileum.[19] Bailey[18] reported the most common areas of intestinal involvement to be rectum and rectosigmoid (88%), sigmoid colon (7%), cecum (3%), and terminal ileum (2%), followed by proximal colon. He noted that other authors have reported small bowel involvement as high as 27%. In most instances, there is only serosal involvement, and the diagnosis is incidentally made at the time of laparotomy for other reasons. Under these circumstances, the patient's state of well-being is not affected, and no treatment is necessary. If intestinal symptoms are present, endometriosis is probably extensive, and resection is almost always required. The diagnosis of small intestinal endometriosis is rarely made prior to operation.[20] A history of colicky abdominal pain might be suggestive.[23]

Patients may be asymptomatic, but a wide variety of intestinal symptoms may occur. These symptoms may include intermittent abdominal crampy pain, rectal or pelvic pain, cyclical rectal bleeding, tenesmus, constipation (especially with menses), decreased stool caliber, bloating, nausea, vomiting, diarrhea, and even bleeding from an umbilical nodule during menses.[17] Extensive intestinal wall involvement can result in occasional bleeding or obstructive symptoms, in which case a diagnosis of neoplasm or inflammatory bowel disease requires exclusion.

The cyclic nature of the symptoms with exacerbations just before or during menstruation yields a clue to the diagnosis. Associated gynecologic symptoms of dysmenorrhea, cyclic lower abdominal and pelvic pain, dyspareunia, menometrorrhagia, infertility, and findings of characteristic tender pelvic nodularity and cul-de-sac induration and thickening during physical examination further point to the diagnosis.[17] Rigid sigmoidoscopy may reveal a flattened or puckered mucosa or rarely a mass secondary to infiltration of the submucosa, along with extrinsic fixation and angulation of the rectosigmoid.[18] In their review of the literature, Croom et al[19] found that endometrial implants in the proximal intestine or appendix may serve as the lead point for intussusception or that associated inflammatory adhesions may produce obstruction by stenosis, kinking, or volvulus. Varras et al[24] reported a case of endometriosis causing extensive intestinal obstruction simulating carcinoma of the sigmoid colon. A point not commonly appreciated is that intestinal endometriosis may produce symptoms long after menopause with an incidence as high as 7%.[18]

Diagnosis

History and Physical Examination

Although physical examination should be the starting point of all investigation, in most cases, physical examination may not be very revealing, especially when disease is located to the abdominal pelvis. In circumstances of pelvic pain, bimanual and rectal examination may reveal nodularity or induration in the rectovaginal septum or anterior cul-de-sac. Palpation of the

ovaries may reveal atypical masses. History is most revealing when associated with cyclical pain or symptoms associated with menses.

Laboratory Evaluation

There are few laboratory correlates with endometriosis; however, CA 125, which is expressed on tissues derived from human coelomic epithelium, may be elevated in moderate to severe endometriosis. Specificity of this test is poor since there may be other etiologies for its elevation. However, in the setting of elevated CA 125 associated with endometriosis, like with carcinoembryonic antigen (CEA) and colon cancer, variations of CA 125 can be associated with gauging response to treatment.

Endoscopy

Although an important adjunct when evaluating the possibility of endometriosis involving the bowel, since lesions are always initially associated with the outside of the bowel, endoscopy is frequently normal, with the exception of severe infiltrating disease and may similarly reveal a stenotic lumen with normal mucosa. A mass or polypoid lesion may be visualized.[25] Dense adhesions may result in kinking or stricturing of the bowel; however, when the submucosa is infiltrated, nodularity and bluish discoloration of the mucosa may result. Endoscopy is often helpful to rule out luminal etiologies that may mimic endometriosis. In addition, flexible and rigid proctoscopy is helpful in assessing the extent of disease in the rectovaginal septum, and may demonstrate fixed rectal wall adhesions and puckering at the site of disease.

Imaging

Ultrasound is an effective and minimally invasive modality used to evaluate endometriosis. Transvaginal ultrasound is a sensitive and specific test and with skilled hands, can identify 90% of ovarian endometriosis. General pelvic ultrasound, however, is minimally effective since the ultrasonographic appearance of endometriosis is highly variable, ranging from highly echogenic to echolucent. Endorectal ultrasound may be more effective in evaluating rectal wall invasion in the cul-de-sac in rectovaginal septum. Doniec et al[26] demonstrated a 97% sensitivity and specificity in diagnosis of endometriosis involving the rectal wall. CT scans are frequently obtained to evaluate abdominal pain; however, sensitivity and specificity for the diagnosis of endometriosis is poor because there are no ways to differentiate it from other pelvic pathology, especially given that lesions of the adnexa may be either solid or cystic or mixed. MRI may be useful because of the ease of multiplanar imaging and the avoidance of radiation. MRI may be more sensitive in diagnosing bowel invasion when there is loss of the fat plane between the rectum and vagina and loss of signal of the anterior bowel wall on T2 images as well as contrast-enhancing masses on T1 images. Sensitivity and specificity of MRI for diagnosing endometriosis is approximately 78 and 98%, respectively.[27,28]

Laparoscopy

Since the diagnosis of endometriosis requires direct visualization, and physical assessment of lesions as well as the opportunity for tissue biopsy, laparoscopy is currently the most sensitive and specific common modality used to confirm diagnosis. Laparoscopic evaluation is 97% sensitive and 77% specific in diagnosing the disease.[29] Especially in unclear circumstances and with larger lesions, biopsy is required for diagnosis and to exclude malignancy. When performing laparoscopy for evaluation of endometriosis it is important to evaluate both ovaries, the entire pelvic peritoneum, the uterus, as well as visualization of the pouch of Douglas, uterosacral ligaments, sigmoid colon, and pelvic sidewalls. Occasional implants can be seen on the appendix and small bowel.

Differential Diagnosis

The differential diagnosis includes primary bowel carcinoma, diverticulosis, other chronic inflammatory bowel diseases, carcinoids, benign intramural neoplasms, metastases from occult intra-abdominal malignancies, pelvic abscess, ischemic stricture, radiation colitis, pelvic (ovarian) and mesenteric neoplasms, and cysts.[19,23]

Treatment

Treatment for endometriosis is reserved for symptomatic patients. As many as 25% of women may have asymptomatic endometriosis, according to a study by Martin et al in a cohort of patients undergoing elective tubal ligation.[30]

Medical Management

The primary goal of medical management is to treat the symptoms of endometriosis, primarily pain and infertility. As opposed to surgery, which can only treat grossly visible disease, medical management is aimed at treating microscopic disease or involvement of critical structures. With successful medical management, sequelae of surgical treatment including pain, lost time at work, and risk of adhesions are avoided. Nevertheless, medical therapy, which is comprised primarily of hormonal manipulation, has a significant disadvantage of side effects from hormonal treatments and the need for prolonged treatment regimens. The primary goal of medical hormonal management is to suppress the cyclical stimulation of endometrial tissue by ovarian estrogen and progesterone. Unfortunately, this treatment does nothing to physically remove sources of endometriosis. Thus, the risk of recurrent symptoms always exists.

Hormonal Therapy

In the late 1950s, the first effective medical therapy was introduced by Kistner,[31] who proposed the use of continuous estrogen and progesterone to induce pseudopregnancy and amenorrhea. Danazol is an effective anti-estrogen agent that functions by lowering peripheral estrogen and progesterone levels via a direct effect on ovarian production of steroid as well as inhibition of pituitary production of follicle-stimulating hormone (FSH) and luteinizing hormone (LH). Unfortunately, the long-term side effect profiles of danazol are poorly tolerated. Early menopause symptoms as well as changes related to rising free testosterone inducing a hyper-androgenic state are common. These problems include hirsutism, weight gain, acne, and voice changes. Gonadotropin-releasing hormone agonists (GnRH-a) emerged as a more

effective alternative primarily by reducing side effects; some examples are leuprolide (Lupron) and nafarelin (Synarel), which have demonstrated equal anti-estrogen activity with fewer side effects. These agents are quite effective in the treatment of small endometrial implants of the peritoneal surfaces but do not have a major impact on large deposits. They are of value in the preoperative preparation of patients for infertility operations because they decrease the vascularity of implants.[18] One of the potential side effects of this class of drugs is the loss of bone mineral density. This problem is minimized with limiting use of the drug to 6 months. Thus, in patients with preexisting osteoporosis, GnRH-a is contraindicated. Aromatase inhibitors are another class of anti-estrogen drugs that function by limiting the conversion of androgens to estrogen. These are commonly used in the treatment of breast cancer and can reduce circulating estrogen to less than 10% of pretreatment levels.[32] Anti-inflammatory medications such as cyclooxygenase inhibitors have been shown in level I studies to reduce pelvic pain and dyspareunia.[33]

Surgical Treatment

When medical management fails, surgical treatment remains the gold standard for intervention. The primary goal of surgical therapy is complete removal or ablation of endometrial implants, as well as oophorectomy in appropriately selected patients. Given the advances in imaging, surgery should no longer be considered primarily for diagnosis rather with the goal of diagnosis and treatment. A thorough understanding of the pathophysiology of endometrial implants that can extend deeply into tissues often surrounded by fibrosis as well as knowledge of the critical abdominal and pelvic structures that may indeed be involved including the ureters and vascular structures is critical for safe surgical management. Therefore, the use of bilateral ureteric catheters can be very helpful.

The most common sites of pelvic endometriosis with intestinal involvement are implants in the rectovaginal septum and pouch of Douglas. Superficial involvement of the posterior vagina and uterosacral ligaments and anterior rectum may be treated with ablation either with electrocautery or with the CO_2 laser. Knowledge of the extent of the disease may help guide the surgeon to the appropriate operative approach. A determination is made of the depth of infiltration of the rectum. Partial-thickness resection should only be performed when the outer longitudinal muscularis is involved and can be peeled mechanically from the inner circular muscularis. The inner muscularis cannot be peeled from the mucosa and any resection will be incomplete. Superficial lesions may also be surgically resected or "shaved" without damaging the rectal mucosa. Careful assessment of the integrity of the bowel wall and repair of partial-thickness defects with Lembert stitches are appropriate. If deeper lesions are suspected or confirmed, bowel resection may be required. If the lesions are isolated to the rectosigmoid colon, primary resection and anastomosis are appropriate. If lesions affect the more distal rectum, and would otherwise require low anterior resection, consideration for disk excision of the affected portion of the rectal wall is the preferred technique. Lesions should be well circumscribed and generally less than 3 cm in diameter to avoid significant stenosis after repair. When more than 50% of the circumference of the bowel wall is included or if there is multicentric disease, disk excision is contraindicated. After full-thickness excision, the defect should be repaired in a transverse fashion. It should be pointed out that the oncologic principles of colon resection and high ligation of the vascular pedicles are not required for the surgical treatment of endometriosis, even if neoplasia is suspected for the endometrial implant. Division of the mesentery close to the bowel wall maximizes perfusion to the remaining segments and minimizes the potential morbidity to pelvic structures. After either shaving of small lesions, disk excision or primary bowel resection, proctoscopic or flexible sigmoidoscopic evaluation with leak testing should be performed.

Koh and Janik[34] evaluated over 400 cases of deep infiltrating endometriosis of the cul-de-sac. Of these, 105 had rectal disease, 22 required laparoscopic colectomy, 17 had full-thickness anterior rectosigmoid resection, and 56 had partial-thickness resection. All cases were laparoscopic except for one colectomy early in the series. Following operation, only one serious complication occurred, rectal perforation, which was treated with a diverting colostomy. A 48% fertility rate was achieved. Kavallaris et al[35] evaluated the microscopic extent of endometriosis in surgical en bloc specimens of 50 patients with intestinal pain, and palpable disease in the rectovaginal septum who underwent combined laparoscopic vaginal en bloc resection of the cul-de-sac with partial resection of the posterior vaginal wall and rectum with reanastomosis by mini-laparotomy. The mean length of the bowel specimen was 7.5 cm. Endometriosis involved the serosa and muscularis propria in all patients, the submucosa in 34% of the patients, and the mucosa in 10% of the patients. After a mean follow-up of 32 months, 90% of the patients reported a considerable improvement or were completely free of symptoms; the rate of recurrence was 4%.

Small bowel endometriosis is much less common than disease involving the rectosigmoid colon or cul-de-sac. However, careful inspection is required. Treatment of superficial lesions can be managed with shaving and local repair, and as with the large bowel, deeper lesions should be treated with segmental resection. Isolated appendiceal involvement can be easily treated with appendectomy.

Malignant Transformation

Only 21.3% of the cases of malignant transformation of endometriosis occur at extragonadal pelvic sites.[36,37] Yantiss et al[37] characterized the clinicopathologic features of neoplasms arising in gastrointestinal endometriosis. They reported 17 cases of gastrointestinal endometriosis complicated by neoplasms (14 cases) or precancerous changes (3 cases). Nine patients had a long history of endometriosis, 11 patients had hysterectomies, and 8 of these patients also had received unopposed estrogen therapy. The lesions involved the rectum (six), sigmoid (six), colon, unspecified (two), and small intestine (three), and comprised eight endometrioid adenocarcinomas, four mullerian adenosarcomas, one endometrioid stromal sarcoma, one endometrioid adenofibroma of borderline malignancy with carcinoma in situ, two atypical hyperplasias, and one endometrioid adenocarcinoma in situ. Up to 2002, 40 cases of endometriosis-associated intestinal carcinoma had been reported in the literature. Of these, 17 cases were primary adenocarcinomas arising in the rectosigmoid colon. In 8 of the 17 case reports, the patients were using unopposed estrogen replacement therapy.

Jones et al[36] reported the ninth case of a patient with malignant transformation of endometriosis in the literature.

Cho et al[38] reported the case of endometrial stromal sarcoma of the sigmoid colon arising in endometriosis with a review of six additional cases of endometrial stromal sarcoma arising in intestinal endometriosis found in the English literature. The patients ranged in age from 36 to 64 years. Presenting symptoms were pain, bloody diarrhea, and tenesmus. Most of the sarcomas arose in the rectosigmoid colon.

37.3 Proctalgia Fugax and Levator Syndrome

Proctalgia fugax may be defined as pain seemingly arising in the rectum that recurs at irregular intervals and is unrelated to organic disease.[39] The term "proctalgia fugax" was first introduced by Thaysen[40] in 1935, and Schuster[41] has provided an excellent description of the clinical presentation. The onset of pain during the day or night is abrupt, and patients may be awakened with pain several hours after falling asleep. The pain appears suddenly mostly at night without any particular warning and disappears completely without any objective traces. The pain varies in severity but often is excruciating. Symptoms last from only a few minutes to less than half an hour, and their duration, although variable from patient to patient, is constant in a given patient. The pain is described variously as gnawing, grinding, cramp-like, sharp, or tight. It is localized in the rectal region above the anus, varying in location from person to person but remaining constant in a given person. Symptoms spontaneously disappear without residue except for a weak, washed-out feeling after particularly severe attacks. There are no associated intestinal disturbances such as alteration in bowel habits, tenesmus, or paresthesias.

The etiology of proctalgia fugax is unknown, although it has been suggested that it is due to spasms of the levator ani muscles.[39] A unique study was reported by Harvey,[42] who obtained intraluminal pressure recordings from the rectum and sigmoid colon in two patients experiencing attacks of proctalgia fugax. In each case, the pain appeared to result from contractions of the sigmoid colon and not from spasm of the levator ani muscles.

Takano[43] reported his experience with 68 patients with proctalgia fugax, among whom 55 patients had tenderness along the pudendal nerve. The location, character, and degree of pain caused by digital examination were confirmed by all of them to be similar to that which they experienced at times of paroxysm. After administration of a nerve block, symptoms disappeared completely in 65% of the patients and decreased in 25%. These data suggest that the pathogenesis of proctalgia fugax is neuralgia of the pudendal nerves.

The condition occurs in approximately 14% of healthy people and is more common in women (17.3%) than in men (8.8%).[44] Between attacks, no consistent physical abnormality is evident. The absence of any objective abnormality suggests that at least a portion, if not all, of these cases are of psychogenic origin. A study of 48 patients with proctalgia fugax by Pilling et al[45] revealed that the majority of the patients had professional or managerial occupations. They were found to be perfectionistic, anxious, and tense; had a relatively high incidence of neurotic symptoms in childhood; and were of above-average intelligence. The authors believed that the tendency of this anxious, perfectionistic group to somatize emotional conflicts by pain in the gastrointestinal tract is strong evidence that proctalgia fugax is of psychogenic origin.

Treatment of this condition is unsatisfactory. Firm upward pressure on the anus can provide relief. Other measures that have been used include taking hot sitz baths, having a bowel movement, inserting a finger into the anus, massaging the muscles, or administering an enema. Such maneuvers probably only pass the time for patients who have a condition in which the duration of pain is self-limited. Inhalation of amyl nitrite or sublingual nitroglycerin has also been used. Eckardt et al[46] conducted a randomized, double-blind, placebo-controlled, crossover trial of inhaled salbutamol in 18 patients with proctalgia fugax and found that salbutamol inhalation shortened the duration of severe pain. Interestingly, in the asymptomatic state, there were no changes in anal resting pressure, anal relaxation during distention, or rectal compliance. Nightly doses of quinine have been recommended for patients who have frequent repeated nocturnal attacks.[40] Anesthetics, sedatives, and spasmolytic agents have been employed.[46] Peleg and Shvartzman[47] described a case where a single dose of an intravenous lidocaine infusion completely stopped pain attacks. Katsinelos et al[48] described a case of proctalgia fugax responding to anal sphincter injection of clostridium botulinum type A toxin. Lowenstein and Cataldo[49] reported a case of proctalgia fugax that responded to 0.3% nitroglycerin ointment. Sinaki et al[50] reported that diazepam was helpful in 40% of their patients.

A closely allied condition, if not a variation of the same theme, is the so-called levator syndrome. Individuals with this syndrome experience a dull ache or pressure in the rectum, sometimes describing the sensation as "sitting on a ball" or "having a ball in my rectum." The pain is worse during sitting and disappears when the patient stands or lies down. Precipitating factors have included the trauma of a long-distance ride in a car, childbirth, lumbar disk surgery, low anterior resection or abdominoperineal resection of the rectum, gynecologic operations, and occasionally sexual intercourse.[51] Often no etiologic factor can be elicited, and a large component of the condition has been attributed to a psychological overlay. The prevalence of this condition has been reported as 6.6% of the general population in the United States[52]

The syndrome occurs more commonly in women, usually in the fourth to sixth decades of life. The diagnosis is made by the demonstration of tenderness and spasm of the affected muscle, which are usually unilateral and on the left side.

Treatment consists of puborectalis muscle massage up to 50 times, performed in a firm manner based on the patient's tolerance and carried out at 3- to 4-week intervals. Warm baths and short-term judicious use of diazepam also can be of value. For patients who do not respond to these measures, Sohn et al[53] first described the use of electrogalvanic stimulation as a treatment. The rationale for this therapy is based on the fact that a low-frequency oscillating current applied to a muscle induces fasciculation and fatigue, which breaks the spastic cycle. The treatment is painless, and no adverse side effects are known. Success rates of 60 to 94% have been reported.[51,53,54,55] Recurrence rates are significant. In the series by Billingham et al,[55] only 25% of the patients remained symptom free. Further improvement can be obtained through retreatment.[54] Less favorable results were reported by Hull et al[56] in

a series of 52 patients; 50% received fewer than four 1-hour treatments, 33% received four to six treatments, and 17% received more than six treatments. The treatment was painless in 77%. With an 88% follow-up with a mean of 28 months, there was symptom relief in 19% of the patients, partial relief in 24%, and no relief in 57%. Total treatment failures may be due to a large psychological component and should be treated accordingly.[51] Hull et al[56] found that misdiagnoses included recurrent pelvic carcinoma and fissure-in-ano. Recognition of this disorder is important to avoid unnecessary and expensive diagnostic investigations, or worse, totally needless operations.

Heah et al[57] assessed the effects of biofeedback on pain relief in 16 consecutive patients (9 men, 7 women, mean age 50 years) with levator ani syndrome. Mean duration of pain was 32.5 months. All underwent a full course of biofeedback using a manometric balloon technique. Mean follow-up was 12.8 months. An independent observer prospectively administered pain scores. After biofeedback, the pain score was significantly improved (median 8 vs. 2). Analgesic requirements were also significantly reduced (all 16 patients needed NSAIDs before biofeedback; only 2 patients needed NSAIDs after biofeedback).

37.4 Melanosis Coli

Melanosis coli is characterized by a deep pigmentation of the mucosa of the colon and rectum caused by the presence of a melanin-like pigment (▶ Fig. 37.2). It may involve the large bowel from the rectum to the ileocecal valve, with a sharp demarcation at this point. This dramatic demarcation is seen at an ileocolic anastomosis (▶ Fig. 37.3). The color of the mucosa varies from shades of yellowish brown to black. It is seen in the appendix but not the terminal ileum. Examination reveals adenomatous polyps and adenocarcinomas rendered strikingly

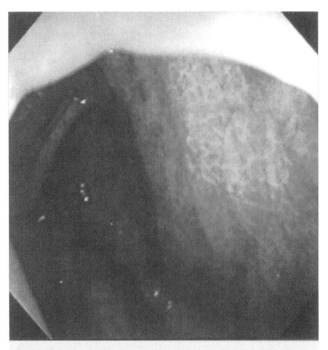

Fig. 37.2 Characteristic appearance of moderately severe melanosis coli.

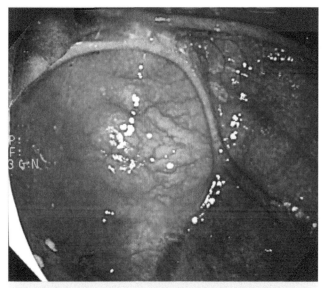

Fig. 37.3 Dramatic demarcation of melanosis coli at an ileocolic anastomosis.

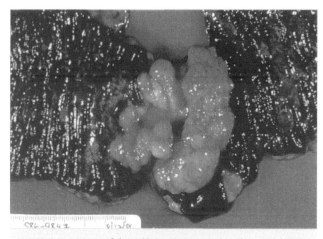

Fig. 37.4 Carcinoma of the colon in a patient with melanosis coli. Note the lack of pigmentation of the neoplastic lesion.

apparent by their lack of pigmentation against the blackish background of the surrounding mucosa (▶ Fig. 37.4).[58] Moreover, nonpigmented areas of mucosa that are not grossly abnormal ultimately prove to be adenomatous hyperplasia. Current data suggest that adenoma detection rate may be increased in the setting of melanosis coli, likely due to enhanced identification made possible by pigmentation differences.[59]

Melanosis may be obvious to the naked eye, but the vast majority of cases are apparent only on microscopic examination. Histologically, the melanin-like pigment is found in histiocytes within the lamina propria and may be seen in the submucosa and even in the regional lymph nodes.[60] There is a lack of inflammatory change in the colon. Walker et al[61] reported an electron microscopic study that showed apoptosis of colonic surface epithelial cells and phagocytosis of resulting apoptotic bodies by intraepithelial macrophages. The latter migrated to the lamina propria where intracellular degradation of the apoptotic bodies resulted in formation of lipofuscin, characteristic of this condition.

Ewing et al[62] reported the case of a patient who underwent a left hemicolectomy for colonic adenocarcinoma and was found incidentally to have melanosis coli associated with long-term use of the herbal laxative Swiss Kriss® (Modern Products, Inc., Mequon, WI) not only in his colonic mucosa, but also in the colonic submucosa and in his pericolic lymph nodes. To their knowledge, the presence of identical pigment in macrophages of pericolonic lymph nodes has been reported in only four other patients in the English literature. Use of a member of the laxative family, which consists of derivatives of anthraquinone (cascara, aloes, rhubarb, senna, and frangula), contributes to this pigmentation.[58]

In most instances, the laxative had been taken almost daily for 1 year or more. This distinct group of cathartics owes its activity to the presence of an irritating anthracene or emodin. The exact mechanism of pigment formation is uncertain. Perhaps the active ingredient of these laxatives contains a pigment or elaborates a pigment within the colon that is phagocytized by the deep mucosal cells.

Pardi et al[63] reported 25 patients with inflammatory bowel disease and melanosis coli, 20% of whom had documented laxative use. Most patients had ulcerative colitis (72%) or Crohn's colitis (24%), and the mean duration of inflammatory bowel disease was more than 7 years. These data raise the possibility that chronic colitis could cause melanosis coli even in the absence of laxative use.

Reports of the incidence of melanosis coli vary from 1 to 5%,[58] and in unselected constipated patients it has been observed in 12 to 31%.[64] Melanosis coli occurs in all races. In a histologic study of 200 autopsy cases, Koskela et al[65] found a prevalence of 60% for melanosis coli, a prevalence that increased with age: 20 to 54 years, 30% and older than 75 years, 71%. Melanosis was more common in the proximal part of the colon: ascending colon, 49%; sigmoid, 18%; and rectum, 6%. Earlier writers suggested that melanosis coli is found in the older age group; however, this, probably, is related to the duration of the ingestion of these laxatives. There is a female preponderance of from 3:1 to 8:1, which probably reflects the greater incidence of constipation and habitual use of laxative agents among women.

Morgenstern et al[58] found that pigment-bearing macrophages are absent from benign and malignant neoplasms and from surrounding normal mucosa. They postulated that the neoplastic epithelium elaborates some substance that inhibits the aggregation or function of macrophages. How this might be related to neoplasia, if at all, is unknown.

Melanosis coli cannot be held responsible for any known symptom complex. A history of constipation is almost universally present, for it is in constipated patients who ingest these laxatives. As a rule, the pigmentation disappears within a period of 4 to 12 months after discontinuation of all anthracene laxatives.

In a colonoscopic study of 2,277 patients, Nusko et al[66] found no significant increase in colorectal carcinoma rate either in laxative users or in patients with melanosis coli.

Subsequently, Nusko et al[67] performed a prospective case-control study to investigate the risk of anthranoid laxative use for the development of colorectal adenomas or carcinomas. A total of 202 patients with newly diagnosed colorectal carcinomas, 114 patients with adenomatous polyps, and 238 patients (controls) who had been referred for total colonoscopy were studied. The use of anthranoid preparations was assessed by standardized interviews, and endoscopically visible or microscopic melanosis coli was studied by histopathological examination. Use of neither anthranoid laxative, even in the long term, nor macroscopic or microscopic melanosis coli was associated with any significant risk for the development of colorectal adenoma or carcinoma.

The associations among colorectal carcinoma and constipation, anthranoid laxative use, and melanosis coli are controversial. Nascimbeni et al[68] investigated the relationship between sigmoid carcinoma and constipation, anthranoid laxative use, and melanosis coli using aberrant crypt foci analysis as an additional tool of investigation. Fifty-five surgical patients with sigmoid carcinoma, 41 surgical patients with diverticular disease, and 96 age- and sex-matched patients without intestinal disease (controls) were interviewed on their history of constipation and anthranoid laxative use. Constipation and anthranoid laxative use were similar between patients with sigmoid carcinoma (30.9 and 32.7%, respectively) and those with diverticular disease (39 and 28.6%) but higher than among controls (18.8 and 8.3%). Melanosis coli was found in 38.2% of the patients with sigmoid carcinoma and 39% of those with diverticular disease. This study confirms the association of aberrant crypt foci frequency with colon carcinoma and does not support the hypothesis of a causal effect relationship of colorectal carcinoma with constipation, anthranoid laxative use, or melanosis coli. Interestingly, melanosis is often difficult to distinguish from certain presentations of mucosal ischemia, and thus clinicians must have a high index of suspicion and keep the diagnosis of melanosis as part of the differential.[69]

37.5 Colitis Cystica Profunda

Colitis cystica profunda (CCP) is a benign disease characterized by varying sizes of mucin-filled cysts located deep at the muscularis mucosae. The chief importance of this entity is its differentiation from colonic mucinous adenocarcinoma. The key feature that distinguishes CCP from malignancy is the fact that the abnormally located glands are normal in histologic appearance. Failure to recognize this benign condition may lead to unnecessary radical operation including possibly stoma.

37.5.1 Age and Sex

The incidence and prevalence of CCP are unknown, but the disease is uncommon. Patients with this condition, once believed to be preponderantly females, usually present in the third and fourth decades.[70,71] However, a review of the world literature disclosed that CCP occurs equally often in men and women.[72]

37.5.2 Etiology

The etiology of CCP remains unclear. This entity is typically found in the setting of internal rectal prolapse in the presence of a solitary rectal ulcer. A plausible explanation is that the condition is the result of invagination of the mucosa during the healing phase of an ulcer. Rutter and Riddell[73] believe that the term "colitis cystica profunda" should be used as a purely descriptive term and should be recognized for what it is: an unusual complication

of several different lesions. The causes of the ulcer might include ulcerative colitis, bacterial colitides, resolution of lymphoid abscesses in the submucosa, radiation, instrumentation, biopsy of the colonic mucosa, polypectomy,[74] and Crohn's disease.[75]

Others consider the lesions to be inverted polyps, either acquired or congenital. If the conditions were congenital, one would expect to find it in pediatric patients, but this has not been the case. Despite the suggestions of those who believe that CCP is of congenital origin, representing hamartomal formation, chronic inflammation has been accepted by most investigators as the primary etiologic factor in its pathogenesis.[76]

37.5.3 Clinical Features

Solitary rectal ulcer syndrome (SRUS) is a fairly rare clinical entity characterized by internal rectal prolapse. Often, the anterior wall of the rectum is the leading edge of the prolapse and as a result chronic trauma and irritation result in the solitary rectal ulcer.[77] Interestingly, true ulcers are only found in 40% of patients. In 20%, these are solitary; the remainder of the lesions may vary in presentation, ranging from hyperemic mucosa to broad-based polypoid lesions. Hematochezia, mucous discharge, diarrhea, tenesmus, and pain (either vague abdominal or perineal) may occur alone or in combination for many months or years before CCP is diagnosed.[71,72,74] Other indications include rectal pain, weight loss, and previous rectal surgery.[76] Involvement may vary from the dentate line to 15 cm from the anal verge, most frequently on the anterior rectal wall from 6 to 7 cm.[71] Rectal examination may reveal single or multiple nodules that frequently have a rubbery consistency. Polypoid masses may be sessile, slightly raised, or pedunculated, and may be single or multiple.[72] When multiple, they may be confluent, with a diameter of several centimeters. Sigmoidoscopy may reveal that the mucosa overlying the cysts has irregularly distributed areas of edema, hyperemia, hypertrophy, and atrophy, with occasional superficial ulceration or central umbilication or a white "cap."[71,72] The mucosa is generally intact, but it may be ulcerated, in which case it may resemble a carcinoma. Stenosis and rectal prolapse have been found, and ulcerative colitis may also be present. An unusual presentation with a complete colonic obstruction due to an intussusception with a rectosigmoid inflammatory mass associated with distal ulcerative colitis has been reported.[78]

37.5.4 Pathology

The mucin-containing cysts in the submucosa of the colon and rectum in a patient with CCP may present as a localized process, a segmental process, or may be diffusely distributed.[79] One hundred and twenty-three of 144 cases reviewed were localized, while 21 were diffusely distributed.[72] Grossly, there are nodular polypoid or plaquelike areas measuring 1 to 3 cm in diameter that are covered by intact mucosa. In the classic lesion, mucus-filled cystic spaces are present, but in the early stages, thickening of the submucosa is present.

Microscopically, the cysts, which are deep at the muscularis mucosae, are lined with normal-appearing columnar epithelium and may be filled with mucus that stains faintly basophilic. The overlying mucosa may be histologically unremarkable or may show focal ulceration. The surrounding submucosa is invariably fibrotic and contains a mixed inflammatory infiltrate of mild to moderate intensity.[74] Differentiating CCP from a well-differentiated mucinous adenocarcinoma may be difficult. Silver and Stolar[80] stressed that multilayering of cystic mucosa with cellular atypia and prominent intraglandular papillation and budding are seen in patients with carcinoma, whereas the mucosal lining of the cysts in patients with CCP is usually unicellular or absent (▸ Fig. 37.5).

Its distribution distinguishes CCP from colitis cystica superficialis, in which multiple tiny mucous cysts are scattered throughout the colon but are confined to the mucosa. The latter condition usually is associated with pellagra.[74]

37.5.5 Diagnosis

The results of barium enema studies may appear normal, or there may be single or multiple radiolucent filling defects of various sizes or longitudinal thickened mucosal folds.[81] Rarely, partial intestinal obstruction may supervene. Endorectal ultrasonography identifies multiple cysts in the rectal submucosa with areas of echorefringent fibrosis between cysts, and confirms the absence of lymph node involvement or invasion of the muscular layer.[82] With CT, the lesion appears as a noninfiltrating entity in the submucosa. With MRI, nodulations produce intense signals that illustrate the mucoprotein content of the cysts. Included in the differential diagnosis are a variety of rectal neoplasms: adenomatous polyps, endometriosis, multiple polyposis, lipoma, leiomyoma, sarcoma, polypoid inflammatory granulomas such as those that occur with schistosomiasis, ulcerative colitis, and Crohn's disease, ischemic proctitis or colitis with submucosal hemorrhage and edema, infectious disorders, drug-induced colitides, and, most importantly, a mucus-producing adenocarcinoma.[72,76] Differentiation among these entities is possible with an adequate biopsy.

Endosonography may also be used to evaluate these lesions in the process of workup for possible malignancy. These areas appear as hypoechoic with systemic or spongy features involving the mucosa and submucosa.[83]

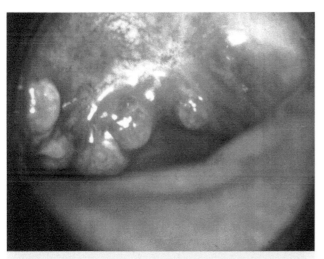

Fig. 37.5 Microscopic appearance of Colitis Cystica Profunda. (Reproduced with permission of the American Society of Colon and Rectal Surgeons.)

Patients may undergo numerous barium enema examinations, sigmoidoscopies, and removal of rectal polyps before CCP is diagnosed. Colonoscopy may aid in the diagnosis of CCP involving the colon. A definitive diagnosis is made based on the typical histologic findings of this disorder and the absence of histologic features of malignancy.[72]

37.5.6 Treatment

Conservative management is initially always attempted. Valenzuela et al[82] reported that re-education of bowel habits aimed at avoiding straining and a high-fiber diet with bulk laxatives can lead to remission of lesions in 6 to 18 months. Similarly, biofeedback has been shown to be helpful. Steroid enemas have been used to treat the condition, but operation is generally the treatment of choice.[72] For patients with associated rectal procidentia, an operation designed to correct the procidentia should be performed. Except in cases of gross procidentia, or refractory symptoms, localized resection should be avoided, and consideration should be given to resection and/or rectopexy. For diffuse involvement, an exceedingly rare situation usually associated with ulcerative colitis, a more extended resection is necessary, with the extent of resection depending on the extent of involvement. Management by diverting colostomy has also been reported.[79]

37.6 Descending Perineum Syndrome

Perineal descent is a normal anatomic result during Valsalva. The anorectal junction descends below the perineal body with normal return. If descent is greater than 3.5 cm, it is considered abnormal.[84] As a result of study of the disordered physiology of patients with rectal prolapse, a distinct condition was recognized in which perineal descent is caused by excessive straining. The pelvic floor muscles are thought to become weakened by repeated straining and stretching, and perineal descent occurs; this condition is referred to as the descending perineum syndrome.[85]

37.6.1 Pathogenesis and Symptomatology

DPS represents a disorder in the normal defecation cycle, which is initiated by pelvic floor weakness. It is the result of a cycle of straining and constipation, which in the setting of a weakened pelvic floor takes weeks to perineal descent (▸ Fig. 37.6). This results in ballooning of the rectum with downward projection of the anterior rectal wall into the anal canal. This leads to a feeling of inadequate emptying, which induces further straining that continues to propagate the cycle. As a result of the chronic straining, pudendal nerve stretching exceeding 20 to 30% of normal length, and subsequent neuropathy, can result. Studies have shown a linear relationship between increased pudendal nerve terminal motor latency (PNTML) and increasing perineal descent; however, these findings do not have uniform acceptance.[86]

Abdominal straining is such a potent inhibitor of pelvic muscle tone that if the individual persists in straining at stool over many years, the effectiveness of the postdefecation reflex

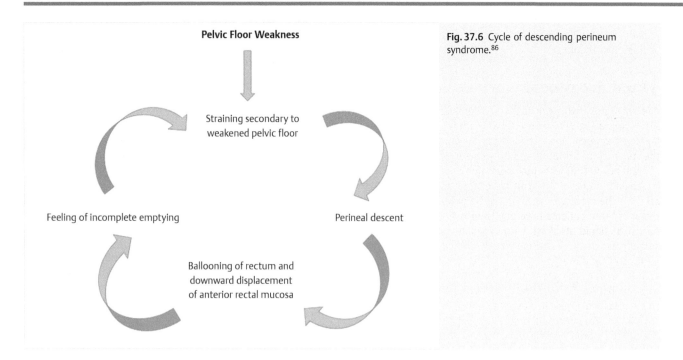

Pelvic Floor Weakness

Straining secondary to weakened pelvic floor

Perineal descent

Ballooning of rectum and downward displacement of anterior rectal mucosa

Feeling of incomplete emptying

Fig. 37.6 Cycle of descending perineum syndrome.[86]

will be reduced considerably. As a result, during the straining effort of defecation, stool is passed, followed by the anterior rectal wall mucosa. Further straining then follows in an effort to pass it. Patients may often describe a feeling of having a rock or a ball in the pelvic area. In advanced cases, prolapsing anterior rectal mucosa becomes so large that it occludes the upper end of the anal canal, giving a feeling of anal blockage and preventing further defecation through straining. The patient typically relates that after partial emptying of the rectum a sense of obstruction develops that cannot be overcome except by ceasing all straining. Indeed, some of these patients develop frank anal obstruction and may pass a finger into the anal canal to temporarily reduce this obstruction and allow defecation. If straining is repeated and prolonged, the anterior rectal wall mucosa will ultimately protrude. Chronic straining may result in prolapsing mucosa, which can result in mucus discharge, bleeding, and pruritus. Partial incontinence also may be present.

In the clinical review by Harewood et al,[87] 39 patients (38 women, 1 man), mean age 53 years, presented with constipation (97%), incomplete rectal evacuation (92%), excessive straining (97%), digital evacuation (38%), and fecal incontinence (15%). Associated features included female gender (96%), multiparity with vaginal delivery (55%), hysterectomy, or cystocele/rectocele repair (74%).

37.6.2 Physical Signs

In the normal individual, the anal margin lies just below a line drawn between the coccyx and the symphysis pubis. In patients with this syndrome, the anal canal is either situated several centimeters below this line or it rapidly descends 3 or 4 cm when a straining effort is made. Digital examination reveals a lack of muscle tone, but the most characteristic change occurs when the patient is asked to strain. The puborectalis muscle descends sharply and can no longer be felt as a separate bar constituting the anorectal ring. Henry et al[88] stated that the descending perineum syndrome could be defined simply as

being present when the plane of the perineum extends beyond that of the ischial tuberosities during a straining effort. On sigmoidoscopy during straining, the anterior wall bulges down into the instrument and follows it as it is withdrawn. Solitary ulceration may be seen on the anterior rectal mucosa in these patients.[73]

37.6.3 Investigations

Anorectal Manometry

Continent patients with the descending perineum syndrome have normal sphincteric pressures, whereas incontinent patients with perineal descent and similar obstructive symptoms exhibit abnormally low pressures.[89] Thus, the obstructive symptoms apparently are not related to the anal tone. The rectal inhibitory reflex is abnormally sensitive in both continent and incontinent patients.[89] Laboratory tests conducted by Harewood et al[87] showed anal sphincter resting pressure was 54 ± 26 mm Hg, and squeeze pressure was 96 ± 35 mm Hg; expulsion from the rectum of a 50-mL balloon required greater than 200 g added weight in 27% of the patients.

Radiologic Studies

Perineal descent may occur in both continent and incontinent patients. Diagnosis is dependent on defecography and correlation with clinical symptoms. Patients with obstructed defecation may have a normal or an obtuse anorectal angle.[89] In patients with the descending perineum syndrome, defecography usually demonstrates a descent of the anal canal greater than 3.5 cm from its resting position at the inferior plane of the ischial tuberosities.[90] Harewood et al[87] found perineal descent was 4.4 ± 1 cm (normal < 4 cm) by scintigraphy. Scintigraphic evacuation, rectoanal angle change during defecation, and perineal descent were abnormal in 23, 57, and 78% of the patients, respectively. The most prevalent abnormality on testing is perineal descent of less than 4 cm; rectal balloon expulsion is an insensitive screening test for the descending perineum syndrome.

37.6.4 Treatment

The chief aim is to prevent further damage by eliminating all straining during evacuation. Conservative measures based on laxatives, suppositories, and enemas in biofeedback constitute the majority of initial treatment maneuvers. Optimizing stool consistency with fiber supplementation may be helpful, though in the later stages of the syndrome, large stool boluses may exacerbate the problem. Laxative may be of limited value because many of these patients have persistently liquid stool; a combination of liquid stool with lax sphincters causes soiling and sometimes partial incontinence. Usually, the most successful method of facilitating rectal emptying is use of a glycerin or bisacodyl irritant suppository. Suppositories are inserted daily, and the patient is instructed to stop straining. The origin of these repeated urges to defecate is explained to the patient, who is told that once the bowel has emptied, all further urges should be ignored. Muscle weakness may be partially corrected by sphincteric exercises, but many weeks may pass before any effect is noted. The utility of biofeedback is varied, with success ranging from 30 to 50%. Some data show that women with a smaller degree of descent respond more favorably to such therapy.[86] Harewood et al[87] reported 17 patients who underwent pelvic floor retraining. At 2-year median follow-up (range, 1–6 years), 12 still experienced constipation or excessive straining; their perineal descent was greater than in patients who responded to retraining. Pelvic floor retraining is a suboptimal treatment for this chronic disorder of rectal evacuation; the extent of perineal descent appears to be a useful predictor of response to retraining.

In patients with large hemorrhoids, an extended hemorrhoidectomy performed to remove the redundant lower rectal mucosa may be of benefit, but the results are rarely sustained.[89]

When severe weakness of the perineal muscles results in anal incontinence, the postanal repair described by Parks may be employed.[88,91] The effect of this operation is to raise the level of the pelvic floor and reduce the anorectal angle. The operation is not the end of the treatment because it is essential that the patient avoid straining during defecation so as not to stretch the repair. Several other operations have been investigated including modified transabdominal sacrocolpopexy, levator plate myorrhaphy as well as transanal stapled approaches; however, there is no consensus that shows that surgical management is an effective option in this syndrome.[86]

37.7 Pneumatosis Coli

The term "pneumatosis coli" (PC) is applied to the condition pneumatosis cystoides intestinalis (PCI) or pneumatosis intestinalis (PI) when it is limited to the large intestine. This rare condition is characterized by cystic accumulations of gas in the submucosa or subserosa of the bowel. The peak incidence is between 40 and 50 years of age.[92] The male-to-female ratio has been reported from 3.5:1 to 1:1.[92,93,94] The condition may be seen in all sections of the gut but is most common in the small intestine. In a collected series, colonic involvement was reported in 36% of the cases.[92] The entire colon and rectum or only a part of the large intestine, more commonly the left side than the right, can be affected. PI can be broadly divided into primary (idiopathic) or secondary types. Secondary PI is the most common and is further subdivided into benign and life-threatening etiologies. Life-threatening etiologies of PC can be caused by intestinal obstruction, volvulus, neutropenic colitis, and intestinal ischemia. Benign etiologies associated with pneumatosis include pulmonary diseases such as asthma, chronic obstructive pulmonary disease (COPD), as well as the use of corticosteroids and chemotherapeutic agents.

37.7.1 Etiology

The etiology of this condition is unknown, but the three most frequent hypotheses are the mechanical, pulmonary, and bacterial theories.[95] Other proposed hypotheses have included biochemical, neoplastic, and nutritional theories, but they have had little support.

Mechanical Hypothesis

It has been suggested that intraluminal gastrointestinal gas, under abnormal pressure because of obstruction, is forced through mucosal defects, enters the submucosal lymphatics, and is distributed distally in the submucosa by peristalsis.[93] Marshak et al[96] reported pneumatosis of the descending colon after sigmoidoscopy without biopsy, and they suggested that the use of instruments in the bowel may produce mucosal defects that lead to localized pneumatosis. Other authors also have reported the development of PC after ulcerations such as a perforated duodenal ulcer, perforated jejunal diverticula, trauma such as colonoscopy, intestinal anastomoses, and jejunoileal bypass.[97,98,99] Smith and Welter[100] reported mucosal ulcerations or necrosis in 45% of their patients, although Koss[93] and others reported that they found no demonstrable mucosal lesions.

Pulmonary Hypothesis

Keyting et al[99] noted an association of PI with chronic pulmonary disease. They postulated that severe coughing produces alveolar rupture and pneumomediastinum. Gas then dissects downward to the retroperitoneum and along perivascular spaces to the bowel wall and accumulates in a subserosal location. Artificial inflation of the lungs is capable of initiating dissection of the air. Asthma and pulmonary fibrosis also have been associated with PCI. The hydrogen content of cystic gas does not support the pulmonary theory since this gas is not present in large quantities in alveoli.

Bacterial Hypothesis

This theory implicates gastrointestinal bacteria as the origin of gas found in the bowel wall. The typical location of gas in patients with pulmonary disease is subserosal, whereas pneumatosis secondary to gastrointestinal disease is linear in distribution and is located in the submucosa. PCI has been produced experimentally in the guinea pig by injecting a mixture of *Escherichia coli, Aerobacter aerogenes,* and *Clostridium welchii* into the bowel wall.[101] Yale and Balish[102] readily produced PCI in the germ-free rat by inoculating its peritoneal cavity with a pure culture of either *C. perfringens* or *C. tertium.* Similar inoculation of the germ-free animal with any one of eight other clostridial species does not result in the formation of PCI. The authors believed, therefore, that the bacterial theory for the formation of at least some cases of PCI has been established and that treatment should be directed at controlling a possible clostridial infection. High hydrogen levels in cysts suggest a bacterial cause since hydrogen is a product of bacterial metabolism.[103]

37.7.2 Associated Conditions

In approximately 15% of the cases, there are no associated medical conditions, and PCI is considered primary. It is estimated that associated abnormalities occur in the remaining 85% of cases and these are considered secondary. Yale[104] listed a large number of conditions that have been found in association with PCI. Included among the pulmonary conditions were chronic lung disease, emphysema, and pneumomediastinum. PCI is more frequently seen in association with gastrointestinal conditions, most commonly with peptic ulceration, carcinoma of the gastrointestinal tract, and pyloric stenosis. Galandiuk and Fazio,[105] in their review of the literature, added the following associated conditions: necrotizing enterocolitis, pseudomembranous enterocolitis, diverticulitis, intestinal strangulation, appendicitis, gallstones, volvulus, Crohn's disease, ulcerative colitis, esophageal stricture, tuberculous enteritis, scleroderma, blunt abdominal trauma, diaphragmatic hernia, and jejunoileal bypass. PCI has been reported as occurring with renal and hepatic transplantation and with the use of lactulose, steroids, and chemotherapeutic regimens.[106] Samson and Brown[107] reported PCI associated with AIDS-associated cryptosporidiosis and suggested that the infection may be pathogenetically involved in the pneumatosis and not merely incidental as the pneumatosis resolved upon treatment of the cryptosporidiosis. Characteristically, the right side of the colon is affected. Colonoscopic polypectomy has been associated with PCI.[108] PCI has been described with needle catheter jejunostomy.[109,110] PCI has also been associated with dermatomyositis,[111] lactulose administration,[112] celiac disease,[113] polymyositis,[114] *C. difficile* pseudomembranous colitis,[115] and previous intestinal anastomosis.[116]

37.7.3 Clinical Features

Symptoms and Signs

The symptomatology and prognosis of PCI are generally attributed to the associated primary condition. The presence of PCI is not associated with any characteristic clinical picture, and when symptoms do occur, they are nonspecific. Manifestations range from the case found incidentally in an asymptomatic individual to the more severe form that may cause partial intestinal obstruction. Bouts of diarrhea, diarrhea alternating with constipation, constipation alone, melena, and flatulence are common. Patients may complain of mucus, colicky lower abdominal pain, incontinence, occasional flecks of bright red blood on the stools, urgency, malabsorption, or weight loss.[105]

Complications of PCI occur in approximately 3% of the cases and include volvulus, pneumoperitoneum, intestinal obstruction, intussusception, tension pneumoperitoneum, hemorrhage, and intestinal perforation.[105]

Physical findings occasionally include an abdominal mass. Rectal examination may reveal cysts in the rectum. The length of the history of a patient with PCI may vary from a few months to a few years.[93]

In adults, the clinical features are usually quite benign, but in children they often are associated with necrotizing enterocolitis, in which case there is usually a fulminant presentation with a high mortality rate.[105,117] Lee et al,[118] in a review of PRI associated with cancer, found that disease confined to the colon was seen in 68% of benign manifestations and in 32% of clinically worrisome pneumatosis. When benign pneumatosis is limited to the colon, the right colon is the most common location.

Radiology

Radiographically, the cysts may be suspected when a plain film of the abdomen reveals radiolucent clusters along the contours of the bowel and in the region of the mesentery. These clusters are more common in the sigmoid mesentery, and they shift in position in different projections. The presence of a pneumoperitoneum in an asymptomatic patient without a clinical perforation syndrome should suggest the disease; indeed, it is almost pathognomonic of the disease. Making a correct diagnosis will prevent an unnecessary operation. The diagnosis can be made from a chest film in which air cysts can be seen in the splenic or hepatic flexure of the colon. Multiple transparent bubbles between the liver and right diaphragmatic dome are called the Moreau–Chilaiditi sign and are present in 15% of the patients with small bowel pneumatosis.[92] Retroperitoneal air may be present beneath the diaphragm bilaterally, showing no shift regardless of the position in which the films are taken, and producing no specific symptoms. Portal vein gas is generally an ominous sign and is often indicative of ischemic bowel, but it can also be a benign condition in adults[116] in association with PCI. Barium enema studies demonstrate large polypoid defects on the wall of the intestine or smooth filling defects that change in shape with distention or compression of the bowel.[96] Sometimes the barium practically obliterates the cysts, and they are not visualized well except on the postevacuation film on which the mucosa appears swollen, suggesting ulcerative colitis. The gas may also be evident as a linear radiolucent strip along the intestinal margin (▶ Fig. 37.7). Streaks of air may separate loops of bowel, and gas may be seen in the portal and mesenteric veins.[105] Sonography shows multiple immobile linear or spotty high echoes in the thickened colonic wall.[119]

CT scanning has been reported as useful in evaluating patients with PCI and distinguishing it from other conditions such as abdominal abscess, mesenteric or biliary air, and bowel infarction.[120] Endoscopic ultrasonography has been used to diagnose colonic pneumatosis.[121] MRI is less sensitive and specific than CT in this setting. CT features that are statistically associated with worrisome PI include automesenteric venous gas, bowel wall thickening, ascites, and mesenteric stranding. Isolated pneumoperitoneum in a clinically stable patient is not associated with worrisome PI.[117]

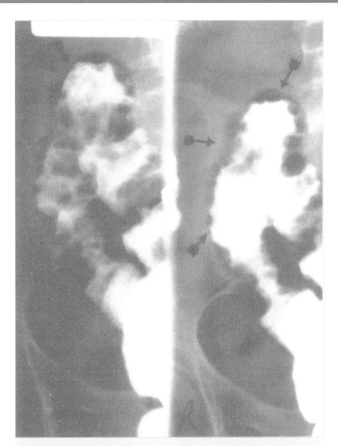

Fig. 37.7 Radiographic appearance of pneumatosis coli with characteristic radiolucent strip along intestinal margin.

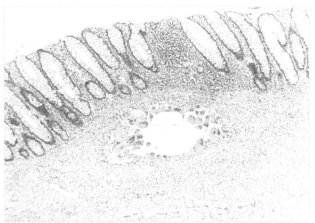

Fig. 37.8 Cystic spaces lying in the submucosa immediately beneath the muscularis mucosae are lined by large macrophages, some of which may be multinucleate with much eosinophilic cytoplasm.

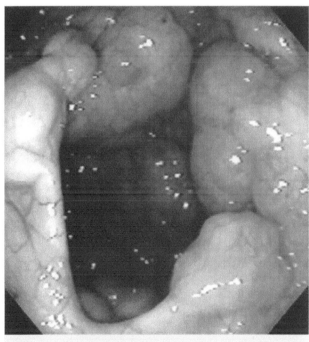

Fig. 37.9 Colonoscopic appearance of pneumatosis coli with multiple protruding cystic lesions of varying size. (This image is provided courtesy of Carol-Ann Vasilevsky, MD.)

Pathology

The cysts vary in size from a few millimeters to a few centimeters in diameter. They may occur either singly or in clusters. Apparently they do not communicate with the intestinal lumen or with each other.

Day et al[122] described the macroscopic appearance of a surgical specimen of cystic pneumatosis as characteristic. The mucosal surface has a coarse cobblestone appearance resulting from a large number of submucosal cysts, the apices of which may show intramucosal hemorrhage. Cysts also project from the serosal surface. The gas appears to be under pressure because rupture of cysts viewed through the sigmoidoscope or in fresh surgical specimens causes a popping sound. Although submucosal cysts predominate in the colon, subserous cysts are frequently found in the small bowel.

Rectal biopsy appearances are distinctive.[122] Cystic spaces lying in the submucosa immediately beneath the muscularis mucosae are lined by large macrophages, some of which may be multinucleate with much eosinophilic cytoplasm (▶ Fig. 37.8). The connective tissue between the cysts, which are often multilobular, shows little or no evidence of inflammation. The covering mucosa is attenuated and sometimes contains small hemorrhages. The appearance is most likely to be confused with that of lymphangioma and oleogranuloma. In a patient with a lymphangioma, there are no macrophages, and the lymphatic spaces are lined by a flattened endothelium without any interstitial inflammation. In a patient with an oleogranuloma,

there is a macrophage response, but also present is much inflammation and fibrosis around fat-filled spaces.

Diagnosis

Very rarely, during examination, a palpable colon may be found. Rectal examination may reveal gaseous cysts. Sigmoidoscopic examination may disclose the clusters of cysts protruding into the bowel's lumen. A simple radiograph of the abdomen may show the very striking appearance of PC. For more proximal involvement, colonoscopic examination will reveal the cysts that project into lumen-like sessile polyps (▶ Fig. 37.9).

This examination might be useful when the diagnosis is in doubt, such as when considering the differential diagnosis of familial adenomatous polyposis.[123] A barium enema study will confirm the diagnosis.

The differential diagnosis with a barium enema study may include familial adenomatous polyposis. Other causes of intestinal perforation in patients presenting with a pneumoperitoneum should be considered. The presence of rectal bleeding may suggest carcinoma. In symptomatic patients with abdominal pain, the condition may be mistaken for appendicitis. Diffuse emphysema is usually distributed in all tissue spaces. Other conditions include enterogenous intestinal cysts, emphysematous gastritis, lymphangioma, and sclerosing lipogranulomatosis.[105]

Careful sigmoidoscopic and radiologic examinations and a biopsy should be performed to avoid errors in diagnosis and thus avoid unnecessary operations.

37.7.4 Treatment

Asymptomatic PCI does not call for any treatment. Indeed, spontaneous remission can occur.[124] Historically, symptomatic patients were treated by operation. The problem of differentiating PC from polyposis and other neoplastic conditions led Calne to favor operation.[123] However, advances in diagnostic modalities have allowed for more subtlety in management.

In the asymptomatic patient with radiographically established PCI (characteristic air-filled cysts in the intestinal wall and free intraperitoneal air), nonoperative management is appropriate.[125] In the absence of an acute abdomen or findings requiring emergency laparotomy, supportive care is adequate. The sole finding of free air with PCI does not mandate exploratory laparotomy.

Therapy for secondary pneumatosis should be directed at the underlying disease process. For example, patients with systemic lupus erythematosus (SLE) have had resolution of their PCI with high-dose steroids, pulse intravenous cyclophosphamide, and octreotide therapy.[126] For patients with PCI secondary to cytotoxic or immunosuppressive treatment for hematologic or oncologic disorders, treatment with broad-spectrum antibiotics and possible parenteral nutrition has been suggested until recovery from the myelosuppression. For patients with PI and AIDS-associated infections—cryptosporidiosis, cytomegalovirus (CMV), and toxoplasmosis, Gelman and Brandt advocated conservative management.[127]

In 1973, Forgacs et al[94] described a method of treatment that was both simple and effective. It consisted of administering oxygen by facemask for a few days. The treatment is based on the theoretical consideration of gas exchange between the cysts and the surrounding tissues. The authors predicted that the cysts could be deflated if the total pressure of gases in venous blood is lowered by the patient's prolonged breathing of a gas mixture containing a high concentration of oxygen. Successful therapy has subsequently been reported by others.[105,128,129,130,131,132,133,134]

The paradoxical persistence of gas-filled cysts in the bowel wall implies that they are replenished at a rate that equals or exceeds the rate of absorption. Since a direct communication with the lumen of the bowel has never been demonstrated, gas presumably enters the cysts by diffusion. The rate of diffusion from bowel gas to cyst and from cyst to capillaries is determined by the partial pressure of gases in each of these compartments, their solubility in tissue fluid, and the dimensions of the diffusing surface represented by the tissues separating them. The object of treatment is to alter the balance between the diffusion of gases into and out of the cysts in favor of absorption. This goal can be accomplished by lowering the total pressure of gases in venous blood by breathing oxygen, thereby increasing the pressure gradient between the cysts and the surrounding tissues. Investigators have described using different quantities of intracystic gaseous constituents. Oxygen content varied from 2.5 to 16%, nitrogen content from 80 to 90%, and carbon dioxide content from 0.3 to 7.5%.[118] Hydrogen content from 2 to 50% has been reported, whereas normal intestinal gas contains 14% hydrogen.[135] Breathing 100% oxygen washes nitrogen out of the lungs and the tissues, leaving only oxygen and carbon dioxide in arterial blood. The tissues metabolize most of the oxygen so that the total pressure of gases at the venous end of the capillary is less than 100 mm Hg and the gas mixture in the cysts remains at or above atmospheric pressure. The pressure gradient, which determines the rate of removal of gases from the cyst, is thus increased severalfold. This approach has been used to hasten reabsorption of gases from a pneumothorax, to relieve postoperative abdominal distention, and to prevent abdominal pain in airmen flying over high altitudes.

A 2-week treatment with an elemental diet also results in cystic resolution and disappearance of symptoms.[133] The rationale of this treatment is that it reduces bacterial hydrogen production. Recurrences are common after a regular diet is resumed. The use of an 8-week course of metronidazole has been reported as an easy ambulatory alternative to high-pressure oxygen therapy. The appropriate dose has not been determined, but doses of 250 to 500 mg three times daily for several months have been used.[126] Successful resolution of the symptomatic and radiologic features of PCI has been documented with the added bonus of avoiding hospitalization and the potential for oxygen toxicity.[131,136,137]

Operation is indicated when PCI is associated with necrosis of the bowel or sepsis or when complications of volvulus, intestinal obstruction, or severe rectal bleeding supervene. A unique case of PC with extensive colon and rectal involvement that did not respond to inhalation oxygen therapy and metronidazole was successfully managed by restorative proctocolectomy.[137] Treatment of obstructive PC has been treated by endoscopic rupture and sclerotherapy with 1 to 2 mL of aethoxysklerol (1%) applied within cysts and cyst walls.[138] Colonoscopic needle deflation alone has been used.[60]

Gagliardi et al[139] reviewed the management of 25 cases treated over a 30-year period. Treatment with antidiarrheals and anti-inflammatory drugs in 14 patients resulted in improvement in 9 cases (64%). Oxygen therapy in nine patients always alleviated symptoms, but there was a high rate of recurrence (78%). Further courses of therapy led to lasting remission in five patients, while two patients underwent colectomy.

37.8 Hidradenitis Suppurativa

Hidradenitis suppurativa, also known as Verneuil's disease, is an acute or chronic infection of the apocrine glands of the skin. In its chronic form, it is an indolent inflammatory disease of the skin and subcutaneous tissue characterized by abscesses and sinus formation. It may be located wherever apocrine sweat glands are found such as at the nape of the neck and in the axilla, mammary, inguinal, genital, perianal, scalp, and periumbilical regions.[140]

37.8.1 Clinical Findings

Hidradenitis suppurativa is a disease characterized by chronic infection of the apocrine glands of the skin. It is essentially a disease of adult life because apocrine glands are activated at the time of puberty.[141] It most often occurs in the third and fourth decades of life and affects both sexes,[140,142] but most authors report that perianal disease is more common in men.[140,143,144,145,146,147] The disease is more prevalent in the black race than in other races.[140,142] Affected individuals frequently have a seborrheic type of skin, are usually overweight, and perspire profusely.

A number of associated abnormalities, including acne vulgaris, diabetes mellitus, hypercholesterolemia, a low basal metabolic rate, interstitial keratitis, anemia, and atopic reactions, have been reported in patients with hidradenitis suppurativa.[148] To these have been added poor personal hygiene, irritation from tight clothing, close shaving, fat skin, excessive sweating, and Cushing's syndrome.[142] In one series, 70% of the patients were smokers.[147] In addition, patients with this infection can be simultaneously affected in other parts of their body.

37.8.2 Etiology

The etiology of the disease is believed to be a result of chronic follicular occlusion resulting in secondary inflammation of the atypical glands.[149]

Terminal dysfunction of the entire follicular pilosebaceous unit (FPSU) leads to follicular rupture and secondary bacterial infection involving the apex and glands. Initially the disease manifests as comedones and tender subcutaneous nodules. This may lead to a chronic and progressive form in which these nodules coalesce, rupture, and drain mucopurulent fluid. This leads to chronic superficial sinus tract formation, and scarring.[149]

Smoking and obesity have been shown to be associated with the disease; conversely, weight loss has been shown to be associated with remission.[150] König et al[151] performed a matched-pair case-control study to evaluate the influence of smoking habits on the manifestation of hidradenitis suppurativa. Sixty-three subjects (27 men, 36 women) were identified; 88.9% were identified as active cigarette smokers and 4.8% of the patients stated to be ex-smokers, while only 6.4% of the subjects had never smoked.

The rate of smokers in the matched-pair control group was 46%. The significantly higher proportion of active smokers among patients with hidradenitis suppurativa can be expressed by an odds ratio of 9.4. The expected smoking prevalence in Germany was 26.7%. Seventy-three percent of their patients had no family history of hidradenitis suppurative, whereas 27% reported at least one affected first-degree relative. From the exceedingly high rate of smokers among patients with this condition, they concluded that cigarette smoking is a major triggering factor of hidradenitis suppurativa.

37.8.3 Bacteriology

Adams and Haisten[152] reported the organisms usually found include *Staphylococcus aureus*, *Streptococcus viridans*, and coliforms. The results of cultures from the series of 104 patients with hidradenitis suppurativa reported by Thornton and Abcarian[140] revealed no growth in 48%, *S. epidermidis* in 44%, *E. coli* in 19%, a-streptococcus in 15%, and other flora in 22%. Proteus species and diphtheroids also have been found.[143] It is uncertain whether the link between *Chlamydia trachomatis* is a direct cause or a predisposing factor.[153]

37.8.4 Diagnosis

Clinically, the diagnosis of hidradenitis suppurativa is made by the above clinical features. One of the key features of hidradenitis suppurativa is multiple sinuses (▶ Fig. 37.10 and ▶ Fig. 37.11). Making the pathologic diagnosis may be difficult because the apocrine glands have been destroyed by abscess formation. The condition may be confused with anal fistulas, Crohn's disease of the perianal skin, furunculosis, and pilonidal disease.[144] An important point of differentiation between a fistulous track of hidradenitis suppurativa and a fistula-in-ano is that the former does not communicate with the intersphincteric plane. Tracking of hidradenitis suppurativa remains superficial to the internal sphincter and bears no relationship to the dentate line. The lack of gastrointestinal symptoms, a normal sigmoidoscopic examination, and negative contrast studies should help in ruling out Crohn's disease. The abscess of hidradenitis suppurativa lacks the necrotic plug or "core" of a furuncle. A lack of midline pits in the coccygeal area should rule out pilonidal disease.

37.8.5 Clinical Course and Associated Conditions

The arthritis associated with hidradenitis suppurativa is rare and most commonly affects the peripheral joints.[154,155] The

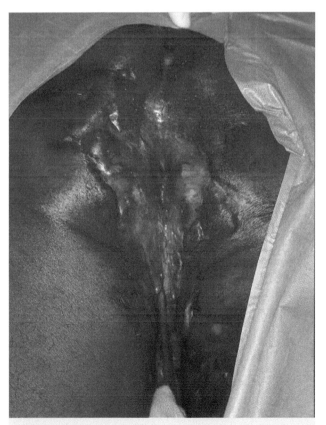

Fig. 37.10 Severe perianal and perineal hidradenitis suppurativa.

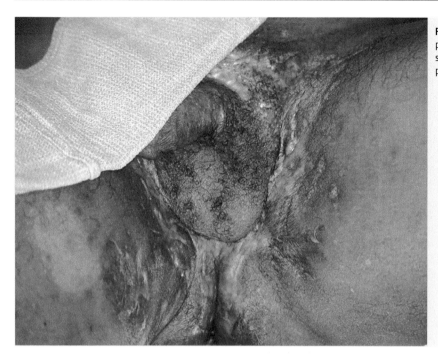

Fig. 37.11 Wide local excision of perianal and perineal hidradenitis suppurativa with partial suture of inguinoscrotal skin. (This image is provided courtesy of Nancy Morin, MD.)

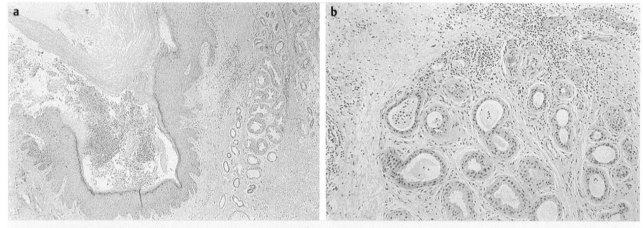

Fig. 37.12 (a) Dilated hair follicle pore with a mixed keratin and inflammatory exudate plug. Dilated apocrine glands (oxyphilic staining) and the darker stained cuboidal cells lining the eccrine glands are noted. **(b)** High power demonstrating a dilated ductal lumen indicating obstruction of the hair follicle and dilated ductules—some filled with inflammatory exudate. There is some distortion of the cellular wall and peristomal inflammation. (These images are provided courtesy of H. Srolovitz, MD.)

axial skeleton is less frequently involved and is often asymptomatic. Hidradenitis suppurativa has been reported in association with Crohn's disease.[156,157] The coexistence of hidradenitis suppurativa and Crohn's disease may affect patient care in three ways.[157] Patients with hidradenitis suppurativa may be mistakenly diagnosed as having Crohn's disease and appropriate operative treatment may be withheld, or inappropriate treatment may be given. Conversely, patients with Crohn's disease may be diagnosed as having hidradenitis suppurativa although this coexistence is unlikely because perianal or perineal Crohn's disease is usually associated with colorectal involvement. Such a misdiagnosis may lead to a more aggressive operation than would be wise. Finally, hidradenitis suppurativa may affect the clinical course of patients with Crohn's disease leading, for example, to persistent perineal skin sepsis after proctectomy. However, conservative treatment of Crohn's disease is generally preferred.

Sepsis stemming from hidradenitis suppurativa justifies a more aggressive approach.

37.8.6 Pathology

This chronic inflammatory condition affects the skin and subcutaneous tissues. The affected area of skin has a red and white blotchy appearance and is thick and edematous, with watery pus draining from multiple openings of sinus tracts. The persistent chronic nature of the disease leads to ulceration and scarring. Lesions may be localized, or they may involve large areas of perianal skin extending onto the buttocks. Microscopic examination of excised specimens shows an inflammatory exudate consisting of plasma cells, lymphocytes, and, occasionally, giant cells of the foreign body type, with the formation of sinus tracts (▶ Fig. 37.12). The tracts become lined by squamous epithelium by down-growth from the surface skin.[122] In long-standing cases, squamous cell carcinoma has been found.[140,152,158,159,160,161]

In their review of the literature, Pérez-Diaz et al[142] found 26 patients with squamous cell carcinoma associated with hidradenitis suppurativa. The average age at diagnosis was 47 years with a predominance of males (77%). The average duration of the disease before carcinoma was 20 years. Wide local excision was the most frequent treatment, but abdominoperineal resections were performed in some patients and some were given radiotherapy. Disease-free survival at 1 year was 31%. Cosman et al[162] described the second case of verrucous carcinoma arising in hidradenitis suppurativa of the anal margin in a nonimmunosuppressed man. The ability of anal and genital hidradenitis suppurativa to form squamous and verrucous carcinomas reinforces the argument for early and complete resection.[162,163]

37.8.7 Treatment

Initially warm baths and cleansing agents are used to maintain hygiene. Both systemic and topical antibiotics have been used based on culture results.[164,165] Jemec and Wendelboe[166] compared topical clindamycin with systemic tetracycline in the treatment of 46 patients with stage 1 or 2 hidradenitis suppurativa in a double-blind, randomized controlled trial. No significant difference was found between the two types of treatment. If the patient presents while she is taking an oral contraceptive, cessation of the medication or a change to an alternative form with greater estrogenic properties may be indicated.[142] Based on their belief that hidradenitis suppurativa is a cutaneous manifestation of variably expressed androgen excess, Mortimer et al[167] have provided a rationale for the treatment of early disease with cyproterone acetate. The use of steroids to decrease inflammation and androgen production and leuprolide acetate to reduce androgen production has been reported.[164]

Sullivan et al[168] noted patients' self-reported disease activity scores for hidradenitis suppurativa were significantly decreased following infliximab infusion treatment for rheumatoid arthritis and psoriasis. This correlated with physician observed clinical improvement. They believe infliximab is a promising agent for the treatment of hidradenitis suppurativa.

The surgical treatment of hidradenitis suppurativa in its acute phase is incision and drainage of a localized abscess. In neither the acute nor the chronic phase are antibiotics considered of value as definitive therapy.[140]

Surgical treatment in the chronic stage may consist of (1) wide excision with the defect left open to granulate and epithelialize, (2) excision and primary closure,[148] (3) excision and split-thickness skin grafting,[141,147,169] and (4) excision and closure with a pedicle flap.[165,170] Each of these procedures has its advocates, and each may have its use, depending on the location and extent of the pathology. In mild chronic cases, unroofing of the area may be considered,[144,158] but in most cases a better and wiser plan would be excision of the diseased skin and subcutaneous tissues. Excision and primary closure are usually suitable for a small wound located in a relatively clean area (i.e., the axilla). Because of the contaminated environment, many surgeons are reluctant to close perineal wounds primarily and they can simply be left open to heal by secondary intention.

If there is extensive infection with abscess formation, incision and drainage may be necessary as a preliminary procedure.

Following this, wide excision should include all sinus and epithelial skin bridges, along with all of the fibrous and inflamed portions of the subcutaneous fat. In the past, split-thickness skin grafts have been applied,[141] but they seldom have been necessary; Bocchini et al[171] presented the results of management of extensive hidradenitis suppurativa in gluteal, perineal, and inguinal areas in 56 patients (93% males) with a mean age of 40 years. Gluteal and perineal diseases were present in 37.6 and 30.6%, respectively. Squamous cell carcinoma and Crohn's disease were observed in one patient each. Wide surgical excision was performed in all. Healing by secondary intention was the choice in 57%, whereas 43% of the patients underwent delayed skin grafting. Diverting colostomy was used in 41% of the patients. Mean time for complete healing in the nongrafted group was 10 weeks and in the skin-grafted group was 6 weeks. New resection was performed in 9% of the patients. Partial graft loss was 38% and recurrence was observed in only one patient.

The establishment of a colostomy, as recommended by some authors, is generally unnecessary.[153] A similar result can be obtained through adequate bowel preparation and placement of the patient on an elemental diet and obstipating medications as described by Gordon.[172]

In fact, Thornton and Abcarian[140] found that even this measure is unnecessary. In an effort to clarify conflicting information and to establish principles of operative treatment, they reviewed the records of 104 patients with perianal and perineal hidradenitis suppurativa who were treated at Cook County Hospital in Chicago. With the patient in the prone jackknife position, their operative procedure consisted of wide excision of the involved area down to normal fat or fascia, with electrocautery used. Wounds were packed with iodoform gauze, and an occlusive dressing was applied. Diverting colostomy or skin grafts were not used routinely, nor were antibiotics administered. In only 1 of their 104 patients was a diverting colostomy deemed necessary. Sitz baths were instituted four times a day, and patients were discharged when comfortable—an average hospital stay of 7.2 days. Average healing times ranged from 3.5 to 7 weeks. Only four patients were operated on for recurrence in the 5-year period of the authors' study. The extensive experience of Thornton and Abcarian and their excellent results indicate that the wide excision along with packing is followed by rapid healing without ancillary measures and is the treatment of choice. Other authors concur[145,147,165] and recommended the use of a Silastic foam dressing to avoid the pain of dressing changes with gauze. Reported recurrence rates after excision of perianal hidradenitis suppurativa have varied from almost nil[173] to 67% of inguinoscrotal skin.[147]

Lapins et al[174] used a carbon dioxide laser technique for stepwise horizontal vaporization in the management of hidradenitis suppurativa in various anatomic locations. In 24 patients followed for an average of 27 months, healing occurred in 4 weeks and only 2 patients developed recurrences. Despite these results, the authors state that in most cases wide local excision is the method of choice. Others have also used this method with success.[175]

37.9 Diversion Colitis

"Diversion colitis" is a term used to describe the clinical entity of nonspecific inflammation of excluded colonic and rectal mucosa. The condition was first described by Glotzer et al[176] in

1981. Its importance lies in the inability to differentiate it from other types of proctitis and may result in inappropriate therapy and reluctance to recommend stoma closure. Of clinical consequence is the fact that there is complete resolution of the inflammatory process when intestinal continuity is restored.

In a study of 53 patients, Whelan et al[177] reported a 91% incidence. Ferguson and Siegal[178] noted that 70% of 20 patients demonstrated diversion colitis. Whelan et al reported that age, type of stoma, or indication for operation plays no role in the incidence of the disease.[177] However, Haas et al[179] found diversion colitis in 25% after operations for carcinoma and 86% after diverticulitis.

The etiology of this condition has not been definitively established, but it is thought to be a deficiency of short-chain fatty acids (SCFA), which are preferred nutrients of the colonic mucosal cell. Butyrate, an SCFA generated by microbial fermentation of dietary substrates, is produced in the colon of humans.[180] Butyrate is absorbed by colonocytes in the proximal colon via passive diffusion and by active transport mechanisms, which are linked to various ion exchange transporters. In the distal colon, the main mechanism of absorption is passive diffusion of the lipid-soluble form. Butyrate and other SCFAs are important for the absorption of electrolytes by the large intestine and may play a role in preventing certain types of diarrhea. The mechanism by which butyrate and other SCFAs exert control over fluid and electrolyte fluxes in the colon is not well delineated, though it may occur through an energy-generated fuel effect, the upregulation of various electrolyte transport systems, as well as possible effects on neuroendocrine factors. Butyrate regulates colonic motility, increases colonic blood flow, and may enhance colonic anastomosis healing. Butyrate may reduce the symptoms from diversion colitis and it may prevent the progression of colitis in general. Harig et al[181] demonstrated low levels of SCFA in the diverted colon and noted that daily irrigation of the diverted segment with a solution of SCFA results in improvement in the endoscopic appearance of the excluded bowel. Bacterial overgrowth by normal colonic flora or invasion by a specific pathogenic organism has been postulated as a cause of diversion colitis. Winslet et al[182] reported that the onset or resolution of diversion proctitis was not associated with any significant changes in colonic cellular proliferation, glycoprotein synthesis, or mucosa-associated or luminal flora.

Rarely has diversion colitis caused clinical problems and for the most part it is seldom clinically significant. The reported frequency of symptoms related to diverted bowel has varied greatly from asymptomatic to 50%.[177,179,180] Whelan et al[177] noted symptoms in only 6% of 53 patients studied. Orsay et al[183] noted that 76% of patients demonstrated mild to severe colitis on an average of 30 weeks following diversion. From the largest series of reported patients with diversion colitis, Haas et al[179] found that almost half of the 85 patients were symptomatic. The most prominent symptom is rectal bleeding, which is usually modest in amount but may be significant enough to require transfusion. Other symptoms include tenesmus, mucous discharge, and abdominal pain. The onset of symptoms may occur any time from 1 month to 22 years after fecal diversion.[184] Diversion colitis is a frequent, persistent, and sometimes problematic complication in patients with myelopathy who have also had colostomies.[173]

Endoscopic examination may reveal abnormal findings in up to 80% of the patients.[185] It may be impossible to distinguish diversion proctitis from inflammatory bowel disease. The simplest procedure to detect underlying disease is flexible fiberoptic sigmoidoscopy. Endoscopic examination reveals a colitic picture ranging from mild to severe. Haas et al[179] found abnormal endoscopic findings in 80% of the patients with diversion colitis, but these included mucous plugs and scybala. In the study by Whelan et al,[177] endoscopic mucosal findings included contact irritation or bleeding (98%), focal erythema (77%), sessile pale polypoid lesions (60%), petechiae (52%), ulcerations (29%), edema (23%), and blood in the lumen (13%). In majority of the patients, the colitis does not uniformly involve the mucosal surface. Instead, patches of inflammation are found interspersed between areas of normal mucosa. In one-fourth of the cases, inflammatory changes are limited to the rectum, whereas in three-fourths of the cases, the inflammatory process involves the rectum and the more proximal diverted colon.[177]

Histologic findings noted in descending order of frequency include mild chronic inflammation, focal inflammation, lymphoid nodule, crypt changes, lymphoid follicle, and glandular atrophy. Other features may include crypt abscesses, epithelial degeneration, crypt regeneration, and aphthoid ulcers.[182] Mucin granulomas are also a histologic feature.[186] It has been suggested that lymphoid hyperplasia is a striking distinctive feature of diversion colitis.[187] Asplund et al[188] reviewed the histologic findings in the defunctioned rectums of 84 consecutive patients. All excised rectal specimens had ulcers and erosions, usually with prominent mucosal lymphoid aggregates, often with mucosal atrophy, diffuse mucin depletion, and marked mucosal architectural distortion. The transmural lymphoid aggregates were identified in 67% and were graded as moderate or marked in 42%. Ten rectal specimens contained non-necrotizing granulomas. No feature in the defunctioned rectum was associated with the original diagnosis or duration of defunctionalization. Granulomas in a defunctioned rectum were associated with an original diagnosis of Crohn's disease. Transmural lymphoid aggregates were common in defunctioned rectums in patients with inflammatory bowel disease and did not indicate Crohn's disease. Nonetheless, biopsies appear to have little or no role in establishing the diagnosis.

The investigation of such patients might include bacterial cultures, search for ova and parasites, and *C. difficile* toxin, but these yield negative results in diversion colitis.

Asymptomatic endoscopic disease requires no pharmacologic treatment. For permanently diverted symptomatic patients, irrigation with a solution of SCFA is recommended twice daily for 2 to 4 weeks. Other less successful treatments have included oral steroids and steroid enemas. Treatment with 5-aminosalicylic acid (5-ASA) enemas has reportedly resulted in both endoscopic and histologic resolution.[185] Definitive treatment consists of stoma closure following which full resolution can be expected. This has been observed in all 21 patients in whom the stoma was closed by Whelan et al[177] and in 34 patients closed by Orsay et al.[183] An increased vascular pattern may persist but is asymptomatic. Winslet et al[182] found macroscopic improvement in all patients after restoration of intestinal continuity, but histologic evidence of disease remained in 50% of the patients. Colostomy closure need not be delayed in these patients.

Patients in whom the diversion is permanent should undergo periodic endoscopic examinations since polyps and malignancy can arise in out-of-circuit large bowel. This is especially true if the original operation was performed for neoplastic disease. In this case, both proximal "discontinuity" bowel and distal "diverted" bowel need inspection. Haas et al[179] underscore the importance of follow-up surveillance. In their series of 85 patients, follow-up detected 4 patients with polyps and 7 cases of carcinoma. Lim et al[189] have suggested that diversion colitis may be a risk factor for the development of ulcerative colitis.

37.10 Segmental or Diverticula-Associated Colitis

A clinical syndrome of chronic colitis unique to the sigmoid colon harboring diverticula has been reported. Peppercorn[190] noted the clinical presentation, endoscopic, radiologic, and pathologic features, and response to therapy in eight patients more than 60 years old who presented with segmental chronic active colitis associated with sigmoid diverticula. Each patient presented with rectal bleeding and mucus and complaints of constipation alternating with loose stools, often with a sense of incomplete evacuation. Crampy lower abdominal pain and excessive flatulence were frequently described, but nausea, vomiting, fever, and weight loss were absent. None of the patients had prior similar complaints, or any symptoms of perirectal disease. Stools for bacterial pathogens, ova and parasites, and *C. difficile* toxin were negative in all eight patients.

Endoscopic appearance consisted of patchy, nonconfluent areas of hemorrhage and exudate limited to the sigmoid colon in an area of multiple diverticula 20 to 50 cm from the anus. The areas of visible inflammation were not contiguous with the diverticular orifices. No gross ulcerations or polypoid lesions were noted. Upper gastrointestinal series and small bowel X-ray studies were normal in all eight patients. From each patient, biopsies of endoscopically involved areas showed focal chronic active colitis without granulomas. Each patient had biopsies from grossly normal-appearing mucosa in the rectum and proximal to the sigmoid colon. The patients were treated with sulfasalazine in doses ranging from 2 to 4 g/d. In each case, there was full resolution of symptoms within 6 weeks of initiating therapy.

Makapugay and Dean[191] analyzed the clinical and pathologic features of 23 patients (age range, 38–87 years; median age, 72 years) with diverticular disease–associated chronic colitis. Nineteen presented with hematochezia, while 4 had abdominal pain. Colonoscopic visualization of the mucosa showed patchy or confluent granularity and friability affecting the sigmoid colon encompassing diverticular ostia. Colonic mucosae proximal and distal to the sigmoid were endoscopically normal. Mucosal biopsy specimens showed features of idiopathic inflammatory bowel disease that included plasma cellular and eosinophilic expansion of the lamina propria (100%), neutrophilic cryptitis (100%) with crypt abscesses (61%), basal lymphoid aggregates (100%), distorted crypt architecture (87%), basal plasmacytosis (61%), surface epithelial sloughing (61%), focal Paneth cell metaplasia (48%), and granulomatous cryptitis (26%). Concomitant rectal biopsies obtained in five patients demonstrated histologically normal mucosa. Fourteen patients treated with high-fiber diet or antibiotics or both improved clinically, as did 9 patients who received sulfasalazine or 5-ASA. Five patients underwent sigmoid colonic resection, three for stricture with obstruction and two for chronic blood loss anemia. Among a control population of 23 age and gender-matched patients with diverticular disease without luminal surface mucosal abnormality, none required resection during the same follow-up period. In addition, three patients developed ulcerative proctosigmoiditis, 6, 9, and 17 months after the onset of diverticular disease–associated colitis. The data indicate that diverticular disease–associated chronic sigmoid colitis expresses morphologic features traditionally reserved for idiopathic inflammatory bowel disease. Its clinical and endoscopic profiles permit distinction from Crohn's disease and ulcerative colitis. Patients with chronic colitis in conjunction with diverticula are at increased risk for sigmoid colonic resection. Diverticular disease–associated chronic colitis may also precede the onset of conventional ulcerative proctosigmoiditis in some cases.

Gore et al[192] described an endoscopic appearance of the sigmoid colon characterized by mucosal swelling, erythema, and hemorrhage strictly localized to the crescentic mucosal folds. In a 5-year period, these changes were seen in 34 of 2,380 colonoscopies and fiberoptic sigmoidoscopies (1.42%). Majority of the patients were middle-aged or elderly. Diverticular disease was present in most (82%), but the abnormalities were confined to the crescentic mucosal folds with sparing of the diverticular orifices. The majority of patients presented with a history of bleeding per anus. Histologically, there was a spectrum of changes varying from minor vascular congestion to florid active inflammatory disease with crypt architectural abnormalities mimicking ulcerative colitis, but rectal biopsies were invariably normal. Three patients later progressed to typical distal ulcerative colitis and two other patients presenting with endoscopic crescentic fold disease had a previous histologically documented history of distal ulcerative colitis. In three patients, the histologic features were of mucosal prolapse. Approximately half of the patients required some form of therapy to control their symptoms. Steroids and/or sulfasalazine were of value, although two patients subsequently underwent sigmoid resection, one to control bleeding and the second for a diverticulosis-associated stricture. Although endoscopic crescentic fold disease represents a specific endoscopic appearance, the clinical and histologic features indicate a wide spectrum of disease.

Imperiali et al[193] evaluated the incidence of segmental colitis associated with diverticula in patients undergoing colonoscopy in a multicenter prospective study. Patients with inflammatory bowel disease–like lesions limited to colonic segments with diverticula were enrolled. Patients were treated with oral and topical 5-ASA until remission was achieved. A total of 5,457 consecutive colonoscopies were recorded at five participating institutions; 20 patients (0.36%) met the endoscopic criteria for segmental colitis associated with diverticula. All patients had lesions in the left colon and one also had lesions in the right colon. Hematochezia was the main clinical feature and no relation with gender, age, or smoking habit was found. Blood chemistries were generally normal and the rectum was spared. The histological features were nondiagnostic and most patients did not complain of any abdominal symptoms 12 months after enrollment.

Guslandi[194] noted that "segmental colitis" often mimics inflammatory bowel disease at histological examination. The observed rectal sparing suggests a possible form of Crohn's disease, but no other similarities between segmental colitis and Crohn's colitis are detectable. Medical treatment for segmental colitis, empirically carried out with drugs such as sulfasalazine and mesalazine, is mostly successful and, when surgery is required, postoperative recurrences are infrequent. Although the existence of segmental colitis as a true clinical entity remains questionable, it appears unlikely that this condition represents an atypical form of inflammatory bowel disease.

In summary, the unusual coexistence of an inflammatory bowel disease and diverticular disease, sometimes with stricturing, suggests a distinct entity. The possible coexistence of Crohn's disease and diverticular disease has been elaborated upon earlier in this chapter.

References

[1] Lirette LS, Chaiban G, Tolba R, Eissa H. Coccydynia: an overview of the anatomy, etiology, and treatment of coccyx pain. Ochsner J. 2014; 14(1):84–87

[2] De Andrés J, Chaves S. Coccygodynia: a proposal for an algorithm for treatment. J Pain. 2003; 4(5):257–266

[3] Kim NH, Suk KS. Clinical and radiological differences between traumatic and idiopathic coccygodynia. Yonsei Med J. 1999; 40(3):215–220

[4] Maroy B. Spontaneous and evoked coccygeal pain in depression. Dis Colon Rectum. 1988; 31(3):210–215

[5] Albrecht S, Hicks MJ, Antalffy B. Intracoccygeal and pericoccygeal glomus bodies and their relationship to coccygodynia. Surgery. 1994; 115(1):1–6

[6] Kane WJ. Fractures of the pelvis. In: Rockwood CA, Green DP, eds. Fractures. 2nd ed. Philadelphia, PA: JB Lippincott; 1984:1124–1125

[7] Marx FA. Coccydynia/levator syndrome. A therapeutic test. Tech Coloproctol. 1996; 4:91

[8] Wray CC, Easom S, Hoskinson J. Coccydynia. Aetiology and treatment. J Bone Joint Surg Br. 1991; 73(2):335–338

[9] Wood GW. Lower back pain and disorders of intervertebral disc. In: Crenshaw AH, ed. Campbell's Operative Orthopedics. 7th ed. St. Louis, MO: CV Mosby; 1987:3289–3299

[10] Grosso NP, van Dam BE. Total coccygectomy for the relief of coccygodynia: a retrospective review. J Spinal Disord. 1995; 8(4):328–330

[11] Doursounian L, Maigne JY, Faure F, Chatellier G. Coccygectomy for instability of the coccyx. Int Orthop. 2004; 28(3):176–179

[12] Hodges SD, Eck JC, Humphreys SC. A treatment and outcomes analysis of patients with coccydynia. Spine J. 2004; 4(2):138–140

[13] Ramsey ML, Toohey JS, Neidre A, Stromberg LJ, Roberts DA. Coccygodynia: treatment. Orthopedics. 2003; 26(4):403–405, discussion 405

[14] Perkins R, Schofferman J, Reynolds J. Coccygectomy for severe refractory sacrococcygeal joint pain. J Spinal Disord Tech. 2003; 16(1):100–103

[15] Chen Y, Huang-Lionnet JHY, Cohen SP. Radiofrequency ablation in coccydynia: a case series and comprehensive, evidence-based review. Pain Med. 2017; 18(6):1111–1130

[16] Snyder MJ. Endometriosis. In: Steele SR, Hull TL, Read TE, Saclarides TJ, Senagore AJ, Whitlow CB, eds. The ASCRS Textbook of Colon and Rectal Surgery, 3rd ed. New York, NY: Springer; 2016:717–733

[17] Gardner GH, Greene RR, Ranney B. The histogenesis of endometriosis. Am J Obstet Gynecol. 1959; 78(2):445–446

[18] Bailey HR. Colorectal endometriosis. Perspect Colon Rectal Surg. 1992; 5:251–259

[19] Croom RD, III, Donovan ML, Schwesinger WH. Intestinal endometriosis. Am J Surg. 1984; 148(5):660–667

[20] Rowland R, Langman JM. Endometriosis of the large bowel: a report of 11 cases. Pathology. 1989; 21(4):259–265

[21] Langlois NE, Park KG, Keenan RA. Mucosal changes in the large bowel with endometriosis: a possible cause of misdiagnosis of colitis? Hum Pathol. 1994; 25(10):1030–1034

[22] Prystowsky JB, Stryker SJ, Ujiki GT, Poticha SM. Gastrointestinal endometriosis. Incidence and indications for resection. Arch Surg. 1988; 123(7):855–858

[23] Singh KK, Lessells AM, Adam DJ, et al. Presentation of endometriosis to general surgeons: a 10-year experience. Br J Surg. 1995; 82(10):1349–1351

[24] Varras M, Kostopanagiotou E, Katis K, Farantos Ch, Angelidou-Manika Z, Antoniou S. Endometriosis causing extensive intestinal obstruction simulating carcinoma of the sigmoid colon: a case report and review of the literature. Eur J Gynaecol Oncol. 2002; 23(4):353–357

[25] Bozdech JM. Endoscopic diagnosis of colonic endometriosis. Gastrointest Endosc. 1992; 38(5):568–570

[26] Doniec JM, Kahlke V, Peetz F, et al. Rectal endometriosis: high sensitivity and specificity of endorectal ultrasound with an impact for the operative management. Dis Colon Rectum. 2003; 46(12):1667–1673

[27] Bazot M, Darai E, Hourani R, et al. Deep pelvic endometriosis: MR imaging for diagnosis and prediction of extension of disease. Radiology. 2004; 232 (2):379–389

[28] Kinkel K, Chapron C, Balleyguier C, Fritel X, Dubuisson JB, Moreau JF. Magnetic resonance imaging characteristics of deep endometriosis. Hum Reprod. 1999; 14(4):1080–1086

[29] Buchweitz O, Poel T, Diedrich K, Malik E. The diagnostic dilemma of minimal and mild endometriosis under routine conditions. J Am Assoc Gynecol Laparosc. 2003; 10(1):85–89

[30] Martin DC, Hubert GD, Vander Zwaag R, el-Zeky FA. Laparoscopic appearances of peritoneal endometriosis. Fertil Steril. 1989; 51(1):63–67

[31] Hall LL, Malone JM, Ginsburg KA. Flare-up of endometriosis induced by gonadotropin-releasing hormone agonist leading to bowel obstruction. Fertil Steril. 1995; 64(6):1204–1206

[32] Soysal S, Soysal ME, Ozer S, Gul N, Gezgin T. The effects of post-surgical administration of goserelin plus anastrozole compared to goserelin alone in patients with severe endometriosis: a prospective randomized trial. Hum Reprod. 2004; 19(1):160–167

[33] Vercellini P, Somigliana E, Viganò P, Abbiati A, Daguati R, Crosignani PG. Endometriosis: current and future medical therapies. Best Pract Res Clin Obstet Gynaecol. 2008; 22(2):275–306

[34] Koh CH, Janik GM. The surgical management of deep rectovaginal endometriosis. Curr Opin Obstet Gynecol. 2002; 14(4):357–364

[35] Kavallaris A, Köhler C, Kühne-Heid R, Schneider A. Histopathological extent of rectal invasion by rectovaginal endometriosis. Hum Reprod. 2003; 18 (6):1323–1327

[36] Jones KD, Owen E, Berresford A, Sutton C. Endometrial adenocarcinoma arising from endometriosis of the rectosigmoid colon. Gynecol Oncol. 2002; 86 (2):220–222

[37] Yantiss RK, Clement PB, Young RH. Neoplastic and pre-neoplastic changes in gastrointestinal endometriosis: a study of 17 cases. Am J Surg Pathol. 2000; 24(4):513–524

[38] Cho HY, Kim MK, Cho SJ, Bae JW, Kim I. Endometrial stromal sarcoma of the sigmoid colon arising in endometriosis: a case report with a review of literatures. J Korean Med Sci. 2002; 17(3):412–414

[39] Douthwaite AH. Proctalgia fugax. BMJ. 1962; 2(5298):164–165

[40] Thaysen TEH. Proctalgin fugax. Lancet. 1935; 2:243–246

[41] Schuster MM. Constipation and anorectal disorders. Clin Gastroenterol. 1977; 6(3):643–658

[42] Harvey RF. Colonic motility in proctalgia fugax. Lancet. 1979; 2 (8145):713–714

[43] Takano M. Proctalgia fugax: caused by pudendal neuropathy? Dis Colon Rectum. 2005; 48(1):114–120

[44] Thompson WG, Heaton KW. Proctalgia fugax. J R Coll Physicians Lond. 1980; 14(4):247–248

[45] Pilling LF, Swenson WM, Hill JR. The psychologic aspects of proctalgia fugax. Dis Colon Rectum. 1965; 8(5):372–376

[46] Eckardt VF, Dodt O, Kanzler G, Bernhard G. Treatment of proctalgia fugax with salbutamol inhalation. Am J Gastroenterol. 1996; 91(4):686–689

[47] Peleg R, Shvartzman P. Low-dose intravenous lidocaine as treatment for proctalgia fugax. Reg Anesth Pain Med. 2002; 27(1):97–99

[48] Katsinelos P, Kalomenopoulou M, Christodoulou K, et al. Treatment of proctalgia fugax with botulinum A toxin. Eur J Gastroenterol Hepatol. 2001; 13 (11):1371–1373

[49] Lowenstein B, Cataldo PA. Treatment of proctalgia fugax with topical nitroglycerin: report of a case. Dis Colon Rectum. 1998; 41(5):667–668

[50] Sinaki M, Merritt JL, Stillwell GK. Tension myalgia of the pelvic floor. Mayo Clin Proc. 1977; 52(11):717–722

[51] Salvati EP. The levator syndrome and its variant. Gastroenterol Clin North Am. 1987; 16(1):71–78

[52] Drossman DA, Li Z, Andruzzi E, et al. U.S. householder survey of functional gastrointestinal disorders. Prevalence, sociodemography, and health impact. Dig Dis Sci. 1993; 38(9):1569–1580

[53] Sohn N, Weinstein MA, Robbins RD. The levator syndrome and its treatment with high-voltage electrogalvanic stimulation. Am J Surg. 1982; 144 (5):580–582

[54] Nicosia JF, Abcarian H. Levator syndrome. A treatment that works. Dis Colon Rectum. 1985; 28(6):406–408

[55] Billingham RP, Isler JT, Friend WG, Hostetler J. Treatment of levator syndrome using high-voltage electrogalvanic stimulation. Dis Colon Rectum. 1987; 30(8):584–587

[56] Hull TL, Milsom JW, Church J, Oakley J, Lavery I, Fazio V. Electrogalvanic stimulation for levator syndrome: how effective is it in the long-term? Dis Colon Rectum. 1993; 36(8):731–733

[57] Heah SM, Ho YH, Tan M, Leong AF. Biofeedback is effective treatment for levator ani syndrome. Dis Colon Rectum. 1997; 40(2):187–189

[58] Morgenstern L, Shemen L, Allen W, Amodeo P, Michel SL. Melanosis coli. Changes in appearance when associated with colonic neoplasia. Arch Surg. 1983; 118(1):62–64

[59] Blackett JW, Rosenberg R, Mahadev S, Green PH, Lebwohl B. Adenoma detection is increased in the setting of Melanosis coli. J Clin Gastroenterol. 2018; 52(4):313–318

[60] Day DW, Jass JR, Price AB, et al, eds. In: Morson and Dawson's Gastrointestinal Pathology. 4th ed. Oxford: Blackwell Scientific Publications; 2003:669–670

[61] Walker NI, Smith MM, Smithers BM. Ultrastructure of human melanosis coli with reference to its pathogenesis. Pathology. 1993; 25(2):120–123

[62] Ewing CA, Kalan M, Chucker F, Ozdemirli M. Melanosis coli involving pericolonic lymph nodes associated with the herbal laxative Swiss Kriss: a rare and incidental finding in a patient with colonic adenocarcinoma. Arch Pathol Lab Med. 2004; 128(5):565–567

[63] Pardi DS, Tremaine WJ, Rothenberg HJ, Batts KP. Melanosis coli in inflammatory bowel disease. J Clin Gastroenterol. 1998; 26(3):167–170

[64] Müller-Lissner SA. Adverse effects of laxatives: fact and fiction. Pharmacology. 1993; 47 Suppl 1:138–145

[65] Koskela E, Kulju T, Collan Y. Melanosis coli. Prevalence, distribution, and histologic features in 200 consecutive autopsies at Kuopio University Central Hospital. Dis Colon Rectum. 1989; 32(3):235–239

[66] Nusko G, Schneider B, Müller G, Kusche J, Hahn EG. Retrospective study on laxative use and melanosis coli as risk factors for colorectal neoplasma. Pharmacology. 1993; 47 Suppl 1:234–241

[67] Nusko G, Schneider B, Schneider I, Wittekind C, Hahn EG. Anthranoid laxative use is not a risk factor for colorectal neoplasia: results of a prospective case control study. Gut. 2000; 46(5):651–655

[68] Nascimbeni R, Donato F, Ghirardi M, Mariani P, Villanacci V, Salerni B. Constipation, anthranoid laxatives, melanosis coli, and colon cancer: a risk assessment using aberrant crypt foci. Cancer Epidemiol Biomarkers Prev. 2002; 11(8):753–757

[69] Ricciuti B, Leone MC, Metro G. Melanosis coli or ischaemic colitis? That is the question. BMJ Case Rep. 2015; 2015:bcr2015212404

[70] Guy PJ, Hall M. Colitis cystica profunda of the rectum treated by mucosal sleeve resection and colo-anal pullthrough. Br J Surg. 1988; 75(3):289

[71] Martin JK, Jr, Culp CE, Weiland LH. Colitis cystica profunda. Dis Colon Rectum. 1980; 23(7):488–491

[72] Guest CB, Reznick RK. Colitis cystica profunda. Review of the literature. Dis Colon Rectum. 1989; 32(11):983–988

[73] Rutter KRP, Riddell RH. The solitary ulcer syndrome of the rectum. Clin Gastroenterol. 1975; 4(3):505–530

[74] Tedesco FJ, Sumner HW, Kassens WD, Jr. Colitis cystica profunda. Am J Gastroenterol. 1976; 65(4):339–343

[75] Madan A, Minocha A. First reported case of colitis cystica profunda in association with Crohn's disease. Am J Gastroenterol. 2002; 97(9):2472–2473

[76] Green GI, Ramos R, Bannayan GA, McFee AS. Colitis cystica profunda. Am J Surg. 1974; 127(6):749–752

[77] Menekse E, Ozdogan M, Karateke F, Ozyazici S, Demirturk P, Kuvvetli A. Laparoscopic rectopexy for solitary rectal ulcer syndrome without overt rectal prolapse. A case report and review of the literature. Ann Ital Chir. 2014:85 (ePub):pii:S2239253X14022208

[78] Freeman HJ. Colitis cystica profunda complicated by complete colorectal obstruction. Can J Gastroenterol. 1994; 8:326–330

[79] Herman AH, Nabseth DC. Colitis cystica profunda: localized, segmental, and diffuse. Arch Surg. 1973; 106(3):337–341

[80] Silver H, Stolar J. Distinguishing features of well differentiated mucinous adenocarcinoma of the rectum and colitis cystica profunda. Am J Clin Pathol. 1969; 51(4):493–500

[81] Rosengren JE, Hildell J, Lindström CG, Leandoer L. Localized colitis cystica profunda. Gastrointest Radiol. 1982; 7(1):79–83

[82] Valenzuela M, Martín-Ruiz JL, Alvarez-Cienfuegos E, et al. Colitis cystica profunda: imaging diagnosis and conservative treatment: report of two cases. Dis Colon Rectum. 1996; 39(5):587–590

[83] Sultan M, Chalhoub W, Gottlieb K, Marino G. Endosonographic Findings in Colitis Cystica Profunda. ACG Case Rep J. 2014; 1(3):122–123

[84] Karasick S, Karasick D, Karasick SR. Functional disorders of the anus and rectum: findings on defecography. AJR Am J Roentgenol.. 1993; 160(4):777–782

[85] Parks AG, Porter NH, Hardcastle J. The syndrome of the descending perineum. Proc R Soc Med. 1966; 59(6):477–482

[86] Chaudhry Z, Tarnay C. Descending perineum syndrome: a review of the presentation, diagnosis, and management. Int Urogynecol J Pelvic Floor Dysfunct. 2016; 27(8):1149–1156

[87] Harewood GC, Coulie B, Camilleri M, Rath-Harvey D, Pemberton JH. Descending perineum syndrome: audit of clinical and laboratory features and outcome of pelvic floor retraining. Am J Gastroenterol. 1999; 94(1):126–130

[88] Henry MM, Parks AG, Swash M. The pelvic floor musculature in the descending perineum syndrome. Br J Surg. 1982; 69(8):470–472

[89] Bartolo D, Roe A. Disorders of the bowel: obstructed defecation. Br J Hosp Med. 1986; 35:225–236

[90] Karasick S, Karasick D, Karasick SR. Functional disorders of the anus and rectum: findings on defecography. AJR Am J Roentgenol. 1993; 160(4):777–782

[91] Browning GG, Parks AG. Postanal repair for neuropathic faecal incontinence: correlation of clinical result and anal canal pressures. Br J Surg.. 1983; 70 (2):101–104

[92] Jamart J. Pneumatosis cystoides intestinalis. A statistical study of 919 cases. Acta Hepatogastroenterol (Stuttg). 1979; 26(5):419–422

[93] Koss LG. Abdominal gas cysts (pneumatosis cystoides intestinalorum hominis). Arch Pathol. 1952; 53:523–549

[94] Forgacs P, Wright PH, Wyatt AP. Treatment of intestinal gas cysts by oxygen breathing. Lancet. 1973; 1(7803):579–582

[95] Reyna R, Soper RT, Condon RE. Pneumatosis intestinalis. Report of twelve cases. Am J Surg. 1973; 125(6):667–671

[96] Marshak RH, Lindner AE, Maklansky D. Pneumatosis cystoides coli. Gastrointest Radiol. 1977; 2(2):85–89

[97] Bryk D. Unusual causes of small-bowel pneumatosis: perforated duodenal ulcer and perforated jejunal diverticula. Radiology. 1973; 106(2):299–302

[98] Ghahremani GG, Port RB, Beachley MC. Pneumatosis coli in Crohn's disease. Am J Dig Dis. 1974; 19(4):315–323

[99] Keyting WS, McCarver RR, Kovarik JL, Daywitt AL. Pneumatosis intestinalis: a new concept. Radiology. 1961; 76:733–741

[100] Smith BH, Welter LH. Pneumatosis intestinalis. Am J Clin Pathol. 1967; 48 (5):455–465

[101] Stone HH, Allen WB, Smith RB, III, Haynes CD. Infantile pneumatosis intestinalis. J Surg Res. 1968; 8(7):301–307

[102] Yale CE, Balish E. Pneumatosis cystoides intestinalis. Dis Colon Rectum. 1976; 19(2):107–111

[103] Read NW, Al-Janabi MN, Cann PA. Is raised breath hydrogen related to the pathogenesis of pneumatosis coli? Gut. 1984; 25(8):839–845

[104] Yale CE. Etiology of pneumatosis cystoides intestinalis. Surg Clin North Am. 1975; 55(6):1297–1302

[105] Galandiuk S, Fazio VW. Pneumatosis cystoides intestinalis. A review of the literature. Dis Colon Rectum. 1986; 29(5):358–363

[106] Janssen DA, Kalayoglu M, Sollinger HW. Pneumatosis cystoides intestinalis following lactulose and steroid treatment in a liver transplant patient with an intermittently enlarged scrotum. Transplant Proc. 1987; 19(2):2949–2952

[107] Samson VE, Brown WR. Pneumatosis cystoides intestinalis in AIDS-associated cryptosporidiosis. More than an incidental finding? J Clin Gastroenterol. 1996; 22(4):311–312

[108] McCollister DL, Hammerman HJ. Air, air, everywhere: pneumatosis cystoides coli after colonoscopy. Gastrointest Endosc. 1990; 36(1):75–76

[109] North JH, Jr, Nava HR. Pneumatosis intestinalis and portal venous air associated with needle catheter jejunostomy. Am Surg. 1995; 61(12):1045–1048

[110] Wolthuis AM, Vanrijkel JP, Aelvoet C, De Weer F. Needle catheter jejunostomy complicated by pneumatosis intestinalis: a case report. Acta Chir Belg. 2003; 103(6):631–632

[111] Selva-O'Callaghan A, Martínez-Costa X, Solans-Laque R, Mauri M, Capdevila JA, Vilardell-Tarrés M. Refractory adult dermatomyositis with pneumatosis cystoides intestinalis treated with infliximab. Rheumatology (Oxford). 2004; 43(9):1196–1197

[112] Goodman RA, Riley TR, III. Lactulose-induced pneumatosis intestinalis and pneumoperitoneum. Dig Dis Sci. 2001; 46(11):2549–2553

[113] Terzic A, Holzinger F, Klaiber C. Pneumatosis cystoides intestinalis as a complication of celiac disease. Surg Endosc. 2001; 15(11):1360–1361

[114] Kuroda T, Ohfuchi Y, Hirose S, Nakano M, Gejyo F, Arakawa M. Pneumatosis cystoides intestinalis in a patient with polymyositis. Clin Rheumatol. 2001; 20(1):49–52

[115] Kreiss C, Forohar F, Smithline AE, Brandt LJ. Pneumatosis intestinalis complicating C. difficile pseudomembranous colitis. Am J Gastroenterol. 1999; 94 (9):2560–2561

[116] Horiuchi A, Akamatsu T, Mukawa K, Ochi Y, Arakura N, Kiyosawa K. Case report: pneumatosis cystoides intestinalis associated with post-surgical bowel anastomosis: a report of three cases and review of the Japanese literature. J Gastroenterol Hepatol. 1998; 13(5):534–537

[117] Weaver TL, Den Beste KA, Frey ES. Benign pneumatosis intestinalis: can we avoid the knife? Am Surg. 2016; 82(9):233–235

[118] Lee KS, Hwang S, Hurtado Rúa SM, Janjigian YY, Gollub MJ. Distinguishing benign and life-threatening pneumatosis intestinalis in patients with cancer by CT imaging features. AJR Am J Roentgenol. 2013; 200(5):1042–1047

[119] Sato M, Ishida H, Konno K, et al. Sonography of pneumatosis cystoides intestinalis. Abdom Imaging. 1999; 24(6):559–561

[120] Quiroz ES, Flannery MT, Martinez EJ, Warner EA. Pneumatosis cystoides intestinalis in progressive systemic sclerosis: a case report and literature review. Am J Med Sci. 1995; 310(6):252–255

[121] Bansal R, Bude R, Nostrant TT, Scheiman JM. Diagnosis of colonic pneumatosis cystoides intestinalis by endosonography. Gastrointest Endosc. 1995; 42(1):90–93

[122] Day DW, Jass JR, Price AB, et al, eds. In: Morson and Dawson's Gastrointestinal Pathology. 4th ed. Oxford: Blackwell Scientific Publications; 2003:636–637

[123] Spigelman AD, Williams CB, Ansell JK, Rutter KR, Phillips RK. Pneumatosis coli: a source of diagnostic confusion. Br J Surg. 1990; 77(2):155

[124] Bloch C. The natural history of pneumatosis coli. Radiology. 1977; 123 (2):311–314

[125] Hwang J, Reddy VS, Sharp KW. Pneumatosis cystoides intestinalis with free intraperitoneal air: a case report. Am Surg. 2003; 69(4):346–349

[126] Boerner RM, Fried DB, Warshauer DM, Isaacs K. Pneumatosis intestinalis. Two case reports and a retrospective review of the literature from 1985 to 1995. Dig Dis Sci. 1996; 41(11):2272–2285

[127] Gelman SF, Brandt LJ. Pneumatosis intestinalis and AIDS: a case report and review of the literature. Am J Gastroenterol. 1998; 93(4):646–650

[128] Born A, Inouye T, Diamant N. Pneumatosis coli: case report documenting time from X-ray appearance to onset of symptoms. Dig Dis Sci. 1981; 26 (9):855–859

[129] Elberg JJ. Oxygen therapy for pneumatosis coli. Symptomatic and radiologic remission of colonic gas cysts after breathing high-concentration oxygen. Acta Chir Scand. 1985; 151(4):399–400

[130] Gillon J, Tadesse K, Logan RF, Holt S, Sircus W. Breath hydrogen in pneumatosis cystoides intestinalis. Gut. 1979; 20(11):1008–1011

[131] Gruenberg JC, Batra SK, Priest RJ. Treatment of pneumatosis cystoides intestinalis with oxygen. Arch Surg. 1977; 112(1):62–64

[132] Masterson JS, Fratkin LB, Osler TR, Trapp WG. Treatment of pneumatosis cystoides intestinalis with hyperbaric oxygen. Ann Surg. 1978; 187(3):245–247

[133] van Leeuwen JCJ, Nossent JC. Pneumatosis intestinalis in mixed connective tissue disease. Neth J Med. 1992; 40(5–6):299–304

[134] Costa M, Morgado C, Andrade D, Guerreiro F, Coimbra J. Pneumatosiscoli treated with metronidazole and hyperbaric oxygen therapy: a successful case. Acta Med Port. 2015; 28(4):534–537

[135] Ecker JA, Williams RG, Clay KL. Pneumatosis cystoides intestinalis: bullous emphysema of the intestine. A review of the literature. Am J Gastroenterol. 1971; 56(2):125–136

[136] Miralbés M, Hinojosa J, Alonso J, Berenguer J. Oxygen therapy in pneumatosis coli. What is the minimum oxygen requirement? Dis Colon Rectum. 1983; 26(7):458–460

[137] Woodward A, Lai L, Burgess B, Beynon J, Carr ND. A case of pneumatosis coli managed by restorative proctectomy and ileal pouch-anal anastomosis. Int J Colorectal Dis. 1995; 10(3):181–182

[138] Johansson K, Lindström E. Treatment of obstructive pneumatosis coli with endoscopic sclerotherapy: report of a case. Dis Colon Rectum. 1991; 34 (1):94–96

[139] Gagliardi G, Thompson IW, Hershman MJ, Forbes A, Hawley PR, Talbot IC. Pneumatosis coli: a proposed pathogenesis based on study of 25 cases and review of the literature. Int J Colorectal Dis. 1996; 11(3):111–118

[140] Thornton JP, Abcarian H. Surgical treatment of perianal and perineal hidradenitis suppurativa. Dis Colon Rectum. 1978; 21(8):573–577

[141] Chalfant WP, III, Nance FC. Hidradenitis suppurativa of the perineum: treatment by radical excision. Am Surg. 1970; 36(6):331–334

[142] Pérez-Diaz D, Calvo-Serrano M, Mártinez-Hijosa E, et al. Squamous cell carcinoma complicating perianal hidradenitis suppurativa. Int J Colorectal Dis. 1995; 10(4):225–228

[143] Broadwater JR, Bryant RL, Petrino RA, Mabry CD, Westbrook KC, Casali RE. Advanced hidradenitis suppurativa. Review of surgical treatment in 23 patients. Am J Surg. 1982; 144(6):668–670

[144] Culp CE. Chronic hidradenitis suppurativa of the anal canal. A surgical skin disease. Dis Colon Rectum. 1983; 26(10):669–676

[145] Harrison BJ, Harding KD, Hughes LE. Surgical management of perianal hidradenitis suppurativa. Br J Surg. 1985; 72 suppl:S143

[146] Day DW, Jass JR, Price AB, et al, eds. In: Morson and Dawson's Gastrointestinal Pathology. 4th ed. Oxford: Blackwell Scientific Publications; 2003:651

[147] Wiltz O, Schoetz DJ, Jr, Murray JJ, Roberts PL, Coller JA, Veidenheimer MC, The Lahey Clinic Experience. Perianal hidradenitis suppurativa. The Lahey Clinic experience. Dis Colon Rectum. 1990; 33(9):731–734

[148] Bell BA, Ellis H. Hidradenitis suppurativa. J R Soc Med. 1978; 71(7):511–515

[149] Micheletti RG. Natural history, presentation, and diagnosis of hidradenitis suppurativa. Semin Cutan Med Surg. 2014; 33(3) suppl:S51–S53

[150] Kromann CB, Ibler KS, Kristiansen VB, Jemec GB. The influence of body weight on the prevalence and severity of hidradenitis suppurativa. Acta Derm Venereol. 2014; 94(5):553–557

[151] König A, Lehmann C, Rompel R, Happle R. Cigarette smoking as a triggering factor of hidradenitis suppurativa. Dermatology. 1999; 198(3):261–264

[152] Adams JD, Haisten AS. Perianal hidradenitis suppurativa. Surg Clin North Am. 1972; 52(2):467–472

[153] Bendahan J, Paran H, Kolman S, Neufeld DM, Freund U. The possible role of Chlamydia trachomatis in perineal suppurative hidradenitis. Eur J Surg. 1992; 158(4):213–215

[154] Bhalla R, Sequeira W. Arthritis associated with hidradenitis suppurativa. Ann Rheum Dis. 1994; 53(1):64–66

[155] Rosner IA, Burg CG, Wisnieski JJ, Schacter BZ, Richter DE. The clinical spectrum of the arthropathy associated with hidradenitis suppurativa and acne conglobata. J Rheumatol. 1993; 20(4):684–687

[156] Tsianos EV, Dalekos GN, Tzermias C, Merkouropoulos M, Hatzis J. Hidradenitis suppurativa in Crohn's disease. A further support to this association. J Clin Gastroenterol. 1995; 20(2):151–153

[157] Church JM, Fazio VW, Lavery IC, Oakley JR, Milsom JW. The differential diagnosis and comorbidity of hidradenitis suppurativa and perianal Crohn's disease. Int J Colorectal Dis. 1993; 8(3):117–119

[158] Brown SC, Kazzazi N, Lord PH. Surgical treatment of perineal hidradenitis suppurativa with special reference to recognition of the perianal form. Br J Surg. 1986; 73(12):978–980

[159] Dufresne RG, Jr, Ratz JL, Bergfeld WF, Roenigk RK. Squamous cell carcinoma arising from the follicular occlusion triad. J Am Acad Dermatol. 1996; 35(3 Pt 1):475–477

[160] Malaquarnera M, Pontillo T, Pistone G, et al. Squamous-cell cancer in Verneciolì's disease. (Hidradenitis suppurativa). Lancet. 1994; 348:1449

[161] Finley EM, Ratz JL. Treatment of hidradenitis suppurativa with carbon dioxide laser excision and second-intention healing. J Am Acad Dermatol. 1996; 34(3):465–469

[162] Cosman BC, O'Grady TC, Pekarske S. Verrucous carcinoma arising in hidradenitis suppurativa. Int J Colorectal Dis. 2000; 15(5–6):342–346

[163] Altunay IK, Gökdemir G, Kurt A, Kayaoglu S. Hidradenitis suppurativa and squamous cell carcinoma. Dermatol Surg. 2002; 28(1):88–90

[164] Rubin RJ, Chinn BT. Perianal hidradenitis suppurativa. Surg Clin North Am. 1994; 74(6):1317–1325

[165] Banerjee AK. Surgical treatment of hidradenitis suppurativa. Br J Surg. 1992; 79(9):863–866

[166] Jemec GB, Wendelboe P. Topical clindamycin versus systemic tetracycline in the treatment of hidradenitis suppurativa. J Am Acad Dermatol. 1998; 39 (6):971–974

[167] Mortimer PS, Dawber RP, Gales MA, Moore RA. A double-blind controlled cross-over trial of cyproterone acetate in females with hidradenitis suppurativa. Br J Dermatol. 1986; 115(3):263–268

[168] Sullivan TP, Welsh E, Kerdel FA, Burdick AE, Kirsner RS. Infliximab for hidradenitis suppurativa. Br J Dermatol. 2003; 149(5):1046–1049

[169] Rosenfeld N, Babar A. Hidradenitis suppurativa of the perineal and gluteal regions, treated by excision and skin grafting. Case report. Plast Reconstr Surg. 1976; 58(1):98–99

[170] Lirón-Ruiz R, Torralba-Martinez JA, Pellicer-Franco E, et al. Treatment of long-standing extensive perianal hidradenitis suppurativa using double rotation plasty, V-Y plasty and free grafts. Int J Colorectal Dis. 2004; 19 (1):73–78

[171] Bocchini SF, Habr-Gama A, Kiss DR, Imperiale AR, Araujo SE. Gluteal and perianal hidradenitis suppurativa: surgical treatment by wide excision. Dis Colon Rectum. 2003; 46(7):944–949

[172] Gordon PH. The chemically defined diet and anorectal procedures. Can J Surg. 1976; 19(6):511–513

[173] Frisbie JH, Ahmed N, Hirano I, Klein MA, Soybel DI. Diversion colitis in patients with myelopathy: clinical, endoscopic, and histopathological findings. J Spinal Cord Med. 2000; 23(2):142–149

[174] Lapins J, Marcusson JA, Emtestam L. Surgical treatment of chronic hidradenitis suppurativa: CO2 laser stripping-secondary intention technique. Br J Dermatol. 1994; 131(4):551–556

[175] Finley EM, Ratz JL. Treatment of hidradenitis suppurativa with carbon dioxide laser excision and second-intention healing. J Am Acad Dermatol. 1996; 34(3):465–469

[176] Glotzer DJ, Glick ME, Goldman H. Proctitis and colitis following diversion of the fecal stream. Gastroenterology. 1981; 80(3):438–441

[177] Whelan RL, Abramson D, Kim DS, Hashmi HF. Diversion colitis. A prospective study. Surg Endosc. 1994; 8(1):19–24

[178] Ferguson CM, Siegel RJ. A prospective evaluation of diversion colitis. Am Surg. 1991; 57(1):46–49

[179] Haas PA, Fox TA, Jr, Szilagy EJ. Endoscopic examination of the colon and rectum distal to a colostomy. Am J Gastroenterol. 1990; 85(7):850–854

[180] Velázquez OC, Lederer HM, Rombeau JL. Butyrate and the colonocyte. Production, absorption, metabolism, and therapeutic implications. Adv Exp Med Biol. 1997; 427:123–134

[181] Harig JM, Soergel KH, Komorowski RA, Wood CM. Treatment of diversion colitis with short-chain-fatty acid irrigation. N Engl J Med. 1989; 320 (1):23–28

[182] Winslet MC, Poxon V, Youngs DJ, Thompson H, Keighley MR. A pathophysiologic study of diversion proctitis. Surg Gynecol Obstet. 1993; 177(1):57–61

[183] Orsay CP, Kim DO, Pearl RK, Abcarian H. Diversion colitis in patients scheduled for colostomy closure. Dis Colon Rectum. 1993; 36(4):366–367

[184] Ona FV, Boger JN. Rectal bleeding due to diversion colitis. Am J Gastroenterol. 1985; 80(1):40–41

[185] Tripodi J, Gorcey S, Burakoff R. A case of diversion colitis treated with 5-aminosalicylic acid enemas. Am J Gastroenterol. 1992; 87(5):645–647

[186] Murray FE, O'Brien MJ, Birkett DH, Kennedy SM, LaMont JT. Diversion colitis. Pathologic findings in a resected sigmoid colon and rectum. Gastroenterology. 1987; 93(6):1404–1408

[187] Yeong ML, Bethwaite PB, Prasad J, Isbister WH. Lymphoid follicular hyperplasia–a distinctive feature of diversion colitis. Histopathology. 1991; 19 (1):55–61

[188] Asplund S, Gramlich T, Fazio V, Petras R. Histologic changes in defunctioned rectums in patients with inflammatory bowel disease: a clinicopathologic study of 82 patients with long-term follow-up. Dis Colon Rectum. 2002; 45 (9):1206–1213

[189] Lim AG, Langmead FL, Feakins RM, Rampton DS. Diversion colitis: a trigger for ulcerative colitis in the in-stream colon? Gut. 1999; 44(2):279–282

[190] Peppercorn MA. Drug-responsive chronic segmental colitis associated with diverticula: a clinical syndrome in the elderly. Am J Gastroenterol. 1992; 87 (5):609–612

[191] Makapugay LM, Dean PJ. Diverticular disease-associated chronic colitis. Am J Surg Pathol. 1996; 20(1):94–102

[192] Gore S, Shepherd NA, Wilkinson SP. Endoscopic crescentic fold disease of the sigmoid colon: the clinical and histopathological spectrum of a distinctive endoscopic appearance. Int J Colorectal Dis. 1992; 7(2):76–81

[193] Imperiali G, Meucci G, Alvisi C, et al. Segmental colitis associated with diverticula: a prospective study. Gruppo di Studio per le Malattie Infiammatorie Intestinali (GSMII). Am J Gastroenterol. 2000; 95(4):1014–1016

[194] Guslandi M. Segmental colitis: so what? Eur J Gastroenterol Hepatol. 2003; 15(1):1–2

Index

W

X